MW01505322

Occupational Therapy for Mental Health

A Vision for Participation

Third Edition

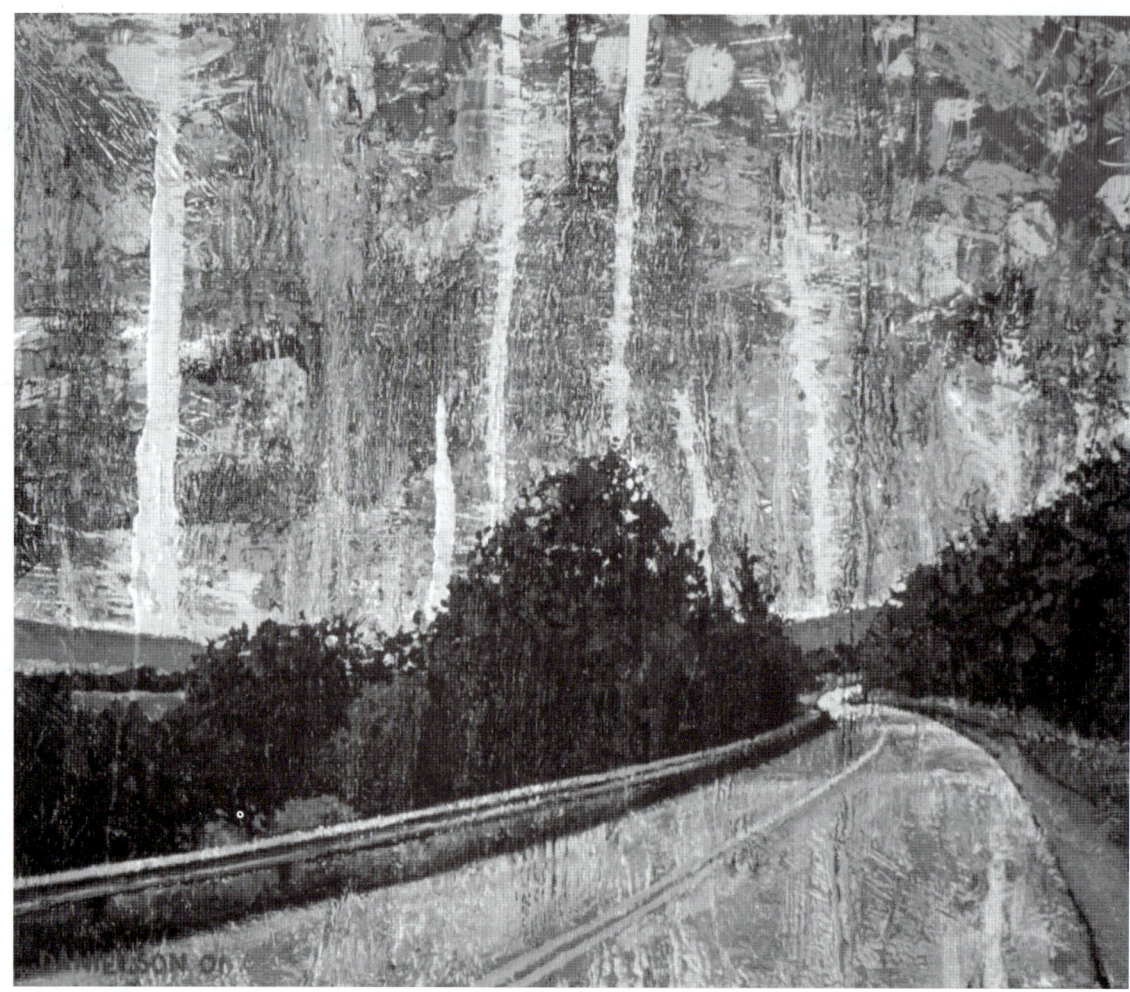

Colours Spring by Frank Danielson

About the Artist

Canadian painter Frank Danielson has been working as a full-time artist since the 1990s. He is presently based in Sudbury, Ontario, where he spent his early years surrounded by the vastness of the iconic Canadian landscape. Frank primarily focuses on the natural beauty of northern Ontario, but his time spent living and working in Toronto and Montreal has also influenced his subject matter.

In 2003, Frank was diagnosed with schizophrenia. Over the past two decades, that diagnosis has led to many difficult periods, but the one constant in his life has been painting. Producing art has provided perspective on the ups and downs of living with mental illness. Although his understanding of the world has been challenged by the onset and recovery from psychosis, the process of working with landscapes in painting has offered Frank an element of stability and predictability.

His work can be seen at www.frankdanielson.com.

Occupational Therapy for Mental Health

A Vision for Participation

Third Edition

Editors:

Catana Brown, PhD, OTR/L, FAOTA
Professor Emerita
College of Health Sciences
Department of Occupational Therapy
Midwestern University–Glendale
Glendale, Arizona, USA

Jaime Phillip Muñoz, PhD, OTR, FAOTA
Independent Practice Scholar
Pittsburgh, Pennsylvania, USA

Virginia C. Stoffel, PhD, OT, FAOTA
Associate Professor Emerita
University of Wisconsin-Milwaukee
School of Rehabilitation Sciences and Technology
Program in Occupational Science, Occupational Therapy
and Technology
Milwaukee, Wisconsin, USA

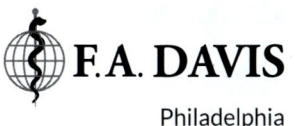

F.A. DAVIS

Philadelphia

F. A. Davis Company
1915 Arch Street
Philadelphia, PA 19103
www.fadavis.com

Copyright © 2025 by F. A. Davis Company

Copyright © 2025 by F. A. Davis Company. All rights reserved. This product is protected by copyright. No part of it may be reproduced, stored in a retrieval system, or transmitted in any form or by any means, electronic, mechanical, photocopying, recording, or otherwise, without written permission from the publisher.

Printed in China

Last digit indicates print number: 10 9 8 7 6 5 4 3 2 1

Publisher: Christa A. Fratantoro
Director of Content Development: George W. Lang
Developmental Editor: Nancy Peterson
Content Project Manager: Julie Chase
Art and Design Manager: Carolyn O'Brien

As new scientific information becomes available through basic and clinical research, recommended treatments and drug therapies undergo changes. The author(s) and publisher have done everything possible to make this book accurate, up to date, and in accord with accepted standards at the time of publication. The author(s), editors, and publisher are not responsible for errors or omissions or for consequences from application of the book, and make no warranty, expressed or implied, in regard to the contents of the book. Any practice described in this book should be applied by the reader in accordance with professional standards of care used in regard to the unique circumstances that may apply in each situation. The reader is advised always to check product information (package inserts) for changes and new information regarding dose and contraindications before administering any drug. Caution is especially urged when using new or infrequently ordered drugs.

Library of Congress Cataloging-in-Publication Data

Names: Brown, Catana, editor. | Muñoz, Jaime Phillip, editor. | Stoffel,
    Virginia, editor.
Title: Occupational therapy for mental health : a vision for participation
    / editors, Catana Brown, Jaime Phillip Muñoz, Virginia Stoffel.
Other titles: Occupational therapy in mental health (Brown)
Description: Third edition. | Philadelphia : F.A. Davis Company, [2025] |
    Preceded by Occupational therapy in mental health. Second edition. 2019.
    | Includes bibliographical references and index.
Identifiers: LCCN 2024038884 (print) | LCCN 2024038885 (ebook) | ISBN
    9781719649667 (hardback) | ISBN 9781719654135 (epub) | ISBN
    9781719654142 (PDF)
Subjects: MESH: Mental Disorders--rehabilitation | Occupational
    Therapy--methods | Patient Participation
Classification: LCC RM735.3 (print) | LCC RM735.3 (ebook) | NLM WM
    450.5.O2 | DDC 615.8/515--dc23/eng/20241105
LC record available at https://lccn.loc.gov/2024038884
LC ebook record available at https://lccn.loc.gov/2024038885

Authorization to photocopy items for internal or personal use, or the internal or personal use of specific clients, is granted by F. A. Davis Company for users registered with the Copyright Clearance Center (CCC) Transactional Reporting Service, provided that the fee of $.25 per copy is paid directly to CCC, 222 Rosewood Drive, Danvers, MA 01923. For those organizations that have been granted a photocopy license by CCC, a separate system of payment has been arranged. The fee code for users of the Transactional Reporting Service is: 978-1-7196-4966-7/25 0 + $.25.

*We dedicate this text to students, practitioners, and educators
who purposefully weave holistic, person-centered occupational therapy that
attends to mind, body, and soul into their everyday practices.
We are inspired by your efforts and advocacy to put mental health
in the foreground of your day-to-day practices.*

We also dedicate this text to our parents.

*To Owen Brown, who modeled a kind intellect, and JoBeth Brown,
who gave me a deep appreciation for nature—Tana*

*To Mary Valdivia, who taught me to be kindhearted and patient,
and Phillip Muñoz, who taught me to work hard and showed me
it is possible to do hard things—Jaime*

*To Trudy Carroll, who taught us all about compassion and how to
cherish family and friend relationships, and to TP (Pop) Carroll, who was
blessed with nine children who brought him love and moved him
beyond grief to a life worth living—Ginny*

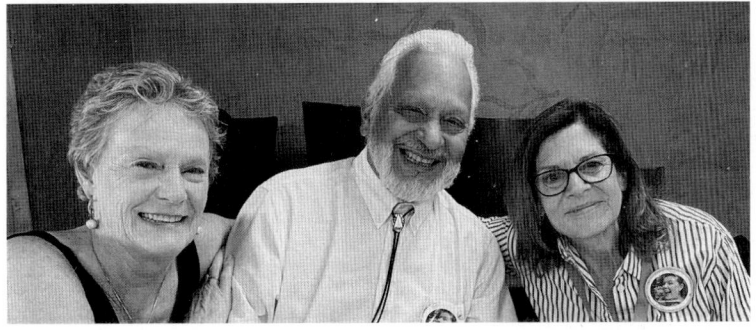

It is almost impossible to talk to someone, go on social media, or watch the news today and not hear or see something about mental or behavioral health. With the ongoing COVID-19 pandemic and the many ripple effects of its presence still manifesting, there is no better time than now for the new edition of this leading occupational therapy textbook. *Occupational Therapy for Mental Health: A Vision for Participation,* Third Edition, continues to be the comprehensive textbook for occupational therapy practice that is mental health focused. More importantly, this new edition is a call to action to recognize that the occupational therapy process and all occupational therapy practitioners (OTPs) are essential to the mental and behavioral health workforce—regardless of practice setting.

This third edition maintains its organizational structure based on the Person-Environment-Occupation (PEO) model and continues to present material so learners and faculty can find practical information on theories, evidence, assessments, and interventions that are crucial to effective occupational therapy practice. It continues to strongly appreciate the lived experience and recovery-oriented perspective that greatly benefits all people with challenges, illnesses, environmental barriers, and diseases that impact occupational engagement and satisfaction.

The editors of this textbook made changes intentionally after seeking feedback and using reflexive thinking to create a roadmap for the third edition that not only highlights occupational therapy practice in mental health today but shows readers where it can and should go moving forward. One notable change in the title, from Occupational Therapy *in* Mental Health to Occupational Therapy *for* Mental Health, shows that language matters, a theme of this text. Most importantly, it shows that occupational therapy as a practice, profession, and scope is applicable for any and all mental health challenges. Occupational therapy exists *for* helping with mental health challenges, not just *in* mental health practice settings.

Another change in this edition is the introduction of a continuum of psychosocial care that occurs for *all* persons across *all* practice settings. It emphasizes that mental health crosses all practice areas, with an intentional examination of occupational therapy practice along a continuum of healthy functioning to mental illness to recovery to flourishing. Occupational therapists and occupational therapy assistants, faculty, students, and practitioners can find evidence of this continuum in the new *Being a Psychosocial OT Practitioner* feature. This feature presents cases that show an OTP's therapeutic reasoning process applied in non–mental health settings. Another new addition is the *Practitioner Profile* feature. With these vignettes, readers can see how a typical day of an OTP in specific settings looks. These profiles provide real-world context and the lived experience of an OTP from a work perspective. Learners, whether first-year students or seasoned clinicians, can feel and imagine a day in their life if they were that practitioner. This is so wonderful because it

further shows the commitment to experiential learning and the tremendous value of lived experience that these editors have consistently presented in this text. Students will love how real the profiles feel, and how well they paint a picture of how occupational therapy practice looks in that context and today's world. The new *Mental Illness in Culture and Society* feature brings in fascinating perspectives on current events, art, books, films, organizations, and/or political issues that concern people with mental illness. Educators will appreciate having all these tools at their disposal to supplement their clinical experience and help them demonstrate how occupational therapy is *for* mental health treatment, anywhere and everywhere.

Overall, these changes help bridge the education and practice worlds such that this textbook not only helps future practitioners learn but supports those in practice with their therapeutic reasoning processes and ability to impact people's mental wellness. For example, as an occupational therapy educator myself, with a background in and a strong commitment to occupational therapy promoting mental wellness, the third edition of this text offers new and innovative ways to teach. I could see myself using the *Being a Psychosocial OT Practitioner* feature to prepare students to meet the psychosocial objectives of any clinical experience before they step foot in a practice setting. I would use this text as a core curricular book that promotes the role of occupational therapy in meeting the needs of all persons, groups, and communities across the continuum of care. This textbook could be used in any practice or process course. At the same time, the videos, The *Lived Experience* vignettes, *PhotoVoices, Apply It Now* activities, and other supplementary resources can help a faculty group put psychosocial wellness and mental health at the forefront of curricular design. A shorter way of saying this is that *Occupational Therapy for Mental Health: A Vision for Participation* is the game-changing tool our occupational therapy educational programs and practice spaces have needed to move the needle in our profession's growth.

It is with tremendous pride and honor that I write this foreword. This textbook will impact many occupational therapy students, practitioners, educators, and researchers in the same way it has me. My career in and passion for occupational therapy all started with the first edition of this text. The editors, Tana Brown, Ginny Stoffel, and Jaime Muñoz, have created a vision again and again that is inclusive of diverse occupational therapy stakeholder groups, the lived experience, and the occupational therapy process and therapeutic reasoning that underpins our great profession. Ginny has brought the perspective of global leadership and policy work to this text over and over again. Her leadership experience in the policy world of mental health has paved the way for so many OTPs and others to see our value. Jaime Muñoz has shown our profession that the issue is rarely the illness or disease, but the systems of care and oppression that make navigating life with mental health issues so tremendously detrimental to individual and societal well-being. Tana Brown has shown us that sensory processing assessment and intervention is our profession's "secret weapon" to promoting mental wellness. And I would be remiss if I didn't mention just how profoundly capable she is of seeing the human in all of us. She taught my first class, day one of my occupational therapy program, and in that moment I knew why I found occupational therapy, and why occupational therapy was better suited for helping those with mental illness than other professions I had considered. These three people have not only changed the educational landscape of mental health occupational therapy, but they have been visionaries, mentors, and stalwart holders of hope for recovery for all persons—and for our profession's place in meeting the mental and psychosocial health needs of people, groups, communities, and society. Together they embody what this text aims to produce: leaders in a continuum of care that emphasizes mental wellness and who see the ways systems can and should change. Last and never ever least, this text and their work have helped us to see that occupational therapy isn't *either* mental health focused *or* not, but it is indeed *both* mental illness *and* overall mental well-being focused.

Halley Read, PhD, OTR/L
Professor of Occupational Therapy and
Doctoral Capstone Coordinator
Western Oregon University Occupational Therapy
Monmouth, Oregon

Beginning with the title, we envisioned a shift in perspective with this third edition. No longer *Occupational Therapy IN Mental Health*, but now *Occupational Therapy FOR Mental Health*, the title speaks to the perspective that all occupational therapy practitioners (OTPs) are mental health practitioners. The title change also speaks to another shift in our presentation. In the third edition, we intentionally examine occupational therapy mental health practice along a continuum of mental illness to recovery and flourishing. OTPs help people and communities achieve their greatest state of mental health and well-being. We maintained the second part of the title: *A Vision for Participation* because our mission remains to promote participation for everyone in all aspects of everyday life.

Trigger Warnings

This text includes sensitive content that could be challenging or distressing for some individuals; however, we have chosen not to include trigger warnings. We trust that instructors will alert learners beforehand to the topics addressed in readings and lectures, and that the titles and headings of the text will allow readers to determine how they choose to approach—or, perhaps in some cases, avoid—material that could be difficult for them.

Guiding Principles

- Each chapter is examined in a holistic and comprehensive manner to ensure that the learner will have a strong grounding in person-centered, occupation-based practices.
- The lived experience of persons experiencing mental health challenges as well as persons in recovery and flourishing is highlighted so that the learner develops a full appreciation for the real people who are recipients of occupational therapy services. The lived experience of the practitioner is also included as a means for presenting the practical, complex, and often messy realities of occupational therapy practice.
- This text recognizes and emphasizes the assertion that practitioners address psychosocial needs for all people in all settings. It includes many examples and features of psychosocial intervention in non–mental health settings.
- The many features of the text translate the content in such a way that the learner can envision real-world applications. In addition, the features facilitate the development of therapeutic reasoning, critical reflection, and therapeutic use of self.

Organizational Structure and Breadth

Occupational Therapy for Mental Health maintains the organizational structure of the Person-Environment-Occupation (PEO) model to ensure a practice that is holistic and comprehensive. Although PEO plays a major role in the text, over 100 practice models and theoretical frameworks are included throughout the text and are listed with their corresponding chapters in Appendix D.

Eight new chapters in the text reflect changes in practice and a more expansive perspective of what practitioners consider when they think of the PEO approach. These chapters are:

- Chapter 1: Occupational Therapy Practice Across the Mental Health Continuum
- Chapter 5: Trauma-Informed Practice
- Chapter 17: Chronic Health Conditions and Mental Health
- Chapter 28: Social Determinants and Mental Health
- Chapter 30: Natural Environments
- Chapter 33: Virtual Environments
- Chapter 44: Addressing Suicide Across the Continuum
- Chapter 49: Connectedness and Belonging

The text is divided into four parts:

1. Part I: Foundations
2. Part II: The Person
3. Part III: The Environment
4. Part IV: Occupation

Part I: Foundations

The introductory part provides information on overarching issues in mental health occupational therapy. *Chapter 1: Occupational Therapy Practice Across the Mental Health Continuum* and *Chapter 2: Recovery and Wraparound Models* set the stage for reflecting on the psychosocial practitioner in all areas of practice and across the full continuum from mental illness to flourishing. The new foundational chapter on *Trauma-Informed Practice* (Chapter 5) acknowledges the importance of this content for all occupational therapy practitioners. Other chapters in Part I provide further perspective and background for mental health occupational therapy practice that is (a) person-centered, (b) occupation-based, (c) grounded in theory, (d) supported by evidence, and (e) based on a comprehensive evaluation.

Part II: The Person

Part II is further divided into Occupational Performance and Selected Conditions sections. The Occupational Performance section addresses underlying skills and abilities that are important for participation. These chapters provide detailed content about the skills addressed, theories related to the skills, and specific information on assessment and intervention. This and subsequent chapters include Therapeutic Reasoning Assessment Tables. In addition, numerous occupational therapy interventions are described that address occupational performance skills.

The Selected Conditions section includes information on the diagnoses based on the *Diagnostic and Statistical Manual of Mental Disorders,* Fifth Edition, Text Revision (*DSM-5-TR*). Although occupational therapy practice is not driven by symptomatology, practitioners can better understand the experience of the individual with mental illness if they are aware of the symptoms the person may be experiencing. In addition, a working knowledge of psychiatric diagnoses is useful when participating on a multidisciplinary team. As an occupational therapy text, a major emphasis of these chapters is the impact of the condition on occupational performance.

The chapters in the Selected Conditions section do provide information on medical interventions such as medications; however, because occupational therapy intervention is not based on diagnoses, the occupational therapy interventions are not included in this section. Rather, each diagnosis chapter includes an Intervention Table that outlines common intervention approaches used to address challenges that individuals with these diagnoses often face. The tables also direct learners to the chapters where these interventions are described in detail. In addition, an Index to Interventions is included in Appendix C at the end of the text. *Chapter 17: Chronic Health Conditions and Mental Health* is a new chapter in this section, illustrating the emphasis of the third edition on psychosocial practice across settings and conditions.

Some content on psychiatric conditions that pertain primarily to children (autism, developmental disabilities, attention deficit hyperactivity disorder [ADHD], etc.) and older adults (e.g., dementia) has been deleted in this edition. Our reasoning is that most faculty and learners turn to other well-established and readily available sources for this information. However, the text maintains a strong life-span focus, and numerous examples and features focus directly on children and older adults. Several chapters, such as *Chapter 36: Early Intervention: A Practice Setting for Early Childhood Mental Health, Chapter 37: School Mental Health,* and *Chapter 50: Play* emphasize the mental health needs of children and youth.

Part III: The Environment

The Environment section of the text provides learners with an explicit understanding of the complex range of socioenvironmental influences and interactions that impact occupational performance. Part III has three sections: Societal Influences, Places, and Mental Health Practice Settings.

The Societal Influences section explores macro factors such as policy, stigma, and families, which directly and indirectly impact populations and individuals. *Chapter 28: Social Determinants and Mental Health* is a new chapter accentuating the powerful role societal factors exert on mental health and recovery. It challenges practitioners to identify and confront these influences in their practice.

The Places section examines influences and interactions in broad environmental contexts such as home environments, neighborhoods, and communities. Two new chapters in this section are *Chapter 30: Natural Environments* and *Chapter 33: Virtual Environments,* providing practitioners with options for evaluating ,and supporting occupational participation and performance in these contexts.

The Mental Health Practice Settings section is devoted to the places where OTPs work, including settings with either a primary or secondary focus on mental health practice. Each chapter includes a description of the setting and details the occupational needs of the population served. The role of occupational therapy is discussed in the context of the team at that setting, and related assessments and interventions are presented. *Chapter 44: Addressing Suicide Across the Continuum,* is a new chapter addressing occupational therapy's role.

Part IV: Occupation

This part of the text covers the familiar occupations of work, self-care, and leisure, but also describes some areas of occupation that are frequently neglected, such as sleep and spiritual occupation. Attention is paid to the character and purpose of different occupations across the life span. Specific evaluations and intervention approaches are included in each of the chapters.

Chapter 49: Connectedness and Belonging, a new chapter in this part, underscores the important role relationships (both human and animal) play in our mental health. The self-care and well-being chapter now includes information on the importance of self-care for the OTP, the play chapter provides more depth around the neuroscience of play, and the leisure chapter is expanded to provide more content on the significance of creative occupations for health and well-being.

Special Features

The features in this text make the content come alive. They apply the information so that the learner can envision how it relates to practice. *Occupational Therapy for Mental Health: A Vision for Participation,* Third Edition, retains several favorite features and includes some new ones that promote deeper understanding and learning and embody the tenet that all occupational therapy practice is mental health practice. The exciting new features are presented first.

Videos

For the first time, this text will include access to videos, most of which were created specifically to accompany the text. These short videos (most are less than 3 minutes) come from three sources: OTPs, occupational therapy students, and individuals with a lived experience that relates to the content of the text. The videos are linked to a primary chapter in which the content is closely related via the Apply It Now section of the chapter, which includes discussion questions associated with the video. Other videos are linked to chapters in the Resources section. The *Instructor's Guide* includes fresh discussion questions for many of the videos and identifies chapters in which the videos can be used as supplemental material.

Being a Psychosocial OT Practitioner

This new feature takes the content from a chapter and illustrates how an OTP applies the information to a person. The feature begins with a brief description of an individual receiving services and that individual's particular occupational wants and needs. It goes through the process of goal setting, assessments used and interpreted, intervention planning and implementation, and the response of the person to the intervention. Many of the features illustrate how the content of the chapter is applied in a non–mental health setting. Most chapters that include intervention content include this feature.

Practitioner Profile

Another new feature found in many of the practice settings chapters is entitled *Practitioner Profile*. This feature provides a first-person narrative from the practitioner's perspective. OTPs tell their story of how it is to provide services in their workplace. This accessible and appealing feature presents the content from a real-world point of view.

Mental Health in Culture and Society

The *Mental Health in Culture and Society* feature occurs primarily in the Selected Conditions chapters. Often provocative, this feature strives to challenge conventional medical and clinical views of mental and physical health. It brings in perspectives on current events, artistic works, books, films, organizations, and/or political issues that concern people with mental illness. It infuses Mad Pride, Mad Studies, Disability Studies, and neurodiversity perspectives into the text.

The following features have been maintained from previous editions.

PhotoVoice

PhotoVoice uses a particular methodology to reveal the voices of individuals who are seldom heard—in this case, individuals with the lived experience of a mental health condition. The individuals who contributed their PhotoVoices to this textbook took or selected a photograph and wrote a corresponding narrative as a way to tell their story. Each *PhotoVoice* includes a reflective question, which allows the reader and/or instructor to more deeply process the message of the story and apply it to the content of the chapter.

The Lived Experience

First-person narratives that reflect the chapters' major concepts and provide the reader with a deeper understanding of the lived experience appear as *The Lived Experience* feature. Most of the narratives are written by individuals with a psychiatric disability, and a few are written by family members or OTPs. In some cases, an interview was conducted to help the person tell their story. We have taken care to maintain each writer's unique voice.

Evidence-Based Practice

Each chapter cites research extensively, and this evidence has been significantly updated in the third edition. *Evidence-Based Practice* boxes highlight important research tied to the chapter topic. In this edition, the *Evidence-Based Practice* boxes have a new, more visually appealing graphic to highlight the content.

Intervention Tables

Intervention Tables are found in the Selected Conditions chapters. As occupational therapy intervention is typically not diagnosis-specific, these tables direct the reader to other chapters in which detailed information is provided about related intervention approaches. Each table provides the following information about an intervention approach: (a) the target of the intervention, (b) a brief synopsis of the approach, and (c) the corresponding chapter with more information. Many new interventions have been added to the third edition.

Therapeutic Reasoning Assessment Tables

The *Therapeutic Reasoning Assessment Tables* were updated for the third edition and present assessment tools that occupational therapists use to evaluate individuals for issues relevant to that particular chapter. The tables are included in most chapters, except for those found in the Foundations and Specific Conditions sections. Therapeutic Reasoning Assessment Tables include the following information about each evaluation: (a) who the tool was designed for, (b) what is required of the person being evaluated, (c) what the tool measures, (d) how long it takes to administer it, (d) where it is administered, and (f) whether the tool is associated with a practice model.

Making the Link

As a comprehensive textbook, it is sometimes difficult to determine where specific content is most appropriately placed. To reduce redundancy, the *Making the Link* feature (look for the icon of the clasped hands) was created to direct the reader to other chapters in which additional or complementary information on a topic can be found.

Here's the Point

Each chapter ends with a bulleted list of key points that capture the essence of the chapter's content. This format for summarizing the content of the chapter links back to the learning outcomes for the chapter. Learners can review these points to determine whether they have grasped the major themes of the chapter.

Apply It Now

At the end of each chapter are experiential learning activities that promote the application of knowledge. The reader can use these activities to enhance their experience, and instructors may choose to assign the activities as assignments within or outside the classroom.

Resources

Each chapter includes a list of additional resources that the student and instructor can use to augment the text and utilize in practice. Examples of resources include books, assessments, intervention manuals, videos, and websites.

Indexes: Assessments, Interventions, and Theories and Practice Models

Readers can find indexes to the assessments, interventions, and theories and practice models covered in the textbook in Appendices B, C, and D, respectively. The Theories and Practice Models Index is included so that readers and instructors can clearly see the extensive inclusion of theoretical content in this text. Although the PEO model serves as the organizing structure of the textbook, many theories and practice models are presented. The assessment and intervention indexes help readers find the relevant information and illustrate the numerous assessments and interventions discussed in the book.

Closing Thoughts

The third edition of *Occupational Therapy for Mental Health: A Vision for Participation* represents an evolution of the text as well as occupational therapy practice. We are excited about the changes and believe that readers and instructors will appreciate the new content and features that update and improve upon the most comprehensive textbook on occupational therapy for mental health. Experts in the field of occupational therapy and in the experience of living with a condition came together to create a textbook that informs the entry level student and more generally the field of mental health practice in occupational therapy. We are hopeful that this work continues to play a significant role in supporting participation in everyday life for all people.

Contributors

Becca Allchin, MAVP Aid and Development, BAppSc Occupational Therapy

Research Fellow, Monash Rural Health, Monash University, Victoria, Australia

FaPMI Coordinator, Eastern Health Mental Health and Wellbeing Program, Victoria, Australia

Rachel Ashcraft, MS, OTR/L, TBRI® Practitioner

Assistant Professor; Program Director: Multitiered Approach to Trauma Graduate Certificate

Department of Occupational Therapy

University of Alabama at Birmingham

Birmingham, Alabama, USA

Monica Ayala, MS, OTR/L

Occupational Therapist

Milwaukee, Wisconsin, USA

Antoine Bailliard, PhD, OTR/L

Associate Professor

Occupational Therapy Doctorate Division

Duke University School of Medicine

Adjunct Professor

Center for Excellence in Community Mental Health

Department of Psychiatry

University of North Carolina at Chapel Hill School of Medicine

Chapel Hill, North Carolina, USA

Skye Barbic, PhD, MSc, BScOT, Reg. OT(BC)

Associate Professor

Occupational Science & Occupational Therapy

University of British Columbia

Vancouver, British Columbia, Canada

Kate Barlow, OTD, OTR/L, IMH-E®

Associate Professor

Occupational Therapy

American International College

Springfield, Massachusetts, USA

Kris Pizur-Barnekow, PhD, OTR/L, FAOTA, IMH-E®

Continuous Quality Improvement Lead, WI-AIMH

Associate Professor Emeritus, University of Wisconsin-Milwaukee

Owner, Families First, LLC

Eagle River, Wisconsin, USA

Susan Bazyk, PhD, OTR/L, FAOTA

Project Director of Every Moment Counts

Professor Emerita, Occupational Therapy, Cleveland State University

Cleveland, Ohio, USA

Meghan Blaskowitz, DrPH, MOT

Associate Professor

Duquesne University

Pittsburgh, Pennsylvania, USA

Janette Boney, OTD, OTR

Clinical Education Support Specialist

Master of Science in Occupational Therapy Program

School of Health Sciences, Stockton University

Galloway, New Jersey, USA

Linda Bowden, BHSc(OT), MHSc(OT), NZROT

Occupational Therapist and 2IC Clinical Manager

Clinical Advisory Services Aotearoa

Auckland, New Zealand

Brent Braveman, OTR, PhD, FAOTA

Director of Rehabilitation Services

MD Anderson Cancer Center

Houston, Texas, USA

Anita C. Bundy, ScD, OTR, FAOTA

Professor and Department Head

Department of Occupational Therapy

Colorado State University

Fort Collins, Colorado, USA

Yu-Wei Ryan Chen, PhD, BSc

Senior Lecturer

Program Director—Master of Occupational Therapy

University of Sydney

Sydney, Australia

Carmen Gloria de las Heras de Pablo, MS, OTR

International Professor and Consultant on Occupational Therapy and Model of Human Occupation

Santiago, Chile

Michelle De Oliveira, OTD, OTR/L, QMHP

Occupational Therapist and Service Coordinator

Washington County Early Assessment and Support Alliance (EASA)

Tigard, Oregon, USA

Elena V. Donoso Brown, PhD, OTR/L
Associate Professor
Duquesne University
Pittsburgh, Pennsylvania, USA

Aaron Eakman, PhD, OTR/L, FAOTA
Associate Professor
Occupational Therapy
Colorado State University
Fort Collins, Colorado, USA

Megan Edgelow, EdD, OT Reg. (Ont.)
Assistant Professor
School of Rehabilitation Therapy
Queen's University
Kingston, Ontario, Canada

Claudette Fette, PhD, OTR
Clinical Professor
Occupational Therapy
Texas Women's University
Denton, Texas, USA

Heidi Fischer, OTD, OTR/L
Clinical Associate Professor, Associate Head,
    Occupational Therapy
Director
OT Self-Management Faculty Practice
College of Applied Health Sciences
University of Illinois-Chicago
Chicago, Illinois, USA

Ellie Fossey, PhD, MSc (Health Psychol), DipCOT (UK)
Professor and Head
Department of Occupational Therapy
Monash University
Victoria, Australia

Jackie Fox, PhD, MSc, BSc (OT)
Lecturer Above the Bar
Occupational Therapy
University of Galway
Galway, Ireland

Valerie Fox, PhD, OTR/L
Occupational Therapist
Durham VA Medical Center
University of North Carolina at Chapel Hill
Durham, North Carolina, USA

Sharon Gartland, OTD, OTR
Clinical Professor, OT Program Director
University of Wisconsin-Madison
Madison, Wisconsin, USA

Maureen Gecht-Silver, MPH, OTD, OTR/L
Assistant Professor of Clinical Family Medicine
Clinical Assistant Professor Occupational Therapy
University of Illinois-Chicago
Chicago, Illinois, USA

Elizabeth Griffin Lannigan, PhD, OTR/L, FAOTA
Occupational Therapy Program
University of New Hampshire
Durham, New Hampshire, USA

Bridget J. Hahn, OTD, OTR/L
Assistant Professor
Department of Occupational Therapy
Rush University
Chicago, Illinois, USA

Mark E. Hardison, PhD, OTR/L
Assistant Professor
Occupational Therapy Graduate Program
University of New Mexico
Albuquerque, New Mexico, USA

Aster Harrison, OTD, PhD
Post-doctoral Scholar
Aix-Marseille Université
Marseille, France

Karen R. Hebert, PhD, OTR/L
Department of Occupational Therapy
University of South Dakota
Vermillion, South Dakota, USA

Christine Helfrich, PhD, OTR/L, FAOTA
Professor & Post-Professional OTD Capstone
    Coordinator
Division of Occupational Therapy
School of Health Sciences
American International College
Springfield, Massachusetts, USA

Kim Hewitt-McVicker, OTReg.Cont
Assistant Clinical Professor (Adjunct)
McMaster University
Hamilton, Ontario, Canada

Janice Hinds, OTD, MS, OTR/L, BCMH
Colorado Mental Health Hospital in Fort Logan
Denver, Colorado, USA

Lisa A. Jaegers, PhD, OTR/L, FAOTA
Associate Professor
Occupational Science and Occupational Therapy
Saint Louis University
Director, Transformative Justice Initiative & OT
    Transition and Integration Services
Saint Louis, Missouri, USA

Nikki Hancock, OTD, OTR/L
Clinical Assistant Professor
Doctoral Capstone Coordinator
Department of Occupational Therapy
East Carolina University
Greenville, North Carolina, USA

Sofia L. Herrera-Jaureguiberry, MOT, OTR/L, COT
Academic Fieldwork Coordinator/Lecturer II
Occupational Therapy Graduate Program
University of New Mexico
Albuquerque, New Mexico, USA

Rebecca Knowles, OTD, OTR/L, RYT
Occupational Therapist
Lockhart, Texas, USA

Terry Krupa, PhD, FCAOT
Professor Emerita
Rehabilitation Therapy
Queen's University
Kingston, Ontario, Canada

Carol Lambdin-Pattavina, OTD, OTR/L, CTP
Associate Professor
Department of Occupational Therapy
Westbrook College of Health Professions
University of New England
Portland, Maine, USA

Shelly J. Lane, PhD, OTR/L, FAOTA
Program Director
Department of Occupational Therapy
Colorado State University
Fort Collins, Colorado, USA

Nadine Larivière, PhD, OTCC
Full Professor
School of Rehabilitation
Université de Sherbrooke
Sherbrooke, Quebec, Canada

Ben Lee, PhD
Postdoctoral Research Associate
University of New Hampshire
Durham, New Hampshire, USA

Bronwyn Lennox Thompson, Msc(Hons), PhD(Cant), DipOccTh(CIT)
Clinical Senior Lecturer
University of Otago
Dunedin, Otago, New Zealand

Adam Lo, PhD, OAM
Senior Mental Health Clinician
Metro South Health
Queensland, Australia

Amy Lynch, PhD, OTR/L, SCFES
Associate Professor of Instruction
Health and Rehabilitation Sciences
Temple University
Philadelphia, Pennsylvania, USA

Lisa Mahaffey, PhD, OTR/L, FAOTA
Professor
Occupational Therapy
Midwestern University - Illinois
Downers Grove, Illinois, USA

Rebecca Mannel, OTD, OTR/L
Assistant Professor of Occupational Therapy
Stockton University
Galloway, New Jersey, USA

Carrie Anne Marshall, PhD, OT Reg. (Ont.)
Associate Professor
School of Occupational Therapy
Director, Social Justice in Mental Health Research Lab
Western University
London, Ontario, Canada

Hilary Marshall, MS, OTR/L
Graduate Research Assistant
Department of Occupational Therapy
University of Illinois-Chicago
Chicago, Illinois, USA

Elizabeth Martin, OTD, MHA, OTR/L, QMHP-C, CCTP-II, SEP™
Clinical Director
Holistic Community Therapy
Portland, Oregon, USA

Amy M. Matilla, PhD, OTR/L
Assistant Professor
Occupational Therapy
Duquesne University
Pittsburgh, Pennsylvania, USA

Beth Mozolic-Staunton, PhD, MS, OTR/L
Associate Professor
Bond University
Casuarina, Australia

Gina Mulanthara, OTD
Occupational Therapist
Sutter Health
San Francisco, California, USA

Justin Newton Scanlan, PhD, MHM, BOccThy
Associate Professor
Occupational Therapy
University of Sydney
Sydney, Australia

Ellen Nicholson, DHSc; M Occ Therapy (UNISA); BHSC(OT); NZROT
Deputy Head of School/Teaching and Learning Lead
School of Clinical Sciences, Auckland University of Technology (AUT)
Auckland, New Zealand

Susan Noyes, PhD, OTR/L, FAOTA
Associate Professor
Department of Occupational Therapy
University of Southern Maine
Portland, Maine, USA

Lauren Parsons, PhD
Research Fellow
Curtin School of Allied Health
Curtin University
Bentley, Perth, Western Australia

Mansi Patel, MSc. OT, OT Reg. (Ont.)
Occupational Therapist
University Health Network
Toronto, Ontario, Canada

Andrew Persch, PhD, OTR/L, BCP, FAOTA
Associate Professor
Department of Occupational Therapy
Colorado State University
Fort Collins, Colorado, USA

Emily Petersen, OTD, OTR/L
Occupational Therapist
Los Angeles, California, USA

Doris Pierce, PhD, OT, FAOTA
Occupational Therapy
Eastern Kentucky University
Richmond, Kentucky, USA

Deborah B. Pitts, PhD, OTR/L, BCMH, CPRP, FAOTA
Professor of Clinical Occupational Therapy
USC Chan Division of Occupational Science and Occupational Therapy
University of Southern California
Los Angeles, California, USA

Evguenia S. Popova, PhD, OTR/L
Assistant Professor
Department of Occupational Therapy
Rush University
Chicago, Illinois, USA

Karen Rebeiro Gruhl, PhD, OT Reg. (Ont.)
Occupational Therapist/Ergothérapeute
Adjunct Professor, School of Kinesiology and Health Sciences
Laurentian University
Sudbury, Ontario, Canada

John V. Rider, PhD, OTR/L, MSCS, CEAS
Associate Professor
School of Occupational Therapy
Touro University Nevada
Henderson, Nevada, USA

Rosa Román-Oyola, PhD, MEd, OTR/L
Associate Professor
University of Puerto Rico Medical Sciences
San Juan, Puerto Rico, USA

Sean Roush, OTD, OTR/L, FAOTA, QMHP
Director of Occupational Therapy| Behavioral Sciences Division
Western Oregon University
Monmouth, Oregon, USA

Adam Sakievich, MOT, OTR/L
EntireCare Rehab & Sports Medicine
Flagstaff Medical Center
Flagstaff, Arizona, USA

Gina Baker, OTD, OTR/L, CTP
Clinical Assistant Professor
University of Kansas Medical Center
Kansas City, Missouri, USA

Jaclyn K. Schwartz, PhD, OTR/L, FAOTA
Assistant Professor of Occupational Therapy and Neurology
Washington University at St. Louis
St. Louis, Missouri, USA

Lauren A. Selingo, PhD, OTR/L
Assistant Professor
University of North Carolina at Chapel Hill
Durham, North Carolina, USA

Lindsay Sinclair, MSc. OT, OT Reg. (Ont.)
Occupational Therapist
Toronto, Ontario, Canada

Josh Skuller, PhD, OTR/L, BCP
Associate Professor
Spalding University
Auerbach School of Occupational Therapy
Louisville, Kentucky, USA

Caitlin Smith, OTD, OTR/L, CLT-UE
Clinical Assistant Professor
Occupational Therapy
University of Illinois-Chicago
Chicago, Illinois, USA

Sara Story, EdD, OTD, OTR/L, BCG, CAPS
Director, Associate Professor of Occupational Therapy
Valparaiso University
Valparaiso, Indiana, USA

Theresa Straathof, BSc. OT, OT Reg. (Ont.)
Occupational Therapist
The Ottawa Hospital
Ottawa, Ontario, Canada

Susan Strong, PhD, OT Reg. (Ont), (C)
Associate Clinical Professor
School of Rehabilitation Science
McMaster University, Ontario
PE/Research Schizophrenia and Community
    Integration Service
St. Joseph's Healthcare
Hamilton, Ontario, Canada

Karen Summers, MS, OTR/L
Staff Occupational Therapist
STRIDE (Supporting Therapeutic Recreation for
    Individuals with Disabilities Everyday)
Winchester, Kentucky, USA

Margaret (Peggy) Swarbrick, PhD, OTR, FAOTA
Associate Director
Center of Alcohol & Substance Use Studies
Research Professor
Graduate School of Applied and Professional Psychology
Rutgers University
New Brunswick, New Jersey, USA

Caitlin E. Synovec, OTD, OTR/L, BCMH
Assistant Director of Medical Respite
National Health Care for the Homeless Council
St. Petersburg, Florida, USA

Jillian Taxman, BS, OTR/L
Occupational Therapist
Milwaukee, Wisconsin, USA

Lauren Thomas, OTD, OTR
Occupational Therapist at Boston Public Schools
Boston, Massachusetts, USA

Ryan Thomure, OTD, OTR/L, LCSW
Clinical Assistant Professor
Academic Fieldwork Coordinator
Occupational Therapy
University of Illinois-Chicago
Chicago, Illinois, USA

Susan Tully, MS, LAMFT, OTR/L
Assistant Professor
Occupational Therapy Program
College of Health Sciences
Midwestern University
Glendale, Arizona, USA

Heather Vrbanac-Cress, MSc. OT, OT Reg. (Ont.)
Occupational Therapist
Regional Mentor and Trainer
CBI Health
Cambridge, Ontario, Canada

Amy Wagenfeld, PhD, OTR/L, SCEM, EDAC, FAOTA
University of Washington
Department of Landscape Architecture and Amy
    Wagenfeld/Design
Seattle, Washington, USA

Valerie Wen, OTD, OTR/L
Occupational Therapist
Oregon State Hospital
Salem, Oregon, USA

Catherine M. White, PhD, OT Reg NB
Prevention Coordinator
Horizon Health Network Addiction and Mental Health
    Services
Fredericton, New Brunswick, Canada

Sarah Wilkes-Gillan, PhD, BAppSc (OT) Hons First Class
Lecturer
Occupational Therapy
University of Sydney
Sydney, Australia

Kermeisha Davenport, MS, OTR/L
Senior Lecturer
Occupational Therapy
Chicago State University
Chicago, Illinois, USA

Amy Kashiwa, OTD, OTR/L
Clinical Associate Professor
Occupational Therapy
University of Puget Sound
Tacoma, Washington, USA

Melissa Khosla, OTD, OTR/L
Assistant Professor, Program Director
Occupational Therapy
Indiana Wesleyan University
Marion, Indiana, USA

Christine Linkie, PhD, MS, OTR/L, CPRP
Clinical Assistant Professor
Department of Rehabilitation Science
School of Public Health and Health Professions
University at Buffalo
Buffalo, New York, USA

Rebecca Mojica, OTD, MS, OTR/L
Clinical Assistant Professor
Occupational Therapy Department
Florida International University
Miami, Florida, USA

De'Andre Nunn, OTD, MSEd, USAW-2, OTR/L
Assistant Professor
Occupational Therapy
Chicago State University
Chicago, Illinois, USA

Katy Schmidt, OTD, OTR/L
Assistant Professor
School of Occupational Therapy
Belmont University
Nashville, Tennessee, USA

Shannon Schoellig, OTD, MS, OTR/L
Assistant Professor
Occupational Therapy
Utica University
Utica, New York, USA

Janeene Sibla, EdD, OTD, OTR/L
Chair of Occupational Therapy Program
Associate Dean of Health Professions
University of Mary
Bismark, North Dakota, USA

Kasey Stepansky, CScD, OTR/L, C/NDT, CBIS
Clinical Assistant Professor
Department of Occupational Therapy
Rangos School of Health Sciences
Duquesne University
Pittsburgh, Pennsylvania, USA

Pam Stephenson, OTD, OTR/L, BCP, FAOTA
Associate Professor
Occupational Therapy Program
Mary Baldwin University
Murphy Deming College of Health Sciences
Staunton, Virginia, USA

Steven D. Taff, PhD, OTR/L, FNAP, FAOTA
Professor, Occupational Therapy and Medicine
Director, Teaching Scholars Program
Washington University in St. Louis
St. Louis, Missouri, USA

Lauren S. Turbeville, SOT, PPOTD
Assistant Professor
Department of Occupational Therapy
East Carolina University
Greenville, North Carolina, USA

Sandra Whisner, OTR, PhD
Program Director and Associate Professor
Entry-Level Doctor of Occupational Therapy Program
TTUHSC School of Health Professions
Lubbock, Texas, USA

Acknowledgments

It is hard to believe that nearly 20 years have passed since this book was conceived, although the "gestation" for the first edition (published in 2011) was the longest (nearly 5–6 years). We are ever so grateful to F.A. Davis for believing that we could produce a text that would be adopted worldwide with contributions by occupational therapy and other mental health practitioners from across the globe. This third edition incorporates ideas generated from readers, thought leaders, students, educators, practitioners, advocates, and persons with lived experiences who help us to illustrate how occupational therapy *for* mental health can be universally applied to promote mental health and well-being, facilitating full participation in everyday life around meaningful occupations. The second edition was published in 2019; since then, we have learned so much from our collective COVID-19 experiences around mental health and its link to everyday life activities, social connectedness, and challenging issues around isolation, anxiety, depression, and despair. We hope that the third edition features such as PhotoVoice, The Lived Experiences, Being a Psychosocial OT Practitioner narratives, Practitioner Profiles, Mental Health in Culture and Society, and our video library offer faculty and students opportunities to learn the creative ways that OTPs address mental health and well-being using their skills to enact therapeutic use of self as a part of skilled interventions for all populations.

Christa A. Fratantoro, Publisher, has been an exceptional advocate for this text from its inception. She helped to create and realize the vision for the text and offered us a skilled developmental editor in Nancy Peterson, who assumed more of a project director role in the third edition, keeping our team on task across many meetings, sometimes weekly, sometimes monthly. Nancy's detailed attention to creating new features was valuable, especially helping us to elicit videos from authors and other contributors and creating the supplemental materials that accompany the videos. Nancy helped us get as many videos as we did because of her diligent efforts. In addition, she generated several new PhotoVoice pieces highlighting caregiving and the challenges to well-being that accompany complex family situations. Julie Chase provided support for ensuring all chapters had the necessary visuals and readied the manuscripts for copyediting so the production team could do its work. How great to have a last name that matches her primary work—she chased us down effectively!

We are grateful for the careful guidance offered by Johnny Rider who took the lead in creating a template for the Being a Psychosocial OT Practitioner feature and coached chapter authors as they developed their respective Being a Psychosocial OT Practitioner features. He was especially reliable and competent in his role. Aster Harrison offered their expertise consistent with our collective vision for the text by pushing boundaries around mental health policy and engaged advocacy. In addition, Aster oversaw the new Mental Health in Culture and Society feature and provided critical guidance on building resources for faculty teaching this content.

We took advantage of being with each other at American Occupational Therapy Association (AOTA) gatherings (which were especially valued after not being able to gather in 2020 and 2021) and used those opportunities to tap into the insights and wisdom of contributors such as Sean Rousch, Halley Read, Amy Mattila, Rondalyn Whitney, Johnny Rider, and Aster Harrison.

We acknowledge Amanda Lind, a student from Midwestern University–Glendale, who helped with the glossary. Margaret J. Bolger, OTR/L, a school-based occupational therapist at Windsor Southeast Supervisory Union in Windsor, Vermont, provided invaluable assistance and enthusiasm in curating this edition's student, practitioner, and lived experience videos. Thanks also to Katie Caspero, MS, OTR/L of OT Graphically in Pittsburgh, Pennsylvania, who helped us envision an infographic presentation for our Evidence-Based Practice feature. We are thankful for all those who contributed to the video library and grateful for those who provided their Practitioner Profile.

We want to recognize the contributors to this text. So many authors contributed, and their effort is nothing short of a labor of love. They worked hard to channel their passion and expertise into the pages of this book—their contributions make this text so awesome.

We acknowledge those professionals who were involved in reviewing chapters, especially those new chapters that were innovated because of your input. We are always thankful for the insights that are shared to help us be sure that we are offering contemporary and evidence-based practice examples, and your reviews provide us with important feedback.

We close with a heartfelt thanks to the people for whom we hope our text offers a message of hope, health, and well-being—those who work to achieve the greatest state of mental health, those who struggle with the stress of everyday life, and those who live with significant disability because of mental health and co-occurring chronic health conditions across all cultures and the life span. We dedicate our work to you and learn with you. We serve you as advocates, humbled by your knowledge and experience, and join you in creating a society that is inclusive, supporting and recognizing all, in building capacity for using occupational therapy *for* building mental health and our "vision for participation" in all the occupations that hold meaning and value to you.

Tana Brown
Jaime Muñoz
Ginny Stoffel

Student, Practitioner, and Lived Experience Videos

We're excited to offer videos to accompany this edition of the text. These short videos (most are less than 3 minutes) were recorded by individuals with a lived experience, occupational therapy students, and occupational therapy practitioners on topics that relate to the content of the text. The videos are referenced in chapters to which they apply and linked to Apply It Now activities or provided as supplemental resources. Videos can be accessed at the online resource center at FADavis.com.

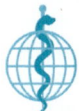 Visit the online resource center at **FADavis.com** to access the videos.

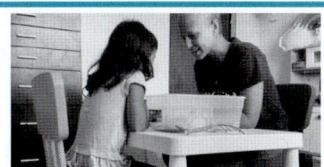 **Videos Showcasing the Lived Experience**

Video Title	Brief Description
Playing for Mother Undergoing Cancer Treatment —*Marylein Serrano and Rosa Román-Oyola, PhD, MEd, OTR/L*	A speech-language pathologist who is a mother of two with several cancer diagnoses discusses with an occupational therapist how her role as mom changed during cancer treatment.
Prioritizing Family During a Mother's Cancer Treatment —*Marylein Serrano and Rosa Román-Oyola, PhD, MEd, OTR/L*	A speech-language pathologist who is a mother of two with several cancer diagnoses discusses with an occupational therapist how friends and extended family helped her prioritize family during treatments.
Will Horowitz: Lived Experience of Autism —*Will Horowitz*	As a child, a young man with autism had a "one-track mind" for trains. He shares how he transformed this interest into a volunteer opportunity as an adult.
Jordan's Lived Experience of Anxiety and Depression —*Jordan Andrews Noah*	An occupational therapist describes her lived experience of anxiety and depression focusing on issues critical to recovery and occupational therapy practice.
Jordan's Lived Experience of Recovery as an Occupational Therapy Practitioner —*Jordan Andrews Noah*	Jordan, an occupational therapist, explains how she blends her own lived experience with anxiety, depression, and recovery into her work as an occupational therapist.
Jennie's Lived Experience of Sensory Processing Differences —*Jennie McDonald*	An occupational therapy degree student with lived experience of sensory differences, anxiety, and depression describes discovering her diagnosis, classroom experiences, and managing her reactions to sensory stimuli.
Mary's Lived Experience as an Unhoused Individual and Her Occupational Therapist's Perspective —*Mary Holsinger and Quinn Tyminski*	Mary provides a first-person account of being unhoused and shares how occupational therapy impacted her life. Mary's occupational therapist describes Mary's journey and transformation.

Video Title	Brief Description
Nicholas's Lived Experience of Schizophrenia —*Nicholas Buekea*	An occupational therapist with lived experience of schizophrenia describes his first episode and how occupational therapy helped him engage, reconnect, and find purpose to support recovery.
Veteran's Caregiver on Advocacy and VA Support —*Nancy Peterson*	The spouse and caregiver of a veteran with early-onset Alzheimer disease shares her experiences and the arduous but important process of applying for VA benefits.
Caregiver of Spouse With Alzheimer Disease on Challenges —*Nancy Peterson*	The spouse of a man with early-onset Alzheimer disease describes his transformation from a person with an exciting career to someone unable to work.
Laura's Experience as a Mother of an Autistic Son —*Laura Horowitz*	A mother describes her son as a baby, observations she and day-care teachers noticed, and her emotions upon learning her loving, talkative, playful child had autism.
Tricks and Techniques From the Mother of an Autistic Son —*Laura Horowitz*	A mother describes creative ways of helping her autistic son succeed and shares "tricks and techniques" from 20 years of experience raising her son.
Aimee's Lived Experience of Substance Use and Autism —*Aimee Klock and Rebecca Knowles*	An occupational therapist with lived experience of substance use disorder, posttraumatic stress disorder, and autism describes how her lived experiences affected her role as an occupational therapy student.
Aster's Lived Experience of Suicidality —*Aster Harrison*	An occupational therapist, educator, and disability researcher shares her experience with major depression and suicidality and shares actions and resources that got them through periods of crisis.

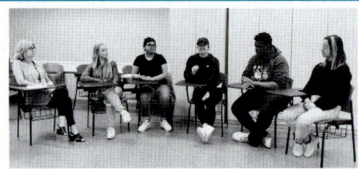

Videos Showcasing the Occupational Therapy Student Experience

Video Title	Brief Description
Fieldwork Experience in Juvenile Correction Setting —*Margaret Bolger*	An occupational therapist reflects on how she felt both prepared and unprepared for her fieldwork experience and the importance of setting boundaries.
Student Panel Discusses Running Groups in Mental Health Settings —*Laurie Knis-Matthews, PhD, OT and Kean University Students*	Occupational therapy students discuss experiences running groups in a psychiatric day program that included feeling intimidated, being welcomed, and their rising confidence running groups.
Student Perceptions of Bias and Stigma —*Quinn Tyminski, Sam Kressman, Mia Pearce, Kendall Johnson, and Anna Brondyke*	Four occupational therapy students share reflections on recognizing and working through personal biases against people who are unhoused and how engagement led to transformative learning.
First Fieldwork Experience in Inpatient Mental Health —*Casey Cushing*	An occupational therapist describes her first fieldwork experience in an inpatient mental health setting. She was nervous, but things turned out well.

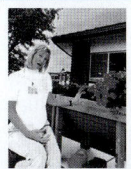

Videos Showcasing the Occupational Therapy Practitioner Experience

Video Title	Brief Description
Child in Crisis —*Brittany Birth*	An occupational therapist describes working in an adolescent unit of a psychiatric hospital with Mikey, an 8-year-old boy who presents with a complex set of challenges.
Positive Mindset Creative Arts Festival —*Adam Lo*	An occupational therapist showcases the Positive Mindset Creative Arts Festival, which promotes positive thinking about mental health and increases help-seeking behaviors using a creative arts focus.
Occupational Therapy Collaboration in Early Head Start —*Joan Ziegler Delahunt and Alison Baker*	An occupational therapist and occupational therapy assistant describe how they work collaboratively to support children, parents, and staff at an Early Head Start program.
Occupational Therapy and Music Therapy in Early Head Start —*Joan Ziegler Delahunt with Cindy Krause*	An occupational therapist and music therapist discuss their group for infants and toddlers emphasizing self-regulation, awareness of self and others, attention, language, and motor function.
Managing a Challenging Behavior in Young Children —*Joan Ziegler Delahunt with Alison Baker*	An occupational therapist and occupational therapy assistant discuss working with children from at-risk families, teachers, and other therapists to identify developmental delays and intervene.
Sensory Garden in Geriatric Psychiatric Unit —*Callie Ward*	An occupational therapist showcases a multisensory garden at an inpatient psychiatric facility and describes how this space impacts arousal levels and has positive effects on residents' participation.
Two Practitioners Discuss Their Work in Suicide Prevention —*Nadine Larivière and Kim Hewitt-McVicker*	Two occupational therapists discuss their work in suicide prevention, sharing reflections and pearls of wisdom gained in years of practice in this area.
Occupational Therapy Approaches in a Shelter for Unaccompanied Refugee Youth —*Claudette Fette*	An occupational therapist shares work in a massive unaccompanied minor shelter. The immigrant minors experienced trauma, a lack of meaningful occupations, bullying, and untrained staff.
Leisure Occupations for Unhoused Individuals —*Kailin Lust*	An occupational therapist working in community mental health and homeless services describes barriers to, and the powerful impact of, participation in leisure for individuals she serves.
Life Skills Groups in an Unhoused Population —*Kailin Lust*	An occupational therapist provides examples of activities used in life skills groups she runs in a women's shelter and describes how group processes facilitate peer-to-peer support.
Using Objects to Promote Engagement —*Jennifer Summers*	An occupational therapist describes discovering an antique wheelchair and how it provided focus, meaning, and purpose for the individuals she worked with in forensic mental health.

Video Title	Brief Description
Civic Engagement Group in an Inpatient Psychiatric Unit —*Jennifer Summers*	The narrator shares experiences working as an occupational therapy assistant in inpatient psychiatry, running civic engagement groups, and how the opportunity to "give back" impacted group members.
Mental Health and Well-Being During COVID —*Caitlin Smith*	An occupational therapist observes how stress and anxiety impacted therapeutic outcomes during the COVID-19 pandemic, reminding her to refocus on mental health challenges in practice.
Person-Centered Interactions in Mental Behavioral Health —*Patrycja Budzyk*	An OTP working in behavioral health describes working with a woman identified as chronically homeless and strategies used to elicit this woman's occupational history.
Cooking Group in a State Mental Hospital —*Samuel Gentile*	An occupational therapist describes a weekly cooking group he runs in a state mental hospital that allows him to assess occupational performance while participants develop functional skills.

Contents in Brief

Contents

Foundations

The introductory section of this text establishes the groundwork for understanding occupational therapy practice in mental health. The first chapter sets the tone for the text by promoting an optimistic and hopeful perspective that acknowledges the continuum of psychosocial care that occurs for *all* individuals across *all* practice settings—in mental health settings and other occupational therapy practice settings. All chapters in the text honor the expertise and point of view of the individual with mental illness by including features that give voice to the diverse individuals who receive occupational therapy services.

In addition to Chapter 1: Occupational Therapy Practice Across the Mental Health Continuum, chapters in this part of the text provide further perspective and background for mental health occupational therapy practice that is (a) person centered, (b) occupation based, (c) grounded in theory, (d) supported by evidence, and (e) cognizant of the historical roots of occupational therapy in mental health. Additionally, chapter contributors intentionally examine occupational therapy mental health practice along the recovery continuum from mental illness to positive, healthy functioning, to flourishing.

PART 1

Occupational Therapy Practice Across the Mental Health Continuum

Skye Barbic

Mental illness is a leading cause of disability worldwide, and it is estimated that nearly one in four people will experience a mental health condition at some point in their lives (GBD 2019 Mental Disorders Collaborators, 2022; Solmi et al., 2022). People of all ages, genders, and backgrounds are affected by mental illness (Patel et al., 2015). The severity of mental health problems can range from mild conditions such as anxiety and depression to more severe conditions such as schizophrenia and bipolar disorder.

Mental illness can affect a person's ability to think, feel, and behave in ways that are consistent with their needs, goals, and values. Stigma, lack of access to mental health care, poverty and social inequality, trauma and conflict, and lack of education and awareness are long-standing factors that contribute to poor mental health across the world (Aguirre Velasco et al., 2020; Radez et al., 2021). Although people often think of mental health specialty practice as occurring in hospital- and community-based settings that serve people with mental illness, occupational therapy practitioners (OTPs) work with people with mental health challenges in all practice settings. In other words, all OTPs are mental health practitioners. **Mental wellness** is the ability to successfully carry out everyday activities, develop supportive relationships, cope with the normal stresses of life, and function productively (Fusar-Poli et al., 2020). OTPs work to promote mental wellness regardless of their practice setting.

This chapter begins by describing current concerns related to the global mental health crisis. Next the profession's history in mental health is presented as a way to understand the unique role occupational therapy plays in providing services across the mental health continuum. There is a key point of emphasis in this third edition of the textbook. The slight change in the title from Occupational Therapy *in* Mental Health to Occupational Therapy *for* Mental Health reflects this new emphasis. This chapter defines the mental health continuum and sets the stage for presenting occupational therapy's role in promoting mental health across the continuum from mental wellness to mental illness throughout the full life span for all people and communities in all settings.

Factors Contributing to the Global Mental Health Crisis

In the past decade, intersecting factors have contributed to what is often described as a global mental health crisis (Solmi et al., 2022). Modern day OTPs must recognize the complex interplay between individual, social, environmental, and spiritual factors that affect the mental health of persons and communities. This includes having a comprehensive understanding of the factors that support an individual's state of well-being, contribute to mental health problems, and impact on a person's ability to recover and live a full and meaningful life.

For example, the isolation, stress, and uncertainty caused by the COVID-19 pandemic are associated with an increase in anxiety, depression, and other mental health problems worldwide (Cénat et al., 2022; *The Lancet Psychiatry*, 2021). Other current factors contributing to mental health concerns include the rising use of social media, which is associated with significant increases in social isolation, bullying, and negative self-comparisons, notably for youth (Kriegel et al., 2021). Substance use and drug toxicity crises are also commonly associated with mental illness and poor outcomes, with a higher prevalence of co-occurrence in cultures in which there is easy access to alcohol and other substances (Marchand et al., 2022; Scheuermeyer et al., 2023).

Increasingly, the impact of climate change is shown to have adverse effects on people's mental health and functioning (Corvetto et al., 2023; Léger-Goodes et al., 2022). The effects of climate change, such as natural disasters, extreme weather events, and loss of biodiversity, can lead to anxiety, depression, posttraumatic stress disorder (PTSD), and other mental health issues that directly affect quality of life and function (Corvetto et al., 2023; Trudell et al., 2021). Climate change is also associated with chronic stress caused by the uncertainty and fear of the future (Léger-Goodes et al., 2022; Trudell et al., 2021). The fear of future disasters, extreme weather, and food insecurity can have long-term mental health effects on the welfare of communities and disrupt long-standing social structures (Léger-Goodes et al., 2022; Trudell et al., 2021). For example, the loss of livelihoods, migration, and displacement create a sense of loss and disconnection.

People at social disadvantage because of stigmatization and a decreased social standing are more likely to experience poor mental and physical health (Boysen et al., 2020). **Minority Stress Theory** posits that stigma results in an increased exposure to stressful life situations (Botha & Frost, 2020; Meyer et al., 2008). At the same time, the people with these increased exposures have fewer resources to mitigate these events. The model takes a social and environmental perspective that the disadvantage is caused by social exclusion and not anything specific to the targeted group. This chapter makes the case that all OTPs have a role in addressing the mental health needs of individuals, communities, and populations. For more information on these factors contributing to a global mental health crisis, see Chapter 27: Mental Health Stigma and Sanism, Chapter 30: Natural Environments, and Chapter 33: Virtual Environments. 🤝

All Occupational Therapy Practitioners Are Mental Health Practitioners

It is critical for OTPs to consider mental health as an essential aspect of overall health and health service delivery and prioritize it accordingly. Mental health refers to the state of an individual's psychological and emotional well-being, including the ability to think, feel, and behave in a way that allows them to function effectively in daily life (Manwell et al., 2015). Similar to physical health, mental health can have a significant impact on an individual's quality of life, relationships, participation in meaningful activities, and overall well-being. Mental health problems, such as anxiety, depression, bipolar disorder, and schizophrenia, can be just as debilitating as physical illnesses and can significantly affect a person's ability to carry out their daily activities.

Moreover, research indicates there is a strong connection between mental and physical health. For instance, people with mental health problems are more likely to have physical health problems, and vice versa. Hence, OTPs treating mental health problems can have a positive impact on physical health, and vice versa. All OTPs play a critical role in understanding the full range of mental health needs of the diverse types of people they work with and providing culturally responsive, evidence-based care where and when needed.

Occupational Therapy's Long and Complex History in Mental Health

With its underlying belief that all people should participate fully in their communities, occupational therapy can play a critical role in leading global health reform for the next century by supporting communities and governments to create systems in which mental health is valued and prioritized and where everyone has access to the care and support they need to live healthy and fulfilling lives. But before discussing the future of the occupational therapy profession, it is important to be familiar with its past.

A Grounding in Mental Health

Occupational therapy in mental health has a long and complex history, dating back to the late 1800s—a time when mental illness was often seen as a moral failing rather than a medical condition. Many people with mental illness at that time were institutionalized in large asylums away from public life. Some researchers suggest that the earliest evidence of using occupation as a therapeutic method for treating people with mental illness can be found in documents dated back to 100 BCE. Greek physicians prescribed treatments of massage, exercise, music, and travel to their patients.

Introduction to the Being a Psychosocial OT Practitioner Feature

As this chapter has asserted, there is an inseparable bond between mental and physical health. Mental health is an essential aspect of overall health and well-being. OTPs address mental health across the continuum of care, in every practice setting, and at all stages of the life span. In an effort to make the concept that all OTPs are psychosocial practitioners tangible, regardless of the population they serve or the practice setting, the editors have created an exciting and innovative special feature, *Being a Psychosocial OT Practitioner*. This feature was designed to help each reader become a competent and caring mental health practitioner.

Throughout the textbook, readers will find practical case studies demonstrating how OTPs identify psychosocial strengths and needs among the people they serve and use a holistic and evidence-based approach to provide effective and compassionate mental health care that meets their unique needs of their patient populations. These case studies describe real clinical scenarios from the perspective of an OTP delivering mental health services across various practice settings, including those commonly viewed as non–mental health settings.

Each special feature draws from the content provided in the corresponding chapter to help readers apply what they have just learned. Each case study ends with reflective questions that encourage readers to consider how they, as OTPs, in collaboration with the person, could contribute to the care plan. These questions promote further exploration of concepts from the chapter by highlighting concerns of the person yet to be addressed and encouraging readers to identify additional interventions or assessments appropriate for the case. Reading the special features and completing the reflective questions will help readers apply the chapter content, develop clinical reasoning skills, and reinforce their role as a psychosocial OTP wherever they work. This special feature and the rest of the textbook provide a foundation in mental health practice principles for all OTPs.

Although it may be clear from reading this textbook and learning from experts in the field that OTPs have a unique and necessary role in mental health care, OTPs can still struggle with their professional identity. Advocating for appropriate mental health care approaches in all settings is difficult. However, OTPs' duty as science-driven, evidence-based health-care providers is to enable people of all ages to participate in daily living or live better with injury, illness, or disability. Doing so includes assessing and treating the full range of mental health needs of the diverse types of people served. This feature demonstrates what skilled OTPs can do in psychosocial practice across all practice settings. Readers should consider the significant role they will have as psychosocial OTPs as they learn how to support and promote the mental wellness of all people.

Unfortunately, these physicians were anomalies of their time. For centuries after, the use of occupation-based interventions for people with mental illness was rare. More commonly, physical and chemical restraints were used as best practice (Farris et al., 2019).

In France in the late 18th century, two pioneering physicians named Drs. Philippe Pinel and Johann Christian

Real proposed significant reforms to hospital-based care for people with mental illness. Instead of heavy physical and chemical restraint, Pinel and Real championed their institution to consider work and leisure activities as ways to enhance the health and quality of life of their patients. This time was branded the Age of Enlightenment, when moral treatment of all individuals was considered a priority. Although not yet formalized as a role, the term "occupational therapy" began to be used across mental health settings as a way to provide patients with meaningful activities and promote their independence and self-worth. The literature of moral treatment discusses examples of specific occupations selected by or for certain patients based on the identified needs of each person (Brigham, 1994; Charland, 2007).

In the United States, Clifford W. Beers, who recovered from psychosis despite the sometimes brutal mental health treatment he received, was a key driver of the **Mental Hygiene Movement** at the turn of the 20th century. His book *A Mind That Found Itself* (Beers, 1908) is one of the earliest first-person accounts of recovery from serious mental illness. Beers collaborated with Adolf Meyer, often identified as the philosophical founder of occupational therapy, who was a prominent psychiatrist in the early 1900s (Purtle et al., 2020). During this time, Meyer was the chief psychiatrist at Johns Hopkins Hospital and the president of the American Psychiatric Association. He established the first occupational therapy department and appointed Eleanor Clarke Slagle as its head. Meyer believed that mental illness was caused by an imbalance of work, rest, and play. At the time, Meyer challenged the belief that an extended convalescence was healing for people with mental illness. Instead, Meyer felt that doing, or involvement in meaningful activity, was essential for well-being. He promoted engagement in occupations as a way to improve mental health.

The **Arts and Crafts Movement** also influenced the developing profession of occupational therapy in the early 1900s. The movement arose in reaction to the industrialization and mechanization of society with the goal of establishing "harmony between architect, designer and craftsman" (Cumming & Kaplan, 1991, p. 6). Followers of the movement placed an emphasis on work done by hand instead of machines, with the important belief that the nature of the work had a positive influence on health. Arts and crafts were soon adopted as therapeutic media in psychiatric hospitals. Arts and crafts projects were useful media, especially in institutions where patients often remained for many years (Fig. 1-1).

For example, Herbert James Hall, MD, established Marblehead Pottery in Marblehead, Massachusetts. The business used persons from the sanitarium as the potters, and their work quickly became some of the most sought-after pottery of its time. Marblehead pottery is still highly valued (Fig. 1-2). In 1905 Hall received a grant to study the use of graded manual occupations for treating neurasthenia, a common diagnosis of the time that was associated with fatigue, anxiety, and depression (Hall, 1905). Four years later he received a second grant to continue his study, which constituted the first systematic research on the effectiveness of therapeutic occupation on the recovery of people with mental health conditions (see the Evidence-Based Practice feature to learn what Hall discovered in this early research).

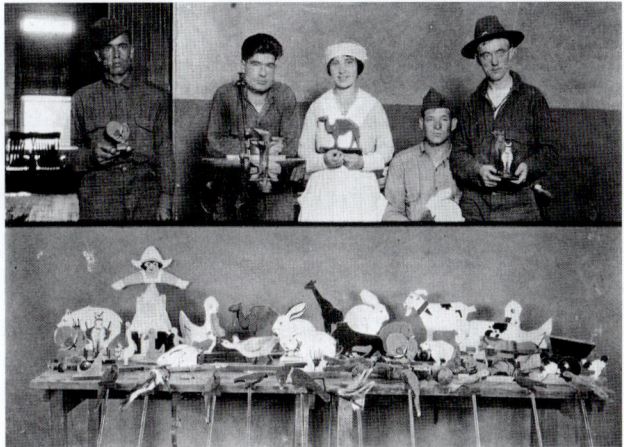

FIGURE 1-1. Toy making for occupational therapy in a psychiatric hospital. World War I era. *Photo courtesy of the Reeve Photograph Collection, National Museum of Health and Medicine, Otis Historical Archives.*

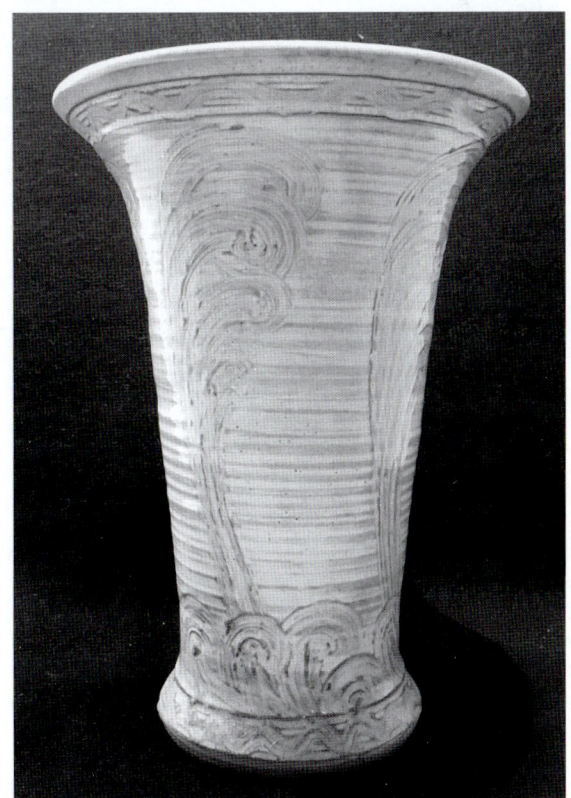

FIGURE 1-2. Marblehead Pottery vase with stylized feather motif. *Photograph courtesy of the Marblehead Museum in Marblehead, MA.*

Arts and crafts are still useful occupational therapy media today, although the economic or vocational benefit might be lower, and the leisure or avocational benefit might be higher. In addition to offering the person the experience of joy and pleasure, they serve as benefits to self-esteem and self-worth. See Chapter 51: Leisure and Creative Occupations.

Evidence-Based Practice

Very Early Example of Evidence-Based Practice

Evidence for the value of occupation existed before occupational therapy was a profession.

RESEARCH
FINDINGS

From 1905 to 1909, Hall followed 100 individuals. Of these, 59 were reported to have "improved," 27 were considered "much improved," and 14 were reported to have "no relief" but without an operational definition of these classifications. Diagnoses included neurasthenia severe, neurasthenia mild, hysteria, psychoses or fixed idea, insanity, and unclassified. All participants were outpatients staying at a boarding home located 500 yards from the Handcraft Shop in Marblehead, Massachusetts. The daily schedule was "a division of the 24 hours into changeable periods of work, rest, and recreation, plenty of air, wholesome food, wise suggestions and such medical treatments as may be indicated" (Hall, 1910, p. 13). Crafts used included pottery, hand weaving, basketry, metalwork, and woodcarving.

APPLICATIONS

➡ OTPs offer their distinct value when they facilitate recovery-oriented programs that structure the person's 24-hour day into those occupations most meaningful to the person, including work, rest, and recreation.
➡ Access to outdoor space, healthy food, and medical care are important considerations in a recovery plan.

REFERENCES

Hall, H. J. (1910). Work cure: A report of five years' experience at an institution devoted to the therapeutic application of manual work. *Journal of the American Medical Association, 54*(1), 12–14. https://doi.org/10.1001/jama.1910.92550270001001d

In 1917, the profession of occupational therapy was founded with the creation of the National Society for the Promotion of Occupational Therapy (Andersen & Reed, 2017). The founding members included William Rush Dunton Jr., Susan Cox Johnson, George Edward Barton, Eleanor Clarke Slagle, Thomas Bessell Kidner, Isabel Gladwin Newton, and Susan Edith Tracy. Many of these founders were working in mental health settings and employing what today would be regarded as "occupation-based" practice. For example, Eleanor Clarke Slagle worked on the mental health unit of Johns Hopkins Hospital with the psychiatrist and philosophical founder of occupational therapy, Adolf Meyer. Together they developed **Habit Training,** a method based on the idea that organizing habits and a well-balanced day of work, games, recreation, and rest was essential to health (Slagle, 1938).

Growth (and Decline) of the Profession

During the early 20th century, advances in medical and psychiatric treatments led to a shift in the focus of mental health care. Once the role of occupational therapy was formalized, OTPs began to play a critical role in team-based care models to work more closely with other health-care providers and became more involved in the treatment of mental illness. This included emphasizing the evidence for activity as a form of therapy to help persons regain skills and abilities that were lost because of their illnesses. During the formative years of the profession, practice in mental hospitals dominated, followed by practice in care of individuals with tuberculosis.

Although the history of the profession reveals that occupation is central to occupational therapy practice, the focus on occupation has been inconsistent over the years (Wong & Fisher, 2015). For a time, the profession, perhaps in a misguided effort to gain credibility, became reductionistic, with a concentration on remediation of person factors (e.g., using exercise to increase grip strength or paper-and-pencil activities to improve cognition). The remedial approaches adopted by OTPs in the 1950s reflected a distinct departure from the early therapeutic use of occupation (Andersen & Reed, 2017).

The **Person-Environment-Occupation (PEO) model,** which serves as the framework of this text, is one of several occupation-focused models that arose out of a need to reclaim occupational therapy's heritage and bring greater attention to the role of the environment in health and occupational performance (Law et al., 1996). See Chapter 3: Person-Environment-Occupation Model. 🤝

In the 1960s and 1970s, the concept of community-based mental health care gained popularity and OTPs began to play a key role in this movement. OTPs supported people transitioning from institutional care to community-based care and worked with them to develop skills needed for daily living and employment. However, treating people with mental illness in the community was still riddled with stigma and a lack of public support. In the United States, deinstitutionalization and the resulting lack of psychiatric beds and reimbursable services resulted in a major decline in the number of OTPs practicing in mental health settings.

The Recovery Movement and Occupational Therapy

In the late 1980s, a new movement called the "Recovery Movement" began (Deegan, 1997). **Recovery** is an approach to mental health treatment that focuses on empowering individuals to take control of their own recovery process (Anthony, 1993). Dr. Deegan, a psychologist and mental health advocate with a history of living with serious mental illness, coined the term and suggested that people could not just live "in the community" but could live full and meaningful lives despite having a mental illness.

The concept of mental health recovery can be traced back to the writings and work of people such as John Thomas Perceval, who wrote of his personal recovery from psychosis in 1840 despite the poor treatment he received from doctors (Bateson, 1961), and Clifford Beers, who worked to reform the treatment of people with mental illness based on his own experiences in mental institutions (Dain, 1980). However, the movement that resulted in recovery-oriented systems of care was initiated in the 1980s by dissatisfied consumers and survivors of a mental health system that focused on symptoms (Davidson et al., 2021).

Leaders in the field included Judi Chamberlin, Fred Frese, and Patricia Deegan. Judi Chamberlin was a political activist whose important work, *On Our Own,* advocated for basic human rights and self-determinism for people with psychiatric disabilities (Chamberlin, 1978). Fred Frese, the director of psychology at the Western Reserve Psychiatric Rehabilitation Center, revealed his diagnosis of schizophrenia during a speech to the American Psychological Association (Frese, 2015). He also served on the board of directors for the American Occupational Therapy Association (AOTA). Dr. Deegan's work focused, and continues to focus, on promoting recovery-oriented approaches to mental health care. This work was instrumental in shifting the mental health field away from a medical model, which focused on symptom management and medication, and toward a recovery model, which emphasizes empowerment, hope, spirituality and meaning, and self-determination (Deegan, 2007; Deegan & Drake, 2006). Dr. Deegan emphasized the importance of listening to the experiences of people with mental illness and incorporating their perspectives into the development of mental health policies and practices.

The Recovery Movement dramatically changed the potential for occupational therapy in the field of mental health. The concept of recovery encouraged a shift from supporting people to live in the community toward supporting people to thrive. The role of occupational therapy soon included supporting individuals in their recovery journey by promoting independence, enhancing quality of life, and facilitating engagement in meaningful activities. In this way, occupational therapy began to play a vital role in the Recovery Movement by empowering individuals to take control of their own recovery process and achieve their personal goals. OTPs also became part of a collective voice in advocating for the rights of people with mental illness, particularly around issues of involuntary treatment and coercion; building inclusive communities for all; working to promote recovery-oriented approaches to mental health care; and advocating for the rights and empowerment of people with mental illness. For more information on the Recovery Movement, see Chapter 2: Recovery and Wraparound Models. 🤝

Current Practice, Barriers and Challenges, and Future Opportunities

Today, occupational therapy is an integral part of mental health care in most parts of the world. In the United States, the profession is making gains in reestablishing the role of its practitioners as mental health practitioners. This includes efforts to receive recognition as qualified mental health providers and qualified behavioral health providers (Wilburn et al., 2021). Occupational therapy is prioritized as a core health service to help people with mental illness of all ages achieve their goals, improve their functioning and independence, and enhance their quality of life.

OTPs work in a range of mental health settings, including hospitals, primary care clinics, corrections facilities, community mental health centers, and schools, among others. OTPs use a variety of interventions, including individual and group therapy, environmental modification, and assistive technology, to help people with mental illness achieve their goals and lead fulfilling lives. OTPs work toward creating awareness and educating the public about mental health conditions, their impact on individuals, and the importance of seeking early treatment. They also work toward preventing mental health conditions, promoting wellness, and building resilience. With the Recovery Movement building a pathway for person-centered care and system reform and global mental health challenges being more prevalent than ever, the need for occupational therapy has never been greater.

Despite occupational therapy's significant role in mental health to promote engagement in meaningful activities, increase social participation, and improve daily functioning in a recovery-oriented movement, several barriers to occupational therapy service delivery in the field of mental health remain. Stigma surrounding mental illness continues to prevent many individuals from seeking help. This is notably true for people who are racialized and marginalized (Castro-Ramirez et al., 2021; Pattison et al., 2021; Rafla-Yuan et al., 2022; Solmi et al., 2022). Access to mental health care is also a barrier for citizens across the world, particularly for people living in rural or low-income areas, where mental health services can be limited or nonexistent (McGorry et al., 2013; Patel et al., 2013). Factors such as cost and language barriers can also play an important role in accessing mental health care (Hickie et al., 2019), including specialized occupational therapy services. The cost of mental health care can be a significant barrier, particularly for people without insurance coverage. Even with insurance, high deductibles and copays can make mental health care unaffordable for many people. Also, in many parts of the world, occupational therapy services for supporting people experiencing mental health challenges might not be covered by public or private insurance.

Perhaps one of the most significant barriers to delivering occupational therapy services for mental health is the lack of a common definition for the term "mental health" itself. Mental health is a complex and multifaceted concept that can be difficult to define across cultures and languages. Mental health is often described as a subjective experience (Manwell et al., 2015), and different people have different views on what constitutes good mental health. What one person considers to be mentally healthy can differ from another person's perspective.

Mental health can also vary depending on cultural factors. For example, some cultures view certain behaviors or emotions as normal or healthy, whereas others consider them abnormal or unhealthy. Mental health also involves multiple factors, including emotions, thoughts, behaviors, and social interactions that affect a person's ability to function. These different factors can interact in complex ways, making it difficult to provide a simple and comprehensive definition. Mental health can also change over time; what might be considered healthy at one point in life might not be the case at another point. For example, some level of anxiety is normal and healthy in certain situations, such as when facing a challenge or danger, but anxiety can become problematic when it persists and interferes with daily functioning. Overall, the difficulty in defining mental health underscores the need for a comprehensive and nuanced approach to occupational therapy's role in mental health, one that takes into account the subjective, cultural, and complex nature of mental health. It also takes an understanding of how society defines the construct of "health."

Health and Mental Health as a Continuum

In 1948, the **World Health Organization** (WHO) defined "health" as "the state of complete physical, mental and social well-being and not merely the absence of disease or infirmity" (WHO, n.d., para. 1). This definition was intended to capture wellness as a fundamental part of health, in addition to and despite having a health condition, disability, or illness. Despite the breadth and ambition of the definition, it has been criticized for its absoluteness, making it an outcome nearly impossible to achieve (Huber et al., 2011). The definition was never considered for adaptation until 2011 (Huber et al., 2011). At that time, a new definition was published in the *British Medical Journal,* which described health as the "ability to adapt and self-manage in the face of social, physical, and emotional challenges" (Huber et al., 2011, p. 235). Although an improvement from 1948, the complexity and subjectivity of the definition continues to pose significant challenges for healthy system providers in the global health community. As many Organisation for Economic

Co-operation and Development (OECD) countries face a paradox of high health-care spending, poor health outcomes, and intense scrutiny for failing to be driven by the full range of needs and priorities of their citizens (Cano & Hobart, 2011; Coulter, 2017), there is a need to reexamine how health is defined and valued in society.

Imagine health as a construct similar to a ruler. At one end of the ruler (0 centimeters/inches) is the worst possible health. At the other end (30 centimeters/12 inches) is the WHO description of *complete* physical, mental, and social well-being. If asked how a person moves from low to high on the ruler, an individual will likely realize that the construct of health is continuous. People of all ages, genders, cultures, and backgrounds have a health journey that is highly influenced and shaped by experiences throughout life. Yet health-care spending for most countries, both per person and as a share of gross domestic product, continues to be mostly dedicated to one side of the definition (i.e., someone is not healthy and requires an acute level of care). For example, in 2021 health spending in the United States was $4.3 trillion, or $12,914 per capita. Approximately 95.6% of spending was allocated to services and costs associated with acute, tertiary, and specialty care services, with only 4.4% of the spending dedicated to government public health activities (Centers for Medicare and Medicaid Services, 2022). It can be argued that health systems across the world were built with a binary definition of health (i.e., either someone is healthy or they are not). For OTPs, this situation can present an opportunity to articulate the roles they can play to support people along the full health continuum, including providing potentially much needed and cost-effective upstream prevention, early intervention, and mental wellness promotion.

Mental health can also be viewed as a continuum. The **mental health continuum** is a model that describes the different states of mental health that a person can experience over time (Keyes, 2002). It is often depicted as a continuum, or a spectrum, with different levels of mental health functioning. Applying the ruler metaphor to the mental health continuum, at one end are states of optimal mental health, where a person feels at peace, is engaged, and is fulfilled in their life. These states are characterized by positive emotions, healthy relationships, and a sense of purpose and meaning. In the middle of the ruler, there are states of moderate mental health, where a person experiences some stress, anxiety, and/or other mental health challenges, but is still able to function and be productive in their daily life. At the other end of the ruler, there are states of poor mental health, where a person experiences severe symptoms of mental illness, such as depression, anxiety, or psychosis. These states can be debilitating and severely affect a person's ability to function in their daily life (see Fig. 1-3).

Because of recent experiences with the global COVID-19 pandemic, fortifying the foundations of health systems is now a priority not only to support healthier populations but to enable substantial economic and societal benefits by avoiding the need for repeated crisis responses. Opportunities exist for OTPs to advocate for how health spending can be allocated along the full range of the health and mental health spectrum, including health promotion, prevention, and early intervention, as well as acute, tertiary, and long-term services—areas of practice in which OTPs have over a century of experience providing evidence-based care.

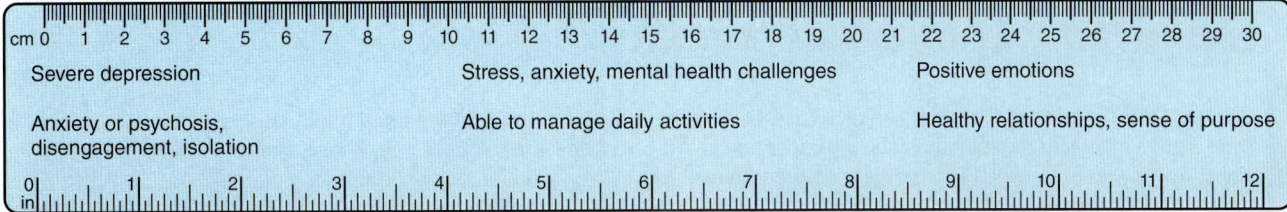

Severe depression	Stress, anxiety, mental health challenges	Positive emotions
Anxiety or psychosis, disengagement, isolation	Able to manage daily activities	Healthy relationships, sense of purpose

FIGURE 1-3. The mental health continuum as a ruler.

The Lived Experience

Max Davenport

Editor's Note: Most chapters in this textbook include a Lived Experience feature to gain the perspective of the person with mental illness. For this first chapter, I chose to include a lived experience by an individual that I believe exemplifies mental wellness. Everyone I know says, "I want to be Max when I grow up." There are many astonishing things about Max, but one of the most remarkable is that in November the bike club will celebrate Max's 94th birthday by riding 94 kilometers with him. —Catana Brown

The way I grew up, I developed my work ethic early on. I always told my boys, "You don't have to be a genius if you are ambitious." I was born in Mt. Pleasant, Michigan, in 1929, three days after the stock market crash. My dad owned a repair shop. We didn't have much money, lived on two acres of land with no electricity or running water. But as a kid I delighted in being in the woods. I would sometimes go in the woods by myself, and I actually liked getting lost because I knew I would find my way out. I had one older brother and two older sisters. I was especially close to the sister nearest in age to me, and everyone remarked on how well we got along. At one point she had a bad accident when she fell off a slide, and I took care of her.

In 1935, on the 4th of July, my father was working under a car in the repair shop and got a piece of steel in his eye. He couldn't get care because of the holiday, and it got infected. Eventually he went to the University of Michigan hospital, where they removed his eye. For three years he was totally blind. He couldn't work and spent most of his time in a dark bedroom. We lived on what my mom could beg from people that owed my dad money. Eventually, my dad was able to go back to work, so he moved to Bloomingdale where he got a job in the oil fields. In 1940, we moved to Bloomingdale to join him.

I was 12 when the United States entered World War II. Those were important years. There were few men in town, so I began working helping the women. At age 13 I was delivering coal in a big truck. I was never hurting for confidence and never wanted to depend on anyone. I told my parents I would buy my own clothes. In 1944, my dad was working in Alberta, Canada, for a British American oil company. My dad said, "Why don't you get four buddies and join me in Alberta for the summer working on the pipeline?" So, we did. At age 16, my buddy and I decided to join the service. They needed new troops because those who had been in combat were coming home. There were two guys working in the recruitment

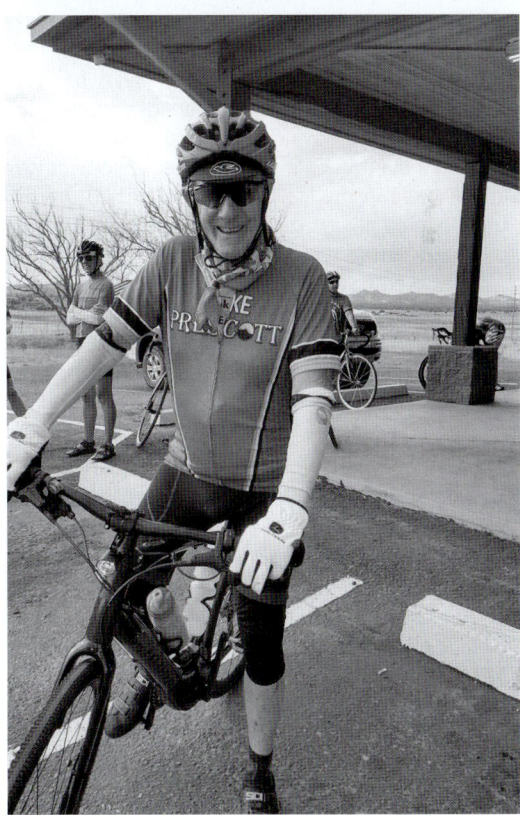

Max after riding 93 kilometers for his 93rd birthday

office on alternate days. We came up with a plan so that I told the first guy I would bring my birth certificate the next day, and then the next day, I told the other guy that I had already brought my birth certificate in, and the first guy must not have marked it down. We first went to Evanston, Illinois, and then went to Biloxi, Mississippi, for basic training in the Army Air Corp. While I was waiting to ship out to Germany, they found out how old I was and sent me home with a regular honorable discharge and recommended further military training when I was old enough.

I started in powerline construction and deferred my requirement for military service until I finished my training to become a journeyman. I re-enlisted in the U.S. Air Force in 1952, and I was put in charge of basic training as a captain of 78 men,

Continued

all from New York City at Sampson Air Force Base. During that time, I put a drill team together that won a competition at West Point. I was made an orderly of the base commander which opened a lot of doors for me. I eventually went to Laughlin Air Force Base and was put in charge of airfield lighting and overhead distribution. It was during this time that I got married. My first son, Kim, was born just before I was sent to England. My wife and I did best when we were struggling together and didn't have much money. Once we had money, we never got along and ended up getting divorced.

After the service I returned to being a journeyman, but it wasn't long till I was a foreman. I eventually became a division manager and then from there worked for the Ball Glass Company as part of their engineering staff. Every few years a plant would be rebuilt, and I would manage the electrical aspects of the rebuilding, moving from factory to factory. I eventually settled in a plant in California. I retired at 59½. It was the best move I made in my life. I wasn't sure I had the money, but I knew I could always make adjustments if I had to. I worked really hard during my career. Now I was out pursuing happiness. I've liked travel and adventure. I traveled all around the U.S. in various RVs.

I moved to Prescott, Arizona, by myself in 1990. At one point I decided to follow the course of Lewis and Clark from St. Louis to the Pacific Ocean. I read everything I could and went to exhibitions, and over the course of three years I covered the trail with four different people. In Prescott I really got into mountain

biking. I raced until I had a bad crash when I was around 70. Since then, I have mostly road biked. I participated in the World Senior Games from the time I was 64–83. When I was 80, 81, and 82 years of age I won the championship in my age group. I raced a few more years till my eyesight forced me to quit racing.

I started losing my vision at about 78 due to macular degeneration. I also have cataracts. I still have peripheral vision, so I have learned to sweep. When riding my bike, I can follow the person in front of me. I'm going to continue riding as long as I can. If I know the area where we are riding, I feel comfortable. I feel a part of the bike club. We enjoy each other. I've always really liked people. I get a big charge of going up to a stranger, like someone working in the grocery store, that's having a bad day and making them smile. God, I love doing that. I've really enjoyed my kids. I like the fact that they are nearby, but it's important that I still live on my own.

One other thing that's helped me enjoy my life. I've learned not to dwell on bad stuff. I've seen other people hold onto bad things for years. I'm able to occupy myself with other things. A person can't help but learn from experiences, and I'm no different. One of the biggest things I've learned is you need to know what makes you happy. I love life and can change when I need to. If life isn't going how you want it to, you need to change. That philosophy may not work for everyone, but it has worked for me.

Supporting People Across the Mental Health Continuum

The mental health continuum is helpful in understanding that mental health is not an all-or-nothing concept. A continuum perspective helps individuals and practitioners realize it is normal for a person's mental health to change. Although everyone has mental health, not everyone has mental health problems. People use occupations to improve their mental well-being and adapt to challenges. Some readers might use yoga and other mindfulness strategies to relax and reduce stress. Others learn something new or engage in art, music, and creative activities. Exercise, connecting with others, and being in nature are other common occupations that help build mental health resiliency. Some people are highly successful at incorporating mental health habits into their routines, whereas others feel considerable inertia when trying to do this.

Occupational therapy can play a crucial role across the mental health continuum. It is a person-centered health profession that focuses on promoting health and well-being using meaningful and purposeful activities. Occupational therapy can be used to promote mental wellness, prevent mental health problems, intervene during an acute episode

of mental illness, and support individuals in their recovery process.

Understanding the mental health continuum of a person, service, community, and population can help OTPs map the range of evidence-based services available to offer. For example, on one end of the mental health continuum (imagine the ruler once again at 12 inches or 30 centimeters). OTPs can specify their assessments and interventions when working with individuals, groups, and communities to promote mental wellness and prevent illness. This could include approaches to support engagement in meaningful occupations, develop healthy relationships, and promote positive emotions. It could also include providing developmentally and culturally relevant education on stress management, coping strategies, harm reduction strategies, and managing life balance. It could include advocating for safe home, school, and workplaces; access to nature and outdoor play spaces; and access to affordable, inclusive, and safe transportation systems.

Moving down the continuum (or mental health ruler), OTPs can also outline how they work with people who require early intervention in an illness trajectory. For example, OTPs can outline a role to support diverse persons of all ages to identify early signs of illness and build in strategies to prevent them from becoming more severe. This could include implementing evidence-based programs such as the Wellness Recovery Action Plan (Copeland, 1997) or Action Over Inertia (Edgelow & Krupa, 2011) to develop strategies to manage symptoms, maintain participation in meaningful activity, and improve quality of life.

OTPs can employ these strategies in all settings. For example, in a rehabilitation setting, individuals with newly acquired physical disabilities are often experiencing mental health challenges. Bullying and social media pressures for children can be addressed in school-based practice. Older adults are often faced with multiple transitions as they manage aging. OTPs work closely with people and their families to understand mental illness and define wellness trajectories that are developmentally and culturally relevant and work together codesigning ways in which occupational therapy can contribute in a good way (Young et al., 2013).

As the illness continuum becomes more acute or severe (moving toward the low end of the ruler), OTPs can work with individuals who are experiencing severe mental health problems in diverse types of settings, such as inpatient care, criminal justice systems, and long-term care. In non–mental health settings, OTPs will also work with individuals experiencing serious mental illnesses. It is not unusual for someone in a physical rehabilitation setting to experience severe depression, anxiety, and/or PTSD. Caregivers of individuals with dementia often deal with their own significant mental health issues. Children and youth in schools and universities can experience high levels of mental illness.

When a person is experiencing mental health symptoms, OTPs can play an important role in supporting individuals to learn about their illness and build a plan to regain their ability to perform daily activities once they are well enough to return to the community. This can include developing skills and habits for self-care, socialization, and productivity. It can also include navigating the transition from acute inpatient care to the community. This is often a vulnerable point of care in a health system, which is often described as fractured because of a lack of funding, lack of training, stigma, workforce issues, and a lack of access to services where and when needed. Further, waitlists for specialized mental health services can be unacceptably long (e.g., greater than 6–12 months) in many jurisdictions (O'Brien et al., 2016). Many services also impose arbitrary limitations on access, such as excluding people with multiple diagnoses or referring individuals to other services, leaving them struggling to navigate a complex system in which they transition among services as their needs evolve (Mathias et al., 2022; Zenone et al., 2021). As experts in supporting individuals through life transitions, OTPs can play a critical role by walking alongside people struggling to navigate this complexity and advocating for improved processes that prioritize rehabilitation and recovery.

For people living in the community with chronic mental health conditions, OTPs can play a key role in supporting individuals to regain their independence and improve their quality of life. This can include developing skills for vocational training, leisure activities, and community integration. In some cases, OTPs can work on specialized mental health teams such as assertive community treatment teams to support individuals to maintain their health in the community while developing strategies for managing symptoms, adapting to changes in their environment, and maintaining social connections.

Overall, occupational therapy can play a significant role in supporting individuals with mental health problems across the continuum of care, from health promotion and prevention to rehabilitation and recovery. This textbook provides core descriptions of best practices and innovations that will lead the profession into the next century. For more detailed descriptions of occupational therapy's role in settings designed to address the needs of individuals with significant mental health challenges, see the chapters in the Mental Health Practice section of this text, such as Chapter 35: Practice Across the Continuum of Service Needs, Chapter 38: Early Psychosis Programs for Adolescents and Young Adults, and Chapter 41: State Hospitals. 🤝

Staying Grounded in the Values of Occupational Therapy

As OTPs evolve in practice and enter complex systems and structures that might not exist in other health settings, it is important to remain grounded in the values of the profession. For a century, the profession has been rooted in values that describe person-centered practice and supporting people to achieve health and quality of life outcomes, through not just occupation but also structured roles and routine. Occupational therapy has consistently played a key role in the mental health field because it prioritizes values that align with movements such as recovery. This includes but is not limited to:

- Person-centered: OTPs prioritize the needs and goals of the people they serve and work closely with diverse populations to codesign treatment plans that are meaningful, culturally sensitive, and holistic.
- Strengths-based: OTPs collaborate to identify and highlight strengths in persons and their environments, as well as the occupations they have mastered and are developing.
- Recovery-oriented: OTPs promote recovery-oriented care, which emphasizes hope, self-determination, and personal responsibility. They encourage people to take an active role in their treatment and focus on their strengths and abilities rather than their deficits and limitations. OTPs understand that recovery does not take place in a vacuum and is instead a complex system of care that creates many barriers to recovery in the first place.
- Developmentally and culturally responsive: OTPs understand the impact of cultural factors on mental health and strive to provide developmentally and culturally responsive care. They recognize and respect cultural differences and adapt their interventions to meet the unique needs of each person.
- Evidence-informed: OTPs use evidence-based practices to guide their assessments, interventions, and evaluations. They ensure that they use interventions that have been shown to be effective and match the needs of the person and their community.
- Ethics: OTPs aim to uphold ethical and professional standards in their practice while maintaining confidentiality and respecting autonomy. They aim to be lifelong learners and understand the potential power dynamics in the practitioner–person relationship and strive to maintain a respectful and collaborative relationship.

■ Justice-focused: OTPs collaborate with persons and communities to identify and address practices and policies that limit or restrain full engagement in occupations or that restrict open access to full participation in everyday life.

By staying grounded in these shared values, OTPs can provide effective and compassionate mental health care that meets the unique needs of each person. The profession of occupational therapy is diverse and innovative, with the underlying value in mental health that people come first. These values guide practitioners to be goal-oriented and to work from the perspective of people seeking care.

Today, opportunity exists for significant investment and innovation in global mental health (Mei et al., 2020). Global mental health transformation refers to the collective effort to improve mental health services and outcomes on a global scale. OTPs can play a key role in a range of activities to improve mental health outcomes and experiences, including addressing the global burden of mental illness, improving access to mental health care, addressing social and commercial determinants of health, and promoting mental health and well-being through initiatives such as mental health education, stress reduction programs, and workplace wellness programs. The role of OTPs in global mental health transformation involves addressing social determinants of mental health through measures such as improving access to education and economic opportunities, reducing social inequalities, and promoting social inclusion and participation.

Here's the Point

■ Gradual change, building on over a century of evidence while adjusting to modern needs of diverse communities, is most likely to support sustainable growth of the occupational therapy profession in mental health over time.
■ Occupational therapy is a profession that focuses on promoting health and well-being through participation in meaningful activities.
■ Understanding the profession's history, evidence, and values is an important starting point for becoming mental health practitioners regardless of the work setting.
■ Mental health can be viewed as a continuum, with one end characterized by positive emotions, healthy relationships, and engagement in meaningful activity, and the other end as serious mental illness, isolation, and a lack of participation.
■ By focusing on the person in the environments in which they live and not just the symptoms of their mental illness, OTPs can help people thrive and contribute to their communities in a meaningful way.
■ Achieving a responsible health-care system that is responsive to the diverse needs of this population will require occupational therapy leadership and innovation over a sustained period of time.

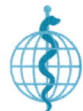 Visit the online resource center at **FADavis.com** to access the videos.

Apply It Now

1. The Occupational Therapy Practitioner as a Mental Health Practitioner

Interview an OTP to gain their perspective on what it means for "every OTP to be a mental health practitioner." Ask them for examples of how they address mental distress as well as mental well-being with the people they serve. Observe them in their everyday practice (such as the first few days of level II fieldwork) and journal about what practices you see them using to meet the mental health needs of those served. Identify ways you think could be effectively used to promote a mentally healthy work environment for those served and the health-care team overall.

2. Video Exercise—First Fieldwork Experience in Inpatient Mental Health

Pair up with another student in your class or form a small group of students. Access and watch the "First Fieldwork Experience in Inpatient Mental Health" video at the online resource center at FADavis.com. Then, discuss and together answer the following questions:
■ Casey shares three things that made her nervous before starting her fieldwork. How do those compare with worries that you have or have had before experiences in a mental health setting? Do they differ from concerns related to experiences in other occupational therapy practice settings? What did she ultimately learn regarding those three concerns?

■ Casey mentions that establishing a therapeutic relationship was very important to her and one of her main priorities as an OTP. What approach did she take to building rapport and facilitating easy interactions that led to deeper conversations and relationships?
■ What do you think of Casey's process of creating and discussing detailed activity proposals before each session? What might they look like? Do you think this preplanning effort affected her group's success and allowed her and her coleader to effectively grade the activity "on the go"? Explain.

3. The Values of Occupational Therapy

Consider the chapter content concerning the values of occupational therapy. Pair up with another occupational therapy student and consider an occupational therapy practice setting that you have observed. Reread the bulleted list of values in the section titled Staying Grounded in the Values of Occupational Therapy. Which values were exemplified in the practice setting? Provide specific examples. Which values were neglected? Do you have ideas how those values might be demonstrated in your chosen setting?

4. Encounters With the Lived Experience of Others

Initiate conversations with individuals who have faced or are currently facing challenges to their physical health or with people who are primary caregivers of such individuals. Inform them you are curious to understand their lived experience of adaptation and coping. Take a ruler as a visual prompt and explain the idea of the mental health continuum. Ask the person how they personally relate to this idea of mental health being on a continuum, and if they are willing, ask them to share examples of when they felt they could place themselves at different points on the continuum.

Resources

- Go to the World Federation of Occupational Therapists (WFOT) website at www.wfot.org and find current resources about global occupational therapy practices such as the following:
  - Current Practice in Occupational Therapy for COVID-19 and Post COVID Condition
  - Occupational Therapy: Resettling Climate Migrants
  - Occupational Therapy: Work With Displaced Persons
  - WFOT Disaster Management
  - Occupational Therapy and Humanitarian Response
    Select one that is of interest to you and access the modules and resources associated with that topic. Review the materials with an eye and ear to how the person/community's mental health needs are identified and integrated into the implementation of occupational therapy services.
- Go to the American Occupational Therapy website at www.aota.org. Do a search of their website and seek out their resources on mental health and well-being. Download the document https://www.aota .org/practice/clinical-topics/ot-mh-non-psychiatric-settings created in 2023 that highlights a variety of ways that occupational therapy integrates a mental health focus in nonpsychiatric settings. Identify which of the resources or documents you might find helpful for your fieldwork or practice setting.
- Listen to the stories of recovery shared by people with mental health challenges on the Recovery International website: https:// www.recoveryinternational.org. Compare and contrast the types of challenges these individuals share and specifically listen for ways they may have used occupation to support their own recovery.
- Watch "Will Horowitz: Lived Experience of Autism" video. In this video, a young adult with autism describes his childhood interest in trains and how it has translated into an adult volunteer opportunity. He explains that, although an individual with autism can seem to have a "one-track mind" about a subject, it can also become an advantage in that they can become very specialized, as has been true for him with the Steam into History project at a local railroad. Access the video at the online resource center at FADavis.com.

References

Aguirre Velasco, A., Cruz, I. S. S., Billings, J., Jimenez, M., & Rowe, S. (2020). What are the barriers, facilitators and interventions targeting help-seeking behaviours for common mental health problems in adolescents? A systematic review. *BMC Psychiatry, 20*(1), 293. https://doi.org/10.1186/s12888-020-02659-0

Andersen, L. T., & Reed, K. (2017). *The history of occupational therapy: The first century.* Slack.

Anthony, W. A. (1993). Recovery from mental illness: The guiding vision of the mental health service system in the 1990's. *Psychosocial Rehabilitation Journal, 16*(4), 11–23. https://doi.org/10.1037/h0095655

Bateson, G. (1961). *Perceval's narrative: A patient's account of his psychosis 1830–1832.* Stanford University Press.

Beers, C. W. (1908). *A mind that found itself.* Longmans.

Botha, M., & Frost, D. M. (2020). Extending the minority stress model to understand mental health problems experienced by the autistic population. *Society and Mental Health, 10*(1), 20–34. https://doi.org/10.1177/2156869318804297

Boysen, G. A., Isaacs, R. A., Tretter, L., & Markowski, S. (2020). Evidence for blatant dehumanization of mental illness and its relation to stigma. *The Journal of Social Psychology, 160*(3), 346–356. https://doi.org/10.1080/00224545.2019.1671301

Brigham, A. (1994). The moral treatment of insanity. *American Journal of Psychiatry, 151*(6, Suppl.), 11–15.

Cano, S. J., & Hobart, J. C. (2011). The problem with health measurement. *Patient Preference and Adherence, 5,* 279–290. https://doi.org/10.2147/PPA.S14399

Castro-Ramirez, F., Al-Suwaidi, M., Garcia, P., Rankin, O., Ricard, J. R., & Nock, M. K. (2021). Racism and poverty are barriers to the treatment of youth mental health concerns. *Journal of Clinical Child and Adolescent Psychology, 50*(4), 534–546. https://doi.org/10.1080/15374416.2021.1941058

Cénat, J. M., Farahi, S., Dalexis, R. D., Darius, W. P., Bekarkhanechi, F. M., Poisson, H., Broussard, C., Ukwu, G., Auguste, E., Nguyen, D. D., Sehabi, G., Furyk, S. E., Gedeon, A. P., Onesi, O., El Aouame, A. M., Khodabocus, S. N., Shah, M. S., & Labelle, P. R. (2022). The global evolution of mental health problems during the COVID-19 pandemic: A systematic review and meta-analysis of longitudinal studies. *Journal of Affective Disorders, 315,* 70–95. https://doi.org/10.1016/j.jad.2022.07.011

Centers for Medicare and Medicaid Services. (2022). *National health expenditure data.* https://www.cms.gov/Research-Statistics-Data-and-Systems/Statistics-Trends-and-Reports/National HealthExpendData/NationalHealthAccountsHistorical

Chamberlin, J. (1978). *On our own: Patient-controlled alternatives to the mental health system.* Haworth Press.

Charland, L. C. (2007). Benevolent theory: Moral treatment at the York Retreat. *History of Psychiatry, 18*(1), 61–80. https://doi.org/10.1177/0957154X07070320

Copeland, M. E. (1997). *Wellness Recovery Action Plan.* Peach Press.

Corvetto, J. F., Helou, A. Y., Dambach, P., Müller, T., & Sauerborn, R. (2023). A systematic literature review of the impact of climate change on the global demand for psychiatric services. *International Journal of Environmental Research and Public Health, 20*(2), 1190. https://doi.org/10.3390/ijerph20021190

Coulter, A. (2017). Measuring what matters to patients. *British Medical Journal, 356,* j816. https://doi.org/10.1136/bmj.j816

Cumming, E., & Kaplan, W. (1991). *The arts and crafts movement.* Thames and Hudson.

Dain, N. (1980). *Clifford W. Beers, advocate for the insane.* University of Pittsburgh Press.

Davidson, L., Rowe, M., DiLeo, P., Bellamy, C., & Delphin-Rittmon, M. (2021). Recovery-oriented systems of care: A perspective on the past, present, and future. *Alcohol Research: Current Reviews, 41*(1), 9. https://doi.org/10.35946/arcr.v41.1.09

Deegan, P. E. (1997). Recovery and empowerment for people with psychiatric disabilities. *Social Work in Health Care, 25*(3), 11–24. https://doi.org/10.1300/J010v25n03_02

Deegan, P. E. (2007). The lived experience of using psychiatric medication in the recovery process and a shared decision-making program to support it. *Psychiatric Rehabilitation Journal, 31*(1), 62–69. https://doi.org/10.2975/31.1.2007.62.69

Deegan, P. E., & Drake, R. E. (2006). Shared decision making and medication management in the recovery process. *Psychiatric Services (Washington, DC), 57*(11), 1636–1639. https://doi.org/10.1176/ps.2006.57.11.1636

Edgelow, M., & Krupa, T. (2011). Randomized controlled pilot study of an occupational time-use intervention for people with serious mental illness. *The American Journal of Occupational Therapy,* *65*(3), 267–276. https://doi.org/10.5014/ajot.2011.001313

Farris, M. S., MacQueen, G., Goldstein, B. I., Wang, J., Kennedy, S. H., Bray, S., Lebel, C., & Addington, J. (2019). Treatment history of youth at-risk for serious mental illness. *Canadian Journal of Psychiatry, 64*(2), 145–154. https://doi.org/10.1177/0706743718792195

Frese, F. J. (2015). Advocacy, stigma, and self-disclosure: A personal perspective. In E. J. Bromet (Ed.), *Long term outcomes in psychopathology research: Rethinking the scientific agenda* (pp. 227–237). Oxford University Press.

Fusar-Poli, P., Salazar de Pablo, G., De Micheli, A., Nieman, D. H., Correll, C. U., Kessing, L. V., Pfennig, A., Bechdolf, A., Borgwardt, S., Arango, C., & van Amelsvoort, T. (2020). What is good mental health? A scoping review. *European Neuropsychopharmacology, 31,* 33–46. https://doi.org/10.1016/j.euroneuro.2019.12.105

GBD 2019 Mental Disorders Collaborators. (2022). Global, regional, and national burden of 12 mental disorders in 204 countries and territories, 1990-2019: A systematic analysis for the global burden of disease study 2019. *The Lancet Psychiatry, 9*(2), 137–150. https://doi.org/10.1016/S2215-0366(21)00395-3

Hall, H. J. (1905). The systematic use of work as a remedy in neurasthenia and allied conditions. *Boston Medical and Surgical Journal, 152*(2), 29–32. https://doi.org/10.1056/NEJM190501121520201

Hall, H. J. (1910). Work cure: A report of five years' experience at an institution devoted to the therapeutic application of manual work. *Journal of the American Medical Association, 54*(1), 12–14. https://doi.org/10.1001/jama.1910.92550270001001d

Hickie, I. B., Scott, E. M., Cross, S. P., Iorfino, F., Davenport, T. A., Guastella, A. J., Naismith, S. L., Carpenter, J. S., Rohleder, C., Crouse, J. J., Hermens, D. F., Koethe, D., Leweke, F. M., Tickell, A. M., Sawrikar, V., & Scott, J. (2019). Right care, first time: A highly personalised and measurement-based care model to manage youth mental health. *The Medical Journal of Australia, 211*(Suppl. 9), S3–S46. https://doi.org/10.5694/mja2.50383

Huber, M., Knottnerus, J. A., Green, L., van der Horst, H., Jadad, A. R., Kromhout, D., Leonard, B., Lorig, K., Loureriro, M. I., van der Meer, J. W., Schnabel, P., Smith, R., van Weel, C., & Smid, H. (2011). How should we define health? *British Medical Journal, 343,* d4163. https://doi.org/10.1136/bmj.d4163

Keyes, C. L. M. (2002). The mental health continuum: From languishing to flourishing in life. *Journal of Health and Social Behavior, 43,* 207–222. https://doi.org/10.2307/3090197

Kriegel, E. R., Lazarevic, B., Athanasian, C. E., & Milanaik, R. L. (2021). TikTok, Tide pods and Tiger King: Health implications of trends taking over pediatric populations. *Current Opinion in Pediatrics, 63*(1), 170–177. https://doi.org/10.1097/MOP.0000000000000989

Law, M., Cooper, B., Strong, S., Stewart, D., Rigby, P., & Letts, L. (1996). The Person-Environment-Occupation model: A transactive approach to occupational performance. *Canadian Journal of Occupational Therapy, 63,* 9–23. https://doi.org/10.1177/000841749606300103

Léger-Goodes, T., Malboeuf-Hurtubise, C., Mastine, T., Généreux, M., Paradis, P. O., & Camden, C. (2022). Eco-anxiety in children: A scoping review of the mental health impacts of the awareness of climate change. *Frontiers in Psychology, 13,* 872544. https://doi.org/10.3389/fpsyg.2022.872544

Manwell, L. A., Barbic, S. P., Roberts, K., Durisko, Z., Lee, C., Ware, E., & McKenzie, K. (2015). What is mental health? Evidence towards a new definition from a mixed methods multidisciplinary international survey. *BMJ Open, 5*(6), e007079. https://doi.org.10.1136/bmjopen-2014-007079

Marchand, K., Fogarty, O., Pellatt, K. M., Vig, K., Melnychuk, J., Katan, C., Khan, F., Turuba, R., Kongnetiman, L., Tallon, C., Fairbank, J., Mathias, S., & Barbic, S. (2022). "We need to build a better bridge": Findings from a multi-site qualitative analysis of opportunities for improving opioid treatment services for youth. *Harm Reduction Journal, 19*(1), 37. https://doi.org/10.1186/s12954-022-00623-7

Mathias, S., Tee, K., Helfrich, W., Gerty, K., Chan, G., & Barbic, S. P. (2022). Foundry: Early learnings from the implementation of an integrated youth service network. *Early Intervention in Psychiatry, 16*(4), 410–418. https://doi.org/10.1111/eip.13181

McGorry, P., Bates, T., & Birchwood, M. (2013). Designing youth mental health services for the 21st century: Examples from Australia, Ireland and the UK. *British Journal of Psychiatry , 202*(Suppl. 54), S30–S35. https://doi.org/10.1192/bjp.bp.112.119214

Mei, C., Fitzsimons, J., Allen, N., Alvarez-Jimenez, M., Amminger, G. P., Browne, V., Cannon, M., Davis, M., Dooley, B., Hickie, I. B., Iyer, S., Killackey, E., Malla, A., Manion, I., Mathias, S., Pennell, K., Purcell, R., Rickwood, D., Singh, S. P., . . . McGorry, P. D. (2020). Global research priorities for youth mental health. *Early Intervention in Psychiatry, 14*(1), 3–13. https://doi.org/10.1111/eip.12878

Meyer, I. H., Schwartz, S., & Frost, D. M. (2008). Social patterning of stress and coping: Does disadvantaged social statuses confer more stress and fewer coping resources? *Social Science & Medicine, 67,* 368–379. https://doi.org/10.1016/j.socscimed.2008.03.012

O'Brien, D., Harvey, K., Howse, J., Reardon, T., & Creswell, C. (2016). Barriers to managing child and adolescent mental health problems: A systematic review of primary care practitioners' perceptions. *The British Journal of General Practice, 66*(651), e693–e707. https://doi.org/10.3399/bjgp16X687061

Patel, V., Belkin, G. S., Chockalingam, A., Cooper, J., Saxena, S., & Unutzer, J. (2013). Grand challenges: Integrating mental health services into priority health care platforms. *PLoS Medicine, 10*(5), e1001448. https://doi.org/10.1371/journal.pmed.1001448

Patel, V., Chisholm, D., Parikh, R., Charlson, F. J., Degenhardt, L., Dua, T., Ferrari, A. J., Hyman, S., Laxminarayan, R., Levin, C., Lund, C., Medina Mora, M. E., Petersen, I., Scott, J., Shidhaye, R., Vijayakumar, L., Thornicroft, G., Whiteford, H., & DCP MNS Author Group. (2015). Addressing the burden of mental, neurological, and substance use disorders: Key messages from disease control priorities, 3rd edition. *Lancet (London, England), 387*(10028), 1672–1685. https://doi.org/10.1016/S0140-6736(15)00390-6

Pattison, R., Puyat, J. H., Giesbrecht, A., Zenone, M., Mathias, S., & Barbic, S. (2021). Examining mental health differences between transgender, gender nonconforming, and cisgender young people in British Columbia. *Frontiers in Psychiatry, 12,* 720681. https://doi.org/10.3389/fpsyt.2021.720681

Purtle, J., Nelson, K. L., Counts, N. Z., & Yudell, M. (2020). Population-based approaches to mental health: History, strategies, and evidence. *Annual Review of Public Health, 41*(1), 201–221. https://doi:10.1146/annurev-publhealth-040119-094247

Radez, J., Reardon, T., Creswell, C., Lawrence, P. J., Evdoka-Burton, G., & Waite, P. (2021). Why do children and adolescents (not) seek and access professional help for their mental health problems? A systematic review of quantitative and qualitative studies. *European Child & Adolescent Psychiatry, 30*(2), 183–211. https://doi.org/10.1007/s00787-019-01469-4

Rafla-Yuan, E., Moore, S., Carvente-Martinez, H., Yang, P., Balasuriya, L., Jackson, K., McMickens, C., & Robles-Ramamurthy, B. (2022). Striving for equity in community mental health: Opportunities and challenges for integrating care for BIPOC youth. *Child and Adolescent Psychiatric Clinics of North America, 31*(2), 295–312. https://doi.org/10.1016/j.chc.2021.11.007

Scheuermeyer, F. X., Lane, D., Grunau, B., Grafstein, E., Miles, I., Kestler, A., Barbic, D., Barbic, S., Slvjic, I., Duley, S., Yu, A., Chiu, I., & Innes, G. (2023). Risk factors associated with 1-week revisit among emergency department patients with alcohol withdrawal. *Canadian Journal of Emergency Medicine, 25*(2), 150–156. https://doi.org/10.1007/s43678-022-00414-w

Slagle, E. C. (1938). Occupational therapy. *Trained Nurse and Hospital Review, 100,* 375–382.

Solmi, M., Radua J., Olivola, M., Croce, E., Soardo, L., Salazar de Pablo, G., Il Shin, J., Kirkbride, J. B., Jones, P., Kim, J. H., Kim, J. Y., Carvalho, A. F., Seeman, M. V., Correll, C. U., & Fusar-Poli, P. (2022). Age at onset of mental disorders worldwide: Large-scale meta-analysis of 192 epidemiological studies. *Molecular Psychiatry, 27*(1), 281–295. https://doi.org/10.1038/s41380-021-01161-7

The Lancet Psychiatry. (2021). COVID-19 and mental health. *The Lancet Psychiatry, 8*(2), 87. https://doi.org/10.1016/S2215-0366(21)00005-5

Trudell, J. P., Burnet, M. L., Ziegler, B. R., & Luginaah, I. (2021). The impact of food insecurity on mental health in Africa: A systematic review. *Social Science & Medicine (1982), 278*, 113953. https://doi.org/10.1016/j.socscimed.2021.113953

Wilburn, V. G., Hoss, A., Pudeler, M., Beukema, E., Rothenbuhler, C., & Stoll, H. B. (2021). Receiving recognition: A case for occupational therapy practitioners as mental and behavioral health providers. *American Journal of Occupational Therapy, 75*(5), 7505090010. https://doi.org/10.5014/ajot.2021.044727

Wong, S. R., & Fisher, G. (2015). Comparing and using occupation-focused models. *Occupational Therapy in Health Care, 29*, 297–314. https://doi.org/10.3109/07380577.2015.1010130

World Health Organization. (n.d.). *Constitution of the World Health Organization.* https://www.who.int/about/accountability/governance/constitution

Young, N. L., Wabano, M. J., Burke, T. A., Ritchie, S. D., Mishibinijima, D., & Corbiere, R. G. (2013). A process for creating the Aboriginal Children's Health and Well-being Measure (ACHWM). *Canadian Journal of Public Health, 104*(2), e136–e141. https://doi.org/10.1007/BF03405677

Zenone, M. A., Cianfrone, M., Sharma, R., Majid, S., Rakhra, J., Cruz, K., Costales, S., Sekhon, M., Mathias, S., Tugwell, A., & Barbic, S. (2021). Supporting youth 12-24 during the COVID-19 pandemic: How foundry is mobilizing to provide information, resources and hope across the province of British Columbia. *Global Health Promotion, 28*(1), 51–59. https://doi.org/10.1177/17579759 20984196

2

Recovery and Wraparound Models

Elizabeth Griffin Lannigan and Claudette Fette

This chapter paints a picture of **recovery** from many perspectives, including those of individuals with the lived experience of recovery. Recovery is a unique and deeply personal experience, driven by the search for active control, or agency, over one's life (Strong & Letts, 2021). True to occupational therapy's **person-centered practice** approach, recovery is guided by the individual's goals, dreams, and strengths. These factors help the person, along with occupational therapy practitioners (OTPs), to create a plan to pursue occupations that matter to them. OTPs can collaborate with individuals in recovery from mental health or substance use challenges by exploring ways to listen to, join in, and reflect on each person's unique recovery experience. As occupational therapy integrates approaches devoted to recovery for adults, **systems of care (SoC)** and **wraparound** for children and youth, and **public health** initiatives, services will better meet the person's needs for greater engagement in occupations and participation. This chapter illustrates the value of extending these approaches to meet the mental health and well-being needs of persons living with psychosocial needs caused by any health challenges across practice areas and settings.

Occupational therapy's overarching purpose is "achieving health, well-being and participation in life through engagement in occupation" (American Occupational Therapy Association [AOTA], 2020, p. 5). This process of engagement happens within many contexts of individuals' lives, including social, physical, cultural, and so on. This essence of occupational therapy directly aligns with the Recovery Model. This chapter and the other chapters of this text aim to support the perspective that, through engagement in each day's needed and desired activities, persons living with mental health and/or substance use challenges can recover.

Definitions of Recovery and Wraparound

The term "recovery" was first used specifically for recovery from alcoholism in 1939 in the first "big book" of Alcoholics Anonymous (Wilson, 1939). Concepts regarding acceptance and peer-to-peer supports would not be incorporated into **mental health recovery** until several decades later during the start of the psychiatric survivors' movement, modeled after the 1950s and 1960s civil rights struggles (Chamberlin, 1977). Psychiatric survivors advanced the understanding that **well-being** and recovery are not dependent upon absence of symptoms, but rather are centered on acceptance of neurodiversity and a focus on living life well. In 2010, the Substance Abuse and Mental Health Services Administration (SAMHSA) gathered a group of people in recovery from substance abuse and/or mental health challenges as well as leaders in the behavioral health field to create what became *SAMHSA's Working Definition of Recovery* (SAMHSA, 2012). This statement asserted:

> Recovery is a process of change through which individuals improve their health and wellness, live a self-directed life, and strive to reach their full potential. (p. 3)

SAMHSA later developed the four dimensions of recovery (Box 2-1).

In addition, SAMHSA identified 10 guiding principles of recovery in its working definition (see Table 2-1):

1. Hope
2. Person-driven
3. Many pathways
4. Holistic
5. Peer support
6. Relational
7. Culture
8. Addresses trauma
9. Strengths/responsibility
10. Respect

BOX 2-1 ■ SAMHSA's Working Dimensions of Recovery

Through the Recovery Support Strategic Initiative, SAMHSA has delineated four major dimensions that support a life in recovery.

1. *Health:* overcoming or managing one's disease(s) or symptoms—for example, abstaining from use of alcohol, illicit drugs, and nonprescribed medications if one has an addiction problem—and for everyone in recovery, making informed, healthy choices that support physical and emotional well-being
2. *Home:* a stable and safe place to live
3. *Purpose:* meaningful daily activities, such as a job, school, volunteerism, family caretaking, or creative endeavors, and the independence, income, and resources to participate in society
4. *Community:* relationships and social networks that provide support, friendship, love, and hope (SAMHSA, 2012)

TABLE 2-1 | The 10 Guiding Principles of Recovery

Principle	Definition
Hope	*Recovery emerges from hope.* Hope is the catalyst of the recovery process.
Person-driven	Self-determination and self-direction are the foundations for recovery as individuals define their own life goals and design their unique path(s) toward those goals.
Many pathways	Recovery pathways are highly personalized. Recovery is nonlinear, characterized by continual growth and improved functioning that may involve setbacks.
Holistic	Recovery includes mind, body, spirit, and community. This addresses self-care practices, family, housing, employment, transportation, education, clinical treatment, services and supports, primary health care, dental care, complementary and alternative services, faith, spirituality, creativity, social networks, and community participation.
Peer support	Peers encourage and engage other peers, providing each other with a vital sense of belonging, supportive relationships, valued roles, and community. Through helping others and giving back to the community, one helps oneself. Peer-operated services and supports are essential resources.
Relational	Family members, peers, providers, faith groups, community members, and other allies form vital support networks. Through these relationships, people engage in new roles that lead to a greater sense of belonging, personhood, empowerment, autonomy, social inclusion, and community participation.
Culture	Services should be culturally grounded, attuned, sensitive, congruent, and competent as well as personalized to meet each individual's unique needs.
Addresses trauma	Services and supports should be trauma-informed to foster safety (physical and emotional) and trust as well as promote choice, empowerment, and collaboration.
Strengths and responsibility	Individuals, families, and communities have strengths and resources that serve as a foundation of recovery. All are responsible for using their strengths to provide opportunities and resources for recovery.
Respect	Community, systems, and societal acceptance and appreciation for people affected by mental health and substance use problems—including protecting their rights and eliminating discrimination—are crucial in achieving recovery.

Adapted from Substance Abuse and Mental Health Services Administration. (2012). SAMHSA's working definition of recovery. Author. https://store.samhsa.gov/sites/default/files/pep12-recdef.pdf

The World Health Organization (WHO, 2022) has shifted beyond a medical definition of mental health and instead seeks to support well-being and mental health at a whole population level. WHO defines **mental health** as "a state of mental well-being that enables people to cope with the stresses of life, to realize their abilities, to learn well and work well, and to contribute to their communities" (p. 8). Box 2-2 presents the alignment of three conceptual views of mental health: (a) SAMHSA's four dimensions of recovery, (b) WHO's definition of mental health, and (c) AOTA's views on health and wellness, as described in the *Occupational Therapy Practice Framework: Domain and Process*, 4th Edition (*OTPF-4*, AOTA, 2020), which incorporated foundational mental health and well-being concepts from the WHO.

As part of a wellness approach to recovery, Swarbrick (2012) stated that recovery is a personal process of regaining physical, mental, emotional, and spiritual balance in the face of illness or trauma. During periods of stress, this process of healing facilitates restoring the balance of well-being throughout individuals' lives. Viewing this healing as a process, Patricia Deegan, one of the first champions of recovery, stated that individuals "experience themselves as recovering a new sense of purpose within and beyond the limits of disability" (Deegan, 1988, p. 11).

These recovery viewpoints emphasize a state of **mental wellness,** "defined as an asset or resource that enables positive states of wellbeing and provides the capability for people to achieve their full potential" (Patel et al., 2018, p. 1562). Mental wellness incorporates well-being in all aspects of people's lives (e.g., physical, social, occupational, spiritual, financial, and environmental), and maintaining mental wellness is

a lifelong process toward realizing a purposeful and satisfying life (Bodeker et al., 2020). For people living with mental health conditions, the distinction between mental wellness and mental disorders is important to understand. People living with symptoms can simultaneously experience mental health or wellness, life satisfaction, flourishing, and reaching their potential (Bodeker et al., 2020).

Galderisi and colleagues (2015) offered a new definition of mental well-being as a "dynamic state of internal equilibrium" (p. 231) in which people are able to use their abilities to express and adjust their own emotions, empathize with others, function in social roles, and demonstrate flexibility and coping with life events. To align with recovery movement perspectives, this definition views recovery as a process toward attaining a fulfilled and valued life. Mental health or well-being consists of emotional (positive feelings and contentment), psychological (meaningful engagement), and social (contribution of one's community or society) components (Chan et al., 2018; Keyes, 2002).

Other terms describing mental health and wellness include "flourishing" and "languishing." Westerhof and Keyes (2010) described "**flourishing** as a state where individuals combine a high level of subjective well-being with an optimal level of psychological and social functioning. Similarly, **languishing** refers to a state where low levels of subjective well-being are combined with low levels of psychological and social well-being" (pp. 111–112). Chan and colleagues (2018) defined flourishing as a state of wholeness that enables satisfactory and fulfilling lives versus languishing, which was defined as experiences of emptiness and stagnation without positive emotionality and meaning. Westerhof and Keyes (2010)

BOX 2-2 ■ Side-by-Side Comparison: Views of Supporting People's Mental Health

World Health Organization (WHO, 2022)	Recovery (SAMHSA, 2012, p. 3)	OTPF-4 (AOTA, 2020, pp. 5–6)
Mental health: state of mental well-being that enables successful coping, being capable across occupations, and contributing to their community Positive mental health supports our ability to: ■ *Thrive:* realize our strengths, feel good, find purpose, and strive for well-being ■ *Cope:* when experiencing stress, adapt to change, make choices, manage emotions ■ *Function:* use cognitive skills, succeed in work and school, make healthy choices, and learn ■ *Connect:* have positive relationships, contribute to communities, feel a sense of belonging, and empathize	Four dimensions: ■ *Health:* overcoming or managing one's disease(s) or symptoms, and making informed, healthy choices that support physical and emotional well-being ■ *Home:* having a stable and safe place to live ■ *Purpose:* conducting meaningful daily activities, such as a job, school volunteerism, family caretaking, or creative endeavors, and the independence, income, and resources to participate in society ■ *Community:* having relationships and social networks that provide support, friendship, love, and hope	Occupational therapy support for mental health: ■ *Health:* "state of complete physical, mental, and social well-being, and not merely the absence of disease or infirmity" (WHO, 2006, p. 1) ■ *Well-being:* "general term encompassing the total universe of human life domains, including physical, mental, and social aspects, that make up what can be called a 'good life'" (WHO, 2006, p. 211) ■ *Participation:* including social participation, occurs naturally when clients are actively involved in carrying out occupations or daily life activities that they find purposeful and meaningful ■ *Engagement in occupation:* performance of occupations as the result of choice, motivation, and meaning within a supportive context (including environmental and personal factors)

In common:

- The importance of health, well-being, purpose, belonging, coping effectively, and thriving
- Participation: "Health is supported and maintained when clients are able to engage in home, school, workplace, and community life" (AOTA, 2020, p. 8).
- Relationships and connection to community are central to mental health and well-being.

---

described a two continua model of mental illness and health, in which one continuum represents the presence or absence of mental illness and the other represents the level of positive mental health. Figure 2-1 illustrates that mental health or well-being is not only the absence of mental illness but includes the existence of social, emotional, and psychological health (Keyes, 2002; Westerhof & Keyes, 2010).

Within these continua, important indicators of well-being emphasize that recovery is aimed at the development of personally valued goals and identity (**personal recovery**) as opposed to improvement in occupational, social, and adaptive functioning (**functional recovery**) or mitigation of clinical symptomatology (**clinical recovery;** Chan et al., 2018). The journey of personal recovery involves individuals reclaiming their autonomy, developing self-worth, and achieving self-determination. Within the recovery vision, one sees hope, empowerment, community inclusion, and full participation driven by choice and everyday solutions. This shows a strong shift from earlier paradigms of mental illness interventions addressing only *clinical recovery* (Slade, 2010). Old emphasis was on pathology and how to reduce symptoms—that is, managing illness through risk management. These more clinical views of mental illness lend themselves to hopelessness and have been stated by people in recovery to hinder the process more than facilitate it (Slade, 2010; Sutton et al., 2012).

The study of positive psychology and its contributions to strengthen mental well-being offers a strengths-based approach to enabling human capacities (Waters et al., 2022). Three positive types of interactions (buffering, bolstering, and building) assist persons to recover and rebuild from adversities. "A **buffering** effect occurs when positive emotions, processes, conditions, and/or relationships serve to diminish or stave off psychological ill health during the crisis" (Waters et al., 2022, p. 304). A **bolstering** effect happens when people act to maintain mental health despite the crisis. A **building** effect means they respond in a transformative way that *builds* new processes and outlooks (e.g., using strengths, self-compassion, or new meaning), increasing future mental health. If practitioners understand where persons are positioned within the dual continua of mental illness and mental health, they are able to integrate positive psychology factors in interventions (meaning in life, coping strategies, self-compassion, courage, gratitude, character strengths, positive emotions, positive interpersonal processes, and high-quality connections). This assists people to maintain mental health as they build new capacities to move beyond mental ill health on their transformation journey. Thus, benefits of strengths-based approaches assist to "reduce mental illness (i.e., buffering), maintain mental health (i.e., bolstering), and strengthen one's psychological resources and capacities (i.e., building)" (Waters et al., 2022, p. 315). By utilizing these approaches, OTPs support persons in recovery in finding meaning, prioritizing self-compassion and optimism, engaging in coping skills, and fostering social connectedness.

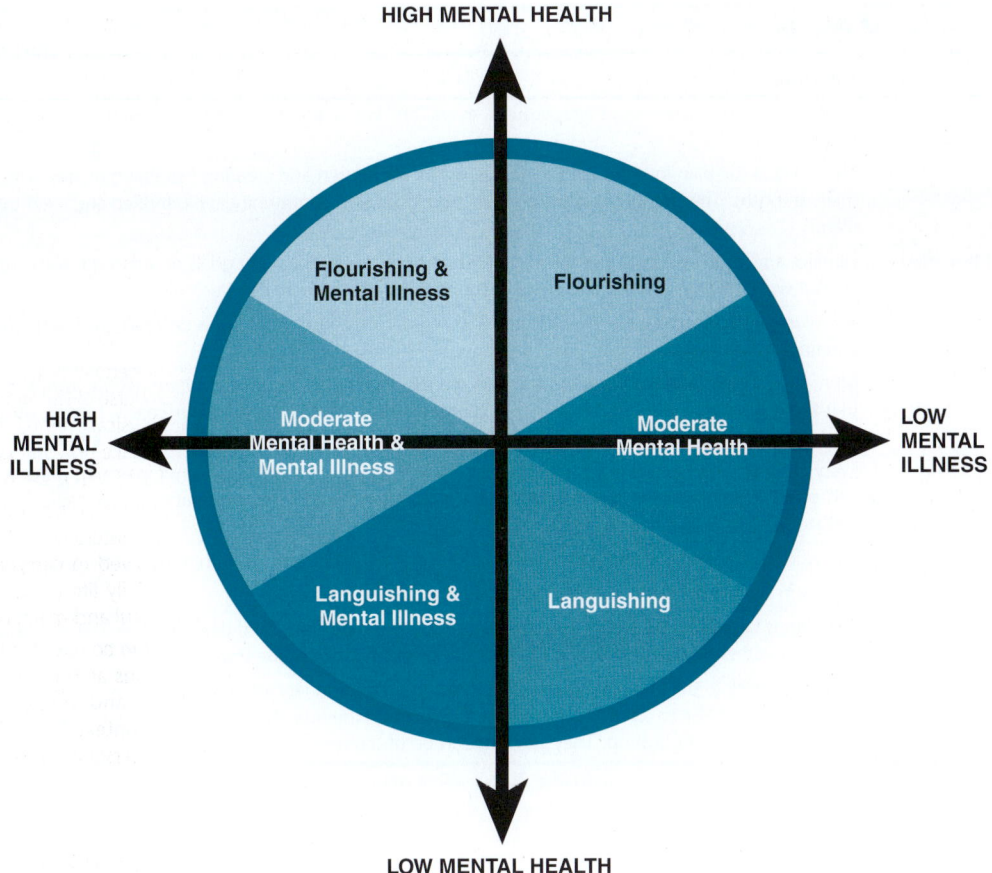

FIGURE 2-1. Dual continua model of mental illness and health. *Reproduced with permission from Keyes, C. L. M. (2014). Mental health as a complete state: How the Salutogenic perspective completes the picture. In G. F. Bauer & O. Hämmig (Eds.),* Bridging occupational, organizational and public health: A transdisciplinary approach *(pp. 179–192). Springer.*

The capacity for resilience predicts better mental health outcomes (Friis-Healy et al., 2022). **Resilience** is the ability to adapt positively to disruptions impacting functioning (Métais et al., 2022). The concept of resilience is described as involving experiences from either of two views (Harms et al., 2018; Métais et al., 2022):

1. **Bouncing back:** recovering from adversities or adapting and bouncing back to previous levels of health
2. **Thriving and rising:** moving beyond just coping with adversities by finding meaning in adversities in order to enhance health and well-being

In promoting well-being, positive psychology emphasizes the orientation of resilience as a process of thriving and moving forward (Métais et al., 2022). Although resilience focuses on personal capacity to bounce back or grow following adversities, people in recovery are seen as transforming themselves from experiencing helplessness and hopelessness into a state of well-being with goals, purpose, meaning, and belonging (Friis-Healy et al., 2022). Resilience-focused intervention can facilitate recovery by enabling people to understand their experiences resulting from stressors and by offering support to lessen potential impacts. Importantly, resilience approaches emphasize using persons' strengths to enable recovery objectives of self-directed meaningful and satisfying lives.

Chan and colleagues (2018) described recovery approaches as shifting away from considering individual progress in terms of clinical services and symptoms and instead moving toward viewing the effectiveness of intervention processes as enabling persons to live life out in the world. That transformation to recovery-oriented service delivery is needed to confront issues around dependency, self-stigma, and hopelessness in order to address critical gaps in services. **Recovery principles** (see Table 2-1) are what practitioners must hold themselves and adult mental health systems accountable to while working to transform from a medical to a recovery paradigm. These systems are called to embrace a focus on increasing health and well-being in the context of safe and stable homes, supportive relationships, and inclusive communities that increase opportunities to contribute and experience purpose. Yet this has proved to be a difficult shift for many across disciplines in the mental health services community (Strong & Letts, 2021).

OTPs can facilitate recovery by supporting increased occupational performance, especially activities of daily living (ADLs) and health management; building health habits and routines; and preventing unhealthy conditions and disease (Cano Prieto et al., 2022; Wastberg et al., 2019). Practitioners can promote physical, mental, and social health and wellness;

TABLE 2-2 | Wraparound Principles

Principle	Definition
Unconditional care	Children are not kicked out of wraparound, ever. They will graduate having succeeded; the team doesn't give up on them.
Strengths-based	The heart of the plan involves identifying strengths of children and creating "enabling niches" where they live their strengths. The strengths of family, team members, and community are identified and used to support the plan.
Family-driven; youth-guided	Families and youth are instrumental in developing their plans, meaning goals or anything related to their plan are not written without them. Family peer support providers are an essential role.
Team-based	The work of the wraparound team occurs in its regular meetings. Nothing is decided outside the team meetings.
Natural supports	More than 50% of the team are not there as professional helpers; rather, they are people from the community that the child and family select (could be extended family, neighbors, teachers, coach, friends, etc.). The plan developed by the team relies heavily on community resources identified by the team members.
Collaboration	Every child-serving agency in which the child is involved agrees to rely on the wraparound process and to be part of this team (so family doesn't have competing agendas and meetings with juvenile justice, school, child welfare, mental health agency, etc.).
Community-based	The work of the wraparound team is focused on creating opportunities within the child's community.
Culturally competent	The team members honor the individual child and family culture.
Individualized	The plan is based on this specific child's needs. Resources are generated based on the strengths and needs of this child, rather than from a set list of strategies or options to choose from.
Outcome-based	This loops back to the first principle of persistent or unconditional care. If something is not working, the team figures out what else to try. Families and youth are not blamed or shamed; the team just develops another strategy. Teams don't give up. They stay focused on outcomes.

Dennis, K. W., & Lourie, I. (2006). Everything is normal until proven otherwise: A book about wraparound services. *Child Welfare League of America.*

hope and satisfaction; and quality of life while facilitating occupational justice and personal recovery (Cano Prieto et al., 2022). This text embraces a recovery philosophy throughout to promote a deep understanding of people; where they live, work, play, learn, laugh, and struggle; and their cherished and needed occupations.

Recovery approaches are designed to address adult populations, but other approaches have been developed for children and youth. The special education eligibility for children in the United States uses the term **"severe emotional disturbance (SED),"** which generally refers to children and youth with significant mental health needs. In child-serving systems, the philosophy of SoC and the principle of wraparound, which is how SoC is operationalized, are the guideposts for working with children and their families (Stroul et al., 2010). SoC began as a response to the lack of mental health care for youth with SED in communities, which resulted in placing large numbers of children in residential facilities with generally poor outcomes (Davis et al., 1995). In SoC, all child-serving agencies are instead asked to come together and develop coordinated strategies to meet the needs of children and youth in their communities. Core values of SoC are that they are:

1. Family-driven and youth-guided
2. Community-based with local child, youth, and family services and support working together rather than in silos
3. Culturally and linguistically competent (Stroul et al., 2010)

SoC sought to use some of the money being spent on institutions to *wrap* supports around these children and youth in

the community (Dennis & Lourie, 2006). In addition to those principles operationalized in wraparound (see Table 2-2), SoC principles include being evidence-informed and developmentally appropriate; protecting the rights of children, youth, and families; and coordinating across systems (Stroul et al., 2010).

Before SoC became the federally funded mechanism for trying to increase resources in communities for children with SED and their families, a few people began developing practices to support children and youth in their homes rather than in institutions. This effort developed into the practice of wraparound, which became the mechanism for supporting these children within the overarching SoCs. You will read more about children and families in Chapter 29: Families. ⬤ Similar to recovery principles, the wraparound principles in Table 2-2 are standards to hold practitioners and systems accountable when working with children, youth, and families.

OTPs are expected to support the mental health and well-being of all people. As practitioners utilizing wraparound or recovery perspectives with a resilience focus, it's essential to avoid using a medical lens, which assumes that there is a therapeutic or restorative benefit to naming and framing illness. Instead, each individual should be viewed from a strengths-based lens, recognizing them as the expert in what they want and need to do and further realizing that their recovery journey is unique to them (many pathways). OTPs are collaborators offering specific knowledge and skills to support people's transformations and assisting them to be resilient in the midst of their challenges, while championing their journeys toward flourishing in roles and communities they choose.

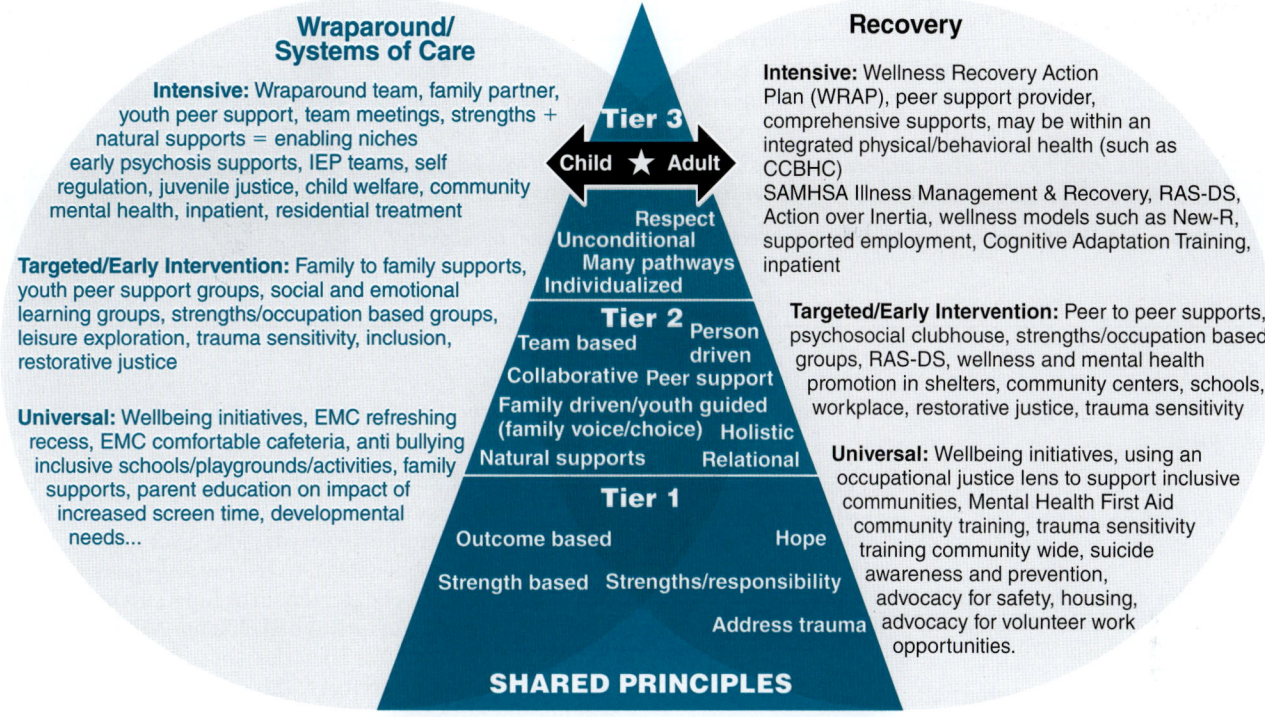

FIGURE 2-2. Recovery—Wraparound intersections. *Copyright Fette, C. (2023, May 8). Mental health from a public health lens.* https://aaron-voices.com/moms-blog/mental-health-from-a-public-health-lens

Public Health Approach

The WHO advocated for a public health approach to mental health, emphasizing promotion, prevention, and intervention (AOTA, 2016; WHO, 2001). Serving individuals across the life span, practitioners need to integrate concepts from SAMHSA's four dimensions of recovery (SAMHSA, 2012) and the philosophy of SoC and wraparound (Stroul et al., 2010) into the public health approach. Figure 2-2 aligns recovery-wraparound principles at three levels:

> *Tier 1: promoting* whole population mental health and well-being (universal tier)
> *Tier 2: preventing* mental ill health for those at risk of developing mental illness (targeted or early intervention level)
> *Tier 3: intensive* services for individuals with identified mental, emotional, or behavioral disorders (intensive level)

Sample interventions supporting person-driven recovery at each level are identified in the figure (AOTA, 2016, 2017). Tier 1/universal interventions include promoting healthy occupations, fostering self-regulation and coping strategies, and promoting mental health literacy across diverse settings. Tier 2/targeted interventions aim to prevent mental health problems for persons at risk from emotional experiences (trauma, abuse), situational stressors (bullying, obesity), genetic risks (family history of mental illness), and other factors. Tier 3/intensive interventions address improving daily functioning, interpersonal relationships, emotional well-being, and coping with challenging daily life. Because occupational therapy is focused on occupation, the objective at each intervention tier is the person's engagement in occupations.

The Lived Experience

People with mental health **lived experience** have long driven efforts to transform mental health services from medical to recovery paradigms, such as members of the psychiatric survivors' movement and families who shaped SoC and wraparound. By valuing lived experience stories within this text, readers can deeply explore just how uniquely and individually recovery is defined and experienced. Furthermore, reflecting on lived experience drives practitioners to create richer and more meaningful interventions, robust SoC, and inclusive communities.

Offering **respect** demands that practitioners value everyone and honor their experiences. **Person-** and **family-driven** pathways are principles of both models. A cornerstone of both is the role of **peer-to-peer support.** Peers are hope personified. For people just beginning their journeys, family and peer support providers offer hope by demonstrating that others, having been in a low place, somehow managed to build a life of substance. Consequently, people currently feeling hopeless can still find hope to craft a life. Peers are guides in unexpected, unfamiliar territory and can be trusted. They have experienced the distress and made their way through it. Connie Wells (2010) shared the following from a parent:

> I felt so alone. When I started to meet other families that had a child like Tara, I started to live again. I had put my feelings on hold for a long time. I never knew who to share with; how much they could understand. Now, I can just say what I mean, and I know I am not the only one who feels that way. (p. 31)

When asked to describe experiences within their program, persons in recovery voiced views that mutual peer support

PhotoVoice

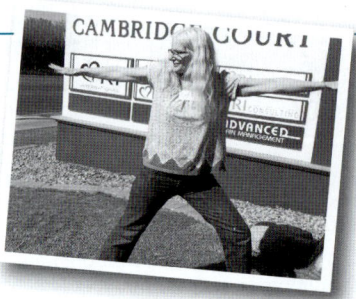

To me, recovery means overcoming my weaknesses and making a future for myself. I have been through a few train wrecks. It has taken me 51 years to start to feel how I did when I was young before I got sick. I look forward to going through training so I can help others who have been through or are going through similar situations. Also because of all the people who have helped me, to show them that the help was not in vain. I am a warrior, and I keep trying.

Which of SAMHSA's recovery principles are reflected in Celia's definition of recovery?

enhanced their social lives and sense of identity (Wastberg et al., 2019):

> I was basically just alone at home before group started, being able to get a foothold on some kind of social life here was fantastic. (p. 376)

> I'm not so afraid, but I used to be even afraid of myself, but I feel quite secure in myself now, which I've not been before, . . . I feel ready for life. (p. 376)

Participants reported growing self-understanding, acceptance, and confidence. They also identified experiences of flow, in which joy in occupation led to the loss of sense of time and all other activity around them (Csikszentmihalyi, 2000). Although the onset of illness led to self-care declines, loss of interests, loneliness, and loss of confidence, they reported that peer and group leader support and individually adapted demands enabled participation (Wastberg et al., 2019). This participation created changes in lifestyle, which occurred from their increased hope, meaning, balance, and engagement in life. Groups and recovery communities support the **relational** recovery principle, meaning that interacting with and supporting others builds well-being for all.

When interviewed regarding views of recovery while attending a clubhouse program, a person spoke to the individuality of recovery:

> Recovery is not a destination, not a fixed place. . . . I think it is part of a journey, our life long journey . . . a process of recovering. I'll always be taking my medications. I'll always visit a psychiatrist a few times a year for check-ins. I'll have a therapist for a period of time while I work on closure for some of the major wounds in my life. But recovery is about becoming and for me, especially, it's about becoming more whole as a person. (Stoffel, 2008, p. 114)

The **many pathways** principle emphasizes that there are many paths to recovery. Setbacks are common, and practitioners must practice acceptance. Holistic supports and serving individualized needs are equally important to identifying individual, family, and community strengths. Strengths-based interventions require each to bring their assets to recovery work.

> The last 10 years has not been easy. There have been hospital stays, numerous medications changes, and major lifestyle changes. All of that has brought me to today where I am in a state of constant recovery. I am fully aware the recovery never ends. As simple as it may sound: I must follow the rules of recovery. . . . I know I am here to defeat my illness. I am not defined by my illness. I am Jason Jepson, and I am recovering.

> Not for the next month or 6 months, but for the rest of my life. (Jepson, 2016, p. 4)

This man shared eloquently that recovery can be an ongoing, active, everyday endeavor. Jepson (2016) made recovery and its strategies a part of his everyday life. Everyday routines, habits, and roles are beneficial to recovery. de Jager and colleagues (2016) found engagement in occupations and activity not only provided structure to daily life but helped motivate persons to move forward. Their daily occupations and activities also helped them connect with others and build a sense of value and purpose again. "It makes me feel as though I'm contributing to something. And I want to feel valuable; I want to feel that I can contribute" (de Jager et al., 2016, p. 1416).

Community is central to both recovery and wraparound. Engaging with others and the community was viewed as an agent of recovery in Jackie Goldstein's (2016) book *Voices of Hope for Mental Illness: Not Against, With*. She explored the power of community culture(s) on recovery. Her message stated that recovery is not just the responsibility of the individual, but of the community at large. Supportive communities have established networks, support systems, and programs that hold members of that community accountable to supporting recovery approaches. When the places people live, work, and love foster the attitude of "not against, with," people living with mental illness find strength not just in themselves but in their families, neighbors, and community at large. Contexts of people's lives impact occupational performance. OTPs can positively affect not just the individual but also groups of people or communities. Creating a fit between the person and environment facilitates function, quality of life, and satisfaction for those in recovery and their supporters.

Lived experience stories paint a picture of life lived in recovery as hard work. Yet with hope, this hard work fosters resilience through skill acquisition, role discovery, and acceptance of life as it is. This man articulates that acceptance is a strength in his recovery:

> In mental illness, we don't fix it, we either accept it, and learn to live with it, or we make it our focus, . . . it's the pebble, the rock in our shoe, . . . in dealing with it, we become better. It hurt in the beginning, but it hurts less and less. I don't feel ill, even though I know I have it—sometimes I feel paranoid or I feel a little suspicious . . . but I'm actually stronger in some ways than others who don't have mental illness are. (Stoffel, 2008, pp. 115–116)

Insight into recovery through experiences shared here builds on definitions discussed at the start of the chapter. Recovery is individually felt and experienced; these individuals share how occupations and the environment either facilitated or hindered recovery. The role of the environment in daily life and recovery is paramount for mental health practitioners to remember.

Exploring the Dimensions of Recovery

SAMHSA's four dimensions of recovery (**health, home, purpose,** and **community**) support a life in recovery. These dimensions are used to guide treatment planning and intervention decision-making for practitioners, communities, and SoC (SAMHSA, 2012). Practitioners begin the occupational therapy process with an occupational profile (AOTA, 2020, 2021), encouraging those in recovery to define what home, health, purpose, and community are for them. The profile enables practitioners to work collaboratively with each person to achieve recovery goals. Additionally, these four dimensions are important to support mental health and well-being at community levels. By addressing these dimensions at the population level, practitioners endorse society-wide universal needs through advocacy to influence policy, regulations, and funding for mental health, well-being, and occupational justice initiatives.

Health

When considering the concept of health through a recovery-oriented lens, the desired outcome is much more than physical health. Health includes "overcoming or managing one's disease(s) or symptoms and for everyone in recovery, making informed healthy choices that support physical and emotional wellbeing" (SAMHSA, 2012, p. 3). This chapter's many shared lived experiences embody health as holistic in nature. Finding balance and maintaining that balance for an ongoing sense of health is desired by many (Anonymous, 2017; Jepson, 2016). Making informed decisions about one's health care requires having the knowledge and tools to make choices that best enable recovery. Recovery-oriented interventions provide opportunities to learn about strategies to manage both emotional and physical wellness.

Using the work of occupational therapist Margaret Swarbrick, SAMHSA (2016) created the Eight Dimensions of Wellness Initiative (see Fig. 2-3) as a method to improve mental and physical health in order to promote recovery.

Swarbrick (2012) described wellness as a deliberate process that involves making choices to enable balance in emotional, environmental, financial, intellectual, occupational, physical, social, and spiritual needs. This balance of eight interconnected dimensions contributes to a lifestyle that holistically supports wellness. See Chapter 45: Self-Care and Well-Being Occupations for recovery-oriented health interventions. 🤝

Home

What does it mean to *have housing* versus *being at home?* Why is home vital to recovery? SAMHSA (2012) defines "home" as "having a stable and safe place to live" (p. 3). Examining this definition, the key words are *stable* and *safe.* For many,

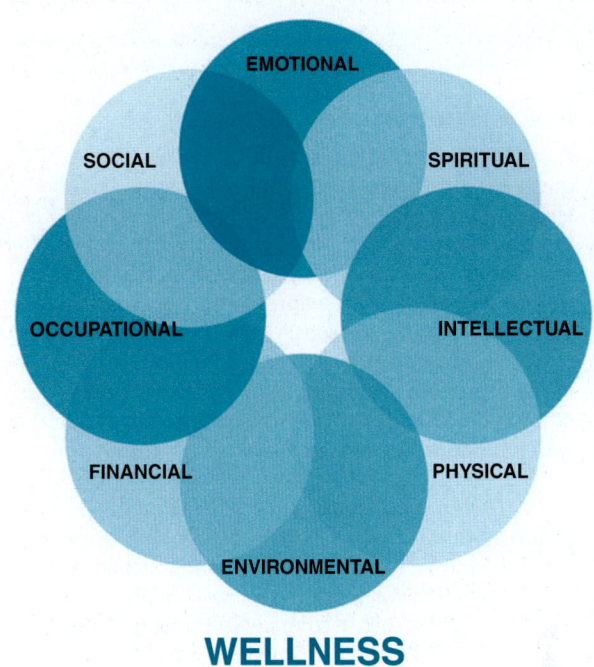

FIGURE 2-3. The Eight Dimensions of Wellness. This SAMHSA initiative works to improve mental and physical health in order to promote recovery. *Reprinted with permission from Substance Abuse and Mental Health Services Administration. (2016).* Creating a healthier life: A step-by-step guide to wellness. *[Workbook.] http://store.samhsa .gov/product/Creating-a-Healthier-Life-c/SMA16-4958*

home is something taken for granted; however, individuals in recovery experience homelessness far too often. Even when housing is available, conditions are frequently substandard and temporary. Home includes a stable and safe community to support persons in recovery. It offers a social group as part of the home and daily activity options, with both contributing to meaningful role development (Goldstein, 2016). However, these concepts are uniquely defined by each person in recovery. What makes a home for one person may be very different from another's experience. For some individuals, living with other people is an important aspect of home, whereas others prefer to have their own place. See Chapter 31: The Home Environment: Permanent Supportive Housing for recovery-oriented home interventions. 🤝

Purpose

The purpose dimension supports recovery because persons strive for their full potential through "meaningful daily activities, such as a job, school, volunteerism, family caretaking or creative endeavors and the independence, income and resources to participate in society" (SAMHSA, 2012, p. 3). Exploring concepts of occupational engagement and participation in meaningful activity, Sutton and colleagues (2012) heard persons in recovery identify a renewed sense of purpose through engaging with others and meeting expectations of resumed valued roles. Many expressed feelings of self-worth and accomplishment when returning to the worker role. Practitioners support persons in recovery journeys to find purpose by assisting their return to valued roles or to find new ones, thus promoting community participation.

The Lived Experience

Mark Freeman: My Recovery

I started experimenting with drugs and alcohol at 14. Frequency of my use increased from Friday nights, to entire weekends, and then progressed to daily use. My drug and alcohol use caused problems in all aspects of my life: strained family relationships, school attendance, and employment, and led to interactions with law enforcement. My accumulated consequences included lost jobs, divorce, and homelessness. The revolving door of frequent incarcerations allowed some breaks in my drug and alcohol use. Unfortunately, I would get out of jail and go back to using. Probation violations led to arrest warrants and soon I was back in jail.

That dark, depressing cycle was my lifestyle for many years. Eventually, I qualified for incarceration in the state prison system. I was in denial. It took 10 months of state custody for my chemically soaked brain to realize what I was doing to myself. Wall posters depicted the physical and mental deterioration that accompanied prolonged use of drugs and alcohol. I realized I had to get sober and stay sober. I was hopeful that treatment would strengthen my ability to recover.

My treatment days started at 5:30 a.m. in a community circle where I'd take my turn sharing my positive affirmations. This was difficult because I focused on the negative facets of my life. Nevertheless, I learned there was always something positive when I looked for it. I was expected to perform structured activities for 13 hours each day. I was also required to actively participate in all my assigned work groups with no isolating, and no incomplete assignments.

The program operated on an accountability model; we were to hold ourselves—and each other—accountable by identifying underlying thinking errors that led to our self-destructive activities. If I acted on a thinking error or committed a rule infraction, I was expected to select an exercise from the "Learning Tree." That was a magazine rack filled with forms for different cognitive learning options. I could complete a gratitude list, use a thinking-error worksheet, write an essay about my flawed thinking, or explain to the entire group how I would think and behave differently in the future. Those exercises taught me the skills necessary to manage myself in society. I took classes in CBT [cognitive behavioral therapy], DBT [dialectical behavior therapy], and MRT [moral reconation therapy]. I learned to pause and think about the consequences of unacceptable behavior, how my thoughts affect my feelings and actions, how to act on rational thinking rather than emotions, how to manage my emotions, and how to apply moral reasoning to my actions to get the results that I really want.

Treatment taught me why I used drugs and alcohol. I was bored, I wanted to shut down my feelings and socialize, and I was thrill-seeking. I understood that this behavior had become a habit. I would have to develop new habits and find other things to do when I was bored. I understood that I would have to practice not giving myself permission to use when I experienced my triggers. I learned to take care of myself, recognize my thinking errors, regulate my emotions, and know that my actions affected others. I had to explore

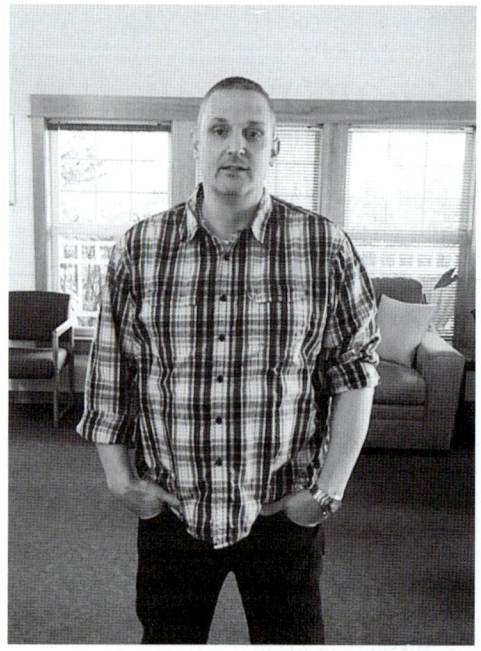

new ways to have fun and learn to socialize sober. I had to control my impulsiveness by stepping back and processing my feelings.

After my release, I went to stay with an aunt who was very supportive of my recovery. I was maintaining good boundaries by not associating with my old acquaintances who were still using. I attended recovery meetings, but I was hesitant to make new friends who were in recovery. After 4 months of isolation, I needed socialization and acceptance. I went to visit my old friends. I relapsed and continued to use. Eight weeks later I was back in prison. I did not practice using my recovery knowledge and tools. It was all new territory. I resolved that I would find new connections in the recovery community.

I knew I would need the influence of good role models and opportunities to strengthen my resolve. I surrendered myself and humbly prayed for help, guidance, and support. I use the term God, for lack of a better word, to describe a concept that I do not fully understand. Wherever love and kindness comes from, that is where I direct my prayers. My prayers were answered. I received a letter from a friend I had known since I was 14.

He was sober, and [said] that if I wanted to walk in recovery with him, he had a place for me by his side. Tears flowed as I read that letter. I responded, immediately. I said, "Yes, I want recovery. I am willing to do whatever it takes to succeed. Please pick me up on my release date!"

He said, "I'm going to help you, and when you're ready, you will help others. That's how this works. We all want recovery, and we need each other to get it and keep it." Later that same day, he helped me get into clean and sober transitional housing and introduced me to my new household. Everyone I met were working their own recovery program, rebuilding their life by repairing their relationships, completing prison

The Lived Experience—cont'd

supervision, and becoming employable again. I longed to add the recovery chapter to my life story. It was such a relief to know I was not alone.

There are no shortcuts. I learned that recovery is a rewarding, frequently inconvenient, day-to-day process. I am free of my addictions and grateful for all the support and guidance that I have received from my recovery network. Recovery is all about people helping one another. I failed when I tried to

do this alone. When I was open to connecting with others, it worked. The people in my recovery community taught me how to repair my shattered relationships and how to form new, healthy ones. I attend four meetings a week, two of them with my sponsor. I meet with my sponsor, and each of my sponsees, once a week to read literature and work on our steps. I'm not perfect, and when I feel myself falling behind, I go back to the basics.

Community

Seen through lived experience reflections in this chapter and the literature, community is one of the most important dimensions of recovery. SAMHSA (2012) defines "community" as "relationships and social networks that provide support, friendship, love and hope" (p. 3). Hope, one of the 10 recovery principles, is a catalyst to recovery and can be fostered by peers, practitioners, and family. Participation is a desired intervention outcome in *OTPF-4* (AOTA, 2020). Occupation-based practice reflects recovery's emphasis on purpose and community participation. **Community integration** is more than spending time in the community; rather, it includes ways persons engage, participate in, and give back to the community. Cano Prieto and colleagues (2022) framed community participation outcomes using *OTPF-4* (AOTA, 2020) as:

1. Increased occupational performance, particularly ADLs and health management
2. Prevention of unhealthy conditions, risky behaviors, and diseases
3. Physical, mental, and social health and wellness
4. Quality of life understood as hope and satisfaction
5. Occupational justice and personal recovery

For people in recovery, these outcomes may be achieved by increasing self-efficacy and their health and wellness through participation in leisure, volunteer, or work activities.

Occupational Therapy Partnerships With Recovery and Wraparound Approaches

This chapter introduced recovery, wraparound, and the public health model. Now is the time to dive still deeper into evidence and examples within occupational therapy practice. Figure 2-4 features models of public health and multi-tiered systems of support (the K–12 application of the public health model; see Chapter 47: Student 🤝) on the far left. The *OTPF-4* (AOTA, 2020) is the prism through which practice is filtered (located in the center), and on the right are occupational therapy roles and practices. The vertical

arrow on the far right indicates that practice is grounded by the use of participation in occupation. This figure highlights intersections of recovery-oriented services and occupational therapy roles and practices across public health model tiers of interventions. Focusing on occupations and participation, occupational therapy has the capacity to support recovery and mental well-being at person, group or community, and population levels (AOTA, 2020; Kelly et al., 2010; Synovec, 2015).

Tier 3: Examples of Occupational Therapy Practices

Tier 3/intensive level intervention services aim at enabling recovery through development or improvement of occupations that people want or need to do. Enabling greater occupational participation leads to people attaining greater satisfaction in their community engagement. OTPs must shift away from the medical model's focus on medications, crisis, and risk management and toward multitiered systems of support, recovery-based practices with adults, and SoC or wraparound and multitiered systems of support with children and youth (Strong & Letts, 2021; Tyminski et al., 2019). Occupational therapy's person-centered, strengths-based approaches support people as they search for meaning and value in their recovery journeys.

Occupation-based interventions are integral to recovery and wraparound approaches by providing settings in which people develop a sense of meaning and purpose, positive self-concept, hope, reestablished routines, coping skills, and social supports (Kelly et al., 2010). Persons increase their self-efficacy and perceived control, which enables their participation in daily occupations, reflecting the person-driven, empowerment, sense of direction dimensions to support the many paths of the recovery journey (Synovec, 2015).

Once people move beyond basic survival stresses, Strong and Letts (2021) recommend that practitioners offer a self-management intervention (see Box 2-3) to support persons reclaiming a satisfying life, as opposed to a medical model approach of disease and risk management.

Recovery—Tier 3

Appreciating the recovery dimensions, OTPs can support *health* within tier 3/intensive level interventions with social

Evidence-Based Practice

Community Integration in Recovery

Researchers looked at the effects of engaging in daily activities on health and well-being outcomes.

RESEARCH FINDINGS

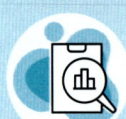

Community integration is important to recovery. For those with mental health or substance use challenges, this can take form in social connections; community roles, such as volunteer or worker; or other participation that facilitates engagement in the mainstream community. Many individuals in recovery tend to spend a significant amount of time sleeping or otherwise disengaged from active participation (inertia).

Action Over Inertia is an occupational therapy intervention (Krupa et al., 2022) that uses strengths-based, person-centered approaches through worksheets facilitating collaboration between person and practitioner. Intervention helps individuals to identify occupational imbalance, explore change, and make plans to engage in meaningful activities. Gewurtz and colleagues (2016) linked effects of engaging in daily activities to health and well-being outcomes, which are crucial for persons living with serious mental illness. Rees and colleagues (2021) identified that Action Over Inertia interventions assisted participants to identify barriers to active engagement in occupations and to understand how time-use relates to well-being, resulting in their making changes to overcome their inertia.

APPLICATIONS

➡ Practitioners can facilitate increased time spent in activity engagement for adults with serious mental illness who experience prolonged disengagement by using Action Over Inertia interventions.

➡ Through supporting community participation in the form of community role engagement, practitioners can increase individuals' sense of belonging and self-efficacy.

REFERENCES

Gewurtz, R. E., Moll, S. E., Letts, L. J., Larivière, N., Levasseur, M., & Krupa T. M. (2016). What you do every day matters: A new direction for health promotion. *Canadian Journal of Public Health, 107*(2), e205–e208. https://doi.org/10.17269/cjph.107.5317

Krupa, T., Edgelow, E., Chen, S.-P., & Mieras, C. (2022). *Promoting activity and participation in individuals with serious mental illness: The Action Over Inertia approach.* Routledge. https://doi.org/10.4324/9781003111368

Rees, E. F., Ennals, P., & Fossey, E. (2021). Implementing an Action Over Inertia group program in community residential rehabilitation services: Group participant and facilitator perspectives. *Frontiers in Psychiatry, 12,* 624803. https://doi.org/10.3389/fpsyt.2021.624803

support groups to build coping skills, develop individualized interventions to help persons create medication management plans, and collaborate with peer wellness coaches to encourage persons to engage in physical activity. Practitioners can address *home* by facilitating the skill development necessary to maintain a home, such as bill paying, home maintenance, and cooking (AOTA, 2020). To support *purpose* and community participation, they can help persons build self-care and personal hygiene, budgeting, and social participation capacity. Additionally, they assist persons in identifying interests and then enabling skill development. Practitioners also contribute by facilitating supportive environments so that individuals can be successful while participating in the *community.*

An occupational therapy intervention that pivots away from a medical model and can be implemented across all three public health tiers is Capabilities, Opportunities, Resources, and Environments (CORE; Pereira & Whiteford, 2022). Built on occupational therapy's core beliefs, this intervention advocates for social and occupational justice to support human rights across various settings, such as supported housing, prisons, homeless shelters, and community centers. Aligning well with recovery, CORE's tenets focus on interventions that support individual strengths, person-driven planning, collaboration, enabling participation in what people want and need to do, building hope, and community-based practices.

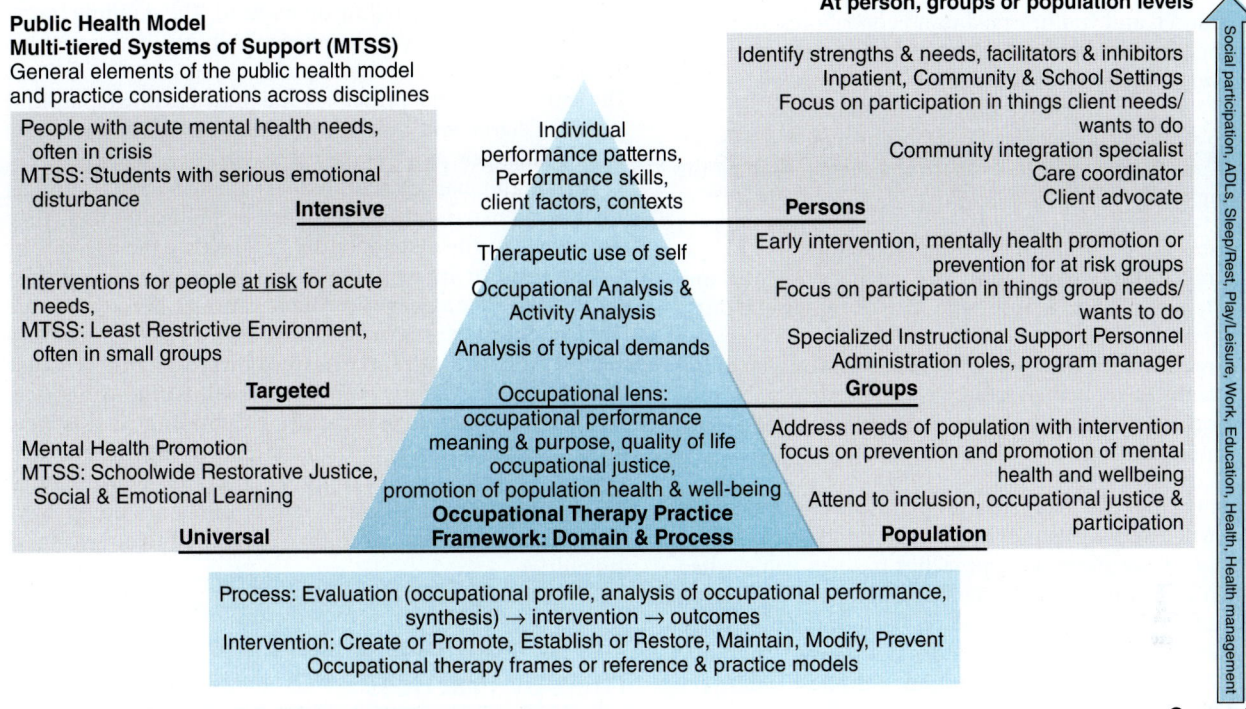

FIGURE 2-4. Intersections of recovery and wraparound. *Copyright Fette, C. (2023, May 8). Mental health from a public health lens. https://aaron-voices.com/moms-blog/mental-health-from-a-public-health-lens*

BOX 2-3 ■ Integrating Occupation-Based Strategies to Support Personal Recovery

Strong and Letts (2021) advocate for strengths-based learning "enmeshed within recovery, health, and building a life" (p. 402) for development of self-management. For people seeking recovery, the ongoing learning process depends on being responsive to individual self-perception, health and illness, strengths and needs, and different learning needs, and must not be time limited. An occupation-based lens is recommended for supporting individuals in learning eight self-management tasks:

1. Reaching a personal understanding of their illness experiences, affirming that they are not alone, and enabling them to build hope

2. Finding medications and client–provider partnerships, offering respect for them as people, and dealing directly with issues of power and control

3. Learning to trust themselves to manage reality testing and self-monitoring

4. Dealing with stigma and discrimination, learning to be kind to themselves, and finding supportive environments

5. Developing and using support networks

6. Discovering ways to deal with the impact of mental illness on daily living activities, as well as developing healthy habits and personal strategies

7. Finding meaningful occupations that fit their views of themselves and enable feeling useful and valued

8. Integrating management of comorbidities and recognizing how conditions impact each other (diabetes, substance use, trauma, brain injury, etc.)

Tier 3/intensive services supporting mental well-being and recovery are utilized for persons with and without identified mental health challenges who are transitioning out of prisons. To accomplish becoming a participating member of society again, people need to build strategies for coping and developing social interaction, positive emotions, sense of self, and self-compassion. Occupational therapy can assist persons to flourish with mental well-being through providing opportunities for valued and meaningful occupational engagement. Recovery approaches can enhance a person's reintegration into the community by supporting individualized pathways, offering respect and acceptance, and assisting them to build peer support.

Systems of Care/Wraparound—Tier 3

With children and youth, wraparound contributes overarching principles (see Table 2-2) that guide best practice, just as recovery principles do with adults. Wraparound itself is generally a tier 3/intensive practice to enable children or youth to attain greater occupational performance. OTPs can serve in many roles within wraparound teams, such as the following:

1. They can be wraparound team facilitators.
2. Practitioners working in any settings not utilizing the wraparound approach can join wraparound teams.
3. Practitioners who serve in any positions enabling youths to apply their strengths can participate by supporting community-based activities that build their strengths.

Understanding the wraparound principles is especially critical when serving as part of a wraparound team. Implementation of wraparound approaches has less value when the team as a whole lacks understanding of the principles. The resulting deterioration of services becomes similar to the case management model, which does not promise the same outcomes as high-fidelity wraparound with these often very challenging youth.

Wraparound principles (see Table 2-2) may be applied in multiple populations and settings. For example, occupational therapy was provided for a second grader, with the pseudonym Charlie, who experienced Friedreich ataxia. He became clumsy when developing symptoms. His friends, made in early childhood, began avoiding him. His family viewed occupational therapy as a resource to improve his abilities and remediate his disability. He and his family pushed themselves hard and were not amenable to energy conservation and compensatory strategies encouraged by their school-based occupational therapist. When losing protective extension reflexes and falling more, Charlie refused to use the standing frame obtained by the physical therapist. His occupational therapist applied wraparound principles, pulling together all school-based team members to brainstorm solutions. Strengths and interests identified using wraparound principles included his attending a well-resourced school with a great team, being a motivated child with a supportive family, maintaining his previous large group of friends, and noting his love of Ferraris. His immediate needs were fall prevention and safety as well as recognition of legitimate needs for accommodations by friends and family. Charlie needed to accept the standing frame. His parents had real difficulty understanding why occupational therapy was not adhering to their initial priority, enabling Charlie to catch up to developmental milestones and remediating his declining coordination and strength. But his parents began to realize the occupational therapist and team's passions to support him to participate in school and began to trust the team.

As the team offered solutions, a teacher reported that her husband worked at a local Ferrari dealership, and the wraparound team hatched a plan. The dealership dipped the standing frame in bright Ferrari yellow paint and fashioned a basket with a real emblem from a Ferrari grill. Suddenly, Charlie was cool! His friends fought over who would help him carry books and supplies. Now willing to use this standing frame, he stopped falling on his head. The standing frame served to cue others that he needed help, but it also met his needs for inclusion. It was acceptable because it was a Ferrari. The team applied the principles and practices of wraparound to meet Charlie and his family's need to adjust to their new set of challenges.

Although Charlie's school district listed wraparound as a tier 3/intensive strategy in their mental health plan, very few people in the district understood either the practice of wraparound or its principles. The occupational therapist demonstrated a leadership role because of her knowledge from facilitating wraparound processes in a community mental health program. She recognized challenges that Charlie and his family were having adjusting to his new set of needs and their difficulty responding to this new set of crises. She brought the school team together to help support Charlie and his family. Wraparound is an effective strategy to support children and families in coping with all kinds of psychosocial challenges related to adjusting to difficulties.

Tier 2: Examples of Occupational Therapy Practices

Tier 2/targeted intervention services for persons at risk aim to prevent mental health challenges from developing or becoming more severe. Through engaging persons in natural occupations, interventions utilizing recovery principles facilitate persons in using their strengths for occupational participation. Enabling healthy occupational engagement can reduce the impacts of personal or environmental factors that put persons at risk.

Doroud and colleagues (2018) challenge OTPs to intervene at both person and population levels. Addressing housing and living environments allows people to have safe, welcoming, and personalized spaces so they can experience freedom, choice, and self-determination. Practitioners enable individuals to choose spaces that match their recovery goals. Their roles include advocating for housing policies to provide living environments and community resources, thereby enabling experiences of community inclusion, recovery, and well-being.

Recovery—Tier 2

Along with one-to-one intervention for persons at the tier 3/intensive level, OTPs can support recovery through creating recovery-oriented workforces and systems that support recovery for intervention at group or population levels, such as through collaboration with peer support specialists (AOTA, 2020; Cano Prieto et al., 2022; Stoffel, 2013; Swarbrick, 2011). To prevent further impacts for at-risk performance and engagement, practitioners can assist by identifying barriers to engagement in daily occupations and community integration. **Relational support** can be created by connecting persons to peers who can guide them in overcoming barriers to support their identified important and meaningful choices. Through partnerships of occupational therapy and peer support specialists, skills gained in occupational therapy tier 3/intensive services can then be maintained or enhanced to prevent additional declines in at-risk performances in community settings.

Supporting the recovery dimension of *health* for groups or communities within the tier 2/targeted level, OTPs might lead school-based small groups in developing emotional regulation and social connectedness for at-risk students, thereby preventing social participation challenges. For persons experiencing an injury or medical disorder, mental health can be facilitated through diabetes support groups, which can prevent experiences of social isolation and loss of sense of self. Another social isolation prevention intervention is providing activities supporting *home,* such as health-promoting social and recreational groups provided in communal living environments. Practitioners can support *purpose* by exploring activities based on individual strengths and interests with groups of people living with mental illness to prevent engagement declines, followed by facilitating opportunities for them to advocate to community boards or with state legislators for resources needed to provide these activities in their community. To support building relationships and *community,* practitioners can facilitate a recovery-oriented community mental health group, creating volunteer opportunities for people living with mental illness to build supportive relationships and reduce risk of isolation. Interventions at the tier 2/targeted level also continue across the tier 3/intensive level.

Occupational therapy approaches supporting recovery and mental well-being are utilized for needs of persons, groups or communities, and populations in non–mental health settings and practice. Regardless of the life-changing consequences of illness, injury, or disorder, OTPs focus on holistic physical, emotional, and psychosocial needs to enable persons to experience meaningful lives. Within the tier 2/targeted level, people living with long COVID are a good example of understanding the needs of an at-risk population (Engels et al., 2021; Lannigan & Tyminski, 2021; Watters et al., 2021). It is critical to be guided by recovery principles when developing mental health promotion and early intervention approaches to support mental well-being needs. Needs include reduced social isolation, decreased leisure participation, and physical as well as mental aftereffects. Providing strategies is necessary to enable essential occupations in spite of cognitive impairments. Boyle and colleagues (2021) urged practitioners to look specifically at occupational impacts of COVID isolation for people living with disability. Consider the question: How do practitioners support people experiencing lingering COVID symptoms to recover using the four dimensions of recovery: health, home, purpose, and community?

Systems of Care/Wraparound—Tier 2

Application of strengths-based and trauma-informed principles at a community level is illustrated by OTPs and students within a massive, temporary shelter for unaccompanied minors fleeing from Central America. The shelter for more than 3,000 boys was quickly organized by administrators and staff, who had no knowledge of trauma-informed practices and little understanding of the trauma experienced by the boys or their need for occupation. It began as a vast sea of cots arranged into pods of approximately 50 youth with one to two adults staffing each pod, spread out across a large convention hall. With limited knowledge of mental health or trauma approaches, staff soon were essentially bullying the boys to move to different locations. Some boys just pulled their blankets over their heads and refused to get up. OTPs and students permitted inside the shelter quickly developed simple trauma training for the staff. Next, they designed strengths-based, culturally relevant activities for the boys and facilitated these in the pods alongside staff members. The anticipated outcome was to prevent retraumatization as the boys were being processed. Wraparound principles were utilized to guide these experiences. The boys were engaged in occupations to support their mental well-being, thus reducing potential impacts of being at risk in these shelters.

OTPs have long been in schools as related services providers for children in special education. Chapter 47: Student 🤝 discusses occupational therapy's role in providing specialized instructional support personnel (SISP), which enables practitioners to support students at risk addressed through interventions at the tier 1/universal and tier 2/targeted levels rather than having to wait until the students are floundering in critical developmental roles and need tier 3/intensive interventions. See Chapter 7: Cognition and Chapter 9: Sensory Processing and the Lived Sensory Experience. 🤝 Practitioners have a responsibility to meet the psychosocial needs of students as well as their sensorimotor and cognitive needs in school. Chapter 38: Early Psychosis Programs for Adolescents and Young Adults 🤝 describes OTPs' roles in early psychosis programs for youth, such as teaching effective strategies and supporting accommodations to enable school success. Early psychosis intervention focuses on preventing or minimizing occupational performance declines.

OTPs serve children and youth in a variety of contexts that are not traditionally thought of as mental health settings, including acute care, outpatient orthopedics, sensory integration clinics, and school-based practice. In these settings, children receiving occupational therapy services experience many mental health needs, such as maintaining their self-concept and esteem after injury or severe illness, coping with loss of important occupations, facing difficulty with social participation and stigma, and needing to acquire and practice social and emotional learning. Provision of tier 2/targeted services before children and youth acquire mental health challenges enables them to maintain and develop age-appropriate occupational participation. Additionally, Chapter 5: Trauma-Informed Practice explains that trauma is a common experience impacting engagement in typical occupations. 🤝 Practitioners serve all individuals, not only children and youth, with histories of trauma across the life span and must attend to supporting the mental health and well-being of people served across populations and settings.

When encountering mental health needs at the person level in any practice setting, services address mental health needs of at-risk groups, such as children with various disabilities, those with trauma histories, and those in marginalized groups. Practitioners can proactively develop small mental health promotion groups to build resilience through exploring and identifying strengths, assisting mutual support, building community, and enabling effective coping strategies.

Tier 1: Examples of Occupational Therapy Practices

Tier 1/universal intervention services are provided for all persons in society, with and without mental health challenges, to promote mental well-being. Through engaging persons in natural occupations, utilization of recovery principles enables practitioners to support individuals and communities to engage in health-promoting behaviors.

Strong and Letts (2021) acknowledge that a significant feature of enabling people's capacity for making "choices" within these models is often inhibited by the current realities of social inequities, resulting in poor support and stigma. They urge practitioners to advocate for provision of resources to meet basic survival needs, so that people have the capacity for recovery. At the tier 1/universal level, practitioners develop and support efforts within schools or communities, such as raising funds for an inclusive playground, advocacy for basic rights and needs for marginalized groups, community education around specific areas of concern, or developing curricula for others to implement. Examples of health and wellness programs developed by OTPs include Nutrition and Exercise for Wellness and Recovery (NEW-R; Brown et al., 2015) to enable healthy eating for people experiencing serious mental illness (promotion of mental health for persons with identified mental health challenges), the Do-Live-Well framework (Gewurtz et al., 2016) to promote healthy living through establishing day-to-day activity patterns associated with health (including mental health) and well-being, or Lifestyle Redesign (Clark et al., 2015) to promote health and well-being for independent-living older adults through engagement in natural occupations. Each of these interventions focused on enhancing healthy behaviors that are beneficial for the mental well-being of all individuals, regardless of whether they are healthy or living with acute or chronic conditions.

Recovery—Tier 1

At the tier 1/universal level for populations, practice examples supporting *health* include building mental health promotion and wellness programs for employees of a high-tech manufacturing plant, providing continuing education on mental health impacts of physical disability for a hospital system, or offering trauma-sensitive training for a school district. Advocating for safe and affordable housing and providing education on adaptive equipment at a local homeless shelter are examples of promotion strategies that address *home*. OTPs can facilitate *purpose* by working with employers to increase awareness of trauma and inclusion of survivors in the workplace. *Community* may be supported by providing mental health first aid education and supporting an antistigma campaign. These benefit persons in recovery as well as members of the entire community.

Occupational therapy interventions benefit from incorporating strategies developed in other disciplines, such as psychology. Within mental health promotion, practitioners can support persons regarding buffering the impact of stressors, bolstering positive mental health to flourish, and building new capacity to grow and transform within the recovery journey (Waters et al., 2022; see Box 2-4). Occupational therapy students will learn and practice skills that will help them

---

BOX 2-4   ■   Mental Health and Flourishing: Integrating Strategies From Other Disciplines to Support Recovery

Waters and colleagues (2022) suggested nine areas of focus to support mental health and flourishing in the era of the COVID pandemic that utilized positive psychology approaches.

1. *Address meaning:* Support persons to explore values for living a meaningful life, counteracting a disrupted sense of self, feelings of powerlessness, and loss of goals; rather, support ways to make a difference for self and others.
2. *Build increased effectiveness for coping with stressors:* Practice positive thoughts (e.g., reframing) and emotions (e.g., gratitude) and use adaptive coping strategies.
3. *Increase self-compassion:* Teach people to give themselves the same kindness and grace that they would give someone else they care about.
4. *Recognize courage:* Encourage self-appraisal and take worthwhile risks despite possible negative consequences.
5. *Practice gratitude:* Recognize benefits received, which helps the giver, receiver, and any onlookers.
6. *Identify and apply strengths:* First explore and use strengths in new ways; second, recognize how to use them in adversity to build capacity for growth.
7. *Use positive emotions in the moment:* Teach strategies and create opportunities for positive emotions to build upon each other.
8. *Teach and practice positive interpersonal processes:* Share laughter, be kind, and express and accept gratitude and other positive interactions.
9. *Create high-quality connections:* Remove distractions and focus on immediate interactions by being curious, being vulnerable, and offering help.

---

effectively support positive mental health at universal, targeted, or intensive levels. Practice examples in this section incorporate strengths-based approaches which include positive psychology components, such as developing self-compassion, coping strategies, and social connections and making meaning in life (Waters et al., 2022).

Systems of Care/Wraparound—Tier 1

An example of tier 1/universal intervention is a student-run wellness center described by Costanzo and colleagues (2022). Local occupational therapy students provided interventions to a local high school during the height of the COVID pandemic. Mental wellness was supported through occupation-based sessions to prevent loss of occupational engagement and offered strategies to maintain participation in typical social and educational tasks. Other tier 1/universal interventions—such as Comfortable Cafeteria and Refreshing Recess programs and other resources developed by Every Moment Counts (n.d.; also see Chapter 47: Student 🤝)—are implemented for schoolchildren and youth of all ages. OTPs teach and practice social and emotional skills with all students to enable them to develop strategies to build their capacity for meeting their mental health needs. Wraparound principles incorporated include offering respect, being strengths-based, and embedding programs with natural supports so that individuals can grow and maintain their mental well-being.

The interventions explored here are just a few examples of methods for supporting mental health and well-being across the public health tiers used by OTPs to provide recovery-oriented services. This textbook includes many other examples. Most important to recovery-oriented practice is that any decisions to try an intervention are reached collaboratively between the person and practitioner. Through hope, support, and empowerment, choices made will facilitate a positive journey and have a lasting effect on recovery. By using recovery and wraparound-oriented perspectives, OTPs can help individuals find hope and respect while choosing their own path based on personal values. This supports individuals to engage in occupations of choice, to build mastery and competence, and to meet their recovery goals as they pursue recovery.

Recovery and Wraparound as Change Agent: Transforming Systems of Care

Recovery is an overarching framework for mental health systems in the United States; however, these systems are affected by where recovery and SoC are situated within the larger mental health system and how services are funded. The overarching federal policy leader in mental health is SAMHSA. Yet, although SAMHSA provides some funding to mental health systems that actually provide services, it typically is in the form of grant initiatives rather than directly providing either capitated or fee-for-services funding for individuals. SAMHSA attempts to shape policy through service expectations attached to its various grant funding opportunities. Serving as a vital source in promoting recovery-oriented services, it has provided resources and grants to grow the behavioral health-care workforce's capacity to deliver recovery-oriented services.

Along with guiding national mental health-care systems and practice, recovery has led to changes in national policy and funding. In the United States, the passage of the Patient Protection and Affordable Care Act (2010; U.S. Department of Health and Human Services, n.d.) moved the system toward an integrated model of care that serves not just behavioral health needs but physical health as well. In March 2014, Congress passed, and the president signed, the Protecting Access to Medicare Act (2014). This piece of legislation included provisions from the Excellence in Mental Health Act that called for demonstration programs aimed at increasing the quality of, and expanding access to, mental health and substance use treatment (SAMHSA, 2023). Already seen as a game changer in community mental health service delivery, the Excellence in Mental Health Act furthered this progress through creating the Certified Community Behavioral Health Clinic (CCBHC) demonstration program. Twenty-four states applied for planning grants; of those, SAMHSA chose eight states to be demonstration grant recipients. Today, those states receive federal monies to

certify behavioral health agencies in their state. Thirty-nine other states are funding CCBHC services through their own Medicaid demonstration programs. CCBHCs meet standards for providing nine required services designed to ensure access to coordinated comprehensive behavioral health care to track those outcomes.

In 2022, President Biden made a commitment to confronting the country's mental health crisis through the Bipartisan Safer Communities Act, the American Rescue Plan, and budget funding (SAMHSA, 2022). To expand access to mental health services in communities that need them most, this funding provided states with revenue to develop and transform CCBHCs, thus expanding access to mental and behavioral health supports and services informed by recovery principles. The Bipartisan Safer Communities Act (BSCA) authorized $15 million in additional funding for CCBHCs.

Not only has recovery demonstrated power in changing the lives of individuals, but it is informing workforce practices and legislative efforts around the world. OTPs can practice daily from a recovery-driven lens and engage in systems change by harnessing the power of recovery and utilizing resources mentioned in this section and throughout this chapter. Applying recovery-driven practices at levels of the person, group or community, and population presents opportunities to make differences in lives of many through impacting quality of services. Greater resources are available to promote mental health and well-being through community activities and population advocacy initiatives. Although recovery approaches grew from the experiences of people living with psychiatric disorders, the application of mental health and well-being approaches have a significant benefit for individuals who live with acute or chronic health concerns and/or lifestyle challenges across the life span. Regardless of practice areas or settings, recipients of occupational therapy are best served with the integration of recovery/wraparound, resilience, and well-being perspectives. It is the challenge and opportunity of not just OTPs but of community members, neighbors, health-care professionals, and society to learn about recovery and build capacity to create the societal, cultural, and economic structures that nurture recovery. As Dr. Goldstein (2016) states,

> We like to say that in this country, everyone has the opportunity to pull themselves up by their bootstraps. The problem is that not everyone has bootstraps. A public investment that provides those bootstraps pays dividends in a with, not against, manner. (p. 129)

Here's the Point

- Recovery is an individual journey that is deeply personal and uniquely experienced by each person.
- Recovery is a means to an end for some and the end itself for others. It can change SoC, empower people, and be the process that allows individuals to discover themselves again.
- Many definitions of recovery have been provided to inform practice, build workforce capacity, and inform public policy.
- The lived experience of persons with mental health or substance use challenges should be listened to by mental health practitioners and community members to build a community understanding of recovery.

- OTPs have a unique role in supporting recovery. Whether for the person or for members in a community, occupation and participation facilitate the recovery process.
- Evidence-based practices in combination with the stories of lived experience are utilized by OTPs to promote recovery.

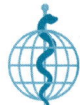

Visit the online resource center at **FADavis.com** to access the videos.

Apply It Now

1. Timeline of Mental Health Treatment From the Perspective of Individuals in Recovery

At the annual Recovery Conference in Wichita, Kansas, in 2000, a timeline of mental health treatment was created based on the perspective of individuals in recovery. Some of these same individuals updated the timeline in 2023. See the timelines below, the first from 2000 and the second from 2023.

How do you think the perspectives of people in recovery might differ from the perspectives of OTPs and other mental health professionals? How do you think society's views have or have not changed over time? Are there important events or perspectives that you think are missing?

This view of mental health treatment shares a person's perspective of recovery. How have mental health services changed over time? How do current perspectives of recovery impact persons now? How have society's views changed over time?

2. Video Exercise–Jordon's Lived Experience of Recovery as an Occupational Therapy Practitioner

Pair up with another student in your class or form a small group of students. Access and watch the "Jordon's Lived

Experience of Recovery as an Occupational Therapy Practitioner" video at the online resource center at FADavis.com. Then, discuss and together answer the following questions:

- Jordon describes struggling with blending the two aspects of herself: an individual with lived experience and an OTP. Do you believe there is a space to blend the practitioner role with that of lived experience? What is the danger of feeling "siloed," and how might that hinder healing and mental wellness?
- Jordon embodies the tools and skills she shares with the people she works with to address mental wellness, and she approaches her recovery and practice from a place of humility, understanding, and compassion. What tools or strategies can OTPs use to help individuals foster self-compassion and mitigate internalized stigma for their own lived experience?
- Jordon claims that, "You can have the perfect assessment or intervention, but it's really meaningless if you can't forge that therapeutic connection." What is her advice to OTPs concerning how to establish that therapeutic connection? Do you agree? What might you add to that advice?
- Jordon explains that, as an individual with lived experience and a practitioner, it is critical to take care of herself

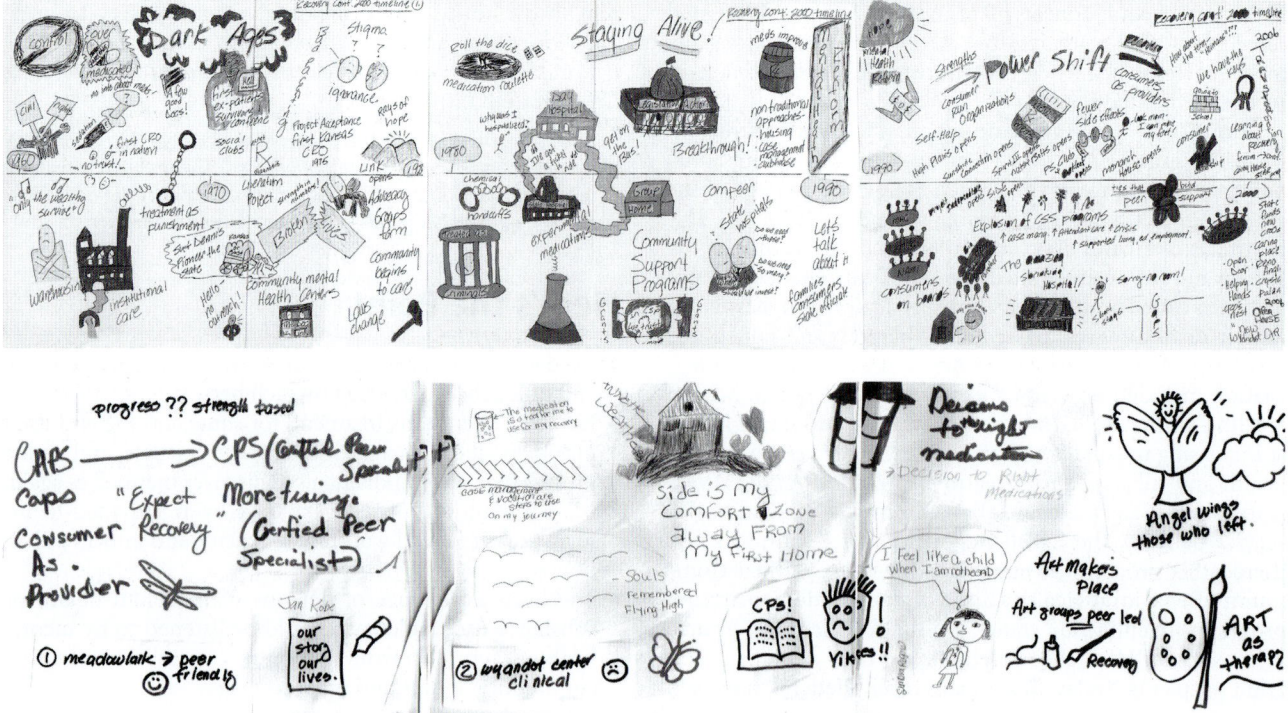

and manage her symptoms. What specific self-care strategies does Jordon describe using in her own life? Do you think the strategies she uses can be helpful for others in recovery? Explain.

3. Reflect on Recovery

Watch the video linked here: https://www.youtube.com/watch?v=IdRMsynXMZY&feature=youtube

Created by Oregon occupational therapy students, this video aimed to show how mental health and substance use challenges connect us more than divide us. How could this video be a catalyst to changing our health-care system? Who would the audience be? How could you measure its impact? What questions would foster discussions on the importance of recovery?

4. Fostering 10 Principles of Recovery: Gould Farms

Watch We Harvest Hope: The Gould Farm Story at https://www.youtube.com/watch?v=uJQODMsY6i4 and explore how a therapeutic community fosters the 10 principles of recovery. Analyze how the four dimensions of recovery are supported by Gould Farms. What aspects of *OTPF-4*'s domain and process do you observe?

Resources

- "Nicholas' Lived Experience of Schizophrenia" video. Nicholas is an occupational therapist living with the lived experience of schizophrenia. In this video, he describes his first episode of psychosis and the crucial role that occupational therapy played in his recovery. Nicholas emphasizes the importance of engaging with other people during rehabilitation and how, through occupational engagement, he discovered reconnection, felt loved, and found a sense of meaning and purpose. Access the video at at the online resource center at FADavis.com.
- Action Over Inertia Intervention: Krupa, T., Edgelow, M., Chen, S.-P., & Mieras, C. (2022). *Promoting activity and participation in individuals with serious mental illness: The Action Over Inertia approach*. Routledge.

   This person-centered, strengths-based occupational therapy intervention promotes mental health and well-being within meaningful activity and participation. Workbook exercises promote engagement through occupational imbalance, goal setting, and meaningful activities.
- Recovery Assessment Scale: Domain and Stages (RAS-DS): https://ras-ds.net.au

   Developed by Australian OTPs, this Australian Partners in Recovery resource includes a free manual, training webinar, and related journal articles plus the downloadable scale. These and the paired *RAS-DS Workbook*, which features recovery exercises, may be used independently by the person or with practitioners.
- Resource Guide to Wraparound: https://nwi.pdx.edu/NWI-book

   This National Wraparound Initiative online book is the definitive work on wraparound.
- National Empowerment Center (NEC): http://www.power2u.org

   Run by consumers, survivors, and ex-patients, NEC's mission is a message of recovery, empowerment, healing, and hope for those with lived experience regarding trauma, extreme states, or other mental health challenges. Their goal is that those with lived experience know that recovery is possible for anyone, regardless of where they are in their personal journey.
- Open Excellence is the Foundation for Excellence in Mental Health Care (FEMHC): https://openexcellence.org

   This foundation—of, by, and for the community of people—addresses improving mental health globally. Grants are used to change and improve how mental health care is conceptualized and provided in order to bring recovery, hope, and support to every community.
- Recovery and Recovery Support: https://www.samhsa.gov/find-help/recovery

   SAMHSA provides approaches for recovery and recovery-oriented practices, with resource links for Guiding Principles, the Four Dimensions of Recovery, the Office of Recovery, Recovery and Resilience Recovery and Relationships, Recovery Support, Cultural Awareness and Competency, and the Office of Behavioral Health Equity.
- Pat Deegan, PhD, & Associates: https://www.patdeegan.com

   This mental health leader has lived experience and seeks to help others in recovery participate in their care and make best treatment decisions. Her Recovery Approach includes the CommonGround Software, Recovery Academy, Medication Empowerment, Certified Personal Medicine Coaching, and the Hearing Distressing Voices Simulation.
- Intentional Peer Support (IPS): https://www.intentionalpeersupport.org/?v=b8a74b2fbcbb

   IPS's framework for thinking about and inviting transformative relationships helps people learn and grow around shared experience. Practitioners use relationships to enable persons to reach alternative views of their experiences, understand personal and relational patterns, and support persons to try new ways of living.
- Saks Institute for Mental Health Law, Policy, and Ethics: http://gould.usc.edu/faculty/centers/saks

   This think tank fosters collaborative research among scholars and policymakers to better the lives of those living with mental health challenges. They research intersections of law, mental health, and ethics to influence policy reform and advocacy actions.
- Mental Health America (MHA): https://mhanational.org

   MHA's work promotes mental health as a significant aspect of overall wellness. Focusing on the goal of recovery, MHA supports prevention for all; early identification and intervention for persons at risk; and integrated care, services, and supports for persons in need.
- Gould Farm: https://www.gouldfarm.org

   As the longest-running U.S. residential therapeutic community, Gould Farm assists adults living with mental illness to transform toward recovery, health, and greater independence through community living, meaningful work, and individual clinical care.
- Aaron's Voices: Resources Page: https://aaron-voices.com/resources

   This website features a collection of links and resources for best practices from wraparound to recovery, including Figures 2-2 and 2-4 used in this chapter.

References

American Occupational Therapy Association. (2016). *Occupational therapy's distinct value: Mental health promotion, prevention, and intervention across the lifespan.* Author. https://www.aota.org/~/media/Corporate/Files/Practice/MentalHealth/Distinct-Value-Mental-Health.pdf?la=en

American Occupational Therapy Association. (2017). Mental health promotion, prevention, and intervention in occupational therapy practice. *American Journal of Occupational Therapy, 71*(Suppl. 2), 7112410035p1–7112410035p19. https://doi.org/10.5014/ajot.2017.716S03

American Occupational Therapy Association. (2020). Occupational therapy practice framework: Domain and process —fourth edition. *American Journal of Occupational Therapy, 74*(Suppl. 2), 7412410010p1–7412410010p87. https://doi.org/10.5014/ajot.2020.74S2001

American Occupational Therapy Association. (2021). Improve your documentation and quality of care with AOTA's updated occupational profile template. *American Journal of Occupational Therapy, 75,* 7502420010p1–7502420010p3. https://doi.org/10.5014/ajot.2021.752001

Anonymous. (2017). My experience with psychiatric services. *Schizophrenia Bulletin, 43*(3), 478–480. https://doi.org/10.1093/schbul/sbv145

Bipartisan Safer Communities Act. Pub. L. No. 117-159, 136 Stat. 1313 (2022). https://www.govinfo.gov/content/pkg/PLAW-117publ159/pdf/PLAW-117publ159.pdf

Bodeker, G., Pecorelli, S., Choy, L., Guerra, R., & Kariippanon, K. (2020, July). Well-being and mental wellness. *In Oxford Research Encyclopedia of Global Public Health.* Oxford University Press. https://doi.org/10.1093/acrefore/9780190632366.013.162

Boyle, P., Stew, G., Galvin, K. T., & Vuoskoski, P. (2021). Living with disability in a COVID-19 world. *British Journal of Occupational Therapy, 84*(10), 603–604. https://doi.org/10.1177/03080226211020993

Brown, C., Read, H., Stanton, M., Zeeb, M., Jonikas, J. A., & Cook, J. A. (2015). A pilot study of the Nutrition and Exercise for Wellness and Recovery (NEW-R): A weight loss program for individuals with serious mental illness. *Psychiatric Rehabilitation Journal, 38*(4), 371–373. https://doi.org/10.1037/prj0000115

Cano Prieto, I., Algado, S. S., & Vigué, G. P. (2022). Peer interventions in severe mental illnesses: A systematic review and its relation to occupational therapy. *Occupational Therapy in Mental Health, 39*(2), 99–136. https://doi.org/10.1080/0164212X.2022.2085645

Chamberlin, J. (1977). *On our own.* National Empowerment Center. https://power2u.org/store/on-our-own

Chan, R. C. H., Mak, W. W. S., Chio, F. H. N., & Tong, A. C. Y. (2018). Flourishing with psychosis: A prospective examination on the interactions between clinical, functional, and personal recovery processes on well-being among individuals with schizophrenia spectrum disorders. *Schizophrenia Bulletin, 44*(4), 778–786. https://doi.org/10.1093/schbul/sbx120

Clark, F. A., Blanchard, J., Sleight, A., Cogan, A., Florídez, L., Gleason, S., Heymann, R., Hill, V., Holden, A., Murphy, M., Proffitt, R., Niemiec, S. S., & Vigen, C. (2015). *Lifestyle redesign: The intervention tested in the USC well elderly studies* (2nd ed.). AOTA Press.

Costanzo, D., Davies, A., Garcia, K., Harvey, S., Pheiffer, B., & Umar, T. (2022). *A school-wide occupational therapy solution to the adolescent mental health crisis.* American Occupational Therapy Association. https://www.aota.org/publications/ot-practice/ot-practice-issues/2022/ot-solution-adolescent-mental-health

Csikszentmihalyi, M. (2000). *Beyond boredom and anxiety: Experiencing flow in work and play.* Jossey-Bass.

Davis, M., Yelton, S., Katz-Leavy, J., & Lourie, I. (1995). Unclaimed children revisited: The status of state children's mental health service systems. *Journal of Mental Health Administration, 22,* 147–166. https://doi.org/10.1007/bf02518755

Deegan, P. E. (1988). Recovery: The lived experience of rehabilitation. *Psychosocial Rehabilitation Journal, 11*(4), 11–19. https://doi.org/10.1037/h0099565

de Jager, A., Rhodes, P., Beavan, V., Holmes, D., McCabe, K., Thomas, N., McCarthy-Jones, S., Lampshire, D., & Hayward, M. (2016). Investigating the lived experience of recovery in people who hear voices. *Qualitative Health Research, 26,* 1409–1423. https://doi.org/10.1177/1049732315581602

Dennis, K. W., & Lourie, I. (2006). *Everything is normal until proven otherwise: A book about wraparound services.* Child Welfare League of America.

Doroud, N., Fossey, E., & Fortune, T. (2018). Place for being, doing, becoming and belonging: A meta-synthesis exploring the role of place in mental health recovery. *Health and Place, 52,* 110–120. https://doi.org/10.1016/j.healthplace.2018.05.008

Engels, C., Segaux, L., & Canoui-Poitrine, F. (2021). Occupational disruptions during lockdown, by generation: A European descriptive cross-sectional survey. *British Journal of Occupational Therapy, 85*(8), 603–616. https://doi.org/10.1177/03080226211057842

Every Moment Counts. (n.d.). *Home page.* https://everymoment-counts.org

Friis-Healy, E. A., Farber, E. W., Cook, S. C., Cullum, K. A., Gillespie, C. F., Marshall-Lee, E. D., Upshaw, N. C., White, D. T., Zhang, S., & Kaslow, N. J. (2022). Promoting resilience in persons with serious mental health conditions during the coronavirus pandemic. *Psychological Services, 19*(Suppl. 1), 13–22. https://doi.org/10.1037/ser0000594

Galderisi, S., Heinz, A., Kastrup, M., Beezhold, J., & Sartorius, N. (2015). Toward a new definition of mental health. *World Psychiatry, 14*(2), 231–233. https://doi.org/10.1002/wps.20231

Gewurtz, R. E., Moll, S. E., Letts, L. J., Larivière, N., Levasseur, M., & Krupa T. M. (2016). What you do every day matters: A new direction for health promotion. *Canadian Journal of Public Health, 107*(2), e205–e208. https://doi.org/10.17269/cjph.107.5317

Goldstein, J. (2016). *Voices of hope for mental illness: Not against, with.* CreateSpace Independent Publishing Platform.

Harms, P. D., Brady, L., Wood, D., & Silard, A. (2018). Resilience and well-being. In E. Diener, S. Oishi, & L. Tay (Eds.), *Handbook of well-being* (pp. 1–12). DEF Publishers.

Jepson, J. (2016). A vets recovery. *Schizophrenia Bulletin, 42*(1), 4. https://doi.org/10.1093/schbul/sbv115

Kelly, M., Lamont, S., & Brunero, S. (2010). An occupational perspective of the recovery journey in mental health. *British Journal of Occupational Therapy, 73*(3), 129–135. https://doi.org/10.4276/030802210X12682330090532

Keyes, C. L. M. (2002). The mental health continuum: From languishing to flourishing in life. *Journal of Health and Social Behavior, 43*(2), 207–222. https://doi.org/10.2307/3090197

Krupa, T., Edgelow, E., Chen, S-P., & Mieras, C. (2022). *Promoting activity and participation in individuals with serious mental illness: The Action Over Inertia approach.* Routledge. https://doi.org/10.4324/9781003111368

Lannigan, E. G., & Tyminski, Q. (2021). Occupational therapy's role in addressing the psychological and social impact of COVID-19. *American Journal of Occupational Therapy, 75*(Suppl. 1), 7511347030p1–7511347030p7. https://doi.org/10.5014/ajot.2021.049327

Métais, C., Burel, N., Gillham, J. E., Tarquinio, C., & Martin-Krumm, C. (2022). Integrative review of the recent literature on human resilience: From concepts, theories, and discussions towards a complex understanding. *Europe's Journal of Psychology, 18*(1), 98–119. https://doi.org/10.5964/ejop.2251

Patel, V., Saxena, S., Lund, C., Thornicroft, G., Baingana, F., Bolton, P., Chisholm, D., Collins, P. Y., Cooper, J. L., Eaton, J., Herrman, H., Herzallah, M. M., Huang, Y., Jordans, M. J. D., Kleinman, A., Medina-Mora, M. E., Morgan, E., Niaz, U., Omigbodun, O., . . . UnÜtzer, J. (2018). The Lancet Commission on global mental health and sustainable development. *Lancet, 392*(10157), 1553–1598. https://doi.org/10.1016/S0140-6736(18)31612-X

Patient Protection and Affordable Care Act. Pub. L. No. 111-148, 124 Stat. 119 (2010). https://www.congress.gov/111/plaws/publ148/PLAW-111publ148.pdf

Pereira, R. B., & Whiteford, G. E. (2022). Enabling inclusive occupational therapy through the Capabilities, Opportunities, Resources, and Environments (CORE) approach. In P. Liamputtong (Ed.), *Handbook of social inclusion* (pp. 1699–1716). Springer. https://link.springer.com/referencework/10.1007/978-3-030-89594-5

Protecting Access to Medicare Act, Pub. L. No. 113-93, 128 Stat. 1040 (2014). https://www.govinfo.gov/content/pkg/PLAW-113publ93/pdf/PLAW-113publ93.pdf

Rees, E. F., Ennals, P., & Fossey, E. (2021). Implementing an Action Over Inertia group program in community residential rehabilitation services: Group participant and facilitator perspectives. *Frontiers in Psychiatry, 12,* 624803. https://doi.org/10.3389/fpsyt.2021.624803

Slade, M. (2010). Mental illness and well-being: The central importance of positive psychology and recovery approaches. *BMC Health Services Research, 10,* 26. https://doi.org/10.1186/1472-6963-10-26

Stoffel, V. C. (2007). Perception of the clubhouse experience and its impact on mental health recovery. *Dissertation Abstracts International Section A: Humanities and Social Sciences, 68* (8~A), 3300.

Stoffel, V. C. (2013). Opportunities for occupational therapy behavioral health: A call to action. *American Journal of Occupational Therapy, 67*(2), 140–145. https://doi.org/10.5014/ajot.2013.672001

Strong, S., & Letts, L. (2021). Personal narratives of learning self-management: Lessons for practice based on experiences of people with serious mental illness. *Australian Occupational Therapy Journal, 68,* 395–406. https://doi.org/10.1111/1440-1630.12748

Stroul, B., Blau, G., & Friedman, R. (2010). *Updating the system of care concept and philosophy.* Georgetown University Center for Child and Human Development, National Technical Assistance Center for Children's Mental Health.

Substance Abuse and Mental Health Services Administration. (2012). *SAMHSA's working definition of recovery.* Author. https://store.samhsa.gov/sites/default/files/pep12-recdef.pdf

Substance Abuse and Mental Health Services Administration. (2016). *Promoting wellness: A guide to community action.* https://store.samhsa.gov/sites/default/files/d7/priv/sma16-4957.pdf

Substance Abuse and Mental Health Services Administration. (2022, October 18). *Biden-Harris administration announces millions of dollars in new funds for states to tackle mental health crisis.* Author. https://www.samhsa.gov/newsroom/press-announcements/20221018/biden-harris-administration-announces-funding-states-tackle-mental-health-crisis

Substance Abuse and Mental Health Services Administration. (2023). *Certified Community Behavioral Health Clinics (CCBHCs).* https://www.samhsa.gov/certified-community-behavioral-health-clinics

Sutton, D. J., Hocking, C. S., & Smythe, L. A. (2012). A phenomenological study of occupational engagement in recovery from mental illness. *Canadian Journal of Occupational Therapy, 79,* 142–150. https://doi.org/10.2182/cjot.2012.79.3.3

Swarbrick, M. (2011). Consumer-operated services. In C. Brown, V. Stoffel, & J. Munoz (Eds.), *Occupational therapy in mental health: A vision for participation* (pp. 503–515). F. A. Davis.

Swarbrick, M. (2012). A wellness approach to mental health recovery. In A. Rudnick (Ed.), *Recovery of people with mental illness: Philosophical and related perspectives* (pp. 30–39). Oxford University Press.

Synovec, C. E. (2015). Implementing Recovery Model principles as part of occupational therapy in inpatient psychiatric settings. *Occupational Therapy in Mental Health, 31*(1), 50–61. https://doi.org/10.1080/0164212X.2014.1001014

Tyminski, Q., Bates, M., & Fette, C. (2019). Building community capacity for mental health program development in underserved populations. *SIS Quarterly Practice Connections, 4*(1), 20–22. https://www.aota.org/publications/sis-quarterly/mental-health-sis/mhsis-2-19

U.S. Department of Health and Human Services. (n.d.). *About the Affordable Care Act.* https://www.hhs.gov/healthcare/about-the-aca/index.html

Wastberg, B. A., Sandstrom, B., & Pooremamali, P. (2019). A turning point towards recovery: An interview study with participants in the culture and health programme for clients with long-term mental health disorders in Sweden. *Issues in Mental Health Nursing, 40*(5), 373–381. https://doi.org/10.1080/01612840.2018.1553002

Waters, L., Algoe, S. B., Dutton, J., Emmons, R., Fredrickson, B. L., Heaphy, E., Moskowitz, J. T., Neff, K., Niemiec, R., Pury, C., & Steger, M. (2022). Positive psychology in a pandemic: Buffering, bolstering, and building mental health. *Journal of Positive Psychology, 17*(3), 303–323. https://doi.org/10.1080/17439760.2021.1871945

Watters, K., Marks, T. S., Edwards, D. F., Skidmore, E. R., & Giles, G. M. (2021). The Issue Is—A framework for addressing clients' functional cognitive deficits after COVID-19. *American Journal of Occupational Therapy, 75*(Suppl. 1), 7511347010p1–7511347010p7. https://doi.org/10.5014/ajot.2021.049308

Wells, C. (2010). *Straight talk: Families speak to families about child and youth mental health.* Axis Group Publishing.

Westerhof, G. J., & Keyes, C. L. M. (2010). Mental illness and mental health: The two continua model across the lifespan. *Journal of Adult Development, 17,* 110–119. https://doi.org/10.1007/s10804-009-9082-y

Wilson, W. G. (1939). *Alcoholics Anonymous: The story of how more than one hundred men have recovered from alcoholism.* Alcoholics Anonymous World Services.

World Health Organization. (2001). *The world health report 2001: Mental health: New understanding, new hope.* Author.

World Health Organization. (2006). *Constitution of the World Health Organization* (45th ed.). https://www.who.int/publications/m/item/constitution-of-the-world-health-organization

World Health Organization. (2022). *World mental health report: Transforming mental health for all (executive summary).* Author. https://www.who.int/publications/i/item/9789240049338

CHAPTER

3

Person-Environment-Occupation Model

Susan Strong and Karen Rebeiro Gruhl

When occupational therapy practitioners (OTPs) and occupational therapy students consider how they can best support people's participation in occupation, the **Person-Environment-Occupation (PEO) model** provides a good starting place. The PEO model is a conceptual framework developed by a group of Canadian occupational therapy clinicians and researchers to provide a systematic way to think about and understand the complex occupational participation issues individuals experience within the context of contemporary occupational therapy practice (Law et al., 1996). The PEO model is the organizing framework for this textbook. This chapter provides an overview of the PEO model as well as a few examples illustrating how the PEO model remains relevant in occupational therapy practice more than 25 years later.

The profession's understanding of the complexity of occupation and occupational therapy practices continues to evolve both locally and globally. OTPs are increasingly expanding their practices within contexts not previously considered with individuals, groups, and organizations. Occupational therapy practices have transitioned beyond solely operating within a rehabilitation framework with people with physical disabilities or mental illnesses, and have moved into primary care, health promotion, and population-based health. Also, OTPs recognize that occupation is context-specific, and that there is a necessity for collaborative practices with a variety of partners to extend the reach and influence of occupational therapy practice (see Rebeiro Gruhl & Lauckner, 2022; Rebeiro Gruhl et al., 2012).

The PEO Model and the Diversity of People and Life

This chapter considers how OTPs might push beyond traditional practices using the PEO model to better address the diversity of individuals, occupations, and environments that reflect today's world. To do so will require OTPs to reflect on how culture, gender identity, race, sexual orientation, differing levels of ability, and varying life circumstances or living conditions impact the **occupational participation** of those seeking occupational therapy services. **Life circumstances** are often referred to in the literature as the sociopolitical determinants of health (Centers for Disease Control and Prevention [CDC], n.d.; Raphael et al., 2019). Life circumstances are important to understand as they can individually and collectively impact the opportunities available for occupational

participation as well as the resources that may be required to do so. The diversity of people who would benefit from OTPs' knowledge of occupation requires occupational therapy to be a profession that not only reflects such diversity but also seeks to understand experiences of varying living conditions and how these impact people's occupational participation. It also requires occupational therapy's theoretical frameworks to be flexible and sufficiently nuanced for the consideration of diversity. The PEO model provides the theoretical and practical nimbleness needed to incorporate diversity and life circumstances within occupational therapy assessment and intervention considerations.

To this end, this chapter systematically considers each aspect of the PEO model to ensure learners develop a strong grounding in occupation-based practices that promote an individual's fullest participation in their everyday lives and within their living environments. OTPs apply therapeutic reasoning skills to help them figure out what is interfering with an individual's occupational participation. For example, there are many reasons why a child might experience difficulty completing homework, so it is important that OTPs do not automatically assume this is a reflection of the person. The child may have attention problems that interfere with focusing on their homework. But OTPs must unpack this further. What might be getting in the way of the child's attention? There may be barriers related to the child's cognitive abilities, which would imply an issue at the level of the person—but keep in mind that this may not be an actual cognitive impairment. Instead, it might reflect inadequate nutrition or uncontrolled diabetes impacting the child's ability to concentrate (again, an issue with the person, but often modifiable).

In addition, there could be family issues or tensions that make doing homework at home difficult, or it might reflect multiple stimuli, such as excessive noise or light or environmental triggers to past trauma experiences. The child may live in poverty and their time is spent on contributing to individual and family survival over homework completion. Learners can appreciate that some environmental issues are more easily rectified than others. And lastly, the occupation itself may present the barrier: The homework may be too difficult or too easy or culturally inappropriate, or the child may not find it interesting or meaningful or engaging. In this scenario, the person, the environment, and the occupation are all likely culprits, and each needs to be considered to remove, mitigate, or manage barriers to the child's full occupational participation with respect to each occupational participation issue.

OTPs focus on individuals' successful participation in occupations of everyday life to support the individuals' development, health, and well-being (Law, 2002). Although success is uniquely defined by the person, the elements that contribute to that success can be understood by the interplay of person, environment, and occupation factors. This interplay is important for OTPs and students to consider and requires an appreciation of some of the theoretical principles that underscore the PEO model:

- Occupation is contextually situated and culturally linked.
- Environments can press or have supporting or constraining effects on occupational participation.
- People are not "one size fits all," but instead are diverse beings having different beliefs, meanings, and cultural connotations about occupation and life experiences.

There are several broad theoretical frameworks in occupational therapy that also consider relationships among the person, environment, occupation, and occupational participation, such as the Person-Environment-Occupation Performance model (Christiansen et al., 2005), the Ecology of Human Performance (Dunn et al., 2003), the Model of Human Occupation (Kielhofner, 2008), and the Canadian Model of Occupational Participation (CanMOP; Egan & Restall, 2022). Although each framework provides a slightly different perspective on these constructs, they all aim to promote the individuals' participation in occupation! The PEO model is parsimonious, appearing on the surface to be simple. Although the dynamic relationships and constructs are complex and multilayered, the central constructs of person, environment, and occupation offer a straightforward system for organizing the material in this text.

Development of the PEO Model

In the 1990s, six Canadian OTPs came together to develop the PEO model in an effort to more comprehensively describe and understand the dynamic complex relationships that impact occupational participation (Law et al., 1996). The PEO model was built on the work of environmental–behavioral theorists who explored the relationships between people and their environments.

Lewin (1933) and Murray (1938), for instance, wrote about the concept of **environmental press**, in which forces in the environment, together with individual needs, evoke variable responses. The environmental press of climate change, for example, may encourage, or press, individuals to alter their behavior or habits, such as the hours they work outdoors, use of public transportation, participation in recycling, or purchasing goods from companies with ethical environmental practices.

The concept of **adaptation** was identified by Lewin (1933) and Murray (1938) as the achievement of a good fit between a person and their environment. In the language of the time, Baker and Intagliata (1982) looked at an individual's perception of their environment and speculated that people actively engage in efforts to achieve a level of comfort or fit between themselves and how they individually viewed their environment. The authors highlighted how individuals bring their past experiences into present situations to foster adaptation.

Lawton's (1986) *Model of Competency* described adaptive and maladaptive behaviors that occurred as the result of environmental press and an individual's competence or ability to meet the demands of that press. Lawton conceptualized **maladaptive behavior** as resulting from someone with too low skills being met with too high challenges or, conversely, someone with too high skills being met with weak or limited challenges. Today, OTPs view **competence** as only one aspect of an individual's personal resources mediated by occupational opportunities and supportive living environments. Further, actions considered to be maladaptive behavior can have survival value as an adaptive response to certain situations.

In general, theories by environmental–behavioral theorists were primarily developed within an interactive framework that simplified the realities of human behavior to cause-and-effect relationships. Also, they did little to inform therapists about occupation, which is the core domain of occupational therapy. What was needed was a transactive model that supported the diversity of therapists' observations of people as occupational beings and reflected how OTPs viewed the world.

In a **transactive model**, relationships are multidirectional and mutually influential across multiple intersections—a change in the occupation can influence change in the person and environment, and iteratively each element can influence each other. The environment can influence the person and vice versa; in the process, the interaction creates both opportunities for and challenges to occupational participation. For example, a parent (person) who is preparing a meal (occupation) for the family creates changes in the food preparation or eating environment, which influence the parent and family perceptions and create a social context for eating together. The reaction of the family then impacts the food preparer. If the family likes the meal and compliments the cook, the parent will feel affirmed and appreciated, and is likely to repeat the experience. However, if a family member complains about the food or misses dinner to attend an event with friends, a different social context is created that affects the parent who prepared the meal and, potentially, subsequent meals together. The experience is laden with personal meaning for everyone involved, and any one change in the person, environment, or occupation of the situation can result in a much different experience and outcome.

The *Theory of Optimal Experience* by psychologists Csikszentmihalyi and Csikszentmihalyi (1988) offers a perspective of people engaging in occupations. In this theory, adaptation is viewed as the congruence between challenges present within an activity and the environment and a person's skills. They coined the term "flow" to describe the experience of losing oneself in an inherently satisfying activity; this can occur when an individual is engaged in an activity in a given environment with the **"just right" challenge** (i.e., when the perceived challenge matches the individual level of skill for that particular activity in that given environment). Rebeiro and Miller-Polgar (1999) considered the relevance of flow theory to occupational engagement and participation. During therapy, therapists create situations of graduated "just right" challenges to encourage engagement, persistence (when faced with new challenges amid accomplishments), and successes.

Theorists who considered influences beyond the individual's immediate environment were also important to the development of the PEO model—reflecting occupational therapy's expanding practice into a variety of roles and settings, and including groups, organizations, communities, and government. Bronfenbrenner's *Ecological Systems model* (1977) provided a useful framework for considering the interdependence of people and **"nested" social systems:** the individual's **microsystem** in the center, surrounded by a **mesosystem** of families and work or school, which is surrounded by an **exosystem** of formal and informal social structures, which in turn is enveloped by a **macrosystem** of institutions in society (e.g., government).

The *Healthy Communities Conceptual Model* (Trainor et al., 1983) considered not only the influence of community, but also that of culture and social policy on the health of an individual. This model conceptually expanded what was considered to be important in the environment and introduced the notion of changing environments rather than changing people to fit the environments.

Evolving Occupational Therapy Lens

The development of the PEO model was influenced by all of these aforementioned ideas and continues to evolve in response to the following contextual changes in larger society, as well as emerging voices within occupational therapy practice and health-care delivery in Canada:

■ Shift in health care to a focus on health promotion and wellness
■ Increased understanding of disabling environments and their impact on occupational participation (Fougeyrollas et al., 1998; Jongbloed & Crighton, 1990)
■ Advanced notions about the importance of social issues as the root cause of disability versus a professional focus on personal problems (Borsay, 1986)
■ A growing consumer movement supported by legislation such as the Americans with Disabilities Act (1990)
■ Consideration of ethical practice within a PEO perspective (Brockett & Dick, 2006)
■ Publication of *Promoting Occupational Participation: Collaborative, Relationship-Focused Occupational Therapy* (Egan & Restall, 2022), which adopted a social model of disability that emphasized contextually situated personal meanings and agency within the context of people's development and history, and therapists' obligations to embed justice, equity, and rights into routine practice
■ Awareness of systemic oppression and colonization in the Truth and Reconciliation Commission of Canada (2017) and the Missing and Murdered Indigenous Women and Girls (Government of Canada, 2019) final reports
■ Understanding how the COVID pandemic and climate crisis have negative impacts on health and well-being, particularly for socioeconomically disadvantaged communities (World Federation of Occupational Therapists [WFOT], 2023)
■ A recognition and appreciation of disability activists' perspectives, such as Lydia X. Z. Brown (n.d.), regarding how disability rights are impacted by a person's **intersecting identities,** and the need for health professionals to consider how race, gender, language, heterosexism, culture, poverty, employment and housing status, ableism, and paternalism impact a person's disability experience and human rights, including access to meaningful occupational opportunities and ongoing participation

All the previously listed ideas, research, and experiences have assisted OTPs to better understand how their practices can support or limit an individual's participation in occupation within their environment. Across various practice settings, OTPs are located within positions of privilege and power that can be leveraged to help, or alternately further contribute to, the systemic inequities and disadvantages that limit individual participation (Whalley Hammell, 2015). From the perspective of **intersectionality,** the OTP addresses systemic oppression and inequities in occupational opportunities while supporting the individual or collective to use participation in occupation to (re)establish their own narratives and create their own life paths with acceptance of their authentic selves. Using an **intersectional lens** of transactive person, environment, and occupation relationships brings into focus all forms of oppression including ableism, ageism, racism, and colonialism.

According to Whalley Hammell (2017), all humans have a right to occupational participation because it contributes to their well-being, which is a human right. Whalley Hammell (2003, 2009) has previously asserted that occupational therapy practice must expand its focus beyond individual impairment to include social, legal, economic, and political environments and to more seriously consider those aspects of the environment identified by persons with disabilities that limit their participation in occupations. Therapists are challenged to redress stigma and the resulting inequities that undermine an individual's recovery and their full social participation (Arboleda-Florez & Stuart, 2012). In routine practice, this requires OTPs to broadly consider the lived experiences of participation as an untapped wealth of information on navigating occupation within different contexts.

Further explanation of the PEO model's early development is found in other research (Law et al., 1996). At this time, occupational therapy was redefining itself within a changing global community and within new understandings of health. Yet, the PEO model remains relevant for guiding, explaining, and defining occupational therapy practice.

Description of the PEO Model

The PEO model describes the transactive, dynamic relationships that occur when people participate in occupations within given environments over time. Environments, occupations, and people have both supporting and constraining effects on one another; they shape each other, change over time, and people ascribe meanings in the process. Change within one part affects the other parts on many levels. Students can consider the transactive relationship involved in working on group projects for school. Diversity in the individuals who make up the group, along with the particular assignment (e.g., familiarity, time frame) and elements of the learning environment (e.g., sense of competition, lighting), can create different supporting and constraining effects. The experience will affect each student's performance differently, and each student's experience will be unique. Furthermore, the transaction across multiple planes or spheres of existence creates a whole that is greater than any of the individual parts. This does not necessarily mean that it is a positive experience, but rather one that is dynamic and complex. The person's experiences over their life span shape performance and vice versa, ascribing ever-changing uniquely personal meanings. The PEO model supports the OTP to conceptualize, analyze, and communicate these dynamic, transactive relationships.

The definitions of the model's main components—person, environment, and occupation—follow in the next section. These constructs reflect the new CanMOP practice guideline, outlined in the publication *Promoting Occupational Participation: Collaborative Relationships-Focused Occupational Therapy* (Egan & Restall, 2022). "Occupational participation" is used throughout this chapter instead of "occupational performance" to reflect the evolving understandings in Canada and within the international occupational therapy community.

Person

The person is a composite of mind, body, and spirit (Law et al., 1996). The person's performance components refer to what the person is feeling (affective), thinking (cognitive), and doing (physical) with regard to what can "contribute to successful engagement in occupation" (Canadian Association of Occupational Therapists [CAOT], 1997, p. 43). More recently, the person refers to the individual or a collective of people receiving occupational therapy services, and the focus is on what can contribute to their successful participation in occupations (Egan & Restall, 2022).

Spirituality is considered to be at the core of all PEO interactions. "Spirituality resides in the person, is shaped by the environment, and gives meaning to occupations" (CAOT, 1997, p. 33). A person's spirituality is imbued with their individual beliefs, values, and goals, all of which guide choices and provide a source of self-determination and personal control. In client-centered (or person-centered) practice, the "client" can be an individual person, a group of individuals, or an organization. The American Occupational Therapy Association (AOTA; 2014) defines "clients" as persons, groups, and populations.

In addition, the personal impact of mental illnesses is presented in Part 2: The Person in Section 1: Occupational Performance and Section 2: Selected Conditions, including assessments and interventions to optimize occupational participation.

Environment

Previously the environment was defined as "the context within which occupational participation takes place" (CAOT, 1997, p. 44). The environment shapes the person's occupational experience and influences the opportunities (or lack of) for occupation. The environment encompasses not only the immediate physical location where an occupation is being performed, but includes local social situations, such as families and neighborhoods. It also includes broader, less tangible influences involving community, provincial or state, and national and international organizations, which are responsible for the allocation of resources and services such as health

TABLE 3-1 | Elements of the Environment

Categories	Aspects
Cultural (shared meanings, expectations, and implicit rules)	• Beliefs • Customs • Traditions • Language
Institutional (organized systems' structures including policies and procedures, resource allocation, and funding structures)	• Legislative bodies • Health-care systems • Social service organizations • Educational institutions • Employment organizations
Social (interpersonal relationships; emotional, instrumental, and structural supports; social inclusion, belonging; stigma, ableism, ageism, racism, colonialism, and other forms of discrimination)	• Friends • Family • Larger social networks
Physical (things that can be seen, touched, and smelled)	• Natural environment • Human-built environment • Physical location (urban or rural)

insurance, transportation systems, and industry or employment opportunities. Elements of the environment have been classified as cultural, institutional, social, and physical.

Table 3-1 outlines aspects of each of these categories. It is important to keep in mind that while classifications such as these can be helpful in breaking down and understanding the inherent complexities of the environment, classifications can also artificially simplify life worlds in the process.

The cultural environment of shared and personally distinct meanings offers implicit expectations and rules that guide occupational behavior. Cultural expectations and rules can support or create barriers to occupational participation through social, political, gendered, and other contextual understandings. It is therefore important for the OTPs to identify the person's own cultural preferences and priorities as well as seek to understand their ascribed meanings. One way to achieve this is to engage in critical reflexivity and coassessments with people and collaboratively codesign and coevaluate interventions (Egan & Restall, 2022).

Therapists consider the structures of institutional environments (e.g., policies and procedures, resource allocation, and funding structures) that express the system's social and political priorities. Institutional structures have wide-ranging impacts on occupational participation through their influence on daily living conditions. Institutional structures systemically support or limit the sociopolitical determinants of health (poverty, inequitable access to health care, lack of education, stigma, and racism). These systemic structures can support or limit an individual's occupational participation. Using an intersectional lens, OTPs can better understand the complexity of these determinants of health and transactional relationships (Hankivsky & Christoffersen, 2008).

The social environment is considered with respect to the capacity to provide emotional (acceptance of authentic self, sense of belonging), instrumental (information, money, food), and structural (reminders, consistency) support. Key elements of a supportive social environment for individuals living with mental illnesses are features that promote social inclusion and a sense of belonging, and counter barriers such as stigmatizing attitudes and discriminatory actions (Rebeiro et al., 2001).

From an OTP's perspective, the physical environment encompasses more than a space filled with natural and human-built materials; rather, it is an environment that is experienced by an individual's senses and interpreted by an individual within the context of their life story and occupational needs. This may include a child living in low-income housing that affords few opportunities for play, or perhaps a senior living in a rural community with few transportation options and, consequently, few opportunities for socialization.

Within the new CanMOP guideline (Egan & Restall, 2022), the environment includes all of the previously mentioned items and considers the environment in terms of nested social systems. As an organizational framework, the OTP is asked to consider relationships within and between the micro (the individual), meso (the group, family, or organization), and macro (the community, societal, or population) levels of environment. The OTP seeks understanding about the context using equity, justice, and rights-based lenses.

Specific aspects of the environment are presented in Part 3: The Environment. The chapters in Section 1: Societal Influences present information on the effect of social environments on occupational participation, whereas Section 2: Places focuses more on the physical environment. Both Sections 1 and 2 include assessments of the environment and interventions aimed at changing the environment or making the best fit to promote occupational participation. The Section 3: Mental Health Practice Settings chapters describe the practice environments in which OTPs work.

Occupation

Occupations have been defined as "clusters of activities and tasks in which people engage while carrying out various roles in multiple" locations and contexts (Strong et al., 1999, p. 125), and as everyday activities that encompass what people need to do and want to do. Historically, OTPs used three classifications of purpose, which were culturally defined: self-care, productivity, and leisure (CAOT, 1997). However, these classifications have been scrutinized as reflecting Caucasian, middle-class, heterosexual, ableist, and Global North assumptions (Laliberte Rudman et al., 2022; Whalley Hammell, 2009). The emphasis has shifted "from categorizing what people do [selfcare, productivity, leisure], based on Global North perspectives, to emphasizing the unique meanings and purposes attributed to the things people need and want to do" (Egan & Restall, 2022, p. 93). OTPs now recognize that occupations are best defined by the particular individual or group involved, that predetermined categories are not particularly useful to their work, and that continuing to use these categories risks excluding important occupations that do not fit these classifications.

Occupations place affective, cognitive, and physical demands on the individual performing the occupation. Examples of an occupation's affective demands include the need for self-regulation (motivation, composure, persistence) when faced with challenges, immediacy of response or feedback, and the delay of gratification or seeing the end result. Cognitive occupational demands involve attention, information processing, conceptualization, planning, organization, reasoning, judgment, and problem-solving. Physical occupational demands include sensory requirements, physical movement, weight, repetition, pace, environmental distractions, and discomfort (noise, temperature). Therapists during return-to-work planning will consult the U.S. Department of Labor's O*Net (https://www.onetonline.org), previously the Dictionary of Occupational Titles, which breaks down job classification by duties and demands. With respect to the affective, cognitive, and physical demands, the OTP considers the occupations' characteristics, duration, structure or patterns of flow, and complexity.

Contemporary guidelines encourage the consideration of occupation as political, as a means for social change or as a way of perpetuating the status quo (e.g., colonization; Egan & Restall, 2022). This view appears compatible with the PEO model depicting occupation within dynamic transactional PEO relationships.

Occupation as a component of the PEO model is further described in Part 4: Occupation. These chapters provide assessments and interventions aimed at improving occupational participation for people dealing with psychosocial concerns. 🤝

Occupational Participation

OTP's understanding of **occupational participation** has changed to reflect new insights about the purpose and focus of occupational therapy—that is, that occupational participation has become the primary focus of occupational therapy. Occupational participation is defined as "having access to, initiating, and sustaining valued occupations within meaningful relationships and contexts" (Eagan & Restall, 2022, p. 76). In the past, focusing predominantly on occupational performance excluded some people's priorities and life circumstances and reinforced the individual being solely responsible for outcomes. The profession has moved toward inclusion and increasing access to occupational opportunities. Therefore, practice goes beyond engagement and performance; successful occupational participation aligns with the individual's or collective's own values, interests, needs, goals, and their situational life conditions (Egan & Restall, 2022).

The new terminology of "occupational participation" is compatible with the PEO model's use of the term "occupational performance." Note, in the PEO model, occupational performance does not reside within the individual; rather, it is the product of person, environment, and occupation relationships. Therefore, substituting the new terminology of occupational participation reflects the product of the dynamic relationships between persons (groups or communities), their environments, and the occupations they wish or need to participate in across the life span. Occupational participation refers to the ability to choose, access, organize, and participate in meaningful and culturally defined occupations to the person's satisfaction within given environments and daily life conditions. Occupational participation may support looking after oneself or someone else, enjoying or sustaining life, or connecting to or contributing to one's family or the larger community.

The transactive relationships among person, environment, and occupation are mutually interdependent, with the result being greater than the sum of these individual elements. The product of these relationships is the quality of a person's experience with regard to being able to satisfactorily participate in meaningful occupations (i.e., occupational participation) as defined by the individuals involved.

Person-Environment-Occupation Fit

In Figure 3-1, the person, environment, and occupation components are represented by three interrelated three-dimensional spheres (shown as Venn diagrams) that move with respect to one another to illustrate the components that dynamically transact over a person's life span. The congruence, or fit, among these components is illustrated by the extent of the overlap of the person, environment, and occupation spheres. The overlap in the center of the spheres represents both the behavior of occupational participation and the dynamic experience of a person engaged in an occupation within an environment over time. The concept of PEO fit describes the elements that support or constrain the individual's or collective's occupational participation.

To illustrate the continuity of these elements transacting throughout life, the three-dimensional components extend into a cylindrical form that reflects the temporal and spatial dimensions of the transactions. Theoretically, the dynamic interactions and forces at play can be examined for a slice in time by making a cross section of the cylinder. The slice allows an analysis of the P × O, O × E, and P × E relationships by examining the fit between each set of components within the context-specific meanings ascribed at that particular point

of time and space. Therefore, discrete moments in an individual's or collective's life can be captured by a series of cross sections at different points in time; each will have a different composition of PEO interplay and a different expression of occupational participation as the person proceeds through time and space. Figure 3-1 includes three cross sections, each with different expressions of occupational participation depicted by different combinations of overlapping spheres.

For example, at one point in time a student may experience satisfaction with their schoolwork; successful participation demonstrates a fit among their abilities, interests, values, goals, and schoolwork's demands (P × O); a fit between the schoolwork's requirements and the school environment's expectations (O × E); and a fit between the student's needs and support given in their micro, meso, and macro levels of environment (P × E). This is illustrated in the first cross section in Figure 3-1. However, at another point in time the same student may have a negative experience and be unable to perform when presented with a new assignment or task that invokes anxiety and expectations of failure (P × O). At that time, the student's environmental supports and resources are not engaged or not helpful for this particular assignment (P × E). The result is poor occupational participation (both experience and behavioral), which is illustrated by limited overlap in the spheres (the second cross section).

At a later point in time, the student asked for help, and useful environmental supports and resources are engaged (P × E). The assignment's instructions are clarified, there is flexibility in the assignment being presented orally or in written form, and the time requirements are altered (P × O). Also, the different manner in which the assignment is to be completed is viewed as acceptable by the school and meets the education system's requirements (O × E). At this point,

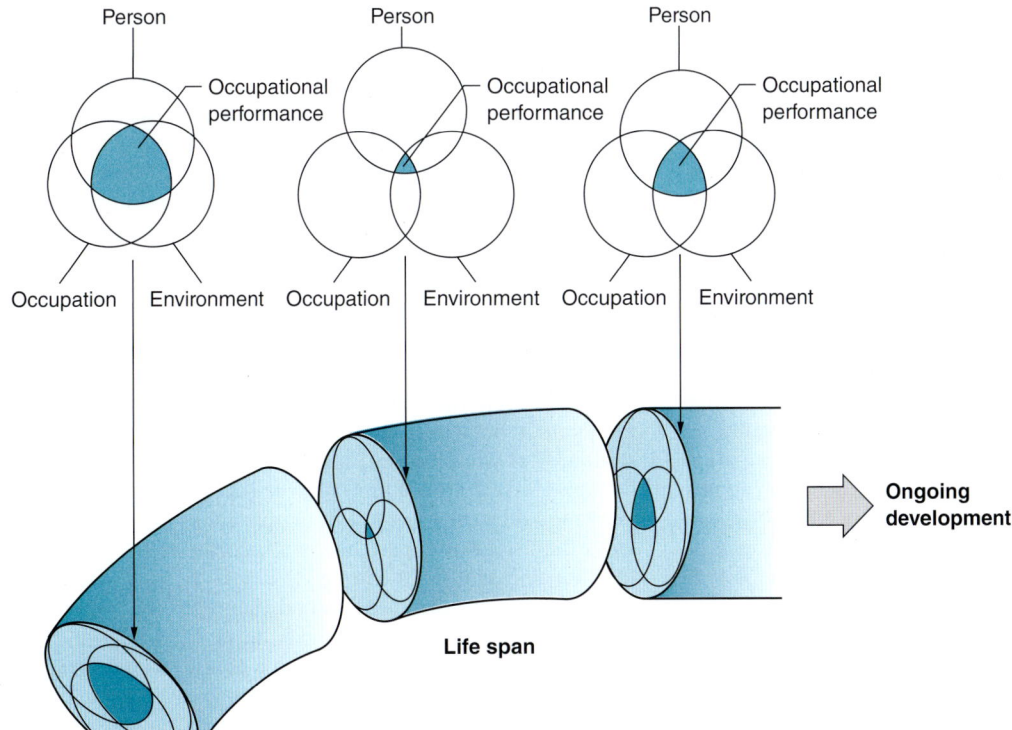

FIGURE 3-1. Depiction of the Person-Environment-Occupation (PEO) model across the life span. The PEO components are represented by three interrelated spheres (Venn diagrams) that illustrate hypothetical changes in occupational participation at three different points in time. *Adapted with permission from Law, M., Cooper, B., Strong, S., Stewart, D., Rigby, P., & Letts, L. (1996). The Person-Environment-Occupation model: A transactive approach to occupational performance. Canadian Journal of Occupational Therapy, 63(1), 9–23. https://doi.org/10.1177/000841749606300103*

PhotoVoice

Hi, my name is John. I have been living with HIV for 9 years. At first, I did not want to live with this diagnosis, so I attempted suicide. Thank God I was not successful! Since then, I have been working on my road to recovery over physical and mental challenges. One group at CHEEERS is "Let's Dish." We cook meals for our fellow participants. It really helps me overcome isolation and it lowers my anxiety! I love to volunteer at CHEEERS and help others that are struggling with their own challenges. I am learning to love my life and the people in it!

What activities do you participate in that help you to overcome isolation and lower anxiety? What aspects of your micro (individual), meso (group, family, organization), and macro (community, society, population) levels of environment support or constrain your participation? What is the transactional relationship among you and those activities? What meanings do these activities hold for you?

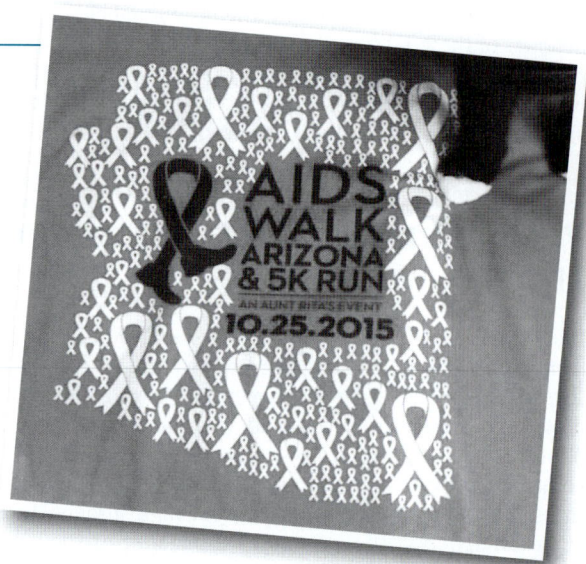

occupational participation is improved, which is illustrated by increased overlap in the spheres (third cross section).

As occupational human beings, people participate in occupations by developing relationships with occupations and environments that are expressed by personal habits, routines, and behaviors. Participation in occupations is experienced sensually, embodied within people's perceptions and their sense of occupational identities, and ascribed meanings as people move through time and space. These relationships are the focus of therapy. In sum, occupational therapy is about improving access to occupational participation for individuals and groups by increasing their PEO fit.

Dimension of Time

The PEO model reflects how individuals grow and change over the course of their lives. For example, when a young adult leaves home, they assume new roles and responsibilities by engaging in additional occupations within new environments, thus expanding the number of layers and dimensions of PEO spheres that transact. There may be added time pressures with fewer environmental supports (i.e., reduced fit between occupation and environment) and, initially, they may have inadequate skills or personal resources to satisfactorily cook meals (i.e., reduced fit between person and occupation). With experience at cooking, as confidence increases and time becomes better managed, there is greater PEO overlap, or congruence, and the experience of occupational participation improves, which is depicted by the enlarged center overlap.

During a person's life span, their roles, occupations, and the meanings ascribed change. For example, as a person ages, being a member of a faith community may have very different meanings: as an adolescent in a youth group trying to find their place in the world, as an isolated parent focused on raising a young child, or as an older adult facing retirement or end-of-life issues. Occupations or roles may be discontinued, which reduces the number of occupation spheres and opportunities for occupational participation. Alternatively, occupations may be restored, depicted by the PEO model as

increases in the number and dimensions within occupation spheres and the corresponding environments.

Time is also an experienced dimension. That is, individuals experience the present while remembering the past and holding ideas of their future. This ability to experience time in three dimensions shapes individuals' perceptions of themselves (e.g., beliefs of what they can and cannot do well), the choices they make, and their evaluation of their own occupational participation. Collectives also have histories together that include the plans, activities undertaken, events experienced, and the ascribed meanings of those joint experiences. Accordingly, it is important for therapists to obtain information about an individual's or collective's occupational history, any changes over time, and perceived impacts on self, occupations, and environments.

Dimension of Space

Space is a further dimension that is experienced by location. Space has an emotional element and attributed meanings. Location refers to the physical aspect of space. People can engage in an occupation in multiple locations. For example, the space in which students choose to study can vary widely. Within the PEO model, this is represented by multiple layers of the environment sphere transacting with the occupation and person spheres (Fig. 3-2). When engaged in occupations, each person has a personally defined use of space and unique standards of what physical space is required to engage comfortably; the extent of fit or congruence can be shown in the PEO model by the extent of PEO overlap. From one point of view, the use of or experience of space can be restrained by functional limitations attributed to illness or aging when only the person component is examined. Alternatively, constraints in space can be considered by examining PEO relationships attributing constraints to inequitable access to environmental resources or occupational opportunities. The second perspective is consistent with disabling environments, whereas the first perspective is aligned with disease-based views. For example, an individual's participation at a location, such as

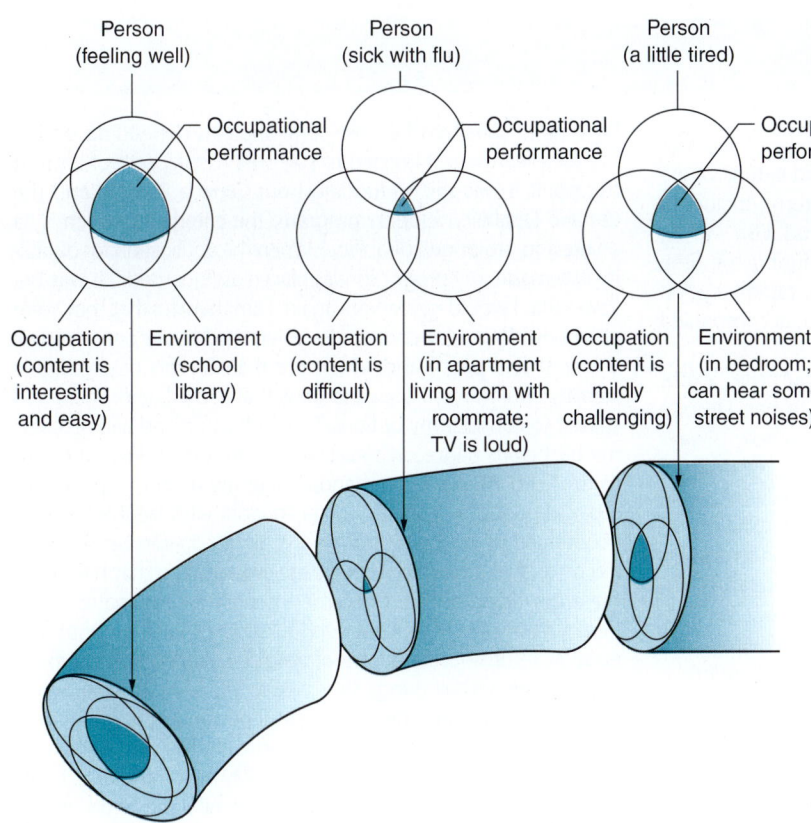

FIGURE 3-2. The Person-Environment-Occupation model in three different situations across time for a person studying (occupation) who prefers a quiet space (environment). *Adapted with permission from Law, M., Cooper, B., Strong, S., Stewart, D., Rigby, P., & Letts, L. (1996). The Person-Environment-Occupation model: A transactive approach to occupational performance. Canadian Journal of Occupational Therapy, 63(1), 9–23. https://doi.org/10.1177/000841749606300103*

an outpatient clinic, can be expanded by creating inviting, supported spaces for their engagement, voice, and collaboration in the care process (e.g., participation in orientations, questionnaires, joint agenda setting worksheets) and the clinic's program development (e.g., user focus groups, user representation on quality improvement committees, monetary payment, transportation support).

Space has emotional connections. Emotional spaces are socially constructed and given meanings by the OTPs and others. For example, OTPs create an accepting, safe space and directly address the power differential in meetings with individuals to support open dialogue and collaborative planning. Depending on the way these sessions are experienced and interpreted, the individual or OTP may or may not label the sessions as person-centered. O'Brien and colleagues (2002) wrote about how the meanings of places and spaces are related to the supporting and constraining features of the environment and whether a person is labeled or inscribed by others as being different. A person's inscription with a diagnosis (e.g., mental illness) and their own ascription of what that diagnosis means mediate a person's use of space. The stigma of mental illness can impact one's use of space, for example, by limiting the opportunities available to them (e.g., preventing an individual from obtaining or even interviewing for a particular job). The same individual may be reluctant to interact with new people because of internalized stigma or, after meeting someone new, may be socially rejected once a diagnosis of mental illness is revealed.

Stigma can also be influenced by one's geography or physical location. Parr (2008) examined the relationship between physical and social space and its effect on the social inclusion of persons with mental illness in rural Scotland. Parr found that an inverse relationship existed between physical and

social space, differentiating urban and rural geographies with respect to social inclusion for persons with a mental illness. In particular, Parr discovered that individuals who lived in close physical proximity to others in urban centers experienced greater social distance from people in the community than their rural cohorts. Despite greater physical distances separating individuals residing in rural places, they experienced greatly reduced social distances, noting that *everybody knows your business*. The meanings of places are dynamic and ever changing, often reflecting one's social identity or the accumulation of life experiences with age, for example.

In the Northern Initiative for Social Action (NISA) study of an occupation-based mental health program (Rebeiro et al., 2001), social space was found to be an important aspect of the environment. Social spaces that fostered an inclusive environment, embraced the authentic selves of participants, and promoted a sense of belonging were found to be particularly important to the individuals' capacity to fully participate in occupations within the space of NISA. To foster belonging, the group created a space that paid attention to diversity and inclusion, to safety (both physical and psychological), and to the importance of self-directed participation—that is, when the person felt safe, accepted for who they are and without the need to apologize for who they are, and in general felt comfortable in the space. Similarly, Nayar and colleagues (2012) highlighted how a sense of comfort and engagement in occupations were shaped by the cultures of private and public spaces for new immigrants to New Zealand. In summary, social aspects of the environment (e.g., inclusion, opportunities, resources) and the person (e.g., internal values, beliefs, citizenship status) can transact with each other to create different opportunities and challenges to occupational participation.

The Lived Experience

Lisa

Lisa is a 45-year-old mother of one who has had extensive experience with mental health services and programs, including several hospital admissions over a 12-year period. Lisa was diagnosed with bipolar affective disorder and, during the time of her involvement with occupational therapy, rapidly cycled between depression and varying levels of mania, accompanied by delusional ideas.

For many years, Lisa identified seeking a purpose, a job, and, specifically, a career as being important to her. Despite the unrelenting nature of her illness, she somehow always persevered with her education and obtained a degree in social work and a diploma in marketing. Lisa held the belief that she would successfully work at some point in the future. She experimented with a variety of jobs, but had difficulty concentrating and was left dissatisfied with many of the jobs. Her career orientation was the reason that Lisa initially sought out involvement with occupational therapy and the NISA (Rebeiro Gruhl et al., 2020), an occupation-based, mental health program.

Lisa's Own Story

I remember a time when I wasn't feeling part of anything. I was standing on a chair, noose around my neck, wishing for the will to push the chair and let myself fall to my death and end the pain that was my daily existence. I had been diagnosed with bipolar disorder and lived with the "highs" of mania and the crashing lows of depression since the age of 13. I was 31 when I started to turn things around for myself.

How does one come back from the depths of such despair to work as a counselor in a nationally recognized program? I believe that several factors came together to bring about this change. A change in medication, becoming drug and alcohol free, lifestyle changes, a refocusing on self-care and routine. Only one thing had to change: everything!!! I became involved in an organization called NISA. NISA is an occupation-based program founded on three essential components of recovery: Being, Belonging, and Becoming needs. It was at NISA that I began to feel that I belonged to society again, that I had something worthwhile to contribute. I contributed a painting to an art show, designed ads, and wrote poetry and articles for the *Open Minds Quarterly Journal,* which was produced by NISA, and much more. In short, I was encouraged to become involved, to participate in occupations of choice, and I felt I was engaged in meaningful occupation. I felt empowered. It was like I was evolving again as a person instead of sitting at a standstill, wasting my life away. I again belonged in this world.

After reaping the benefits of my new-found sense of worth for almost a year, I became pregnant with my first child. I gave birth to my son and, subsequently, to another purpose for my life. Routine, such an important factor in my recovery, became paramount. I stayed with my father and stepmother for 1.5 months after my son was born. I was blessed with a child who slept through the night at 2 months and had a regular feeding schedule. We both returned home very content. I slipped into the role of mother like a glove. Now, I was not only staying well for myself, but for my son. I chose to be proactive with illness management, and consciously decided to take steps to not decompensate, or

become hospitalized because someone was depending on me . . . for everything. I needed to stay well to take care of him. At this point, I was still on funding from Canada Pension and the Ontario Disability Support program, the criteria for which is "a severe and prolonged disability." When the application for disability was made, my prognosis was placed as "guarded." It was believed that I would never work again. I am thankful that they were all wrong! With the confidence given me by my occupational therapist and peers, and with more than 2 years of psychiatric stability behind me, I began to think that I could work again and started to consider my options. I was educated and had received my bachelor's degree in social work. Dare I think I could return to my field? At the recommendation of my doctor, I applied for a part-time job as a social worker to work with troubled youth. I continued to work with troubled youth for 5 years before moving on and returning to work for the organization that had given me a new lease on life. I became a program coordinator there. I enjoyed my time but continued to struggle with burnout and episodic returns to the depths of despair. I needed balance for all things work and all things life. I needed to learn to help others as an occupation and help myself as a person at the same time. Balancing the needs of those I worked with, my son, my family, and myself presented a challenge I am only now mastering. I was, and continue to be, in need of balance for all things work and all things life. We are all seeking that balance continuously and I am no different than any other in that aspect. Perhaps if there is a difference, it is a difference in the strength of my determination to find and maintain that healthy balance and wellness. The cost of not maintaining that focus is too great for me.

Lifestyle changes including becoming drug and alcohol free, a regular routine including a consistent sleep/wake schedule, eating a more balanced and nutritious diet, working physical activity into my daily routine, bringing both my surroundings and my physical self-care up to a better standard, and a change in medication all helped to move me along in my recovery.

After yet another burnout while working in residential services, I decided to try my hand at running my own business of providing creativity and mental health workshops in my home community. Having control over hours and the freedom afforded by this position was beneficial. I could back off when I felt the need and move forward as good mental health allowed. The financial uncertainty and the stress of it, however, caused me to rethink my work life and I sought employment part time in my field. I was successful in obtaining employment as a social worker with the Canadian Mental Health Association and I am currently employed there. For certain, if I was not introduced to meaningful occupation, my ongoing recovery from the mental health crisis that plagued my life would not be possible. I have meaning, purpose, and a wonderful life with a 12-year-old son and a fiancé I love. I am so grateful to everyone who was and is part of my ongoing recovery from what is called mental illness. It cannot be underestimated the importance of occupation even for those who seemingly are beyond hope. There is always meaningful occupation when that very meaning is defined by those who are participating in their own lives and recovery, and there is always, always hope.

(Readers can find more information about Lisa's perspectives on client-centered occupational therapy in Bibyk, B., Day, D. G., Morris, L., O'Brien, M. C., Rebeiro, K. L., Seguin, P., Semeniuk, B., Wilson, B., & Wilson, J. (1999). Who's in charge here? The client's perspective on client-centred care. *Occupational Therapy Now, Sept/Oct,* 11–12.)

The PEO Model in Occupational Therapy Psychosocial Practice

The focus of occupational therapy is occupational participation; supporting people or collectives to have access to, initiate, and sustain valued occupations within meaningful relationships and situated contexts (Egan & Restall, 2022). The PEO model can guide OTPs to understand these complex relationships and how maximizing the PEO fit can optimize attainment of this professional focus (Fig. 3-3). In collaboration with individuals, OTPs (a) coassess the supports and constraints to occupational participation, and (b) partner to codesign interventions to address meso- and macro-level factors preventing or fostering meaningful occupational participation. The PEO model can be a tool for building these collaborative relationships, facilitating critical reflexive practice, and guiding intervention plans and evaluations. The PEO model is a platform for such collaborative work: offering space for people to be heard; a Venn diagram for communication, shared understanding within context, and joint problem-solving; and a means of facilitating reflection to codesign and coevaluate interventions for collective change.

The PEO fit is critical to successful occupational therapy processes and outcomes. In the situation of supporting employment for people living with mental illnesses, the OTPs can leverage strategies that focus on the person, the environment, or the occupation. For example, with respect to the environment, the individual may be offered a quiet place to retreat and use self-management strategies when feeling overwhelmed. Supervisors and coworkers can be engaged in a discussion about mental illness, challenging misconceptions and generating strategies for creating a more accepting work environment. The OTP may partner with management and the union to facilitate opportunities for socializing outside the workplace to foster positive work relationships for all. The occupation is targeted when specific job duties are adapted or modified to increase successful participation. These approaches may be fruitless if the PEO fit is compromised by an unrealistic expectation, such as a fast-paced work environment in which an individual is experiencing high job anxiety or when the work being done is not valued by the worker or by people in the work environment. An examination of PEO relationships with the individual and management constructing Venn diagrams together would support effective communication and joint planning.

Using the PEO model, OTP and individual or collective can coanalyze and explain how different PEO relationships can influence occupational participation. This information supports personally tailored intervention plans. Discussions focus on reflections of the fit (or lack of fit) between a person's personal resources, the demands of the occupation, and the environmental conditions in which the occupation takes place. In this way, the model can illustrate the current PEO relationships surrounding a particular occupational participation issue and how changes to components can support improvements in occupational participation.

For example, as shown in Figure 3-4, if changes were made to a person's environment (e.g., eliminated time pressures) that improved the $P \times E$ congruence and the $O \times E$ congruence, these changes could be depicted by moving the environment sphere inward to increase its overlap with the person and occupation spheres, resulting in the increased overlap in the center, which depicts improved occupational participation. The model illustrates how a single intervention or intervention focused solely on one component will not result in optimal participation. If the intervention only influenced the $P \times E$ transaction and not the $O \times E$ transaction, the E sphere would not be moved uniformly toward the center; rather, it would move toward the P sphere to increase the P-E overlap and not the P-O overlap in spheres, depicting improved but not optimal occupational participation. Similarly, interventions could be focused on the person component or on the occupation component to improve the congruence with one or all components of the model.

The PEO model is effective in mental health practice because it promotes people's full participation in their everyday lives in several ways:

■ It embodies the promotion of occupational participation within a collaborative process. OTPs are most effective when their practice is informed by the experiences and expertise of the people they serve. The PEO model facilitates an understanding of valued occupations and occupational participation issues from people's lived experiences by providing a platform for co-reflection

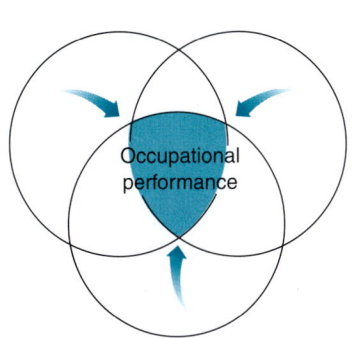

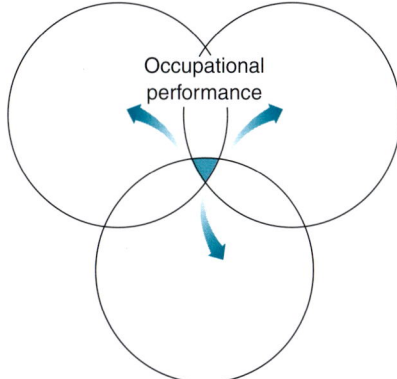

Maximizes fit
and therefore maximizes occupational performance

Occupational performance

Minimizes fit
and therefore minimizes occupational performance

Occupational performance

Occupational performance

FIGURE 3-3. Changes to occupational participation as a consequence of variations in person, environment, and occupation fit. *Adapted with permission from Law, M., Cooper, B., Strong, S., Stewart, D., Rigby, P., & Letts, L. (1996). The Person-Environment-Occupation model: A transactive approach to occupational performance.* Canadian Journal of Occupational Therapy, 63(1), 9–23. *https://doi.org/10.1177/000841749606300103*

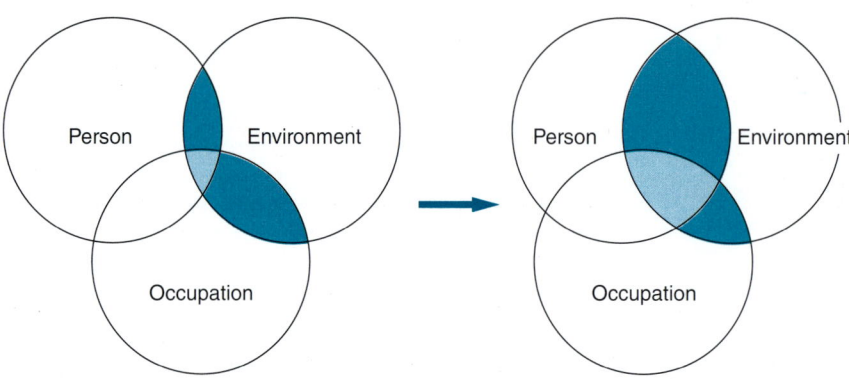

FIGURE 3-4. Effect of intervention to change the environment on occupational participation. *Adapted with permission from Law, M., Cooper, B., Strong, S., Stewart, D., Rigby, P., & Letts, L. (1996). The Person-Environment-Occupation model: A transactive approach to occupational performance.* Canadian Journal of Occupational Therapy, 63(1), 9–23. *https://doi.org/10.1177/000841749606300103*

of the situation, codesign of interventions, and coevaluation of outcomes. A shared understanding of issues and priorities supports a strong therapeutic relationship and effective working partnerships. It also fosters OTPs' practices to be grounded in the daily realities of people's lives, experiences, histories, and life stages.

■ It operationalizes rights-based, individually determined ethical practice principles. The product of the PEO model is the human right to occupational participation. Further, the outcome of successful participation is defined by the individual and their experience of occupational participation. The outcome is the result of transactive PEO relationships, including relationships of inclusion and exclusion, belonging and marginalization, and acceptance and oppression. The PEO model supports consideration of culture, justice, and equity as part of occupational therapy practice. OTPs reflect upon the socioeconomic, legal, and political factors within environmental structures (cultural, institutional, social, and physical) that impact occupational opportunities to access, choose, and sustain valued occupations.

■ It supports critically reflective evidence-based practice. The PEO model offers a systematic approach to the analysis of occupational participation issues. It promotes the gathering of evidence, reflection, and the use of clinical reasoning.

■ It supports OTPs to see both the "forest and the trees." Using the PEO model as a conceptual framework assists OTPs in reaching a more comprehensive understanding of the complexities of human performance and experiences, while considering influential relationships at the micro, meso, and macro levels.

■ It expands options for intervention. The PEO model broadens the focus of the therapist's formulation and offers guidance regarding potential areas for intervention that involve the environment and occupation, and not solely the person. The PEO model fosters consideration of interventions not only focused on the individual or group, but also examining the occupational demands and the influence of organizations, local environments, communities, and various macro-level systems of the broader society and government.

■ It frames the scope of practice. The PEO model provides OTPs with a framework that helps them to define the scope of occupation-based practice. OTPs have historically used this model in a variety of roles (e.g., direct service provider, consultant, manager, and advocate)

and settings (e.g., community, hospitals, businesses, schools) to advocate for occupational therapy services.

■ It facilitates communication of practice within and outside occupational therapy practice. The PEO model is easily understood by other health-care professionals, non–health-care professionals, families, and community members. Its broad application in multiple contexts has illustrated the fact that the model can be used with other theories and combined with other perspectives. Also, constructive teamwork is facilitated by focusing discussions on the shared PEO fit issues rather than placing responsibility on any one person or organization, thus reducing potential feelings of defensiveness.

■ It supports advances in the occupational therapy profession. By clearly articulating occupational therapy theory and practical application, the PEO model supports therapists to systematically evaluate practice and engage in research. Researchers have used the PEO framework for data collection, analysis, and interpretation of findings.

Formulating Occupational Participation

The relationships among the PEO components are examined systematically by reflecting on the elements that influence the fit and the lack of fit between the models' main components (P × O, O × E, P × E) individually and as a whole. The fit is considered within the ascribed meanings, situational relationships, and within the context of the particular occupational participation issue. This analysis involves looking at different layers of relationships and then synthesizing the understandings into a formulation as a whole to identify options for improving the PEO fit. It is understood that the OTP acts in collaboration with the people being served in each step of formulation. The relationships are systematically examined in the context of the identified occupational participation issue and the opportunities or challenges to select, initiate, and sustain the valued occupations by the following:

1. Assess the important elements that influence the individual's or collective's identified occupational participation issue(s) in the context of the particular individual's living situation with respect to each of the three main components: person, environment, and occupation.

2. Assess the PEO transactions by reflecting on the P × O, O × E, and P × E relationships, as well as the supports or demands, resiliencies or pressures, opportunities or systemic oppressions, and inequities within each pairing of components.

3. Recognize and understand from the individual's or collective's perspective the meanings ascribed for engaging in the occupation in the given environment across time and space, particularly the influence of gender, race, history, and culture. Using an intersectional lens, the OTP examines how experiences such as ableism, ageism, racism, colonialism, and other forms of discrimination impact occupational participation.

4. Consider the whole, all three components and the transactional relationships, to help ascertain what factors support and constrain occupational participation for this individual or collective to select, initiate, and sustain participation in the identified occupation within the given environment. The OTP validates and elaborates upon the formulation by discussing their understanding with the individual or collective, perhaps by drawing a Venn diagram to illustrate the lack of PEO fit.

5. In collaboration with the individual or collective, draw Venn diagrams to envision and develop strategies to improve occupational participation by identifying and addressing barriers and constraints through devising new or expanded occupational opportunities and creating supports to improve the quality of the PEO fit.

It is important to examine relationships from the individual's perspective and life experiences in order to properly recognize the ascribed meanings. For example, Bejerholm and Eklund's (2006) study of people with schizophrenia found that engagement in occupations provided rhythm and meaning to their days. Even quiet activities that can be easily dismissed as "just passing time" were ascribed different meanings to these individuals within the supportive or constraining home environments. While working with a group living with serious mental illnesses to pursue work goals, Nagle and colleagues (2002) studied individuals making occupational choices related to personal perceptions of how the occupation supported their health and social connections in the life context of restricted social and economic resources. In another similar unemployed sample, everyday occupations engendered feelings of competence and helped participants manage their illness symptoms (Argentzell et al., 2012). For plans to be relevant and effective, OTPs consider the situational realities of the particular individual's daily life and the context within which the occupational participation issue is situated.

An ethnographic study of individuals with schizophrenia who worked at an affirmative business highlighted how the meaning of occupation was personal and changed over time (Strong, 1998). The meaning ascribed to work changed with the person's relationship to their own illness and recovery. For example, when illness was the main focus in individuals' lives, work was a bolster against the daily battle with illness and a buffer for dealing with society's negative attitudes. When workers viewed themselves as becoming capable people with a future, work took on the meaning of providing concrete evidence that they were more than just an illness and may have a future. When workers were actively engaged in their recovery and getting on with their lives, work became

the modality to practice and develop the interests, skills, and habits necessary for being a worker and friend. When finding a place in the world was considered important, work was a means to feel valued and offered a place to belong.

Example of PEO Analysis in Practice

Figure 3-5 illustrates the use of the PEO model to systematically analyze an occupational participation issue for a fictitious individual. Donald Shivay, a 21-year-old self-identified male, was referred to occupational therapy to help him become more involved in the community. Shivay views himself as a first generation Canadian of Indian heritage who grew up in a Hindu household. Shivay was given a diagnosis of schizophrenia, as well as attention deficit-hyperactivity disorder (ADHD). Shivay's goal is to eventually obtain employment. Shivay completed grade 11 but had difficulty with concentration. According to his father, he is also socially awkward, often interrupting others and lacking boundaries regarding personal information. With Shivay's consent, the OTP arranged for him to work as a volunteer to repair and recycle computers at the Working Centre (www.theworkingcentre.org). The Working Centre is a nonprofit organization created as a community development project in response to local unemployment and poverty.

The PEO model can be used for ongoing analysis, shared understanding, and joint intervention planning. In the example of Shivay, the job placement went well initially, and Shivay wanted to spend all of his time volunteering. He began to make friends. Over time, he was observed to spend more time socializing and less time working on computers. The therapist met with Shivay and reaffirmed with him his goal to obtain employment and that he continued to see volunteering at the Working Centre as a step to achieving his goal by learning how to recycle and repair computers. The OTP, using the PEO model, was able to explore with Shivay the situation and how he experienced volunteering at the Centre. The therapist drew Venn diagram circles and placed notes using Shivay's words to depict the transactional relationships and ascribed meanings. Shivay commented he was learning "the ways of work" (work routines, habits, social norms) and "how to tear down and rebuild computers" (skills). He proudly spoke of the work he was doing. He expressed feeling a sense of belonging, something he had not felt in high school. He felt he could talk to people and could check with his supervisor about what was going on when he was unsure of what to make of social situations. He spoke of learning when not to talk to some of the workers who were less accepting of him and enjoying the company of people who worked beside him. He acknowledged lately spending more time socializing and less time getting work done.

By examining Shivay's volunteer experiences using the PEO model, the therapist and Shivay were able to explore Shivay's need to feel accepted, to socialize and develop friendships, to have a sense of belonging, and to obtain employment at this stage of his life in the context of his own personal history. When the therapist asked about the social tensions he feels when volunteering and how he usually deals with them, the therapist was surprised to learn about an additional role of socializing with coworkers. Shivay explained that in his Hindu household, his family valued peace and harmony, which meant conflict was avoided or prevented. To

Donald's Identified Occupational Performance Issue
• Obtain employment

Assessment of Main Components Impacting Occupational Performance

Occupation—Computer Recycle and Repair
- Requires: Knowledge of computer hardware and software and hand tools. Abilities: inspect and test electronic equipment and assemblies; diagnose and locate circuit, component, and equipment faults; adjust, align, replace, or repair electronic equipment and assemblies; complete work orders, tests, and maintenance reports
- Basic skills: Reading text; document use; numeracy; writing; communication; working with others; problem-solving; decision-making; critical thinking; job task planning and organizing; significant use of memory; finding information; continuous learning
- Employers require basic security clearance (criminal record check).
- Industry standard is completion of high school, CompTIA A+ certification.

Person	**Environment**
• Motivated to work and be like others his own age • Desires to contribute and help others • Socially awkward • Negative experiences at school, grade 11 education, limited life experience • Developing sense of self, own values • Engaged in therapy, taking medication • Difficulties with concentration, processing verbal information, and planning • Disorganized with unfamiliar tasks • No legal involvement or criminal record • Physically healthy	• Work is highly valued by parents and society • Interpersonal relationships are restricted to family and health care • Lives with parents • Uses public transportation • The Working Centre (www.theworkingcentre.org) is a nonprofit organization created in response to unemployment and poverty for self-help and community development.

Assessment of Person-Environment-Occupation Transactions

Person-Occupation (P × O)	**Occupation-Environment (O × E)**	**Person-Environment (P × E)**
• Donald is interested in computers and has experience with games. • ADHD symptoms are better controlled in 1:1 situations and when focusing on enjoyable activities. • Visual and tactile information facilitates learning.	• Working Centre provides education and hands-on training in computer recycling and repair. • Work is organized at Donald's own pace, and 1:1 instruction is available. • Expectation is to work a minimum of 1 hour per shift.	• Working Centre supports individuals with little experience to obtain the skills, computer fundamentals, and confidence for future courses. • Donald interrupts others, inappropriately discloses personal information, and is easily distracted and taken off task.

Formulation of Occupational Performance Issue (P × E × O)

Lacking life experience and challenged by the impact of schizophrenia and ADHD on occupational performance, Donald needs a supportive, flexible work environment to build on his strengths, experience success, develop sense of self and self-efficacy, and learn the fundamental computer knowledge and other work skills required to take future certification training to meet his goal.

Theoretical Approaches to Guide Intervention

- Neurocognitive behavioral theories: to understand the impact of schizophrenia and ADHD on learning and working; guide cognitive behavioral therapy
- Environmental theories: for identifying supportive work environment; guide provision of accommodation
- Psycho-emotional theories: for understanding the need for social support; guide counseling

Recommendations/Plan to Improve Occupational Performance (the PEO Fit)

- Supported volunteer placement at the Working Centre
- Weekly counseling to support problem-solving, action planning of arising on-the-job issues, and long-term career planning

FIGURE 3-5. Example of a systematic analysis of an occupational participation issue using the Person-Environment-Occupation model.

Shivay, socializing on the job was a way of maintaining harmony within the workplace organization. He had placed the expectation on himself as a duty to maintain the harmony. This opened a conversation of how to harmonize workplace needs, coworkers' needs, and Shivay's needs. The diagrams were used as the basis for a discussion with Shivay, and this visual helped him to focus and to participate in collaborative decision-making. Further, the PEO model enriched the therapist's understanding of how Shivay experienced the situation, as well as the contributions of workplace relationships to occupational opportunities and outstanding needs.

With Shivay's permission, the therapist arranged for a meeting with his supervisor to review Shivay's progress. His supervisor spoke of what Shivay had learned to do, how he had become an important member of the Centre, and how his socializing on the job had increased such that work was not getting done. With the therapist's new understanding of the meaning of socializing at work, the therapist was able to facilitate a negotiation of expectations and needs. The supervisor was asked if they identified social tensions at the Centre and what was being done or could be done to reduce tensions. The supervisor acknowledged tensions arising from a group of people with different work and communication styles and, with prompting, agreed discrimination toward people of color existed. Shivay and his supervisor both agreed Shivay's opportunities related to his work goal were not restricted at the Centre. The supervisor expressed belief that those individuals who expressed discriminatory behavior would find themselves restricted in today's workplaces and that racism and discriminatory behavior were not tolerated at the Centre. The supervisor identified that in this setting it was everyone's responsibility to support each other and do what they could to get along with each other; this was not only Shivay's responsibility. The supervisor recognized the workflow did not have a formal 15-minute break time for everyone to break together and socialize; rather, individually they were encouraged to work at their own pace and then stop and refresh as needed. The supervisor saw the potential benefits for doing both and agreed to pursue the idea with the Centre's director. After the supervisor meeting, the therapist explored with Shivay additional ways to socialize and to make friends outside of volunteering. Shivay also recognized his need for support and structure to achieve his work goals. Regular sessions with the therapist to review progress were used to help Shivay to stay on track and to support Shivay's problem-solving of on-the-job issues as they arose at his volunteer work.

For further examples, readers are directed to view an article by Strong and colleagues (1999), in which the PEO model is described as a practical analytical tool for the analysis of occupational participation issues, intervention planning and evaluation, and communication of occupational therapy practice to others. In this article, three scenarios illustrate the application of the model to common situations encountered in different occupational therapy practice settings: an older man wanting to return home from a hospital after a hip fracture, a child with cerebral palsy feeling frustrated with written work at school, and a man with schizophrenia expressing that he cannot return to a transitional work placement.

Integrating PEO Into the Occupational Therapy Process

Incorporating the constructs of the PEO model is useful throughout the occupational therapy process. It begins with the initial evaluation and is carried out through the intervention. The following scenario illustrates the steps involved in applying the PEO framework in the occupational therapy treatment process. The example includes what is often considered a physical or medical condition to illustrate the emotional management and mental health considerations that are inherent in all aspects of occupational therapy practice. OTPs working with individuals living with chronic diseases focus on supporting their **self-management** occupations in order to live well with chronic condition(s) by gaining the knowledge, skills, and confidence to manage the medical, role, and emotional aspects of the disease (Adams et al., 2004).

Mental health considerations for people with chronic conditions are further described in Chapter 17: Chronic Health Conditions and Mental Health, including the emotional issues commonly experienced by people with chronic conditions and the impact of these issues on occupational participation.

Identifying a Priority Occupational Participation Issue

Sheryl, a 33-year-old working single mother, was referred to occupational therapy at the bariatric clinic providing follow-up after gastric surgery. The clinic staff asked her to consider her eating as an addiction and a chronic disease. Sheryl was living with diabetes and obesity, and she experienced many failed attempts to lose the 95 pounds she had gained since her first pregnancy and later divorce. Sheryl described her life as progressively restricted and isolated because of her weight gain. Sheryl stated: "I can't keep up with the things I need to do! I'm exhausted all the time." She reported experiencing her days as repetitive routines of getting the children off to school as best she can, dragging herself to work, doing her best to get through her day, arriving home with the children too tired to cook, serving whatever she had on hand, bathing the children, and going to bed. On the weekends she rested. Sheryl received complaints about her performance at work, and she worried that her job was threatened. She blames herself for her children being ridiculed by the children at school for having a "fat" mother. Sheryl expressed feeling hopeless, sad, and disempowered. The therapist learned that Sheryl's most important occupational participation issue is regularly providing healthy meals for her two young children.

Exploring Factors That Influence PEO

As the interview continued, the therapist and Sheryl collaboratively explored her priority occupational participation issue with respect to influential person, environment, and occupation factors. Sheryl told the therapist about herself, including her interests, values, cultural beliefs, self-concept, what she was able to do and not do, and the challenges she frequently faced. Together they identified the strengths and challenges of her situation surrounding meal preparation (Table 3-2).

Examining Relationships Among the PEO Components

Next, the relationships among the PEO components were examined by reflecting on the fit or lack of fit among the transactions (P × O, O × E, and P × E) while identifying ascribed meanings and considering the influence of time and space. It is important that the analysis goes deeper to gain understanding of relationships and the quality of those relationships rather than stopping at the previous step.

Person-Occupation Transactions

■ Sheryl values meal preparation for her children and is motivated to address this area.

TABLE 3-2 | **PEO Components Related to Meal Preparation—Strengths and Challenges**

Occupation Component

- It is imbued with meaning related to being a "good" mother; it is an expression of love.
- Healthy meals are necessary for living well.
- Healthy meals require knowledge for healthy choices.
- It demands planning, organization, decision-making, and problem-solving abilities and energy.
- It involves stress related to procuring food and preparing healthy meals.
- It requires equipment, space, and time.
- It requires adequate finances.

Person Component

Physical	• Body mass index (BMI) of 38 kg/m^2 • Shortness of breath upon walking six stairs and one city block • Daily pain in knees and right hip on movement; osteoarthritis • Not sleeping well with sleep apnea and early morning wakening • Numbness in her feet and frequent urinary infections re: diabetes
Affective	• Frustrated with feeling exhausted • Overwhelmed by household activities not getting done • Worried about children's needs and potential loss of job • Frightened about what the future will hold • Feels as if nothing she has done has worked
Cognitive	• Tires easily, which affects her concentration and memory • Some knowledge of what is involved in healthy eating, being active; limited knowledge of managing obesity and diabetes • Aware of potential negative outcomes to her health and quality of life if no changes are made in her life • Frequent negative self-talk and limited coping strategies
Spiritual	• Time spent with her children gives her strength and provides meaning to her life. • She views providing healthy meals and being a positive role model as important to being a good mother.

Environment Component

Cultural	• Her own mother and positive childhood experiences provide a strong sense of motherhood and healthy living. • Internalized societal stigmatizing attitudes toward obesity: She is to blame and just needs to eat properly and get exercise. • North American culture emphasizes thin female body image, attached to self-worth.
Physical	• Lives in a two-bedroom townhouse • Takes public transit to work • Shares a vehicle with her mother for shopping
Institutional	• She inconsistently receives some child support from father. • Children's school sent home note and information sheets requesting children be sent to school with healthy lunches and snacks. • Breakfast program available at school for selected economically disadvantaged children; those who attend are marginalized at school.
Social	• She is divorced; ex-husband is not involved in their lives. • Siblings live some distance away; occasional phone calls. • Her mother provides some instrumental support limited by her own failing health. • Sheryl no longer has contact with past friends made through work.

- Eating her prepared meals together is a family time that she cherishes, and these experiences provide her with strength to keep going.
- There is a mismatch between her current abilities and the physical, affective, and cognitive demands of meal preparation.

Occupation-Environment Transactions

- The kitchen physically supports meal preparation with respect to space and sufficient equipment.
- Limited income restricts food purchases.
- The kitchen is mainly stocked with inexpensive prepared foods for quick meal assembly that offer limited variety and high-calorie meals.
- The children's school expects parents to provide healthy lunches and snacks, and assistance is limited to reminder letters that perpetuate blame and a breakfast program that contributes to marginalization.
- There is no computer at home, but she has an iPhone to support healthy meal preparation.
- The children are not involved in meal preparation.

Person-Environment Transactions

- Sheryl is isolated with limited emotional and instrumental supports for daily living and for managing her chronic illnesses of obesity and diabetes.
- She has internalized societal stigmatizing attitudes toward obesity, believes she is to blame and largely copes through negative self-talk that perpetuates poor self-image and low self-efficacy.
- She views her family doctor's comments about needing to lose weight and notes home from her children's school as not helpful and further evidence of her inadequacies, which are contributing to her stress.

Formulating a Plan

Upon examining the relationships among the PEO components, the therapist further explored with Sheryl key potential barriers and supports to healthy meal preparation. The therapist's initial assessment of PEO fit was shared with Sheryl in order to validate, confirm, elaborate, refine, or refocus key issues. Together, Sheryl and the therapist developed an intervention plan to improve the PEO fit. The plan used feasible strategies to eliminate or reduce the barriers and increase support to improve occupational participation. Given that occupational participation is influenced by complex transactional processes among the person, environment, and occupation, OTPs need to direct interventions at all three components.

Sheryl admitted that she had internalized stigmatizing attitudes toward being overweight. She felt alone and needed help with limited personal resources. Going to the bariatric clinic was her first step to getting assistance and to taking charge of her health by learning to manage obesity and diabetes as chronic diseases. Sheryl reiterated that learning how to prepare healthy meals for her children was her main priority, and at the clinic she was learning how to have a new and healthier relationship with food. The main barriers to participation in meal preparation were identified as limited access to healthy ingredients and foods and also the intersection of Sheryl's current mental and physical endurance. The extent to which mood, joint pain, management of blood sugar levels, and poor sleeping might be contributing to Sheryl's occupational participation was unknown.

Completion of the Beck Depression Inventory–II (Beck et al., 1996), a depression screening tool used in psychiatric services, indicated that Sheryl would benefit from a referral to psychiatry services. The therapist and Sheryl formulated a plan of reengaging in healthy self-care routines. Cognitive behavioral therapy (CBT) strategies were used to assist Sheryl to reframe her negative self-talk and to consider alternative behavioral responses to her occupational challenges. The therapist suggested Sheryl write her reflections on her progress at the end of each day with statements of gratitude. The PEO model is supportive of CBT by helping the individual to view things differently and respond differently, especially where the person is unable to change the past (e.g., trauma).

The extent to which diabetes and joint pain influenced Sheryl's fears of complications was unknown. Sheryl supported experimenting with a range of strategies once the potential depression was addressed. Sheryl was introduced to energy conservation and joint protection principles and was provided with assistance to apply them to her daily activities. She was also assisted in reorganizing her kitchen to have all the materials routinely used nearby. Sheryl was supported to put into action what she has learned in her sessions with the dietitian and diabetes educator. While losing weight, she was given a supervised exercise program in conjunction with stretching to safely become more active. As she managed better, her fears lessened, and as she lost weight, her diabetes and chronic pain were more controlled. When she had more energy, the therapist talked with Sheryl about participating in a neighborhood garden program for families, which involved growing food together and the sharing of resources and cooking events. With permission from the gardening committee, the therapist met with the school principal to talk about the letters sent home to parents and to leave information about the neighborhood gardening program.

Interventions, Ongoing Evaluation, and Modifications

Implemented interventions were evaluated by both Sheryl and the therapist by examining changes in the occupational participation of the priority occupational participation goal(s). For Sheryl, the plans were evaluated with respect to whether they helped her to routinely prepare healthy meals for her children and the quality of her experiences with meal preparation.

Initially, interventions focused on her mental and physical endurance while providing support before refining meal preparation practices and lifestyle routines. Each intervention in turn (linking with psychiatrist, energy conservation, joint protection, structured exercise, and cognitive behavioral strategies to manage obesity, diabetes, and chronic pain) was evaluated with the individual to examine progress, address any challenges, and readjust plans to meet her changing life situation (e.g., a child home sick for a few weeks). The PEO model provided a framework for joint analysis, communication, and codesigning implementation of plans. The therapist drew circle or Venn diagrams to explain the lack of PEO fit

and the intentions of interventions relating to the PEO relationships. The PEO model was helpful to facilitate Sheryl to move away from blaming herself for what she viewed as a lack of progress and focus on aspects of her occupation and environment, areas over which she had some control, while waiting for depression medications to take effect, experiencing gradual weight loss, and building cardiovascular capacity. For the therapist, the PEO model was helpful in identifying the contributing factors and relationships between those factors, and to refrain from oversimplification or focusing solely on the individual.

After some progress, Sheryl experienced a setback with new pain from a soft tissue injury in her foot. After seeing her family doctor, Sheryl and her therapist revised her activity and exercise levels to support a 5- to 6-week healing period that used low-impact activities such as swimming or bicycle riding to maintain her gains. Then, together, they designed a plan to build Sheryl's endurance using graduated activity in her daily routines within her own ratings of pain and self-efficacy. Sheryl maintained an activity log and rated her pain and confidence. In this way, Sheryl engaged in self-monitoring and made daily adjustments to improve the PEO fit. The therapist suggested using a phone app, such as *MyFitnessPal* or *Foodility,* to further support self-monitoring of her net calories, nutrition, and exercise levels. Each of these tailored interventions was targeted to improve the PEO fit and support her participation in taking charge of her health.

Application of the PEO Model

Internationally, the PEO model has been applied in a variety of settings and contexts, from direct service and consultation to teaching students, research, and advocacy, while working with individuals, groups, or organizations.

Occupational therapy academic programs continue to teach the PEO model as a tool for OTPs to use in the systematic analysis and formulation of occupational participation issues. Not only is the PEO model cited as a framework for planning, evaluating, and making recommendations for individual and collective interventions, but it is also used for the planning and development of occupational therapy services. For example, in a discussion paper, Molineux (2004) used the PEO model to substantiate the position that OTPs working in inpatient psychiatry benefit from a lived experience understanding of how each individual experienced boredom, which facilitated individuals to develop more adaptive time use and effective coping skills. In a health policy call to action paper, Virginia Stoffel (2013) recognized the fit between SAMHSA's perspective on health, purpose, home, and community and the PEO concepts, and suggested using the PEO model to communicate the unique knowledge and skills of occupational therapy when advocating for services in integrated care.

In research, the PEO model is cited as a framework for research design, for developing data collection measures and methods to capture occupational participation, and for organizing data analysis and interpretation of findings. For example, it provided the theoretical basis for developing the Profiles of Occupational Engagement in people with Schizophrenia (POES; Bejerholm et al., 2006). The POES is

Evidence-Based Practice

The PEO Model's Utility and Validity

Research reveals the diversity of PEO use and its utility and validity.

RESEARCH FINDINGS

A scoping review by Rigby and colleagues (2015) found 473 peer-reviewed journal articles that cited the PEO publications. Collectively, these citations illustrated the diversity of PEO use and provided evidence of the PEO model's utility and validity. The citations involved descriptions of interventions, the development of theory or practice principles, and research that examined practice and theory across the breadth of occupational therapy.

APPLICATIONS

➡ OTPs can use the PEO framework in intervention planning to identify factors that contribute to an individual's occupational participation concerns.

➡ The Venn diagram of the PEO model can be used to explain the particular areas that will be targeted in interventions.

➡ The evidence supports the validity of PEO concepts and relationships. OTPs can use the model to develop interventions.

REFERENCES

Rigby, P., Stewart, D., & Law, M. (2015, May). *Exploring the theoretical assumptions of the PEO model: Preliminary results.* PowerPoint presentation at the Canadian Association of Occupational Therapists' Annual Conference. Winnipeg, MB, Canada.

---

an assessment tool to identify the occupational barriers and facilitators upon which to base interventions. The POES consists of a log of occupations and self-reflections coupled with a semistructured interview for examining what has influenced occupational patterns. Another version of the POES was created to target work settings, the Profiles of Occupational Engagement in people with Severe mental illness: Productive occupations (POES-P; Tjornstrand et al., 2013). The POES-P has an occupational log and self-rating of eight dimensions of occupational participation in work-type settings. Studies using the POES, the POES-P, and the Canadian Occupational Performance Measure (COPM), another data collection tool with underpinnings from the PEO model, illustrate the utility and validity of the PEO model.

The following are a few examples of PEO citations focused on understanding the occupational lives of individuals living with mental illness:

■ Using a mixed-methods design, Bejerholm and Eklund (2006) examined the engagement and experience of daily occupations within context over time for a Swedish group of men and women with schizophrenia to reveal how this group could have meaningful lives, experience pleasure, and enjoy life.

■ In New Zealand, McWha and colleagues (2003) compared the perceptions of a group of women living in late life with depression to a health-care team's perceptions with respect to the impact of a group activity and the environment on rehabilitation outcomes.

■ An exploration of the meaning and experience of occupational engagement for persons with mental illness at a Canadian occupation-based program highlighted key elements of social environments that OTPs need to address to avoid creating handicapping environments (Rebeiro, 2001).

■ An ethnographic study examining the meaning of work and the role of work in recovery used the PEO model to answer why the experience at a consumer-run business was satisfying and successful for some individuals but not for others (Strong, 1998).

■ A case study of the individual placement and support approach with five individuals over 1 year used the PEO model as a framework with POES-P to job match and plan support and accommodation interventions (Lexen et al., 2013).

■ Personal narratives of individuals living with serious mental illness reveal learning self-management serendipitously over many years. The PEO model can be used to frame targeted self-management conversations of life challenges and identify barriers or supports for occupational participation (Strong & Letts, 2021).

Criticisms of the PEO Model and Counterstrategies

The PEO model has been criticized for being culturally biased. Pongsaksri's (2004) study identified how OTPs in Thailand perceived the PEO model as not matching their culture's emphasis on collectivism, viewing the PEO model as a Western tool focused on the individual. Similarly, Iwama (1999, 2007) reflected on the Japanese culture; questioned Western notions of individual agency and self-efficacy, as well as the global relevance of person-centered practice; and offered the Kawa model to reflect Eastern worldviews. It is true the original PEO model authors are North American centric. However, the three main components—person, environment, and occupation—were broadly defined, and users are invited to tailor the tool to support its application more broadly. In some situations, it may be helpful to interpret the "person" not as an individual but rather a family or societal group for the PEO model to be more relevant. Vrkljan (2006) provided an example of relabeling the "person" as both the driver and copilot when she applied the PEO model to analysis of the use of in-vehicle navigation technology among older drivers.

The PEO analysis process artificially separates the person, environment, and occupation at a cross section in time to assist the therapist's conceptualization and support a logical manipulation of concepts for planning, which could lead to overly simplistic thinking. OTPs are cautioned against reductionist thinking, given the fact that behavior and occupation can never be fully understood in isolation of the conditions in which they take place (Aldrich, 2008). The human occupational experience must be understood within the symbolic richness of personal meanings and a person's life course perspective (Eakman, 2007). Bertilsson and colleagues (2015) pointed out the PEO's "slices of understanding" were removed from context. This is why it is so important for the OTP to provide a formulation of the "whole" within the presenting life circumstances.

To counter these tendencies, it is important to consider transactional relationships, ascribed personal meanings based on a life span of experience, and the complexity of daily living in multiple contexts as intended by the PEO model. Egan and colleagues (2010) suggested using the model as a framework and supplement it with work from anthropology, sociology, and human geography.

Ultimately, the PEO model is a tool that is only as good as its user. OTPs are reminded of the importance of critical self-reflection and the need to ensure that their practices demonstrate respect for individuals; their strengths, experiences, culture, chosen identity, and knowledge; and their right to make choices and to engage in collaborative relationships with individuals (Whalley Hammell, 2013).

Here's the Point

- The PEO model represents how OTPs view humans as complex occupational beings engaged in occupations in given environments over time and represents the occupational therapy tenet that participation in meaningful occupation is essential to people's development, health, and well-being.

- Six OTPs built upon the work of prominent theorists, concepts, and models to create a model to describe and understand the complex, dynamic nature of occupational participation.

- The PEO model is illustrated by three spheres (person, environment, and occupation) transacting through space and time. The product or outcome from the spheres' interwoven, dynamic, transactional relationships is the quality of the occupational participation. Occupational participation involves both the person's occupational experience and the performance of the occupation within a given environment. Success is uniquely defined by the individual and living circumstances.

- Environments, occupations, and people have both supporting and constraining effects on one another. They shape each other, changing over time. We ascribe meaning in the process of our occupational experiences. Environments, including the people in those environments, can constrain or be a barrier to a person's engagement and full participation; in other words, they can be disabling environments.

- In practice, an OTP focuses on the PEO fit with the intent to maximize the fit for optimal occupational participation with respect to the identified occupational participation issue.

- Analysis of occupational participation issues involves identifying and assessing model elements, relationships, and ascribed meanings that support and constrain optimal occupational participation.

- Based on a synthesis of analysis findings, in collaboration with the individual, barriers and supports are identified as a focus for intervention. Guided by selected theoretical approaches, an intervention plan is formulated for discussion with the individual with the aim to eliminate or limit barriers and build upon supports and strengths. Implemented interventions are monitored and evaluated by the individual and OTP by examining changes in occupational participation. In this way, the PEO model is used throughout the occupational therapy process.

- The PEO model supports psychosocial occupational therapy practice by being a tool to support OTPs' systematic analysis of occupational participation in a way that assists OTPs to "see the forest for the trees" while expanding options for intervention beyond the person and broadening the scope of practice. By representing the occupational therapy lens, the model articulates practice and advocates for the role and value of occupational therapy. In this manner, the PEO model facilitates communication within and outside the profession.

- The model's generic, parsimonious constructs and flexible heuristic depiction have allowed OTPs internationally to use the PEO model for a variety of practice roles, as well as for education and research purposes. OTPs are encouraged to guard against reductionist thinking and take time to consider the transactional relationships in the context of an individual's dynamic, complex occupational lives at the depth of their experiences.

- Now OTPs are applying an intersectional lens within the PEO model in order to identify and critically consider how people's various identities create differing opportunities for occupational participation.

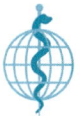 Visit the online resource center at FADavis.com to access the videos.

Apply It Now

1. Your Experience of PEO Fit

Choose an activity that you really enjoy. Reflect on what makes it a successful experience for you. Identify how the PEO transactions are congruent at this time. Has this activity always been a positive experience for you?

Next, think about a negative experience with an activity. What was different at that time? Was there a fit with your skills, abilities, values, demands of the occupation, and the environmental conditions?

2. A Clinical Experience of PEO Fit

Think of a clinical situation (placement) that you felt went well or observed to be a positive experience. Identify the PEO transactions and their congruency. Reflect upon what made this a successful clinical intervention and discuss it with a peer. Similarly, think of a clinical situation that did not go as well as you had hoped (or had observed). Identify the PEO transactions and see if you can identify how you might improve the experience for the individual and optimize the intervention given your understanding of the PEO model.

3. Video Exercise–Using Objects to Promote Engagement

Pair up with another student in your class or form a small group of students. Access and watch the "Using Objects to Promote Engagement" video at the online resource center at FADavis.com. Then, discuss and together answer the following questions:

- When working in forensic/criminal justice settings, there are often restrictions concerning what supplies and materials practitioners may bring into the facility. How did this occupational therapist take something that might have been considered junk and turn it into a multifaceted, therapeutic object? What clinical skills did she use to turn the wheelchair into something with meaning and purpose to a variety of the individuals she worked with?
- How did this wheelchair bring a sense of connection and belonging to the residents of this facility? Think about what the wheelchair might have represented, especially for the population this occupational therapist was working with (i.e., those aging in place in a forensic mental health facility). How might the wheelchair have connected them to residents from generations before them, as well as with their peers?
- How did the wheelchair facilitate the coming together of the person, the environment, and the occupation in this story? Describe the person factors, the environmental factors, and the occupations that led to occupational engagement and participation.

4. Using the PEO Model to Communicate the Occupational Therapy Perspective

Explain to a friend the focus of occupational therapy using the PEO model in your own language with Venn diagrams. When describing the model, use as an example someone who experiences a mental health problem. Explain what can happen to the ability to choose, organize, and satisfactorily perform culturally and personally meaningful occupations.

Reflective Questions
- What examples did you include in your description?
- Was it easier to describe the person, environment, occupation, or occupational participation constructs?
- How did you explain the transactional nature of the model?
- Do you think your friend understood your explanation?
- Would you use the model with an individual as a communication tool and to support development of a partnership?

5. Using the PEO Model to Understand Occupational Participation Issues

Reexamine Figure 3-5. Considering only the information in the first part of the table (i.e., Assessment of Main Components Impacting Occupational Performance) and isolating it from the other information, what picture do you form in your mind of this person and his circumstance? Next, looking at the latter half of the information (i.e., Assessment of Person-Environment-Occupation Transactions), in what way does this information provide a new understanding of this person and their occupational participation issue?

Reflective Questions
- What personal meanings do you now understand?
- What can this information tell you about time and space?
- What else would you want to know? How could you obtain further information about both the subjective experience of engaging in an occupation in a given environment and the observable performance?

6. Using the PEO Model to Understand Lisa's Lived Experience With Recovery

Revisit the story of Lisa in this chapter's The Lived Experience narrative and complete a PEO analysis using the template in Appendix A of this textbook to further examine Lisa's experiences with both the mental health system and with NISA.

Additional background information is shown in the accompanying table.

Occupation Component

- Lisa views herself as both a professional and a social worker.
- Lisa has attempted other careers, including marketing, but found that they were not stimulating to her, nor did this kind of work provide her with a sufficient sense of satisfaction with her work.
- In addition, Lisa has used both art and writing as ways to express her experiences of health and illness, and Lisa recognized that these occupations were primarily therapeutic. Lisa understood that in order to participate as a helping professional, she would need to better manage her own illness and health issues.
- Her occupations met the needs of others and the organization.
- Her later transition to self-employment, while assisting with work–home balance, increased her financial stress.

Person Component

Physical	• Physically capable, but lacking fitness for an 8-hour workday • Keeping up with the care needs of a young child before and after work • Sleeping well • Smoker
Affective	• Excited to fulfill her career goals that had previously been placed on hold because of illness, and later because of having a baby. • Fearful that she may be triggered by others' experiences. Lisa grew up in an abusive family environment, punctuated by alcohol use and abuse. She is personally sensitive to many of the issues dealt with by her profession, such as abuse, alcoholism, and dysfunctional relationships. • Nervous about leaving work to attend to child's appointments or school—finding it hard to have a balance between work and home.
Cognitive	• Long days contribute to her becoming easily fatigued, which affects her concentration and memory. • She is concerned about the effects of medication on her concentration. • She endorses the steps required to reestablish her career.
Spiritual	• Time spent with her son helps to motivate her • Good support from family and friends • No specific religious affiliation

Environment Component

Cultural	• For her recovery, at the beginning she needed a place that not only felt safe but also offered the flexibility for her to make choices. • Working at NISA among other peers, Lisa was able to experiment with a variety of occupations without fear of failure or social rejection. • Mistakes were handled in a low-key, matter-of-fact manner, and she was given the opportunity to make corrections. • The environment was accommodating of Lisa's parenting role and responsibilities.

Environment Component (continued)

Physical	• Work involves a 40-km return drive from the workplace and is not located near the day care. • Public transit is not available where Lisa lives and she must rely on an older vehicle to get to work. • Parking is available at work and Lisa shares an office with another employee.
Institutional	• Lisa is a recipient of provincial disability funding and must declare her employment earnings on a monthly basis. If she earns above a certain amount, she will lose her drug coverage. • Lisa maintains regular appointments with her psychiatrist.
Social	• Lisa has a fiancé whom she finds supportive and understanding of her working. • Lisa's father and stepmother live close, are supportive, and help out financially and with babysitting. • Her peers expressed their belief in her and held the hope for a better life for her when she could not do so for herself. • Lisa's social life revolves mostly around her son and fiancé.

Reflective Questions

■ What is noteworthy from an OTP's perspective with respect to the environment? The occupation?

■ What are the theoretical underpinnings of the intervention?

■ At NISA, was the person the focus of the intervention, or was the environment, or was the occupation? Did anything really change with the person to improve Lisa's health and well-being? In your opinion, what made the difference for Lisa's recovery? What are the implications for an occupation-based practice?

Resources

Books and Journal Articles

• Law, M., Baum, C. M., & Baptiste, S. (2002). *Occupation based practice: Fostering performance and participation.* Slack, Inc.
• Law, M., Cooper, B., Strong, S., Stewart, D., Rigby, P., & Letts, L. (1996). The Person-Environment-Occupation model: A transactive approach to occupational performance. *Canadian Journal of Occupational Therapy, 63*(1), 9–23. https://doi.org /10.1177/000841749606300103
• Letts, L., & Rigby, P. (2003). *Using environments to enable occupational performance.* Slack, Inc.
• Strong, S., & Rebeiro, K. (2003). Creating supportive work environments for people with mental illness. In L. Letts, P. Rigby, & D. Stewart (Eds.), *Using environment to enable occupational performance* (pp. 137–154). Slack, Inc.
• Strong, S., Rigby, P., Stewart, D., Law, M., Cooper, B., & Letts, L. (1999). Application of the Person-Environment-Occupation model: A practical tool. *Canadian Journal of Occupational Therapy, 66*(3), 122–133. https://doi.org/10.1177 /000841749906600304
• Strong, S., & Shaw, L. (1999). A client-centred framework for therapists in ergonomics. In K. Jacobs & C. M. Bettencourt (Eds.), *Ergonomics for therapists* (2nd ed., pp. 22–46). Butterworth-Heinemann.

Video

• "Mental Health and Wellbeing During COVID" video. Caitlin is an OTP who has worked in outpatient settings with both adults and children. In this video, she talks about how occupational therapy practice during the COVID-19 global pandemic allowed her to see in a new way the effects of stress and anxiety on patient outcomes. She discusses how she incorporates mental health and well-being into her practice and her belief that it promotes successful healing and recovery. Access the video at the online resource center at FADavis.com.

Measurement and Evaluation

- Bejerholm, U., Hansson, L., & Eklund, M. (2006). Profiles of occupational engagement in people with schizophrenia, POES: Development of a new instrument based on time-use diaries. *British Journal of Occupational Therapy, 69*(2), 58–68. https://doi.org/10.1177/030802260606900203
- Canadian Occupational Performance Measure. http://www.thecopm.ca [video example, resources, tool purchase]
- Egan, M. Y., Kubina, L.-A., Lidstone, R. I., Macdougall, G. H., & Raudoy, A. E. (2010). A critical reflection on occupational therapy within one assertive community treatment team. *Canadian Journal of Occupational Therapy, 77*(2), 70–79. https://doi.org/10.2182/cjot.2010.77.2.2
- Hamera, E., & Brown, C. E. (2000). Developing a context-based performance measure for persons with schizophrenia: The test of grocery shopping skills. *American Journal of Occupational Therapy, 54*(1), 20–25. https://doi.org/ 10.5014/ajot.54.1.20
- Lexen, A., Hofgren, C., & Bejerholm, U. (2013). Support and process in individual placement and support: A multiple case study. *Work: A Journal of Prevention, Assessment & Rehabilitation, 44*(4), 435–448. https://doi.org/10.3233/WOR-2012-1360
- Peloquin, S. M., & Ciro, C. A. (2013). Self-development groups among women in recovery: Client perceptions of satisfaction and engagement. *American Journal of Occupational Therapy, 67*(1), 82–90. https://doi.org/10.5014/ajot.2013.004796
- Tjornstrand, C., Bejerholm, U., & Eklund, M. (2013). Psychometric testing of a self-report measure of engagement in productive occupations. *Canadian Journal of Occupational Therapy, 80*(2), 101–110. https://doi.org/10.1177/0008417413481956

References

Adams, K., Greiner, A., & Corrigan, J. (2004). *Report of a summit: The 1st annual cross the quality chasm summit: A focus on communities.* National Academies Press.

Aldrich, R. M. (2008). From complexity theory to transactionalism: Moving occupational science forward in theorizing the complexities of behavior. *Journal of Occupational Science, 15*(3), 147–156. https://doi.org/10.1080/14427591.2008.9686624

American Occupational Therapy Association. (2014). Occupational therapy practice framework: Domain and process (3rd ed.). *American Journal of Occupational Therapy, 68*(Suppl. 1), S1–S47. https://doi.org/10.5014/ajot.2014.682006

Americans with Disabilities Act, Pub. L. 101-336, 104 Stat. 327 (1990). https://www.govinfo.gov/content/pkg/STATUTE-104/pdf/STATUTE-104-Pg327.pdf

Arboleda-Florez, J., & Stuart, H. (2012). From sin to science: Fighting the stigmatization of mental illness. *Canadian Journal of Psychiatry, 57*(8), 457–463. https://doi.org/10.1177/070674371205700803

Argentzell, E., Hakansson, C., & Eklund, M. (2012). Experience of meaning in everyday occupations among unemployed people with severe mental illness. *Scandinavian Journal of Occupational Therapy, 19*, 49–58. https://doi.org/10.3109/11038128.2010.540038

Baker, F., & Intagliata, J. (1982). Quality of life in the evaluation of community support systems. *Evaluation and Program Planning, 5*, 69–79. https://doi.org/10.1016/0149-7189(82)90059-3

Beck, A. T., Steer, R. A., Ball, R., & Ranieri, W. (1996). Comparison of Beck Depression Inventories–IA and –II in psychiatric outpatients. *Journal of Personality Assessment, 67*(3), 588–597. https://doi.org/10.1207/s15327752jpa6703_13

Bejerholm, U., & Eklund, M. (2006). Engagement in occupations among men and women with schizophrenia. *Occupational Therapy International, 13*(2), 100–121. https://doi.org/ 0.1002/oti.210

Bejerholm, U., Hansson, L., & Eklund, M. (2006). Profiles of occupational engagement in people with schizophrenia, POES: Development of a new instrument based on time-use diaries. *British Journal of Occupational Therapy, 69*(2), 58–68. https://doi.org/10.1177/030802260606900203

Bertilsson, M., Love, J., Ahlborg, G., & Hensing, G. (2015). Health care professionals' experience-based understanding of individuals' capacity to work while depressed and anxious. *Scandinavian Journal of Occupational Therapy, 22*(2), 126–136. https://doi.org/ 10.3109/11038128.2014.985607

Borsay, A. (1986). Personal trouble or public issue: Towards a model of policy for people with physical and mental disabilities. *Disability & Society, 1*(2), 179–196. https://doi.org/10.1080/02674648666780181

Brockett, M., & Dick, R. (2006). *The Canadian framework for ethical occupational therapy practice.* Canadian Association of Occupational Therapists. https://learnethics.files.wordpress.com/2016/03/ethicalframeworkjuly2006.pdf

Bronfenbrenner, U. (1977). Toward an experimental ecology of human development. *American Psychologist, 32*, 513–531. https://doi.org/10.1037/0003-066X.32.7.513

Brown, L. X. Z. (n.d.). *Welcome.* https://autistichoya.net

Canadian Association of Occupational Therapists. (1997). *Enabling occupation: An occupational therapy perspective.* CAOT Publications.

Centers for Disease Control and Prevention. (n.d.). *Social determinants of health at CDC.* https://www.cdc.gov/about/sdoh/index.html

Christiansen, C. H., Baum, C. M., & Haugen, J. B. (2005). *Occupational therapy: Performance, participation and well-being.* Slack, Inc.

Csikszentmihalyi, M., & Csikszentmihalyi, I. S. (1988). *Optimal experience: Psychological studies in flow in consciousness.* Cambridge University Press.

Dunn, W., Brown, C., & Youngstrom, M. J. (2003). Ecological model of occupation. In P. Kramer, J. Hinojosa, & C. B. Royeen (Eds.), *Perspectives in human occupation: Participation in life* (pp. 222–263). Lippincott William & Wilkins.

Eakman, A. (2007). Occupation and social complexity. *Journal of Occupational Science, 14*(2), 82–91. https://doi.org/10.1080/14427591.2007.9686588

Egan, M., Kubina, L., Lidstone, R., Macdougall, G., & Raudoy, A. (2010). A critical reflection on occupational therapy within one assertive community treatment team. *Canadian Journal of Occupational Therapy, 77*(2), 70–78. https://doi.org/10.2182/cjot.2010.77.2.2

Egan, M., & Restall, G. (Eds.). (2022). *Promoting occupational participation: Collaborative, relationship-focused occupational therapy.* CAOT Publications ACE.

Fougeyrollas, P., Noreau, L., Bergeron, H., Cloutier, R., Dion, S. A., & St-Michel, G. (1998). Social consequences of long-term impairments and disabilities: Conceptual approach and assessment of handicap. *International Journal of Rehabilitation Research, 21*, 127–141. https://doi.org/10.1097/00004356-199806000-00002

Government of Canada. (2019). *Reclaiming power and place: The final report of the National Inquiry Into Missing and Murdered Indigenous Women and Girls.* https://www.mmiwg-ffada.ca/final-report

Hankivsky, O., & Christoffersen, A. (2008). Intersectionality and the determinants of health: A Canadian perspective. *Critical Public Health, 18*(3), 271–283. https://doi.org/10.1080/09581590802294296

Iwama, M. (1999). Are you listening? Cross-cultural perspectives on client-centred occupational therapy practice: A view from Japan. *Occupational Therapy Now, 1*(6), 4–6. https://doi.org/10.1177/000841740407100203

Iwama, M. (2007). Culture and occupational therapy: Meeting the challenge of relevance in a global world. *Occupational Therapy International, 14*(4), 183–187. https://doi.org/10.1002/oti.234

Jongbloed, L., & Crighton, A. (1990). A new definition of disability: Implications for rehabilitation practice and social policy. *Canadian Journal of Occupational Therapy, 57*, 32–38. https://doi.org/10.1177/000841749005700107

Kielhofner, G. (2008). *Model of Human Occupation: Theory and application* (4th ed.). Lippincott Williams & Wilkins.

Laliberte Rudman, D., Aldrich, R. M., & Kiepek, N. (2022). Evolving understandings of occupation. In M. Egan & G. Restall (Eds.), *Promoting occupational participation: Collaborative relationship-focused occupational therapy* (pp. 11–30). CAOT Publications ACE.

Law, M. (2002). Participation in the occupations of everyday life, 2002 Distinguished Scholar Lecture. *American Journal of Occupational Therapy, 56,* 640–649. https://doi.org/10.5014/ajot.56.6.640

Law, M., Cooper, B., Strong, S., Stewart, D., Rigby, P., & Letts, L. (1996). The Person-Environment-Occupation model: A transactive approach to occupational performance. *Canadian Journal of Occupational Therapy, 63*(1), 9–23. https://doi.org/10.1177/000841749606300103

Lawton, M. P. (1986). *Environment and aging* (2nd ed.). The Center for the Study of Aging.

Lewin, K. (1933). *Dynamic theory of personality.* McGraw-Hill.

Lexen, A., Hofgren, C., & Bejerholm, U. (2013). Support and process in individual placement and support: A multiple case study. *Work, 44,* 435–448. https://doi.org/ 10.3233/WOR-2012-1360

McWha, J. L., Pachana, N. A., & Alpass, F. M. (2003). Exploring the therapeutic environment for older women with late life depression: An examination of the benefits of an activity group for older people suffering from depression. *Australian Occupational Therapy Journal, 50,* 158–169. https://doi.org/10.1046/j.1440-1630.2003.00373.x

Molineux, M. (2004). Occupation in occupational therapy: A labour in vain? In M. Molineux (Ed.), *Occupation for occupational therapists* (pp. 79–88). Blackwell.

Murray, H. (1938). *Explorations in personality.* Oxford University Press.

Nagle, S., Valient Cook, J., & Polatajko, H. (2002). I'm doing as much as I can: Occupational choices of persons with a severe and persistent mental illness. *Journal of Occupational Science, 9*(2), 72–81. https://doi.org/10.1080/14427591.2002.9686495

Nayar, S., Hocking, C., & Giddings, L. (2012). Using occupation to navigate cultural spaces: Indian immigrant women settling into New Zealand. *Journal of Occupational Science, 19*(1), 62–74. https://doi.org/10.1080/14427591.2011.602628

O'Brien, P., Dyck, I., Caron, S., & Mortenson, P. (2002). Environmental analysis: Insights from sociological and geographical perspectives. *Canadian Journal of Occupational Therapy, 69*(4), 229–238. https://doi.org/10.1177/000841740206900407

Parr, H. (2008). *Mental health and social space: Towards inclusionary geographies?* Blackwell Publishing Ltd.

Pongsaksri, A. (2004). *A trans-cultural study of practice of occupational therapists in Thailand and Australia: Reframing theories of practice.* [Doctoral dissertation]. Curtin University of Technology, Thailand.

Raphael, D., Bryant, T., & Rioux, M. (2019). *Staying Alive: Critical perspectives on health, illness, and health care.* Canadian Scholars Press.

Rebeiro, K. L. (2001). Enabling occupation: The importance of an affirming environment. *Canadian Journal of Occupational Therapy: Revue Canadienne d'Ergotherapie, 68*(2), 80–89. https://doi.org/10.1177/000841740106800204

Rebeiro, K. L., Day, D. G., Semeniuk, B., O'Brien, M. C., & Wilson, B. (2001). NISA: An occupation-based, mental health program. *American Journal of Occupational Therapy, 55,* 493–500. https://doi.org/10.5014/ajot.55.5.493

Rebeiro, K. L., & Miller-Polgar, J. (1999). Enabling occupational participation: Optimal experiences in therapy. *Canadian Journal of Occupational Therapy, 66*(1), 14–22. https://doi.org/10.1177/000841749906600102

Rebeiro Gruhl, K. L., Boucher, M., & Lacarte, S. (2020). Evaluation of an occupation-based, mental-health program: Meeting being, belonging and becoming needs. *Australian Occupational Therapy Journal, 68*(1), 78–89. https://doi.org/10.1111/1440-1630.12707

Rebeiro Gruhl, K. L., Kauppi, C., Montgomery, P., & James, S. (2012). Employment services for persons with SMI in northeastern Ontario: The case for partnerships. *WORK: A Journal of Prevention, Assessment & Rehabilitation (IOS Press), 43*(1), 77–89. https://doi.org/10.3233/WOR-2012-1449

Rebeiro Gruhl, K., & Lauckner, H. (2022). Promoting occupational participation with groups. In M. Egan & G. Restall (Eds.), *Promoting occupational participation: Collaborative, relationship-focused occupational therapy* (pp. 167–197). CAOT Publications ACE.

Rigby, P., Stewart, D., & Law, M. (2015, May). *Exploring the theoretical assumptions of the PEO model: Preliminary results.* PowerPoint presentation at the Canadian Association of Occupational Therapists' Annual Conference. Winnipeg, MB, Canada.

Stoffel, V. (2013). Opportunities for occupational therapy behavioral health: A call to action. *American Journal of Occupational Therapy, 67*(2), 140–145. https://doi.org/10.5014/ajot.2013.672001

Strong, S. (1998). Meaningful work in supportive environments: Experiences with the recovery process. *American Journal of Occupational Therapy, 52,* 31–38. https://doi.org/10.5014/ajot.52.1.31

Strong, S., & Letts, L. (2021). Personal narratives of learning self-management: Lessons for practice based on experiences of people with serious mental illness. *Australian Occupational Therapy Journal, 68*(5), 395–406. https://doi.org/10.1111/1440-1630.12748

Strong, S., Rigby, P., Stewart, D., Law, M., Cooper, B., & Letts, L. (1999). The Person-Environment-Occupation model: A practical intervention tool. *Canadian Journal of Occupational Therapy, 66,* 122–133. https://doi.org/10.1177/000841749906600304

Tjornstrand, C., Bejerholm, U., & Eklund, M. (2013). Psychometric testing of a self-report measure of engagement in productive occupations. *Canadian Journal of Occupational Therapy, 80*(2), 101–110. https://doi.org/10.1177/0008417413481956

Trainor, J., Pomeroy, E., & Pape, B. (1983). *A new framework for support for people with serious mental health problems.* Canadian Mental Health Association.

Truth and Reconciliation Commission of Canada. (2017). *Truth and Reconciliation Commission of Canada: Calls to action.* https://ehprnh2mwo3.exactdn.com/wp-content/uploads/2021/01/Calls_to_Action_English2.pdf

Vrkljan, B. H. (2006). *In-vehicle navigation systems and driving safety: The occupational performance of older drivers and passengers—A mixed methods approach.* [Doctoral dissertation]. Rehabilitation Science, University of Western Ontario, Ontario, Canada.

Whalley Hammell, K. (2003). Changing institutional environments to enable occupation among people with severe physical impairments. In L. Letts, P. Rigby, & D. Stewart (Eds.), *Using environments to enable occupational performance* (pp. 35–49). Slack, Inc.

Whalley Hammell, K. (2009). Self-care, productivity, and leisure, or dimensions of occupational experience? Rethinking occupational "categories." *Canadian Journal of Occupational Therapy, 76*(2), 107–114. https://doi.org/10.1177/000841740907600208

Whalley Hammell, K. (2013). Client-centred occupational therapy in Canada: Refocusing on core values. *Canadian Journal of Occupational Therapy, 80,* 141–149. https://doi.org/10.1177/0008417413497906

Whalley Hammell, K. (2015). Client-centred occupational therapy: The importance of critical perspectives. *Scandinavian Journal of Occupational Therapy, 22,* 237–243. https://doi.org/10.3109/11038128.2015.1004103

Whalley Hammell, K. (2017). Opportunities for well-being: The right to occupational engagement. *Canadian Journal of Occupational Therapy (1939), 84*(4-5), 209–222. https://doi.org/10.1177/0008417417734831

World Federation of Occupational Therapists. (2023). *WFOT disaster preparedness and risk reduction manual.* Author. https://wfot.org/resources/wfot-disaster-preparedness-and-risk-reduction-manual

CHAPTER

4

Person-Centered Evaluation

Elena V. Donoso Brown and Jaime Phillip Muñoz

Evaluation is the initial step in the occupational therapy process. Determining who the person is and if there is a need for occupational therapy is the starting point for delivering services. Effective evaluation in mental health practice requires a practitioner to be person-centered in all relationships and to investigate a broad range of factors that may impact occupational functioning (American Occupational Therapy Association [AOTA], 2020d; Canadian Association of Occupational Therapists [CAOT], 2021; World Federation of Occupational Therapists [WFOT], 2016). Person-centered evaluation requires practitioners to intentionally cultivate a manner of thinking, doing, and being that ensures people and their families are acknowledged as the experts in their own lives with a critical voice in the decision-making that informs interventions.

Although a variety of assessments are used as examples, the intent of this chapter is not to provide an exhaustive inventory of assessment tools. Many of the subsequent chapters in this text provide examples of data gathering methods that are specific to the setting or population being discussed in those chapters. In this chapter, the focus is on describing a person-centered evaluation process. The term "practitioner" is used throughout this chapter in accordance with the role and responsibilities outlined by AOTA with the initiation and direction of the evaluation process being the primary role of occupational therapy practitioners (OTPs), with certified occupational therapy *assistants* supporting and collaborating throughout the process (AOTA, 2020b).

Purpose of Evaluation

OTPs can only implement occupational therapy interventions after they complete an evaluation. A practitioner's first task is to understand the person from an occupational perspective in order to then use this understanding to generate an intervention plan and collaborate with the person regarding the outcomes of intervention (AOTA, 2020d). Unless someone is extremely adventurous, they would not take a trip to a foreign place by starting without a map or by jumping on any plane without knowing the plane's destination. In the same way, a practitioner would not begin intervention without an idea of the person's identity and goals. Therefore, the critical first step in the occupational therapy process is to complete a person-centered evaluation.

Within the occupational therapy literature, the terms "evaluation," "assessment," and "outcomes measurement" are often used interchangeably (Kramer & Grampurohit, 2020;

Laver-Fawcett, 2013). For example, the Canadian Practice Process Framework identifies "assess and evaluate" as one action point in the occupational therapy process, during which the practitioner identifies factors that may be challenging the person's occupational performance. The evaluation of outcomes is a separate but related action step in this framework and involves the practitioner making a determination of whether the occupational therapy interventions worked and established goals were met (Polatajko, Craik, et al., 2007; Townsend & Polatajko, 2013).

This chapter utilizes terminology provided in the AOTA *Occupational Therapy Practice Framework (OTPF)*. The *OTPF* defines **evaluation** as the process of data gathering and suggests that evaluation methods vary, but include assessments that measure occupational performance via interviews, self-reports, and direct assessment of specific performance areas (AOTA, 2020d). In the *OTPF*, the measurement of outcomes is defined as the judgment of intervention effectiveness. Table 4-1 provides definitions for common terms used in the evaluation process.

Evaluation is a complex, iterative, multistep process, and each step presents unique challenges to the practitioner. The *OTPF* articulates two key components in this process: an occupational profile and an analysis of occupational performance. The generation of an **occupational profile** begins when the practitioner initiates contact with the person in order to summarize the person's occupational history. Patterns of time use and daily living, roles, goals, values, interests, and culture are some of the lived experiences that influence each person's occupational profile (AOTA, 2020d).

In order to produce an **analysis of occupational performance,** a practitioner may choose to employ a variety of assessment tools including but not limited to interviews, self-reports, and performance assessments to determine the person's current level of occupational performance. An evidence-based practitioner applies therapeutic reasoning skills at multiple decision points throughout the evaluation process (Pépin & Kielhofner, 2017). After gathering data in these areas it is essential that the practitioner interpret and synthesize these data to support personalized recommendations and next steps (AOTA, 2020d).

The overall purpose of evaluation is to generate the most complete and accurate understanding of an individual's occupational profile and performance capabilities. In order to accomplish this, practitioners can structure their initial therapeutic reasoning by answering the guiding questions presented in Box 4-1.

This approach can help a practitioner construct an individual's occupational profile, choose which areas of occupational performance to focus on during the evaluation, and help establish a baseline from which to document progress and reason about the person's prognosis and potential for improvement.

TABLE 4-1 | Key Terms in Evaluation

Term	Definition
Evaluation	An ongoing process that consists of two components, the occupational profile to identify what the person needs and wants to do and the analysis of occupational performance that identifies what the person can do and what barriers to occupational performance exist (AOTA, 2020d)
Assessment	A tool that is designed to support the evaluation process through observation, inquiry, and measurement (AOTA, 2020d)
Outcome measurement	A process designed to capture what resulted from occupational therapy intervention. The *OTPF* outlines several general categories that can be considered outcomes for occupational therapy practice. These include occupational performance, prevention, health and wellness, quality of life, participation, role competence, well-being, and occupational justice (AOTA, 2020d)
Reevaluation	Process used to determine the amount of change a person has made (AOTA, 2020d)
Reassessment	The use of nonstandardized or standardized assessments after initial evaluation to determine current performance (Kramer & Grampurohit, 2020)
Therapeutic reasoning	A process of synthesizing information about the person's identity, occupations, and environments to design occupational therapy interventions that are creative and meaningful to the individual (Clifford O'Brien et al., 2023)

BOX 4-1 ■ Guiding Questions When Initiating the Evaluation Process

- What is this person's identity and occupational history (i.e., life story, experiences, cultural background, current and past life roles)?

- What concerns or challenges to engaging in occupations bring this person to occupational therapy?

- What factors in the environment support what this person is doing, being, or becoming?

- What barriers in the environment get in the way of participation?

- What does this person most want and need to do? What are this person's key priorities?

- Would this person benefit from occupational therapy?

Evaluation as a Process

Evaluation is a process of continuous information gathering, as in a single meeting the OTP will only learn a part of a person's story and abilities. Initiating an evaluation process always goes before intervention planning (AOTA, 2020d; Chisholm & Boyt Schell, 2014); however, the evaluation process rarely goes in a linear manner, and many factors influence the process. The evaluation process requires practitioners to reflect on their interactions with a person and synthesize data from a variety of assessments to allow their understanding of the person to become fuller and more nuanced.

In the evaluation process, art and science are present in the practitioner's abilities to pick the right tool at the right time for the right reason based on their synthesis of what is known and unknown about the person they are working with (Mattingly, 1991; Rogers, 1983). The artistry is seen when practitioners use tacit knowledge and imagination when deciding how to proceed with a particular person and when collaboratively envisioning the next chapter with the person (Mattingly, 1991). Scientific reasoning can be seen when practitioners apply practical knowledge, evidence, and occupational therapy theories into the evaluation process. The consideration of multiple factors that are often changing is the primary reason the evaluation process does not always proceed in a clear linear fashion. The factors that can influence the evaluation process are illustrated in Figure 4-1.

To illustrate these factors, consider this scenario. Imagine that a practitioner works in a locked, acute psychiatric unit that has an average length of stay of 7 days, during which the focus of intervention is to evaluate, titrate medications as appropriate, reduce symptomatology, and facilitate discharge to the most appropriate, least restrictive intervention setting. Xiaoyu is a 23-year-old international male college student from China who demonstrates significant paranoid

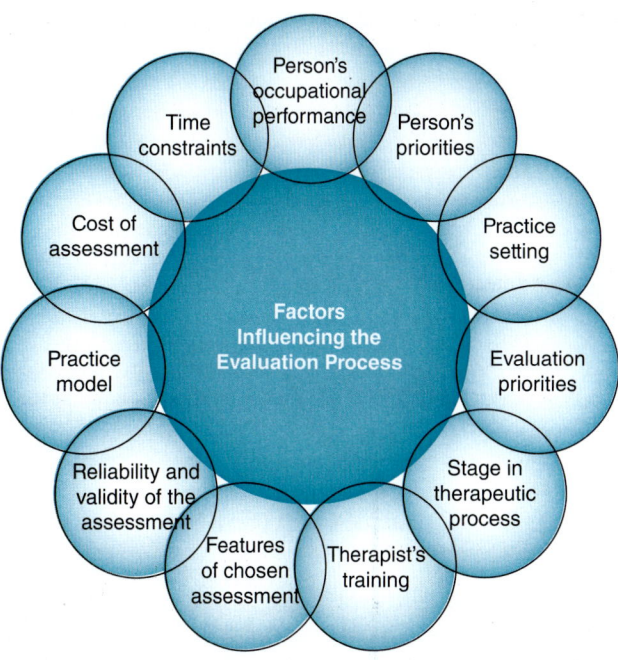

FIGURE 4-1. Factors influencing the evaluation process. Because multiple factors that are often changing must be considered, the evaluation process does not always proceed in a clear linear fashion.

symptoms. He has been placed on constant observation because of his suicidal ideation. In this example, multiple factors could influence the evaluation process. Some of these include the practice setting; the focus of intervention within this setting; occupational therapy's role within the multidisciplinary team; personal factors such as age, language capacities, and culture of Xiaoyu; and his presenting symptomatology.

More specifically, the practice setting influences the amount of time a practitioner has to complete an evaluation. In addition, Xiaoyu's personal factors will influence the assessment tools selected, as the practitioner will want to ensure validity in a similar population.

Evaluation begins when the person is referred to the practitioner and ends with discharge and the cessation of all follow-up interventions. Although the logistics and mechanics of the evaluation process depend on the practice setting, the process often unfolds in a predictable pattern (Chisholm & Boyt Schell, 2014; Shotwell, 2014). A visual depiction of the key steps in the evaluation process is provided in Figure 4-2.

From the beginning, the practitioner should consider what data exist, what data are needed to understand the person and begin intervention, and what data can be collected that will help measure outcomes of the intervention for this person and the program. When those elements are clear, evaluation can proceed. The practitioner then chooses evidence-based and person-centered assessments and begins the evaluation process with the goal of creating an occupational profile of the person. With a clearer picture of the person, more information on the analysis of occupational performance is gathered, in which case the practitioner chooses additional assessments to gain information on specific areas of occupational performance.

A synthesis of all available data and collaboration with the person helps set goals and form the initial intervention plan. Finally, after some amount of intervention, the practitioner reevaluates the plan as appropriate. Each step of the evaluation process in Figure 4-2 is expanded upon in the following sections, and key considerations and therapeutic reasoning questions for each step are discussed.

Screen Data to Guide Therapeutic Reasoning

When initiating the occupational therapy process, some of the first questions a practitioner will ask are: "Who is this person?" and "What information about this person do I already have?" The practitioner begins to answer these questions by screening the existing data. In settings in which written data exist, a practitioner may review these data before meeting the person. In a hospital setting, this often includes a review of the medical record, which may include the person's medical, psychiatric, social, and family history. In a school setting, a review of the individualized education plan (IEP) or school file can be a logical place to begin the data gathering process. In a community-based setting, the comprehensiveness of record-keeping may vary widely, but can include demographic, social history, and/or program eligibility data.

In some situations, abundant data may be available, and a practitioner's plan for evaluation can be tailored to address specific gaps in the data that, if collected, would help create a more robust picture of the person's occupational profile. It is just as likely, however, that there is limited data available or a review of the existing data leads the practitioner to question whether occupational therapy is warranted or whether the person can effectively participate in the evaluation process. In such situations, a brief in-person screening may help the practitioner determine the best evaluation plan.

In mental health practice, an informal screening can be as simple as the practitioner stopping by the room for a quick introduction and closely observing social, cognitive, emotional, and physical cues. In some situations, it may include observing the person completing a task. For example, consider this scenario. Mauve was just admitted to a neurocognitive unit specializing in addressing the needs of older adults.

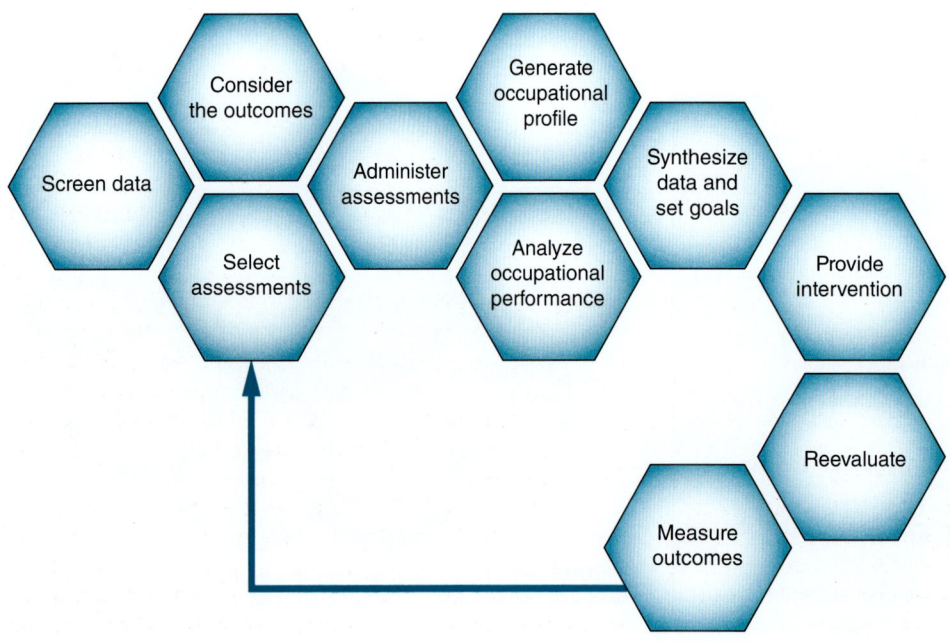

FIGURE 4-2. Key steps in the evaluation process. The logistics and mechanics of the evaluation process depend on the individual and the practice setting, but the process often unfolds in a predictable pattern.

Mauve is a 67-year-old widow with a diagnosis of depression and with suspected dementia. A review of her records includes some data on her past and current medical diagnoses. There are no data describing Mauve's social history or her current or past role performances. Her records provide no information regarding her expected discharge environment. After identifying the gaps related to information about her occupational profile and performance, it would be important to screen Mauve to determine whether her current symptomatology prohibits her from active participation in the evaluation process.

One way to do this is through a deeper dive into the chart and seeing if any screening or evaluation has already occurred. Upon chart review, it is seen that the neuropsychologist has met with Mauve already and completed the Montreal Cognitive Assessment (MoCA), a short screening that assesses several cognitive domains (Nasreddine et al., 2005). The Beck Depression Inventory-Second Version (BDI-II), which is a screening designed to measure the severity of depression (Beck et al., 1996), was also completed. Mauve's scores reflect mild cognitive impairment and moderate levels of depression.

Even with these additional data about cognition and affect, it is difficult to create a comprehensive picture of Mauve's occupational profile and performance. A practitioner who was thinking about using an interview to begin the evaluation process would review these new data and instead decide to use an in-person screening to determine the next steps in the evaluation process.

Based on the previously presented therapeutic reasoning, the practitioner wants to first get to know Mauve by using a screen to determine if an interview would be appropriate. This begins with an informal observation of Mauve on the unit and discussion with the team. Through these screening mechanisms it appears that she is improving, likely because of the structure and routine of the acute hospital unit. Mauve is experiencing a decrease in depressive symptomatology and improvements in global cognitive functioning. Next, the OTP meets directly with Mauve and confirms that an interview can be a useful way to gain information. Therefore, the practitioner uses an informal interview to build rapport and gain a comprehensive understanding of Mauve's occupational profile and historical occupational performances.

As one can see through this story, the evaluation process requires consideration of multiple factors. The use of therapeutic reasoning to determine the next steps is critical to determining the choice of assessments. Also of note is the use of formal (i.e., MoCA, BDI-II) and informal screening tools (i.e., informal observations, team conversations) as they supported therapeutic reasoning throughout the evaluation initiation.

Consider Key Outcomes

From the start, it is important for the practitioner to identify areas that stand out as particular concerns voiced by the individual and to consider what end results therapy can achieve. Creek provides a simple, person-centered definition that states **outcomes** are an "agreed, clearly defined, expected or desired result of intervention" (2003, p. 56). At the beginning of the evaluation process the practitioner should consider the key areas that will be the focus for outcome evaluation

in order to select tools that are appropriate for measuring these outcomes and monitoring change. The *OTPF* provides guidance on this subject and identifies common areas of outcome evaluation for OTPs, such as gains in occupational performance and improvements in quality of life (AOTA, 2020d).

Specific areas of outcome evaluation can also be identified within a practice setting. For example, in an inpatient mental health setting that treats persons with severe and persistent mental illness, an occupational therapy program may focus on improvements in cognition, activities of daily living (ADLs) and instrumental activities of daily living (IADLs), physical health, and/or personal goal attainment. These outcomes may be relevant for a majority of individuals in this setting and may be areas the occupational therapy program specifically addresses before discharge. Considering key outcomes early in the evaluation process facilitates the selection of tools for evaluation that can capture data needed to assess both individual and program level outcomes.

Select Assessments

Assessments are tools, and a critical step in the practitioner's therapeutic reasoning is choosing the right tools—the right tool for the right reason at the right time. Readers can likely recall a time when they needed a hammer but one was not available, so instead of using a hammer they used something else, such as a shoe, rock, or stapler. These alternatives may have worked but likely not as effectively as a hammer. The point is that there are several valid and reliable tools for practitioners to use to gather data. The task is to choose the tool that is designed to gain the needed data and, if possible, demonstrate the effectiveness of occupational therapy practice.

There are typically three elements that should be considered when selecting an assessment for use in an evaluation: utility, validity, and reliability. **Utility** is a practitioner's judgment as to whether a particular assessment tool is useful in a particular setting for a particular person and whether the practitioner has the skill sets to competently administer and interpret the results of the assessment. Utility is often one of the first components considered when choosing assessments. This is because if a tool is impractical, because of factors such as time constraints, cost, or the practitioner's experience with the tool, it likely won't be a good choice.

The characteristics of the person can also influence the utility of an assessment. Think back to the story of Mauve. On admission, she presented with significant confusion and depressive symptomatology; therefore, a tool requiring an element of self-awareness would have poor utility. Culture is another characteristic of the person that can influence utility. When choosing an assessment tool, a practitioner needs to consider whether the tool is consistent with the person's cultural background. If it is an assessment using normative scoring processes, it is useful only if it has been validated using a representative sample inclusive of people similar to the individual the OTP is evaluating.

When choosing an assessment, the practitioner should consider a tool's **validity** to ensure the assessment has demonstrated the ability to measure the desired construct. In other words, choosing a valid tool is important because if the OTP is looking to measure a person's cognition, choosing

Evidence-Based Practice

Montreal Cognitive Assessment (MoCA)

The MoCA proves to be an effective tool for identifying individuals with mild cognitive impairment.

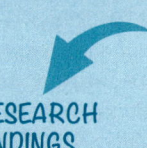

RESEARCH FINDINGS

The MoCA is a performance-based assessment that was developed to screen individuals for mild cognitive impairment. It was originally paper-and-pencil based but now also has an electronic version (MoCA Cognition, 2023). The MoCA has been examined for its validity and diagnostic accuracy and has been tested in populations with mental health conditions such as dementia (Islam et al., 2023), schizophrenia (e.g., Ramírez et al., 2014), depression (e.g., Blair et al., 2016), and substance use (e.g., Ko et al., 2022). As the MoCA is a screening tool, if an individual scores below the cutoff of 26, additional assessment with a more robust cognitive assessment may be utilized to better understand the nature of the cognitive impairment. It is also important to note that in order to ensure the integrity of administration of the paper-based test, creators of the MoCA require completion of the official training and certification (MoCA Cognition, 2023).

APPLICATIONS

➡ The MoCA is a quick, performance-based screening tool that can indicate if an individual is experiencing mild cognitive impairment.

➡ The sensitivity and specificity of the MoCA as well as its predictive properties have been studied in certain populations with mental health issues.

➡ Completing the required training will ensure that the assessment is administered correctly and that the screening provides the most accurate information.

REFERENCES

Blair, M., Coleman, K., Jesso, S., Desbeaumes Jodoin, V., Smolewska, K., Warriner, E., Finger, E., & Pasternak, S. H. (2016). Depressive symptoms negatively impact Montreal Cognitive Assessment performance: A memory clinic experience. *The Canadian Journal of Neurological Sciences, 43*(4), 513–517. https://doi.org/10.1017/cjn.2015.399

Islam, N., Hashem, R., Gad, M., Brown, A., Levis, B., Renoux, C., Thombs, B. D., & McInnes, M. D. (2023). Accuracy of the Montreal Cognitive Assessment tool for detecting mild cognitive impairment: A systematic review and meta-analysis. *Alzheimer's & Dementia, 19*(7), 3235–3243. https://doi.org/10.1002/alz.13040

Ko, K. Y., Ridley, N., Bryce, S. D., Allott, K., Smith, A., & Kamminga, J. (2022). Screening tools for cognitive impairment in adults with substance use disorders: A systematic review. *Journal of the International Neuropsychological Society, 28*(7), 756–779. https://doi.org/10.1017/S135561772100103X

MoCA Cognition. (2023). *Training and certification.* https://mocacognition.com/training-certification

Ramírez, L. R., Saracco-Álvarez, R., Escamilla-Orozco, R., & Orellana, A. F. (2014). Validity of the Montreal Cognitive Assessment scale (MoCA) for the detection of cognitive impairment in schizophrenia. *Salud Mental, 4*(37), 517–522. https://doi.org/10.17711/SM.0185-3325.2014.062

a tool that measures mood or sensory perception would be an inappropriate choice that would not support effective intervention planning.

In addition, considering a tool's **reliability** is especially crucial when choosing assessments because a practitioner wants to be confident that the tool selected is a precise measure. There are several types of reliability that can be considered when choosing an assessment. Consideration of how the tool is going to be used in practice can help determine which properties of reliability may be the most important to one's therapeutic reasoning. Table 4-2 outlines properties to consider when choosing an assessment.

Also see Chapter 6: Evidence-Based Practice for more detailed information on evaluating evidence related to assessments. 🤝

Consideration of utility, validity, and reliability when choosing assessments to include in an evaluation will ensure that a practitioner is able to obtain an accurate measurement of the desired construct using a method that is a good fit for the person and setting. As the evaluation process unfolds, a practitioner's intentional choice of the right assessments will help construct a robust description of the person's occupational profile and current occupational performance. This then supports the generation of goals that are most

TABLE 4-2 | Psychometric Properties to Consider When Choosing an Assessment

Intended Use of Tool	Property of Reliability	Rationale for Use
Intake measure	Internal consistency	Shows that all the items in a tool are measuring a single construct
	Rater reliability (inter and intra)	Can be confident the information the OTP is getting at intake is reliable regardless of who completes the assessment
Outcome measure	Test-retest reliability	Can be confident a measure is stable over a time when change is not expected
	Rater reliability (inter and intra)	Can be confident the information the OTP is getting at intake is reliable regardless of who completes the assessment
	Responsiveness	Can be confident the measure will show a change after intervention, if a change has occurred
	Standard error of measurement	Can identify how much error is likely present in this observed score
	Minimal clinically important difference (MCID)	Can identify if a change is clinically important
Diagnostic tool	Internal consistency	Shows that all the items are measuring a single construct
	Sensitivity/Specificity	Demonstrates the tool's ability to diagnose a condition
Use by multiple therapists	Interrater reliability	Useful when it is important or essential that two or more therapists assign similar ratings to performance

Note: Detailed descriptions of these types of reliability may be found in several of the references provided in the Resources section at the end of this chapter.

Brown, C. (2022). The evidence-based practitioner: Applying research to meet client needs (2nd ed.). F.A. Davis.

Law, M. C., & MacDermid, J. (Eds.). (2014). Evidence-based rehabilitation: A guide to practice (3rd ed.). Slack, Inc.

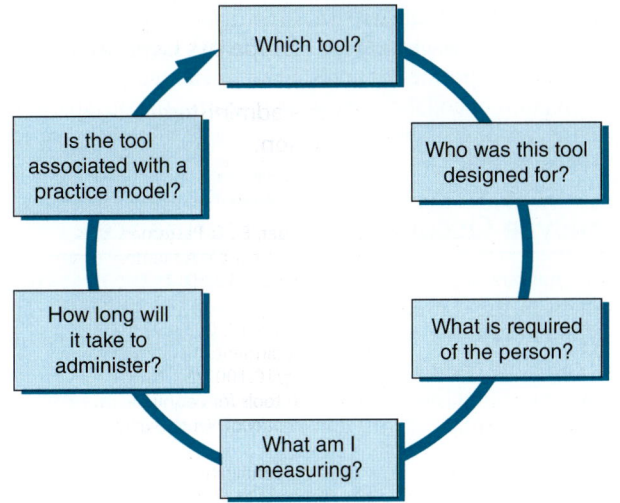

FIGURE 4-3. Choosing an assessment tool. As the evaluation process unfolds, a practitioner's intentional choice of the right assessment tools will help construct a person's occupational profile and current occupational performance, which will then support the generation of meaningful goals.

meaningful to the person. Figure 4-3 provides some questions to consider when selecting an assessment tool.

Administer Assessments

After a tool has been selected, a practitioner must ensure competency in the administration of the tool before using it. If training is required to administer the tool, this should be done as directed by the assessment developer. If no formal training is required, the practitioner should first read the manual and observe a competent practitioner administer the tool. This should be followed by several practice administrations and scorings. Finally, a novice evaluator should be observed by a practitioner competent in the administration of the tool. Observation can help determine if competency has been achieved and allow the observer to provide feedback to the novice administrator. The process of establishing competency in a tool is an ethical responsibility of the evaluator. If a practitioner is not competent in administering an assessment, the analysis of the data and the recommendations made based on the data gathered from that tool may be faulty and lead to poor intervention planning.

Once competency is established, another ethical component of assessment delivery is to obtain consent from the person being assessed. The principle of autonomy in the AOTA *Code of Ethics* (AOTA, 2020c) addresses consent, stipulating that, relative to assessment, it is the practitioner's responsibility to ensure that the person is informed of the assessment's purpose, its procedures, and how the information will be used. This needs to be done in language the person will understand, and the right to decline the assessment must be respected. If an individual is not capable of understanding or making those decisions, the person responsible, such as a spouse, partner, or family member with the power of attorney, should be provided with the same information and allowed to make the decision on behalf of the person.

Once competency and consent are established, the practitioner can prepare to administer the assessment. The initial steps in preparation are to set up the testing environment and gather any materials needed for the assessment. When delivering standardized assessments it is important that the practitioner be prepared to follow the procedures outlined in the manual, which may include providing only a certain amount of verbal or behavioral cues or following a script. A practitioner who is well prepared to deliver an assessment can facilitate smooth data gathering and decrease elements of error related to the environment or improper administration or scoring.

Being prepared for assessment administration requires the practitioner to anticipate factors that could impact administration. For example, if the person has begun a new medication that may cause drowsiness, the practitioner can adjust the assessment schedule to improve the opportunity for valid data gathering. However, it is not always possible to predict every potential complication.

The practitioner must be prepared to manage and adapt as needed to accommodate unexpected occurrences. For example, the practitioner may wish to gather an occupational profile and perceived occupational performance using a semi-structured interview tool, but during administration the interviewee may struggle to generate occupational challenges independently. The practitioner has several different options to manage this situation including providing choices of occupations to the person, switching to a different tool, or making the data gathering more informal. The practitioner will need to make a decision quickly in these situations and consider many of the factors listed previously in Figure 4-1.

Another key component of effective assessment administration is the practitioner's capacity to elicit a person's active engagement in the evaluation process. It is important that the practitioner develop a strong rapport with the person in order to allow for assessment tools to be successfully delivered. This is especially important when using tools such as interviews or self-reports. In order to establish rapport, the practitioner should be aware of the nonverbal signs and signals being sent to the person. Extrinsic signs of professionalism that can support the evaluation process and development of rapport include maintaining an open and welcoming posture, eye contact, and active listening (DeIuliis, 2017). Effective use of these approaches will support communication and enhance the evaluation process. Figure 4-4 illustrates nonverbal behaviors that can facilitate engagement in the evaluation process and those that can act as barriers to the process.

After an assessment is administered, it is scored. The score(s) is then interpreted by an OTP. A competent practitioner will have practiced scoring the chosen assessments; however, a good practice for the evaluator is to constantly be vigilant for the possibility of scoring error. Scoring errors can include a rater being too lenient, too severe, or inconsistent in

the use of a scoring protocol (Kramer & Grampurohit, 2020). Procedures for scoring and measurement scales vary by assessment. Again, ethical practice requires a practitioner to study assessment manuals, practice, and ensure competency in scoring and interpretation of assessment results.

Generate an Occupational Profile

After administering, scoring, and interpreting the assessment(s), the OTP considers all the collected data to generate an occupational profile. According to the *OTPF* a complete occupational profile presents a picture of the person's unique values, beliefs, roles, habits, and routines and is an essential component of every evaluation (AOTA, 2020d). Through the construction of an occupational profile the practitioner gains an understanding of a person's identity and occupations of importance. In addition, the person and the practitioner can begin to identify intervention priorities and the key desired outcomes of therapy.

To support practitioners in developing this key piece of an evaluation, AOTA created an occupational profile template that includes essential components drawn from the *OTPF* (AOTA, 2020a). This template structures the process to ensure the profile a practitioner generates elicits the person's report; gathers data about the person's environment; elicits the person's goals; and considers cultural, personal, temporal, and virtual contexts that support or create barriers to occupational engagement (AOTA, 2020a). Generation of the occupational profile supports person-centered practice and the creation of collaborative goals. Data for the occupational profile can be gathered using a variety of methods that are discussed in the last section of this chapter.

Analyze Occupational Performance

The analysis of occupational performance is the next component in the evaluation process defined by the *OTPF*. The *OTPF* (AOTA, 2020d) identifies several methods to gather data for this component of evaluation; however, one of the first tools a practitioner can use to generate data is observation of performance. For example, recall in the story of Mauve

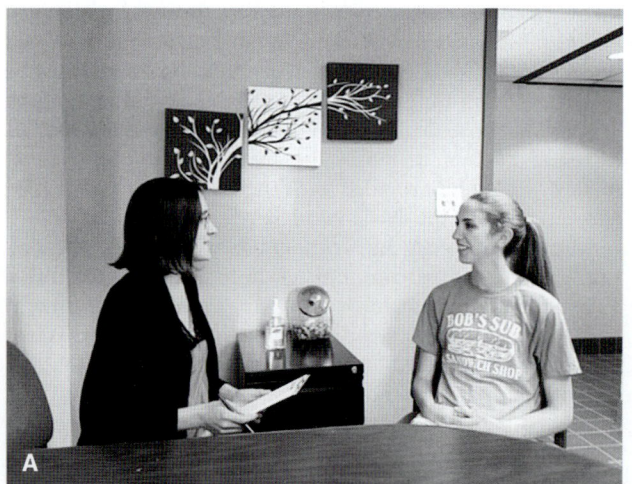 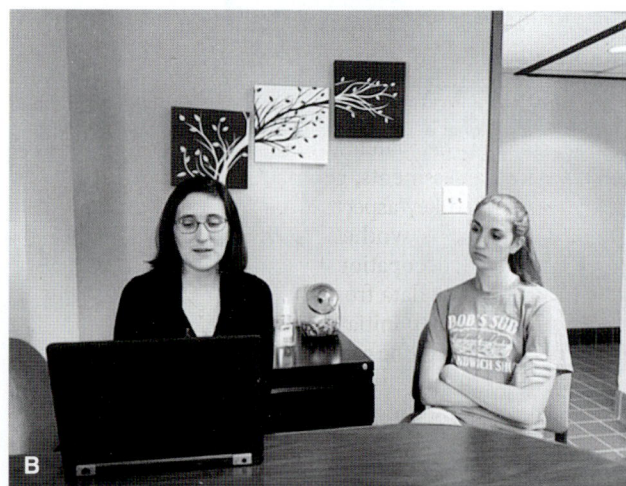

FIGURE 4-4. Nonverbal behaviors in the administration of an assessment tool. (A). The use of nonverbal behaviors that facilitate engagement in the evaluation process (e.g., eye contact, positive facial expression, and open body posture). (B). Nonverbal behaviors that can act as barriers (e.g., body turned away from person, engagement with device instead of person, and no eye contact).

that the practitioner used ongoing informal observations to assess changes in Mauve's cognitive and emotional functioning and that one of the reasons for Mauve's admission was to rule out dementia. Recall also that the evaluation process can be considered both an art and a science. Practitioners synthesizing these initial cues could reason that cognition, ability to care for self, and her surroundings and safety may all be areas to target in an evaluation with Mauve.

A critical aspect of therapeutic reasoning in this stage of the evaluation process is the practitioner's decision-making regarding which components of a person's occupational performance are most likely to impact participation in occupations. A focused analysis of these occupational performance areas ensures that the practitioner identifies those areas that (a) are most important to the person and (b) may benefit most from occupational therapy intervention. In Mauve's story we learned that, on admission, her cognitive functioning was screened with the MoCA. To complete a deeper evaluation of cognition a practitioner may choose a more robust functional assessment such as the Allen Cognitive Level (Allen et al., 2007), the Executive Function Performance Test (Baum & Edwards, 1993), or the Performance Assessment of Self-care Skills (PASS; Chisholm et al., 2014).

On the other hand, if it became clear that Mauve would return to live alone and the team wanted to be confident that Mauve could safely live independently and manage daily living tasks, then the OTP might select an assessment such as the Kohlman Evaluation of Living Skills (Kohlman Thompson & Robnett, 2016), which was designed as a quick screening of a person's independence when performing a variety of living skills. Other options include the Test of Grocery Shopping Skills (Brown et al., 2009), which is designed to examine performance and cognitive functioning in a natural community environment, or the Texas Functional Living Scale (Cullum et al., 2009), an observation-based rating scale designed to evaluate a person's independence when performing IADLs.

Ultimately, the information a practitioner is able to analyze regarding occupational performance is highly dependent upon what tools were selected earlier in the process. The information gained through the scoring and interpretation of scores requires therapeutic reasoning and shapes how all the pieces of information gained during the evaluation are put together in the next step.

Synthesize Data and Set Goals

At this stage in the evaluation process the practitioner has administered assessments, generated the occupational profile, and analyzed key aspects of occupational performance. These data must be synthesized to inform the creation of person-centered, occupation-focused goals and intervention plans. Synthesizing data from multiple sources is a complex task. In general, when initiating a synthesis of the data it may be useful to return to the guiding questions posed in Box 4-1.

Recall that these questions were designed to help a practitioner initiate the process of formulating an occupational profile. Synthesis of data is supported when the practitioner considers the person's strengths and areas in which occupational performance is challenged, including the identification of specific skills, factors, and contexts that impact performance. This process of summarizing the person's performance is enhanced when a theoretical model is used to support the organization of key pieces of data about the person's occupational profile, current occupational performance, and environmental and social context. The use of models to support the evaluation process is discussed in detail later in this chapter. An effective synthesis of the data informs goal setting and, subsequently, intervention planning.

Goals within occupational therapy should be relevant, valued by the person, and focused on function to ultimately improve an individual's occupational performance, well-being, and participation. It is also important that these goals be measurable so that progress toward them can be monitored. Goal setting is evidence of a complete initial evaluation and should reflect the data that were gathered while generating an occupational profile and analyzing occupational performance. A framework that is commonly used by a variety of health-care professionals, including OTPs, is to write goals using the SMART goal model (Bailey, 2019). In this method, S = Specific, M = Measurable, A = Attainable, R = Relevant, and T = Time. Constructing SMART goals can help practitioners document the intended outcomes of therapy and help engage the person in a goal-setting process that provides a roadmap for collaboration in therapy.

For example, if a person with depression wants to reengage in former leisure pursuits related to art, a practitioner could write: "In two weeks, Jo will make art for at least 60 minutes/week with no more than two verbal cues." The goal is SMART as it is clear, because it indicates what leisure activity is of interest, and it states the parameters that are needed to be met in order to say this goal was accomplished.

However, before the practitioner can establish a goal with the person, the focus of the intervention must be defined. Novice practitioners are sometimes concerned when their synthesis of the assessment data reveals multiple areas that may simultaneously need intervention. The challenge is where to begin. Person-centered goal setting begins with the person. A skillful therapist can collaboratively define the specific outcome for goal attainment by engaging the person in a conversation in which the person answers questions such as (Egan, 2006):

- How will it look when this problem situation is being managed more effectively?
- What will you be doing or not doing that will help manage this situation better?
- What habits or patterns of doing will be in place that are not in place now?
- What will you be doing differently in the relationships in your life?
- What changes in your current lifestyle are you most willing to commit to?

The reflective questions in Table 4-3 can also help guide a practitioner's therapeutic reasoning and support the prioritization of intervention goals.

Provide Intervention and Reevaluate

Completion of an initial evaluation and identification of goals is not the end of the evaluation process. Evaluation continues throughout the occupational therapy process. The *OTPF* (AOTA, 2020d) states that periodic reevaluation is a key step for monitoring a person's response to intervention. The results of a reevaluation can lead to a change in the intervention

TABLE 4-3	Prioritizing Goals Using Therapeutic Reasoning
Goal Component	**Therapeutic Reasoning Questions**
Urgency	• Is the problem situation urgent? • Does it cause a high level of distress? • Does it occur frequently?
Importance	• Is this a problem situation the person feels is so important? • Is the person motivated to act on it?
Timing	• Is this a problem situation that can be managed now? • Does the person currently have the resources to address this situation now?
Complexity	• Is this a complex problem situation with many parts? • Can the situation be divided into more manageable parts?
Success	• Is there a high probability that addressing this problem situation can lead to success?
Spread effect	• Which of the problem situations, if it was managed, could lead to improvements in other parts of the person's life situation?
Control	• Is this a problem situation that is under the person's control? • Does action to address this situation require that someone other than the person take action?
Cost/Benefits	• Do the benefits of working on this problem outweigh the costs in time, stress, effort, or impact on relationships?

plan. Reevaluating also helps the practitioner develop a deeper understanding of the person through continued development of the occupational profile and further analysis of occupational performance.

Each time a practitioner engages the person there is an opportunity for formal or informal assessment. That is, in some therapy sessions the practitioner may choose an assessment that can focus on a specific performance skill to determine progress. In other situations, a more informal interactive assessment approach can be used within therapy to gather more information about an individual's occupational history, current roles, and routines, or to determine the impact of cognitive and environmental cues on a person's occupational performance. The key point is that each therapeutic encounter offers an opportunity to add to what was gained in the initial evaluation. Reevaluation requires an ongoing synthesis of all available data and ensures the practitioner is constantly building a deeper understanding of the person, which in turn influences intervention.

The reevaluation process is especially important when individuals are not able to provide a complete occupational profile or analysis of performance during the initial screen or evaluation. In these situations, practitioners use data from the initial evaluation to springboard intervention but then continue building on the occupational profile and comparing the analysis of occupational performance with what was completed in the initial evaluation. In this way, the initial evaluation also acts as a reference point for comparison

during these subsequent analyses of performance during the intervention review.

Measure Outcomes

Outcome measurement is another critical part of the evaluation process. This step determines whether the intervention is effective for the person or if a new strategy needs to be implemented in the intervention phase to affect change. In short, reliable outcome measurement justifies the interventions the practitioner is using. In addition, through the use of reliable and valid outcome measures, practitioners are able to build the body of evidence that supports occupational therapy practice (Law et al., 2016).

Recall that one of the initial steps in the evaluation process is to consider key outcomes. The use of reliable and valid assessments in the evaluation process supports outcome measurement. These practices allow for the measurement of change over time and provide one form of evidence that can support practice. OTPs have recognized the key importance of outcomes measurement for a long time. Christensen, as cited in Kielhofner, stated, "Without the development of a research base to refine and provide evidence about the value of its practice, occupational therapy simply will not survive, much less thrive as a health profession" (2006, p. 4). For this reason, many chapters in this text present a variety of tools that can be implemented within mental health practice to not only create occupational profiles and assess occupational performance, but to measure outcomes related to interventions for occupational performance. Measuring outcomes is a critical aspect of the evaluation process that must be engaged in by all practitioners.

Applying Therapeutic Reasoning During the Evaluation Process

Earlier in this chapter, multiple factors that can impact a practitioner's decision-making during the evaluation process were presented. Throughout this chapter, consideration of these factors is discussed as an element of the practitioner's decision-making process and is described as **therapeutic reasoning.** Multiple definitions of clinical reasoning exist in the occupational therapy literature, but the term therapeutic reasoning is intentionally used here for two reasons. First, the term therapeutic reasoning highlights a person-centered approach derived from an interaction process between the practitioner and the person that is grounded in mutuality and collaboration (Clifford O'Brien et al., 2023). It emphasizes that therapeutic interactions are those that prioritize the person's circumstances and wishes. The term therapeutic reasoning is also used in place of clinical reasoning because much of occupational therapy mental health practice does not occur in a clinic; for some practitioners, the term clinical is associated with a medical model and diagnostic reasoning processes.

On the other hand, the term therapeutic reasoning implies the practitioner's intentional use of a practice model to guide decision-making and "use theory to understand a client and to develop, implement and monitor a plan of therapy with a client" (Forsyth, 2017, p. 159). Kielhofner (1992) argued that

TABLE 4-4 | Therapeutic Reasoning Throughout the Evaluation Process

Component	Purpose	Guiding Questions for Therapeutic Reasoning
Screen data	• Establish if the person can participate in the evaluation process and benefit from occupational therapy.	• Does the referral list specific concerns? • Have there been recent changes in occupational performance, living situation, or health status? • Does this person need occupational therapy services?
Consider key outcomes	• Establish indicators that reflect therapy-influenced positive change.	• What are the target areas of intervention for this person? • What data do I need to provide evidence of program effectiveness? • What outcome areas are present for a majority of our patients that we want to measure?
Choose assessment(s)	• Intentionally choose assessments based on the person, setting, and circumstances of therapy.	• What data from the screening help define my approach to the person? • Given the person and the context, which valid and reliable assessments could elicit the occupational performance data I need the most? • Do these tools take into account the person's culture or cultural identities? • Is this tool practical for use in my current practice setting?
Administer assessment(s)	• Effectively and efficiently collect valid and reliable data.	• Am I qualified to administer the assessment? • Have I obtained the consent necessary to complete this assessment? • Are there precautions to consider? • Is the testing environment set up to support success of the person and reduce error?
Generate an occupational profile	• Establish a synopsis of the person's occupational history and patterns of performance.	• Who is this person? • Are there other relevant sources of data (e.g., caregivers, spouse or partner, other professionals/staff) that I need to consider? • What are this person's patterns of occupational performance through time? • What are key occupations of priority?
Analyze occupational performance	• Determine a person's capacities.	• In order to understand this person, what key areas of occupational performance do I most need to know about? • What performance abilities may interfere the most with this person's most valued occupations?
Synthesize data and set goals	• Use data from assessments, in collaboration with the person, to make informed decisions about therapy.	• Have I adequately identified the person's strengths, areas of need, and priorities for intervention? • What practice model is guiding my therapeutic reasoning around intervention planning? • What, if any, referrals to other professionals should be considered?
Provided intervention and reevaluate	• Reevaluate or reassess the person after a certain period of time of intervention to monitor the progress or increase understanding of the person.	• Have more recent observations led me to believe a deeper understanding of a particular construct is needed? • Are there components of the occupational profile that require expansion? • Are there areas of occupational performance that need further in-depth analysis to determine the root cause?
Measure outcomes	• Compare findings of tools across time with support adjustments in individual plans of care as well as programmatic changes.	• Do the tools used have established reliability and validity for the populations we see most often at my setting? • How do we build outcome measures into our processes to ensure reliable data gathering?

a key measure of the usefulness of an occupational therapy practice model was the ability of the model to guide a practitioner's decisions, including the provision of assessment tools that supported reasoning with the model's constructs.

Again, the evaluation process is not linear. Each aspect of the evaluation process requires the OTP to reason therapeutically so that the outcome of evaluation is that the practitioner understands the person—even individuals who may be nonverbal or currently unable to engage in the evaluation or actively collaborate in the development, implementation, and monitoring of the intervention plan. Table 4-4 reviews components of the evaluation process and provides questions for a practitioner to use as a therapeutic reasoning guide.

Validating Therapeutic Reasoning

Recall that gathering a complete occupational picture of an individual is an ongoing part of the therapeutic process that begins with looking at available records on an individual. The following are three key strategies that an OTP can use to increase the clarity of that picture: triangulating the data, performing validity checks, and using valid and reliable tools.

Triangulating Data

Triangulation is a strategy often used in qualitative research that requires a researcher to complete data collection or data analysis in a way that gathers multiple perspectives. In occupational therapy evaluation, triangulation can be completed by putting together the data from the individual's medical chart, data collected with the person during the initial evaluation, and information collected from a family member, friend, or another member of the health-care team. By putting all these pieces of information together from multiple vantage points, an OTP is more likely to gain greater insight into the person's identity and occupational performance and understand where pieces of this picture may be unclear or missing.

Performing Validity Checks

The second strategy that can be implemented also stems from qualitative research and involves validity checks, which are part of a process of interpretation, reflection, and questioning that allows the OTP to ensure that what is being observed is accurate (Kielhofner & Forsyth, 2001). In practice, this can occur after an OTP has observed an individual completing an activity, such as money management, in which the person continues to repeat the same mistake on multiple trials. The practitioner through observation notes that the individual is repeatedly making the same error and reasons that this is because of difficulty organizing the information. This is the OTP's interpretation. Upon reflection, the OTP recognizes a possible pattern in behavior, noting that in other types of tasks this person also struggles with organization, for example, getting through the morning routine.

The final step in the process of validity checking is posing this interpretation to the person for a response. An OTP might say, "Casey, I have noticed that in doing your daily routines you seem to have trouble organizing the materials to get the job done. Do you think that is an accurate picture of what is happening?" Using a phrase such as this allows Casey the chance to respond and provide input on the OTP's interpretation.

This strategy may not be as effective with an individual who lacks awareness; however, it still might provide a practitioner with an understanding of the person's perspective and can inform the evaluation.

Using Valid and Reliable Tools

Another method that can help validate therapeutic reasoning and ensure a complete occupational picture is using tools that are valid and reliable. As discussed previously, it is important that both elements be present in order for a practitioner to ensure accurate measurement of the construct. It is important to note that the properties of reliability and validity are not static, but are highly dependent on to whom and how the tool is administered. For example, if a practitioner uses a tool with a person whose primary diagnosis is schizophrenia, and that tool has only been used with individuals who have depression, the properties related to reliability and validity in the literature are not usable because the tool may function differently in individuals with schizophrenia than in those with depression.

This does not mean that the tool cannot be implemented, but rather that the information gained from that measurement may be less valuable because the practitioner cannot be certain the tool is measuring the same construct accurately in this new population. Similarly, if proper training on the administration of a tool is not completed, it is likely that inter- and intrarater reliability will not be consistent with what is in the literature. For these reasons, it is critical that practitioners understand the assessments that they are using from both a theoretical and practical standpoint in order to ensure that the information they are gathering is reliable and valid.

Using Practice Models

During the evaluation process, OTPs gain valuable information about the individual that informs therapeutic reasoning and future intervention. Because occupational therapy is a profession that takes a holistic view of the individual, a holistic approach must be reflected in the evaluation process. This requires that the practitioner consider multiple factors during the evaluation process.

Selecting an occupational therapy practice model can provide the practitioner with a holistic lens to view the multiple characteristics and factors considered during the evaluation process. For example, by using the Model of Human Occupation (MOHO) as a guide, a practitioner would be cued to assess volition, what matters and motivates the person (i.e., values, goals, interests). In addition, the use of MOHO would encourage assessment of habituation, or how a person's occupations are organized (i.e., roles, habits, and routines), and what the person can do by assessing performance skills (i.e., physical function, cognition, interpersonal skills, etc.). This model would also direct the practitioner to look at the person's environments, which can include social and economic contexts, culture, and political conditions (Taylor et al., 2023). Using an occupational therapy model to guide the evaluation can help ensure that the practitioner is gathering data on all components that could impact an individual's occupational performance.

The concept of holistic evaluation is beginning to expand to other professions, and it is important for practitioners to be able to communicate their distinct occupational perspective across professions. One framework that aims to assist health professionals in doing this is the *International Classification of Functioning, Disability and Health* (*ICF;* World Health Organization [WHO], 2002). This framework was created to provide clinicians from all disciplines with a common language to talk about health and disability (Fig. 4-5).

This framework can also be used to organize different areas to include in an evaluation. For example, the *ICF* does contain elements that are internal to the person, specifically body structure and body function, and individual factors. The *ICF* also includes the environment as a factor that is external to the person and should be considered when thinking about health and disability.

Although the *ICF* can assist in interprofessional communication, practitioners developing their evaluation skills would be best served to identify an occupational model of practice to support a complete understanding of an individual's occupational performance. The *ICF* does not completely define characteristics under personal factors, which would be necessary for a holistic occupational therapy evaluation.

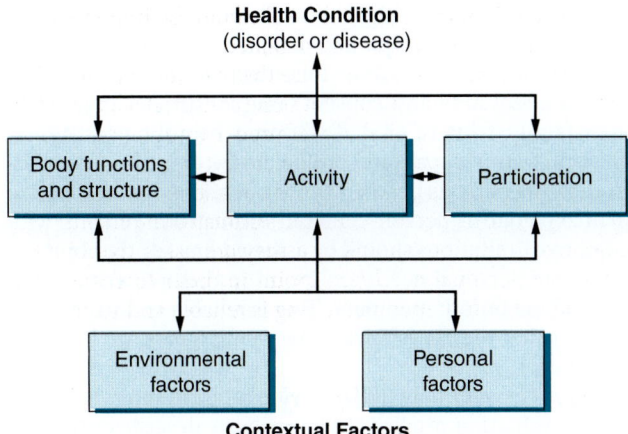

Health Condition
(disorder or disease)

Body functions
and structure

Activity

Participation

Environmental
factors

Personal
factors

Contextual Factors

FIGURE 4-5. *International Classification of Functioning, Disability and Health.* This framework was created to provide clinicians from all disciplines with a common language to talk about health and disability. *Modified from World Health Organization. (2002).* Towards a common language for functioning, disability and health. *Author. https://www .who.int/publications/m/item/icf-beginner-s-guide-towards-a-common -language-for-functioning-disability-and-health*

Assessment Methods

Just as a master woodcrafter has a workshop full of tools, with each having a purpose, practitioners have a variety of tools for data gathering. Similar to the woodcrafter, some tools are highly specialized with one, singular purpose, whereas other tools can be used for a variety of situations. Choosing the right tool at the right time for the right purpose is a critical skill to learn and practice, as has been emphasized in the previous section. Earlier in this chapter, a variety of factors influencing the evaluation process were identified (review Fig. 4-1); each of them influences the practitioner's therapeutic reasoning. After consideration of these factors, a practitioner can choose a method that supports effective and efficient data gathering. Review the questions in Figure 4-3 to further support these reasoning processes.

OTPs have a myriad of choices when selecting assessments. Primary methods of data gathering in psychosocial practice settings include informant-based methods, such as interviews or self-reported questionnaires, and performance-based assessments. Some tools combine these methods. For the most part, each of these methods of data gathering can be completed informally.

For example, imagine a practitioner is working in an afterschool program. The practitioner arrives early and finds a spot overlooking the playground and begins making informal, but directed observations of the children in the program who are playing outside. Specifically, the practitioner attends to the students' peer interactions and physical capacities in this context. A different practitioner works as part of a community outreach team and is engaged in a one-on-one cooking task in a person's home. As the activity unfolds, the practitioner observes that the person has considerable culinary skills and initiates a conversation about food preparation. An intervention goal for this individual is employment, so the practitioner might shift the conversation to learn about the person's vocational interests and work experience in food service jobs.

In these examples, spontaneous data gathering informs the practitioner's therapeutic reasoning. In many ways, a practitioner's ability to make informal but systematic observations and to elicit a person's perspectives constitute the most basic assessment tools. An effective practitioner uses these tools throughout the occupational therapy process. In this chapter, however, the focus is on the practitioner's intentional use of published, valid, and reliable assessment tools to gather data.

Interviews

Interviews are effective ways to gather data that help a practitioner generate an occupational profile and gain information about a person's perceived occupational performance. A common characteristic of a skilled practitioner is the ability to build rapport by engaging individuals in a relaxed conversation about themselves and their situations. Effective interviews are conversations with a purpose. There are a variety of specific interview tools that a practitioner may choose to use. These vary in terms of format, content, and purpose.

Some interviews were developed for use with a specific occupational therapy practice model. For example, there are at least five interviews, each with a distinct format and purpose, that support a practitioner in applying the MOHO. These include the Occupational Performance History Interview-II (OPHI-II; Kielhofner et al., 2004), which helps a practitioner generate a broad-based occupational profile inclusive of the person's perceived past occupational performance, and the Occupational Circumstances Assessment Interview and Rating Scale (Forsyth et al., 2005), which is designed to determine the person's perception of current occupational performances.

The School Setting Interview (Hemmingsson et al., 2014) helps examine the impact of the school environment for students with disabilities, whereas the Worker Role Interview (Braveman et al., 2005) and the Work Environment Interview Scale (Moore-Corner et al., 1998) both focus on work, vocational history, worker role identity, and the impact of the work environment on a person's performance using the MOHO lens.

Another interview commonly used in psychosocial practice and associated with a specific practice model is the Canadian Occupational Performance Measure (COPM; Colquhoun et al., 2012; Gustafsson et al., 2012; Law et al., 2014; Nieuwenhuizen et al., 2014). This tool is used to elicit a person's perceived performance and satisfaction in self-care, work, and leisure occupations and is based on the Canadian Model of Occupational Performance and Engagement (Polatajko, Townsend, et al., 2007). Each of these interviews provides a set of semistructured questions that guide the interview process and each has a rating scale designed to help practitioners assess the data they gather.

The Kawa River Model (Iwama, 2006) uses the metaphor of life as a river to elicit the individual's perceived life circumstances and the impact of the social and physical environment on the person's life story. The practitioner guides the individual through an interview process to create an image of a river that represents the person's life situation and current priorities. The banks of the river represent the person's social and physical environment and contexts that influence occupational engagement and performances. Rocks within the person's river of life characterize challenging situations or problems that are obstacles for the person, whereas driftwood exemplifies factors that influence the person's life flow. Finally, opportunities for growth and potentially increasing one's life flow are symbolized by the spaces between the rocks (Iwama, 2006). Figure 4-6 displays the key components of the Kawa River Model.

Teoh and Iwama (2015) stipulate that the Kawa interview does not need to unfold in a particular order as the practitioner engages the person in a discussion of these Kawa components. Therefore, when using the Kawa interview, eliciting a person's explanations and experiences of everyday life is a goal that supersedes the interview procedure. A set of guiding questions that give a practitioner examples of common questions that can be asked and how questions might be phrased has been developed to support the use of this tool (Teoh & Iwama, 2015).

The use of metaphor in the Kawa interview process highlights an issue a practitioner must consider regardless of which interview tool is selected. Exploration of the components in the Kawa interview process requires the person to think in analogies (i.e., a rock represents a problem situation). An interview of this nature may not be the best choice for a person with cognitive impairments or with symptoms that interfere with higher order cognitive processing (i.e., awareness or insight into deficits).

In some situations, after following worksite procedures for confidentiality and consent, the practitioner may interview family, friends, or staff who may help the practitioner construct an occupational profile. To be clear, it is essential to elicit the person's perspective; this remains a preferred and primary goal in person-centered evaluation. Persons with cognitive limitations should be assessed first for the ability to articulate personal needs and priorities before asking proxies such as family members. Two examples of images produced using the Kawa River interview process are included in Figure 4-7.

A practitioner may utilize a wide range of interview tools in the evaluation process. The previously described tools reflect a few commonly used options. There are a variety of other interview assessments within and outside the occupational therapy profession that may be appropriate choices. One of the most important tools in the evaluation process practitioners have is their own therapeutic reasoning and therapeutic use of self. Table 4-5 lists examples of commonly used interview tools and is structured using therapeutic reasoning questions that practitioners would consider when deciding whether or not to select the interview tool.

Self-Report Assessments

The recovery model in psychosocial practice emphasizes that people with mental illness can be in control of their lives even when experiencing symptoms that are, at times, seemingly beyond their control. A key guiding principle of the Substance Abuse and Mental Health Services Administration (SAMHSA, 2023) in the United States stresses that recovery is person driven (i.e., recovery is a process that is built on a foundation of self-direction and making informed decisions that help individuals gain or regain control of their lives). A recovery perspective acknowledges the person's lived experience and expertise.

Although interviews typically provide an opportunity for a practitioner to generate a broad understanding of a person's occupational profile, self-report tools, including questionnaires, checklists, and surveys, represent a method of data gathering that also acknowledges the person's lived illness experience. A **self-report tool** is an assessment that requires

FIGURE 4-6. Basic features of the Kawa model process. Circles are rocks representing problem situations. Wavy lines reflect the flow of the river and outline the river banks, which represent the social and physical environment. In this image, positive (+) aspects of the environment are represented in the top section and negative (-) aspects are represented in the bottom section. The tubular shapes represent driftwood, which are resources a person may draw upon to help them manage problem situations.

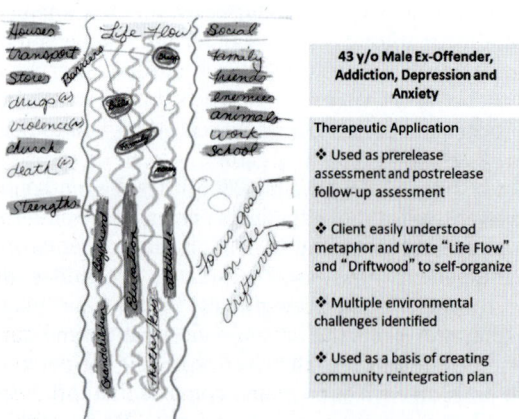
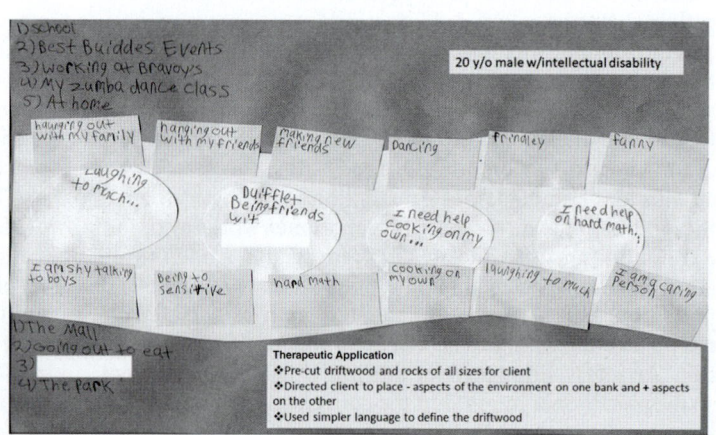

FIGURE 4-7. Examples of the Kawa River model.

TABLE 4-5 | Therapeutic Reasoning Assessment Table: Interview Assessments

Which Tool?	Who Was This Tool Designed For?	What Is Required of the Person? Can They Use the Tool?	What Am I Measuring?	How Long Does It Take and Where Do I Administer This Assessment?	Is the Tool Associated With a Practice Model?
Canadian Occupational Performance Measure (COPM) (Law et al., 2014)	Children older than 8 years of age to adults with mental illness; persons with neurological or orthopedic conditions	Person can communicate what areas are difficult when performing tasks and prioritize concerns using rating scales	A person's perceived problems in self-care, work, and leisure; person quantitatively rates perceived occupational performance and satisfaction with performance	Around 20 to 30 minutes for initial assessment, shorter for readministration; can administer in any space where the person and practitioner can discuss privately	Canadian Model of Occupational Performance
Kawa model (Iwama, 2006)	Can be used with children to adults or families, as well as with groups and organizations	Individual must be able to communicate and reason at a basic level with the metaphors in this approach	A person's perceptions of problem situations, personal strengths and attributes, and environmental supports that aid or undermine performance	Varies depending on the abilities of the person, but a drawing can be made in fewer than 20 minutes with 15 to 20 minutes of discussion to understand the person's perspectives	Kawa model
Work Environment Impact Scale (Braveman et al., 2005)	Persons with mental illness	Person is aware of and can communicate the environmental impact on the worker's role performance	Elicits person's perspectives of any environmental factors impacting a return to work	Around 20 to 30 minutes to interview, but requires practitioner to gather chart data and observe performance	Model of Human Occupation

a person to read an item and select or compose a response. Naturally, this basic description can be modified as the situation dictates. For example, items may be read to the person or the person may select or compose a response by a variety of means; in some cases, the report may occur by proxy, meaning that someone knowledgeable about the person completes the assessment for the person. In other cases, the practitioner may reconstruct the survey as a card sort activity that mimics the items and response choices.

When using self-report tools, the practitioner is providing an opportunity for information sharing about the person's feelings, perspectives, attitudes, beliefs, life circumstances, environmental contexts, and performance (Kramer et al., 2017). To a greater or lesser degree, all self-report assessments inherently provide an expectation and an opportunity for the person to engage in self-reflection. For example, if the tool focuses on occupational roles, the person may be given the opportunity to reflect specifically on current and past roles, the balance or lack of balance manifest in current life roles, and how to prioritize personal roles and goals. If an assessment focuses on sensory processing, the tool could provide an opportunity for individual reflection on perceived responses to environmental situations, which could lead the person or the practitioner to notice patterns of behavioral responses when engaging in different environments.

For the practitioner, using a self-report tool often creates an opportunity to begin or extend a conversation about specific areas of occupational functioning. But, the most important tool is the practitioner's therapeutic reasoning, so that the choice of tool is made with intention and reflects an understanding of the person's needs and priorities. In addition, the right tool will illustrate a clear purpose and elicit data in an area that helps build a more robust picture of the person's occupational profile and occupational functioning.

There is a vast array of self-report assessment tools that are useful in psychosocial practice. Some of these have been developed by OTPs, but many tools that were developed outside the profession are useful and relevant. This chapter describes only a few self-report assessments commonly used in psychosocial practice. Many of the subsequent chapters include descriptions of self-reports a practitioner will find useful in specific settings, when working with specific populations, or when addressing specific occupational performance components.

The Role Checklist is a good example of a self-report assessment. It is a paper-and-pencil checklist originally developed to measure a person's past and current participation in 10 common roles (worker, caregiver, student, homemaker, etc.). The person is also asked to project what pattern of participation in these same roles might be in the future and to prioritize the importance of these 10 roles by assigning a value from *not valuable* to *very valuable* (Oakley et al., 1986). The tool was designed to apply the MOHO and to assist the practitioner in collaborating with the person to address habituation (roles and habits) based on the person's perceived role participation (Oakley et al., 1986).

Practitioners have used the results of this tool to open a conversation with the person about role functioning. This is done by comparing past, present, and projected future roles; the number of roles the person participates in; and what this information indicates about the person's participation in society (Dickerson, 2008). Other topics that can be discussed are how the priority and value designations placed on the different roles relate to role balance, role overload, or an absence of roles (Liu et al., 2004). It has also been used to initiate a conversation about the connection between role participation and time use (Dickerson, 2008).

The newest version of the Role Checklist, called the Role Checklist Version 3 (RCv3), is a modification of the original 1986 version (Oakley et al., 1986). This version looks specifically at what roles are currently engaged in, satisfaction with current roles, and what roles the person is interested in doing in the future. The same 10 roles from previous versions are used. One difference in this version is that it can be delivered electronically. In initial testing of this version it was found to have acceptable test-retest reliability and was recommended for use by 75% of the participants who completed the study (Scott et al., 2019).

The Child Occupational Self-Assessment (COSA; Kramer et al., 2014) is a children's version of the Occupational Self-Assessment (OSA; Baron et al., 2006; Kielhofner et al., 2009). Both self-assessments were designed to be person-directed assessments that gather data on a person's values and sense of competence when completing everyday ADLs. Notably, each of these tools was created to deliberately engage the person in setting priorities for intervention (Baron et al., 2006; Kramer et al., 2014). Despite the fact that these tools were engineered with widely different age groups and populations in mind, parallel processes are used in the administration, scoring, and interpretation of results.

The COSA is used to assess two things based on the child's self-report: perceived level of competence when completing everyday activities ("I have a big problem with this," "I have a little problem with this," "I do this OK," "I am really good at this.") and the importance the child places on these activities ("Not really important to me," "Important to me," "Really important to me," "Most important of all to me"; Kramer et al., 2014). The daily activities are listed in plain words that are at a reading level consistent with the expected reading level of a child. Example activities include "keep my body clean," "dress myself," "buy something for myself," and "follow classroom rules."

The text-based rating scales are accompanied by visual scales featuring stars and happy or sad faces. The practitioner may choose to use a paper-and-pencil checklist or a card sort format when administering this tool; the choice is based on the practitioner's therapeutic reasoning about the child's abilities. Regardless of the format, this tool is used to gather data while maximizing the child's opportunity to identify and engage in planning for how to address prioritized and meaningful occupations.

Another self-report tool with both adult and child versions focuses specifically on the sensory processing that may impact occupational functioning. The Adolescent/Adult Sensory Profile (A/ASP; Brown & Dunn, 2002) can be used with persons ages 11 to 90, whereas the Sensory Profile 2 (Dunn, 2014) is designed to assess sensory processing patterns in children from birth to 14 years of age. The A/ASP is a self-report assessment designed to measure a person's sensory processing preferences and responses to sensory events that occur in everyday life. This 60-item tool includes items that seek to examine the person's sensory processing profile when participating in activities including reactions to taste, smell, vision, touch, or auditory or kinesthetic input.

The items in the A/ASP portray a variety of responses to sensory stimuli (e.g., "I like to go to places that have bright lights and are colorful"; Brown & Dunn, 2002), which are then rated by the person using the response set of *nearly never, seldom, occasionally, frequently,* or *almost always.* A person's responses are interpreted using Dunn's Model of Sensory Processing, which hypothesizes that an individual's behavioral responses can be categorized into one or more of four different quadrants: sensation seeking, sensation avoiding, sensory sensitivity, and low registration (Dunn, 1997).

The A/ASP is intentionally designed as a self-report and ideally is completed by the person you are working with as opposed to an informant. This does not mean a caregiver with close, regular interaction with the person could not complete the self-report by proxy, but a practitioner would have to cautiously interpret the results and look for patterns in the responses as opposed to making intervention decisions based solely on calculated scores.

The Sensory Profile 2 has versions specific to infants, toddlers, and children and consists of a battery of questionnaires. This version of the tool is an example of assessment by proxy, because it is completed by parents, caregivers, teachers, and other professionals based on their observations and interactions with the child (Dunn, 2014).

Table 4-6 lists selected commonly used self-report tools outlined by questions to support a practitioner's therapeutic reasoning about the evaluation process. The use of self-report assessments is consistent with person-centered evaluation processes because self-reports gather data directly from the person's perspective. For this reason, self-report assessments support a collaborative understanding of the person's life situation and challenges to occupational functioning.

Performance Assessments

An assessment tool for measuring occupational performance that practitioners always carry with them are their observation skills. Practitioners observe people perform a variety of tasks from the mundane activity of washing one's face to the skilled orchestration of culinary skills required to successfully use a complex recipe to prepare a dinner of beef bourguignon. Astute observation of people using their skills to complete a set task—whether simple or complicated—is a method of data collection that supports the practitioner's assessment of a person's performance capacities.

Performance assessment, especially in natural environments, can help practitioners to assess the frequency, strength, and pervasiveness of both positive and problem behaviors. As previously discussed, much can be gleaned from informal observation. However, this discussion focuses on tools that apply specific rubrics that allow for assessment of performance using observational processes that are structured, consistent, and often repeated. The use of specific performance assessment tools allows the practitioner to set a baseline of performance and compare a person's performances through time or compare one person's performance with that of a larger group or against a benchmark that constitutes skilled performance.

Unlike interviews or self-reports, performance assessments are tools that do not require the person to communicate a response either verbally or in writing. Similarly, there are no demands for the person to have insight or the capacity to reflect on current or past performances. Performance assessments are far more likely to be used to analyze occupational performance, whereas self-reports and interviews

TABLE 4-6 | Therapeutic Reasoning Assessment Table: Self-Report Assessments

Which Tool?	Who Was This Tool Designed For?	Is This a Type of Tool My Patient Can Do? What Is Required of the Person?	What Am I Measuring?	How Long Does It Take and Where Do I Administer This Assessment?	Is the Tool Associated With a Practice Model?
Occupational Self-Assessment OSA 2.2 and OSA Short Form (Kramer et al., 2014; Popova et al., 2019)	People older than 12 years of age diagnosed with a wide range of disabilities	Persons can concentrate to rate occupational performance, self-reflect, and participate in goal planning	Self-perceived competence of performance, value attributed to occupational performance and environmental situations	Around 10 to 15 minutes to administer checklist and 15 to 20 minutes to review, probe responses, and set priorities for intervention	Model of Human Occupation
Role Checklist, Version 3 (Scott et al., 2019)	Developed for adults 18 – 65+; can be used with adolescents and older adults in a variety of settings	Person can concentrate to self-rate participation, satisfaction, and quality of performance in 10 common occupational roles; person needs to have a sense of time	Person's perception of role participation, level of satisfaction with current roles and interest in roles not currently held	10 to 15 minutes to administer the checklist and 15–20 minutes to interview person, identify priorities, and review and probe responses	Model of Human Occupation
Adolescent Adult Sensory Profile (Brown & Dunn, 2002)	Age 11 to older adult	Self-report completed by the person independently or OTP can read items and circle responses	Person's perceived response to sensory information from the environment	60 questions completed in 20–30 minutes at home or in the practice setting	Dunn's model of sensory processing

typically support the practitioner's efforts to construct the overall occupational profile. Seeing the person do something provides fundamentally different data than hearing the person's self-reported perception of performance.

A variety of performance assessments are available, each with a unique focus, structure, or process for making and recording observations. Some common characteristics of these tools have been defined by de las Heras de Pablo and colleagues (2017, p. 225):

- They can be completed in natural or contrived environments.
- They can be completed in a noninvasive manner.
- The procedures for making observations and ratings are defined.
- The rating scales offer quantifiable data that complement other methods of data collection.
- They guide therapeutic reasoning.

The Allen Cognitive Level Screen (ACLS-5) is a test of functional cognition designed to help a practitioner apply the Cognitive Disabilities Model (Allen et al., 2007). A core assumption of this model is that global cognitive functioning can be inferred by observing a person's functional performance (McCraith et al., 2011). The ACLS-5 was designed to provide a quick screening of functional cognition using a series of three visual motor tasks. A practitioner offers directives in a graded fashion beginning with visual demonstration and verbal instruction and moving to asking the person to complete the task using only a visual model. When using this tool, the practitioner systematically observes the person's performance on three increasingly complex leather-lacing stitches.

These observations are then compared with the ACLS-5 scoring rubric that matches a person's performance with the ACLS. This ordinal scale features six levels of cognitive function and is hypothesized to reflect a hierarchy of increasingly complex cognitive ability such that someone functioning at cognitive level 1 represents the least and most simplistic cognitive abilities and a person functioning at cognitive level 6 does not demonstrate cognitive limitations (Allen & Blue, 1992).

An oversized version of this assessment, the Large Allen Cognitive Level Screen (LACLS), is designed to accommodate individuals whose visual acuity is limited or who may have fine motor problems (Allen et al., 2007). As the name implies, these are screening tools; thus, continued assessment with this and other tests of cognitive processing are required to determine specific areas of dysfunction and monitor changes in cognitive functioning.

Practitioners can also assess performance by making observation in naturalistic environments. The PASS is an example of a performance-based, criterion-referenced, and person-centered observational tool. There are 26 tasks in the PASS, but the assessment is flexible, and practitioners can choose which of the tasks are most relevant to the person being evaluated. Some PASS tasks are used to assess functional mobility, and a few assess basic ADLs. However, most tasks assess IADLs, with a few of these tasks emphasizing physical performance and most of them emphasizing cognitive performance (Chisholm et al., 2014). All tasks used in the PASS are administered in a standardized way, including how the practitioner places objects used in the task. In addition, task-specific instructions are provided to the individual. Prompts are provided only if necessary and are graded to offer the least amount of assistance first.

Each task on the PASS is rated for independence, the ability to complete a task without assistance and with few or no prompts; safety, the ability to complete tasks without risks to the person or environment; and adequacy, which is an assessment of the overall efficiency of the performance and quality of the end product (Chisholm et al., 2014). The PASS is designed to be completed in the person's own natural task environment, though a clinical version of the PASS also exists. The home version uses materials in the person's own home for the tasks (Raina et al., 2007).

The Volitional Questionnaire (VQ) was originally designed to assess volition in older children who could not participate in interviews or self-reports because of cognitive, physical, or verbal impairments (de las Heras et al., 2007), but it has been used with any older child or adult who is not able to participate in interviews or self-reports. The Pediatric VQ was developed to address similar concerns in any child between the ages of 2 and 6 (Basu et al., 2008), but it may also be used with older children exhibiting significant developmental delays (de las Heras de Pablo et al., 2017). In the same way that Allen posited that global cognitive functioning can be inferred by observing a person's functional performances (Allen et al., 2007), de las Heras and colleagues (2007) asserted that people who cannot verbally communicate nonetheless express their values, interests, and goals in their actions.

A practitioner uses the structured observational rating tool of the VQ to systematically make observations. The rating form is composed of 14 different items that assess actions reflecting the person's intrinsic motivation, sense of competence, interests, and values. The person's behavior in these environments is rated as passive, hesitant, involved, or spontaneous. Behaviors indicative of high motivation would be observable in the person who shows pride in accomplishment, is curious about the environment, takes appropriate risks or seeks a new challenge, or is someone who is motivated to try to solve a problem, fix an error that has been made, or stick with a challenging activity until completion. Observations are made in at least two different environments and can be as brief as 15 minutes or as long as a half an hour.

It is important to note that the focus of the observation is not on what environmental supports may be necessary to elicit behavior, but rather on how the spontaneously exhibited behaviors reflect the person's volition.

The performance assessments reviewed here are each different in terms of the scope of occupational performance they focus on and the level of practitioner training needed to competently employ these tools. Yet, they reflect an essential aspect of effective performance assessments by providing a specific and structured process for making consistent ratings in a systematic way. Observation is an essential tool for OTPs, but similar to any tool it must be maintained to remain sharp and ready when needed. Practitioners must practice using their observation skills in order to improve their capacities and build confidence in their therapeutic reasoning.

Performance assessments and specifically the habitual use of structured rubrics that guide systematic observation of performance are vital tools for every practitioner to have and hone. Table 4-7 reviews several performance assessments

TABLE 4-7 | Therapeutic Reasoning Assessment Table: Performance Assessments

Which Tool?	Who Was This Tool Designed For?	Is What Is Required of the Person? Can They Use the Tool?	What Am I Measuring?	How Long Does It Take and Where Do I Administer This Assessment?	Is the Tool Associated With a Practice Model?
Executive Function Performance Test (Baum et al., 2008)	Adults with psychiatric disorders and people with neurological conditions	Complete four IADL tasks: paying bills, medication management, use of telephone, and a cooking task; graded cues are provided as needed	Assesses executive function skills including safety, organization, sequencing, initiation, and judgment; used to define level of assistance for functional tasks	Typically 60–90 minutes; requires access to a space for cooking; can be used in home, clinical, or community settings	No specific model, but consistent with several models that include an emphasis on functional performance
Performance Assessment of Self-Care (Holm & Rogers, 2008)	Can be used with adolescents and adults with cognitive, physical, or behavioral impairments	Completes Performance Assessment of Self-Care Skills (PASS) tasks that are selected based on relevance to the person's life situation	Person's ability to live independently and safely in the community by assessing performance on various ADLs and IADLs	Can use tasks that are accessible within the space/setting; may not be private space to assess basic activities of daily living; requires OTP to have several types of items on hand; must be able to self-develop tasks that fit within setting	No specific model, but consistent with several models that include an emphasis on functional performance
Test of Grocery Shopping Skills (Hamera et al., 2002)	Developed for use with individuals with schizophrenia	Cognitive, communication, and executive functioning skills to efficiently find items from a list in a grocery store environment	Person's ability to efficiently locate and effectively select the lowest priced grocery within the natural environment of a grocery store	This is a timed test taking 20–30 minutes in a grocery store	No specific model, but consistent with several models that include an emphasis on functional performance

that are commonly used in psychosocial practice. Additional performance assessments that are useful in specific settings or with specific populations are included in subsequent chapters.

Here's the Point

■ Evaluation is all about choices: choosing the right tool at the right time for the right reason. Choose wisely.

■ Evaluation is a complex process but one of the practitioner's most critical responsibilities. It should always be a person-centered process.

■ Different mental health practice settings may dictate different approaches to evaluation, but overall the process of evaluation unfolds in a predictable pattern of steps: screen data to guide therapeutic reasoning, consider key outcomes, choose assessments, administer assessments, generate an occupational profile, analyze occupational performance, synthesize data and set goals, reevaluate, and measure outcomes.

■ Each step in the evaluation process requires the practitioner to apply therapeutic reasoning processes. The practitioner who intentionally reflects on each step in the process is more likely to maintain an evidence-based, occupation-focused, and person-centered approach to evaluation.

■ Validation of therapeutic reasoning can occur with triangulating data, performing validity checks, and using valid and reliable tools.

■ A variety of valid reliable assessment tools exist and a practitioner must choose intentionally so that the data collected informs key outcomes for the individual and for occupational therapy programming.

■ Effective assessment methods include interviews, self-report tools, and performance assessments.

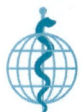 Visit the online resource center at **FADavis.com** to access the video.

Apply It Now

1. Framing Assessment Selection

Use the *OTPF* to fill in the following table with a component of the identified construct (e.g., construct = occupation; named area = education). Then identify what type of tool you might use in an evaluation to assess this area (e.g., interview, observation of performance, or self-report).

OTPF Construct	Named Area	Type of Tool
Occupation		
Person factors		
Performance skills		
Performance patterns		
Context & environment		

2. Choosing the Right Tool for Sue

Scenario: Sue is a 29-year-old Black female who was recently discharged from the hospital after having suicidal ideations secondary to major depressive disorder. She has been referred to your practice setting with goal areas in IADLs.

Sue is a married mother of one 2-year-old child. She is a stay-at-home mom who before her onset of depression enjoyed spending time outside with her family as well as baking.

You want to select a tool that would allow you to assess Sue's occupational performance in several IADL areas.

Your task is to identify a tool that can provide a comprehensive picture of Sue's performance in IADL tasks that are important to her roles as a mother and wife. It would be administered in an outpatient setting where a typical evaluation

lasts 90 minutes. Use the Rehabilitation Measures Database (https://www.sralab.org/rehabilitation-measures) to identify at least two tools that could be used in Sue's evaluation.

Use the following questions from the Guiding Therapeutic Reasoning Table to support your evaluation of these tools.

■ What data from the screening helps define my approach to the person?

■ Given the person and the context, which valid and reliable assessments could elicit the occupational profile and performance data I need the most?

■ Does the person's current occupational functioning allow for effective participation in the evaluation process?

■ Do these tools take into account the individual's culture or cultural identities?

■ Am I using valid and reliable tools and methods to generate data?

3. Using Triangulation in Evaluation

Xavier is a 34-year-old Hispanic male with a diagnosis of generalized anxiety who speaks English as a second language. He has been referred to the clubhouse where you are a staff therapist. You were able to see him for an initial evaluation, at which time you completed the OSA to identify occupations that Xavier felt were challenging.

■ What are two strategies that you could use to triangulate the findings from the OSA?

■ How would the addition of the two strategies with the data from the OSA help you feel more confident in your therapeutic reasoning related to Xavier's occupational profile?

4. Video Exercise–Occupational Therapy and Music Therapy in Early Head Start

Pair up with another student in your class or form a small group of students. Access and watch the "Occupational Therapy and Music Therapy in Early Head Start" video at the online resource center at FADavis.com. Then, discuss and together answer the following questions:

■ The occupational and music therapist explain that they identified where the infants were when they started and where they wanted to go. What assessments did they use, and what specifically were they assessing?
■ Why is it important to use assessment results when developing a new group?
■ Make a case for other assessments you are familiar with that you might use in this situation. Are there informal means of evaluation that you would also employ?
■ One of the overall outcomes from the music therapy group was improved social engagement with adults and peers. What is the mechanism by which music helped facilitate improved social engagement?
■ What did the music therapist mean when she said, "Music and occupational therapy blend together" to support goals? Give one example.

Resources

Evidence-Based Rehabilitation: A Guide to Practice

• Law, M. C., & MacDermid, J. (Eds.). (2014). *Evidence-based rehabilitation: A guide to practice* (3rd ed.). Slack, Inc.
  In this book, additional resources for critiquing assessments' psychometric properties and summaries of tools are presented. Additionally, forms and guidelines for appraising clinical measurement studies are included to support application in practice.

Health and Psychosocial Instruments (HaPI)

• This reference database contains the records of 190,000 assessment tools in the areas of health fields and psychosocial sciences. The database was designed to support the searching of assessments for measurement in both clinical and research settings.

MOHO Clearinghouse

• http://moho-irm.uic.edu
  This is a website that a clinician could use to search for assessments that fit with the MOHO practice model. The tools can be searched by using a variety of strategies and are then stratified by age. Some of the tools are available for free with registration to the MOHO Clearinghouse.

PROMIS

• http://www.healthmeasures.net/explore-measurement-systems/promis
  The PROMIS was a project funded by the National Institute of Health to coordinate several research sites in the United States aimed at developing patient self-reported outcome measures to be used by clinicians and researchers. All measures have a short-form, computer-assisted version for use. There are several domains of PROMIS measures including physical functions, perceived cognitive functions, fatigue, pain, anxiety, depression, sleep, anger, spiritual health, social support, role function, and so on. These measures are available for free on the website.

Shirley Ryan Ability Lab Assessment Measures Database

• https://www.sralab.org/rehabilitation-measures
  This website provides summaries of administration procedures and psychometric properties for more than 500 assessment tools for a variety of diagnoses. It was developed in collaboration with rehabilitation professionals to provide a resource when selecting assessments. When possible, the assessment is provided.

The Evidence-Based Practitioner

• Brown, C. (2022). *The evidence-based practitioner: Applying research to meet client needs* (2nd ed.). F.A. Davis.

In this textbook, specific chapters have been written to support a clinician's ability to evaluate measurement studies and select appropriate tools, which has been identified in this chapter as a critical piece of the evaluation process.

References

Allen, C. K., Austin, S. L., David, S. K., Earhart, C. A., McCraith, D. B., & Riska-Williams, L. (2007). *Allen Cognitive Level Screen-5 (ACLS-5)/Large Allen Cognitive Level Screen-5 (LACLS-5)*. ACLS and LCLS Committee.

Allen, C. K., & Blue, T. (1992). *Occupational therapy treatment goals for the physically and cognitively disabled*. American Occupational Therapy Association.

American Occupational Therapy Association. (2020a). *AOTA occupational profile template*. https://www.aota.org/practice/practice-essentials/documentation/improve-your-documentation-with-aotas-updated-occupational-profile-template

American Occupational Therapy Association. (2020b). Model state regulation for supervision, roles, and responsibilities during the delivery of occupational therapy services. *American Journal of Occupational Therapy, 74*(Suppl. 3), 7413410020p1–7413410020p6. https://doi.org/10.5014/ajot.2020.74S3004

American Occupational Therapy Association. (2020c). Occupational therapy code of ethics. *American Journal of Occupational Therapy, 74*(Suppl. 3), 7413410005p1–7413410005p13. https://doi.org/10.5014/ajot.2020.74S3006

American Occupational Therapy Association. (2020d). Occupational therapy practice framework: Domain and process (4th ed.). *American Journal of Occupational Therapy, 74*(Suppl. 2), 7412410010p1–7412410010p87. https://doi.org/10.5014/ajot.2020.74S2001

Bailey, R. R. (2019). Goal setting and action planning for health behavior change. *American Journal of Lifestyle Medicine, 13*(6), 615–618. https://doi.org/10.1177/1559827617729634

Baron, K., Kielhofner, G., Iyenger, A., Goldhammer, V., & Wolenski, J. (2006). *The Occupational Self-Assessment* (Version 2.2). Model of Human Occupation Clearinghouse, Department of Occupational Therapy, College of Applied Health Sciences, University of Illinois at Chicago.

Basu, S., Kafkes, A., Schatz, R., Kiraly, A., & Kielhofner, G. (2008). *A user's manual for the Pediatric Volitional Questionnaire* (2.1 ed.). Model of Human Occupation Clearinghouse, Department of Occupational Therapy, College of Applied Health Sciences, University of Illinois at Chicago.

Baum, C. M., Connor, L. T., Morrison, T., Hahn, M., Dromerick, A. W., & Edwards, D. F. (2008). Reliability, validity, and clinical utility of the Executive Function Performance Test: A measure of executive function in a sample of people with stroke. *American Journal of Occupational Therapy, 62*(4), 446–455. https://doi.org/10.5014/ajot.62.4.446

Baum, C. M., & Edwards, D. F. (1993). Cognitive performance in senile dementia of the Alzheimer's type: The Kitchen Task Assessment. *American Journal of Occupational Therapy, 47*(5), 431–436. https://doi.org/10.5014/ajot.47.5.431

Beck, A. T., Steer, R. A., & Brown, G. K. (1996). *BDI-II: Beck Depression Inventory manual* (2nd ed.). Psychological Corporation.

Blair, M., Coleman, K., Jesso, S., Desbeaumes Jodoin, V., Smolewska, K., Warriner, E., Finger, E., & Pasternak, S. H. (2016). Depressive symptoms negatively impact Montreal Cognitive Assessment Performance: A memory clinic experience. *The Canadian Journal of Neurological Sciences, 43*(4), 513–517. https://doi.org/10.1017/cjn.2015.399

Braveman, B., Robson, M., Velozo, C., Kielhofner, G., Fisher, G., Forsyth, K., & Kershbaum, J. (2005). *Worker role interview* (Version 10.0). Model of Human Occupation Clearinghouse, Department of Occupational Therapy, College of Applied Health Sciences, University of Illinois at Chicago.

Brown, C. (2022). *The evidence-based practitioner: Applying research to meet client needs* (2nd ed.). F.A. Davis.

Brown, C., & Dunn, W. (2002). *Adolescent/Adult Sensory Profile.* Psychological Corporation.

Brown, C., Rempfer, M., & Hamera, E. (2009). *The test of grocery shopping skills.* AOTA Press.

Canadian Association of Occupational Therapists. (2021). *Competencies for occupational therapists in Canada.* https://acotroacore.org/sites/default/files/uploads/ot_competency_document_en_hires.pdf

Chisholm, D., & Boyt Schell, B. A. (2014). Overview of the occupational therapy process and outcomes. In B. A. Boyt Schell, G. Gillen, & M. Scaffa (Eds.), *Willard and Spackman's occupational therapy* (12th ed., pp. 266–280). Lippincott Williams & Wilkins.

Chisholm, D., Toto, P., Raina, K., Holm, M., & Rogers, J. (2014). Evaluating capacity to live independently and safely in the community: Performance assessment of self-care skills. *British Journal of Occupational Therapy, 77*(2), 59–63. https://doi.org/10.4276/030802214X13916969447038

Clifford O'Brien, J., Patnaude, M. E., & Garcia Ready, T. (2023). *Therapeutic reasoning in occupational therapy: How to develop critical thinking for practice.* Elsevier.

Colquhoun, H., Letts, L. J., Law, M. C., MacDermid, J. C., & Missiuna, C. A. (2012). Administration of the Canadian Occupational Performance Measure: Effects on practice. *Canadian Journal of Occupational Therapy, 79,* 121–128. https://doi.org/10.2182/cjot.2012.79.2.7

Creek, J. (2003). *Occupational therapy defined as a complex intervention.* College of Occupational Therapists.

Cullum, C. M., Weiner, M. F., & Saine, K. (2009). *Texas Functional Living Scale.* Pearson.

DeIuliis, E. D. (2017). Definitions of professionalism. In E. D. DeIuliis (Ed.), *Professionalism across occupational therapy practice* (pp. 3–42). Slack, Inc.

de las Heras, C. G., Geist, R., Kielhofner, G., & Li, Y. (2007). *The Volitional Questionnaire* (Version 4.1). Model of Human Occupation Clearinghouse, Department of Occupational Therapy, College of Applied Health Sciences, University of Illinois at Chicago.

de las Heras de Pablo, C., Cahill, S. M., Raber, C., Moody, A., & Kielhofner, G. (2017). Observational assessments. In R. R. Taylor (Ed.), *Kielhofner's Model of Human Occupation: Theory and application* (pp. 225–247). Wolters Kluwer.

Dickerson, A. E. (2008). The Role Checklist. In B. J. Hemphill-Pearson (Ed.), *Assessment in occupational therapy mental health: An integrative approach* (2nd ed., pp. 251–258). Slack, Inc.

Dunn, W. (1997). The impact of sensory processing abilities on the daily lives of young children and their families: A conceptual model. *Infants and Young Children, 9,* 23–35.

Dunn, W. (2014). *Sensory Profile 2.* Pearson.

Egan, G. (2006). *Essentials of skilled helping: Managing problems, developing opportunities.* Brooks Cole.

Forsyth, K. (2017). Therapeutic reasoning: Planning, implementing and evaluating the outcomes of therapy. In R. R. Taylor (Ed.), *Kielhofner's Model of Human Occupation: Theory and application* (pp. 159–172). Wolters Kluwer.

Forsyth, K., Deshpande, S., Kielhofner, G., Henriksson, C., Haglund, L., Olson, L., Skinner, S., & Supriya, K. (2005). *The Occupational Circumstance Assessment Interview and Rating Scale* (Version 4.0). Model of Human Occupation Clearinghouse, Department of Occupational Therapy, College of Applied Health Sciences, University of Illinois at Chicago.

Gustafsson, L., Mitchell, G., Fleming, J., & Price, G. (2012). Clinical utility of the Canadian Occupational Performance Measure in spinal cord injury rehabilitation. *British Journal of Occupational Therapy, 75*(7), 337–342. https://doi.org/10.4276/030802212X13418284515910

Hamera, E., Brown, C., Romper, M., & Davis, N. C. (2002). Test of Grocery Shopping Skills: Discrimination of people with and without mental illness. *Psychiatric Rehabilitation, 6*(3), 296–311. https://doi.org/10.1080/10973430208408440

Hemmingsson, H., Egilson, S., Lidström, H., & Kielhofner, G. (2014). *The School Setting Interview* (SSI) [Version 3.0]. Sveriges Arbetsterapeuter.

Holm, M. B., & Rogers, J. C. (2008). The Performance Assessment of Self-Care Skills (PASS). In B. J. Hemphill-Pearson (Ed.), *Assessments in occupational therapy mental health* (2nd ed., pp. 101–112). Slack, Inc.

Islam, N., Hashem, R., Gad, M., Brown, A., Levis, B., Renoux, C., Thombs, B. D., & McInnes, M. D. (2023). Accuracy of the Montreal Cognitive Assessment tool for detecting mild cognitive impairment: A systematic review and meta-analysis. *Alzheimer's & Dementia, 19*(7), 3235–3243. https://doi.org/10.1002/alz.13040

Iwama, M. (2006). *The Kawa model: Culturally relevant occupational therapy.* Elsevier.

Kielhofner, G. (1992). *Conceptual foundations of occupational therapy.* F.A. Davis.

Kielhofner, G. (2006). The necessity of research in a profession. In G. Kielhofner (Ed.), *Research in occupational therapy: Methods of inquiry for enhancing practice* (pp. 1–9). F.A. Davis.

Kielhofner, G., & Forsyth, K. (2001). Measurement properties of a client self-report for treatment planning and documenting therapy outcomes. *Scandinavian Journal of Occupational Therapy, 8*(3), 131–139. https://doi.org/10.1080/110381201750464485

Kielhofner, G., Forsyth, K., Kramer, J., & Iyenger, A. (2009). Developing the occupational self assessment: The use of Rasch analysis to assure internal validity, sensitivity, and reliability. *British Journal of Occupational Therapy, 72*(3), 94–104. https://doi.org/10.1177/030802260907200302

Kielhofner, G., Mallison, T., Crawford, C., Nowak, M., Rigby, M., Henry, A., & Walens, D. (2004). *Occupational Performance History Interview–II* (Version 2.1). Model of Human Occupation Clearinghouse, Department of Occupational Therapy, College of Applied Health Sciences, University of Illinois at Chicago.

Ko, K. Y., Ridley, N., Bryce, S. D., Allott, K., Smith, A., & Kamminga, J. (2022). Screening tools for cognitive impairment in adults with substance use disorders: A systematic review. *Journal of the International Neuropsychological Society, 28*(7), 756–779. https://doi.org/10.1017/S135561772100103X

Kohlman Thompson, L., & Robnett, R. (2016). *Kohlman evaluation of living skills* (4th ed.). AOTA Press.

Kramer, J., Forsyth, K., Lavedure, P., Scott, P., Shute, R., Maciver, D., ten Velden, M., Suman, M., Nakamura-Thomas, H., Yamada, T., Keponen, R., Pan, A.-W., & Kielhofner, G. (2017). Self-reports: Eliciting client's perspectives. In R. R. Taylor (Ed.), *Kielhofner's Model of Human Occupation: Theory and application* (pp. 248–274). Wolters Kluwer.

Kramer, J., ten Velden, M., Kafkes, A., Basu, S., Fedrico, J., & Kielhofner, G. (2014). *The Child Occupational Self-Assessment* (Version 2.2). Model of Human Occupation Clearinghouse, Department of Occupational Therapy, College of Applied Health Sciences, University of Illinois at Chicago.

Kramer, P. & Grampurohit, N. (2020). *Hinojosa and Kramer's evaluation in occupational therapy: Obtaining and interpreting data* (5th ed.). AOTA Press.

Laver-Fawcett, A. (2013). Assessment, evaluation and outcome measurement. In E. Cara & A. MacRae (Eds.), *Psychosocial occupational therapy: An evolving practice* (pp. 600–642). Delmar Cengage Learning.

Law, M., Baptiste, S., Carswell, A., McColl, M. A., Polatajko, H., & Pollock, N. (2014). *Canadian Occupational Performance Measure* (5th ed.). CAOT Publications.

Law, M., Baum, C., & Dunn, W. (2016). *Measuring occupational performance: Supporting best practice in occupational therapy* (3rd ed.). Slack, Inc.

Law, M., & MacDermid, J. (Eds.). (2014). *Evidence-based rehabilitation: A guide to practice* (3rd ed.). Slack, Inc.

Liu, L. T., Chen, T. J., Chung, L., & Pan, A. W. (2004). Role Checklist: The reliability and validity study for psychiatric patients in Taiwan. *Formosan Journal of Medicine, 5,* 630–638.

Mattingly, C. (1991). What is clinical reasoning? *American Journal of Occupational Therapy, 45*(11), 979–986. https://doi.org/10.5014/ajot.45.11.979

McCraith, D., Austin, S., & Earhart, C. (2011). The cognitive disabilities model. In N. Katz (Ed.), *Cognition, occupation, and participation across the life span: Neuroscience, neurorehabilitation, and models of intervention in occupational therapy* (3rd ed., pp. 386–406). AOTA Press.

MoCA Cognition. (2023). *Training and certification.* https://mocacognition.com/training-certification

Moore-Corner, R. A., Kielhofner, G., & Olson, L. (1998). *Work Environment Impact Scale* (Version 2.0). Model of Human Occupation Clearinghouse, Department of Occupational Therapy, College of Applied Health Sciences, University of Illinois at Chicago.

Nasreddine, Z. S., Phillips, N. A., Bédirian, V., Charbonneau, S., Whitehead, V., Collin, I., Cummings, J. L., & Chertkow, H. (2005). The Montreal Cognitive Assessment, MoCA: A brief screening tool for mild cognitive impairment. *Journal of the American Geriatrics Society, 53*(4), 695–699. https://doi.org/10.1111/j.1532-5415.2005.53221.x

Nieuwenhuizen, M. G., de Groot, S., Janssen, T. W., van der Maas, L. C., & Beckerman, H. (2014). Canadian Occupational Performance Measure performance scale: Validity and responsiveness in chronic pain. *Journal of Rehabilitation Research and Development, 51*(5), 727–746. https://doi.org/10.1682/JRRD.2012.12.0221

Oakley, F., Kielhofner, G., Barris, R., & Reichler, R. K. (1986). The Role Checklist: Development and empirical assessment of reliability. *Occupational Therapy Journal of Research, 6*(3), 157–170. https://doi.org/10.1177/153944928600600303

Pépin, G., & Kielhofner, G. (2017). Therapeutic reasoning guidelines. In R. R. Taylor (Ed.), *Kielhofner's Model of Human Occupation: Theory and application* (pp. 217–221). Wolters Kluwer.

Polatajko, H. J., Craik, J., Davis, J., & Townsend, E. A. (2007). Canadian process practice framework. In E. A. Townsend & H. J. Polatajko (Eds.), *Enabling occupation II: Advancing an occupational therapy vision for health, well-being, & justice through occupation* (pp. 229–246). CAOT Publications.

Polatajko, H. J., Townsend, E. A., & Craik, J. (2007). Canadian model of occupational performance and engagement (CMOP-E). In E. Townsend & H. Polatajko (Eds.), *Enabling occupation II: Advancing an occupational therapy vision of health, well-being and justice through occupation* (pp. 22–36). CAOT Publications.

Popova, E. S., Ostrowski, R. K., Wescott, J. J., & Taylor, R. R. (2019). Development and validation of the Occupational Self-Assessment–Short Form (OSA-SF). *The American Journal of Occupational Therapy, 73*(3) 7303205020p1–7303205020p10. https://doi.org/10.5014/ajot.2019.030288

Raina, K. D., Rogers, J. C., & Holm, M. B. (2007). Influence of the environment on activity performance in older women with heart failure. *Disability and Rehabilitation, 29*(7), 545–557. https://doi.org/10.1080/09638280600845514

Ramírez, L. R., Saracco-Álvarez, R., Escamilla-Orozco, R., & Orellana, A. F. (2014). Validity of the Montreal Cognitive Assessment scale (MoCA) for the detection of cognitive impairment in schizophrenia. *Salud Mental, 4*(37), 517–522. https://doi.org/10.17711/SM.0185-3325.2014.062

Rogers, J. C. (1983). Clinical reasoning: The ethics, science and art. *American Journal of Occupational Therapy, 37*(9), 601–616. https://doi.org/10.5014/ajot.37.9.601

Scott, P. J., McKinney, K. G., Perron, J. M., Ruff, E. G., & Smiley, J. L. (2019). The revised Role Checklist: Improved utility, feasibility, and reliability. *OTJR: Occupation, Participation and Health, 39*(1), 56–63. https://doi.org/10.1177/1539449218780618

Shotwell, M. P. (2014). Evaluating clients. In B. A. Boyt Schell, G. Gillen, & M. Scaffa (Eds.), *Willard and Spackman's occupational therapy* (12th ed., pp. 281–301). Lippincott Williams & Wilkins.

Substance Abuse and Mental Health Services Administration. (2023, April). *Substance Abuse and Mental Health Services Administration draft strategic plan.* https://www.samhsa.gov/sites/default/files/draft-strategic-plan-2023.pdf

Taylor, R. R., Bowyer, P., & Fisher, G. (2023). *Kielhofner's Model of Human Occupation: Theory and application* (6th ed.). Wolters Kluwer.

Teoh, J. Y., & Iwama, M. K. (2015). *The Kawa model made easy: A guide to applying the Kawa model in occupational therapy practice* (2nd ed.). http://www.kawamodel.com/download/KawaMadeEasy2015.pdf

Townsend, E. A., & Polatajko, H. J. (2013). *Enabling occupation II: Advancing an occupational therapy vision for health, well-being and justice through occupation.* Canadian Association of Occupational Therapists.

World Federation of Occupational Therapists. (2016). *Minimum standards for the education of occupational therapists.* https://wfot.org/assets/resources/COPYRIGHTED-World-Federation-of-Occupational-Therapists-Minimum-Standards-for-the-Education-of-Occupational-Therapists-2016a.pdf

World Health Organization. (2002). *Towards a common language for functioning, disability and health.* Author. https://www.who.int/publications/m/item/icf-beginner-s-guide-towards-a-common-language-for-functioning-disability-and-health

Trauma-Informed Practice

Rachel Ashcraft and Amy Lynch

This chapter invites the reader to consider trauma as a theme that permeates across all occupational therapy settings for individuals, coworkers, organizations, and practitioners. This chapter defines trauma and its impact on occupation, contextualizes the Substance Abuse and Mental Health Services Administration (SAMHSA) principles of **trauma-informed care (TIC)** to occupational therapy practice, and invites readers to consider their own roadmap to becoming more trauma informed.

This chapter also represents current evidence-based practice, combining insights from occupational therapy and cognitive, developmental, and neurological psychology; neuroscience; restorative justice; and theories including life course health development (Halfon & Hochstein, 2002), ecological systems (Briggs et al., 2021; Bronfenbrenner, 1989), family systems theory (Laszloffy, 2002), and dynamic systems theory (Thelen & Smith, 2006). However, it also represents the ancient wisdom that peoples of many cultures have long understood. Fundamentally, this chapter is about how the events of readers' past influence their present and shape their futures, the power of relationships to heal or harm, the responsibility of individuals and systems to act justly to resist trauma, and the hope found in occupationally just and TI practices.

Defining Trauma and Levels of Trauma

Trauma is multifaceted and can be considered in terms of individual trauma, family and community trauma, and collective trauma.

Individual Trauma

SAMHSA (2014, p. 7) defines **trauma** as "a single event, multiple events, or a set of circumstances that is experienced by an individual as physically and emotionally harmful or threatening and that has lasting adverse effects on the individual's physical, social, emotional, or spiritual well-being." The landmark **adverse childhood experiences (ACEs)** study (Felitti et al., 1998; see Evidence-Based Practice box) brought awareness to the impact of childhood trauma on an individual. Since that initial study, scholars have expanded ACE categories, established awareness of trauma occurrences in adulthood, further contextualized the impact of community

and historical trauma on individuals, and defined compassion fatigue, vicarious trauma, and secondary traumatic stress. Chapter 25: Trauma- and Stressor-Related Disorders discusses individual trauma and stress-related disorders in further detail, but a cursory understanding is necessary to ground the remaining content of this chapter. 🤝

Individualized experiences of trauma can occur at any point in the life span, from in utero to the end of life. A traumatic event(s) occurring at any time in a person's life has the potential to be life altering; however, adversity that occurs in childhood and while the child's brain is still developing generally has more detrimental effects on both the individual and their family (Atchison & Suarez, 2021; Willis-Hepp & Ashcraft, 2021).

It is important to note that the experience of trauma and the resulting stress response is highly influenced by the individual resiliency factors (van der Kolk, 1989) that a person has available to them to cope with that event. Examples of individual resiliency factors include safe housing, access to health care, support systems, performance patterns, and individual factors. Chapter 10: Coping and Resilience elaborates on coping and resilience and is applicable to considerations of trauma. 🤝

Trauma has a pervasive impact on body function, thinking, acting, and emoting (Lynch & Mahler, 2021). Essentially, trauma for an individual occurs when an event or set of harmful events occurs and the individual is therefore fundamentally changed.

Trauma Within Community and Family Systems

Ellis and colleagues (2022) expanded on the idea of individual ACEs by adding community ACEs as depicted in Figure 5-1. The Pair of ACEs Model depicts the interactional relationship among adverse community experiences and ACEs. Community trauma in this context primarily refers to identified experiences of trauma within a specific geographical area. Community-level experiences such as neighborhood violence, widespread poverty, and difficulty accessing safe and affordable housing are examples of trauma. The model suggests these community-level experiences combine with individual-level experiences of trauma such as untreated caregiver mental health needs, abuse, neglect, and interpersonal violence (IPV) within the home.

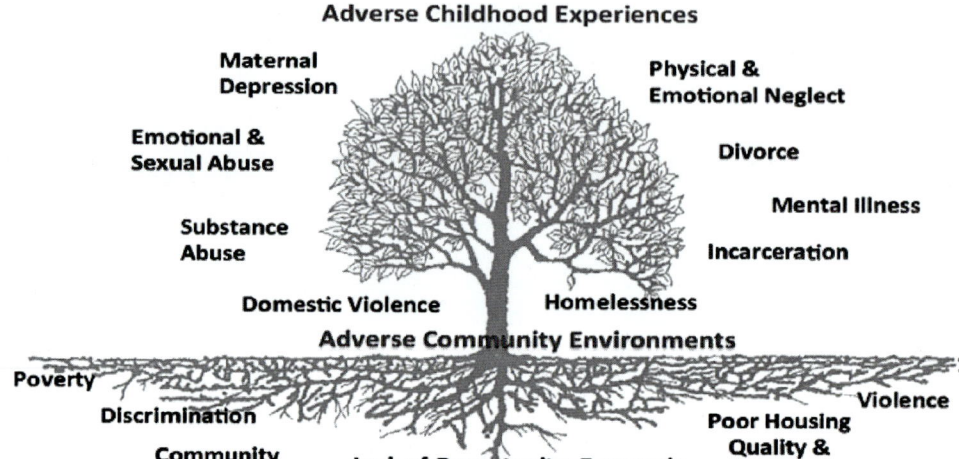

Adverse Childhood Experiences

Maternal Depression

Physical & Emotional Neglect

Emotional & Sexual Abuse

Divorce

Mental Illness

Substance Abuse

Incarceration

Domestic Violence

Homelessness

Adverse Community Environments

Poverty

Violence

Discrimination

Community Disruption

Lack of Opportunity, Economic Mobility & Social Capital

Poor Housing Quality & Affordability

FIGURE 5-1. In the "Pair of ACEs Tree," adverse community environments can foster adverse childhood experiences.

The coactional relationship among community level and individual level in the Pair of ACEs Model suggests that the presence of experiences at multiple levels exacerbates the potential for negative outcomes, restricts the potential for resilience, and increases the risk of perpetuating trauma within and across generations. Community experiences of trauma can be expanded within the Pair of ACEs Model to include subcommunities within geographical regions such as family systems, educational systems, and employment systems.

Family Systems

Trauma and related physical and mental health difficulties must also be considered within the context of family. The definition of family varies among people and cultures (see Chapter 29: Families 🤝). All families are influenced by the larger population and cultural contexts where they exist (Willis-Hepp & Ashcraft, 2021). A uniting feature of families is the concept of shared histories and shared futures, often translated through caregiving practices, attitudes, values, and beliefs.

Families often, but not always, have shared biology. All people have shared biology with ancestors regardless of whether those relations consider themselves as family. Therefore, the shared biology of trauma and related experiences such as mental health and substance use is relevant, as it impacts the family structure regardless of how family is defined and established. For example, a child who is adopted will be influenced by the caregiving of their adoptive parents as well as the biology of their first family. (*Note*: "First family" is used instead of birth or biological family because it is considered more affirming.)

It is within the interwoven relationship between nurture and biology that practitioners must recognize how and where trauma influences play out for members of the family and across the family system itself. Family factors can act as either adverse or protective factors in the life course; therefore, occupational therapy practitioners (OTPs) should consider the familial factors related to trauma and mental health.

A family is usually the first social system a person encounters in their life. The caregiving that a child receives in their first year of life informs what attachment style that person

will adopt (Ainsworth et al., 1978; Bowlby, 1982). Attachment style is a pattern of relating to others. There are both secure and insecure attachment styles (Ainsworth, 1978; Bowlby, 1982). According to attachment theory, a person will develop a secure attachment style if their primary caregiver(s) is available to them and able to meet their needs. Quality caregiving occurs across all socioeconomic categories and cultures with community support and extended relative support playing a role in attachment opportunities (Howes & Guerra, 2009; Wassell, 2014; Watts, 2017).

Individual and family trauma may be experienced because of historical and contemporary systemic trauma (Heberle et al., 2020). For example, having an incarcerated family member is an individual ACE. Historical and contemporary trauma experienced through systemic racism and mass incarceration may be the underlying reason a family member is incarcerated.

Epigenetic research in recent years has revealed that gene expression and biological functioning are guided by inherited DNA markers as well as environmental factors. The way that DNA is expressed or "turned on and off" is linked to the experiences of trauma by prior generations (Jiang & He, 2019). For example, the children of Holocaust survivors have been found to have specific gene expressions that resulted not from their own lived experience but from the trauma their parents experienced during the Holocaust (Bierer et al., 2020; Yehuda et al., 2016).

The anchor of a family system can ground and support the family members as they explore the world and inevitably confront various life challenges both internal and external to the family system. Conversely, family systems can serve as a barrier, holding family members back from needed growth. The role and makeup of families varies across peoples and cultures, but all families hold the power to be a source of healing or harm. The answer to the age-old question of nurture versus nature turns out to be both.

Educational Systems

Educational systems in the United States include early childhood education (birth through preschool), lower education (kindergarten through 12th grade), and higher education (college and graduate level education). OTPs in educational settings can support positive mental health using a TI lens (Lynch et al., 2020; Whiting, 2018; Whiting et al., 2021).

Early Childhood Education and Lower Education

Traumatization within the school setting can occur through different means: trauma that occurs at school (e.g., bullying, gun violence), the school's inability to recognize and respond appropriately to children who have histories of trauma, and the school's responding to medical and mental health diagnoses in a way that is traumatizing. On the other hand, TI school-based approaches can create childhood educational spaces that promote healing and can buffer the impact of trauma. The school-based OTP can be a powerful mental health provider for children. (See Box 5-1 for examples, as well as Chapter 36: Early Intervention: A Practice Setting for Early Childhood Mental Health and Chapter 37: Student Mental Health 🤝)

Higher Education: College

The college experience can be challenging for individuals with a trauma history. This section is framed in the context of occupational therapy education, because it will be particularly relatable to the readers of this text.

The OTP and occupational therapy assistant (OTA) in a school setting can provide powerful experiences where students can form new social support networks within the context of a shared passion. This may also be a time of increased challenges. As a profession that seeks to include practitioners of diverse lived experiences, OTPs must consider how students with histories of trauma are supported within their occupational therapy programs.

Clinical coursework involves learning about difficult topics. For example, perhaps someone is reading this chapter and realizing their own history is impacting the way they participate in school. Do they need to stop and take a moment for their own safety and regulation? What occupational therapy–based coping strategies might the person need to use for themselves? If they are doing a capstone project and chose to study an ACE that they also experienced such as divorce, adoption, or foster care, do they and their advisor have a safety plan to ensure the person's own mental health is protected in the process? Are there faculty in their program that have diverse lived experiences and identities that they can connect with?

Practitioners begin their journey as OTPs in higher education and therefore TI teaching of occupational therapy and consideration of students' positive mental health are crucial for students' emotional safety to learn (Carello & Butler, 2014).

Employment Systems

Employers can largely impact society's capacity to embed TI practices and approaches into the cultural landscape. Conversely, employers can be among the main barriers to societal progress toward a more TI culture.

In some workspaces, including occupational therapy practice settings, trauma for employees can also occur as secondary traumatic stress or vicarious trauma (National Child Traumatic Stress Network, Secondary Trauma Stress

---

BOX 5-1 ■ Examples of Trauma-Informed Practice in the School Setting

Responding to a Child With a History of Childhood Trauma

Sanyu is a child who does not have a recognized medical diagnosis to receive an individualized education plan (IEP) but has needs related to handwriting and attention to task. Sanyu is currently in foster care, with a history of neglect, food insecurity, intergenerational trauma, and loss of first family. The school reports Sanyu has poor attention abilities, sensory seeking behaviors that can be perceived as playing too rough and being aggressive, flight behaviors making him an elopement risk, and he also steals and hoards food.

Sanyu will likely experience retraumatization at school if he is responded to in a way that stigmatizes and punishes behavior instead of recognizing and meeting the underlying need. A TI school-based OTP would be able to explain and advocate for him. The OTP would recognize that Sanyu's sensory processing needs are consistent for children who have experienced neglect (Cross et al., 2019). The OTP would recognize that elopement behaviors are not misbehavior but rather a fear-driven flight response (Kavanaugh et al., 2015) and invite the team to problem-solve where felt safety may be lacking. The TI OTP could also explain food insecurity and advocate for universal interventions supporting felt safety such as having healthy snacks and water available at all times in the classroom.

Responding to a Child With a Diagnosis in a Way That Does Not Cause Trauma

Andrea is an autistic girl in a school-based setting. She has a supportive family who affirms her neurodivergent diagnosis as a strength. At school, however, she receives interventions in which her sensory needs are not consistently met; rather, she receives a pom-pom for every 30 minutes she does not flap her hands. Instead of acknowledging sensory stimulating behaviors as regulatory, she is taught at school to dissociate from her body signals, to mask her regulation needs, and to value herself as "good" only when she is not acting in concordance with her authentic self.

Andrea could benefit from interoception awareness building interventions (Lynch & Mahler, 2021) but instead is taught neuromajority-driven social skills using color scales that label behavioral expressions as "good" and "bad," further jeopardizing her self-worth. She uses a communication device effectively, but school personnel speak to her as if she is cognitively delayed, which she is not. Neurodivergent students are often othered and shamed. In this way, Andrea is being traumatized by nonneurodivergent-affirming school-based practices.

A TI school-based OTP would realize that the school system is causing trauma to Andrea through shaming approaches that don't provide body-based felt safety. The OTP would recognize that stimming is a meaningful activity for Andrea and utilize a workload approach where intervention at a classroom level would include educating teachers on stimming and finding neurodivergent affirming ways to incorporate a student's need to stim into the learning environment. The OTP could also intervene at a systems level to incorporate sensory supportive environments school wide that would benefit Andrea as well as many other students.

Committee, 2011). This occurs when a provider begins to experience the negative health effects of trauma as if they experienced it themselves (Cain & Gautreaux, 2022). For example, after a child discloses sexual abuse within an occupational therapy session, the OTP may experience headache, gastrointestinal disruption, and difficulty sleeping, and may become withdrawn in social interactions. Occupational therapy can also be a part of this solution by advocating for TI workplaces, which are discussed in more detail later in this chapter.

Collective Trauma

Entire groups of people can experience collective trauma. This can occur within geographical regions, as in the case of natural disasters, hostile leadership, forced migrations, and active war. Collective trauma also occurs among systematically oppressed groups of people, often based on identity and lived experience (e.g., race, gender, orientation, religion, and class), as well as collective experiences of disease within populations. Sonu and colleagues (2021) expand on the Pair of ACEs Model (Ellis et al., 2022) by adding that the soil in the tree illustration represents experiences of systemic and collective trauma, which feed into the roots of the tree.

Sometimes these collective traumatic experiences can intersect when a group or population experiences multiple collective traumas. When that happens, the negative impacts of collective trauma can increase. Systemic trauma, natural disasters, and disease all have implications for occupational therapy practice.

Systemic Trauma

Systemic oppression is trauma and is referred to in this chapter as **systemic trauma**. Stigma, prejudice, and discrimination are linked to physical and mental health needs (Sonu et al., 2021). Meyer (2003) introduced this concept through the Minority Stress Model, explaining it is the experience of being *systemically minoritized* and not a minority status itself that results in negative health outcomes. For example, racism (not race) is the risk factor for trauma-related health disparities (Abou-Arab, 2021). Systemic trauma experienced by people identifying within LGBTQIA+ (lesbian, gay, bisexual, transgender, queer (and in some cases, questioning), intersex, and asexual) communities is a risk factor for poor health, not someone's sexual or gender identity (Neumann et al., 2021).

Systemic trauma results in the prolonged activation of the biological stress response because of a chronic sense of being and feeling unsafe (Sarno et al., 2020). Health disparities such as cardiovascular disease, hypertension, depression, anxiety, cancer, and obesity are linked to experiences of systemic trauma (Centers for Disease Control and Prevention [CDC], 2021). This means that there is an increased likelihood that people receiving occupational therapy in medical settings have a history of systemic trauma (e.g., cancer and cardiovascular units within a hospital and mental health settings). In the context of occupational therapy practice, systemic trauma and oppression are recognized as barriers that need to be dismantled to optimize occupational participation (Lavalley & Johnson, 2022).

Natural Disasters

Natural disasters can lead to displacement of living, loss of life, loss of workplace and sustainable income, exposure to disease, and devastation to land. Natural disasters do not discriminate based on identity and class but can reveal systemic inequity. For example, systemic oppression such as access to basic needs, housing stability, employment opportunities, transportation, and infrastructure support is likely to increase the potential devastation of a natural disaster (Zoraster, 2010). The effects of natural disasters can cause rapid and involuntary shifts in individual and community habits, roles, routines, and occupations. Occupational therapy has a role in both proactive and reactive responses to natural disasters, such as advocating for accessible emergency community planning and working with people to reestablish meaningful occupation following displacement (Creek et al., 2021).

Disease

Disease is a collective experience of trauma that can be geographically isolated (endemic) or global as experienced in the COVID-19 pandemic (World Health Organization [WHO], 2022). Illness can impact an individual's ability to engage in occupation. Death from disease impacts survivors through individual and community grief as well as changing roles and routines. During the COVID-19 pandemic, people experienced disruption to their work, interpersonal relationships, leisure, and roles (Taff et al., 2021). Nonfrontline health-care workers in health-care facilities were at additional risk of secondary traumatic stress (Hou et al., 2020).

OTPs working in medical, school, and community settings were challenged to navigate their own life disruptions while providing interventions to others impacted by COVID-19 either directly or indirectly. As of the writing of this chapter, over 1 million Americans have died from COVID-19 (CDC, 2023), which is more than the combined American war-related deaths from 1775 to 1991 (Veterans Affairs, 2019). The collected traumatic experience of disease, most recently the COVID-19 pandemic, increased occupational disruption as well as the number of Americans experiencing grief because of the loss of a loved one. OTPs can utilize a trauma-informed care (TIC) framework using occupation-based strategies and interventions to address grief (Borio & Sood, 2022) as well as support individuals and communities in reestablishing meaningful roles and occupation (Taff et al., 2021). Disease is another collective trauma experience which disproportionately impacts those who experience systemic oppression (Taff et al., 2021).

Intersectionality of Trauma Experiences

Trauma can intersect and compound as demonstrated in the Pair of ACEs Model, with the soil, roots, and branches intertwining individual and community trauma. Kimberlé Crenshaw first coined the term "intersectionality," referring to the compounding effects when one experiences simultaneous racial and gender inequality (Crenshaw, 1991). The impact of trauma compounds as various individual, systemic, and collective trauma experiences occur. For example, a Black, trans woman with a disability could experience prejudice because of any of those identities and therefore will likely experience increased trauma (Neumann et al., 2021).

Another example is provided when considering the impact of Hurricane Katrina in New Orleans. Before the hurricane in 2005, systemic injustice impacted those who were impoverished, experienced racial or ethnic minoritization, and were populations with disabilities (Zoraster, 2010). Minoritized groups based on race, income status, and disability were less likely to have the opportunity to evacuate when Hurricane Katrina hit New Orleans. Populations that had already experienced systemic trauma then experienced additional trauma, as these communities experienced decimation by flooding, lost access to basic needs in the immediate aftermath of the storm, and were more likely to be permanently displaced (Logan, 2007; Zoraster, 2010). See Debra's story of complex posttraumatic stress disorder in this chapter's The Lived Experience feature.

Impact of Trauma

OTPs understand that people's occupational performance is shaped by the dynamic interaction between the person, environment, and occupation (Law et al., 1996) throughout their life. Trauma has the potential to impact all these domains. See Table 5-1 for examples.

Resilience and Posttraumatic Growth

Facing the negative and pervasive impacts of trauma can feel overwhelming. It is important to recognize the extent to which trauma permeates individuals, communities, and society to then advocate for change and healing. The chapter

The Lived Experience

My Life With Complex Posttraumatic Stress Disorder–Debra Guckenheimer, PhD

My life has been chockful of trauma after trauma–emotional abuse by my dysfunctional family, acquaintance rape, the murder of a neighbor while I was home and possibly also unsuccessfully targeted, and one ableist blunder after another. On top of that add the intergenerational trauma of being an Ashkenazi Jew whose ancestors narrowly escaped Nazis and pogroms, a mother bullied, and a father who served in the Vietnam War. And then there's climate change, white supremacy, and a global pandemic. It is no wonder that I have complex posttraumatic stress disorder (CPTSD).

As I try to write this, my brain gets distracted by the loud train horn and plane flying overhead outside my door. The noises start setting off an alarm system in my nervous system, and I focus on sending my brain the corrective signal that there is no danger. I try to focus on my body, but there's too much pain there. I try repeating to myself the mantra, "I am safe."

That's what some health practitioners have instructed me to do; however, that's gaslighting myself. Because I'm not safe. The memory of having told myself that I'm safe as I was traumatized again and again makes that tactic not work, especially when it comes to accessing health care. The world is absurd pandemonium, especially for single, disabled, queer moms like me.

"Every medical practitioner is my enemy," a friend of mine who also experiences severe chronic pain shared in a support group as we described our weekly fiascos trying to get health care including insensitive comments blaming us for our illness, insurance denials, and medical crises because of unresponsive providers. Add to that the fact that what a medical professional writes in their notes about us can determine whether or not we lose the disability benefits that we rely on to live. The government and insurance companies are always looking for an excuse to deny disability benefits. I get anxiety before just about any medical appointment, sometimes requiring me to take a benzo just to go to the appointment. At a lot of medical appointments, traumatic things are happening. My anxiety is

a tool to survive when I know how to harness it, despite the danger surrounding me.

It's no wonder that I get anxiety with medical professionals. Let's take my last surgery. I brought a letter from my pain management doctor outlining a plan to control my pain since this is usually an issue. Still, the postsurgical pain was 10/10, causing my body to go into a trauma response of playing dead. My pain improved for a few weeks, and then became intense. When I contacted my surgeon's office, I got the message, "See your headache specialist." I responded, "I don't have a headache specialist." The nurse let me know that was code for he wouldn't even talk to me. I was left alone with horrific pain, symptoms, and a bill for $20,000 that my insurance wouldn't cover because the hospital wouldn't apply for authorization despite my many calls. I only got it resolved when I used my platform to tweet at the hospital after a year had passed and my insurance said it was too late to get any coverage.

Medical professionals commonly withhold health care from me on the presumption that my physical symptoms are psychosomatic, like the time my ovary twisted up and died when I was 18. The ER doctor refused to check anything, saying: "It's stressful to be a young woman in college, and this is just anxiety." A surgeon later told me that if that doctor had ordered an ultrasound, which was the standard procedure, they would have caught it and been able to save my ovary with surgery. This was before I had a PTSD diagnosis, but any mental health diagnosis is not a valid excuse to skip standard testing.

Having multiple complex chronic illnesses and undergone countless major surgeries, I have worked with OTPs many times to try to increase my ability to do activities of daily living. Some of these OTPs horrifically made my CPTSD worse. My worst experience was after I asked my GP for help getting a wheelchair to try to get out of my house more. The OTP I was referred to required an in-person visit during the pandemic. I wanted to help my ex not take more time off work by driving myself to the appointment. The disabled parking was limited and taken. By the time that I got to the OTP's office with just my cane, I was in horrific pain and dizzy like I might pass out. The OTP walked me what felt like across the building, only to tell me after a few

Continued

The Lived Experience—cont'd

minutes that she couldn't help me. I begged her to try to do something for me. It took so long to get that appointment, and I would have to rest for days to recover from it.

I saw the OTP because I could use help finding adaptations to become more independent. She referenced my CPTSD, which she made clear she doesn't treat, and sent me on my way with a card for another office to have a new referral sent (even though my GP, this OTP, and the other OTP are all a part of the same health system).

Other OTP experiences have been empowering, improving my physical and mental health. My best experiences were through an organization for disabled parents and children called Through the Looking Glass. Their OTP, Sharon, asked about the specific tasks that I am struggling with as a disabled parent, then suggested practical adaptations, including lending me adaptive equipment. The only time she mentioned my mental health was in relation to a support group for disabled parents that the organization was starting. And even then, she did not harp on my mental health as a problem, but instead spoke about the strains that any disabled parent experiences and the ways in which we can support each other.

I use a lot of adaptive equipment including an electric reclining wheelchair, a cane, a walker, an adaptive crib, and a grabber. Insurance has paid for none of it. I either buy the equipment myself or get it for free from a friend or the Center for Independent Living. I'm told my wheelchair would have cost $10,000 and it cost me over $40,000 to get a ramp put on a van. There's probably a lot more that I could do with more adaptive equipment and techniques, but I can't afford the time, money, or trauma.

But adaptive equipment and finding adaptations for the way that I usually do things are my tickets to freedom. I am generally housebound and spend about 18 to 20 hours per day in bed. I spent a lot of time away from my kids until my OTP Sharon suggested that I put a bed in the playroom. Be that person who makes your patient's life better and not the person who traumatically wastes her time. If your patient has a mental health diagnosis and that is not the reason for them coming to you for help, realize that it's none of your business and does not negate your patient's need for support.

I am not ashamed of having CPTSD. When I found a couple of mental health practitioners who could hold the dangers that I live with and allow me to acknowledge them, then I started

to learn how to accept the absurdity of the world and start to heal. Now, when I notice a trauma response, I can feel the fear, prepare for what I can the best I can, and learn how to let go of what I cannot control. My trauma response shows me when people and institutions are not safe, and now I can listen and remove from my life that which does not serve me.

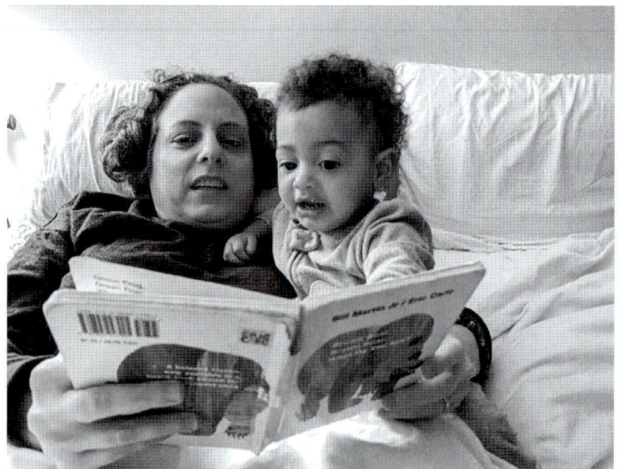

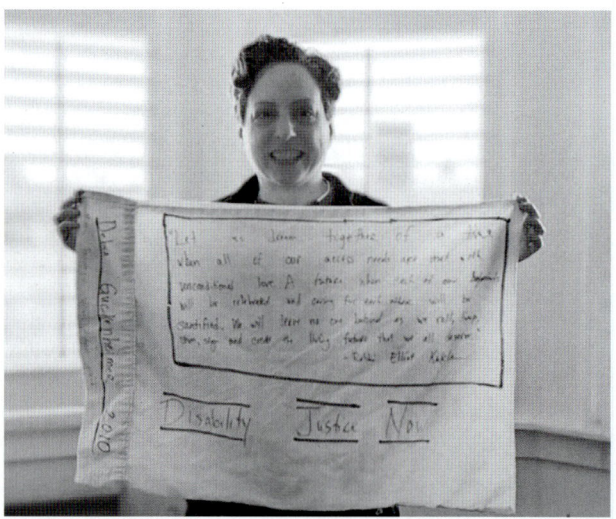

now shifts from the negative impacts of trauma to considering pathways to healing that can lead to joy and hope.

Van der Kolk (1989) described resilience in terms of internal and external resiliency factors. Internal resiliency factors include what OTPs would consider performance patterns (examples: meaningful life role, functional habits and predictable routines, valued rituals), performance skills (examples: executive functioning, emotional regulation, praxis, social interaction skills), and individual factors (examples: values, beliefs, and spirituality; cardiovascular function; brain structures and function). External resiliency factors include what OTPs would consider to be environmental factors (examples: mental health supports; access to food, water, and safe housing; positive social opportunities). Within the context of trauma, OTPs can consider internal and external resiliency factors as points of intervention to address a deficit or build on a strength. Increasing resiliency factors support a person's opportunities to experience **posttraumatic growth (PTG)**. See Chapter 10: Coping and Resilience. 🤝

The term "posttraumatic growth" was coined by Tedeschi and Calhoun (1998) and is defined as "positive psychological

TABLE 5-1 | Impact of Trauma

Person

Physical health
- Prolonged elevation of stress hormones (reduced memory making, insight, & problem-solving; Duffy et al., 2018)
- Increased risk of cardiovascular disease, cancer, diabetes, and obesity (Alcalá et al., 2017; Felitti et al., 2019; Godoy et al., 2021; Holman et al., 2016; Zhu et al., 2022)
- Decreased interoception awareness, which impairs body awareness and emotion regulation (Lynch & Mahler, 2021)
- Increased sensory processing differences causing difficulty regulating arousal for occupation (Lynch & Mahler, 2021). Specific subtype patterns of sensory processing differences are associated with the type of ACE (example: neglect vs. physical abuse) a child experienced (Howard et al., 2020).

Mental health
- Changes in brain structures, including the amygdala, insula, hippocampus, and prefrontal cortex (Duffy et al., 2018)
- Childhood trauma (including insecure attachment) is linked with impaired vagal activity in borderline personality disorder (Back et al., 2022).
- Increase in stress hormone cortisol and overactivation of the hypothalamic-pituitary-adrenal (HPA) axis, which results in a heightened fight, flight, or freeze response (Lu et al., 2016)
- Early childhood adversity can contribute to anxiety and depression (Duffy et al., 2018).

Environment

In the Person-Environment-Occupation (PEO) model, the environment corresponds to the physical, cultural, institutional, social, and socioeconomic environment. Each of these domains can serve as a source of healing or harm.

If any of these domains are a source of harm and trauma, then OTPs can conceptualize their impact using the Pair of ACEs tree illustration (Ellis et al., 2022; Sonu et al., 2021). Trauma's impact on environment is represented through the
- "roots" or community trauma in the Pair of ACEs Model (Ellis et al., 2022) as well as the
- "soil" (Sonu et al., 2021) or collective trauma such as systemic trauma, natural disasters, and disease (Abou-Arab, 2021; Meyer, 2003; Neumann et al., 2021).

Occupation

Trauma has the potential to negatively impact occupational participation for all areas of occupation.

Area	Example	Explanation
ADLs	Dressing and grooming	A person may experience retraumatization in a hospital setting if ADL dressing and grooming interventions are not affirming of their gender identity. A Black person in the hospital may not have access to appropriate hair care supplies (Abou-Arab, 2021).
IADLs	Parenting	The attachment style used to parent is impacted by the parenting a person received as a child (Kim et al., 2019). Caregivers who experienced child abuse themselves may desire to break the cycle but lack practical resources for parenting, which is exacerbated by a distrust of health-care providers and child welfare agencies (Herbell & Bloom, 2020).
Health management	Management of chronic disease	People with histories of trauma are more likely to have higher chronic health issues and so health management may play a significant role in their occupations (Anda et al., 2004).
Rest and sleep	Sleeping in new environments, nightmares	A child who was abused during the night and placed in foster care may have difficulty falling asleep in the new foster home or experience nightmares (Kovachy et al., 2013; Rischard & Cromer, 2019).
Education	School	A child who has experienced multiple ACEs will have more difficulty in both the academic as well as social components of school (Frieze, 2015).
Work	Work stability	A person who has a history of childhood trauma may have difficulty navigating workplace stress and demands. This person may have difficulty sustaining employment (Liu et al., 2013). Transgendered people experience increased discrimination, harassment, and mistreatment in the workplace, with one study reporting that over 50% of individuals reported not being hired, being fired, or being overlooked for a promotion because of their gender identity (Grant et al., 2011).
Play	Development of play	A child who experienced chronic neglect may not have developmental play skills associated with their age. They may lack joy and pleasure in play, avoid play, or reenact trauma through play (Terradas & Asselin, 2022).
Leisure	Traumatic reenactment	An adult may consciously or unconsciously create a present-day leisure experience that mimics a childhood trauma and therefore experience negative thoughts and feelings instead of feelings of relaxation and joy often associated with leisure (Griffin, 2005). A child who watched someone commit suicide by jumping off a bridge becomes focused as an adult on bungee jumping but finds the activity brings feelings of hopelessness. They continue this form of leisure despite a lack of joy associated with the activity.
Social participation	Dissatisfaction with friendship in adulthood	A person who experienced ACEs may have decreased ability to develop and maintain friendships in adulthood because of possible symptoms associated with ACEs such as impulsivity, mistrust, and low self-esteem (Herrenkohl et al., 2012). Adults with histories of psychological abuse are likely to have increased feelings of dissatisfaction with friendships in adulthood (Sheikh, 2018).

changes experienced as a result of the struggle with trauma or highly challenging situations" (Tedeschi et al., 2018, p. 504). This does not mean that people initially react positively to trauma or that the negative impacts of trauma are minimized. Nor does PTG excuse or celebrate experiences that are innately harmful and traumatic such as childhood abuse. Instead, PTG represents a reclaiming of oneself despite traumatic events. Tedeschi and Calhoun (2004, p. 58) note that "growth occurs from the struggle with coping and not from the trauma itself." A focus on growth will be effective only when coexisting alongside empathy for the pain of trauma survivors (Tedeschi & Calhoun, 2004).

PTG represents both a process and an outcome (Tedeschi et al., 2018). PTG outlines five major domains that can be outcomes of the PTG process: (1) personal strength, (2) relating to others, (3) new possibilities, (4) appreciation of life, and (5) spiritual and existential change. These domains align with occupational therapy practices. The **Person-Environment-Occupation (PEO) model** is helpful in considering the relevance of the five PTG domains to occupational therapy practice.

OTPs can be mindful of the five domains of PTG and utilize their own therapeutic use of self to attune to signs and language that someone may be processing through one of the PTG domains. The practitioner who utilizes TIC approaches to occupational therapy fosters an environment conducive to PTG for the person. Finally, it is important to note that PTG may not always result as a part of the healing process, which does not negate the value of their experience or the extent to which they have experienced healing.

Tedeschi and Calhoun (2004, p. 58) state, "Posttraumatic growth is neither universal nor inevitable. Although a majority of individuals experiencing a wide array of highly challenging life circumstances experience posttraumatic growth, there are also a significant number of people who experience little or no growth in their struggle with trauma. This sort of outcome is quite acceptable–we are not raising the bar on trauma survivors, so that they are to be expected to show posttraumatic growth before being considered recovered."

Regardless if PTG occurs for the person or not, accessing occupational therapy through TI systems creates avenues of service that promote safety and reduce retraumatization.

Trauma-Informed Care

"Trauma-informed care" is a term used by different people and within different contexts to mean different things. At the time of publication, there is no one uniformly agreed on definition. Therefore, it is important to establish how the term "trauma-informed care" is used within this text. SAMHSA (2014, p. 9) describes TIC as follows: "A program, organization, or system that is trauma-informed realizes the widespread impact of trauma and understands potential paths for recovery; recognizes the signs and symptoms of trauma in clients, families, staff, and others involved with the system; and responds by fully integrating knowledge about trauma into policies, procedures, and practices, and seeks to actively resist re-traumatization."

Within this framework, practitioners may deliver trauma-specific assessments and interventions. However, services are considered "trauma informed" only when the entire system meets the definition provided from SAMHSA. This is a tall order and one that most organizations will continually move toward. **Trauma Informed Oregon (TIO)** is a helpful model for practitioners to consider when seeking to identify next steps in their own learning and as an agent of change within their organization.

Trauma Informed Oregon

TIO is a model that outlines steps to progress a workplace, health-care setting, community center, school, or any system to a TI culture (TIO, 2016). TIO outlines four major steps that a system will move through in the progression toward becoming trauma informed: (1) trauma aware, (2) trauma sensitive, (3) trauma responsive, and (4) trauma

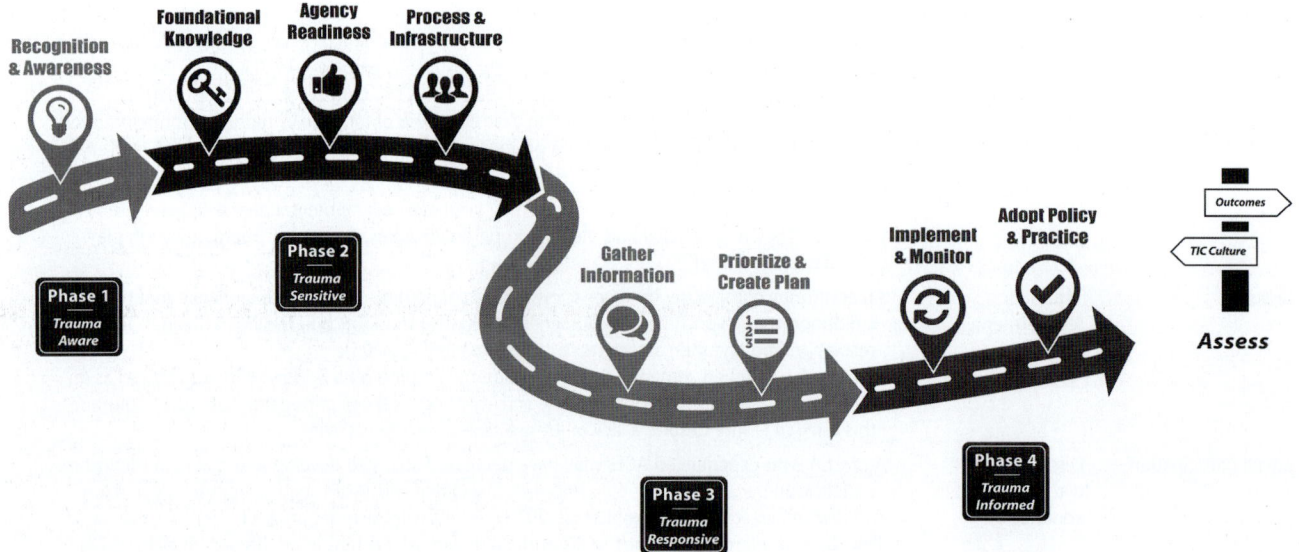

FIGURE 5-2. Trauma-informed roadmap. *From traumainformedoregon.org.*

informed (Fig. 5-2). It is important to note that within this framework, one expert in an organization championing the need for TIC themselves only places the organization at the first level, trauma aware. At the final TI level, the next step is ongoing reassessment. In this way, this model recognizes that the quest for being trauma informed is ongoing work and requires organizational commitment throughout dynamic systems.

Essentially, "trauma informed" is not an endpoint but represents ongoing commitment to continual growth. Practitioners wishing to set their own pathway to becoming a TI practitioner can utilize the TIO interactive online model. This includes a screening tool and interactional, translatable strategies for moving an organization through the four phases. A link to TIO can be found in Table 5-4.

Readers of this textbook chapter will likely find themselves in the "trauma aware" phase, as they are aware of some basic implications of trauma and the need for TIC. Additionally, they understand how trauma impacts providers and the individuals who receive occupational therapy services. Therefore, the rest of the chapter is devoted to foundational knowledge which students and practitioners can utilize at a **trauma-sensitive** level as practitioners become agents of change within their workplace. Trauma-sensitive OTPs will utilize strengths-based approaches and begin incorporating the SAMHSA principles of TIC.

Trauma-sensitive OTPs also realize the need for self-reflection and self-accountability for their own professional growth and can act as change agents within their organization. Person-focused and trauma-sensitive assessment and intervention considerations are provided as a launch point. Readers of this chapter are encouraged to explore in depth evidence, resources, and TI models recommended in the Resources section of this chapter.

Strengths-Based Approach

Strengths-based approaches seek to prioritize and promote the strengths of individuals as opposed to a focus on deficits. This is a relevant consideration within the conversation surrounding trauma as any discussion of trauma inherently centers on the negative experiences over the strengths of an individual. Dr. Shawn Ginwright calls for a shift from TIC to "healing centered engagement" (Ginwright, 2016). He notes that even though understanding needs through the lens of trauma is necessary, each person is also more than the worst things that have happened to them. Further, he notes the importance of addressing trauma not just at an individual level but at a societal one, stating, "A healing-centered approach views trauma not simply as an individual isolated experience, but rather highlights the ways in which trauma and healing are experienced collectively."

Dr. Ginwright notes that, "A healing centered approach to addressing trauma requires a different question that moves beyond 'what happened to you?' to 'what's right with you?' and views those exposed to trauma as agents in the creation of their own well-being rather than victims of traumatic events." This approach centers on the idea of collective well-being. Some research suggests outcomes of a healing-centered approach may reduce anxiety and depression as well as increase the perception of leadership, self-esteem, and resilience (Maleku et al., 2022). Strengths-based approaches

TABLE 5-2	**Strengths Profile for "S"**

Person

Performance patterns: S values role of mother. Family had predictable daily routines, which can be reestablished.
Performance skills: S is able to recognize and label emotions of herself and others; S is funny and demonstrates good safety insight.
Individual factors: S finds meaning in daily prayer, S believes that she can recover, and S has intact sensory motor functions.

Environment

Environmental factors: One-level home with social support to install a ramp if needed for a two-step entrance. Family culture includes supportive extended family members who are offering to assist with transportation, home modifications, and child care. Access to rehabilitation services is available to identify strengths and address needs to support a successful transition home.
Personal factors: S is a 37-year-old person with no known physical chronic health conditions before injury. S identifies as Latinx. S's culture is a source of pride for S and her family. Cultural and family stories of resilience are significant to S. S has health insurance and support from her work for paid Family and Medical Leave Act (FMLA) leave, thus reducing the financial stress of traumatic events on the family. S is a second-grade teacher.

which consider "what is right with you?" are consistent with supporting resiliency and PTG.

The OTP can support a person's meaningful occupational engagement as they work together to identify and build on strengths. Strengths are a vital component of the occupational profile and can include internal and external resiliency factors as previously noted. Strengths can also be organized using the PEO model and language for person and environment. See Table 5-2 for an example of an adult evaluated for occupational therapy in a rehabilitation setting following a motor vehicle accident with multiple broken bones and concussion.

SAMHSA Trauma-Informed Principles

TIC principles serve as a guiding lens through which to apply the practice of occupational therapy. Thus, trauma informed is not something someone "does" as much as "how someone is." The principles of TIC as defined by SAMHSA, when combined with strengths-based and culturally respectful approaches such as Ginwright's "healing centered engagement," clearly align with best practices in occupational therapy.

SAMHSA (2014) introduces four assumptions and six key principles that guide the application and approach to TIC. These assumptions and principles align with the *Occupational Therapy Practice Framework,* Fourth Edition (*OTPF-4*), which states "Occupational therapy practitioners recognize the importance and impact of the mind-body-spirit connection on engagement and participation in daily life" (American Occupational Therapy Association [AOTA], 2020, pp. 6–7).

SAMHSA (2014) introduces the four assumptions as foundational to TIC, stating, "A program, organization, or system that is trauma-informed realizes the widespread impact of trauma and understands potential paths for recovery; recognizes the signs and symptoms of trauma in clients, families, staff, and others involved with the system; and responds by fully integrating knowledge about trauma into policies, procedures, and practices, and seeks to actively resist re-traumatization" (SAMHSA, 2014, p. 9). These "four R's" of realize, recognize, respond, and resist align with the occupational therapy process. Occupational therapy assessment will include realizing and recognizing the impact of trauma on occupational participation. Responding with TI intervention planning and resisting retraumatization through person-centered care aligns with TIC considerations of treatment.

SAMHSA expands on the components that must be present in order for the "four R's" to be addressed. These are summarized through SAMHSA's six principles of TIC: (1) safety; (2) trustworthiness and transparency; (3) peer support; (4) collaboration and mutuality; (5) empowerment, voice, and choice; and (6) consideration for cultural, historical, and gender issues. TI assessment and interventions which align with SAMHSA TI principles through occupational therapy practice are further discussed in the text that follows. However, before discussing the application of TI occupational therapy practices, practitioners must begin with the assessment and intervention needed for them to become a TI practitioner.

Becoming a Trauma-Informed Practitioner

The process of becoming a TI practitioner is exactly that, a process. It is a commitment to lifelong learning and growth. Dynamic and ongoing professional growth is required as humanity's understanding of trauma at individual and systemic levels continues to expand. This journey starts with self-reflection and leads to action and accountability (Fig. 5-3).

Self-Reflection

Self-reflection serves as a foundation for effective occupational therapy practice. To become a TI practitioner, readers should consider the trauma of their own individual past and how those experiences shaped the unique perspective they brought to the world. In addition to asking "What happened to me?" ask "What is right with me?" (Ginwright, 2016). In this way, practitioners will be able to honestly reflect on how harm within their past as well as their unique strengths have shaped and continue to shape them. Taylor's (2008) Intentional Relationship Model and Iwama's (2006) Kawa model

are helpful tools for students and practitioners to use in self-reflection.

Once a practitioner is able to honestly consider their own story, they can reflect on how they have intersected with the stories of others and society at large (Ashcraft & Lynch, 2021). Are there systems of trauma and inequity within society that the practitioner is unequally harmed by or unequally benefits from? How might these experiences shape the perspective that they bring to the practice of occupational therapy, for better or worse? Safety, which is necessary to TIC, cannot be achieved when systems of power and othering are sustained as status quo.

Action and Accountability

Self-reflection does not stop at reflection, but continues with action and then **self-accountability.** There is work that the TI therapist does outside school and work hours for their own healing. This work will often be self-directed, uncomfortable, and sometimes painful in the way that meaningful growth is always painful. The TI OTP will commit to healing work from their individual past trauma so that they are able to bring their healthiest and most regulated self to the occupational therapy process.

Self-accountable practitioners recognize that the ability to create safety and support the cultivation of healing communities requires commitment to actively learn from those with lived experiences outside their own. This is not a linear or one-time process. Instead, this is a continual cycle of growth necessary to resist retraumatization within occupational therapy practice. Self-accountability is essential work requiring personal commitment and development of cultural humility. Cultural humility (as opposed to cultural competence) involves lifelong self-reflection and accountability with openness and respect for cultural differences and a willingness to challenge and dismantle power imbalances (Markey et al., 2021; Tervalon & Murray-Garcia, 1998).

Implementation and Continued Learning

A practitioner engaged in self-reflection and self-accountability is ready to begin implementation of trauma-sensitive practices as they move to becoming more of a TI practitioner. The trauma-sensitive practitioner will identify areas of continued learning needed within their own practice setting.

Multiple evidence-based models of TI practice exist; they emphasize different areas of practice and concerns and can support practitioners in moving beyond entry level knowledge. For example, the Trust-Based Relational Intervention® (TBRI®) was developed with a specific emphasis on intervention sequences for children who have histories of early adversity (Purvis et al., 2013). The Neurosequential Model of Therapeutics™ (NMT™) and Polyvagal Theory are rooted in developmental processes of neurology and apply across the life span (Perry, 2006; Porges, 2022). The interoception curriculum (Mahler, 2019) is an occupation-based approach to trauma-sensitive interoception practice that has application across the life span. The OTP is encouraged to consider the additional resources that follow when considering which next steps of learning might be most applicable to their area of practice.

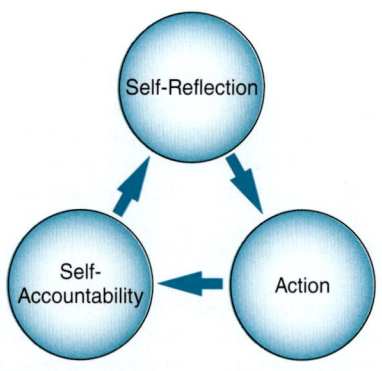

FIGURE 5-3. Self-reflection.

The following assessment and intervention considerations are provided as a starting point for trauma-sensitive practice for entry level practitioners to consider across settings.

Trauma-Sensitive Assessment Considerations

Trauma-sensitive practices can be considered as "universal mental health precautions." Universal precautions in physical terms refer to policies such as treating all blood as having the potential to contain a blood-borne pathogen. Therefore, gloves are recommended anytime a health-care provider interacts with another person's blood. In this example, there is no harm to always using gloves even if not needed, and sometimes gloves are imperative. Trauma-sensitive practices are "universal mental health precautions" in a similar way. All people have the potential to have trauma in their history, but this will not always be readily known to the OTP.

Additionally, in many cases it may not be appropriate to ask about a trauma history in an initial evaluation to determine if a trauma-sensitive approach is needed. Instead, assessment for all people should be completed in a trauma-sensitive way. Trauma-sensitive practices can benefit all people but are imperative for those with trauma histories.

Occupational Profile

Fortunately, the occupational therapy process of assessment aligns easily with trauma-sensitive assessment practices. This begins with the occupational profile. Trauma-sensitive assessments will include ensuring the person feels validated and safe before providing instructional information (Perry, 2006; Purvis et al., 2013). The occupational profile provides the opportunity to connect and build rapport with a person before providing instructional information such as administering a range of motion assessment or setting goals. Taylor's Intentional Relationship Model (2008) can provide crucial guidance to OTPs wanting to develop a trauma-sensitive therapeutic use of self. Taylor's model aligns with SAMHSA guidance for TIC as it provides practical guidance needed to meet the "four R's" of TIC, such as developing empathy, understanding the strengths and needs of a practitioner's therapeutic modes, and foundational skills needed to build person-centered communication within occupational therapy practice.

Readers will likely notice that trauma-sensitive practices readily align with best occupational therapy practices. Strategies for a trauma-sensitive therapeutic use of self may include the following:

- Ensuring safety and encouraging the person to collaborate as a part of the occupational therapy process by positioning oneself at the level of the person instead of standing over them. For example, in the hospital setting, this may include kneeling beside a wheelchair or hospital bed if the practitioner is able. In a pediatric setting, this might include positioning oneself at or below eye level to assume an inviting posture.
- Safety is a particular concern when working with children as the caregiver may need to contribute relevant information for the occupational profile that is not safe for the child to hear. For example, a child who is asked to sit and complete a task while the OTP interviews the caregiver and the caregiver shares negative behaviors of the child or trauma history is essentially being asked to self-regulate alone while the hardest parts of their history are being discussed. This is counter to trauma-sensitive care and TIC. Instead, the caregiver can be informed ahead of time that negative discussions in front of the child will not take place and those questions related to the child's trauma history will be addressed without the child present. This can be done through intake paperwork or by having the OTA administer standardized testing in another room while the OTP completes the caregiver portion of the occupational profile interview.
- Ensure trustworthiness and transparency by taking the time to introduce yourself, explain why the person is seeing you or was referred to you, validate their concerns, and be honest about how the occupational therapy process will be conducted using terms that can be understood at the person's level. For example, consider a child who is referred to occupational therapy secondary to occupational disruption related to attention deficit-hyperactivity disorder (ADHD). The practitioner could say something such as, "Did you know a lot of kids have trouble with grown-ups telling them all the time to 'Pay attention!' when they really are already trying their best to pay attention? I help kids be able to not feel so frustrated at school with stuff like that. Does that sound like something you'd like me to help you with?"
- Provide collaboration and mutuality by involving the person in identifying their own priorities and goals.
- Consider cultural, historical, and gender issues during evaluation by ensuring the most inclusive language possible is being used. For example, it is not uncommon for a person to be admitted to the hospital with a wristband that does not match their chosen name and pronouns. In this case, the OTP ensures they address the person by asking about their chosen name and pronouns.

The occupational profile will also consider the contexts of a person's occupational participation. Assessment, intervention, and discharge planning across occupational therapy settings consider the support systems a person has. Family is often a part of those support systems. As noted earlier, family has the potential to be a strength or barrier (and sometimes a little bit of both!) for the person receiving occupational therapy services.

The OTP has the expertise to consider trauma within the context of family occupations, habits, routines, rituals, and roles that can be the lived expressions of a family's trauma story. These become powerful points of occupational therapy intervention to help families develop or to help leverage strengths in these areas (Willis-Hepp & Ashcraft, 2021). This may involve inclusion of the family in therapy or involve employing therapeutic use of self to stay nonjudgmental when family topics may be triggering. Two examples are included here to illustrate this concept:

1. *Pediatric example:* A child in foster care is referred to occupational therapy services with the court requirement of first family attendance as part of a reunification plan. The OTP discovers in the assessment that

the child in foster care and first family have different routines surrounding morning and bedtime. The child might have sensory processing needs that the foster care home or first family misinterpreted as a behavior problem. The OTP can work with both the first and foster families to establish predictable routines across settings so that the child experiences predictable routines as first family home visits increase; help establish interventions to have sensory needs met within both family contexts; and include the first family within the treatment setting to build parenting skills. These skills could be related to playing with their child; developing strategies to work through sensory needs; and establishing meaningful rituals, roles, and routines. In this way, occupational therapy can be a powerful part of reunification planning and implementation in foster care.

2. *Adult example:* An adult in an inpatient mental health setting is referred to occupational therapy as part of treatment for borderline personality disorder. The evaluating OTP cannot assume the person's history. However, the OTP using trauma-sensitive "universal mental health precautions" recalls a correlation with borderline personality disorder, insecure attachment style, and childhood trauma (Back et al., 2022). The OTP will also recall that impairment in interoception awareness is linked to many mental health diagnoses. If the person becomes dysregulated or demonstrates a "fight, flight, or freeze" response during the initial assessment, the OTP knows that this person's response to them and the initial assessment might have nothing to do with the person's motivation or feelings toward occupational therapy; rather, it is rooted in that person's attachment style and interoceptive awareness. A person with a trauma history can feel unsafe and have difficulty establishing trust (Levy et al., 2010; Quilty et al., 2017). The trauma-sensitive OTP modifies the interview as needed through therapeutic use of self-tools and recognizes that a "fight, flight, or freeze" trauma-based response does not mean the person is not motivated.

Analysis of Occupational Performance

Analysis of occupational performance will involve considering the occupational profile content to determine what occupations and contexts should be addressed as well as what assessments are appropriate. The assessments chosen will be dependent on the person and their goals. Activity and occupational analysis can be ideal assessment methods as they can be graded to ensure that the person feels safe and supported throughout the process.

Analysis Considerations: Standardized Assessment

Standardized assessments provide valuable insight for goal setting and intervention planning. Administration of standardized assessments requires some trauma-sensitive considerations such as the following:

■ Adherence to a standardized assessment script may not always provide the most inclusive, transparent, or

supportive language to the person. Scripts may feel impersonal and demanding. In this case, the OTP can note where modifications were made in the assessment process for the purpose of safety.

■ Standardized assessments are often focused on identifying deficits in individual factors and performance skills. This means that the person may feel the OTP is repeatedly asking them to fail at something, especially in assessments that require a ceiling for errors before stopping the assessment. Identifying that this may happen before the assessment can alleviate stress. For example, when administering a standardized assessment to an 8-year-old, the OTP might say, "Look at the front of this, do you see that it says for ages 2 through 100? That means even grown-ups as old as 100 do this. So, if it feels tricky don't worry because it gets tricky for grown-ups too. Just try your best."

Analysis Considerations: Consent

Consent is crucial, especially when the OTP is completing analysis that requires the person to be touched. The OTP provides empowerment, voice, and choice by always ensuring the person can consent to the extent they are able for each part of the assessment process and give choices when possible. For example, in a rehabilitation setting, an OTP could say, "Part of what I'm going to assess today is active range of motion or how your joints are moving on their own and then I'll be looking at the strength of your muscles for those movements. Is it okay if I touch your shoulder?" If a person does not consent to an assessment approach, the OTP can utilize therapeutic use of self-skills to modify the assessment or investigate the barriers.

An attitude of staying curious is consistent with trauma-sensitive practice. Therefore, an OTP may document "person did not consent to having shoulder touched and upon further investigation revealed they were afraid of being hurt. OTP worked with person to modify testing in a way that felt safe to the person and results are explained below" instead of noting, "person refused manual muscle and range of motion testing."

Analysis Considerations: Interoception

Interoception is an important consideration for mental health and trauma. Interoception refers to a person's physiological sense of their body (Craig, 2003). This includes homeostatic interoception (examples: hunger, thirst, pain, temperature) as well as affective interoception (examples: how one's body feels when angry, happy, joyful, sad; Mahler, 2019). Disrupted interoceptive processing is associated with many mental health diagnoses including anxiety disorders, mood disorders, eating disorders, addictive disorders, and somatic symptom disorders (Khalsa et al., 2018). Increasing evidence supports that those with experiences of trauma are likely to have impaired interoception awareness (Schaan et al., 2019). Interoception awareness is also linked with adult attachment styles and emotional regulation (Ferraro & Taylor, 2021).

OTPs as mental health practitioners can implement interoceptive assessment and interventions. Interoception intervention requires a holistic view of the person that recognizes the inseparable relationship between mental and physical health, which aligns with the *OTPF-4* (AOTA, 2020).

Interoception can be assessed using the Comprehensive Assessment of Interoceptive Awareness (Mahler, 2016). For more information on interoception see Chapter 9: Sensory Processing and the Lived Sensory Experience.

Analysis Considerations: Assessing for Strengths

Assessing for strengths is another critical component of a trauma-sensitive occupational therapy assessment. Assessment of **positive childhood experiences (PCEs)** may feel counterintuitive in many current medical and educational systems, which were built around evaluation and intervention

for deficits and impairments. However, at the core of TIC is the understanding that individuals, families, communities, and systems are far more than their deficits and impairments. In fact, Ginwright (2016) supports the identification of and leveraging of strengths as vital to posttraumatic healing. Ginwright's perspective is congruent with emerging research about the presence of PCEs to mitigate outcomes in light of trauma.

Understanding PCE experiences also aligns with the profession of occupational therapy's aim to be strengths focused. Supporting a person's identification of strengths as part of TI intervention propels practitioners to better support individuals in PTG. See the "Being a Psychosocial OT Practitioner" feature for an example of applying TI practices.

Being a Psychosocial OT Practitioner

Providing Trauma-Informed Services in a School Setting

Identifying Psychosocial Strengths and Needs

OTPs using a TI lens build on strengths and identify needs related to personal and contextual factors to support occupational engagement. Consider the story of Andrea, an autistic 9-year-old girl in a school setting. She has a supportive family who affirms her neurodivergent diagnosis as a strength. They explain that Andrea dances around the living room as if she was a butterfly (flapping her wings), enjoys physical activity and being outside (jumping on a trampoline), assembles puzzles with great focus with her grandmother (excelling at edges), and loves sitting with her mom's arm around her shoulders to complete above grade level math homework.

At school, however, Andrea's education team describes Andrea as unable to stay seated to engage in academic tasks (typically standing up and walking and bouncing up on her toes in the back of the room) and having difficulty with eating in the cafeteria (usually flapping her hands and covering her ears). During recess, she struggles with peers (constantly touching other students' clothing or standing very close and leaning into them).

The education team develops a functional behavior plan for Andrea. She receives candy every 20 minutes she stays on task with a tabletop educational activity and a pom-pom for every 10 minutes in the cafeteria she does not flap her hands. Andrea sits with an aide at a separate table from her neuromajority-aligned peers and earns outside time if she eats all of her lunch. She is permitted to play with peers only on the swings so that she can keep her distance and not be close enough to touch her peers.

The OTP determines Andrea is not feeling seen, heard, or understood by her education team and that Andrea does not feel a sense of belonging to her peers. Every time Andrea is asked not to flap, not to stand, or not to cover her ears, she is essentially told that she is broken and needs to be the same as others; every time fellow students see Andrea given candy or a pom-pom or sit at a separate table in the cafeteria, Andrea experiences othering. These are traumatizing experiences that compound upon one another. Instead of acknowledging sensory stimming behaviors as regulatory, the current school plan is teaching Andrea to dissociate from her body signals, to mask her regulation needs, and to value herself as "good" and "belonging in a social play circle" only when she is not acting in concordance with her authentic self.

Using a Holistic Occupational Therapy Approach

The OTP completes an evaluation that includes an interest and activities satisfaction assessment with the Children's Assessment of Participation and Enjoyment and Preferences for Activities of Children (CAPE/PAC; King et al., 2004), a motor assessment with the Bruininks Oseretsky Test of Motor Proficiency 2 (Bruininks & Bruininks, 2005), a sensory assessment with the Sensory Profile 2 (Dunn, 2014; Licciardi & Brown, 2021), and the Comprehensive Assessment of Interoception Awareness-3rd Edition (Mahler, 2023). Andrea's identified interests include music, dancing, puzzles, math, taking care of pets, and gardening. She has motor coordination dilemmas that make navigating group spaces, organized group sports, or other group play activities challenging. Andrea struggles with auditory processing (hyperresponsive) and processing multiple simultaneous and unexpected sound sources (such as the cafeteria). Auditory discrimination is a strength used for properly identifying sounds quickly. She seeks vestibular and proprioception input (hyporesponsive). Andrea presents with interoception strengths and challenges. Her strengths include identifying body signals related to temperature and urge to go to the bathroom and affective body signals related to being happy and scared. Interoception challenges include difficulty with signals related to thirst, hunger, satiety, and the affective body signals related to being sad and angry.

The OTP determines that Andrea's interoception, sensory, motor, and social needs are not being met through her current behavior plan. In fact, these intersecting needs are making things more difficult for her. For example, Andrea has difficulty with hunger and satiety cues, which impact her ability to eat. She is overwhelmed in the cafeteria from a sensory standpoint (especially auditory), making it more difficult to attune to hunger and satiety cues. Further, because she is isolated at lunch and working to "earn" regulated outside time, she feels sad. However, she has difficulty interpreting and verbalizing this while simultaneously feeling auditorily overwhelmed and trying to override her body cues related to hunger and satiety. In an effort to regulate herself, she engages in stimming and therefore does not finish her lunch. Therefore, she loses access to regulated outside time.

The OTP establishes that the school and Andrea would benefit from a multitiered TI approach and proposes building-wide, classroom, peer group, and individual-level strategies. At a building-wide level, the OTP suggests that morning announcements include a school song where everyone is invited to dance to a specific sequence of movements that include fast, slow, and just right speeds, followed by a school cheer. This provides movement for all students for regulation and connection. Within

Continued

Being a Psychosocial OT Practitioner—cont'd

the classroom, the OTP suggests the educator have structured movement breaks three times a day at predictable intervals and two check-in "this or that"-type choice questions (nonemotional and no answer is wrong), once after morning announcements and once right after lunch. The OTP will guide multiple peer groups during academic station times, ensuring Andrea is with the same peers for the first half of the school year to promote social engagement and group problem-solving skills.

The OTP suggests Andrea could benefit from interoception awareness building interventions (Lynch & Mahler, 2021), such as inviting students to explore their own interoception, homeostatic (thirst, hunger, satiety, etc.), and affective cues (happy, sad, angry, etc.) using focused interoception experiments such as those in Mahler's (2023) interoception curriculum. The OTP further advocates for the education team to reframe their understanding of Andrea by shifting away from extinguishing behaviors to a goal of meeting her unmet needs and building on strengths. The OTP educates school staff about Andrea's capacity to perceive the emotional tone of others and her social pragmatic communication dilemma suggesting empathy and speech language pathology referral. A culture of coregulation is recommended for the classroom using a "partner peace corner" where students who have self-regulation skills may "partner" with a student needing the peace corner for coregulation. In this way, a buddy system engages all students and does not use the "peace corner" as a "time out" but as a peer support coregulation station.

Reflective Questions

1. What other sensory motor strategies might be useful to explore with Andrea that she could utilize in her classroom individually? As part of her whole class?

2. How might the OTP specifically address the school staff's perception of Andrea's strengths, capacities, and desires to feel a part of the group?

3. How would an OTP design a treatment session to provide Andrea with a mastery experience to advocate for group engagement and set the scene for positive interactions with others and a foundation upon which to establish a sense of self-worth?

References

Bruininks, R. H., & Bruininks, B. D. (2005). *Bruininks-Oseretsky Test of Motor Proficiency second edition—Users manual.* Pearson.

Dunn, W. (2014). *Sensory Profile 2—Users manual.* Pearson.

King, G., Law, M., King, S., Hurley, P., Rosenbaum, P., Hanna, S., Kertoy, M., & Young, N. (2004). *Children's Assessment of Participation and Enjoyment and Preferences for Activities of Children (CAPE/PAC)—Users manual.* Pearson.

Licciardi, L., & Brown, T. (2021). An overview & critical review of the Sensory Profile–second edition. *Scandinavian Journal of Occupational Therapy, 30*(6), 1–13. https://doi.org/ 10.1080 /11038128.2021.1930148

Lynch, A., & Mahler, K. (2021). Chapter 2: Trauma impact upon neurobiological, social emotional, and motor function: Implications for occupation. In A. Lynch, R. Ashcraft, & L. Tekell, *Trauma, occupation, and participation: Foundations and population considerations for occupational therapy* (pp. 19–40). AOTA Press.

Mahler, K. (2023). *Interoception curriculum publications.* Mahler Autism Services. https://www.kelly-mahler.com/product -category/publications

Trauma-Sensitive Interventions

Bruce Perry's NMT™ provides a helpful framework to consider not only the interventions involved in trauma-sensitive care but the sequencing of interventions (Perry, 2006). The goal of this model is to guide clinical reasoning through a neurodevelopmental lens designed to create safety and build individual capacity. NMT™ is not designed to be utilized as a replacement to other models but as a complement to other evidence-based models (MacKinnon, 2012). The OTP can combine the NMT™ approach with other clinical reasoning tools and frameworks such as the *OTPF-4* (AOTA, 2020), PEO model (Law et al., 1996), Kawa model (Iwama, 2006), Model of Human Occupation (MOHO; Kielhofner, 1995), and SAMHSA principles of TIC (SAMHSA, 2014).

As readers progress toward becoming more trauma informed, NMT™ offers additional training opportunities (see link in the Resources section). Perry offers a helpful framework to structure interventions in sequences that align with neurological processing. In this model, neurological regulatory networks are considered in the hierarchical framework of brainstem, diencephalon and cerebellum, limbic system, and cortex (Perry & Winfrey, 2021). Perry outlines that a person must have lower brain functioning needs met before they are able to process higher level cognitive reasoning demands (Gaskill & Perry, 2017). In this way, it is not simply the intervention itself that is trauma sensitive but the sequence of the intervention.

Perry outlines that a person must **regulate** at a physiological level including sensory needs before they are able to **relate**

in relationship to others as well as to themselves. Only when a person has lower brain functioning needs of regulation and relationship (brainstem, diencephalon and cerebellum, and limbic system) met are they able to truly access the cerebral cortex functions of **reason** (Perry & Winfrey, 2021). An intervention may be appropriate for a person at a reasoning level (an example would be to utilize executive functioning support strategies when cooking) but only once their regulation and relationship needs have been met. Their regulation needs will include basic homeostatic and interoceptive needs (hunger, thirst, sleep, etc.). Their relationship needs include their ability to relate to themselves and others and establish a therapeutic relationship with the OTP. Reasoning needs include the teaching of new skills related to occupational performance, language-based instruction and learning, and executive functioning.

An example of how this might relate within a mental health setting would be if a practitioner was leading a social skills group. The OTP would first ensure participants' basic needs were met, then complete a sensory regulation activity that provides an opportunity for the group to connect with each other, followed by the building of safety and connection among participants, and finally the teaching of social skills strategies that require higher level cognitive functioning.

This framework of regulate, relate, and reason parallels with interventions at each of the six SAMHSA principles of TIC. Table 5-3 provides examples of occupational therapy considerations within the context of the regulate, relate, and reason framework alongside the SAMHSA principles of TIC.

TABLE 5-3 | Occupational Therapy Interventions Using the Regulate, Relate, Reason Sequencing

SAMHSA Six Principles	NMT Sequence of Clinical Reasoning		
	Regulate	*Relate*	*Reason*
Safety	Proactively consider the social and physical environment and reduce potential triggers. Example: In a residential treatment facility, consider modifications to "family visit" days so that those without family support systems are not as likely to be triggered. This may include staggering visitation opportunities instead of having one family visit day for everyone.	Employ the power of co-occupation by participating with the person in preparatory regulating interventions. Example: Instead of instructing or providing handouts on a regulating technique, join the individual and participate in deep breathing or progressive muscle relaxation as a coregulating activity.	Explain actions before and during assessment or intervention. Example: During an interoception awareness building activity using Mahler's interoception curriculum, explain that all interoception experiments are optional and there is no right or wrong answer.
Trustworthiness and Transparency	Predictability and trustworthiness build regulation over time. Example: If you promise a person you will "do a requested intervention next session," or "that was the last one," then you must make every effort to hold true to that.	Within appropriate boundaries you may "therapeutically disclose" your experiences. Example: In the pediatric setting you may say, "Whew, this rain is making me feel sleepy and that makes it hard to work. Do you feel that way too? I wonder what we could do to wake ourselves up?"	Explain honestly and to the extent the person has cognitive capacity to process why something is happening or why you are asking the person to do something. Example: A person finishes a task quicker than expected. Instead of saying, "You did that so fast let's do it again!" say "Wow, our time is supposed to go until 2:15 and it's only 2:05. You are getting stronger! We really do need to work together another 10 minutes; let me tell you some ideas we could try."
Peer Support	Peers can be powerful sources of coregulation for children and adults. Example: A child who may become easily dysregulated during a school assembly is paired with a student "buddy" who can offer coregulation during the event.	Support groups related to a shared traumatic experience can offer powerful peer support. Example: Alcoholics Anonymous (AA), a spinal cord injury support group, or autistic peer group may develop surrounding a special interest.	Peer support groups can offer problem-solving ideas to new challenges based on shared lived experiences. Example: Adult autistic support groups may include problem-solving ways to navigate challenging situations.
Collaboration and Mutuality	Recognition is given in the value of all organizational members to support a regulating environment. The OTP empowers team members including support staff in TI practices. Example: In a school setting, cafeteria staff can be crucial members of the team with the OTP to implement Every Moment Counts Comfortable Cafeteria (Bazyk et al., 2018).	Person receiving occupational therapy is included as a collaborator in their own care. Hierarchies in treatment where the clinician is seen as the expert over the individual is counter to collaboration and mutuality. Example: The OTP has devoted time to learning the Intentional Relationship Model therapeutic modes and adjusts their therapeutic use of self to ensure the person they are supporting has an active voice in their treatment.	A system-based intervention to offer a community support system involves those with lived experience and active community members as crucial experts. Example: An OTP developing a trauma-sensitive vocational service program in a prison setting includes a formerly incarcerated person in program development.
Empowerment, Voice, and Choice	Check in with person to determine if their basic needs for regulation have been met before beginning a treatment session. Example: Before we get started, do you need anything to eat or drink?	Active listening: Listen to understand instead of listening to respond. Use of "echo" in which you may restate something to ensure you are understanding. Example: A person receiving occupational therapy following a spinal cord injury may say, "I don't want to use that sliding board, I'm going to fall," and you repeat back, "You are worried you will fall if we use the sliding board. Is that right?"	Offer choices in interventions. Choices include options in which both are reasonably expected to be acceptable to the person. Example: If a practitioner knows that a person hates painting, then the choices cannot be painting or yoga. Instead, the practitioner offers occupation-based choices that match the person's interests.

Continued

TABLE 5-3 | Occupational Therapy Interventions Using the Regulate, Relate, Reason Sequencing—cont'd

SAMHSA Six Principles	NMT Sequence of Clinical Reasoning		
	Regulate	**Relate**	**Reason**
Cultural, Historical, and Gender Issues	Effort is made to identify and reduce potential triggers within the social and physical environment that might result in a hypervigilant stress response. Example: A school-based OTP works with school administration to identify and modify assignments that would violate safety and cause dysregulation for a child with early adversity such as "my life story timeline" or "family tree" activities.	OTP is intentional in learning about lived experiences outside themselves and is mindful of the language, assessments, and interventions they choose. Example: An OTP working in an inpatient mental health unit would be educated on gender-affirming ADLs and be prepared to support a person's gender expression within meaningful occupations.	The OTP will be aware of their own potential biases and recognize that racism and systemic oppression are frequent risk factors to occupational participation (i.e., racism, not race, is a risk factor for health disparities linked to trauma experiences; Abou-Arab, 2021). Example: In an addiction treatment center, the OTP will not use judgment-based descriptions of a person that are likely rooted in bias such as describing an individual as "unmotivated" or "noncompliant." Instead, the OTP will self-reflect if there is a barrier to occupational participation that may be rooted in systemic injustice.

Advocating for Trauma-Informed Practice

OTPs can advocate for TI practice within the profession of occupational therapy as well as within an OTP's individual organization and setting. All areas within the profession of occupational therapy can benefit from a commitment to TI practice. In addition to advocacy for TIC at the professional level, OTPs can advocate specifically for TIC within their individual setting and organization. OTPs can utilize the TIO roadmap to guide their advocacy toward more TI organizational practices. The following are examples of advocacy that an OTP might engage in using the TIO roadmap:

Phase 1: Trauma Aware

- Recognition and Awareness:
  - The OTP recognizes and brings awareness to ways in which trauma may be impacting the people served within that community or setting.
  - The OTP invites others to learn alongside them through shared learning such as lunchtime journal club, book club, or podcast discussion group.
  - The OTP is intentional about sharing knowledge that they are gaining with others through formal and informal sharing of knowledge such as providing a company-based education event as well as in informal conversations.
  - The OTP advocates with leadership to gather information and data regarding the relevance of TIC to their practice setting and the populations they serve.

Phase 2: Trauma Sensitive

- Foundational Knowledge
  - The OTP researches TI models that apply to their setting and seeks out advanced training.
  - The OTP assists in training others within the organization.
- Agency Readiness
  - The OTP who has received advanced training in TIC can serve as a leader in this area within the

organization and support leadership understanding of the need for TIC. TIC is considered for both the people receiving occupational therapy services as well as the work culture and management of OTPs themselves.

- The OTP advocates for organization supports to mitigate the impact of secondary traumatic stress and vicarious trauma in staff.
- The OTP models TIC in the way they engage with consumers, coworkers, and the community at large.
- Process and Infrastructure
  - The OTP advocates for a workgroup or committee within the organization focused on TIC application within their setting.
  - The OTP serves as an agent of change within the organization, infusing knowledge to others in formal and informal ways.
  - The OTP uses advocacy skills to call out non–TI policy and practice, which includes power structures.
  - The OTP utilizes activity and occupational analysis skills to develop a communication plan that can be effective within providers' workday.

Phase 3: Trauma Responsive

- Gather Information and Identify Opportunities
  - OTP participates in or leads within the workgroup established at Phase 2.
  - Workgroup reviews all organizational policies and procedures using a trauma lens that considers the "four R's" and six principles of TIC that all consumers and employees experience within a setting.
  - The organization has a process for consulting with staff as well as service users to receive ongoing feedback in a way that feels safe for the person providing feedback.
- Prioritize and Create a Work Plan
  - The workgroup that the OTP is a part of has a system to prioritize needs and actions based on what policies and procedures are identified to need modification or support.

■ Implementation of prioritized changes occurs with the TI committed workgroup collecting ongoing data.

Phase 4: Trauma Informed

■ Implement and Monitor
   ■ Implementation of needed changes and interventions has begun and a method of tracking effectiveness is in place. The OTP can contribute to this initiative by implementing TI practices within their setting as well as supporting systemic changes needed at an organizational level.
■ Adopt Policy or Practice
   ■ The OTP brings their unique holistic lens and understanding of contexts to help the workgroup evaluate processes and adopt those that are effective.

Evidence-Based Practice

The Adverse Childhood Experiences Study

Increased harm in childhood results in increased challenges throughout the life span.

RESEARCH FINDINGS

The understanding that traumatic events experienced within childhood led to poor quality of life throughout the life span gained broader recognition following the Kaiser Permanente ACE study (Felitti et al., 1998). This study was first conducted among about 17,000 Southern California residents in a relatively homogeneous sample group. Participants were given a questionnaire containing 10 questions. Each of these questions sought to identify experiences of early adversity the individual may have had. The original 10 questions addressed three categories: Abuse, Neglect, and Household Dysfunction. A score of 1 was given for each affirmative answer to each question where a particular childhood adverse experience occurred.

Participants were also asked about their mental and physical health and overall quality of life. Findings from this initial study showed a strong link between harm experienced as a child and lasting chronic mental and physical health outcomes. This study propelled further scientific investigation of trauma and early childhood adversity. Similar studies have been repeated in less homogeneous groups and across cultures (John-Henderson et al., 2020; Wade et al., 2016) and the findings consistently showed that increased harm in childhood resulted in increased challenges throughout the life span. As more research continued, the recognition of community ACEs and historical trauma was added to the ACE pyramid published by the CDC (2021).

APPLICATIONS

➡ All OTPs, regardless of practice setting, should identify where they are in the process of becoming trauma informed in terms of self-reflection, accountability, and action.
➡ OTPs can be change agents in their practice settings to make sure that the organization is implementing trauma-informed practices.

REFERENCES

Centers for Disease Control and Prevention. (2021). *About the CDC-Kaiser ACE study.* https://www.cdc.gov/violenceprevention/aces/about.html

Felitti, V. J., Anda, R. F., Nordenberg, D., Williamson, D. F., Spitz, A. M., Edwards, V., Koss, M. P., & Marks, J. S. (1998). Relationship of childhood abuse and household dysfunction to many of the leading causes of death in adults. The adverse childhood experiences study. *American Journal of Preventive Medicine, 14,* 245–258. https://doi.org/10.1016/s0749-3797(98)00017-8

John-Henderson, N. A., Henderson-Matthews, B., Ollinger, S. R., Racine, J., Gordon, M. R., Higgins, A. A., Horn, W. C., Reevis, S. A., Running Wolf, J. A., Grant, D., & Rynda-Apple, A. (2020). Adverse childhood experiences and immune system inflammation in adults residing on the Blackfeet Reservation: The moderating role of sense of belonging to the community. *Annals of Behavioral Medicine, 54*(2), 87–93. https://doi.org/10.1093/abm/kaz029

Wade, R., Cronholm, P. F., Fein, J. A., Forke, C. M., Davis, M. B., Harkins-Schwarz, M., Pachter, L. M., & Bair-Merritt, M. H. (2016). Household and community-level Adverse Childhood Experiences and adult health outcomes in a diverse urban population. *Child Abuse & Neglect, 52,* 135–145. https://doi.org/10.1016/j.chiabu.2015.11.021

Here's the Point

- Trauma has the potential to negatively impact all people at individual, family, community, and societal levels.
- If left unaddressed, trauma is likely to negatively impact all areas of occupations.
- The impact of childhood trauma permeates into adulthood and is therefore relevant to OTPs in all practice settings.
- Simply because trauma has happened does not mean that a person's trajectory is doomed. PTG and posttraumatic healing are possible. Occupational therapy can be an important part of that healing.
- The OTP must engage in self-reflection and self-accountability to ensure they are trauma sensitive in their occupational therapy practice.
- It's not necessary for people to know they are receiving trauma-sensitive care to provide trauma-sensitive care.

This is similar to universal health precautions and can be considered "universal mental health precautions."
- SAMHSA's six principles can be combined with occupational therapy theory and other TI models and theories to support best practice.
- TIO is a public health model providing systemic steps for organizations. The OTP can be a change agent within their organization.
- There is no one "right" model of TIC training; instead, practitioners can pull from extensive evidence and choose models that apply to their specific population and setting.

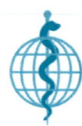 Visit the online resource center at **FADavis.com** to access the videos.

Apply It Now

1. Safety in Trauma-Informed Care

Safety is the first principle of SAMHSA's TIC and is the foundation of TI models such as the NMT, Trust-Based Relational Intervention, Mahler's interoception curriculum, and polyvagal theory.

What are three strategies that you could use in treatment to promote safety?

2. Using the Trauma Informed Oregon Roadmap

Utilize the online TIO roadmap and assess your workplace, a fieldwork setting, or a community setting using these criteria. Using the roadmap steps, what would this organization's next step be in the journey toward becoming more trauma informed?

3. Review Your History

Reflect on your own life story. What feelings come up for you when reading this chapter? What challenges do you have in remaining regulated in occupational therapy settings when working with others? How might your history be related to your present-day challenges?

4. Video Exercise–Child in Crisis

Pair up with another student in your class or form a small group of students. Access and watch the "Child in Crisis" video at the online resource center at FADavis.com. Then, discuss and together answer the following questions:
- How do you think Mikey's personal history of ACEs affected his behavior in the group setting?
- Why was it important for Brittany to go beyond Mikey's labels (e.g., homicidal, suicidal, defiant, disruptive) when working with Mikey? How did that contribute to her success with this child?
- Trauma-informed care is reflected in actions such as giving voice and providing choice, collaborating, ensuring safety, being trustworthy, and encouraging self-help and peer support. Did Brittany take a trauma-informed approach with Mikey? Why, or why not?

Resources

- Table 5-4 is included with additional resources to support the readers' continued learning.
  - **"Fieldwork Experience in Juvenile Correction Setting" video.** In this video, occupational therapist Maggie reflects on how she felt prepared and unprepared for her fieldwork experience. She touches on topics such as trauma, emotional regulation, and sensory processing, and emphasizes the need to be aware of her own self-care by setting boundaries. Access the video at the online resource center at FADavis.com.
  - **"Life Skills Groups in an Unhoused Population" video.** Kailin is an occupational therapist who works in community mental health and homeless services. In this video, she describes the impactful life skills groups she runs in a women's shelter and how the use of a group facilitates peer-to-peer

support. Kailin offers several creative examples of life skill group activities. She emphasizes the need to employ trauma-informed practices and harm-reduction strategies in this population, meeting people where they truly are. Access the video at the online resource center at FADavis.com.
  - **"Managing Challenging Behaviors in Young Children" video.** In this video, an occupational therapist and OTA discuss the OTA's work in an Operation Breakthrough program within Head Start. The OTA works with young children from at-risk families; together with teachers and other therapists, she helps to catch any developmental delays and intervene as necessary. She describes a particularly challenging behavior in one child and the strategies she uses to help him feel comfortable, safe, and loved, allowing him to better participate in the classroom and individual sessions. Access the video at the online resource center at FADavis.com.

- **"Prioritizing Family During a Mother's Cancer Treatment" video.** Marylein Serrano is a mother of two children and a speech language therapist who has had several cancer diagnoses. In this video, she discusses how she worked to prioritize her family during cancer treatment, with the help of friends and extended family. She also shares her fears and how she made the most of her time with her husband and children. Access the video at the online resource center at FADavis.com.
- **"Occupational Therapy Approaches in a Shelter for Unaccompanied Refugee Youth" video.** In this video, occupational therapist Claudette Fette shares the impactful work she, volunteer students, and staff performed in a massive unaccompanied minor shelter in Texas in 2021. Many of the minors, mostly from Central America, had histories of trauma, and the conditions in the shelter were dismal–lack of meaningful occupations, bullying, untrained staff, and so on. Claudette describes her approach to assessing the environment, training staff, recruiting volunteers, responding to the minors' trauma responses, and creating and supporting occupations and leisure activities. Access the video at the online resource center at FADavis.com.

TABLE 5-4 | Additional Trauma-Informed Resources

Resource	Description	Reference and Website Links
Substance Abuse and Mental Health Services Administration (SAMHSA)	SAMHSA is a beneficial resource regarding trauma and TI approaches. This is a robust website with research and guidance on many trauma considerations.	www.samhsa.gov https://www.samhsa.gov/trauma-violence https://www.samhsa.gov/child-trauma https://store.samhsa.gov/product/SAMHSA-s-Concept-of-Trauma-and-Guidance-for-a-Trauma-Informed-Approach/SMA14-4884
Trauma Informed Oregon (TIO)	TIO's website has accessible and practical guidance to screen and intervene at systems levels toward TIC.	https://traumainformedoregon.org
Chapter 25: Trauma- and Stressor-Related Disorders	Chapter 25 of this text provides increased details regarding trauma and considerations for the OTP including additional helpful resources.	Chapter 25. Author: Megan Edgelow
Trauma Occupation and Participation: Foundations and Population Considerations in Occupational Therapy *Disclaimer: The authors of this chapter are editors of this text.	This AOTA-published text is devoted entirely to considerations of trauma within the field of occupational therapy.	https://myaota.aota.org/shop_aota/product/900599
Interoception by Kelly Mahler	Dr. Kelly Mahler's work in interoception provides occupation- and evidence-based strategies related to interoception.	https://www.kelly-mahler.com
Trust Based Relational Intervention® (TBRI®)	TBRI® is an attachment-based TI approach that is beneficial when working with children and families with histories of trauma.	https://child.tcu.edu/about-us/tbri
Neurosequential Model of Therapeutics™ (NMT™)	The NMT™ is a biologically respectful approach rooted in neurobiology to support children, families, and communities.	https://www.neurosequential.com
Polyvagal Theory Safe and Sound Protocol	The safe and sound protocol is an auditory intervention for children and adults based on polyvagal theory.	https://integratedlistening.com/polyvagal-theory
Somatic Experiencing™ International	SE™ provides a body-focused model to support healing from trauma and other stress disorders.	https://traumahealing.org
Healing Centered Engagement	Healing centered engagement provides organization-level approaches that confront racial inequity through addressing individual beliefs, interpersonal relationships, and relationships to dynamic systems.	https://flourishagenda.com
Every Moment Counts (EMC)	EMC is a mental health promotion initiative developed to help all children and youth become mentally healthy in order to succeed in school, at home, and in the community.	EveryMomentCounts.org

References

Abou-Arab, A. (2021). Chapter 13: Trauma-informed care: Historical and modern implications of racism and the engagement in meaningful activities. In A. Lynch, R. Ashcraft, & L. Tekell (Eds.), *Trauma, occupation, and participation: Foundations and population considerations in occupational therapy* (pp. 223–243). AOTA Press.

Ainsworth, M. S., Blehar, M. C., Waters, E., & Wall, S. (1978). *Patterns of attachment: A psychological study of the strange situation.* Lawrence Erlbaum.

Alcalá, H. E., Tomiyama, A. J., & von Ehrenstein, O. S. (2017). Gender differences in the association between adverse childhood experiences and cancer. W*omen's Health Issues, 27*(6), 625–631. https://doi.org/10.1016/j.whi.2017.06.002

American Occupational Therapy Association. (2020). Occupational therapy practice framework: Domain and process (4th ed.). *American Journal of Occupational Therapy, 74*(Suppl. 2), 7412410010p1–7412410010p87. https://doi.org/10.5014/ajot .2020.74S2001

Anda, R. F., Fleisher, V. I., Felitti, V. J., Edwards, V. J., Whitfield, C. L., Dube, S. R., & Williamson, D. F. (2004). Childhood abuse, household dysfunction, and indicators of impaired adult worker performance. *The Permanente Journal, 8*(1), 30. https://doi.org/10.7812 /tpp/03-089

Ashcraft, R., & Lynch, A. (2021). Chapter 6: Becoming a trauma informed practitioner. In A. Lynch, R. Ashcraft, & L. Tekell (Eds.), *Trauma, occupation, and participation: Foundations and population considerations in occupational therapy* (pp. 89–102). AOTA Press.

Atchison, B., & Suarez, M. (2021). Chapter 1: Introduction to trauma and the role of occupational therapy. In A. Lynch, R. Ashcraft, & L. Tekell (Eds.), *Trauma, occupation, and participation: Foundations and population considerations in occupational therapy* (pp. 3–18). AOTA Press.

Back, S. N., Schmitz, M., Koenig, J., Zettl, M., Kleindienst, N., Herpertz, S. C., & Bertsch, K. (2022). Reduced vagal activity in borderline personality disorder is unaffected by intranasal oxytocin administration, but predicted by the interaction between childhood trauma and attachment insecurity. *Journal of Neural Transmission, 129*(4), 409–419. https://doi.org/10.1007 /s00702-022-02482-9

Bazyk, S., Demirjian, L., Horvath, F., & Doxsey, L. (2018). The comfortable cafeteria program for promoting student participation and enjoyment: An outcome study. *The American Journal of Occupational Therapy, 72*(3), 7203205050p1–7203205050p9. https:// doi.org/10.5014/ajot.2018.025379

Bierer, L. M., Bader, H. N., Daskalakis, N. P., Lehrner, A., Provençal, N., Wiechmann, T., Klengel, T., Makotkine, I., Binder, E. B., & Yehuda, R. (2020). Intergenerational effects of maternal Holocaust exposure on FKBP5 methylation. *American Journal of Psychiatry, 177*(8), 744–753. https://doi.org/ 10.1176/appi.ajp.2019.19060618

Borio, J., & Sood, D. (2022). Understanding the current role of school-based occupational therapy practitioners in addressing childhood grief and loss and identifying next steps to expand their current practice. *Journal of Occupational Therapy, Schools, & Early Intervention, 15*(4), 374–389. https://doi.org/10.1080 /19411243.2021.2003735

Bowlby, J. (1982). Attachment and loss: Retrospect and prospect. *American Journal of Orthopsychiatry, 52*(4), 664–678. https://doi .org/10.1111/j.1939-0025.1982.tb01456.x

Briggs, E. C., Amaya-Jackson, L., Putnam, K. T., & Putnam, F. W. (2021). All adverse childhood experiences are not equal: The contribution of synergy to adverse childhood experience scores. *American Psychologist, 76*(2), 243–252. https://doi.org/10.1037 /amp0000768

Bronfenbrenner, U. (1989). Ecological systems theory. *Annals of Child Development, 6,* 187– 249.

Bruininks, R. H., & Bruininks, B. D. (2005). *Bruininks-Oseretsky Test of Motor Proficiency second edition—Users manual.* Pearson.

Cain, C., & Gautreaux, K. (2022). Reducing secondary traumatic stress and fueling knowledge of child maltreatment among health care providers. *Journal of Trauma Nursing, 29*(1), 41–46. https:// doi.org/10.1097/JTN.0000000000000630

Carello, J., & Butler, L. D. (2014). Potentially perilous pedagogies: Teaching trauma is not the same as trauma-informed teaching. *Journal of Trauma & Dissociation, 15*(2), 153–168. https://doi.org /10.1080/15299732.2014.867571

Centers for Disease Control and Prevention. (2021). *About the CDC-Kaiser ACE study.* https://www.cdc.gov/violenceprevention /aces/about.html

Centers for Disease Control and Prevention. (2023). *COVID data tracker weekly review.* https://www.cdc.gov/coronavirus /2019-ncov/covid-data/covidview/index.html

Craig, A. D. (2003). Interoception: the sense of the physiological condition of the body. *Current Opinion in Neurobiology, 13*(4), 500–505. https://doi.org/10.1016/S0959-4388(03)00090-4

Creek, J., Moore, T., & Sinclair, K. (2021). Chapter 15: Trauma-informed occupational therapy for displaced persons. In A. Lynch, R. Ashcraft, & L. Tekell (Eds.), *Trauma, occupation, and participation: Foundations and population considerations in occupational therapy* (pp. 275–290). AOTA Press.

Crenshaw, K. (1991). Mapping the margins: Intersectionality, identity politics, and violence against women of color. *Stanford Law Review, 43*(6), 1241–1279. https://doi.org/10.2307/1229039

Cross, D., Call, C. D., Howard, A., & Lynch, A. (2019). Sensory processing in children with a history of maltreatment. *American Journal of Occupational Therapy, 4,* (Suppl 1), 7311505163. https:// doi.org/10.5014/ajot.2019.73S1-PO6012

Duffy, K. A., McLaughlin, K. A., & Green, P. A. (2018). Early life adversity and health-risk behaviors: Proposed psychological and neural mechanisms. *Annals of the New York Academy of Sciences, 1428*(1), 151–169. https://doi.org/10.1111/nyas.13928

Dunn, W. (2014). *Sensory Profile 2—Users manual.* Pearson.

Ellis, W., Dietz, W. H., & Chen, K.-L. (2022). Community resilience: A dynamic model for public health 3.0. *Journal of Public Health Management and Practice, 28*(Suppl. 1), S18–S26. https:// doi.org/10.1097/PHH.0000000000001413

Felitti, V. J., Anda, R. F., Nordenberg, D., Williamson, D. F., Spitz, A. M., Edwards, V., Koss, M. P., & Marks, J. S. (1998). Relationship of childhood abuse and household dysfunction to many of the leading causes of death in adults. The adverse childhood experiences study. *American Journal of Preventive Medicine, 14,* 245–258. https://doi.org/10.1016/s0749-3797(98)00017-8

Felitti, V. J., Anda, R. F., Nordenberg, D., Williamson, D. F., Spitz, A. M., Edwards, V., Koss, M. P., & Marks, J. S. (2019). Relationship of childhood abuse and household dysfunction to many of the leading causes of death in adults: The adverse childhood experiences (ACE) study. *American Journal of Preventive Medicine, 56*(6), 774–786. https://doi.org/10.1016/j.amepre.2019.04.001

Ferraro, I. K., & Taylor, A. M. (2021). Adult attachment styles and emotional regulation: The role of interoceptive awareness and alexithymia. *Personality and Individual Differences, 173,* 110641. https://doi.org/10.1016/j.paid.2021.110641

Frieze, S. (2015). How trauma affects student learning and behaviour. *BU Journal of Graduate Studies in Education, 7*(2), 27–34.

Gaskill, R. L., & Perry, B. D. (2017). Chapter 3: A neurosequential therapeutic approach to guided play, play therapy, and activities for children who won't talk. In C. A. Malchiodi & D. Crenshaw (Eds.), *What to do when children clam up in psychotherapy interventions to facilitate communication* (pp. 38–66). Guilford Press.

Ginwright, S. (2016). *Dare to disrupt keynote.* National Summer Learning Association. https://childcareta.acf.hhs.gov/ncase -resource-library/2016-dare-disrupt-keynote-shawn-ginwright-phd

Godoy, L. C., Frankfurter, C., Cooper, M., Lay, C., Maunder, R., & Farkouh, M. E. (2021). Association of adverse childhood experiences with cardiovascular disease later in life: A review. *JAMA Cardiology, 6*(2), 228–235. https://doi.org/10.1001/jamacardio.2020.6050

Grant, J. M., Mottet, L. A., Tanis, J., Harrison, J., Herman, J. L., & Keisling, M. (2011). *Injustice at every turn: A report of the National Transgender Discrimination Survey.* National Center for Transgender Equality and National Gay and Lesbian Task Force.

Griffin, J. (2005). Recreation therapy for adult survivors of childhood abuse: Challenges to professional perspectives and the evolution of a leisure education group. *Therapeutic Recreation Journal, 39*(3), 207–228.

Halfon, N., & Hochstein, M. (2002). Life course health development: An integrated framework for developing health, policy, and research. *The Milbank Quarterly, 80*(3), 433–479. https://doi.org/10.1111/1468-0009.00019

Heberle, A., Obus, E., & Gray, S. (2020). An intersectional perspective on the intergenerational transmission of trauma and state-perpetrated violence. *Journal of Social Issues, 76*(4), 814–834. https://doi.org/10.1111/josi.12404

Herbell, K., & Bloom, T. (2020). A qualitative metasynthesis of mothers' adverse childhood experiences and parenting practices. *Journal of Pediatric Health Care, 34*(5), 409–417. https://doi.org/10.1016/j.pedhc.2020.03.003

Herrenkohl, T. I., Klika, J. B., Herrenkohl, R. C., Russo, M. J., & Dee, T. (2012). A prospective investigation of the relationship between child maltreatment and indicators of adult psychological well-being. *Violence and Victims, 27*(5), 764–776. https://doi.org/10.1891/0886-6708.27.5.764

Holman, D. M., Ports, K. A., Buchanan, N. D., Hawkins, N. A., Merrick, M. T., Metzler, M., & Trivers, K. F. (2016). The association between adverse childhood experiences and risk of cancer in adulthood: A systematic review of the literature. *Pediatrics, 138*(Suppl. 1), S81–S91. https://doi.org/10.1542/peds.2015-4268L

Hou, T., Zhang, R., Song, X., Zhang, F., Cai, W., Liu, Y., Dong, W., & Deng, G. (2020). Self-efficacy and fatigue among non-frontline health care workers during COVID-19 outbreak: A moderated mediation model of posttraumatic stress disorder symptoms and negative coping. *PLoS One, 15*(12), e0243884. https://doi.org/10.1371/journal.pone.0243884

Howard, A. R. H., Lynch, A. K., Call, C. D., & Cross, D. R. (2020). Sensory processing in children with a history of maltreatment: An occupational therapy perspective. *Vulnerable Children and Youth Studies, 15*(1), 60–67. https://doi.org/10.1080/17450128.2019.1687963

Howes, C., & Guerra, A. G. W. (2009). Networks of attachment relationships in low-income children of Mexican heritage: Infancy through preschool. *Social Development, 18*, 896–914. https://doi.org/10.1111/j.1467-9507.2008.00524.x

Iwama, M. K. (2006). *The Kawa model: Culturally relevant occupational therapy.* Churchill Livingstone Elsevier.

Jiang, B., & He, D. (2019). Repetitive transcranial magnetic stimulation (rTMS) fails to increase serum brain-derived neurotrophic factor (BDNF). *Neurophysiologie Clinique, 49*(4), 295–300. https://doi.org/10.1016/j.neucli.2019.05.068

John-Henderson, N. A., Henderson-Matthews, B., Ollinger, S. R., Racine, J., Gordon, M. R., Higgins, A. A., Horn, W. C., Reevis, S. A., Running Wolf, J. A., Grant, D., & Rynda-Apple, A. (2020). Adverse childhood experiences and immune system inflammation in adults residing on the Blackfeet Reservation: The moderating role of sense of belonging to the community. *Annals of Behavioral Medicine, 54*(2), 87–93. https://doi.org/10.1093/abm/kaz029

Kavanaugh, B., & Holler, K. (2015). Brief report: Neurocognitive functioning in adolescents following childhood maltreatment and evidence for underlying planning & organizational deficits. *Child Neuropsychology, 21*(6), 840–848. https://doi.org/10.1080/09297049.2014.929101

Khalsa, S. S., Adolphs, R., Cameron, O. G., Critchley, H. D., Davenport, P. W., Feinstein, J. S., Feusner, J. D., Garfinkel, S. N., Lane, R. D., Mehling, W. E., Meuret, A. E., Nemeroff, C. B., Oppenheimer, S., Petzschner, F. H., Pollatos, O., Rhudy, J. L., Schramm, L. P., Simmons, W. K., Stein, M. B., . . . von Leupoldt, A. (2018). Interoception and mental health: A roadmap. *Biological Psychiatry: Cognitive Neuroscience and Neuroimaging, 3*(6), 501–513. https://doi.org/10.1016/j.bpsc.2017.12.004

Kielhofner, G. (1995). *A Model of Human Occupation* (2nd ed.). Williams & Wilkins.

Kim, D. H., Kang, N. R., & Kwack, Y. S. (2019). Differences in parenting stress, parenting attitudes, and parents' mental health according to parental adult attachment style. *Journal of the Korean Academy of Child and Adolescent Psychiatry, 30*(1), 17–25. https://doi.org/10.5765/jkacap.180014

King, G., Law, M., King, S., Hurley, P., Rosenbaum, P., Hanna, S., Kertoy, M., & Young, N. (2004). *Children's Assessment of Participation and Enjoyment and Preferences for Activities of Children (CAPE/PAC)—Users manual.* Pearson.

Kovachy, B., O'Hara, R., Hawkins, N., Gershon, A., Primeau, M. M., Madej, J., & Carrion, V. (2013). Sleep disturbance in pediatric PTSD: Current findings and future directions. *Journal of Clinical Sleep Medicine, 9*(5), 501. https://doi.org/10.5664/jcsm.2678

Laszloffy, T. (2002). Rethinking family development theory: Teaching with the systemic family development (SFD) model. *Family Relations, 51*(3), 206–214. https://doi.org/10.1111/j.1741-3729.2002.206098.x

Lavalley, R., & Johnson, K. R. (2022). Occupation, injustice, and anti-black racism in the United States of America. *Journal of Occupational Science, 29*(4), 487–499. https://doi.org/10.1080/14427591.2020.1810111

Law, M., Cooper, B., Strong, S., Stewart, D., Rigby, P., & Letts, L. (1996). The Person-Environment-Occupation model: A transactive approach to occupational performance. *Canadian Journal of Occupational Therapy, 63*, 9–23. https://doi.org/10.1177/000841749606300103

Levy, K., Ellison, W., Schott, L., & Bernecker, S. (2010). Attachment style. *Journal of Clinical Psychology, 67*(2), 193–203. https://doi.org/10.1002/jclp.20756

Licciardi, L., & Brown, T. (2021). An overview & critical review of the Sensory Profile–second edition. *Scandinavian Journal of Occupational Therapy, 30*(6), 1–13. https://doi.org/10.1080/11038128.2021.1930148

Liu, Y., Croft, J. B., Chapman, D. P., Perry, G. S., Greenlund, K. J., Zhao, G., & Edwards, V. J. (2013). Relationship between adverse childhood experiences and unemployment among adults from five US states. *Social Psychiatry and Psychiatric Epidemiology, 48*(3), 357–369. https://doi.org/10.1007/s00127-012-0554-1

Logan, J. R. (2007). *The impact of Katrina: Race and class in storm-damaged 48 neighborhoods. Spatial structures in the social sciences, Hurricane Katrina Project.* Brown University.

Lu, S., Gao, W., Huang, M., Li, L., & Xu, Y. (2016). In search of the HPA axis activity in unipolar depression patients with childhood trauma: Combined cortisol awakening response and dexamethasone suppression test. *Journal of Psychiatric Research, 78*, 24–30. https://doi.org/10.1016/j.jpsychires.2016.03.009

Lynch, A., Ashcraft, R., Mahler, K., Cameron Whiting, C., Schroeder, K., & Weber, M. (2020). Using public health model as a foundation for trauma-informed care for occupational therapists in school settings. *Journal of Occupational Therapy, Schools, & Early Intervention, 13*(3), 219–235. https://doi.org/10.1080/19411243.2020.1732263

Lynch, A., & Mahler, K. (2021). Chapter 2: Trauma impact upon neurobiological, social emotional, and motor function: Implications for occupation. In A. Lynch, R. Ashcraft, & L. Tekell, *Trauma, occupation, and participation: Foundations and population considerations for occupational therapy* (pp. 19–40). AOTA Press.

MacKinnon, L. (2012). The Neurosequential Model of Therapeutics: An interview with Bruce Perry. *Australian and New Zealand Journal of Family Therapy, 33*(3), 210–218. https://doi.org/10.1017/aft.2012.26

Mahler, K. (2016). *The Comprehensive Assessment of Interoceptive Awareness.* Autism Asperger Publishing Company.

Mahler, K. (2019). *The interoception curriculum: A step-by-step guide to develop mindful self-regulation.* https://www.kelly-mahler.com/product/the-interoception-curriculum-a-step-bystep-guide-to-developing-mindful-self-regulation

Mahler, K. (2023). *Interoception curriculum publications.* Mahler Autism Services. https://www.kelly-mahler.com/product-category/publications

Maleku, A., Subedi, B., Kim, Y. K., Haran, H., & Pyakurel, S. (2022). Toward healing-centered engagement to address mental well-being among young Bhutanese-Nepali Refugee women in the United States: Findings from the cultural leadership project. *Journal of Ethnic & Cultural Diversity in Social Work, 1*–19. https://doi.org/10.1080/15313204.2022.2161684

Markey, K., Prosen, M., Martin, E., & Repo Jamal, H. (2021). Fostering an ethos of cultural humility development in nurturing inclusiveness and effective intercultural team working. *Journal of Nursing Management, 29,* 2724–2728. https://doi.org/10.1111/jonm.13429

Meyer, I. H. (2003). Prejudice, social stress, and mental health in lesbian, gay, and bisexual populations: Conceptual issues and research evidence. *Psychological Bulletin, 129*(5), 674–697. https://doi.org/10.1037/0033-2909.129.5.674

National Child Traumatic Stress Network, Secondary Trauma Stress Committee. (2011). *Secondary traumatic stress: A fact sheet for child-serving professionals.* National Center for Child Traumatic Stress.

Neumann, M., Neu, D., & Christian Ungco, J. (2021). Chapter 12: Addressing LGBTQIA+ trauma: Your role and your responsibility. In A. Lynch, R. Ashcraft, & L. Tekell (Eds.), *Trauma, occupation, and participation: Foundations and population considerations in occupational therapy* (pp. 195–221). AOTA Press.

Perry, B. D. (2006). Applying principles of neurodevelopment to clinical work with maltreated and traumatized children: The Neurosequential Model of Therapeutics. In N. B. Webb (Ed.), *Social work practice with children and families. Working with traumatized youth in child welfare* (pp. 27–52). Guilford Press.

Perry, B. D., & Winfrey, O. (2021). *What happened to you? Conversations on trauma, resilience, and healing.* Flatiron Books.

Porges, S. (2022). Polyvagal theory: A science of safety. *Frontiers in Integrative Neuroscience, 16,* 871227. https://doi.org/10.3389/fnint.2022.871227

Purvis, K., Cross, D., Dansereau, D., & Parris, S. (2013). Trust Based Relational Intervention (TBRI): A systemic approach to complex developmental trauma. *Child and Youth Services, 34,* 360–386. https://doi.org/10.1080/0145935X.2013.859906

Quilty, L. C., Taylor, G. J., McBride, C., & Bagby, R. M. (2017). Relationships among alexithymia, therapeutic alliance, and psychotherapy outcome in major depressive disorder. *Psychiatry Research, 254,* 75–79. https:doi/org/10.1016/j.psychres.2017.04.047

Rischard, M. E., & Cromer, L. D. (2019). The role of executive function in predicting children's outcomes in a cognitive behavioral treatment for trauma-related nightmares and secondary sleep disturbances. *Journal of Child & Adolescent Trauma, 12*(4), 501–513. https://doi.org/10.1007/s40653-019-00252-6

Sarno, E. L., Newcomb, M. E., & Mustanski, B. (2020). Rumination longitudinally mediates the association of minority stress and depression in sexual and gender minority individuals. *Journal of Abnormal Psychology, 129*(4), 355–363. https://doi.org/10.1037/abn0000508

Schaan, V. K., Schulz, A., Rubel, J. A., Bernstein, M., Domes, G., Schächinger, H., & Vögele, C. (2019). Childhood trauma affects stress-related interoceptive accuracy. *Frontiers in Psychiatry, 10,* 750. https://doi.org/10.3389/fpsyt.2019.00750

Sheikh, M. A. (2018). Psychological abuse, substance abuse distress, dissatisfaction with friendships, and incident psychiatric problems. *Journal of Psychosomatic Research, 108,* 78–84. https://doi.org/10.1016/j.jpsychores.2018.03.001

Sonu, S., Marvin, D., & Moore, C. (2021). The intersection and dynamics between COVID-19, health disparities, and adverse childhood experiences: Intersection/dynamics between COVID-19, health disparities, and ACEs. *Journal of Child & Adolescent Trauma, 14*(4), 517–526. https://doi.org/10.1007/s40653-021-00363-z

Substance Abuse and Mental Health Services Administration. (2014). *SAMHSA's concept of trauma and guidance for a trauma-informed approach* (p. 9). HHS Publication No. (SMA) 14-4884. U.S. Department of Health and Human Services.

Taff, S. D., Russell-Thomas, D. C., Tyminski, Q., Wilson, A., Barco, P., & Berg, C. (2021). Chapter 7: Occupational therapy in the pandemic: Facing challenges, building resilience, and sparking innovation. In A. Lynch, R. Ashcraft, & L. Tekell (Eds.), *Trauma, occupation, and participation: Foundations and population considerations in occupational therapy* (pp. 105–121). AOTA Press.

Taylor. R. (2008). *The intentional relationship: Occupational therapy and use of self.* F.A. Davis Company.

Terradas, M. M., & Asselin, A. (2022). Episodic experiences of child physical abuse, early relational trauma and post-traumatic play: Theoretical considerations and clinical illustrations. *Journal of Child and Adolescent Trauma, 16,* 365–379. https://doi.org/10.1007/s40653-022-00489-8

Tedeschi, R. G., & Calhoun, L. (1998). Posttraumatic growth: Future directions. In R. G. Tedeschi, C. L. Park, & L. G. Calhoun (Eds.), *Post-traumatic growth: Positive changes in the aftermath of crisis* (pp. 93–102). Lawrence Erlbaum.

Tedeschi. R. G., & Calhoun, L. (2004). Posttraumatic growth: A new perspective on psychotraumatology. *Psychiatric Times, 21*(4), 58.

Tedeschi, R. G., Shakespeare-Finch, J., Taku, K., & Calhoun, L. G. (2018). *Posttraumatic growth: Theory, research, and application.* Routledge. https://doi.org/10.4324/9781315527451

Tervalon, M., & Murray-Garcia, J. (1998). Cultural humility versus cultural competence: A critical distinction in defining physician training outcomes in multicultural education. *Journal of Health Care Poor Undeserved, 9*(2), 117–125. https://doi.org/10.1353/hpu.2010.0233

Thelen, E., & Smith, L. B. (2006). Dynamic Systems Theories. In R. M. Lerner & W. Damon (Eds.), *Handbook of child psychology: Theoretical models of human development* (6th ed., pp. 258–312). John Wiley & Sons.

Trauma Informed Oregon. (2016). *Roadmap to trauma informed care.* https://traumainformedoregon.org/implementation/implementation-and-accountability-overview/roadmap-to-trauma-informed-care

van der Kolk, B. A. (1989). The compulsion to repeat the trauma. Re-enactment, revictimization, and masochism. *The Psychiatric Clinics of North America, 12*(2), 389–411.

Veterans Affairs. (2019, November). *America's wars fact sheet.* https://www.va.gov/opa/publications/factsheets/fs_americas_wars.pdf

Wade, R., Cronholm, P. F., Fein, J. A., Forke, C. M., Davis, M. B., Harkins-Schwarz, M., Pachter, L. M., & Bair-Merritt, M. H. (2016). Household and community-level adverse childhood experiences and adult health outcomes in a diverse urban population. *Child Abuse & Neglect, 52,* 135–145. https://doi.org/10.1016/j.chiabu.2015.11.021

Wassell, E. (2014). *The influence of family care leave policy on the long-term wellbeing outcomes of children.* ProQuest Dissertations Publishing.

Watts, K. S. (2017). *Families with low incomes and the search for child care: An exploration of factors influencing search actions and choices.* Available from ProQuest Dissertations & Theses Global. https://login.ezproxy3.lhl.uab.edu/login?url=https://www.proquest.com/dissertations-theses/families-with-low-incomes-search-child-care/docview/2013203133/se-2

Whiting, C. C. (2018). Trauma and the role of the school-based occupational therapist. *Journal of Occupational Therapy, Schools, & Early Intervention, 11*(3), 291–301. https://doi.org/10.1080/19411243.2018.1438327

Whiting, C. C., Ochsenbein, M., Schoen, S., & Spielmann, V. (2021). A multi-tiered and multi-dimensional approach to intervention in schools: Recommendations for children with sensory integration and processing challenges. *Journal of Occupational Therapy, Schools, & Early Intervention, 15*(3), 314–327. https://doi.org/10.1080/19411243.2021.1959486

Willis-Hepp, B., & Ashcraft, R. (2021). Chapter 3: Trauma across the lifespan and family systems theory: Considerations for occupational therapy. In A. Lynch, R. Ashcraft, & L. Tekell (Eds.), *Trauma, occupation, and participation: Foundations and population considerations in occupational therapy* (pp. 41–51). AOTA Press.

World Health Organization. (2022). *WHO coronavirus (COVID19) dashboard.* https://covid19.who.int

Yehuda, R., Daskalakis, N., Bierer, L., Bader, H., Klengel, T., Holsboer, F., & Binder, E. (2016). Holocaust exposure induced intergenerational effects on FKBP5 methylation. *Biological Psychiatry, 80*(5), 372–380. https://doi.org/10.1016/j.biopsych.2015.08.005

Zhu, S., Shan, S., Liu, W., Li, S., Hou, L., Huang, X., Liu, Y., Yi, Q., Sun, W., Tang, K., Adeloye, D., Rudan, I., Song, P., & Global Health Epidemiology Research Group. (2022). Adverse childhood experiences and risk of diabetes: A systematic review and meta-analysis. *Journal of Global Health, 12.* https://doi.org/10.7189/jogh.12.04082

Zoraster, R. (2010). Vulnerable populations: Hurricane Katrina as a case study. *Prehospital and Disaster Medicine, 25*(1), 74–78. https://doi.org/10.1017/S1049023X00007718

CHAPTER
6

Evidence-Based Practice

Catana Brown

When it comes to understanding the people occupational therapy practitioners (OTPs) serve, making predictions about outcomes, and selecting useful assessments and interventions, the research evidence is an important source of information for OTPs, who are expected to use evidence to make therapeutic decisions. The evidence in evidence-based practice comes from research, practitioner experience, and the values and preferences of the person. All three components should be taken into account when making decisions; however, this chapter focuses on the component of evidence-based practice that comes from scientific research.

In today's health-care environment, OTPs are often asked to justify their decisions from several sources. For example, when an OTP recommends an intervention in a team meeting, professionals from other disciplines may ask about the research evidence before providing support. People often present information from internet searches and ask for a professional opinion. Insurance companies may deny payments for services that are not grounded in the research evidence. Most importantly, the research evidence provides a source of information that helps OTPs partner with individuals to make the best decisions.

This chapter describes evidence-based practice and explains the different types of research evidence, including the purpose of each type. In addition, it provides information on how to evaluate the quality of each type of research. A table of research studies is provided with each type of research to offer examples of psychosocial practice from the occupational therapy literature.

The Use of Evidence in Professional Reasoning

The most widely cited definition of **evidence-based medicine** comes from David Sackett, a pioneer of evidence-based medicine, and his colleagues (1996): "Evidence based medicine is the conscientious, explicit and judicious use of current best evidence in making decisions about the care of individual patients" (p. 71). **Evidence-based practice** in occupational therapy is based on these principles of evidence-based medicine. However, the use of evidence in practice does not mean that practice becomes a rote process or that the research evidence is the only source of information. The concept of evidence-based practice has evolved to recognize

that therapeutic reasoning is a more complex process that includes scientific evidence, practitioner experience, and the values and preferences of the person.

Occupational therapy practice is both an art and a science. Each individual situation is unique. The use of research studies is just one component of therapeutic reasoning. The OTP will also draw on their knowledge of theories and practice models, the story they've acquired from the individual during the occupational profile, and pragmatic considerations related to resources (Schell, 2019).

The Process of Using Research in Practice

Implementing research into practice can seem daunting; however, a five-step process can make this important task less overwhelming. The five steps can be viewed as a cycle (Fig. 6-1) and are described in greater detail in the text that follows.

The first step involves *identifying a problem.* Perhaps OTPs are interested in the effectiveness of a particular intervention, or they want to know if a specific assessment is reliable when multiple therapists are going to use it. This step guides the process toward the next step, which is *identifying the relevant*

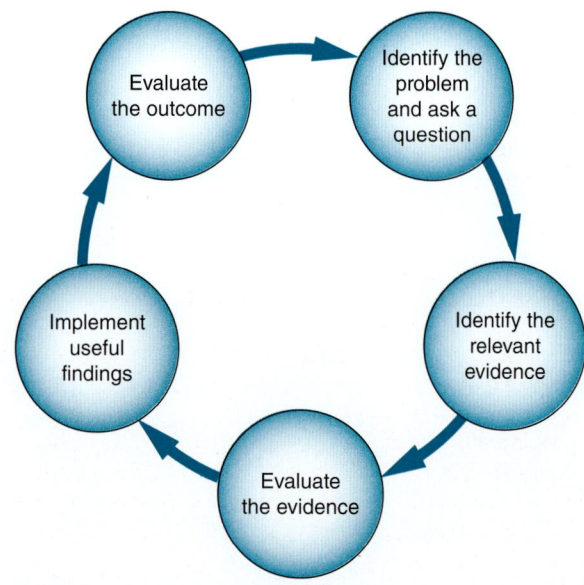

FIGURE 6-1. The cycle of evidence-based practice.

The Lived Experience

Editor's Note: This lived experience differs from those in other chapters in that it captures the experience of the therapy practitioner instead of the person or family member with a mental health concern.

When the Person's Feedback Is Your Evidence
—Halley Read, MOT, OTR/L, QMHP

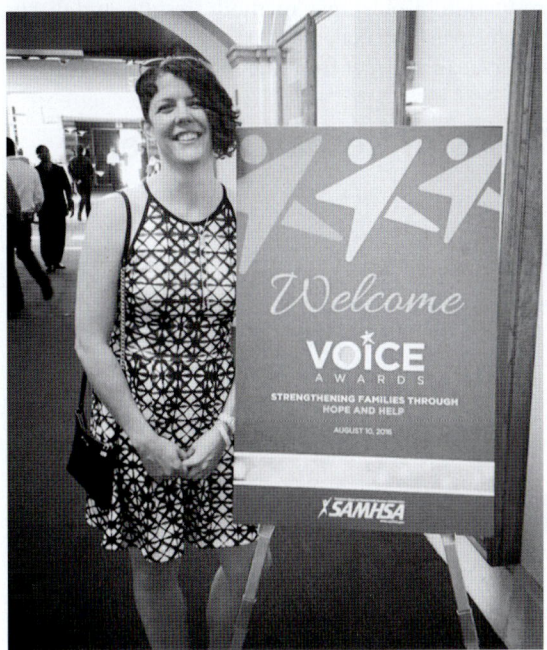

Halley represented AOTA at the SAMHSA Voice Awards, which recognizes individuals and the media for positive portrayals of individuals with mental illness.

When first using evidence to inform my practice I remember thinking to myself, "OK, what environment or tools need to be set up to ensure the best outcome using this literature?" Or, "Can I make some adaptations to implementing this, but still use the results of this evidence-based outcome?" The more I served people in my community mental health occupational therapy role, the more I began to see that a clinician who uses evidence-based practice is not just repeating study methodologies for similar results. It is a delicate combination of evidence and the person's experience to inform the occupational therapy process, clinical reasoning, evaluation tools, and treatment team planning. Evidence-based practice, I believe now, never was about solely focusing on what research or literature says MUST happen, but is about focusing on what CAN happen to help a person reach his or her goals.

In clinical practice I worked on the Early Assessment Support Alliance (EASA). EASA is an evidence-based model program that provides community-based wraparound services to those young people at risk for a psychotic illness, or those having their first episode of psychosis. Meant for those youth and young adults, ages 14 to 25, it is built on the evidence that suggests the longer the duration of untreated psychosis, the more chronic or long term the illness can become, and the fewer opportunities for positive life outcomes these folks can have. Integrating ideas from other evidence-based models, such as Assertive Community Treatment,

EASA provides 2 years of case management, occupational therapy, supported employment and education, counseling, family therapy, and community support and integration to ensure these young people still reach their typical young adult milestones, all while learning what helps them find and maintain recovery.

My time with EASA, both clinically and program development-wise, taught me the importance of using evidence to inform the treatment, but, more importantly, that the people's and their family's lived experience and feedback were the most important form of evidence. Using the EASA model to inform my clinical decisions taught me that I was most effective at best practice when I combined evidence with the people's input, feedback, and experiential evidence.

Similar to other fidelity-based models, this program tracks outcomes, asks for quarterly data, and ensures that each EASA team in the state is meeting strong fidelity, based on a yearly review of the team against the fidelity scale. For example, the fidelity guidelines helped when I was new to the team and practice, to understand my role as the OTP, what my teammates' roles were, and what the overall goal of the EASA participation is for these young folks and their families. In this way, this evidence-based practice model helped me learn my job, and inspired me to function on my team in a transdisciplinary way.

My experience with EASA and other evidence-based work has taught me about the other "evidence" to use in my clinical decisions: the person's lived experience and feedback. EASA asks its teams to regularly seek feedback from people in formal and informal ways. Formally, team members use a rating scale, again based on evidence, to get input from people on how the session went for them along with overall satisfaction in the areas of school, work, social life, and stress in their lives.

Another tenet of this model that showed me the power of using lived experience as evidence was the requirement to perform regular 90-day reviews with the person, their family or support network, and the treatment team. Yes, I used best occupational therapy practice to build independent living skills; yes, I promoted sensory modulation strategies; and sure, I built community integration skills for these young folks, and used the most evidence-based occupational therapy assessments, but I never used that evidence alone. It was always in combination with or informed by the person's input, feedback, and lived experience of his or her illness, strengths, and challenges.

Community mental health occupational therapy work has taught me that best practice is when evidence-based practice, research outcomes, data, and literature combine with the participants' feedback and their recovery experience to inform the treatment planning and care coordination for them. This, to me, has been so wonderfully empowering because this is also the distinct value of occupational therapy. We harness our therapeutic use of self to review the evidence, take the knowledge to our patients, and create a person-centered plan. Evidence-based practice work has shown me that evidence is sometimes the person whom you are serving's story more than what the data from research shows. And, to see recovery happen for the people you serve, combine therapeutic use of self, data, and individual feedback.

For more information about EASA you can go to: easacommunity.org.

Find EASA on Facebook!

evidence. Based on the problem that was elucidated, OTPs can use key words to search relevant evidence. Once the evidence is found, they need to *evaluate the evidence.* Not all studies are created equal, and some research designs are better than others in providing strong evidence. These concepts are discussed in greater detail in the next sections.

Once OTPs are familiar with the evidence they can then *implement this information into practice.* In other words, they will use the evidence to make decisions about what intervention or assessment to use, or the evidence may help them better understand an individual's situation. Finally, *the outcomes of the implementation should be evaluated.* The reflective practitioner does not take the research at face value but draws upon their experience and the individual's to make decisions. This might lead the OTP to identify new problems and begin the evidence-based process again. Read this chapter's The Lived Experience feature to see how one OTP incorporated the research evidence into her practice and, in doing so, listened closely to the evidence that emerged from the people she served.

When reading the research evidence, it is helpful to know the typical organizational structure of a research article. The four main components of a research article are the introduction, the methods, the results, and the discussion. The introduction provides background information that explains why the study is important. The introduction typically ends with a purpose statement that explains the aims of the study and includes a research question or hypothesis. The methods section explains the processes used to conduct the research, such as the methods used to recruit participants, the measures used, and the statistical analysis. The results section provides the findings based on the statistical analysis or, in the case of qualitative research, the thematic analysis. This section also includes tables or graphs to present the results. The discussion summarizes the findings but also provides an explanation. The discussion may also include information on implications for practice as well as limitations of the study design.

All research studies will begin with an abstract. An abstract provides a very brief summary of the study organized around the four sections that were presented previously: introduction or objective, methods, results, and discussion or conclusions (Tanaka et al., 2022). Figure 6-2 provides an example of an abstract from the research literature.

Types of Research Evidence

There are many types of research that can inform OTPs in their practice. This chapter organizes research into five categories:

1. Descriptive research
2. Predictive research
3. Efficacy research
4. Assessment research
5. Qualitative research

Abstract

BACKGROUND:

Mood and adjustment disorders are two major causes of long-term sick leave among employees, leading to large social losses. Therefore, a return to work (RTW) intervention was attempted, targeting patients with mood and adjustment disorders.

OBJECTIVE:

This study aimed to investigate the outcome of an interdisciplinary RTW intervention including occupational therapy implemented within the Japanese healthcare framework.

METHODS:

An interdisciplinary RTW intervention including occupational therapy was conducted five times a week for approximately 3 months, targeting individuals with mood and adjustment disorders who took a leave of absence. Their mental symptoms, cognitive functioning, job performance, temperament, social adaptation, psychosocial state, and readiness to RTW before and after the intervention were evaluated. Full-time RTW ratios at 3, 6, 12, 18, and 24 months from baseline were followed up and compared with those of prior studies.

RESULTS:

A total of 30 individuals completed the intervention. After the intervention, participants' psychological symptoms, cognitive function, vocational aptitude, temperament, social adaptation, psychosocial state, and readiness to RTW improved ($p \leq 0.001$–0.0279). The ratios of RTW at 3, 6, 12, 18, and 24 months from the baseline were 6.7%, 46.7%, 73.3%, 77.8%, and 82.6%, respectively, reflecting a higher pattern than prior reports.

CONCLUSIONS:

The interdisciplinary RTW intervention including occupational therapy has the potential to improve not only depressive symptoms but also cognitive functioning, job performance, social adaptation, and readiness to RTW. They can also raise RTW ratios.

FIGURE 6-2. Example of a research abstract. *From Tanaka, S., Kuge, R. I., Nakano, M., Inukai, S., Hamamoto, M., Terasawa, M., Nakamura, T., Sugiyama, N., Kobayashi, M., & Washizuka, S. (2022). Outcomes of an interdisciplinary return to work intervention including occupational therapy for mood and adjustment disorders: A single-arm clinical trial. Work, 74(2), 515–530. https://doi.org/10.3233/WOR-211144*

This Text's Evidence-Based Practice Feature

One of the special features included in each chapter of this text is the Evidence-Based Practice feature. Using infographics as a way to display the information, one or more studies are described that relate to the chapter topic. Each Evidence-Based Practice feature includes a summary statement, a summary of the research findings, applications for OTPs, and the study citation(s). By reading the feature, you can learn how to take information from the research and apply it to your own practice.

Most research is **quantitative research,** meaning that numbers are used to present the findings. In quantitative research, a **hypothesis** is tested. The hypothesis proposes an expected finding, and the statistical analysis determines if the hypothesis is supported. For example, a researcher may start with a hypothesis that positive affect is associated with a larger social network. The researcher assesses both positive affect and social network size and then conducts a statistical analysis to determine if a statistically significant relationship exists. Descriptive, predictive, efficacy, and assessment research are all quantitative in nature. **Qualitative research,** on the other hand, uses a much different approach to collecting the data and presents the findings in the form of quotes, narratives, and themes.

Each type of research is described in the following sections, using examples of research from occupational therapy to illustrate each type of research. In addition, information on how to evaluate the quality of each type of research is provided. Although evidence-based OTPs use research from a wide variety of disciplines, this chapter uses occupational therapy examples to show the breadth of evidence supplied by the profession. Check out the box titled "This Text's Evidence-Based Practice Feature" to understand how this text is using this feature to promote evidence-based practice.

Descriptive Research

Descriptive studies provide information about psychiatric conditions, practice settings, and the practitioners who work in mental health. Descriptive studies use observational methods to depict situations and conditions as they exist. For this reason, descriptive studies may also be called **nonexperimental** because there is no manipulation of the situation (e.g., participants are not randomly assigned to groups).

Prevalence and incidence studies (more broadly described as epidemiological research) fall into the category of descriptive research. These studies furnish information about the number of individuals with a particular condition. **Epidemiology** is the study of the frequency and distribution of health conditions. **Prevalence** is the proportion of a population with a condition. For example, one study with 1,320 participants found that 11% of OTPs experienced bullying in the workplace (Bolding et al., 2021). **Incidence** is the number of new cases of a condition within a specified period of time. For example, Östergren, Canivet, and Agardh (2022) followed 7,759 volunteers for 1 year to identify the incidence of sexual harassment. They found the highest incidence of 17.5% was identified in women ages 18 to 34. They also found that sexual harassment was associated with poor mental health. (This additional finding would be an example of predictive research, which is discussed in the text that follows.)

OTPs are often interested in descriptive research to better understand the occupational performance needs of certain populations. Descriptive research can help them learn more about person factors, environmental conditions, and occupational performance. For example, a study comparing adults with and without intellectual disability found that despite similar orthopedic procedures, those with intellectual disability had longer lengths of stay and were less likely to be discharged home (Bathje et al., 2021).

Survey research is a common method used for collecting data in some, but not all, descriptive studies. Survey research has the advantage of expedience, as it is possible to collect a large amount of data relatively quickly with a survey. In a survey of meaningful activities during the COVID-19 lockdown in Belgium, the researchers found that in-home activities such as doing chores in and around the house remained the same, that some activities were modified in terms of how and where they were done (e.g., 65% did work in a different environment), and still other activities were abandoned (e.g., 37.4% discontinued social activities outdoors; Cruyt et al., 2021).

Descriptive studies may also collect data using standardized assessments. Oftentimes, nonexperimental group comparison studies are used to compare individuals with a disability with individuals without a disability to describe differences between the two groups. For example, the Difficulties in Emotion Regulation Scale was used to measure emotion dysregulation in children with attention deficit-hyperactivity disorder (ADHD; Ben-Dor Cohen et al., 2021). The study found children with ADHD had greater levels of emotion dysregulation than children without ADHD.

Appraising Descriptive Studies

Important considerations in appraising descriptive studies include sample size, response rates, and representativeness of the sample. Although **sample size** (the number of participants in a study) is important in most types of quantitative research, it is particularly important in epidemiological studies designed to provide an accurate estimate of population numbers and characteristics of a population. For example, the Centers for Disease Control and Prevention reports the prevalence rate of autism as 1 in 44 children (Maenner et al., 2021). This number was determined after evaluating 220,281 children located in 11 different settings. If the same study were conducted with a small number of children, it might underestimate or overestimate the prevalence based on chance.

One challenge with survey research is receiving an adequate response. The **response rate** is the number of surveys returned divided by the number of surveys that were distributed. When the response rate is low, it is possible that the individuals who completed the survey were not representative of the entire sample that was given the survey. Descriptive studies using other methods can also suffer from poor representativeness. It is useful for the authors of a study to provide information in their results section comparing the sample characteristics with the known characteristics of the population. Returning to the autism study mentioned previously, boys are 4.2 times more likely than girls to be diagnosed with autism (Maenner et al., 2021). Therefore, a representative

TABLE 6-1 | Examples of Descriptive Studies in Occupational Therapy in Mental Health

Author/Date	Research Design	Study Purpose	Findings
Chan et al. (2022)	Survey	Examine the attitudes and practices of OTPs regarding assistive dogs.	Over 60% of OTPs found it within their scope of practice to assess and refer people for assistive dogs, but two-thirds had not had the opportunity to do so.
Engel-Yeger (2022)	Group comparison	Compare depression, anxiety, and quality of life for women with and without ADHD during COVID-19.	Women with ADHD had higher levels of anxiety and lower levels of physical and psychological quality of life compared with women without ADHD. There was no difference in depression between the two groups.
Gaber et al. (2019)	Group comparison	Compare the use of technology when participating in public spaces for people with and without dementia.	People without dementia visited more places and used more technology than people with dementia; however, there were many public places where people with dementia still participated equally as people without dementia.
Kao et al. (2021)	Retrospective analysis of data set	Describe the timing of the shift of responsibility for daily tasks from parent to child.	Shifting tasks from parent to child occurred over a period of years, with many tasks having an interval of 5 years and more risky and complex tasks taking 15 years.
Koenig & Williams (2017)	Survey	Describe the viewpoints of autistic adults regarding their preferred interests as children and adults.	Autistic adults viewed their preferred interests as strengths with positive and calming effects. Retrospectively, they saw their parents as supportive of their interests and teachers as discouraging.
Ip et al. (2022)	Survey	Describe dating practices among young adults and compare dating activities in Australia and Hong Kong.	In Australia, participants were introduced to people to date through other people, whereas in Hong Kong participants met dates at school or work. The most common first dates involved dining, but Australian participants were more likely to report drinking, walking, and intimate activities during first dates, whereas those in Hong Kong were more likely to go shopping.
Rotenberg & Dawson (2022)	Group comparison with normative sample	Describe the functional cognitive impairments of older adults experiencing subjective cognitive decline.	When compared with normative samples, participants had less satisfaction with memory, more difficulty with everyday tasks that involved working memory, and worse performance on complex daily life tasks.
Wright et al. (2022)	Survey	Examine the use of sensory approaches in mental health care in Australia.	Most settings used sensory interventions to reduce anxiety and assist in emotional regulation. Sensory groups were rarely used.

sample of children with autism would include many more boys than girls.

Examples of Descriptive Studies

Table 6-1 provides several examples of descriptive studies in mental health occupational therapy. Several of the studies use a group comparison approach in which they examine similarities and differences between people with and without a condition. Other studies use a survey approach to gather descriptive data, and one study used existing data to describe a population.

Predictive Research

Another type of nonexperimental study is **predictive research.** In this type of observational study, at least two variables are measured to determine if they are related. **Correlational study designs** provide information about the relationship between the variables. These study designs are also typically **cross-sectional** because the data are collected at one point in time. In some predictive studies, the strength of the relationship between two sets of variables is determined (basic correlation), whereas in other predictive studies multiple variables are examined to determine which variable best predicts a particular outcome.

When multiple variables are entered into the same equation, a **regression analysis** is typically employed. A regression analysis provides additional information that allows the researcher to determine which variables are most important in predicting an outcome. OTPs are often interested in how person or environmental variables are related to occupational performance. For example, one simple correlational design study found in children with autism, oral sensory sensitivity, was related to food refusal and food selectivity (Chistol et al., 2018). Another study used a regression analysis to examine the relationships of adverse childhood experiences (ACEs), depression, and physical activity (Royer & Wharton, 2022). ACEs were associated with depression, but physical activity helped to alleviate depression among adults with high levels of ACEs.

Predictive studies may also use **group comparison designs,** such as a case control design, retrospective cohort design, or prospective cohort design. In all these designs one group with a condition is compared with a group without the condition. Different variables are examined as possible contributors or results of the condition. In a **case control design,** the two groups, one with a condition and one without, are compared at a single point in time. For example, Al-Kader and colleagues (2022) found greater rates of depression and anxiety in adults with a history of traumatic brain injury when compared with healthy controls.

TABLE 6-2 | Examples of Predictive Studies in Occupational Therapy in Mental Health

Author/Date	Research Design	Study Purpose	Findings
Brown et al. (2020)	Review of multiple cross-sectional studies	Determine the sensory processing preferences of people with psychiatric disabilities.	A general pattern of greater sensory sensitivity, sensation avoiding, and low registration with less sensation seeking was common across conditions.
Segev-Jacubovski et al. (2022)	Cross-sectional, correlation	Identify psychological factors associated with functional ability and participation after hip fracture.	Optimism predicted functional ability and hope predicted participation at the 6-month follow-up visit for older adults with a hip fracture.
Shin et al. (2022)	Cross-sectional, linear regression	Identify predictors of burnout for OTPs in the United States.	Lower burnout was associated with a greater perceived level of supervisor support, satisfaction with income, and higher educational attainment.
Tan et al. (2020)	Cross-sectional, regression	Examine associations between occupational competence, occupational identity, and personal recovery for people with schizophrenia.	Occupational competence had stronger associations with personal self-efficacy than actual functional ability. Depressive symptoms and hope predicted occupational identity.
Toth et al. (2022)	Cross-sectional, correlation	Examine relationships between cognitive function and performance of instrumental activities of daily living for older adults.	The strongest relationships were found between immediate memory and paying bills, delayed memory and following emergency procedures and paying bills, and executive functioning and making and keeping medical appointments.
Waldman-Levi et al. (2022)	Cross-sectional, correlation	Understand relationships between a father's own playfulness, supportiveness of playfulness, and the child's playfulness.	The father's own playfulness was not related to the child's playfulness. However, the father's supportiveness was related to the child's playfulness.
Zetler et al. (2022)	Cross-sectional, correlation	Examine the relationship of repetitive and restricted behaviors and interests (RRBIs) and sensory processing patterns for children with autism.	RRBIs were most strongly associated with sensory hyperresponsiveness, but also with sensory seeking behaviors.

A **retrospective cohort study** follows people through time, but does so after the fact. In many cases, the data were collected through typical health-care services and then the researcher goes back and looks at existing records. A study that looked at different types of dementia and caregiver burden found that caregiver burden was greatest with Lewy body disease (Huang et al., 2022). Other factors associated with caregiver burden included severity of the dementia, neurological symptoms, and being cared for by more than two caregivers.

A **prospective cohort study** follows people through time, but it does so before something occurs to potentially identify predictors of a condition or situation. For example, the long-term nurses' health study used a prospective cohort design. Participants in this study are followed for decades; this particular analysis covered a 5-year time frame. The study found that women who attended religious services at least once a week were five times less likely to commit suicide than women who attended fewer or no religious services (VanderWeele et al., 2016).

Appraising Predictive Studies

The design of a study has a significant impact on the strength of the evidence for making a prediction. In order of strength, a prospective cohort study provides the best evidence for making a prediction. This is followed by a retrospective cohort study, a case control study, and then a correlational design. However, one should not conclude that correlations or relationships indicate causation. Well-designed efficacy studies are intended to answer questions of causation and

are discussed in greater detail later. Still, predictive studies do provide evidence about the likelihood that two or more things will occur together.

As in most research, sample size is an important consideration when appraising predictive studies. Although there is no universally agreed upon acceptable number, generally speaking the more predictors included in a study, the larger the sample size.

Examples of Predictive Studies

Table 6-2 provides several examples of predictive studies in mental health occupational therapy. Most of the studies are cross-sectional, which is not surprising because this design is simpler to carry out; data are collected at a single point in time. One longitudinal study followed participants through time. All the studies looked at factors that were associated with different aspects of occupational performance, such as sensory processing, symptoms, and the use of everyday technology.

Efficacy Research

Efficacy research provides information about the usefulness of a particular intervention. Therefore, these studies are particularly important for evidence-based practice because they provide OTPs with information that they can share with the people they work with to make decisions about intervention. The best efficacy studies are designed so that they can imperfectly provide information about causation (e.g., did the intervention cause an improvement in a desired outcome?). "Imperfectly" is important, because no study is perfect and alternative explanations are possible. However, a strong study limits alternative explanations.

Efficacy studies typically use **experimental designs** in which the groups are manipulated such that one group receives an intervention and another group either receives no intervention or a comparison intervention. There can be more than two groups offering different types of comparisons. The difference between an experimental group comparison and a nonexperimental or observational comparison (e.g., a case control or cohort study) is that in an experimental design the participants are assigned to groups instead of comparing already existing groups.

The randomized controlled trial is the gold standard of efficacy studies. In a **randomized controlled trial** participants are randomly assigned to one of at least two groups. For example, a study examining a yoga-based program for eating disorders compared the randomly assigned intervention participants to a waitlist control group (Estey et al., 2022). When compared with the control group, participants in the yoga group experienced greater decreases in eating disordered behaviors, depression, and difficulties regulating emotions.

In a **nonrandomized controlled trial,** participants are assigned to one of at least two groups but their assignment is not random. For example, one classroom may receive a new intervention and another a traditional intervention. In a nonrandomized controlled trial examining the efficacy of psychoeducation for individuals with serious mental illness, some residential facilities offered the psychoeducation program, whereas others provided treatment as usual (Magliano et al., 2016). The study found that there were greater improvements in global functioning among the individuals who received psychoeducation. These results also suggest that the intervention caused the improvements, but there are more limitations with this design because there could be differences in the residential facilities that could account for the intervention outcomes.

Other efficacy designs with fewer protections against bias include the pretest-posttest design without a control and single-subject designs. In a **pretest-posttest design without a control,** there is only one group, so it is difficult to ascertain whether participants would have improved without treatment. A **single-subject design** also compares a baseline with performance during or after an intervention, but it does not combine participant scores; rather, each participant is considered separately. For example, in a single-subject design study with three children, the Cog-Fun intervention was used to improve executive function for children with ADHD (Kim et al., 2020). All three children made significant improvements on tests of executive function.

Appraising Efficacy Studies

When appraising efficacy studies, an important concept involves threats to validity. **Threats to validity** are confounding factors that suggest the conclusions of a study may be inaccurate. A threat to validity with an efficacy study implies that something other than the intervention caused the result. For example, in an uncontrolled study, it is possible and even likely that the natural healing process resulted in at least some degree of improvement and that this improvement would have occurred without the intervention.

The concept of levels of evidence is often used to examine the quality of efficacy studies. The randomized controlled

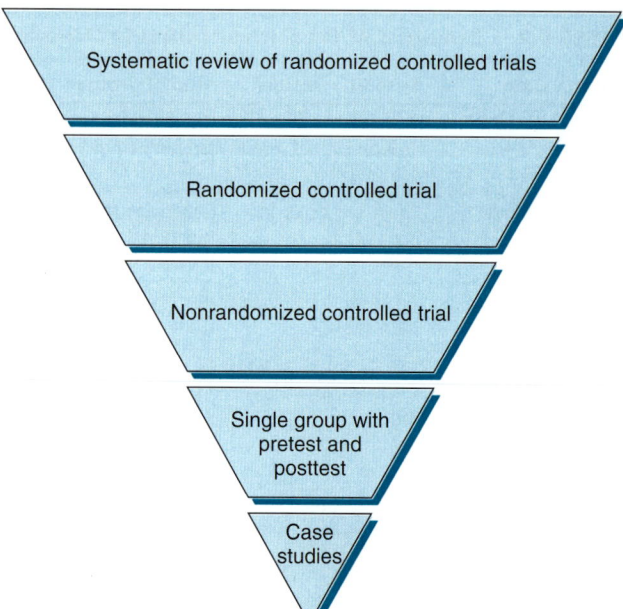

FIGURE 6-3. Levels of evidence for efficacy studies.

trial is the best single-study design for determining whether an intervention actually caused the outcome, because it is the best design for controlling many (but not all) threats to validity. Random assignment to groups and the inclusion of a control or comparison group make the randomized controlled trial a strong design. Evidence hierarchies are based primarily on study design. There are many versions of evidence hierarchies with slight variations similar to the one presented in Figure 6-3, but most are derived from the Oxford Levels of Evidence 2 (Center for Evidence-Based Medicine, 2009) and Sackett and colleagues' hierarchy (2000).

Level I evidence is provided from systematic reviews that include at least two randomized controlled trials. **Systematic reviews** examine multiple studies on a single topic; therefore, their inclusion of randomized controlled trials means the review is based on individual studies with strong research designs. **Level II evidence** comes from a single randomized controlled trial. A nonrandomized controlled trial provides **Level III evidence.** This design, which may also be described as a quasi-experimental study, has the benefit of a control group but is weaker because of the lack of random assignment. **Level IV evidence** comes from a single group design without a control group. This design may also be described as a pretest-posttest without a control. This study design is weak because it is difficult to determine if the intervention or some other factor contributed to the outcomes found. Finally, **Level V evidence** is based on case studies or expert opinion.

Another important consideration when appraising efficacy studies is sample size. A larger sample makes it more likely that the researcher will be able to detect the effects of the intervention if they do exist. **Generalizability** is another consideration. Sometimes efficacy studies are designed so carefully to manage threats to validity that they lose applicability to real-life practice. Studies in which the participants, therapists administering the intervention, and the intervention itself are similar to current practice situations are more generalizable.

TABLE 6-3 | Examples of Efficacy Studies in Occupational Therapy in Mental Health

Author/Date	Research Design	Study Purpose	Findings
Brown et al. (2022)	Randomized controlled trial	Examine the efficacy of a weight loss intervention (NEW-R) for individuals with psychiatric disability.	The intervention group improved more than the control group in perceived competence for exercise and healthy eating and behaviors related to nutrition and spiritual growth. NEW-R participants in supportive settings lost more weight than participants in the control condition in the same settings.
Cahill et al. (2020)	Systematic review	Identify evidence for occupational therapy interventions for children and youth with mental health concerns.	A large body of high-quality studies exists to support the use of activity and occupation-based interventions to address the mental health concerns of children and youth.
Chung et al. (2022)	Randomized controlled trial	Determine the efficacy of Zentangle®, a repetitive, mindful art approach, on affective well-being.	The Zentangle® participants experienced significantly greater reductions in anxiety and improvements in self-compassion when compared with the control group.
Gunnarsson et al. (2022)	Randomized controlled trial	Examine the long-term outcomes of the tree theme method compared with traditional occupational therapy for people with anxiety or depression.	Both groups had significant improvements in participation in everyday occupations, but one group did not improve more than the other.
Gutman et al. (2020)	Randomized controlled trial	Determine if a tailored occupational therapy intervention could reduce stress and ADHD symptoms and enhance daily role functioning for adult women with ADHD.	The intervention group improved more than the control group in terms of perceived stress, ADHD symptoms, and performance of and satisfaction with daily activities.
Omairi et al. (2022)	Randomized controlled trial	Examine the efficacy of Ayres Sensory Integration® for autistic children in Brazil.	Children in the intervention group scored higher on outcomes measures of self-care, social function, and goal attainment when compared with the control group.
Peters et al. (2022)	Randomized controlled trial	Assess preliminary efficacy of an equine therapy program for youth with autism.	Children in the equine therapy group improved more than the control group in goal attainment.
Pisegna et al. (2022)	Systematic review	Determine what interventions within the occupational therapy scope of practice are effective at addressing depression and anxiety in physical disability rehabilitation.	There is limited high-quality evidence available, but there is support for cognitive and behavioral strategies.
Vizzotto et al. (2021)	Randomized controlled trial	Test the efficacy of the occupational goal intervention (OGI) method for improving executive function in treatment-resistant schizophrenia.	Compared with the control group, the OGI group had greater improvements in executive function.

Examples of Efficacy Studies

Table 6-3 provides several examples of efficacy studies in mental health occupational therapy. All the studies examine the efficacy of an intervention that includes occupational therapy to some degree. A promising development in creating this table was the greater availability of high-level evidence for occupational therapy interventions as compared with the same table for the earlier edition of this textbook. All of the studies in this table are either a systematic review or randomized controlled trial.

Assessment Research

Assessment research examines the reliability and validity of tests as well as their usefulness in practice and research. Assessment studies can help OTPs identify the most appropriate tests for a specific practice situation. **Reliability** refers to the consistency and stability of a test. It is important that test scores not fluctuate through time unless there has been a change in an individual. Stability in testing through time is referred to as **test-retest reliability.** Another desirable

characteristic is **interrater reliability,** which indicates the degree to which two or more testers will arrive at the same score. Reliability is typically measured on a scale of 0 to 1.0, with higher numbers indicating greater reliability. For example, a study of a new comprehensive functional measure named the Vellore Occupational Therapy Evaluation Scale found strong evidence for both test-retest reliability of 0.928 and interrater reliability of 0.928 (Samuel et al., 2016).

Validity denotes the extent to which a test measures what it is intended to measure. For example, measures of attention and memory sometimes involve a list learning task in which an individual must remember a list of words. If the person taking the assessment is required to read the words, then reading or visual acuity may come into play and interfere with a valid assessment of attention and memory. A common method of examining validity is to correlate the index measure with a gold standard. Another way that validity is often measured is to determine if a measure distinguishes between individuals who should possess a specific trait and those who should not. These studies provide **discriminant validity** evidence. In other words, the measure can accurately discriminate between different types of people. In another type of validity study, **predictive validity** is investigated by determining how well a measure predicts an outcome.

The different types of validity come together to support the overall **construct validity** of a test. The greater the cumulative evidence, the more confidently one can determine whether an assessment measures the intended construct.

For example, evidence was collected for the construct validity of the Satisfaction with Daily Occupations Scale (SDO-13) by associating this measure with global occupational satisfaction and general health (Wastberg et al., 2016). Convergent validity was supported as both measures were significantly correlated with the SDO-13; however, discriminant validity was not supported as the measure was ineffective in distinguishing between people with and without a psychiatric disability.

Another important consideration in assessment studies is **responsiveness,** which indicates the ability of a measure to detect change. This characteristic is particularly important when an OTP wants to use a measure before and after treatment to determine if the individual has progressed. Floor or ceiling effects can interfere with a measure's responsiveness. If a measure has a **floor effect,** too many individuals score at the bottom range of the scale and the measure is not effective at detecting lower scores. In the case of a **ceiling effect,** many individuals score at the high range of the scale, leaving little range for improvement. A responsive measure will not have a floor or ceiling effect and will also find a difference before and after an intervention if a change took place. A sound method for judging responsiveness is to determine if the index measure identifies the same degree of change as an existing measure with known responsiveness qualities.

Appraising Assessment Studies

Criteria for appraising assessment studies is less well established than for efficacy studies, but important concerns include issues with (a) missing items, (b) the similarity of conditions when relationships are examined, and (c) the use of **hypotheses testing** in validity studies. A hypothesis indicates which direction the researcher expects the results to go. Many assessment tools include multiple items, and it is possible that when an assessment is completed during the research process some items will be missing. This could be because of negligence, or the respondent may refuse or be unable to respond to a particular item. Assessment studies should report the percentage of missing data. Large amounts of missing data would suggest that there are limitations to the study.

In studies in which relationships are examined, it is important that conditions are similar. For example, in a test-retest reliability study, factors such as time of day, level of fatigue of the test taker, and administration procedures of the test should be similar for both administrations of the measure. Also, if two different measures are related to one another, the study will be stronger if the contextual factors (e.g., time, place, and administration) are the same for both measures.

Finally, in validity studies the direction of the relationship or the differences between groups should be specified beforehand in a hypothesis. For example, if two measures are expected to be similar in response for the same participant, the hypothesis would indicate an expectation of convergence. On the other hand, if the two measures are expected to be unrelated, the hypothesis would be one of divergence.

Examples of Assessment Studies

Table 6-4 provides several examples of assessment studies in psychosocial practice. Each study examined a different assessment and had a unique focus. The examples represent a wide range of reliability and validity studies.

Qualitative Research

Qualitative research answers questions about meaning and experience by collecting in-depth data from the perspective of individuals with the lived experience of interest. One important way that qualitative research is distinguished from quantitative research is its use of inductive reasoning. Instead of beginning with a hypothesis and designing a study to determine if the evidence supports the hypothesis (deductive reasoning), qualitative research moves from the specific to the general (inductive reasoning). Very specific information is collected from interviews, observations, and the examination of documents or other artifacts, and the qualitative researcher looks for themes in the data.

In qualitative research, data are typically collected on a few individuals (sometimes only one). Qualitative research emphasizes discovery instead of confirmation. Extensive information is collected so that the researcher has a thorough understanding of the phenomenon in question. Data collection is often based on lengthy open-ended interviews but may also include observations of participants or the collection of artifacts such as personal records, diaries, or photographs. Once the data are collected, the analysis identifies recurring themes within the data.

Qualitative research is a broad term that encompasses several different designs, such as phenomenology, grounded theory, and narrative research. **Phenomenology** is a very common qualitative method that uses the lived experience of individuals to better understand a phenomenon. For example, in a phenomenological study of OTPs working in long-term care facilities during COVID-19, themes were found related to the proximity of death and losses associated with living and dying in a long-term care facility (Figueiredo et al., 2022). The challenge of trying to address isolation and other losses while preventing contagion was especially difficult for the therapists.

The purpose of **grounded theory** is to collect qualitative data so that a new theory can be developed from that data. For example, researchers examined the professional reasoning of OTPs when selecting activities together with older adults with dementia (Schumacher et al., 2022). The resulting theory indicates that OTPs should consider personal elements such as interests and opportunity for autonomy, functional elements such as the match of the activity to the person's skills, and finally interpersonal elements including building a sense of trust and partnership.

Narrative research takes a storytelling approach and often describes a single individual's experience during an extended period of time. In a study of an elite athlete with an eating disorder, the stories of the athlete and parents were told to reveal that family difficulties occurred when family members had contrasting stories (Papathomas et al., 2015).

In **participatory research,** efforts are made to equalize the positions of researchers and participants. The participants become collaborators and take an active role in the research process. In addition, some participatory studies involve an action component in which results of the study are utilized

TABLE 6-4 | Examples of Assessment Studies in Occupational Therapy in Mental Health

Author/Date	Research Design	Study Purpose	Findings
Al-Heizan et al. (2022)	Sensitivity/Specificity and validity	Examine sensitivity and specificity and concurrent validity of the menu task, a test of executive function.	Sensitivity = 0.89 was greater than specificity = 0.58. Concurrent validity was supported by relationships with the weekly calendar planning activity.
Boone et al. (2022)	Validity	Assess the concurrent validity of the electronic version of the Activity Card Sort (ACS3).	High correlations were found between the subscales of the Activity Card Sort and the electronic version of the Activity Card Sort.
Chui et al. (2022)	Internal consistency, test-retest reliability, and discriminant validity	Compare the psychometric properties of three depression measures, the Center for Epidemiologic Studies Depression Scale (CES-D), Beck Depression Inventory-II (BDI-II), and Geriatric Depression Scale (GDS), for people with stroke.	All three measures had good internal consistency. The CES-D was better at discriminating between different levels of disability for people with stroke. The GDS had the best test-retest reliability.
Keleman et al. (2022)	Predictive validity	Determine if an instrumental activities of daily living (IADL) questionnaire or a performance-based IADL measure was better at predicting preclinical Alzheimer disease.	The performance-based measures (specifically the Performance Assessment of Self-Care Skills) had a stronger association with biomarkers of Alzheimer disease than the IADL questionnaire.
Lee et al. (2022)	Item development, reliability, validity	Identify the best-fitting items and preliminary reliability and validity for assessing implied meaning/theory of mind in schizophrenia.	The researchers identified 14 items with good Rasch reliability and found that participants with schizophrenia had lower scores than participants without schizophrenia.
Rojo-Mota et al. (2021)	Internal consistency and convergent and discriminant validity	Determine the internal consistency and validity of the Spanish version of the Executive Function Performance Test (EFPT) in people with substance addiction.	Internal consistency was adequate and the EFPT correlated as expected with neuropsychological tests supporting convergent validity.
Somerville et al. (2019)	Validity	Examine the construct validity of the In-Home Medication Management Performance Evaluation (HOME-Rx).	Validity of the HOME-Rx was supported by statistically significant relationships as predicted with two related measures.

PhotoVoice

The pandemic has included a lot of different emotions and changes in daily life, making life very stressful and hard to balance (especially interacting with different people). One thing I have learned: I need my time alone as well as with my husband. One of our favorite things to do is road trips: Enjoying the open road and not allowing circumstances to hinder the excitement of life. Another pleasure is pulling off and resting.

What did you learn about yourself and your needs from your experience during the COVID pandemic?

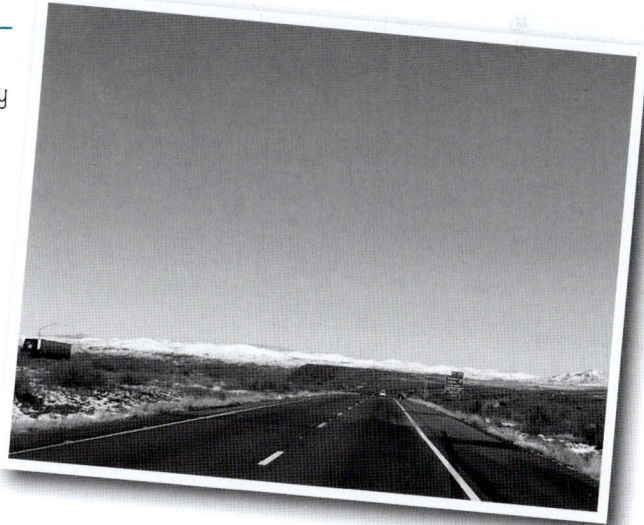

to enact change. Participatory research typically uses qualitative approaches but may use quantitative methods as well. **PhotoVoice** is a methodology that is used as a participatory approach as a way to give voice directly to the research participants (Wang & Burris, 1997). For example, a study using PhotoVoice advocated for the creation of sensory-friendly public spaces because of the distressing feelings autistic children reported in certain spaces (Clément et al., 2022). Similarly, PhotoVoice is used throughout this text to give voice to

people whose voices are often unheard. The PhotoVoice example in this chapter was taken from a study examining the lived experience of therapists during the COVID pandemic.

Appraising Qualitative Studies

The appraisal of qualitative research is based on trustworthiness, which comprises four characteristics: credibility, transferability, dependability, and confirmability (Lincoln & Guba, 1985). **Trustworthiness** means that the data presented in a qualitative study accurately reflect the phenomena of interest.

The first characteristic, **credibility,** reflects a study's authenticity (i.e., it is an accurate representation of the participants' experiences). To enhance credibility, it is important that the data and findings are corroborated from multiple sources, which may mean that several researchers come to a consensus or that the researchers and participants agree with the findings.

The second component of trustworthiness is **transferability,** which is based on the extent to which qualitative research can be applied to other situations. Detailed depictions of the experience, including quotes from the participants, allow for greater transferability.

Trustworthiness is also supported by **dependability** or the extent to which qualitative data are consistent. The use of multiple coders during data analysis can promote dependability; in this method, more than one individual codes the data for themes and then the coders get together to compare results.

Finally, **confirmability** is the extent to which the findings of a qualitative study can be corroborated by others. **Audit trails,** which collect the documents from the study for outside sources to review, provide one method of confirmability.

Examples of Qualitative Studies

Table 6-5 provides several examples of qualitative studies in mental health occupational therapy. Several different designs are represented, including narrative, phenomenology, and grounded theory.

Resources for Accessing Research in Occupational Therapy and Mental Health

A major challenge to evidence-based practice is the time and resources required to access and appraise the available research; however, there are many resources that have done much of the work already. Following is a description of

TABLE 6-5 | Examples of Qualitative Studies in Occupational Therapy in Mental Health

Author/Date	Research Design	Study Purpose	Findings
Dixon et al. (2022)	Phenomenology	Explore women's experiences in a women-only preventive and recovery care service.	Women with mental health issues valued women-only service because they felt understood and safer, and it was easier to talk about difficult topics.
Kalingel-Levi et al. (2022)	Phenomenology	Illuminate aspects of the pain experience by adults with autism spectrum disorder.	The experience of physical pain, coping strategies, participation outcomes, and suggestions for health-care providers were described from the perspective of the participants.
Krishnakumaran et al. (2022)	Phenomenology	Explore the role of occupational therapy with forced migration in Canada.	Themes included engaging individuals in new environments, translating the everyday, connecting and networking, and advocating for occupational justice.
LeBlanc-Olmstead & Kinsella (2023)	Ethnography	Scrutinize the potential risks, challenges, and complexities when including service users as storytellers for health education.	Themes elucidated both the benefits of service user storytelling as well as complexities and risks, such as the emotional labor involved and the performance expectations.
Pèrez-Corrales et al. (2022)	Phenomenology	Describe the experience of people with serious mental illness engaged in volunteer work.	Volunteer work enhanced recovery and was perceived as a process of mutual support.
Rabaey et al. (2021)	Participatory	Understand advocacy messages of caregivers of children with disabilities.	Themes included that children with disabilities (a) should be shown love, (b) should be well taken care of, and (c) need help because they have different needs.
Roberts & Skipsey (2022)	Phenomenology	Explore the recovery experiences of women with bulimia nervosa.	Participants described occupation emerging through committed action, not doing what fueled the condition, adopting new ways of living, prioritizing self-care, connecting with others, and creating supportive environments.
Smith et al. (2020)	Grounded theory	Understand family experiences during mealtime for families with school-age children.	The family meal model identified influences (e.g., way I was raised, not enough time, importance, don't feel like it, not really thinking about it) and benefits (enjoyment of being together, having conversations, staying connected).
Takata et al. (2020)	Phenomenology	Explore the experience of individuals receiving mind-body interventions within hand therapy.	Participants had positive experiences as indicated by the following themes: insight on the body, relaxation and relief, I am in control, and mindfulness as a meaningful activity.

several evidence-based practice resources that are applicable to occupational therapy in mental health.

Occupational Therapy-Specific Resources

The American Occupational Therapy Association (AOTA) provides many evidence-based practice resources to its members. Some are free of charge, whereas others involve a cost. These resources can be found by going to the practice section of the AOTA website, www.aota.org, and then going to the section titled "Evidence-Based Practice and Knowledge Translation." One of the most helpful resources is the practice guidelines series. AOTA practice guidelines include a systematic review that provides a summary and critique of the evidence. In addition, and perhaps most importantly for the busy practitioner, practice guidelines provide the practitioner with specific recommendations based on the existing evidence. Currently, AOTA has the following practice guidelines available for a fee:

- Productive Aging for Community-Dwelling Older Adults
- Adults With Serious Mental Illness
- Adults With Alzheimer Disease and Related Major Neurocognitive Disorders
- Mental Health Promotion, Prevention, and Intervention for Children and Youth
- Individuals With Autism Disorder

Readers can access the practice guidelines at http://www.aota.org/Practice/Researchers/practice-guidelines.aspx.

The AOTA evidence-based practice section has organized an extensive list of systematic reviews published in the *American Journal of Occupational Therapy* within the last 5 years. These reviews are more specific than the practice guideline subjects. A sample of a few topics of note for the psychosocial practitioner include interventions to address depression and anxiety in the physical disability inpatient rehabilitation setting (Pisegna et al., 2022); home-based occupational therapy for adults with dementia and their informal caregivers (Raj et al., 2021); early intervention in mental health for adolescents and young children (Read et al., 2018); occupational therapy intervention with employment and education for adults with serious mental illness (Noyes et al., 2018); and specific sensory techniques and sensory environmental modifications for children and youth with sensory integration difficulties (Bodison & Parham, 2018).

Substance Abuse Mental Health Services Administration

The Substance Abuse Mental Health Services Administration (SAMHSA) provides an Evidence-Based Practices Resource Center that provides information and tools for practitioners. Readers can either search for a particular intervention or identify interventions that target a particular outcome or population. Examples of resources include "Prevention and Treatment of Anxiety, Depression, and Suicidal Thoughts and Behaviors Among College Students," "Trauma-Informed Care in Behavioral Health Services," and "Permanent Supportive Housing Evidence-Based Practices." Each resource is similar to a practice guideline providing very user-friendly information. The resource includes background on a topic, information about the research related to that topic, and detailed information about implementing interventions with real-world examples and additional resources. Readers can access the resources at https://www.samhsa.gov/resource-search/ebp.

Shared Decision-Making

This chapter has explained the importance of incorporating research into the professional decision-making process; however, the person who ultimately drives the decision-making is the individual receiving occupational therapy services. From a person-centered perspective, OTPs highly regard the expertise the person brings to the situation in the form of the lived experience. As mentioned previously, a key component of evidence-based practice is the values and experiences of the individual. A model for combining the research evidence, the therapist's experience, and the individual's situation and perspective is known as **shared decision-making.**

In shared decision-making, both parties impart information related to their areas of expertise. The therapist contributes their professional experience and knowledge of the available research. The person receiving services, in contrast, provides expertise related to their situation, lived experience, values, and preferences. They also might have their own knowledge of the research evidence. The two parties then work together to arrive at a plan for moving forward.

The following is a list of considerations for implementing shared decision-making:

1. Many people referred to occupational therapy will expect the therapist to conduct an assessment and prescribe a treatment. For this reason, the OTP will need to begin the process by educating the individual about shared decision-making.
2. Talk to the person about the role they want to take in the decision-making process. At one end of the continuum is the individual who wants to receive information about the research evidence and the practitioner's experience and then independently make a decision about the direction of their care. At the other end is the individual who prefers that the therapist take control of the decision-making process. However, even at this end of the continuum it is essential that the therapist gathers information about the person's situation, values, and preferences when developing an intervention plan.
3. During the shared decision-making process, there can be times when there are multiple treatment options available. In other cases, the choices can be very limited. Even when there is only one viable treatment choice, it is important to remember that declining treatment is always an option for the person.

Here's the Point

- Evidence-based practice provides OTPs and the individual with information that allows for better decision-making.

- Research evidence consists of many types of studies including descriptive, predictive, efficacy, assessment, and qualitative.
- OTPs should not only familiarize themselves with research studies but should also appraise the quality of the evidence provided in each study.
- There are many resources available to OTPs, particularly those who are members of national associations, which make accessing research evidence easier.

- It is essential that OTPs engage individuals in a shared decision-making process in which case both parties can communicate their knowledge in the process of coming to an agreement about future services.

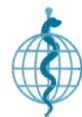 Visit the online resource center at **FADavis.com** to access the video.

Apply It Now

1. Find Additional Research Conducted by Occupational Therapy Practitioners

Find a study that includes occupational therapy researchers addressing a psychosocial issue for each of the five types of research identified in the chapter. Fill in the following table describing the five studies.

Author/Date	Research Design	Study Purpose	Findings
Descriptive			
Relational/Predictive			
Efficacy			
Assessment			
Qualitative			

Reflective Questions
- How challenging was it to find additional research?
- Which areas of research seemed to have more studies and which had less?
- Generally speaking, how would you describe the quality of the research?
- What did you learn by going through this process?

2. Complete a Critically Appraised Paper (CAP)

AOTA provides an opportunity for students with a faculty mentor to critically appraise a research paper and then share that information on their website. This could be a project in which students work in small groups with a faculty mentor to complete the CAP and could be undertaken after you have taken an evidence-based practice course in your program that prepares you to evaluate the evidence. A CAP uses an established format to describe and evaluate a study and, perhaps most importantly, identify a "clinical bottom line" for the OTP. A published article that is relevant to occupational therapy practice is selected and then analyzed. Information on this process is provided at http://www.aota .org/Practice /Researchers/Evidence-Exchange/MH.aspx.

Resources

- AOTA Practice Guidelines
  http://www.aota.org/Practice/Researchers/practice-guidelines
  .aspx
- AOTA Critically Appraised Papers
  http://www.aota.org/Practice/Researchers/Evidence
  -Exchange/MH.aspx
- National Registry of Evidence-Based Interventions From the Substance Abuse and Mental Health Services Administration
  www.samhsa.gov/resource-search/ebp
- **"Child in Crisis" video.** In this video, occupational therapist Brittany shares her experience working in a psychiatric rehab hospital's adolescent unit with Mikey, an 8-year-old boy presenting with a complex set of challenges. Diagnosed at birth with fetal alcohol syndrome, Mikey has a history of multiple ACEs. On admission, he presented with suicidal and homicidal ideation and symptoms consistent with posttraumatic stress disorder (PTSD). Brittany describes how she did her own research, learned more about Mikey, and developed an intervention that worked well for him and the other children in the group. Access the video at the online resource center at FADavis.com.

References

Al-Heizan, M. O., Marks, T. S., Giles, G. M., & Edwards, D. F. (2022). Further validation of the menu task: Functional cognition screening for older adults. *OTJR: Occupation, Participation and Health, 42*(4), 286–294. https://doi.org/10.1177/15394492221110546

Al-Kader, D. A., Onyechi, C. I., Ikedum, I. V., Fattah, A., Zafar, S., Bhat, S., Malik, M. A., Bheesham, N., Qadar, L. T., & Sajjad Cheema, M. (2022). Depression and anxiety in patients with a history of traumatic brain injury: A case-control study. *Cureus, 14*(8), e27971. https://doi.org/10.7759/cureus.27971

Bathje, M., Conrad, S., Medick, M., Ross, M., & Fogg, L. (2021). Differences in hospital-based care for patients with intellectual and developmental disabilities. *American Journal of Occupational Therapy, 75*(3), 7503180080. https://doi.org/10.5014 /ajot.2021.046508

Ben-Dor Cohen, M., Eldar, E., Maeir, A., & Nahum, M. (2021). Emotional dysregulation and health related quality of life in young adults with ADHD: A cross sectional study. *Health and Quality of Life Outcomes, 19*(1), 270. https://doi.org/10.1186 /s12955-021-01904-8

Bodison, S. C., & Parham, L. D. (2018). Specific sensory techniques and sensory environmental modifications for children and youth with sensory integration difficulties: A systematic review. *American Journal of Occupational Therapy, 72*(1), 7201900040p1–7201190040p11. https://doi.org/10.5014/ajot.2018.029413

Bolding, D. J., McCallister, C., Poisson, K., Pufki, D. M., Ramirez, A., Rickly, C., & Scattini, V. (2021). Incivility in the occupational therapy workplace: A survey of practitioners. *American Journal of Occupational Therapy, 75*(3), 7503205020. https://doi.org/10.5014/ajot.2021.046698

Boone, A. E., Wolf, T. J., & Baum, C. M. (2022). Development and initial testing of the Electronic Activity Card Sort (ACS3) among community-dwelling adults. *American Journal of Occupational Therapy, 73*(3), 7603345030. https://doi.org/10.5014/ajot.2022.047522

Brown, C., Cook, J. A., Jonikas, J. A., Steigman, P. J., Burke-Miller, J., Hamilton, M. M., Rosen, C., Tessman, D. C., & Santos, A. (2022). Nutrition and exercise for wellness and recovery: A randomized controlled trial of a community-based health intervention. *Psychiatric Services, 74*, 463–471. https://doi.org/10.1176/appi.ps.202200038

Brown, C., Karim, R., & Steuter, M. (2020). Retrospective analysis of studies examining sensory processing preferences in people with a psychiatric condition. *American Journal of Occupational Therapy, 74*(4), 7404205130p1–7404205130p11. https://doi.org/10.5014/ajot.2020.038463

Cahill, S. M., Egan, B. E., & Seber, J. (2020). Activity and occupation-based interventions to support mental health, positive behavior, and social participation for children and youth: A systematic review. *American Journal of Occupational Therapy, 74*(2), 7402180020p1–7402180020p28. https://doi.org/10.5014/ajot.2020.038687

Center for Evidence-Based Medicine. (2009). *Levels of evidence.* http://www.cebm.net/oxford-centre-evidence-based-\medicine-levels-evidence-march-2009

Chan, K. W., Young, J., Williams, L. J., & Nottle, C. (2022). Assistance dogs in occupational therapy practice: A survey of Australian occupational therapists' experiences and recommendations. *Australian Occupational Therapy Journal, 69*(2), 129–139. https://doi.org/10.1111/1440-1630.12775

Chistol, L. T., Bandini, L. G., Must, A., Phillips, S., Cermak, S. A., & Curtin, C. (2018). Sensory sensitivity and food selectivity in children with autism spectrum disorder. *Journal of Autism and Developmental Disorders, 48*(2), 583–591. https://doi.org/10.1007/s10803-017-3340-9

Chui, E. C., Chen, Y. J., Wu, W. C., Chou, C. X., & Yu, M. Y. (2022). Psychometric comparisons of three depression measures for patients with stroke. *American Journal of Occupational Therapy, 76*(4), 7604205140. https://doi.org/10.5014/ajot.2022.049347

Chung, S. K., Ho, F. Y. Y., & Chan, H. C. Y. (2022). The effects of Zentangle* on affective well-being among adults: A pilot randomized controlled trial. *American Journal of Occupational Therapy, 76*(5), 7605205060. https://doi.org/10.5014/ajot.2022.049113

Clément, M. A., Lee, K., Park, M., Sinn, A., & Miyakje, N. (2022). The need for sensory-friendly "zones": Learning from youth on the autism spectrum, their families, and autistic mentors using a participatory approach. *Frontiers in Psychology, 13,* 883331. https://doi.org/10.3389/fpsyg.2022.883331

Cruyt, E., De Vriendt, P., De Letter, M., Vlerick, P., Calders, P., De Pauw, R., Oostra, K., Rodriguez-Bailón, M., Szmalec, A., Merchán-Baeza, J. A., Fernández-Solano, A. J., Vidaña-Moya, L., & Van de Velde, D. (2021). Meaningful activities during COVID-19 lockdown and association with mental health in Belgian adults. *BMC Public Health, 21*(1), 622. https://doi.org/10.1186/s12889-021-10673-4

Dixon, K., Fossey, E., & Petrakis, M. (2022). Using PhotoVoice to explore women's experiences of a women-only prevention and recovery care service in Australia. *Health and Social Care in the Community, 30,* e5839–e5847. https://doi.org/10.1111/hsc.14015

Engel-Yeger, B. (2022). Emotional status and quality of life in women with ADHD during COVID-19. *OTJR: Occupation, Participation and Health, 42*(3), 219–227. https://doi.org/10.1177/15394492221076516

Estey, E., Roff, C., Kozlowski, M. B., Rovig, S., Guyker, W. M., & Cook-Cottone, C. P. (2022). Efficacy of Eat Breathe Thrive: A randomized controlled trial of a yoga-based program. *Body Image, 42,* 427–439. https://doi.org/10.1016/j.bodyim.2022.07.009

Figueiredo, C. S., Giacomin, K. C., Gual, R. F., de Almeida, S. C., & Assis, M. G. (2022). Death and other losses in the COVID-19 pandemic in long-term care facilities in older adults in the perception of occupational therapists: A qualitative study. *Omega,* 302228821086169. https://doi.org/10.1177/00302228821086169

Gaber, S. N., Nygård, L., Brorsson, A., Kottorp, A., & Malinowsky, C. (2019). Everyday technologies and public space participation among people with and without dementia. *Canadian Journal of Occupational Therapy, 86*(5), 400–411. https://doi.org/10.1177/0008417419837764

Gunnarsson, A. B., Håkansson, C., Hedin, K., & Wagman, P. (2022). Outcomes of the tree theme method versus regular occupational therapy: A longitudinal follow-up. *Australian Occupational Therapy Journal, 69*(4), 379–390. https://doi.org/10.1111/1440-1630.12796

Gutman, S. A., Balasubramanian, S., Herzog, M., Kim, E., Swirnow, H., Retig, Y., & Wolff, S. (2020). Effectiveness of a tailored intervention for women with attention deficit hyperactivity disorder (ADHD) and ADHD symptoms: A randomized controlled study. *American Journal of Occupational Therapy, 75*(1), 74012050p1–74012050p11. https://doi.org/10.5014/ajot.2020.033316

Huang, W. C., Chang, M. C., Wang, W. F., & Jhang, K. M. (2022). A comparison of caregiver burden for different types of dementia: An 18-month retrospective cohort study. *Frontiers in Psychology, 12,* 798315. https://doi.org/10.3389/fpsyg.2021.798315

Ip, I. M. H., Honey, A., & McGrath, M. (2022). 'Doing' dating: A cross-sectional survey of young adults (18–35 years) in Australia and Hong Kong. *Australian Occupational Therapy Journal, 69*(3), 233–242. https://doi.org/10.1111/1440-1630.12785

Kalingel-Levi, M., Schreuer, N., Granovsky, Y., Bar-Shalita, T., Weissman-Fogel, I., Hoffman, T., & Gal, E. (2022). "When I'm in pain, everything is overwhelming": Implications of pain in adults with autism on their daily living and participation. *Frontiers in Psychology, 13,* 911756. https://doi.org/10.3389/fpsyg.2022.911756

Kao, Y. C., Coster, W., Cohn, E. S., & Orsmond, G. I. (2021). Preparation for adulthood: Shifting responsibility for management of daily tasks from parents to their children. *American Journal of Occupational Therapy, 75*(2), 7502205050. https://doi.org/10.5014/ajot.2020.041723

Keleman, A. A., Bollinger, R. M., Wisch, J. K., Grant, E. A., Benzinger, T. L., Ances, B. M., & Stark, S. L. (2022). Assessment of instrumental activities of daily living in preclinical Alzheimer disease. *Occupational Therapy Journal of Research, 42*(4), 277–285. https://doi.org/10.1177/15394492221100701

Kim, M. J., Park, H. Y., Yoo, E. Y., & Kim, J. R. (2020). Effects of a cognitive-functional intervention method on improving executive function and self-directed learning in school-aged children with attention deficit hyperactivity disorder: A single-subject design study. *Occupational Therapy International, 2020,* 1250801. https://doi.org/10.1155/2020/1250801

Koenig, K. P., & Williams, L. H. (2017). Characterization and utilization of preferred interests: A survey of adults on the autism spectrum. *Occupational Therapy in Mental Health, 33,* 129–140. https://doi.org/10.1080/0164212X.2016.1248877

Krishnakumaran, T., Bhatt, M., Kiriazis, K., & Giddings, C. E. (2022). Exploring the role of occupational therapy and forced migration in Canada. *Canadian Journal of Occupational Therapy,* *89*(3), 238–248. https://doi.org/10.1177/00084174221084463

Leblanc-Olmstead, S., & Kinsella, E. A. (2023). "Come and share your story and make everyone cry": Complicating service user educator storytelling in mental health professional education. *Advances in Health Sciences Education, 28,* 387–410. https://doi.org/10.1007/s10459-022-10157-z

Lee, S. D., Chen, K. W., Huang, C. Y., Li, P. C., Hsieh, T. L., Lee, Y. C., & Hsueh, I. P. (2022). Development of a Rasch-calibrated test for assessing implied meaning in patients with schizophrenia. *American Journal of Occupational Therapy, 76*(4), 7604205020. https://doi.org/10.5014/ajot.2022.047316

Lincoln, Y. S., & Guba, E. G. (1985). *Naturalistic inquiry.* Sage.

Maenner, M. J., Shaw, K. A., Bakian, A. V., Bilder, D. A., Durkin, M. S., Esler, A., Furnier, S. M., Hallas, L., Hall-Lande, J., Hudson, A., Hughes, M. M., Patrick, M., Pierce, K., Poynter, J. N., Salinas, A., Shenouda, J., Vehorn, A., Warren, Z., Constantino, J. N., . . . Cogswell, M. E. (2021). Prevalence and characteristics of autism spectrum disorder among children aged 8 years–Autism and Developmental Disabilities Monitoring Network, 11 sites, United States, 2018. *Morbidity and Mortality Weekly Report, 70*(11), 1–16. https://doi.org/10.15585/mmwr.ss7011a1

Magliano, L., Puviani, M., Rega, S., Marchesini, N., Rossetti, M., & Starace, F. (2016). Feasibility and effectiveness of a combined individual and psychoeducational group intervention in psychiatric residential facilities: A controlled, non-randomized study. *Psychiatry Research, 235,* 19–28. https://doi.org/10.1016/j.psychres.2015.12.009

Noyes, S., Sokolow, H., & Arbesman, M. (2018). Evidence for occupational therapy intervention with employment and education for adults with serious mental illness: A systematic review. *American Journal of Occupational Therapy, 72,* 7205190010. https://doi.org/10.5014/ajot.2018.033068

Omairi, C., Mailloux, Z., Antoniuk, S. A., & Schaaf, R. (2022). Occupational therapy using Ayres Sensory Integration˚: A randomized controlled trial in Brazil. *American Journal of Occupational Therapy, 76*(4), 7604205160. https://doi.org/10.5014/ajot.2022.048249

Östergren, P. O., Canivet, C., & Agardh, A. (2022). One-year incidence of sexual harassment and the contribution to poor mental health in the adult general population. *European Journal of Public Health, 32*(3), 360–365. https://doi.org/10.1093/eurpub/ckab225

Papathomas, A., Smith, B., & Lavallee, D. (2015). Family experiences of living with an eating disorder: A narrative analysis. *Journal of Health Psychology, 20,* 313–325. https://doi.org/10.1177/1359105314566608

Pèrez-Corrales, J., Huertas-Hoyas, E., Garcìa-Bravo, C., Güeita-Rodriguez, J., & Palacios-Ceña, D. (2022). Volunteering as a meaningful occupation in the process of recovery from serious mental illness: A qualitative study. *American Journal of Occupational Therapy, 76*(2), 7602205090. https://doi.org/10.5014/ajot.2022.045104

Peters, B. C., Wood, W., Hepburn, S., & Moody, E. J. (2022). Preliminary efficacy of occupational therapy in an equine environment for youth with autism spectrum disorder. *Journal of Autism and Developmental Disorders, 52*(9), 4114–4128. https://doi.org/10.1007/s10803-021-05278-0

Pisegna, J., Anderson, S., & Krok-Schoen, J. (2022). Occupational therapy interventions to address depressive and anxiety symptoms in the physical disability inpatient rehabilitation setting? A systematic review. *American Journal of Occupational Therapy, 76,* 76101180110. https://doi.org/10.5014/ajot.2022.049068

Rabaey, P., Hepperlen, R., Manley, H., & Ament-Lemke, A. (2021). Empowering caregivers of children with disabilities in Zambia: A PhotoVoice study. *American Journal of Occupational Therapy, 75*(4), 7504180030. https://doi.org/10.5014/ajot.2021.045526

Raj, S. E., Mackintosh, S., Fryer, C., & Stanley, M. (2021). Home-based occupational therapy for adults with dementia and their informal caregivers: A systematic review. *American Journal of*

Occupational Therapy, 75, 7501205060p1–7501205060p27. https//doi.org/10.5014/ajot.2020.040782

Read, H., Roush, S., & Downing, D. (2018). Early intervention in mental health for adolescents and young adults: A systematic review. *American Journal of Occupational Therapy, 72,* 7205190040p1–7205190040p8. https://doi.org/10.5014/ajot.2018/033118

Roberts, E., & Skipsey, J. (2022). Exploring occupation in recovery from bulimia nervosa: An interpretive phenomenological analysis. *British Journal of Occupational Therapy, 85*(7), 487–495. https://doi.org/10.1177/03080226211045289

Rojo-Moto, G., Pedrero-Pèrez, E. J., Verdugo-Cuartero, I., Blanco-Elizo, A. B., Aldea-Poyo, P., Alonso-Rodrìguez, M., Leòn-Frade, I., & Morales-Alonso, S. (2021). Reliability and validity of the Spanish version of the Executive Function Performance Test (EFPT) in assessing people in treatment for substance addiction. *American Journal of Occupational Therapy, 75*(2), 7502205080. https://doi.org/10.5014/ajot.2020.041897

Rotenberg, S., & Dawson, D. R. (2022). Characterizing cognition in everyday life of older adults with subjective cognitive decline. *OTJR: Occupation, Participation and Health, 42*(4), 269–276. https://doi.org/10.1177/15394492221093310

Royer, M. F., & Wharton, C. (2022). Physical activity mitigates the link between adverse childhood experiences and depression among U.S. adults. *PLoS One, 17*(10), e0275185. https://doi.org/10.1371/journal.pone.0275185

Sackett, D., Rosenberg, W. M. C., Gray, J. A. M., Haynes, R. B., & Richardson, W. S. (1996). Evidence based medicine: What it is and what it isn't. *British Medical Journal, 312,* 71–72. https://doi.org/10.1136/bmj.312.7023.71

Sackett, D., Straus, S. E., & Richardson, W. S. (2000). *How to practice and teach evidence-based medicine* (2nd ed.). Churchill Livingstone.

Samuel, R., Russell, P. S., Paraseth, T. K., Ernest, S., & Jacob, K. S. (2016). Development and validation of the Vellore Occupational Therapy Evaluation Scale to assess functioning in people with mental illness. *International Journal of Social Psychiatry, 62,* 616–626. https://doi.org/10.1177/0020764016664754

Schell, B. A. B. (2019). Professional reasoning in practice. In B. A. B. Schell & G. Gillen (Eds.), *Willard and Spackman's occupational therapy* (13th ed., pp. 482–497). Wolters Kluwer.

Schumacher, T. P., Andresen, M., & Fallahpour, M. (2022). Clinical reasoning of occupational therapists in selecting activities together with older adults with dementia to postpone further development of cognitive decline. *Scandinavian Journal of Occupational Therapy, 30*(1), 98–108. https://doi.org/10.1080/11038128.2022.2112282

Segev-Jacubovski, O., Magen, H., & Maeir, A. (2022). Psychological factors predicting functional ability and participation after hip fracture. *American Journal of Occupational Therapy, 76*(3), 7603205080. https://doi.org/10.5014/ajot.2022.047365

Shin, J., McCarthy, M., Schmidt, C., Zellner, J., Ellerman, K., & Britton, M. (2022). Prevalence and predictors of burnout among occupational therapy practitioners in the United States. *American Journal of Occupational Therapy, 76*(4), 7604205080. https://doi.org/10.5014/ajot.2022.048108

Smith, S. L., Ramey, E., Sisson, S. B., Richardson, S., & DeGrace, B. W. (2020). Influences on family mealtime participation. *OTJR: Occupation, Participation and Health, 40*(2), 138–146. https://doi.org/10.1177/1539449219876878

Somerville, E., Massey, K., Keglovits, M., Vouri, S., Hu, Y. L., Carr, D., & Stark, S. (2019). Scoring, clinical utility, and psychometric properties of the In-Home Medication Management Performance Evaluation (HOME-Rx). *American Journal of Occupational Therapy, 73*(2), 7302205060p1–7302205060p8. https://doi.org/10.5014/ajot.2019.029793

Takata, S. C., Hardison, M. E., & Roll, S. C. (2020). Fostering holistic hand therapy: Emergent themes of client experiences of mind–body interventions. *OTJR: Occupation, Participation and Health, 40*(2), 122–130. https://doi.org/10.1177/1539449219888835

Tan, B. L., Lim, M. W. Z., Xie, H., Li, Z., & Lee, J. (2020). Defining occupational competence and occupational identity in the context of recovery in schizophrenia. *American Journal of Occupational Therapy, 74*(4), 7404205120p1–7404205120p11. https://doi.org/10.5014/ajot.2020.034843

Tanaka, S., Kuge, R. I., Nakano, M., Inukai, S., Hamamoto, M., Terasawa, M., Nakamura, T., Sugiyama, N., Kobayashi, M., & Washizuka, S. (2022). Outcomes of an interdisciplinary return to work intervention including occupational therapy for mood and adjustment disorders: A single-arm clinical trial. *Work,* 515–530. https://doi.org/10.3233/WOR-211144

Toth, C., Tulliani, N., Bissett, M., & Liu, K. P. (2022). The relationship between cognitive function and performance in instrumental activities of daily living in older adults. *British Journal of Occupational Therapy, 85*(2), 120–129. https://doi.org/10.1177/03080226211008722

VanderWeele, T. J., Li, S., Tsai, A. C., & Kawachi, I. (2016). Association between religious service attendance and lower suicide rates among US women. *JAMA Psychiatry, 73,* 845–851. https://doi.org/10.1001/jamapsychiatry.2016.1243

Vizzotto, A., Celestino, D., Buchain, P., Oliveira, A., Oliveira, G., Di Sarno, E., Napolitano, I., & Elkis, H. (2021). Occupational goal intervention method for the management of executive dysfunction in people with treatment-resistant schizophrenia: A randomized controlled trial. *American Journal of Occupational Therapy, 75*(3), 7503180050. https://doi.org/10.5014/ajot.2021.043257

Waldman-Levi, A., Cope, A., & Olson, L. (2022). Understanding father-child joint play experience using a convergent mixed-methods design. *American Journal of Occupational Therapy, 76*(5), 7605205070. https://doi.org/10.5014/ajot.2022.046573

Wang, C., & Burris, M. A. (1997). PhotoVoice: Concept, methodology, and use for participatory needs assessment. *Health Education & Behavior, 24*(3), 369–387. https://doi.org/10.1177/109019819702400309

Wastberg, B. A., Persson, E. B., & Eklund, M. (2016). The Satisfaction with Daily Occupations (SDO-13) Scale: Psychometric properties among clients in primary care in Sweden. *Occupational Therapy in Health Care, 30,* 29–41. https://doi.org/10.3109/07380577.2015.1048036

Wright, L., Meredith, P., & Bennett, S. (2022). Sensory approaches in psychiatric units: Patterns and influences of use in one Australian health region. *Australian Occupational Therapy Journal, 69*(5), 559–573. https://doi.org/10.1111/1440-1630.12813

Zetler, N. K., Cermak, S. A., Engel-Yeger, B., Baranek, G., & Gal, E. (2022). Association between sensory features and higher-order repetitive and restricted behaviors and interests among children with autism spectrum disorder. *American Journal of Occupational Therapy, 76*(3), 7603205010. https://doi.org/10.5014/ajot.2022.048082

PART 2

The Person

The Person, Part 2 of the text, is divided into sections on occupational performance and selected conditions.

Section 1: Occupational Performance addresses skills and abilities that are important for participation. These chapters provide detailed content about the skills addressed, theories related to those skills, and specific information on diagnoses that are associated with impairments in those skill areas. In addition, these chapters provide information on specific assessments and interventions that target occupational performance skills. Therapeutic reasoning assessment tables are included in each of the occupational performance chapters for easy reference to the relevant assessment tools.

It is important for occupational therapy practitioners (OTPs) to have a thorough understanding of the conditions of the individuals they work with. For this reason, major psychiatric diagnoses are presented in Section 2, with a focus on symptoms, etiology, impact on occupational performance, and when appropriate, medications used to treat the condition. This section also includes chapters on acquired physical disabilities and chronic conditions, focusing on the psychosocial implications associated with these conditions.

Although occupational therapy practice is not driven by symptomatology, practitioners can better understand the lived experience of individuals with psychiatric conditions when they are aware of symptoms those individuals might be experiencing. In addition, a working knowledge of psychiatric diagnoses is useful when participating on a multidisciplinary treatment team. Because occupational therapy practice is not symptom-based, specific information on occupational therapy interventions is not included in these chapters; however, intervention tables have been added to refer readers to the relevant chapters that do comprehensively address the relevant interventions.

PART 2

Occupational Performance

SECTION **1**

CHAPTER

7

Cognition

Catana Brown

Cognition as a performance skill and person factor is necessary for all occupational participation, be it daily activities, work, socialization, leisure, and so on. For many people with a mental health diagnosis, cognition is a challenge. Even when people are feeling just a little bit anxious, or depressed, or angry, it is likely that their cognitive abilities will be compromised to some degree. The environment and occupation also contribute significantly to the cognitive demands of a situation. Some environments and occupations are cognitively complex, whereas other environments and occupations are simple or may have features that reduce the cognitive load. Occupational therapy practitioners (OTPs) are concerned with how people use their cognitive abilities to perform occupations in real-world environments, in other words, functional cognition.

This chapter describes the components of cognition and explains how cognition and mental health conditions intersect. When discussing the role of OTPs in assessment and intervention, the chapter focuses on functional cognition. The assessment section reviews specific performance-based assessments that evaluate cognition within the context of occupational performance. The intervention section also takes a functional cognition stance and examines practice models that help OTPs create interventions so that people can successfully carry out the occupations they need and want to perform in their real lives.

Cognition and Psychiatric Disabilities

Cognitive impairments are common in many psychiatric disabilities; for some persons, these impairments represent the core feature of their disorder. For example, dementia is distinguished by a significant deterioration in cognitive functioning. Alzheimer dementia, the most common form of the disease, begins with impairments in recall memory and progresses to a total decline in cognitive and occupational performance (Jahn, 2013). Normal aging also results in decrements in cognitive ability. Attention deficit-hyperactivity disorder (ADHD) is considered a cognitive impairment; in addition to attentional problems, the disorder is characterized by deficits in working memory, inhibitory control, and the executive functions of planning and organization (Pievsky & McGrath, 2018).

The *Diagnostic and Statistical Manual of Mental Disorders,* Fifth Edition (*DSM-5;* American Psychiatric Association [APA], 2013), made an important change in terminology from "mental retardation" to "intellectual disability." In addition, the *DSM-5* places less emphasis on IQ cut-off scores and more emphasis on specific cognitive abilities, such as verbal comprehension, working memory, and adaptive reasoning in academic learning, social understanding, and practical understanding (Harris, 2013).

Other psychiatric disabilities that are characterized primarily by mood or psychotic symptoms are nevertheless associated with significant cognitive impairments. Cognitive impairment is extensively studied in schizophrenia. An umbrella review of systematic reviews found that people with schizophrenia had impairments in memory, verbal fluency, processing speed, social cognition, and executive function (Gebreegziabhere et al., 2022) with the strongest evidence for impairments in processing speed, verbal memory, and working memory. These impairments can interfere with successful community living, employment, and socialization (Nuechterlein et al., 2014).

There are similar cognitive impairments in individuals with bipolar disorder (Kravariti et al., 2005). The obsessive thoughts inherent in obsessive-compulsive disorder (OCD) can be characterized as cognitive inflexibility and difficulty with switching sets (Gruner & Pittenger, 2017). In addition, individuals with OCD have difficulty switching attention and are challenged with decision-making because of an intolerance of uncertainty.

The evidence suggests that the cognitive impairments in schizophrenia occur early in the course of the condition and persist, but do not decline over time (Gebreegziabhere et al., 2022). In contrast, the cognitive impairments in depression primarily involve difficulties with concentration and decision-making and seem to be most intense during acute phases of the illness, although for some individuals the impairments may persist (Trivedi & Greer, 2014). OTPs need to be familiar with the cognitive impairments associated with psychiatric disabilities so that these barriers to occupational performance can be addressed.

The Lived Experience

Just Easily Distracted

Lauren Berman

When I was asked to write about my experience living with ADHD, I told my mom that I would *gladly* share my story with the world. I was kind of surprised when she asked me to contribute to this book because giving me a platform to share my experience with ADHD also kind of puts her on the spot. You see, my mom is Dr. Catana Brown, you may have seen her name displayed prominently on this textbook? And since getting diagnosed with ADHD at the age of 34, I have teased my mom for not catching it sooner and getting me diagnosed as a child.

In fairness, I was (am) a quirky person, so it's hard to point out which of my quirks are just "me" and which are related to my ADHD. To paint a more accurate picture: I am a theatre person. In my experience, neurodivergence and musical theatre go together like peanut butter and jelly. Think about the theatre kids from your high school, they're often hard to ignore. At least at my school, we were generally very high energy (loud), intensely passionate about our craft and the theatre world in general, and constantly learning new skills like speaking with accents or learning how to juggle. This aligns beautifully with the ADHD brain: hyperactivity, hyperfocus, and novelty.

One time in high school, I was grounded for getting bad grades and my parents told me I couldn't do the school play. I'm not sure if you know this, Mom, but I still auditioned. Oops. Thankfully for all involved, I didn't end up getting cast in the play, because there was no way I was going to hide the fact that I suddenly had rehearsals every day after school. This was a pretty typical pattern for me, impulsive decisions, avoiding my responsibilities, and facing dire consequences only to do it all again. I guess it's a good thing my hyperfixation was theatre and not something more dangerous like drag racing.

It was a running joke with my friends that I was grounded almost every other week. I was constantly getting in trouble for bad grades or my messy room. Simple tasks like putting my laundry away would take constant reminders, and the threat of missing out on my social life for another weekend still wasn't enough to motivate me to do it. My grades were only good enough to get me into college because I work well under pressure and have a natural aptitude for writing papers and taking tests. But doing my homework, studying, and paying attention in class were of zero interest to me. As soon as I got home from school, any homework that wasn't interesting to me immediately disappeared from my brain.

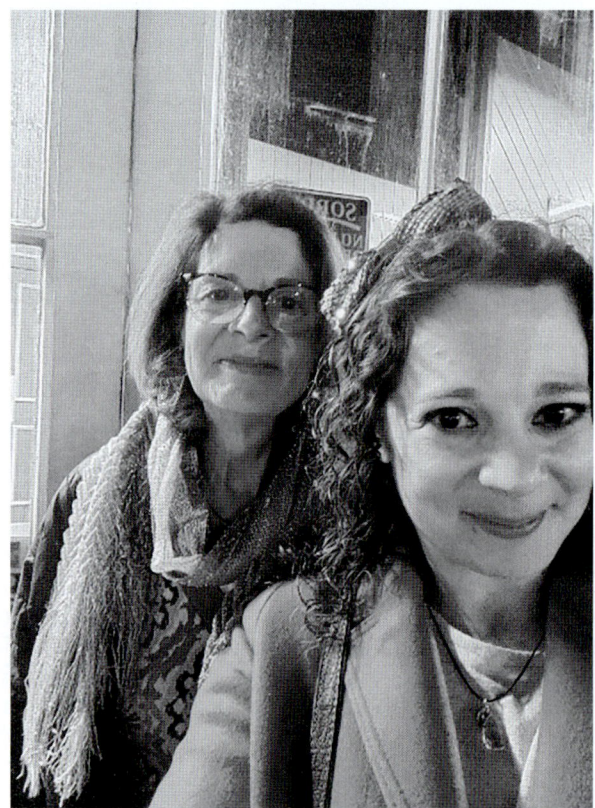

My parents met with my teachers and school counselors to try and figure out a solution for my lack of focus on schoolwork (to my knowledge, none of my teachers or counselors suspected ADHD either). They got me tutors, arranged appointments with my teachers to catch up on missing work, made sure I wrote my assignments in my planner every day, and helped me organize my backpack which was often stuffed with loose, crumpled up worksheets and exams. It was basically where all my schoolwork went to die.

At one point I had to have progress reports sent home each week to be signed by my parents. But I eventually figured out a loophole and started forging my mom's signature, which of course I didn't get away with more than once. In one especially dramatic attempt to hide a D on my report card, I intercepted the mail before my parents got home and painstakingly cut and pasted letters to make it look like I'd actually received a C in the class. And that's the story of how I ended up being grounded

The Lived Experience—cont'd

for my 16th birthday. I was lucky to grow up in an era before parents could check their children's grades online at all times.

You might be thinking "if she's willing to go to such lengths to cover up her bad grades, why wouldn't she just spend that same time and energy on her schoolwork instead and just avoid the drama?!" That's a great question, and one I never really asked myself at the time. To be honest, I just thought I was lazy. Or dumb. My grades on standardized tests were apparently above average at a young age, but I still assumed I just wasn't as smart as the other students who seemed to have no problem turning in assignments or paying attention in class. At one point I asked my mom if she thought I had ADHD, and she laughed and said, "No, you just have trouble paying attention." I bring that up as often as possible since my official diagnosis.

I love to give my mom a hard time for not recognizing the traits of ADHD that seem so obvious now. But the truth is, my situation is not unique. I've learned that inattentive ADHD often goes undiagnosed, especially in women. The traits most commonly associated with ADHD that catch the attention of teachers and parents are the ones that are disruptive: constant fidgeting, blurting things out in class, inability to sit still, etc. These traits are more specific to hyperactive-impulsive ADHD, which is more common in men. As a result, many women don't get diagnosed until later in life, if at all.

And now we've come full circle back to my diagnosis. Despite my struggles in high school, I ended up doing fine in college. Lucky for me, I was able to follow my passion and study music, so I was more motivated to complete my assignments because I actually cared about the subject matter. And while there were a few classes I couldn't bring myself to care about (looking at you, Calculus), my course load was so full as a Music Education major that I still graduated with a 3.6 GPA. I went on to do a master's degree in Voice Performance, and ultimately completed my Doctor of Musical Arts in 2017 with a 3.96 GPA. Occasionally I even take community college classes for fun. Turns out, I love school when it's something I'm interested in!

So, I made it through higher education without a diagnosis, accommodations, or medication and I was doing great! I spent my time teaching voice lessons out of my house, performing as frequently as I could, and working as adjunct faculty at both the local university and community college. And then, about two years ago, I decided to start a business. I got a commercial space that would eventually become a multi-teacher voice studio, and I had about a month to get everything set up. I was spending long hours at the studio oscillating between administrative tasks, getting the space ready, finding students, and learning how to run a business and suddenly I hit a wall.

I was exhausted, unfocused, struggling to accomplish the simplest tasks, emotionally drained, and realizing I couldn't run a business like this. I didn't know exactly what had caused everything to come crashing down so suddenly, but I knew I needed answers, or my business would never survive. I got in with a therapist who diagnosed me with ADHD, and as I learned about how my brain works, I found answers for so many questions I didn't realize I had. Understanding ADHD has helped me create systems that help me stay on top of tasks. It has also validated so many of my experiences which has done wonders for my overall self-esteem. While preventing the kind of overwhelm that led to burnout when I was starting my business two years ago.

Better yet, understanding my ADHD has helped me realize that just because my brain works differently, doesn't mean that I function at a lower level than other people. Hyperfixation can be draining, but I've also learned that I absorb information and progress quickly when I'm hyperfixated on a specific task or learning a new skill. Being talkative (an ADHD trait especially associated with women) may have been annoying to my teachers in school (remember those comments on my report cards, Mom?), but as my communication skills have developed, it has helped me to build bonds and connect with people quickly and has turned out to be a great networking tool. Plus seeing the world a little differently from neurotypical people seems to be a pretty great thing in creative fields like music and theatre. So, I guess I turned out ok. And I *guess* that's largely due to the support I received when I was growing up. But don't worry Mom, I'm still going to heckle you about this.

Components of Cognition

Cognition involves mental processes that are associated with perceiving, making sense of, and using information. It is helpful to understand the components of cognition, but OTPs always consider cognition within the context of occupational participation. Cognition is often described as having three major components (and their related subcomponents): attention, memory, and executive function. There are general strategies OTPs can consider for addressing impairments in each of these areas of cognition, as outlined in Table 7-1. The intervention section of this chapter provides more detailed information on functional cognition approaches used by OTPs.

Attention

Today's world is exploding with information. For a minute, consider a unique environment. What are the sights, sounds, and feelings that are available to someone in that environment? When people pause to pay attention, do they notice things that they were previously unaware of, such as the ticking of a clock, the color of the carpet, and the feel of clothing against their skin?

There is so much information available to people at any given moment that it is impossible to attend to everything. **Attention** involves efficiently using cognitive resources to take in the information needed to accomplish a task. To be efficient, you must allocate cognitive resources to the entity

TABLE 7-1 | Strategies for Addressing Specific Areas of Cognitive Impairment

Area of Cognitive Impairment	Intervention Strategy
Selective attention	• Remove irrelevant stimuli. • Enhance and intensify important information. • Use auditory and visual cues. • Address internal distractions such as anxiety and auditory hallucinations.
Divided attention	• If possible, separate tasks so that the individual does not need to divide attention. • Work toward making one or more tasks automatic. • Practice doing the two tasks together.
Vigilance	• Incorporate breaks. • Slow down the rate at which information is presented. • Make stimulus easy to detect. • Schedule difficult tasks when individual is well rested and during preferred times of day.
Memory	• Chunk items together. • Create mnemonics. • Ask questions about the information. • Apply information to oneself. • Use memory aids such as calendars, checklists, and alarm clocks.
Working memory	• Simplify tasks. • Provide devices that can substitute or assist in the manipulation of information (e.g., calculators, maps).
Concept formation and categorization	• Provide cue sheet with categories and exemplars. • Provide real-world experiences to practice with concepts and categories.
Schemas and scripts	• Write out or use pictures to show the steps of a task. • Create simple maps that include steps of the task. • Order objects (e.g., clothing for the day) in the sequence in which the task is carried out. • Repeatedly practice the sequence of a task.
Problem-solving	• Provide and practice problem-solving heuristics. • Prevent or eliminate common problems that occur with specific tasks.
Decision-making	• Limit the number of options. • Teach individual about potential biases in decision-making. • Teach individual to step back and think through important decisions. • Ask other individuals for input when making important decisions.
Metacognition	• Create questions for individual to ask self before engaging in task. • Have individual evaluate performance after completing a task.

that provides the most useful input. This process can be challenging for anyone.

Distractions in the environment interfere with the ability to focus on relevant information, screen out what is irrelevant, and maintain attention through time. For example, suppose someone may be trying to study while their roommate is watching TV or talking loudly on the telephone. The person notices that their attention wanders from the study material to the television program. Or they may be tired or preoccupied and unable to focus on the textbook that they are trying to read for tomorrow's class. The person also keeps thinking about an argument that they had with a friend earlier that day.

Many things in the external environment and internal to the person compete for attentional resources. Selective attention, divided attention, and vigilance are specific aspects of attention.

Selective attention involves sorting out and focusing on the relevant sensory stimuli in the environment. This process is involved in just about everything people do and is absolutely essential; without it, a person would be completely overwhelmed by all the competing available input. The execution of daily occupations is more effective and efficient when an individual can attend to the relevant input and screen out what is irrelevant.

One of the earliest descriptions of selective attention comes from Broadbent's (1958) **filter theory**, which suggests that there is a limit to the amount of information a person can attend to at any one point in time. Therefore, individuals use an "attentional filter" that lets in some information and blocks the rest. Only the information that is allowed in can be used later. The attentional filter prevents people from experiencing information overload. However, for the filter to be effective, it must correctly select the important or relevant information and block what is not needed.

Distracters can be external or internal. Noises and movement in the environment can distract a person's attention, as can thoughts, daydreams, and anxiety. Individuals with psychosis face another internal distraction: hallucinations. Auditory hallucinations or "voices" can be very difficult to inhibit and, therefore, present a significant attentional challenge. Obsessions and rumination represent a different type of internal distraction common to OCD and depression.

Reducing distractions is important to support improved attention; however, this may do little to diminish the interference of internal distractions. It is important to consider interventions that limit internal as well as external distractions. For example, mindfulness exercises may reduce feelings of anxiety and improve focus (Lueng et al., 2014).

Selective attention implies that people work on one task at a time; however, everyday people frequently engage in one or more tasks simultaneously, a process that is often referred to as "multitasking." **Divided attention** is the ability to pay attention to more than one task at a time. For example, a mother might change her infant's diaper and, at the same time, watch her toddler play. When playing sports, a strong athlete can take a shot at the basket while still attending to where the other players are located on the court. Much consideration has been given to the divided attention required to drive and talk on a cell phone.

For the most part, individuals do better when focused on a single task. However, people can better manage two tasks at once when at least one of the tasks is automatic or when the two tasks have been practiced together. In a classic study by Spelke et al. (1976), individuals were asked to perform two controlled tasks: (1) reading for comprehension and (2) writing down dictated words. Participants practiced these tasks for 85 sessions. Eventually, the participants were able to perform both tasks simultaneously at the same level at which they had initially performed each task alone. However, it took 85 sessions to reach this proficiency.

The research on divided attention has implications for practice. For individuals with attentional impairments, tasks that require divided attention should be avoided. When divided attention tasks cannot be avoided, additional time is necessary, although this time may be reduced if extensive practice is provided.

Vigilance refers to the ability to sustain attention through time. It is similar to attention span and requires that the individual maintain a readiness to respond to a target stimulus. For example, a lifeguard must maintain attention to the activity in a pool to identify dangerous situations. When cooking, vigilance is necessary to watch what is happening to the food that is on the stove and make sure that it does not burn.

Vigilance, or the sensitivity to the desired information, wanes under certain conditions; for example, the passage of time results in deteriorating performance. Think about how a person's ability to pay attention becomes more difficult the longer a lecture goes. Fatigue plays a large role in vigilance, and individuals perform best when well rested and during their optimal time of day (Lara et al., 2014). Consequently, it is best for a "night person" to study at night. Also, the rate at which information is presented affects the ability to respond to information. If stimuli are presented very rapidly, an individual will miss more of the information. For example, if someone recites an unfamiliar phone number very rapidly, the listener may miss some of the numbers. However, if the information presented occurs extremely infrequently, vigilance may also be impaired.

Strategies to support vigilance include incorporating frequent breaks, optimizing the rate at which information is presented, making the stimulus obvious, and limiting the area in which the stimulus can take place.

Memory

Similar to attention, memory is one of the most basic cognitive functions that is employed in virtually every daily life activity. Sometimes people are very cognizant of the fact that they are drawing on their memory resources, such as while taking a test or recalling a telephone number. Other times use of memory is less obvious, but still critical. For example, memory is essential to reading a sentence and typing on a keyboard. Memory can be categorized in terms of semantic, episodic, procedural, short-term, and long-term memory.

Semantic memory is memory regarding facts. Semantic memory tends to be created and forgotten with relative ease.

However, there are many strategies that can be used to help people retain information. Shallow rehearsal, or repeating information, is the least effective method for remembering. **Deep processing**, which involves finding meaning in facts, results in better remembering. Examples of deep processing include answering questions about the information to be remembered (Craik & Tulving, 1975), identifying distinctiveness (Friedman, 1979), and relating information to oneself (Rogers et al., 1977).

Episodic memory is memory for events that have happened to you. It is organized temporally, or by when it occurred. When you recall something that happened to you, you may not remember the exact date, but you think of it in terms of the time and place it happened. Memories about a spring break vacation, a trip to the emergency room, or even what you had for dinner last night are all examples of episodic memory.

Procedural memory is memory about how to do something, such as how to ride a bike or bake a cake. Procedural memory takes longer to create and is less susceptible to errors. Procedural memory is also more implicit, meaning it is less consciously accessible. For example, it is difficult to describe how to ride a bike. Much of an OTP's work involves helping people establish procedural memories, whether new motor patterns or self-care tasks such as toothbrushing.

Short-term memories are held for only a matter of seconds or minutes. The classic paper by Miller (1956) indicated that most adults have a **short-term memory** capacity for about seven items, plus or minus two. Chunks of items can often be remembered as a single item, allowing people to recall more information. For example, a person may remember a phone number in terms of three separate chunks of information: XXX-XXX-XXXX. If not rehearsed, information in short-term memory is lost in approximately 20 seconds (Peterson & Peterson, 1959). The capacity for **long-term memory** is unknown, but includes the accumulation of information during a lifetime.

Executive Function

The term **executive function** is commonly used to refer to higher-order cognitive skills; however, a specific definition for executive function is somewhat elusive. Executive function skills can be distinguished from reflexive or automatic responses. They require a level of awareness and conscious effort. Executive function is required in situations that are new, conflicting, or complex (Godefroy, 2003), and includes skills such as working memory, concept formation and categorization, schemas and scripts, problem-solving, and decision-making.

Working memory involves short-term memory storage and active manipulation of new information; that is, the person is temporarily "working with" the information. Working memory allows a person to hold several bits of information in their mind at the same time so that the information can be processed. If someone has $10 in their pocket and orders from a menu at a fast food restaurant, in their head they figure out which items they want to eat among the list, how much it will cost, and whether their selection fits within their budget.

The person may have to adjust their choices if their selection costs too much. They go through these steps not to memorize the menus, but so that they can accomplish the temporary daily living activity of placing an order within their budget. This is an example of working memory in action.

Concept formation and **categorization** are also higher order skills that involve putting things into groups. Humans present knowledge in words and symbols. The basic unit of knowledge is the concept. There are concrete concepts (e.g., table, cat, and grass) and abstract concepts (e.g., democracy, hope, and creativity). Concepts establish order to a person's knowledge base. When confronted with new information, people relate new objects or ideas to previously existing concepts.

Knowledge is further organized by grouping concepts into categories. For example, table falls into the category of furniture, whereas democracy may be categorized as a form of government. When creating categories, people define features of the category around prototypes (Sternberg, 2003). For example, when defining the category of bird, features such as it has feathers, it flies, and it lays eggs can be noted. However, exceptions can challenge these rules. For example, people think of an ostrich as a bird, yet it does not fly. These exceptions allow categories to remain flexible.

Concept formation and categorization are important skills for many daily life activities. For example, it is essential to know what is edible and safe to eat versus what is poisonous or toxic. When doing laundry, clothes are sorted into whites, delicates, and darks, and there can be consequences if a mistake is made such as adding bleach to the dark-colored clothes. People also categorize clothing in terms of what is worn when it is cold versus hot and what is appropriate to wear to work versus going out on a Friday night.

Most of the concept formation and categorization people do is implicit. However, when working with individuals with cognitive impairments, OTPs may need to make concepts and categories more explicit. For example, teaching grocery shopping skills may incorporate information on how items are categorized in the grocery store. The person may be taught what types of items are found in the section labeled dairy.

Schemas are mental representations that create structure out of related concepts. Schemas go beyond categories in that they include information about the relationship of a concept. For example, a person's schema about an airport might include the terminals, the check-in counters, and security. A **script** is a type of schema that describes the sequence of events that a person would expect to occur in a familiar activity (Schank & Abelson, 1977). If someone is a frequent traveler, they have a schema for getting to the airport, checking in and receiving their boarding pass, going through security, boarding the plane, and finding their seat. Depending on the airports they have been through, they may or may not know how the process varies slightly according to the location.

Schemas and scripts help people integrate information and organize memories. However, schemas and scripts can result in memory mistakes, especially through time, because people tend to recall material in such a way that it is consistent with their schema (Wynn & Logie, 1998). In other words, people create inferences that may or may not be accurate. For example, a person may remember a classmate being present during a particular lecture because this classmate is typically there; however, on that particular day, the classmate was sick and not present.

In intervention, OTPs can create explicit scripts to help people with cognitive impairments sequence and negotiate the steps of complex activities. For example, a person might write out the steps for preparing a frozen dinner in a microwave and post this list on the microwave itself.

The cognitive skill of **problem-solving** is what someone uses when they want to reach a certain goal, but they cannot immediately figure out the best pathway to that goal (Matlin, 2005). Problem-solving is a mental process that involves overcoming obstacles that interfere with goal attainment. The steps to problem-solving include the following:

1. Recognizing that there is a problem
2. Understanding the problem
3. Identifying strategies or solutions to resolve the problem
4. Evaluating the strategies
5. Selecting and carrying out a strategy
6. Evaluating the outcome

These steps can be applied to the following example of buying a textbook for a college course. A student realizes there is a problem when they go to the college bookstore and find that the bookstore has sold out of a required textbook. The problem is that they have a quiz in 2 weeks based on a reading assignment from the book that is unavailable. The student imagines several different solutions, including asking the bookstore to order them a copy of the book, getting a digital version online, or asking another student if they can borrow the book. The bookstore could take up to 2 weeks to get the book, and borrowing the book would only be a short-term solution. The student learns that they can get the book immediately if they order it online. The student decides to order online, get the book, complete the reading, and get an A on the quiz. They did a good job of problem-solving that situation; however, next time they may go to the bookstore earlier in the semester if they want a hard copy of the text.

Although individuals may have impairments in the skill of problem-solving per se, the ability to solve a particular problem is highly dependent on domain expertise. In other words, how much experience and knowledge does someone have related to the specific situation? For example, someone with cooking expertise may be able to figure out how to substitute for missing key ingredients in a recipe, whereas a new cook may just have to abandon the task.

OTPs can help people with problem-solving difficulties by teaching the steps of the problem-solving process and working toward establishing expertise in a content area.

Decision-making is the process of making a choice when several options are available. Kahneman and Tversky (1996) suggested people use a small number of heuristics to guide decision-making. **Heuristics** are simple "rules of thumb" that help people make decisions quickly; unfortunately, heuristics can also lead to biased or incorrect decisions.

The **representativeness heuristic** suggests that people make decisions when something resembles a prototype or model they have come to expect. A person might make decisions about what the weather is going to be by looking outside the window or have expectations about the taste of an apple based on their prototype of an apple. The **availability heuristic** is used when people estimate frequency or make decisions based on how easy it is to think of an example. For example, if a person was recently sick after eating a particular food, they would probably not eat that same food the next day, but they might make a different decision in another 5 years.

In the **anchoring and adjustment heuristic,** people start with an anchor and then make adjustments with additional information. For example, someone might start out estimating that it will take 4 hours to write a paper, but once 3 hours have passed and they are still researching the background, they make an adjustment to the estimate. People also use the anchoring and adjustment heuristic when making judgments about people. Heuristics usually lead to accurate decisions; however, people can make better decisions when inherent biases are known. OTPs can use techniques to help persons consider all possible options. When decision-making is overwhelming, it can be helpful to limit the number of options available.

Functional Cognition

Functional cognition is the application of cognition within the context of everyday activities; consequently, functional cognition is what OTPs are most concerned with. It can be tempting to assess the cognitive components described previously and then make predictions about what a person can and cannot do. However, this is a dangerous practice because it does not consider other factors that impact occupational performance and make up functional cognition such as strategy use, habits and routines, and environmental resources (Wesson & Giles, 2019).

For example, a person may perform poorly on a memory test but is able to manage many daily activities because they use lists and calendars as a compensatory strategy. In another example, driving or taking public transportation to a familiar location, such as work, may be so routinized that a person has no trouble getting there; however, that same person may find getting to a new location extremely difficult. The environment is also taken into account with functional cognition.

As a case in point, a quiet, nonbusy environment may be more beneficial for someone with attentional issues. When observing an activity from a functional cognition perspective, the OTP will consider factors such as the initiation of the task, organization, sequencing, identification of errors, problem-solving, judgment, safety, and quality of the task completion. OTPs collectively consider the components of cognition, strategy use, habit and routines or experiences, and environmental resources when analyzing occupational participation.

Metacognition is an element of functional cognition (Wesson & Giles, 2019). Defined in a circular fashion, **metacognition** is cognition about one's own cognition. Metacognition is an awareness of what a person knows and what they do not know. It includes anticipating one's abilities to cognitively manage situations and recognizing errors as they occur. Metacognition is an important regulatory mechanism that helps people match their abilities with their desired occupations. Individuals with difficulty with functional cognition may lack metacognition, resulting in a lack of awareness of what occupations may give them difficulty.

People can learn to approach tasks more metacognitively. A list of questions can be provided that promote a reflective approach (e.g., What should I do first? Am I going too fast or too slow? How am I doing?).

Assessment

OTPs may obtain assessment information about cognition from observation of performance, reports of the person or caregiver, neuropsychological reports, and administration of standardized measures. Functional cognition is best assessed with the use of performance-based measures (Giles et al., 2019). Performance measures not only provide information about functional cognition and occupational performance; they may also provide information about the ways the person engages in the task, the strategies they use, and their awareness of errors and response to those errors.

Furthermore, there is evidence that performance-based functional cognition assessment is better than neuropsychological paper-and-pencil tasks at predicting participation in everyday activities (Arieli et al., 2022, Morrison et al., 2015). This section will describe assessments used by OTPs with an emphasis on measures that assess cognition using functional tasks or everyday objects (Table 7-2).

Allen Cognitive Level Screen-5

The Allen Cognitive Level Screen (ACLS)-5 uses a leather lacing task as a screening tool to determine the cognitive level based on Allen's Cognitive Disability Practice Model (Allen et al., 2007). Participants are instructed to make three stitches, which the OTP demonstrates. Two errors are created for the person to fix. Participants are rated on a scoring rubric that corresponds to the levels associated with the Cognitive Disabilities Model. Penny et al. (1995) found the ACLS to be related to social competence in people with schizophrenia.

In another study of schizophrenia, Seacrest et al. (2000) found relationships between the ACLS and the Wisconsin Card Sorting test, and the ACLS was associated with the Shipley Institute of Living scale in another sample of people with psychiatric disabilities (David & Riley, 1990). Another study found the ACLS-5 was useful for assessing functional cognition for people with addiction (Rojo-Mota et al., 2017).

Cognitive Performance Test

The Cognitive Performance Test (CPT; Burns, 2018) was designed for use with the Cognitive Disabilities Reconsidered Model. This assessment is specific to individuals with dementia. Individuals are observed while performing up to seven everyday activities (managing medications, dressing, shopping, toasting, making phone calls, washing, and traveling). If the individual has difficulty completing the task, the tester provides standardized cues. Scoring is based on the amount of cueing required to complete the task. The scores from the CPT are converted into a cognitive level based on the Cognitive Disabilities Model for Dementia (Levy, 2018). The CPT assesses memory and executive functioning as components of instrumental activities of daily living (IADL) performance.

One study found that the content validity of the CPT was supported by similar outcomes on the Short Mini Mental Status Examination and the Assessment of Motor and Process Skills (Douglas et al., 2012). Another study found the CPT was useful for assessing fitness to drive for people with cognitive impairment (Burns et al., 2018).

TABLE 7-2 | Therapeutic Reasoning: Assessment Table: Cognitive Skills

Which Tool?	Who Was This Tool Designed For?	Is This a Type of Tool This Person Can Do? What Is Required of the Person?	What Am I Measuring?	How Long Does It Take and Where Do I Administer This Assessment?	Is the Tool Associated With a Practice Model?
Allen Cognitive Level Screen (ACLS; Allen et al., 2007) • Large Allen Cognitive Level Screen (LACLS)	Adults with psychiatric disorders, adults with dementia, people with disruption in cognitive processing skills; use LACLS for visually impaired	Leather lacing task requires person to follow verbal and/or visual directions.	Global cognition as it affects occupational performance. Corresponds to the Allen Scale of Cognitive Performance Levels 3.0 to 5.8.	Can be administered in the clinic in 10–20 minutes to screen possible limitations in information processing impacting function; results of screening should be verified with other tools.	Cognitive Disabilities Model
Cognitive Performance Test (CPT; T. Burns, 2018)	Adults with dementia or suspected dementia	The individual completes up to seven everyday life activities such as making toast and setting up a medication box.	Cognition as it affects occupational performance. The score is converted to a cognitive disabilities reconsidered model level.	It takes approximately 30 minutes to administer (depending on the number of tasks) and can be administered in a clinic or home.	Cognitive Disabilities Reconsidered Model
Contextual Memory Test (CMT; Toglia, 1993)	Adults with brain injury or psychiatric conditions	Questionnaire of person's awareness of memory and ability to recall pictures of everyday objects	Assesses awareness of memory problems and recall memory. Includes a dynamic component to determine if individual can learn strategies to improve performance.	Takes 10–20 minutes to measure; administered in a clinical setting	Toglia's Dynamic Interactional Approach
Do-Eat (Josman et al., 2010)	Children at a chronological or behavioral age of 5 to 8	Complete three tasks: make a sandwich, prepare chocolate milk, and fill out a certificate of performance.	Three areas are measured: performance of the tasks, sensory motor skills, and executive function.	Administered in a home environment, classroom, or clinic and takes approximately 20 minutes	Metacognitive model for children with atypical brain development
Executive Function Performance Test (EFPT; Baum & Wolfe, 2013)	Adults with neurological or psychiatric conditions	Person performs four IADLs— cooking, telephone use, medication management, and bill paying, with graded cues as needed.	Executive impairment effect on capacity for independent functioning and level of assistance needed. Executive function areas measured include initiation, organization, sequencing, judgment, safety, and completion.	Administered in a clinical or home setting with cooking space and takes approximately 1 to 1½ hours to administer	No, but places an emphasis on assessing what the person can do and the level of assistance needed
Menu Task (Al-Heizan et al., 2020; Edwards et al., 2019)	Individuals with suspected mild cognitive impairments	Person follows specific rules for selecting items on a hospital menu.	Ability to initiate and complete a complex task with specific rules	Typically administered in a hospital setting; takes about 4 minutes	No
Multiple Errands Test (Shallice & Burgess, 1991) • Multiple Errands Test— Simplified Version • Multiple Errands Test—Revised	Adults with brain injury, stroke, or psychiatric conditions	Person must perform simple tasks such as purchasing items and making a phone call while adhering to specific rules.	Executive function as performed in a natural environment scored in terms of rule breaks, inefficiencies, task failure, and interpretation failure.	Administered in a shopping center or hospital and takes approximately 30–45 minutes	No, but it is based on the theory that executive dysfunction may be better detected in natural environments (as opposed to controlled assessment environments)

TABLE 7-2 | **Therapeutic Reasoning: Assessment Table: Cognitive Skills—cont'd**

Which Tool?	Who Was This Tool Designed For?	Is This a Type of Tool This Person Can Do? What Is Required of the Person?	What Am I Measuring?	How Long Does It Take and Where Do I Administer This Assessment?	Is the Tool Associated With a Practice Model?
Weekly Calendar Planning Activity (Toglia, 2015)	People with subtle cognitive impairments including those with mental health conditions (ages 12–older adults)	The person needs to follow instructions to fill out a weekly calendar.	Memory impairment, executive function, ability to recognize and correct errors, follow rules and employ strategies	The short form takes 10–15 minutes, and the long form takes 20–40 minutes. It can be administered in any setting.	Toglia's Dynamic Interactional Approach

Contextual Memory Test

The Contextual Memory Test (CMT; Toglia, 1993) includes a subjective assessment of the individual's awareness of their memory ability (metacognition) and an objective assessment of memory. The awareness component asks the individual to predict their score. This is done at the beginning of the assessment and at different points throughout.

Part I of the objective assessment is the static assessment of memory. The test uses 20 drawings with either a restaurant or morning routine theme to assess recall memory. Each picture is presented for 90 seconds. After all 20 pictures are presented, the individual is asked to recall as many items as possible. After 15 to 20 minutes, the individual is asked to recall the items again. If the individual does poorly on Part I, then Part II, the dynamic assessment, is administered. The alternate theme of either restaurant or morning routine is presented. The individual is given cues about the theme of the pictures and instructed to analyze the overall context before attending to the specifics of each picture. Dynamic assessment is useful for determining if an individual can benefit from strategy training.

Several studies of the CMT examined discriminant validity. On the awareness component of the test, individuals with brain injury tend to overestimate their memory capacity and base their abilities on functioning before the brain injury (Toglia, 1993). The CMT did discriminate individuals with Alzheimer disease (Gil & Josman, 2001) and children with brain injury (Josman et al., 2000).

Do-Eat

The Do-Eat is a performance-based assessment for children 5 to 8 years of age either chronologically or behaviorally (Josman et al., 2010). It is intended to be administered in natural surroundings such as a home kitchen or classroom but can be administered in a clinic. The child completes three tasks: making a sandwich, preparing chocolate milk, and filling out a certificate of performance. A dynamic assessment approach is used such that predetermined cues are provided to assist children who have difficulty.

The Do-Eat is scored in three areas: performance of the task, sensory motor skills, and executive function. The scoring considers the level and amount of cueing required to complete the tasks. A study of the Do-Eat found that the assessment had good interrater reliability and internal consistency and was able to distinguish between children with and without developmental coordination disorder (Josman et al., 2010). The Do-Eat was also adapted to use washing hands as the task (Washy); a study indicated that the measure was good at discriminating between children with and without autism, and that it was strongly correlated with the Pediatric Evaluation of Disability Inventory (Levy-Dayan et al., 2023).

Executive Function Performance Test

The Executive Function Performance Test (EFPT) is a performance-based standardized assessment of cognition and executive function (Baum & Wolf, 2013). The Kitchen Task Assessment, an earlier performance-based assessment test designed by Baum and Edwards (1993), was used as the prototype in developing the EFPT. The EFPT includes four standardized IADL tasks (cooking, telephone use, medication management, bill paying), which the person performs with graded cues provided by the OTP.

The EFPT serves three purposes: to determine which executive function components are deficient (i.e., initiation, organization, sequencing, judgment and safety, or completion); determine an individual's capacity for independent functioning; and determine the type of assistance necessary for task completion. The EFPT has been validated in studies of individuals with stroke, multiple sclerosis, schizophrenia, and traumatic brain injury (TBI; Baum et al., 2008, 2017; Goverover et al., 2005; Katz et al., 2007). The Performance Assessment of Self-Care Skills (Rogers et al., 2016) and the Test of Grocery Shopping Skills (Brown et al., 2009) use a similar process as the EFPT.

These performance-based tests include standardized administration and ratings of cognitively complex IADLs, but because the ratings emphasize IADL performance these measures are discussed in greater detail in Chapter 46: Activities of Daily Living, Instrumental Activities of Daily Living, and Health Management Occupations.

Menu Task

The Menu Task is intended for use as a screening tool of functional cognition (Edwards et al., 2019). It takes only 4 minutes to administer, but a more extensive measure should be administered if concerns are identified with the Menu Task. Participants are asked to select choices from a hospital menu including three meals and two snacks. Specific rules regarding the selection are included such as selecting at least two heart healthy options and not talking to the examiner during administration. The measure is scored on completion, initiation, and inhibition. There is evidence supporting the measure's interrater reliability, internal consistency, and construct validity (Al-Heizan et al., 2020; Edwards et al., 2019).

Multiple Errands Test

The Multiple Errands Test (MET; Shallice & Burgess, 1991) is a measure of executive function that is administered in a hospital or shopping mall. Simple tasks are assigned, such as getting information about the times a particular service is available, purchasing items in a store, and getting oneself to an identified location at a prearranged time. In addition, specific rules are established, such as "No shop should be entered other than to buy something." This measure is designed to test strategy use in an ecologically valid setting.

Shallice and Burgess (1991) studied individuals with brain injury who performed well on IQ tests and laboratory measures of executive function and found that these individuals did poorly on the MET. They argue that tests such as the MET are more sensitive to subtle impairments of executive function that are common in neurological disorders. There is a simplified measure of the test (Alderman et al., 2003) and a revised measure that can be administered in a hospital setting (Knight et al., 2002). The test has good interrater reliability, and both the simplified and hospital versions distinguished people with and without brain injury.

The MET-Revised is but one version of a modified MET with over 20 versions created for specific settings (Rotenberg et al., 2020). Although adjustments are often necessary to meet the needs of a setting, this does call into question the integrity of these adaptations. The team of Scarff and colleagues (2022) provide guidelines for developing site-specific modifications that stay true to the intentions of the original MET.

Weekly Calendar Planning Activity

The Weekly Calendar Planning Activity is another example of a performance-based assessment (Toglia, 2015). The participant is given a list of either 17 (adult version) or 18 (youth version) appointments or errands and is asked to enter these into a calendar. Additional rules are provided, such as leaving a day free or not responding to questions from the examiner. The measure is scored in terms of accuracy, efficiency, time, rules followed, and planning time. The task requires that the person keep track of rules, avoid conflicts, monitor the passage of time, and inhibit distractions. The measure is suitable for populations with executive function impairments including mental health conditions such as schizophrenia, substance abuse, and mood disorders (Lussier et al., 2019). Studies indicate it has good discriminant validity for community and at-risk youth (Toglia & Berg, 2013) and college students with and without ADHD (Lahav et al., 2018).

Intervention: Models and Techniques for Cognitive Impairment

In occupational therapy intervention, there are two primary approaches for addressing cognitive impairment: remediation and compensation. In the **remediation approach,** the

cognitive impairment is targeted, and intervention is directed at improving a specific skill or teaching strategy. In the **compensatory approach,** the OTP adapts the environment, task, or teaching method to compensate for the cognitive impairment. The separation between the two approaches is not always clear cut, and some interventions combine both strategies.

This section presents several models of intervention that are relevant for occupational therapy practice, including Cognitive Remediation, Multicontext Approach, Cognitive Adaptation, Cognitive Orientation to Daily Occupational Performance (CO-OP), Metacognitive Reflection and Insight Therapy (MERIT), Cognitive Disabilities Model, Cognitive Disabilities Model for Dementia, Errorless Learning, Cognitive Functional Intervention, and the Unstuck and On Target method.

Cognitive Remediation

Cognitive Remediation is aimed at improving or restoring specific cognitive skills, such as attention, memory, and problem-solving, so that the individual can more successfully engage in everyday occupations. Neuroplasticity provides the scientific rationale behind Cognitive Remediation (Kaneko & Keshavan, 2012). It is now understood that the brain can adapt and change structure, function, and connectivity in response to experience at any age.

Cognitive Remediation is used as an intervention to give individuals experiences and practice with cognitive skills to promote changes in the brain. The intervention techniques utilized in Cognitive Remediation incorporate computer-based training, paper-and-pencil tasks, and group exercises that are incrementally graded for improving cognitive processes (Barlati et al., 2013). Repetition and rehearsal are essential characteristics of Cognitive Remediation; consequently, the approach is more effective when intervention sessions are frequent and provided during extended time periods (several times a week for many months) and often include homework exercises.

Cognitive Remediation should target those cognitive areas that are known to be impaired (Averbuch & Katz, 2011). Because the type and severity of impairment can vary significantly among individuals with psychiatric disabilities, it is important that a careful assessment is conducted initially to identify the targets of intervention. Activities are selected that challenge the impaired cognition; then, as performance improves, the exercises become more difficult. For example, a letter cancellation task such as the one shown in Box 7-1 may be used to address selective attention and vigilance.

The OTP then records both the amount of time it takes to complete the task and the number of errors (both missing the "b" and crossing out the incorrect letter). The OTP can also observe how the person goes about the task—for example, does the person use a systematic approach to scanning? If not, the OTP can provide the person with feedback on how to systematically scan from left to right.

BOX 7-1 ■ Letter Cancellation Task

Cross out each letter "b"

d f r s b h q r s l t u b m n v b f a s b c t r o l b h a f h l b b o
  p r s t u v

l m j b o r s l f q r s b e w q o h t u v w s m u b l b n m b w u
  y x y t o

The exercise is repeated until the individual becomes competent, at which point increasingly complex exercises are added. For example, the letter cancellation may involve only letters that are similar to the target, such as

b p p d q b p d q p b b d d p b q q d p b q d p b q d b p p d q b q p d b d d

Different tasks can be used to address other areas of attention, memory, and executive function. There are many commercially available packages providing Cognitive Remediation activities (see Resources).

Cognitive Remediation is widely studied in schizophrenia. Results consistently indicate that the intervention is effective in improving basic cognitive skills and that these improvements are maintained through time (Vita et al., 2021). There is also substantial support for Cognitive Remediation in eating disorders (Tchanturia et al., 2014) and bipolar disorder (Tsapekos et al., 2020). When Cognitive Remediation comprises simply drill and practice, improvements in cognition are found, but these skills do not generalize to everyday life (Medalia & Saperstein, 2013). Cognitive Remediation is most

effective and improvements are generalized to daily functioning when the approach is used in combination with other interventions that target occupational participation such as work or independent living (Wykes et al., 2011).

Occupation-based practice is grounded in the premise that intervention occurs within the context of occupational performance; therefore, OTPs using Cognitive Remediation should always consider the importance of generalizing the improvements of cognitive skills to occupational performance. Utilizing the earlier letter cancellation task as an example, the strategies developed with this paper-and-pencil task may then be applied to grocery shopping, and the person may be asked to search through the products on a store shelf to find strawberry yogurt.

An expert working group identified the core techniques that should be included in Cognitive Remediation for schizophrenia (Bowie et al., 2020). These core techniques include the following: (a) Cognitive Remediation should be facilitated by a practitioner who has a working knowledge of cognitive processes and how cognitive abilities affect everyday functioning; (b) intensive training is required for meaningful effects,

Evidence-Based Practice

Choosing Wisely Initiative

When using Cognitive Remediation interventions, OTPs should adopt approaches that embed the training in everyday life activities.

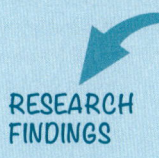
RESEARCH FINDINGS

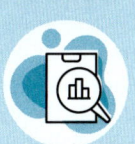

AOTA's initial participation with the Choosing Wisely initiative identified five things that patients and providers should question when receiving occupational therapy services (American Occupational Therapy Association [AOTA], 2018). One of those things reads, "Don't provide cognitive-based interventions (e.g., paper-and-pencil tasks, table-top tasks, cognitive training software) without direct application to occupational performance." This recommendation is consistent with research indicating cognitive-based interventions provided with direct application to employment are effective in improving employment outcomes for people with schizophrenia. Participants receiving Cognitive Remediation in addition to employment services were more likely to stick with their jobs, work more hours, and earn more wages when compared with a group that only received employment services (Burns & Erickson, 2022; Teixeira et al., 2018).

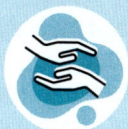
APPLICATIONS

➡ When using Cognitive Remediation interventions, the OTP should adopt approaches that embed the training in everyday life activities.
➡ When targeting an occupation such as employment, education, or IADLs, outcomes may be augmented with the inclusion of Cognitive Remediation, particularly for individuals with known cognitive impairments.

REFERENCES

American Occupational Therapy Association. (2018). *Choosing Wisely, five things patients and providers should question.* https://www.choosingwisely.org/societies/american-occupational-therapy-association-inc

Burns, A., & Erickson, D. H. (2022). Adding Cognitive Remediation to employment support services: A randomized controlled trial. *Psychiatric Services,* appips202100249. https://doi.org/10.1176/appi.ps.202100249

Teixeira, C., Mueser, K. T., Rogers, E. S., & McGurk, S. R. (2018). Job endings and work trajectories of persons receiving supported employment and Cognitive Remediation. *Psychiatric Services, 69*(7), 812–818. https://doi.org/10.1176/appi.ps.201700489

with 40 or more hours being common, (c) Cognitive Remediation should include strategy training; and (d) the training should include techniques for transfer to real-world activities.

Multicontext Approach

The **Multicontext Approach** is based on the Dynamic Interactional Model of Cognition (Toglia & Foster, 2021). The approach focuses on strategy training and the ability to use these strategies in real-world occupational participation (Steinberg & Zlotnik, 2019). The Multicontext Approach considers the interplay of the person, activity, and environment. The focus of this approach is not on cognitive subskills, such as attention and memory, but on the functional information processing capacity of the individual. This capacity is modifiable and varies as the activity, environment, and person change. In other words, cognition is dynamic. Structured activities are chosen that elicit the types of performance challenges the person needs to work on. The activities should be relevant and interesting to the person. Repeated practice is encouraged by providing activities with similar cognitive demands.

In this approach, intervention focuses on processing strategies and self-monitoring skills (Steinberg & Zlotnik, 2019). Using a metacognitive framework, the OTP has a preactivity and postactivity discussion with the person by asking open-ended questions that prompt the person to consider strategies. For example, "What can you do to remember to pay your bill on time?" The goal is for the person to generate strategies, but initially they may need more help from the OTP.

The Multicontext Approach facilitates generalization by working on a strategy across different activities and situations that gradually change. For example, the strategy of anticipation can be taught to an individual who tends to engage in tasks impulsively. The person is taught to think about an activity before starting it and possibly answer questions such as, "What problems might this create for me, and what might I do if I run into difficulty?" This strategy would be practiced with increasingly difficult activities and in increasingly dissimilar environments. For an individual who is easily distracted, the strategy could involve underlining, bolding, or listing the most important information.

The Multicontext Approach was originally designed for people with TBI, but it has been applied to people with schizophrenia and children with learning disabilities and ADHD (Josman, 2005).

Cognitive Adaptation

Cognitive Adaptation involves strategies that adapt the environment or task to compensate for cognitive impairments. Because of the limitations of Cognitive Remediation, compensatory approaches are often used instead of or in addition to remedial strategies. Compensatory strategies include the use of adaptive devices and thinking techniques. A day planner is an example of an adaptive device, and the use of a memory mnemonic is a thinking technique. The use of thinking strategies is generally more effective if the individual has some awareness of their cognitive impairment. The person must also have the cognitive ability to learn and remember the steps of the strategy.

Adapting Tasks and Environments

Task analysis and environmental assessment are the first steps toward developing environmental adaptations. By

Toothbrushing

1. Remove the cap of the toothpaste.
2. Squeeze a pea-size ball of toothpaste on your toothbrush.
3. Wet the toothbrush under running water in your sink.
4. Brush your teeth for 2 minutes (use your timer).
5. Remember to brush front and back teeth and all surfaces, including your gums.
6. Rinse your mouth and the toothbrush.
7. Check your face in the mirror to make sure you've rinsed away all toothpaste.
8. Replace the cap on the toothpaste.
9. Return toothpaste and toothbrush to the medicine chest.

FIGURE 7-1. Sample script for toothbrushing.

understanding the components of a task, it is often possible to modify it to compensate for cognitive impairments. For example, cooking tasks can be adapted by using prechopped ingredients, prepared foods, and simple recipes with limited steps and ingredients. Alternate methods may also be used to accomplish a task; for example, money management may be simplified by using direct deposit and automatic bill paying systems. Scripts can be created to help an individual sequence the steps of a task (Fig. 7-1).

Environmental adaptations often include the use of cues such as labels, signs, symbols, alarms, and beepers. Cabinets and drawers can be labeled to indicate contents. Signs that provide reminders can be placed in relevant locations; for example, a sign stating "don't forget your keys" may be placed on the inside of the door. Phones, watches, and timers are used by most people to wake up in the morning or to time the baking of a cake, but more sophisticated systems are also available to remind individuals to take their medication, follow a self-care routine, and alert a caregiver that someone has left the house (see Resources).

Calendars and day planners can be used to help provide reminders of appointments and daily schedules. Checklists are useful in helping establish routines. For example, individuals who have difficulty organizing housecleaning or feel overwhelmed by the task can use a weekly checklist to make housecleaning more manageable (Fig. 7-2). A meta-analysis of cognitive compensatory interventions for people with psychosis found a medium effect for functioning and evidence that the improvements were maintained over time (Allott et al., 2020).

Organizational strategies can be particularly useful in school-based practice for children with cognitive impairments such as ADHD or learning disabilities. One OTP has created a system for keeping the student's desk organized by using a template placed in the storage section of the desk with labels for placement of the school-related objects such as books, pencil case, binders, and so on (Gary Groening, personal communication, 2005).

Weekly Housecleaning Checklist

⬤ Sunday	Wash dishes	✘
Monday	Wash dishes	✘
	Take out garbage	✘
Tuesday	Wash dishes	✘
	Clean bathrooms	
⬤ Wednesday	Wash dishes	✘
	Dust	✘
Thursday	Wash dishes	
	Vacuum and sweep floors	
Friday	Wash dishes	✘
Saturday	Wash dishes	✘
⬤	Laundry	

FIGURE 7-2. Sample weekly checklist for housecleaning.

Social supports provide another powerful compensatory tool. Family members or peers can provide reminders or cues. These same individuals may also perform a task alongside the person to act as a model. Naturally occurring community supports should also be considered. A friendly bus driver may be willing to help someone recognize their stop, a classmate can be a study partner, and the clerks at the grocery store may be available to help people locate items.

Cognitive Adaptation Training

Cognitive Adaptation Training is a manualized program developed by a psychologist with initial input from occupational therapy (Velligan et al., 1996). The program uses a different set of strategies for apathetic versus disinhibited behaviors in people with schizophrenia. Strategies to address apathetic behaviors focus on prompts and cues, such as creating checklists, using labels, and placing everyday objects such as toothbrushes within eyesight. Strategies to address disinhibited behavior involve the removal of distractions and organization of materials, such as removing out-of-season clothes from the closet and using colored bins to sort the laundry. A randomized controlled trial of Cognitive Adaptation Training found that, at the end of the study period, individuals in the Cognitive Adaptation Training group had higher levels of global functioning and lower relapse rates (Velligan et al., 2000). Cognitive Adaptation Training has also been used in the early intervention of psychosis (Allott et al., 2016) and as a family intervention (Kidd et al., 2014) with positive outcomes.

Cognitive Orientation to Daily Occupational Performance

The **Cognitive Orientation to Daily Occupational Performance (CO-OP)** approach uses functional cognition to promote the acquisition of functional skills (Gimeno et al., 2019). It was initially developed for children with developmental coordination disorder, but since then it has been applied to many populations including children with ADHD and developmental disabilities as well as adults with neurological conditions. An extensive body of research indicates that CO-OP is effective in skill acquisition, as well as generalization and transfer to untrained goals. It borrows from the work of Donald Meichenbaum (1979), an early developer of compensatory thinking strategies who used self-talk as a strategy to help the individual attend to the task, think through the steps before acting on them, and with repeated practice support the development of automatic processing.

In addition to strategy training, the OTP engages in a dynamic performance analysis to determine where the performance is breaking down. In CO-OP, a global four-step strategy is taught to help the individual work through motor tasks (Polatajko et al., 2011):

1. Goal—What do you want to do?
2. Plan—How will you go about doing it?
3. Do—Carry out the plan.
4. Check—Did the plan work? Does it need to be modified?

A domain-specific strategy is then created to support the particular goal of the person. The OTP guides the person in developing specific strategies to help with carrying out the task. For example, Nancy wants to be able to pump up her bicycle tires so that she does not have to rely on others when she wants to go for a ride (Goal). She has trouble remembering all the steps and finds it physically difficult to fill the tires. The OTP then helps Nancy identify the domain-specific strategies that will be useful in carrying out the task (Plan). Perhaps the steps are written down in a script, and Nancy reminds herself to hold the pump with both feet, pull all the way up, and push all the way down with the pump. After implementing these strategies (Do), Nancy decides whether or not it is working (Check) and whether new strategies should be implemented.

A review of CO-OP included 27 studies of children with developmental coordination disorder and found the intervention was effective in helping the children achieve their goals and increase their satisfaction with performance of desired occupations (Scammell et al., 2016).

Metacognitive Reflection and Insight Therapy

Metacognitive Reflection and Insight Therapy (MERIT) was designed as a metacognitive approach that can be used by practitioners with different backgrounds and in conjunction with other approaches (Lysaker et al., 2020). MERIT is focused on the therapeutic relationship as a means for addressing everyday problems. Wasmuth and colleagues (2022) described how this approach can be used by OTPs in mental health practice. The MERIT guidelines are divided into three types of therapeutic elements: content elements, process elements, and superordinate elements. The four content elements address current wishes and challenges and are described in the list that follows:

■ *The agenda:* The OTP uses occupation-based assessments such as the Occupational Circumstances Assessment Interview and Rating Scale (OCAIRS)

PhotoVoice

I think the calendar is a wonderful idea for the MARC Center. The calendar lets you know the different activities on different days that will be taking place at the MARC Center. What a wonderful idea for the monthly calendar to help keep me alert of certain activities that may be going on that day.

It is likely that most individuals attending the MARC Center have a smartphone. How might you use the calendar app to promote occupational performance for individuals with serious mental illness with cognitive impairments?

(Forsyth et al., 2005) to guide conversations that explore potential agendas. The agenda is based on the wishes and needs of the person

- *Insertion of the therapist's mind:* The OTP partners with the person and reflects observation related to valued roles, task completion, and occupational engagement.
- *Eliciting the narrative episode:* Using an occupational history, the OTP elicits a narrative from the person that examines current experiences and relates them to prior events. For example, if the person is concerned about being evicted the OTP would discuss previous times when they have maintained or lost an apartment.
- *Defining the psychological problem:* The OTP and the person identify psychological barriers to occupational engagement.

The two process elements are based on reflection of the context:

- *Reflecting on the therapeutic relationship:* The OTP can use the Intentional Relationship Model (Taylor, 2020) and reflect with the person about their experiences with interpersonal interactions.
- *Reflecting on progress:* The OTP uses a combination of performance-based assessments and self-reports to promote conversation about the person's progress.

The final two superordinate elements involve OTP interventions that meet the level of the person:

- *Stimulating self-reflection and awareness of others:* Through occupational engagement and conversation interventions, the OTP helps the person identify changes in metacognition.
- *Stimulating mastery:* The OTP finds opportunities for occupational engagement that match the person's capacity.

Overall, the MERIT model is about engaging in a shared reflection in which the OTP recognizes the person as an expert in their own life and shows a sincere interest and appreciation for their story. In addition, the OTP believes in the person's recovery and sets up situations in which the person can experience mastery.

Cognitive Disabilities Model

Claudia Allen (1985) suggested that Cognitive Remediation is not a reasonable goal for people with serious cognitive impairments and developed the **Cognitive Disabilities Model** as a framework for OTPs to use to create situations in which individuals with cognitive impairments can be successful. Modifications to the activity and environment form the basis for intervention.

OTPs can use this model to explain patterns of behavior and performance using the six hierarchical levels of cognitive functioning (McCraith & Earhart, 2018) outlined in Table 7-3. These six levels are further broken down into sublevels, such as Level 1.1, 1.2, and so on, which make up the Allen Cognitive Levels (ACL) scale.

When applying the model to intervention, the OTP begins with a detailed and multifaceted assessment. This typically includes an interview with the person and caregivers, observation of performance, and administration of standardized tests such as the ACLS-5 (Allen et al., 2007) and the Allen Diagnostic Module, 2nd Edition (Earhart, 2006). This information is used for determining the individual's cognitive level. Therapists are encouraged to use multiple sources of information to obtain a more accurate estimate.

The intervention then focuses on creating the best fit for the individual to promote participation in valued occupations (McCraith & Earhart, 2018). Intervention planning considers what the person "can do," "will do," and "may do." Occupations the individual "can do" are those that are cognitively realistic for the individual to perform. Occupations that the individual "will do" are those that are interesting and desired, and occupations that the individual "may do" are those that the environment supports.

The emphasis in the Cognitive Disabilities Model is on interventions aimed at modifying occupations and environments. Previous sections in this chapter that discuss environmental modification can be used for guidance. The model does not exclude the use of restorative interventions that target cognitive capacities. Using the model, OTPs provide

TABLE 7-3 | Cognitive Disability Frame of Reference—Hierarchical Levels of Cognitive Functioning

Cognitive Disability Level	Individual Characteristics	OTP Responses
Level 1: Automatic actions	• Impaired awareness, but person is conscious and has reflexive responses • Able to perform only very basic habits such as eating and drinking • Responses are primarily instinctive	• Use one-word commands. • Provide familiar cues (e.g., place plate of food within view and hand individual a fork).
Level 2: Postural actions	• Aware of movements of their own muscles and joints • Watches movements of others • Seeks movements that are pleasurable or comfortable • May be resistive or easily agitated	• Imitate gross motor actions and simultaneously provide simple verbal directions (e.g., watch me, and then you try it). • Focus is on gross motor movements.
Level 3: Manual actions	• Able to attend to the external environment, particularly tactile cues • Can use hands to manipulate materials • May include seemingly purposeless actions • Easily distracted	• Imitate manipulation of objects (e.g., brushing teeth). • Provide repetitive practice of routine tasks. • Use manually guided instruction.
Level 4: Goal-directed actions	• Can respond to visual motor cues • Attention is directed toward one cue at a time • Actions are more goal directed • Has difficulty correcting errors • Can attend a 1-hour group	• Provide visual demonstration. • Limit instruction to one step at a time. • Make all objects clearly visible. • Provide visual comparisons so that individual knows what they are working toward. • Situation-specific training is useful.
Level 5: Exploratory actions	• Concrete relations are understood, although they have trouble with abstraction • Uses exploratory actions, as well as trial-and-error problem-solving • Does not anticipate problems	• Accompany visual demonstration with verbal explanation. • Select or modify tasks to reduce problem-solving requirements. • Use concrete explanations and examples. • Assist with planning ahead.
Level 6: Planned actions	• Can make sense of symbolic cues and abstraction • Can plan ahead • Anticipates errors and engages in mental problem-solving • Pauses to think about potential problems	• Use verbal and written instruction, diagrams, and drawings. • Can carry out instructions from previous sessions.

activities in which the individual can succeed, with the goal of creating an environment that allows the individual the least restrictions while maintaining safety.

Often, OTPs using the Cognitive Disability Frame of Reference create therapeutic groups based on cognitive levels. For example, persons at Level 3 might work with familiar tools and materials to create basic craft products.

Allen's Cognitive Disabilities Model was combined with Reisberg's Theory of Retrogenesis in the design of an interdisciplinary dementia program in a long-term care facility (Warchol, 2004). The OTP works directly with the person and also consults with and provides training to other staff members so that they can implement strategies and supports that allow the individual to participate more successfully in the activities and dining programs.

Research related to this model suggests that the cognitive levels may be related to other cognitive measures, social competence, and community living status (Penny et al., 1995; Secrest et al., 2000; Wilson et al., 1989). There is limited research on the efficacy of the model as an intervention approach. A small pilot study of individuals with schizophrenia compared an intervention group that received treatment according to Allen's Cognitive Disabilities Model with a control group at a community activity center (Raweh et al., 1999). The intervention group improved significantly more on the ACL, although both groups improved on the routine task inventory.

Cognitive Disabilities Model for Dementia

The **Cognitive Disabilities Model for Dementia** focuses on the individual's capacities (Levy, 2018). The ACLs are reconceptualized (ranging from 1.0 to 5.6); that is, the levels are described in terms of the functional decline associated with dementia, with the lowest level being unresponsive and the highest normal functioning. The levels are determined by using the CPT (Burns, 2018). The ability to participate in activities of daily living (ADLs) and IADLs as well as the level and type of assistance required is described for each level. For example, the level of assistance may be a verbal cue or actual hand-over-hand assistance.

During the assessment, an occupational profile identifies valued occupations, after which the CPT is used to identify the impact of cognitive impairment on occupational performance. This process includes an assessment of safety concerns.

Intervention involves maximizing the individual's strengths and creating an enabling environment that supports

TABLE 7-4 | Cognitive Disabilities Model for Dementia—Hierarchical Levels of Functioning

Cognitive Disability Level	Individual Characteristics	OTP Responses
Level 1.0 Very severe functional decline	• Minimal response. Attention limited to basic cues such as pain and hunger.	• Comforting interventions are useful such as wrapping the individual in a blanket, passive exercise, and massage. Caregivers need assistance with end-of-life decisions.
Level 2.0 Very severe functional decline	• Confusion is typical even in familiar settings. Responds to touch and sound. Participation is passive.	• Simple repetitive activities are often comforting such as rocking, music, and the provision of objects to hold. Need total support for ADLs with possible exception of feeding. Support for the caregiver is important and in-home care or placement in long-term care setting often occurs at this level.
Level 3.0 Severe functional decline	• Minimal attention. Memory is severely impaired such that individual may forget their own children. Individual will often appear confused and often mistake past for present events. Most actions are devoid of goal direction. Simple motor planning is impaired.	• Caregiver instruction includes removal of hazards and fall prevention programs may be helpful. Help individual to continue to use familiar objects after set-up and with simple verbal and tactile cues for basic ADLs such as feeding.
Level 4.0 Moderate to moderately severe functional decline	• Significant difficulties with executive function such as planning ahead, problem-solving, and new learning. May be disoriented to time or place. Performance declines in even basic ADLs. Much more supervision is required to maintain safety. Behavioral concerns may become more challenging. Problems develop with carrying on a conversation.	• Caregiver training is often essential as caregiver will need to provide structure and assistance by maintaining routines, setting up tasks, removing distractions, and initiating activities. Caregivers need to know to expect inconsistency and errors. Driving is a common concern and the caregiver may need assistance in recognizing the risk and restricting driving. OTPs can help caregivers with breaking down tasks and identifying activities where the individual can be successful. Structured day programs may be helpful.
Level 5.0 Mild functional decline	• Beginning deficits in executive functioning and processing of abstract information develop. Information processing is slower. ADLs are retained. Difficulties develop with IADLs, particularly for individuals who are still working or engaged in complex activities.	• Modify IADLs or identify replacement activities if necessary. Individuals and caregiver may need support for adjusting to new diagnosis of dementia as well as increased awareness for potential safety issues. • Responds well to direct, concrete, and visible cues such as lists.
Level 5.6 Absence of functional-cognitive disability	• Absence of cognitive disability. Individual is capable of planning, problem-solving, and learning.	• OTP can help person learn new occupations or activities as needed.

performance in desired occupations. For example, at a cognitive disability level of 3 the individual has severe impairments in attention and memory but can still typically engage in parts of basic ADLs. At this level, the OTP might teach the caregiver how to provide set up with cues for toothbrushing. The caregiver can set out the toothbrush and toothpaste in front of the sink and then provide step-by-step cues as needed. Table 7-4 describes the CPT levels and the OTP's responses to each level. Included in the description is caregiver training.

Errorless Learning

Individuals with cognitive impairments such as Alzheimer's disease, schizophrenia, intellectual disabilities, and learning disabilities often have difficulty learning new information. Learning is made more difficult by the inability to self-monitor. In other words, they may have difficulty recognizing mistakes and using feedback about these errors to change future performance. In this situation, the errors can intrude on a correct response. For example, a person may have had the experience of mistakenly learning the incorrect name for an individual. It then becomes more difficult to correct that mistake, and the person has a tendency to still call that person by the wrong name. **Errorless Learning** compensates for self-monitoring problems and prevents intrusive or perseverative (making the same mistake again and again) errors.

When using Errorless Learning, the training process is structured so that mistakes are minimized or not allowed to occur. The process has four parts (Kern et al., 2005):

1. The task is broken down into simple components.
2. The training starts with simple tasks with a high likelihood of success.
3. Increasingly difficult tasks are added, but prompts, cues, and guided instruction are used at each level until a high level of proficiency is attained.
4. Performance at each level is overlearned using repetition, successful practice, and positive reinforcement.

These steps are similar to many other rehabilitation strategies; the main difference is that mistakes are avoided.

Errorless Learning is most easily applied to discrimination tasks such as learning names. For example, in a day treatment program for individuals with Alzheimer disease, a goal may be established for group members to learn the names of the OTP and the four other people in the treatment group. In an "effortful" learning situation, the OTP might ask a group member to go around the circle and state the names of everyone in the group. However, this is likely to result in mistakes.

In an Errorless Learning approach, the OTP may use several strategies to help group members learn the names: going around the circle with each person saying their name aloud, having each person hold up a sign with their name on it so the group members can say the names aloud, showing photographs of the group members so the OTP can say each name aloud and ask each group member to repeat the name, and so on. Once the OTP believes that an individual has learned a name, she might show a picture and say, "Don't guess if you're not sure, but if you do know, tell me the name of this person."

Studies of Errorless Learning have demonstrated the efficacy of this approach in individuals with dementia for improving more complex skills. For example, one study found Errorless Learning was effective in increasing food intake for institutionalized individuals with dementia (Wu et al., 2014) and another found Errorless Learning effective in improving IADLs (Thivierge et al., 2014). Still another study found Errorless Learning was effective in improving ADLs for individuals with dementia, but it was no more effective than a trial-and-error approach (Voigt-Radloff et al., 2017).

Furthermore, Errorless Learning has been successfully applied in schizophrenia to more complex activities such as work tasks (Kern et al., 2002) and social problem-solving (Leshner et al., 2013). Giles (2005) described using Errorless Learning in occupational therapy practice to teach washing and dressing skills. Tasks that are more difficult to teach using Errorless Learning strategies include those in which several behaviors or options are available, those for which the best response is highly dependent on previous responses, and those for which situational and contextual factors are variable and influence the preferred response. For example, teaching someone how to address an envelope is much easier using an Errorless Learning approach than teaching someone how to write a letter.

Being a Psychosocial OT Practitioner

Addressing Cognitive Concerns on a General Medical Unit

Kelli Chen, MS, OTR/L, and Bobby Walsh, DBH, OTR/L, BCMH

Editor's Note: The contributors of this feature are OTPs at The Johns Hopkins Hospital in Baltimore, MD. They are part of a proactive consultation-liaison psychiatry program, along with psychiatrists, nurses, and social workers, that focuses on patients on medical units who face the complex intersection of psychiatric and general medical conditions. Kelli and Bobby serve as liaisons for patients on medical units who experience cognitive, psychological, emotional, or behavioral concerns that co-occur or are secondary to medical illness. They facilitate the early detection of problem situations and collaborate with patients and staff to develop intervention strategies that promote meaningful occupational engagement. In occupational therapy, it is crucial to understand and recognize the vital link between general medical and mental illnesses. This approach acknowledges the interconnected nature of these conditions and aims to address their profound impacts on overall functional cognition, well-being, and quality of life.

Identifying Psychosocial Strengths and Needs

OTPs commonly treat individuals with cognitive difficulties experiencing emotional distress and behavioral challenges in the hospital setting. Consider the example of Cheryl, a 67-year-old female with a history of a cerebral vascular accident and recent experience of vascular dementia. She was admitted to the hospital after being found walking alone outside her assisted living facility (ALF) following one of many elopements. She historically reported suicidal ideation related to losing her previous housing. She is experiencing an extended period of hospitalization because of worsening symptoms of vascular dementia, iron deficiency anemia, other medical complications, discharge barriers involving guardianship election, and difficulty with placement in a safe living setting geared toward dementia care. The team consulted an OTP to provide treatment appropriate for individuals with dementia with a behavioral component.

Cheryl ambulates independently and has good static and dynamic balance. To better understand Cheryl's functional cognition, the OTP observed Cheryl's performance in ADLs and IADLs and administered the ACLS-5. Cheryl's ACL was 3.8, indicating significant limitations in attention, memory, judgment, and safety, and she requires supervision and assistance for most ADL and IADL participation. In initial sessions, the OTP often found Cheryl disheveled in appearance, wearing many layers of clothing, and mishandling food items (for example, mixing jelly and butter into coffee). She has a history of leaving the stove on, experiences frequent disorientation, and often wanders or becomes lost when not directly supervised. The OTP determined that Cheryl eloped from her ALF because of continued discontent with losing her home, disliking her roommate, and "wanting to get out and go shopping," her preferred hobby.

Using a Holistic Occupational Therapy Approach

The OTP engages in patient advocacy and provides nursing education for dementia-specific care. The OTP educates and directs the nursing staff to consider Cheryl's cognitive limitations and provide increased supervision or assistance during ADLs, simplify tasks, provide a limited number of options (e.g., when ordering meals), present one task at a time, and promote slowing down of tasks with breaks included. Additionally, the OTP recommended environmental modifications to promote decreased sensory stimuli (e.g., less clutter, fewer medical tools, decreased noise, and low lighting).

The OTP focuses on providing Cognitive Adaptations and relies on a compensatory approach for ADL engagement. The OTP works with Cheryl to complete a checklist for ADLs as a memory aid and practices using it on multiple occasions, thereby engaging in repetitive tasks in the hospital setting to promote new procedural memories. The OTP also targeted emotional identification strategies. Cheryl is presented with cards depicting simplified emotions and demonstrates the ability to read through each. She is then presented with varied prompts related to personal experiences and is asked to say or hold up the card with the word describing how she feels about the prompt provided. For example, when the OTP asks Cheryl about "being in the hospital," she responds with "sad," and when asked about "family," she responds with "loving." This activity is repeated over multiple sessions to open dialogue about Cheryl's internal experience.

Continued

Being a Psychosocial OT Practitioner—cont'd

The OTP determines that Cheryl engages in minimal activity while hospitalized and attempts to elope from her hospital room when not mentally stimulated. Along with shopping, Cheryl enjoys completing crafts, Bible study, listening to music, and emotionally benefits from reminiscing about her past. The OTP allows participation in preferred tasks that provide cognitive stimulation and IADL engagement to reduce distress, including bracelet making, shopping in the hospital gift shop, performing sensory activities (e.g., aromatherapy, lotion application with self-massage), cleaning and organizing tasks, and reminiscing activities with music and photos. The OTP holds sessions in the early afternoon, Cheryl's most alert and energized time of day.

The OTP also uses an Errorless Learning approach for Cheryl to help her use the television remote to turn to two specific channels to view church services/Bible study and listen to music. The OTP integrates the following Errorless Learning methods into treatment sessions.

No Guessing	Cheryl is encouraged not to guess the channels as a strategy to locate them; if she hesitates or offers the incorrect channel number, the correct channel number is immediately provided.
Verbal Instruction	The OTP verbalizes all steps of the task while modeling.
Visual Instruction	The OTP adheres a piece of contrast tape to the remote with the correct channels written on the tape.
Modeling	The OTP demonstrates each task step—first locating the remote using the connected cable, then turning on the TV, then utilizing the remote to turn to the desired channel. Cheryl is invited to repeat each step immediately following the therapist's modeling.
Verbal Instruction	The OTP verbalizes all steps of the task while modeling.

Stepwise Approach	Cheryl first masters locating the remote, then turning on the television, then masters turning to one specific channel at a time.
Vanishing Cues	The OTP grades assistance by providing fewer cues as the task steps are mastered.
Spaced Retrieval	The OTP incorporates increasing delays as Cheryl demonstrates initial mastery of the task. If hesitation or incorrect response occurs, the OTP provides the correct answer. The recall interval is again reduced and gradually built until Cheryl can turn to the desired channel without cues within an appropriate interval (in this case, the two days between occupational therapy sessions).

As Cheryl becomes more active in her hospital room and nursing provides increased support and decreased extemporaneous stimuli, elopement attempts cease. Cheryl stops reporting dissatisfaction and does not identify any suicidal ideation. The OTP shifts their focus to transition preparation with graded exposure to off-unit activity and documentation of strategies developed to share with staff at the discharge setting.

Reflective Questions

1. What other cognitive strategies from the chapter might be helpful to explore with Cheryl? How can you ensure these strategies are tailored to her needs and preferences?
2. How might adding mindfulness-based approaches or relaxation techniques support Cheryl in managing her emotional distress, improving her attention, and promoting her overall well-being?
3. What other intervention or assessment approaches might address Cheryl's needs and strengths, and how might these approaches be tailored to her specific cognitive and emotional limitations and her preferences and interests?

Cognitive-Functional Therapy for People With Attention Deficit-Hyperactivity Disorder

The **Cognitive-Functional (Cog-Fun)** intervention was originally designed to help young people with ADHD acquire executive strategies and self-efficacy so that they can engage more successfully in occupational performance (Maeir et al., 2014). More recently, Cog-Fun has been expanded for use with adolescents and adults (Maeir et al., 2018. It is a manualized intervention that uses four main change mechanisms: (1) metacognitive learning, (2) environmental supports, (3) occupation-centered assessment and intervention, and (4) positive engagement. The metacognitive training borrows from Toglia's multicontext treatment approach described earlier in this section (Steinberg & Zlotnik, 2019) with an emphasis on strategy training for task performance.

When strategy use is not sufficient, tasks and environments are modified to support performance. Modifying the environment can increase success and decrease frustration while the person learns new skills. Assessments and interventions should be occupation based, meaning both should utilize occupational performance and active engagement in real-world occupations. Positive engagement means that the therapy sessions should highlight the person's strengths, be fun, and be interesting.

The strategies match the targeted age group. For example, a child-friendly activity uses a red light/green light approach for developing inhibition skills. The therapeutic setting is created using principles from Taylor's (2020) Intentional Relationship Model. Therapeutic use of self- and family-centered principles are employed to establish a rapport. The primary principle of the intervention is the creation of a playful environment for intervention. For children, parents play a central role; they are included in the therapy sessions, and a weekly communication with the parents occurs between sessions. For adults, there is an emphasis on self-management with the inclusion of strategies related to acceptance and self-compassion. A randomized controlled crossover study examined the efficacy of Cog-Fun with 100 children age 7 to 10 (Hahn-Markowitz et al., 2017) with positive outcomes related to child and parent self-efficacy as well as executive function and participation of children.

Unstuck and On Target

Unstuck and On Target is a manualized intervention designed to improve flexibility, planning, and organization in autistic children (Cannon et al., 2021). It is typically taught within a small group format. Content lessons that include information on vocabulary, routines, and scripts are arranged around experiments or applications that include videos, discussion, and activities. For example, one lesson focuses on whether different scenarios are a big deal or a little deal. A 1 to 10 scale is created using masking tape on the floor. As different scenarios are read (e.g., you stub your toe, you have a fight with your friend), the child moves to the corresponding number on the scale. Skills are also taught with games and role-play. Discussion includes identifying characteristics that make something a little deal or a big deal. The children also problem-solve how to turn a big deal into a little deal.

The manual includes information on strategies teachers and parents can use to help the child with a particular concept or skill and provides prompts or questions to help the child develop a script around the topic. Parents receive a manual so that they can reinforce the skills at home. A randomized controlled trial of autistic third to fifth graders found that children in the Unstuck and On Target group had greater improvement in problem-solving, flexibility, and planning or organization when compared with the group that received social skills training (Kenworthy et al., 2014).

Here's the Point

- OTPs are primarily concerned with functional cognition, which is the use of cognition in everyday occupations.
- The primary components of cognition include attention, memory, and executive function. Each of these components is made up of subcomponents.
- There is great variability in the type of cognitive impairment associated with a particular mental illness and within individuals.
- Careful assessment is important to determine an individual's cognitive strengths and impairments, as well as the ways in which cognition affects occupational performance.
- OTPs assess functional cognition using performance-based measures.
- A variety of intervention approaches are available to OTPs. Some focus on remediating cognitive impairments, or teaching strategies, whereas others adapt the environment or instructional method. Many combine techniques.
- All cognitive occupational therapy interventions are concerned with functional cognition and address occupational performance and participation.

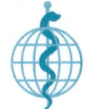 Visit the online resource center at **FADavis.com** to access the videos.

Apply It Now

1. Contextualizing Cognitive Remediation

This chapter discusses the importance of applying Cognitive Remediation activities to real-life activities. In the chapter, the letter cancellation task is applied to finding items on a grocery shopping shelf. In the left column of the following table is a list of several different types of Cognitive Remediation tasks that are done on either a computer or as a paper-and-pencil exercise. For each task, list a real-life activity in which a person could perform the same skill.

Task	Real-Life Activity
Remembering the third word in a list of five words	
Sorting lists of items into categories	
Pressing a button every time a word that starts with "S" appears	
Ignoring a conversation while solving a simple math problem	

2. Applying Multiple Cognitive Strategies

OTPs typically use more than one approach when providing treatment for a particular person. Consider the following situation:

Oliver is 15 years old and wants to set up an Instagram account and learn how to use it so that he can interact with others through social media. Cognitive evaluation indicates Oliver has difficulties with selective attention, problem-solving, and decision-making but has good memory skills and is very good at taking photos. The ACLS indicates he is at a Level 4.

Utilize the following table to identify strategies you could use in this situation based on the different approaches.

Approach	Strategy
Cognitive disabilities	
Cognitive Orientation to Daily Occupational Performance	
Errorless Learning	

Resources

Videos

- "Sensory Garden in Geriatric Psychiatric Unit" video. In this video, occupational therapist Callie Ward showcases the sensory garden at an inpatient psychiatric facility. The multisensory garden was designed for occupational therapy groups with a goal of helping participants identify the effects the garden and its related tasks have on their level of arousal. Callie offers specific examples of the many positive effects of the garden on residents, such as collaborating on tasks, problem-solving, encouraging routines, working on cognition, and assisting with self-regulation, among others. She explains how she uses it for active and passive group interventions and in one-to-one sessions. Access the video at the online resource center at FADavis.com.
- "Cooking Group in a State Mental Hospital" video. In this video, occupational therapist Samuel Gentile describes an extremely meaningful therapeutic group he runs in a state mental hospital. Samuel's weekly cooking group allows him to assess individuals' occupational performance and physical health, as well as help them develop functional skills. He shares why the experience is so powerful for the hospital residents and what it has taught him as an OTP. Access the video at the online resource center at FADavis.com.

Intervention Resources

Cognitive Adaptation Training

- CAT Manual: https://iceebp.uthscsa.edu/tpii/cat-resources/cat-manual-01-13.pdf

Cognitive Disabilities Model

- allencognitive.com

Cognitive Orientation to Daily Occupational Performance in Occupational Therapy

- Dawson, D. R., McEwen, S. E., & Polatajko, H. J. (2017). *Cognitive Orientation to Daily Occupational Performance in occupational therapy.* AOTA Press.

Metacognitive Reflection and Insight Therapy

- Lysaker, P. H., & Klion, R. E. (2017). *Recovery, meaning-making, and severe mental illness: A comprehensive guide to Metacognitive Reflection and Insight Therapy.* Routledge.

Multicontext Treatment Approach

- multicontext.net

Cog-Fun

- https://medicine.ekmd.huji.ac.il/en/occupationalTherapy/research/cogfun/Pages/default.aspx

Unstuck and On Target

- Cannon, L., Kenworthy, L., Alexander, K. C., Werner, M. A, & Anthony, L. G. (2021). *Unstuck and On Target! An executive functioning curriculum to improve flexibility, planning and organization* (2nd ed.). Brookes Publishing. unstuckandontarget.com

Cognitive Remediation Programs

- Frontal/Executive program: http://www.fep-lab.jp/en/program.html
- Attention Process Training (APT3): https://lapublishing.com/apt3-attention-process-training
- Medalia, A., Herlands, T., Saperstein, A., & Revheim, N. (2017). *Cognitive Remediation for psychological disorders.* Oxford University Press.

Compensatory Devices

- Rehab Store: rehab-store.com

Cognitive Measures

- Allen Cognitive Level Screen: https://www.therapro.com/Browse-Category/Cognitive-Assessments/Allen-Cognitive-Level-Screen-5_10.html
- Cognitive Performance Test: https://blog.therapro.com/an-overview-of-the-cognitive-performance-test
- Contextual Memory Test: cmt.multicontext.net
- Do-Eat: https://blog.therapro.com/the-do-eat-an-assessment-of-adl-iadls
- Executive Function Performance Test: https://www.ot.wustl.edu/about/resources/executive-function-performance-test-efpt-308
- Menu Task: https://kinesiology.education.wisc.edu/research/dorothy-edwards-research/the-menu-task
- Multiple Errands Test Revised: https://www.astate.edu/college/conhp/departments/occupational-therapy/files/F_MET%20Revised%20examiners%20packet%20_2016.pdf
- Weekly Calendar Planning Activity: Toglia, J. (2015). *Weekly calendar planning activity.* AOTA Press

General Information

- Katz, N., & Toglia, J. (2018). *Cognition, occupation, and participation across the life span: Neuroscience, neurorehabilitation, and models of intervention in occupational therapy* (4th ed.). AOTA Press
- Wolf, T. J., Edwards, D. E., & Giles, G. M. (2019). *Functional cognition and occupational therapy: A practical approach to treating individuals with cognitive loss.* AOTA Press.

References

Alderman, N., Burgess, P. W., Knight, C., & Henman, C. (2003). Ecological validity of a simplified version of the Multiple Errands Shopping Test. *Journal of the International Neuropsychological Society, 9,* 31–44. https://doi.org/10.1017/s1355617703910046

Al-Heizan, M. O., Giles, G. M., Wolf, T. J., & Edwards, D. F. (2020). The construct validity of a new screening measure of functional cognitive ability: The menu task. *Neuropsychological Rehabilitation, 30*(5), 961–972. https://doi.org/10.1080/09602011.2018.1531767

Allen, C. K. (1985). *Occupational therapy for psychiatric diseases: Measurement and management of cognitive disabilities.* Little, Brown, and Company.

Allen, C. K., Austen, S. K., David, S. K., Earhart, C. A., McCraith, D. B., & Williams, L. R. (2007). *Manual for the Allen Cognitive Level Screen 5 and Large Cognitive Level Screen.* S & S Worldwide.

Allott, K., Killackey, E., Sun, P., Brewer, W. J., & Velligan, D. I. (2016). Feasibility and acceptability of Cognitive Adaptation Training for first episode psychosis. *Early Intervention in Psychiatry, 10,* 476–484. https://doi.org/10.1111/eip.12207

Allott, K., van-der-El, K., Bryce, S., Parrish, E. M., McGurk, S. R., Hetrick, S., Bowie, C. R., Kidd, S., Hamilton, M., Killackey, E., & Velligan, D. (2020). Compensatory interventions for cognitive impairments in psychosis: A systematic review and meta-analysis. *Schizophrenia Bulletin, 46*(4), 869–883. https://doi.org/10.1093/schbul/sbz134

American Occupational Therapy Association. (2018). *Choosing Wisely, five things patients and providers should question.* https://www.choosingwisely.org/societies/american-occupational-therapy-association-inc

American Psychiatric Association. (2013). *Diagnostic and statistical manual of mental disorders* (5th ed.). American Psychiatric Publishing. https://doi.org/10.1176/appi.books.9780890425596

Arieli, M., Agmon, M., Gil, E., & Kizony, R. (2022). The contribution of functional cognition screening during acute illness hospitalization of older adults in predicting participation in daily life after discharge. *BMC Geriatrics, 22,* 739. https://doi.org/10.1186/s12877-022-03398-5

Averbuch, S., & Katz, N. (2011). Cognitive rehabilitation: A retraining model for clients with neurological disabilities. In N. Katz (Ed.), *Cognition and occupation, and participation across the lifespan: Models for intervention in occupational therapy* (pp. 277–298). AOTA Press.

Barlati, S., Deste, G., De Peri, L., Ariu, C., & Vita, A. (2013). Cognitive Remediation in schizophrenia: Current status and future perspectives. *Schizophrenia Research and Treatment, 2013,* 156084. https://doi.org/10.1155/2013/156084

Baum, C. M., Connor, L. T., Morrison, M. T., Hahn, M., Dromerick, A. W., & Edwards, D. F. (2008). The reliability, validity, and clinical utility of the Executive Function Performance Test: A measure of executive function in a sample of people with stroke. *American Journal of Occupational Therapy, 62*(4), 446–455. https://doi.org/10.5014/ajot.62.4.446

Baum, C. M., & Edwards, D. F. (1993). Cognitive performance in senile dementia of the Alzheimer's type: The Kitchen Task Assessment. *American Journal of Occupational Therapy, 47,* 431–436. https://doi.org/10.5014/ajot.47.5.431

Baum, C. M., & Wolf, T. J. (2013). *Executive Function Performance Test manual.* Washington University in St. Louis.

Baum, C. M., Wolf, T. J., Wong, A. W. K., Chen, C. H., Walker, K., Young, A. C., Carlozzi, N. E., Tulsky, D. S., Heaton, R. K., & Heinemann, A. W. (2017). Validation and clinical utility of the Executive Function Performance Test in persons with traumatic brain injury. *Neuropsychological Rehabilitation, 27*(5), 603–617. https://doi.org/10.1080/09602011.2016.1176934

Bowie, C. R., Bell, M. D., Fiszdon, J. M., Johannesen, J. K., Lindenmayer, J. P., McGurk, S. R., Medalia, A. A., Penades, R., Saperstein, A. M., Twamley, E. W., Ueland, T., & Wykes, T. (2020). Cognitive Remediation for schizophrenia: An expert working group white paper on core techniques. *Schizophrenia Research, 214,* 49–53. https://doi.org.10.1016/j.schres.2019.10.047

Broadbent, D. E. (1958). *Perception and communication.* Pergamon Press.

Brown, C., Rempfer, M., & Hamera, E. (2009). *The Test of Grocery Shopping Skills.* AOTA Press.

Burns, A., & Erickson, D. H. (2022). Adding Cognitive Remediation to employment support services: A randomized controlled trial. *Psychiatric Services,* appips202100249. https://doi.org/10.1176/appi.ps.202100249

Burns, T. (2018). *The Cognitive Performance Test Revised manual.* Maddak.

Burns, T., Lawler, K., Lawler, D., McCarten, J. R., & Kuskowski, M. (2018). Predictive value of the Cognitive Performance Test (CPT) for staging function and fitness to drive in people with neurocognitive disorders. *American Journal of Occupational Therapy, 72,* 7204205040. https://doi.org/10.5014/ajot.2018.027052

Cannon, L., Kenworthy, L., Alexander, K. C., Werner, M. A., & Anthony, L. G. (2021). *Unstuck and On Target! An executive functioning curriculum to improve flexibility, planning and organization* (2nd ed.). Brookes Publishing.

Craik, F., & Tulving, E. (1975). Depth of processing and the retention of words in episodic memory. *Journal of Experimental Psychology: General, 104,* 268–294. https://doi.org/10.1037/0096-3445.104.3.268

David, S. K., & Riley, W. T. (1990). The relationship of the Allen Cognitive Level test to cognitive abilities and psychopathology. *American Journal of Occupational Therapy, 44,* 493–497. https://doi.org/10.5014/ajot.44.6.493

Douglas, A., Letts, L., Eva, K., & Richardson, J. (2012). Use of the Cognitive Performance Test for identifying deficits in hospitalized older adults. *Rehabilitation Research and Practice, 2012,* 638480. https://doi.org/10.1155/2012/638480

Earhart, C. A. (2006). *Allen Diagnostic Module 2nd edition: Manual.* S & S Worldwide.

Edwards, D. F., Wolf, T. J., Marks, T., Alter, S., Larkin, V., Padesky, B. L., Spiers, M., Al-Heizan, M. O., & Giles, G. M. (2019). Reliability and validity of a functional cognition screening tool to identify the need for occupational therapy. *American Journal of Occupational Therapy, 73*(2), 7302205050p1–7302205050p10. https://doi.org/10.501/ajot.2019.028753

Forsyth, K., Deshpande, S., Kielhofner, G., Henriksson, C., Haglund, L., Olson, L., Skinner, S., & Kukarni, S. (2005). *The Occupational Circumstances Assessment Interview and Rating Scale (OCAIRS) Version 4.0 assessment manual.* University of Illinois at Chicago.

Friedman, A. (1979). Framing pictures: The role of knowledge in automatized encoding and memory for gist. *Journal of Experimental Psychology: General, 108,* 316–355. https://doi.org/10.1037//0096-3445.108.3.316

Gebreegziabhere, Y., Habatmu, K., Mihretu, A., Cella, M., & Alem, A. (2022). Cognitive impairment in people with schizophrenia: An umbrella review. *European Archives of Psychiatry and Clinical Neuroscience, 272*(7), 1139–1155. https://doi.org/10.1007/s00406-022-01416-6

Gil, N., & Josman, N. (2001). Memory and metamemory performance in Alzheimer's disease and healthy elderly: The Contextual Memory Test (CMT). *Aging Clinical Experimental Research, 13,* 309–315. https://doi.org/10.1007/BF03353427

Giles, G. M. (2005). A neurofunctional approach to rehabilitation following severe brain injury. In N. Katz (Ed.), *Cognition and occupation across the lifespan: Models for intervention in occupational therapy* (pp. 139–165). AOTA Press.

Giles, G. M., Wolf, T. J., & Edwards, D. F. (2019). Principles of functional-cognitive assessment. In T. J. Wolf, D. F. Edwards, & G. M. Giles (Eds.), *Functional cognition and occupational therapy: A practical approach to treating individuals with cognitive loss* (pp. 31–38). AOTA Press.

Gimeno, H., Dittman, K., Polatajko, H., & McEwen, S. (2019). Cognitive Orientation to Daily Occupational Performance. In T. J. Wolf, D. F. Edwards, & G. M. Giles (Eds.), *Functional cognition and occupational therapy: A practical approach to treating individuals with cognitive loss* (pp. 201–218). AOTA Press.

Godefroy, O. (2003). Frontal syndrome and disorders of executive function. *Journal of Neurology, 250,* 1–6. https://doi.org/10.1007/s00415-003-0918-2

Goverover, Y., Kalmar, J., Gaudino-Goering, E., Shawaryn, M., Moore, N. B., Halper, J., & DeLuca, J. (2005). The relation between subjective and objective measures of everyday life activities in persons with multiple sclerosis. *Archives of Physical Medicine and Rehabilitation, 86,* 2303–2308. https://doi.org/10.1016/j.apmr.2005.05.016

Gruner, P., & Pittenger, C. (2017). Cognitive inflexibility in obsessive-compulsive disorder. *Neuroscience, 345,* 243–255. https://doi.org/10.1016/j.neuroscience.2016.07.030

Hahn-Markowitz, J., Berger, I., Manor, I., & Maeir, A. (2017). Impact of the Cognitive-Functional (Cog-Fun) intervention on executive functions and participation among children with attention deficit hyperactivity disorder: A randomized controlled trial. *American Journal of Occupational Therapy, 71,* 7105220010p1–710522001p9. https://doi.org/10.5014/ajot.2017.022053

Harris, J. C. (2013). New terminology for mental retardation in *DSM-5* and *ICD-11. Current Opinions in Psychiatry, 26,* 260–262. https://doi.org/10.1097/YCO.0b013e32835fd6fb

Jahn, H. (2013). Memory loss in Alzheimer's disease. *Dialogues in Clinical Neuroscience, 15,* 445–454. https://doi.org/10.31887/DCNS.2013.15.4/hjahn

Josman, N. (2005). The dynamic interactional model in schizophrenia. In N. Katz (Ed.), *Cognition and occupation across the lifespan: Models for intervention in occupational therapy* (pp. 169–186). AOTA Press.

Josman, N., Berney, T., & Jarus, T. (2000). Evaluating categorization skills in children following severe brain injury. *Occupational Therapy Journal of Research, 20,* 241–255. https://doi.org/10.1177/153944920002000402

Josman, N., Goffer, A., & Rosenblum, S. (2010). Development and standardization of a "Do-Eat" activity of daily living performance test for children. *American Journal of Occupational Therapy, 64,* 47–58. https://doi.org/10.5014/ajot.64.1.47

Kahneman, D., & Tversky, A. (1996). On the reality of cognitive illusions. *Psychological Review, 103,* 582–591. https://doi.org/10.1037/0033-295x.103.3.582

Kaneko, Y., & Keshavan, M. (2012). Cognitive Remediation in schizophrenia. *Clinical Psychopharmacology and Neuroscience, 10,* 125–135. https://doi.org/10.9758/cpn.2012.10.3.125

Katz, N., Felzen, B., Tadmor, I., & Hartman-Maeir, A. (2007). Validity of the Executive Function Performance Test (EFPT) in persons with schizophrenia: An occupational performance test. *Occupational Therapy Journal of Research, 27,* 44–51. https://doi .org/10.1177/153944920702700202

Kenworthy, L., Anthony, L. G., Naiman, D. Q., Cannon, L., Wills, M. C., Luong-Tran, C., Werner, M. A., Alexander, K. C., Strang, J., Bal, E., Sokoloff, J. L., & Wallace, G. L. (2014). Randomized controlled effectiveness trial of executive function intervention for children on the autism spectrum. *Journal of Child Psychology and Psychiatry, and Allied Disciplines, 55*(4), 374–383. https://doi .org/10.1111/jcpp.12161

Kern, R. S., Green, M. F., Mitchell, S., Kopelowicz, A., Mintz, J., & Liberman, R. P. (2005). Extensions of Errorless Learning for social problem solving deficits in schizophrenia. *American Journal of Psychiatry, 162,* 513–519. https://doi.org/10.1176/appi.ajp.162.3.513

Kern, R. S., Liberman, R. P., Kopelowicz, A., Mintz, J., & Green, M. F. (2002). Applications of Errorless Learning on improving work performance in persons with schizophrenia. *American Journal of Psychiatry, 159,* 1921–1926. https://doi.org/10.1176/appi .ajp.159.11.1921

Kidd, S. A., Kaur, J., Virdee, G., George, T. P., McKenzie, K., & Herman, Y. (2014). Cognitive Remediation for individuals with psychosis in a supported education setting: A randomized controlled trial. *Schizophrenia Research, 157,* 90–98. https://doi .org/10.1016/j.schres.2014.05.007

Knight, C., Alderman, N., & Burgess, P. W. (2002). Development of a simplified version of the Multiple Errands Test for use in hospital settings. *Neuropsychological Rehabilitation, 12,* 231–256. https:// doi.org/10.1080/09602010244000039

Kravariti, E., Dixon, T., Frith, C., Murray, R., & McGuire, P. (2005). Association of symptoms and executive function in schizophrenia and bipolar disorder. *Schizophrenia Research, 74,* 221–231. https:// doi.org/10.1016/j.schres.2004.06.008

Lahav, O., Ben-Simon, A., Inbar-Weiss, N., & Katz, N. (2018). Weekly calendar planning activity for university students. Comparison of individuals with and without ADHD by gender. *Journal of Attention Disorders, 22,* 368–378. https://doi .org/10.1177/1087054714564621

Lara, T., Madrid, J. A., & Correa, A. (2014). The vigilance decrement in executive function is attenuated when individual chronotypes perform at their optimal time of day. *PLoS One, 19,* e88820. https://doi.org/10.1371/journal.pone.0088820

Leshner, A. F., Thom, S. R., & Kern, R. S. (2013). Errorless Learning and social problem solving ability in schizophrenia: An examination of the compensatory effect of training. *Psychiatric Research, 206,* 1–7. https://doi.org/10.1016/j.psychres.2012.10.007

Levy, L. L. (2018). Neurocognition and function: Intervention in dementia based on the Cognitive Disabilities Model. In N. Katz & J. Toglia (Ed.), *Cognition, occupation, and participation across the life span: Neuroscience, neurorehabilitation and models of intervention in occupational therapy* (4th ed., pp. 500–522). AOTA Press.

Levy-Dayan, H., Josman, N., & Rosenblum, S. (2023). Basic activity of daily living evaluation of children with autism spectrum disorder: Do-Eat Washy adaptation preliminary psychometric characteristics. *Children, 10*(3), 514. https://doi.org/10.3390 /children10030514

Lueng, N. T., Lo, M. M., & Lee, T. M. (2014). Potential therapeutic effects of meditation for treating affective dysregulation. *Evidence Based Complementary and Alternative Medicine: eCAM, 2014,* 402718. https://doi.org/10.1155/2014/402718

Lussier, A., Doherty, M., & Toglia, J. (2019). Weekly calendar planning activity. In T. J. Wolf, D. F. Edwards, & G. M. Giles (Eds.), *Functional cognition and occupational therapy: A practical approach to treating individuals with cognitive loss* (pp. 75–90). AOTA Press.

Lysaker, P. H., Gagen, E., Klion, R., Zalzala, A., Vohs, J., Faith, L. A., Leonhardt, B., Hamm, J., & Hasson-Ohayon, I. (2020). Metacognitive Reflection and Insight Therapy: A recovery-oriented treatment approach for psychosis. *Psychological Research and Behavior Management, 2*(13), 331–341. https://doi.org/10.2147 /PRBM.S198628

Maeir, A., Bar-Ilan, R. T., Kastner, L., Fisher, O., Levanon-Erez, N., & Hahn-Markowitz, J. (2018). An integrative Cognitive-Functional (Cog-Fun) intervention for children, adolescents, and adults with ADHD. In N. Katz & J. Toglia (Ed.), *Cognition, occupation, and participation across the life span: Neuroscience, neurorehabilitation and models of intervention in occupational therapy* (4th ed., pp. 335–351). AOTA Press.

Maeir, A., Fisher, O., Bar-Ilan, R. T., Boas, N., Berger, I., & Landau, Y. E. (2014). Effectiveness of Cognitive-Functional (Cog-Fun) occupational therapy intervention for young children with attention deficit hyperactivity disorder: A controlled study. *American Journal of Occupational Therapy, 68,* 260–267. https://doi.org/10.5014 /ajot.2014.011700

Matlin, M. W. (2005). *Cognition* (6th ed.). John Wiley & Sons.

McCraith, D. B., & Earhart, C. A. (2018). Cognitive Disabilities Model: Creating fit between functional cognitive abilities and cognitive activity demands. In N. Katz & J. Toglia (Eds.), *Cognition, occupation, and participation across the life span: Neuroscience, neurorehabilitation and models of intervention in occupational therapy* (4th ed., pp. 469–495). AOTA Press.

Medalia, A., & Saperstein, A. M. (2013). Does Cognitive Remediation for schizophrenia improve functional outcomes? *Current Opinion in Psychiatry, 26,* 141–157. https://doi.org/10.1097 /YCO.0b013e32835dcbd4

Meichenbaum, D. (1979). *Cognitive behavior modification: An integrative approach.* Plenum Press.

Miller, G. A. (1956). The magical number seven, plus or minus two: Some limits on our capacity for processing information. *Psychological Review, 63,* 81–97. https://doi.org/10.1037/0033-295x .101.2.343

Morrison, M. T., Edwards, D. F., & Giles, G. M. (2015). Performance-based testing in mild stroke: Identification of unmet opportunity for occupational therapy. *The American Journal of Occupational Therapy, 69*(1), 6901360010p1–6901360010p5. https://doi.org/10.5014/ajot.2015.011528

Nuechterlein, K. H., Ventura, J., Subotnik, K. L., & Bartzokis, G. (2014). The early longitudinal course of cognitive deficits in schizophrenia. *Journal of Clinical Psychiatry, 75,* 25–29. https:// doi.org/10.4088/JCP.13065.su1.06

Penny, N. H., Mueser, K. T., & North, C. T. (1995). The Allen Cognitive Level test and social competence in adult psychiatric patients. *American Journal of Occupational Therapy, 49,* 420–427. https:// doi.org/10.5014/ajot.49.5.420

Peterson, L. R., & Peterson, M. J. (1959). Short-term retention of individual items. *Journal of Experimental Psychology, 58,* 193–198. https://doi.org/10.1037/h0049234

Pievsky, M. A., & McGrath, R. E. (2018). The neurocognitive profile of attention-deficit/hyperactivity disorder: A review of meta-analyses. *Archives of Clinical Neuropsychology, 33*(2), 143–157. https://doi.org/10.1093/arclin/acx055

Polatajko, H. J., Mandich, A., & McEwen, S. E. (2011). Cognitive Orientation to Daily Occupational Performance (CO-OP): A cognitive-based intervention for children and adults. In N. Katz (Ed.), *Cognition, occupation, and participation across the life span: Neuroscience, neurorehabilitation and models of intervention in occupational therapy* (3rd ed., pp. 299–322). AOTA Press.

Raweh, D. V., Holon, R., & Katz, N. (1999). Treatment effectiveness of Allen's Cognitive Disabilities Model with adult schizophrenia outpatients: A pilot study. *Occupational Therapy in Mental Health, 14,* 65–77. https://doi.org/10.1300/J004v14n04_04

Rogers, J. C., Holm, M. B., & Chisholm, D. (2016). *Performance assessment of self-care skills – Version 4.1.* University of Pittsburgh.

Rogers, T., Kuiper, N., & Kirker, W. (1977). Self-reference and the encoding of personal information. *Journal of Personality and Social Psychology, 35,* 677–688. https://doi.org/10.1037 //0022-3514.35.9.677

Rojo-Mota, G., Pedrero-Pérez, E. J., Huertas-Hoyas, E., Merritt, B., & MacKenzie, D. (2017). Allen Cognitive Level Screen for the classification of subjects treated for addiction. *Scandinavian Journal of Occupational Therapy, 24*(4), 290–298. https://doi.org/10.3109/11038128.2016.1161071

Rotenberg, S., Ruthralingam, M., Hnatiw, B., Neufeld, K., Yuzwa, K. E., Arbel, I., & Dawson, D. R. (2020). Measurement properties of the Multiple Errands Test: A systematic review. *Archives of Physical Medicine and Rehabilitation, 101*(9), 1628–1642. https://doi.org/10.1016/j.apmr.2020.01.019

Scammell, E. M., Bates, S. V., Houldin, A., & Polatajko, H. J. (2016). The Cognitive Orientation to Daily Occupational Performance (CO-OP): A scoping review. *Canadian Journal of Occupational Therapy, 83*, 216–225. https://doi.org/10.1177/0008417416651277

Scarff, S. M., Nalder, E. J., Gullo, H. L., & Fleming, J. (2022). The Multiple Errands Test: A guide for site-specific version development. *Canadian Journal of Occupational Therapy, 90*(3), 280–296. https://doi.org/10.1177/00084174221142184

Schank, R. C., & Abelson, R. P. (1977). *Scripts, plans, goals and understanding.* Erlbaum.

Secrest, L., Wood, E. W., & Tapp, A. (2000). A comparison of the Allen Cognitive Level test and the Wisconsin Card Sorting test in adults with schizophrenia. *American Journal of Occupational Therapy, 54*, 129–133. https://doi.org/10.5014/ajot.54.2.129

Shallice, T., & Burgess, P. W. (1991). Deficits in strategy application following frontal lobe damage in man. *Brain, 114*, 727–741. https://doi.org/10.1093/brain/114.2.727

Spelke, E., Hirst, W., & Neisser, U. (1976). Skills of divided attention. *Cognition, 4*, 215–230. https://doi.org/10.2466/pms.1985.61.1.236

Steinberg, C. J., & Zlotnik, S. (2019). The Multicontext Approach. In T. J. Wolf, D. F. Edwards, & G. M. Giles (Eds.), *Functional cognition and occupational therapy: A practical approach to treating individuals with cognitive loss* (pp. 219–229). AOTA Press.

Sternberg, R. J. (2003). *Cognitive psychology* (3rd ed.). Wadsworth.

Taylor, R. R. (2020). *The intentional relationship: Occupational therapy and the use of self* (2nd ed.). F.A. Davis.

Tchanturia, K., Lounes, N., & Holttum, S. (2014). Cognitive Remediation in anorexia nervosa and related conditions: A systematic review. *European Eating Disorders Review, 22*, 454–462. https://doi.org/10.1002/erv.2326

Teixeira, C., Mueser, K. T., Rogers, E. S., & McGurk, S. R. (2018). Job endings and work trajectories of persons receiving supported employment and Cognitive Remediation. *Psychiatric Services, 69*(7), 812–818. https://doi.org/10.1176/appi.ps.201700489

Thivierge, S., Jean, L., & Simard, M. (2014). A randomized crossover controlled study on cognitive rehabilitation of instrumental activities of daily living in Alzheimer disease. *American Journal of Geriatric Psychiatry, 22*, 1188–1199. https://doi.org/10.1016/j.jagp.2013.03.008

Toglia, J. P. (1993). *Contextual Memory Test.* Psychological Corporation.

Toglia, J. (2015). *Weekly calendar planning activity: A performance test of executive function.* AOTA Press.

Toglia, J., & Berg, C. (2013). Performance-based measure of executive function: Comparison of community and at-risk youth. *American Journal of Occupational Therapy, 67*, 515–523. https://doi.org/10.5014/ajot.2013.008482

Toglia, J., & Foster, E.R. (2021). *The Multicontext Approach to cognitive rehabilitation: A metacognitive intervention to optimize functional cognition.* Gatekeeper Press.

Trivedi, M. H., & Greer, T. L. (2014). Cognitive dysfunction in unipolar depression: Implications for treatment. *Journal of Affective Disorders, 152–154*, 19–27. https://doi.org/10.1016/j.jad.2013.09.012

Tsapekos, D., Seccomandi, B., Mantingh, T., Cella, M., Wykes, T., & Young, A. H. (2020). Cognitive enhancement interventions for people with bipolar disorder: A systematic review of methodological quality, treatment approaches, and outcomes. *Bipolar Disorders, 22*(3), 216–230. https://doi.org/10.1111/bdi.12848

Velligan, D. I., Bow-Thomas, C. C., Huntzinger, C., Ritch, J., Ledbetter, N., Prihoda, T. J., & Miller, A. L. (2000). Randomized controlled trial of the use of compensatory strategies to enhance adaptive functioning in outpatients with schizophrenia. *American Journal of Psychiatry, 157*, 1317–1323. https://doi.org/10.1176/appi.ajp.157.8.1317

Velligan, D. I., Mahurin, R. K., True, J. E., Lefton, R. S., & Flores, C. V. (1996). Preliminary evaluation of Cognitive Adaptation Training to compensate for cognitive deficits in schizophrenia. *Psychiatric Services, 47*, 415–417. https://doi.org/10.1176/ps.47.4.415

Vita, A., Barlati, S., Ceraso, A., Nibbio, G., Ariu, C., Deste, G., & Wykes, T. (2021). Effectiveness, core elements and moderators of response of Cognitive Remediation for schizophrenia: A systematic review and meta-analysis of randomized clinical trials. *JAMA Psychiatry, 78*(8), 848–858. https://doi.org/10.1001/jamapsychiatry.2021.0620

Voigt-Radloff, S., de Werd, M. M., Leonhart, R., Boelen, D. H., Olde Rikkert, M. G., Fliessbach, K., Klöppel, S., Heimbach, B., Fellgiebel, A., Dodel, R., Eschweiler, G. W., Hausner, L., Kessels, R. P., & Hüll, M. (2017). Structured relearning of activities of daily living in dementia: The randomized controlled REDALI-DEM trial on Errorless Learning. *Alzheimer's Research & Therapy, 9*(1), 22. https://doi.org/10.1186/s13195-017-0247-9

Warchol, K. (2004). An interdisciplinary dementia program model for long-term care. *Topics in Geriatric Rehabilitation, 20*, 59–71. https://doi.org/10.1097/00013614-200401000-00008

Wasmuth, S., Horsford, C., Mahaffey, L., & Lysaker, P. H. (2022). "Metacognitive Reflection and Insight Therapy" (MERIT) for the occupational therapy practitioner. *Canadian Journal of Occupational Therapy, 90*(4), 333–343. https://doi.org/10.1177/00084174221142172

Wesson, J., & Giles, G. M. (2019). Understanding functional cognition. In T. J. Wolf, D. F. Edwards, & G. M. Giles (Eds.), *Functional cognition and occupational therapy: A practical approach to treating individuals with cognitive loss* (pp. 7–20). AOTA Press.

Wilson, D., Allen, C. K., McCormack, G., & Burton, G. (1989). Cognitive disability and routine task behaviors in a community-based population with senile dementia. *Occupational Therapy Practice, 1*, 58–66.

Wu, H. S., Lin, L. C., Su, S. C., & Wu, S. C. (2014). The efficacy of space retrieval combined with Errorless Learning in institutionalized elders with dementia: Recall performance, cognitive status and food intake. *Alzheimer's Disease and Associated Disorders, 28*, 333–339. https://doi.org/10.1111/jan.12352

Wykes, T., Huddy, V., Cellard, D., McGurk, S. R., & Czobor, P. (2011). A meta-analysis of Cognitive Remediation for schizophrenia: Methodology and effect sizes. *American Journal of Psychiatry, 168*, 472–485. https://doi.org/10.1176/appi.ajp.2010.10060855

Wynn, V. E., & Logie, R. H. (1998). The veracity of long-term memories—Did Bartlett get it right? *Applied Cognitive Psychology, 12*, 1–20. https://doi.org/10.1002/(SICI)1099-0720(199802)12:1‹3.0.CO;2-M

CHAPTER
8

Cognitive Beliefs

John V. Rider

Is the glass half full or half empty? This common question may be asked to gauge someone's worldview in general or specific situations. It refers to whether an individual's perspective and beliefs are more optimistic (glass half full) or pessimistic (glass half empty). As a metaphor, it suggests that there is more than one way to perceive, think about, feel, and behave depending on individuals' beliefs about themselves, others, the world, and the future.

In a convincing argument on the importance of addressing beliefs as a psychosocial factor in rehabilitation, Rosenfeld (1997), an occupational therapy practitioner (OTP), recounts using this metaphor in an occupational therapy intervention with an older woman who was receiving treatment following hip replacement surgery.

> She made slow but steady progress in her rehabilitation. Despite improvements, however, she always focused on how much she still could not do. Her discouragement diminished her energy and effort. I pointed out her "glass half empty" way of seeing things. The woman readily admitted this, but felt she could not change. With a contract to try, and persistent monitoring and substitution of more positive cognitions and statements, the patient was able to describe and to feel "the glass half full." "I just need a little assistance with the last 6 inches down to sitting, now," she said. "Six weeks ago, I needed two people to carry me from the wheelchair to the toilet." (Rosenfeld, 1997, p. 35)

Rosenfeld discusses how and why the therapist's approach effectively facilitated the woman's ability to attain her goal. Her mood, efforts, and occupational performance abilities improved dramatically because of the therapist's willingness to listen to her thoughts about her performance and progress. The therapist brought the impact of the woman's negative thinking to her attention, educated her about substituting more positive thoughts and self-statements for her negative thoughts, and supported her in self-monitoring her thoughts about her progress. This collaborative approach acknowledged the impact of her thoughts and cognitive beliefs on her feelings and behavior, including her occupational performance. Using cognitive behavioral strategies as part of her ongoing rehabilitation helped her modify her thoughts, attitudes, and beliefs about her abilities and progress in therapy. In turn, this contributed to modifying her mood and effort related to achieving her rehabilitation and occupational performance goals.

This occupational therapy psychosocial intervention introduces the primary focus and topics in this chapter, which include the relationship between cognitive beliefs and occupational performance; the nature of cognitive beliefs; the role of cognitive beliefs in psychiatric conditions, rehabilitation, and recovery; an overview of belief-oriented Cognitive Behavioral Therapy (CBT) and Acceptance and Commitment Therapy (ACT); and the use of CBT and ACT methods for occupational therapy assessment and intervention to address cognitive beliefs and their impact on occupational performance and participation in daily activities.

Cognitive Beliefs and Occupational Performance

The *Occupational Therapy Practice Framework: Domain and Practice,* 4th Edition *(OTPF-IV)* defines **cognitive beliefs** as "something that is accepted, considered to be true, or held as an opinion" (American Occupational Therapy Association [AOTA], 2020, p. 51). The *OTPF-IV* classifies cognitive beliefs as a person factor that "resides within the client and influences the client's performance in occupations" (p. 51). (This text uses the term *person* rather than *client*.) Cognitive beliefs are "affected by the presence or absence of illness, disease, deprivation, and disability, as well as by life stages and experiences" (AOTA, 2020, p. 15). Along with values and spirituality, beliefs influence a person's motivation to engage in occupations and give life meaning (AOTA, 2020). The *OTPF-IV* reminds OTPs that beliefs are "affected by occupations, contexts, performance patterns, and performance skills" (p. 15). Cognitive beliefs, among other person factors, should be identified and discussed as part of the occupational profile, measured within the analysis of occupational performance, and addressed as part of the intervention process (AOTA, 2020). The *OTPF-IV* also highlights how beliefs and feelings about oneself and whether one can move toward a goal influence a person's quality of life (AOTA, 2020). Furthermore, the *OTPF-IV* description of cognitive beliefs is consistent with the World Health Organization's (WHO, 2001) *International Classification of Functioning, Disability and Health.*

OTPs frequently work with individuals whose beliefs about themselves, others, the world, and the future may positively or negatively influence their occupational performance and quality of life. Hope and a belief in possible recovery for persons with psychiatric conditions are critical for successful therapy outcomes (Corrigan et al., 2014). Therefore, it is essential to identify, address, and document cognitive beliefs throughout the occupational therapy process. OTPs can address cognitive beliefs within occupation-based interventions to enable successful participation in valued occupations.

The Nature of Cognitive Beliefs

Several psychiatric, psychological, and learning theories, grounded in cognitive tradition, recognize cognitive beliefs as basic to learning, mental and physical health, effective performance, and overall functional well-being. Although these theories differ in various aspects, there is general agreement regarding some basic assumptions about the nature of beliefs and their significance for human functioning, including occupational performance. A better understanding of these assumptions will help OTPs recognize their own cognitive beliefs and those of the people they work with, allowing the practitioner to examine the influence of those beliefs and interaction with occupational performance. These assumptions are listed in Box 8-1 and explained in the following text. For simplicity, this chapter uses the terms "cognitive beliefs" and "beliefs" interchangeably.

BOX 8-1 ■ Theoretical Assumptions About the Nature of Cognitive Beliefs

1. Core beliefs that operate at a deep structural level influence the more surface structure of our thoughts, as well as our emotions, behavior, and physiological arousal.
2. Beliefs and their dynamic interaction with behavior (including occupational performance.), emotions, physiological reactions, and the environment comprise human functioning.
3. Beliefs are instrumental in how people perceive, appraise, and attach meaning to information from within ourselves and the external environment.
4. Beliefs that are true or held to be true for the believer often act as self-fulfilling prophecies.
5. Beliefs start to develop in early childhood and continue to develop throughout adulthood.
6. Beliefs affect relationships, group affiliations, and society at large; in turn, these social contexts also affect beliefs.

Levels of Beliefs

Assumption 1: Core beliefs that operate at a deep structural level influence the more surface structure of people's thoughts, as well as their emotions, behavior, and physiological arousal.

Beliefs are often conceptualized as a continuum of overlapping levels (J. S. Beck, 2011). **Automatic thoughts** comprise the outermost or surface level of a person's thoughts. These thoughts, consisting of words, images, and self-talk that pass through a person's mind, typically arise in reaction to external situations or internal personal experiences. They are considered to be most accessible, flexible, and specific to a situation or person. The innermost or deepest level is the storehouse for an individual's most fundamental or **core beliefs** and philosophies, sometimes referred to as schemas (A. T. Beck, 1976; J. S. Beck, 2011). **Schemas** serve as cognitive templates of absolutes about how individuals see themselves, others, the world, and the future. Although accessible if focused on in an effortful manner, these deeply rooted beliefs usually operate outside conscious awareness. They are characterized as being more rigid, entrenched, and global. As such, they impact a person's internal and external experience, behavior, and emotions. Various constructs, such as assumptions, attitudes, and values, are typically used to label the intermediate level of thoughts and beliefs. Referred to as rules for living, they tend to fit a conditional, "if . . . then" format (e.g., "If I do not do what others want me to do, then they won't like me," or "If I can't walk again, I will be of no use to anyone"). The levels of beliefs are summarized in Table 8-1 with examples. As readers review these examples, they should consider their own levels of beliefs, their dynamic relationship, and how they have changed throughout their life.

In a dynamic feedback loop, core beliefs generate an individual's intermediate and surface thoughts and beliefs. In turn, surface thoughts often serve as a window to underlying rules for living and the deeper, core beliefs. Surface and intermediate thoughts and beliefs also strengthen and reinforce core beliefs. This dynamic relationship is illustrated in Figure 8-1.

TABLE 8-1 | **Levels of Beliefs**

Levels of Beliefs		Example Situation: Student A and Student B Do Poorly on a Test		Example Situation: Person A and Person B Are Rejected After a Job Interview	
Level	*Description*	*Student A*	*Student B*	*Person A*	*Person B*
Automatic thoughts	Surface, peripheral; spontaneous, flexible, accessible, situational; arise from core beliefs	"I'm a failure." "Of course, I failed; why bother?" "I'll never pass this class."	"I did poorly because I didn't prepare." "I'd better study harder next time." "I know I can do better."	"I am a loser." "This was a waste of time." "I knew I wouldn't get the job; I should never have applied."	"I didn't do my best, but now I have some experience." "I better practice some interview questions to be more prepared next time."
Assumptions or rules for living	Intermediate assumptions, values, conditional "if . . . then . . ." rules; easier to test; arise from core beliefs	"If I don't do good on a test, then I must not be smart enough to be in this class."	"If I work hard and put in the time, then I can be successful in this class."	"If I get rejected from a job, then I must not be good enough to get any job."	"If I keep preparing for job interviews, then I will get a good job eventually."
Core beliefs or schemas	Template of absolutes about self, others, world; rigid, global, entrenched	"I am incompetent."	"I am competent."	"I am incapable."	"I am capable."

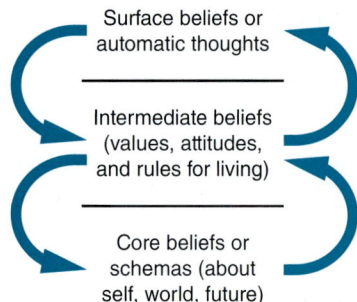

FIGURE 8-1. Levels of beliefs: A dynamic relationship.

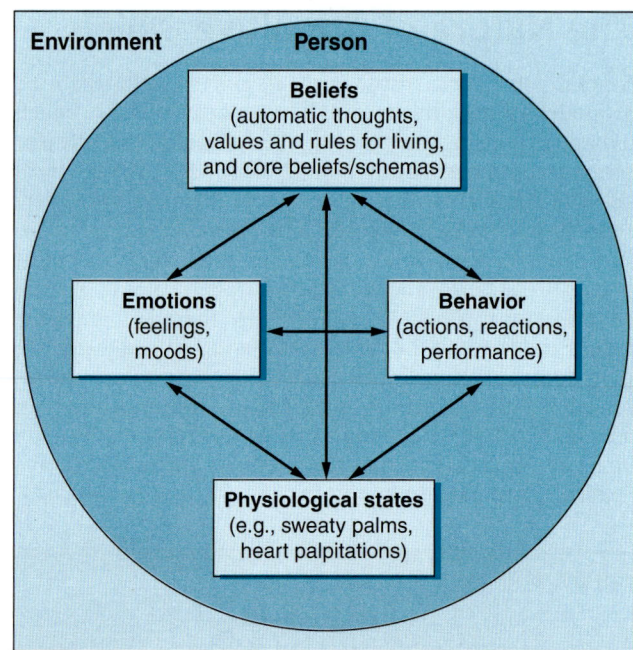

FIGURE 8-2. The dynamic, interactive relationship between the external environment and personal factors, including cognitive beliefs, emotions, and physiological states.

The terms "beliefs" and "thoughts" are used interchangeably in this chapter unless the author intends to specifically distinguish core beliefs from more surface, automatic thoughts or from intermediate beliefs or rules for living.

Dynamic Interaction

Assumption 2: Beliefs and their dynamic interaction with behavior (including occupational performance), emotions, physiological states, and the environment comprise human functioning.

Internal personal factors (e.g., beliefs, emotions, physiological states), behavior (e.g., actions, reactions, performance), and external environmental factors (e.g., cultural, social, spiritual, physical contexts, and situations) all interact dynamically and thus influence, and are influenced by, one another (A. T. Beck, 1976; J. S. Beck, 2011). Figure 8-2 illustrates this dynamic interaction between the external environment and personal factors, including beliefs, emotions, behavior, and physiological states. Although not explicit in the figure, it is important to recognize the influence of traumatic experiences on all levels of beliefs. Trauma can challenge assumptions and rules for living that help individuals navigate life and perform daily activities (Substance Abuse and Mental Health Services Administration, 2014). More information can be found in Chapter 5: Trauma-Informed Practice.

Beliefs and Information Processing

Assumption 3: Beliefs are instrumental in how people perceive, appraise, and attach meaning to information from within ourselves and the external environment.

Beliefs, stored in memory, act as filters for the cognitive processing of information and events that individuals experience. Beliefs filter what people perceive (see, hear, feel, smell) and how people appraise, interpret, and give meaning to the myriad of situations and experiences they encounter in the environment. The interpreted information is synthesized and triggers emotional responses, including moods and feelings; behavior in the form of actions, reactions, and performance; and physiological reactions, such as sweaty palms and rapid heart rate. In turn, emotions, behavior, and physiological responses provide feedback that impacts beliefs and triggers new information processing. From this perspective, although other people and external situations and events can impact how individuals feel and act, they are not the major determinants. Rather, how individuals perceive and process situations and events, determined significantly by their beliefs,

albeit frequently subconsciously or unconsciously, determines how they feel and act (Friedman et al., 2008). This complex relationship is illustrated in Figure 8-3.

Beliefs as Self-Fulfilling Prophecies

Assumption 4: Beliefs that are true or held to be true for the believer often act as self-fulfilling prophecies.

Beliefs represent one alternative among many rather than the one true fact or rule agreed upon by all. Although beliefs are not facts, one's beliefs often carry the weight of facts, and individuals may find it hard to distinguish between the two without assistance. Regardless of what one believes, it is human nature to try to create consistency between one's life experience and one's beliefs. Once individuals believe something to be true, they tend to ignore counterexamples and options, perceiving and accepting only those events that verify their beliefs. Through time, as individuals generate more evidence from what they perceive and process, beliefs can become increasingly entrenched and can appear more real, thus leading to their own fulfillment, sometimes referred to as a "self-fulfilling prophecy" (Madon et al., 2011).

Consider the following scenario: Joe oversleeps and predicts, "Now, I'm probably going to be late and have a lousy day." Therefore, he feels irritable. When he gets to work, he is unusually argumentative and demanding with his coworkers, who become annoyed with him, thus making his prediction of a lousy day come true. His actions have fulfilled his prediction. In contrast, Elizabeth, who espouses a positive prediction (e.g., "I'm going to have a great day!"), is more likely to act in ways that might make her prediction true. Even when individuals recognize that some beliefs have a fragile contact with any known larger reality, they are rarely motivated to challenge or change them unless they contribute to significant distress in their daily lives.

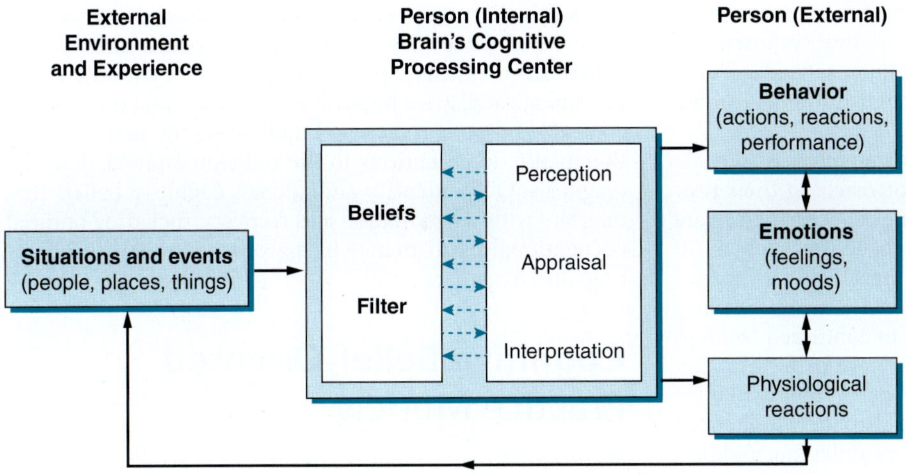

External Environment and Experience

Person (Internal) Brain's Cognitive Processing Center

Person (External)

FIGURE 8-3. Beliefs act as a central filtering function for information processing. Beliefs, stored in memory, filter what and how situations and events in the external environment are perceived, appraised, and interpreted by the brain's processing center. Beliefs also function as a major mediator or determinant of behavior and emotions. Behavior and emotions influence each other and become part of situations and events that influence behavior.

Development of Beliefs

Assumption 5: Beliefs start to develop in early childhood and continue to develop throughout adulthood.

From birth, infants absorb life experiences from interactions in the world and with other people, particularly primary caregivers. Because very young children have limited ways in which to choose or evaluate the accuracy and functionality of these early life experiences, they typically accept much of what they are told or experience about themselves (e.g., "You are dumb and incompetent" or "You can achieve whatever you choose"). These experiences lead to certain "understandings" that become organized as core beliefs or schemas about the self that carry the weight of truths for the person. For example, core beliefs are a significant determinant of whether individuals consider themselves worthy of respect or worthless, competent or incompetent, fairly treated or victimized, independent or helpless, and so on. In time, individuals also absorb and form beliefs about relationships with others, the world, and the future. These early experiences and core beliefs contribute significantly to developing personality and adult views. Beliefs continue to form and change throughout the adult years through the influence of internal and external factors, such as family and other role models, cultural and ethnic values, trauma, spiritual orientation, and the many different contexts and environments in which people function. However, unlike young children, adults can choose, evaluate, modify, and replace beliefs when they no longer meet their needs and interests (A. T. Beck, 1976; J. S. Beck, 2011).

Beliefs, Social Contexts, and Relationships

Assumption 6: Beliefs affect relationships, group affiliations, and society at large; in turn, these social contexts also affect beliefs.

Humans function in many social contexts and relationships, such as interactions with family, friends, colleagues, and acquaintances at work, school, and leisure activities. At a broader level, individuals also function as members of their primary cultural and ethnic group, communities, and society, affiliating with groups based on their beliefs and the collective beliefs conveyed by the group. These affiliations

and social transactions impart cultural, spiritual, relational, political, and many other beliefs, values, and attitudes that shape views of oneself, others, and society at large, as well as emotions and behaviors, both individual and collective. Similarly, one's beliefs influence affiliation with persons and groups. Thus, beliefs are both uniquely individual and, at the same time, inseparably interrelated with the beliefs of others and society (Bandura, 1986).

Consider this example adapted from Dr. Judith Beck (2011). Imagine several students reading this book as part of an occupational therapy course assignment. In this context, each student has a unique emotional, behavioral, and physiological response to this assigned activity (environmental event) based on their automatic thoughts as they begin the reading assignment. For example:

■ Reader A thinks, "This book really makes sense. Finally, I have a guide for what I need to know and do to work in a mental health setting as an occupation-based OTP!" Reader A feels excited and eagerly becomes engrossed in the assigned readings, making notes on key points.
■ Reader B thinks, "There's so much information to learn. If I don't learn everything, I'll never be a good OTP." Feeling anxious and overwhelmed, Reader B breaks out in a sweat whenever they think about completing the assignment and puts off doing it. When this reader finally begins, they take meticulous notes but do not finish on time. This behavior further contributes to this reader's emotional and physiological distress.

These student readers have different emotional, behavioral, and physiological responses to the assignment associated with their perceptions and thoughts, leading to different potential consequences. Each reader's response is likely mediated or influenced, often subconsciously or unconsciously, by one or more rules for living, as well as by underlying core beliefs developed early in life. Reader B may hold fast to a core belief that they are incompetent, which gives rise to the rule that "If I don't do everything perfectly, then I might as well not do it at all." This belief also triggers the psychological and physiological response of anxiety. This reader is unlikely to be aware of this relationship between their psychological and physiological responses and this core belief or its self-fulfilling nature. By putting off the assignment until able to do it "perfectly," Reader B sets themself up to fail, reinforcing the core belief of being incompetent. Because this dysfunctional pattern will likely repeat for other assignments, Reader B's belief may become more entrenched and self-fulfilling, leading to more significant consequences.

Reader A's thoughts support a more adaptive or flexible emotional and behavioral response for reaching their professional goals. They may have a core belief that they are competent, which gives rise to a rule for living, such as, "If I complete assignments as best I can, then I will be successful." Although both desire to do well, Reader A is more likely to have beliefs and thoughts that lead to continued feelings, actions, and thoughts that fulfill their core belief of being competent. This will likely enhance Reader A's ability to meet their professional goals. Each reader is also likely influenced by past academic experiences, peer group affiliation, and personal or environmental factors, such as cultural background, upbringing, study environment, and previous academic success. If someone were to question the truth of these readers' automatic thoughts or core beliefs, it is probable that both would strongly defend their position.

Cognitive Beliefs and Psychiatric Conditions

The mental health field has witnessed a growing interest in theory and research on the role of cognition and beliefs in understanding psychopathology and psychotherapeutic approaches to psychiatric conditions and psychological and behavioral challenges. Dr. Aaron Beck (1967) introduced a cognitive model for understanding the underlying influence of cognitive beliefs in depression. From this perspective, emotions and behavior are influenced or mediated by distorted and dysfunctional beliefs, information processing biases, and distorted interpretations of environmental experiences. These cognitive influences can create a vulnerability to various psychiatric disorders and other psychological and behavioral challenges and contribute to their maintenance and resistance to intervention. For example, the basic cognitive model of substance use disorders assumes that certain internal or external events (e.g., anxiety, interpersonal conflicts) trigger fundamental drug-related beliefs and automatic thoughts related to substance use (e.g., "Drinking helps me focus," or "Drinking makes me more comfortable in social situations"). These beliefs and thoughts strengthen a person's urges and cravings to use alcohol or other substances. A. T. Beck et al. (1993) hypothesized that at least three types of beliefs contribute to substance use and abuse: anticipatory, relief-oriented, and facilitative beliefs. **Anticipatory beliefs** "involve some expectation of reward" (p. 169), for example, "I know tonight's party will be a blast because there will be lots of booze on hand." **Relief-oriented beliefs** refer to "assumptions that using a substance will alleviate discomfort" (p. 169), such as "This has been a rough day at work. I will feel less stressed and be able to relax if I have a drink." **Facilitative beliefs** are permissive and view substance use as "acceptable despite the potential consequences" (p. 169), for example, "Just one won't hurt me" or "I have a great tolerance for alcohol, and I know when to stop."

Profiles of core beliefs and dysfunctional thoughts have been proposed for various psychiatric conditions, such as the previously discussed one regarding substance use disorders. However, there are also significant differences among core beliefs of individuals experiencing psychiatric conditions and psychological distress because of the substantial influence of contexts and person factors, highlighting the need to tailor therapeutic interventions to the individual rather than the diagnosis. OTPs identify and address cognitive beliefs that interfere with rehabilitation and recovery, including optimal occupational performance in daily activities across all settings and diagnoses.

Cognitive Belief-Oriented Practice Models

The predominant practice models OTPs use to address cognitive beliefs are subsumed within what has come to be known as **Cognitive Behavioral Therapy (CBT)**. Traditional CBT is one of the most widely used and researched models for addressing cognitive beliefs that support or hinder recovery for persons with various psychiatric conditions and psychological challenges (A. T. Beck, 2005; Fordham et al., 2021; Hofmann et al., 2012). The multiple approaches within the scope of CBT integrate cognitive and behavioral theories and therapies to varying degrees. These different CBT models share the same theoretical perspective, which assumes that the processes called "thinking" or cognition, including cognitive beliefs, are accessible and can be evaluated, monitored, and changed. Furthermore, these cognitive processes can have a strong mediational or deterministic influence on behavior and emotions. CBT theorists hypothesize that changes in cognition can alter behavior and emotions just as behavior and emotions can impact cognition. Thus, cognition and behavior are the two primary indicators of change related to CBT outcomes, with emotions and physiological states also recognized as indicators of change to a lesser degree.

CBT approaches can be classified based on what aspects of cognition are addressed to enact behavioral change. For example, some approaches focus on restructuring the content of cognitions, such as thoughts, attitudes, and beliefs; others emphasize acquiring cognitive skills, such as coping skills or psychological flexibility; and others center on developing problem-solving strategies. Because this chapter is about cognitive beliefs, theories and therapies that address beliefs, or the content of cognition, are emphasized and referred to as belief-oriented CBT. Most belief-oriented CBT approaches view dysfunctional beliefs as the problem impacting occupational participation and performance and causing psychological distress. Traditional CBT methods consider the dysfunctional thought to be the problem and, therefore, attempt to restructure or alter thoughts or cognitions. In contrast, ACT methods view the struggle with the dysfunctional thought, not the thought itself, as the problem and instead attempt to alter a person's relationship with those thoughts. Multiple treatment approaches exist within the scope of CBT, which can confuse students and new practitioners; however, most approaches share the theoretical perspective that assumes cognitive events (e.g., thoughts) mediate behavior change (Dobson & Dozois, 2010). Therefore, in some manner, all belief-oriented CBTs assess beliefs and their influence on behavior and seek to address both through the development of cognitive skills such as coping strategies, problem-solving approaches, or cognitive restructuring methods (Dobson & Dozois, 2010). This chapter introduces cognitive beliefs and their influence on occupational performance and participation; however, additional reading and training are necessary for competence in applying belief-oriented CBT approaches in clinical practice.

Evidence for Cognitive Behavioral Therapy

An extensive review of meta-analyses on the efficacy of CBT (Hofmann et al., 2012) documented the substantial and impressive body of research on its effectiveness as a primary or adjunctive therapeutic intervention for a wide range of psychiatric conditions and psychological challenges. Fordham and colleagues (2021) completed an updated metareview, demonstrating consistent evidence for CBT across many physical and psychological conditions. Table 8-2 provides information about evidence concerning CBT applications and evidence for specific psychiatric conditions and related beliefs.

TABLE 8-2	Evidence Reviews of Cognitive Behavioral Therapy and Various Psychiatric Conditions
Psychiatric Conditions	**CBT Evidence**
Anxiety disorders	CBT is effective for various anxiety disorders and appears to be as effective as exposure therapy (Kaczkurkin & Foa, 2015). CBT also effectively treats anxiety disorders in children and adolescents and lowers recurrence rates (Pegg et al., 2022).
Bipolar disorder	CBT explicitly designed for bipolar disorder effectively improves mood and reduces relapse rates (Chiang et al., 2017; Swartz & Swanson, 2014).
Depression (unipolar)	CBT is the most studied nonpharmacological intervention for depression. It is effective for reducing depression, and combining CBT with medication is more effective than medication alone (Cuijpers et al., 2013). CBT is also effective for children and adolescents with depression (Oud et al., 2019).
Eating disorders	CBT-enhanced (CBT-E) targets the underlying pathology associated with eating disorders and is effective for a wide range of eating disorders (Atwood & Friedman, 2019; Murphy et al., 2010).
Posttraumatic stress disorder (PTSD)	CBT has large effects on PTSD (Cusack et al., 2016). Trauma-focused CBT, which directly addresses memories of the traumatic event or related thoughts and feelings, also has a large evidence base for treating PTSD (Watkins et al., 2018).
Substance abuse	CBT is effective for substance use but is typically combined with motivational and skill-building approaches (McHugh et al., 2010).
Schizophrenia	CBT appears to have only a small effect on positive and negative symptoms of schizophrenia (Jauhar et al., 2014). However, it may be effective for addressing specific aspects of functioning, such as low self-esteem or work performance (Lysaker et al., 2009).

Occupational therapy and CBT share important therapeutic principles relevant to belief-oriented assessment and intervention. Interventions are present-oriented, time-limited, and solution-focused (J. S. Beck, 2011; Duncombe, 2005). A person-centered, collaborative relationship in which therapists actively listen, role model, offer encouragement, and provide feedback is central to the intervention process, which is grounded in theory and evidence. Both combine educational and systematic empirical cognitive processes to gain new insights and skills, test them with active behavioral experimentation, and apply them in daily life. Furthermore, practitioners of occupational therapy and CBT value successful engagement in meaningful activities as a critical, evidence-based strategy for modifying distorted or dysfunctional beliefs related to one's performance abilities.

Acceptance and Commitment Therapy

ACT (pronounced as the word "act," not as the individual letters), developed by Steven Hayes over 40 years ago, is a newer form of CBT falling under the umbrella of belief-oriented CBT approaches (Hayes, 2016; Hayes et al., 1999; 2012). ACT uses mindfulness and acceptance strategies to address cognitive beliefs and help people make valued changes. This chapter briefly introduces the theoretical basis of ACT, focusing more on the therapeutic processes OTPs utilize.

ACT's philosophical roots are in functional contextualism, which views psychological events as "ongoing actions of the whole person, interacting in and with historically and situationally defined contexts" (Hayes et al., 2006, p. 4). In other words, functional contextualism considers how behavior functions in different contexts, such as the context of the person's life. ACT is based on a behavioral account of human language and cognition called Relational Frame Theory (RFT; Hayes et al., 2006). RFT integrates a wide range of psychological phenomena into a theory of language based on contextual relationships, and an in-depth description is beyond the scope of this chapter. In simple terms, RFT proposes that relating one concept to another (i.e., relational framing) is the foundation of all human language (Hayes et al., 2013). The arbitrary development of relating concepts in life to each other leads to various levels of beliefs, such as rules for living, and individuals get "stuck" in these rules, which may negatively influence behavior. Becoming "stuck" on these assumptions or rules for living can lead to psychological inflexibility, demonstrated by rigid attempts to control psychological reactions and discomfort at the expense of value-guided actions. Psychological inflexibility and being stuck, in turn, leads to experiential avoidance, described as attempts to avoid or escape thoughts, feelings, memories, physical sensations, or other internal experiences (Harris, 2019). Experiential avoidance keeps individuals from what they genuinely desire, leading to further distress and dysfunction.

From an ACT perspective, the form or content of cognitive beliefs is not directly troublesome unless the contextual features lead the beliefs to regulate action in unhelpful ways. ACT suggests that it is not the negative thoughts, emotions, feelings, or sensations that are problematic but how one responds to them that can cause difficulties and psychological distress. This perspective differs from traditional CBT, which views the negative or dysfunctional thought as the problem and attempts to restructure or alter the thought. ACT conceptualizes psychological suffering as primarily caused by cognitive entanglement, experiential avoidance, and the resulting psychological inflexibility that impedes one's ability to take steps or act in ways consistent with their core values (Hayes et al., 2013). Instead of altering the content or frequency of cognitions, ACT seeks to change the individual's psychological relationship with those thoughts, feelings, emotions, or sensations to promote greater psychological flexibility and allow individuals to engage in occupations according to their values (Hayes et al., 2013; White et al., 2011).

For example, consider an individual who values friends and building relationships but reports that they are depressed. This person may often feel ignored in social situations, leading to significant social anxiety. To avoid the resulting anxiety, the person stays home and watches television alone rather than going out with family, friends, and colleagues. They believe that by avoiding social situations, they can avoid unpleasant thoughts, feelings, emotions, and sensations. Although this behavior allows them to avoid the anxiety of being in social situations, they are "stuck" because they lack the social relationships they want and need and continue to be entangled by unpleasant thoughts, feelings, and sensations despite avoiding social situations. Their anxiety is replaced with more severe loneliness and depression, leading to further psychological distress and reduced participation in meaningful occupations. In ACT, this is called experiential avoidance, which is comparable with occupational withdrawal. Psychological inflexibility is demonstrated because the individual tries to "control" psychological reactions at the expense of meaningful occupational engagement. In this scenario, developing psychological flexibility would involve examining values and cognitive beliefs; accepting the apprehension that comes with stepping into social situations; and moving toward, rather than away from, those situations. An ACT approach in this scenario would help the individual recognize what they value in life, learn skills to become aware of their beliefs surrounding social situations, and acknowledge that it is okay to have those automatic thoughts and feelings. Furthermore, a clinician using ACT could assist the individual with strategies to "defuse" or become "unstuck" from their thoughts, feelings, and emotions and return to the present moment so they can make a conscious decision to participate in social situations that will help them build the relationships they value. ACT approaches often include self-compassion, mindfulness training, and graded activity exposure toward person-centered behavioral goals. OTPs can use ACT to offer an alternative to experiential avoidance through various therapeutic interventions that help individuals learn to reduce the impact and influence of unwanted thoughts and feelings and engage in meaningful occupations (Harris, 2006). ACT emphasizes changing an individual's awareness of and relationship to their thoughts, emotions, and behaviors to do what matters most (Hayes & Duckworth, 2006). Moreover, because ACT does not seek to change thoughts, just the relationship with them, it may be a better fit for situations when individuals are experiencing psychosis, where challenging thoughts is often ineffective and may increase paranoia.

The overarching focus of ACT is to increase psychological flexibility, or the ability to contact the present moment more fully as a conscious human being, and to change or persist in behavior when doing so serves valued ends

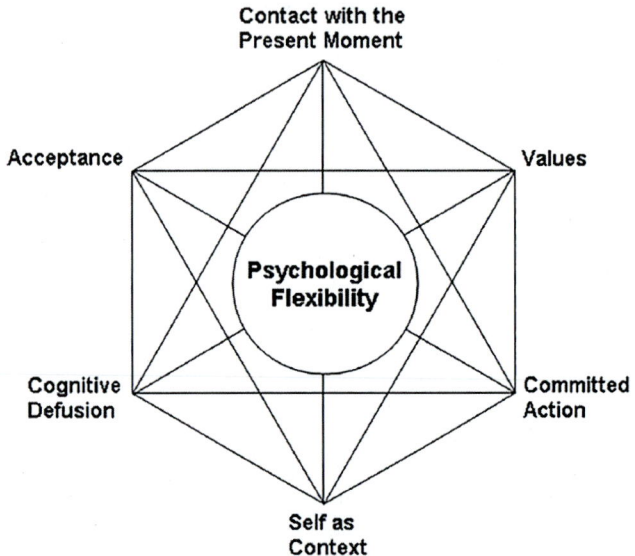

FIGURE 8-4. The "Hexaflex" demonstrates the six interconnected core processes of ACT that form the structure of case formulation and guide treatment, with the goal of developing increased psychological flexibility. *Copyright Steven C. Hayes. Used with permission.*

(Hayes et al., 2006; 2013). Psychological flexibility is established through six core ACT processes, as shown in Figure 8-4.

Each area is conceptualized as a positive psychological skill, not merely a method of avoiding psychopathology, and can be addressed through therapeutic interventions. In general, these core processes work together through mindfulness and acceptance skills, leading to a commitment and behavior change process. The acceptance and mindfulness processes assist individuals in lessening the effect of inner experiences that make following their values difficult, whereas the behavior change processes involve determining directions for behavior change and utilizing supported techniques to facilitate that change (Hayes et al., 2006; Twohig & Levin, 2017). Russ Harris (2019) has further simplified ACT's core processes through the ACT Triflex, highlighting three main concepts necessary for psychological flexibility: opening up, being present, and doing what matters (see Fig. 8-5). Consider how these key concepts are also emphasized throughout occupational therapy intervention approaches. ACT uses metaphors, stories, and activities to teach core processes. As this is only an introduction to ACT, additional resources for continued training, examples of metaphors and stories, and application in clinical practice are provided at the end of this chapter.

Core Processes of ACT

Acceptance (I can approach challenges instead of avoiding them): Acceptance is taught to people as an alternative to experiential avoidance and involves opening up and making room for unpleasant feelings, sensations, urges, and other private experiences, allowing them to come and go without struggling, fighting, running from, or giving them undue attention (Harris, 2019). Contrary to what many may think when they hear the word, acceptance is not giving in, resigning, or tolerating; it is an action and an ongoing process (Twohig & Levin, 2017). Acceptance is a willingness to

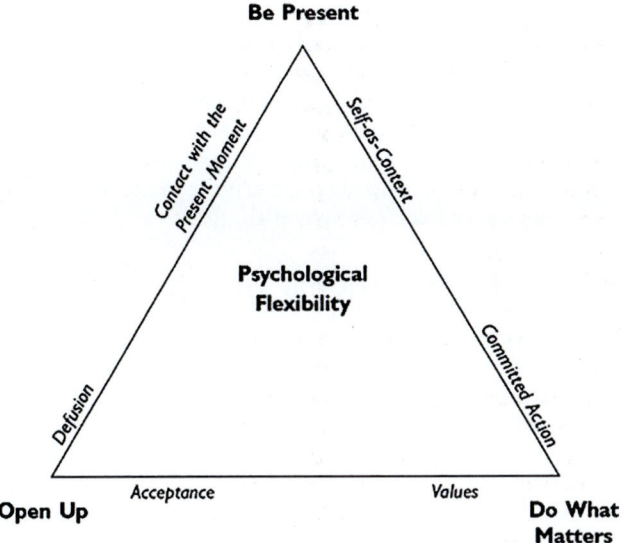

Be Present

Contact with the Present Moment

Self-as-Context

Psychological Flexibility

Defusion

Committed Action

Acceptance

Values

Open Up

Do What Matters

FIGURE 8-5. The ACT Triflex focuses on three functional skills: being present, opening up, and doing what matters. This model demonstrates how the six core ACT processes can be used to develop these skills and increase psychological flexibility. *Harris, R. (2019). ACT made simple: An easy-to-read primer on Acceptance and Commitment Therapy (2nd ed.). New Harbinger Publications, Inc.*

experience thoughts and feelings (nonjudgmentally) even when unwanted or not enjoyable, rather than struggling to control or suppress them. Intervention approaches to increase acceptance often focus on opening up, recognizing thoughts and feelings, and embracing them for what they are—just thoughts and feelings. ACT emphasizes that control is the problem, not the solution, and the struggle to control one's thoughts and feelings often increases suffering.

Cognitive defusion (It is just a thought, let it pass): Cognitive defusion is about taking a step back and looking *at* thoughts rather than *from* thoughts and letting them come and go rather than holding on to them. Harris (2006) described this as, "Learning to perceive thoughts, images, memories, and other cognitions as what they are—nothing more than bits of language, words, and pictures—as opposed to what they can appear to be—threatening events, rules that must be obeyed, objective truths and facts" (p. 7). It is recognizing that personal thoughts and beliefs are just one of many viewpoints, and becoming "fused" with those thoughts and beliefs often causes psychological distress. One example of the many techniques developed to defuse from unhelpful thoughts is for people to thank their mind for the thought and label the process of thinking. For example, when an unhelpful thought, such as "I am not good enough," pops into one's mind, they should say, to themself, verbally or in their mind, "I am having the thought that I am not good enough. Thank you, mind." Doing so reduces the literal quality of the thought, weakens the tendency to believe what the thought refers to ("I am not good enough."), and helps individuals see these thoughts for what they are—just automatic thoughts passing through (Harris, 2019; Hayes et al., 2006).

Contact with the present moment (mindfulness): Being present or in contact with the present moment is similar to mindfulness. It involves "bringing full awareness to the hear-and-now experiences, with openness, interest, and receptiveness; and focusing on and engaging fully in whatever you are

doing" (Harris, 2006, p. 7). The goal is to experience the world more directly and be attentive and responsive to what is happening in the present moment so behavior is more flexible, and thus actions will be more consistent with values (Hayes et al., 2006; Twohig & Levin, 2017). For example, suppose a person seems distant, disengaged, and disconnected from their thoughts and feelings. They are easily distracted, lack self-awareness, and are in need of grounding. They miss important aspects of daily experiences and are fused with their unhelpful beliefs. In that case, OTPs can help them enhance awareness and be more present to perceive more accurately what is happening and gather important information about whether to change or persist in their behavior. Often, when someone is experiencing a panic attack, they are naturally drawn to focus on their physiological sensations. Although this may be useful in certain circumstances, paying attention to the other interesting and meaningful stimuli in one's environment is also beneficial, as it can help individuals refocus and act according to their values (Twohig & Levin, 2017). OTPs can help individuals develop skills to engage (engage fully in their current activity or connect deeply with whomever or whatever is involved), savor (savor, enjoy, and appreciate their current activity if it is something pleasurable), and focus (focus entirely on whatever aspects of their current activity are most important) through various mindfulness activities (Harris, 2019). By developing skills to contact the present moment, OTPs can help individuals be more present, acknowledge their thoughts, and return to fully engaging in the occupation.

Self-as-context (What am I thinking and doing?): ACT recognizes that there are two distinct components of the mind: a part that thinks and a part that notices. ACT suggests that people are not the content of their thoughts or feelings; instead, they are the consciousness experiencing or observing those thoughts and feelings. People need to recognize the part of their mind that can observe thoughts, feelings, and sensations as they occur. Self-as-context is a viewpoint from which people can step back and observe thoughts and feelings and a psychological space where thoughts and feelings can move around (Harris, 2019). It is a safe place to observe their experience without being caught up or entangled. People access this psychological space by noticing that they are noticing their thoughts and feelings or becoming conscious of their consciousness (Harris, 2019). OTPs can facilitate defusion and acceptance by helping individuals develop greater awareness of their thoughts and behaviors through self-as-context and the observing or noticing of self. Self-as-context is fostered in ACT by mindfulness exercises, metaphors, and experiential processes.

Values (What do I stand for? What is important to me?): Values in ACT are not about what a person wants to get or achieve. Instead, they are about how the person wants to behave or act at any given moment and on an ongoing basis (Harris, 2019). ACT helps individuals clarify their values so they can use them for inspiration, motivation, and guidance. In the *OTPF IV*, values, beliefs, and spirituality are person factors that influence motivation to engage in occupations and give life and existence meaning (AOTA, 2020). Aligned with occupational therapy literature, ACT looks at the degree of consistency or inconsistency between values and daily actions. The greater the discrepancy between values and actions, the more likely an individual will have psychological distress. In contrast, greater consistency between the two leads to increased happiness, well-being, quality of life, and so on (Gaudiano et al., 2020). OTPs can help individuals identify their values and explore ways to live them by engaging in meaningful occupations guided by their values. In ACT, values are often compared with a compass. If one's values are the compass point by which they want to guide their life's journey, then their goals are the road map that can lead them there. Consider the following question adapted from Harris (2019) to help people explore and clarify their values:

> Imagine I had a magic wand that I could wave, and all your painful thoughts, feelings, and memories would no longer have any impact on you. What would you do with your life? What would you start, stop, or do more or less of? How would you behave differently? If I watched you on a video, what would I see and hear that would show me the magic wand was successful?

There are many ways to clarify values. OTPs can help people use artistic methods to paint, draw, or sculpt values; discuss role models and personal strengths or qualities they admire; or review checklists of common values to help people identify and clarify their values.

Committed action (I can do what matters to me even if it is difficult): Lastly, "ACT encourages the development of larger and larger patterns of effective action linked to chosen values" (Hayes et al., 2012, p. 187). In this perspective, ACT resembles traditional behavior therapy. Almost any behavior change method fits into an ACT approach, including graded exposure, skills acquisition, shaping methods, goal setting, and so on (Hayes et al., 2012). Flexible action is at the heart of committed action: "readily adapting to situational challenges and persisting with or changing behavior as required while living chosen values" (Harris, 2019, p. 238). Consistent with occupational therapy practice, ACT encourages the development of achievable, concrete goals guided by a person's values. Additionally, ACT almost always involves work outside of therapy leading to short- and long-term behavior change goals (Hayes et al., 2012). Behavior change efforts inevitably lead to contact with psychological barriers addressed through other ACT processes, such as acceptance and defusion, requiring people to utilize skills from the core processes of ACT. Committed action is a goal-directed pursuit and how individuals *live life to the fullest*. OTPs can help translate values into effective patterns of occupational engagement (i.e., committed action) through effective goal setting, action planning, problem-solving, skills training, role-playing, graded exposure, behavioral activation, and other evidence-based behavioral interventions (Harris, 2019). Through formal goal setting and using "SMART" or "COAST" goals, OTPs can help individuals set appropriate, values-guided behavioral goals. The most common skills taught through committed action are problem-solving, goal setting, and action planning, skills in which OTPs have extensive training.

Evidence for ACT

Evidence for the efficacy of ACT across multiple psychological conditions is growing. To date, there are over 1,000 randomized controlled trials on ACT. A recent review of meta-analyses by Gloster and colleagues (2020) found ACT effective at treating many conditions, including depression, anxiety, substance use, eating disorders, and stress. Based on 20 meta-analyses, this review found efficacy for ACT in improving quality of life, psychological flexibility, measures of well-being, functioning, and disability across multiple psychiatric conditions and psychological problems (Gloster et al., 2020). Although less is known about using ACT with children, current evidence suggests that ACT significantly improves most self- and clinician-reported outcomes across psychological problems (Swain et al., 2015).

ACT and Occupational Therapy

The concept of psychological flexibility underpins the occupational therapy domain to support occupational engagement and participation to optimize health (AOTA, 2020). OTPs can support participation (i.e., committed action in ACT) in meaningful occupations (i.e., values in ACT) by addressing the core processes of ACT and supporting the development of psychological flexibility. Although ACT has been effective as an overall treatment for many conditions, a meta-analysis also supports the utility of each core process to enact change on its own, outside the larger ACT therapy context (Levin et al., 2012). For example, consider a person who shares with the OTP that they get stuck on particular thoughts and often feel as if they can't move forward or do anything meaningful when they have these unhelpful thoughts. OTPs can utilize components of ACT, such as helping the person recognize when they are getting caught up in a specific thought (e.g., cognitive fusion) and teaching them applicable defusion and self-compassion skills to "unhook" from those thoughts and engage in meaningful occupations. Although interdisciplinary evidence for ACT continues to grow, examples within occupational therapy are also increasing (AOTA, 2022; Clarke et al., 2012; Gaudiano et al., 2020; Rider & Smith, 2023; Rider & Tay, 2022; Thompson, 2013).

Assessment of Cognitive Beliefs

Within the context of belief-oriented CBT, the assessment of cognitive beliefs is typically an individualized, collaborative process focused on identifying which situations or events trigger cognitive thoughts and beliefs and how these thoughts and beliefs influence individuals' behavior and emotions, as well as identifying performance strengths and deficits that may be impacting beliefs about one's abilities (J. S. Beck, 2011). OTPs typically gather this assessment information as part of developing an occupational profile and analyzing occupational performance to determine intervention goals, methods, and outcomes (AOTA, 2020). Wright and colleagues (1993) stressed that, as an interdisciplinary team member in belief-oriented CBT intervention programs, the expertise of OTPs enables them to contribute valuable assessment information related to occupational and skill performance strengths and deficits and provide task analysis and occupational and skill training to support positive adaptive cognitive beliefs. The first critical skill is recognizing cognitive beliefs, such as automatic thoughts, and their impact on their occupational performance. The awareness and recognition of thoughts and emotions may be enough for the person to start addressing their thoughts or the relationship with them throughout their daily activities. This chapter organizes instruments and strategies for assessing cognitive beliefs according to their structure, yielding a continuum of instruments and strategies ranging from structured, to semistructured, to unstructured.

Structured Assessments

Clinical researchers in psychology and psychiatry have led the way in developing several structured psychometric assessment instruments and techniques, such as questionnaires and self-report inventories, for evaluating cognitive beliefs. For the most part, these psychometric tools are used to validate theoretical constructs, identify the cognitive beliefs associated with various psychiatric diagnoses, and evaluate outcomes of cognitive behavioral interventions. Although beyond the scope of this chapter, Dunkley and colleagues (2010) have reviewed some of these psychometric instruments to assess beliefs and intervention outcomes for persons with anxiety and depression. Several scales and questionnaires have also been developed as research measures of beliefs related to **self-efficacy**, the belief in one's ability to succeed in specific situations or to accomplish a task (Bandura, 2006). With limited exceptions, very few structured instruments and techniques developed for research are used in clinical practice (Dunkley et al., 2010).

The occupational therapy literature includes a few structured assessment tools for assessing cognitive thoughts and beliefs and their impact on occupational performance. Van Huet and Williams (2007) found the Pain Self-Efficacy Questionnaire (PSEQ; Asghari & Nicholas, 2001; Nicholas, 2007) and the performance and satisfaction scales of the Canadian Occupational Performance Measure (COPM; Law et al., 2005) to be reliable and valid measures of changes in self-efficacy beliefs and occupational performance following a 3-week CBT intervention for managing chronic pain. The COPM is a semistructured assessment interview but is included in this section on structured assessments as part of the Van Huet and Williams study. Gage and colleagues (1994) developed the Self-Efficacy Gauge to examine self-efficacy beliefs in the context of occupational performance. As in psychology and psychiatry, a review of the occupational therapy literature suggests that most structured, psychometric measures of cognitive beliefs are used infrequently in practice.

Multiple questionnaires have been developed to measure psychological flexibility or inflexibility, a focus of ACT interventions. Although these structured assessments are not readily found in the occupational therapy literature, they may be helpful for OTPs employing ACT-based approaches. The Acceptance and Action Questionnaire II (AAQ-II; Bond et al., 2011), the Brief Experiential Avoidance Questionnaire (BEAQ; Gámez et al., 2014), and the Multidimensional Psychological Flexibility Inventory (MPFI; Rolffs et al., 2018) are a few questionnaires that measure psychological inflexibility and experiential avoidance. ACT-congruent questionnaires for beliefs surrounding specific areas addressed by OTPs are also available, such as the Psychological Inflexibility in Pain Scale (PIPS; Wicksell et al., 2010), the Chronic Pain Acceptance Questionnaire–Revised (CPAQ-R; McCraken et al., 2004), and the Body Image Psychological Inflexibility Scale (BIPIS; Callaghan et al., 2015). Most are available for free online.

Semistructured Assessments

Several semistructured assessments have more clinical utility because they can be incorporated into a collaborative, individualized interaction between the person and the therapist as part of an initial assessment and the ongoing assessment and intervention process (J. S. Beck, 2011). **Socratic questioning with guided discovery**, the process of asking a series of questions that promotes reflection and self-awareness, is a hallmark of this type of semistructured belief-oriented CBT methodology that can be incorporated into a clinical interview by OTPs (J. Beck, 2011). J. S. Beck's thought record (J. S. Beck, 2011), Burns's TIC-TOC technique (Burns, 1993), and Ellis's ABC Model (Ellis, 1994) are additional examples of semistructured CBT strategies that can be integrated into the assessment process. Because these strategies are also integral to belief-oriented CBT interventions, they are described in more detail in the intervention section.

In occupational therapy practice, the assessment focuses on identifying how individuals' cognitive beliefs and occupational performance influence each other and impact participation needs and desires. OTPs might conduct a semistructured clinical interview guided by the following questions, tailored to individual needs and contexts, and asked using lay terminology.

- What thoughts or beliefs are getting in the way of living the life you want to?
- What situations or circumstances trigger thoughts and beliefs interfering with your desired occupational performance and participation in daily activities?
- What are your thoughts and beliefs about your abilities to successfully address your occupational performance and participation needs and desires?
- What environmental (e.g., limited money or transportation) and social (e.g., others' opinions or values) factors might facilitate or hinder achieving your desired occupational performance needs and goals for successful participation? Do these factors confirm or disconfirm your thoughts and beliefs about your desired occupational performance, participation goals, and expectations?
- What physiological (e.g., sweaty palms, rapid breathing, feeling faint) and emotional reactions (e.g., sadness, anger) trigger beliefs that might facilitate or hinder achieving your goals for occupational performance and participation in your daily life? What thoughts or feelings trigger physiological and emotional reactions that might facilitate or hinder achieving your desired goals?

Unstructured Assessments

A more unstructured approach to assessing beliefs may occur when embedded within the ongoing intervention process by focusing on real-time or concurrent thoughts and beliefs related to occupational performance as they naturally arise in the therapy process (J. S. Beck, 2011). When this occurs, the person also benefits by actively identifying and addressing interfering beliefs and behaviors that mirror the same self-management process they might use in real life. This more unstructured, real-time assessment approach embedded in the therapy process is illustrated in the

TABLE 8-3 | Therapeutic Reasoning Assessment Table–Cognitive Beliefs

Which Tool?	Who Was This Tool Designed For?	Is This a Type of Tool This Person Can Do? What Is Required of the Person?	What Am I Measuring?	How Long Does It Take and Where Do I Administer This Assessment?	Is the Tool Associated With a Practice Model?
Structured Assessments (Research and use in practice documented in the literature)					
Pain Self-Efficacy Questionnaire (Nicholas, 2007)	Adults with chronic pain	Complete a 6-point Likert scale survey of 10 items about confidence in ability to perform tasks	Confidence (beliefs in ability) to perform tasks (e.g., self-care, social, leisure, and work despite pain)	Paper-and-pencil survey takes approximately 10 minutes to complete in institutional or home setting	Bandura's (1986) Model of Self-Efficacy Beliefs; part of Social Cognitive Theory
Self-Efficacy Gauge (Gage et al., 1994)	Adults with occupational performance dysfunction with a range of diagnoses and disabilities	Complete a 10-point Likert scale survey of 27 items about confidence in ability to perform tasks	Confidence (beliefs in ability) to competently perform occupational performance tasks	Paper-and-pencil survey takes approximately 20 minutes to complete in institutional or home setting	Bandura's (1986) Model of Self-Efficacy Beliefs; part of Social Cognitive Theory
Semistructured Assessments (Research and use in practice documented in the literature)					
Socratic Questioning (J. S. Beck, 2011; Padesky, 1993)	School-age children, adolescents, and adults with range of diagnoses, disabilities, and occupational performance problems	Collaborate in semistructured dialogue with therapist; respond to open-ended, guiding questions to discover beliefs impacting occupational performance	Beliefs that facilitate or hinder occupational performance and goal attainment	Open-ended dialogue process may be tailored to time available in any setting conducive to conversation	Cognitive Behavior Theory and Therapy
Dysfunctional Thought Records (J. S. Beck, 2011; p. 193)	Adolescents and adults with a range of diagnoses, disabilities, and occupational performance problems	Collaboratively or independently complete a three- to five-column worksheet to self-evaluate automatic thoughts	Automatic thoughts related to distressing occupational performance situations	Paper-and-pencil worksheet takes approximately 10 minutes to complete in any setting	Cognitive Behavior Theory and Therapy
TIC-TOC Technique (Burns, 1993)	Adolescents and adults	Collaboratively or independently complete a three-column worksheet to self-evaluate and redefine beliefs	Beliefs that interfere with and support engagement in desired tasks	Paper-and-pencil worksheet takes 10–15 minutes to complete in any setting	Cognitive Behavior Theory and Therapy
Identifying ABCs (Ellis, 1994)	Adolescents and adults	Collaboratively or independently complete a three- to five-column worksheet to identify events, irrational beliefs, and consequences related to sources of distress in life	Activating events, irrational beliefs, emotional and behavioral consequences related to sources of distress in life	Paper-and-pencil worksheet takes about 15 minutes to complete in any setting	ABC Model of Emotional Distress as part of Rational Emotive Therapy

description of the woman receiving occupational therapy following hip replacement surgery at the beginning of this chapter. Table 8-3 outlines cognitive belief-oriented assessment instruments and processes.

Intervention

In clinical practice, belief-oriented CBT approaches typically integrate cognitive, behavioral, and social cognitive theories and intervention methods because they work synergistically to effectively achieve intervention outcomes focused on cognitive content, specifically cognitive beliefs (J. S. Beck, 2011). For example, many people with depression have low energy and activity levels. Often, their inactivity reinforces depression. Continued inactivity may strengthen the struggle with dysfunctional beliefs (e.g., life is meaningless, or I am incompetent) and lead to more inaction and, ultimately, more psychological distress. Developing strategies to modify cognitive beliefs or the relationship with those beliefs can help individuals behave differently because they are no longer constrained by dysfunctional beliefs or struggling with them. Once having behaved differently—for example, by increasing involvement in meaningful daily activities—new self-enhancing cognitive beliefs (e.g., I can do some things well or find some activities meaningful) are formed and strengthened. Self-enhancing beliefs and strategies to increase psychological flexibility lead to an increased ability to enter the present moment fully and either change or persist in behavior guided by values, further increasing meaningful occupational engagement. At the same time, people who develop behavioral strategies (e.g., increasing engagement in meaningful activity) to manage depression or anxiety, for example, learn that they can better self-manage their distress and other related problems. This encourages adaptive beliefs and the use of cognitive coping skills that support continued engagement in similar adaptive behavioral strategies. And, in the case of a psychiatric condition such as depression or anxiety, which has a strong component of emotional distress, persons typically experience less emotional distress.

In general, approaches addressing cognitive beliefs are moving toward an overall model that emphasizes being open, centered, mindful, and actively pursuing values, which is congruent with all aspects of occupational therapy practice. OTPs aware of the fundamental approaches to address cognitive beliefs within the context of occupational engagement can better identify which approach may be more appropriate during the assessment process. OTPs can apply interventions in this chapter across psychiatric conditions and modify them for various ages and practice settings.

Cognitive Restructuring With CBT Methods

The cognitive theories and therapies developed by Aaron Beck (1967, 1976), a psychiatrist, and Albert Ellis (1962, 1994), a psychologist, are the prototypes of traditional CBT approaches that use **cognitive restructuring methods** to directly target cognitive beliefs for persons with psychiatric conditions and other psychological problems. These methods involve identifying, reframing, and replacing cognitive distortions, perceptions, and appraisals of life events with more realistic and adaptive appraisals, automatic thoughts, attitudes, and core beliefs.

Beck's Cognitive Therapy

In A. T. Beck's cognitive therapy (1976), described in detail by his daughter, J. S. Beck (2011), the therapist and person collaboratively reflect on the responses or outcomes of cognitive restructuring processes and use these reflections to revise existing beliefs or create new beliefs and hypotheses that they can test with behavioral experiments. For this approach to be effective, the outcome must reflect a change in cognitive beliefs and behavior. Cognitive restructuring relies heavily on Socratic questioning and guided discovery.

Socratic Questioning and Guided Discovery

Socratic questioning involves strategically using open-ended, guiding questions that avoid interpretation. *Guided discovery* involves the strategic and collaborative process between the person and the therapist that leads to uncovering information relevant to an issue being discussed and alternative options for addressing the issue. When used together and appropriately, Socratic questioning and guided discovery create a person-centered process that encourages individuals to reflect on and reevaluate dysfunctional beliefs and information-processing errors that are impacting their behavior and emotions so that they can apply new insights to either revise existing beliefs or create new beliefs to be more adaptive (Padesky, 1993).

In addition, Socratic questioning and guided discovery may also be incorporated into other cognitive restructuring techniques such as thought records, the use of self-talk and affirmations, and the TIC-TOC technique, described in the following text. For OTPs, using Socratic questioning and guided discovery facilitates person-centered discovery and clarification of beliefs and thoughts that may support or hinder occupational performance in meaningful daily activities.

Padesky (1993) identified four phases of questioning that may proceed in a stepwise fashion and shift from one to another depending on how the dialogue unfolds. Table 8-4 outlines each phase with examples of relevant questions that a therapist might ask.

Table 8-5 illustrates the use of three Socratic questions to facilitate guided discovery as part of what is sometimes formalized as the *three-question technique* (J. S. Beck, 2011). In this example, the Socratic questions guide the person to reframe their situation and, in so doing, discover how helpful

---

TABLE 8-4 | **Four Phases of Socratic Questioning and Examples**

Phase	Examples of Questions
1. Ask *informational questions* that the person can answer to help make concerns explicit and for the person to feel heard.	*What are you thinking or feeling when you do _____?* *Could you give me an example? Elaborate?* *What do you mean when you say _____?* *How long have you felt or believed this way?*
2. Ask *questions that reflect empathic listening* and summarize issues related to the problem.	*Let me see if I understand; do you mean _____?* *When you say ___, are you implying ____?* *Let me summarize: Are you thinking ____? Or feeling ____?*
3. Ask *questions that draw the person's attention to information relevant* to the issue being discussed but may be outside the person's current focus.	*What evidence do you have to support or refute that view?* *In a similar situation, what did you do? How did that turn out?* *What might someone who disagrees say?*
4. Ask *analytic or synthesizing questions* that guide the person toward new information to reevaluate a previous conclusion or construct a new idea.	*How could you find out if that is true or not?* *How does this information fit with _____?* *What are the advantages and disadvantages?* *Are there alternative explanations?*

TABLE 8-5 | Three-Question Technique Illustrating the Use of Socratic Questions for Guided Discovery

Situation: An individual has recently lost their job and presents with significant stress and anxiety about their future.

Belief: I will never work again.

Socratic, Guiding Questions	Example
What is the *evidence* for and against the belief?	For: *I was fired from my job. I won't be able to get a reference from my boss.* Against: *I've found work in the past. There are others I can use as a reference. I have received positive work evaluations in the past. My resume will help me.*
What are the *alternative explanations* of the event or situation?	*My boss and I got off to a bad start and were never able to develop a good working relationship. It wasn't a good fit for me, and it was time for me to find a new job anyway.*
What are the real *implications* or consequences if the belief is correct?	*It's possible that I won't get work in my field, but I could always do something else. I may need to look at other skills I have and consider multiple options for work.*

TABLE 8-6 | Examples of Thought Distortions or Errors in Thinking

All-or-nothing thinking	Viewing a situation as absolute, black or white, or in extremes
Magnifying or minimizing	Exaggerating things way out of proportion to what is reasonable or assuming things are much less important than they are
Catastrophizing or fortune-telling	Arbitrarily predicting the worst-case scenario without considering what is most likely to occur
Mental filter	Focusing only on the negative and ignoring the positive
Emotionalizing or emotional reasoning	Presuming that feelings are facts and ignoring or discounting evidence to the contrary
Personalizing	Blaming yourself for everything even when there is no evidence that you are at fault

their beliefs are, if at all, for meeting their needs and goals. This opens new options and the possibility of revising or creating new beliefs that are more realistically oriented toward addressing problematic situations and related emotions and, for occupational therapy interventions, occupational performance and participation needs and goals.

Thought Records

Aaron Beck (1976) recognized that when distressed, a person's perceptions and automatic thoughts and how they are processed are often distorted and dysfunctional. He identified several **core cognitive distortions** or errors in thinking that reflect dysfunctional cognitive beliefs. Table 8-6 describes examples of these cognitive distortions or thinking errors.

The thought record is a worksheet that helps individuals organize and evaluate their thoughts, beliefs, and emotional responses when distressed by a situation they encounter (J. S. Beck, 2011). Comprising three to five columns, a thought record usually includes the date and columns for describing a distressing situation (e.g., where, what, when); related emotional responses (e.g., what, intensity rating); and automatic thoughts (e.g., what, strength of belief rating). Additional columns may be included for identifying thought distortions, an alternative response (e.g., other views, explanations, positive

reframing of distortion), and outcomes (e.g., follow-up rating of emotional intensity and belief strength; J. S. Beck, 2011). In its simplest form, a thought record might be set up as illustrated in Figure 8-6 with additional rows for subsequent situations. From an ACT perspective, a thought record consistent with ACT concepts may be set up with the following columns: situation (e.g., describe the distressing situation), feelings (e.g., what feelings do you notice, emotions, sensations, etc.), thoughts (e.g., what thoughts do you have when you are in this situation), present-moment awareness (e.g., identify and practice a present-moment awareness exercise, such as a form of mindfulness, and write down any responses), values (e.g., what values are important in this situation), and action (e.g., choose an action or response consistent with the person's values).

TIC-TOC Technique

The **TIC-TOC technique,** developed by Burns (1993), a colleague of Beck, is particularly appropriate for occupational therapy interventions because it focuses on identifying and reframing task-interfering cognitions (TICs) and replacing them with task-oriented cognitions (TOCs). First, the person identifies a task they want or need to do but is avoiding or resisting. Then the person completes a three-column worksheet that includes identifying TICs, related thought distortions, and new, reframed TOCs related to the problematic task. As with similar techniques, this worksheet is used to "discover" new options for achieving desired goals and is most effective when both the person and the therapist reflect collaboratively on the options. Figure 8-7 illustrates this technique. Please also refer to the Being a Psychosocial Practitioner feature for an example of an OTP addressing cognitive beliefs in home health with the TIC-TOC activity.

Self-Talk and Affirmations

Self-talk is the term used to describe the process in which human beings continually talk to themselves out loud or as part of an inner dialogue stream experienced both on the conscious and unconscious levels. This self-talk or self-dialogue can be positive and self-affirming or negative and self-negating, and it often reflects a person's automatic thoughts and beliefs. For example, athletes often use self-talk to control or modify certain psychological states, including cognitive beliefs and performance outcomes (Weinberg & Gould, 2015). Similarly, positive self-talk helps restructure or modify

Thought Record						
Date/Time	Situation	Emotion	Automatic Thought	Thoughts/ Distortions	Alternative Thought/ View	Outcome
7/13/24 7 a.m.	Forgot to set alarm. Overslept and ended up late for work.	Angry, anxious. Emotional intensity: 90%	I'll be fired. I always mess up. I'm an idiot. Belief strength: 90%	Fortune-telling; magnifying	Late once before, and I wasn't fired. I can offer to stay late to make up time. I need to be sure to set my alarm.	Emotional intensity: 40% Belief strength: 20%

FIGURE 8-6. Sample thought record, illustrating how alternative thoughts can change the intensity and strength of negative emotions. OTPs can then use this to further discuss the impact of the person's thoughts on occupational performance and explore cognitive and coping strategies.

Being a Psychosocial OT Practitioner

Using Cognitive Behavioral Strategies to Address Fear of Falling

Identifying Psychosocial Strengths and Needs

OTPs in home health encounter people whose psychosocial challenges, such as anxiety, can impair participation and lead to further functional decline. Consider the story of Estele, an older adult living alone. While vacuuming, she tripped on the cord, fell, and broke her hip. She is now recovering at home from a total hip arthroplasty. Appropriate home modifications are in place, and Estele has a safety alert system in case of an emergency. She also has supportive family and friends nearby who are willing to help as needed and check on her daily.

Estele demonstrates no cognitive impairments, has good static and dynamic balance, and safely ambulates with a front-wheeled walker. She participates in seated activities, such as dressing and self-care, and is willing to do therapeutic exercises while seated and standing in front of a chair. However, she becomes fearful when encouraged to progress in occupational therapy and reengage in chores and community mobility. She relies on family and friends for help with housework, meal preparation, and shopping. Estelle reports to her OTP that she has not left the house since returning home from the hospital or resumed basic home management tasks, which she indicated were important to her during the initial evaluation.

Despite her physical progress, Estele perceives herself as still being "weak" and "old." She fears "another fall is inevitable." She ruminates about falling again and often expresses fear, anxiety, lack of confidence, and poor self-efficacy during therapy.

The OTP determines that Estele's fear of falling has led to a pattern of activity avoidance. She believes Estele is at high risk for further functional decline and social isolation.

Using a Holistic Occupational Therapy Approach

Through a semistructured interview about her fear of falling and avoidance behavior, Estele's OTP helps her identify what cognitive beliefs are affecting her occupational performance.

To encourage self-reflection, the OTP asks Estele about factors that predisposed the problem, what factors precipitated the current problem, and what factors might be perpetuating the problem in terms of cognitive, behavioral, emotional, physical, and social factors.

Estele shares a history of anxiety that began when she was a young adult. She feels her ability to manage her anxiety disappeared after her recent fall. She shares stories about friends who have fallen and lived the rest of their lives in nursing homes. Estele recognizes that she often imagines worst-case scenarios (i.e., magnification) and can't stop thinking about falling again and returning to the hospital (i.e., rumination). Despite the OTP's assessment of functional ambulation and balance, Estele shares that she doesn't feel physically ready to walk more than the distance from her bed to the bathroom, and the idea of cleaning her house or making a meal terrifies her.

With Estele's permission, the OTP explores TICs. Using the TIC-TOC technique, the OTP helps her explore some common thought distortions and how they could be contributing to her fear of falling and avoidance behavior. With the OTP's encouragement, Estele is able to identify and begin to reframe TICs and replace them with TOCs.

TIC-TOC Activity

Activity: Home management tasks

Task-Interfering Cognitions (TICs)	Thought Distortions	Task-Oriented Cognitions (TOCs)
• I will never be able to walk like I used to. • I am old and weak and will just fall again and end up on the floor. • If I fall again, it will be so much worse, and I will have to go to the hospital for a long time. • If I fall, my kids might put me in a nursing home, and I don't want to end up like my friend.	• All-or-nothing thinking • Catastrophizing: magnifying and ruminating • Fortune telling • Mental filter	• I might not walk as fast as I used to, but I can still walk with a walker. • I have overcome a lot of things in my life, and I can keep making progress. • I might still be afraid of falling, but I can start small by walking with my OTP or a family member to be safe. • I don't know what will happen in the future, but I know I want to stay in my home and do as much as I can for myself. • I have made my home as safe as I can and have a safety alert button if I need help.

Continued

Being a Psychosocial OT Practitioner—cont'd

Together, Estele and her OTP make a plan to slowly integrate more home-management tasks into therapy through graded exposure. The OTP teaches Estele fall recovery techniques and includes family and friends in therapy to increase Estele's confidence in herself and her support system. Using behavioral activation strategies, the OTP helps Estele schedule specific activities to increase the likelihood that she will participate in graded home-management tasks and remove decision-making as an obstacle to engagement. Together, Estele and the OTP continue to explore cognitive beliefs and apply cognitive behavioral strategies. Estele reports that thought records are helpful as a homework activity, and she begins applying cognitive restructuring

strategies to other automatic thoughts. Finally, the OTP ensures that each session includes graded activity exposure designed to support mastery experiences, raise self-efficacy, and affirm TOCs.

Reflective Questions

1. What other cognitive behavioral strategies might be useful to explore with Estele?
2. How might the OTP specifically address Estele's magnifying and ruminating thoughts about falling?
3. How would you design a treatment session with the goal of providing Estele with a mastery experience to raise her self-efficacy beliefs regarding her functional abilities in the home?

TIC-TOC Activity		
Task-Interfering Cognitions (TICs)	**Thought Distortions**	**Task-Oriented Cognitions (TOCs)**
I have nothing to do all weekend. I just lie around all day doing nothing. I'm worthless. It doesn't do any good to do anything.	All-or-nothing thinking	I don't feel like doing anything, but it won't hurt me to try to do some things I used to like to do. I might even feel better.

FIGURE 8-7. Sample TIC-TOC activity, showing how changing thoughts can promote doing.

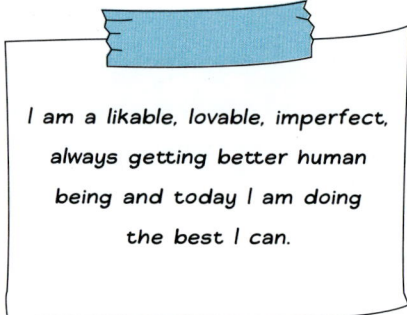

I am a likable, lovable, imperfect, always getting better human being and today I am doing the best I can.

FIGURE 8-8. Example of an affirmation.

thoughts and beliefs to facilitate engagement in occupational performance; for example, repeating a TOC to oneself (e.g., "If I go for a walk, I will feel less stressed about my upcoming job interview," or "If I get out of bed and take a shower, I will have more energy to do something today").

An **affirmation**, a written or oral statement that confirms or reinforces something as true, is a form of positive self-talk that helps to counteract negative self-scripts or beliefs. Affirmations can help achieve specific goals, including occupational performance and participation goals. For example, when undertaking a difficult task that has been avoided, an individual might encourage themself to engage in the task by using an affirmation such as, "I can do whatever I set my mind to do" or "I am a success story." For a person whose self-talk focuses on negative thoughts about the self, an affirmation such as, "I am superior to my negative thoughts" might be helpful. It is also helpful for the person and therapist to collaboratively script affirming thoughts; select prescripted quotations that fit the person's specific situation; and reflect adaptive, affirming thoughts and beliefs. These may be written down and posted in visible places as frequent affirmative reminders, as illustrated in Figure 8-8. For persons using smartphones, many apps provide scripted and unique affirmations on their phones at specified frequencies.

Ellis's Rational Emotive Behavior Therapy

Ellis's (1962, 1994) **Rational Emotive Behavior Therapy (REBT)** is based on his cognitive model of emotional response. The core tenet of this model is that irrational beliefs

about how things "must" and "should" be for an individual to be happy lead to unhappiness.

Ellis (1962, 1994) devised the **ABC Model** as an acronym to explain this view of emotional disturbance. It provides a cognitive restructuring framework to identify the activating events (A), irrational beliefs (B), and emotional and behavioral consequences (C) related to specific situations, beliefs, or emotions that are interfering with a person's well-being. This method highlights the irrational beliefs that can be the source of emotional distress and maladaptive behavior, including occupational performance and participation problems, in contrast to the situations that the individual often thinks are the source of their distress. In REBT, persons are taught to use the ABC Model to identify, evaluate, and actively challenge the irrational beliefs at the core of their emotional problems. They are encouraged to restructure or replace irrational beliefs with more realistic, rational beliefs, initially with a therapist's guidance and, eventually, on their own. The ABC Model is illustrated in Figure 8-9 with an example.

Behavior/Learning-Oriented CBT Methods

When using interventions based on behavioral and learning theories within the context of belief-oriented CBT, the focus is on taking action by testing, changing, or acquiring new behaviors to support adaptive cognitive beliefs. With many psychiatric conditions and psychological challenges, behavior- and learning-oriented interventions can also positively impact negative emotions. This chapter highlights several intervention methods that are typically part of belief-oriented CBT interventions (J. S. Beck, 2011) and applicable

A—Activating Event	B—Beliefs (often irrational)	C—Consequences
(What was the event or situation that triggered your thoughts, actions, and feelings?)	(What thoughts went through your head when the activating event occurred?)	(How did you act and feel after you had those thoughts?)
	Irrational Beliefs:	
My friend doesn't ask me to go to the movies with him.	• He is rejecting me. • Rejection means he doesn't like me. • I am not worthy of being liked.	Actions—I don't answer his phone call the next time he calls. Emotions—I feel hurt, angry, and rejected.
	Replace Irrational Beliefs With Rational Beliefs:	
	• My friend may have his own reasons for not asking me. • I know he likes me. • I am a worthy and likable person.	Actions—I answer the phone when my friend calls. He apologizes for not inviting me and explains his cousin was in town and they went together. Emotions—I feel liked, connected, and satisfied.

FIGURE 8-9. Example illustrating Ellis's ABC Model.

PhotoVoice

Victory After Storm
Donisha

On the left, there is a storm with rain and a flower. The storm represents the struggle in our life, and the flower represents me. As you can see, the flower is frail and weak and seems to be beat upon by the storm, but still holds a certain beauty. On the right, as you can see, I have overcome both the storm and the struggle. One may think a storm or struggle is a bad thing, but look at the flower on the right. As you can see, the storm added more beauty, character, and strength, which brings sunshine and a rainbow with promise of victory.

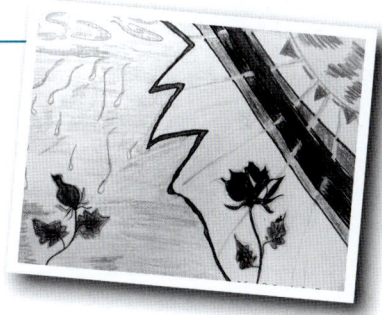

Can you identify a struggle that added beauty, character, and/or strength to your life?

to occupational therapy interventions designed to address cognitive beliefs as part of achieving desired occupational performance and participation.

Behavioral Experiments

Behavioral experiments involve a collaborative strategy in which the therapist and the person create opportunities to actively test thoughts, attitudes, beliefs, and related behaviors as part of discovering their relative utility or validity. Behavioral experimentation is an essential behavioral strategy within CBT's methodology for facilitating change in beliefs, behavior, and emotions that interfere with functional well-being (J. S. Beck, 2011). The typical behavioral experiment involves developing a belief-related hypothesis to test; predicting the outcome; undertaking the behavioral test or experiment, which typically includes taking an action or doing something; evaluating the result; and then using this feedback to revise or create new beliefs as appropriate. This powerful process is critical to belief change, particularly when combined with cognitive restructuring strategies. For example, a student might believe their classmates will think they are stupid if they ask for help with an assignment. The student might test this belief in a behavioral experiment by asking classmates if they would think they are stupid if they asked for help or by asking the teacher for help and observing their classmates' responses. The outcome of this experiment provides feedback on the validity of the student's belief, an important aspect of restructuring dysfunctional beliefs and developing more adaptive ones.

Behavioral Activation and Activity Scheduling

For many psychiatric conditions, inactivity or avoidance of activities is related to negative cognitive beliefs about one's competence or worth and contributes to psychological

Evidence-Based Practice

Efficacy of Thought Records and Behavioral Experiments

Use of thought records and behavioral experimentation as part of occupation-based interventions can facilitate optimal attainment of occupational performance and participation outcomes.

RESEARCH FINDINGS

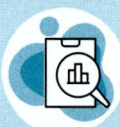

In a study with a nonclinical sample of 91 participants that examined the relative efficacy, in comparison with a control condition, of thought records and behavioral experiments, the findings confirmed the usefulness of both interventions with a slight advantage of behavioral experiments over thought record interventions for effecting belief change sooner and with greater generalization (McManus et al., 2012). Although more research is needed with different belief changes in varied situations, these findings have several important implications for OTPs:

APPLICATIONS

➡ OTPs should be aware of and assess cognitive beliefs that can interfere with achieving occupation-based outcomes.
➡ Occupation-based intervention approaches that address beliefs related to occupational performance frequently include behavioral experimentation; these interventions can also
➡ contribute significantly to a change in cognitive beliefs that interfere with recovery for persons with various psychiatric conditions.
➡ Use of thought records in combination with behavioral experimentation as part of occupation-based interventions can facilitate optimal attainment of occupational performance and participation outcomes in occupational therapy.

REFERENCES

McManus, F., Van Doorn, K., & Yiend, J. (2012). Examining the effects of thought records and behavioral experiments in instigating belief change. *Journal of Behavior Therapy and Experimental Psychiatry, 43*(1), 540–547. https://doi.org/10.1016/j.jbtep.2011.07.003

distress. As described in the example at the beginning of this intervention section, the interaction of dysfunctional cognitive beliefs and inactivity can become a vicious cycle that maintains the emotional problems associated with various psychiatric conditions, such as depression or anxiety. **Behavioral activation** is a strategy with the purpose of increasing positive reinforcement through engagement in activity (Martell et al., 2010). Typically, behavioral activation incorporates **activity scheduling,** which involves making a list, chart, or calendar of daily and weekly activities and committing to engage in them. Creating a schedule helps to increase the likelihood that people will engage in desired activities and removes decision-making as an obstacle to engagement.

Self-Monitoring
Behavioral experimentation, behavioral activation, and activity scheduling rely on **self-monitoring**, a cognitive behavioral self-regulatory or self-management process that involves paying deliberate attention to specific aspects of one's beliefs,

emotions, and behavior. Typically, it includes recording and tallying the frequency of behaviors and associated thoughts and feelings for a designated period of time (e.g., on an hour-by-hour basis for 1 week). It may also involve monitoring and rating one's thoughts and feelings or the degree of mastery or pleasure associated with each action, activity, or behavioral experiment performed (e.g., on a scale from 0 to 100, where 0 is the worst one has ever felt or the most negative and 100 is the best or most positive; Cohen et al., 2013).

For example, suppose a person believes they do nothing all day. As homework, the OTP might have them self-monitor their behavior by keeping a record of what they do every half hour for several days to evaluate if, in fact, they are doing nothing 24 hours a day. This concrete feedback provides evidence for the person to evaluate and revise their beliefs. In addition to basic charts that involve recording and tallying daily activities, the Occupational Experience Profile (OEP) developed by Karen Atler provides another option for detailed information on recorded activities and experience patterns from the person's perspective. The OEP is an occupation-focused assessment that helps people become aware of what they do and experience daily and reflect on how their daily activities and experiences impact their health and well-being (Atler et al., 2015).

This information can be used to guide the selection and scheduling of appropriate activities and monitor actual engagement in activities and the impact on beliefs and emotions. Types of scheduled activities may include (a) those that are associated with pleasure, increased energy, mastery, or a good mood; (b) those that have been meaningful or rewarding in the past but are not currently being engaged in by the person; (c) new activities that are important for reaching desired rehabilitation or recovery goals; and (d) those involving behavioral experiments for testing and evaluating cognitive beliefs. A successful experience provides contradictory evidence to negative or distorted cognitive beliefs, supporting more adaptive beliefs and improving emotional well-being. Follow-through or failure to follow through also provides a basis to discuss the beliefs and thoughts that may be supporting or interfering with performance and strategies to improve follow-through. For occupational therapy interventions, combining behavioral strategies such as behavioral experiments, behavioral activation, activity scheduling, and self-monitoring with a cognitive restructuring technique such as the TIC-TOC technique can be a powerful use of CBT methods for addressing cognitive beliefs and achieving occupational performance outcomes.

Brief ACT Interventions

OTPs can use metaphors and activities on the core processes of ACT to help individuals understand and apply ACT principles. For example, OTPs can share the ACT "Tug-of-War" metaphor, easily found online and in ACT resources, to explore acceptance and help the person recognize that the struggle is the problem, not the solution, and lead into a discussion of things that are outside the person's control (e.g., the vast majority of emotions, feelings, thoughts, and sensations people experience) and within their control (e.g., how they respond to their emotions, feelings, thoughts, and sensations). Next, the OTP can do the ACT "Hands as Thoughts and Feelings" exercise (developed by Russ Harris, 2019, and available online; see the Resources section) to help the person understand the rationale for and benefits of developing defusion skills. ACT interventions work toward increasing psychological flexibility, and OTPs help individuals translate cognitive skills into behavior changes, such as improved participation and performance in meaningful occupations. The following exercises briefly introduce ACT interventions within the scope of occupational therapy and highlight examples that can be applied within occupational therapy sessions across settings and diagnoses.

Defusion Skills

From an ACT perspective, the biggest issue people face is cognitive fusion—the tendency to get attached to thinking patterns to the point where people cannot separate themselves from their thoughts or feelings. When this happens, cognitions (e.g., unhelpful thoughts, beliefs, and feelings) dominate their behavior. Cognitive fusion may then lead to decisions about occupational engagement based on the struggle with their unhelpful thoughts and feelings rather than what is really going on in the world. This often leads to experiential avoidance and further distress. Cognitive defusion is sometimes called "deliteralization," because the goal is to see thoughts and feelings for what they are—simply thoughts and feelings—not as what they say they are. The "Hands as Thoughts and Feelings" metaphor by Russ Harris (2019) can introduce fusion and defusion. In addition to this metaphor, there are many skills that OTPs can teach to help individuals defuse from cognitions. Here are a few examples OTPs can use to help persons defuse from unhelpful thoughts and feelings.

- "I'm having the thought that. . . ." Identify a negative self-judgment that you may struggle with and that hinders doing things that are meaningful, and phrase it in the form of "I am _____." For example, "I am not good enough." Take a moment and try to fuse with this thought. Get caught up in it and believe it as much as you can. Think of how it has negatively impacted you in your life. Now, in your head or aloud, say, "I'm having the thought that. . . ." For example, "I'm having the thought that I am not good enough." Now, replay it again, but say, "I notice that I am having the thought that. . . ." For example, "I notice that I am having the thought that I am not good enough." (Adapted from Harris, 2019; Hayes et al., 1999.) This is one of many exercises to help individuals notice a sense of separation or distance from the thought.
- Other ideas used by ACT practitioners include taking the negative self-judgment and silently singing the thought to the tune of "Happy Birthday" or a favorite tune; thanking your mind for the thought (e.g., "Thank you mind, for the thought that I am not smart enough to be in this class"); saying or imagining the thought in silly or famous voices; imagining the thought written on a computer screen and playing around with the formatting, font, and color; imagining the unhelpful thoughts and feelings as leaves floating on a stream and watching them float by; and so on. Each of these exercises aims to distance people from unwanted thoughts or feelings and see them as they are, just a thought or a feeling that they can let come and go without "fusing" or getting entangled by them.

As with all interventions, OTPs should ensure ACT-based interventions are person-centered and support individuals in practicing the exercises or activities in their daily lives to ensure carryover and increase participation in meaningful occupations. For example, a session can include learning about cognitive fusion, identifying when cognitive fusion hinders or negatively impacts meaningful occupational engagement, experimenting with cognitive defusion techniques, and identifying and practicing how to apply them outside of therapy to improve occupational participation. The person could then keep a journal of how they incorporated the techniques, what helped and what didn't help, and any difficulties encountered for discussion and further training in their next occupational therapy session.

Contacting the Present Moment

The "dropping anchor" exercise developed by Dr. Russ Harris can help individuals become more fully present and engage in what they are doing, allowing them to regain control over their actions and occupational performance to focus on what is important here and now (Harris, 2019). It is an excellent exercise for individuals interested in mindfulness or those who want to get better at "unhooking" from difficult thoughts and feelings. The following metaphor is helpful in introducing this exercise and considering how the person may feel when they are overwhelmed by unhelpful thoughts or feelings and "fused" within the moment. After the individual has shared how it feels when overwhelmed by difficult thoughts, feelings, emotions, or memories, the OTP can share a version of the following metaphor (adapted from Harris, 2019).

> You have all these thoughts spinning around your head and all these feelings whirling around in your body. It's like an emotional storm happening inside you. Imagine that you are in a sailboat during a massive storm. While that storm is sweeping you away, there is nothing effective you can do. You are at the mercy of the elements. Now, suppose your boat is sailing into the harbor just as the huge storm begins. What is your top priority? (Allow the person to answer.) It might be to drop the anchor as fast as possible. It is the same with us. When an emotional storm begins, the person must first "drop their anchor." Dropping the anchor won't make the storm go away. Anchors don't control the weather. However, dropping the anchor will hold the person steady until the storm passes.

An anchor can be anything in the present moment that is not part of the storm; for example, anything a person can see, hear, touch, taste, or smell, as well as their breathing, their posture, what they are doing with their arms or legs, and so on. Anything that can help the person stay present, grounded, and in contact with where they are and what they are doing can be an anchor amid their emotional storm and allow them to refocus and act guided by their values. Dropping one's anchor is similar to what some may call "grounding techniques."

Dr. Harris (2019) suggests three steps to help people in dropping their anchor, and they follow the acronym ACE:

A–*Acknowledge one's thoughts and feelings:* OTPs can help individuals acknowledge thoughts, feelings, emotions, memories, sensations, or urges that are present. Guide the person to acknowledge whatever thoughts or feelings arise silently and kindly. Teach them to observe their inner experience curiously and nonjudgmentally.

C–*Come back into one's body:* Assist the person in coming back into and connecting with their physical body. It is important to help the person find their preferred way of achieving this, but utilizing body scans and movement techniques is often helpful. For example, have the person move, stretch, change posture, sit upright, stand, walk, slow down their breathing, push their feet onto the floor, straighten their back, and so on. In ACT, the goal of this exercise is not to distract a person from their thoughts and feelings; instead, it is to remain aware of their thoughts and feelings, acknowledge their presence, and simultaneously come back and connect with their body (Harris, 2019). Simply put, this exercise teaches people to "expand their focus" so they have room for more than unhelpful thoughts and feelings.

E–*Engage in the world:* At this point, the goal is to help the person expand their awareness. Engage in what you are doing. Help the person refocus their attention by noticing where they are, what you are doing, and what they can see, hear, touch, taste, and smell. Have the person look around and notice something they can see, hear, touch, and so on. This is not to distract them from their thoughts and feelings but to help them notice what else is there (Harris, 2019).

After teaching this skill to individuals, OTPs can help them identify how to use it in their own lives when they become caught up in an emotional storm. After dropping their anchor, the goal is to be more present and aware and have more control over responses and actions. This exercise is designed to be person-centered and allows for creativity and modifications. Collaboratively identify ways for the person to acknowledge their thoughts and feelings, come back into their body, and engage in their world to increase psychological flexibility.

The Choice Point

The Choice Point is an ACT tool that OTPs can use to help people quickly map out problems, identify sources of suffering, and collaboratively formulate an ACT approach to handling them (Harris, 2019). The Choice Point was first developed by Ciarrochi and colleagues (2014) and later expanded into version 2.0 by Dr. Russ Harris (2017). It can be used at any stage of the recovery process and for many purposes. OTPs can use it to explain the overall spirit of ACT, utilize and reinforce specific core processes, set an agenda for a treatment session, summarize a session, and/or gather information during the assessment process for goal development.

The Choice Point is commonly used as an activity to illustrate and connect the person to the two main options they have in any given situation: The person can move toward or away from what matters to them. In the Choice Point 2.0 (Harris, 2017), "away moves" are considered ineffective, values-incongruent actions. In lay terms, they are things that move us away from the person we want to be or the life we want to build (Harris, 2019). Often, away moves are caused by experiential avoidance or fusion with thoughts, feelings, emotions, or memories (Harris, 2017). In contrast, "toward moves" are values-congruent actions or things that move us toward the person we want to be and the life we want to live. These "moves" are always from the individual's perspective. For example, if they see their behavior as life-enhancing, acting effectively, and behaving similar to the person they want to be, it is considered a toward move. If necessary, values can be revisited compassionately and respectfully explored in future occupational therapy sessions to see if certain moves (behaviors) are truly values-congruent (Harris, 2017). Additionally, a behavior may be toward or away depending on the context. For example, watching the television mindlessly to avoid going to the gym or procrastinating homework would be classified as an away move. However, watching a favorite show with a partner as a conscious, values-guided choice that enriches life can be classified as a toward move.

See Figure 8-10 for an example of the Choice Point adapted from Harris (2017). OTPs can draw this figure in a treatment session and add responses from the person to help them identify key ACT concepts, such as their values; what thoughts, feelings, or situations "hook" them; what "away" and "toward" moves look like; and so on. For example, the OTP can start with the "Choice Point" at the bottom and identify situations, thoughts, and feelings that might be distressful, highlighting that we can either get entangled in them

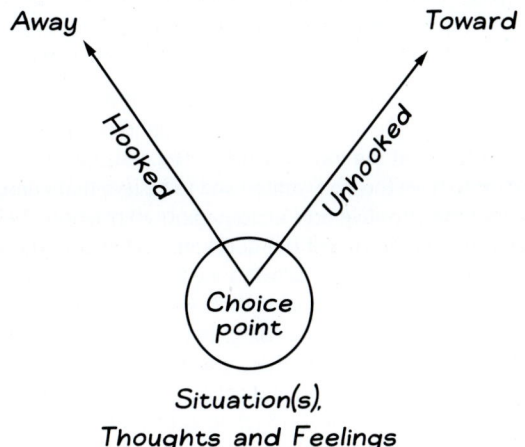

FIGURE 8-10. The Choice Point activity.

or act in a way that moves us away or toward what matters. If the person identifies an automatic thought or belief they are often fused with, it would be written at the bottom of the figure. The OTP would then facilitate a discussion about the person's "away" and "toward" moves and what it looks like when they are "hooked" versus "unhooked," as well as strategies to "unhook," and write them along the arrows. The person's values would be written at the top of the image. This image becomes a visual representation of what the person can do whenever they experience situations, thoughts, or feelings that can "hook" them and how to "unhook" and keep working toward the life they want to live (i.e., their values). Multiple videos and worksheets for the Choice Point are available online. See Harris (2017; 2019) for more detailed examples of how to use this in practice.

Self-Efficacy Beliefs and Performance

Albert Bandura's (1986, 1997) social cognitive theory, also called social learning theory, emphasizes the critical roles of social and cognitive factors and behavior and environment in his theory of human learning and behavior change. For this reason, it is sometimes referred to as a bridge between cognitive and behavioral theories. Although social cognitive theory covers many topics, self-efficacy beliefs and their relationship to successful performance are particularly relevant in belief-oriented CBT and occupational therapy interventions. **Self-efficacy beliefs**, the beliefs people have regarding their capabilities to succeed in a specific situation or in accomplishing a desired task, play a significant motivational role in whether persons "will attempt certain behaviors, how much effort they will expend, and how long they will stick with the behavior, particularly if problems or obstacles arise" (Bandura, 1981, p. 85). They also influence "how persons will feel about what they are doing and ultimately whether or not they will succeed" (Bandura, 1997). Conversely, successful occupational performance and participation positively impact cognitive beliefs. Gage and Polatajko (1994) emphasize the importance of the reciprocal relationship between self-efficacy beliefs and occupational performance for effective occupation-based intervention outcomes. OTPs must design interventions that allow individuals to experience

occupational performance successes and accomplishments, as these typically raise self-efficacy beliefs; in contrast, performance failures tend to affirm dysfunctional or distorted beliefs and lower self-efficacy beliefs (Bandura, 1986). Bandura (1986) identified mastery experiences, vicarious experiences, social modeling, and social persuasion as important sources of influence for enhancing self-efficacy beliefs, which can positively impact occupational performance and participation, emotional well-being, and mental health. For more information on self-efficacy, please see Chapter 11: Motivation. 🤝

In this chapter's The Lived Experience feature, Martha shares how integrating peer support, engagement in meaningful activities and occupation, cognitive restructuring strategies, and behavioral experiments were critical to her recovery. They helped her counter dysfunctional thoughts and beliefs, strengthen her self-efficacy beliefs, and focus on acquiring the skills she needed to live the life she wanted, including participation in meaningful, productive work and engagement in social and parenting occupations. For more information on the Wellness Recovery Action Plan shared by Martha and commonly utilized by OTPs, you can visit https://www.wellnessrecoveryactionplan.com.

Other Educational/Learning Methods

Cognitive belief-oriented approaches, such as CBT and ACT, aim to educate or teach people to self-manage their beliefs, thoughts, feelings, and actions in their daily lives, emphasizing relapse prevention (Greenberger & Padesky, 2016; Hayes et al., 2012). Two explicit educational or learning methods are considered essential, not optional, elements of the intervention process: psychoeducation and homework (J. S. Beck, 2011; Friedman et al., 2008). Skilled psychoeducation can relate directly to belief-oriented concepts or to the successful performance that supports altering beliefs, the relationship with them, or both. When optimally designed, skilled psychoeducation on belief-oriented concepts (e.g., cognitive restructuring in CBT or cognitive defusion in ACT) enhances performance, and successful performance supports positive and adaptive beliefs.

Psychoeducation involves teaching relevant psychological principles, knowledge, and skills to the individual receiving services. This may include any concepts discussed in this chapter that are relevant to the person and their recovery. Collaborative psychoeducation and engagement in the intervention process empower people to develop skills for self-managing their beliefs, emotions, and behavior to improve their quality of life and well-being.

Psychoeducation may take the form of "minilectures," demonstrations, recommended books, workbooks, activities or exercises, or audiovisual resources such as those listed in the Resources section at the end of this chapter. It also may be incorporated into the ongoing therapeutic, collaborative dialogue between the therapist and the person. Incorporating psychoeducation into a group therapy context also takes advantage of the opportunities that social support and modeling play in facilitating change in beliefs, emotions, and behavior. The psychoeducational process takes place both within therapy sessions and outside them as homework. Combining psychoeducation with behavioral experiments and practice related to circumstances and contexts that are personally significant to the individual has been shown to

The Lived Experience

Martha's Story

Recovery from mental illness isn't a straight-line trajectory to wellness. I was a veterinarian in the Air Force when I fell and ended up with a head injury. I became very depressed and suicidal and was in the hospital for more years than I care to remember. Finally, after returning to school for 2 years and then working for over 2 years, I thought I had beaten the "beast"—the overwhelming depression that left me chronically suicidal. Unfortunately, this was not the case. Life happens and I found myself very depressed and made another attempt on my life. The next several months in the hospital were brutal. The negative self-talk and belief that I was worthless and that people would be better off without me was back with a vengeance. I could have resigned myself to a life of chronic depression and disability. Some professionals even thought I just needed to accept that as my lot in life.

Fortunately, I found the power of peer support. This started through my introduction to WRAP (Wellness Recovery Action Plan; Copeland, 2011) by an OTP. WRAP starts by having you describe your traits when you are well. This was a novel idea for me because previously I had concentrated on how not to be sick. There is a big difference between focusing on being well and focusing on not being sick. My goal to "maintain and keep my symptoms in check" now became "how can I live the life I want?" Instead of believing I was a sick person who needed to learn how to manage my symptoms, I gradually started believing that I could be a recovering person learning skills for living the life I wanted to live. Of course, I first had to convince myself to believe that there was a life out there for me where I could feel successful and satisfied and be a productive member of society. Instead of feeling as if I was a failure because I couldn't work as a veterinarian, I had to begin believing that I could find something new and meaningful for work if I wanted to.

During the next few years I found that life through the power of sharing my story and working on my WRAP and gaining inspiration from others who shared their stories with me. I became a certified peer specialist (CPS), supporting and giving hope to others who might not yet have found the light at the end of the tunnel. Some of the tools I learned and now teach to others include overcoming fear of failing and negative self-talk and beliefs. I had to really work on countering negative self-talk with self-talk that reminded me of my successes and of what I could do to have the life I wanted and to believe that I deserved it. Sometimes positive and encouraging affirmations helped. Other times asking myself the question, "What would I do if I was not afraid of failing?" allowed me to get in touch with my hopes and dreams that I had pushed aside so long ago. I could imagine a different life doing things that I actually enjoyed such as satisfying work, helping others, doing fun things, and taking care of myself by exercising and eating healthy. Actually acting "as if" and just taking action such as exercising or walking my dog would help to rekindle hope. And, once that flicker of hope was there, it got easier to build on it.

I had to learn that taking a risk was a good thing and that it was okay to fail. Previously failure meant relapse, which meant suicidal thoughts and negative self-talk. I had to learn to embrace failure as a learning experience, as a way to refine what I needed to do to live the life I wanted, and, most importantly, as a part of experiencing life to the fullest. All this was about coming to believe that I wasn't worthless and that I could accomplish worthwhile things. Another tool I learned that has proven invaluable came from the physical rehab world: Skills + Supports = Success and Satisfaction. I posted this on my wall and said it to myself as a reminder.

Once I had that dream of a better life I could look at what skills I had or that I could learn to help me get to where I wanted to be in life. Attending the training to be a CPS was a big step for me. I also learned that supports are crucial. What people, places, and things do I have in my life or need to have to help me to live the life I want to live? I used to believe that asking for help was a weakness. I had to learn that NOT asking for support was really the weakness. My family has always been central to my recovery and they continue to support me in every way. This is where I also found the power of peer support. Talking to others who have been there and gotten through it is truly inspirational. I also must put in a plug for my pets. Their unconditional love, even on my worst days, gives me a reason to take another step.

---

support effective belief-oriented CBT outcomes based on an extensive literature review by Lukens and McFarlane (2004).

Homework, another essential educational component of belief-oriented approaches, involves doing assignments outside therapy sessions. These assignments encourage individuals to experiment with, apply, practice, and supplement what is addressed in occupational therapy. Most of the strategies and techniques presented in this chapter could be assigned as homework. Table 8-7 lists various types of homework with examples. Homework assignments are typically most effective when they are determined collaboratively between the therapist and person and reviewed together after the homework is completed (J. S. Beck, 2011). Many of the workbooks in the Resources section provide worksheets that can be used as homework assignments outside occupational therapy sessions.

The following example illustrates an occupational therapy session incorporating psychoeducation, cognitive restructuring, behavior activation, and experimentation with homework for a person who attended a day program in the community 5 days a week. The person was diagnosed with major depressive disorder. Through Socratic questioning with guided discovery, the person expressed the belief that they were worthless because they did not do anything but lie around all day watching the television. To help the person understand that their inactivity might be more about their condition than their character, the OTP explained that inactivity is a symptom of depression and gave them a pamphlet to read about depression. The OTP also explained how engaging in activities helps to counter self-deprecating beliefs and decrease emotional distress. The OTP and the person

TABLE 8-7 | Homework Types and Methods

Types of Homework	Methods
Psychoeducation	Reading books, watching videos, or listening to podcasts about psychiatric conditions, CBT, ACT, and other topics related to beliefs and emotional distress
Data collection	Completing thought records, keeping a journal, self-monitoring daily activities
Test the validity of thoughts and beliefs	Carrying out behavioral experiments
Defuse from thoughts and feelings	Practicing various defusion skills when unhelpful thoughts or feelings arise
Contacting the present moment	Practicing various mindfulness activities
Experiment with new behaviors	Practicing various cognitive and behavioral strategies
Behavior activation	Scheduling and engaging in meaningful activities
Review therapy session or prepare for the next session	Keeping therapy notes, creating an agenda

Homework

Check each assignment when completed.

1. Read pamphlet about depression.
2. Each day of weekend, read TIC and TOC and affirmation created in OT session.
3. Schedule and do three activities before Monday:
   Physical exercise: Go for a walk
   Social support: Call sister
   Calming activity: Color a picture
4. Keep a record of when you do each activity and list thoughts and feelings before and after doing each activity.
5. Bring record of activities, thoughts, and feelings to next session.

FIGURE 8-11. Example of homework assignments to test task-oriented cognition.

collaborated in completing the TIC-TOC technique related to their belief (see Fig. 8-7). The person also created an affirmation they could refer to when feeling discouraged about themself (see Fig. 8-8). Then, the person and the OTP collaboratively planned several homework assignments to test the TOC that trying to do some things the person used to do wouldn't make things worse and might even help them feel better. The person wrote the homework in a notebook, as Figure 8-11 illustrates.

The next step in this person's intervention program would involve a collaborative review of their homework with the OTP as the basis for setting the agenda for the next therapy session.

Other Assessment and Intervention Considerations

Thus far, the selection of intervention methods that integrate behavioral, social learning, and cognitive strategies that meet the person's needs and abilities has been recommended to ensure optimal intervention outcomes related to cognitive beliefs and occupational performance. However, in taking the specific needs and abilities of individuals into account, two additional person factor considerations may impact the selection of intervention methods: the metacognitive demands of belief-oriented strategies and cultural differences and norms regarding beliefs, emotions, and behavior.

Metacognitive Demands of CBT

Cognitive restructuring strategies and techniques that directly target cognitive beliefs require various **metacognitive reasoning abilities**, such as the ability to reflect on one's thinking, identify and evaluate the validity of one's beliefs, differentiate between beliefs and reality, and grasp the critical influence of beliefs on feelings and behavior. However, when individuals have temporary or permanent metacognitive limitations or impairments, they may find the cognitive restructuring methods of traditional CBT overwhelming or excessively demanding of time and effort. When people are experiencing psychosis, changing or challenging thoughts during psychotic episodes may be ineffective and may even increase paranoia. Using behavioral and social cognitive strategies may be more appropriate for these individuals than cognitive restructuring strategies. ACT-based approaches may be a better fit for situations where thoughts cannot be challenged or changed, such as when individuals are experiencing psychosis or may have impaired metacognitive reasoning abilities (Gaudiano et al., 2020).

In addition, some cognitive behavior therapists recommend emphasizing behavioral strategies early in therapy with more severely symptomatic persons, such as those with intense depression, bipolar symptoms, or schizophrenia (Kingdon & Turkington, 2005). These recommendations are also suggested for mental health professionals working with children (Crawley et al., 2010) and adults with temporary or permanent cognitive limitations (Dagnan et al., 2007; Duncombe, 2005).

Culture, Cognitive Beliefs, and Belief-Oriented Approaches

Hays and Iwamasa (2006), the editors of *Culturally Responsive Cognitive Behavioral Therapy,* point out that CBT research and clinical applications have focused primarily on European American perspectives and assumptions. They recognize that CBT's nonjudgmental focus on strengths and an educational approach, as well as awareness of the importance of social context, support the appropriateness of CBT for people of diverse cultural identities. Their publication focuses on the applicability, limitations, and "use of CBT with ethnic cultures, including people of Native, Latino, Asian, and African American heritage, as well as people of Arab and Orthodox Jewish heritage." In this valuable resource, they also "address the use of CBT with people of non-ethnic minority groups: older adults, people with disabilities, and sexual minorities" (p. 13).

ACT is a pragmatic, experiential, and collaborative approach based on connecting people to their values. Because values are flexible, diverse, and identified by the person, ACT interventions allow for culturally adaptable modifications. ACT literature shows evidence of culturally adapted ACT interventions with positive outcomes (Woidneck et al., 2012). A comprehensive review of published ACT outcome research demonstrates that ACT has been implemented and researched across multiple countries worldwide and with diverse populations, suggesting that ACT is effective among diverse groups (Woidneck et al., 2012).

In particular, **acculturation**, the process of adopting another group's cultural traits or social patterns, is an essential construct concerning the psychological functioning of immigrants and ethnic minorities (Tanaka-Matsumi et al., 2002). Information about the person's language(s), social supports, and participation in ethnic and cultural activities provides important data regarding the possible relationship between cultural adjustment difficulties, presenting problems, traditions, and beliefs. Pride in one's cultural identity; culture-specific beliefs that help one cope, such as healing rituals; and cultural icons, which can serve as role models, may offer critical perspectives and support for reframing beliefs to be more adaptive.

Ultimately, the greater the OTP's knowledge of the person's cultural definitions of beliefs, emotions, and behavior; what makes a belief irrational or rational, inappropriate or appropriate, or maladaptive or adaptive; and the cultural norms regarding change strategies and the change agents, the more accurate and useful assessment and intervention will be (Okazaki & Tanaka-Matsumi, 2006; Pantalone et al., 2009). OTPs must continue to move toward a practice of cultural humility when utilizing belief-oriented approaches.

Here's the Point

- Cognitive beliefs about oneself, other people, the world, and the future are part of the content of a person's internal cognitive processes and are often held to be true by the believer.

- Cognitive beliefs develop beginning in early childhood and are viewed as a continuum of overlapping layers that range from surface thoughts to intermediate rules for living to deep core beliefs or schema.
- Cognitive beliefs are dynamically interrelated with emotions, physiological states, behavior, and social environments and contexts.
- Distortions in how persons perceive, appraise, and process information about themselves and the environment lead to dysfunctional beliefs that can be self-fulfilling.
- Dysfunctional beliefs and the struggle with those beliefs are associated with psychiatric conditions and psychological problems and often interfere with rehabilitation and recovery.
- CBT, an umbrella term for several evidence-based approaches, offers assessment and intervention strategies for addressing cognitive beliefs compatible with occupational therapy practice in mental health.
- ACT, a newer form of CBT, seeks to increase psychological flexibility by changing an individual's relationship with their unhelpful thoughts and feelings; its core processes are compatible with occupational therapy practice in mental health.
- Belief-oriented CBT approaches typically integrate cognitive, behavioral, and social cognitive intervention methods because they work synergistically to most effectively achieve outcomes related to cognitive content, specifically cognitive beliefs.
- Evidence suggests that regardless of method, for CBT to be an effective intervention for reframing dysfunctional cognitive beliefs to be more adaptive, outcomes need to reflect observable changes in behavior and cognition.
- Occupational therapy assessment should include an assessment of persons' cognitive beliefs to evaluate how they support or interfere with persons' mental health, occupational performance, and participation needs and desires.
- Belief-oriented intervention approaches typically focus on restructuring the content of cognitions, such as thoughts, attitudes, and beliefs; or on acquiring cognitive skills, such as coping skills or psychological flexibility; or on developing problem-solving strategies.
- OTPs can use numerous evidence-based belief-oriented CBT and ACT interventions to target cognitive beliefs and help individuals experiencing psychological distress achieve desired occupational performance and participation outcomes across diagnoses and practice settings.

Apply It Now

1. Application of Martha's Lived Experience

Reread The Lived Experience feature concerning Martha. Divide a piece of paper into three columns with the following headings:

Dysfunctional Beliefs	Functional Beliefs	Impact on Occupational Performance Behavior

List Martha's dysfunctional beliefs in the first column and then list how she restructured those beliefs to be more adaptive in the middle column. In the third column, describe how restructuring each belief impacted her occupational performance and participation goals.

Next, divide a piece of paper into three columns with the following headings:

Cognitive	Behavioral	Social Cognitive

List the cognitive, behavioral, and social cognitive methods Martha identified as useful for modifying and self-managing her dysfunctional cognitive beliefs and achieving her desired occupational performance and participation outcomes.

2. Personal Reflection

Reflect on a situation in which empowering thoughts and beliefs have given you the strength and courage to accomplish an important task or goal. Then, reflect again, this time selecting a situation when worry, procrastination, self-criticism, or other negative self-talk affected your mood and derailed you from achieving your goal.

Reflective Questions

■ Describe the thoughts that were associated with each situation. What thoughts and beliefs supported or interfered with working toward and achieving your goal?
■ What environmental or performance factors helped or hindered you? What people and skills supported you or interfered with the process? Were there other environmental supports or barriers, such as finances, scheduling, or geography?
■ What intervention(s) provided in this chapter to address unhelpful thoughts and feelings are you interested in trying and why?

3. Practice Using CBT Strategies and Techniques

Based on the problematic situation you reflected on previously or another situation of your choosing, try out several of the cognitive, behavioral, and social cognitive methods described in the intervention section for identifying and restructuring dysfunctional beliefs (e.g., thought record, ABC method, TIC-TOC technique, behavioral experiments, activity scheduling, affirmations).

Reflective Questions

■ How did the method(s) facilitate or hinder your understanding of the beliefs and thoughts that affect your feelings and behavior related to the situation?

■ What do you think it would take for you to change your problematic belief? What are the challenges involved?
■ Restructure your belief(s) to support you more appropriately in a challenging situation.

4. Practice Using ACT Strategies and Techniques

Based on the problematic situation you reflected on previously or another situation of your choosing, try out several of the ACT interventions described in the intervention section to increase psychological flexibility (e.g., cognitive defusion techniques, contacting the present moment, dropping your anchor, Choice Point).

Reflective Questions

■ How did the method(s) facilitate or hinder your understanding of the beliefs and thoughts that affect your feelings and behavior related to the situation?
■ What do you think it would take for you to implement these strategies in your daily life? What are the challenges involved?
■ Identify what strategies you can use to "drop your anchor" and acknowledge your thoughts and feelings, come back into your body, and engage in the world when caught up in an emotional storm.

5. Practical Application

Select a person in your fieldwork diagnosed with depression, anxiety, or another condition for which evidence supports using CBT or ACT interventions. Read about this condition and how belief-oriented theories have been applied to understand the condition and intervention.

Reflective Questions

■ What insights have you gained about this person because of your reading?
■ How would you enhance or alter your occupational therapy intervention with this person using belief-oriented interventions based on this information?

Resources

Organizations With Books, Audiovisual, and Other Resources and Courses

- The Albert Ellis Institute provides training and resources for REBT: www.rebt.org
- The Beck Institute for Cognitive Therapy and Research provides training and resources for CBT: https://beckinstitute.org
- The British Association for Behavioural and Cognitive Psychotherapies provides training and resources for CBT: www.babcp.com
- Dr. Pat Deegan shares her inspiring story about how she found a way out of her despairing and hopeless beliefs about her life and went on to become a leading force in the recovery and disability rights movement; visit her blog at: https://www.patdeegan.com
- Dr. Russ Harris shares free audio clips, videos, articles, worksheets, handouts, and workshops, and hosts ACT interest groups on his website: www.actmindfully.com.au
- The Association for Contextual Behavioral Science provides training and resources for ACT: www.contextualscience.org

- Psychwire provides a platform to ask questions and take courses from world-leading experts in behavioral science, including CBT, ACT, motivational interviewing, and more: www.psychwire.com

Workbooks

- There are numerous resources available with cognitive behavior exercises that can be adapted for belief-oriented occupational therapy interventions. Following is a sampling of these resources:
  - Bourne, E. J. (2020). *The anxiety and phobia workbook* (7th ed.). New Harbinger Publications, Inc.
  - Burns, D. B. (1999). *Ten days to self-esteem.* HarperCollins.
  - Clark, D. A., & Beck, A. (2012). *The anxiety and worry workbook: The cognitive behavioral solution.* Guilford Press.
  - Forsyth, J. P. (2016). *The mindfulness and acceptance workbook for anxiety: A guide to breaking free from anxiety, phobias, and worry using Acceptance and Commitment Therapy* (2nd ed.). New Harbinger Publications, Inc.
  - Greenberger, D., & Padesky, C. A. (2016). *Mind over mood: Change how you feel by changing the way you think* (2nd ed.). Guilford Press.

- Knaus, W. J., & Ellis, A. (2012). *The cognitive behavioral workbook for depression: A step by step program* (2nd ed.). New Harbinger Publications, Inc.
- McKay, M., Davis, M., & Fanning, P. (2007). *Thoughts and feelings: Taking control of your moods and your life.* New Harbinger Publications, Inc.
- McKay, M., Greenberg, M., & Fanning, P. (2020). *The ACT workbook for depression and shame: Overcome thoughts of defectiveness and increase well-being using Acceptance and Commitment Therapy.* New Harbinger Publications, Inc.
- Stallard, P. (2002). *Think good and feel good: A cognitive behavioral therapy workbook for children.* John Wiley & Sons.
- Suro, G. (2019). *Learning to thrive: An Acceptance and Commitment Therapy workbook.* Rockridge Press.

Books

- Beck, J. S. (2011). *Cognitive behavior therapy: Basics and beyond* (2nd ed.). Guilford Press.
- Black, T. D. (2022). *ACT for treating children: The essential guide to Acceptance and Commitment Therapy for kids.* New Harbinger Publications, Inc.
- Dobson, K. S. (2010). *Handbook of cognitive-behavioral therapies* (3rd ed.). Guilford Press.
- Hayes, S. C. (2005). *Get out of your mind and into your life: The new Acceptance and Commitment Therapy.* New Harbinger Publications, Inc.
- Hayes, S. C., Strosahl, K. D., & Wilson, K. G. (2012). *Acceptance and Commitment Therapy: The process and practice of mindful change* (2nd ed.). Guildford Press.
- Harris, R. (2008). *The happiness trap: How to stop struggling and start living.* Trumpeter Books.
- Harris, R. (2019). *ACT made simple: An easy-to-read primer on Acceptance and Commitment Therapy* (2nd ed.). New Harbinger Publications, Inc.
- Harris, R. (Ed.). (2021). *Trauma-focused ACT: A practitioner's guide to working with mind, body, and emotion using Acceptance and Commitment Therapy.* Context Press.

References

American Occupational Therapy Association. (2020). Occupational therapy practice framework: Domain and process (4th ed.). *American Journal of Occupational Therapy, 74*(Suppl. 2), 7412410010. https://doi.org/10.5014/ajot.2020.74S2001

American Occupational Therapy Association. (2022). Role of occupational therapy in pain management. *American Journal of Occupational Therapy, 75*(Suppl. 3), 7513410010. https://doi.org/10.5014/ajot.2021.75S3001

Asghari, A., & Nicholas, M. K. (2001). Pain self-efficacy beliefs and pain behaviour: A prospective study. *Pain, 94,* 85–100. https://doi.org/10.1016/S0304-3959(01)00344-x

Atler, K., Eakman, E., & Orsi, B. (2015). Enhancing construct validity evidence of the Daily Experiences of Pleasure, Productivity, and Restoration Profile. *Journal of Occupational Science, 23*(2), 278–290. https://doi.org/10.1080/14427591.2015.1080625

Atwood, M., & Friedman, A. (2019). A systematic review of enhanced cognitive behavioral therapy (CBT-E) for eating disorders. *International Journal of Eating Disorders, 53*(3), 311–330. https://doi.org/10.1002/eat.23206

Bandura, A. (1981). Self-referent thought: A developmental analysis of self-efficacy. In J. H. Flavell & L. Ross (Eds.), *Social cognitive development: Frontiers and possible futures* (pp. 200–239). Cambridge University Press.

Bandura, A. (1986). *Social foundations of thought and action: A social cognitive theory.* Prentice Hall.

Bandura, A. (1997). *Self-efficacy: The exercise of control.* W.H. Freeman.

Bandura, A. (2006). Guide for constructing self-efficacy scales. In F. Pajares & T. Urdan, *Self-efficacy beliefs of adolescents* (pp. 307–337). Information Age Publishing.

Beck, A. T. (1967). *Depression: Causes and treatment.* University of Pennsylvania Press.

Beck, A. T. (1976). *Cognitive therapy and the emotional disorders* (4th ed.). International University Press.

Beck, A. T. (2005). The current state of cognitive therapy: A 40-year retrospective. *Archives of General Psychiatry, 62,* 953–959. https://doi.org/10.1001/archpsyc.62.9.953

Beck, A. T., Wright, F. D., Newman, C. F., & Liese, B. S. (1993). *Cognitive therapy of substance abuse.* Guilford Press.

Beck, J. S. (2011). *Cognitive behavior therapy: Basics and beyond* (2nd ed.). Guilford Press.

Bond, F. W., Hayes, S. C., Baer, R. A., Carpenter, K. M., Guenole, N., Orcutt, H. K., Waltz, T., & Zettle, R. D. (2011). Preliminary psychometric properties of the Acceptance and Action Questionnaire–II: A revised measure of psychological inflexibility and experiential avoidance. *Behavior Therapy, 42,* 676–688. https://doi.org/10.1016/j.beth.2011.03.007

Burns, D. D. (1993). *Ten days to self-esteem.* HarperCollins.

Callaghan, G. M., Sandoz, E. K., Darrow, S. M., & Feeney, T. K. (2015). The Body Image Psychological Inflexibility Scale: Development and psychometric properties. *Psychiatry Research, 226*(1), 45–52. https://doi.org/10.1016/j.psychres.2014.11.039

Chiang, K. J., Tsai, J. C., Liu, D., Lin, C. H., Chiu, H. L., & Chou, K. R. (2017). Efficacy of cognitive-behavioral therapy in patients with bipolar disorder: A meta-analysis of randomized controlled trials. *PloS One, 12*(5), e0176849. https://doi.org/10.1371/journal.pone.0176849

Ciarrochi, J., Bailey, A., & Harris, R. (2014). *The weight escape: How to stop dieting and start living.* Shambhala Publications.

Clarke, S., Kingston, J., Wilson, K. G., Bolderston, H., & Remington, B. (2012). Acceptance and Commitment Therapy for a heterogeneous group of treatment-resistant clients: A treatment development study. *Cognitive and Behavioral Practice, 19*(4), 560–572. https://doi.org/10.1016/j.cbpra.2012.03.001

Cohen, J. S., Edmund, J. M., Brodman, D., & Kendall, P. C. (2013). Using self-monitoring: Implementation of collaborative empiricism in cognitive-behavioral therapy. *Cognitive and Behavioral Practice, 20*(4), 419–428. https://doi.org/10.1016/j.cbpra.2012.06.002

Copeland, M. E. (2011). *The Wellness Recovery Action Plan* (5th ed.). Peach Press Inc.

Corrigan, P., Druss, B., & Perlick, A. (2014). The impact of mental illness stigma on seeking and participating in mental health care. *Psychological Science and Public Interest, 15*(2), 37–70. https://doi.org/10.1177/1529100614531398

Crawley, S. A., Podell, J. L., Beidas, R. S., Braswell, L., & Kendall, P. C. (2010). Cognitive-behavioral therapy with youth. In K. S. Dobson (Ed.), *Handbook of cognitive-behavioral therapies* (3rd ed., pp. 375–410). Guilford Press.

Cuijpers, P., Berking, M., Andersson, G., Quigley, L., Kleiboer, A., & Dobson, K. S. (2013). A meta-analysis of cognitive-behavioural therapy for adult depression, alone and in comparison with other treatments. *Canadian Journal of Psychiatry, 58*(7), 376–385. https://doi.org/ 10.1177/070674371305800702

Cusack, K., Jonas, D. E., Forneris, C. A., Wines, C., Sonis, J., Middleton, J. C., Feltner, C., Brownley, K. A., Olmsted, K. R., Greenblatt, A., Weil, A., & Gaynes, B. N. (2016). Psychological treatments for adults with posttraumatic stress disorder: A systematic review and meta-analysis. *Clinical Psychology Review, 43,* 128–141. https://doi.org/10.1016/j.cpr.2015.10.003

Dagnan, D., Jahoda, A., & Kroese, B. S. (2007). Psychosocial interventions for persons with intellectual disabilities and mental ill-health. *Current Opinion in Psychiatry, 20*(5), 456–461. https://doi.org/10.1097/YCO.0b013e3282ab9963

Dobson, K. S., & Dozois, D. J. (2010). Historical and philosophical bases of the cognitive-behavioral therapies. In K. S. Dobson (Ed.), *Handbook of cognitive-behavioral therapies* (3rd ed., pp. 3–38). Guilford Press.

Duncombe, L. (2005). The cognitive-behavioral model in mental health. In N. Katz (Ed.), *Cognition and occupation across the life span: Models for intervention in occupational therapy* (2nd ed., pp. 187–80). AOTA Press.

Dunkley, D. M., Blankstein, K. R., & Segal, Z. V. (2010). Cognitive assessment: Issues and methods. In K. S. Dobson (Ed.), *Handbook of cognitive-behavioral therapies* (3rd ed., pp. 133–171). Guilford Press.

Ellis, A. (1962). *Reason and emotion in psychotherapy.* Lyle Stuart.

Ellis, A. (1994). *Reason and emotion in psychotherapy, revised and updated.* Carol Publishing Group.

Fordham, B., Sugavanam, T., Edwards, K., Stallard, P., Howard, R., das Nair, R., Copsey, B., Lee, H., Howick, J., Hemming, K., & Lamb, S. E. (2021). The evidence for cognitive behavioural therapy in any condition, population or context: A meta-review of systematic reviews and panoramic meta-analysis. *Psychological Medicine, 51*(1), 8–29. https://doi.org/10.1017/S0033291720005292

Friedman, E. S., Thase, M. E., & Wright, J. H. (2008). Cognitive and behavioral therapies. In A. Tasman, J. Kay, J. A. Lieberman, M. B. First, & M. Maj, *Psychiatry* (3rd ed., pp. 1920–1947). John Wiley & Sons, Ltd.

Gage, M., Noh, S., Polatajko, H. J., & Kaspar, B. (1994). Measuring perceived self efficacy in occupational therapy. *American Journal of Occupational Therapy, 48,* 783–790. https://doi.org/10.5014/ajot.48.9.783

Gage, M., & Polatajko, H. (1994). Enhancing occupational performance through an understanding of perceived self-efficacy. *American Journal of Occupational Therapy, 48,* 452–461. https://doi.org/10.5014/ajot.48.5.452

Gámez, W., Chmielewski, M., Kotov, R., Ruggero, C., Suzuki, N., & Watson, D. (2014). The Brief Experiential Avoidance Questionnaire: Development and initial validation. *Psychological Assessment, 26*(1), 35–45. https://doi.org/10.1037/a0034473

Gaudiano, B., Zamor, A., Ostrove, B., & Hill, J. (2020). *Acceptance and Commitment Therapy for occupational therapy practitioners* [Online course]. AOTA Continuing Education.

Gloster, A. T., Walder, N., Levin, M. E., Twohig, M. P., & Karekla, M. (2020). The empirical status of Acceptance and Commitment Therapy: A review of meta-analyses. *Journal of Contextual Behavioral Science, 18,* 181–192. https://doi.org/10.1016/j.jcbs.2020.09.009

Greenberger, D., & Padesky, C. A. (2016). *Mind over mood* (2nd ed.). Guilford Press.

Harris, R. (2006). Embracing your demons: An overview of Acceptance and Commitment Therapy. *Psychotherapy in Australia, 12*(4), 2–8.

Harris, R. (2017). The Choice Point 2.0: A brief overview. ACT-Mindfully. https://www.actmindfully.com.au/free-stuff/worksheets-handouts-book-chapters

Harris, R. (2019). *ACT made simple: An easy-to-read primer on Acceptance and Commitment Therapy* (2nd ed.). New Harbinger Publications, Inc.

Hayes, S. C. (2016). Acceptance and Commitment Therapy, Relational Frame Theory, and the third wave of behavioral and cognitive therapies—Republished article. *Behavior Therapy, 47*(6), 869–885. https://doi.org/10.1016/j.beth.2016.11.006

Hayes, S. C., & Duckworth, M. P. (2006). Acceptance and Commitment Therapy and traditional cognitive behavior therapy approaches to pain. *Cognitive and Behavioral Practice, 13,* 185–187. https://doi.org/10.1016/j.cbpra.2006.04.002

Hayes, S. C., Levin, M. E., Plumb-Vilardaga, J., Villatte, J. L., & Pistorello, J. (2013). Acceptance and Commitment Therapy and contextual behavioral science: Examining the progress of a distinctive model of behavioral and cognitive therapy. *Behavior Therapy, 44*(2), 180–198. https://doi.org/10.1016/j.beth.2009.08.002

Hayes, S. C., Luoma, J. B., Bond, F. W., Masuda, A., & Lillis, J. (2006). Acceptance and Commitment Therapy: model, processes and outcomes. *Behaviour Research and Therapy, 44*(1), 1–25. https://doi.org/10.1016/j.brat.2005.06.006

Hayes, S. C., Strosahl, K. D., & Wilson, K. G. (1999). *Acceptance and Commitment Therapy: An experiential approach to behavior change.* Guilford Press.

Hayes, S. C., Strosahl, K. D., & Wilson, K. G. (2012). *Acceptance and Commitment Therapy: The process and practice of mindful change.* Guilford Press.

Hays, P. A., & Iwamasa, G. Y. (Eds.). (2006). *Culturally responsive cognitive-behavioral therapy: Assessment, practice, and supervision.* American Psychological Association.

Hofmann, S. G., Asnaani, A., Vonk, I., Sawyer, A. T., & Fang, A. (2012). The efficacy of cognitive behavioral therapy: A review of meta-analyses. *Cognitive Therapy Research, 36*(5), 427–440. https://doi.org/10.1007/s10608-012-9476-1

Jauhar, S., McKenna, P. J., Radua, J., Fung, E., Salvador, R., & Laws, K. R. (2014). Cognitive-behavioural therapy for the symptoms of schizophrenia: Systematic review and meta-analysis with examination of potential bias. *British Journal of Psychiatry, 204,* 20–29. https://doi.org/ 10.1192/bjp.bp.112.116285

Kaczkurkin, A. N., & Foa, E. B. (2015). Cognitive-behavioral therapy for anxiety disorders: An update on empirical evidence. *Dialogues in Clinical Neuroscience, 17*(3), 337–346. https://doi.org/10.31887/DCNS.2015.17.3/akaczkurkin

Kingdon, D. G., & Turkington, D. (2005). *Cognitive therapy of schizophrenia.* Guilford Press.

Law, M., Baptiste, S., Carswell, A., McColl, M. A., Polatajko, H., & Pollock, N. (2005). *Canadian Occupational Performance Measure* (4th ed.). Canadian Association of Occupational Therapists.

Levin, M. E., Hildebrandt, M. J., Lillis, J., & Hayes, S. C. (2012). The impact of treatment components suggested by the psychological flexibility model: A meta-analysis of laboratory-based component studies. *Behavior Therapy, 43*(4), 741–756. https://doi.org/10.1016/j.beth.2012.05.003

Lukens, E. B., & McFarlane, W. F. (2004). Psychoeducation as evidence-based practice: Considerations for practice, research, and policy. *Brief Treatment and Crisis Intervention, 4*(3), 205–225. https://doi.org/10.1093/brief-treatment/mhh019

Lysaker, P. H., Davis, L. W., Bryson, G. J., & Bell, M. D. (2009). Effects of cognitive behavior therapy on work outcomes in vocational rehabilitation for participants with schizophrenia spectrum disorders. *Schizophrenia Research, 107*(2-3), 186–191. https://doi.org/10.1016/j.schres.2008.10.018

Madon, S., Willard, J., Guyll, M., & Scherr, K. C. (2011). Self-fulfilling prophecies: Mechanisms, power, and links to social problems. *Social and Personality Psychology Compass, 5,* 578–590. https://doi.org/10.1111/j.1751-9004.2011.00375.x

Martell, C. R., Dimidjian, S., & Herman-Dunn, R. (2010). *Behavioral activation for depression: A clinician's guide.* Guilford Press.

McCraken, L. M., Vowles, K. E., & Eccleston, C. (2004). Acceptance of chronic pain: Component analysis and a revised assessment method. *Pain, 107,* 159–166. https://doi.org/10.1016/j.pain.2003.10.012

McHugh, R. K., Hearon, B. A., & Otto, M. W. (2010). Cognitive-behavioral therapy for substance use disorders. *Psychiatric Clinics of North America, 33*(3), 511–525. https://doi.org/10.1016/j.psc.2010.04.012

McManus, F., Van Doorn, K., & Yiend, J. (2012). Examining the effects of thought records and behavioral experiments in instigating belief change. *Journal of Behavior Therapy and Experimental Psychiatry, 43*(1), 540–547. https://doi.org/10.1016/j.jbtep.2011.07.003

Murphy, R., Straebler, S., Cooper, Z., & Fairburn, C. G. (2010). Cognitive behavioral therapy for eating disorders. *Psychiatric Clinics of North America, 33*(3), 611–627. https://doi.org/10.1016/j.psc.2010.04.004

Nicholas, M. K. (2007). The Pain Self-Efficacy Questionnaire: Taking pain into account. *European Journal of Pain, 11*(2), 153–163. https://doi.org/10.1016/j.ejpain.2005.12.008

Okazaki, S., & Tanaka-Matsumi, J. (2006). Cultural considerations in cognitive-behavioral assessment. In P. A. Hays & G. Y. Iwamasa (Eds.), *Culturally responsive cognitive-behavioral therapy: Assessment, practice, and supervision* (pp. 247–266). American Psychological Association.

Oud, M., de Winter, L., Vermeulen-Smit, E., Bodden, D., Nauta, M., Stone, L., van den Heuvel, M., Taher, R. A., de Graaf, I., Kendall, T., Engels, R., & Stikkelbroek, Y. (2019). Effectiveness of CBT for children and adolescents with depression: A systematic review and meta-regression analysis. *European Psychiatry, 57,* 33–45. https://doi.org/10.1016/j.eurpsy.2018.12.008

Padesky, C. (1993). *Socratic questioning: Changing minds or guided discovery? (Keynote address).* European Congress of Behavioural and Cognitive Therapies, September 24, London, England. Retrieved from https://padesky.com/wp-content/uploads/2012/11/socquest.pdf

Pantalone, D. W., Iwamasa, G. Y., & Martell, C. R. (2009). Adapting cognitive-behavioral therapies to diverse populations. In K. S. Dobson (Ed.), *Handbook of cognitive behavioral therapies* (3rd ed., pp. 445–464). Guilford Press.

Pegg, S., Hill, K., Argiros, A., Olatunji, B., & Kujawa, A. (2022). Cognitive behavioral therapy for anxiety disorders in youth: Efficacy, moderators, and new advances in predicting outcomes. *Current Psychiatry Reports, 24,* 853–859. https://doi.org/10.1007/s11920-022-01384-7

Rider, J., & Smith, K. (2023). Persistent pain. In S. Dahl-Polizio, K. Smith, M. Day, S. Muir, & W. Manard, *Primary care occupational therapy: A quick reference guide* (pp. 387–400). Springer Publishing Company.

Rider, J. V., & Tay, M. C. (2022). Increasing occupational engagement by addressing psychosocial and occupational factors of chronic pain: A case report. *The Open Journal of Occupational Therapy, 10*(3), 1–12. https://doi.org/10.15453/2168-6408.2027

Rolffs, J. L., Rogge, R. D., & Wilson, K. G. (2018). Disentangling components of flexibility via the Hexaflex model: Development and validation of the multidimensional psychological flexibility inventory (MPFI). *Assessment, 25*(4), 458–482. https://doi.org/10.1177/1073191116645905

Rosenfeld, M. A. (Ed.). (1997). *Motivational strategies in geriatric rehabilitation.* American Occupational Therapy Association.

Substance Abuse and Mental Health Services Administration. (2014). *Trauma-informed care in behavioral health services.* Author.

Swain, J., Hancock, K., Dixon, A., & Bowman, J. (2015). Acceptance and Commitment Therapy for children: A systematic review of intervention studies. *Journal of Contextual Behavioral Science, 4*(2), 73–85. https://doi.org/10.1016/j.jcbs.2015.02.001

Swartz, H. A., & Swanson, J. (2014). Psychotherapy for bipolar disorder in adults: A review of the evidence. *Focus (American Psychiatric Association Publication), 12*(3), 251–266. https://doi.org/10.1176/appi.focus.12.3.251

Tanaka-Matsumi, J., Higginbotham, H. N., & Chang, R. (2002). Cognitive-behavioral approaches to counseling across cultures: A functional analytic approach for clinical applications. In P. B. Pedersen, W. J. Lonner, J. G. Draguns, & J. E. Trimble (Eds.), *Counseling across cultures* (5th ed., pp. 337–354). SAGE.

Thompson, B. (2013). Occupational therapy's ACTions: Using ACT within occupational therapy for people with chronic pain. *Ngau Mamae: New Zealand Pain Society,* 4–10.

Twohig, M. P., & Levin, M. E. (2017). Acceptance and Commitment Therapy as a treatment for anxiety and depression: A review. *The Psychiatric Clinics of North America, 40*(4), 751–770. https://doi.org/10.1016/j.psc.2017.08.009

van Huet, H., & Williams, D. (2007). Self-beliefs about pain and occupational performance: A comparison of two measures used in a pain management program. *Occupational Therapy Journal of Research: Occupation, Participation, and Health, 27*(1), 4–12. https://doi.org/10.1177/153944920702700102

Watkins, L. E., Sprang, K. R., & Rothbaum, B. O. (2018). Treating PTSD: A review of evidence-based psychotherapy interventions. *Frontiers in Behavioral Neuroscience, 12,* 258. https://doi.org/10.3389/fnbeh.2018.00258

Weinberg, R. S., & Gould, D. (2015). *Foundations of sport and exercise psychology* (6th ed.). Human Kinetics.

White, R., Gumley, A., McTaggart, J., Rattrie, L., McConville, D., Cleare, S., & Mitchell, G. (2011). A feasibility study of Acceptance and Commitment Therapy for emotional dysfunction following psychosis. *Behaviour Research and Therapy, 49*(12), 901–907. https://doi.org/10.1016/j.brat.2011.09.003

Wicksell, R. K., Lekander, M., Sorjonen, K., & Olsson, G. L. (2010). The Psychological Inflexibility in Pain Scale (PIPS)—Statistical properties and model fit of an instrument to assess change processes in pain related disability. *European Journal of Pain, 14*(7), 771.e1–771.e7714. https://doi.org/10.1016/j.ejpain.2009.11.015

Woidneck, M. R., Pratt, K. M., Gundy, J. M., Nelson C. R., & Twohig, M. P. (2012). Exploring cultural competence in Acceptance and Commitment Therapy outcomes. *Professional Psychology: Research and Practice, 43*(3), 227–233. https://doi.org/10.1037/a0026235

World Health Organization. (2001). *International classification of functioning, disability and health (ICF).* Author.

Wright, J., Thase, M., Ludgate, J., & Beck, A. T. (1993). The cognitive milieu: Structure and process. In J. Wright, M. Thase, J. Ludgate, & A. T. Beck, *Cognitive therapy with inpatients: Developing a cognitive milieu* (pp. 61–87). Guilford Press.

Sensory Processing and the Lived Sensory Experience

Antoine Bailliard, Ben Lee, and Valerie Fox

Barb and Joan are friends who like to go to the same exercise class; however, when they get to the gym they position themselves in different corners of the room. Barb likes to be in a spot where a large fan blows directly on her, whereas Joan locates herself where she can't feel the wind from any of the fans in the room.

Two children, Joshua and Aaron, attend the same preschool. Joshua digs right into the finger paints, play dough, and mud piles outside, whereas Aaron dislikes getting his hands dirty. He really enjoys the building blocks and puzzles at the school.

Allison and Sarah are college roommates. Allison likes to stay in the busy dormitory and study in the room with the radio playing or the TV turned on. Sarah finds this too distracting and has found a quiet study room in the library.

These individuals are all successfully engaging in important occupations, but their preferences and ways of expressing their occupations differ, in part because they have different sensory systems and sensory habits that create a different relationship with the world. Most people intuitively choose activities and modify their environments to support their sensory preferences without thinking about it. However, people's sensory preferences for seeing, smelling, and hearing significantly affect what they do in their daily lives and how they feel about those activities.

Sometimes individuals have sensory processing systems or sensory habits that do not match the demands of their sensory environments and have difficulty in adjusting their actions or environments to improve the match. When a person is not able to adjust their environment to accommodate their sensory preferences and support their participation in occupation, they may experience a restriction in their occupational participation. In these situations, occupational therapy practitioners (OTPs) can use their knowledge about sensory processing and the lived sensory experience to design interventions that support individuals to engage in important occupations, regardless of their sensory preferences or sensory health.

The purpose of this chapter is to describe how sensory processing and the lived sensory experience affect the occupations of people with mental illness and occupational therapy in mental health. The chapter begins with an overview of sensory processing and the lived sensory experience to introduce different perspectives for understanding how the senses are involved in occupational performance. Next, readers are introduced to the different sensory modalities, how atypical sensory processing can lead to disruptions in occupation, and how sensory processing is related to psychiatric conditions in children and adults. The chapter ends with an overview of occupational therapy assessment and intervention related to sensory processing and mental health.

Overview of Sensory Processing and the Lived Sensory Experience

Sensory processing and the **lived sensory experience** are two distinct ways of looking at how individuals use their senses to live in the world through their bodies. Traditional theories of sensory processing have been developed and expanded upon in the medical and biological fields and, therefore, embrace many biomechanical assumptions inherent to those fields. Theories regarding the lived sensory experience have also been developed and expanded upon in other fields such as anthropology, sociology, geography, and occupational science. Therefore, these theories about the lived sensory experience embrace a different worldview regarding how humans use their senses to operate in the world. Both views are complementary and important for OTPs to understand persons and when performing assessments and interventions that target a person's sensory health.

Sensory processing is conceptualized as a sequence of steps for obtaining information about the world and the body. Sensory processing involves multiple steps at both the neural and behavioral levels. It includes noticing a stimulus, recognizing or classifying the stimulus, and then understanding or giving meaning to the stimulus. After the stimulus is processed, a behavioral response can occur (Bagby et al., 2012). For example, when driving, a person may startle at a loud and unexpected auditory stimulus and respond by looking in the rearview mirror. After recognizing that the origin of the noise is an ambulance rapidly approaching from behind, the person then decides to let the ambulance pass and begins the process of pulling over to the side of the road.

Sensory processing is frequently described as a linear process; it begins with a sensory stimulus that is detected by sensory receptors, the peripheral ends of the nervous system. There are many different types of receptors that capture different types of sensory information. For example, chemoreceptors detect chemicals in the environment and are used in taste and smell, whereas mechanoreceptors detect changes in pressure, position, and acceleration and are used in vestibular and proprioceptive perception (explained in the text that follows). Sensory receptors (e.g., chemoreceptors, mechanoreceptors) are concentrated on sensory organs (e.g., taste buds of the tongue).

When a neural receptor is stimulated, it fires an electric impulse. When the stimulus is strong (e.g., loud noises, bright lights, intense flavors), neurons tend to respond with more intensity (e.g., more respond, for longer, with higher frequency). The increased intensity of neural sensory activity is more likely to rise to the level of a person's conscious awareness (i.e., they are more likely to notice the stimulus because of a more significant neuronal response). A weak stimulus results in impulses that are slower, shorter in duration, or involve fewer receptors. Such stimuli are less likely to be noticed by people because they cause low intensity neural activity.

There is tremendous variability among people's sensory capacities. Receptor sensitivities vary significantly between sensory systems and among individuals based on each person's unique threshold for detecting specific stimuli. It is common for people to experience situations when one person notices a smell, sound, or visual stimulus that another person in the same situation does not detect. Humans demonstrate significant variability in their receptor sensitivities and sensory capacities without any detrimental impact to their health or participation in meaningful occupations. However, some individuals may respond too intensely (i.e., **hyperresponsive**) or too mildly (i.e., **hyporesponsive**) to their sensory environments, contributing to poor health and difficulties participating in meaningful or necessary occupations.

People's nervous systems are constantly active and in the process of coupling with their sensorial environments. The traditional stimulus-response paradigm tends to take those phases of action out of context from the real-world flow of everyday action and stimulation. People experience sensory stimuli as they are already engaged in the flow of daily occupations. They do not receive sensory stimuli passively in a vacuum devoid of other stimuli, meanings, and actions.

As the nervous system continuously couples with the dynamic sensorial environment, the body and brain recognize or classify stimuli that were encountered. For example, the pitch and volume of a sound are deciphered into human speech, or a chemical in the environment is translated by the olfactory bulb as the smell of coffee brewing. Once a stimulus is identified, individuals typically attribute meaning to that information (e.g., words are not just sounds but can tell a story or provide a warning) and assimilate that information into what they are doing at the time. The meanings people associate with their sensations contribute to the ongoing experiences of doing occupations and therefore affect the meanings of their occupations.

A person's behavioral response to a collection of stimuli is a complex reaction that occurs both consciously and unconsciously and usually includes cognitive and motor processing. For example, after smelling coffee, a person may consciously note the smell and react by seeking a mug and pouring themself a cup because it smells pleasurable. Conversely, people may reflect on their interoceptive state (explained in the text that follows) and decide that they have already had too much caffeine for the day and the smell does not seem as appealing to them.

Unconsciously, the lived experience of drinking the coffee is a complex intersection of stimuli with various meanings that generate a gestalt or whole lived sensory experience of drinking the coffee in that moment. Drinking the coffee in a travel mug in a classroom while listening to a lecture generates a very different lived experience of the sensory qualities of the coffee than drinking the same coffee in a hand-crafted mug while sitting on a tropical beach watching the sun rise. Lived sensory experiences are **polysensorial** (i.e., involve more than one sensation) and reflect a dynamic intersection of numerous stimuli that are mutually affecting the person's momentary experience of any singular stimulus (Bailliard et al., 2023).

OTPs are concerned with all aspects of sensory processing and the lived sensory experience because of their critical role in the performance of occupation. Although most of the activity involved in sensory processing occurs at the neural level, therapists infer what is happening in the nervous system based on behavioral observation (Lane et al., 2000) including how a person's lived sensory experience in the moment is affected by past sensory experiences and sociocultural factors from their occupational profile (e.g., past trauma, cultural traditions). It is important to recognize that inferences related to someone's lived sensory experience may be incorrect at times.

For example, if an individual stiffens and makes a disgusted face when receiving a hug, the therapist may interpret their response as tactile defensiveness, indicating the stimuli are too intense for them. However, this assumption may be incorrect; the individual could be responding this way because they may have previously experienced trauma or it may come at a time when sociocultural norms dictate it is inappropriate and it therefore feels wrong to the person. Indeed, sociocultural differences and different norms regarding what behaviors are acceptable can also have an impact on the lived sensory experience. Because there are so many reasons that could stimulate such a behavioral response, it is critical that OTPs engage in collaborative practices to explore those responses.

Understanding how neurological sensory systems, sensory habits, and sociocultural norms for expressing sensory needs combine to generate the lived sensory experience provides important information to guide occupational therapy assessment and intervention. It is therefore critical for therapists to go beyond biomedical understandings of sensory processing to also be mindful of life experiences and sociocultural backgrounds and their effect on sensory experiences during occupation.

Framework for Understanding the Lived Sensory Experience

The Sensory Health: A Relational and Embodied (SHARE) Framework for Occupation (Bailliard, 2022) complements the biomedical Model of Sensory Processing and provides OTPs with a framework for understanding how sociocultural and historical factors affect a person's lived sensory experiences. The framework proposes that people are born with biological systems and sensory capacities that are nurtured and/or extinguished as they develop through their sociocultural environments. A person's lived sensory experience in a moment is significantly influenced by their past experiences and the various environments they have lived through.

SHARE is a research-based framework that describes the lived sensory experiences as (a) selective and focused, (b) prereflective and habitual, (c) embodied and emplaced, (d) relational, (e) polysensorial, (f) aesthetic, and (g) political.

Selective and focused: Research has demonstrated that people are not passive recipients to sensory stimuli (Bailliard, 2013; Bailliard et al., 2023). Instead, people are active sensory beings who are already engaged with a sensory environment that is overflowing with stimuli and the body orients itself to different features of that sensory environment (Hass, 2008). For example, when hearing the ambulance siren in the previously noted example, the driver experienced the auditory stimulus differently than hearing the same stimulus when sitting in their office working.

Prereflective and habitual: As a person develops through their contexts, they acquire habits for sensing their environments (Bailliard, 2015). For example, as a child develops, their caregivers frequently orient their attention to different aspects of their environment (e.g., listening to bird sounds when walking in the woods) and the child becomes accustomed to attending to those sensory features over others (e.g., listening for birds when outside).

Embodied and emplaced: As a person repeatedly performs occupations in similar contexts, recurring sensory experiences become embodied as sensory expectations (Bailliard, 2013, 2015). The lived sensory experience is emplaced because a person relies on the presence of sensory anchors (i.e., sensations that inform the person an action is proceeding as intended; Bailliard, 2015; Bailliard et al., 2023) to perform occupations successfully. These sensory anchors connect a person's sensory capacities with the sensory environment. For example, a person walking on a treadmill will subconsciously monitor sensory anchors (e.g., the sensation of stepping correctly on the treadmill) while watching a television show to pass the time.

Relational: Sensory habits are often developed through participation in a social world. As a person develops through meaningful occupations with others, they learn to attune their sensory orientation with others (Bailliard et al., 2018). For example, people of different cultures develop different gustatory habits and preferences for foods based on participation in social occupations and rituals that repeatedly expose them to certain tastes.

Polysensorial: Sensory stimuli are never experienced in isolation. The meaning and experience of any particular stimulus is affected by the intersection of that stimulus with other stimuli the person experiences in that situation (Bailliard et al., 2023). For example, the smell of bleach may not be bothersome when cleaning, but it is very aversive when coupled with eating.

Aesthetic: Repeated sensory experiences that are coupled with affective memories can become embodied as aesthetic preferences and orientations to the world (Bailliard, 2013; 2015; Bailliard et al., 2023). For example, people often prefer meals prepared in ways they repeatedly experienced as children or prefer to perform occupations in ways they originally learned them. The lived sensory experience is aesthetic because it is imbued with feelings of how something should feel.

Political: Embodied sensory habits and sensory processing patterns can lead to the exclusion of people from meaningful occupations and built environments that assume a normative expectation for sensory processing (Bailliard, 2022). For example, a child who needs a lot of movement to self-regulate and stay focused on a task will be reprimanded and marginalized in classrooms that expect students to stay seated at their desks without movement for extended periods.

The seven tenets of the SHARE framework remind OTPs that the lived sensory experience is far more than a biomechanical production of the sensory modalities transmitting sensory data to the brain; it is also an affective and aesthetic experience that is historical because it is shaped by a person's sociocultural experiences. It is useful to keep this perspective in mind when using a biomedical frame of reference for sensory processing to maintain a holistic understanding of sensory processing and the lived sensory experience.

Sensory Modalities

When asked to identify **sensory modalities**, people generally think of the five senses: vision, hearing, touch, taste, and smell. However, there are three additional senses that are important. The proprioceptive, vestibular, and interoceptive senses also provide information that is essential to function. The next section briefly describes each of the sensory modalities using a biomechanical framework for sensory processing.

Visual System

Humans rely heavily on the **visual system** to function in the world. The visual system provides information about the physical properties of the environment and the objects in it, such as their shape, size, color, and proximity to the person and other objects. The lens of the eye is responsible for focusing vision and, therefore, relates to visual acuity (the ability to discriminate between shapes and the details of things from a distance). The **visual field** is the area an individual can see from their position in an environment. In humans, the visual field of each eye overlaps to create **binocular vision** that enables humans to see depth and three-dimensional images.

Photoreceptors in the eye convert light into electrical signals and are connected to the optic nerve. There are two types of photoreceptors: **cones** and **rods**. Rods are best at detecting motion and are more prominent on the periphery of the retina. Cones allow for the perception of color and produce sharp images in bright light. According to Schneider (1969), there are two visual systems: One system detects movement (location of something) and the other detects form (what something is). The parallel processing of these two visual systems (i.e., for form and movement) is supported by clinical evidence (Kandel et al., 2012). For example, a lesion of the cerebral cortex can result in loss of vision for movement but not vision for form.

Auditory System

Similar to the visual system, the **auditory system** is important for locating objects in the environment, such as the presence of threats and objects of interest. The auditory system also plays a critical role in detecting and deciphering the auditory stimuli that constitute speech including variations in tone that also communicate meaning (sarcasm, mood, etc.). Humans have complex neurological abilities to selectively attend to some auditory stimuli while "tuning out" other auditory stimuli. For example, individuals can decide to listen to one conversation over another or ignore ambient sounds in the background of noisy environments with numerous competing auditory stimuli.

Auditory stimuli are vibrations that move through elastic mediums (i.e., gases, liquids, solids) in the form of **sound waves** that can be measured in **amplitude** and **frequency**. When a sound's amplitude and frequency are within a range detectable by the auditory system, a person hears it and has a sensation. The amplitude of a sound refers to its loudness and is measured by the height of a sound wave (i.e., number of molecules that are displaced by the vibration). The frequency of a sound refers to its pitch and is measured by the total number of waves produced in 1 second.

The hearing process begins when sound waves pass from the outer ear to vibrate the **eardrum** in the middle ear. These vibrations pass through the **ossicles** (three small bones) in the middle ear and then create pressure waves in the inner ear (fluid-filled **cochlea**). In the cochlea, the vibrations stimulate small hair cells that convert the vibrations to electrical signals that travel to the brain.

People can also hear through bone conduction, such as when individuals hear themselves speak or chew. This form of hearing explains why people sound different when listening to themself speak on a recording. When they speak, they hear themself both through bone and air conduction, whereas they only hear themself through air conduction during a recording.

Tactile System

The **tactile system** consists of a variety of sensory receptors in the skin. Some of the receptors are close to the surface of the skin, whereas others are found in the deeper subcutaneous tissue. Some of the receptors respond to light touch, which is an arousing sensation that causes individuals to pay attention and notice something in the environment. Another type of receptor responds to pressure and contributes to **discriminative touch** (i.e., where and what a person is touching). The skin also contains thermoreceptors that recognize hot and cold and nociceptors that detect pain. There is an uneven concentration of tactile receptors over different areas of the body. Generally, a person's skin is more sensitive in distal parts of the body (e.g., fingers, toes) than proximally (e.g., shoulders, trunk). The face is particularly sensitive to pressure.

The tactile system can habituate itself to stimuli so that a person can stop detecting or being aware of a tactile stimulus if a steady pressure is applied to the skin. People are less likely to habituate to weaker stimuli that are experienced intermittently. This explains why **deep pressure** is comforting and **light touch** is arousing, and why people are generally not constantly aware of the feel of their clothing until their movement rubs it against the skin.

The tactile system is also an important component of food preferences. In addition to the taste of a food, individuals are keenly aware of the texture or feel of foods. People will often dislike a particular food because of its tactile qualities rather than its taste (e.g., slimy meat of raw oysters or the fuzzy skin of a peach).

Gustatory and Olfactory Systems

Smell (**olfactory system**) is the only sense that connects directly to the **amygdala** and **hippocampus** before going to the **thalamus**. The amygdala and hippocampus are associated with emotional responses and the consolidation of memories, which may explain why smell is so strongly associated with feelings and memories (Herz, 2016). Smells often "take people back" to a specific place and point in time. For this reason, odors can be used to evoke positive memories and moods. Historically, smells have also been used to stigmatize and marginalize deprivileged groups of people to label them as dirty and undesirable (Classen, 1992).

The gustatory and olfactory systems are chemical sensory systems that are highly connected. In the case of smell, airborne molecules enter the nasal cavity and are detected by olfactory receptors that extend into the nostril as **cilia** or hair. With taste (gustatory), a chemical (typically in the form of food) is placed directly on the tongue to activate the receptors in the taste buds. However, many of the nuances associated with taste are actually attributed to olfaction because when people taste food, they typically smell it. Taste and smell are very important in food selection and food avoidance. These senses can help identify unsafe or unpleasant foods. Although humans can detect the presence of an odor with low levels of the stimulus, their ability to recognize odors (i.e., name the smell) is poor.

Proprioceptive System

Proprioception is the awareness of the body's position in space and is required for all activities requiring body movement, such as walking. Proprioceptive receptors detect changes in the position of muscles and joints, which provide information about the relative position of the body in space. **Muscle spindles** act as sensory receptors and provide information about muscle length and velocity of stretch. In addition, **Golgi tendon** organs provide information at the site where the tendon meets the muscle. Together, these sensory receptors let a person know when they have raised their arm, including the arm's approximate location in relation to the rest of the body. Proprioception is especially important when performing movements without visual input (e.g., touch typing).

Vestibular System

Of all the senses, people are typically least aware of the **vestibular system**—unless it becomes dysfunctional and causes unpleasant sensations of dizziness and nausea. The vestibular system supports a person's ability to balance their body by detecting their head's position and movement in space. Vestibular receptors are in the **semicircular canals** of the inner ear and are positioned along three different planes of bodily movement. As the head moves in any direction, the receptors detect its movement along those planes. The vestibular system allows a person to keep their body balanced during activities and also enables a person to keep their eyes fixed on a particular point in space as their body moves around.

Interoceptive System

Interoception is generally understood as the sensory perception of internal bodily states and organ function (Barrett et al., 2004). The interoceptive system plays a significant role in typical daily functioning and affects a person's decision-making, learning, emotional capabilities (Brewer et al., 2021), and social skills (Arnold et al., 2019). There is no consensus regarding models for understanding interoception and there is a lack of conceptual clarity among the various terms that have emerged in this body of research, such as interoceptive awareness and interoceptive accuracy (Mehling et al., 2018).

Recent research shows that interoception consists of a complex integration across different modalities, including exteroceptive modalities (Quigley et al., 2021) in an ever-changing internal and external environment (Schmitt & Schoen, 2022). In other words, there is increasing evidence that interoception and exteroception intimately affect each other as the environment also constantly fluctuates. Therefore, assessing interoception is complex and important because of its critical role in everyday functioning, mental and physical health, and well-being.

When Sensory Processing Disrupts Occupation

Sensory systems do not work independently and are critical for occupational performance. For example, when a student takes notes in a class, the vestibular system keeps them balanced in their chair and helps them move their eyes from the instructor to their paper. In addition, there is the sensation of hearing the lecture, the use of visual input to keep writing on the lines, and a great deal of tactile and proprioceptive sense to hold the pen and form the letters. Imagine how difficult note taking would become without the input of just one of those sensory modalities. Indeed, occupational performance is polysensorial—it involves the body's sensory systems simultaneously and the lived experience of any specific sensory modality is affected by other sensory modalities (Bailliard et al., 2023).

People often take their senses for granted unless there is a problem. Research has shown that children and adults with psychiatric diagnoses often have atypical sensory processing patterns that interfere with daily life (Andersson et al., 2021; Bailliard & Whigham, 2017). Atypical sensory modulation has been identified as a potential risk factor for mental illnesses (Bar-Shalita & Cermak, 2016). Occupational therapy experts have created a nosology to identify specific sensory processing patterns that disrupt occupation (Miller et al., 2007). These conditions may or may not exist concurrently with other psychiatric conditions.

Sensory modulation refers specifically to the brain's ability to respond appropriately to the sensory environment and to remain at the appropriate level of arousal or alertness. Research suggests that demographic factors, such as age and level of educational attainment, may affect a person's sensory processing patterns (Machingura et al., 2019) as does a person's historical sociocultural background (Bailliard, 2022). Therefore, OTPs need to pay close attention to how a persons' sensory processing patterns have been influenced by their sociocultural positionality and how they may have changed across the life course.

There are three primary types of sensory modulation disorders:

- **Overresponsivity:** an exaggerated response of the nervous system to sensory stimuli. For example, people who get motion sick easily are overresponding to

vestibular experiences (the sensation of movement). The nervous system goes into fight-or-flight mode even when no real danger exists.
- **Underresponsivity:** a lack of response, or insufficient response to the sensory environment. People with underresponsivity may appear to be daydreaming or unfocused on what is happening around them. They may also have difficulty with coordination and the development of motor skills.
- **Sensory seeking:** A sensory-seeking nervous system pursues intense sensory input. A person with a sensory-seeking nervous system will engage in occupations and behaviors that provide intense sensory experiences.

The following section describes the atypical sensory processing patterns that are often associated with specific psychiatric diagnoses.

Sensory Processing and Children With Psychiatric Conditions

As children develop, their sensory systems also develop, and they learn to relate to their sensory experiences through their sociocultural environments. During this part of the life course, children will experience opportunities to experiment with and refine their sensory capacities. When walking into any preschool, OTPs can observe children reveling in sensory experiences, such as creating art with finger paints, diving into sand, or splashing on water tables. There will also be children who are cautiously observing these activities from a distance.

Children can be unaware that specific sensory experiences can cause them anxiety, distractibility, or even anger. Children with sensory processing challenges are often unable to articulate or understand what is upsetting to them. In some cases, extreme reactions to sensory experiences can result in behaviors that are disruptive to the child's daily life and sometimes to those around them. Teachers and parents are often unaware that there may be underlying sensory challenges and may attempt to respond to disruptive reactions through a strictly behavioral approach. Interventions that fail to address the underlying sensory challenges of disruptive behaviors will not be successful and may lead to worse outcomes (O'Donnell et al., 2012).

The following sections explain sensory processing patterns that are associated with three psychiatric and/or developmental disorders: attention deficit-hyperactivity disorder (ADHD), autism spectrum disorder (ASD), and developmental trauma disorder.

Attention Deficit-Hyperactivity Disorder

Children diagnosed with ADHD tend to have atypical sensory processing patterns (Dellapiazza et al., 2021). It is a common misconception that children with ADHD simply do not have the ability to attend to information. Children with ADHD also experience difficulty with filtering out extraneous sensory stimuli. Research has shown that children with ADHD can be both overresponsive and underresponsive to

BOX 9-1 ■ Sensory Features of ADHD in the Classroom

Creating an Optimal Sensory Environment in the Classroom for Tyler

An OTP was providing services to Tyler, a first grader with ADHD who was placed in a highly structured classroom. The teacher had a strict behavioral program in place that significantly limited movement in the classroom. The first graders had individual trash receptacles placed at their desks, and there were no out-of-seat activities for a large portion of the morning. Even activities such as pencil sharpening occurred only at designated times. The team believed that this type of structure would be the answer for Tyler, who seemed to be in constant motion. Although the program was successful in limiting Tyler's out-of-seat behavior, he grew more anxious each day in the classroom.

After Tyler spent a few days in the classroom, the OTP went to check with the teacher to see how things were going. This visit occurred during one of the designated movement times. The teacher reported successfully eliminating unnecessary movement, although task completion was still an issue. The children filed off to the restroom. As Tyler began walking down the hall, pieces of his clothing fell to the floor. By the time he had reached the restroom, most of his jeans and a large portion of his shirt were missing. Although Tyler had not been out of his seat all morning,

he had been cutting his clothing rather than completing the group art project.

Although this story represents an extreme case of ADHD, it illustrates the fact that behavioral approaches can be ineffective in extinguishing sensory processing difficulties. Using a sensory frame of reference, the OTP can provide insight to the types of sensory problems that interfere with daily performance and offer strategies to reduce the negative reactions to the sensory experiences. For Tyler, allowing periods of movement was critical to his ability to concentrate on the task at hand. When he was required to sit for long periods of time, he was less likely to attend to classroom tasks and still as likely to seek sensory stimuli in ways that detracted from his focus on the class.

Tyler's team reconvened, and a different classroom was selected that gave Tyler increased opportunities for movement throughout his day and a vestibular disk placed on his chair for in-seat activities. When movement strategies were incorporated into his classroom routine, his productivity increased. It is important to note that, in addition to sensory issues that interfered with performance, Tyler had cognitive challenges as well. It was the combination of adaptations in the cognitive demands, such as removing distractors and creating the optimal sensory environment, that led to more success in academic performance.

---

sensory information when compared with children without ADHD (Shimizu et al., 2014).

Children with ADHD have higher rates of low registration, sensory sensitivity, and sensation seeking than typical children (Delgado-Lobete et al., 2020) and these atypical sensory processing patterns persist into adulthood ADHD (Kamath et al., 2020). A study using the Sensory Processing Measure (SPM) found that children with ADHD scored differently than children without ADHD on all seven subtests (Pfeiffer et al., 2015). These findings suggest that modulation of sensation is an issue for children with ADHD and that they respond differently to different situations. For example, in some situations they will seek sensation by moving their bodies or making loud noises, whereas at other times they may find sensations, such as touch, aversive and avoid tactile input.

These atypical sensory processing patterns often lead to behavioral challenges at home and in school. In Box 9-1, Tyler illustrates how the sensory features of his ADHD became problematic in the classroom.

Autism Spectrum Disorder

Sensory processing impairments have long been recognized as a core component of ASD, but it was not until the criteria for the diagnosis were revised for the *Diagnostic and Statistical Manual of Mental Disorders*, Fifth Edition *(DSM-5)* that these impairments were included as a symptom of the condition. The *DSM-5* now states one of the symptoms of autism as "hyper or hypo reactivity to sensory input in sensory aspects of the environment" (American Psychiatric Association [APA], 2013).

A review of research integrating the symptom and neural literature found evidence of both hypo- and

hyperresponsiveness to sensory stimuli in ASD (Schauder & Bennetto, 2016). However, there tends to be greater hyporesponsiveness in infants and toddlers and greater hyperresponsiveness in adolescents and adults. The sensory modalities most affected appear to be in the auditory, visual, and tactile (including oral tactile sensitivity) systems. In a meta-analysis of sensory symptoms in ASD, Ben-Sasson and colleagues (2019) confirmed that sensory overresponsivity, sensory underresponsivity, and sensory seeking were atypical in ASD compared with typical controls; however, they also found that sensory overresponsivity was the only core feature of ASD that was significant compared with other clinical groups.

Temple Grandin (2000), an adult with ASD, described her experiences as a child in a paper entitled "My Experiences With Visual Thinking Sensory Problems and Communication Difficulties." Temple had an extreme hypersensitivity to touch and auditory stimulation. She described the following account from her childhood:

> When I was a child, I feared the ferry boat that took us to our summer vacation home. When the boat's horn blew, I threw myself on the floor and screamed. Autistic children and adults may fear dogs or babies because barking dogs or crying babies may hurt their ears. Dogs and babies are unpredictable, and they can make a hurtful noise without warning. . . . (p. 1)

Grandin's seminal paper illustrated that aversive sensory stimuli are not just upsetting to some children with atypical sensory processing, but they can also be painful. Grandin's example illustrates the critical importance of addressing the impact of atypical sensory processing on the occupations, health, and well-being of children.

A significant challenge in working with autistic children is that it is difficult to shed one's sensory habits of perception to understand the fundamental differences in their sensory processing patterns and how they impact their functioning. People often make assumptions about how an autistic child is interpreting information based on how they would interpret it. A classic example is the general assumption that, when a child is not visually attending to a person or an activity, they are not engaged in the task. However, in the case of ASD, eye contact during conversation can be difficult and does not indicate whether they are paying attention to a person talking.

This is especially problematic when interventionists impose their expectations for how certain skills or occupations should be performed. Such interventions amount to oppression, especially when they interfere with strategies the child has developed for living with their sensory processing differences. For example, an interventionist may focus on teaching an autistic child to make eye contact because of their social expectations, but the child may avoid eye contact to regulate their sensory system to attend to the ongoing conversation.

Autistic children experience many challenges in managing their classroom sensory environments. For example, an autistic child may be better equipped to attend to a classroom task if they are allowed to move to another part of the room when noise levels increase. Classrooms are typically sensory-rich environments that can overwhelm children who are sensory sensitive. When confronted with a situation with overwhelming sensory stimuli, autistic children may respond with disruptive behaviors because of a lack of control in implementing coping strategies.

Working with autistic people to enhance their control over the sensory environment is a useful strategy to enhance occupational participation. Similar challenges with learning environments often continue into adolescence and adulthood. For example, a study of adolescents found that sensory issues, particularly hyperresponsiveness to auditory stimuli in the classroom, resulted in physical discomfort and difficulties concentrating (Howe & Stagg, 2016).

Another area of daily life that is often impacted by the sensory features of autism is food selectivity. Many autistic children have restricted diets because of food intolerances that are sensory-based. Therefore, some autistic children are at potential risk for nutritional deficiencies (Cermak et al., 2010). This sensory pattern also continues into adulthood with a strong preference for familiar foods and a strong dislike for foods with undesirable textures and flavors (Kuschner et al., 2015).

Developmental Trauma Disorder

Child abuse and neglect are critical public health issues. In the United States in 2020, approximately 618,000 children were victims of abuse and neglect, resulting in 1,750 deaths (U.S. Department of Health & Human Services et al., 2022). It is estimated that one of every seven children experienced some form of abuse and this number is likely an underestimate because of underreporting. Chronic childhood trauma interferes with the capacity to integrate sensory, emotional, and cognitive information, and can lead to negative coping mechanisms and reduced ability to respond adaptively to stress.

According to attachment theory, infants begin to develop their ability to manage physiological arousal through the presence of a stable attachment figure (Pisoni et al., 2014). Through reciprocal multisensory exchanges between the infant and caregiver, the infant's arousal is balanced using a combination of soothing and stimulating sensory experiences. The child experiences increases and decreases in arousal as they alternate between exploring their environment and returning to their caregivers. When a child frequently does not receive caregiving that modulates their arousal, they may experience difficulties in learning how to play, process, integrate, and categorize what they are experiencing. Indeed, different parenting styles have been shown to affect young adults' regulation of emotional distress, with consequences for their interoceptive awareness (Oldroyd et al., 2019).

Adverse childhood experiences (ACEs) are forms of childhood trauma or neglect and are shown to interfere with brain development and poor long-term health outcomes (Petruccelli et al., 2019). Approximately 61% of adults report experiencing at least one ACE and almost one in six adults report experiencing four or more types of ACEs; however, during COVID-19 nearly three out of four high school students reported at least one ACE and 7.8% reported four or more (Anderson et al., 2022). Research suggests that experiencing four or more ACEs places individuals at an especially high risk for poor mental and physical health outcomes (Felitti et al., 1998; Ippen et al., 2011).

Trauma is highly associated with posttraumatic stress disorder (PTSD), substance use disorders, and other mental illnesses via changes in the limbic system, the hypothalamic-pituitary-adrenal axis, and dysregulation of neurotransmitters (Substance Abuse and Mental Health Services Administration, 2014). Neglect contributes to deprivation and a lack of sensory input, and abuse leads to impairments in fear learning (McLaughlin et al., 2014).

Children who have experienced trauma often experience fluctuations between hyperarousal and numbed depression and withdrawal. They may have difficulty coping with stress, regulating their level of arousal, and can respond to stressors with significant emotional intensity. For example, a child who has experienced trauma may find physical contact unbearable and therefore exhibits extreme reactions when touched.

OTPs can work with caregivers to help children who have experienced trauma to feel competent and safe. These children often respond favorably to predictability, stability, and environments that make them feel safe. It is also helpful to identify trauma-related triggers and allow children opportunities to learn how to manage their triggers in a controlled, safe environment. Although there is a lack of empirical research that evaluates the effectiveness of trauma-informed and sensory-based interventions for children with traumatic experiences, research suggests it leads to promising outcomes for this population group (Dowdy et al., 2020; Fraser et al., 2017). Box 9-2 provides an example of a child who experienced trauma and is receiving sensory-based intervention.

Also see Chapter 5: Trauma-Informed Practice, Chapter 25: Trauma- and Stressor-Related Disorders, and Chapter 36: Early Intervention: A Practice Setting for Early Childhood Mental Health. 🤝

BOX 9-2 ■ Creating a Safe Environment to Meet Zack's Sensory-Seeking Needs

Zack came to the United States after his adoption by Mary and Jane, his moms. Zack and his twin sister, Nicole, were born in Romania and lived their first 2 years of life in a Romanian orphanage. Zack met his OTP via his school district that was seeking a preschool assessment. The school team consisted of an OTP, speech language pathologist, and a school psychologist.

Upon meeting Zack, the OTP noted he was an extremely small 3-year-old (failure to thrive) but he ran faster than lightning and unfortunately without purpose. If a door was open, he exited quickly and would climb anything in sight: walls, fences, and playground equipment. His motor development was within normal limits and actually above typical developmental levels for activities such as running, climbing, and jumping, except he did not seem to do any movement with purpose, it appeared.

But to Zack, this excessive movement had a purpose and met a sensory need for him. Zack had no affect: no smiles, did not cry when hurt, no laughing, and no eye contact with children or adults. He was just beginning to have a relationship with his moms where he would allow them to hold him and comfort him but for very limited amounts of time. His play was robust gross motor play only, with no play involving toys or any objects or tools. He ate a very limited diet that consisted of pureed type foods and resisted any variance of texture or temperature. His sleep patterns were greatly disrupted as he would awaken nightly at 2 a.m. and remain awake until 5 or 6 a.m. From the assessments as a school-based team, it was determined that Zack would best benefit from a home-based program to assist this family with his sensory-seeking behaviors, play challenges, and lack of attention for school readiness.

Working very closely with a local clinical psychologist, the home-based therapy team employed a developmental individual-difference relationship (DIR)/floortime approach with Zack. For 6 months twice weekly, the OTP played with Zack in a darkened, very small room where he sat on a sit-and-spin and used flashlights to localize and pay attention. He loved this game and attended up to 15 minutes at a time. He began to laugh as the

therapist lit up animal pictures and made the animal sound. Upon seeing this affect—smiles, laughter—the team decided to create social and emotional goals that considered his sensory profile (SP) of sensory-seeker and combined this with play and cognitive tasks. He demonstrated that in a safe environment that honored his sensory-seeking needs, he could begin to play with an object and toys appropriately and began to be more involved with his self-care needs: feeding himself, bathing, and toileting.

As Zack approached 5 years of age, Zach's team recommended to his parents that they try him in a special education preschool. Out of the demands of the preschool that wanted him in a table-and-chair environment, it was discovered that his behavior deteriorated from the time he was in a home-based setting with a program that honored his sensory-seeking profile. His home-based program included both an indoor and outdoor jungle gym, swing set, and sandbox with music provided for both indoor and outdoor activities. His new school environment was a large classroom with table and chairs and an imagination room but no outlet for his need for movement. It was obvious to his OTP that his educational environment needed to honor his sensory needs.

It took the parents the entire school year to get the school to agree to create a sensory modulation section for the classroom that included a jumping mattress, small trampoline, and a music-and-headphone section. The staff was trained to use this area for his cognitive or academic lessons. They discovered that as he jumped he could repeat the alphabet or his numbers, or name colors. Movement and rhythmicity were calming to Zack, allowing for his learning to occur.

It was not until the age of 8 that the school could even consider Zack to be in a table-and-chair environment, and once he was successful in that environment he still needed the sensory body breaks. Zack's parents advocate for his sensory needs; upon meeting a new teacher, therapist, physician, or other service provider, they are prepared to discuss their son's sensory needs. It became obvious that once Zack felt safe and honored, he could participate.

Sensory Processing and Adults With Psychiatric Conditions

Several psychiatric disabilities that are prevalent in adults also involve atypical sensory processing patterns. However, there is a lack of peer-reviewed research and evidence-based interventions that target the effects of atypical sensory processing on the daily lives of people living with psychiatric conditions (Bailliard & Whigham, 2017). When data are available, scores from the Adolescent/Adult Sensory Profile (A/ASP) are presented for specific diagnoses. Figure 9-1 shows that psychiatric conditions (schizophrenia, bipolar disorder, depression, PTSD, and obsessive-compulsive disorder [OCD]) are associated with distinct sensory processing patterns.

In general, sensory processing difficulties are a nonspecific transdiagnostic phenotype that is associated with many psychiatric conditions (van den Boogert, 2022). Individuals across all psychiatric diagnoses tend to have higher scores for sensory sensitivity, low registration, and sensation avoiding and lower scores for sensation seeking than the general population (Brown et al., 2020); however, there is emerging evidence of distinct patterns of atypical sensory processing for different diagnoses (Brown et al., 2020).

Schizophrenia and Schizoaffective Disorders

There is a growing body of neuroscience research demonstrating that adults with schizophrenia spectrum disorders experience atypical sensory processing patterns (Bailliard & Whigham, 2017). Adults with schizophrenia have atypical sensory gating (as measured by the brain's electrophysiological response to a stimulus) that interferes with their ability to filter out extraneous and redundant auditory stimuli (Javitt & Freedman, 2015; Wan et al., 2008).

Research has also found that this group has atypical mismatch negativity, which interferes with their ability to recognize changes in predictable patterns of auditory stimuli (Jahshan et al., 2013; Javitt & Freedman, 2015). Therefore, they tend to have more difficulty discriminating sounds and tend to be more affected by distractions when compared with controls (Javitt & Sweet, 2015). Self-reports from people with schizophrenia have described sensory experiences as sometimes overwhelming (e.g., noises were too loud or it seemed there was too much information at a time; McGhie & Chapman, 1961).

Visual processing impairments in schizophrenia include difficulty perceiving motion and the speed of a moving object,

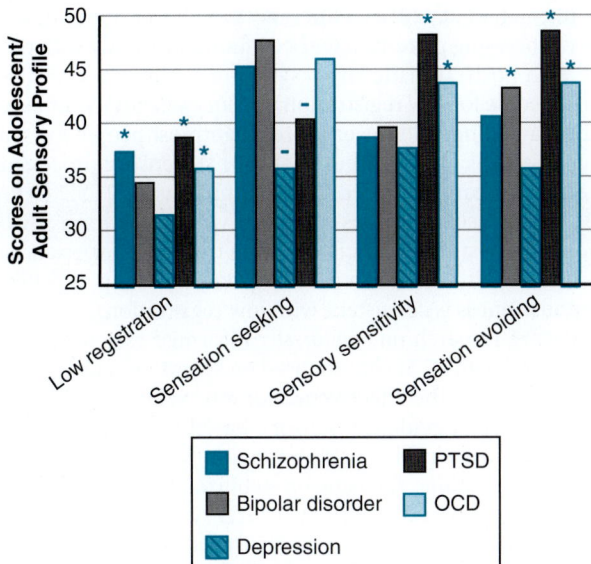

FIGURE 9-1. Sensory processing preferences in adults with psychiatric conditions. Data regarding schizophrenia and bipolar disorder from Brown and colleagues (2002); data on depression from Engel-Yeger, Muzio, and colleagues (2016); data regarding PTSD from Engel-Yeger and colleagues (2013); and data regarding OCD from Rieke and Anderson (2009). Scores are the reported mean score in the study along with the categorization according to the standardization sample. In all studies, the participants were adults.
* *indicates statistically significantly higher than the standardization sample.*
- *indicates statistically significantly lower than the standardization sample*

lack of smooth eye tracking (e.g., reading the lines in a paragraph), and difficulty organizing the parts of a visual stimulus into a coherent whole (Yoon et al., 2013). Visual processing impairments are important because they have been related to community functioning (Butler & Javitt, 2005) and can be barriers to many necessary and meaningful occupations.

In addition to visual and auditory perceptual anomalies, research has found that other senses such as olfaction (Bunney et al., 1999; Takahashi et al., 2018) and interoception vary for this group. Emerging research on interoception with this population suggests that people with schizophrenia have reduced interoceptive accuracy (Ardizzi et al., 2016; Koreki et al., 2021) and altered interoceptive sensibility (Koreki et al., 2021).

Because of these differences, adults with schizophrenia frequently experience challenges in communicating their emotions and in interpreting the emotional expressions of others. Atypical sensory processing in this group often leads to difficulties with social cognition (Green et al., 2005) including perceiving sarcasm (Kantrowitz et al., 2014) and detecting and interpreting the meaning of intonation and rhythm of speech (Javitt & Sweet, 2015). Likewise, impairments in basic visual processing are associated with difficulties interpreting facial expressions (Chen & Ekstrom, 2015).

Behaviorally, individuals with schizophrenia report higher scores on low registration and sensation avoiding, and lower scores on sensation seeking on the SP than individuals without mental illness, which suggests they are not receiving adequate information about their environment and their own bodies (Brown et al., 2002). Not only do people with schizophrenia miss input, but also, when they do detect sensory stimuli, they can find it unpleasant and engage in behaviors to

avoid the sensation (Andersson et al., 2021). Experiences of repetitive and unwanted sensations in daily life among people living with schizophrenia negatively affect their participation in everyday activities (Andersson et al., 2021; Landon et al., 2016), as well as their capability to live independently in the community (Light & Braff, 2005).

OTPs have a history of incorporating sensory-based interventions in psychiatric settings. Although there is evidence that these interventions have been effective in preparing persons for participation in occupations, more research is needed to develop systematic intervention protocols and strategies that are evidence-based (Machingura et al., 2021).

The topic of schizophrenia is covered in detail in Chapter 23: Schizophrenia Spectrum and Psychotic Disorders.

Mood Disorders

There is evidence supporting a relationship between mood and sensory processing patterns. In typical adults, sensory sensitivity, sensation avoiding, and low registration have been associated with negative mood, whereas sensation seeking was associated with positive mood (Engel-Yeger & Dunn, 2011). Other studies have found that sensory sensitivity is associated with anxiety (Liss et al., 2005; Neal et al., 2002), depression (Liss et al., 2005), and negative mood (Brown et al., 2001). Likewise, depression and anxiety have been linked to sensory defensiveness (Kinnealey & Fuiek, 1999).

In individuals with a diagnosed mood disorder, a lack or disinterest in sensation seeking was associated with depression (Engel-Yeger, Gonda, et al., 2016). In a similar study (Engel-Yeger, Muzio, et al., 2016), people diagnosed with mood disorders were more likely to struggle with adapting to different sensory environments, resulting in impaired functioning. Although bipolar disorder is characterized by risk-taking behaviors, one study found that individuals with bipolar disorder had preferences for sensation avoiding (Brown et al., 2002). This may reflect a period when the individual with bipolar disorder is experiencing a depressive episode. These findings are consistent with the understanding that individuals experiencing negative moods are more likely to withdraw and less likely to participate in daily occupations.

A common co-occurring issue in individuals with depression is physical pain, which adds another complicated layer to understanding associated sensory processing patterns. People who experience depression and pain concurrently are more likely to experience problems with work and daily activities (Vietri et al., 2015). Studies of individuals with sensory modulation disorder find that people who are overresponsive to a wide range of sensory stimuli also experience pain more intensely (Bar-Shalita et al., 2012). People who demonstrate an exaggerated negative response to pain experiences tend to have higher levels of sensory sensitivity and sensation avoiding (Meredith et al., 2015).

Furthermore, the impacts of pain in people with atypical sensory processing may go beyond the individual and include their families. Research with families of typically developing children found that parents' sensory sensitivity affected their parenting style (e.g., permissive or authoritarian regarding which sensory stimuli are exposed to their children) and how they mediated their children's sensory environments (Branjerdporn et al., 2019). Although sensory processing patterns of children experiencing chronic pain did not correlate with parent functioning, researchers have suggested investigating whether children's sensory processing patterns correlate with those of their parents (Kerley et al., 2021).

Also see Chapter 15: Pain and Chapter 20: Mood Disorders.

Posttraumatic Stress Disorder

One of the symptoms of PTSD is reexperiencing the trauma, often with vivid sensory stimuli, such as visual hallucinations or intrusive memories of sounds, smells, or visual images (APA, 2013). Children continuously exposed to traumatic incidents may be at risk of developing sensory processing differences, with the possibility of developing both under- and overresponsivity to sensory stimuli (Yochman & Pat-Horenczyk, 2020). Studies indicate that individuals with PTSD are more likely to notice sensory stimuli that is related to their experienced trauma (Kleim et al., 2012).

For example, veterans with PTSD tend to have intense responses to the smell of burning rubber whereas veterans without PTSD who experienced similar trauma do not

(Wilkerson et al., 2018). Differences in all four types of sensory processing patterns have been found in a study with people with posttraumatic stress symptoms: higher scores than most people for low registration, sensory sensitivity, and sensation avoiding; and lower scores than most people for sensation seeking (Engel-Yeger et al., 2013). Sensory processing preferences can be related to the symptoms of PTSD (APA, 2013). Increased arousal is consistent with sensory sensitivity, avoidance of stimuli associated with a traumatic experience is consistent with sensation avoiding, and numbing of general responsiveness is consistent with low registration.

Recent research on sensorially informed care for people diagnosed with PTSD has focused on symptom management and measuring the effectiveness of interventions. Although there is limited evidence, sensory-based interventions have been noted as helpful in preparation for facilitating participation in occupations, focusing on stabilization, and developing a sense of safety and security (McGreevy & Boland, 2020).

Also see Chapter 5: Trauma-Informed Practice and Chapter 25: Trauma- and Stressor-Related Disorders.

The Lived Experience

Suzette

I am an OTP who has struggled with sensory integrative dysfunction since childhood. Being an OTP hasn't given me the magical ability to "cure" myself, but it has provided many tools that make what I experience manageable so that I can live a full life, experiencing ability instead of disability.

I was in my mid-30s before receiving a diagnosis on the autism spectrum. At that point, I had been diagnosed with a myriad of other things, including a generalized anxiety disorder, major depression, schizoaffective disorder, anorexia nervosa, and complex partial seizures. For me, these diagnoses bear dysfunctional sensory elements (although this may not be true for others), and I have grown to look at diagnoses as stepping stones along a pathway of discovery.

At the time I received the autism diagnosis, life had been filled with challenges. I'd come to believe most were "emotionally based" and that I'd done something spiritually wrong. I spent much of my childhood and young adult years feeling frightened and overwhelmed—even within the safety of my home. I quickly felt dizzy, off-balance, and anxious, and this affected nearly everything I did. When I was at school, in crowds, on the playground, at a medical appointment, on family vacations, sleeping over at a friend's, riding horses, grocery shopping, playing my cello—I was prone to episodes where my equilibrium was challenged . . . and disrupted.

Things that others don't seem to notice could make it impossible for me to concentrate or remain in a room—I felt tossed about and overstimulated so much of the time that I'd often leave a class early (causing me to get in trouble) or stay home from school entirely (causing missed assignments and social isolation). From an early age, I dreaded going to school but couldn't vocalize why—I knew it sounded "crazy" so I worked to keep the sensations I experienced quiet. I loved the

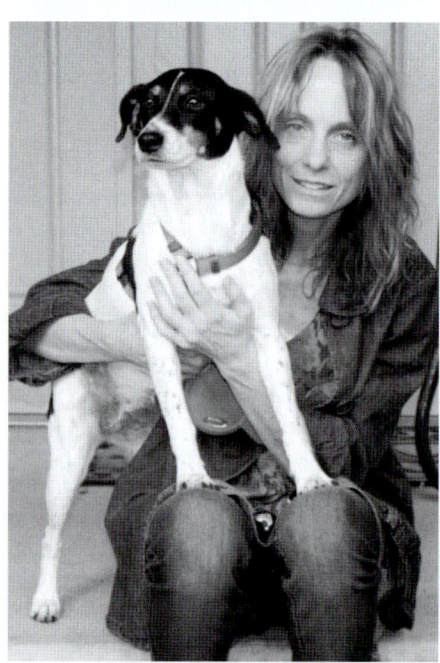

"thinking" part of school, but the sensory overwhelm I experienced frequently ruined the adventure.

From early on, I couldn't eat foods with chunks or strange textures in them. I had episodes where parts of my body felt too big, and I felt frightened and hypervigilant, worrying about when it might happen again. I was extremely introverted, seeming to lack the inner initiative to interact with others, although hanging out with one friend at a time was perfect. I preferred being in quiet places (or outside) to avoid feeling anxious and overwhelmed. Although most kids love breaks

The Lived Experience—cont'd

from school, I found the change in routine very difficult. I had a good childhood—but it was a constant effort to try and fit into the "mold" of a world that created so much disharmony for me. I developed intricate routines to follow to maintain inner order and stability—routines that later transformed into a serious eating disorder and other obsessive-compulsive behaviors that have taken years to overcome.

The rigid routines and beliefs helped me feel in control in a body and world that felt out of control, but they interfered deeply with developmental milestones and just being able to do the "normal" things in life.

Almost every day presented challenges—but I didn't necessarily realize it wasn't that way for others. You have to take life where it's at for you—finding ways to remain hope filled and grateful, and to reach the goals you set for yourself. My parents have always been huge encouragers—without them I would never have gone as far as I have. Strength does come from the support and love of others—those who help you face challenges with determination and an attitude of success. Another tool I've always used is my spiritual life and the inspiration of people I admire. Helen Keller's quote, "Keep your face to the sun and you will not see the shadows" is one of my personal mottos!

I grew from being a child with a dysregulated nervous system into an adult with a dysregulated nervous system. It seemed as if the wrong things got in, and in return, the wrong things resulted. I am proof that children with sensory integrative dysfunctions can become adults with them. Some of the behaviors and life concerns might change, but the core issues remain pretty steady.

It is through my personal journey of discovery that I stumbled on the field of occupational therapy. I was enthralled by the things OTPs did to help people with sensory challenges, and was amazed at their approach to people who had autism, traumatic brain injuries, learning disabilities, cerebral palsy, and Parkinson's disease. I wanted to be part of this world! An OTP worked with me during one of my hospitalizations, and we looked at the impact my health was having on a "circle of life domains" chart. It was the first time I realized there was a profession that took a whole-person, whole-life approach when treating people like me. OTPs were always looking beyond the clinical environment (or taking treatment right into real life environments), examining how someone's challenges affected the quality of life in all life's domains. I began to understand what purposeful living meant and to learn new personal tools toward obtaining this.

I rejoiced when I was accepted to Colorado State University's Occupational Therapy Program, and graduated from it in 1994. School was difficult for me for the reasons I've already described. I underachieved at the goals I'd set, but in the midst of feeling discouraged, I began learning about accommodations and the Americans with Disabilities Act. I was blessed to receive accommodations that allowed me the chance to complete some assignments alternatively, as well as to succeed at all my fieldwork placements. In classes, these included taking tests alone, being allowed to sit in the back, having note takers, and presenting work to smaller groups. In fieldwork, these included working fewer hours and drawing the experiences out for longer time periods, getting frequent breaks, doing some of my paperwork in a quiet environment, and doing local placements so I didn't have to travel far or relocate.

At this time, I was still mostly carrying the stigma of having many psychiatric diagnoses. It was embarrassing to tell others why I needed accommodations, and I didn't have the vocabulary to fully explain what I needed. I was determined to become an OTP—but my inability to self-advocate often got in the way.

In 2000, an astute doctor gave me the autism diagnosis and helped me better understand what I experience as a syndrome that begins in my nervous system. This was a huge turning point for me. He was the one who really helped me understand the strong interplay among genetics, environment, and the neurophysical and neurochemical pieces when it comes to sensory disorders. For once, I stopped blaming myself and began to find new ways to engage in the life I desired—adopting a lifestyle that didn't include so many self-defeating challenges and negative inner voices.

As humans, OTPs, physicians, whoever we are, we must be very careful to not make assumptions about people's health based only on their past, or their age. I was doing fairly well in life until a few years ago when I began to suffer from severe headaches, vertigo (very different from being dizzy), fatigue, joint pain, episodic fevers, and other neurological problems. After several doctors tried to (mis)label me as mentally ill, an astute doctor diagnosed me with Lyme disease. Unfortunately, an early diagnosis is less likely to lead to chronic symptoms, and Lyme disease has inched its pervasive fingers into the areas where I was already vulnerable, particularly my vestibular system.

I have had to work through anger and frustration regarding my health, things I can no longer do, and issues with dismissive health-care attitudes. Through this I am learning better how to live in the moment and to make each day count, to not compare my abilities with others', and to stay grounded inside of me—within my own spiritual self—because nothing, not even illness/disease/injury, will take that from me. It's also what keeps me centered and focused on the positives when I feel angry at systems I cannot change.

Hope, encouraging words, realistic goals, and nonlabeling are vital to give to those struggling to sing their song in this world. Within our uniqueness lies that common thread called humanity, and it is what weaves us together as we discover (and rediscover) our own purposes for living. From birth until death, we are ever-evolving, and occupational therapy is such an awesome field because of its unique focus on purpose, and giving people that prolific chance at "YES"!

Obsessive-Compulsive Disorder

Research has also examined sensory processing differences in OCD. Sensory phenomena (i.e., uncomfortable invasive sensations) are core aspects of the diagnosis that drive repetitive behaviors (Brown et al., 2019). These sensory urges are associated with activation in the somatosensory cortex and insula and are experienced as sensory-based compulsions that cannot be ignored. In psychophysiological studies of the startle response, individuals with OCD are more likely to startle at an unexpected auditory stimuli and less likely to inhibit their startle reflex (Ahmari et al., 2012). This finding has been linked to a more general difficulty with filtering sensory information and inhibiting responses.

Using the A/ASP, Rieke and Anderson (2009) found that individuals with OCD tended to have scores higher than most people in the areas of sensory sensitivity, sensation avoiding, and low registration. Sensory abnormalities are likely to exist among children with OCD and anxiety disorders, but more evidence is needed to make firm conclusions (Houghton et al., 2020). Researchers are suggesting that sensory overresponsivity is a core sensory feature of OCD (Van Hulle et al., 2019). Because distress is frequently associated with compulsive behaviors and sensory overresponsivity, interventions aimed at distress tolerance may be helpful (Castle et al., 2023). One distress tolerance intervention, TIPP (Temperature, Intense exercise, Paced breathing, Paired muscle relaxation), uses intentional sensory input of cold to alert the sensory system to reduce the effects of an overwhelmed emotional state. This allows an individual to recenter and regain control of their thoughts and behaviors and more effectively problem-solve situations and use their established coping skills.

OCD is explored in greater detail in Chapter 21: Obsessive Disorders. 🤝

Comparing Psychiatric Conditions and Sensory Processing Patterns Using the A/ASP

The sensory processing preferences of people with psychiatric conditions are different from those of people without mental health diagnoses, and these differences are condition-specific (Brown et al., 2020). In general, individuals across all psychiatric diagnoses tend to have higher scores for sensory sensitivity, low registration, and sensation avoiding and lower scores for sensation seeking than the general population (Brown et al., 2020). Although all the sensory processing preferences have positive and negative attributes, in general, sensory seeking is the most adaptive preference, whereas extreme sensory sensitivity, sensation avoiding, and low registration are more detrimental to participation.

As previously mentioned, only sensory seeking is associated with positive affect (Engel-Yeger & Dunn, 2011). In adults with serious mental illness, high scores in low registration and sensory sensitivity were associated with less participation, and high scores in sensory seeking were associated with higher levels of participation (Pfeiffer et al., 2014). This suggests that missing sensory information or feeling overwhelmed by sensory stimuli interferes with occupational performance.

Based on the studies with the A/ASP presented in Figure 9-1, PTSD resulted in the most detrimental sensory processing patterns, with "more than typical" scores for low registration, sensory sensitive, and sensation avoiding, and "less than typical" scores for sensation seeking (Engel-Yeger et al., 2013). Research has found similar trends in OCD, except study participants had similar scores in sensation seeking to people without a psychiatric condition (Rieke & Anderson, 2009). In addition, the scores in low registration, sensory sensitivity, and sensation avoiding were not as extreme for OCD as they were for PTSD.

In schizophrenia, the only difference outside of the A/ASP standardization sample was in the area of low registration (Brown et al., 2002). Low registration appears to be a prominent feature of schizophrenia; however, it is possible that other characteristics of the condition (e.g., disorganization, cognitive impairments) are contributing to this measurement. Individuals with depression have lower sensation seeking scores than most people, which suggests that, although they do not avoid sensory stimuli, they do not seek it out. Bipolar disorder had the highest sensation seeking scores of any group and they also had high sensation avoiding scores. Both of these scores indicate a person is inclined to actively engage their environments through seeking or avoiding behaviors.

Assessment

In occupational therapy, assessment of sensory processing typically uses rating scales to ask about experiences related to sensory processing in daily life. Several sensory processing assessments are described in the text that follows and included in Table 9-1. A thorough assessment would also include observations of the person's occupations in natural contexts.

Clinical Observations of Sensory Processing Patterns

An important tool for assessing a person's sensory processing patterns is to observe them participating in occupations in their natural contexts and to look for their responses to sensory stimuli. Although standardized assessments provide important information for clinical decision-making and measuring progress, skilled systematic observations can provide a granular analysis of a person's occupational participation in a specific context.

When using observations to assess sensory processing, an expert OTP will consider behaviors that indicate whether a person is aware of relevant sensory stimuli, whether they appear to enjoy it or find it aversive, whether they can filter out competing extraneous stimuli, and any other sensory factors that affect the person's participation, health, and well-being.

Questions the OTP might ask when making observations of a person's sensory processing patterns include:

- Does the person notice relevant stimuli?
- Can the person filter out or habituate to irrelevant information?
- Can the person identify a sensory stimulus correctly?
- Is the person able to communicate their sensory preferences and needs?
- Does the person use sensory information effectively to better understand the environment, their participation, or their own body?

TABLE 9-1 | Therapeutic Reasoning Assessment Table—Sensory Processing

Which Tool?	Who Was This Tool Designed For?	Is This a Type of Tool the Person Can Do? What Is Required of the Person?	What Am I Measuring?	How Long Does It Take and Where Do I Administer This Assessment?	Is the Tool Associated With a Practice Model?
Infant Sensory Profile 2 (Dunn, 2014)	Birth to 6 months	Caregiver completes the form based on observation and caregiving experiences.	Sensory processing preferences as observed through participation in daily life	30 minutes at home or clinic	Dunn Model of Sensory Processing
Toddler Sensory Profile 2 (Dunn, 2014)	7–35 months	Caregiver completes the form based on observation and caregiving experiences.	Sensory processing preferences as observed through participation in daily life	30 minutes at home or clinic	Dunn Model of Sensory Processing
Short Sensory Profile 2 (Dunn, 2014)	3–14 years	Caregiver completes the form based on observation and caregiving experiences.	Sensory processing preferences as observed through participation in daily life	10 minutes at home or in the clinic	Dunn Model of Sensory Processing
School Companion 2 (Dunn, 2014)	3–14 years	Teacher completes the form based on observation and teaching experiences.	Sensory processing preferences as observed through participation in daily life	30 minutes at school	Dunn Model of Sensory Processing
Adolescent Adult Sensory Profile (Brown & Dunn, 2002)	Age 11 to older adult	Self-report completed by the participant independently or therapist can read items and circle responses.	Sensory processing preferences as observed through participation in daily life	30 minutes at home or clinic	Dunn Model of Sensory Processing
Sensory Processing Measure (Miller-Kuhaneck et al., 2007)	Ages 3–12	Caregiver or teacher completes the form based on observation.	Sensory responses and sensory processing disorders	15–20 minutes at home or school	Ayres Sensory Integration
Highly Sensitive Person Scale (Aron & Aron, 1997)	Adults	Self-report completed by the individual.	Awareness and creativity in response to the sensory environment	15 minutes at home or in the clinic	None
Sensory Profile Interoception (SPI) (Dunn et al., 2022)	Age 11 to older adult	Self-report completed by the participant independently or therapist can read items and circle responses.	How interoception manifests in everyday life behaviors, particularly related to self-care, eating, and daily routines	30 minutes at home or clinic	Dunn Model of Sensory Processing

■ How do a person's responses to sensory stimuli affect their health and well-being?

■ How do the person's responses to sensory stimuli affect their participation and inclusion in social occupations?

■ Does the person implement effective sensory strategies to respond to challenges in sensory processing?

■ Does the person come from a different cultural background in which English is not their first language? If so, what sensory norms and values do they have that might not be recognized in their host country?

■ Does the person have a history of ACEs or trauma? If so, how is that impacting their current sensory processing?

■ Are specific combinations of sensory stimuli barriers to occupation?

■ Is the time of day (e.g., morning, after a meal, after physical activity) relevant to the person's observed sensory processing and level of arousal?

■ How do a person's responses to sensory stimuli affect their participation, health, and well-being?

Sensory Profiles

The SPs are assessments based on Dunn's (1997) Model of Sensory Processing (described in more detail in the following Intervention section). The SPs assess an individual's response to sensory events in their everyday life and categorize these responses into four sensory preferences: sensory sensitivity, sensation avoiding, low registration, and sensation seeking. There are several versions of the SP that are intended for specific age groups. The Sensory Profile 2 assessments are completed by parents and teachers and include the Infant Sensory Profile 2 (birth to 6 months), the Toddler Sensory Profile 2 (7 to 35 months), the Short Sensory Profile 2 (3 to 14 years), and the School Companion Sensory Profile 2 (3 to 14 years). The A/ASP is a self-reported version of the measure that is designed for individuals age 11 and over. The Sensory Profile Interoception (SPI) scale measures how high or low levels of interoception can affect participation in activities.

Sensory Processing Measure

The **Sensory Processing Measure** (SPM) is based on sensory integration theory. It is a behavioral rating scale for children ages 2 to 12 that assesses their different sensory modalities while also identifying sensory vulnerabilities in the areas of under- and overresponsivity, sensory seeking, and perceptual problems (Miller-Kuhaneck et al., 2007). It can be used to assess sensory responses in the home, school, and community environments and includes teacher and parent rating scales.

Highly Sensitive Person Scale

The Highly Sensitive Person Scale, which was developed by psychologists (Aron & Aron, 1997), is a 27-item self-reported Likert scale assessment that asks respondents how they relate to environmental features such as noise, taste, and other people's moods. It contains several items that reflect greater interest and sensitivity to creative stimuli such as music and art.

Intervention

Based on Jean Ayres's (1972) innovative work in sensory integration, OTPs have been pioneers in health care in implementing interventions addressing sensory health. Ayres's focus on the relationship between sensory processing and occupation encouraged the development of additional theoretical understandings of sensory processing in occupational therapy and associated clinical approaches. This section presents several different interventions that target the sensory processing of children and adults.

Sensory Integration

Sensory integration theory is based on A. Jean Ayres's theory of Sensory Integration (1972). Ayres Sensory Integration (ASI) theory was originally based on her study of motor difficulties in children with mild to moderate learning problems. The theory has evolved as additional measures have been developed, and the approach has been applied to different populations (Mailloux & Miller-Kuhaneck, 2014) including extensive use with autistic children.

ASI uses a child-directed approach that prioritizes the child's needs and responses in the selection of activities. In ASI, OTPs use play activities to target specific senses to elicit an adaptive response (Parham & Mailloux, 2010). Core tenets of ASI include supporting optimal arousal and maximizing the child's success. Accordingly, play activities must be individualized, child-directed, and based on assessment that identifies sensory integration needs.

ASI proposes that when a child receives the necessary sensory input, they are more able to organize information and successfully participate in desired occupations. ASI interventions often occur in specialized clinics that provide (through equipment) various forms of sensory input to meet the child's sensory needs. ASI tends to focus on three sensory processing systems: tactile, vestibular, and proprioceptive systems. For example, a child with tactile defensiveness may be encouraged to play in a ball pit, pack peanuts, or locate toys within a container of rice. A child with a need for vestibular input may be encouraged to play with scooter boards or swings.

The Ayres Sensory Integration Fidelity Measure (ASIFM) was developed to ensure consistency in ASI interventions. The measure evaluates the structure and process of occupational therapy interventions that espouse ASI intervention principles (Parham et al., 2011). For an intervention to be classified as ASI, the intervention must include specific processes that introduce a range of sensory experiences that challenge motor control, motor planning, and organization, while creating a safe environment that promotes optimal alertness, ensures success, and involves collaboration to harness a child's intrinsic motivation. The ASIFM also requires that therapists are trained in the method and that the clinical environment is sufficiently equipped to deliver the intervention.

Sensory-Based Interventions

Sensory-based interventions (SBIs) are different from ASI and are directed by a therapist or caregiver. These interventions target sensory modulation challenges (i.e., when a person has difficulty self-regulating their level of arousal to the demands of the situation). For example, an individual's hyperarousal may make it difficult or impossible for them to pay attention in class or at work. SBIs are provided in a person's natural environment (e.g., at home, in school, at work) and generally use sensory input through occupation to stabilize their level of arousal to meet the demands of the situation. Specific SBIs presented in the text that follows are Zones of Regulation, the Alert Program, and Deep Pressure Touch Strategies.

Zones of Regulation

The **Zones of Regulation** intervention is designed to help individuals with sensory modulation difficulties develop their skills for self-regulation (Kuypers, 2011). The intervention helps individuals identify their level of arousal using four categories or zones that range from low alertness to hyperarousal. Each category is assigned a color and sign. The green zone indicates the individual is in an optimal state of arousal and is ready to proceed with activities. The yellow zone suggests the individual is beginning to experience hyperarousal and should pause to assess the situation and regulate their level of arousal. The red zone indicates the individual is in a state of hyperarousal and needs to take a break to use self-regulation strategies to stabilize their level of arousal. The blue zone is a rest area where the person can reenergize but may also experience boredom and sadness. Table 9-2 outlines the zones with strategies that can be used by individuals to better control their emotions and manage their sensory needs.

Evidence-Based Practice

Efficacy of the Ayres Sensory Integration (ASI) Intervention

Sensory integration has the potential to improve children's motor skills, sensory processing, behaviors, and academic performance.

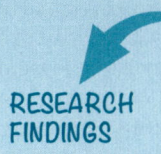

RESEARCH FINDINGS

Over the years, there have been many systematic reviews on the efficacy of ASI intervention (e.g., May-Benson & Koomar, 2010; Schaaf et al., 2018; Schoen et al., 2019). However, many of those reviews are inaccurate and misrepresentative of the efficacy of ASI because of methodological concerns in selecting studies to review (i.e., many studies that were reviewed did not actually implement ASI principles; Schoen et al., 2019).

In Schaaf and colleagues' (2018) review of research between 2007 and 2015, only three studies met inclusion criteria for their review (i.e., their research methods were sufficiently rigorous and they adhered to ASI principles). There was strong evidence that ASI leads to positive outcomes in achieving person-generated goals, moderate evidence that it leads to improvements in caregiver assistance for self-care and in autistic behaviors, and emerging but insufficient evidence that ASI improves outcomes in play, sensory-motor, and language skills and caregiver assistance for social skills.

Schoen and colleagues (2019) used the Council for Exceptional Children (CEC) Standards for Evidence-Based Practices in Special Education to review studies on the efficacy of ASI from 2006 to 2017. After two stages of review, only three studies remained; the others were excluded because of major methodological flaws and inconsistencies with the core principles of ASI. The remaining three studies met 100%, 85%, and 50% of the CEC criteria for an evidence-based practice, respectively. Therefore, according to Schoen and colleagues (2019), ASI is an evidence-based practice when it is applied with fidelity to the intervention criteria—which is often not the case.

APPLICATIONS

➡ Sensory integration is designed to target children with sensory processing and sensory integration needs.
➡ When using sensory integration in practice, OTPs should be faithful to the basic tenets of the approach.
➡ Sensory integration has the potential to improve children's motor skills, sensory processing, behaviors, and academic performance.
➡ Sensory integration appears especially effective in helping parents meet their identified goals for their children.

REFERENCES

May-Benson, T. A., & Koomar, J. A. (2010). Systematic review of the research evidence examining the effectiveness of interventions using a sensory integrative approach for children. *American Journal of Occupational Therapy, 64,* 403–414. https://doi.org/10.5014/ajot.2010.09071

Schaaf, R., Dumont, R., Arbesman, M., & May-Benson, T. (2018). Efficacy of occupational therapy using Ayres Sensory Integration: A systematic review. *American Journal of Occupational Therapy, 72*(1), 7201190010p1–7201190010p10. https://doi.org/10.5014/ajot.2018.028431

Schoen, S., Lane, S., Mailloux, Z., May-Benos, T., Parham, D., Roley, S., & Schaaf, R. (2019). A systematic review of Ayres Sensory Integration intervention for children with autism. *Autism Research, 12*(1), 6–19. https://doi.org/10.1002/aur.2046

The Alert Program

The **Alert Program** is very similar to the Zones of Regulation intervention in that it targets self-regulation skills for managing levels of alertness or arousal; however, instead of signs and zones, it uses the metaphor of "How does your engine run?" (Williams & Shellenberger, 1996). The metaphor encourages individuals to view their level of arousal as an engine: Sometimes an engine runs too fast, sometimes too slow, and

TABLE 9-2 | Zones of Regulation

Zone	How It Feels	Strategies to Manage
Blue	• Sad • Bored • Lonely	• Think happy thoughts. • Listen to music. • Get a drink of water.
Green	• Happy • Calm • Focused	• Work on goals, help others, and complete work.
Yellow	• Nervous • Hyper • Frustrated • Excited	• Talk to an adult. • Take a walk. • Use positive self-talk.
Red	• Angry • Terrified • Out of control • Elated	• Take deep breaths. • Engage in physical activity such as running. • Take a break. • Use cold temperature (i.e., TIPP method).

Source: Adapted from Kuypers, L. M. (2011). The Zones of Regulation: A curriculum designed to foster self-regulation and emotional control. *Social Thinking Publishing.*

sometimes just right. The Alert Program is a manualized 12-week intervention that consists of three stages. During Stage 1 the person learns to identify and label the engine levels. In Stage 2 they practice using sensory strategies to change the engine level to a more optimal level of arousal, and in Stage 3 the person learns how to choose strategies that match their needs.

Deep Pressure Touch Strategies

Deep pressure can provide a calming sensation by activating the parasympathetic nervous system and can be used when individuals are feeling restless, anxious, or out of control (Chen et al., 2016). Deep pressure uses tactile sensory input such as firm holding, hugging, and squeezing. One method for applying a consistent deep pressure is to wear a device that allows the individual to move around and engage in desired activities while receiving the desired calming input. The weighted vest offers one form and typically comes with a range of weights that can be used to provide the desired amount of proprioceptive input. The Tjacket is another example of a deep pressure garment that uses air pressure to adjust the amount of input. There are also weighted blankets that can be used to provide similar input.

A critical review of research on the Alert Program was performed by Gill and colleagues (2018). A total of six articles met their inclusion criteria. Using the Effective Public Health Practice Project Quality Assessment Tool, the authors found weak to moderate evidence supporting efficacy. Using the U.S. Department of Education, Elementary and Secondary Education Act guidelines, the authors found strong to promising evidence that the program improves self-regulation. The Alert Program has been used to improve self-regulation in children with fetal alcohol spectrum disorder (Nash et al., 2015). The results of Nash and colleagues' study indicated that children receiving the intervention improved their ability to inhibit undesirable behaviors and had better ability to understand social cues. Parents reported a reduction in behavior problems and better emotion regulation. Improvements were maintained at 6-month follow-up.

Dunn Model of Sensory Processing

The Dunn (1997) Model of Sensory Processing provides a theoretical framework for understanding how individuals respond to sensory stimuli. This data-driven model was based on a factor analysis of 1,037 SPs of typically developing children. The factor analysis revealed that the items on the SP were best grouped according to particular patterns of sensory processing (e.g., sensory sensitivity or low registration) rather than sensory modalities (e.g., visual or auditory). The Dunn model is composed of four quadrants that are formed by the intersection of a neurological threshold continuum and a behavioral response/self-regulation continuum.

The neurological threshold continuum runs from low (sensitization) to high (habituation). A low threshold indicates that it takes less sensory stimuli or less intense stimuli for the nervous system to fire and take notice of a stimulus, whereas a high threshold requires more or an increased intensity of the stimuli. A very low threshold is equated with hypersensitivity, and a very high threshold is equated with hyposensitivity.

The other continuum, behavioral response/self-regulation, ranges from passive to active responses. An active response involves intentionally controlling, choosing, or changing environments to manage sensory input, whereas a passive response occurs when the individual responds in accordance with their threshold. The intersection of the two continua results in the four quadrants of the Dunn model.

Four Quadrants

The four quadrants of the Dunn model and their corresponding processing preferences are:

1. Low threshold and passive response = sensory sensitivity
2. Low threshold and active response = sensation avoiding
3. High threshold and passive response = low registration
4. High threshold and active response = sensation seeking

People with **sensory sensitivity** notice things that others do not notice. This can lead to a heightened awareness of the environment and more information with which to make decisions. In contrast, people who are sensory sensitive can be highly distractible and more likely to experience discomfort in high-intensity environments.

People with **sensation avoiding** create or choose environments that reduce sensory input. They can do well in low stimulus situations or settings that others find dull. In addition, people with sensation avoiding tend to be skilled at adapting environments to meet their needs. Conversely, these individuals may miss important information and become distressed in situations in which they cannot control the environment.

People with **low registration** tend to miss input that others notice. They may be slow to respond or require repetition and cues. Yet, these individuals are highly flexible because they tend to not be bothered by sensory stimuli and can typically manage distracting environments very well.

People with **sensation seeking** actively engage with their environment to meet their sensory needs. They change the environment or select environments to obtain higher levels of sensory input. Sensation seekers are easily bored or frustrated in environments that do not meet their elevated needs for sensation.

Intervention Based on the Dunn Model of Sensory Processing

The primary intervention approach using the Dunn (1997) model involves designing environments to meet an individual's sensory processing preferences. This involves understanding how environmental features match a person's sensory processing preferences. An environment that is a good match for someone with sensory sensitivity will likely be very different than an environment that is a good match for a person with low registration. This section describes how OTPs can evaluate the sensory features of environments and create environments that are aligned with an individual's sensory preferences.

In some instances, the OTP will modify environments to help the person be successful, whereas in other cases they will help identify an environment that is the best match. For example, if someone really enjoys their current work situation but is having sensory difficulties in that setting, an environmental modification might be appropriate. However, someone interested in exploring work opportunities for the first time or who is transitioning to a new job would benefit from finding an existing work environment that is a good fit with their sensory preferences.

The following sensory features of the environment should be considered:

- Intensity—the strength of the stimuli
- Amount—how much of the stimuli is present
- Repetition/frequency—how often the stimuli occurs
- Competing stimuli—whether or not there are other stimuli that compete for attention
- Predictability—whether stimuli can be anticipated
- Familiarity—whether a stimuli is known
- Speed—how fast the stimuli appears
- Contrast—how much the stimuli stands out from other forms of stimuli

These features are described differently across the sensory modalities. For example, intensity in the auditory modality is described as loudness, whereas intensity of the visual environment is characterized by colors and brightness. Table 9-3 provides descriptions of the different characteristics of each sensory modality.

Guidelines for fitting the environment to sensory processing preferences follow and are depicted in Figure 9-2. Box 9-3 provides examples of strategies for managing different sensory processing needs in the workplace.

Sensory Sensitivity

A person with sensory sensitivity will benefit from strategies that improve the organization of stimuli and eliminate extraneous or irrelevant stimuli. The environment should be adjusted to decrease the intensity of available sensations, with particular attention given to the reduction of competing stimuli. Examples of simple interventions include having a student sit at the front of the class, an employee work in a quiet space, or a distracted driver turn off the radio. In some

TABLE 9-3 | Characteristics of the Sensory Environment

Sensory Modalities	Features				
	Auditory	*Visual*	*Tactile*	*Taste/Smell*	*Vestibular/ Proprioceptive*
Intensity	• Quiet or loud	• Brightness • Colors	• Light or deep pressure • Irritating or soothing feelings	• Spiciness • Temperature • Strength of taste and smells	• Small or large movement • Gentle or pounding movements
Amount	• Intermittent or constant	• Number of objects	• Body surface affected	• May or may not even be part of the experience	• Activity level
Repetition	• Rhythmic	• Clean lines • Patterns	• Soothing or annoying touch	• All foods taste the same	• Rhythmic • Cadenced movement
Competing stimuli	• Background noise • Multiple conversations	• Clutter	• Ambient environment (e.g., fans, temperature)	• Foods mixed together • Unpleasant smells	• Movement that cannot be controlled (e.g., elevators, vehicles)
Predictability	• Startle	• Organized movement	• Handshake vs. being touched from behind	• Taste/smell is what is expected	• Can anticipate movement and body in space
Familiarity	• Accents • Garbled speech	• Recognizable	• Recognizable	• Have eaten or smelled before	• Established motor patterns
Speed	• Rate of speech/ sounds	• Static vs. moving (e.g., when riding in vehicle)	• Fast or slow	• Savor vs. devour	• Slow/quick
Contrast	• Distinguish voices	• Clarity • Legibility	• Distinguish boundaries of self and others	• Tastes/smells can be distinguished	• Body awareness

Low Registration		Sensory Seeking	
↑ Intensity and **contrast**		↑ **Intensity, amount,** and speed	
↓ Predictability, familiarity, and **speed**		↓ **Consistency**, predictability, and familiarity	
Sensory Sensitivity		Sensation Avoiding	
↑ Predictability and familiarity		↑ **Consistency, predictability**, and familiarity	
↓ Intensity, amount, and **competing stimuli**		↓ **Intensity**, amount, and speed	

FIGURE 9-2. Changing the sensory environment to address sensory processing preferences. Up arrow indicates increase; down arrow indicates decrease; bolded strategies are the most important for that particular preference.

BOX 9-3 ■ Applying Sensory Strategies in the Workplace

Actual cases of individuals with distinct sensory processing preferences are presented as examples of how the Dunn Model of Sensory Processing can be used to guide the intervention process in specific workplace situations.

Harold—Sensory Sensitivity

Harold worked at a café that employed individuals with psychiatric disabilities and was run by an OTP. Harold's sensory sensitivity caused him to become agitated if he was overwhelmed and easily distracted. On the other hand, Harold noticed when things were dirty and was meticulous about cleaning. Although it took some trial and error problem-solving on the part of the OTP, eventually it was determined that running the industrial dishwasher was the perfect job. The position of the dishwasher meant that Harold's back was turned to the busy activity in the kitchen and allowed him to focus on his task at hand. His visual sensitivity made him successful in inspecting his work.

John—Sensation Avoiding

An OTP was asked to evaluate John, an adult with schizophrenia who was having difficulty with his janitorial job. The A/ASP was administered, and there were clear patterns of sensation avoiding. However, the relationship between these sensory processing patterns and problems at work was not apparent until the OTP observed John at work. John was avoiding a major part of his job: vacuuming. When asked, John explained that the sounds of the vacuum cleaner were overwhelming and also triggered auditory hallucinations. Once this was known, job reassignments were made so that he was not required to vacuum, and John was once again successful at work.

James—Low Registration

James was employed in the same café where Harold worked, but his issues with low registration required a very different set of strategies. He was assigned the job of setting the tables, but his low registration resulted in his not noticing important information, such as the salt and pepper shakers being empty. The OTP intervened by creating a checklist that James used successfully to make sure that all the necessary items were full and were placed on the table before the dinner started.

Wilhelmina—Sensation Seeking

Wilhelmina participated in a community program for individuals with psychiatric disabilities and was interested in finding a part-time job. She often felt that she did not fit in at the community program because she found herself to be louder and more energetic than many of the other participants. After administering the A/ASP, the OTP discovered that despite her diagnosis of schizophrenia, Wilhelmina scored "more than most people" in sensation seeking. The OTP was able to work with a senior residence to create a job for Wilhelmina that involved teaching an exercise class in which Wilhelmina was able to expend her energy and use her outgoing personality to her advantage.

---

instances, OTPs can leverage an individual's ability to notice sensory information to enhance occupational performance. For example, sensory sensitivity can help a person notice details that others could miss and is a significant strength for tasks that require attention to detail.

Sensation Avoiding

Interventions for sensation avoiding involve reducing the amount and intensity of stimuli and increasing their predictability and familiarity. Established predictable routines that offer predictable forms of stimuli are generally helpful for individuals with sensation avoiding. In addition, allowing for breaks or providing a quiet space can be helpful, as well as giving the individual more control over the sensory stimuli they are exposed to.

Low Registration

For individuals with low registration, it is important to enhance relevant sensory stimuli so that the individual notices what they need to function. This might include increasing the intensity or amount of a sensory stimulus or reducing the speed at which information is presented so the person has time to take in the information. Cues such as signs or alarms can be helpful for a person with low registration. It is also helpful to reduce the predictability or familiarity of the input, so signs may need to be changed regularly, and the individual may benefit from a change in setting.

Sensation Seeking

People with sensation seeking tend to enjoy variety, intensity, and unpredictability in their environment, and will benefit from opportunities to explore and take control of the environment to create sensations. Sensations that may be distracting to others might be helpful for people who are sensation seeking to maintain their arousal and focus. If a person with sensation seeking is required to be in a low stimulus environment, they may need breaks to get up and move around, talk, or spend time engaged in a higher level of activity.

Being a Psychosocial OT Practitioner

Using Sensory Strategies to Support an Adult With Schizophrenia at Home and Work

Identifying Psychosocial Strengths and Needs

OTPs in all practice settings encounter people with different sensory processing capacities and patterns. In school-based and mental health settings, it is very common for OTPs to work with individuals who have sensory processing patterns that interfere with their occupations, social inclusion, and well-being. To illustrate a common scenario encountered by adults with schizophrenia, consider the story of Gary, a 22-year-old adult with schizophrenia who recently dropped out of college after experiencing a first episode of psychosis that required hospitalization in an inpatient psychiatric unit for 2 weeks.

Gary always excelled at school and was very well liked by his peers. Growing up, he enjoyed participating in sports like soccer and basketball and took every opportunity to be outdoors in nature. His dream was to be a traveling medic for the World Health Organization to help people who are marginalized and vulnerable get access to basic health care.

Gary was on the premed track at his university and hoped to attend med school immediately after college. During his last year in college, the stress of school began to weigh more on Gary, and he began to feel different. He was having trouble focusing and started wondering whether his roommates were stealing money from his wallet at night. As time passed, Gary felt increasingly disorganized and was having more and more trouble focusing on his schoolwork and other basic tasks, such as doing his laundry or cleaning his living space. Things just felt overwhelming. While using a stethoscope during an internship at a local outpatient clinic, Gary could not tune out all the ambient sounds to focus on his patient's heartbeat. His hearing was good, but he could not ignore other sounds to focus on what he needed. All noisy environments were becoming increasingly stressful and difficult for him to manage, so he began avoiding social spaces he used to enjoy.

Gary's roommates were aware of his increasing disorganization and lack of attention to household chores. They also became concerned by Gary's withdrawal from social activities. He would no longer go out with them at night and was frequently isolated in his room. After failing to pay his part of the bills or complete his assigned chores for a couple of weeks, Gary's roommates reached out to his parents to ask for their intervention. Gary reacted very angrily to his parents and accused them and his roommates of betrayal and working behind his back to undermine him. He grew increasingly belligerent and threatened to assault his father. His parents called the police, and Gary's reaction to their arrival was so violent that he was committed to an inpatient psychiatric unit.

After his discharge back to the community, Gary began seeking outpatient therapy, including occupational therapy. He lives with his parents and has a good relationship with them but wants to move out to live independently in his own home. Gary intentionally avoids going out to certain places (e.g., malls, grocery stores, parks) on weekends or during peak periods because he dislikes crowds and noisy environments, even though he enjoys walking around and being active. He is a volunteer at a local health clinic to gain health-care experience and wants to return to school to work in health care.

Using a Holistic Occupational Therapy Approach

Through collaborative assessment and goal identification, the OTP and Gary identified the following three areas to address to lead him toward his goal of living independently in the community:

1. Develop sensory strategies to manage auditory sensitivities that interfere with his occupations.
2. Develop a monthly budget to manage finances independently.
3. Develop an effective morning routine to prepare for work, school, or volunteering.

To help with focus and attention, the OTP collaborated with Gary to identify and develop person-centered cognitive scaffolds (e.g., schedules, checklists, step-by-step visuals to guide task performance) that could help him stay on-task and complete the necessary occupations to move him toward his goals. To increase the likelihood he would use those cognitive scaffolds, Gary and his OTP decorated them with logos of his favorite club soccer team.

To address his auditory sensitivities, Gary and his OTP problem-solved to develop a sensory diet and environmental modifications that would help him maintain optimal sensory health throughout the day to complete his occupations without feeling hypersensitive, hyposensitive, or anxious. Gary's sensory diet included calming occupations during his morning routine and throughout the day to ensure he could manage loud auditory environments when needed. Gary's sensory diet begins with calming walks around his neighborhood immediately after waking up. He ensures his home environment is quiet and no longer listens to the television as he gets ready to avoid creating too much ambient noise.

Gary also changed his shower head because the old one made a lot of noise, which was unpleasant and distracting. Gary wears noise-canceling headphones during his commute to prevent hearing too many competing auditory stimuli. This works better than earplugs or regular headphones that muffle sounds but don't eliminate multiple competing auditory stimuli. At his volunteer job, he has asked his manager to work in a quieter space and listens to his favorite music with noise-canceling headphones. The OTP and Gary also identified a sensory toolkit to respond to acute moments of distress. Instead of the sensory diet that aims to create healthy patterns of sensory health to prevent distress, the sensory toolkit is meant to respond to acute moments of distress that are not predictable.

Gary's toolkit consists of a weighted vest, peppermint gum, an instant cold pack, and a few hand fidgets. Gary keeps his toolkit in a quiet closet near his workspace where he can take a quick break to regulate his sensory health. With these cognitive structures and sensory strategies in place, Gary is able to move toward his life goals and feel a part of his community. He and the OTP continue to collaborate to adjust his strategies and scaffolds to ensure the just right challenge and maximize his satisfaction with his occupations.

Reflective Questions

1. What other sensory strategies might be useful to explore with Gary?
2. How might the OTP use sensory strategies to support Gary's participation in social occupations?
3. Imagine Gary obtained paid employment in a noisy and busy environment with many people. What sensory strategies might the OTP and Gary identify to optimize his ability to work in that environment successfully?

Sensory Environments and Sensory Rooms

Sensory environments and sensory rooms are utilized in treatment settings to provide desired sensory stimuli to individuals with atypical sensory needs. Snoezelen environments are typically used with individuals with significant cognitive impairments to reduce agitation and increase engagement. Sensory rooms are often used to manage anxiety and reduce disruptive behaviors.

Snoezelen Environments

The Snoezelen environment was first developed by Jan Hulsegge and Ad Verheul (1987) in Holland. The term comes from the Dutch verbs "snuffelen," which means to seek, and "doezelen," which means to relax. Unlike other sensory approaches, the intent of the Snoezelen environment is not to develop skills or sensory modulation strategies; it is to create a room that allows individuals to explore sensory features to reduce agitation and anxiety, as well as promote relaxation. There are two essential variables for Snoezelen: the environment, which provides sensory stimulation for exploration and control, and the staff members who guide the person to experience stimuli available in the environment.

The Snoezelen environment has been used most frequently with individuals with severe impairments that limit communication and result in disruptive behaviors, particularly individuals with dementia (Strom et al., 2016). The Snoezelen environment consists of a multimedia space of sensory experiences, with different areas used for different sensory modalities, such as headphones for music, comfortable

---

BOX 9-4 ■ Making "Sense" Out of Addiction Recovery: A Novel Program Introducing Sensory Modulation to Adolescents in Addiction Recovery High School

Jennifer Gardner, OTD, OTR; Geraldine Pagoa-Cruz, MS, OTR; Thais K. Petrocelli, MHA, OTR

The Department of Occupational Therapy, in collaboration with the Kean University Occupational Therapy Community Cares Clinic (KUOT-CCC), partnered with the Raymond J. Lesniak Experience, Strength and Hope (ESH) Recovery High School in New Jersey.

The ESH High School mission is to provide a recovery-oriented learning environment for teenagers in addiction recovery. Based upon emerging evidence and unique knowledge of this population, the Department of Occupational Therapy initiated and implemented sensory-based group programming in collaboration with the staff and educators of ESH High School.

The sensory-based programming was initially structured around a 7-week time frame, with the end goal of developing an onsite sensory modulation room. Graduate occupational therapy students, under the supervision of licensed faculty and staff, were responsible for the development and implementation of the programming. To gain understanding of the high school students' sensory preferences, each student completed the A/ASP during week 1. Staff/educators, as well as the high school students, were then counseled as to what the results of the profile meant, particularly in regard to occupational engagement. This resultant discussion also served as an opportunity to introduce the idea of developing a customized onsite sensory modulation room to the high school students.

The remaining weeks primarily focused on providing education of the various sensory systems and how one's arousal level can be regulated through engagement in various materials and/or activities. The education included ample opportunity for the high school students to explore varying sensory-based materials and activities to learn of sensory preferences and potential self-regulatory strategies to support recovery. The high school students were also empowered to make decisions related to the name of the room, as well as the materials and activities to be accessed and available for continued exploration. The role of the staff and educators of the ESH High School was to order the list of materials and activities as generated by the high school students, as well as solicit donations for the sensory modulation room. The last group session culminated in the official opening of the sensory modulation room with a ribbon cutting ceremony during which the high school students were able to express to invited guests how access to the sensory modulation room positively impacted their recovery. Figure 9-3 shows the room before and after the project.

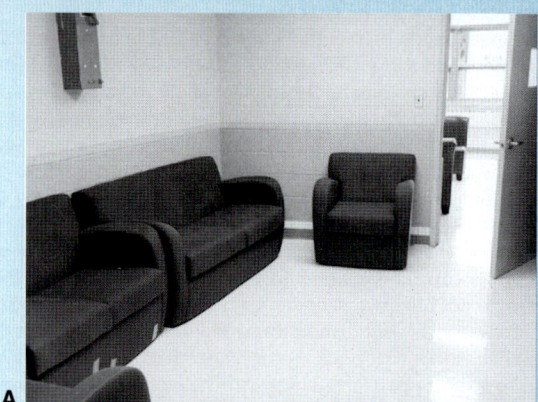

A

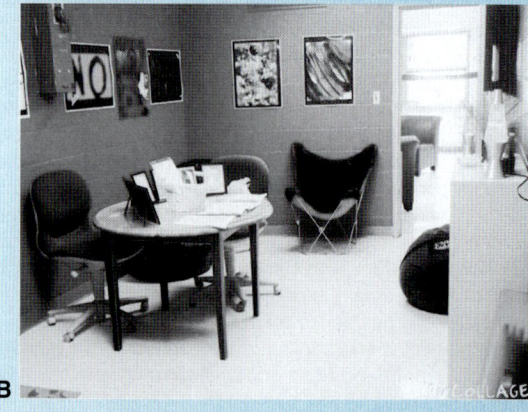

B

FIGURE 9-3. Adolescent sensory room. (A) Before. (B) After. These photos illustrate the sensory features selected by the adolescents to meet their sensory needs.

Although the sensory room was developed in the spring of 2015, the sensory-based collaboration with ESH High School continued with facilitation of in-depth modules connected to each of the sensory systems in the fall of 2015. These modules were designed to reinforce learning, as well as provide continued exploration of preferred sensory strategies to support recovery. Preliminary outcomes of this collaborative intervention include curriculum that continues to integrate the use of the sensory modulation room within the ESH High School learning environment and culture.

cushions, vibrating pads, mirror balls, and bubble machines. A therapist is expected to be in close contact with the person in the Snoezelen environment and promote exploration and enrichment.

Most research with the Snoezelen environment has been with people with dementia. Evidence suggests Snoezelen environments are effective in reducing agitation and improving depression and anxiety; however, they may not be more effective than other interventions (Bauer et al., 2015; Solé et al., 2022; Strom et al., 2016). A qualitative systematic review found that, despite potential benefits, existing Snoezelen environments were often underused in settings, partially because of a lack of staff training (Collier & Jakob, 2016). This suggests that OTPs could train other staff in the use of Snoezelen environments and other sensory approaches.

Sensory Rooms

Sensory rooms are increasingly used in inpatient psychiatric settings as a way for individuals to self-regulate and as a method for reducing seclusion and restraints. Pioneers Tina Champagne (an OTP) and Nan Stromberg (a nurse; 2004) advocated for the inclusion of sensory approaches in their contributions to a task force on reducing seclusion and restraints in institutions in Massachusetts. Champagne and Stromberg's work highlighted the importance of meeting sensory needs to reduce behaviors that result in the use of restraints and seclusion, which can be traumatic and have long-lasting negative effects on individuals.

In general, they recommended approaches that use activities to provide individuals with necessary sensory input for them to maintain a desirable level of arousal that promotes healthy participation in a setting. Depending on the individual and the specific situation, calming activities might involve exercise against resistance, rocking, using a weighted blanket, deep breathing, and chewing gum. In other situations, such as self-harm associated with anxiety, activities that are alerting and orienting, such as snapping a rubber band on the wrist or biting into a lemon, may be recommended.

Champagne also advocates for the development of an individual crisis prevention plan before a crisis occurs. It is important for a person to learn how to use a crisis plan effectively when they are calm before attempting to do so when experiencing a crisis. A crisis plan specifies what types of sensory approaches the individual prefers and finds effective in regulating their level of arousal. With this plan, staff members know what strategies have worked in the past and can effectively support a person with sensory strategies when needed to avoid a crisis that might lead to seclusion and restraint. Therefore, an important component of this approach involves training staff to understand sensory processing theory and how individuals would benefit from sensory approaches.

According to a report by the National Association of State Mental Health Program Directors, implementing environmental changes to include "comfort and sensory rooms" is part of six core strategies for reducing seclusion and restraint (Huckshorn, 2006, p. 7). This report has set the standard for inpatient settings in the United States and therefore has increased the adoption of sensory approaches. OTPs have a nuanced understanding of sensory processing and its relationship to health outcomes. Therefore, they can play an important role in the adoption and effective implementation of sensory approaches in their settings. Box 9-4 presents an example of how OTPs worked with adolescents in their treatment setting to design a sensory room based on their choices.

Here's the Point

- Effective processing of sensory information is necessary for individuals to learn about their world.
- People are born with different sensory processing capacities that are extinguished and/or nurtured through participation in meaningful occupations with others in different sociocultural environments.
- People develop different habits of sensing and sensory anchors based on their sociocultural background and past participation in meaningful occupations.
- There is significant variation in sensory processing patterns among healthy individuals.
- Children and adults with psychiatric conditions often experience atypical sensory processing patterns that have a detrimental impact on their occupational participation, health, and well-being.
- Expert OTPs use both a biomedical understanding of sensory processing and an understanding of the lived sensory experience to implement effective assessment and intervention.
- There are several occupational therapy assessments that can be used to identify and understand sensory processing differences.
- OTPs can utilize a variety of interventions to help individuals manage their sensory experiences so that they can more successfully engage in desired occupations.
- Some approaches that target children are designed to expose children to sensory experiences so that their nervous system can better integrate sensory information and use it adaptively.
- Other interventions help individuals better self-regulate their level of arousal.
- There are intervention approaches for both children and adults that aim to provide the desired sensory input so that the individual can meet their sensory needs to successfully participate in occupational performance.

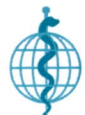 Visit the online resource center at **FADavis.com** to access the videos.

Apply It Now

1. Video Exercise–Jenny's Lived Experience of Sensory Processing Differences

Pair up with another student in your class or form a small group of students. Access and watch the "Jenny's Lived Experience of Sensory Processing Differences" video at the online resource center at FADavis.com. Then, discuss and together answer the following questions:

Reflective Questions

■ How did seeking occupational therapy services for her sensory processing differences support Jenny as a student and in her other occupational roles?

■ Based on Jenny's additional, self-reported mental health diagnoses of anxiety and depression, how might her sensory processing differences intersect with and contribute to her overall mental well-being? As an OTP, what strategies would you recommend to manage her symptoms for improved mental health?

■ How did Jenny take her insight and knowledge about sensory processing differences and turn them into an advocacy skill for herself and peers? What were her recommendations to OTPs with regard to people with sensory processing differences? How will her lived experience benefit her as an OTP?

■ Jenny points out that everyone has sensory processing preferences. What strategies do you use to support your success as a student based on your own sensory needs?

2. Applying the Dunn Model of Sensory Processing to Studying

As an occupational therapy student, you do a lot of studying. Consider the strategies that you employ to help you be successful with studying. Make a list of those strategies.

Reflective Questions

■ What do you consider to be your sensory processing preferences?

■ Are your current strategies for studying consistent with your preferences?

■ Now that you are familiar with the approaches OTPs take to help people meet their sensory needs, what additional or different strategies might be useful for your particular situation and sensory preferences?

3. Analyzing the Sensory Features of an Environment

This exercise is designed to help you identify the most salient sensory features of an environment. Think of one environment that you enjoy and then think of another environment that you find unpleasant. Using Table 9-3, identify the sensory characteristics that are the most prominent in that environment. To do so, think about which sensory systems are the most engaged when in this environment.

Identify what it is about the one environment that makes it a good match for you and why the other one is a poor match. How could you change the environment that is a poor match to meet your sensory health needs?

4. Helping Individuals Manage Their Hyperarousal

Many individuals with psychiatric conditions, both children and adults, experience hyperarousal. This chapter describes many strategies for helping individuals manage their hyperarousal such as use of a weighted blanket or self-monitoring using the Zones of Regulation approach. OTPs can help individuals who have trouble self-regulating by providing options. Brainstorm at least 20 activities or strategies for children and 20 activities or strategies for adults to help someone either prevent hyperarousal or reduce hyperarousal. Consider other chapters in this text that might provide additional insights (e.g., Chapter 8: Cognitive Beliefs, Chapter 10: Coping and Resilience, and Chapter 12: Emotion Regulation 🤝).

Resources

Videos

• "Fieldwork Experience in Juvenile Correction Setting" video. In this video, occupational therapist Maggie reflects on how she felt prepared and unprepared for her fieldwork experience. She touches on topics such as trauma, emotional regulation, and sensory processing, and emphasizes the need to be aware of her own self-care by setting boundaries. Access the video at the online resource center at FADavis.com.

• "Sensory Garden in Geriatric Psychiatric Unit" video. In this video, occupational therapist Callie Ward showcases the sensory garden at an inpatient psychiatric facility. The multisensory garden was designed for occupational therapy groups with a goal of helping participants identify the effects the garden and its related tasks have on their level of arousal. Callie offers specific examples of the many positive effects of the garden on residents, such as collaborating on tasks, problem-solving, encouraging routines, working on cognition, and assisting with self-regulation, among others. She explains how she uses it for active and passive group interventions and in one-to-one sessions. Access the video at the online resource center at FADavis.com.

Websites

• Alert Program: https://www.alertprogram.com
• Ayres Sensory Integration˚:
  • Ayres, A. J. (1979). *Sensory integration and the child.* Western Psychological Services—a classic text written for parents
  • Training in Ayres Sensory Integration: http://www.zoemailloux.com/workshops.html
• OT Innovations—Website describing Tina Champagne's sensory programs addressing trauma-informed care, sensory modulation, and reduction of seclusion and restraints: www.ot-innovations.com
• Sensory Processing Disorder Foundation: http://www.spdfoundation.net
• Sensory Profile Measures: www.sensoryprofile.com
• Snoezelen Environments: www.flaghouse.com/SnoezelenAL.asp and http://www.snoezelen.info
• Tjacket: www.mytjacket.com
• Zones of Regulation: Kuypers, L. M. (2011). *The Zones of Regulation: A curriculum designed to foster self-regulation and emotional control.* Social Thinking Publishing.

References

Ahmari, S. E., Risbrough, V. B., Geyer, M. A., & Simpson, H. B. (2012). Impaired sensorimotor gating in unmedicated adults with obsessive-compulsive disorder. *Neuropsychopharmacology, 37*, 1216–1223. https://doi.org/10.1038/npp.2011.308

American Psychiatric Association. (2013). *Diagnostic and statistical manual of mental disorders* (5th ed., text revision). American Psychiatric Publishing. https://doi.org/10.1176/appi.books.9780890425596

Anderson, K., Swedo, E., Trinh, E., Ray, C., Krause, I., Verlenden, J., Clayton, H., Villaveces, A., Massetti, G., & Niolon, P. (2022). Adverse childhood experiences during the COVID-19 pandemic and associations with poor mental health and suicidal behaviors among high school students—Adolescent behaviors and experiences survey, United States, January–June 2021. *Morbidity and Mortality Weekly Report, 71*(41), 1301–1305. https://doi.org/10.15585/mmwr.mm7141a2

Andersson, H., Sutton, D., Bejerholm, U., & Argentzell, E. (2021). Experiences of sensory input in daily occupations for people with serious mental illness. *Scandinavian Journal of Occupational Therapy, 28*(6), 446–456. https://doi.org/10.1080/11038128.2020.1778784

Ardizzi, M., Ambrosecchia, M., Buratta, L., Ferri, F., Peciccia, M., Donnari, S., & Gallese, V. (2016). Interoception and positive symptoms in schizophrenia. *Frontiers in Human Neuroscience, 10*, 379. https://doi.org/10.3389/fnhum.2016.00379

Arnold, A. J., Winkielman, P., & Dobkins, K. (2019). Interoception and social connection. *Frontiers in Psychology, 10,* Article 2589. https://doi.org/10.3389/fpsyg.2019.02589

Aron, E., & Aron, A. (1997). Sensory processing sensitivity and its relation to introversion and emotionality. *Journal of Personality and Social Psychology, 73*, 345–368. https://doi.org/10.1037//0022-3514.73.2.345

Ayres, A. J. (1972). Improving academic scores through sensory integration. *Journal of Learning Disabilities, 5*(6), 338–343. https://doi.org/10.1177/002221947200500605

Ayres, A. J. (1979). *Sensory integration and the child.* Western Psychological Services.

Bagby, M. S., Dickie, V. A., & Baranek, G. T. (2012). How sensory experiences of children with and without autism affect family occupations. *American Journal of Occupational Therapy, 66*(1), 78–86. https://doi.org/10.5014/ajot.2012.000604

Bailliard, A. L. (2013). The embodied sensory experiences of Latino migrants to Smalltown, North Carolina. *Journal of Occupational Science, 20*(2), 120–130. https://doi.org/10.1080/14427591.2013.774931

Bailliard, A. L. (2015). Habits of the sensory system and mental health: Understanding sensory dissonance. *The American Journal of Occupational Therapy, 69*(4), 6904250020p1–8. https://doi.org/10.5014/ajot.2015.014977

Bailliard, A. L. (2022, October 15). *Sensory Health: A Relational and Emplaced (SHARE) framework of occupation* [Symposium session]. 2022 STAR Sensory Symposium, Denver, CO. https://sensoryhealth.org/basic/welcome-to-2022-star-sensory-symposium

Bailliard, A. L., Carroll, A., & Dallman, A. (2018). The inescapable corporeality of occupation: Integrating Merleau-Ponty into the study of occupation. *Journal of Occupational Science, 25*(2), 222–233. https://doi.org/10.1080/14427591.2017.1397536

Bailliard, A. L., Lee, B., & Bennett, J. (2023). Polysensoriality, aesthetics and agency: The lived sensory experiences of adults with serious mental illness. *Canadian Journal of Occupational Therapy, 90*(1), 103–113. https://journals.sagepub.com/doi/10.1177/00084174221145811

Bailliard, A. L., & Whigham, S. C. (2017). Linking neuroscience, function, and intervention: A scoping review of sensory processing and mental illness. *The American Journal of Occupational Therapy, 71*(5), 7105100040p1–7105100040p18. https://doi.org/10.5014/ajot.2017.024497

Barrett, L. F., Quigley, K. S., Bliss-Moreau, E., & Aronson, K. R. (2004). Interoceptive sensitivity and self-reports of emotional experience. *Journal of Personality and Social Psychology, 87*(5), 684–697. https://doi.org/10.1037/0022-3514.87.5.684

Bar-Shalita, T., & Cermak, S. A. (2016). Atypical sensory modulation and psychological distress in the general population. *The American Journal of Occupational Therapy, 70*(4), 7004250010. https://doi.org/10.5014/ajot.2016.018648

Bar-Shalita, T., Vatine, J. J., Parush, S., Deutsch, L., & Seltzer, Z. (2012). Psychophysical correlates in adults with sensory modulation disorder. *Disability and Rehabilitation, 34*, 943–950. https://doi.org/10.1016/j.physbeh.2009.09.020

Bauer, M., Rayner, J. A., Tang, J., Koch, S., While, C., & O'Keef, F. (2015). An evaluation of Snoezelen* compared to "common best practice" for allaying the symptoms of wandering and restlessness among residents with dementia in aged care facilities. *Geriatric Nursing, 36*, 462–466. https://doi.org/10.1016/j.gerinurse.2015.07.005

Ben-Sasson, A., Gal, E., Fluss, R., Katz-Zetler, N., & Cermak, S. (2019). Update of meta-analysis of sensory symptoms in ASD: A new decade of research. *Journal of Autism and Developmental Disorders, 49*, 4974–4996. https://doi.org/10.1007/s10803-019-04180-0

Branjerdporn, G., Meredith, P., Strong, J., & Green, M. (2019). Sensory sensitivity and its relationship with adult attachment and parenting styles. *PLoS One, 14*(1): e0209555. https://doi.org/10.1371/journal.pone.0209555

Brewer, R., Murphy, J., & Bird, G. (2021). Atypical interoception as a common risk factor for psychopathology: A review. *Neuroscience and Biobehavioral Reviews, 130*, 470–508. https://doi.org/10.1016/j.neubiorev.2021.07.036

Brown, C., Cromwell, R. L., Filion, C., Dunn, W., & Tollefson, N. (2002). Sensory processing in schizophrenia: Missing and avoiding information. *Schizophrenia Research, 55*, 187–195. https://doi.org/10.1016/s0920-9964(01)00255-9

Brown, C., & Dunn, W. (2002). *Adolescent/adult sensory profile.* Psychological Corp.

Brown, C., Karim, R., & Steuter, M. (2020). Retrospective analysis of studies examining sensory processing preferences in people with a psychiatric condition. *American Journal of Occupational Therapy, 74*(4), 7404205130p1–7404205130p11. https://doi.org/10.5014/ajot.2020.038463

Brown, C., Shahab, R., Collins, K., Fleysher, L., Goodman, W., Burdick, K., & Stern, E. (2019). Functional neural mechanisms of sensory phenomena in obsessive-compulsive disorder. *Journal of Psychiatric Research, 109*, 68–75. https://doi.org/10.1016/j.jpsychires.2018.11.018

Brown, C., Tollefson, N., Dunn, W., Cromwell, R., & Filion, D. (2001). The Adult Sensory Profile: Measuring patterns of sensory processing. *American Journal of Occupational Therapy, 55*, 75–82. https://doi.org/10.5014/ajot.55.1.75

Bunney, W. E., Hetrick, W. P., Bunney, B. G., Patterson, J. V., Jin, Y., Potkin, S. G., & Sandman, C. A. (1999). Structured Interview for Assessing Perceptual Anomalies (SIAPA). *Schizophrenia Bulletin, 25*, 577–592. https://doi.org/10.1093/oxfordjournals.schbul.a033402

Butler, P. D., & Javitt, D. C. (2005). Early-stage visual processing deficits in schizophrenia. *Current Opinion in Psychiatry, 18*, 151–157. https://doi.org/10.1097/00001504-200503000-00008

Castle, D., Feusner, J., Laposa, J. M., Richter, P. M. A., Hossain, R., Lusicic, A., & Drummond, L. M. (2023). Psychotherapies and digital interventions for OCD in adults: What do we know, what do we need still to explore? *Comprehensive Psychiatry, 120*, 152357. https://doi.org/10.1016/j.comppsych.2022.152357

Cermak, S. A., Curtin, C., & Bandini, L. G. (2010). Food selectivity and sensory sensitivity in children with autism spectrum disorder. *Journal of the American Dietetic Association, 110*, 238–246. https://doi.org/10.1007/s10803-017-3340-9

Champagne, T., & Stromberg, N. (2004). Sensory approaches in inpatient psychiatric settings: Innovative alternatives to seclusion and restraint. *Journal of Psychosocial Nursing and Mental Health Services, 42*, 34–45. https://doi.org/10.3928/02793695-20040901-06

Chen, H. Y., Yang, H., Meng, L. F., Chan, P. S., Yang, C. Y., & Chen, H. M. (2016). Effect of deep pressure input on parasympathetic system in patients with wisdom tooth surgery. *Journal of the Formosan Medical Association, 115*(10), 853–859. https://doi.org/10.1016/j.jfma.2016.07.008

Chen, Y., & Ekstrom, T. (2015). Visual and associated affective processing of face information in schizophrenia: A selective review. *Current Psychiatry Review, 11*, 266–272. https://doi.org/10.2174/1573400511666150930000817

Classen, C. (1992). The odor of the other: Olfactory symbolism and cultural categories. *Ethos, 20*, 133–166. https://doi.org/10.1525/eth.1992.20.2.02a00010

Collier, L., & Jakob, A. (2016). The multisensory environment in dementia care. *HERD: Health Environments Research and Design Journal, 10*, 39–51. https://doi.org/10.1177/1937586716683508

Delgado-Lobete, L., Pértega-Díaz, S., Santos-del-Riego, S., & Montes-Montes, R. (2020). Sensory processing patterns in developmental coordination disorder, attention deficit hyperactivity disorder and typical development. *Research in Developmental Disabilities, 100*, 103608. https://doi.org/10.1016/j.ridd.2020.103608

Dellapiazza, F., Michelon, C., Vernhet, C., Muratori, F., Blanc, N., Picot, M., & Baghdadli, A. (2021). Sensory processing related to attention in children with ASD, ADHD, or typical development: Results from the ELENA cohort. *European Child & Adolescent Psychiatry, 30*, 283–291. https://doi.org/10.1007/s00787-020-01516-5

Dowdy, R., Estes, J., Linkugel, M., & Dvornak, M. (2020). Trauma, sensory processing, and the impact of occupational therapy on youth behavior in juvenile corrections. *Occupational Therapy in Mental Health, 36*, 373–393. https://doi.org/10.1080/0164212X.2020.1823930

Dunn, W. (1997). The impact of sensory processing abilities on the daily lives of young children and their families: A conceptual model. *Infants and Young Children, 9*(4), 23–35. https://doi.org/10.1097/00001163-199704000-00005

Dunn, W. (2014). *Sensory Profile 2: User's manual*. Psychological Corp.

Dunn, W., Brown, C., Breitmeyer, A., & Salwei, A. (2022). Construct validity of the Sensory Profile Interoception scale: Measuring sensory processing in everyday life. *Frontiers in Psychology, 13*. https://doi.org/10.3389/fpsyg.2022.872619

Engel-Yeger, B., & Dunn, W. (2011). Exploring the relationship between affect and sensory processing patterns in adults. *British Journal of Occupational Therapy, 74*, 456–464. https://doi.org/10.4276/030802211X13182481841868

Engel-Yeger, B., Gonda, X., Muzio, C., Rinosi, G., Pompili, M., Amore, M., & Serafini, G. (2016). Sensory processing patterns, coping strategies and quality of life among patients with unipolar and bipolar disorders. *Revista Brasileira de Psiquiatria, 38*, 207–215. https://doi.org/10.1590/1516-4446-2015-1785

Engel-Yeger, B., Muzio, C., Rinosi, G., Solano, P., Geoffroy, P. A., Pompili, M., Amore, M., & Serafini, G. (2016). Extreme sensory processing patterns and their relation with clinical conditions among individuals with major affective disorders. *Psychiatry Research, 236*, 112–118. https://doi.org/10.1016/j.psychres.2015.12.022

Engel-Yeger, B., Palgy-Levin, D., & Lev-Wiesel, R. (2013). The sensory profile of people with post-traumatic stress symptoms. *Occupational Therapy in Mental Health, 29*, 266–278. https://doi.org/10.1080/0164212X.2013.819466

Felitti, V. J., Anda, R. F., Nordenberg, D., Williamson, D. F., Spitz, A. M., Edwards, V., & Koss, M. P. (1998). Relationship of childhood abuse and household dysfunction to many of the leading causes of death in adults: The adverse childhood experiences (ACE) study. *American Journal of Preventive Medicine, 14*(4), 245–258. https://doi.org/10.1016/s0749-3797(98)00017-8

Fraser, K., MacKenzie, D., & Versnel, J. (2017). Complex trauma in children and youth: A scoping review of sensory-based interventions. *Occupational Therapy in Mental Health, 33*, 199–216. https://doi.org/10.1080/0164212X.2016.1265475

Gill, K., Thompson-Hodgetts, S., & Rasmussen, C. (2018). A critical review of research on the alert program. *Journal of Occupational Therapy, Schools, & Early Intervention, 11*(2), 212–228. https://doi.org/10.1080/19411243.2018.1432445

Grandin, T. (2000). *My experiences with visual thinking sensory problems and communication difficulties*. http://web.archive.org/web/20080430021634/http://www.autism.org/temple/visual.html

Green, M. F., Olivier, B., Crawley, J. N., Penn, D. L., & Silverstein, S. (2005). Social cognition in schizophrenia: Recommendations from the Measurement and Treatment Research to Improve Cognition in Schizophrenia New Approaches Conference. *Schizophrenia Bulletin, 31*, 882–887. https://doi.org/10.1093/schbul/sbi049

Hass, L. (2008). *Merleau-Ponty's philosophy*. Indiana University Press.

Herz, R. S. (2016). The role of odor-evoked memory in psychological and physiological health. *Brain Science, 6*(3), piiE22. https://doi.org/10.3390/brainsci6030022

Houghton, D. C., Stein, D. J., & Cortese, B. M. (2020). Exteroceptive sensory abnormalities in childhood and adolescent anxiety and obsessive-compulsive disorder: A critical review. *Journal of the American Academy of Child & Adolescent Psychiatry, 59*, 78–87. https://doi.org/10.1016/j.jaac.2019.06.007

Howe, F. E., & Stagg, S. D. (2016). How sensory experiences affect adolescents with an autism spectrum condition within the classroom. *Journal of Autism and Developmental Disorders, 46*, 1656–1668. https://doi.org/10.1007/s10803-015-2693-1

Huckshorn, K. A. (2006). *6 core strategies to reduce the use of seclusion and restraint: Planning tool*. http://www.nasmhpd.org/sites/default/files/Consolidated%20Six%20Core%20Strategies%20Document.pdf

Hulsegge, J., & Verheul, A. (1987). *Snoezelen: Another world*. Rompa.

Ippen, C. G., Harris, W. H., van Horn, P., & Lieberman, A. F. (2011). Traumatic and stressful events in early childhood: Can treatment help those at highest risk? *Child Abuse and Neglect, 35*(7), 504–513. https://doi.org/10.1016/j.chiabu.2011.03.009

Jahshan, C., Wynn, J. K., & Green, M. F. (2013). Relationship between auditory processing and affective prosody in schizophrenia. *Schizophrenia Research, 143*, 348–353. https://doi.org/10.1016/j.schres.2012.11.025

Javitt, D. C., & Freedman, R. (2015). Sensory processing dysfunction in the personal experience and neuronal machinery of schizophrenia. *American Journal of Psychiatry, 172*, 17–31. https://doi.org/10.1176/appi.ajp.2014.13121691

Javitt, D. C., & Sweet, R. A. (2015). Auditory dysfunction in schizophrenia: Integrating clinical and basic features. *National Review of Neuroscience, 16*, 535–550. https://doi.org/10.1038/nrn4002

Kamath, M., Dahm, C., Tucker, J., Huang-Pollock, C., Etter, N., & Neely, K. (2020). Sensory profiles in adults with and without ADHD. *Research in Developmental Disabilities, 104*, 103696. https://doi.org/10.1016/j.ridd.2020.103696

Kandel, E. R., Schwartz, J. H., Jessell, T. M., Siegelbaum, S. A., & Hudspeth, A. J. (2012). *Principles of neural science* (5th ed.). McGraw-Hill. https://neurology.mhmedical.com/content.aspx?bookid=1049&sectionid=59138139

Kantrowitz, J. T., Hoptman, M. J., Leitman, D. I., Silipo, G., & Javitt, D. C. (2014). The 5% difference: Early sensory processing predicts sarcasm perception in schizophrenia and schizo-affective disorder. *Psychological Medicine, 44*, 25–36. https://doi.org/10.1017/S0033291713000834

Kerley, L., Meredith, P. J., Harnett, P., Sinclair, C., & Strong, J. (2021). Families of children in pain: Are attachment and sensory processing patterns related to parent functioning? *Journal of Child and Family Studies, 30*, 1554–1566. https://doi.org/10.1007/s10826-021-01966-8

Kinnealey, M., & Fuiek, M. (1999). The relationship between sensory defensiveness, anxiety, depression, and perception of pain in adults. *Occupational Therapy International, 6,* 195–296. https://doi.org/10.1002/oti.97

Kleim, B., Ehring, T., & Ehlers, A. (2012). Perceptual processing advantages for trauma-related visual cues in post traumatic stress disorder. *Psychological Medicine, 42,* 173–181. https://doi.org/10.1017/S0033291711001048

Koreki, A., Funayama, M., Terasawa, Y., Onaya, M., & Mimura, M. (2021). Aberrant interoceptive accuracy in patients with schizophrenia performing a heartbeat counting task. *Schizophrenia Bulletin, 2*(1), sgaa067. https://doi.org/10.1093/schizbullopen/sgaa067

Kuschner, E. S., Eisenberg, I. W., Orionzi, B., Simmons, W. K., Kenworthy, L., Martin, A., & Wallace, G. L. (2015). A preliminary study of self-reported food selectivity in adolescents and young adults with autism spectrum disorder. *Research in Autism Spectrum Disorder, 15/16,* 53–59. https://doi.org/10.1016/j.rasd.2015.04.005

Kuypers, L. M. (2011). *The zones of regulation: A curriculum designed to foster self-regulation and emotional control.* Social Thinking Publishing.

Landon, J., Shepherd, D., McGarry, M., Theadom, A., & Miller, R. (2016). When it's quiet, it's nice: Noise sensitivity in schizophrenia. *American Journal of Psychiatric Rehabilitation, 19*(2), 122–135. https://doi.org/10.1080/15487768.2016.1162758

Lane, S. J., Miller, L. J., & Hanft, B. E. (2000). Toward a consensus in terminology in sensory integration theory and practice: Part 2: Sensory integration patterns of function and dysfunction. *Sensory Integration Special Interest Section Quarterly, 23*(2), 1–3.

Light, G. A., & Braff, D. L. (2005). Mismatch negativity deficits are associated with poor functioning in schizophrenia patients. *Archives of General Psychiatry, 62,* 127–136. https://doi.org/10.1001/archpsyc.62.2.127

Liss, M., Timmel, L., Baxley, K., & Killingsworth, P. (2005). Sensory processing sensitivity and its relation to parental bonding, anxiety and depression. *Personality and Individual Differences, 39,* 1429–1439. https://doi.org/10.1016/j.paid.2005.05.007

Machingura, T., Kaur, G., Lloyd, C., Mickan, S., Shum, D., Rathbone, E., & Green, H. (2019). An exploration of sensory processing patterns and their association with demographic factors in healthy adults. *Irish Journal of Occupational Therapy, 48,* 3–16. https://doi.org/10.1108/IJOT-12-2018-0025

Machingura, T., Lloyd, C., Murphy, K., Goulder, S, Shum, D., & Green, H. (2021). Views about sensory modulation from people with schizophrenia and treating staff: A multisite qualitative study. *British Journal of Occupational Therapy, 84,* 550–560. https://doi.org/10.1177/0308022620988470

Mailloux, Z., & Miller-Kuhaneck, H. (2014). From the desk of the guest editors—Evolution of a theory: How measurement has shaped Ayres Sensory Integration*. American Journal of Occupational Therapy, 68,* 495–499. https://doi.org/10.5014/ajot.2014.013656

May-Benson, T. A., & Koomar, J. A. (2010). Systematic review of the research evidence examining the effectiveness of interventions using a sensory integrative approach for children. *American Journal of Occupational Therapy, 64,* 403–414. https://doi.org/10.5014/ajot.2010.09071

McGhie, A., & Chapman, J. (1961). Disorders of attention and perception in early schizophrenia. *British Journal of Medical Psychology, 34,* 103–116. https://doi.org/10.1111/j.2044-8341.1961.tb00936.x

McGreevy, S., & Boland, P. (2020). Sensory-based interventions with adult and adolescent trauma survivors: An integrative review of the occupational therapy literature. *Irish Journal of Occupational Therapy, 48,* 31–54. https://doi.org/10.1108/IJOT-10-2019-0014

McLaughlin, K. A., Sheridan, M. A., & Lambert, H. K. (2014). Childhood adversity and neural development: Deprivation and threat as distinct dimensions of early experience. *Neuroscience and Biobehavioral Review, 47,* 578–591. https://doi.org/10.1146/annurev-devpsych-121318-084950

Mehling, W. E., Acree, M., Stewart, A., Silas, J., & Jones, A. (2018). The Multidimensional Assessment of Interoceptive Awareness, version 2 (MAIA-2). *PloS One, 13*(12), e0208034. https://doi.org/10.1371/journal.pone.0208034

Meredith, P. J., Rappel, G., Strong, J., & Baily, K. J. (2015). Sensory sensitivity and strategies for coping with pain. *American Journal of Occupational Therapy, 69,* 6904240010. https://doi.org/10.5014/ajot.2015.014621

Miller, L. J., Anzalone, M. E., Lane, S. J., Cermak, S. A., & Osten, E. T. (2007). Concept evolution in sensory integration: A proposed nosology for diagnosis. *American Journal of Occupational Therapy, 61,* 135–140. https://doi.org/10.5014/ajot.61.2.135

Miller-Kuhaneck, H., Henry, D. A., Glennon, T. J., & Mu, K. (2007). Development of the Sensory Processing Measure–School: Initial studies of reliability and validity. *American Journal of Occupational Therapy, 61,* 170–175. https://doi.org/10.5014/ajot.61.2.170

Nash, K., Stevens, S., Greenbaum, R., Weiner, J., Koren, G., & Rovet, J. (2015). Improving executive functioning in children with fetal alcohol spectrum disorders. *Child Neuropsychology, 21,* 191–209. https://doi.org/10.1080/09297040802385400

Neal, J. A., Edelmann, R. J., & Glachan, M. (2002). Behavioural inhibition and symptoms of anxiety and depression: Is there a specific relationship with social phobia? *British Journal of Clinical Psychology, 41,* 361–374. https://doi.org/10.1348/014466502760387489

O'Donnell, S., Deitz, J., Kartin, D., Nalty, T., & Dawson, G. (2012). Sensory processing, problem behavior, adaptive behavior, and cognition in preschool children with autism spectrum disorder. *American Journal of Occupational Therapy, 66,* 586–594. https://doi.org/10.5014/ajot.2012.004168

Oldroyd, K., Pasupathi, M., & Wainryb, C. (2019). Social antecedents to the development of interoception: Attachment related processes are associated with interoception. *Frontiers in Psychology, 10,* 712. https://doi.org/10.3389/fpsyg.2019.00712

Parham, L. D., & Mailloux, Z. (2010). Sensory integration. In J. Case-Smith, A. S. Allen, & P. N. Pratt (Eds.), *Occupational therapy for children* (pp. 356–411). Elsevier.

Parham, L. D., Smith-Roley, S., May-Benson, T. A., Koomar, J., Brett-Green, B., Burke, J. P., Cohn, E. S., Mailloux, Z., Miller, L. J., & Schaff, R. C. (2011). Development of a fidelity measure for research on the effectiveness of the Ayres Sensory Integration Intervention. *American Journal of Occupational Therapy, 65,* 442–449. https://doi.org/10.5014/ajot.2011.000745

Petruccelli, K., Davis, J., & Berman, T. (2019). Adverse childhood experiences and associated health outcomes: A systematic review and meta-analysis. *Child Abuse & Neglect, 97,* 104127. https://doi.org/10.1016/j.chiabu.2019.104127

Pfeiffer, B., Brusilovskiy, E., Bauer, J., & Salzer, M. S. (2014). Sensory processing, participation and recovery in adults with serious mental illnesses. *Psychiatric Rehabilitation Journal, 37,* 289–296. https://doi.org/10.1037/prj0000099

Pfeiffer, B., Daly, B. P., Nicholls, E., & Gullo, D. F. (2015). Assessment of sensory processing problems in children with and without attention deficit hyperactivity disorder. *Physical and Occupational Therapy in Pediatrics, 35*(1), 1–12. https://doi.org/10.3109/01942638.2014.904471

Pisoni, C., Garagoli, F., Tzialla, C., Orcesi, S., Spinillo, A., Politi, P., Balottin, U., Manzoni, P., & Stronati, M. (2014). Risk and protective factors in maternal-fetal attachment development. *Early Human Development, 90*(Suppl. 2), S45–S46. https://doi.org/10.1016/S0378-3782(14)50012-6

Quigley, K. S., Kanoski, S., Grill, W. M., Barrett, L. F., & Tsakiris, M. (2021). Functions of interoception: From energy regulation to experience of the self. *Trends in Neurosciences, 44*(1), 29–38. https://doi.org/10.1016/j.tins.2020.09.008

Rieke, E. F., & Anderson, D. (2009). Adolescent/Adult Sensory Profile and obsessive-compulsive disorder. *American Journal of Occupational Therapy, 63,* 138–145. https://doi.org/10.5014/ajot.63.2.138

Schaaf, R., Dumont, R., Arbesman, M., & May-Benson, T. (2018). Efficacy of occupational therapy using Ayres Sensory Integration: A systematic review. *American Journal of Occupational Therapy, 72*(1), 7201190010p1–7201190010p10. https://doi.org/10.5014/ajot.2018.028431

Schauder, K. B., & Bennetto, L. (2016). Toward an interdisciplinary understanding of sensory dysfunction in autism spectrum disorder: An integration of the neural and symptom literatures. *Frontiers in Neuroscience, 10,* 268. https://doi.org/10.3389/fnins.2016.00268

Schmitt, C. M., & Schoen, S. (2022). Interoception: A multi-sensory foundation of participation in daily life. *Frontiers in Neuroscience, 16,* 875200. https://doi.org/10.3389/fnins.2022.875200

Schneider, G. E. (1969). Two visual systems. *Science, 163,* 895–902. https://doi.org/10.1126/science.163.3870.895

Schoen, S., Lane, S., Mailloux, Z., May-Benos, T., Parham, D., Roley, S., & Schaaf, R. (2019). A systematic review of Ayres Sensory Integration intervention for children with autism. *Autism Research, 12*(1), 6–19. https://doi.org/10.1002/aur.2046

Shimizu, V. T., Bueno, O. F., & Miranda, M. C. (2014). Sensory processing abilities of children with attention deficit hyperactivity disorder. *Brazilian Journal of Physical Therapy, 18*(4), 343–352. https://doi.org/10.1590/bjpt-rbf.2014.0043

Solé, C., Celdrán, M., & Cifre, I. (2022). Psychological and behavioral effects of Snoezelen rooms on dementia. *Activities, Adaptation & Aging.* Advance online publication. https://doi.org/10.1080/01924788.2022.2151805

Strom, B. S., Ytrehus, S., & Grov, E. K. (2016). Sensory stimulation for persons with dementia: A review of the literature. *Journal of Clinical Nursing, 25,* 1805–1834. https://doi.org/10.1111/jocn.13169

Substance Abuse and Mental Health Services Administration. (2014). *Trauma-informed care in behavioral health services.* Author.

Takahashi, T., Nakamura, M., Sasabayashi, D., Komori, Y., Higuchi, Y., Nishikawa, Y., Nishiyama, S., Itoh, H., Masaoka, Y., & Suzuki, M. (2018). Olfactory deficits in individuals at risk for psychosis and patients with schizophrenia: Relationship with socio-cognitive functions and symptom severity. *European Archives of Psychiatry and Clinical Neuroscience, 268*(7), 689–698. https://doi.org/10.1007/s00406-017-0845-3

U.S. Department of Health & Human Services, Administration for Children and Families, Administration on Children, Youth and Families, Children's Bureau. (2022). *Child maltreatment 2020.* http://www.acf.hhs.gov/programs/cb/research-data-technology/statistics-research/child-maltreatment

van den Boogert, F., Klein, K., Spaan, P., Sizoo, B., Bouman, Y. H. A., Hoogendijk, W. J. G., & Roza, S. J. (2022). Sensory processing difficulties in psychiatric disorders: A meta-analysis. *Journal of Psychiatric Research, 151,* 173–180. https://doi.org/10.1016/j.jpsychires.2022.04.020

Van Hulle, C. A., Esbensen, K., & Goldsmith, H. H. (2019). Co-occurrence of sensory overresponsivity with obsessive-compulsive symptoms in childhood and early adolescence. *Journal of Developmental and Behavioral Pediatrics, 40*(5), 377–382. https://doi.org/10.1097/DBP.0000000000000671

Vietri, J., Otsuby, T., Montgomery, W., Tsuji, T., & Harada, E. (2015). The incremental burden of pain in patients with depression: Results of a Japanese study. *BMC Psychiatry, 15,* 104. https://doi.org/10.1186/s12888-015-0488-8

Wan, L., Friedman, B. H., Boutros, N. N., & Crawford, H. J. (2008). P50 sensory gating and attentional performance. *International Journal of Psychophysiology, 67,* 91–100. https://doi.org/10.1016/j.ijpsycho.2007.10.008

Wilkerson, A. K., Uhde, T. W., Leslie, K., Freeman, W. C., LaRowe, S. D., Schumann, A., & Cortese, B. M. (2018). Paradoxical olfactory function in combat veterans: The role of PTSD and odor factors. *Military Psychology: The Official Journal of the Division of Military Psychology, American Psychological Association, 30*(2), 120–130. https://doi.org/10.1080/08995605.2018.1425063

Williams, M. S., & Shellenberger, S. (1996). *"How does your engine run?" The leader's guide to the Alert Program® for self regulation.* TherapyWorks.

Yochman, A., & Pat-Horenczyk, R. (2020). Sensory modulation in children exposed to continuous traumatic stress. *Journal of Child & Adolescent Trauma, 13,* 93–102. https://doi.org/10.1007/s40653-019-00254-4

Yoon, J. H., Sheremata, S. L., Rokem, A., & Silver, M. A. (2013). Windows to the soul: Vision science as a tool for studying biological mechanisms of information processing deficits in schizophrenia. *Frontiers in Psychology, 4,* 681. https://doi.org/10.3389/fpsyg.2013.00681

Coping and Resilience

Adam Lo and Catana Brown

Coping involves the process, strategies, and behaviors that individuals use to adapt, adjust, and manage the challenges and stressful demands of daily life. Coping can be adaptive or maladaptive and contributes to the overall resilience of individuals over time (Hoge et al., 2007).

Resilience refers to the ability of individuals to adapt to challenges, trauma, and life changes in order to maintain well-being, productivity, and meaning in their everyday life. Resilience is a dynamic process that involves the development and strengthening of various factors within each unique individual and includes adaptive coping skills, self-efficacy, cognitive flexibility, and levels of emotional regulation and mindfulness (Lavis, 2014).

Occupational therapy, through its emphasis on helping people address the performance demands of life tasks, assists individuals to develop resilience and overcome challenges associated with moving, thinking, sensing, and/or feeling to promote independence, overall well-being, and quality of life (Unger & Theron, 2019).

This chapter provides an overview of concepts pertinent to stress, coping, and resilience; describes the relationships between mental illness and resilience; and provides foundational information on evaluation and intervention strategies related to stress, coping, and the promotion of resilience.

Models of Stress and Coping

Stress is a natural response to challenges and stressors, which can be internal or perceived (such as examination worries) or come from external sources (such as an aggressive person). It can motivate people to study for examinations or protect them from danger by triggering a protective response. There are many different models that explain how people respond to stress. These models help occupational therapy practitioners (OTPs) better understand behaviors that might indicate a coping response, and they can assist OTPs in designing interventions for promoting adaptive responses and resilience.

The Acute Stress/Fear Response: Fight, Flight, Freeze, or Fawn

The acute stress response involves a physiological reaction to a real or a perceived threat and is believed to be evolutionary in nature (Kozlowska et al., 2015). When a person is confronted with a fear, the sympathetic nervous system is activated, resulting in a release of cortisol. This causes a cascade of physiological responses such as an increase in heart rate, rapid breathing, muscles tensing, slowed digestion, and bladder relaxation. The ultimate objective is to avoid or manage the threat and return the individual to some level of homeostasis or calm. When a person experiences fear, the amygdala is activated and the individual makes a quick decision (which can be unconscious) as to how to respond. These responses include fight, flight, freeze, or fawn (see Fig. 10-1).

The **fight** response involves confronting the threat with a physical reaction. If a person doesn't think they can successfully fight off the threat, they can try to avoid the danger with **flight**. With **freeze**, they are still and quiet until the danger passes. It is an attempt to avoid detection. More recently, **fawn** has been added to describe a response wherein a person tries to please the person who is triggering the fear (Walker, 2013). This response is common in trauma survivors to avoid being hurt by an abuser. In some situations, the person may move through different responses. Perhaps they freeze initially but then either fight back or flee.

Although these responses are often helpful in protecting people from harm, they can also bring negative consequences if triggered inappropriately or excessively. In addition, the acute stress response is useful for managing situational challenges, but people must also be able to turn off the stress response or else long-term physical and mental health damage will occur (Floriou-Servou et al., 2021).

Diathesis-Stress Model

The nature versus nurture debate is often used in trying to understand the development of mental illness. The debate centers around biological factors or social and environmental causes (Christiansen, 2007). The Diathesis-Stress Model, developed by Adolf Meyer, explains that mental illness is caused by the interaction between biological susceptibility and environmental stressors (A. Meyer, 1921). This means that people with a genetic vulnerability will develop a condition when triggered by certain stressors and environmental conditions. The model helps explain why some people with a biological predisposition do not necessarily develop a mental illness and, likewise, why some individuals undergoing extreme stress remain mentally healthy.

Research on identical twins suggests that both nature and nurture play a role in the development of mental illness, as identical twins do not always develop the same disorders despite sharing the same genetic makeup. For example, in a very

The Acute Stress Response

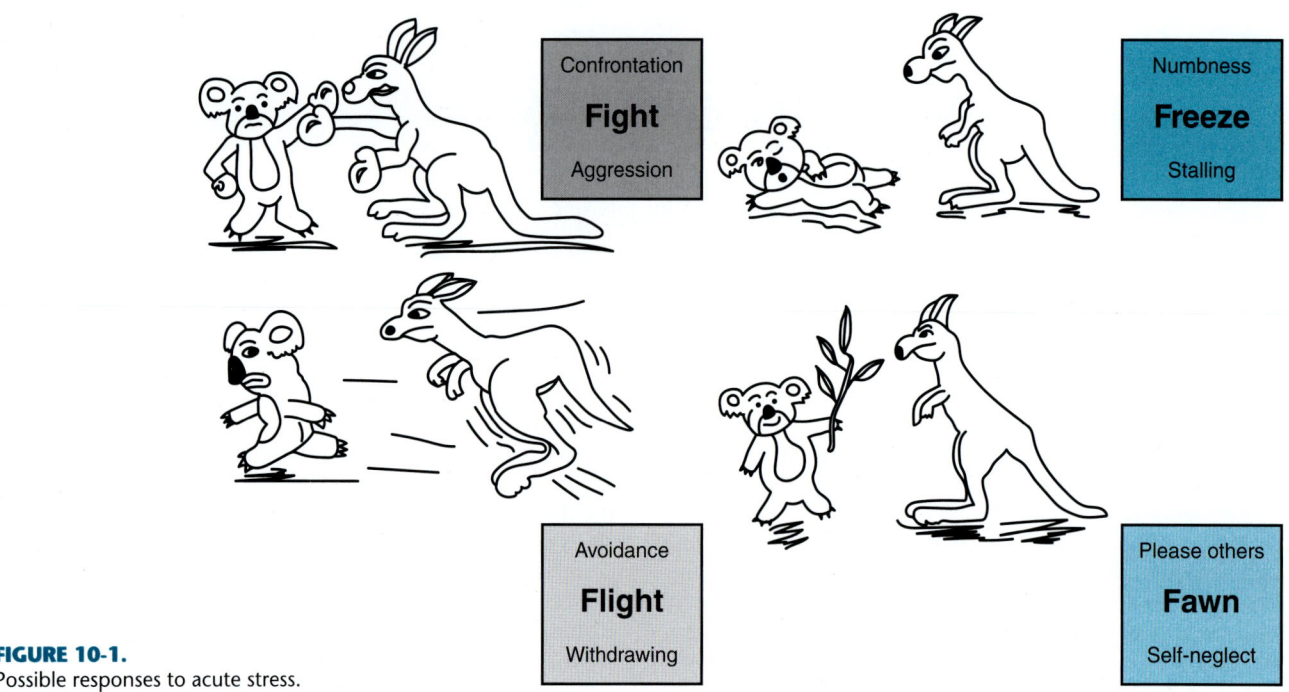

FIGURE 10-1.
Possible responses to acute stress.

large twin study, the concordance rate (the probability that both twins will develop the same disorder) for schizophrenia is approximately 33% for identical twins and only 7% for nonidentical twins (Hilker et al., 2017).

Transactional Model of Stress and Coping

The **Transactional Model of Stress and Coping** developed by Lazarus and Folkman (1984) describes the process by which people deal with stressful situations. People are constantly appraising their environment. When they detect a threat or stressor, coping strategies are initiated to manage the situation. The person then reappraises the situation and determines if the coping strategy was successful or if a different strategy is needed.

Appraisal is an important concept in the model. As a cognitive process, the person ascribes meaning to a situation and deems whether a situation is benign-positive, irrelevant, harmful, or challenging. Although both harmful and challenging situations can be stressful, harmful appraisals elicit negative emotions whereas challenging situations have the potential for rewards and growth. If a situation is deemed harmful or challenging, a coping response is needed to mitigate the stress.

According to Folkman and Lazarus (1988), there are two primary types of coping that can be employed: emotion-focused coping and problem-focused coping. With **emotion-focused coping**, the person uses strategies that reduce negative emotions associated with a stressor. With **problem-focused coping**, the person resolves the stressful situation or alters the source of stress. Initial views of the model suggested that emotion-focused coping was maladaptive, whereas problem-focused coping was effective. However, current applications suggest that the coping strategies are not inherently effective or ineffective; rather, it depends on how well the coping strategy corresponds with the current situation (Biggs et al., 2017).

The Ways of Coping Questionnaire, which is based on the Transactional Model, includes eight subscales or different methods of coping (see Table 10-1).

Salutogenesis and Sense of Coherence

Some people experience extreme stress and still manage to stay mentally well. The **Salutogenic Model** focuses on understanding health instead of disease to explain how some people adapt and survive in the face of adversity (Antonovsky, 1979). The model was developed by Aaron Antonovsky, who studied Holocaust survivors. The Salutogenic Model was key in establishing health as a continuum and is consistent with the emphasis in this text that there is a continuum of mental health that ranges from languishing to flourishing.

An important construct in the Salutogenic Model is **sense of coherence** (Moksnes, 2021). People can better manage stress when they can make sense of, and have confidence that they can deal with, the stressful situation. There are three components to the sense of coherence: comprehensibility, manageability, and meaningfulness. **Comprehensibility** is the degree to which a situation is understandable and predictable for the person. **Manageability** is the degree to which the person believes they can handle the situation and have the necessary resources to do so. **Meaningfulness** is the belief that the situation is worth engaging in and that the person cares about what will happen. Successful coping with stress is highly dependent on having a strong sense of coherence. OTPs can use the Salutogenic Model to make difficult life situations more comprehensible, manageable, and meaningful.

TABLE 10-1 | Coping Strategies

Coping Strategy	Type of Coping	Example
Planful problem-solving	Problem-solving	Your plane was canceled so you rent a car to get to your destination.
Confrontive coping	Problem-solving	You tell your boss that you are unhappy with the most recent schedule.
Seeking social support	Problem-solving	You join a support group after receiving a cancer diagnosis.
Accepting responsibility	Emotion focused	You acknowledge to your roommate that you forgot to pay the utility bill and say that you will cover the cost of the late fee.
Escape-avoidance	Emotion focused	You spend long hours at work so that you don't have to deal with difficult situations at home.
Distancing	Emotion focused	You make a conscious effort to not think about a fight with your boyfriend while taking a final examination.
Self-controlling	Emotion focused	You decide not to buy something you really want because you want to stick to your budget.
Positive reappraisal	Emotion focused	After a serious health scare, you find greater appreciation for life, friends, and family.

Resilience

There is a lack of consensus regarding the definition of **resilience** and a unifying theory to explain it (Robinson et al., 2022; Young et al., 2019) though resilience is generally thought of as the ability to bounce back from difficulties or a form of resistance to adversity. Much research has investigated factors associated with resilience. Factors that are malleable, in other words, can be modified and can serve as targets for intervention (E. C. Meyer et al., 2019).

One of the most studied malleable factors is psychological flexibility. As described in the context of Acceptance and Commitment Therapy (ACT; see Chapter 8: Cognitive Beliefs 🤝), psychological flexibility involves persistence in changing behavior based on what the situation affords and consistent with the person's goals and values (Hayes et al., 2006). Other psychological factors associated with resilience include self-efficacy and optimism. Self-efficacy provides the individual with the agency to address problems while they arise; similarly, optimism may provide the individual with confidence.

Environmental variables also play a role in resilience. Social connectedness is an important predictor of resilience, as is having a strong, positive bond with a caregiver during development (Pastorelli et al., 2016). In addition, having exposure to manageable stress during development allows for the development of coping skills and emotion regulation for dealing with future stressors (Tottenham, 2014).

Coping and Psychiatric Conditions

The Diathesis-Stress Model suggests that environmental events or stressors contribute to the development of psychiatric conditions when a person is biologically vulnerable (A. Meyer, 1921). Coping models suggest that the ways a person reacts to or understands stressful situations impact their mental health (Antonovksy, 1979; Lazarus & Folkman, 1984). Although maladaptive coping is rarely identified as a symptom per se, based on these models it follows that all psychiatric conditions are associated with some breakdown in coping. However, certain conditions are more directly associated with stress.

Trauma- and Stressor-Related Disorders

In the *Diagnostic and Statistical Manual of Mental Disorders,* Fifth Edition, Text Revision (*DSM-5-TR;* American Psychiatric Association, 2022), exposure to trauma or stress is a prerequisite for a diagnosis of a trauma- or stressor-related disorder. The conditions in this category of diagnoses include reactive attachment disorder, disinhibited social engagement disorder, posttraumatic stress disorder (PTSD), acute stress disorder, and adjustment disorders. A lack of adequate caregiving is a requirement for a diagnosis of the two childhood disorders: (1) attachment disorder and (2) disinhibited social engagement disorder. With reactive attachment disorder, the child becomes emotionally withdrawn with minimal social responsiveness. Conversely, in disinhibited social engagement disorder the child approaches and interacts with unfamiliar adults without hesitation.

PTSD may be diagnosed in children or adults and requires the presence of intrusive symptoms associated with a traumatic event, avoidance of stimuli associated with the traumatic event, an alteration in cognitions or mood after the traumatic event, and alterations in arousal associated with a traumatic event. Acute stress disorder is the development of PTSD symptoms within 3 days to 1 month after the trauma exposure. With adjustment disorder, the person experiences marked distress that is out of proportion to the severity or intensity of a stressor. The research into protective and vulnerability factors for trauma and stressor disorders has led to evidence-based intervention that promotes resilience (Horn & Feder, 2018).

Anxiety Disorders

Anxiety is closely linked to stress, which is triggered by external events and can include physical and mental responses. Anxiety is often an internal phenomenon that may continue even after the stressor is gone or may be present when there is no immediate threat. Worries and other thoughts such as self-criticism or shame bring on feelings of discomfort referred to as anxiety. People with anxiety disorders tend to have a heightened sensitivity to threats (Penninx et al., 2021) though the particular sensitivity can differ. For example, an individual with social anxiety will be highly threatened by having to speak in public, whereas someone with agoraphobia will be more fearful when exposed to crowds or a confined environment. Anxiety disorders are the most common type of mental condition in childhood, and with many adults a heightened stress response has been present since childhood.

Avoidance is a coping strategy commonly used in anxiety disorders. Although avoiding dangerous stimuli is necessary for survival, in anxiety disorders maladaptive avoidance means the individual stays away from relatively safe situations (Ball & Gunaydin, 2022). Consequently, the avoidance behavior is reinforced as it temporarily relieves the anxiety. Over time, avoidance becomes a dominant coping response that prevents the individual from confronting overly sensitive threat beliefs and results in decreased participation in desired occupation.

Assessment

OTPs work collaboratively with individuals to explore areas of current stress and personal coping in the context of their impact on quality of life and occupational performance. Family and significant others are often included in the process. Measures of stress, trauma, coping, and resilience might include checklists, self-appraisal tools, physiological measures, observations, and interviews (Table 10-2). Factors to consider when selecting a measure include the individual's cognitive level, potential for insight, motivation, cultural appropriateness, and the time and cost required to complete the assessment (Kato, 2015).

Self-Report Measures

Assessment tools in which the person provides their own perspective are the most common method of assessing stress and coping. Some measures assess the stressors that the individual is experiencing, such as the Recent Life Changes Questionnaire (Rahe, 1975) and the Social Readjustment Scale (Holmes & Rahe, 1967); some evaluate the type of coping method used, such as the Coping Responses Inventory (Moos, 1990), and the Ways of Coping Checklist-Revised (Folkman & Lazarus, 1988); and others assess both stressors and coping methods, such as the Stress Management Questionnaire (Stein & Cutler, 2002) or the Occupational Stress Inventory Revised (Osipow & Spokane, 1998), which looks specifically at stressors and coping in the workplace. There are many resilience measures available including the Resilience Factor Inventory (Reivich & Shatte, 2002).

Based on age, context, and developmental stage, children's experience of stress and coping may differ from that of adults. Assessment for adults often includes items that are not relevant for children and adolescents, but fortunately there are many stress and coping scales available for children and adolescents, such as the Adolescent Perceived Events Scale (Compas et al., 1987). There are also specific assessment tools designed for measuring the stress associated with parenting such as the Parenting Stress Index (Abidin, 2011).

Stress and coping instruments are simple to administer but additional information can be gained from other methods. This can include other evaluation techniques using observation, interview, history-taking, and formal task assessment.

Observation

Observing a person's occupational performance in various settings, both natural and structured, can provide valuable insights (Law et al., 2005). Task-based assessments allow therapists to observe how a person copes with stress and unexpected difficulties, as well as their problem-solving capacity, frustration tolerance levels, and adaptive coping skills. It is important to consider factors that may affect the person's ability to complete assessments, such as their emotional state at the time, physical health status, age, cognition, level of therapeutic alliance, effects of medication, and even the testing environment itself.

Observations of the person's response to task demands provide valuable information regarding the person's occupational performance. Areas for observation in stress and coping include:

- Reaction to occupational performance in expected daily activities
- Relationship and interactions with significant others (e.g., spouse, children)
- Person factors such as emotional state, reaction to stress, and ability to cope
- Appraisal of the situation by the person as compared with actual facts

Interviews

Interviews serve to expand on information gained from inventories and allow the therapist to use clinical reasoning for further inquiry. Interviews can be conducted on a formal or informal basis and may include the use of structured interview guides (Patton, 2014), an open-ended interview, or specific interview tools such as the Family Stress and Coping Interview (Nachshen et al., 2003).

Occupation-based tools such as the Canadian Occupational Performance Measure (Law et al., 1998) and the Occupational Case Analysis Interview and Rating Scale (Kaplan & Kielhofner, 1989) are helpful to provide a person-centered focus on perceptions of occupational performance as related to stress, coping, and quality of life.

Stress Diaries

Another approach to measuring stress and coping, the stress diary (Linehan, 1993), provides a means for the person and the OTP to track stress and coping over time. Various forms of stress diaries exist; they generally involve a journal or recording of the times and events surrounding stress, personal reactions to events, and coping strategies used. One common form of the stress diary, Linehan's (1993) diary card, is used with dialectical behavioral therapy (see Chapter 12: Emotion Regulation 🤝). The diary card can be used to derive an initial baseline on maladaptive coping strategies used (e.g., alcohol, self-harm), as well as track the use of adaptive coping skills. The diary card serves as a means to provide feedback, increase insight into stressors that evoke maladaptive coping, and record skills that may be used to more positively work through the stress.

Other types of activity and sleep diaries can be used to help increase understanding of personal stress and coping (e.g., Shafer & Bader, 2013). These instruments track daily activities and sleep patterns and help the individual and practitioner understand the stress response related to what is going on in an individual's life.

TABLE 10-2 | Therapeutic Reasoning Assessment Table: Stress Measurement and Coping Skills

Which Tool?	Who Was This Tool Designed For?	What Is Required of the Person? Can They Use the Tool?	What Am I Measuring?	How Long Does It Take and Where Do I Administer This Assessment?	Is the Tool Associated With a Practice Model?
Adolescent Coping Scale-2 (Frydenberg, 2012)	Adolescents (12–18 years)	Adolescent must have ability to self-assess and reflect (with help of a professional)	Analyzes types of coping and facilitates strategies for coping skill development	Varies based on adolescent skill/ reading level; may take up to an hour	No, but could be used with CBT
Adolescent Perceived Events Scale (Compas et al., 1987)	Adolescents (generally 10–18 years)	Ability to self-reflect	Rates perceived stress on life events	Fewer than 30 minutes—varies based on skill/ reading level	No, but could be used with CBT
Baruth Protective Factors Inventory (BPFI; Baruth & Caroll, 2002)	Adolescents and adults with capacity for insight	Ability to participate in a self-report inventory	Examines four protective factors: adaptable personality, supportive environments, fewer stressors, compensating experiences	Fewer than 30 minutes	Social-ecological framework
Children's Coping Strategies Checklist (Ayres et al., 1996)	Research was done on 9- to 13-year-olds for the tool's development.	Basic reading ability— may need assistance from therapist or trusted adult	Measures coping strategies	Up to an hour depending on the level of the child	Comes from dimensional coping models but would fit with CBT
Connor-Davidson Resilience Scale (CD-RISC; Connor & Davidson, 2003)	Designed for adults, though may be appropriate for older teens	Ability to participate in a self-report inventory	Measures five resilience factors: personal competence, tolerance of negative affect, positive acceptance of change and secure relationships, control, and spiritual influences	Fewer than 30 minutes	Developed based on theories of resilience
Coping Responses Inventory (Moos, 1990)	Two inventories, one for adults, one for youth 12–18	Ability to participate in a self-report inventory	Measures coping strategies in youth and adults	20–40 minutes— shorter version is available	No, although follows theories and models related to stress and coping
Diary Cards (Linehan, 1993)	Adolescents and adults	Ability to self-reflect	Individual identifies stressful events and coping mechanisms used as they happen	10 minutes	Dialectical Behavior Therapy
Family Stress and Coping Interview (Nachshen et al., 2003)	Originally designed for parents of a child with developmental conditions; has been used with families in the general population	Ability to self-reflect	Measures stress and coping related to caregiving	Fewer than 30 minutes	No, but relates to stress-response theories
KidCOPE (Spirito et al., 1988)	Children and adolescents from ages 7–18	Ability to self-reflect	Rates the frequency and efficacy of various coping strategies in children	Fewer than 30 minutes	No, but aligns well with stress and coping models as well as CBT
Life Events Checklist (J. H. Johnson & McCutcheon, 1980)	Children 13–18	Ability to self-reflect	Rates events and perceived stress related to each event	Fewer than 30 minutes	No, but relates to stress-response theories

Continued

TABLE 10-2 | Therapeutic Reasoning Assessment Table: Stress Measurement and Coping Skills—cont'd

Which Tool?	Who Was This Tool Designed For?	What Is Required of the Person? Can They Use the Tool?	What Am I Measuring?	How Long Does It Take and Where Do I Administer This Assessment?	Is the Tool Associated With a Practice Model?
Life Events Coping Inventory for Children (Dise-Lewis, 1988)	Children and teens	Ability to self-reflect	Measures coping strategies in youth	20–30 minutes	No, but relates to stress-response theories
Occupational Stress Inventory Revised (Osipow & Spokane, 1998)	Working adults/those seeking a job	Ability to self-reflect	Measures three domains of occupational adjustment (occupational stress, psychological strain, coping resources)	30 minutes	Fits into occupation-based models
Parenting Stress Index, 4th ed. (Abidin, 2011)	Parents of children (special identification of children 0–12 years)	Ability to participate in a self-inventory and reflect on results	Measures stress related to parenting	20–45 minutes, depending on the reading and processing of the parent (120 questions)	No, but aligns well with stress and coping models as well as CBT and occupation-based approaches for skill development
Recent Life Changes Questionnaire (Rahe, 1975)	Adults	Ability to participate in a self-inventory	Measures stress impact of recent life events (1 year)	Fewer than 30 minutes	No, although cognitive behavioral in nature
Resilience Factor Inventory (Reivich & Shatte, 2002)	Adults	Ability to participate in a self-inventory and reflect on results	Trait inventory designed to measure levels of resilience	Fewer than 30 minutes	Developed based on theories of resilience; fits into CBT
Resilience Scales for Children and Adolescents: A Profile of Personal Strengths (Prince-Embury, 2006, 2008)	Youth 9–18 years	Third-grade reading level and ability to participate in self-reflection	Measures resilience based on four scales	Fewer than 30 minutes— about 5 minutes/scale	Developed based on theories of resilience; fits into CBT
Response to Stress Questionnaire (Connor-Smith et al., 2000)	Used most often with adolescents (validated for use in several cultures)	Participation in self-report—some studies have also involved parents	Coping response styles (differing categories than many other tools: voluntary/involuntary processes and engagement and disengagement	20–40 minutes	Volitional coping model
Social-Emotional Assets and Resilience Scales (SEARS) (Jones et al., 2018)	Designed for children and adolescents 8–18 years; SEARS consists of two scales: the Social-Emotional Assets Scale (SEAS) and the Resilience Scale (RS).	Ability to participate in self-report and self-reflections; can be completed by parents, teachers, or the children themselves	The SEAS measures social-emotional competencies in children and adolescents, including self-awareness, self-management, social awareness, relationship skills, and responsible decision-making. The RS measures resilience.	20–30 minutes	Based on the framework of the Collaborative for Academic, Social, and Emotional Learning (CASEL), which outlines five core social-emotional competencies: self-awareness, self-management, social awareness, relationship skills, and responsible decision-making.
Social Readjustment Scale (Holmes & Rahe, 1967)	Adults	Ability to read and fill out form (or with assistance)—does not require much self-reflection	Stress events occurring in an individual's life over the past year	Fewer than 30 minutes	Psychoimmunology stress and health theories

TABLE 10-2 | Therapeutic Reasoning Assessment Table: Stress Measurement and Coping Skills—cont'd

Which Tool?	Who Was This Tool Designed For?	What Is Required of the Person? Can They Use the Tool?	What Am I Measuring?	How Long Does It Take and Where Do I Administer This Assessment?	Is the Tool Associated With a Practice Model?
Stress Management Questionnaire (Stein & Cutler, 2002)	Adults	Ability to self-reflect	Three categories measured: stress symptoms, stressors, and ways of coping	30 minutes	Biopsychosocial emphasis that fits into CBT approaches
Stress Symptom Checklist (Schlebusch, 2004)	Adults (may eventually be adapted for other populations)	Ability to participate in self-report and self-reflection	Checklist of major symptoms often corresponding to stress	Fewer than 20 minutes	None specified, although authors emphasize a biopsychosocial focus; also fits with CBT
Ways of Coping (WOC) Checklist-Revised (Folkman & Lazarus, 1988)	Adults	Ability to participate in self-report—some need skill to self-reflect	Self-appraisal of situations and coping styles	20–40 minutes	No, but fits well with CBT and occupation-based approaches for skill development

Physiological Measures

Whereas sophisticated physiological methods of measuring stress (e.g., cortisol levels) are often used for research purposes, many simple tools are currently available, especially with the advent of tracking devices that can provide biofeedback in the form of heart rate and blood pressure. Individuals can work with the OTP to identify baseline physiological data as well as experiment with stress-relieving activities and identify the ones that result in the desired physiological response. Tracking devices can be useful when teaching the person to self-regulate physiological responses to stress.

Intervention

Regardless of the practice setting, OTPs often incorporate interventions that target stress and coping. Intervention can focus on developing adaptive coping skills, promoting resilience, processing stress and trauma, or creating supportive environments.

Cognitive Behavioral Therapy

Cognitive behavioral therapy (CBT) addresses the tenet that distorted thinking leads to unpleasant emotions and maladaptive behaviors (Hofmann et al., 2012). The intervention uses cognitive restructuring to replace negative thought patterns such as catastrophizing or overgeneralization with more balanced thinking. Another component of CBT is behavioral activation. Through engaging in activities that promote positive emotions and a sense of mastery, even when feeling low or unmotivated, the person develops better coping. The goal is to increase positive experiences and build a sense of achievement and momentum. (See Chapter 8: Cognitive Beliefs.)

For example, an occupational therapy student might express the fear that they are 100% certain they will fail an examination. The OTP could challenge the student's assumption by noting that this is likely an overestimate and provide evidence to the contrary such as past positive outcomes on similar examinations. Extensive research indicates that CBT is effective for many mental health and chronic physical conditions and is considered a gold-standard treatment for anxiety and stress-related disorders (Curtiss et al., 2021). When used with anxiety disorders, exposure therapy is often included as a component of the intervention. With exposure, the individual faces the feared object or situation and uses strategies to reduce the stress reaction (Jørstad-Stein & Heimberg, 2009). However, a study of people with social phobia found that exposure alone was less effective than exposure with social skills training (Beidel et al., 2014). This has important implications for OTPs, as our interventions are more likely to integrate CBT approaches within the context of occupational performance such as socializing with others.

Acceptance and Commitment Therapy

ACT is aimed at enhancing psychological flexibility (Hayes et al., 2011). As mentioned earlier in this chapter, psychological flexibility is a hallmark of adaptive coping and resilience. Psychological flexibility involves being fully present and having the ability to change consistent with what the situation demands. Psychological flexibility also requires that the person persist in behavior that is consistent with one's values. Specifically, the ACT framework supports individuals to develop psychological flexibility by accepting difficult thoughts and emotions and responding flexibly; building mindfulness skills to help regulate emotions; promoting values-based action by identifying and pursuing meaningful goals and purposes; and developing compassion to oneself to foster a sense of self-worth and self-efficacy through kindness and understanding (Kashdan & Rottenberg, 2010). (For more information about ACT see Chapter 8: Cognitive Beliefs.)

Creative Activities

Occupational therapy interventions for stress and coping often involve creative expression through media such as writing, art, and drama. A recent scoping review conducted in Australia (A. Johnson et al., 2022) identifies the potential benefits of arts-as-therapy in occupational therapy mental health practice; these include self-expression and discovery, a sense of mastery, improved self-esteem, and better mental and physical health. Art-as-therapy conducted in a group setting promoted belongingness. A systematic review of using art to reduce anxiety symptoms found that although the evidence was limited, the working mechanisms of art included the promotion of relaxation, access to traumatic memories that led to cognitive processing, and improved emotion regulation (Abbing et al., 2018). Read The Lived Experience to get a sense of how music and other arts were integral to Glenn developing an authentic and satisfying life.

The Lived Experience

Glenn

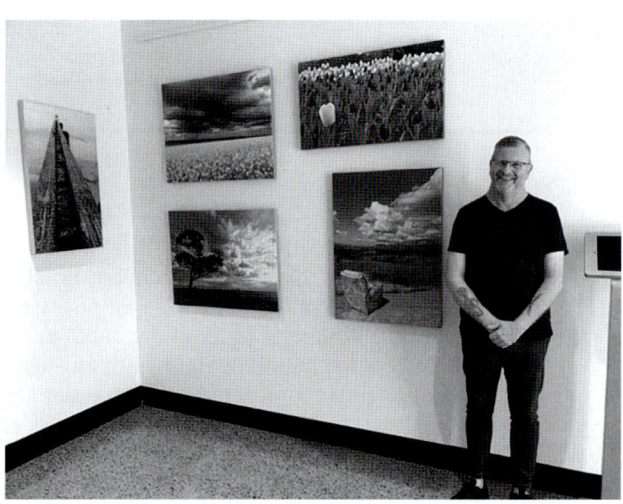

Editor's Note: The following narrative communicates the difficulties of coping with a mental illness and the importance of meaningful occupation in the recovery process.

Glenn's childhood was an ever-swaying pendulum between the male role models in his life. It swung from having to play the role of protector for his mother and siblings against his father's domestic abuse to witnessing great compassion from his stepfather. It was a childhood marked by abuse and trauma.

However, born with a gift of musical ability, Glenn was enveloped in a sense of joy when he was surrounded by music and singing. Unfortunately, it was a gift discouraged and ridiculed within his family. He endured mockery from influential figures and became locked in a lifetime of denial of his talent. Yet, his grandma's words to him, at 8 years old, rang strong and helped him maintain a grip on what would eventually bring him his greatest contentment. "Glenn, you have an amazing gift. Never stop singing," she said.

In 1974, his family was seemingly destroyed when his mother placed Glenn and his brothers into the Church of England Homes for Children at Carlingford, Sydney, just months after Glenn had sung as a boy soprano at the opening concerts at the Sydney Opera House. Although his mother attempted to dig her way out of destitution, an industrial accident later rendered her unable to work.

Fate intervened again, but this time fortuitously. Glenn's mother met a World War II Navy veteran who fell in love with the remnants of his long-suffering mother. He opened his heart to Glenn's mother and supported her to the extent that she could retrieve her children from the home. They later married. It was during his ensuing teen years that Glenn continued to develop maladaptive "survival" skills to deal with years of trauma, but was otherwise afforded the safety and normalcy of a healthy relationship with his new stepfather. Glenn credits this as a central reason he didn't slip completely into emotional and social dysfunction.

Tragically, in 1987, Glenn and his brothers were orphaned a second time when his mother and stepfather died, just 8 weeks apart. Glenn, still a young man and struggling with a difficult family culture that hindered his emotional healing, sacrificed a professional music career to move back into the family's Housing Commission home, working two jobs to help guide his brothers into careers.

At 26, Glenn joined the Royal Australian Air Force and it was the first time that he felt a lightening of the burden of being responsible for others. This was a pivotal moment where he could attempt to put his unfortunate life behind him and look toward a positive future. Although his trauma followed him, his energy to move on from his unfortunate background allowed him to focus enough to hold leadership positions in the Air Force. Glenn valued the structure of military life that had been absent from his childhood and made friends for life. However, he was also exposed to instances of unacceptable behavior during his service, which furthered his plunge into complex PTSD.

Having been married for 29 years, Glenn's focus has been on the nurturing of his three children, keeping them safe from the traumas of the childhood that he had endured. His own experience as a victim/survivor of abuse has also led Glenn to become an active ambassador and, eventually, state chair for an Ambassadors Network for White Ribbon Australia, which advocates for women who experience domestic violence. Glenn proudly declares that he is a feminist, which helps him show the empathy he developed for women whilst witnessing his mother's abuse journey. These days, having been denied his creative life as a child and masking it in the military, Glenn felt it was time for him to finally allow his creative self its full expression. Glenn's story has been published in a book that celebrates veteran artists, and his portrait tours Australia in a veteran artists exhibition. His creative life is on the verge of flourishing. With the support of psychological therapy, his writing, music, and photography, he now has the opportunity to appreciate and develop himself as an artist. Glenn is finally, and fittingly, a respected artist who continues to explore how the arts and his gifts can help him transcend his struggle with trauma.

Various studies demonstrate the effectiveness of therapeutic writing techniques, suggesting that personal reflection in response to stress and trauma improve overall health and well-being (Haertl, 2014; Martin et al., 2018, Pennebaker & Chung, 2011). In a study of pain reduction for fibromyalgia and Emotion Awareness and Expression Therapy, intervention included therapeutic writing and other strategies such as role-playing to express and address avoided emotions (Lumley et al., 2017). The study found that the intervention was more effective than CBT for reducing fibromyalgia symptoms and pain.

There are many different approaches to therapeutic writing. Journaling, for example, is a common form of expressive writing. Typically, people who keep a journal find a regular time to write about their feelings. Journaling is a low-risk activity, and though the results are varied, there is a general consensus that journaling can improve mental health symptoms such as anxiety and depression (Sohal et al., 2022). A more specific and structured form of expressive writing was developed by James Pennebaker, who has studied the benefits of therapeutic writing (Pennebaker & Chung, 2011). In this writing experience, people write for several days in a row about things that are bothering them. The writer is encouraged to describe their feelings about the situation. Research indicates that following this approach, there is a significant reduction in both mental and physical health problems. For more information about the Pennebaker Protocol, see Box 10-1.

Most people keep their journals private, and the Pennebaker Protocol also encourages privacy. Another form of therapeutic writing or storytelling is done to share one's experiences with others. Recovery narratives have become an important feature of the recovery movement and are used as an educational tool, a method of self-discovery, a way of offering peer support, and, perhaps most importantly, as an advocacy device (Llewellyn-Beardsley et al., 2019). In fact, lived experience stories have been used as a way to give voice to people in recovery in this textbook.

However, not all people benefit from sharing their story, and one group in particular may be survivors of sexual violence (Delker et al., 2020). One study found that the people in stories of survivors of sexual abuse, when compared with the people in stories of survivors of natural disasters, were perceived as less desirable. This is consistent with the victim blaming and stigma that is associated with sexual abuse survivors. OTPs should help individuals decide if there may be some risk involved in sharing their story.

Visual arts provide another therapeutic creative outlet. Visual arts can be useful when verbal expression is difficult. Individuals may be able to draw pictures or paint, take pictures, or use other visual media to represent thoughts and feelings when words are lacking. As an example, this textbook uses PhotoVoice as a method to see and hear from people in recovery. Typically carried out in a group, PhotoVoice brings together people with shared experiences to display photographs and brief personal narratives around a theme (Kile, 2022). It is used as a tool to give voice to people who are seldom heard.

Another method of visual storytelling is the Tree Theme Method developed by an OTP as a way to manifest the concepts of doing (painting a picture), being (reflecting on it afterward), and becoming (promoting the development of a self-image; Gunnarsson et al., 2006). The Tree Theme Method uses a tree to symbolize oneself. The intervention takes place over five sessions. In each session the person paints a tree representing

---

BOX 10-1 ■ Pennebaker Expressive Writing Protocol

The following is a summary of the instructions given for writing about a difficult situation using the Pennebaker Protocol (Pennebaker & Evans, 2014).

- Write for 4 days (preferably in a row). You can write about the same topic or choose a different topic every day.
- Pick a topic that is emotionally upsetting but don't choose something that may be too traumatic. Choose an event or situation that you can handle.
- Write for 15 to 20 minutes without stopping. Don't worry about spelling or grammar. If you run out of things to say, repeat what you have already written.
- It is important to share your deepest feelings and thoughts when writing.
- Write only for yourself. Don't intend to share your writing with others so that you can be more honest. You can destroy or hide what you have written after you finish.
- You may feel sad after writing. This typically lasts only a few minutes or a few hours.
- Writing is not for everyone. If you feel as if it is not helping you, try something else. You may want to seek professional mental health advice.

For additional information on the Pennebaker Protocol go to:

Pennebaker, J. W., & Evans, J. H. (2014). *Expressive writing: Words that heal.* Idyll Arbor. https://liberalarts.utexas.edu/psychology/faculty/pennebak

---

different life phases: (a) present life situation, (b) childhood, (c) adolescence, (d) adulthood, and (e) the future.

During the painting phase, the person is encouraged to remain silent. After painting, the picture is hung on the wall and the storytelling begins. The person is asked to describe how the tree represents themselves while the OTP interjects with questions to encourage more description and reflection. The OTP helps the individual identify themes including strengths and limitations presented in everyday life. At the end of each session, the individual identifies a personal task to complete before their next session that relates to their problems and needs in everyday life. During the last session, the first four trees are reviewed and serve as a starting point to develop strategies to cope with future everyday occupations.

A randomized controlled trial (Gunnarsson et al., 2022) examined the efficacy of the Tree Theme Group and an occupational therapy as usual group for people with depression and anxiety. Both groups had significant improvements in performance and satisfaction of daily occupations, occupational balance, and a reduction in depression and anxiety symptoms. Based on the person's needs and interests, the Tree Theme Method can have positive outcomes for people with anxiety and/or depression. For more about creative activities see Chapter 51: Leisure and Creative Occupations.

An example of using creative arts as an occupation to enhance resilience and well-being in children is shown in Box 10-2.

Mindfulness

Mindfulness practice refers to the intentional and non-judgmental awareness of present-moment experiences, thoughts, and feelings. It involves paying attention to the present moment without distraction from other events or

BOX 10-2 ■ Example of Creative Arts as an Occupation to Promote Mental Health

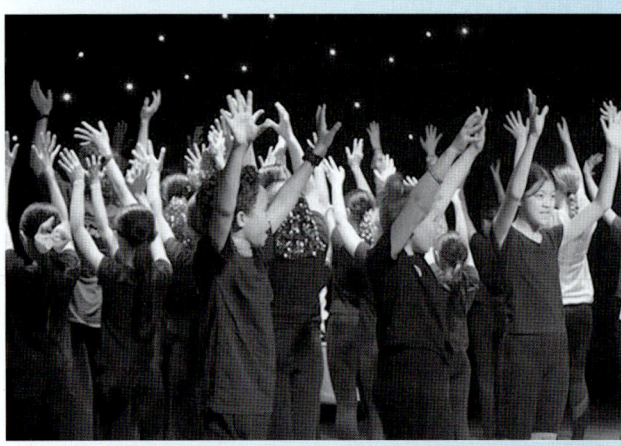

The Positive Mindset Creative Arts Festival promotes positive mental health, reduces stigma, and enhances mental health literacy by promoting engagement with the creative arts occupation in school communities. It proved itself to be a useful alternative to traditional teaching methods such as the use of books and classrooms. It utilizes drama, music, dance, visual art, and media art outside the classrooms to teach students about resilience, coping strategies, help-seeking behaviors, and understanding mental illness. This is particularly useful for students who learn more effectively through experiential and multisensory modalities. The creative arts also bring additional purpose, identity, and role that is unique for each individual participant in the festival (Lo, 2020). Students can be a dancer, performer, singer, painter, observer, volunteer, or a member of the audience in their engagement with the festival, and be able to benefit in the following identified key areas based on feedback surveys collected:

1. Enhanced awareness of mental health literacy
2. Reduction of stigmatized assumptions on mental illness and addiction issues
3. Enhanced awareness of appropriate services available for mental well-being
4. Recognition of the significance of mental health needs in the community

thoughts. Rooted in Buddhist meditation practices, it has been adapted for use in a variety of settings to reduce stress, anxiety, and depression, and to promote well-being and resilience (Kabat-Zinn, 1994). Mindfulness practice can be diverse and includes mindful breathing exercises, body scans, and mindful movement practices such as yoga and tai chi.

Mindfulness meditation is a widely used and well-studied technique in mental health practice, with many systematic reviews finding positive outcomes. For example, a large systematic review and meta-analysis found moderate evidence that mindfulness meditation was effective in reducing anxiety, depression, and pain (Goyal et al., 2014). Another review found that mindfulness-based programs for health-care students were effective in decreasing anxiety, stress, and depression (Parsons et al., 2022). Mindfulness training was also found to reduce job burnout in health-care practitioners and teachers (Luken & Sammons, 2016).

Mindfulness can be practiced alone or with other activities such as yoga or tai chi. It can involve focusing on an object or breath or the person's surroundings. There are many resources for developing mindfulness skills including books, websites, and apps. Similar to most skills, it takes practice to develop the ability to be fully present, and maybe even more challenging is the skill of observing without judgment.

Mindfulness and meditation are explored in greater detail in Chapter 12: Emotion Regulation and Chapter 45: Self-Care and Well-Being Occupations.

Resiliency Training

Several programs have been developed with the goal of enhancing resilience and adaptation for individuals who are experiencing stress or trauma. These programs operate with the understanding that resilience is something that can be acquired and typically integrate the previously discussed strategies such as CBT and mindfulness.

One program called Stress Management and Resiliency Training (SMART) has been studied with health professionals (Magtibay et al., 2017; Sood et al., 2011) and people with physical and mental health conditions (Loprinzi et al., 2011). The SMART program includes 12 modules. With each module there is a reading assignment, a self-assessment, and a video introducing the topic and exercises to apply the concepts into daily life. The training uses principles associated with mindfulness along with cognitive reframing focused on gratitude, compassion, acceptance, and forgiveness.

An example of resilience training that targets a specific population is FOCUS: Families OverComing Under Stress (Lester et al., 2011). This program teaches strategies for better communication and problem-solving for military children, families, and couples. The FOCUS program is typically six to eight sessions and within the program the family tells its story to build on strengths and enhance cohesion.

Special Considerations for Specific Populations

Considerations to enhance coping and resilience for several identified at-risk groups are highlighted here. This includes the child and youth population, children of parents/families with a mental illness (COPMI), older persons, the culturally and linguistically diverse (CALD) population including Indigenous people, and the LGBTQIA+ (lesbian, gay, bisexual, transgender, queer [and in some cases, "questioning"], intersex, and asexual) population.

Child and Adolescent Intervention

Occupational therapy can play a significant role in promoting coping skills and resilience in children and youth, ensuring full participation in their daily lives, including school, home, and community settings. Some of the ways occupational therapy can promote mental health in children and youth include:

1. Occupational therapy can teach children and youth techniques and coping strategies to manage stress and

Evidence-Based Practice

Art Supports Health and Wellness

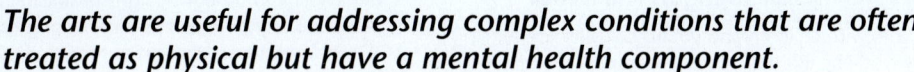

The arts are useful for addressing complex conditions that are often treated as physical but have a mental health component.

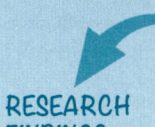

RESEARCH FINDINGS

A recent scoping review by the World Health Organization (Fancourt & Finn, 2019) examined global evidence from over 3,000 studies and identified crucial evidence for the arts in the promotion of health and management of illness across the life span, including mental illness. A theme identified in this review is that the arts are often useful for addressing complex conditions that are often treated as physical but have a mental health component. For example, children and adolescents taking part in social circus arts programs demonstrated improved levels of well-being, socialization, and resilience (Stevens et al., 2019).

APPLICATIONS

➡ OTPs commonly work with individuals experiencing stress and trauma and can provide creative activities to express and process emotions.
➡ Application of expressive techniques should be grounded in theory and matched to the individual.

REFERENCES

Fancourt, D., & Finn, S. (2019). *What is the evidence on the role of the arts in improving health and wellbeing? A scoping review (Health Evidence Network synthesis report 67).* World Health Organisation. https://apps.who.int/iris/handle/10665/329834
Stevens, K., McGrath, R., & Ward, E. (2019). Identifying the influence of leisure-based social circus on the health and well-being of young people in Australia. *Annals of Leisure Research, 22*(3), 305–322. https://doi.org/10.1080/11745398.2018.1537854

anxiety, such as relaxation and mindfulness techniques (Forman, 1993). To help reduce feelings of overwhelm, consideration for a graded person-centered approach, adapting for the child's age and developmental level, is essential (Rew et al., 2012).

2. Use a strengths-based approach and provide positive feedback, praise, and encouragement to reinforce helpful and adaptive coping behaviors, as well as the development of self-esteem and self-efficacy (Lavis, 2014; Murthi et al., 2023).

3. Provide support to engage in meaningful activities that they enjoy, such as sports, music, or art. This promotes a meaning and purpose, which improves their overall well-being (Collins et al., 2014).

4. Build living skills to help individuals manage their daily routines and self-care such as hygiene, grooming, and meal preparation. These skills can promote a sense of competence and independence (Laverdure & Beisbier, 2021).

5. Develop social skills needed to interact positively with others and navigate social situations (Chen et al., 2009, Yuen et al., 2023). This can help reduce social isolation and promote a sense of belonging (Gilbert & Mirawski, 2005).

6. Collaborate with families and other professionals to create supportive environments (Cahill & Beisbier, 2020).

As indicated in Box 10-3, when working with children, a comprehensive assessment of personal and environmental factors involving significant others and stakeholders across both the home and school contexts will provide a more

---

BOX 10-3 ■ Example of a Pediatric Coping Intervention

Jeremy, an 8-year-old boy with fetal alcohol syndrome and conduct disorder, had a history of aggression, poor social skills, and low self-esteem. His mother complained that he did not have any friends and that all he ever wanted to do was play video games. On admission, the therapist conducted a comprehensive evaluation, including assessment of his developmental level, sensory processing, and perceived stress. A home observation and interview of the parents was also completed. Results indicated that Jeremy had difficulty not only with coping, but also with poor sensory processing, emotional dysregulation, and ineffective social skills.

In addition to play therapy and sensory-based approaches, the therapist used expressive media, storytelling, and role-play in order to teach Jeremy about social situations. Jeremy was initially resistant to engage in therapy and discuss social scenarios, but this changed when the therapist incorporated a puppet of one of Jeremy's favorite cartoon characters. Through the use of puppetry, Jeremy projected onto the character his own feelings in situations and was able to learn basic coping techniques, such as deep breathing, to deal with stressful situations.

Being a Psychosocial OT Practitioner

Helping an Overwhelmed and Anxious High School Senior

Identifying Psychosocial Strengths and Needs

OTPs often work with children and young people experiencing distress and mental health difficulties that impact their daily lives. OTPs also work with families, significant others, and relevant stakeholders to provide person-centered, comprehensive care to the young person. A major role of the OTP is to help individuals develop the mental health literacy and coping skills they need to manage their mental well-being, enhance their stress management competency, and allow them to participate fully in daily activities to live healthy and purposeful lives.

Consider the lived experience of Tom, a multitalented and high-performing 17-year-old student in his final year of high school. He was also a popular student among his peer groups and held student leadership roles. However, over the past 6 months, Tom started to exhibit various changes in his mood and behavior. His teachers, coaches, and peers noticed the changes and were concerned. The basketball coach first noticed Tom's declining performance during practice, training, and games. Tom started missing more practices and appeared tired and disinterested when he did attend. Teachers also noted his social withdrawal during class and break and that he fell asleep often. Tom's close friends were concerned about his increasing irritability, moodiness, and reduced appetite.

Tom was referred to the OTP and student well-being officer at the school. Tom expressed feeling overwhelmed, unable to cope with his responsibilities and daily activities, and anxious about not meeting expectations. He worried extensively about school, sports, and other people's opinions. In trying to cope with the distress, Tom started drinking alcohol every night.

Using a Holistic Occupational Therapy Approach

The OTP completed a comprehensive assessment using concepts from the Model of Human Occupation (MOHO) to gain a holistic perspective and insight into Tom's experiences. The assessment included Tom's developmental and occupational history, values, interests, and current strengths, as well as his stressors and difficulties (at the personal, social, and environmental levels), coping styles, and strategies used. The OTP also explored issues relating to his physical health, past traumas, evidence of neurodiversity experiences, cognitive and learning barriers, and any family history of mental illness.

The OTP also conducted a mental health examination to explore specific mental illness symptoms, including his appearance, thoughts, behaviors, speech, perceptions, insight, concentration, attention, and somatic symptoms, such as his sleep patterns, appetite, and energy levels. The OTP incorporated occupational and functional assessments to understand functioning and occupational performance across different activities of daily living, work, and leisure. With Tom's consent, additional information

was collected from his significant others and stakeholders (e.g., parents, family doctor, teachers, and peers). Finally, the OTP conducted a risk assessment for nonsuicidal self-injury behaviors and thoughts; signs of suicidal ideation, intent, and/or plan; and any potential risks of causing harm to others.

This holistic assessment approach provided a comprehensive understanding of Tom's situation and presentation. It revealed that Tom was having difficulties coping with various life stressors and was probably experiencing mixed episodes of anxiety and depression. Tom also had poor sleep hygiene and low mental health literacy. There was no immediate safety concern for Tom or others at the time of the assessment.

Based on the assessment, the OTP collaborated with Tom and, when appropriate, his significant others and stakeholders to set realistic and meaningful goals that align with his values and priorities. These goals included reducing alcohol consumption, developing healthy coping strategies, and improving overall occupational functioning through several codesigned activities and interventions, including:

- Developing better daily routines
- Improving sleep hygiene
- Exploring new engagement or reengagement in social activities and physical activities
- Developing more suitable, helpful coping skills and strategies relevant to Tom's needs and preferences (e.g., mindfulness and relaxation techniques)
- Enhancing Tom's mental health literacy through psychoeducation
- Offering parent/caregiver education and training on how to support and assist Tom in his recovery
- Providing CBT to develop skills to manage negative thoughts and emotions
- Collaborating with the multidisciplinary team for referrals to relevant professionals (e.g., a psychiatrist for further evaluation and prescription medications if needed)
- Referrals to other suitable community programs and support services (e.g., drug and alcohol programs to address Tom's substance misuse)

The OTP monitored Tom's progress, and they continuously reevaluated the effectiveness of the intervention together throughout the school year, allowing modifications to be made to the treatment plan as needed.

Reflective Questions

1. What other therapies might be helpful to explore with Tom?
2. How might the OTP involve each of the other stakeholders in supporting Tom, such as his coaches, teachers, and student peers?
3. How would you develop an intervention plan for Tom if he identifies creative arts as a potential coping strategy?

accurate picture of the presentation and intervention needs (Cahill & Beisbier, 2020). Lifestyle patterns, thoughts, and cognitions affect how individuals and family systems react to stress and function in society (Thompson et al., 2014). Please refer to the Being a Psychosocial OT Practitioner feature on this page for a specific example of how psychosocial OTPs can work holistically with children and young people experiencing distress and mental health difficulties that impact their daily lives.

Culturally and Linguistically Diverse Population

When working with the CALD population, including Indigenous peoples, it is important for OTPs to recognize and respect cultural differences and to provide culturally responsive care. CALD individuals often encounter unique challenges because of language barriers and cultural differences in health beliefs and practices, as well as racism and discrimination (Levy-Fenner et al., 2022). OTPs can work with these individuals to identify their needs, preferences, and strengths, and to develop a plan of care that is culturally appropriate and sensitive.

For Indigenous or First Nations people, occupational therapy can play a role in promoting cultural revitalization, supporting the appropriate use of traditional healing practices, and acknowledging the impacts of colonization and other trauma experienced over generations. OTPs can also work with First Nations/Native communities to identify their unique needs and to develop culturally appropriate interventions (Kirmayer et al., 2011).

In both cases, OTPs might need to adapt their assessment and treatment approaches to accommodate different cultural practices and values. For example, an OTP working with a First Nations community could incorporate traditional healing practices, such as smoking ceremonies or drumming, into their treatment plan. When working with CALD communities, it is important to recognize that different meanings and perceptions might exist for certain occupations and activities.

LGBTQIA+ People

OTPs can support LGBTQIA+ people in a variety of ways. These groups may experience additional stressors and barriers to participation because of discrimination or lack of access. OTPs can work with individuals to identify their strengths, interests, and goals, and help them develop skills and strategies to overcome challenges and achieve their objectives. OTPs can provide education and advocacy to help promote inclusion and understanding in the wider community and in the service systems where OTPs work (McNair & Bush, 2016).

OTPs need to be comfortable discussing any specific health or wellness needs related to sexual participation and gender identity. This can involve support in accessing sexual orientation and gender-affirming health care, joining a support group, addressing mental health concerns related to stigma and discrimination, and providing education and resources related to sexual health and wellness (Puckett et al., 2019).

Here's the Point

- Different models are available to explain stress, coping, and resilience. These models can help guide occupational therapy intervention.
- Stressors are associated with all psychiatric conditions, but they are at the core of anxiety and trauma- and stressor-related disorders.
- There are numerous coping and resilience assessments that use self-report, observation, interview, diary, and physiological approaches.
- OTPs provide interventions that help individuals develop adaptive coping skills, promote resilience, process stress and trauma, and create supportive environments.
- OTPs should be sensitive to the special considerations associated with addressing different age groups, culturally and linguistically diverse populations, and LGBTQIA people.

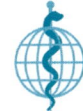 Visit the online resource center at **FADavis.com** to access the videos.

Apply It Now

1. Personal Assessment of Coping

Select and complete a self-assessment stress inventory and coping tool (either online or available from your instructor). Sample links:
- Coping and Stress Management Test: http://psychologytoday.tests.psychtests.com/take_test.php?idRegTest=3200
- Link to Various Stress Assessments: http://www.nysut.org/~/media/files/nysut/resources/2013/april/social-services/socialservices_stressassessments.pdf?la=en

Reflective Questions
Following completion of the self-assessment tools, answer the following:
- What areas of your life currently cause you the most stress?
- What means of coping do you use to deal with stressors?
- If you were a therapist designing an intervention for yourself, what approaches would you take and why?
- Can you identify three realistic goals for yourself?
- What barriers do you anticipate in achieving your goals? How could you be proactive in addressing these barriers?

- In evaluating your experience related to your self-assessment, how did it feel? Was it difficult? What did you learn?

2. Expressive Writing and Journaling

Choose and complete one of the journaling approaches described in the list that follows for a period of 7 days. At the conclusion of the period, reflect on the process and any noticeable changes in your feelings, thoughts, and behaviors. Try another approach for another period of 7 days if time permits. If you were able to try two different approaches, which did you prefer and why?
- *Daily thoughts and feelings:* At the end of each day, before going to bed, write and reflect on events and activities of the day, noting any associated emotions or feelings.
- *Gratitude diary:* During the course of a 24-hour day, note down at least three things that you are grateful for and consider to be positive, regardless of how big or small they are. This practice encourages our mind to focus on positive aspects of our life and enhances resilience when negative things occur.

■ *Art journaling:* This type of journaling involves expressive writing that incorporates drawings, photos, diagrams, graphs, collage of paper clippings, tickets and objects, and so on. This approach provides an outlet for mixed medium creativity and an opportunity to process emotions and situations. Use your creativity to enhance your writing with other art forms.

■ *Relationship journaling:* This approach focuses on relationships that are important to you. Write about the highlights of your relationship today, including what you did for, or with, one another. How did it make you feel? What are you grateful for and is there anything that can be changed or improved upon?

Resources

Websites

- Ardell Wellness Stress Test: https://premierespeakers.com /donald-ardell/posts/the-ardell-wellness-stress-self-assessment
- Be You Resources: https://beyou.edu.au/resources
- Beyond Blue: https://www.beyondblue.org.au
- Every Moment Counts: https://everymomentcounts.org/calm-moments-cards https://everymomentcounts.org/embedded-strategies
- FOCUS: Resilience Training for Military Families: https:// focusproject.org
- Headspace Mindfulness Interactive Activity: https://headspace .org.au/online-and-phone-support/interactive-tools/activities /mindfulness
- SAMHSA Evidence-Based Practices Kits (order a hard copy or download PDF):https://www.samhsa.gov/resource/ebp /supported-employment-evidence-based-practices-ebp-kit
- SAMHSA Trauma-Informed Care Information: http://www.samhsa.gov/nctic/trauma-interventions https://store.samhsa.gov/product/samhsas-concept -trauma-and-guidance-trauma-informed-approach/sma14-4884
- Scoring for the Holmes-Rahe Social Readjustment Scale: https://www.mindtools.com/avn893g /the-holmes-and-rahe-stress-scale
- Ways of Coping Questionnaire. Mind Garden, Inc.: http://www .mindgarden.com/products/wayss.htm

Videos

- "Playing for Mother Undergoing Cancer Treatment" video. Marylein Serrano is a mother of two children and a speech language therapist who has had several cancer diagnoses. In this video, she discusses how her role as a mother changed during cancer treatment. She describes how playing with her daughter became therapy for herself as well and helped connect her to her role as a mom. She demonstrates her resilience as she describes how she adapted and learned to reconnect with herself, her life, and her children. Access the video at the online resource center at FADavis.com.
- "Jordan's Lived Experience of Recovery as an Occupational Therapy Practitioner" video. In this video, occupational therapist Jordan describes her lived experience of anxiety and depression. She touches on many issues critical to recovery and occupational therapy practice, including social determinants of health, peer support, and how mental health labels can adversely affect an individual's medical treatment. Importantly, she explains how she has learned to blend her lived experience with her work as an occupational therapist, while ensuring she takes care of herself and manages her symptoms. Jordan also offers priceless words of wisdom to practitioners regarding establishing a therapeutic connection with individuals with whom they practice. Access the video at the online resource center at FADavis.com.

- "Mary's Lived Experience as an Unhoused Individual and Her Occupational Therapist's Perspective" video. In this video, Mary provides a first-person account of being unhoused and the tremendous impact occupational therapy services have had on her life. In addition, occupational therapist Quinn Tyminski describes working with Mary and shares her perspective on Mary's journey and transformation, including her improved conflict resolution and emotion regulation skills. Access the video at the online resource center at FADavis.com.
- "Veteran's Caregiver on Advocacy and Veterans Affairs (VA) Support" video. Nancy is the spouse and caregiver of a veteran with early-onset Alzheimer disease. In this video, she shares about his diagnosis and the arduous process of applying for VA benefits. In her case, the application was successful, and she describes how critical those resources have been for her and her husband. Nancy urges OTPs to work with social workers to ensure families of veterans receive the benefits they have earned. Access the video at the online resource center at FADavis.com.

Books

- Creative Use of Activities in Occupational Therapy
  - Evetts, C., & Peloquin, S. M. (2017). *Mindful crafts as therapy.* F.A. Davis.
  - Huri, M. (2018). *Occupational therapy: Therapeutic and creative use of activity.* Intechopen.
- Diary Cards and Dialectical Behavior Therapy Skills Training
  - Linehan, M. (2014). *DBT skills training.* Guilford Press.
- General Stress and Coping
  - Collins, K. M., Onwuegbuzie, A. J., & Jiao, Q. G. (Eds.). (2010). *Toward a broader understanding of stress and coping.* Information Age Publishing.
  - Kabat-Zinn, J. (2013). *Full catastrophe living.* Bantam Books.
  - Lazarus, R. S., & Folkman, S. (1984). *Stress appraisal and coping.* Springer Publishing Company.
- Resilience
  - Reivich, K., & Shatte, A. (2002). *The resilience factor: 7 keys to finding your inner strength and overcoming life's hurdles.* Three Rivers Press.
- Mindfulness Meditation
  - Chaskalson, M. (2014). *Mindfulness: Weeks 1-2 of your eight week plan.* Harper Collins.
  - Harp, D. (2011). *Mindfulness on the go: How to meditate while you are on the move.* New Harbinger Publications.
  - Kabat-Zinn, J. (1994). *Wherever you go there you are: Mindfulness meditation in everyday life.* Hyperion.
- Writing Techniques in Occupational Therapy
  - Haertl, K. H. (2020). Journaling as an assessment tool in mental health occupational therapy. In B. Hemphill-Pearson & C. K. Urish (Eds.), *Assessment in occupational therapy mental health* (2nd ed., pp. 95–115). Slack, Inc.
  - Pennebaker, J. W., & Evans, J. H. (2014). *Expressive writing: Words that heal.* Idyll Arbor.

References

Abbing, A., Ponstein, A., van Hooren, S., de Sonneville, L., Swaab, H., & Baars, E. (2018). The effectiveness of art therapy for anxiety in adults: A systematic review of randomised and non-randomised controlled trials. *PloS One, 13*(12), e0208716. https://doi.org/10.1371/journal.pone.0208716

Abidin, R. R. (2011). *Parenting stress index manual* (4th ed.). Pediatric Psychology Press.

American Psychiatric Association. (2022). *Diagnostic and statistical manual of mental disorders* (5th ed., text rev.). American Psychiatric Publishing. https://doi.org/10.1176/appi.books.9780890425787

Antonovsky, A. (1979). *Health, stress, and coping*. Jossey-Bass.

Ayres, T. S., Sandler, I. N., West, S. G., & Roosa, M. W. (1996). A dispositional and situational assessment of children's coping: Testing alternative models of coping. *Journal of Personality, 64,* 923–958. https://doi.org/10.1111/j.1467-6494.1996.tb00949.x

Ball, T. M., & Gunaydin, L. A. (2022). Measuring maladaptive avoidance: From animal models to clinical anxiety. *Neuropsychopharmacology, 47,* 978–986. https://doi.org/10.1038/s41386-021-01263-4

Baruth, K. E., & Caroll, J. J. (2002). A formal assessment of resilience: The Baruth Protective Factors Inventory. *The Journal of Individual Psychology, 58*(3), 235–244.

Be You. (2023). *Growing a mentally healthy generation*. https://beyou.edu.au

Beidel, D. C., Alfano, C. A., Kofler, M. J., Rao, P. A., Scharfstein, L., & Wong Sarver, N. (2014). The impact of social skills training for social anxiety disorder: A randomized controlled trial. *Journal of Anxiety Disorders, 28*(8), 908–918. https://doi.org/10.1016/j.janxdis.2014.09.016

Biggs, A., Brough, P., & Drummond, S. (2017). Lazarus and Folkman's psychological stress and coping theory. In C. L. Copper & J. C. Quick (Eds.), *The handbook of stress and health: A guide to research and practice* (pp. 351–364). Wiley Blackwell.

Cahill, S. M., & Beisbier, S. (2020). Occupational therapy practice guidelines for children and youth ages 5–21 years. *American Journal of Occupational Therapy, 74,* 740439701p1–p48. https://doi.org/10.5014/ajot.2020.744001

Chen, H., Cohen, P., Johnson, J. G., & Kasen, S. (2009). Psychiatric disorders in adolescence and relationship with peers from age 17–27. *Social Psychiatry and Psychiatric Epidemiology, 44,* 223–230. https://doi.org/10.1007/s00127-008-0421-2

Christiansen, C. H. (2007). Adolf Meyer revisited: Connections between lifestyles, resilience and illness. *Journal of Occupational Science, 14,* 63–76. https://doi.org/10.1080/14427591.2007.9686586

Collins, S., Woolfson, L. M., & Durkin, K. (2014). Effects on coping skills and anxiety of a universal school-based mental health intervention delivered in Scottish primary schools. *School Psychology International, 35,* 85–100. https://doi.org/10.1177/0143034312469157

Compas, B. E., Davis, G. E., Forsythe, J., & Wagner, B. M. (1987). Assessment of major and daily stressful events during adolescence: The Adolescent Perceived Events Scale. *Journal of Consulting and Clinical Psychology, 4,* 534–541. https://doi.org/10.1037/0022-006X.55.4.534

Connor, K. M., & Davidson, J. R. T. (2003). Development of a new resilience scale: The Connor-Davidson Resilience Scale (CD-RISC). *Depression and Anxiety, 18,* 76–82. https://doi.org/10.1002/da.10113

Connor-Smith, J. K., Compas, B. E., Wadsworth, M. E., Thomsen, A. H., & Saltzman, H. (2000). Responses to stress in adolescence: Measurement of coping and involuntary stress responses. *Journal of Consulting and Clinical Psychology, 68,* 976–992. https://doi.org/10.1037/0022-006X.68.6.976

Curtiss, J. E., Levine, D. S., Ander, I., & Baker, A. W. (2021). Cognitive-behavioral treatments for anxiety and stress-related disorders. *Focus, 19,* 184–189. https://doi.org/10.1176/appi.focus.20200045

Delker, B. C., Salton, R., McLean, K. C., & Syed, M. (2020). Who has to tell their trauma story and how hard will it be? Influence of cultural stigma and narrative redemption on the storying of sexual violence. *PloS One, 15*(6), e0234201. https://doi.org/10.1371/journal.pone.0234201

Dise-Lewis, J. E. (1988). The life events and coping inventory: An assessment of stress in children. *Psychosomatic Medicine, 50,* 484–499. https://doi.org/10.1097/00006842-198809000-00005

Fancourt, D., & Finn, S. (2019). *What is the evidence on the role of the arts in improving health and wellbeing? A scoping review (Health Evidence Network synthesis report 67)*. World Health Organisation. https://apps.who.int/iris/handle/10665/329834

Floriou-Servou, A., von Ziegler, L., Waag, R., Schläppi, C., Germain, P. L., & Bohacek, J. (2021). The acute stress response in the multiomic era. *Biological Psychiatry, 89*(12), 1116–1126. https://doi.org/10.1016/j.biopsych.2020.12.031

Folkman, S., & Lazarus, R. S. (1988). *Manual for the ways of coping*. Consulting Psychology Press.

Forman, S. G. (1993). *Coping skills interventions for children and adolescents*. Jossey-Bass.

Frydenberg, E. (2012). *Adolescent Coping Scale-2: Administrator's manual*. Acer Press.

Gilbert, J. N., & Mirawski, C. (2005). Stress coping for elementary school children: A case for including lifestyle. *Journal of Individual Psychology, 61,* 314–328.

Goyal, M., Singh, S., Sibinga, E. M., Gould, N. F., Rowland-Seymour, A., Sharma, R., Berger, Z., Sleicher, D., Maron, D. D., Shihab, H. M., Ranasinghe, P. D., Linn, S., Saha, S., Bass, E. B., & Haythornthwaite, J. A. (2014). Meditation programs for psychological stress and well-being: A systematic review and meta-analysis. *JAMA Internal Medicine, 174*(3), 357–368. https://doi.org/10.1001/jamainternmed.2013.13018

Gunnarson, A. B., Hakansson, C., Hedin, K., & Wagman, P. (2022). Outcomes of the Tree Theme Method versus regular occupational therapy: A longitudinal follow-up. *Australian Occupational Therapy Journal, 69,* 379–390. https://doi.org/10.1111/1440-1630.12796

Gunnarsson, A. B., Jansson, J., & Eklund, M. (2006). The Tree Theme Method in psychosocial occupational therapy: A case study. *Scandinavian Journal of Occupational Therapy, 13,* 229–240. https://doi.org/10.1080/11038120600772908

Haertl, K. L. (2014). Writing and the development of the self-heuristic inquiry: A unique way of exploring the power of the written word. *Journal of Poetry Therapy, 2,* 55–68. https://doi.org/10.1080/08893675.2014.895488

Hayes, S. C., Luoma, J. B., Bond, F. W., Masuda, A., & Lillis, J. (2006). Acceptance and Commitment Therapy: Model, processes and outcomes. *Behaviour Research and Therapy, 44,* 1–25. https://doi.org/10.1016/j.brat.2005.06.006

Hayes, S. C., Strosahl, K. D., & Wilson, K. G. (2011). *Acceptance and Commitment Therapy: The process and practice of mindful change* (2nd ed.). Guilford Press.

Hilker, R., Helenius, D., Fagerlund, B., Skytte, A., Christensen, K., Werge, T. M., Nordentoft, M., & Glenthoj, B. (2017). Heritability of schizophrenia and schizophrenia spectrum based on the Nationwide Danish Twin Register. *Biological Psychiatry, 83*(6), 492–498. https://doi.org/10.1016/j.biopsych.2017.08.017

Hofmann, S. G., Asnaani, A., Vonk, I. J. J., Sawyer, A. T., & Fang, A. (2012). The efficacy of cognitive behavioral therapy: A review of meta-analyses. *Cognitive Therapy and Research, 36*(5), 427–440. https://doi.org/10.1007/s10608-012-9476-1

Hoge, E. A., Austin, E. D., & Pollack, M. H. (2007). Resilience: Research evidence and conceptual considerations for posttraumatic stress disorder. *Depression and Anxiety, 24*(2), 139–152. https://doi.org/10.1002/da.20175

Holmes, T. H., & Rahe, R. H. (1967). The Social Readjustment Rating Scale. *Journal of Psychosomatic Research, 11,* 213–218. https://doi.org/10.1016/0022-3999(67)90010-4

Horn, S., & Feder, A. (2018). Understanding resilience and preventing and treating PTSD. *Harvard Review of Psychiatry, 26*(3), 158–174. https://doi.org/10.1097/HRP.0000000000000194

Johnson, A., Ashby, S., & Lawry, M. (2022). A scoping review exploring the use of art-making-as-therapy in adult mental health occupational therapy practice. *The Open Journal of Occupational Therapy, 10*(4), 1–18. https://doi.org/10.15453/2168-6408.1947

Johnson, J. H., & McCutcheon, S. (1980). Assessing life events in older children and adolescents: Preliminary findings with the life events checklist. In I. G. Sarason & C. D. Spielberger (Eds.), *Stress and anxiety* (Vol. 7, pp. 111–125). Hemisphere.

Jones, S. M., Brush, K., House, S. N., Gross, J. M., Strangeway, M. J., & Merrell, K. W. (2018). *Social-emotional assets and resilience scales (SEARS): Technical manual.* University of Oregon. https://doi.org/10.25656/01:7054

Jørstad-Stein, E. C., & Heimberg, R. G. (2009). Social phobia: An update on treatment. *The Psychiatric Clinics of North America, 32*(3), 641–663. https://doi.org/10.1016/j.psc.2009.05.003

Kabat-Zinn, J. (1994). *Wherever you go there you are: Mindfulness meditation in everyday life.* Hyperion Books.

Kaplan, K., & Kielhofner, G. (1989). *Occupational Case Analysis Interview and Rating Scale.* Slack, Inc.

Kashdan, T. B., & Rottenberg, J. (2010). Psychological flexibility as a fundamental aspect of health. *Clinical Psychology Review, 30*(7), 865–878. https://doi.org/10.1016/j.cpr.2010.03.001

Kato, T. (2015). Frequently used coping scales: A meta-analysis. *Stress and Health, 31*(4), 315–323. https://doi.org/10.1002/smi.2557

Kile, M. (2022). Uncovering social issues through PhotoVoice: A comprehensive methodology. *HERD, 15,* 29–35. https://doi.org/10.1177/19375867211055101

Kirmayer, L. J., Dandeneau, S., Marshall, E., Phillips, M. K., & Williamson, K. J. (2011). Rethinking resilience from Indigenous perspectives. *The Canadian Journal of Psychiatry, 56*(2), 84–91. https://doi.org/10.1016/j.cpr.2010.03.001

Kozlowska, K., Walker, P., McLean, L., & Carrive, P. (2015). Fear and the defense cascade: Clinical implications and management. *Harvard Review of Psychiatry, 23*(4), 263–287. https://doi.org/10.1097/HRP.0000000000000065

Laverdure, P., & Beisbier, S. (2021). Occupation- and activity-based interventions to improve performance of activities of daily living, play and leisure for children and youth ages 5 to 21: A systematic review. *American Journal of Occupational Therapy, 75,* 7501205050p1–p24. https://doi.org/10.5014/ajot.2021.039560

Lavis, P. (2014). Resilience and results: How promoting children's emotional and mental well being helps improve attainment. *Education and Health, 32,* 30–34.

Law, M., Baptiste, S., Carswell, A., McColl, M., Polatajko, H., & Pollock, N. (1998). *Canadian Occupational Performance Measure* (3rd ed.). Canadian Association of Occupational Therapy.

Law, M., Baum, C. M., & Dunn, W. (2005). *Measuring occupational performance: Supporting best practice in occupational therapy* (3rd ed.). Slack, Inc.

Lazarus, R. S., & Folkman, S. (1984). *Stress, appraisal, and coping.* Springer.

Lester, P., Mogil, C., Saltzman, W., Woodward, K., Nash, W., Leskin, G., Bursch, B., Green, S., Pynoos, R., & Beardslee, W. (2011). Families overcoming under stress: Implementing family-centered prevention for military families facing wartime deployments and combat operational stress. *Military Medicine, 176*(1), 19–25. https://doi.org/10.7205/milmed-d-10-00122

Levy-Fenner, E., Colucci, E., & McDonough, S. (2022). Lived experiences of mental health recovery in persons of culturally and linguistically diverse (CALD) backgrounds within the Australian context. *Journal of Psychosocial Rehabilitation and Mental Health, 11,* 7–32. https://doi.org/10.1007/s40737-022-00319-y

Linehan, M. (1993). *Skills training manual for treating borderline personality disorder.* Guilford Press.

Llewellyn-Beardsley, J., Rennick-Egglestone, S., Callard, F., Crawford, P., Farkas, M., Hui, A., Manley, D., McGranahan, R., Pollock, K., Ramsay, A., Sælør, K. T., Wright, N., & Slade, M. (2019). Characteristics of mental health recovery narratives: Systematic review and narrative synthesis. *PloS One, 14*(3), e0214678. https://doi.org/10.1371/journal.pone.0214678

Lo, A. (2020). Using the occupation of the creative arts to promote mental health in young people: Positive Mindset Creative Arts Festival. *World Federation of Occupational Therapists Bulletin, 77*(1), 28–32. https://doi.org/10.1080/14473828.2020.1834256

Loprinzi, C. E., Prasad, K., Schroeder, D. R., & Sood, A. (2011). Stress Management and Resilience Training (SMART) program to decrease stress and enhance resilience among breast cancer survivors: A pilot randomized clinical trial. *Clinical Breast Cancer, 11,* 364–368. https://doi.org/10.1016/j.clbc.2011.06.008

Luken, M., & Sammons, A. (2016). Systematic review of mindfulness practice for reducing job burnout. *The American Journal of Occupational Therapy: Official Publication of the American Occupational Therapy Association, 70*(2), 7002250020p1–7002250020p10. https://doi.org/10.5014/ajot.2016.016956

Lumley, M. A., Schubiner, H., Lockhart, N. A., Kidwell, K. M., Harte, S. E., Clauw, D. J., & Williams, D. A. (2017). Emotional awareness and expression therapy, cognitive behavioral therapy, and education for fibromyalgia: A cluster-randomized controlled trial. *Pain, 158*(12), 2354–2363. https://doi.org/10.1097/j.pain.0000000000001036

Magtibay, D., Chesak, S., Coughlin, K., & Sood, A. (2017). Decreasing stress and burnout in nurses. *JONA: The Journal of Nursing Administration, 47*(7/8), 391–395. https://doi.org/10.1097/NNA.0000000000000501

Martin, L., Oepen, R., Bauer, K., Nottensteiner, A., Mergheim, K., Gruber, H., & Koch, S. C. (2018). Creative arts interventions for stress management and prevention—A systematic review. *Behavioral Sciences, 8*(2), 28. https://doi.org/10.3390/bs8020028

McNair, R. P., & Bush, R. (2016). Mental health help seeking patterns and associations among Australian same sex attracted women, trans and gender diverse people: A survey-based study. *BMC Psychiatry, 16,* 209. https://doi.org/10.1186/s12888-016-0916-4

Meyer, A. (1921). The contributions of psychiatry to the understanding of life's problems. In E. E. Winters (Ed.), *The collected papers of Adolf Meyer* (pp. 1–16). The Johns Hopkins University Press.

Meyer, E. C., Kotte, A., Kimbrel, N. A., DeBeer, B. B., Elliott, T. R., Gulliver, S. B., & Morissette, S. B. (2019). Predictors of lower-than-expected posttraumatic symptom severity in war veterans: The influence of personality, self-reported trait resilience, and psychological flexibility. *Behaviour Research and Therapy, 11,* 1–8. https://doi.org/10.1016/j.brat.2018.12.005

Moksnes, U. K. (2021). Sense of coherence. In G. Haugan & M. Eriksson (Eds.), *Health promotion in health care—Vital theories and research* (Ch. 4, pp. 35–46). Springer. https://doi.org/10.1007/978-3-030-63135-2_4

Moos, R. H. (1990). *Coping responses inventory manual.* Center for Health Care Evaluation, Stanford University and Department of Veterans' Administration Medical Centers.

Murthi, K., Chen, Y.-L., Shore, S., & Patten, K. (2023). Strengths-based practice to enhance mental health for autistic people: A scoping review. *American Journal of Occupational Therapy, 77,* 7702185060. https://doi.org/10.5014/ajot.2023.050074

Nachshen, J. S., Woodford, L., & Minnes, P. (2003). The Family Stress and Coping Interview for families of individuals with developmental disabilities: A lifespan perspective on family adjustment. *Journal of Intellectual Disability Research, 47,* 28. https://doi.org/10.1046/j.1365-2788.2003.00490.x

Osipow, S. H., & Spokane, A. R. (1998). *Occupational Stress Inventory Manual (Professional Version).* Psychological Assessment Resources.

Parsons, D., Gardner, P., Parry, S., & Smart, S. (2022). Mindfulness-based approaches for managing stress, anxiety and depression for health students in tertiary education: A scoping review. *Mindfulness, 13*(1), 1–16. https://doi.org/10.1007/s12671-021-01740-3

Pastorelli, C., Lansford, J. E., Kanacri, B. P. L., Malone, P. S., Di Giunta, L., Bacchini, D., Bombi, A. S., Zelli, A., Miranda, M. C., Bornstein, M. H., Tapanya, S., Tirado, L. M. U., Alampay, L. P., Al-Hassan, S. M., Chang, L., Deater-Deckard, K., Dodge, K. A., Oburu, P., Skinner, A. T., & Sorbring, E. (2016). Positive parenting and children's prosocial behavior in eight countries. *Journal of Child Psychology and Psychiatry, 57,* 824–834. https://doi.org/10.1111/jcpp.12477

Patton, M. Q. (2014). *Qualitative research and evaluation methods: Integrating theory and practice* (4th ed.). Sage.

Pennebaker, J. W., & Chung, C. K. (2011). Expressive writing and its links to mental health and physical health. In H. S. Friedman (Ed.), *Oxford handbook of health psychology* (pp. 417–437). Oxford University Press.

Pennebaker, J. W., & Evans, J. H. (2014). *Expressive writing: Words that heal.* Idyll Arbor.

Penninx, B. W., Pine, D. S., Holmes, E. A., & Reif, A. (2021). Anxiety disorders. *Lancet (London, England), 397*(10277), 914–927. https://doi.org/10.1016/S0140-6736(21)00359-7

Prince-Embury, S. (2006). *Resilience scales for children and adolescents: A profile of personal strengths.* Pearson.

Prince-Embury, S. (2008). The Resilience Scales for Children and Adolescents–Psychological status and clinical status in adolescents. *Canadian Journal of School Psychology, 23,* 41–56. https://doi.org/10.1177/0829573509335475

Puckett, J. A., Matsuno, E., Dyar, C., Mustanski, B., & Newcomb, M. E. (2019). Mental health and resilience in transgender individuals: What type of support makes a difference? *Journal of Family Psychology, 33*(8), 954–964. https://doi.org/10.1037/fam0000561

Rahe, R. H. (1975). Epidemiological studies of life changes and illness. *International Journal of Psychiatry in Medicine, 6,* 133–146. https://doi.org/10.2190/JGRJ-KUMG-GKKA-HBGE

Reivich, K., & Shatte, A. (2002). *The resilience factor: 7 essential skills for overcoming life's inevitable obstacles.* Broadway Books.

Rew, L., Principe, C., & Hannah, D. (2012). Changes in stress and coping during late childhood and pre-adolescence. *Journal of Childhood and Adolescent Psychiatric Nursing, 25,* 130–140. https://doi.org/10.1111/j.1744-6171.2012.00336.x

Robinson, M., McGlinchey, E., Bonanno, G. A., Spikol, E., & Armour, C. (2022). A path to post-trauma resilience: A mediation

model of the flexibility sequence. *European Journal of Psychotraumatology, 13*(2), 2112823. https://doi.org/10.1080/20008066.2022.2112823

Schlebusch, L. (2004). The development of a stress symptom checklist. *South African Journal of Psychology, 34,* 327–349. https://doi.org/10.1177/008124630403400301

Shafer, V., & Bader, K. (2013). Relationship between early life stress load and sleep in psychiatric outpatients: A sleep diary and actigraphy study. *Stress & Health, 29,* 177–189. https://doi.org/10.1002/smi.2438

Sohal, M., Singh, P., Dhillon, B. S., & Gill, H. S. (2022). Efficacy of journaling in the management of mental illness: A systematic review and meta-analysis. *Family Medicine and Community Health, 10*(1), e001154. https://doi.org/10.1136/fmch-2021-001154

Sood, A., Prasad, K., Schroeder, D., & Varkey, P. (2011). Stress management and resilience training among Department of Medicine faculty: A pilot randomized clinical trial. *Journal of General and Internal Medicine, 26,* 858–861. https://doi.org/10.1007/s11606-011-1640-x

Spirito, A., Stark, L. J., & Williams, C. (1988). Development of a brief coping checklist for use with pediatric populations. *Journal of Pediatric Psychology, 13*(4), 555–574. https://doi.org/10.1093/jpepsy/13.4.555

Stein, F., & Cutler, S. (2002). *Psychosocial occupational therapy: A holistic approach* (2nd ed.). Singular Publishing Group.

Stevens, K., McGrath, R., & Ward, E. (2019). Identifying the influence of leisure-based social circus on the health and well-being of young people in Australia. *Annals of Leisure Research, 22*(3), 305–322. https://doi.org/10.1080/11745398.2018.1537854

Thompson, S. F., Zalewski, M., & Lengua, L. J. (2014). Appraisal and coping styles account for the effects of temperament on pre-adolescent adjustment. *Australian Journal of Psychology, 66,* 122–129. https://doi.org/10.1111/ajpy.12048

Tottenham, N. (2014). The importance of early experiences for neuro-affective development. *Current Topics in Behavioral Neuroscience, 16,* 109–129.

Ungar, M., & Theron, L. (2019). Resilience and mental health: How multisystemic processes contribute to positive outcomes. *Lancet Psychiatry, 7*(5), 441–448. https://doi.org/10.1016/s2215-0366(19)30434-1

Walker, P. (2013). *Complex PTSD: From surviving to thriving.* Azure Coyote.

Young, C., Roberts, R., & Ward, L. (2019). Application of resilience theories in the transition to parenthood: A scoping review. *Journal of Reproductive and Infant Psychology, 37*(2), 139–160. https://doi.org/10.1080/02646838.2018.1540860

Yuen, H. K., Spencer, K., Edwards, L., Kirklin, K., & Jenkins, G. R. (2023). A magic trick training program to improve social skills and self-esteem in adolescents with autism spectrum disorder. *American Journal of Occupational Therapy, 77,* 7701205120. https://doi.org/10.5014/ajot.2023.049492

Motivation

Carmen Gloria de las Heras de Pablo

Motivation is intrinsically linked to occupation. It is the source of energy that moves people to explore and participate in meaningful occupations by themselves and with others and to sustain participation over time. This chapter reviews motivational theories and approaches from psychology and occupational therapy from a person-centered perspective. It describes how occupational therapy practitioners (OTPs) can address individuals' motivation with the most frequently used assessments and intervention methods to evaluate and facilitate people's motivation to participate in occupations.

Motivation and Occupational Therapy

Historically, motivation is recognized in occupational therapy practice as one of the most important aspects to consider as a potential facilitator or barrier to occupational participation (de las Heras de Pablo et al., 2019; Kielhofner, 1983, 2008).

Although OTPs and academicians recognize motivation as a key element to consider in practice, one sensitive issue that merits reflection is the tendency of OTPs to import techniques from the psychology discipline to address individuals' motivation. Often, when working on an individual's motivation, OTPs choose to use extrinsic motivation approaches, mainly **operant conditioning** (an approach in which behavior is conditioned by either rewards or punishment; Bruce & Borg, 2002; Cooper et al., 2019). However, the operant conditioning approach hinders **intrinsic motivation** (the personal drive to explore oneself and the environment and to feel competent and satisfied with what one achieves with their own actions) and self-determination and therefore is not consistent with contemporary occupational therapy values (Boyt Shell & Gillen, 2019; Kielhofner, 2009; Peloquin, 2005).

Occupation-focused models and approaches, such as the Model of Human Occupation (MOHO; Kielhofner, 2008; Taylor et al., 2023), the Canadian Model of Occupational Performance and Engagement (CMOP-E; Polatajko et al., 2007; Townsend et al., 2002), Person-Occupation-Environment (PEO) model (Boyt Shell & Gillen, 2019; Law et al., 1996; Letts et al., 2003), Ecological Model of Human Performance (EHP; Dunn et al., 1994), Participative Occupational Justice Frame of Reference (POJF; Whiteford & Townsend, 2011; Whiteford et al., 2017), and Person-Environment-Occupation-Performance Model (PEOP; Baum et al., 2015), share their focus on PEO interaction processes to promote people's well-being and quality of life. They view people as unique individuals, with a particular motivation for occupation and needs of self-determination, social connectedness, belonging, and personal dignity.

These models all support working in collaboration with individuals (i.e., being person-centered) and their environments as essential for personal occupational fulfillment. They also highlight the importance of supporting people in their natural environments of participation.

The CMOP-E, PEOP, PEO, EHP, and POJF promote people's motivation by working with individuals and collectives toward their goals, addressing personal and environmental factors that could promote or interfere with satisfactory and dignifying occupational performance and participation. In addition, MOHO's theory and practice explain and address the motivation for occupation in detail, providing assessment and intervention processes that enable practitioners to work systematically with people who have severe motivational challenges.

Complexity of Motivation Problems

Motivation is a complex phenomenon, and motivational difficulties cannot be explained by considering only one cause. A myriad of factors that are part of individuals and their environments cause motivational challenges:

- Central nervous system (CNS) morphological and chemical alterations
- Acquired chronic physical illness (e.g., immunological diseases, neurological consequences of spinal cord injuries or stroke, and amputations)
- Personal social and physical losses because of environmental physical and sociopolitical catastrophic events, such as wars, forced emigration, the global economic crisis, hurricanes, earthquakes, and other natural phenomenon
- Persistent emotional and physical stress caused by PEO misfit, such as overloaded routines, unsatisfactory lifestyles, consistent experiences of failure, being unemployed, and lacking dignifying occupational opportunities
- Personal traumatic events, such as the loss of loved ones, sexual abuse, continued psychological and/or physical abuse, and bullying

- Professional negligence in mental health, such as reductionist vision, lack of empathy and connectedness with people, directive approaches, and selfishness
- External stigma and internalized stigma

Stigma is one of the most significant factors influencing motivation in people with mental illnesses. Stigma can be defined as a misconception about a phenomenon or circumstance that leads to social discrimination. Stigma does not emerge spontaneously; rather, it develops over time in relationship to the predominant culture, which imbues social groups with values, beliefs, and positions that influence behavior when encountering human realities that are perceived as "not being part of the norm." These misconceptions are usually generated from misinformation, which over time leads to convictions, until relevant knowledge from different sources is generated and socialized or, in extreme cases, until these situations or phenomena occur in one's personal life (de las Heras de Pablo, 2015).

Both people who discriminate and people who are discriminated against internalize these convictions as part of their thinking, feeling, and doing. **Internalized stigma** affects discriminated people's perceptions about themselves, creating vicious cycles of interaction that can decrease motivation and cause people to withdraw from social interactions (de las Heras de Pablo, 2015; Kielhofner et al., 2011; Whiteford & Townsend, 2011). In addition, internalized stigma from some health-care professionals at hospitals and in the community, family, and other relevant social groups are responsible in part for stigma and discrimination.

Discrimination can happen in any place. It derives from dismissing and ignoring people's motivational needs and potentials, creating an ongoing incompatibility between the individual's occupational needs and the social demands and opportunities of participation provided to others, providing too low or too high expectations or demands, or being meaningless or unworthy. This continuous process can invalidate people, producing a sense of inefficacy, boredom, or passivity, and leading to feelings of little or no personal meaning in life (de las Heras de Pablo, 2015).

See Chapter 27: Mental Health Stigma and Sanism or a more comprehensive discussion of the concept of stigma.

Common Conditions Affecting Motivation

Some motivational problems are successfully solved with an appropriate intervention provided at the right time and lasting just the necessary time. Other motivational problems result from a person's typical ways of responding to obstacles and environmental challenges, which are not effective and might even be self-destructive, for example, the actions taken by people with substance abuse or bulimia and anorexia nervosa. In addition, some health conditions are long-standing and affect motivation because their causes involve alterations in the CNS. This is true for schizophrenia and major mood disorders, two mental health conditions in which the CNS directly affects motivation. Both conditions severely impact the individuals' usual motivational condition that underlies occupational participation; consequently, either they find it impossible or difficult to engage and persist in goal-directed activity, or they have an extreme urge to engage in too many activities, thoughts, and actions.

Schizophrenia

Schizophrenia is a disease that affects the limbic system and its connections with the frontal lobe. Motivational impairments in schizophrenia have been associated with abnormalities of the brain morphology and to a dysfunctional dopamine system in the cortical striatal pathway (Crow, 1990; Meltzer, 1990; Strauss et al., 2014). These abnormalities in the CNS explain the alteration in **volition** as being a core feature of schizophrenia. Volition is influenced by the negative symptoms of the disease, symptoms that include apathy, social withdrawal, poverty of thought, dullness of emotions, slowness of movements, and lack of *energy,* causing severe difficulties in people's daily participation. Chapter 23: Schizophrenia Spectrum and Psychotic Disorders includes a more comprehensive discussion of these disorders.

To understand motivation in people with schizophrenia, the Scale for the Assessment of Negative Symptoms can be used to determine the degree of symptomatology. The scale lists **avolition** (a decrease in motivation to initiate and perform self-directed, purposeful activities) as one

The Lived Experience

Forever Ignored

The following poem was written by a man with schizophrenia. His mother found it among hundreds of other poems, after years of trying to understand her son's feeling of helplessness at not being understood by others (Bouricius, 1989, pp. 201–208):

> Who is the lonely dreamer who was thrown away from his own dreams? His soul is broken and he cries overflowing. His desires are still here, with more faith than eternity, stronger than death and hell. I am a lonely "nothing", a being, but ignored. Forever ignored. My afflictions fill the place that was meant to share love. Why can't

> I laugh and cry with others?. . . Why am I full of sorrow?. . . I have tried to evade it, but now I look selfish, dependent, horrible. That is what I observe. I have no life, I have pain. . . . I have the immensity and beauty of my dreams and desires, and conflicts that make everything impossible. I want to love. I envy those who can relate to others. . . . Only in the mental hospital I know others who walk near me. . . . I have lost feelings I had, all the joy and good times are no longer here. . . . I try to be good to myself and show everyone else that I am correct and special. They [the hospital workers] don't come close to me, they don't understand me, they reject me. Why do I always have to prove that I am worthy?

of five negative symptoms (Andreasen, 1984). On this scale, avolition includes lack of attention to grooming and hygiene, difficulty persisting at work or school activities, and physical inertia.

Supporting people's subjective experiences with empirical findings, a study about the determinants of motivational deficits in people with schizophrenia affirms that the impact of internalized stigma is a stronger determinant of intrinsic motivation than avolition itself, and it persists from the early stage to the extended stage of the illness, suggesting OTPs should be involved in early intervention to support improving this group of people's intrinsic motivation (Firmin et al., 2018). For more information about early intervention see Chapter 38: Early Psychosis Programs for Adolescents and Young Adults. 🤝

From a psychological perspective, people with schizophrenia have difficulties initiating goal-directed behaviors. This finding is associated with people having self-efficacy problems, which results in low expectations about themselves (Bentall et al., 2010, de las Heras de Pablo et al., 2019). Past experiences in which others have undermined their capabilities and caused them to internalize the stigma can lead some individuals with schizophrenia to be less motivated to engage in activities because they expect to fail.

Major Mood Disorders

Major depression is often a chronic mood disorder that causes extreme feelings of sadness and hopelessness, anhedonia, slow mental activity, and problems in concentration, memory, eating, and sleeping. Motivation is seriously affected in this disorder. People often lose their sense of pleasure in activities of interest, their self-efficacy, and feelings of worth. Subjectively, some people have referred to major depression as having the most difficult time ever.

Bipolar disorder causes intense fluctuations in mood, energy, thinking, and behavior. Fluctuations in mood include depressive episodes and hypomanic or manic episodes. Manic episodes are the opposite of depressive episodes. They are characterized by people having extremely high levels of optimism; increased activity, energy, or agitation; exaggerated feelings of well-being and self-efficacy (euphoria); reduced need for sleep; unusual talkativeness; and being full of ideas and also distracted. Subjectively, some people who have had these episodes described them as having the best time in their lives, because they felt they were able to do anything they could imagine. However, it is also difficult when they realize the consequences of their actions on themselves and others (e.g., losing jobs, wasting money, losing friends, and harming their family life). Thus, their self-efficacy lowers, and they feel shame and loneliness. See Chapter 20: Mood Disorders for a more complete description of these disorders. 🤝

Theories of Motivation

This section reviews five psychological theories of motivation that have in common their principles based on people's intrinsic motivation.

- Maslow's Hierarchy of Needs
- Self-Determination Theory
- Flow Theory
- Self-Efficacy Theory
- Transtheoretical Model of Change

This section also includes the MOHO, an occupational therapy theory that underlies the profession's philosophy and praxis.

Maslow's Hierarchy of Needs

Abraham Maslow (1943) developed one of the earliest and most enduring models of motivation: the hierarchy of needs.

Theoretical Foundations

Maslow's theory provides a categorization system that reflects the universal needs that motivate people to pursue some actions and activities to satisfy unmet needs, and the hierarchical patterns in which human needs and motivations generally follow.

The most basic needs recognized by Maslow (1943) are physiological, such as food, water, air, urination, excretion, and sleep. The next stage of needs is safety and security needs, which involve feeling protected and feeling physically and emotionally secure. The third stage of needs involves love and belonging needs. Belonging includes feelings of comfort and connectedness to others, feelings that emanate from being accepted, respected, and loved. The next stage of needs is related to esteem, involving needs of self-respect (i.e., needs for feeling competence, autonomy, confidence) and recognition and approval from others. The highest stage of needs is self-actualization, which involves the desire to become the most that one can be, leading to feelings of self-fulfillment and realization of one's potential and personal growth.

Maslow's hierarchy of needs involves two key themes: individualism and prioritization of needs. Individualism recognizes that each individual's needs are unique, as is their intrinsic worth (i.e., their own interests, values, goals). Prioritization explains that, for motivation to arise at the next stage, each prior stage must be satisfied by an individual (Maslow, 1943, 1954).

Maslow also acknowledged the possibility that the different levels of motivation could overlap or occur at any time in the human mind, implying the hierarchy is dynamic. Also, in his latest work, Maslow (1971) introduced transcendental, or spiritual, needs as needs that were beyond all other human needs, yet could exist with any of the other needs in the hierarchy. Furthermore, culture places an important influence on how people prioritize their needs, as important differences exist between the Eastern and Western worlds (Koltkol-Rivera, 2006). Figure 11-1 illustrates the latest conceptualization of Maslow´s hierarchy of needs.

Assumptions About Facilitating Motivation

According to Maslow's Hierarchy of Needs, the lowest level of needs that has not been met must be addressed or satisfied before the individual can move onto higher level needs. The hierarchy of needs stages are used as an evaluation tool, allowing a step-by-step process by which self-actualization is achievable.

Relationship to Occupation

Understanding that each level of unmet needs influences what people do in order to satisfy them, OTPs and students can

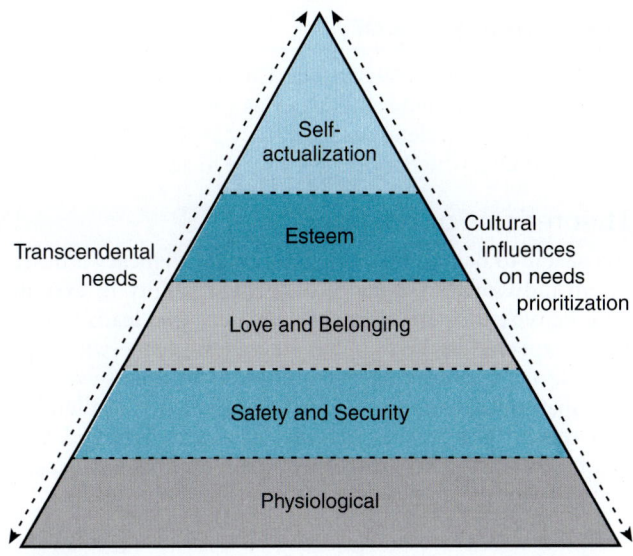

FIGURE 11-1. Maslow's latest conceptualization of the hierarchy of needs.

contextualize the appropriateness of their person-centered services to the unique circumstances of individuals' basic and personal growth needs.

Self-Determination Theory

Self-Determination Theory (SDT) is a theory of human motivation, personality development, and well-being that focuses on self-determined behavior and the social and cultural conditions that promote it (Deci & Ryan, 2012; Ryan, 2009); SDT was first articulated by Edward Deci and Richard Ryan in 1985, based on the evidence of several studies that explained the differences between intrinsic and extrinsic motivation, the effects that intrinsic and extrinsic motivational approaches had on people, and the impact that an extrinsic motivation approach had on decreasing motivation when people were already participating in intrinsically motivating activities (Deci, 1975; Deci & Ryan, 1985).

Theoretical Foundations

SDT is an evidence-based, holistic theory of motivation that asserts that human beings are active organisms that seek psychological growing and well-being. The active nature of human beings is explained through intrinsic motivation or "the natural tendency manifested from birth to seek out challenges, novelty and opportunities to learn" (Ryan, 2009, p. 1). SDT affirms that *specific supports from one's social environment* are necessary for people to achieve personal growth, integrity, and well-being. These supports satisfy three fundamental psychological needs for self-determination: autonomy, competence, and relatedness.

- *Autonomy*: The need of being able to take direct action that will result in real change
- *Competence*: The need to gain mastery of tasks and feel self-efficacy, which is essential to determining own goals, and being active to look for more opportunities of learning
- ***Connection or relatedness***: The need to experience a sense of belonging and connectedness to other people

SDT also explains that extrinsically rewarding versus intrinsically satisfying outcomes have differential effects on well-being and performance. Intrinsically satisfying goals make people continue to work toward their accomplishment, whereas extrinsically motivated goals vanish with time as people realize they are not personally gratifying.

Assumptions About Facilitating Motivation

Deci and Ryan (2012) state that intrinsic motivation, well-being, and personal growth can be fostered by establishing close, empathetic, and affectionate relationships and interactions with people. Acknowledging people's feelings, encouraging them, and providing positive feedback about their task performance are all necessary to facilitate autonomy and competence. Environments that provide this kind of positive social climate and opportunities for active participation in activities that are inherently enjoyable are identified as best to enhance self-determination.

SDT recognizes the need for sustained support when developing and internalizing autonomy and competence. More specifically, autonomy is supported when there are opportunities for self-initiated action, choice, and self-direction. Conversely, controlling environments with rigid deadlines, threats, and pressure hinders autonomy. Positive feedback, the absence of harsh criticism, and optimal challenge are all conducive to feelings of competence (self-efficacy).

Relationship to Occupation

SDT relates to occupation in many ways. Motivation for occupation is conceived as both self-driven and socially constructed. People's self-competence, autonomy, and self-determination are the main concerns of OTPs. Principles of the profession highlight the people OTPs serve as protagonists of their occupational lives; therefore, OTPs must provide individuals with diverse opportunities of participating in meaningful and dignifying occupations that offer an optimal challenge and possibilities for exploration and decision-making.

Flow Theory

The concept of "flow" as a subjective experience was coined by the psychologist Mihaly Csikszentmihalyi (2000). **Flow** is the experience of participation in an activity that is so intrinsically rewarding that the person "loses" themselves in the process.

Theoretical Foundations

Flow Theory explains the phenomenon of the optimal personal experience that occurs while participating in any intrinsically motivating activity, whether it is recreational, work- or education-related, or an activity of daily living.

Flow experience is explained by the dynamics of the relationship between people's subjective perception of their skills and the challenges posed by a particular activity. People in a state of flow function at their full capacity when there is a balance between perceived capacity and action opportunities.

That is, the state of flow emerges when activity/environments provide the optimal level of challenge; the activity must be challenging enough to elicit an internal feeling of capacity, but not so challenging that the individual anticipates failure. When performing the activity, this optimal level of challenge increases the potential of skills that individuals already have, offering immediate feedback from their own expected performance. This in turn provides an experience of joy that is maintained by engaging in more challenging actions. Therefore, the intensity of flow experience is directly related to the match of challenge and skills (Nakamura & Csikszentmihalyi, 2002).

Nakamura and Csikszentmihalyi (2002) described the following characteristics of a state of flow:

- State of intense and focused concentration on an activity
- Merging of action and awareness (i.e., the person does not have to think about what they are doing, but at the same time remains intensely alert to the action)
- Loss of self-consciousness (i.e., the person does not worry about being watched or judged by others)
- Deep sense of control
- Distortion in time (i.e., the individual loses all track of time, and hours seem as if they are minutes)
- Absence of anxiety
- Activity is fully perceived as motivating in and of itself

Assumptions About Facilitating Motivation

Flow Theory has been tested in different settings of participation, finding that environments that offer opportunities of collaboration and self-determination facilitate flow. School environments that promote flow in students use active pedagogy, such as cooperative learning, instead of passive pedagogy, in which students are recipients of content taught by professors. Work environments that promote flow in workers consider workers to be active members of the workplace; the work standards of performance are flexible to match workers' skills, and management is open to workers' proposals for new practices and ideas based on their knowledge and experience. This environment maximizes the match between challenges and skills, and thus promotes self-efficacy and satisfaction.

Nakamura and Csikszentmihalyi (2002) explain that people's flow experiences can be facilitated both in daily activities they usually perform and in activities during which they once experienced flow. As the Flow Theory explains, to continue experiencing flow, people must engage progressively in more complex challenges. To foster experiences of flow, this theory involves a system of graded challenges, which is able to accommodate to people's continued and deepening enjoyment as their skills increase.

Relationship to Occupation

Flow Theory involves providing opportunities to participate in intrinsically motivating activities that provide the right challenge according to the person's subjective perception of their own capacity and of what they conceive as challenging. This matches with the occupational therapy profession's philosophy and practice of facilitating individuals to find their maximum satisfaction in doing the things they like and value. Having knowledge of people's subjective perception of their capacities and valued occupations and interests allows OTPs to promote individuals' self-efficacy, and therefore their performance skills, by structuring the physical, occupational, and social environmental conditions that allow the individual to progressively find flow in occupation or regain flow experiences.

Self-Efficacy Theory

Similar to White (1959) and de Charms (1968), Bandura (1999) also identified self-efficacy as the primary driver of humans. Bandura defines self-efficacy as the belief in one's own capability, which motivates people to act.

Theoretical Foundations

According to Bandura (2006), perceived self-efficacy is based on an individual's judgment of their capability to execute specific types of performances, judgment that leads to personal expectations of possible outcomes. People with high self-efficacy are more likely to set goals for themselves and anticipate relative success, persist longer when challenged, and remain resilient to failures. Bandura identified four sources of self-efficacy: mastery, modeling, social persuasion, and somatic/emotional states:

- *Mastery* is the strongest and most enduring source of self-efficacy. When individuals experience success, this leads to a positive belief about their own skills and abilities. In contrast, failure can undermine self-efficacy.
- *Modeling* is a source of self-efficacy in which people are motivated by other individuals, mostly by those who are seen as similar to themselves, such as peers. For example, a shy adolescent who wants to get to know her classmates would be motivated by a friend who invites her to go together to a group gathering after school, rather than an adult who is a social leader in their community.
- *Social persuasion* refers to verbal encouragement. Verbal encouragement can positively influence self-efficacy when practitioners do it thoughtfully, considering, among other factors, matching an individual's personality and their specific self-efficacy needs. In this theory, positive feedback is considered part of social persuasion. Reversely, feedback in the form of harsh criticism can erode a person's beliefs in their capability.
- *Somatic/emotional states,* or the physical and emotional response to an activity, can either encourage or dishearten an individual. For example, extreme anxiety related to taking an oral examination in front of a group of professors might cause some students to avoid the situation or freeze when questioned. Other students might feel excited about the opportunity to probe their abilities in front of others.

Agentic Perspective

"To be an agent is to intentionally make things happen by one's actions. Agency embodies the endowments, belief systems, self-regulatory capabilities, and distributed structures and functions through which personal influence is exercised" (Bandura, 2001, p. 2).

Self-efficacy is not solely an individualistic notion. Bandura (2002) discussed three types of agency or ways in which people meet goals: personal agency, proxy agency, and collective agency. *Personal agency* is exercised individually, as when a person joins a gym after making a New Year's resolution to lose weight and designs a schedule to exercise independently three times a week. *Proxy agency* is demonstrated when the individual looks for others to act on their behalf. Hiring a personal trainer would be an example of proxy agency, because the individual is using the trainer for motivation. *Collective agency* involves people working together to shape their future. For example, everyone at a work site might agree to go for a walk together over the lunch hour three times a week.

Self-efficacy is required for both personal and collective agencies. In collective agency, the individual must believe that they can work with others and contribute to the collective. People often use proxy agency when concerned about their own self-efficacy.

The pursuit of goals and the type of agency exercised occurs within a cultural context (Bandura, 2002). Although a culture may value collective agency over personal agency or vice versa, it is important to avoid stereotyping individuals and to, instead, assess the unique nature of each person.

Assumptions About Facilitating Motivation

Self-Efficacy Theory proposes general action guidelines to facilitate motivation. The understanding of the sources of self-efficacy can guide practitioners when creating interventions to enhance self-efficacy.

Relationship to Occupation

Self-Efficacy Theory provides information about the sources of motivation for occupation, which is crucial for people to participate as an agent of change in their own occupational journey. Perceived self-efficacy is an important element in the MOHO, which is described in more detail at the end of the theory section.

Transtheoretical Model of Change

Theoretical Foundations

The Transtheoretical Model of Change (TTC; Prochaska & DiClemente, 1982, 2005; Prochaska & Velicer, 1997) is a widely used approach to health behavior change. The TTC focuses on changing unhealthy behaviors, such as smoking, lack of exercise, alcohol abuse, weight gain, risky sexual practices, and drug abuse, and promoting the adoption of health behaviors such as exercise and taking prescribed medications (Velicer et al., 1998). The TTC facilitates intentional change, focusing on promoting individuals' decision-making as active participants of their own processes. The model views people's change as a process that occurs over time and not as an immediate reaction to a personal desire or social mandate.

Assumptions About Facilitating Motivation

The TTC is a stage model; that is, practitioners promote people to move across five stages of change: precontemplation, contemplation, preparation, action, and maintenance.

In *precontemplation,* the individual is not even thinking about or intending to make a change in the near future. They might not realize that their behavior is problematic or that it produces negative consequences. Or, because they have tried to change before without success, they focus more on the reasons not to change the behavior than the advantages of doing so.

Contemplation is the stage at which people intend to change in the near future. They are more aware of the pros of changing, but they still feel a deep ambivalence about taking action, which prevents them from advancing further in their process of change.

Preparation is the stage during which people intend to take action in the near future, usually within a period of 1 month. They have an action plan to take small steps, such as getting social supports, engaging in self-education, or engaging daily in meaningful activities that provide them with a sense of capacity and self-worth.

Action is the stage at which people make the desired change. They have made specific modifications in their lifestyle within the past 6 months and intend to keep moving forward. *Maintenance* is the stage at which people have sustained their behavior change for more than 6 months and make efforts to maintain the behavior change on an ongoing basis. People at this stage work to prevent relapse to earlier stages.

Consistent with its assumptions about motivation, this model does not see relapse as a failure, but rather as a common part of the process. Thus, people are welcomed to reengage at earlier stages to make new attempts at change, usually moving back and forth within the stages.

To promote progress through the stages, this model identifies seven processes that specifically support people in the first stages of change (Prochaska & DiClemente, 2005; Prochaska & Velicer, 1997):

1. *Consciousness raising,* or increasing awareness about the healthy behavior
2. *Dramatic relief,* or emotional arousal about the health behavior
3. *Self-reevaluation,* or self-reappraisal to realize the healthy behavior is part of who they want to be
4. *Environmental reevaluation,* or social reappraisal to realize how their unhealthy behavior affects others
5. *Social liberation,* or the environmental opportunities that exist to show society is supportive of the healthy behavior
6. *Self-liberation,* or commitment to change behavior based on the belief that achievement of the healthy behavior is possible
7. *Helping relationships,* or finding supportive relationships that encourage the desired change

TTC is utilized together with other approaches and theories of motivation, for example, with the Motivational Interviewing (MI) approach and Self-Efficacy Theory, to support people in their processes during the precontemplation and contemplation stages.

Relationship to Occupation

The TTC promotes behavioral change to enhance healthy lifestyles, taking into consideration where the person is in the decision-making process. Occupational therapy promotes health through occupation by facilitating people's participation in meaningful and satisfying routines, thereby fostering their choice making and self-determination. Thus, TTC and occupational therapy are complementary. See Table 11-1 for strategies practitioners can use to promote change.

Model of Human Occupation

The MOHO was introduced to occupational therapy in 1980. MOHO is an intercultural, evidence-based, and integrative occupational and person-centered conceptual model of practice that can be applied across all populations, ages, and occupational therapy practice settings, focusing on people's occupational

TABLE 11-1 | Stages of Change: Strategies to Promote Change

Stage of Change	Strategies
Precontemplation	• Provide gentle encouragement and information. • Avoid lecturing and intensive approaches. • Express belief in the person's ability to make a change.
Contemplation	• Help the person weigh the pros and cons for changing and elicit reasons that promote change. • Provide feedback to resolve the person's ambivalence.
Preparation	• Help the person realistically assess the difficulties related to making a change. • Provide options for ways to go about change. • Help the person think creatively about the most effective plan.
Action	• Provide support for behavior. • Listen and affirm that the person is doing the right thing. • Help the person make changes in the plan if difficulties arise.
Maintenance	• Continue to provide support. • Recognize that people need time to make long-term changes. • Be prepared for the possibility of relapse.

needs rather than the impairments people have. Its general goal is to promote individuals' and collectives' occupational participation to achieve meaningful and satisfying lifestyles that support their well-being and quality of life (Kielhofner, 2008, 2009).

Theoretical Foundations

MOHO is grounded in the beliefs that (a) participation in occupation is a central aspect of the human experience that has a unique personal, historical, and social meaning; and (b) individuals and their environments are inseparable and interdependent. Thus, MOHO explains the concepts and dynamics of the following four occupational elements that in continued interaction conform and transform our participation in occupation: volition, habituation, performance capacity, and environment.

Habituation refers to the internalized patterns or ways people do things and organize their participation. Individuals learn these patterns by experience and repetition under similar circumstances, allowing them to interact semiautomatically with their habitual contexts of participation. MOHO conceptualizes habits, internalized roles, and their mutual influences as the main elements that predispose individuals to organize their occupational participation and performance in patterns and routines, which conform to their own lifestyles.

Performance capacity considers the extent to which underlying abilities from the internal mind-body systems (e.g., muscle strength, range of motion, sensory processing abilities, and cognitive abilities) facilitate or inhibit occupational performance and participation, and includes the subjective mind-body experiences. The environment includes the cultural, political, economic, social, and physical characteristics that interact dynamically and constantly with individuals'

volition, habituation, and underlying capacities, providing opportunities, resources, demands, and challenges for participating in occupation.

Through continued participation in occupation, individuals develop their occupational identity, occupational competence, and occupational adaptation. **Occupational identity** refers to one's own perception of who they are and who they wish to become. **Occupational competence** refers to the extent to which individuals maintain a meaningful and satisfactory lifestyle (i.e., a lifestyle that reflects their occupational identity). Finally, **occupational adaptation** is achieved when one has a clear occupational identity and a lifestyle that represents it.

Assumptions About Motivation

Volition, or motivation for participating in occupation, is defined as the thoughts and feelings individuals hold about themselves as participants in their daily lives, which evolve as they experience, interpret, anticipate, and choose what they do. These volitional thoughts and feelings relate to what one considers important (values), what one perceives as personal capacity and efficacy (personal causation), and what one finds pleasurable (interests; Kielhofner, 2008; Taylor, 2017, Taylor et al., 2023).

How do people get motivated to do things? Why and how do they make this or that decision, choice of activities, or selection of life projects? How do they perceive themselves as participants in their occupational life, and who do they want to become as such? What occupational circumstances give them meaning and pleasure, and why? Volition answers these questions and explains their inherent dynamics as follows.

Thoughts and feelings about personal competence and the sense of pleasure and meaning are always intertwined. People experience participation in occupations by feeling different amounts of pleasure, meaning, and capacity. They reflect on these feelings by interpreting the experiences (e.g., How did I do this? Did I have a good time? Does it make sense to my life?), and accordingly, they anticipate their future participation and make their occupational and activity choices. The continuous cycle of experiencing, interpreting, anticipating, and choosing constitutes the volitional process. Figure 11-2 illustrate the continuous **volitional process.**

The intertwined dimensions of volition, personal causation, interests, and values explain people's feelings and

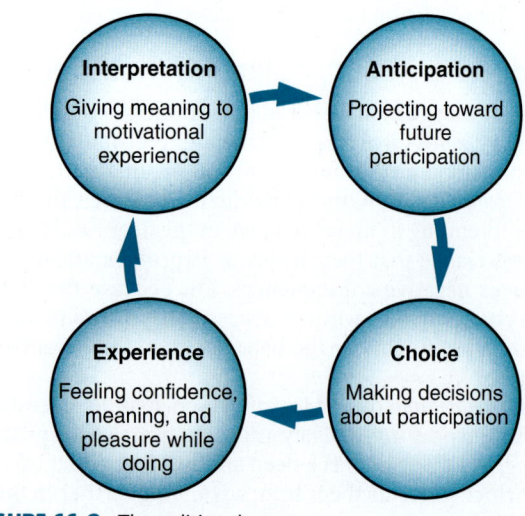

FIGURE 11-2. The volitional process.

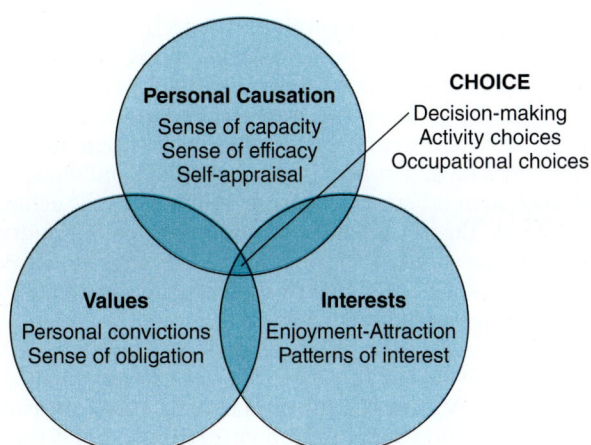

FIGURE 11-3. Intertwined essential aspects of values, interests, and personal causation in the choice-making processes.

thinking about themselves as occupational and human beings through the volitional process, constituting the essence of occupational identity (Who I am, how I perceive myself, and what I want to become). Figure 11-3 illustrates the intertwined essential aspects of values, interests, and personal causation in the process of making choices.

Personal causation refers to one's own sense of competence or efficacy. Personal causation can be expressed in actions such as daring to make decisions, taking initiative, facing challenges and problems, accepting personal mistakes, and accepting constructive criticism.

MOHO conceptualizes a continuum in personal causation development, identifying the **sense of capacity** as its most basic manifestation, this being the personal acknowledgment of one's abilities. **Self-efficacy**, a more complex and stronger manifestation of personal causation, is the personal conviction that one's abilities and skills are useful to achieve one's daily occupational purposes. This personal conviction makes people feel in control over their participation and believe in the impact of their efforts for achieving desired results and personal goals. Thoughts and feelings about personal capacity and efficacy develop through continuous exploration and participation in occupation, evolving in one's **self-appraisal** about their strengths and weaknesses.

Values are tied to individuals' cultural and social contexts from which they learn and develop certain customs, beliefs, and rituals. Values are defined as a group of personal convictions about what is important in life and give meaning or performance standards to occupations. Values are unique to each person and entail a wide range of convictions about spirituality, religion, social relationships, family, politics, goodness, money, love and being loved, effort, work, faith, friendship, and so on.

Values are manifested in the priorities people assign to their occupations and in the responsibility to pursue their occupational choices. When values are strong, they can support motivation and persistence to complete life projects or activities and tasks, despite the difficulties or challenges encountered.

Interests refer to what one enjoys doing. In MOHO, pleasure is conceived as coming from participating in any occupation (Box 11-1). A sense of pleasure comes from a wide

---

BOX 11-1 ■ MOHO Analysis of Ralph's Volition

Because of a traumatic accident while skiing, Ralph, a 34-year-old adult, sustained serious damage in his spinal cord at the C6 level. His neurological damage inhibited his mobility and other body functions. He learned that his acquired patterns of performance and routines weren't useful for him anymore; he needed to explore many new ways of performing and organizing to reinvent his lifestyle. One might expect Ralph's volition to be negatively affected by these challenges. However, Ralph's personal history involved overcoming many other challenges since he was 10 years old and lost his mother. Therefore, he was able to maintain a positive attitude toward living. He made extra efforts to pursue his occupational goals while helping his father raise his two younger siblings. He was a young man who organized his time to volunteer in his community accompanying children who were homeless and work as the administrator of his father's business. His faith, love for life, and his desire to do things the best he could gave him the strength to face the challenge of making the changes he needed to make to meet his occupational purposes.

Ralph also had many people who appreciated him, including his father and siblings who loved him. He also had those with whom he participated in community projects, who offered him and his family emotional and practical support. So, in his unique occupational experience, although his abilities diminished and impacted negatively on his occupational performance and his ways of doing, Ralph's volition and social network (environment) strengthened, supporting his participation.

It is important for OTPs to recognize that not all occupational elements change synergically under certain circumstances. They adjust in interaction as a whole toward the development of renewed participation. Figure 11-4 illustrates Ralph's process of change.

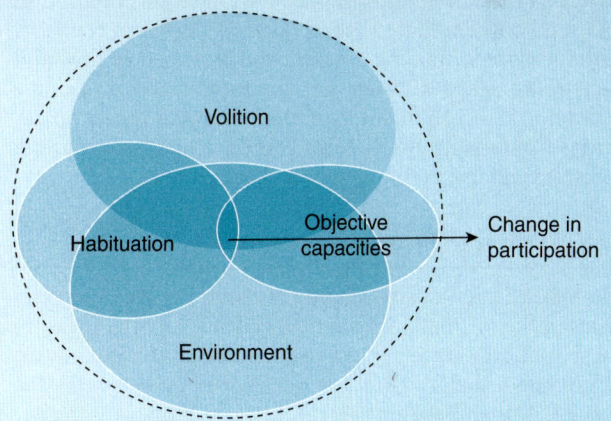

FIGURE 11-4. Ralph: Dynamics of his occupational change.

After reading Ralph's story, review the MOHO theory and answer the following questions:

1. Which MOHO concepts can be identified in Ralph's story? You can go back and forth from the story to the theory.
2. How would you describe Ralph's volition, considering the elements included in MOHO theory?
3. Reflect on Ralph's history. What do you think he would have decided to do if he had not been supported by the community residents, and why?
4. Take time to reflect on yourself and identify your volitional strengths and weaknesses. When, where, with whom, and while doing what do you feel your volition strengthening?

range of factors associated with doing things. For example, some individuals may be attracted to riding a bicycle because of enjoying the feeling of their body working out, whereas another individual may be attracted to it because the air against their body makes them feel free and relaxed. Also, people have *patterns of interests*, which means they tend to prefer certain ways of carrying out activities, such as a tendency to prefer solitary or social activities or a tendency to prefer physical or intellectual activities.

Assessment

This section describes the most relevant assessments and evaluation approaches supported by psychological motivational theories and MOHO.

Flow Theory

The Flow Questionnaire (Csikszentmihalyi & Csikszentmihalyi, 1988; Nakamura & Csikszentmihalyi, 2002) is a paper-and-pencil measure of flow that evaluates the dimensions of flow experienced. This tool has several sections to describe the flow state in terms of the person's experience, the level of intensity of these experiences, their frequency, and the activities in which flow is experienced.

The Experience Sampling Method (ESM) is a technique that collects data about the subjective experience of people while they participate in daily activities performed within their natural settings (Csikszentmihalyi & Rathunde, 1993). The ESM evaluates flow experiences several times during the day, with participants describing their most recent activity, the context in which it took place, and their subjective experience at the time. Csikszentmihalyi used this method to study and develop Flow Theory. The ESM has been used as a valid measure to understand repeated moments of flow and their relationships with relevant environments as a resource to develop motivation and facilitate full involvement in activities (Csikszentmihalyi & Rathunde, 1993; Nakamura & Csikszentmihalyi, 2002).

Self-Efficacy Theory

The Self-Efficacy Scales (Bandura, 2006), a set of several scales in the form of paper-and-pencil self-reports, measure the self-efficacy beliefs of children. adolescents, and adults. To complete the Self-Efficacy Scales, the person rates the strength of their belief in their ability to comply with the demands of particular tasks on a 100-point scale, ranging in 10-unit intervals from 0 ("cannot do") to 50 ("moderately can do") to 100 ("highly certain can do").

Self-Determination Theory

The AIR Self-Determination Scales (SDS; Wolman et al., 1994) come in three forms of paper-and-pencil self-reports: a form for students, a form for parents, and a form for teachers. For this chapter, the form for students has been selected as an example.

The AIR SDS, Form for Students consists of two sections with a list of statements representing self-determination actions in which students engage (What I do); feelings and

thoughts students experience (How I feel); and two sections with statements representing what other people do at school and at home (What happens at school, What happens at home). The students rate each statement using a Likert scale from 1 to 5 to assess how often they engage in their actions, how often they have particular feelings and thoughts, and how often others at school and at home do the actions mentioned. The test has a narrative section for the student to answer questions about their goals and plans to achieve them. Finally, the practitioner uses the ratings to create the AIR Self-Determination Profile.

Similar to the AIR SDS for students, the ARC SDS (Wehmeyer, 1995) and the ChoiceMaker Self-Determination Assessment (Martin & Huber Marshall, 1994) measure self-determination skills and opportunities to build those skills in adolescent students with disabilities, serving as a guide to facilitate students' active involvement in educational planning as part of educational outcomes. The assessments are administered by educators.

The SDS (Sheldon & Deci, 1993) is a paper-and-pencil self-report that captures the exemplar of a self-determined adult. The SDS is a 10-item scale, with two 5-item subscales. The first subscale relates to awareness of oneself, and the second relates to perceived choice in one's actions. For each item there are two statements (A and B) for the person to determine which one feels more true, using a 1 to 9 rating scale, where "Only A feels true" represents rating 1 and "Only B feels true" represents rating 9. The subscales can be used separately or combined into an overall SDS score.

Model of Human Occupation

This section describes the most frequently used assessments of volitional process and occupational identity development.

The Modified Interest Checklist (Kielhofner & Neville, 1983) is a widely used MOHO self-report suited for adolescents, adults, and older adults. The Modified Interest Checklist consists of a list of 66 activities and an item for "others that are not listed." For each activity, people check their level of interest during the past 10 years and during the past year using a three-point rating scale, their present participation in these activities, and their desire to participate in the activities or explore some new activities in the future.

After completing the form, the practitioner and the person engage in a collaborative analysis or interview to understand the characteristics of attraction, the unique pattern of activities identified as pleasurable, the extent of environmental opportunities, and the person's strengths that support participation in these activities. This information is then considered for joint goal setting and planning. The Modified Interest Checklist has been adapted in some countries to match people's cultural backgrounds.

The Pediatric Interest Profiles (PIP; Henry, 2000) is a MOHO self-report measure that evaluates children and adolescents' interest in a variety of games and leisure activities, using questions regarding their participation and frequency of participation in the activities, enjoyment, sense of competence, and social interactions during their participation. For children's profiles, stick figures are used to represent each item.

The assessment includes three different profiles designed for specific age ranges: The Kid Play Profile (50 activities), Pre-Teen Play Profile (59 activities), and Adolescent

Leisure Interest Profile (83 activities). After completing the self-report, the therapist does a narrative interview. The PIP guides therapeutic reasoning to facilitate satisfactory participation and enhance volition in recreational activities.

The Role Checklist (v.1.0; Oakley et al., 1986) is a widely used MOHO self-report for older adolescents and adults that is designed to understand individuals' perception about their participation in valued roles across life history and of their occupational balance. This self-report has three sections.

In the *first section,* the person identifies the roles in which they have participated in the past, participate in the present, and plan to participate in sometime in their future. In the *second section,* the person rates the extent in which they value each role using a three-point rating scale. The *third section* consists of *the joint analysis of information and conclusions* around the presence or absence of significant roles, the congruence between the roles performed and the value assigned to them, and the personal feelings of efficacy with role performance and how these factors impact on their occupational balance. The environmental and personal occupational characteristics that have favored or limited their participation in significant roles are also considered for goal setting and planning.

The Occupational Performance History Interview–Second Version (OPHI-II; v.2.1; Kielhofner et al., 2004) is a valid and reliable semistructured interview (Kielhofner et al., 2001) designed for adolescents, adults, and older adults.

This interview uses a narrative approach to understand people's occupational identity, occupational competence, and the environmental impact on occupational adaptation through the continuity of life.

The OPHI-II consists of three parts: the interview, the rating of three scales (occupational identity scale, occupational competence scale, and occupational behavior settings scale), and the completion of a life history narrative with qualitative information and features of the individual's life story.

The interview is designed to be very flexible to facilitate the flow of the person's narrative. Practitioners need to relate naturally and respectfully; be empathic, active listeners; ask open-ended questions; validate and affirm the person's unique strengths, values, efforts, and resources; use summary statements based on the person's story and its meaning; share their own experiences; occasionally use a person's meaningful objects to help that person retrieve their experiences; reflect on themselves; and narrate these experiences as stories. This interview prioritizes obtaining specific types of information in five thematic areas (activity/occupational choices, critical life events, daily routine, occupational roles, and occupational behavior contexts), which can be covered in any successive order or by moving back and forth between them.

The rating of 29 items on the three scales is completed by matching each item's criteria statements with the person's narrative and using a four-point rating scale that indicates the extent to which the items positively or negatively affect occupational adaptation. Practitioners share the three scales with the person for their review, and to encourage engagement in joint reasoning. The joint analysis of a graphic in which the therapist plots the person's life story is the final step to complete the life history narrative form and make joint conclusions, set goals, and create an action plan.

The Occupational Self-Assessment (OSA; Baron et al., 2006) is a valid and reliable MOHO self-report (Kielhofner et al., 2007) designed for adolescents, adults, and older adults to evaluate their self-perception of their occupational competence for daily participation in occupations and the value the persons assigned to them in order to set priorities and goals for therapy.

The OSA consists of two parts. The first part (Myself) consists of a list of 21 statements related to a variety of daily tasks and actions linked with the domains of volition, habituation, and occupational performance. Individuals complete the form following three consecutive steps, in which they rate the extent of how well they perceive they perform each task or action and how important each task/action is to them, using four-point rating scales. Individuals finish completing this form by choosing four items perceived as a priority to change.

The second part (My environment) is for people, using a four-point rating scale, to rate the extent to which the physical and social domains of different settings support their participation in occupations, and how important each environmental aspect is for them. After the forms are completed, the therapist and the person do a joint analysis of the answers, identify the person's strengths and difficulties, and discuss priorities to facilitate goal setting and planning.

The Child Occupational Self-Assessment (COSA; Version 2.2; Kramer et al., 2014) is a valid and reliable measure (Kramer et al., 2010) that is similar to the OSA and designed for use with young children and youth up to age 17. The COSA uses 26 statements concerning daily tasks and actions and four-point rating scales that are age-appropriate. The COSA comes in three versions: a youth rating form with symbols; a youth rating scale without symbols, and a card sort option. The instrument has also been adapted for younger children and children who can only choose between options. As with the OSA, children have the opportunity to review their answers and concerns, identify strengths and difficulties, and review priorities with their therapist to set goals and planning. Both the OSA and COSA provide a follow-up form to evaluate outcomes of the plan developed together with the OTP.

The Volitional Questionnaire (VQ; Version 4.1; de las Heras et al., 2007) and the Pediatric Volitional Questionnaire (PVQ; Version 2.2; Basu et al., 2008) are valid and reliable MOHO observational assessments (Anderson et al., 2005; Chern et al., 1996; Li & Kielhofner, 2004) that have been widely applied to people of all ages, conditions, and abilities to measure their motivation for participating in occupations and the effects of impact that the physical, occupational, and social characteristics of different contexts have on their volition. The VQ and PVQ provide specific information about a person's values, personal causation, interests, decision-making, and activity choices, as well as the relationships between them and their consistency and variation across different occupations and environmental contexts.

The VQ consists of 14 items that are represented by behaviors that reflect volition in a continuum of progress or change through the stages of exploration, competency, and achievement. Before administration, practitioners perform an initial evaluation to gain knowledge about the person's occupational profile. Administration of the VQ and PVQ consists of a systematic observation of the person's volition while participating in different activities in different contexts.

Observation in multiple contexts ensures the understanding and fair conceptualization and contextualization of a person's volition. Practitioners' subtlety, attention to multiple factors, naturalness, and use of self-care are all important for the administration of these assessments.

After each session of observation, practitioners complete the rating forms, rating each volitional behavior using a four-point scale to measure the spontaneity of the emergence of volition versus the amount of support, encouragement, and structure the person needs to express the behaviors (4: Spontaneous; 3: Involved [minimal support is needed]; 2: Hesitant [substantial/constant support is needed]; 1: Passive [despite all support given, volition remains inhibited], and N/O [not observed]). Practitioners add comments to support the ratings assigned to each item and complete the environmental form for the session. Table 11-2 summarizes the assessments discussed that are most frequently used to evaluate motivation.

TABLE 11-2 | Therapeutic Reasoning Assessment Table: Motivation

Which Tool?	Who Was This Tool Designed For?	What Is Required of the Person? Can They Use the Tool?	What Am I Measuring?	How Long Does It Take and Where Do I Administer This Assessment?	Is the Tool Associated With a Practice Model?
Experience Sample Method (ESM; Csikszentmihalyi & Rathunde, 1993)	Adolescents and adults	People describe activities, the context in which they took place, and their subjective experience at the time.	People's subjective experience of flow while engaging in daily activities	People take 10–15 minutes to record each experience.	Flow Theory
Self-Efficacy Scales (Bandura, 2006)	Children, adolescents, and adults Scales: • Self-Efficacy to Regulate Exercise • Self-Efficacy to Regulate Eating Habits • Driving Self-Efficacy • Children Self-Efficacy Scales • Self-Efficacy for Mathematics • Collective Self-Efficacy for Reading and Mathematics • Teacher Self-Efficacy Scales • Parental Self-Efficacy Scales • Collective Family Self-Efficacy	Filling out the self-report scales to record the strength of their efficacy beliefs for each task's demand on a 100-point scale, ranging in 10-unit intervals from 0 ("Cannot do") to 100 ("Highly certain can do")	Self-efficacy beliefs related to different tasks' demands. Scales are designed for different age groups, listing the specific tasks and their demands.	Filling out scale forms could take from 10–40 minutes.	Self-Efficacy Theory (Bandura)
Modified Interest Checklist (Kielhofner & Neville, 1983)	Young adults, adults, and older adults	• People fill out a form that lists 66 activities. For each, they indicate their level of interest during the past (10 year and the past year) using a three-point rating scale. They also indicate their participation or not in the present, and if they want to pursue them or not in the future. • They participate in a joint analysis and interview, goal setting, and planning.	Identification, attraction, and pattern of activities of interest in the past and present, and the desire to pursue them in the future	Filling out the self-report, doing the analysis/interview, and setting goals and planning can take 40 minutes.	MOHO
The Pediatric Interest Profile (PIP; Henry, 2000)	Children 6–9, 9–12, and adolescents (12–21); the PIP includes three different profiles: • The Kid Play Profile • The Pre-Teen Play • The Adolescent Leisure Interest Profile For children's profiles, stick drawing figures are used to represent each item.	They fill out the forms appropriate to their age by marking the options of responses to questions that each activity item provides. • After filling out the forms, the therapist does a narrative interview with the kid or adolescent.	Identification of interests in a variety of games and leisure activities; considering participation and frequency of participation in the activities; amount of enjoyment felt; sense of competence and social interactions during their participation	Filling out the self-report and participating in the interview can take 45 minutes.	MOHO

TABLE 11-2 | Therapeutic Reasoning Assessment Table: Motivation—cont'd

Which Tool?	Who Was This Tool Designed For?	What Is Required of the Person? Can They Use the Tool?	What Am I Measuring?	How Long Does It Take and Where Do I Administer This Assessment?	Is the Tool Associated With a Practice Model?
Occupational Self-Assessment (OSA; Baron et al., 2006) Child Occupational Self-Assessment (COSA; v.2.2; Kramer et al., 2014) Similar to the OSA in its format and procedures, but with adapted content to be age-appropriate	Adolescents, adults, older adults Children and youth, 5–17 Versions: • A youth rating form with symbols • A youth rating scale without symbols • A card sort option	People use a four-point rating scale to indicate how well they do each task and action and how important these tasks and actions are for them and choose four items perceived as the priority items to improve. • They rate the environmental items following the same steps. • They participate in joint analysis and design of an action plan.	Individuals' self-perception of their occupational competence when doing a variety of daily tasks and actions, and their assigned value to them. It measures the extent in which the physical and social environment support their occupational identity and competence.	Filling out the self-report, doing joint analysis, and devising the action plan can takes 45 minutes to an hour.	MOHO
Role Checklist (v.1.0; Oakley et al.,1986)	Adolescents, adults, older adults	People fill out two forms of 10 listed occupational roles, marking the temporality in which they have participated in each role, and they assign value to each one by using a three-point rating scale. • They participate in joint analysis through an interview, goal setting, and design of an action plan.	Person's self-perception of occupational balance and their satisfaction with occupational participation. • It informs about people's participation in occupational roles in the past and present, and their desire of participating or not in their future.	Filling out the self- report, doing the interview, and developing the joint design of the action plan can take 40 minutes.	MOHO
Occupational Performance History Interview (OPHI-II; v.2.1; Kielhofner et al., 2004)	Adolescents, adults, older adults	Within an empathic and open social context, people participate in a narrative interview with the OTP, sharing their lived experiences about their participation in occupation in their continuum of life, giving meaning to it through their volitional interpretation of events and circumstances. • People participate on reviewing the criteria and the rating of scales' items, previously filled out by the OTP, engaging in a joint reasoning that is represented in a graphic showing their life narrative in progress. • They participate in goal setting and designing an action plan.	People's occupational adaptation in three interrelated dimensions: occupational identity, occupational competence, and occupational settings. • The OPHI-II provides information about people's subjective appreciation of their occupational identity in relationship with their occupational competence and the environments where they participate in the continuum of their past, present, and projected future. • Occupational identity, occupational competence, and occupational behavior settings scales allow individuals to identify items' specific criteria that best match with the person's narrative, and to rate the items using a four-point rating scale.	The interview and rating of the scales takes 45 minutes to an hour. The shared reasoning, analysis, and goal setting takes another 30–45 minutes. The whole process can be done in three sessions.	MOHO

Continued

TABLE 11-2 | Therapeutic Reasoning Assessment Table: Motivation—cont'd

Which Tool?	Who Was This Tool Designed For?	What Is Required of the Person? Can They Use the Tool?	What Am I Measuring?	How Long Does It Take and Where Do I Administer This Assessment?	Is the Tool Associated With a Practice Model?
The Volitional Questionnaire (VQ; v.4.1; de las Heras et al., 2007) The Pediatric Volitional Questionnaire (PVQ; v.2.1; Basu et al., 2008)	Children age 7 to older adults with a myriad of abilities Children age 2–7 Similar to the VQ in its format and procedures, but with content of items adapted to be age-appropriate to younger children	Individuals participate in different activities within different contexts.	People's volition (values, personal causation, interests, decision-making) and the extent in which the physical, occupational, and social features of different contexts of participation facilitate or inhibit volition Following systematic observation of a person's volition while participating in different activities or tasks within different contexts, OTPs rate the 14 VQ items using a four-point rating scale to indicate the extent in which the person spontaneously displays the volitional behaviors versus the amount of encouragement, support, and structure they need to do so. An environmental form is also filled out for each setting where observations took place.	Time for observation usually varies from 15 to 30 minutes. Filling out the scale and the environmental form takes 20 minutes.	MOHO

Intervention

Motivational Interviewing

MI is "a collaborative, goal-oriented style of communication with particular attention to the language of change. It is designed to strengthen personal motivation for and commitment to a specific goal by eliciting and exploring the person's own reasons for change within an atmosphere of acceptance and compassion" (Miller & Rollnick, 2013, p. 29).

The MI technique is particularly useful when people feel ambivalent and confused about change, they have low self-efficacy regarding their ability to change, they are unsure about their desire to make a change, or there is uncertainty about the benefits of change or the disadvantages of their current situation. Thus, MI is differentiated into two phases: The first phase focuses on increasing motivation for change, and the second focuses on consolidating commitment for change (Miller & Rollnick, 2013; Hettema et al., 2005).

Assumptions About Facilitating Motivation

MI has a strong relationship to Carl Rogers's persons-centered approach, evidencing the efficacy of many of Rogers's techniques and attitudes toward people, including considering people as unique human beings who need to be understood and respected in their perspectives, supported in their autonomy, and viewed as experts, using empathy and acceptance, a collaborative style, and having confidence in their ability to change (Csillik, 2013; Miller & Moyers, 2017; Miller & Rollnick, 2017, Rogers, 1961). The spirit of MI reflects these elements in the four facets of partnership, acceptance, evocation, and compassion.

Partnership means that the therapist and person collaborate as experts (Miller & Rollnick, 2013). The individual is an expert in their own life, and the therapist is an expert in their discipline. MI is done "with" someone and not "to" someone. It helps the person identify their own reasons for change.

Acceptance means accepting people as they are (Miller & Rollnick, 2013). Acceptance includes absolute worth, or the sincere belief and respect for a person's natural desire to change in a positive direction. It also includes empathy, or the practitioner's capacity to take the person's perspective and collaborate truthfully with them. The practitioner's role is to recognize and support the person's capacity for self-direction and for making their own choices, as well as recognizing the person's strengths and efforts.

Evocation means eliciting from the person their own goals and values regarding change (Miller & Rollnick, 2013). Evocation is the process of drawing out the wisdom and experience of the person to facilitate a discussion about change.

Compassion is considered an essential component of the spirit of MI (Miller & Rollnick, 2013). A compassionate attitude is the OTP's genuine dedication to promote and prioritize individuals' welfare and well-being. None of the other three facets of the MI spirit could be effective without the selfless commitment of the practitioner.

MI ensures practitioners develop skills that promote the effectiveness of its application. To best accomplish this purpose, practitioners use the Motivational Interviewing Target Scheme (MITS; Allison et al., 2012) for supervisor's feedback. MI core skills include:

- *Asking open-ended questions* to explore the person's experiences, perspectives, and ideas. Open-ended questions encourage a person to explain, narrate, and reflect on their own situations (i.e., How would you go about solving that situation now? How would you explain this in more detail to me? Describe the circumstances in which you could . . .).
- *Offering information within the structure of open-ended questions.* OTPs generate a dialogue with the person by drawing out the person's knowledge first, respectfully offering the practitioner's knowledge, and continuing to elicit the person's thoughts and experiences (Elicit-Inform-Elicit).
- Reflective *listening* is used to maintain an empathic attitude and true understanding of what people need to communicate. In reflective listening, the practitioner carefully listens to what people need to express and, at the right moments, expresses their understanding of it. Practitioners do this by rephrasing, repeating, or offering a deeper interpretation about what the person is communicating, and always soliciting the person's feedback about their interpretation.
- Affirmation refers to practitioners making honest statements or gestures that acknowledge people's strengths, efforts, and past successes to help build the person's hope and self-efficacy in their ability to change.
- Making *summary statements* serves to summarize what has been discussed to ensure a shared understanding and emphasize the key points made by the person.
- *Eliciting change talk* refers to attending progressively to the language of change, taking into consideration the extent to which people are ready for change or ambivalent about deciding to change. First, the practitioner recognizes what is being said as either against or in favor of change. The OTP encourages change talk when possible and the person's reflection of how change can be meaningful or possible. Together, the person and practitioner collaborate to make a plan change.

MI has been widely applied across a range of settings, such as health, human services, and education; across different treatment formats, such as individually or in groups; and to approach different concerns, such as health, nutrition, risky sex, substance abuse and other addictions, and illegal behaviors.

The Remotivation Process

The Remotivation Process (RP) is a MOHO protocol-based intervention for people whose volition inhibits or restricts their participation in occupations. The RP improves motivation by promoting a gradual increase in sense of self-worth, effectiveness, and belonging. It involves collaborative efforts between the individual and the practitioner, as well as the person's meaningful social network in relevant contexts.

The RP was developed and has been clinically studied since 1988, in response to the lack of intervention strategies for people who had very low volition, some of whom were undermined or ignored by practitioners who viewed them as being "unreachable," "difficult to manage or to work with," or "not interested in doing." Since its first publication (de las Heras et al., 2003), the RP has been widely used and researched in different cultures.

Recall that the volitional process is the foundation of volitional change. The RP evidence shows that people can experience their volitional process in different ways, according to the cycle of personal development, abilities, and the opportunities or restrictions of the environment. Some people can simply experience feelings of worth and pleasure while being part of certain occupational circumstances, whereas others can experience volition and make choices, or go through the complete cycle (de las Heras de Pablo et al., 2017, 2019).

The volitional process is socially constructed. Through others' recognition of individuals as human beings, they develop personal meaning. Through the others' expressions of their thoughts and feelings about individuals, they learn and internalize how they perceive themselves. Through social opportunities of exploration and participation in meaningful occupation, people develop and reaffirm their interests, personal causation, and values (de las Heras de Pablo et al., 2019).

Thus, the volitional process is embedded with the environmental characteristics of one's relevant settings of participation. The extent to which the environment facilitates or inhibits people's volition depends on the interaction between individual characteristics of volition and the environment. Figure 11-5 illustrates this relationship and the environmental impact on volition.

Implications for Practitioners

The RP requires practitioners to:

- Deeply appreciate each individual's subjective experience
- Maintain self-awareness and effective use of self
- Be aware of the unique variations of experience within different occupations and environmental contexts and the qualities of their dimensions
- Remain flexible at the moment of selecting and implementing interventions that are appropriate to individuals' unique personal and environmental realities

When facilitating volition, practitioners must generate an exploratory context—that is, a social climate of openness, collaboration, and trust that makes individuals feel comfortable with exploring, trying, and discovering or rediscovering their own interests, values, goals, capacities, initiatives, environmental demands, and opportunities. They must focus on the person's

Evidence-Based Practice

The Remotivation Process for Women With Lymphedema

OTPs can offer a unique contribution in addressing chronic conditions.

RESEARCH FINDINGS

Rubio and colleagues (2022) discovered the positive effects of the RP on changing the daily performance of lymphedema management techniques and on the individual's manifestation of breast cancer–related lymphedema (BCRL). A within-subject quasi-experimental design with a repeated measure of volition and weekly performance of the symptom management program (SMP) was implemented as the dependent variable. Eleven females age 18 or older participated in the study.

The RP was implemented in the form of one-on-one weekly discussions with each participant through Zoom for 4 weeks with a follow-up discussion during the eighth week. A set of open-ended guided questions corresponding to each stage of the RP were used to facilitate each participant's reflection of their experience when performing the SMP, as well as their perception of BCRL in the context of daily activities during the week. Field notes recorded the observations during the discussion, determined each participant's level of motivation during the week, and framed the discussion according to the participant's volitional stage of the RP. The study used the VQ, frequency count of SMP, and circumferential measurement as outcome measures. The statistical analysis revealed that participants showed significant improvements in volition, an increase in adherence to the SMP, and a decrease in the size of the corresponding upper extremity at the end of the study.

APPLICATIONS

➡ The study showed that the RP, used as an occupational therapy intervention, can have a positive effect on the participant's motivation.
➡ The study demonstrated that OTPs can offer a unique contribution in addressing chronic conditions.

REFERENCES

Rubio, K., Bowyer, P., Hite, S., Pingale, V., Freysteinson, W., Hersch, G., & Raber, C. (2022). Promoting self-management of breast cancer-related lymphedema through the Remotivation Process. *The Open Journal of Occupational Therapy, 10*(4), 1–13. https://doi.org/10.15453/2168-6408.1911

Physical Dimension/Objects
Availability
(presence and distribution)
Meaning
Adequacy
(fit with abilities)
Versatility
Sensory features

Occupational Dimension/Tasks
Availability
(valuable, interesting, fits abilities)
Structural flexibility
Temporal features
Social connotation
(individual or in group, private or public)

CULTURE

Person —— *Environmental Impact*

Social Dimension
(persons/groups)
Availability
Interaction/relationships
Social climate/attitudes
Occupational expectations

Physical Dimension/Spaces
Accessibility
(safe entrance and navigation within it)
Adequacy
(size, distribution, privacy)
Personalization
Sensory features

FIGURE 11-5. Relationship between personal occupational characteristics and the features of contexts of participation: environmental impact on volition.

intentions and their gradual processes of self-knowledge and self-determination, while providing the "just right" volitional support when needed (de las Heras de Pablo et al., 2019).

Because the RP is often implemented by a variety of persons along with the OTP, including other team members, staff, family members, friends, peers, and other individuals, participatory social education, guidance, and support are crucial throughout the process.

The MOHO assessments that are more frequently utilized during the RP are the ones previously described in this chapter (see Table 11-2). The VQ and PVQ guide the detailed intervention through the whole process. The other MOHO assessments are incorporated according to individuals' needs, when their sense of capacity shows the proper readiness for participating in an interview or a self-assessment, and their abilities allow them to do it. Figure 11-6 shows the volitional continuum provided by the VQ.

Phases, Stages, Steps, and Procedures

The RP involves an interwoven sequence of three phases of intervention that relate to the three stages of volitional process development: exploration, competence, and achievement.

Thus, for assuring a valid application of the RP, practitioners must have in mind that the phase, stages, and steps of the process, as well as the time it takes to move through each phase and stage or through the entire process, depends on each individual's development of their volitional process. That volitional continuum is dynamic, not rigid; phases and stages can interrelate or overlap at any given point. Figure 11-7 shows the interwoven phases and stages.

Read the Being a Psychosocial OT Practitioner feature and consider what phases Olivia and the OTP are going through.

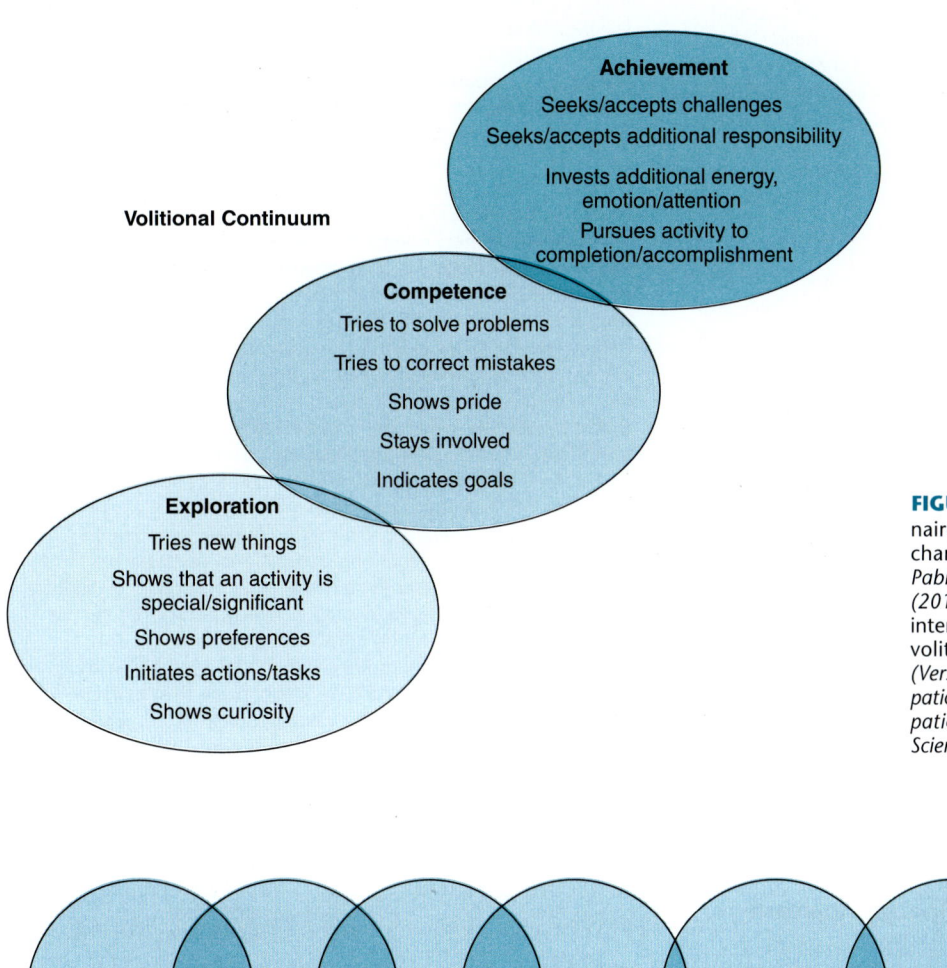

FIGURE 11-6. The Volitional Questionnaire and the volitional continuum of change. *Modified from de las Heras de Pablo, C. G., Llerena V., & Kielhofner, G. (2019). Remotivation Process: Progressive intervention for people who have severe volitional challenges. A user's manual (Version 2.0). The Model of Human Occupation Clearinghouse, Department of Occupational Therapy, College of Applied Health Sciences, University of Illinois at Chicago.*

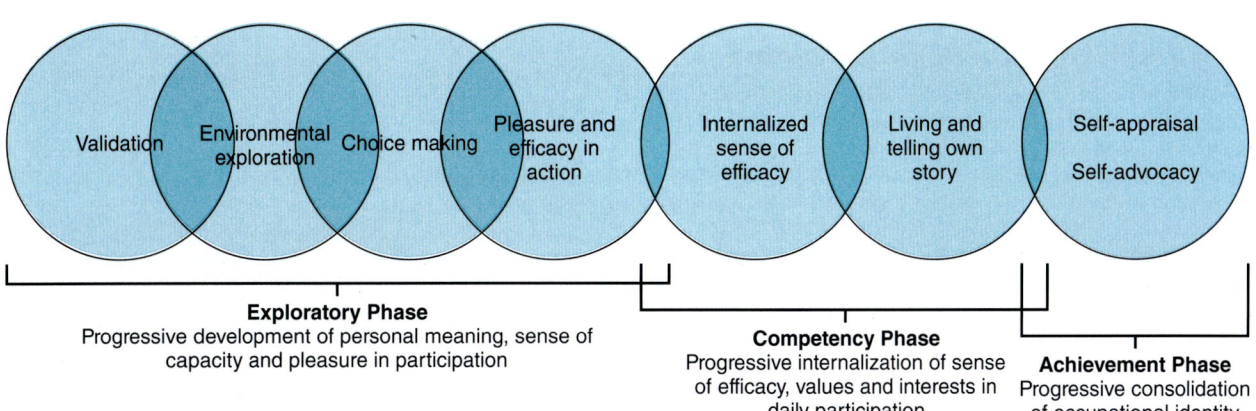

FIGURE 11-7. The Remotivation Process: Interwoven phases and stages.

Being a Psychosocial OT Practitioner

Olivia and her OTP Recognize Olivia's Desire to Live a Simple, Comfortable Life

Identifying Psychosocial Strengths and Needs

OTPs can use the principles of the MOHO RP to focus on a person's uniqueness and relevant environments to facilitate volition through *feeling, thinking, and doing with* them instead of deciding for them. Consider the story of Olivia, a 52-year-old woman living with her mother in an apartment. Olivia was diagnosed with schizophrenia at age 24 and is currently taking medications for symptom management. She was referred to occupational therapy by her psychiatrist, who is concerned that Olivia is not leaving her apartment and lacks engagement and motivation for participation in daily activities.

The OTP met Olivia at her mother's apartment. Because of her discomfort meeting someone unknown, the OTP greeted her affectionately and waited for Olivia to indicate where she should sit. The OTP spoke kindly as she gathered an occupational profile and information about her personal needs. This generated an atmosphere of trust and respect that allowed the OTP to explore Olivia's experiences, interests, and social contexts and to decide which evaluation methods would be the most appropriate to use with her. In this first meeting, informal conversation and participant observation sufficed. In a second meeting, the OTP decided to use the OPHI-II, MOHO's narrative interview.

Olivia worked as an executive secretary from the age of 20 to 25. She valued that job and felt it was compatible with her skills. She reported enjoying life with her parents, brothers, and nephews; meeting with friends; playing cards and board games; watching television; and shopping.

Olivia assigned great importance to the affection given by her parents, being cared for by others, and doing a job well, highlighting the period of time in which she worked as the most satisfying in her life. However, Olivia portrays herself as a shy person and dependent on the affection and recognition of others to feel satisfied. She refers to a significant break in her occupational narrative beginning at the age of 40 with the death of her father because of cancer. Her mother also has health problems including dementia, so Olivia's mother relies on paid assistance for all housework.

Although Olivia sees herself in life roles as "having been a good worker and a good aunt and responsible for her medical treatment," she hesitates to identify her strengths and weaknesses, tending to hold others responsible for her actions and decisions. Despite having resources and opportunities to engage in many activities at home with family members, she is "bored and without a desire to do things either at home or outside of it" and she is dissatisfied with her lifestyle, but has no intention of changing it.

Using a Holistic Occupational Therapy Approach

By facilitating a shared experience during the initial interview, a therapeutic relationship was established and confirmed the OTP's decision to use the OSA, MOHO's self-assessment, to further facilitate Olivia's active participation and sense of control in determining her strengths and weaknesses related to her occupational competence, and to collaborate on short-term goals. Olivia's appraisals and the feedback from the OTP resulted in more in-depth information about Olivia's values, sense of responsibility, self-efficacy, perception of her routines, and expectations of support from her relatives.

Based on Olivia's interests, the OTP and Olivia jointly participated in card playing. The OTP used the VQ to gather data on motivation through observation. While playing cards, they talked about past situations that gave meaning and pleasure to Olivia, facilitating the collaborative exploration of other activities (e.g., walking through the building's garden among the trees and returning to the apartment to continue with her preferred routines). While engaged in participation, decision-making was facilitated around choosing what else to do, how to carry out the activities, and when to do them.

Once Olivia began showing initiative, trying new things, making decisions during her participation, and making activity choices spontaneously, the OTP invited her to explore activities that gave her the most pleasure and meaning. She readily chose to have a coffee and treat at her favorite pastry shop she frequented with her friends when she used to work. Just before leaving the apartment, Olivia regretted the plan, explaining that she hoped the OTP would take her in her car. She said, "I do not like public transportation, but I'll go if you take me in your car." However, facing the reality that public transportation was her only option moving forward, Olivia worked through her concerns and went to the pastry shop on three occasions. While at the pastry shop, Olivia was cheerful, spontaneous, determined, and open to new conversations.

These experiences opened her interest in returning to the hairdresser four blocks from her apartment. Responding to her purpose, the OTP and Olivia agreed on her going to the hairdresser independently on Saturday mornings, just as she did before. However, Olivia didn't follow through. During weekly occupational consultation, Olivia assertively told the OTP that her self-knowledge acquired during therapy helped her realize that she prefers to live a simple, comfortable life. Her family had always taken her by car to the hairdresser and social gatherings and assisted her at home. She was habituated to others doing things for her, and at this point in her life she did not want to change this. Her reflections and making this decision demonstrated Olivia's desires regarding occupational participation. Olivia had rediscovered and internalized her occupational identity and chosen the lifestyle she wished to reincorporate into her life.

During the weekly family consultation meeting, the OTP updated her brother and mother about Olivia's evolution and decision-making process and gave feedback on their expectations of Olivia's doing. The OTP validated their future goals as a family and their feelings of relief and reassurance from knowing she was stable and satisfied. The OTP provided a written and verbal report to the attending psychiatrist. The psychiatrist responded, "It is clear that Olivia is confident and content. Her passivity is not a consequence of negative symptoms."

Reflective Questions

1. What other assessments could you explore to understand Olivia's self-determination?
2. Would you continue to address Olivia's hesitation to participate in meaningful activities, given that she doesn't want to take on any additional responsibility to pursue them? If so, how? If not, why not?
3. Considering this chapter's content, reflect on Olivia's narrative and decision about her future lifestyle. What would you have thought, felt, and done under these circumstances?

The *exploratory phase* of the RP is used to support people who experience major difficulties in self-initiated actions, are fearful of interacting with their environments, or lack a sense of meaning in life. Many of these individuals have a long history of remaining in a negative cycle of interaction with their social contexts.

In this phase, the practitioner concentrates on helping the person rebuild their volitional experience by providing repeated opportunities of positive experiences through four sequenced and related stages. The practitioner needs to go where the person feels comfortable and secure, following a slow and progressive validation process with gradual steps and strategies for environmental exploration; initiating actions; participating in activities; and performing tasks of a meaningful collective occupational project. Along with the practitioner's immediate feedback, this approach promotes a sense of connectedness, belonging, and capacity in decision-making. At the end of this phase, individuals can make activity choices and show pleasure during their participation. They can accept more demands and opportunities when given substantial volitional support.

The RP *competency phase* focuses on the internalization of the sense of efficacy, one's own values and interests. Practitioners support the person gradually to accept or seek more challenges within meaningful participation and to accept and feel comfortable with personal and environmental changes and with increased personal and environmental performance demands.

In the first stage of the competency phase, people are progressively supported toward full participation in meaningful collective occupational projects (with peers, friends, family members, classmates, or other groups) as well as peer support educational groups. Practitioners promote the individuals' continued active participation in planning, sharing, problem-solving, and taking on responsibilities with others. At the same time, practitioners facilitate the development of critical performance skills to enrich the individuals' self-efficacy, thus opening anticipation for taking on their own personal occupational projects.

In this stage, practitioners guide the person to link their volitional experiences with their interpretation. The immediate feedback provided by practitioners expands into a more specific process that invites people to pay special attention to their volitional experiences through asking key open-ended questions that elicit their thoughts and feelings about themselves. As people progress in self-knowledge, there is an affirmation of interests and values, along with participation in more challenging occupational opportunities. This results in learning new occupational performance skills.

In the second stage of the competency phase, people's practice of reflecting on their volitional experience and its interpretation supports them to project toward the future. Through occupational consulting, individuals are invited to narrate their experiences of participation and reflect with the OTP on their efforts toward attaining their weekly activity goals. Together, they analyze the challenges and opportunities of establishing occupational goals and plan and review their process of participation in personal occupational projects. At the end of this phase, individuals achieve a sense of efficacy and responsibility in their daily participation. They can negotiate between personal and environmental expectations in a variety of familiar contexts according to their occupational goals.

At the RP achievement phase, people seek challenges, establishing goals of achieving balance between their occupational identity and their lifestyle (occupational competence). This involves individuals negotiating with themselves and maximizing or accepting a range of opportunities and demands that their environments provide. Therefore, the intervention process focuses on facilitating consistency between self-appreciation and participation, which leads to autonomous self-advocacy under diverse circumstances. Thus, the OTP's main role is being a consultant.

Practitioners facilitate choice in the face of new challenges by providing positive feedback. They facilitate exploration through identifying existing social resources, such as friends, family members, or peers, as well as the use of volitional self-monitoring strategies. At the end of this phase, individuals naturally continue improving their lifestyles and developing new strategies to seek and confront new challenges. Box 11-2 summarizes the reconstruction of a man's volitional process using the RP intervention.

BOX 11-2 ■ Remotivation Process: Intervention in Action

G. was a Chilean singer-songwriter who had lived abroad for 15 years. Since puberty, he had been interested in music, learning and mastering the use of wind, percussion, and string instruments. He actively participated in folkloric musical development and taught others to interpret it. G. participated in numerous musical festivals in Asia, Latin America, and Spain.

In his mid-40s, G. reported continuously getting into arguments and confrontations with his friends and colleagues. He explained: "I felt very impatient and accelerated, and also forgot my song lyrics before going on stage! Thanks to God that I managed to interpret them by improvising. . . . But I lost everything. . . . I lost them all." After this episode, G. suffered a severe depression. "My friends took me in their arms and sent me back to Chile with my guitar and my trunk."

G. was received at home by his family. His mother, a widow, supported his medical treatment after he was diagnosed with bipolar disorder. His depression was severe, and he didn't have access to new generation medications until 10 years after his return. Fifteen years passed, and he continued isolating himself in his bedroom. His mother turned to a community integration center ("Reencuentros") to ask for help. From interviewing her, the OTP learned important information about G.'s occupational narrative and his volition. "Music was his world, and he has not touched his guitar for 15 years. I don't know what to do."

Because of G.'s conditions, the occupational therapist decided to start by approaching him at his home. Based on the narrative interview with his mother, she decided to evaluate his volition with the VQ in different circumstances at home to decide how, when, and where to start working with him and address his motivation. G. needed substantial support to receive the therapist and initiate actions. He was in his room, where his guitar remained in a corner in its case, and he spent most of his time sitting on his bed, looking sadly at the guitar case and smoking cigarettes.

Upon the respectful greeting of the therapist and her comments about music, G. responded with a gentle smile. Taking this response into consideration, the therapist decided to express her intention of knowing him better and, if he accepted, also sharing her experiences with music.

Continued

BOX 11-2 ■ Remotivation Process: Intervention in Action—cont'd

They met twice a week. Following the first steps of the RP *exploratory phase's* validation stage, the therapist began validating G.'s attachment to the music by briefly commenting about her experiences with her guitar and bringing some music magazines of his interest. After six sessions, G. showed more confidence in the therapist, responding with a smile to her comments while still looking at his guitar case. He demonstrated interest in listening to the therapist's musical experiences and soon began to smile when looking at his guitar case. These were signs of him anticipating to open the guitar case and look at it again.

Two weeks later and with substantial volitional support, G. opened the guitar case and showed it to her. As she and G. commented about it, he agreed to take it out of its case. From that day on, G. kept the guitar out of its case and instead placed it hanging over his bed. With the therapist's validation and after touching his guitar, G. opened up and briefly recounted a few positive experiences from his past. In 3 more weeks, with his permission, the occupational therapist took his guitar and sang a Latin American folk song to him, requesting his feedback as an expert on that matter.

Following that, the therapist invited G. to meet in his living room to play the guitar, instead of meeting in his bedroom. The meetings with G. consisted of commenting on musical events, the therapist playing the guitar, and reviewing folk and popular music magazines together, like they did in his bedroom.

G.'s personal storage trunk, which he had not opened since he arrived in Chile, was in the living room. During the following four meetings, the occupational therapist took a seat close to the trunk, commenting on its beautiful wooden design while waiting for G. to express interest in the trunk.

G. began to respond to her comments, explaining its origin and qualities. This was a sign for the occupational therapist to ask him respectfully about the things he kept inside. G. explained, "My trunk keeps my history . . . all my compositions, news clippings, photos of each of my musical activities and friends." He could not face opening it since his return home. Listening to his narrative, the therapist reaffirmed his feelings and suggested they open it together, "just as we did with the guitar case," with no other expectation than to know more about his talent. Together, they explored, cleaned, and rearranged the objects and musical compositions. This event was critical for G.'s volition. He spontaneously began to choose his best compositions and take them off the trunk "until I feel ready to sing them to you and my mother."

Observing the initial emergence of some volitional indicators of the competence stage of change in this context, the occupational therapist expanded the environmental exploration stage of the *exploratory phase* out of his home, inviting him to go with her to "Reencuentros." There, he could help her evaluate the needs for improvement and innovation of the Musical Group, a collective occupational project with the goal of bringing monthly musical experiences to children and older adults living at sheltered residences. For G., this implied a new meaningful, but also challenging, opportunity.

After a few attempts to get out of his home, G. decided to walk arm in arm with the therapist to the center. This experience marked the beginning of the RP *competency phase.* He met the members of the Musical Group and participated in their rehearsals. After receiving his enthusiastic professional feedback, the therapist offered him the role of group monitor, inviting him first to explore this role in collaboration with another group member until he made a decision. In the process of exploring his responsibilities in this role. G. showed spontaneity on the VQ exploratory volitional indicators and some competence with minimal support, although he still required substantial volitional support for facing mistakes and problems when participating. After 3 weeks, G. accepted the therapist's proposal and began to participate in this project.

Soon, G. was transitioning the first stage of the RP *competency phase* in every context. He participated in the OPHI-II and in occupational consulting, establishing with the occupational therapist weekly goals and plans to extend his participation in other roles at home, in the community center, and in the community by attending musical events with a peer's company.

G. agreed to participate in another collective occupational project as part of the organizational committee of a major fundraising musical event, in which he collaborated with a well-known singer-songwriter. As the event came closer, his enthusiasm grew, so the occupational therapist asked him to help test the microphone and audio equipment of the venue's auditorium with a peer, a sound engineer and musician, and herself.

As G. stepped on stage with his guitar and stood in front of the microphone, he began to flow excitedly, singing and playing his guitar just as he did years ago. When he finished, he smiled and commented, "Look at this sunset. Isn't it wonderful?" Since then, his occupational goals became clear. With substantial volitional support from his peers, and working with his therapist, he planned, prepared, and delivered his curriculum vitae, rehearsed, and went to auditions. Overcoming these challenges, G. began to transition the RP *achievement phase.* He started to sing in various cultural centers of Santiago, returning progressively to his world: the music, the stage, and himself.

After reading G.'s RP and the content of this intervention in the chapter, answer the following reflective questions:

1. What do you think were the most important elements the OTP considered when supporting G.'s volition in their first meetings at his home?

2. Identify who was part of the team for the progressive facilitation of G.'s volition and the ways in which they did it.

3. Reflect on your experience with a person you have supported who has been challenging for you because of having important motivation difficulties. What actions did you take that were of benefit to facilitate this person's motivation? Which aspects and general procedures of the RP do you think could have been useful to facilitate this person's motivation?

4. What do you think would be strengths you could use to apply the RP? What do you think are the skills you would need to develop before the application of the RP?

Here's the Point

- OTPs consider intrinsic motivation as a critical element to address and support participation in occupation.
- Individuals' subjective experiences are crucial to understanding their motivation.
- Individuals with psychiatric conditions can experience different types of motivational challenges.
- Internalized stigma is one of the major factors that decreases motivation in people with severe psychiatric conditions.

- Maslow's hierarchy of needs suggests that lower-level needs must be met before higher-level needs are considered.
- SDT indicates that it is not just competence (e.g., self-efficacy) that drives motivation, but also autonomy and relatedness.
- Flow experiences involve a "just right" match between the individual's subjective perception of their own abilities and of the challenges occupation and environments provide.
- Individuals will be more motivated to engage in occupations in which they feel self-efficacy.
- The MOHO explains volition, or motivation for occupation, as the feelings and thoughts about ourselves as participants in occupation, related to our personal interests, values, and personal causation/self-efficacy and their interaction in the process of choice making.

- The TTC suggests that individuals can be at different points along a continuum of change.
- The MI technique provides person-centered strategies to communicate with people who are reluctant to make a change.
- The MOHO RP provides OTPs with a progressive and detailed intervention to facilitate motivation with people who have severe volitional challenges, enhancing occupational performance and participation.

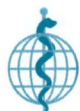 Visit the online resource center at **FADavis.com** to access the videos.

Apply It Now

1. "The Best Chef"–A Flow Experience

Sara, an older woman, told her OTP: "Every afternoon, I put on my apron and I transform myself into the best chef. I organize myself in the morning to finish with all household chores, so I have the afternoon for cooking. . . . I love cooking. . . . I cook all afternoon. . . . I make two or three different dishes at the same time, some for my husband and I, and some for my children to pick up. . . . Believe me, they are delicious! . . . I do not need to follow recipes. . . . I add things as I smell the need. . . . I feel like creating something new every time, you know? . . . I do not even know what time it is until my husband comes back home from work. . . . My husband tells me all the time that I should do things for fun, but this is too much fun for me!"

Reflective Questions

After reading Sara's experience:
- Note what story of yours comes into your mind first.
- Identify the characteristics of a flow state.
- Reflect on your story and identify characteristics of a flow state that you have experienced.

2. Applying Motivational Theories

Identify an occupation that you engage in regularly and that gives you pleasure. Describe the activity. How often do

you participate in it? How long have you been doing it? Is it something you do alone or with others? Consider the different theories of motivation and how they might apply to your motivation to participate in this occupation.

Reflective Questions
- Maslow's hierarchy of needs—Which type of need is met by this occupation? Have there been occasions when you could not participate in this occupation because you had to meet lower-level needs?
- Self-determination—Does the occupation promote competence (self-efficacy), autonomy (you are in control), and relatedness (connection to others)?
- Flow—Is this a flow experience; for example, do you lose yourself in the occupation? Lose track of time? Feel the "just right" challenge?
- Self-efficacy—Do you feel skillful/competent when performing this occupation? How did you learn to do this occupation? Who are your role models?
- TTC—Where are you in terms of your level of change? Are there times when you have been less action oriented?
- MOHO—Is this occupation a reflection of your interests, values, and sense of efficacy?

Resources

Books and Websites
- Csikszentmihalyi, M. (1998). *Finding flow: The psychology of engagement in everyday life.* Basic Books.
- Csikszentmihalyi, M. (2000). *Beyond boredom and anxiety: Experiencing flow in work and play.* Jossey-Bass.
- Csikszentmihalyi's Ted Talk: http://www.ted.com/speakers/mihaly_csikszentmihalyi
- Model of Human Occupation Resources—All MOHO assessments manuals, the Remotivation Process (Version 2.0), and other intervention manuals can be obtained at the Model of Human Occupation Clearinghouse. The website also provides a reference list of publications: www.moho-irm.uic.edu

- Motivational Interviewing—Miller, W. R., & Rollnick, S. (2013). *Motivational Interviewing: Helping people change* (3rd ed.). Guilford Press.
- Self-Determination Theory—Information, publications, and resources, including assessments related to SDT: www.psych.rochester.edu/SDT
- Self-Efficacy Theory—Albert Bandura's website with access to publications and videos: https://albertbandura.com/albert-bandura-academic-publications.html
- Transtheoretical Stages of Change Model—Carlo DiClemente's website at the University of Maryland Baltimore County includes information about the Transtheoretical Stages of Change Model and a current list of resources: http://habitslab.umbc.edu

Videos

- "Will Horowitz: Lived Experience of Autism" video. In this video, a young autistic adult describes his childhood interest in trains and how it has translated into an adult volunteer opportunity. He explains that, although an autistic individual can seem to have a "one-track mind" about a subject, it can also become an advantage in that they can become very specialized, as has been true for him with the Steam Into History project at a local railroad. Access the video at the online resource center at FADavis.com.

- "Using Objects to Promote Engagement" video. Jennifer is an OTP who works in a forensic mental health facility. She tells a charming story of discovering an antique wheelchair in a storage closet. It unexpectedly became an object with great meaning and purpose in her practice and for the individuals she worked with. Jennifer's story is a real-life example of the power of objects for engaging people in occupations. Access the video at the online resource center at FADavis.com.

References

Allison. J., Bes, R., & Rose, G. (2012). *Motivational Interviewing Target Scheme/MITS 2.1. An* instrument *for practitioners, trainers, coaches and researchers. Explanation & Guidance.* MiCampus.

Anderson, S., Kielhofner, G., & Lai, J. S. (2005). An examination of the measurement properties of the Pediatric Volitional Questionnaire. *Physical and Occupational Therapy in Pediatrics, 25*(1/2), 39–57.

Andreasen, N. C. (1984). *Scale for the assessment of negative symptoms.* University of Iowa.

Bandura, A. (1999). Self-efficacy: Toward a unifying theory of behavioral change. In R. F. Baumeister (Ed.), *The self in social psychology* (pp. 285–298). Psychology Press.

Bandura, A. (2001) Social cognitive theory: An agentic perspective. *Psychology Annual Reviewers, 52,* 1–26. https://doi.org/10.1146/annurev.psych.52.1.1

Bandura, A. (2002). Social cognition theory in cultural context. *Applied Psychology: An International Review, 51,* 269–290. https://doi.org/10.1111/1464-0597.00092

Bandura, A. (2006). Guide for constructing self-efficacy scales. In F. Pajares & T. Urdan (Eds.) *Self-efficacy beliefs of adolescents* (pp. 307–337). Information Age Publishing.

Baron, K., Kielhofner, G., Iyenger, A., Goldhammer, V., & Wolensky, J. (2006). *The Occupational Self-Assessment (OSA)* (Version 2.2). Model of Human Occupation Clearinghouse, Department of Occupational Therapy, College of Applied Sciences, University of Illinois at Chicago.

Basu, S., Kafkes, A., Geist, R., Killery, A., & Kielhofner, G. (2008). *The Pediatric Volitional Questionnaire* (Version 2.1). Model of Human Occupation Clearinghouse, Department of Occupational Therapy, College of Applied Sciences, University of Illinois at Chicago.

Baum, C. M., Christiansen, C. H., & Bass, J. D. (2015). The Person-Environment-Occupation-Performance Model (PEOP). In C. H. Christiansen, C. M. Baum, & J. D. Bass (Eds.), *Occupational therapy: Performance, participation, and well-being* (4th ed., pp. 49–56). Slack, Inc.

Bentall, R. P., Simpson, P. E., Lee, D. A., Williams, S., Elves, S., Brabbins, C., & Morrison, A. P. (2010). Motivation and avolition in schizophrenia patients: The role of self-efficacy. *Psychosis: Psychological, Social and Integrative Approaches, 2,* 12–22. https://doi.org/10.1080/17522430903505966

Bouricius, J. K. (1989). Negative symptoms and emotions in schizophrenia. *Schizophrenia Bulletin, 15*(2), 201–208. https://doi.org/10.1093/schbul/15.2.201

Boyt Shell, B, & Gillen, G. (2019). *Willard & Spackman's occupational therapy* (13th ed.). Wolters Kluwer.

Bruce, M., & Borg, B. (2002). *Psychosocial frames of reference.* Slack, Inc.

Chern, J., Kielhofner, G., de las Heras, C., & Magalhaes, L. (1996). The Volitional Questionnaire: Psychometric development and practical use. *American Journal of Occupational Therapy, 50,* 516–525. https://doi.org/10.5014/AJOT.50.7.516

Cooper, J. O., Heron, T. E., & Heward, W. L. (2019). *Applied behavior analysis* (3rd ed.). Pearson Education.

Crow, T. J. (1990). Temporal lobe asymmetries as the key to the etiology of schizophrenia. *Schizophrenia Bulletin, 16,* 433–443. https://doi.org/10.1093/schbul/16.3.433

Csikszentmihalyi, M. (2000). *Beyond boredom and anxiety: Experiencing flow in work and play.* Jossey-Bass.

Csikszentmihalyi, M., & Csikszentmihalyi, I. S. (Eds.). (1988). *Optimal experience: Psychological studies of flow in consciousness.* Cambridge University Press.

Csikszentmihalyi, M., & Rathunde, K. (1993). The measurement of flow in everyday life: Toward a theory of emergent motivation. In J. E. Jacobs (Ed.), *Nebraska symposium on motivation, 1992: Developmental perspectives on motivation* (pp. 57–97). University of Nebraska Press.

Csillik, A.S. (2013). Understanding Motivational Interviewing effectiveness: Contributions from Rogers' client-centered approach. *The Humanistic Psychologist, 41,* 350–363. https://doi.org/10.1080/08873267.2013.779906

de Charms, R. E. (1968). *Personal causation: The internal affective determinants of behavior.* Academic Press.

Deci, E. L. (1975). *Intrinsic motivation.* Plenum.

Deci, E. L., & Ryan, R. M. (1985). *Intrinsic motivation and self-determination in human behaviour.* Plenum.

Deci, E. L., & Ryan, R. M. (2012). Motivation, personality, and development within embedded social contexts: An overview of Self-Determination Theory. In R. M. Ryan (Ed.), *Oxford handbook of human motivation* (pp. 85–107). Oxford University Press.

de las Heras, C. G., Geist, R., Kielhofner, G., & Li, Y. (2007). *The Volitional Questionnaire (VQ)* (Version 4.1). Model of Human Occupation Clearinghouse, Department of Occupational Therapy, College of Applied Sciences, University of Illinois at Chicago.

de las Heras, C. G., Llerena, V., & Kielhofner, G. (2003). *Remotivation Process: Progressive intervention for people who have severe volitional challenges. A user´s manual* (Version 1.0). Model of Human Occupation Clearinghouse, Department of Occupational Therapy, College of Applied Health Sciences, University of Illinois at Chicago.

de las Heras de Pablo, C. G. (2015). *Modelo de ocupación humana.* Editorial Síntesis, S.A.

de las Heras de Pablo, C. G., Fan, Ch. W., & Kielhofner G. (posthumous). (2017). Dimensions of doing. In Renée Taylor, *Kielhofner's Model of Human Occupation* (Ch. 8, pp. 107–122). Wolters Kluwer.

de las Heras de Pablo, C. G., Llerena V., & Kielhofner, G. (2019). *Remotivation Process: Progressive intervention for people who have severe volitional challenges. A user´s manual* (Version 2.0). The Model of Human Occupation Clearinghouse, Department of Occupational Therapy, College of Applied Health Sciences, University of Illinois at Chicago.

Dunn, W., Brown, C., & McGuigan, A. (1994). The ecology of human performance: A framework for considering the effect of context. *American Journal of Occupational Therapy, 48,* 595–607. https://doi.org/10.5014/ajot.48.7.595

Firmin, R. L., Luther, L., Lysaker, P., & Vohs, J. (2018). Internalized stigma has a stronger relationship with intrinsic motivation compared to amotivation in early phase and prolonged schizophrenia. *Schizophrenia Bulletin, 44*(Suppl. 1), S319–S319. https://doi.org/10.1093/schbul/sby017.778

Henry, A. D. (2000). *The Pediatric Interest Profile: Surveys of play for children and adolescents.* Model of Human Occupation Clearinghouse, Department of Occupational Therapy, University of Illinois at Chicago.

Hettema, J., Steele, J., & Miller, W. (2005). Motivational Interviewing. *Clinical Psychology Annual Review, 1,* 91–111. https://doi.org/10.1146/annurev.clinpsy.1.102803.143833

Kielhofner, G. (Ed.) (1983). *Health through occupation.* F. A. Davis Company.

Kielhofner, G. (Ed.) (2008). *Model of Human Occupation: Theory and application* (4th ed.). Wolter Kluwer/Lippincot Williams & Wilkins.

Kielhofner, G. (2009). Conceptual foundations of occupational therapy practice (4th ed.). F.A. Davis.

Kielhofner, G., de las Heras, C. G., & Suarez-Balcazar, Y. (2011). Human occupation as a tool for understanding and promoting social justice. In F. Kronenberg, N. Pollard, & D. Sakellariou (Eds.), *Occupational therapies without borders—Volume 2: Towards an ecology of occupation-based practices* (pp. 269–278). Elsevier.

Kielhofner, G., Forsyth, K., Kramer, J., & Iyenger, A. (2007). Developing the Occupational Self-Assessment: The use of Rasch Analysis to assure internal validity, sensitivity, and reliability. *British Journal of Occupational Therapy, 72*(3), 94–104. https://doi.org/10.1177/030802260907200302

Kielhofner, G., Mallinson, T., Crawford, C., Nowak, M., Rigby, Henry, A., & Walens, D. (2004). *The Occupational Performance History Interview OPHI-II* (Version 2.1). Model of Human Occupation Clearinghouse, Department of Occupational Therapy, College of Applied Sciences, University of Illinois at Chicago.

Kielhofner, G., Mallinson, T., Forsyth, K., & Lai, J. S. (2001). Psychometric properties of the second version of the Occupational Performance History Interview (OPHI-II). *The American Journal of Occupational Therapy, 55,* 260–267. https://doi.org/10.5014/ajot.55.3.260

Kielhofner, G., & Neville, A. (1983). *The Modified Interest Checklist.* Model of Human Occupation Clearinghouse, Department of Occupational Therapy, University of Illinois at Chicago.

Koltko-Rivera, M. (2006). Rediscovering the later version of Maslow's hierarchy of needs: Self-transcendence and opportunities for theory, research, and unification. *Review of General Psychology. American Psychological Association, 10*(4), 302–317. https://doi.org/10.1037/1089-2680.10.4.302

Kramer, J., Kielhofner, G., & Smith, E. (2010). Validity evidence of the Child Occupational Self-Assessment. *The American Journal of Occupational Therapy, 64,* 621–632. https://doi.org/10.5014/ajot.2010.08142

Kramer, J., ten Velden, M., Kafkes, A., Basu, S., Federico, J., & Kielhofner, G. (2014). *The Child Occupational Self-Assessment* (Version 2.2). Model of Human Occupation Clearinghouse, Department of Occupational Therapy, College of Applied Sciences, University of Illinois at Chicago.

Law, M., Cooper, B., Strong, S., Stewart, D., Rigby, P., & Letts, L. (1996). The Person-Environment-Occupation model: A transactive approach to occupational performance. *Canadian Journal of Occupational Therapy, 63*(1), 9–23. Sage Publications. https://doi.org/10.1177/000841749606300103

Letts, L., Rigby, P., & Stewart, D. (2003). *Using environments to enable occupational performance.* Slack, Inc.

Li, Y., & Kielhofner, G. (2004). Psychometrics of the Volitional Questionnaire's third version. *Israel Journal of Occupational Therapy, 13*(3), E85–E98. http://www.jstor.org/stable/23468864

Martin, J. E., & Huber Marshall, L. H. (1994). *ChoiceMaker self-determination transition assessment and curriculum.* University of Colorado at Colorado Springs, Center for Educational Research.

Maslow, A. H. (1943). A theory of human motivation. *Psychological Review, 50,* 370–396. https://doi.org/10.1037/h0054346

Maslow, A. H. (1954). *Motivation and personality.* Harper Press.

Maslow, A. H. (1971). *The farther reaches of human nature.* Arkana/Penguin Books.

Meltzer, H. Y. (1990). Biology of schizophrenia subtypes: A review and proposal for method of study. *Schizophrenia Bulletin, 16*(3), 460–473. https://doi.org/10.1093/SCHBUL/5.3.460

Miller, W. R., & Moyers, T. B. (2017). Motivational Interviewing and the clinical science of Carl Rogers. *Journal of Consulting and Clinical Psychology, 85*(8), 757–766. https://doi.org/10.1037/ccp0000179

Miller, W. R., & Rollnick, S. (2013). *Motivational Interviewing: Helping people to change* (3rd ed.). Guilford Press.

Miller, W. R., & Rollnick, S. (2017). Ten things that MI is not. *Behavioural and Cognitive Psychotherapy, 37,* 129–140. https://doi.org/10.1017/S1352465809005128

Nakamura, J., & Csikszentmihalyi, M. (2002). The concept of flow. In C. R. Snyder & S. J. Lopez (Eds.), *Handbook of positive psychology* (pp. 89–105). Oxford University Press.

Oakley, F., Kielhofner, G., Barris, R., & Reichler, R. K. (1986). The Role Checklist: Development and empirical assessment of reliability. *Occupational Therapy Journal of Research, 6,* 157–170. https://doi.org/10.1177/153944928600600303

Peloquin, S. M. (2005). The 2005 Eleanor Clarke Slagle Lecture—Embracing our ethos, reclaiming our heart. *American Journal of Occupational Therapy, 59,* 611–625. https://doi.org/10.5014/AJOT.59.6.611

Polatajko, H. J., Townsend, E. A. & Craik, J. (2007). Canadian Model of Occupational Performance and Engagement (CMOP-E). In E. Townsend & H. J. Polatajko (Eds.), *Enabling occupation II: Advancing an occupational therapy vision of health, well-being, & justice through occupation* (pp. 22–36). CAOT Publications ACE.

Prochaska, J. O., & DiClemente, C. C. (2005). The transtheoretical approach. In J. C. Norcross & M. R. Goldfried, *Handbook of psychotherapy integration* (2nd ed., Ch. 7, pp. 147–171). Oxford University Press, Inc.

Prochaska, J. O, & Velicer, W. F. (1997). The Transtheoretical Model of Health Behavior of Change. *American Journal of Health Promotion, 12*(1), 38–48. https://doi.org/10.4278/0890-1171-12.1.38

Rogers, C. (1961). *On becoming a person: A therapist view of psychotherapy.* Houghton Mifflin Company.

Rubio, K., Bowyer, P., Hite, S., Pingale, V., Freysteinson, W., Hersch, G., & Raber, C. (2022). Promoting self-management of breast cancer-related lymphedema through the Remotivation Process. *The Open Journal of Occupational Therapy, 10*(4), 1–13. https://doi.org/10.15453/2168-6408.1911

Ryan, R. M. (2009). Self-determination and wellbeing. *Wellbeing in Developing Countries (WeD).* Centre for Development Studies University of Bath. www.welldev.org.uk

Sheldon, K. M., & Deci, E. (1993). *Self Determination Scale (SDS)* [Database record]. APA PsycTests. https://doi.org/10.1037/t53985-000

Strauss, G. P., Waltz, J. A., & Gold, J. M. (2014). A review of reward processing and motivational impairment in schizophrenia. *Schizophrenia Bulletin, 40*(Suppl. 2), S107–S116. https://doi.org/10.1093/schbul/sbt197

Taylor, R. R. (Ed.). (2017). Kielhofner's Model of Human Occupation: Theory and application (5th ed.). Wolters Kluwer.

Taylor, R. R., Fisher, G., & Scott, P. (Eds.). (2023). *Kielhofner's Model of Human Occupation: Theory and application* (6th ed.). Wolters Kluwer.

Townsend, E., Stanton, S., Law, M., Polatajko, M., Baptiste, S., Thompson-Franson, T., Kramer, C., Swedlove, F., Brintnell, S., & Campanile, L. (2002). *Enabling occupation, an occupational therapy perspective (Rev. ed.).* CAOT Publications ACE.

Velicer, W. F., Prochaska, J. O., Fava, J. L., Norman, G. J., & Redding, C. A. (1998) Smoking cessation and stress management: Applications of the Transtheoretical Model of behavior change. *Homeostasis in Health and Disease, 38,* 216–233.

Wehmeyer, M. L. (1995). *The ARC's Self-Determination Scale: Procedural guidelines.* Arc of the United States.

White, R. W. (1959). Motivation reconsidered: The concept of competence. *Psychological Review, 66*(5), 297–333. https://doi.org/10.1037/h0040934

Whiteford, G., Townsend, E., Bryanton, O., Wicks, A., & Pereira, R. (2017). The Participatory Occupational Justice Framework: Salience across contexts. In D. Sakellariou & N. Pollard (Eds.), *Occupational therapy without borders: Integrating justice and inclusion with practice* (2nd ed., pp. 163–174). Elsevier.

Wolman, J., Campeau, I., DuBois, P. A., Mithaug, D. E., & Stolarski, V. S. (1994). *AIR Self-Determination Scale and user guide.* American Institute for Research.

Emotion Regulation

Karen R. Hebert

Emotions are a core element of the human experience that are essential to survival. Strong emotions such as fear, love, and happiness add texture to people's daily lives. Millions of people around the world experience emotion-related disorders such as anxiety and depression, with varying degrees of challenge in their daily life, such as difficulty maintaining healthy relationships, functioning effectively in work and school, and enjoying life. Emotions play a critical role in what people pay attention to, and they influence decisions they make about their behavior and activities in daily life. Without emotional highs and lows, people would struggle to make sense of the world and their place in it.

Human beings begin developing skills in emotion regulation from infancy, and these early experiences form the basis for emotion regulation in adulthood. The inability to regulate emotions in an adaptive way can have a significant negative impact on people's ability to function in society.

Occupational therapy practitioners (OTPs) can help individuals develop emotional awareness and skillful emotion regulation strategies to improve their occupational performance and positive, adaptive, quality engagement in life. This chapter describes emotions in terms of experience, behavior, and neurophysiology; provides a framework for understanding emotion regulation and dysregulation; and describes how to apply evidence-based approaches to assessment and intervention. The intention is to enhance the ability of OTPs in multiple practice areas to foster effective emotion regulation skills within people across the life span.

Theories of Emotion

Although a uniform definition is difficult to find, an **emotion** is largely agreed to reflect a subjective thought process that is associated with expressive behaviors, including the facial expressions people make and the words that they say, as well as physiological and neurological changes (Gross, 1998). Much theoretical debate exists regarding how emotions are experienced, including the number of basic emotional categories, how individuals understand and label their emotions, the types and ranges of behaviors associated with emotions, and whether all cultures experience emotions in the same way.

Disagreement exists regarding the basic number of emotions, with estimates running from two to 10 primary emotions (Ortony & Turner, 1990). In addition to the primary categories, individuals experience a range of secondary emotions (for example, jealousy and contentment) that involve combinations across categories. Most theories organize all emotional states into the two larger categories of positive and negative emotions (Fig. 12-1). Following the biological basis of approach and avoidance motivations, early theorists frequently considered positive and negative emotions to sit on opposite ends of a continuum (Kring & Bachorowski, 1999). From this perspective, individuals experience either high positive affect *or* high negative affect.

More current theories recognize the independence of positive and negative affect and the ability of individuals to experience high or low rates of both positive and negative emotions at the same time (Diener & Emmons, 1984). This recognition of the independence of positive and negative affect has led to important conceptualizations of the role of emotional processing in psychological diagnoses as well as assessments and interventions that target specific emotional states.

Emotions can be distinguished from feelings and mood states. **Feelings** reflect the purely conscious mental understanding of an emotional state (Damasio, 2004). They are what occurs when an individual recognizes that their physiology (racing heart), behavior (smiling wide and reaching out a hand), and subjective thought process ("Wow, this person standing in front of me is so famous!") means that they are having a specific emotion (excitement). **Mood states**, such as depression and cheerfulness, represent a more comprehensive emotional state that persists for a longer period of time. In mood states, there is typically no specific situation that the individual can identify as triggering the emotions.

According to the **Modal Model of Emotions** (Gross, 1998), emotions can be described as unfolding in four basic phases that involve a recursive relationship between the person and the situation in the context of a specific goal. These phases involve the Situation → Attention → Appraisal → Response, with the response feeding back into the situation in a process that continues until the goal is either accomplished or modified (see Fig. 12-2).

An example of a negative emotion could occur when a teacher takes a toy from the ground in front of a child (situation), the child notices that the toy is missing (attention), they realize that the removal of the toy has prevented their goal of playing with the toy (appraisal), and the child begins to scream (response). In a recursive process, the child's screaming (response) could result in the teacher placing the toy back in front of the child (modified situation); the return of the toy

	Negative Emotions			Positive Emotions	
Fear	**Anger**	**Sadness**	**Disgust**	**Happiness**	**Surprise**
Anxiety	Annoyance	Grief	Shame	Love	Amazement
Terror	Rage	Remorse	Guilt	Joy	Interest
Apprehension	Jealousy	Regret	Boredom	Serenity	Enthusiasm
Worry	Resentment	Loneliness	Contempt	Pride	Optimism
Nervousness	Irritation	Melancholy	Dislike	Confidence	Hopeful

FIGURE 12-1. Negative and positive emotions. Dark-colored boxes are primary emotions, while light-colored boxes are secondary emotions.

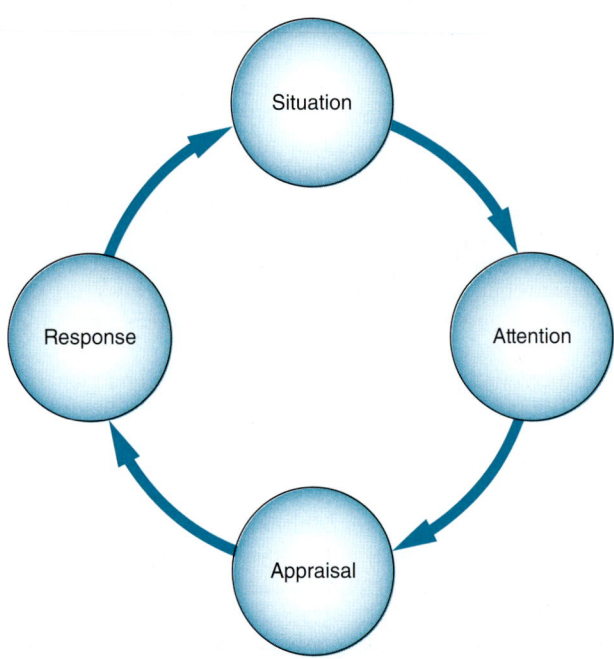

FIGURE 12-2. The Modal Model of Emotions.

allows the child to now accomplish the goal of playing with the toy, and the child might stop screaming (response).

Note that in this situation the two middle steps (attention and appraisal) are still required for the emotional experience to resolve. For example, the child could fail to notice that the toy has been returned (attention), or their goal might have changed to wanting to be held and comforted, in which case the return of the toy will not provide comfort (appraisal) and the crying (response) may continue.

Emotional Function in Daily Life: Emotion Regulation and Dysregulation

The *Occupational Therapy Performance Framework*, 4th Edition *(OTPF-4)*, highlights the importance of emotional expression, management, and regulation as skills necessary for successful occupational performance (American Occupational Therapy Association [AOTA], 2020). **Expresses emotions** is identified as a necessary social interaction performance skill that is defined as "displays affect and emotions in a socially appropriate manner" (p. 48). **Emotional performance** including the "regulation and range of emotions, appropriateness of emotions, and lability of emotions" (p. 52) is identified as a person factor relevant to occupational therapy practice.

Additionally, the *OTPF* identifies social and emotional health promotion and maintenance as part of improving quality of life as a health management occupation. This occupation of emotional health management and the identification of self-regulation as an area of occupational therapy intervention (AOTA, 2020) highlights the importance of addressing emotion regulation skills for OTPs.

In the same way the definition of emotion remains elusive, it is difficult to clearly define **emotion regulation**, although it involves an individual's ability to utilize strategies to manage their emotional states (Gross, 1998). Multiple factors affect a person's ability to successfully utilize emotion regulation in their daily life. First, an individual must be aware that a situation is occurring that is likely to lead to an emotional response. Researchers have argued that emotion regulation can only be understood in the context of goal performance. That is, no emotional experience is inherently negative; rather, the frequency, intensity, duration, speed of onset, and ability to recover from certain emotions can prevent the completion of an individual's goals (R. A. Thompson, 1994). Individuals also have a range of strategies that can be used to regulate their emotions. The ability to successfully select and utilize these strategies varies based on the specific situation as well as the individual's previous experiences and capabilities.

The **Process Model of Emotional Regulation** (Gross, 1998) follows closely with the Modal Model of Emotion (Gross, 1998) and identifies how strategies can be employed to modulate an emotional experience as it is unfolding (Fig. 12-3). Before an emotional event, an individual can use **situation selection** to increase the likelihood that a specific emotion will occur. Although often overlooked in treatments for emotion regulation, this is a key step in which careful activity scheduling can be used by OTPs to increase the frequency of positive situations available throughout the day.

The next opportunity is **situation modification**, in which environmental and social factors can be modified as the situation unfolds to impact the resulting emotional experience. OTPs with their training in activity analysis and the effect of the environment on occupational performance are particularly well suited to help individuals identify and implement strategies at this stage.

Attentional deployment describes how individuals pay attention to aspects of the situation that trigger a specific emotional response (Gross, 1998). For example, an individual might ignore a friend's expression of hello and only pay attention to

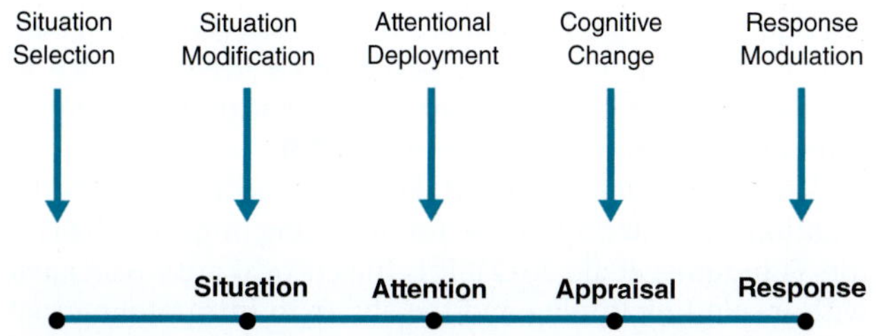

FIGURE 12-3. The Process Model of Emotional Regulation. The circles represent the stages of an emotional event whereas the arrows indicate what strategies can be applied to regulate emotions at each stage of the unfolding event. *Adapted from Gross, J. J. (2013). Emotion regulation: Taking stock and moving forward. Emotion, 13(3), 359–365. https://doi.org/10.1037/a0032135; Gross, J. J. (2015). Emotion regulation: Current status and future prospects. Psychological Inquiry, 26, 1–26. https://doi.org/10.1080/1047840X.2014.940781; Gross, J. J., & Thompson, R. A. (2007). Emotion regulation: Conceptual foundations. In J. J. Gross (Ed.), Handbook of emotion regulation (pp. 3–4). Guilford Press.*

their closed-off body language. Cognitive Behavioral Therapies (CBTs) are designed to help individuals redirect attention to the salient positive features of the situation.

Cognitive reappraisal refers to deliberately challenging and reinterpreting our automatic emotional response to a situation. For example, a traffic accident that makes you late to a party might lead to the thought, "I can't be late. I have the cake, and everyone will be angry at me," resulting in feelings of anxiety and anger. A cognitive reappraisal of the situation involves challenging the thought and thinking, "These are my friends, and they will understand that things happen and will just be happy to see me." Cognitive reappraisal is a positive emotion regulation strategy with extensive evidence supporting its success in managing emotional situations (Webb et al., 2012).

The final stage for strategy use is **response modulation**, which occurs after the emotion has unfolded and typically involves efforts to suppress the emotion. Emotion suppression strategies include actively suppressing the expression of an emotion (i.e., keeping a neutral face), as well as suppressing the experience of the emotion and the thoughts associated with the event (Webb et al., 2012). Evidence suggests that suppression of emotional expression can result in short-term changes in the ability to complete goals despite the presence of the emotion, although over time this strategy is associated with an increase in dysregulation (Webb et al., 2012).

Significant cross-cultural differences exist in how often and how useful the strategies of cognitive reappraisal and emotional suppression are in the management of emotions (Matsumoto et al., 2008). For example, individuals who live in other-oriented cultures such as China and Japan are more likely to engage in emotional suppression strategies than individuals in the United States. Not only is emotional suppression more frequently utilized in these cultures, but it serves as a positive adaptive strategy, with fewer negative outcomes related to well-being and social functioning (Matsumoto et al., 2008).

Emotion dysregulation describes emotional responses that are not adapted to the current situation (R. A. Thompson, 1994). Typically, emotion dysregulation occurs when negative emotions interfere with the completion of goal-directed activity. This interference involves unsuccessful strategy use and can be classified in at least two different ways:

emotion regulation failures and emotional misregulation (Gross & Jazaieri, 2014).

Emotion regulation failures occur when an individual fails to engage in a strategy that would be helpful in the situation. For example, they fail to use cognitive reappraisal of the situation to help reduce feelings of anger when a stranger accidentally bumps into them on a crowded street. **Emotional misregulation** occurs when an individual uses an emotion regulation strategy that is poorly matched to the current situation. For example, an individual suppresses feelings of frustration when speaking with their boss, resulting in an argument later that evening in which they yell at their spouse.

Alexithymia is a related concept that focuses on difficulties with the awareness of emotions. Individuals with alexithymia have trouble identifying, describing, and differentiating emotions and difficulty recognizing the physical sensations (such as a racing heart) associated with emotions. They display a tendency to focus on external facts instead of internal experiences (Bagby et al., 1994). The concept of alexithymia was independently developed in psychosomatic medicine and shares many features of emotion regulation. The term "alexithymia" is frequently employed in literature focused on emotional processing in children and adults with physical or neurological conditions.

Neuroscience of Emotion Regulation

A cluster of physiological, behavioral, and cognitive responses are involved in experiencing an emotion. Individuals differ in the strength of their physiological response to emotional events. The **hypothalamic-pituitary axis (HPA)** is a key component of the autonomic nervous system response. Variability in HPA responsiveness to stress appears to play an important role in the influence of childhood adversities on the development of mental illness (Koss & Gunnar, 2018). Exposure to adversity in childhood leads to an abnormally heightened short-term stress response that over time evolves into chronic underresponsiveness to stress. Abnormal responding in the HPA is seen both in children and adolescents with externalizing problems (e.g., conduct disorder, substance abuse, impulsive behavior) and internalizing conditions (e.g., depression, anxiety).

Occupation-based sensory processing interventions use sensory techniques to modify physiological symptoms of over- and underarousal (Dunn, 2007). When working with children, OTPs frequently use techniques that address sensory processing, emotion regulation, and behavioral control in a comprehensive manner, as development of these skills is intertwined. In adulthood, sensory strategies that address the physiological symptoms of arousal are an important component of interventions designed to improve emotion regulation skills. Also see Chapter 9: Sensory Processing and the Lived Sensory Experience. 🤝

Accumulating evidence suggests that emotions are not represented in the brain as discrete categories (for example, there is no sadness center of the brain) but rather as a distributed network (Aldao et al., 2016; Lindquist et al., 2012; Martin & Ochsner, 2016). This network includes subcortical areas (i.e., amygdala, insula, ventral striatum, and hippocampus) that are involved in being aware of an emotional event. Higher cortical areas (i.e., prefrontal cortex, orbitofrontal cortex, and anterior cingulate cortex [ACC]) are activated when individuals use specific strategies to modify the experience and expression of emotions.

Dysfunctions in brain area activation and balance have been documented in conditions including depression, anxiety, posttraumatic stress disorder (PTSD), bipolar disorder, substance abuse disorder, and attention deficit-hyperactivity disorder (ADHD; Amstadter, 2008; Davidson et al., 2002; Kober, 2014; Lanius et al., 2011; Shaw et al., 2014; Urosević et al., 2008). The explosion of interest in affective neuroscience and mental health has led to important new conceptualizations of how clinical symptoms should be understood and spurred the development of new interventions targeting specific symptom clusters.

Subcortical structures including the amygdala and insula appear to be more responsive to negative emotions, whereas the ventral striatum is associated with positive emotions, although significant overlap exists. The amygdala is the primary subcortical area involved in identifying the social and environmental emotional cues that occur in a situation (Lindquist et al., 2012). Although early research focused on the role of the amygdala in negative emotions, especially fear, it is now well accepted that it is also active in positive emotions such as pleasure and reward.

The insula responds to visceral sensations from the body that are associated with emotions, such as the hollow feeling in the stomach when afraid or the physical recoil associated with disgust. The ventral striatum is involved in learning which cues predict a rewarding outcome (Martin & Ochsner, 2016). These cues are often social in nature (e.g., a smiling face) but can also be tangible objects such as the bath soap or favorite candle associated with a relaxing bath.

The hippocampus is a key subcortical area involved in long-term memory storage and retrieval. Because emotions provide important cues to survival and social functioning, events that cause a strong emotional response are more likely to be stored in memory (Davidson et al., 2002). Functioning in hippocampus is responsible for the feelings associated with a specific place or situation (Lanius et al., 2011); for example, a feeling of calm happiness when one enters a loved one's home, or stress and anxiety when entering a classroom where they recently failed an examination. The intensity of these feelings is influenced by specific memories and varies greatly among individuals. The classroom that causes intense anxiety for some students can be associated with feelings of mastery for a student who recently gave a well-received speech in the same space.

Higher order cortical brain areas are associated with executive functions, including problem-solving, planning, directing attention, and impulse control (Lindquist et al., 2012). During emotional responding, these areas are involved in using cognitive skills and strategies to regulate emotions. The prefrontal cortex modulates activity in subcortical structures such as the amygdala and ventral striatum (Davidson et al., 2002) and is involved in tracking the positive and negative aspects of a situation in a goal-dependent manner. For example, a soft pile of blankets might be positive if someone's goal is watching a movie on the couch, but negative if the goal is folding the laundry and tidying the living room. The prefrontal cortex is particularly active during the emotion regulation strategy of cognitive reappraisal (Ochsner et al., 2012), although not during less beneficial strategies such as emotional suppression. For more information on executive functions see Chapter 7: Cognition.

The **orbitofrontal cortex (OFC)** is a key component of the emotional circuit responsible for inhibiting impulsive behaviors (Lindquist et al., 2012). It is the cortical area associated with insula functioning and the ability to integrate internal feelings (e.g., butterflies in the tummy) with the external context (e.g., my teacher is talking about a test) to guide behavior (e.g., start studying for the examination). Individuals with damage to the OFC display significant impairments in regulating emotions and using emotions to guide successful decision-making (Damasio, 2004). Damage in this area is associated with risk tasking and difficulty with delaying immediate rewards as needed to meet long-term goals.

The OFC also plays a crucial role in regulating impulsive outbursts associated with anger and aggression (Lindquist et al., 2012). Deficits in OFC activation appear to increase the likelihood that an individual will respond to interpersonal conflict with aggression. This tendency to respond aggressively to conflict is a key feature of externalizing disorders such as intermittent explosive disorder and conduct disorder, as well as personality disorders including antisocial personality disorder.

Finally, the ACC is involved in managing cognitive conflict (Lindquist et al., 2012). This brain area has classically been associated with sadness and the experience of depression. When presented with emotional information, it is involved in determining its importance and regulating an individual's response. In depression, it becomes hypersensitized to negative cues and no longer manages conflicting emotional information appropriately. Damage to the ACC results in significant emotional lability, suggesting that this area helps control the natural variations of emotional highs and lows that occur throughout the day.

Development of Emotion Regulation Across the Life Span

Temperament describes how an infant is predisposed to react to the environment as well as their ability to self-regulate core responses. Parents often describe their infant's temperament as easygoing, slow-to-warm, active, or fussy. Temperament is an important predictor of a child's success and struggles throughout the school years and adolescence. Many theories argue that temperament is a precursor to emotion regulation and represents a genetic vulnerability to approaching situations with a specific affective style (Southam-Gerow & Kendall, 2002). Interactions between temperament and environmental factors play a role in the development of psychopathology across the life span.

Emotion regulation abilities are not fully present in young children and develop over time. The ability to manage negative and positive emotions in the pursuit of goals appears to develop along separate timelines in children (Martin & Ochsner, 2016). The prefrontal cortex regions develop at a slower rate than the subcortical structures and do not reach full maturation until early adulthood. The resulting imbalance between subcortical and cortical activation could contribute to the heightened emotional reactivity seen in children and adolescents.

Evidence suggests that the ability to control negative emotions is particularly poor throughout adolescence, whereas the ability to experience and regulate positive emotions is a relative strength among this age group (Martin & Ochsner, 2016). Environmental influences including the presence of loving caregivers, peers, and high stress negative events and traumas all impact the degree to which an individual can develop skills in emotion regulation.

Children who undergo adverse childhood experiences (ACEs), including traumatic events such as being exposed to violence in the family or community or family members with mental illness or substance abuse diagnoses, experience worse physical and mental health outcomes as adults (Rudenstine et al., 2019). When a child is exposed to a chronic stressor such as high rates of violence in the community, they develop hypervigilance to perceived threats, which interferes with the brain's ability to manage stress and regulate emotions over time (Aldao et al., 2016). Factors such as the age of the child when the stressor was experienced and the length of the stressful events affect the degree to which it influences adult performance.

The impact of chronic stressors is cumulative with children who experience four or more ACEs, and they report worse functioning as adults. Emotion regulation abilities appear to mediate the impact of ACEs, and children who have difficulties with emotion regulation experience greater rates of psychological distress as adults (Rudenstine et al., 2019). This fact suggests that interventions to help children develop emotion regulation skills could be beneficial in reducing the negative impact of traumatic experiences on later development. Also see Chapter 5: Trauma-Informed Practice and Chapter 25: Trauma- and Stressor-Related Disorders.

The presence of supportive caregivers affects the development of emotion regulation skills through multiple avenues. Children observe and model the emotion regulation style of loving caregivers as well as experiencing the overall emotional climate of their families (Morris et al., 2017). In general, families that are warm and supportive with secure child–caregiver relationships and clear rules regarding behavior facilitate the development of emotion regulation abilities. Caregivers model specific techniques, including emotional socialization for young children (e.g., focusing attention on something else, providing comfort) and emotional coaching (e.g., solving emotional problems, labeling emotions) for adolescents.

Cross-cultural differences exist in how parents model, discuss, and react to their children's emotions (Yang & Wang, 2019). Although Western parents use facial expressions to model and guide children in the expression of positive emotions, Eastern parents are more likely to use verbal expressions to guide emotional understanding. In general, Western parents help their children learn to manage emotions by elaborating on their feelings and guiding them through emotional coaching strategies. Although Eastern parents were less likely to teach their children specific emotional coping strategies, there was also less of a relationship between parental coaching and positive child well-being (Yang & Wang, 2019).

Adolescence is a time of heightened risk for the onset of disorders related to emotion regulation (Southam-Gerow & Kendall, 2002). A general increase in the frequency and intensity of negative emotions is seen during this stage. The developmental demands of adolescence are complex and include increased levels of conflict with parents, independence in the school environment, and new peer and romantic relationships (Farley & Kim-Spoon, 2014).

Peer and romantic relationships present unique emotional challenges, with evidence suggesting that adolescents use different emotion regulation strategies around their parents than peers. Bidirectional development occurs, with a child's emotional skills influencing the quality of peer and romantic relationships while success in these relationships helps further skill development. These findings suggest that adolescence is a key time for interventions that support emotional skill development and community- and school-based programs that support the development of peer relationships more broadly. For more information on school-based programs see Chapter 37: School Mental Health.

Emotion regulation skills tend to solidify during early and middle adulthood, with individuals able to modify their approach to different emotional states (e.g., anger vs. fear) as appropriate (Zimmermann & Iwanski, 2014). The ability to accomplish personal and life goals tend to dominate this phase of life, and emotion regulation skills are deployed to support these goals. Individuals use social support seeking and passive avoidance in situations that evoke sadness, while dysfunctional levels of rumination are still seen in relation to anger.

Adults are more effective at using social support from peers, friends, and romantic relationships to help manage negative emotions than adolescents, indicating continued growth in this area. Greater skills in emotion regulation are associated with better quality of life, well-being, and more success in work and romantic relationships during this phase of life.

The relationship between emotions and functioning in older adulthood is complex. Overall emotions tend to become more positive with age, with adults in their 60s and 70s reporting more positive affect and less negative affect than individuals in their 20s and 30s (Isaacowitz et al., 2017). In part, this is thought to reflect changes in life goals and social networks, with older adults more focused on maintaining social networks and engaging in life review activities than younger adults (Charles & Carstensen, 2010). Social engagement is an important source of positive emotions that contributes to health and well-being across the life span. Also see Chapter 49: Connectedness and Belonging.

Older adults report less intensity and greater predictability in the emotions that they experience on a daily basis, which results in less fear and anger and more pleasant calmness over time. Given their rich life history and experience, older adults are better able to regulate emotions in the early phases by identifying and choosing situations that support their goals of social cohesion and enjoyment (Isaacowitz et al., 2017). Although these changes are not universal and are impacted by a person's health, social, and environmental history, they do suggest that older adulthood is characterized by relative emotional calm.

Changes across the life span in emotional responding also vary across cultures, with individuals in Eastern societies not demonstrating the same reduction in the intensity of negative emotions experienced (Grossmann et al., 2014). Older adults in these cultures are still more likely to show positive emotions in unpleasant situations than younger adults. OTPs working with older adults should be careful to avoid assumptions that age-related declines in physical and cognitive abilities are associated with heightened negative emotions. Instead, careful evaluation of an individual's emotional experiences and self-regulation skills in the context of their life history and current functional goals is warranted.

Emotion Dysregulation and Mental Illness

The central importance of emotion regulation in mental illness has been highlighted by several research reviews that classify mental health conditions according to difficulties with emotional responding (Aldao et al., 2016; Gross & Jazaieri, 2014; Sloan et al., 2017). Developmental theories categorize psychological symptoms along an internal/external dimension that is fundamentally emotional in nature (Aldao et al., 2016; Kring & Bachorowski, 1999). Internalizing disorders activate the behavioral inhibitory system and involve negative emotions (e.g., depression and anxiety). Externalizing disorders include impulsive behaviors (e.g., substance abuse, disordered eating, and risk-taking) that cause high positive affect. Although the clinical conditions outlined in the text that follows involve difficulties with multiple psychological processes, emotion regulation skills play a prominent role.

Depression

Individuals with depression experience high rates of negative affect *as well as* low levels of positive affect (Kring & Bachorowski, 1999). Rumination, in which individuals attempt to deal with worry by repetitively dwelling on past mistakes, regrets, and shortcomings, is typical in depression (Aldao et al., 2016). Although sadness is the emotion most associated with depression in popular understanding, it is **anhedonia** (a reduced ability to experience pleasure) and low rates of happiness and joy that appear to be unique to the clinical diagnosis of depression.

Low positive affect results in difficulties with goal-directed behavior, trouble responding to positive emotional cues, and an inability to use positive situations to shift into a positive emotional state. These biases are seen in both occupational and social environments, with individuals with depression paying more attention to negative events, being more likely to remember negative events, and having trouble identifying positive emotions displayed by others (LeMoult & Gotlib, 2019). Over time, these biases toward negative events and away from positive events cause the individual to withdraw from previously valued activities and develop a sense of hopelessness regarding the future.

A biological model of depression highlights the brain basis of these emotion regulation factors. Studies of individuals with depression identify overresponding of the amygdala to neutral or mildly negative cues, underresponding of the ventral striatum to positive cues, and underactivation of the prefrontal cortex during attempts to regulate negative emotions (Davidson et al., 2002). Treatments such as behavioral activation, which are designed to increase the frequency of pleasant activities in daily life, can be utilized by OTPs; these individuals directly use occupations to increase the rates of positive affect in individuals with depression. Also see Chapter 20: Mood Disorders.

Anxiety

Anxiety disorders involve excessive negative affect, especially related to the emotion of fear. Although fear responses are often appropriate and protective, in individuals with anxiety, the timing and intensity of this fear response often do not match the situation (Amstadter, 2008). The fear response often continues long after the situation has ended, affecting a person's sleep and ability to return to a calm state.

Physiologically, individuals with anxiety display hyperarousal with an increased heart rate in response to stressful situations and hypervigilance to threats cues. Situations that are seen as threatening vary and can include specific phobias related to flying, public speaking, and social situations. A tendency to view most situations as potentially threatening underlies generalized anxiety disorder.

Individuals with anxiety frequently use suppression, an unsuccessful coping strategy that involves ignoring the emotion, which paradoxically results in higher psychological distress. Engagement in avoidance strategies can occur because individuals with anxiety tend to view fear as an unacceptable emotion that cannot be tolerated. Mindfulness and acceptance-oriented therapies such as Dialectical Behavior Therapy (DBT; Linehan, 2020) and Acceptance and Commitment Therapy (ACT; Hayes et al., 2011), which focus on observation and radical acceptance of negative emotions, can be effective for treating anxiety conditions. Also see Chapter 18: Anxiety Disorders.

Bipolar Disorder

Bipolar disorder is a mood disorder in which individuals experience depression and at least one episode of mania, which involves extreme positive affect or sometimes irritability (American Psychiatric Association [APA], 2022). A biological model of bipolar disorder involves dysregulation in the **behavioral approach system (BAS)**, with an increased orientation toward rewards and achieving goals (Katz et al., 2021). In this model, the BAS is activated when the person experiences a rewarding event, such as studying for an examination, meeting an attractive person, or going to a party. The BAS is deactivated when rewards are lost or when failures occur (e.g., loss of a friend, job, failure on an examination).

Individuals with bipolar disorder experience a greater magnitude of BAS activation and deactivation during typical daily rewards and losses. This results in impulsivity, and the person engages in behaviors with a higher potential for reinforcement without careful consideration of the risks and consequences of the behavior. Emotion regulation difficulties occur because it is difficult for the individual to manage the magnitude of BAS changes, resulting in a failure to avoid highly positive emotional states during mania and manage negative states during depression. Dysregulation of the BAS is also thought to contribute to the development of substance abuse and eating disorders, as outlined in the text that follows. Also see Chapter 20: Mood Disorders.

The Lived Experience

Marian Schienholz

Since the early years of adolescence, I have experienced symptoms of a mood disorder that affected my growth, development, and ability to function. One set of these symptoms with which I have struggled repeatedly over the years has been suicidal thoughts and ideas.

The first time I attempted suicide, I was 16. By then I had been experiencing undiagnosed depression for several years. The incident that preceded my suicide attempt involved a bell, a priest, and an adult religious education class—a very strange incident that retrospectively caused me shame and a deep sense of the worthlessness of my situation and my life. I awoke the next day and went to school without telling my family or friends. I did confide what I had done to another priest, who served as a counselor at my school. He listened and sent me to the school nurse—when I told her I didn't feel well, she offered me an aspirin. What the priest did not do was refer me for further counseling or intervention, nor did he suggest I tell my family and ask for their help.

This story exemplifies how my emotional responses to situations were significantly colored by my predominantly depressive moods and beliefs about the world. My illness was complicated because I have bipolar II disorder. This meant that I had fluctuating moods and functioning, so much of the time I was able to hide my impairment. In fact, I excelled academically, but my self-esteem was severely impaired, and I experienced a sense of hopelessness and dread. I avoided many social situations and was fearful of opportunities that might result in failure. During adolescence, I spent a great deal of time isolated in my bedroom and secretly crying. I now attribute the cause of this to genetic predisposition to clinical depression, a highly critical family, and a series of traumatic life events.

From my upbringing I learned to suppress emotions, and I often turned anger and frustration inward and experienced them as depression. I did get help eventually for my illness when I entered graduate school at age 25 and experienced severe depression after a painful breakup. It has taken many years of therapy, medication, and using alternative methods for me to reach my current state of stability. I have been able to work for most of this time, although I was hospitalized for suicidal intentions several times. Because of ongoing issues, I also found myself in some dangerous situations where I experienced violence. I also experienced trauma during one of my psychiatric hospitalizations when I was admitted to a hospital of very poor quality. In addition, I have had some other serious medical problems and I lost my husband to cancer after only 6 years of marriage. But I have survived . . . and thrived thanks to the time, love, and patience of my family, friends, and mental health providers.

My Recovery

After nearly 35 years of living with a psychiatric disability, I have a regime that enables me to have a productive and satisfying life, and I do believe I am achieving my goal of contributing something worthwhile to others. I am recovering from my illness through personal exploration, coping mechanisms, and a relationship with a supportive significant other and supportive friends, reasonable medical intervention, and ongoing therapy.

But I do still experience periods of increased symptoms—even occasional suicidal thoughts—to this day. This happens to me, especially during periods when my depressive symptoms are exacerbated because of external stress, anniversaries of difficult events, and hormonal fluctuations. Stressors include relationship issues, work pressures, and family difficulties.

I would like to share what has been important to my recovery and how I cope with the stress and periodic occurrence of symptoms in my daily life. I am sharing some of the things that have helped me, although I believe each *individual* must determine what works best for them. In my research into the theory and techniques of dialectical behavioral therapy (DBT) I was struck with the similarity of much of the model to my own emotional "pain management" strategies.

These strategies are not listed in a particular order of importance; established external resources (mental health professionals and support groups) are at the end of the list, but not necessarily more or less helpful. The other ideas can help in time between contact with these resources and as ongoing preventive/recovery strategies.

■ *Alternative activities:* Identify several activities that ease the feelings or provide distraction. The activities should be meaningful to the person. These should range in degree of concentration and energy needed for engagement. These are very individual, but some of the ones that I use are taking a walk; having a bath; reading a magazine or an interesting, but not too complex, book; calling, e-mailing, or texting a friend/family member; going to a support group; visiting a bookstore or library; gardening; crocheting; and playing with my cats. Outdoor activities have been particularly helpful to me such as hiking in the woods, sitting by a lake or at the beach, or visiting a park. I think they bring a sense of peace and connection with nature.

■ *Rational thought:* I have a list of rational reasons why I feel depressed or think about suicide—things that challenge thinking "I'm an awful/bad/unlucky/stupid, etc. person" or "life is too much trouble, not worthwhile, too painful/difficult" or "no one really cares about me or loves me." This can include identifying the current stressors or anniversaries of stressful events. The list should include projections of how/when the stressor will abate.

I keep a list of the alternative activities and rational thoughts posted at home and/or carry it along with me when I am experiencing symptoms. Consulting the list when concentration or initiative is lacking is helpful.

■ *Journaling:* This is a special type of "alternative activity" that I find very helpful. It's a way to pour out negative thoughts and feelings, and then try to challenge them or reflect how they have diminished in the past. It is useful to journal the good times as well and reread these passages when one is feeling especially down.

Continued

The Lived Experience—cont'd

- *Relaxation:* I find progressive relaxation and deep breathing helps ease the painful feelings. I sometimes use a guided relaxation tape if I am having difficulty concentrating. Visualizing a peaceful place I have enjoyed during vacation enhances the effect for me. I am also now using a sound machine to relax. The sound of ocean surf, rain, and thunderstorms are relaxing to me.

- *Creative activities:* I find writing poetry to be helpful in expressing my feelings in a constructive way. I often do this as part of my journaling. I share some of my poetry with others and some I don't. Dancing and doing crafts also relax and distract me. However, this can backfire if the activity is too complex. It is important to identify and pursue activity appropriate for one's state of mind.

- *Identify a reason to go on:* Make it simple. It should be important and specific to the individual and does not necessarily have to make sense or be important to others. For example, I have used the thought that I need to continue living to take care of and love my cats.

- *Structure:* During times of distress it is important to follow a normal daily schedule of structured activities even if one is unable to engage in some routines such as work or school.

- *Exercise:* This is a critical part of my plan for recovery. Finding the motivation to exercise may be a problem but I find that little tricks such as thinking "I will take a 5 minute walk" can often get the sneakers on and enable me to do more.

- *Reward system:* It is important to give oneself congratulations for getting through simple daily tasks such as personal hygiene and getting dressed. They take energy and concentration. They are an accomplishment when one is feeling depressed or having suicidal thoughts.

- *Talk to someone:* For a very long time I had difficulty calling my doctor or therapist in times of distress. I have weekly appointments, but at times I needed help in between. I am now better at this and have found the contact very helpful. If a person is feeling suicidal, mental health professionals can assess the degree of danger as well as the need for immediate intervention. Two hotline resources are Trans Lifeline (https://translifeline.org) or the 988 National Suicide and Crisis Line (https://988lifeline.org).

- *Self-help or support groups:* Such groups can provide persons who will listen, support, and share their experience in dealing with suicidal thoughts and urges. The Depression and Bipolar Support Alliance (https://www.dbsalliance.org), the National Alliance on Mental Illness (www.nami.org), and Alcoholics Anonymous (www.aa.org) have established chapters and support groups in many areas of the United States. The program, fellowship, and encouragement of seeing others have been very helpful. Resources are also available through Fireweed Collective (https://fireweedcollective.org), Project LETS (https://projectlets.org), and Mental Health America (https://mhanational.org).

Finally, for those who are experiencing mental illness, have *hope.* Think about it, read about it, talk about it. Plan to do something that you want to do that is important to you and will make you happy. Believe it can and will happen. Keep a mental or written list of the times you hoped for something and it came true. This is what keeps us all alive after all—the hope for a better life, the continuation of current happiness, and the belief that things will turn around as the cycles of the seasons and all living things do.

Substance Use Disorder

Individuals who use substances such as alcohol and drugs, despite the occurrence of significant negative consequences, are diagnosed with substance use disorders (APA, 2022). Hallmarks of the disorder include the inability to reduce rates of use despite a desire to stop and a loss of control over cravings. Individuals with substance use disorders display higher rates of negative mood, emotion dysregulation, and impulsivity (Kober, 2014).

Throughout development, individuals use substances to reduce underlying negative mood states, as most abusive substances induce a feeling of positive affect or euphoria. This sets up a cycle in which withdrawal from the substance leads to a rebound of the intense negative mood, which reinforces the use of the substance to escape the negative feelings (Shadur & Lejuez, 2015). For this reason, substance use disorders frequently develop and are diagnosed in individuals with clinical conditions involving negative affective states, such as depression and anxiety.

Environmental and situational cues, such as attending a celebration, meeting a friend who is a substance abuser, or driving by a liquor store, trigger cravings in individuals with substance abuse disorders (Kober, 2014). Cravings are a unique source of intense negative affect that is a key contributor to drug use and relapse. Strong BAS activation, in conjunction with positive expectations that the drug will make them feel better, results in cravings. Brain areas including the amygdala and ventral striatum mediate cravings, with the prefrontal cortex responsible for regulating craving-related behavior and preventing relapse.

Individuals with substance use disorders can benefit from learning specific emotion regulation skills to manage their intense cravings. CBTs and mindfulness-based therapies have been successfully used to teach skills and reduce relapse rates in individuals with substance abuse (Bowen et al., 2010). Interventions that involve developing new social relationships and identifying new activities that don't involve substances are also important components of long-term relapse prevention. Also see Chapter 24: Substance-Related and Addictive Disorders.

Eating Disorders

Anorexia nervosa (AN) is characterized by restricted calorie intake and significantly low weight, whereas bulimia nervosa (BN) involves binge eating and compensatory behaviors (e.g., purging, excessive exercise) with a normal weight profile (APA, 2022). Both conditions include high rates of co-occurring mood and anxiety disorders. Evidence suggests that underlying deficits in emotion regulation are similar across eating disorders, although the behaviors that occur because of the lack of emotional control (e.g., restrictive eating vs. binging/purging) vary (Prefit et al., 2019). Individuals with eating disorders experience high negative emotionality, alexithymia, and trouble with awareness of emotions. Significant difficulties with distress tolerance occur, with nonacceptance of negative emotions and strong beliefs that negative emotions should be avoided at all costs. These beliefs might arise in part from heightened punishment sensitivity, which results in strong avoidance of negative situations.

More broadly, many individuals eat to help manage negative emotions. Individuals with low sensory awareness and high sensory sensitivity are more likely to eat when stressed or presented with an environmental cue to eat, such as walking by a bakery (Hebert, 2018). This use of food consumption, including binge eating and restricted eating, as a maladaptive strategy to manage intense negative emotions involves BAS activation. Because eating is a necessary daily activity that both increases negative affect and serves as a means of emotion regulation in vulnerable individuals, it is particularly resistant to treatment and requires intensive intervention to address. Also see Chapter 19: Eating Disorders.

Borderline Personality Disorder

Borderline personality disorder (BPD) is the personality disorder most associated with emotion dysregulation. The diagnostic criterion for BPD specifically includes symptoms of reactivity of mood as well as inappropriate, intense anger or difficulty controlling anger (APA, 2022). Individuals with BPD have difficulty in five areas associated with emotion: emotion sensitivity, greater intensity of negative emotions, greater lability of negative emotions, a lack of appropriate regulation strategies, and an excess of maladaptive regulation strategies (Carpenter & Trull, 2013).

Linehan's biosocial theory (Crowell et al., 2009) suggests a developmental approach to BPD in which predisposed individuals are sensitive to emotions as infants and then experience high rates of negative emotions over time. This combination results in difficulties with developing appropriate emotion regulation strategies. The role of traumatic and invaliding environments and the frequency of abuse in the clinical history of individuals with BPD are also highlighted by Linehan's theory. Although high rates of negative emotions occur in multiple psychiatric conditions, it is the instability of the emotional picture and the tendency of anger and hostility to rapidly increase without warning that are unique to BPD (Carpenter & Trull, 2013).

Individuals with BPD also have difficulty with emotional awareness and the ability to accurately label emotions. This results in problems in identifying and using adaptive coping strategies, such as situation modification and cognitive reappraisal, to manage feelings of anger. Extreme maladaptive regulation strategies such as suicidal and self-injurious behaviors are sometimes used as attempts to manage negative emotions. Impulsive behaviors, including disordered eating, substance abuse, impulsive buying,

and other risk-taking activities, are also frequently seen. Dialectical behavioral therapy was developed specifically for individuals with BPD to address both the underlying emotion dysregulation and the significant behavioral impulsivity that characterizes this disorder (Linehan, 2020). Also see Chapter 22: Personality Disorders.

Posttraumatic Stress Disorder

PTSD is unique among the anxiety disorders because it involves experiencing a traumatic situation that results in a pattern of abnormal emotional, physical, and psychosocial responding. Individuals typically display an intense and prolonged startle response to threatening cues (e.g., loud noises) as well as flashbacks and reexperiencing of the traumatic event. Research suggests that two subtypes of PTSD exist, based on emotional responding; in the first, individuals are hyperresponsive to threat situations, and in the second, individuals shut down in the face of intense emotions and experience emotional numbing and alexithymia (Lanius et al., 2011).

Factors such as the type of trauma, age at which the trauma was experienced, cumulative nature of the trauma, and ability to avoid environmental cues related to the trauma likely affect how an individual responds emotionally. Although both subtypes involve an imbalance in the prefrontal-cortex control of the amygdala, effective treatments are likely to vary based on the type of emotion dysregulation experienced by the individual. Also see Chapter 25: Trauma- and Stressor-Related Disorders.

Attention Deficit-Hyperactivity Disorder

The primary impairments in ADHD are cognitive, with difficulties in paying attention (inattentive subtype) and controlling behavior (hyperactive-impulsive subtype) dominating the clinical picture. A prominent role for emotion dysregulation has long been recognized with this disorder, although debate exists about whether the cognitive difficulties are simply being applied to emotional situations (inattention to emotional cues) or if the emotional symptoms are a separate deficit (Shaw et al., 2014).

Children with ADHD have trouble regulating irritability and are often diagnosed with conditions that involve the expression and control of anger, aggression, and irritability, such as oppositional defiance disorder and conduct disorder. Developmental studies suggest that children with ADHD often display a difficult temperament as infants with frequent and intense negative emotional displays (Southam-Gerow & Kendall, 2002). Hyperactivity in the amygdala and underactivity in the ventral striatum likely contribute to this temperament style. Mood lability with rapid changes from positive to negative moods, especially involving aggression, are frequently seen during childhood.

Importantly, these difficulties with emotional control have a greater impact on the well-being of individuals with ADHD than the inattentive and hyperactive symptoms. Psychostimulant medications designed to treat the cognitive symptoms have been shown to reduce emotional lability and irritability in some children and adults with ADHD, suggesting a common pathway between these features.

Autism

Core symptoms of autism, including difficulties with language and communication, theory of mind, and sensory processing deficits, play a role in emotion dysregulation and the frequent additional diagnosis of psychiatric disorders (APA, 2022). Alexithymia is of particular interest, as it is identified in about 50% of autistic individuals (Poquerusse et al., 2018). This includes difficulties in interpreting and regulating one's *own emotions* as well as interpreting and responding to *others' emotions*.

Emotion interpretation difficulties in autism might stem from impairments in **interoception**, the ability to correctly identify and describe physiological processes. For example, a feeling of discomfort in the stomach could be associated with hunger or feelings of anxiety. The insula is the integration center in the brain responsible for associating bodily sensations (e.g., gnawing in the stomach) and feelings (e.g., anxiety). Imaging studies show that autistic individuals have atypical function and connectivity in the insula cortex (Nomi et al., 2019).

Broad deficits in sensory perception are characteristic of autistic individuals and atypical interoceptive awareness, highlighting the importance of sensory processing in emotional experiences. These findings suggest that sensory interventions that include identifying and understanding sensory processes and interoception can help improve emotion regulation in autistic individuals (Mahler et al., 2022). OTPs are well skilled in the use of sensory interventions to promote performance and should consider the specific impact of sensory modifications on emotional awareness and control.

Assessment

When working with individuals with emotion dysregulation, OTPs can draw from a range of assessments that examine emotional experiences, emotion regulation skills, and related coping and self-regulation abilities. See Table 12-1.

TABLE 12-1 | Therapeutic Reasoning Assessment Table: Emotion Regulation

Which Tool?	Who Was This Tool Designed For?	What Is Required of the Person? Can They Use the Tool?	What Am I Measuring?	How Long Does It Take and Where Do I Administer This Assessment?	Is the Tool Associated With a Practice Model?
Emotional Experiences in Activities of Daily Living Scale (EEADLs; Hebert & Ricker, 2022)	Adults	The EEADLs involves rating how often a person experiences five emotions in 25 occupations in a paper-based questionnaire. Only occupations that are completed on a weekly basis are rated.	The EEADLs measures the frequency of positive and negative emotional experiences during daily occupations.	The EEADLs can be administered in 15–20 minutes in a clinic or home environment. It works best with the therapist guiding the completion.	No
Emotion Regulation Scale for Adolescents (Strauss et al., 2016)	Adolescents	Person rates how often they engage in 39 occupations in response to a specific emotion in a paper-based questionnaire.	The scale measures the use of occupations when managing unpleasant emotions.	The scale can be administered in 10–15 minutes in a clinic or home environment.	No
Difficulties in Emotion Regulation Scale (DERS; Gratz & Roemer, 2004)	Adolescents and adults	The DERS involves rating 36 items related to individuals' awareness of and difficulty using strategies to regulate emotions in a paper-based questionnaire.	The DERS measures emotion regulation capacity and skill use.	The DERS can be administered in 10–15 minutes in a clinic or home environment.	No, but DERS emphasizes assessing the individual's skill level in recognizing, acknowledging, and responding to emotional needs.
Emotion Regulation Skills Questionnaire (ERSQ; Berking & Znoj, 2008)	Adults and adolescents	The ERSQ involves rating 27 items related to individuals' use of regulation skills in the previous week in a paper-based questionnaire.	The ERSQ assesses the use of eight different adaptive emotion regulation skills (e.g., awareness/mindfulness, acceptance, tolerance, and modifying emotions).	The ERSQ can be administered in 10–15 minutes in a clinic or home environment.	Affect Regulation Training (ART)

TABLE 12-1 | Therapeutic Reasoning Assessment Table: Emotion Regulation—cont'd

Which Tool?	Who Was This Tool Designed For?	What Is Required of the Person? Can They Use the Tool?	What Am I Measuring?	How Long Does It Take and Where Do I Administer This Assessment?	Is the Tool Associated With a Practice Model?
Profile of Emotional Competence (PEC; Brasseur et al., 2013)	Adults	The PEC involves rating 50 items related to how individuals use emotional competency skills when responding to their own as well as others' emotions.	The PEC assesses competency in using skills to manage interpersonal and emotional situations.	The PEC can be administered in 15–20 minutes in a clinic or home environment.	No
Emotion Regulation Questionnaire (ERQ; Gross & John, 2003)	Adults	The ERQ requires completion of a 10-item paper questionnaire	The ERQ measures individual differences in the habitual use of two emotion regulation strategies: cognitive appraisal and suppression of emotional expression.	The ERQ can be administered in about 5 minutes in a clinic or home environment.	No
Emotion Regulation Questionnaire for Children and Adolescents (ERQ-CA; Gullone & Taffe, 2012)	Children and adolescents	The ERQ-CA requires completion of a 10-item paper questionnaire. Questions are revised to be appropriate for children.	The ERQ-CA measures individual differences in the habitual use of two emotion regulation strategies: cognitive appraisal and suppression of emotional expression.	The ERQ-CA can be administered in about 5 minutes in a clinic or home environment.	No
Toronto Alexithymia Scale (TAS-20; Bagby et al., 1994)	Adults	The TAS-20 requires completion of a 20-item paper questionnaire.	The TAS-20 measures awareness of emotions and the ability to identify and describe feelings.	The TAS-20 can be administered in about 5–10 minutes in a clinic or home environment.	No
Five Facet Mindfulness Questionnaire (FFMQ; Baer et al., 2006)	Adults	The FFMQ requires self-report of 39 items related to knowledge and skills in mindfulness practice.	The FFMQ measures five facets of mindfulness: observing, describing, acting with awareness, nonjudging inner experience, and nonreactivity to inner experience.	The FFMQ takes about 10 minutes to complete at home or in the clinic.	No
Preschool Self-Regulation Assessment (PSRA; Smith-Donald et al., 2007)	Preschool children	The child will participate in simple situations that require self-regulation (for example, being able to wait to eat a snack).	The PSRA measures self-regulation of emotion, attention, and behavior through skilled observation and teacher report.	The PSRA takes about 50 minutes to complete in the clinic environment.	No

Occupation-Based Assessments

The Emotional Experiences in Activities of Daily Living Scale (EEADLs) directly measures how frequently individuals experience specific emotions when performing typical occupations (Hebert & Ricker, 2022). This scale assesses the frequency with which an individual experiences five discrete emotional states (engagement, excitement, frustration, overwhelm, and fatigue) in 25 occupations, which are divided into three categories of activities of daily living (ADLs; self-care, simple instrumental activities of daily living [IADLs], and complex IADLs). The emotional states included in this scale draw on flow psychology and reports of the importance of daily hassles and uplifts on long-term mental health. Individuals only rate occupations that they complete at least weekly to ensure that responses reflect current experiences and not expectations of how an activity should make them feel.

Responses are summarized into two emotional subscales (positive affect and negative affect). Because occupational items are rated on all five emotions, it is possible to identify activities that are associated with positive emotions, negative emotions, or both types of emotional affect. Individuals typically rate complex IADLs as more intense across the affective spectrum with higher rates of both positive and negative emotions being experienced.

Findings from this scale highlight the importance of occupations in an individual's emotional life. Occupations that cause negative affect can be reduced in frequency or modifications can be made to the activity or environment to reduce the negative impact. By incorporating principles of behavioral activation, OTPs can help people identify ways to increase engagement in occupations associated with positive affect.

The Emotion Regulation Scale for Adolescents was developed by occupational therapists to identify how individuals use occupations as a coping mechanism to manage emotions (Strauss et al., 2016). A self-report measure of occupational strategies used by adolescents, this 39-item scale assesses strategy use in five categories (comfort and sharing, antisocial behavior, creative activities, physical activities, and eating) in response to a specific emotional state (e.g., anger) in adolescents. In contrast to other scales that examine emotion regulation skills, the strategies identified are behaviorally oriented occupations (e.g., creative activities such as painting or sharing with a friend on social media). This focus on the use of occupations to *manage* emotions is helpful for OTPs who work with individuals with emotion dysregulation.

Emotion Regulation and Dysregulation Assessments

The Difficulties in Emotion Regulation Scale (DERS) is a self-report measure of emotion regulation (Gratz & Roemer, 2004). This 36-item scale measures regulation in six domains: acceptance of negative emotions, engagement in goal-directed behavior, control of impulsive behavior, emotion regulation strategy use, emotional awareness, and emotional clarity. Higher scores indicate greater difficulty with emotion regulation. This scale has high internal consistency and reliability. It is frequently used by clinicians to determine an individual's overall difficulty with managing their emotions and has been used in multiple treatment studies to measure improvements following therapy (Sloan et al., 2017).

The Emotion Regulation Skills Questionnaire (ERSQ) is a self-report measure of how frequently individuals use emotion regulation skills (Berking & Znoj, 2008). This 27-item scale measures the use of skills during the previous week in nine areas: awareness of emotions, ability to identify/label emotions, ability to interpret emotion-related body sensations, ability to understand emotional prompts, ability to support oneself in distressing situations, ability to modify negative emotions, ability to accept emotions, ability to tolerate negative emotions, and ability to confront situations to attain important goals. Clinical samples of individuals with mental health conditions had less mastery of these nine skills than healthy controls (Berking et al., 2008). Furthermore,

the ERSQ was used to measure the impact of CBT interventions on emotion regulation skills in several clinical populations.

The Profile of Emotional Competence (PEC) is a self-report measure of competency in regulating emotions in daily life (Brasseur et al., 2013). This 50-item scale measures how much an individual identifies using emotional competency skills in five categories: identification, understanding, expression, regulation, and use of emotions. This scale is unique in that it examines these five competency skills in how the individual addresses their own emotions as well as the emotions of others, resulting in an intrapersonal as well as an interpersonal subscale. The interpersonal scale is particularly valuable in helping identify an individual's competency in responding to others' emotions, which plays a large role in social situations and peer support.

The Emotion Regulation Questionnaire for Children and Adolescents (ERQ-CA) is a brief, 10-question self-report measure of the frequency with which children engage in the emotion regulation strategies of cognitive reappraisal and emotional suppression (Gullone & Taffe, 2012). This scale is derived from the well-validated Emotion Regulation Questionnaire (Gross & John, 2003), which assesses the frequency of strategy use in adults. The questions in the ERQ-CA were simplified and reworded to be appropriate for children and adolescents. The creation of scales that are designed to assess emotion regulation in children has been lacking, despite the prominence of symptoms in several developmental psychopathology conditions. Scales specifically designed for children are of value for OTPs working in the school system when developing interventions to improve strategy use.

The primary use of self-report assessments in occupational therapy practice is to help individuals identify current difficulties with specific components of emotional processing. Assessment results provide guidance for the development of occupational therapy–based interventions that are targeted to individual skills. For example, an individual with difficulty in interpreting emotion-related body sensations using the ERSQ might benefit from interventions designed to increase awareness of sensory processing and interoception. This individual might also benefit from a sensory diet or other modifications to the environment designed to support sensory processing. An adolescent who frequently suppresses negative emotions based on their ERQ-CA results could be taught alternative strategies based in self-regulation, coping, and mindfulness to increase their tolerance of negative emotions.

The unique role of occupational therapy can be to help ground these techniques in daily occupations through the identification of frequently experienced emotional situations and active practice of emotional occupations utilizing self-regulation strategies.

Assessments Related to Emotion and Emotion Awareness

Emotions are core mental processes that are intricately tied to a range of successful outcomes, including academic and social performance and broad measures of well-being. For this reason, emotion and emotional awareness form a component of many assessments that are not directly concerned with regulation skills. Additional assessments that provide insight into emotion-related skills are of value to OTPs working with people across the life span.

As an important component of emotion regulation, alexithymia is often addressed independently in therapy. Specific difficulties with awareness of emotions are often assessed utilizing the Toronto Alexithymia Scale (TAS-20; Bagby et al., 1994). This 20-item shortened version of the original scale assesses performance in three areas: difficulty identifying feelings, difficulty describing feelings, and externally oriented thinking. This scale can be particularly helpful for OTPs working with individuals who seem to lack the ability to recognize when emotional situations are occurring or the impact of those situations on their current feelings. People who can identify emotional experience in their daily life but are unable to manage those emotions to achieve personal goals would be better assessed using emotion regulation questionnaires.

Multiple questionnaires exist that assess an individual's knowledge and skills in mindfulness practice. The Five Facet Mindfulness Questionnaire (FFMQ) is a self-report measure of the ability to be mindful (Baer et al., 2006). This 39-item survey examines mindfulness in five areas: nonreactivity, observing, acting with awareness, describing/labeling, and nonjudging of an experience. Mindfulness assessments are valuable for OTPs who plan to utilize Mindfulness-Based Interventions (MBIs), but they also can provide a broader picture of an individual's approach to mental experiences.

Although questionnaires developed to assess emotion regulation skills focus on the ability to observe, identify, and *control* emotions, mindfulness assessments focus on the complementary ability to observe, identify, and *purposefully not engage* with emotions. Nonreactivity to emotional experiences is a core feature of Dialectical Behavioral Therapy (DBT; Linehan, 1993) and Mindfulness-Based Stress Reduction (Kabat-Zinn, 1990), treatments that utilize an alternative approach to coping with intense emotions.

The Preschool Self-Regulation Assessment (PSRA) measures self-regulation in emotion, attention, and behavior domains (Smith-Donald et al., 2007). This assessment allows for direct observation of a young child's skills with self-regulation (e.g., while waiting for a signal to eat a snack or waiting to touch a wrapped present), as well as reports of socioemotional adjustment. Clinician reports of performance in the areas of social competence, externalizing behaviors, and internalizing behaviors in the testing situation are identified. Unlike self-report measures, the use of direct observation of skills in challenging situations allows for this assessment to be utilized with young children who are unable to verbally respond to questions. The tasks in this assessment are easy to perform in the classroom or clinic environment and involve typical activities that a young child would encounter in daily life.

Intervention

As awareness has grown that both negative and positive emotions independently contribute to an individual's overall life satisfaction, interventions have emerged that address various aspects of the process model of emotion. This section of the chapter highlights interventions that take two different approaches: (1) interventions that teach skills and techniques to manage intense negative emotions and (2) interventions that directly introduce positive situations and emotions.

Interventions That Regulate Negative Emotions

Dialectical Behavioral Therapy

DBT is a mindfulness-based approach involving individual psychotherapy and psychosocial skills training (Linehan, 1993, 2020). Originally developed to address suicidal and parasuicidal behaviors in individuals with BPD, DBT is now used to treat emotion dysregulation and impulsive behavior in a range of externalizing conditions, including substance use disorders, suicidal adolescents, eating disorders, and ADHD (Robins & Chapman, 2004).

DBT is a modified form of standard CBT and incorporates many of the same techniques, including skills training and behavioral analysis, to address symptoms. Its focus on the **dialectic**, which involves considering and integrating contradictory facts and ideas, forms the core of DBT (Linehan, 1993, 2020). In DBT, the primary dialectic is the balance between acceptance of an individual's severe negative emotions and embracing strategies to change these emotions.

DBT skills training involves teaching new strategies for addressing intense emotions in a group format (Linehan, 1993, 2020). Evidence suggests that skills training can be effective as a stand-alone treatment in improving emotion regulation for individuals with depression, ADHD, substance abuse, and in forensic populations, among others (Valentine et al., 2015). OTPs, with their background in psychoeducation and group dynamics, typically participate in DBT interventions through leading skills training groups.

DBT includes four modules of training: mindfulness, interpersonal effectiveness, emotional modulation, and distress tolerance (Linehan, 1993, 2020). Mindfulness is taught first as a core emotion regulation skill and involves learning to direct attention toward the current moment in an observant and nonjudgmental manner. Interpersonal effectiveness training focuses on improving the interpersonal problem-solving, assertiveness, and social skills needed to successfully navigate the social situations that cause intense negative emotions.

Emotional modulation training focuses on increasing the ability to identify and label emotions, recognize obstacles to changing emotions, and reduce vulnerability to strong emotions. Distress tolerance skills involve the ability to experience a negative emotional state without attempting to change it in the moment. These skills can include engagement in occupations that help an individual distract from the intense emotion, self-soothe, and improve their current feelings. Distress tolerance skills uniquely rely on engagement in activities to help tolerate negative emotions instead of using psychological and cognitive processes to manage the emotional experience.

DBT is an intensive intervention that is often provided in inpatient treatment settings including residential treatment facilities for eating disorders and forensics mental health settings that also employ OTPs.

PhotoVoice

This is a photo of the lake with the city of Milwaukee in the distance. This is my attempt to escape the chaos of the city. There is always so much going on in Milwaukee—festivals, construction, violence; sometimes I need to get away. There are times when I am on campus and feel this need. There are young people everywhere, riding skateboards, bikes, and listening to headphones, not paying attention to or caring about who they are running over. Don't get me wrong, I love that they are able to be young and carefree. However, sometimes I need an escape. Heading out to the lake gives me the space I need to decompress.

How do you use escape as a means of emotion regulation? When is escape useful, and when is it detrimental?

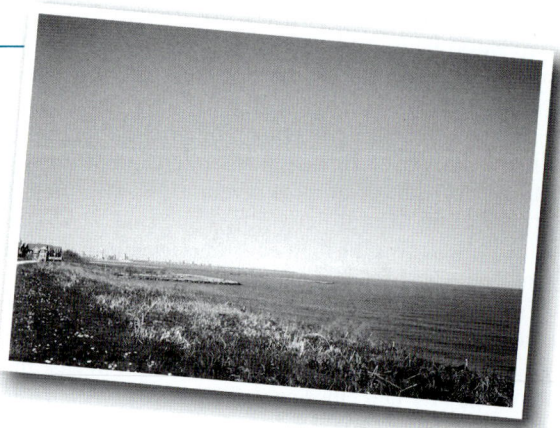

Mindfulness-Based Therapies

Mindfulness is a state of mind achieved by bringing one's awareness to the present moment, observing, and accepting one's feelings, thoughts, and bodily sensations (Kabat-Zinn, 1990). Although the concept of mindfulness is ancient and has its roots in Eastern Buddhist religious and meditation practices, the current widespread interest in its therapeutic benefits traces back to Jon Kabat-Zinn's introduction of Mindfulness-Based Stress Reduction (MBSR) as a complementary treatment for individuals with chronic pain (Kabat-Zinn, 1990).

Since the original introduction of MBSR, mindfulness concepts and techniques have been integrated into various psychological treatment approaches, with Mindfulness-Based Cognitive Therapy (MBCT; Segal et al., 2002) and ACT (Hayes et al., 2011) being the most prominent. Emotion regulation skills have emerged as one of the primary areas targeted by MBIs. The fact that emotion regulation skills are improved by a variety of therapies across multiple clinical conditions supports the idea that emotion regulation is a core psychological function implicated across psychopathology (Sloan et al., 2017).

Mindfulness-Based Occupational Therapy (MBOT) is an emerging approach that seeks to integrate mindful approaches into occupational therapy practice. The value of occupational engagement in providing specific opportunities for mindful awareness and flow states has been highlighted (Reid, 2011). Further, it has been argued that mindfulness has a natural fit with occupations, given its focus on awareness in the present moment, a factor that occurs naturally during heightened engagement with activities (Elliot, 2011). A scoping review of mindfulness interventions in physical rehabilitation settings found that, although only two of the studies included an OTP as the primary provider, all the reviewed interventions fit within the occupational therapy scope of practice (Hardison & Roll, 2016).

The emerging interest in MBOT is also seen in several pilot studies exploring the role of OTPs in providing MBIs in a variety of settings. For example, an occupational therapist led a mindfulness-based yoga program for children with concussions that was found to improve self-efficacy in academic, social, and emotional domains (Paniccia et al., 2019). An 8-week occupational therapist–led MBSR program for community-dwelling individuals with chronic conditions improved somatic awareness and the development of healthy habits and routines (B. Thompson, 2009).

A particular avenue for OTPs interested in this area can be the integration of sensory processing and mindfulness approaches to occupational performance. Individuals who score low in mindfulness and experience more mind wandering and distraction in daily life have sensory processing patterns characterized by poor awareness (Hebert, 2016). Interventions in interoception, sensory awareness, and mindfulness could help individuals bring mindful attention to occupational and social activities, leading to improvements in the quality of emotional experiences.

Emotional Awareness Training in Neurological Rehabilitation

Individuals treated in inpatient neurorehabilitation units with diagnoses including traumatic brain injury, stroke, multiple sclerosis, and Parkinson disease often demonstrate difficulties processing emotions, which can result in high rates of anxiety and depression as well as alexithymia and emotion dysregulation (Ricciardi et al., 2015). Interventions have been developed to teach psychoeducational skills in this population, including identification and description of emotions, building emotional vocabularies, differentiating between emotions, and identifying changes in physical sensations (Neumann et al., 2017).

A particular focus has been on teaching emotional awareness and coping skills to individuals with traumatic brain injuries, given the substantial impact of these deficits on successful community integration. Although it was previously believed that the cognitive impairments following an acquired brain injury would prevent a person from being able to learn new emotional skills, increases in emotional self-awareness and regulation have been found following individual and group-based training (Neumann et al., 2017). Pilot work also supports group-based CBT and stress management interventions to improve emotion regulation in individuals with multiple sclerosis (Yu & Mathiowetz, 2014). Although still in the early stages of development, emotional awareness training as a part of neurological rehabilitation is an important example of how OTPs can address psychosocial factors across practice settings. Also see Chapter 16: Acquired Physical Disability and Mental Health.

Evidence-Based Practice

Mindfulness Practices and Emotion Regulation

OTPs skilled in mindfulness practices can teach the techniques to people to support better emotion regulation and overall wellness.

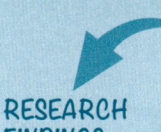

RESEARCH FINDINGS

A meta-analysis of MBIs explored the impact of standardized mindfulness treatments on aspects of emotional processing and mental health (Hoge et al., 2021). MBSR and MBCT programs were delivered in a group format with sessions lasting approximately 2.5 hours per week for a minimum of 8 weeks. Emotional processing was assessed through self-report questionnaires, interviews, and physiological measures. Individuals with clinical diagnoses including medical conditions, anxiety, and depression, as well as healthy individuals reporting high levels of stress, were included in the studies. Significant improvements in overall emotion-related processing, depression, anxiety, mental health, and stress were found following treatment.

APPLICATIONS

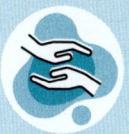

➡ Many individuals treated by OTPs could benefit from group-based mindfulness practice to improve emotional processing and mental health.
➡ OTPs who are skilled in mindfulness practices can teach mindfulness to people to support better emotion regulation and overall wellness.

REFERENCES

Hoge, E. A., Acabchuk, R. L., Kimmel, H., Moitra, E., Britton, W. B., Dumais, T., Ferrer, R. A., Lazar, S. W., Vago, D., Lipsky, J., Schuman-Olivier, Z., Cheaito, A., Sager, L., Peters, S., Rahrig, H., Acero, P., Scharf, J., Loucks, E. B., & Fulwiler, C. (2021). Emotion-related constructs engaged by Mindfulness-Based Interventions: A systematic review and meta-analysis. *Mindfulness (N.Y.), 12*(5), 1041–1062. https://doi.org/10.1007/s12671-020-01561-w

Emotion Regulation Interventions in the Classroom

OTPs have adapted programs designed to improve emotion regulation skills for the classroom environment. These community-based programs take a preventive approach by teaching skills to children who are at high risk for developing psychopathology associated with emotion dysregulation.

For example, the Alert Program (Williams & Shellenberger, 1996) is a self-regulation intervention developed for school-age children that uses cognitive learning and sensory activities to change a child's alertness level and increase participation in classroom activities. It has been adapted by OTPs for children enrolled in specialized classrooms for individuals with emotional disturbances (Barnes et al., 2008). The 8-week long adaptation focuses on recognizing arousal states and increasing self-regulation skills using the Alert Program format. Preliminary findings suggest that this program improves sensory processing and self-regulation skills in the classroom environment (Barnes et al., 2008).

Another classroom-based program, the Interoception Curriculum, was designed by an occupational therapist to address issues with interoception and alexithymia in autistic children (Mahler et al., 2022). This 25-week program involves teaching body mindfulness strategies, including the ability to notice body signals, identify the unique emotion associated with each body signal, and explore actions and activities that increased comfort with each body signal. Autistic children demonstrated improvements in interoception as well as emotional, cognitive, and behavioral regulation following the intervention.

These programs suggest that OTPs working in the school setting have a role in developing preventive programs to improve emotion regulation in high-risk children. Also see Chapter 37: School Mental Health.

Interventions That Increase Positive Emotions

Behavioral Activation and Occupational Engagement

Behavioral activation is an effective treatment for depression (Cuijpers et al., 2007) that is also used in other conditions with high rates of negative emotions. This technique draws on principles of activity scheduling to help individuals identify and increase the frequency of pleasant activities in daily life. Behavioral activation differs from other CBT techniques because it uses a direct approach to quickly increase an individual's experience of positive emotions, instead of focusing on modifying the thought processes associated with negative emotions. Behavioral activation principles are uniquely well suited to be applied by OTPs because they rely on techniques already incorporated in multiple treatment settings.

Key components of behavior activation include identification and analysis of activities to identify pleasant experiences, time management and scheduling to increase the opportunity for activities, and modifications of activities as needed to ensure successful performance. Although the relationship between occupational engagement and behavioral activation has not received much research analysis, this area is an important example of using occupations to directly address psychosocial concerns. The Being a Psychosocial OT Practitioner feature in this chapter provides an in-depth example of using behavioral activation principles in conjunction with occupational engagement in an outpatient day program.

Creative Therapies in Mental Health Practice

Creative activities, such as drawing, painting, pottery, craftwork, music, and drama, have been utilized by OTPs in mental health settings since the beginning of the profession (Griffiths & Corr, 2007). The use of these modalities has waxed and waned over time in part because of the lack of systematic research on their efficacy. Although it has often been assumed that part of the value of these activities is to increase mood, little research has been done to directly examine this impact.

Being a Psychosocial OT Practitioner

An Occupation-Based Approach to Managing Negative Affect and Increasing Opportunities for Positive Affect

Identifying Psychosocial Strengths and Needs

OTPs working in adult neurological rehabilitation are responsible for the assessment and treatment of individuals whose emotion regulation skills are impacted by their condition. Consider the story of Stacy, a 44-year-old woman who is being seen in a comprehensive outpatient day program for 4 weeks following a right cerebral vascular accident. Stacy lives with her husband and three high school–age children in a small single-story home.

Stacy presents with moderate left side numbness and weakness that is worse in the upper extremity and hand. She has poor static and dynamic balance and uses a hemi-walker when ambulating short distances. She demonstrates moderate deficits in attention, working memory, and problem-solving that are evident when completing therapeutic activities and occupations in the clinic. Stacy also presents with emotional lability with frequent episodes of crying and laughing during sessions that she describes as "coming out of nowhere, I don't know why they happen." These episodes alternate with periods of flat affect where she has difficulty engaging in conversation. Upon interview, she acknowledges that before the stroke, she had a history of "flying off the handle" and getting really upset when she felt things weren't turning out as she expected.

Since discharge from the hospital, Stacy has been relying on her family to complete the housework, cooking, and shopping. Her mother has been coming over daily to help Stacy with personal care activities, especially dressing and showering, as well as household tasks, a situation that Stacy finds very frustrating as she reports that "I don't get along that well with my mother, she always wants things done her way which isn't my way."

Stacy identifies that she wants to begin completing more occupations at home but is overwhelmed by the idea and doesn't know where to start. The OTP determines that Stacy's physical and cognitive impairments and high expectations about how tasks should be performed put her at risk for emotional outbursts when performing occupations.

Using a Holistic Occupational Therapy Approach

The OTP working with Stacy decides to utilize the EEADLs to help identify daily occupations that are a source of significant negative emotions and activities that provide an opportunity for positive enjoyment.

Out of 25 possible occupations, Stacy consistently participates in five personal care activities, one simple IADL, and two complex IADLs, which is a significant reduction from the 20 occupations she engaged in before her stroke. Highlighted in the table that follows are specific occupations where she reports either *often* or *almost always* feeling the associated emotions before her diagnosis.

Emotional Experiences in Activities of Daily Living Scale

	Negative Affect (Frustration and Overwhelm)	Positive Affect (Engagement and Excitement)	Fatigue
Personal care		Cell phone/computer use, eating on the go	
Simple IADLs	Cleaning		Laundry, getting the mail
Complex IADLs	Planning a meal, complex cooking, paying bills	Shopping, driving	Caring for a child, indoor exercise

Since discharge from the hospital, she reports feeling negative affect and fatigue when completing most personal care activities (bathing, getting dressed, grooming, and using a cell phone). She also reports rarely participating in previously enjoyable activities, such as shopping or eating on the go. In conjunction with her OTP, Stacy identifies a few low negative affect occupations in which she wants to increase her participation at home. These activities include washing the dishes and simple meal preparation. She also wants to improve her ability to use her cell phone to keep up with friends on social media as this used to be a highly positive occupation.

The OTP also helps Stacy identify the physical, cognitive, and emotional demands associated with her high negative affect occupations. For example, Stacy shares that cooking dinner for the family has always been frustrating because there are multiple recipes and steps that must be managed, everything needs to be done at the same time, and her family often doesn't seem to appreciate the final meal.

Stacy and her OTP make a plan to address her emotional lability and negative affect during occupational engagement in therapy sessions. The OTP begins by introducing emotional awareness techniques that include describing emotions and identifying physical changes in the body associated with negative emotions. Using mindfulness-based strategies, the OTP helps Stacy use deep breathing, direct attention to task components, and positive imagery to increase her tolerance of unexpected labile and negative emotions. Behavioral activation principles, in conjunction with the results of the EEADLs, are employed to

alternate occupations across sessions so that frustrating activities are followed by relaxing and enjoyable activities. Finally, guided reflection helps Stacy anticipate episodes of dysregulation and evaluate the success of her emotion regulation strategies.

Reflective Questions

1. How might the Process Model of Emotional Regulation be applied to the excitement Stacy previously experienced while shopping?
2. How might the cognitive impairments outlined in this case contribute to the episodes of emotion dysregulation observed when completing simple meal preparation tasks?
3. How would you design a treatment session with the goal of using mindfulness techniques to manage her distress when using social media apps on her cell phone?

A study completed by occupational therapists utilized creative artful kits to help individuals manage emotions (Sokmen & Watters, 2016). Individuals created a personalized self-soothing kit that involved items related to music, journaling, painting, jewelry making, drawing, and other tasks in group-based sessions. Use of the kits varied across individuals from daily to weekly use and were introduced in conjunction with mindfulness techniques. Improvements in awareness of emotions, a reduced tendency to suppress negative emotions, and overall increased mood was noted following intervention. Although this study introduces the use of these kits for individuals in an outpatient mental health setting, similar kits could easily be incorporated into physical health practice settings with individuals struggling with chronic stress or emotion dysregulation.

Positive Psychology Interventions in Chronic Health Conditions

There has been increased interest in techniques designed to increase happiness and positive emotions by addressing the five stages in Gross's (1998) Process Model of Emotional Regulation (Quoidbach et al., 2015). Treatments are wide ranging and include well-being therapy, quality of life therapy, solution-focused coping, and mindfulness-based techniques to cultivate positive emotions. Short-term increases in positive emotions have been found using techniques that target attentional deployment, cognitive change, and response modulation. Long-term improvements following skills training in situation selection during the event and attentional deployment before, during, and after the event are well supported by the literature.

As an example of attentional deployment, consider someone planning an upcoming dinner with friends or family. The person could visualize specific aspects of the event, including where the person plans to go to dinner and what they plan to order (anticipation–before), the fun conversation and delicious food they enjoyed (experience–during), and specific aspects of the dinner such as a funny joke someone told or how the dessert looked on the plate (reminiscence–after). Because these interventions involve focusing cognitive resources on specific components of an event, often in conjunction with

modifications to the environment in which the event occurs, therapeutic skills in activity analysis and modification are particularly valuable.

Peer Groups and Community-Based Interventions

Because of the importance of social relationships and peer groups in the development and maintenance of mental health, interventions have been designed that utilize peer coaching to effect change in emotional performance. Community-based peer mentoring programs that pair individuals with severe mental illness with trained peer coaches who also have a mental health diagnosis are successful in improving self-regulation skills and quality of life (Cabassa et al., 2017).

Peer mentoring programs have become increasingly common in school settings and are used to address self-regulation skills through engagement in group activities (Petosa & Smith, 2014), although the efficacy of school-based programming remains mixed. Although the coaching focus and techniques used vary across programs, frequent engagement in positive social interactions with the identified peer is a core component. OTPs can help develop peer-based programming designed to increase positive emotional experiences throughout the life span and across multiple practice settings.

Here's the Point

- People's daily lives are filled with emotions that can be regulated by strategies that are applied before and during occupations and social situations.
- There is a neurological basis to emotion regulation skills, which develop and mature across the life span. Social situations and environments can have a substantial impact on brain development and the ability to use emotion regulation strategies.
- Emotion dysregulation has been identified as a core impairment in psychological disorders as diverse as depression, anxiety, BPD, substance abuse, eating disorders, ADHD, and autism.

■ OTPs can use newer occupation-specific assessments as well as questionnaires that draw from the broader psychological literature to identify emotion dysregulation.

■ Interventions including mindfulness-based practice, DBT, and awareness training can be used by OTPs to assist individuals in the developmental of regulation skills. Interventions designed to increase the frequency of positive experiences in daily life are an important supplement to skills training.

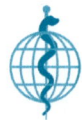

Visit the online resource center at **FADavis.com** to access the videos.

Apply It Now

1. Consider Your Own Emotion Regulation

Think of a recent experience when you had a strong emotional reaction. Analyze the experience using the Modal Model of Emotions (Gross, 1998):

■ Describe the situation.
■ What factors drew your attention to the emotion (e.g., bodily sensations)?
■ What was your cognitive appraisal of the situation?
■ How did you respond?

Reflective Questions

■ Was your emotional response in proportion to the situation?
■ Were you able to be in the situation and have a nonjudgmental experience or did you evaluate your feelings as it was happening?
■ Would you handle the situation differently if it were to happen again? If so, how?

2. Emotional Awareness of Occupational Performance

Think of a household occupation that you complete each day (e.g., cooking, washing the dishes, shopping). Identify how often you feel engaged, excited, overwhelmed, frustrated, and fatigued while completing this activity.

Reflective Questions

■ Which aspects of the occupation are associated with each emotion?
■ Does the environment in which the occupation occurs affect the emotions you experience? If so, how?
■ How could you modify the occupation to reduce the negative emotions experienced?

3. Mindfulness Techniques

Engage in one of the mindfulness practices described in the interventions section.

Reflective Questions

■ How was the experience for you?
■ Mindfulness is a skill that requires practice. How might you integrate mindfulness into your daily routines? How might it become a regular practice for you?
■ How do you think mindfulness could help a person with emotion dysregulation?

4. Video Exercise: Laura's Experience as a Mother of an Autistic Son.

Pair up with another student in your class or form a small group of students. Access and watch the "Laura's Experience as a Mother of an Autistic Son" at the online resource center at FADavis.com. Then, discuss and together answer the following questions.

Reflective Questions

■ Laura openly describes her journey of moving from being a parent of a "big, healthy, snuggly baby" who met all his developmental milestones to learning to be a parent of an autistic child. What were some of the signs that Laura and the teachers at Will's day care noticed that eventually led to his evaluation and diagnosis?
■ Laura mentioned that Will's day-care providers were a powerful part of his care team and that they used his strengths to help him succeed. From her description of Will, what strengths do you think those were, and how could they have been used to adapt and learn how to better regulate his emotions?
■ Laura describes a graded-entry approach for Will into day care due to severe separation anxiety. Do you think the approach was effective? Why or why not? In what other areas might a graded approach be helpful with Will and other autistic children?
■ What accommodations did the teachers at Will's day care create to accommodate and support Will's free play of lining up cars in a row? What other situations in the daily flow of preschool might Will potentially find challenging, and what accommodations might you recommend to the teachers?

5. Video Exercise: Managing Challenging Behaviors in Young Children

Pair up with another student in your class or form a small group of students. Access and watch the "Managing Challenging Behaviors in Young Children" video at the online resource center at FADavis.com. Then, discuss and together answer the following questions.

Reflective Questions

■ What is Allison's primary approach to working with children with difficult behavior as a result of poor self-regulation? Why is this approach particularly important for children who have experienced and/or are experiencing trauma?
■ The occupational therapy assistant (OTA) described using a feelings tool to check in with the children she works with. Why is interoception and emotional literacy foundational for self-regulation?
■ Why are transitions so difficult for children and adults with emotion regulation challenges? What strategies does the OTA use to signal the transition and help the child manage the transition?
■ What are some universal trauma-informed strategies that the OTA can share with the staff at the Early Head Start

program to support the population of children she works with and reduce their challenging behaviors?

■ Allison described consistency as key and shares how she creates rituals and routines in her occupational therapy space that help children know what to expect, to manage

transitions, and to self-regulate. What are ways that these same strategies might be used more universally in these children's classrooms by their teachers? Or individualized in the home setting with parents or caregivers?

Resources

Mindfulness Training

- Center for Mindfulness in Medicine, Health Care, and Society at University of Massachusetts Memorial Medical Center, Shaw Building, Worcester, MA 01655-0267, or access the website at: https://www.ummhealth.org/center-mindfulness
- Duke Integrative Medicine, Health & Well-Being Programs, Durham, NC: https://dhwprograms.dukehealth.org/programs-training

Dialectical Behavior Therapy Resources

- DBT worksheets can be found online at: www.dbtselfhelp.com
- Training in DBT: Marsha Linehan Behavioral Tech Research Inc. are found at: www.behavioraltech.org

Interoceptive Awareness Training

- Resources related to interoceptive awareness and teaching self-regulation are found at: www.kelly-mahler.com/interoception-for-professionals

Positive Psychology Resources

- Resources including assessments, tools, and techniques related to positive psychology are found at: www.PositivePsychology.com

Videos

- "Fieldwork Experience in Juvenile Correction Setting" video. In this video, occupational therapist Maggie reflects on how she felt prepared and unprepared for her fieldwork experience. She touches on topics such as trauma, emotion regulation, and sensory processing, and emphasizes the need to be aware of her own self-care by setting boundaries. Access the video at the online resource center at FADavis.com.
- "Positive Mindset Creative Arts Festival" video. This video showcases the Positive Mindset Creative Arts Festival, held at the Queensland Children's Hospital in Australia. This annual children's festival promotes positive thinking about mental health and increases help-seeking behaviors with a creative arts focus. It is a notable example of how OTPs can contribute to community health efforts. The emphasis is on art as an occupation and creating space in the community to encourage and celebrate mental health. In addition, the event promotes the idea of social connection and belonging centered around self-expression of feelings across the mental health continuum and how that ultimately encourages the sense of connection and belonging with people and communities. Access the video at the online resource center at FADavis.com.
- "Sensory Garden in Geriatric Psychiatric Unit" video. In this video, occupational therapist Callie Ward showcases the sensory garden at an inpatient psychiatric facility. The multisensory garden was designed for occupational therapy groups with a goal of helping participants identify the effects the garden and its related tasks have on their level of arousal. Callie offers specific examples of the many positive effects of the garden on residents, such as collaborating on tasks, problem-solving, encouraging routines, working on cognition, and assisting with self-regulation, among others. She explains how she uses it for active and passive group interventions and in one-to-one sessions. Access the video at the online resource center at FADavis.com.

- "Occupational Therapy and Music Therapy in Early Head Start" video. In this video, an occupational therapist and music therapist discuss their unique and effective collaboration in a Head Start program. Running an 8-week group for infants and toddlers, the therapists assessed the children and established preventive goals linked to developmental milestones in areas such as self-regulation, awareness of self and others, attention, language, and motor movements. Access the video at the online resource center at FADavis.com.
- "Mary's Lived Experience as an Unhoused Individual and Her Occupational Therapist's Perspective" video. In this video, Mary provides a first-person account of being unhoused and the tremendous impact occupational therapy services have had on her life. In addition, occupational therapist Quinn Tyminski describes working with Mary and shares her perspective on Mary's journey and transformation, including her improved conflict resolution and emotion regulation skills. Access the video at the online resource center at FADavis.com.
- "Tricks and Techniques From the Mother of an Autistic Son" video. In this video, Laura describes her and her family's creative and adaptive ways of helping their autistic son, Will, succeed. Giving several specific examples of solutions to common problem behaviors and challenges, Laura shares practical wisdom, "tricks and techniques" from 20 years of experience as the mother of a son with autism, with a focus on recognizing and focusing on Will's strengths. Access the video at the online resource center at FADavis.com.
- "Aimee's Lived Experience With Substance Use and Autism" video. Aimee is an occupational therapist with the lived experience of substance use disorder. In this video, Aimee shares that she was diagnosed with childhood PTSD and that she also realized that she is autistic. She describes the behaviors that led her to that conclusion, her coping strategies, and how her lived experience affected her role as student in graduate school. Access the video at the online resource center at FADavis.com.

References

Aldao, A., Gee, D. G., Los Reyes, A. D., & Seager, I. (2016). Emotion regulation as a transdiagnostic factor in the development of internalizing and externalizing psychopathology: Current and future directions. *Development and Psychopathology, 28*(4pt1), 927–946. https://doi.org/10.1017/S0954579416000638

American Occupational Therapy Association. (2020). Occupational therapy practice framework: Domain and process (4th ed.). *American Journal of Occupational Therapy, 74*(Suppl. 2), 7412410010. https://doi.org/10.5014/ajot.2020.74S2001

American Psychiatric Association. (2022). *Diagnostic and statistical manual of mental disorders* (5th ed., text rev.). American Psychiatric Publishing. https://doi.org/10.1176/appi.books.9780890425787

Amstadter, A. (2008). Emotion regulation and anxiety disorders. *Journal of Anxiety Disorders, 22*(2), 211–221. https://doi.org/10.1016/j.janxdis.2007.02.004

Baer, R. A., Smith, G. T., Hopkins, J., Krietemeyer, J., & Toney, L. (2006). Using self-report assessment methods to explore facets of mindfulness. *Assessment, 13*(1), 27–45. https://doi.org/10.1177/1073191105283504

Bagby, R. M., Parker, J. D., & Taylor, G. J. (1994). The twenty-item Toronto Alexithymia Scale—I. Item selection and cross-validation of the factor structure. *Journal of Psychosomatic Research, 38*(1), 23–32. https://doi.org/10.1016/0022-3999(94)90005-1

Barnes, K. J., Vogel, K. A., Beck, A. J., Schoenfeld, H. B., & Owen, S. V. (2008). Self-regulation strategies of children with emotional disturbances. *Physical & Occupational Therapy in Pediatrics, 28*(4), 369–387. https://doi.org/10.1080/01942630802307127

Berking, M., Wupperman, P., Reichardt, A., Pejic, T., Dippel, A., & Znoj, H. (2008). Emotion-regulation skills as a treatment target in psychotherapy. *Behavior Research and Therapy, 46*(11), 1230–1237. https://doi.org/10.1016/j.brat.2008.08.005

Berking, M., & Znoj, H. (2008). Entwicklung und Validierung eines Fragebogens zur standardisierten Selbsteinschätzung emotionaler Kompetenzen. [Development and validation of a self-report measure for the assessment of emotion-regulation skills]. *Zeitschrift für Psychiatrie, Psychologie und Psychotherapie, 56*(2), 141–152. https://doi.org/10.1024/1661-4747.56.2.141

Bowen, S., Chawla, N., & Marlatt, G. A. (2010). *Mindfulness-based relapse prevention for addictive behaviors: A clinician's guide.* Guilford Press.

Brasseur, S., Grégoire, J., Bourdu, R., & Mikolajczak, M. (2013). The Profile of Emotional Competence (PEC): Development and validation of a self-reported measure that fits dimensions of emotional competence theory. *PloS One, 8*(5), e62635. https://doi.org/10.1371/journal.pone.0062635

Cabassa, L. J., Camacho, D., Vélez-Grau, C. M., & Stefancic, A. (2017). Peer-based health interventions for people with serious mental illness: A systematic literature review. *Journal of Psychiatric Research, 84,* 80–89. https://doi.org/10.1016/j.jpsychires.2016.09.021

Carpenter, R. W., & Trull, T. J. (2013). Components of emotion dysregulation in borderline personality disorder: A review. *Current Psychiatry Reports, 15*(1), 335. https://doi.org/10.1007/s11920-012-0335-2

Charles, S. T., & Carstensen, L. L. (2010). Social and emotional aging. *Annual Review of Psychology, 61,* 383–409. https://doi.org/10.1146/annurev.psych.093008.100448

Crowell, S. E., Beauchaine, T. P., & Linehan, M. M. (2009). A biosocial developmental model of borderline personality: Elaborating and extending Linehan's theory. *Psychology Bulletin, 135*(3), 495–510. https://doi.org/10.1037/a0015616

Cuijpers, P., Van Straten, A., & Warmerdam, L. (2007). Behavioral activation treatments of depression: A meta-analysis. *Clinical Psychology Review, 27*(3), 318–326. https://doi.org/10.1016/j.cpr.2006.11.001

Damasio, A. R. (2004). Emotions and feelings. In A.S.R. Manstead, N. Frijda, & A. Fischer (Eds), *Feelings and emotions: The Amsterdam symposium* (pp. 49–57). Cambridge University Press.

Davidson, R. J., Pizzagalli, D., Nitschke, J. B., & Putnam, K. (2002). Depression: Perspectives from affective neuroscience. *Annual Review of Psychology, 53,* 545–574. https://doi.org/10.1146/annurev.psych.53.100901.135148

Diener, E., & Emmons, R. A. (1984). The independence of positive and negative affect. *Journal of Personality and Social Psychology, 47*(5), 1105–1117. https://doi.org/10.1037/0022-3514.47.5.1105

Dunn, W. (2007). Supporting children to participate successfully in everyday life by using sensory processing knowledge. *Infants & Young Children, 20*(2), 84–101. https://doi.org/10.1097/01.IYC.0000264477.05076.5d

Elliot, M. L. (2011). Being mindful about mindfulness: An invitation to extend occupational engagement into the growing mindfulness discourse. *Journal of Occupational Science, 18*(4), 366–376. https://doi.org/10.1080/14427591.2011.610777

Farley, J. P., & Kim-Spoon, J. (2014). The development of adolescent self-regulation: Reviewing the role of parent, peer, friend, and romantic relationships. *Journal of Adolescence, 37*(4), 433–440. https://doi.org/10.1016/j.adolescence.2014.03.009

Gratz, K. L., & Roemer, L. (2004). Multidimensional assessment of emotion regulation and dysregulation: Development, factor structure and initial validation of the Difficulties in Emotion Regulation Scale. *Journal of Psychopathology and Behavioral Assessment, 26,* 41–54. https://doi.org/10.1023/B:JOBA.0000007455.08539.94

Griffiths, S., & Corr, S. (2007). The use of creative activities with people with mental health problems: A survey of occupational therapists. *British Journal of Occupational Therapy, 70*(3), 107–114. https://doi.org/10.1177/030802260707000303

Gross, J. J. (1998). The emerging field of emotion regulation: An integrative review. *Review of General Psychology, 2*(3), 271–299. https://doi.org/10.1037/1089-2680.2.3.271

Gross, J. J., & Jazaieri, H. (2014). Emotion, emotion regulation, and psychopathology: An affective science perspective. *Clinical Psychological Science, 2*(4), 387–401. https://doi.org/10.1177/2167702614536164

Gross, J. J., & John, O. P. (2003). Individual differences in two emotion regulation processes: Implications for affect, relationships, and well-being. *Journal of Personality and Social Psychology, 85*(2), 348–362. https://doi.org/10.1037/0022-3514.85.2.348

Grossmann, I., Karasawa, M., Kan, C., & Kitayama, S. (2014). A cultural perspective on emotional experiences across the life span. *Emotion, 14*(4), 679–692. https://doi.org/10.1037/a0036041

Gullone, E., & Taffe, J. (2012). The Emotion Regulation Questionnaire for Children and Adolescents (ERQ–CA): A psychometric evaluation. *Psychological Assessment, 24*(2), 409–417. https://doi.org/10.1037/a0025777

Hardison, M. E., & Roll, S. C. (2016). Mindfulness interventions in physical rehabilitation: A scoping review. *The American Journal of Occupational Therapy, 70*(3), 7003290030p1–7003290030p9. https://doi.org/10.5014/ajot.2016.018069

Hayes, S. C., Strosahl, K. D., & Wilson, K. G. (2011). *Acceptance and Commitment Therapy: The process and practice of mindful change.* Guilford Press.

Hebert, K. R. (2016). The association between sensory processing styles and mindfulness. *British Journal of Occupational Therapy, 79*(9), 557–564. https://doi.org/10.1177/0308022616656872

Hebert, K. R. (2018). Sensory processing styles and eating behaviors in healthy adults. *British Journal of Occupational Therapy, 81*(3), 162–170. https://doi.org/10.1177/0308022617743708

Hebert, K. R., & Ricker, T. J. (2022). Reliability of the Emotional Experiences in Activities of Daily Living Scale. *OTJR: Occupation, Participation and Health, 43*(2), 271–279. https://doi.org/10.1177/15394492221085288

Hoge, E. A., Acabchuk, R. L., Kimmel, H., Moitra, E., Britton, W. B., Dumais, T., Ferrer, R. A., Lazar, S. W., Vago, D., Lipsky, J., Schuman-Olivier, Z., Cheaito, A., Sager, L., Peters, S., Rahrig, H., Acero, P., Scharf, J., Loucks, E. B., & Fulwiler, C. (2021). Emotion-related constructs engaged by Mindfulness-Based Interventions: A systematic review and meta-analysis. *Mindfulness (N.Y.), 12*(5), 1041–1062. https://doi.org/10.1007/s12671-020-01561-w

Isaacowitz, D. M., Livingstone, K. M., & Castro, V. L. (2017). Aging and emotions: Experience, regulation, and perception. *Current Opinion in Psychology, 17,* 79–83. https://doi.org/10.1016/j.copsyc.2017.06.013

Kabat-Zinn, J. (1990). *Full catastrophe living: Using the wisdom of your body and mind to face stress, pain and illness.* Bantam Books.

Katz, B. A., Naftalovich, H., Matanky, K., & Yovel, I. (2021). The dual-system theory of bipolar spectrum disorders: A meta-analysis. *Clinical Psychology Review, 83,* 101945. https://doi.org/10.1016/j.cpr.2020.101945

Kober, H. (2014). Emotion regulation in substance abuse disorders. In J. J. Gross (Ed.), *Handbook of emotion regulation* (2nd ed., pp. 428–446). Guilford Press.

Koss, K. J., & Gunnar, M. R. (2018). Annual research review: Early adversity, the hypothalamic–pituitary–adrenocortical axis, and child psychopathology. *Journal of Child Psychology and Psychiatry, 59*(4), 327–346. https://doi.org/10.1111/jcpp.12784

Kring, A. M., & Bachorowski, J. (1999). Emotions and psychopathology. *Cognition and Emotion, 13*(5), 575–599. https://doi.org/10.1080/026999399379195

Lanius, R. A., Bluhm, R. L., & Frewen, P. A. (2011). How understanding the neurobiology of complex post-traumatic stress disorder can inform clinical practice: A social cognitive and affective neuroscience approach. *Acta Psychiatrica Scandinavica, 124*(5), 331–348. https://doi.org/10.1111/j.1600-0447.2011.01755.x

LeMoult, J., & Gotlib, I. H. (2019). Depression: A cognitive perspective. *Clinical Psychology Review, 69*, 51–66. https://doi.org/10.1016/j.cpr.2018.06.008

Lindquist, K. A., Wager, T. D., Kober, H., Bliss-Moreau, E., & Barrett, L. F. (2012). The brain basis of emotion: A meta-analytic review. *Behavioral Brain Science, 35*(3), 121–143. https://doi.org/10.1017/S0140525X11000446

Linehan, M. M. (1993). *Skills training manual for treating borderline personality disorder.* Guilford Press.

Linehan, M. M. (2020). *Dialectical Behavior Therapy in clinical practice.* Guilford Publications.

Mahler, K., Hample, K., Jones, C., Sensenig, J., Thomasco, P., & Hilton, C. (2022). Impact of an interoception-based program on emotion regulation in autistic children. *Occupational Therapy International, 2022*, Article ID 9328967. https://doi.org/10.1155/2022/9328967

Martin, R. E., & Ochsner, K. N. (2016). The neuroscience of emotion regulation development: Implications for education. *Current Opinions in Behavioral Science, 10*, 142–148. https://doi.org/10.1016/j.cobeha.2016.06.006

Matsumoto, D., Yoo, S. H., & Nakagawa, S. (2008). Culture, emotion regulation, and adjustment. *Journal of Personality and Social Psychology, 94*(6), 925–937. https://doi.org/10.1037/0022-3514.94.6.925

Morris, A. S., Criss, M. M., Silk, J. S., & Houltberg, B. J. (2017). The impact of parenting on emotion regulation during childhood and adolescence. *Child Development Perspectives, 11*(4), 233–238. https://doi.org/10.1111/cdep.12238

Neumann, D., Malec, J. F., & Hammond, F. M. (2017). Reductions in alexithymia and emotion dysregulation after training emotional self-awareness following traumatic brain injury: A phase I trial. *Journal of Head Trauma Rehabilitation, 32*(5), 286–295. https://doi.org/10.1097/HTR.0000000000000277

Nomi, J. S., Molnar-Szakacs, I., & Uddin, L. Q. (2019). Insular function in autism: Update and future directions in neuroimaging and interventions. *Progress in Neuro-Psychopharmacology and Biological Psychiatry, 89*, 412–426. https://doi.org/10.1016/j.pnpbp.2018.10.015

Ochsner, K. N., Silvers, J. A., & Buhle, J. T. (2012). Functional imaging studies of emotion regulation: A synthetic review and evolving model of the cognitive control of emotion. *Annals of the New York Academy of Sciences, 1251*(1), E1–E24. https://doi.org/10.1111/j.1749-6632.2012.06751.x

Ortony, A., & Turner, T. (1990). What's basic about basic emotions? *Psychological Review, 97*(3), 315–331. https://doi.org/10.1037/0033-295X.97.3.315

Paniccia, M., Knafo, R., Thomas, S., Taha, T., Ladha, A., Thompson, L., & Reed, N. (2019). Mindfulness-based yoga for youth with persistent concussion: A pilot study. *The American Journal of Occupational Therapy, 73*(1), 7301205040p1–7301205040p11. https://doi.org/10.5014/ajot.2019.027672

Petosa, R. L., & Smith, L. H. (2014). Peer mentoring for health behavior change: A systematic review. *American Journal of Health Education, 45*(6), 351–357. https://doi.org/10.1080/19325037.2014.945670

Poquerusse, J., Pastore, L., Dellantonio, S., & Esposita, G. (2018). Alexithymia and autism spectrum disorder: A complex relationship. *Frontiers in Psychology, 9*, 1196. https://doi.org/10.3389/fpsyg.2018.01196

Prefit, A. B., Candea, D. M., & Szentagotai-Tătar, A. (2019). Emotion regulation across eating pathology: A meta-analysis. *Appetite, 143*, 104438. https://doi.org/10.1016/j.appet.2019.104438

Quoidbach, J., Mikolajczak, M., & Gross, J. J. (2015). Positive interventions: An emotion regulation perspective. *Psychological Bulletin, 141*(3), 655–693. https://doi.org/10.1037/a0038648

Reid, D. (2011). Mindfulness and flow in occupational engagement: Presence in doing. *Canadian Journal of Occupational Therapy, 78*(1), 50–56. https://doi.org/10.2182/cjot.2011.78.1.7

Ricciardi, L., Demartini, B., Fotopoulou, A., & Edwards, M. J. (2015). Alexithymia in neurological disease: A review. *Journal of Neuropsychiatry and Clinical Neuroscience, 27*, 179–187. https://doi.org/10.1176/appi.neuropsych.14070169

Robins, C. J., & Chapman, A. L. (2004). Dialectical Behavior Therapy: Current status, recent developments, and future directions. *Journal of Personality Disorders, 18*(1), 73–89. https://doi.org/10.1521/pedi.18.1.73.32771

Rudenstine, S., Espinosa, A., McGee, A. B., & Routhier, E. (2019). Adverse childhood events, adult distress, and the role of emotion regulation. *Traumatology, 25*(2), 124–132. https://doi.org/10.1037/trm0000176

Segal, Z. V., Williams, J. M. G., & Teasdale, J. D. (2002). *Mindfulness-Based Cognitive Therapy for depression: A new approach to preventing relapse.* Guilford Press.

Shadur, J. M., & Lejuez, C. W. (2015). Adolescent substance use and comorbid psychopathology: Emotion regulation deficits as a transdiagnostic risk factor. *Current Addiction Reports, 2*(4), 354–363. https://doi.org/10.1007/s40429-015-0070-y

Shaw, P., Stringaris, A., Nigg, J., & Leibenluft, E. (2014). Emotion dysregulation in attention deficit hyperactivity disorder. *American Journal of Psychiatry, 171*(3), 276–293. https://doi.org/10.1176/appi.ajp.2013.13070966

Sloan, E., Hall, K., Moulding, R., Bryce, S., Mildred, H., & Staiger, P. K. (2017). Emotion regulation as a transdiagnostic treatment construct across anxiety, depression, substance, eating and borderline personality disorders: A systematic review. *Clinical Psychology Review, 57*, 141–163. https://doi.org/10.1016/j.cpr.2017.09.002

Smith-Donald, R., Raver, C. C., Hayes, T., & Richardson, B. (2007). Preliminary construct and concurrent validity of the Preschool Self-Regulation Assessment (PSRA) for field-based research. *Early Childhood Research Quarterly, 2*(2), 173–187. https://doi.org/10.1016/j.ecresq.2007.01.002

Sokmen, Y. C., & Watters, A. (2016). Emotion regulation with mindful arts activities using a personalized self-soothing kit. *Occupational Therapy in Mental Health, 32*(4), 345–369. https://doi.org/10.1080/0164212X.2016.1165642

Southam-Gerow, M. A., & Kendall, P. C. (2002). Emotion regulation and understanding: Implications for child psychopathology and therapy. *Clinical Psychology Review, 22*(2), 189–222. https://doi.org/10.1016/S0272-7358(01)00087-3

Strauss, M., Raubenheimer, J. E., Campher, D., Coetzee, C., Diedericks, A., Gevers, H., Green, K., & van Niekerk, S. (2016). The development of an emotional regulation scale for adolescents. *South African Journal of Occupational Therapy, 16*(3), 41–48. https://doi.org/10.17159/2310-3833/2016/v46n3a8

Thompson, B. (2009). Mindfulness-Based Stress Reduction for people with chronic conditions. *British Journal of Occupational Therapy, 72*(9), 405–410. https://doi.org/10.1177/030802260907200907

Thompson, R. A. (1994). Emotion regulation: A theme in search of definition. *Monographs of the Society for Research in Child Development, 59*(2), 25–52. https://doi.org/10.2307/1166137

Urosević, S., Abramson, L. Y., Harmon-Jones, E., & Alloy, L. B. (2008). Dysregulation of the behavioral approach system (BAS) in bipolar spectrum disorders: Review of theory and evidence. *Clinical Psychology Review, 28*, 1188–1205. https://doi.org/10.1016/j.cpr.2008.04.004

Valentine, S. E., Bankoff, S. M., Poulin, R. M., Reidler, E. B., & Pantalone, D. W. (2015). The use of Dialectical Behavior Therapy skills training as a stand-alone treatment: A systematic review of the treatment outcome literature. *Journal of Clinical Psychology, 71*(1), 1–20. https://doi.org/10.1002/jclp.22114

Webb, T. L., Miles, E., & Sheeran, P. (2012). Dealing with feeling: A meta-analysis of the effectiveness of strategies derived from the process model of emotion regulation. Psychological Bulletin, 138(4), 775–808. https://doi.org/10.1037/a0027600

Williams, M., & Shellenberger, S. (1996). *How does your engine run? A leader's guide to the Alert Program for self-regulation.* Therapy Works.

Yang, Y., & Wang, Q. (2019). Culture in emotional development. In V. LoBue, K. Pérez-Edgar, & K. A. Buss (Eds.), *Handbook of emotional development* (pp. 569–594). Springer. https://doi.org/10.1007/978-3-030-17332-6_22

Yu, C.-H., & Mathiowetz, V. (2014). Systematic review of occupational therapy-related interventions for people with multiple sclerosis: Part 2. Impairment. *American Journal of Occupational Therapy, 68*(1), 33–38. http://dx.doi.org/10.5014/ajot.2014.008680

Zimmermann, P. & Iwanski, A. (2014). Emotion regulation from early adolescence to emerging adulthood and middle adulthood: age differences, gender differences, and emotion-specific developmental variations. *International Journal of Behavioral Development, 38*(2), 182–194. https://doi.org/10.1177/0165025413515405

Communication and Social Skills

Sarah Wilkes-Gillan, Yu-Wei Ryan Chen,
and Lauren Parsons

Communication and social interaction skills develop across the life span and enhance human connection. Successful social interactions boost personal relationships, build a sense of self-efficacy, and contribute to a positive self-concept.

A person's ability to effectively interact with others is dependent on the development and interplay of a wide array of cognitive, perceptual, and language abilities that form the basis for communication and social skills. A person engaged in social interaction must be aware of their motivation and the message that they intend to communicate. They must be able to appreciate the context of the interaction, understand the behavior and perspective of their conversational partner, and have an awareness of social rules and boundaries to respond appropriately (Matthews et al., 2018).

For all people, social interaction can be compromised by a multitude of factors, such as a lack of clarity or logical content of the message, poor perceptual awareness of others, misinterpretation of body language and tone of voice, inability to comprehend the message conveyed, insensitivity to others' needs and interests, and poor understanding of the rules of conversation (Lezak et al., 2012). But for people challenged by communication and social skills, the impact on social participation can be far reaching.

Occupational therapy practitioners (OTPs) recognize that communication and socialization are essential to occupational performance and that difficulties in these areas are associated with decreased meaningful interaction, challenges in occupational role functioning, loss of confidence, social withdrawal, isolation, and depression (Sheets & Kraines, 2014). OTPs can help to improve an individual's social participation through the provision of skilled interventions that facilitate the acquisition and practice of such skills or by structuring environments and adapting occupations in order to maximize an individual's social participation and occupational performance.

This chapter explores components of communication and social skills required for social interaction, explains various theories underlying communication and social skills, and describes how some mental health conditions (including autism, attention deficit-hyperactivity disorder [ADHD], trauma and stress-related disorders, anxiety disorders, schizophrenia, personality disorders, and substance use disorders) can impact an individual's ability to succeed in social interactions. Methods of assessing communication and social skills, and several intervention approaches OTPs can use to strengthen and expand a person's social repertoire, are presented.

Components of Communication and Social Skills

Communication and socialization involve at least one other person, which increases the complexity of this aspect of performance, as each person, situation, and environment involves unique and dynamic demands. This section uses the *Occupational Therapy Practice Framework: Domain and Process,* 4th Edition (*OTPF-4;* American Occupational Therapy Association [AOTA], 2020), to discuss the factors, performance skills, and social context that make up the person's communication and socialization.

Person Factors

The *OTPF-4* (AOTA, 2020) describes some of the relevant capacities that underlie one's ability to communicate effectively with others as **client factors**, or capacities that reside within the person that influence their performance in occupations. Client factors that directly influence a person's ability to communicate and socialize include mental functions and language. However, by describing client factors that underlie socialization and communication, OTPs do not intend to imply that these factors should be the sole target of occupational therapy intervention.

There are situations in which a person can benefit from approaches that focus on skill acquisition, but equally important is the provision of interventions that create structured environments or adapted occupations that promote social interaction and connectedness. Nevertheless, it is still important to understand the client factors that contribute to socialization and communication to determine the best intervention approach, whether it targets the person, environment, or the occupation.

Mental Functions

Mental functions are cognitive, affective, and perceptual skills that influence performance in occupations. Those most relevant to communication and socialization fall within the **specific mental functions** designation of the *OTPF-4* (AOTA, 2020) and can be classified into cognitive functions and emotional functions.

Cognitive functions consist of *higher-level cognitive functions* (e.g., planning, mental flexibility, judgment and impulse control, perspective taking), *attention,* and *memory* (e.g., working memory), and contribute to an individual's ability to communicate socially. For example, topic management in conversation requires a person to process information at a speed to follow the ongoing interaction, maintain attention throughout the discourse, plan and organize language to communicate an intended message, utilize working memory to avoid repetition and respond accurately, apply judgment to avoid irrelevant responses, and exercise inhibitory control to suppress one's own perspective or response (Abbot-Smith et al., 2023).

Emotional functions connected to communication and social skills include **emotion perception**, **empathy**, and **emotional regulation**. *Emotion perception* includes the recognition and interpretation of emotional signals that are part of social communication. Relevant information about another person's emotional state is usually perceived via facial expressions, gestures, posture of the body, and tone of voice. An ability to interpret these cues provides important insight into another person's state of mind, enhances awareness of others, and aids in comprehension of the message conveyed. However, there is considerable variability in the way different individuals perceive, interpret, and respond to emotional signals (Brooks et al., 2019), and emotion perception is often challenging for individuals with psychiatric conditions.

Empathy is a complex construct of emotion perception that encompasses the perception of emotion in both oneself and other people, understanding what another person is thinking or feeling, self-awareness, and the regulation of one's own emotional state. Empathy is influenced by a person's temperament and personality and derived in part from complex cognitive skills such as insight, judgment, cognitive flexibility, and self-regulation. These higher order cognitive skills enable a person to be aware of and understand their own thought processes.

Self-awareness is essential to *emotional regulation*. For example, a person must have an awareness of their own internal somatic states (e.g., nervousness, irritation, calm) and the ability to identify and describe their emotions in order to accurately perceive their emotional experience *before* being able to control it effectively (Schwarzer et al., 2021). That is, the ability to analyze and verbalize one's own feelings is a precursor to being able to understand the emotional experience of another person. The ability to understand another's mental state, appreciate it as separate from one's own, and respond with appropriate emotion is the basis for empathic, prosocial behavior (Hein et al., 2018).

For example, a teacher may feel empathy for a nervous student who is having trouble getting through a presentation. The teacher is not feeling anxious but identifies the signs of nervousness in the student. The teacher then responds by providing the student with supportive comments to help the student regain composure. An individual without empathy would not be able to relate to the student's experience.

Language

Language, including voice and speech functions designated in the *OTPF-4* (AOTA, 2020), is inextricably linked to the specific mental functions discussed previously. Conversation underpins much of our socialization as humans, and the ability to conceptualize, formulate and plan, produce, and comprehend language is critical to conversing with others.

To organize and produce language that another person can comprehend, people rely on a complex combination of verbal language structures that follow implicitly agreed upon rules among speakers of the same language. Violations of these rules can have varying degrees of impact on one's ability to communicate and socialize with others. For example, selecting a word that is imprecise but not inaccurate may lead to minor confusion or misunderstanding. However, if there are missing or substituted speech sounds in several words of the sentence, a communication breakdown is the likely outcome. This is especially true if the listener is challenged by decoding the spoken language.

When communicating with another, the spoken words and sentences form part of a larger discourse. Organizing words and sentences effectively ensures coherence and relevance to the broader discourse, while also making sense to the audience. Language that is disconnected, missing critical information, or disorganized is difficult for another to follow and can also lead to communication breakdowns.

The communication skills required for social participation reach far beyond language comprehension and production. The ability to notice and interpret the nonverbal cues that enhance and deepen the meaning of the spoken message is also critical, as well as the ability to integrate these verbal and nonverbal communication behaviors with the social and emotional context of the social interaction. In other words, what people say is important, but *how they say it and matching it to the context of the interaction is just as critical.*

Nonverbal communication cues contribute to the richness of interpersonal communication. **Gesture**, **facial expression**, and **body posture** are nonverbal means of conveying emotion or adding emphasis to the verbal language tools people use to communicate. **Vocal prosody**, which includes the intonation, tone, stress, and rhythm of voice, is important in signaling the form of the utterance (e.g., vocal inflection varies depending on whether a person is uttering a statement, question, or command, and it aids the regulation of conversational interaction by providing cues to indicate when a speaker is inviting the listener to make a contribution to the conversation (Cole, 2015).

Prosody is often used to reflect the speaker's emotional state or attitude toward what is being said. For example, a speaker's tone of voice may rise if they are anxious or fearful; the speaker may put stress on words, slow down the rhythm of speech, or add pauses to emphasize a point; and/or the speaker may vary the speech intentionally in order to indicate humor or sarcasm. Together, these nonverbal cues enable a person to convey emotion, emphasize thoughts, and expand and personalize the array of verbal tools one has to contribute to and punctuate social exchanges.

Performance Skills

Social interaction skills are occupational performance skills that are observed during the ongoing stream of a social interaction and underlie one's ability to participate in desired occupations (AOTA, 2020). The term **pragmatics** is used to refer to the social interaction skills that combine to facilitate participation in social interactions. Recent definitions of pragmatics encompass behaviors related to the communicative, social, and emotional aspects of social communication (Adams et al., 2005; Cordier et al., 2019). This definition refers to an

BOX 13-1 ■ Behaviors Related to Pragmatics

- Introducing suitable conversation topics in appropriate ways
- Responding to the communication of others with contingent utterances that build on the social interaction
- Maintaining and changing topics appropriately
- Repairing conversation breakdowns
- Using and interpreting gesture, facial expressions, body posture, and distance to promote social interactions
- Perspective taking
- Recognizing and responding to the emotional state of others
- Regulating one's own emotions and behaviors
- Adapting language and behaviors to the social situation
- Maintaining engagement in a social interaction that is mutually beneficial
- Employing ways to express emotions and resolve disagreements so that a positive interaction is maintained

Data from Cordier, R., Munro, N., Wilkes-Gillan, S., Speyer, R., Parsons, L., & Joosten, A. (2019). Applying Item Response Theory (IRT) modelling to an observational measure of childhood pragmatics: The Pragmatics Observational Measure-2. *Frontiers in Psychology, 10*, 408. https://doi.org/10.3389/fpsyg.2019.00408

individual's ability to use specific mental functions (e.g., high-level cognitive functions, attention, memory, emotion perception and regulation) effectively while also adhering to the rules of social language that dictate acceptable ways to communicate in different social contexts (Bosco et al., 2017). Pragmatic competence is important for successful social participation and occupational role performance across the life span.

Pragmatic skills include more than the use of polite language (e.g., "please" and "thank you"); turn-taking in conversation; use of eye contact, gestures, and other expressive behavior to communicate engagement; respect for another's personal space; and use of acceptable strategies to gain attention, interject comments, and ask questions. See Box 13-1 for examples of behaviors related to pragmatics. Pragmatic competence also encompasses one's sensitivity to the violation of social norms, ability to convey sincerity and use humor appropriately, and to offer and respond to expressions of affection appropriately.

Social Context and Environment

Often the context or environment in which a social interaction occurs determines the social norms or rules for communicating. The ability to communicate effectively within a social interaction relies on a person's ability to adjust their language and communicative behavior based on the social environment and context (Cordier et al., 2019), or for the social environment or context to be adjusted to meet the social needs of the individual.

According to the *OTPF-4* (AOTA, 2020), the term **environment**, when applied to social interactions, refers to the physical surroundings where an interaction occurs as well as the social environment. The social environment is considered to involve the relationships with and expectations of those with whom people interact. **Context** refers to the elements surrounding and within an individual that influence performance; it can be examined in terms of cultural, personal, temporal, and virtual contexts, which underpin how an individual interacts with others.

Given that the environments and contexts of social interactions can be thought of across multiple dimensions, adapting communicative behavior to a social environment or context is complex; it requires an understanding of the relationship between the conversational partners, knowledge of the co-conversant's emotional state, an understanding of shared knowledge with the co-conversant(s), an understanding of cultural norms within the co-conversant(s)' culture, background knowledge about the setting and topic, and general knowledge of the world around them (Matthews et al., 2018).

For example, the implicit and explicit norms of communicating are different depending on whether one is speaking with a small child, a close friend, a potential employer, or a stranger on the street. Or a speaker may choose to omit information if they know there is a shared topic or general knowledge between themselves and conversational partners. Increasingly, the virtual context is important for social interactions across the life span.

Discussion of communication and social interaction thus far within the chapter has focused on in-person spoken interactions occurring in real-time. Technology-facilitated interactions that occur in virtual contexts also determine the modification of communication behaviors. For example, the topic an individual may select to initiate with another is likely to vary depending on whether that interaction is occurring via the telephone, direct message on a social media platform, or a videogame console.

For some individuals, certain modes of communication via technology may be more comfortable and promote better communication and social interaction. Similarly, certain social settings or people will foster interpersonal connectedness. For example, some individuals thrive in large social settings, whereas others can interact and communicate better with another individual. Everyone has people that they find easier to communicate with than others. OTPs must recognize environmental features that can support the people they serve.

Theories Underlying Communication and Social Interaction

Theories underlying communication and social interaction help explain how individuals develop skills in communicating and interacting with others. The theories discussed in this section can help OTPs understand why some individuals have difficulty with social situations. *Social cognition theory* proposes that basic cognitive abilities underlie our ability to understand and appropriately respond to social situations. *Social learning theory* explains that much of what people learn about social situations is based on observing others and then modeling that behavior. *Language theories* describe how partners in conversation work together to make shared meaning. *Attachment theory* describes how bonding early in life affects mental representations of social interactions and experiences in relationships later in life.

Social Cognition Theory

Social cognition refers to the psychological processes that are involved in processing social information. As an individual develops from childhood to adulthood, the requirements for social interaction become increasingly complex. Social cognition allows the individual to manage different social situations and different contexts with flexibility.

Social cognition can be divided into subprocesses (Green et al., 2017). One subprocess, **perception of social cues**, involves the nuanced and complicated process of perceiving and making sense of the information provided through facial expressions, voice inflection, gestures, and physical proximity. These cues provide information about feelings and can also impart additional content that adds to the spoken word. For example, pointing might indicate a direction, and facial expression and vocal inflection are often used to indicate someone is joking.

Mentalizing is another subprocess of social cognition related to understanding the mental states of others. This process, also described as theory of mind (Baron-Cohen et al., 1985), involves being able to attribute beliefs, intents, and desires to oneself and others, and recognizing that one's own and others' mental states can differ (Matthews et al., 2018). For example, someone with healthy mentalizing and theory of mind knows that a work colleague is unaware of what they did the night before, whereas someone without a strong mentalizing process may begin to talk about the previous night as if the person were there.

Central coherence is a third subprocess used to describe social processing, particularly in relation to explaining differences in the way social information is processed by autistic and nonautistic individuals (Skorich et al., 2016). The process is underpinned by the idea that many pieces of social information are pulled together in a drive for coherence or sense making within a social situation. Central coherence, for example, allows an individual to enter a discussion about certain players and teams and recognize that his friends are talking about an upcoming basketball game. Conversely, someone with weak central coherence may get caught up with a particular player's name and miss the main point of the conversation.

Social cognition recognizes that the process of interacting with others is highly complex. The concept of social cognition has received a great deal of attention in the literature concerning schizophrenia (Javed & Charles, 2018); however, the term or similar terms are also used in conceptualizing social functioning in autism and intellectual disabilities.

As a theory, social cognition posits that difficulties in social interactions are caused by impairments in specific cognitive processes that are necessary for effective communication. The social impairments that are common in many psychiatric conditions may be explained by difficulties in cognitively processing social information. Interventions from a social cognition perspective may include the development of skills, such as being able to recognize emotions in facial expressions, or may include compensatory strategies, such as utilizing a cue sheet and checklist for interactions that occur during a doctor's visit.

Social Learning Theory

Social learning theory posits that most learning occurs by observing others in a social context (Bandura, 1977). For example, a child does not have to manipulate a faucet to learn how to turn it on. Instead, the child can watch others doing it and then use the same process. People choose to imitate the behavior of others they see as models, and they are more likely to choose a model when that person is similar. For example, some musical instruments tend to have gender associations that appear to be based on their vocal register and the gender most associated with playing that instrument historically. Consequently, when choosing an instrument in elementary school, girls are more likely to choose a flute, whereas boys are more likely to choose the trumpet.

Although there are always exceptions, some modeling will likely occur based on gender expectations. Similarly, a new supervisor with a democratic style may look to other supervisors of a similar temperament when seeking role models in the workplace, as opposed to looking for an autocratic leader as a role model.

Once a behavior is exhibited, it may be reinforced or punished. Individuals will repeat behaviors that are reinforced and avoid behaviors that are punished. OTPs use positive responses to encourage the development of new skills. These positive responses can be as simple as eye contact or a smile, but often involve very specific feedback, such as, "When you asked your friend for her opinion, it showed that you cared about her."

According to Bandura (1977), there are four prerequisites for social learning to occur: (1) attention, (2) retention, (3) reproduction, and (4) motivation (Fig. 13-1). OTPs can intervene with any prerequisite. For example, an OTP may help the person with focus by encouraging them to attend to facial expressions when trying to read emotion. OTPs also may provide strategies for remembering by using cues or lists. Skill development involves role-play and practice, whereas motivation is enhanced through positive reinforcement of desired behaviors.

Language Theories

The theorization of language for social use emerged from the fields of linguistics, philosophy, and psychology. Different theories have emerged to explain language more broadly, but the two theories presented here pertain to the ways that language is used in conversation. They are based on an implicit agreement between conversation partners that conversations are a cooperative act, and language is used to achieve certain goals.

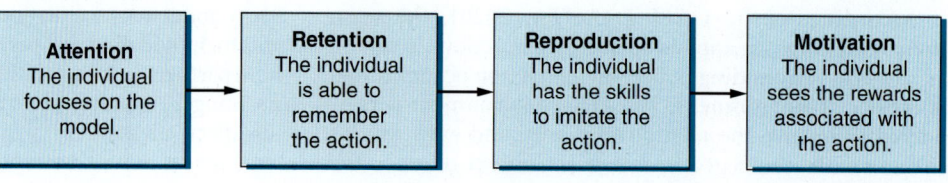

FIGURE 13-1. Process of social learning. There are four prerequisites for social learning to occur: attention, retention, reproduction, and motivation.

| Attention The individual focuses on the model. | → | Retention The individual is able to remember the action. | → | Reproduction The individual has the skills to imitate the action. | → | Motivation The individual sees the rewards associated with the action. |

Speech act theory posits that language is used to achieve goals or tasks, and speech acts are units of communication with specific intentions. The theory has helped shed light on the complex relationship between language and action, and it has contributed to people's understanding of how language shapes their social reality. Everything people say can be classified into one of several categories of speech acts, based on the underlying intention and the social context in which the utterance is spoken. Examples of speech acts can include requests, suggestions, comments, commands, or responses.

The development of speech acts begins in early childhood as children learn to communicate and interact with others. Initially, children use language primarily to make requests and convey their basic needs, such as asking for food or expressing discomfort. As their language skills develop, they begin to use language to perform a wider range of speech acts, such as making statements, asking questions, and expressing opinions. Understanding the intended effects of language use beyond the literal meaning of the words is also critical to successful communication. For example, the utterance "Can you open the window?" in one instance might be a very literal question about another's ability to open a window, whereas in another circumstance the underlying intention may be a request that the listener open a nearby window.

Relevance theory for effective communication conversation began with a set of principles for conversation proposed by Grice (1989). Conversational partners expect each other to follow a set of four maxims (or rules) to ensure smooth communication. These rules state that turns within a conversation must be informative, relevant, truthful, and clear (Grice, 1989). The importance of these rules becomes clear when examples of their violation are highlighted. For example, a student telling their friend "Class was absolutely fascinating today" has violated the maxim of truthfulness if they in fact found their class boring that day.

Sperber and Wilson (1995) then extended upon Grice's maxims to develop relevance theory. Relevance theory attempts to explain how people interpret and understand language in communication. The theory proposes that communication is most effective when the information conveyed is relevant to the listener's goals and expectations. It argues that people process information in a selective manner, attending to the most relevant aspects of a message while ignoring irrelevant or redundant information.

Relevance theory also suggests that communication involves a joint effort between the speaker and the listener, with both parties engaging in inferential processes to arrive at a mutually understood meaning. This means that the speaker should provide enough contextual clues and information to enable the listener to make inferences and understand the intended meaning. The listener, on the other hand, should be able to use their own background knowledge and context to make inferences and arrive at the intended meaning.

Attachment Theory

Attachment theory, developed by Bowlby in 1969, has greatly influenced our understanding of how emotional connections develop between infants and caregivers. It is often used to explain the negative impact of deprivation, neglect, and maltreatment on young children. Attachment theory is applied in infant mental health, but it is also used to explain

problems that older children and adults experience with relationships later in life. The theory posits a child needs to feel that their needs will be met to develop a sense of security and confidence, and that needs are met through the complementary relationship between infant and caregiver. The mother is often described as the primary attachment figure in early writings, but the individual who serves as the primary attachment figure can be any individual who serves this role. This person serves as a source of comfort and is the one the individual turns to when feeling fear or anxiety.

Four attachment styles have been described and linked to social behaviors throughout the life span, particularly as they relate to peer and romantic relationships: (1) secure attachment, (2) insecure–avoidant attachment, (3) insecure resistant/ambivalent attachment, and (4) disorganized/disoriented attachment (Hazen & Shaver, 1987).

Attachment experiences are thought to shape mental representations of social relationships, and these representations are used to organize and process social information (Bowlby, 1969/1982). In this way, attachment is thought to lay the foundation for emotional responses, recognition and understanding of emotions, and emotional regulation. Secure attachment may also be foundational in facilitating organized conversations about emotions between children and attachment figures that support empathy and attunement to the emotions of others (Stern & Cassidy, 2018).

Attachment theory is particularly useful when designing preventive interventions. At-risk parents may be taught parenting skills that allow for the development of secure attachment. Foster and adoptive parents can also benefit from understanding the attachment needs of children who have not developed secure attachment. Interventions for older children and adults focus on adaptive coping strategies and emotion regulation.

Communication and Social Skills in Individuals With Mental Health Conditions

Mental health conditions can result in impairments in communication and social skills; in fact, in some cases, these impairments are a core manifestation of the condition. The following section describes some mental health conditions for which communication and social skills present significant challenges.

Autism

Autism is characterized by social communication difficulties and restricted or repetitive behaviors or interests (American Psychiatric Association [APA], 2022). Inherent in the diagnostic criteria of autism are differences in the way individuals communicate and read cues in social settings; these differences are apparent in early childhood and persist into adulthood.

Early studies observed some children on the autism spectrum tended to use gestures, initiate conversations, and respond to questions with less frequency than nonautistic children (Bartak et al., 1975). There is a tendency for some to use a narrowed range of communicative acts to have their needs met (Casenhiser et al., 2015) and omit relevant information or be overly verbose during social interactions (Tager-Flusberg et al., 2005). Recognizing and responding to the emotional states of others are also areas of social difficulty for some autistic individuals (Kinnaird et al., 2019).

Adults on the autism spectrum attribute a sense of discomfort with participating in social interactions to difficulties understanding implied meanings, interpreting and using nonverbal cues, making socioemotional inferences, and producing impromptu responses (Müller et al., 2008), attesting to the lasting nature of pragmatic language difficulties for individuals on the autism spectrum. All domains of pragmatics are impacted (i.e., introduction and responsiveness, nonverbal communication, social-emotional attunement, executive function, negotiation), so it is imperative that interventions for autistic children and adults can address this broad range of skills.

Various theories have been used to explain the social interaction differences of individuals on the autism spectrum. From the perspective of social cognition theory, some have hypothesized that difficulties with theory of mind can explain difficulties in conversation and social interaction, particularly within groups of people when there are multiple perspectives and mind states to track (Baron-Cohen et al., 1985; Wu et al., 2020). Weak central coherence has also been used to explain some of the social difficulties for those on the autism spectrum.

Individuals on the autism spectrum tend to have strengths related to detecting specific information. For example, autistic individuals often perform well on tasks that involve searching for an object within a set of objects. Conversely, they may have trouble integrating information into a whole. This pattern is described as a preference for local over global processing. When applied to a social interaction, information of interest might be processed over the more salient information needed for sense making in an interaction.

Attention Deficit-Hyperactivity Disorder

ADHD is a neurodevelopmental disorder characterized by symptoms of inattention, hyperactivity, and impulsivity that can interfere with daily functioning (APA, 2022). Individuals with ADHD may interrupt frequently, have trouble following a conversation, or struggle to listen attentively. They may also be more impulsive and struggle to regulate their emotions, which can impact their ability to empathize and interact effectively with others.

One of the key challenges individuals with ADHD can face is maintaining attention and focus during conversations. Difficulty with impulse control may also result in behaviors that are perceived as inappropriate or disruptive, such as interrupting, blurting out inappropriate comments, or failing to take turns. Therefore, people with ADHD may miss important details, struggle to understand the context of a conversation, or be perceived as rude or disrespectful by others. This in turn can impact their ability to build and maintain relationships, as others may perceive them as uninterested or unengaged. In addition to these challenges, individuals with ADHD may struggle with regulating their emotions, which

may result in becoming easily frustrated or overwhelmed, which can lead to outbursts or social withdrawal (Ros & Graziano, 2018).

Trauma and Stressor-Related Disorders

Trauma and stressor-related disorders, such as posttraumatic stress disorder (PTSD) and attachment disorders, can result from experiencing or witnessing a traumatic event or series of events, such as abuse, neglect, or exposure to violence (APA, 2022). Trauma can affect an individual's sense of safety, trust, and well-being, and is a substantial risk factor for mental health problems across the life span.

PTSD is characterized by symptoms such as intrusive thoughts or memories, avoidance, negative changes in mood or thinking, and changes in physical and emotional reactions (APA, 2022). A history of maltreatment is associated with an elevated risk of language and social skills difficulties for some school-age children (Lum et al., 2018) and increased problems with social skills during adolescence (Pierce et al., 2022).

By definition, attachment disorders are conditions that include difficulties with social relationships with attachment figures and others (APA, 2022). Reactive attachment disorder and disinhibited social engagement disorder are both related to severe neglect, but they manifest in different ways. With reactive attachment disorder, a child might exhibit internalizing or externalizing behaviors, have difficulty with empathy, or be emotionally withdrawn. With disinhibited social engagement disorder, the child approaches unfamiliar adults in an overly familiar way. Children with attachment disorders also tend to have basic impairments in communication. For example, one study found that children with reactive attachment disorder had impairments in use of language and reciprocal social interaction that was comparable to autistic children (Sadiq et al., 2012).

Although the research is only beginning to examine the long-term impact of trauma and stressor-related disorders on communication and social skills, there is promising data indicating that most children with reactive attachment disorder and some children with disinhibited social engagement disorder will no longer have symptoms after receiving adequate care (Zeanah & Gleason, 2015). Therefore, OTPs can work with parents to develop parenting skills that promote attachment—be it with the child's biological parents or the adoptive or foster parents of a child with an attachment disorder.

With appropriate care from a mental health practitioner, the psychological symptoms of PTSD can be reduced. OTPs are well placed to address the associated social difficulties given that the principles of occupational therapy align with trauma-informed principles for practice (Fette et al., 2019; see Chapter 5: Trauma-Informed Practice and Chapter 25: Trauma- and Stressor-Related Disorders).

Anxiety Disorders

Anxiety disorders are a group of mental health conditions characterized by excessive and persistent feelings of fear, worry, and unease that are out of proportion to the actual danger or threat (APA, 2022). Specific anxiety disorders include generalized anxiety disorder, panic disorder, and social anxiety disorder. Social anxiety disorder is characterized by a fear of interacting or talking with others, which interferes with daily routines, relationships, and other activities such as work or school.

Social anxiety is associated with social and communication difficulties and is a common co-occurrence with autism. Anxiety symptom severity has also been associated with lower levels of social skills in young people with ADHD (Bishop et al., 2019). Although social communication difficulties are not universal among those with social anxiety, longitudinal research suggests that social communication difficulties underlie social anxiety for some children (Pickard et al., 2017). A recent meta-analysis also found that social cognition, specifically theory of mind, rather than emotion recognition accounted for elevated social anxiety in nonautistic children (Pearcey et al., 2021; see Chapter 18: Anxiety Disorders).

Schizophrenia

The socialization challenges experienced by individuals with schizophrenia appear to be associated with cognitive ability; however, the actual impairments in schizophrenia often are more subtle than those on the autism spectrum. Relative to individuals without schizophrenia, persons with schizophrenia can be challenged by tasks requiring emotional recognition across a range of sensory modalities, including the recognition of negative emotions such as fear and sadness in facial expressions and vocal inflection (Tseng et al., 2013).

The presence of schizophrenia symptoms (i.e., hallucinations, delusions, and disorganized thoughts) has also been associated with emotional processing difficulties, such as difficulty identifying pleasant or happy emotions, which researchers believe may be because of the tendency of persons with psychosis to attribute fear or sadness to any stimulus.

Individuals with schizophrenia also appear to have relatively intact social reciprocity and language but are limited in their ability to use social cues to provide information about social exchanges (Green, 2016). An individual with schizophrenia may engage in a conversation but fail to notice or misinterpret facial and other nonverbal cues that indicate, for example, that the person is becoming angry or wants to disengage from the conversation. These challenges result in significant social disconnection, such as restricted friendships and family relationships, minimal participation in social activities, and significant loneliness (Green et al., 2017; see Chapter 23: Schizophrenia Spectrum and Psychotic Disorders).

Personality Disorders

Individuals with personality disorders are often described by others in terms such as "difficult to deal with," "touchy," "manipulative," or "self-centered." These interpretations speak to the impact of the person's challenging behaviors on their interpersonal relationships. Some of the cognitive factors associated with personality disorders can negatively impact social behavior. For instance, persons with personality disorders tend to exhibit an egocentric view of their circumstances, which may limit their ability to empathize with the feelings of others. A lack of insight into one's behavior renders the person unable to realize the role that their own behavior plays in creating interpersonal difficulties, and thus the person may blame others for conflicts they experience and therefore be resistant to change.

Cognitive inflexibility, sometimes referred to as "black and white thinking," is common in individuals with personality disorders and can make it difficult to self-correct behaviors. Cognitive inflexibility may also result in limited emotional response flexibility, with predictable behaviors such as shutting down or escalating behaviors when experiencing strong feelings. Difficulties with emotion regulation, such as poor impulse control and outbursts, may lead others to question the individual's character, rather than attributing the inconsistency of interactions to the disorder itself, often resulting in interpersonal relationships characterized by distress and distrust (Tyrer et al., 2015; see Chapter 22: Personality Disorders).

Substance Use Disorders

Rather than considering substance use as deviant or risky behavior, the normalization thesis of drug use posits that some individuals are more likely to use illicit substances when their use is widespread (Williams, 2016). The initiation and perpetuation of substance use appears to be at least partially related to one's peer group; that is, individuals are more likely to use drugs and alcohol when their peer group endorses a particular substance. Whether or not this use becomes a disorder is dependent on several factors; however, peer group use and cultural acceptance are potential precipitating factors. There is some evidence that perceived use as compared with actual use has a greater impact on substance abusers (Deutsch et al., 2015). Substance abusers tend to overestimate the amount of substances their peer group uses (e.g., for adolescent cigarette and marijuana use).

Consequently, one of the challenges for individuals with substance abuse who are working toward recovery is disengaging from friends or family members who encourage substance use. Specific communication and socialization issues for this population include developing assertiveness skills to refuse offers of substances and finding alternative venues and activities for socialization that do not involve using (see Chapter 24: Substance-Related and Addictive Disorders).

Assessment of Communication and Social Skills

Communication and socialization are dynamic and multifaceted processes that can be challenging to assess. People should consider how they moderate their own communication and social skills as they interact with family, friends, acquaintances, supervisors, and teachers. They should also reflect on how many interactions occur regularly with a variety of community members, such as store employees, neighbors, government officials, and health-care professionals, as well as how their ability to interact effectively may vary

The Lived Experience

Leah Berman

The last time I wrote about my experience with autism spectrum disorder, I was just graduating high school (6 years ago), and I didn't have as much knowledge and insight about my diagnosis as I do now. I was also dealing with undiagnosed depression and anxiety, though I didn't fully understand that I was depressed/anxious at the time. Six years ago, I was having great difficulty socializing, which is pretty classic for autistic children and adults, and I'm thankful to say that socializing is becoming a lot easier for me these days, though it can still be difficult sometimes.

As a child, my mom was the first one to pick up on my autism. I showed classic signs as a young child; I wouldn't respond to my parents if they called for me (I actually ended up getting my hearing checked later on in the second grade because of this). Other signs were that when people would come over, I'd hide behind the couch so that I wouldn't have to interact with them, and I didn't have much of an interest in talking to people who weren't my close friends and family members.

I was clinically diagnosed with ASD at 4 years old, and I vaguely remember sitting in a doctor's office at our local Children's Hospital with my parents while my pediatric doctor talked to us about the diagnosis. I received treatment soon after in the form of RDI (Relational Development Intervention), which heavily involved my family members in my socialization to put me back onto a "typical" developmental path. I also saw an RDI specialist for about 3 or 4 years, and though I don't remember what we did together, I remember feeling frustrated that I had to keep going to see her. I wanted to know why I was being treated differently since I just wanted to be like every other kid. I didn't understand what was happening to me, and it was exhausting to experience that.

High school was a pretty challenging time for me, and it became more important than ever to have a group of close friends nearby. At the end of grade 10, I joined a new group of friends, after having spent the first 2 years with one group of people. I loved my new friends, we always ate lunch together and in grade 12, we decided we would try a new restaurant and get bubble tea every Friday.

It was fantastic to have that group, but I still struggled a lot with interacting with people who I didn't know/acquaintances, and there were many times where I would remain completely (or almost completely) silent around classmates and people I didn't know well, because I genuinely didn't know how to make conversation with them, and because my mind would go completely blank. It was an awful experience to go through, and I found I was constantly rating my social interactions as either wins, or fails. Every win felt great, but didn't last long, and every fail felt crippling, and like the embarrassment of it would last forever. I don't judge myself quite as harshly these days, but I do notice myself doing this behavior sometimes.

I still struggle with socializing in certain scenarios. It can feel like everyone has a manual of social norms and expectations, and my copy got lost in the mail, and I find myself being silent in many conversations that I would actually like to contribute to. Oftentimes, I find that hanging out with people for extended periods of time can be really draining, and if I don't take necessary breaks to recharge my social battery, I will get very tired and irritable.

The thing I struggle with the most nowadays in social situations is my own personal confidence. I'm often scared I will say something stupid, or a joke I have made won't land, or that I'll sound like a know-it-all if I correct someone or clarify something that I know about. And you know what? That does happen sometimes. Sometimes I make jokes that don't land, sometimes I ask something and ask myself later "why did I say that?", and sometimes I feel I can be a bit of a know-it-all. But the people who love and accept me love and accept me in spite of that.

Something I've struggled with for a long time is my own autistic identity, and whether I'm "autistic enough" (if such a thing even exists). I find myself saying "well, most people can't tell that I'm autistic, maybe I'm just putting on a show" and even "maybe the doctors were wrong, maybe I don't really have autism." I know that thinking like this isn't productive, because everyone on the autism spectrum is different. But it's difficult to live a life when you know that you have autism, but most people can't tell that you do. I have felt like an imposter for a good chunk of my life due to this, and it's frustrating knowing you are something, but people don't see you that way. Sometimes I even feel like I need to prove to others that I'm autistic. At the end of the day though, I don't need to prove myself to anyone, not even myself.

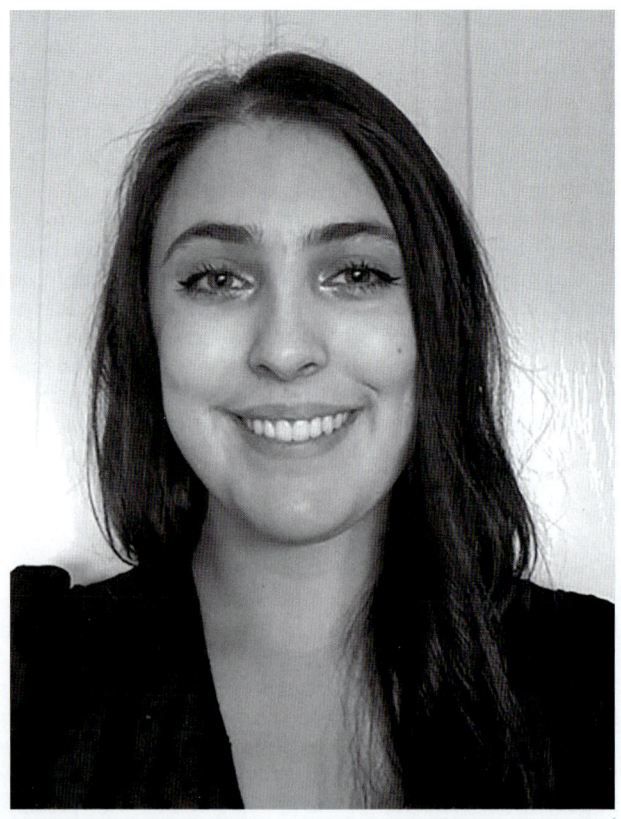

The Lived Experience—cont'd

I've gotten a therapist since the last time I wrote about having ASD, and she's helped me in ways that I didn't even think were possible. I started going after my first break-up to deal with depression and anxiety, and I've learned that it's important to be myself, no matter what people have to say about that. I feel more at peace with my identity, and less of an imposter as I grow up and become my own person.

You may be wondering, how am I doing now? I'm graduating university with my Bachelor's Degree of Arts, I've gotten some excellent job opportunities with the cooperative education program through my university, I have great friends (who I miss dearly, as our schedules never seem to line up), and I have a really great boyfriend, who is super supportive and is continuing to learn how to support my needs. I do still deal with a fair bit of anxiety, and some depression (though I'm not struggling with depression nearly as much as I used to), but I have faith that one day, I'll be able to deal with things that I struggle with in a healthier way.

depending on the situation. To evaluate a person's communication and social skills, it is important to examine how they can utilize these skills to achieve positive outcomes across a range of social contexts.

There are various ways to evaluate communication and social skills, including self-report, rating scales completed by others, and in-context observation. Each method has its benefits and limitations. Assessment that relies on reports from the person or others are straightforward to conduct, offer convenience for OTPs, and require little training to both administer and interpret. However, the accuracy of the information gathered from the person is determined by the person's cognitive ability and interest in completing questionnaires, which can be influenced by age, mental health status, or motivation. Conversely, relying on rating scales completed by others (e.g., parents) may be constrained by the fact that they may be aware of the person's social interaction behaviors only in a particular setting (e.g., home). This can lead to challenges in fully capturing the breadth of social and communication skills.

Observation, on the other hand, provides information on behaviors during social exchanges and can be conducted in natural or contrived contexts. Frequently, OTPs can conduct observations in a specific social context that requires intervention. For instance, an OTP may observe the child interacting with peers or teachers if they are struggling in a school setting. Alternatively, the OTP may observe the individual engaging in real-life interactions with a spouse or friend if the challenges arise within personal relationships. However, it is noteworthy that the observed behaviors are limited to specific social contexts and circumstances, such as social interactions within the home, school, or workplace, as well as the individuals with whom one interacts.

In addition, follow-up discussions help understand the perspective of all parties after the observation occurs. For example, the OTP may notice that a person tends to share overly personal information that appears to make others uncomfortable. The OTP can check in with both the individual and those they are conversing with to ensure that these observations are accurate.

Table 13-1 provides a summary of selected assessment tools for the evaluation of social and communication skills. As evident, assessing social and communication skills is complicated because it entails evaluating numerous distinct, interrelated skills used in various social situations with different individuals across diverse contexts. It is therefore difficult for a single assessment tool to comprehensively measure all aspects of social and communication skills (Cordier et al., 2015).

In addition to the assessment tools listed in Table 13-1, there are other measures involving social and communication skills as components of the assessment. For example, the Test of Playfulness (ToP; Skard & Bundy, 2008) is used to evaluate a child's playfulness via direct observation or video recordings of a child's free play with peers in natural play settings. The ToP can provide useful information regarding the child's social and communication skills, including engagement, initiation, negotiation, supporting others, sharing in social play, and the ability to read and respond to social cues. Another example is the Vineland Adaptive Behavior Scale-3 (Vineland-3; Sparrow et al., 2016), which evaluates the adaptive behaviors of individuals across all ages. In addition to assessing daily living and motor skills, it can examine communication skills and socialization.

For individuals with a diagnosis of autism, two assessment tools are available for evaluating social and communication skills associated with the autistic characteristics—the Social Communication Questionnaire (SCQ; Rutter et al., 2003) and the Social Responsiveness Scale–Second Edition (SRS-2; Constantino, 2012). These tools can help identify specific areas of socialization that are challenging for individuals on the autism spectrum and can be targeted for intervention (Bölte et al., 2011). The SCQ is designed for children age 4 years and older to assess social interaction, communication, and repetitive behavior patterns.

The SCQ Lifetime Form is used for diagnostic screening of autism, whereas the Current Form is used to track changes in behavior over time. Similarly, the SRS-2 is used to identify social impairment associated with autism and quantify severity. It includes four forms for different age groups: Preschool Form (ages 2.5 to 4.5 years), School-Age Form (4 to 18 years), Adult Form (ages 19 and up), and Adult Self-Report Form (ages 19 and up). The first three forms can be administered by adults familiar with the person, and input from multiple perspectives (such as parents and teachers) is beneficial. The total score reflects the severity of social impairment, and five treatment subscale scores are provided: social awareness, cognition, communication, motivation, and restricted interests and repetitive behavior.

TABLE 13-1 | Therapeutic Reasoning Assessment Table: Communication and Social Skills

Which Tool?	Who Was This Tool Designed For?	What Is Required of the Person? Can They Use the Tool?	What Am I Measuring?	How Long Does It Take and Where Do I Administer This Assessment?	Is the Tool Associated With a Practice Model?
Preschool and Kindergarten Behavior Scales–2nd Edition (PKBS-2; Merrell, 2003)	Children ages 3–6 years	Scales completed by a variety of behavioral informants, such as parents, teachers, and other caregivers	To evaluate social skills and problem behaviors of young children: • Social skills: social cooperation, social interaction, social independence • Problem behaviors: externalizing/explosive, attention problems/overactive, antisocial/aggressive and internalizing (social withdrawal), and anxiety/somatic problems	8–12 minutes; can be completed at home, at school, or in the clinic	N/A
Social Skills Improvement System–Rating Scales (SSIS-RS; Gresham & Elliott, 2008)	Individuals or small groups ages 3–18 years	Three forms: self-report (ages 8–18 only), parent-report, and teacher-report	To measure social skills and problematic behaviors: • Social skills: communication, cooperation, assertion, responsibility, empathy, engagement, and self-control • Problem behaviors: externalizing, internalizing, hyperactivity/inattention, autism spectrum, and bullying • Academic competence: reading, math, motivation, parent support, general impressions of cognitive functioning	10–25 minutes; can be completed at home or school	N/A
Evaluation of Social Interaction (ESI; Fisher & Griswold, 2014)	People over 2 years of age into older adulthood at any level of social interaction	An observational instrument during natural social exchanges with typical social partners	Social interaction skills in natural context with typical social partners during occupations: • Social skills that relate to initiating and ending a social interaction, producing the interaction, physically supporting the interaction, shaping the content and maintaining the flow of the interaction, verbally supporting the interaction, and adapting to problems that might arise during the interaction	Less than 1 hour for administration and scoring in the familiar environment (clinical or community)	Occupational Therapy Intervention Process Model (Fisher, 2009)
Home and Community Social Behavior Scales (HCSBS; Merrell & Caldarella, 2000) & School Social Behavior Scales –2nd Edition (SSBS-2; Merrell, 2002)	Children and youth ages 5–18 years	HCSBS completed by parents, group home supervisors, and other community-based raters; SSBS-2 completed by teachers	To evaluate students' social competence and antisocial behaviors across the school (SSBS-2), home, and community settings (HCSBS)" • Social competence regarding adaptive and positive social behavior (e.g., cooperates with peers in a variety of situations, remains calm when problems arise, behaves appropriately in a variety of situations) • Antisocial behavior (e.g., blames others for their problems, gets into fights, teases and makes fun of others)	<10 minutes; can be completed at home, community, and school	N/A

TABLE 13-1 | Therapeutic Reasoning Assessment Table: Communication and Social Skills—cont'd

Which Tool?	Who Was This Tool Designed For?	What Is Required of the Person? Can They Use the Tool?	What Am I Measuring?	How Long Does It Take and Where Do I Administer This Assessment?	Is the Tool Associated With a Practice Model?
Assessment of Communication and Interaction Skills (ACIS; Forsyth et al., 1998)	Children through older adults	Person is observed in a natural context that involves interaction	To measure social interaction and communication during context of carrying out an occupation: • Physicality: nonverbal communication such as eye contact and gestures • Information exchange: language/ conversational skills (ability to articulate and initiate and sustain a conversation) • Relations: skills in developing a connection with others (social norms and establishing rapport)	1 hour for administration and scoring in the real-life environment (home, school, work)	Model of Human Occupation (Kielhofner, 1995)
Pragmatics Observation Measure (POM; Cordier et al., 2019)	Children ages 5–11 years	The children in peer–peer interactions during free and uninterrupted play are videoed	To evaluate childhood pragmatic language skills: • Introduction/ responsiveness (introducing communication and being responsive to social interactions with peers) • Nonverbal communication (interpreting and using nonverbal communication) • Social-emotional attunement (understanding and using emotional reactions and intentions of peers) • Executive function (higher level thinking in interactions) • Negotiation (appropriate negotiation techniques when interacting with peers)	15–20 minutes for scoring and rating on the video-recorded interaction	N/A
Children's Communication Checklist, Second Edition (CCC-2; D. V. M. Bishop, 2006)	Children and youth ages 4–16 years	Checklist completed by an adult who has regular contact with the child, usually a parent, teacher, therapist, or other professional	To screen communication skills of children: • Language: speech, syntax, semantics, coherence • Pragmatics: initiation, scripted language, context, nonverbal communication, social relations, interests	5–10 minutes; can be completed at home, school, or clinic	N/A
Triple C: Checklist of Communication Competencies (Bloomberg & West, 2009)	Adolescents and adults (20–70 years) who have severe or multiple disabilities	Checklist completed by support workers and caretakers who are familiar with the person	To evaluate cognitive and early communication skills at five stages: • Unintentional passive (e.g., awareness of sounds, voices) • Unintentional active (e.g., reaches or moves toward familiar people in familiar situations) • Intentional informal (e.g., uses people to get objects) • Symbolic: basic (e.g., gives or shows an object to a person to obtain an action) • Symbolic: established (e.g., cause/effect relationships)	A few days for observation in person's home or day service during daily routines. A speech pathologist or other communication specialist scores the checklist to determine the person's communication level.	Developmental model

Intervention

An array of intervention approaches are available to support the social and communication needs of people on the autism spectrum, as well as those with ADHD and other mental health conditions. This section aims to explore psychosocial interventions across the life span, from childhood to adulthood, and to consider the current evidence for these interventions. This section also considers the role of OTPs in implementing these intervention approaches. Some interventions target the environment to enable social and communication skills, whereas other interventions directly target building these skills.

In most cases, it is likely that OTPs will need to consider using a combination of environmental and person-focused individual or group interventions. OTPs should also be guided by evidence-based practice when seeking to support a person's social and communication needs. This includes understanding the evidence of the intervention approach they are implementing, considering their practice context and resources and the person's unique skills and circumstances, while using outcome measures to monitor process before and after an intervention is provided (Cordier & Wilkes-Gillan, 2021).

Interventions for Children and Youth

A large body of research is dedicated to the investigation of interventions targeting the social and communication skills of children and youth. Eleven systematic reviews containing 256 studies are summarized in the text that follows. These systematic reviews evaluated *social skills training (SST) interventions* for children with ADHD (Storebø et al., 2019) and on the autism spectrum (Tanner et al., 2015), *peer-mediated interventions (PMIs)* for autistic children and children with ADHD (Aldabas, 2020; Chang & Locke, 2016; Cordier et al., 2018), *play-based interventions* for autistic children (Kent et al., 2020; O'Keeffe & McNally, 2021) and children with ADHD (Cornell et al., 2018), *communication interventions* for autistic children (Parsons et al., 2017), and *occupation-based* (Cahill et al., 2020) and *social participation-based interventions* (Tanner et al., 2015).

Social Skills Training

Social skills training (SST) is based on principles from social learning theory, positing social skills can be learned from observation, modeling, reinforcement, and generalization (Bandura, 1977). SST is led by a therapist and usually occurs in groups of children with similar difficulties or the same diagnoses. Group sessions are preferred as they allow for more interaction and practice with others. The goal of SST is to develop specific skills used to interact and communicate with others but to also enhance overall functioning and reduce social difficulties (Storebø et al., 2019).

Having stronger social skills can make success in many areas of occupational performance easier to achieve; for example, enhanced social skills are important for team sports, playing on the playground, and getting along with others in the classroom. SST are often conducted in clinic-based settings and involve 50- to 90-minute sessions for 8 to 12 weeks. Parent groups often run concurrently to give parents the opportunity to assist their children in learning and applying the skills taught (Storebø et al., 2019).

SST typically involves the following sequence presented in Table 13-2, which describes the process for each step in SST (Bellack et al., 2012). A core principle of SST is the importance of repeated practice for a skill to become established. Building a person's confidence in their ability to actually use the skill before implementing it outside the group is an important aspect of SST.

Although SST is often used for children with ADHD, a systematic review of 25 randomized controlled trials (RCTs) found it was not an effective intervention for this population (Storebø et al., 2019). However, Tanner and colleagues (2015) reported strong evidence for social skills groups for autistic children.

For children on the autism spectrum, group-based SST in a clinic setting was found to increase social communication and positive interactions. Moreover, group-based SST in schools or summer camps had medium to large effect sizes and was found to increase children's social skills and joint engagement on the playground (Tanner et al., 2015). These findings are further supported by three systematic reviews that found clinic-based and contextual SST groups improved the social competency and social participation of children with a diagnosis of autism (Rao et al., 2008; Schreiber, 2011; White et al., 2007; see Table 13-3).

Peer-Mediated Interventions

Peer-mediated interventions (PMIs) are an extension of peer involvement in interventions, whereby the peer is a key and active agent of change within the intervention. In PMIs, peers are trained to provide instruction and to facilitate social interactions with selected children (Cordier et al., 2018).

An advantage of PMIs is that they can be incorporated into a child's natural, everyday social context and involve children they regularly interact with. Usually typically developing peers are selected for PMIs and are nominated by a teacher or therapist on the basis of having well-developed social and communication skills as well as similar interests to the child receiving the intervention (Cordier et al., 2018). Peers are then provided with strategies relevant to the intervention and engage in role-play with the teacher or therapist. Peers learn strategies such as how to approach another child and invite them to play, share a toy, talk about what they are doing, and promote interaction (Chang & Locke, 2016).

A specific example of a PMI is Stay, Play, Talk. This particular approach is used with preschoolers. The peer is taught to stay next to a friend, play with their friend or use similar toys, and talk to the friend by asking questions, making comments, or giving compliments (Barber et al., 2016).

Although PMIs are an emerging intervention approach for use with children with ADHD, they have been more frequently implemented for autistic children. Tanner and colleagues (2015) reported PMIs to have moderate evidence for children on the autism spectrum, reporting on six RCTs where gains in social skills were found. In a systematic review of PMIs, Chang and Locke (2016) also found strong evidence that this approach can result in improvements in language and social skills for children on the autism spectrum. These are similar findings to those reported by Aldabas (2020), where PMIs were also found to improve the social skills of autistic children. Although no PMIs were found in the review by Cordier and colleagues (2018), findings indicated

TABLE 13-2 | Steps in Social Skills Training

Skill Step	Process	Example
Identify the skill.	• Provide a rationale for why the skill is important. • This step typically includes asking participants for suggestions.	• Joining an ongoing conversation
Discuss the steps of the skill.	• Skill is broken down into components. • Steps are posted or provided in a handout so participants can follow. • Steps may also be shown in a video clip with model demonstrating desired and undesired skills in an appropriate scenario.	• Stand close by and listen to the conversation, then wait for a break in the conversation. • Move closer once you know the topic of the conversation. • Make a comment that is relevant to the conversation.
Model the skill.	• Leaders model the skill in a role-play.	• As the role-play takes place, group members are encouraged to watch for the steps and give feedback.
Practice the skill.	• Each group member practices the skill in a role-play.	• Typically, a group member participates in a role-play with a leader(s). • It is useful to have someone who is relatively skilled go first. • Peers then practice with each other within the group.
Provide positive reinforcement.	• Provide specific feedback about what the participant did well. • This step includes eliciting feedback from group members.	• "I really like how you looked toward the other people as you joined the conversation." • "Great job identifying the topic of 'movies' and talking about the new releases at the movies."
Provide corrective feedback.	• Provide brief, nonjudgmental, and specific feedback. • Focus on one or two things that are most important. • This step also includes eliciting feedback from group members.	• "You could present yourself with more confidence when asking to join the group. For example, speak in a tone of voice that is easy to hear." • "You could pretend to read a book or have a drink of water while you stand by and listen in on the topic of conversation."
Assign homework.	• Participants are given an assignment to practice the skill before the next group meeting. • The assignment can include asking individuals to identify a particular situation in which they will try out the skill. • The assignment may require participants to complete a worksheet after completing homework.	• "During the next week, find an opportunity to practice joining a conversation. When might there be a situation in which you could practice this skill next week?"
Review homework.	• In the subsequent session, homework is reviewed. • Ask participants for specific information about implementation of the skill with positive reinforcement and corrective feedback provided as needed.	• Provide positive feedback for participants who successfully completed homework and encouragement and problem-solving to participants who did not.

moderate improvement in social skill outcomes for children with ADHD following peer inclusions interventions. See Being a Psychosocial OT Practitioner and Table 13-3.

Communication Interventions

The interventions described in the text that follows are examples of interventions that aim to promote children's communication in the context of social interactions and play. These interventions are most commonly provided to young children on the autism spectrum and focus on two-way communication skills. These interventions target children's ability to communicate their needs, their joint and shared attention, and their nonverbal and socioemotional communicative skills.

Joint Attention Training

One of the most basic skills of reciprocity in communication involves joint attention. Joint attention is often a skill that distinguishes very young children on the autism spectrum (Warreyn et al., 2014). Joint attention can include a parent and child looking at the same page in a book, and the child pointing with the expectation that the parent will look.

One manualized joint attention program is Joint Attention in Symbolic Play for Engagement and Regulation (JASP/ER). This intervention gives parents and teachers strategies for promoting joint attention (Lawton & Kasori, 2012). Intervention involves setting up the play environment, engaging the child in play, modeling and promoting joint attention, and encouraging eye contact.

In a systematic review of pragmatic language interventions for autistic children (Parsons et al., 2017) that reported a small-medium intervention effect, JASP/ER was the most frequently researched intervention ($n = 6$). Joint attention interventions have also been reported to have strong evidence (Tanner et al., 2015; see Table 13-3).

Developmental Individual-Differences Relationship-Based (DIR) Floortime

The DIR Floortime model was developed by Greenspan and Wieder in the 1980s. The intervention is most often used with

TABLE 13-3 | Systematic Reviews of Psychosocial Interventions to Improve Social and Communication Skills in Children and Youth

Study/Aim	Included Studies	Participants/Outcomes	Interventions	Main Results/Conclusions
Cornell et al. (2018) Play-based interventions	• Seven studies (single subject design excluded) • Three interventions across seven studies	• 127 *ADHD children ages 5–11 years* • Social play (n = 3) • ADHD symptoms (n = 3) • Pragmatic language (n = 2)	• Clinic-based play therapy (8, 2x weekly, 45 minutes) • School-based play therapy (16, 1x weekly, 30 minutes) • Clinic play-based intervention (7, 1x weekly, 1 hour)	• Positive outcomes reported in all seven studies. • Cannot yet be considered an evidence-based practice, but it is a promising practice.
Kent et al. (2020) Interventions to improve play skills	• 19 studies • All RCTs (inclusion RCT design only) • Meta-analysis (n = 11)	• 1,149 *autistic children ages 2–12 years* • Play outcome (n = 19) • Parent-report (n = 1) • Observations of child's behavior (n = 18)	• Preschool/school-based (n = 10) • Community-based (n = 1) • Clinic-based (n = 5) • Home-based (n = 2) • Clinic and home (n = 1)	• Small significant effect • Significant improvement (n = 15); not significant (n = 4) • Findings support play-based interventions with focus on social environments
O'Keeffe & McNally (2021) Play-based interventions in educational contexts	• Nine studies • RCT (n = 3) • Multiple baseline (n = 3) • AB single case (n = 2) • Within subject (n = 1)	• 107 *autistic children* • 43 *autistic children waitlist control groups* • Ages 3–13 years • Outcomes: social communication outcomes (n = 9)—inclusion criteria	• Special schools (n = 3) • Mainstream schools (n = 6) • Within classroom play (n = 4); nonclass/playground (n = 5) • Average 21 minutes for 2–34 weeks) • Social play with peers (n = 6) • Guided, adult involved (n = 9)	• Promising evidence for social communication skills through play in education • Positive findings (n = 3) • Mixed findings (n = 6) • Research gaps in interventions in naturalistic educational settings
Storebø et al. (2019) Evidence of SST	• 25 RCTs (across 45 reports)	• *ADHD children and youth ages 5–18 years* • 2,690 participants Outcomes: • Social skills, behavior, emotional competence	• SST • Cognitive behavioral therapy • Multimodal psychosocial • Child life and attention skills • Challenging horizon program • Metacognitive training • Behavior therapy	• No clinically relevant treatment effect of interventions on teacher rated: *social skills, emotional competencies, or general behavior*
Parsons et al. (2017) Pragmatic language interventions	• 21 studies (reporting on 18 interventions)	• *Autistic children/youth* • 925 participants • 21 months to 14 years • No studies had participants age 15–18 years	• Various modifications of JASP/ER (n = 4) • Building Blocks program • Emotion recognition • Mind reading computer program • Group setting (n = 9) • Clinic setting (n = 15)	• Effect sizes ranged from 0.16–1.29 in pre-/postintervention within group's analysis • 24% large effect • 29% medium effect • 29% small effect • 18% < 0.2 effect size
Boshoff et al. (2020) Child outcomes—DIR/Floortime	• Nine studies • RCT (n = 3) • Pretest/posttest (n = 5) • Single case design (n = 1)	• *Autistic children* • N = 392 • 2–12 years Outcomes: • Social, communication, autism symptoms	• DIR/Floortime (n = 9); 6–52 weeks • With speech therapy, sensory integration (n = 1) • Six studies average >10 hours per week (DIR recommended minimum is 2–5 hours per day)	• Outcomes: mostly improved socio-emotional skills • Evidence is emerging. Use should be supported by sound clinical reasoning, fidelity, and valid outcome measures.

TABLE 13-3 | Systematic Reviews of Psychosocial Interventions to Improve Social and Communication Skills in Children and Youth—cont'd

Study/Aim	Included Studies	Participants/Outcomes	Interventions	Main Results/Conclusions
Chang & Locke (2016) Peer-mediated interventions	• Five studies • Four RCTs • One pretest/posttest design	• Autistic children (preschool to high school) • N = 260 Outcomes: social skills	• School setting (n = 4) • Camp setting (n = 1) • Four studies in classroom and one on playground	• All studies reported improved social skills. • Two studies reported effect sizes on social outcomes: effect sizes were small (d = 0.23) to large (d = 0.74)
Aldabas (2020) PMI for autistic children	• 16 studies • All multiple-baseline design	• Autistic (n = 51) 3–14 years • Peer participants (n = 78) Outcomes: • Engagement (n = 2) • Social skills (n = 8) • Social interaction (n = 8) • Communication (n = 3)	• Peer-mediated (n = 5) • Peer training (n = 5) • Peer network strategy (n = 2) • Buddy system (n = 1) • Socialization opportunity (n = 2) • Peer tutoring (n = 1)	• Positive results for 11 of 12 studies that measured social skills suggest PMI effective • Four studies measured communication skills and reported improvements
Cordier et al. (2018) Peer inclusion interventions for ADHD children	• 17 studies • RCTs and controlled quasi-experimental studies	• 2,567 participants ages 6–16 years • ADHD participants (n = 2,284) Outcome: • Social functioning (n = 17)	• SST (n = 7) • Behavioral treatment (n = 3) • Behavioral and SST (n = 2) • Multimodal (n = 5) • Peer use: Peer-mediated (n = 0), peer involvement (n = 16), peer proximity (n = 1)	• Limited evidence to support or contest efficacy • Pre/post-effect sizes ranged from 0.17 (small) to 1.34 (large) • Moderate improvement in social skills following peer inclusion interventions
Cahill et al., (2020) Occupational therapy interventions for mental health, behavior, and social participation	• 62 studies with activity- and occupation-based interventions	• 5,222 Children and youth with/at risk for mental health concerns or controls • 5–21 years Outcomes: mental health or positive behavior or social participation	• Outdoor groups/camps (n = 8) • Video/computer games (n = 8) • Productive occupations and life skills (n = 4) • Yoga (n = 11), meditation (n = 6) • Animal-assisted (n = 6) • Creative arts (n = 5) • Play (n = 8), sports (n = 6)	• Moderate to strong evidence for use of yoga and sports • Moderate-strength evidence for use of play, creative arts • Low-strength evidence for animal-assisted intervention, meditation, video/computer games, and productive occupations
Tanner et al. (2015) Interventions for social participation, play, leisure, and restricted and repetitive behaviors	• 66 studies • Systematic review (n = 17) • RCT (n = 21) • Nonrandomized (n = 7) • Pretest/posttest (n = 10) • Multiple baseline (n = 1)	• Autistic children Outcomes: • Social skills (n = 36) • Social communication (n = 19) • Play (n = 4) • Leisure (n = 4) • Restricted and repetitive behaviors (n = 4)	• Social skills groups • PMIs • Activity-based interventions • Computer-based intervention • Social stories • PECS • Parent-mediated • Sensory motor interventions • Joint attention interventions • DIR-Floortime • Social-pragmatic intervention	• Strong evidence for social skills groups, PECS, joint attention, and parent-mediated interventions for social participation • Moderate evidence for peer-mediated and naturalistic behavior interventions • Mixed evidence for social stories • DIR mixed evidence, small gains, or no effect

Being a Psychosocial OT Practitioner

Using Peer Mediation to Facilitate Positive Experiences on the Playground

Identifying Psychosocial Strengths and Needs

OTPs in private pediatric practice often work with children at school who have difficulty with handwriting and other fine motor skills related to class-based work, such as cutting with scissors, which impacts their in-class participation. Some children may also have psychosocial needs like impulse control and pragmatic language use. These psychosocial needs can impact their social participation on the playground, peer play, and friendships.

Consider the story of Harry, a first-grade student in mainstream school. Harry is an only child and has a supportive family and teacher. He plays weekly soccer on a community team with five other children from his class. His school has a teacher and staff on duty as playground monitors. They also have a "find a friend bench" where children can sit if they need help finding peers to play with. Because of his challenges with engaging in fine motor activities during class, he attends weekly fine motor occupational therapy sessions at his school.

Harry often acts impulsively, swinging his legs while sitting on his chair and accidentally kicking or bumping his OTP in sessions. He talks off-topic and needs excessive prompting to listen and respond to what his OTP asks him. He also has difficulty noticing and responding to nonverbal cues given by his OTP, such as folding arms, serious tone of voice, sighing, or tapping his table as if "waiting" for him to listen. On the other hand, Harry reported to his OTP that other children don't want to play with him at lunchtime and run away from him. He also reported teachers told him on the playground to go and play somewhere else when he tried playing on the equipment and didn't understand why.

Harry's IQ is above average, and his academic achievement across all areas is average. After a recent pediatrician review, Harry was found to have elevated ADHD symptoms but did not meet the criteria for a formal ADHD diagnosis. Harry's teacher reports that in class, Harry is interested in his peers and clowns to get their attention and often talks to them to try to make friends. However, he often does this at inappropriate times (such as during a spelling test). His teacher reported that she is not usually on playground duty. However, she has noticed peers become annoyed by Harry when he talks off-topic or acts impulsively, such as grabbing and throwing their hats when they wait in the class line.

Using a Holistic Occupational Therapy Approach

Harry's OTP decides to conduct a playground observation at lunchtime, using the Pragmatics Observational Measure (POM) and ToP to understand better Harry's social play and communication skills on the playground.

While on the playground, Harry's OTP observed that he enjoyed playing, regularly approached his peers, and was interested in their games and conversations. He even rushed eating his lunch to be ready to run onto the playground as soon as eating time was over (reflecting the ToP element—*intrinsic motivation*). When using the equipment, Harry pushed past children and refused to take turns on the slide—running back up the slide as soon as he'd gone down (ToP element—*internal control*). When playing tag, he grabbed at children's shirts and pulled them rather than tapping them, and he pushed others in front of him so others didn't tag him. When his peers screamed "Ouch!" and put their hands up in front of them or turned away, he didn't seem aware he was being too rough and did not change his actions in response to their cues (ToP element–*skills related to framing*; POM area—*nonverbal communication*).

When one of Harry's peers tagged him lightly and said "You're it," Harry responded aggressively, trying to push him and saying, "Liar!" (POM areas—*social-emotional attunement* and *negotiation*). As the bell rang, one of Harry's peers said, "*Tomorrow we could make tag more fun by having a safe zone and playing stuck in the mud tag.*" Harry replied, "*Once I ran so fast, I beat everyone in a running race—that's how fast I am at running*" (POM area—*introduction/responsiveness*).

The OTP explored how play-based interventions using typically developing playmates could support Harry's social participation on the playground at school. The OTP collaborated with Harry's teacher to ensure the strategies suggested fit within their usual class routine and that the strategies wouldn't be too time-consuming for his teacher. The OTP came up with the following plan:

Applying Play-Based Intervention Involving Peer Mediation

Activity: Applying a clinical intervention to a school setting

Teacher's Role	Peers' Role	Playground Monitor Role
• Whole class discussion about what "green play" (great play—Keep going!) should be on their playground and what "red play" (stop and think) should be. • Teacher to help the class to come up with "three things to remember" while they play (e.g., [1] Tell our friend "Too rough" if the play is rough. [2] Call a teacher for help if needed. [3] Share ideas about the rules). • Have the discussion just before lunch 3 days of the week to help children remember just before they go out to play. • Have a class discussion straight after lunch as a feedback session of what went well and what needs to be remembered or changed for tomorrow when playing together.	• OTP asks the teacher to select three class peers to have a special role. • Peers need to have well-developed social and communication skills and similar interests to Harry. • Peers are trained by OTP to "help make play fun for everyone" on the playground. • Peers are trained to negotiate rules of a game, give clear messages with their voices and body actions, and call a teacher if play gets too rough. • Remind friends to do "green play" and show them how.	• Approach a group of children if their play appears to be similar to "red play." • Involve the children in a problem-solving discussion about how to make it "green play" again. Get them to come up with the steps (e.g., combine ideas so everyone is happy with the rules, then start a new game). • Help the children understand the perspective of another (e.g., why did you think your friend was lying?).

Reflective Questions

1. How would you justify the importance of developing Harry's social and communication skills to his parents (given they originally came to you for fine motor support)?

2. How could you also work individually with Harry and his parents to build his knowledge of social skills? Which social skills intervention approach would you consider for application?

3. How could you help Harry's parents generalize these strategies to his weekly soccer games?

Evidence-Based Practice

Play-Based Interventions for Children With ADHD

Play is a promising intervention approach for children with ADHD.

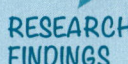

RESEARCH FINDINGS

In a systematic review of play-based interventions for children with ADHD, positive intervention outcomes were reported in all studies. The authors concluded play is a promising intervention approach for children with ADHD (Cornell et al., 2018). For autistic children, Kent and colleagues (2020) found play-based interventions had a small but significant treatment effect. When evaluating play-based interventions in education contexts for children with autism, O'Keeffe and McNally (2021) concluded there is promising evidence for using play-based interventions to promote socialization for autistic children in educational settings. For children and youth with mental health concerns, play interventions had moderate-strength evidence for supporting social participation (Cahill et al., 2020).

APPLICATIONS

➡ OTPs should strongly consider using play-based interventions for autistic children and children with ADHD.

➡ When utilizing a play-based approach, outcome measures should be implemented, and other evidence-based intervention components should also be included such as parent training and involvement.

REFERENCES

Cahill, S. M., Egan, B. E., & Seber, J. (2020). Activity- and occupation-based interventions to support mental health, positive behavior, and social participation for children and youth: A systematic review. *The American Journal of Occupational Therapy, 74*(2), 7402180020p1–7402180020p28. https://doi.org/10.5014/ajot.2020.038687

Cornell, H. R., Lin, T. T., & Anderson, J. A. (2018). A systematic review of play-based interventions for students with ADHD: Implications for school-based occupational therapists. *Journal of Occupational Therapy, Schools, & Early Intervention, 11*(2), 192–211. https://doi.org/10.1080/19411243.2018.1432446

Kent, C., Cordier, R., Joosten, A., Wilkes-Gillan, S., Bundy, A., & Speyer, R. (2020). A systematic review and meta-analysis of interventions to improve play skills in children with autism spectrum disorder. *Review Journal of Autism and Developmental Disorders, 7*(1), 91–118. https://doi.org/ 10.1007/s40489-019-00181-y

O'Keeffe, C., & McNally, S. (2021). A systematic review of play-based interventions targeting the social communication skills of children with autism spectrum disorder in educational contexts. *Review Journal of Autism and Developmental Disorders, 10*(1), 51–81. https://doi.org/10.1007/s40489-021-00286-3

autistic children. DIR Floortime takes a developmental approach based on emotions, which are considered essential for language, cognitive, social, and motor development. Sessions are child-led, focusing on joint and shared attention, pretend play, and conversations, and can involve sensory activities. There is an emphasis on parent–child interactions, which are supported by a therapist. DIR Floortime guidelines recommend a minimum of 2 to 5 hours per day of treatment (Boshoff et al., 2020).

Although DIR Floortime is often readily used in private pediatric practice, little research has been conducted. In a systematic review of nine studies (Boshoff et al., 2020), three studies reported a significant improvement on one aspect of socioemotional development and three studies reported a significant improvement on one aspect of communication. The results of the review were mixed, with not all children making improvements and several nonsignificant improvements reported. Compared with other interventions, studies in this systematic review reported a high number of therapy hours per week, with six studies reporting an average of over 10 hours per week.

The authors conclude that higher quality research into this intervention is urgent and needed to determine its evidence base. Because of the quality and number of studies, they also recommend that use of this approach is supported by sound clinical reasoning and use of valid and reliable outcome measures. These recommendations, and the fact that 10 hours of therapy per week may not be feasible for a majority of families, need to be an important consideration for OTPs implementing this model (see Table 13-3).

Picture Exchange Communication System

The **Picture Exchange Communication System (PECS)** is a widely used, protocol-driven method that allows individuals

PhotoVoice

Communication

Sometimes the perception of children on the autism spectrum is that they are cognitively unable to be independent and are always unable to understand the world outside of theirs, but that is not always the case. The ability to communicate, and to figure out how to get the information taken in by the autistic individual, is most of the time the issue. Branden uses a book (yellow) called the PECS Book to ask for food, his sippy cup, juice or milk, and the cars picture either for his toys or to go for a ride; that one he knows very well. When he was in the hospital, I wanted to make sure that any of the health-care workers walking in the room knew that Branden has some verbal skills.

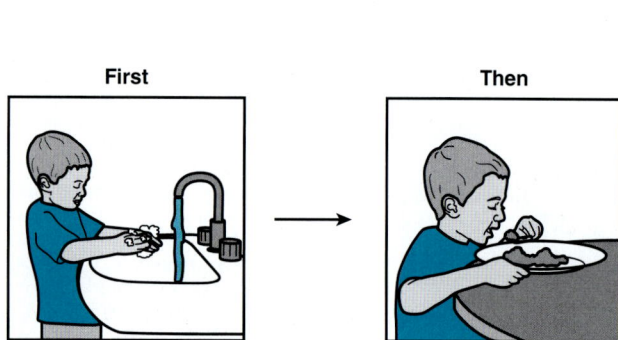

I have Autism.

I have some verbal skills.

I understand some verbal commands.

Ask me "What do you want?" then give me a few seconds to respond physically or verbally, if you need to ask me again.

If you start by saying "I want" usually I will respond.

I love my aunt and she loves me more. (Written by my sister)

It was important for me to make sure everyone knew how to communicate with Branden, without me having to say it all the time. —Veronica

How might health-care workers have responded differently to Branden if his mother had not provided the list of bullet points?

---

with limited verbal communication to use pictures to express their wants or needs (Bondy & Frost, 1998). This augmentative and alterative communication (AAC) tool includes extensive training for the individual who will be using the system. A card with a picture or symbol of the intended message is given to another individual to initiate a social contact and to communicate a want or need. For example, a picture of a computer may indicate the person wants to get on the computer. The process for learning to use PECS is divided into six phases:

1. *How to communicate:* The individual exchanges a picture with another individual to indicate that they want something.
2. *Distance and persistence:* The individual learns how to generalize the system to different people and places and to be persistent when communicating.
3. *Picture discrimination:* The individual chooses pictures, which are then placed in a communication book for use in communication.
4. *Sentence structure:* Pictures are used together to make a sentence, such as an "I want" picture with a drink picture to indicate "I want a drink."
5. *Answering questions:* Pictures are used to answer the question, "What do you want?"
6. *Commenting:* Questions are expanded to things such as "What do you see?" with sentence answers such as "I see a dog."

Visual supports were used to prepare autistic children before undergoing dental procedures, with most able to tolerate dental procedures including fillings (Cagetti et al., 2015). Two systematic reviews found strong evidence for PECS in improving communication and social interaction for individuals on the autism spectrum (Iacono et al., 2016; Tanner et al., 2015) and that it was particularly helpful for young children

FIGURE 13-2. First–Then communication board for washing hands before eating. Visual supports can prepare the individual for new situations by communicating what will happen.

(preschool-age) and autistic individuals with a co-occurring intellectual disability (see Table 13-3).

Additional Strategies to Support Communication

Visual supports use pictures or text to promote communication with individuals who have limited verbal language. For example, a First–Then communication board depicts a two-step sequence, as shown in Figure 13-2. After a two-step sequence is mastered, more steps are added to communicate the steps to a routine. A bedtime routine can be communicated by including pictures for (a) brushing teeth, (b) putting on pajamas, (c) reading a story, and (d) sleeping.

Social stories use a written format to introduce and teach appropriate behavior to children on the autism spectrum (Kokina & Kern, 2010). Social stories are typically used to prepare a child before they enter a difficult situation, such as riding a school bus, going to a doctor, or attending a birthday party. A social story must include the following statements:

1. *Descriptive:* communicates the situation and people involved in it
2. *Perspective:* describes the reactions, feelings, and responses of others
3. *Directive:* explains the appropriate action
4. *Cooperative:* describes what others will do to help
5. *Affirmative:* validates the values of a culture
6. *Control:* provides strategies for using appropriate behaviors; statement developed by the child

Different types of visual supports are rarely implemented in isolation and usually form one component of an intervention. There is mixed evidence to support social stories (Tanner et al., 2015; see Table 13-3).

Interventions for Youth and Adults

As individuals reach adolescence and adulthood, the focus of interventions shifts to meet their changing occupational needs. For older youth and young adults, interventions expand in their aims to support social functioning in the context of academic achievement and employment. Interventions also aim to build and strengthen individuals' social network, through group-, peer-, and family-supported interventions. For individuals in older adulthood, interventions focus on enhancing social participation and quality of life and reducing loneliness.

Seven systematic reviews or literature reviews containing 175 intervention studies are summarized in the text that follows. These reviews include *SST* (Dubreucq et al., 2022) and *nonpharmacological interventions* for autistic adults and adults with other mental health conditions such as schizophrenia (Speyer et al., 2022; Webber & Fendt-Newlin, 2017). The reviews also include *early intervention* to improve performance in occupations (Read et al., 2018), *social participation* (Webber & Fendt-Newlin, 2017), *social network* (Brooks et al., 2022), *group peer support* (Lyons et al., 2021), and *occupational therapy* (Kirsh et al., 2019) interventions for people experiencing mental health conditions.

Social Skills Training

SST for adolescents and adults follows the same format as SST interventions provided to children. The **Program for the Education and Enrichment of Relational Skills (PEERS)** is an example of an evidence-based SST program focused more explicitly on the making and keeping of friends for autistic adolescents and young adults (Laugeson et al., 2015). Some of the topics included in the program include use of humor, handling teasing, participating in social media, asking someone on a date, and handling rejection. This manualized program of 16 sessions is similar to other social skills programs in its didactic teaching of a skill, use of role-play, feedback, and homework.

A unique aspect of the PEERS program is the inclusion of caregivers who act as coaches to promote the practice and implementation of skills taught. Caregivers attend a separate but concurrent session and learn how to provide the coaching tailored specifically to the needs of the adolescent or young adult. Caregivers include parents, job coaches, life coaches, and peer mentors. Also unique to PEERS is an ecologically valid approach to identifying the steps of skills through obtaining data from individuals who demonstrate these skills successfully. One example would be to address verbal bullying behavior through a range of data-informed steps, one of which includes a short and smart verbal comeback, rather than ignoring the bully.

Although few studies exist evidencing SST for adolescents and adults with ADHD, SST has been more extensively researched for autistic adolescents and adults. In a systematic review of 41 nonpharmacological interventions for autistic adults (Speyer et al., 2022), social functioning interventions were the most studied. Further, the PEERS program was found to have the strongest evidence for social skills improvement. Individual studies also demonstrate that parents participating in the intervention had greater self-efficacy regarding their skills as a parent of an autistic young person (Karst et al., 2015). The study also found that the intervention reduced parental stress and family chaos. These findings are supported by a systematic review of SST interventions for autistic adults that reported an overall positive effect of the intervention (Dubreucq et al., 2022; see Table 13-4).

Cognitive behavioral social skills training (CBSST) is a manualized intervention example of a cognitive SST approach. CBSST is designed to facilitate the acquisition of social skills for individuals with schizophrenia (Granholm et al., 2016). CBSST is based on recovery principles and combines cognitive skills training and problem-solving skills training with SST.

Each area of training consists of a module, each of which includes six sessions, for a total of 18 sessions. The developers recommend that participants progress through the intervention once and then be offered a second opportunity to participate, to allow for more practice and consolidation of the skills. The cognitive component of this intervention uses a cognitive behavioral approach and focuses on helping participants develop more positive ways of thinking. The social skills model uses role modeling, role-play, positive reinforcement, corrective feedback, shaping, and homework assignments to promote skill acquisition and application to real-life situations. The problem-solving module teaches a systematic strategy to help participants solve immediate problems and prepare to manage future problems.

In a systematic review of nonpharmacological interventions for autistic adults (Speyer et al., 2022), 11 studies were cognitive skills training interventions. Most studies reported significant outcomes following intervention. Three studies reported significant, large intervention effects and one a significant moderate effect for improving quality of life. A systematic review of interventions to improve performance in occupations for youth and young adults with mental health conditions concluded cognitive strategies can be implemented by OTPs to enhance socialization (Read et al., 2018).

Efficacy studies of CBSST for schizophrenia have compared the intervention to supportive group therapy focused on goal attainment for life skills (Granholm et al., 2013, 2014). Compared with supportive group therapy, CBSST was most distinctive in terms of reducing self-defeatist attitudes; in fact, participants with these attitudes benefited most from the intervention. For older adults, both approaches were effective in improving functioning and reducing symptom distress (Granholm et al., 2013). In young and middle-aged adults, CBSST was more effective than supportive group therapy for improving functioning and negative symptoms (Granholm et al., 2014; see Table 13-4).

TABLE 13-4 | Reviews of Psychosocial Interventions to Improve Social and Communication Skills in Youth and Adults

Study/Aim	Included Studies	Participants/Outcomes	Interventions	Main Results/ Conclusions
Dubreucq et al. (2022) Social skills training—Autism *Systematic review*	• 18 studies (five were randomized controlled trials [RCTs])	Autism spectrum disorder ($n = 676$) Social outcomes: • Vocational SST • Social knowledge • Empathy • Social contact frequency • Loneliness/psychiatric symptoms	• Four of the RCTs used a 14–16 session adult adaptation of the PEERS intervention • Two interventions for interview skills or job-based social skills • One combined CBT and SST, one social cognition and SST, and one romantic relationships social skill	• Five studies in meta-analysis ($n = 145$ adults - Overall nonsignificant positive effect of SST of 0.93 ($p = 0.39$) • > 15 sessions = small moderating effects on SST effectiveness • Five studies delivered in enriched environments (i.e., social learning in context and promotes skill generalization)
Speyer et al. (2022) Nonpharmacological intervention—Autism *Systematic review*	• 41 studies • All RCTs compared with one waitlist control ($n = 21$; 2) alternate intervention ($n = 13$; 3) treatment as usual ($n = 7$)	• Adults with autism ($n = 846$) • Controls ($n = 819$) • Mean age above 30 years ($n = 8$) • Inclusion of adults over 65 years ($n = 1$) Outcomes: • Social functioning • Behavior • Employment skills	Intervention categories: • Social functioning and language skills ($n = 20$) • Vocational rehabilitation outcomes ($n = 10$) • Cognitive skills training ($n = 7$) • Independent living skills ($n = 1$)	• Social functioning was the most studied intervention. • *PEERS for young adults* and *Project SEARCH plus ASD* support interventions had the strongest evidence (for social skills and employment, respectively). • Only two studies focused on language skills.
Read et al. (2018) Early intervention for performance in occupations—Mental health *Systematic review*	• 30 studies • Systematic review ($n = 6$) • RCTs ($n = 19$) • Pretest/posttest ($n = 5$)	• Youth and young adults (12–35 years) • With or at risk of serious mental illness (psychosis, depression, or anxiety) Social outcomes: • Social attainment ($n = 2$) • Social functioning ($n = 5$) • Social and occupational functioning ($n = 5$) • Constructive communication ($n = 1$)	• Cognitive remediation ($n = 7$) • Cognitive-behavioral therapy ($n = 9$) • Supported employment and supported education ($n = 6$) • Family psychoeducation (FPE; $n = 8$)	• Moderate to strong evidence for supported employment/supported education to improve social and occupational outcomes in employment and academics • Cognitive strategies can be implemented in occupational therapy to enhance socialization • OTPs to facilitate FPE because of training in promoting social and occupational functioning.
Webber & Fendt-Newlin (2017) Social participation interventions—Mental health conditions *Literature review*	• 19 studies • RCT ($n = 6$) • Nonrandomized control ($n = 4$) • Single group pre/post ($n = 5$) • Qualitative study ($n = 2$) • Case study ($n = 2$)	• Adults • Sample size not reported • Schizophrenia ($n = 5$) • Chronic/severe mental health problems ($n = 6$) • Depression ($n = 3$) • Psychoses ($n = 4$) Outcomes: • Social networks • Social relationships • Social functioning • Social-related QoL	• Individual SST • Groups skills training • Supported community engagement • Group-based community activities • Employment interventions • Peer support interventions	• Social network gains appear strongest for supported community engagement intervention • Overall, evidence was limited. • All studies reported improvements. • Significant improvement on at least one social outcome ($n = 6$). • Improvement on at least one social outcome ($n = 13$)

TABLE 13-4 | **Reviews of Psychosocial Interventions to Improve Social and Communication Skills in Youth and Adults—cont'd**

Study/Aim	Included Studies	Participants/Outcomes	Interventions	Main Results/ Conclusions
Brooks et al. (2022) Social network interventions—Mental health conditions *Systematic review*	• Nine studies • All RCTs	• 2,226 adult participants • Mean age 35.7 years • Schizophrenia or psychosis ($n = 4$) • Major depressive disorder ($n = 1$) • All types of mental health diagnoses ($n = 4$) Outcomes: • Enhanced social networks	• Intervention delivered in the community face-to-face ($n = 9$) • Health professional delivered ($n = 5$), duration 3–12 months Intervention categories: • Supported social activity ($n = 2$) • Peer support ($n = 2$) • Assertive community treatment ($n = 3$) • One-to-one intervention ($n = 2$)	• The current evidence base is of unclear quality. • Interventions that focused on supporting social activities appear to hold the most promise for enhancing social networks. • Effect sizes reported in four studies ranged from small (0.39) to medium (0.65)
Lyons et al. (2021) Group peer support interventions—Mental health conditions *Systematic review*	• Eight studies • All RCTs	• 2,131 participants • Common mental health conditions • Adults aged 18 years or over Outcomes: • Personal recovery • Clinical recovery • Acute mental health service use • Social outcomes (employment, social support, and social network)	• Interventions 3 weeks to 12 months Intervention categories: • Mutual support groups • Peer support groups Subintervention categories: • Antistigma ($n = 3$) • Self-management ($n = 4$)	• Meta-analyses are only possible for peer support groups. • Group peer support may make small improvements to overall recovery (not hope, clinical symptoms, or empowerment). • Evidence for effectiveness for outcomes which could not be meta-analyzed was mixed. • Most social outcomes were absent in the literature—only one study reported social outcomes, with no evidence of intervention effect.
Kirsh et al. (2019) Occupational therapy interventions—Mental health conditions *Literature review*	• 50 studies (13 RCTs, 9 other control groups, 15 pre/ post, 7 qualitative, 2 single case, 4 mixed methods)	• Psychiatric diagnosis Social outcomes: • Intrapersonal skills ($n = 1$) • School behavior ($n = 2$) • Interpersonal skills ($n = 1$) • Social functioning ($n = 3$) • Social activities ($n = 1$) • Social interaction and communication ($n = 2$)	• Seven categories of interventions • Employment/education • Psychoeducation • Creative occupations/ activity • Time use/occupational balance • Skills/habit development • Group/family approaches • Animal-assisted therapy	• Majority (68%) addressed occupation-based outcomes. • Only 10 studies reported a social outcome. • Most successful interventions are supported employment (SE) and individual placement and support (IPS); these enable vocational skills and competitive employment.

Social Participation Interventions

Social participation interventions for adults with mental health conditions focus on an additional component of building quality social connections, contacts, and relationships, as well as developing meaningful roles within the community. These interventions are delivered through individual SST, groups skills training, supported community engagement, group-based community activities or peer support interventions with an emphasis on quality of relationships, and having meaningful social roles outside mental health-care services (Webber & Fendt-Newlin, 2017).

One literature review (Webber & Fendt-Newlin, 2017) found there was limited evidence to support a social participation outcome from current intervention approaches,

finding some studies reported a significant improvement on at least one social outcome. More recent systematic reviews agreed the evidence base requires greater quality (Kirsh et al., 2019; Lyons et al., 2021), while also finding interventions that focused on supporting social activities appeared to hold the most promise for enhancing social networks (Brooks et al., 2022; see Table 13-4).

Here's the Point

■ Social and communication skills are influenced by person factors such as cognition, emotion, and language, as well as acquisition of specific performance skills and opportunities for interactions.

- Acquisition of social and communication skills can be partially explained by understanding the impact of cognition on social skills, importance of observation and modeling for skill attainment, bonding experience of infants, and the conversational functions of language use.
- Social and communication skill impairments are the predominant characteristic of autism and are common in other psychiatric conditions such as ADHD, trauma and stress-related disorders, anxiety disorders, schizophrenia, personality disorders, and substance use disorders.
- A single assessment tool is unlikely to measure all aspects of social and communication skills. Observation in a variety of settings, coupled with information from the person and/or others, will help understand communication and social skills comprehensively.
- Some interventions that address social and communication skills use environmental supports in the form of peer mediators or peer supports.
- Other interventions target the development of new skills using skills training approaches and therapeutic groups.

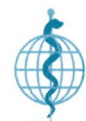 Visit the online resource center at **FADavis.com** to access the videos.

Apply It Now

1. Self-Assessment

Therapeutic use of self is a basic approach to SST. When a therapist is able to effectively model good communication in a variety of social settings, people actively learn. They should begin by assessing their own communication and social interaction skills, using the following guiding questions:

Reflective Questions
- What are your strengths and weaknesses as a communicator? What is your comfort level in social situations? What is your comfort level in leading groups? What is your comfort level in meeting new people?
- What interpersonal skills do you need to further develop? How do you plan to do so?
- How comfortable are you with collaborating with a person who is angry or agitated? Depressed?

- How will these communication skills be important in your future practice as an OTP.

2. Designing Visual Supports

Select a common self-care routine and design a First–Then communication board. Then create a larger visual schedule with multiple steps for the routine.

3. Beginning Steps to Design a Social Skills Training Module

Refer to Table 13-2 and examine the first two steps. Pick a social skill that is different from the example used in the table. Identify the skill (step 1) and then break the skill down into parts and create a handout that lists the components of the skill (step 2). Choosing a skill that is relatively simple and observable will make this task simpler.

Resources

General
- www.autismspeaks.org: This site has many resources for understanding communication issues in autism and strategies for communicating with autistic individuals.
- http://www.attachmentparenting.org: This site contains information and resources for developing effective parenting skills to promote secure attachment.
- https://www.samhsa.gov/recovery/peer-support -social-inclusion: This site has information and resources for peer support services for individuals with mental illness.

Interventions
- Program for the Education and Enrichment of Relational Skills (PEERS)
  - The UCLA PEERS intervention requires certification to provide. More information is available at http://www2.semel .ucla.edu/peers.
- Picture Exchange Communication System
  - Pyramid Education Consultants provides training and resources on the PECS: http://www.pecsusa.com.
- Stay, Play, Talk—Peer-Mediated Intervention
  - Ledford, J. R., Osborne, K., & Chazin, K. T. (2016). *Evidence-based instructional practices for young children with autism and other disabilities: Stay, play, talk procedures.* https://ebip .vkcsites.org/stay-play-talk-procedures

- Visual Supports
  - http://card.ufl.edu/resources/visual-supports
  - https://theautismprogram.illinois.edu/category/visual-supports

Videos
- "Child in Crisis" video. In this video, occupational therapist Brittany shares her experience working in a psychiatric rehab hospital's adolescent unit with Mikey, an 8-year-old boy presenting with a complex set of challenges. Diagnosed at birth with fetal alcohol syndrome, Mikey has a history of multiple ACEs. On admission, he presented with suicidal and homicidal ideation and symptoms consistent with PTSD. Brittany describes how she did her own research, learned more about Mikey, and developed an intervention that worked well for him and the other children in the group. Access the video at the online resource center at FADavis.com.
- "Occupational Therapy and Music Therapy in Early Head Start" video. In this video, an occupational therapist and music therapist discuss their unique and effective collaboration in a Head Start program. Running an 8-week group for infants and toddlers, the therapists assessed the children and established preventive goals linked to developmental milestones in areas such as self-regulation, awareness of self and others, attention, language, and motor movements. Access the video at the online resource center at FADavis.com.
- "Mary's Lived Experience as an Unhoused Individual and Her Occupational Therapist's Perspective" video. In this video, Mary provides a first-person account of being unhoused and the

tremendous impact occupational therapy services have had on her life. In addition, occupational therapist Quinn Tyminski describes working with Mary and shares her perspective on Mary's journey and transformation, including her improved conflict resolution and emotion regulation skills. Access the video at the online resource center at FADavis.com.

- "Laura's Experience as a Mother of an Autistic Son" video. Laura is the mother of an adult son, Will, who was diagnosed with autism at age 3. In this video, she describes what Will was like as a baby and what signs she and day-care teachers first noticed. She explains what the evaluation process was like and how it felt when she learned that her loving, talkative, playful child had autism. Occupational therapy, social skills therapy, speech therapy and other services—as well as intensely involved parents—laid the groundwork for Will to succeed in school and go on to fulfill his occupational dream as a young adult. Access the video at the online resource center at FADavis.com.
- "Tricks and Techniques From the Mother of an Autistic Son" video. In this video, Laura describes her and her family's creative and adaptive ways of helping their autistic son, Will, succeed. Giving several specific examples of solutions to common problem behaviors and challenges, Laura shares practical wisdom, "tricks and techniques" from 20 years of experience as the mother of an autistic son, with a focus on recognizing and focusing on Will's strengths. Access the video at the online resource center at FADavis.com.

References

Abbot-Smith, K., Dockrell, J., Sturrock, A., Matthews, D., & Wilson, C. (2023). Topic maintenance in social conversation: What children need to learn and evidence this can be taught. *First Language, 43*(6), 614–642. https://doi.org/10.1177/01427237231172652

Adams, C., Baxendale, J., Lloyd, J., & Aldred, C. (2005). Pragmatic language impairment: Case studies of social and pragmatic language therapy. *Child Language Teaching and Therapy, 21*(3), 227–250. https://doi.org/10.1191/0265659005ct290oa

Aldabas, R. (2020). Effectiveness of peer-mediated interventions (PMIs) on children with autism spectrum disorder (ASD): A systematic review. *Early Child Development and Care, 190,* 1586–1603. https://doi.org/10.1080/03004430.2019.1580275

American Occupational Therapy Association. (2020). Occupational therapy practice framework: Domain and process—Fourth edition. *American Journal of Occupational Therapy, 74*(Suppl. 2), 7412410010p1–7412410010p87. https://doi.org/10.5014/ajot.2020.74S2001

American Psychiatric Association. (2022). *Diagnostic and statistical manual of mental disorders* (5th ed, text revision). American Psychiatric Publishing.

Bandura, A. (1977). *Social learning theory.* Prentice Hall.

Barber, A. B., Saffo, R. W., Gilpin, A. T., Craft, L. D., & Goldstein, H. (2016). Peers as clinicians: Examining the impact of Stay Play Talk on social communication in young preschoolers with autism. *Journal of Communication Disorders, 59,* 1–15. https://doi.org/10.1016/j.jcomdis.2015.06.009

Baron-Cohen, S., Leslie, A. M., & Frith, U. (1985). Does the autistic child have a theory of mind? *Cognition, 21,* 37–46. https://doi.org/10.1016/0010-0277(85)90022-8

Bartak, L., Rutter, M., & Cox, A. (1975). A comparative study of infantile autism and specific development receptive language disorder. I. The children. *British Journal of Psychiatry, 126,* 127–145. https://doi.org.10.1192/bjp.126.2.127

Bellack, A. S., Mueser, K. T., Gingerich, S., & Agresta, J. (2012). *Social skills training for schizophrenia: A step by step guide.* Guilford Press.

Bishop, C., Mulraney, M., Rinehart, N., & Sciberras, E. (2019). An examination of the association between anxiety and social functioning in youth with ADHD: A systematic review. *Psychiatry Research, 273,* 402–421. https://doi.org/10.1016/j.psychres.2019.01.039

Bishop, D. V. M. (2006). *The Children's Communication Checklist* (2nd ed.). Pearson.

Bloomberg, K., & West, D. (2009). *The Triple C: Checklist of communication competencies.* SCOPE Vic. Ltd.

Bölte, S., Westerwald, E., Holtmann, M., Freitag, C., & Poustka, F. (2011). Autistic traits and autism spectrum disorders: The clinical validity of two measures presuming a continuum of social communication skills. *Journal of Autism and Developmental Disorders, 41,* 66–72. https://doi.org/10.1007/s10803-010-1024-9

Bondy, A. S., & Frost, L. A. (1998). The Picture Exchange Communication System. *Seminars in Speech and Language, 19,* 373–388. https://doi.org/10.1055/s-2008-1064055

Bosco, F. M., Parola, A., Sacco, K., Zettin, M., & Angeleri, R. (2017). Communicative-pragmatic disorders in traumatic brain injury: The role of theory of mind and executive functions. *Brain & Language, 168,* 73–83. https://doi.org/10.1016/j.bandl.2017.01.007

Boshoff, K., Bowen, H., Paton, H., Cameron-Smith, S., Graetz, S., Young, A., & Lane, K. (2020). Child development outcomes of DIR/Floortime™-based programs: A systematic review. *Canadian Journal of Occupational Therapy, 87*(2), 153–164. https://doi.org/10.1177/0008417419899224

Bowlby, J. (1969/1982). *Attachment and loss*: Vol. 1. *Attachment* (Original ed. 1969; 2nd ed. 1982). Basic Books.

Brooks, H., Devereux-Fitzgerald, A., Richmond, L., Bee, P., Lovell, K., Caton, N., Cherry, M. G., Edwards, B. M., Downs, J., Bush, L., Vassilev, I., Young, B., & Rogers, A. (2022). Assessing the effectiveness of social network interventions for adults with a diagnosis of mental health problems: A systematic review and narrative synthesis of impact. *Social Psychiatry and Psychiatric Epidemiology, 57*(5), 907–925. https://doi.org/10.1007/s00127-022-02242-w

Brooks, J. A., Chikazoe, J., Sadato, N., & Freeman, J. B. (2019). The neural representation of facial-emotion categories reflects conceptual structure. *Proceedings of the National Academy of Sciences, 116*(32), 15861–15870. https://doi.org/10.1073/pnas.1816408116

Cagetti, M. G., Mastroberardino, S., Campus, S., Olivari, B., Faggioli, R., Lenti, C., & Strohmenger, L. (2015). Dental care protocol based on visual supports for children with autism spectrum disorders. *Medicina Oral Patologia Oral y Cirugia Bucal, 20,* e596–e604. https://doi.org/10.4317/medoral.20424

Cahill, S. M., Egan, B. E., & Seber, J. (2020). Activity- and occupation-based interventions to support mental health, positive behavior, and social participation for children and youth: A systematic review. *The American Journal of Occupational Therapy, 74*(2), 7402180020p1–7402180020p28. https://doi.org/10.5014/ajot.2020.038687

Casenhiser, D. M., Binns, A., McGill, F., Morderer, O., & Shanker, S. G. (2015). Measuring and supporting language function for children with autism: Evidence from a randomized control trial of a social-interaction-based therapy. *Journal of Autism and Developmental Disorders, 45,* 846–857. https://doi.org/10.1007/s10803-014-2242-3

Chang, Y. C., & Locke, J. (2016). A systematic review of peer-mediated interventions for children with autism spectrum disorder. *Research in Autism Spectrum Disorder, 27,* 1–10. https://doi.org/10.1016/j.rasd.2016.03.010

Cole, J. (2015). Prosody in context: A review. *Language, Cognition and Neuroscience, 30*(1-2), 1–31. https://doi.org/10.1080/23273798.2014.963130

Constantino, J. N. (2012). *Social Responsiveness Scale™—Second Edition.* Western Psychological Services.

Cordier, R., Munro, N., Wilkes-Gillan, S., Speyer, R., Parsons, L., & Joosten, A. (2019). Applying Item Response Theory (IRT) modelling to an observational measure of childhood pragmatics: The Pragmatics Observational Measure-2. *Frontiers in Psychology, 10,* 408. https://doi.org/10.3389/fpsyg.2019.00408

Cordier, R., Speyer, R., Chen, Y. W., Wilkes-Gillan, S., Brown, T., Bourke-Taylor, H., Doma, K., & Leicht, A. (2015). Evaluating the psychometric quality of social skills measures: A systematic review. *PLoS One, 10*(7), e0132299. https://doi.org/10.1371/journal.pone.0132299

Cordier, R., Vilaysack, B., Doma, K., Wilkes-Gillan, S., & Speyer, R. (2018). Peer inclusion in interventions for children with ADHD: A systematic review and meta-analysis. *BioMed Research International, 2018,* 7693479. https://doi.org/10.1155/2018/7693479

Cordier, R., & Wilkes-Gillan, S. (2021). Evidence-based practice in occupational therapy. In T. Brown, H. M. Bourke-Taylor, S. Isbel, R. Cordier, & L. Gustafsson (Eds.), *Occupational therapy in Australia: Professional and practice issues* (2nd ed., pp. 183–200). Routledge.

Cornell, H. R., Lin, T. T., & Anderson, J. A. (2018). A systematic review of play-based interventions for students with ADHD: Implications for school-based occupational therapists. *Journal of Occupational Therapy, Schools, & Early Intervention, 11*(2), 192–211. https://doi.org/10.1080/19411243.2018.1432446?scroll=top&needAccess=true

Deutsch, A. R., Chernyavskiy, P., Steinley, D., & Slutske, W. S. (2015). Measuring peer socialization for adolescent substance use: A comparison of perceived and actual friends' substance use effects. *Journal of the Studies on Alcohol and Drugs, 76,* 267–277. https://doi.org/10.15288/jsad.2015.76.267

Dubreucq, J., Haesebaert, F., Plasse, J., Dubreucq, M., & Franck, N. (2022). A systematic review and meta-analysis of social skills training for adults with autism spectrum disorder. *Journal of Autism and Developmental Disorders, 52*(4), 1598–1609. https://doi.org/10.1007/s10803-021-05058-w

Fette, C., Lambdin-Pattavina, C., & Weaver, L. L. (2019). Understanding and applying trauma-informed approaches across occupational therapy settings. *OT Practice Magazine,* CE1–CE9.

Fisher, A. G. (2009). *Occupational Therapy Intervention Process Model: A model for planning and implementing top–down, client-centered, and occupation-based interventions.* Three Star Press.

Fisher, A. G., & Griswold, L. A. (2014). *Evaluation of social interaction* (3rd ed.). Three Star Press.

Forsyth, K., Salamy, M., Simon, M., & Kielhofner, G. (1998). *The Assessment of Communication and Interaction Skills (Version 4.0).* Model of Human Occupation Clearinghouse, Department of Occupational Therapy, College of Applied Health Sciences, University of Illinois at Chicago.

Granholm, E., Holden, J., Link, P. C., & McQuaid, J. R. (2014). Randomized clinical trial of cognitive behavioral social skills training for schizophrenia: Improvement in functioning and experiential negative symptoms. *Journal of Consulting and Clinical Psychology, 82,* 1173–1185. https://doi.org/10.1037/a0037098

Granholm, E., Holden, J., Link, P. C., McQuaid, J. R., & Jeste, D. V. (2013). Randomized controlled trial of cognitive behavioral social skills training for older consumers with schizophrenia: Defeatist performance attitudes and functional outcome. *American Journal of Geriatric Psychiatry, 21,* 251–262. https://doi.org/10.1016/j.jagp.2012.10.014

Granholm, E. L., McQuaid, J. R., & Holden, J. L. (2016). *Cognitive-behavioral social skills training for schizophrenia: A practical treatment guide.* Guilford Press.

Green, M. F. (2016). Impact of cognitive and social cognitive impairment on functional outcomes in patients with schizophrenia. *Journal of Clinical Psychiatry, 77*(Suppl 2), 8–11. https://doi.org/10.4088/JCP.14074su1c.02

Green, M. F., Horan, W. P., Lee, J., McCleery, A., Reddy, L. F., & Wynn, J. K. (2017). At issue: Social disconnection in schizophrenia and the general community. *Schizophrenia Bulletin, 15,* 242–249. https://doi.org/10.1093/schbul/sbx082

Gresham, F. M., & Elliott, S. N. (2008). *Social Skills Improvement System (SSIS)—Rating scales.* Pearson Assessments.

Grice, H. (1989). *Studies in the way of words.* Harvard University Press.

Hazen, C., & Shaver, P. R. (1987). Romantic love conceptualized as an attachment process. *Journal of Personality and Social Psychology, 52,* 511–524. https://doi.org/10.1037/0022-3514.52.3.511

Hein, S., Röder, M., & Fingerle, M. (2018). The role of emotion regulation in situational empathy-related responding and prosocial behaviour in the presence of negative affect. *International Journal of Psychology, 53*(6), 477–485. https://doi.org/10.1002/ijop.12405

Iacono, T., Trembath, D., & Erickson, S. (2016). The role of augmentative and alternative communication for children with autism: Current status and future trends. *Neuropsychiatric Disease and Treatment, 19,* 2349–2361. https://doi.org/10.2147/NDT.S95967

Javed, A., & Charles, A. (2018). The importance of social cognition in improving functional outcomes in schizophrenia. *Frontiers in Psychiatry, 9,* 157. https://doi.org/10.3389/fpsyt.2018.00157

Karst, J. S., Van Hecke, A. V., Carson, A. M., Stevens, S., Schohl, K., & Dolan, B. (2015). Parent and family outcomes of PEERS: A social skills intervention for adolescents with autism spectrum disorder. *Journal of Autism and Developmental Disorders, 45,* 752–765. https://doi.org/10.1007/s10803-014-2231-6

Kent, C., Cordier, R., Joosten, A., Wilkes-Gillan, S., Bundy, A., & Speyer, R. (2020). A systematic review and meta-analysis of interventions to improve play skills in children with autism spectrum disorder. *Review Journal of Autism and Developmental Disorders, 7*(1), 91–118. https://doi.org/10.1007/s40489-019-00181-y

Kielhofner, G. (1995). *A Model of Human Occupation: Theory and application* (2nd ed.). Williams & Wilkins.

Kinnaird, E., Stewart, C., & Tchanturia, K. (2019). Investigating alexithymia in autism: A systematic review and meta-analysis. *European Psychiatry, 55,* 80–89. https://doi.org/10.1016/j.eurpsy.2018.09.004

Kirsh, B., Martin, L., Hultqvist, J., & Eklund, M. (2019). Occupational therapy interventions in mental health: A literature review in search of evidence. *Occupational Therapy in Mental Health, 35*(2), 109–156. https://doi.org/10.1080/0164212X.2019.1588832

Kokina, A., & Kern, L. (2010). Social Story™ interventions for students with autism spectrum disorders: A meta-analysis. *Journal of Autism and Developmental Disorders, 40,* 812–826. https://doi.org/10.1007/s10803-009-0931-0

Laugeson, E. A., Gantman, A., Kapp, S. K., Orenski, K., & Ellingsen, R. (2015). A randomized controlled trial to improve social skills in young adults with autism spectrum disorder: The UCLA PEERS® Program. *Journal of Autism and Developmental Disorders, 45,* 3978–3989. https://doi.org/10.1007/s10803-015-2504-8

Lawton, K., & Kasori, C. (2012). Teacher implemented joint attention intervention: Pilot randomized controlled study for preschoolers with autism. *Journal of Consulting and Clinical Psychology, 80,* 687–693. https://doi.org/10.1037/a0028506

Lezak, M. D., Howieson, D. B., Bigler, E. D., & Tranel, D. (2012). *Neuropsychological assessment* (5th ed.). Oxford University Press.

Lum, J. A. G., Powell, M., & Snow, P. C. (2018). The influence of maltreatment history and out-of-home-care on children's language and social skills. *Child Abuse & Neglect, 76,* 65–74. https://doi.org/10.1016/j.chiabu.2017.10.008

Lyons, N., Cooper, C., & Lloyd-Evans, B. (2021). A systematic review and meta-analysis of group peer support interventions for people experiencing mental health conditions. *BMC Psychiatry, 21,* 315. https://doi.org/10.1186/s12888-021-03321-z

Matthews, D., Biney, H., & Abbot-Smith, K. (2018). Individual differences in children's pragmatic ability: A review of associations with formal language, social cognition, and executive functions. *Language Learning and Development, 14*(3), 186–223. https://doi.org/10.1080/15475441.2018.1455584

Merrell, K. W. (2002). *School Social Behavior Scales: Second Edition.* Assessment- Intervention Resources.

Merrell, K. W. (2003). *Preschool and Kindergarten Behavior Scales: Second Edition (PKBS-2).* Pro-Ed.

Merrell, K. W., & Caldarella, P. (2000). *Home and Community Social Behavior Scales.* Assessment-Intervention Resources.

Müller, E., Schuler, A., & Yates, G. B. (2008). Social challenges and supports from the perspective of individuals with Asperger syndrome and other autism spectrum disabilities. *Autism, 12,* 173–190. https://doi.org/10.1177/1362361307086664

O'Keeffe, C., & McNally, S. (2021). A systematic review of play-based interventions targeting the social communication skills of children with autism spectrum disorder in educational contexts. *Review Journal of Autism and Developmental Disorders, 10*(1), 51–81. https://doi.org/10.1007/s40489-021-00286-3

Parsons, L., Cordier, R., Munro, N., Joosten, A., & Speyer, R. (2017). A systematic review of pragmatic language interventions for children with autism spectrum disorder. *PloS One, 12*(4), e0172242. https://doi.org/10.1371/journal.pone.0172242

Pearcey, S., Gordon, K., Chakrabarti, B., Dodd, H., Halldorsson, B., & Creswell, C. (2021). Research review: The relationship between social anxiety and social cognition in children and adolescents: A systematic review and meta-analysis. *Journal of Child Psychology and Psychiatry, 62*(7), 805–821. https://doi.org/10.1111/jcpp.13310

Pickard, H., Rijsdijk, F., Happé, F., & Mandy, W. (2017). Are social and communication difficulties a risk factor for the development of social anxiety? *Journal of the American Academy of Child & Adolescent Psychiatry, 56*(4), 344–351. https://doi.org/10.1016/j.jaac.2017.01.007

Pierce, H., Jones, M. S., & Holcombe, E. A. (2022). Early adverse childhood experiences and social skills among youth in fragile families. *Journal of Youth and Adolescence, 51*(8), 1497–1510. https://doi.org/10.1177/0044118X21996378

Rao, P. A., Beidel, D. C., & Murray, M. J. (2008). Social skill intervention for children with Asperger's syndrome or high-functioning autism: A review and recommendations. *Journal of Autism and Developmental Disorders, 38*, 352–361. https://doi.org/10.1007/s10803-007-0402-4

Read, H., Roush, S., & Downing, D. (2018). Early intervention in mental health for adolescents and young adults: A systematic review. *The American Journal of Occupational Therapy, 72*(5), 7205190040p1–7205190040p8. https://doi.org/10.5014/ajot.2018.033118

Ros, R., & Graziano, P. A. (2018). Social functioning in children with or at risk for attention deficit/hyperactivity disorder: A meta-analytic review. *Journal of Clinical Child & Adolescent Psychology, 47*(2), 213–235. https://doi.org/10.1080/15374416.2016.1266644

Rutter, M., Bailey, A., & Lord, C. (2003). *The Social Communication Questionnaire*. Western Psychological Services.

Sadiq, F. A., Slator, L., Skuse, D., Law, J., Gillberg, C., & Minnis, H. (2012). Social use of language in children with reactive attachment disorder and autism spectrum disorders. *European Child and Adolescent Psychiatry, 21*, 267–276. https://doi.org/10.1007/s00787-012-0259-8

Schreiber, C. (2011). Social skills interventions for children with high-functioning autism spectrum disorders. *Journal of Positive Behavior Interventions, 13*, 49–62. https://doi.org/10.1177/1098300709359027

Schwarzer, N. H., Nolte, T., Fonagy, P., & Gingelmaier, S. (2021). Mentalizing and emotion regulation: Evidence from a nonclinical sample. *International Forum of Psychoanalysis, 30*(1), 34–45. https://doi.org/10.1080/0803706X.2021.1873418

Sheets, E., & Kraines, M. (2014). Personality disorder traits as a moderator of poor social problem-solving skills and depressive symptoms. *Journal of Individual Differences, 35*(2), 103–110. https://doi.org/10.1027/1614-0001/a000132

Skard, G., & Bundy, A. (2008). A Test of Playfulness. In L. D. Parham & L. S. Fazio (Eds.), *Play in occupational therapy for children* (pp. 71–94). Mosby Elsevier.

Skorich, D. P., May, A. R., Talipski, L. A., Hall, M. H., Dolstra, A. J., Gash, T. B., & Gunningham, B. H. (2016). Is social categorization the missing link between weak central coherence and mental state inference abilities in autism? Preliminary evidence from a general population sample. *Journal of Autism and Developmental Disorders, 46*, 862–881. https://doi.org/10.1007/s10803-015-2623-2

Sparrow, S. S., Cicchetti, D. V., & Saulnier, C. A. (2016). *Vineland Adaptive Behavior Scales, Third Edition (Vineland-3)*. Pearson.

Sperber, D., & Wilson, D. (1995). *Relevance: Communication and cognition* (2nd ed.). Blackwell.

Speyer, R., Chen, Y. W., Kim, J. H., Wilkes-Gillan, S., Nordahl-Hansen, A. J., Wu, H. C., & Cordier, R. (2022). Non-pharmacological interventions for adults with autism: A systematic review of randomised controlled trials. *Review Journal of Autism and Developmental Disorders, 9*(2), 249–279. https://doi.org/10.1007/s40489-021-00250-1

Stern, J. A., & Cassidy, J. (2018). Empathy from infancy to adolescence: An attachment perspective on the development of individual differences. *Developmental Review, 47*, 1–22. https://doi.org/10.1016/j.dr.2017.09.002

Storebø, O. J., Elmose Andersen, M., Skoog, M., Joost Hansen, S., Simonsen, E., Pedersen, N., Tendal, B., Callesen, H. E., Faltinsen, E., & Gluud, C. (2019). Social skills training for attention deficit hyperactivity disorder (ADHD) in children aged 5 to 18 years. *Cochrane Database of Systematic Reviews, 6*(6), CD008223. https://doi.org/10.1002/14651858.CD008223.pub3

Tager-Flusberg, H., Paul, R., & Lord, C. (2005). Language and communication in autism. In F. R. Volkmar, R. Paul, A. Klin, & D. Cohen (Eds.), *Handbook of autism and pervasive developmental disorders: Diagnosis, development, neurobiology, and behavior* (3rd ed., pp. 335–364). John Wiley & Sons, Inc.

Tanner, K., Hand, B. N., O'Toole, G., & Lane, A. E. (2015). Effectiveness of interventions to improve social participation, play, leisure and restricted and repetitive behaviors in people with autism spectrum disorder: A systematic review. *American Journal of Occupational Therapy, 69*, 6905180010p1–6905180010p12. https://doi.org/10.5014/ajot.2015.017806

Tseng, H.-H., Chen, S.-H., Liu, C.-M., Howes, O., Huang, Y.-L., Hsieh, M. H., Liu, C.-C., Shan, J.-C., Lin, Y.-T., & Hwu, H.-G. (2013). Facial and prosodic emotion recognition deficits associate with specific clusters of psychotic symptoms in schizophrenia. *PLoS One, 8*(6), e66571. https://doi.org/10.1371/journal.pone.0066571

Tyrer, P., Reed, G. M., & Crawford, M. J. (2015). Classification, assessment, prevalence, and effect of personality disorder. *The Lancet, 385*(9969), 717–726. https://doi.org/10.1016/S0140-6736(14)61995-4

Warreyn, P., van der Paelt, S., & Roeyers, H. (2014). Social-communicative abilities as treatment goals for preschool children with autism spectrum disorder: The importance of imitation, joint attention and play. *Developmental Medicine and Child Neurology, 56*, 712–716. https://doi.org/10.1111/dmcn.12455

Webber, M., & Fendt-Newlin, M. (2017). A review of social participation interventions for people with mental health problems. *Social Psychiatry and Psychiatric Epidemiology, 52*, 369–380. https://doi.org/10.1007/s00127-017-1372-2

White, S. W., Keonig, K., & Scahill, L. (2007). Social skills development in children with autism spectrum disorders: A review of the intervention research. *Journal of Autism and Developmental Disorders, 37*, 1858–1868. https://doi.org/10.1007/s10803-006-0320-x

Williams, L. (2016). Muddy waters?: Reassessing the dimensions of the normalisation thesis in twenty-first century Britain. *Drugs: Education, Prevention and Policy, 23*(3), 190–201. https://doi.org/10.3109/09687637.2016.1148118

Wu, H. C., Biondo, F., O'Mahony, C., White, S., Thiebaut, F., Rees, G., & Burgess, P. W. (2020). Mentalising and conversation-following in autism. *Autism, 24*(8), 1980–1994. https://doi.org/10.1177/1362361320935690

Zeanah, C. H., & Gleason, M. M. (2015). Annual research review: Attachment disorders in early childhood—Clinical presentation, causes, correlates and treatment. *Journal of Child Psychology and Psychiatry, 56*, 207–222. https://doi.org/10.1111/jcpp.12347

Time Use and Habits

Justin Newton Scanlan

The ways in which humans use their time and structure their days through routines and habits provide a unique insight into individuals' daily lives, occupational engagement, and strategies they use to maintain well-being. This chapter introduces the concepts of time use and habits and explains how occupational therapy practitioners (OTPs) can effectively understand an individual's occupational experience by exploring time use. It also explores what is understood about the time use of people living with psychiatric disabilities and how this compares with the time use of the general population. A range of assessment methods that can be used to explore time use are described and analyzed, as well as intervention approaches that can support individuals in developing new habits and achieving occupational balance through improving the way they use their time.

Time Use and Occupational Balance

The way individuals use their time is influenced by their roles, interests and values, environments, history, and the future they desire for themselves. One of the primary ways in which OTPs understand time use and its relationship to well-being is through the concept of "occupational balance." A pioneer of occupational therapy, Adolf Meyer, described the human need for a satisfying balance of work, rest, play, and sleep (Meyer, 1922/1983), and several other occupational therapy theorists and occupational scientists have further developed the concept.

At a basic level, **occupational balance** is simple to understand: Every human seeks a variety of activities and occupations to meet their various occupational needs. However, understanding the concept of occupational balance in the context of each individual's life is much more complex. First, there is no one "correct" mix of activities. Although it is tempting to seek simple, "one size fits all" solutions (e.g., 8 hours each of work, rest/sleep, and play), this approach is not practical or possible.

Occupational balance can only be defined subjectively, and similar patterns of activity can be experienced in significantly different ways by different people. For example, the pattern of 12 hours of employment-related activity and 7 hours of sleep interspersed with 5 hours of other activities might seem "unbalanced" at first glance. However, for an individual without family commitments who derives an immense sense of satisfaction and value from their work,

this pattern could be experienced as very "balanced." On the other hand, for an individual who derives little pleasure from work, has young children, is caring for an aging parent, and does not have enough time to play their favorite sport, this pattern of time use would feel significantly imbalanced.

More than simply avoiding multiple demands on one's time, occupational balance incorporates a variety of factors. One model of occupational balance, referred to as "lifestyle balance," has been proposed by Matuska and Christiansen (2008). In this model, **lifestyle balance** is defined as "a satisfying pattern [congruence between actual participation and desired participation] of daily occupation that is healthful, meaningful, and sustainable to an individual within the context of their current life circumstances" (p. 11). The authors further suggest that a balanced lifestyle should support five occupational needs (p. 11):

1. Meet basic instrumental needs necessary for sustained biological health and physical safety.
2. Have rewarding and self-affirming relationships with others.
3. Feel engaged, challenged, and competent.
4. Create meaning and a positive personal identity.
5. Organize time and energy in ways that enable the meeting of important personal goals and renewal.

Despite the widespread use of existing models of occupational balance, they have been criticized as being too "Western" in perspective. Criticisms include being too focused on the individual and failing to consider concepts such as balance with natural, social, and cultural contexts (Liu et al., 2021b). As an alternative, the Model of Occupational Harmony (Liu et al., 2021a, 2021b) has been proposed. This model, based on concepts from traditional Chinese philosophy, proposes that balance is achieved when there is (Liu et al., 2021b):

- Equilibrium between physical and mental engagement, quiet and active engagement, and individual and social engagement
- Harmony among five dimensions of occupational engagement
- Overall harmony between human–environment transactions over time

Habits and Routines

Habits and the routines that link habits together help people to organize their time and support efficient occupational performance. **Habits** are patterns of doing activities that are

PhotoVoice

As my husband's caregiver, I often put pressure on myself to guide him to spend his time productively. However, Alzheimer's disease makes it really difficult for him to do the things he used to do so well. I have to remember that what's meaningful to him now might not seem meaningful to me, but that's *my* problem. For example, he will spend hours picking leaves out from between the cracks of our deck and, you know what? It makes him happy and leaves him feeling as though he has accomplished something important. So now I encourage that.

Is there an activity you enjoy that other people might not consider meaningful? What meaning does the activity hold for you?_____

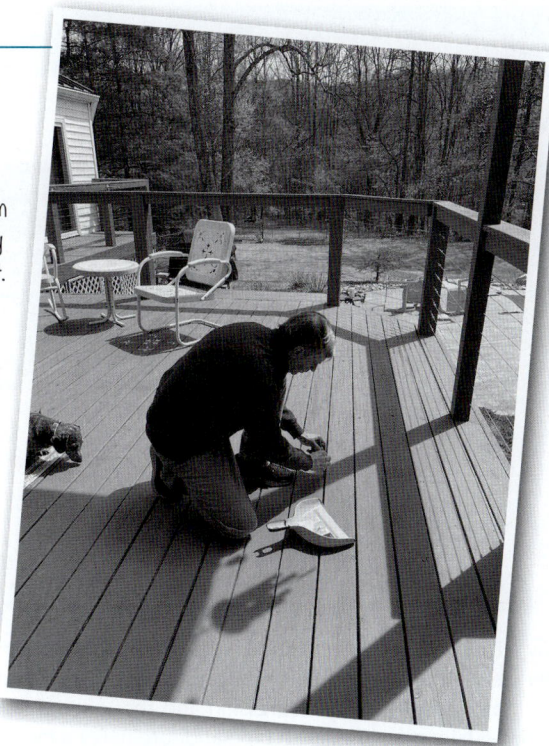

so familiar that they become essentially automatic. When undertaking habitual activities, there is less need for individuals to consciously plan or organize their actions. Habits prevent the need to make thousands of decisions every day. For example, imagine if a person had to think through the process of brushing their teeth or making a cup of coffee every time they did it.

Routines are the patterns of activity that comprise habits and the typical sequence in which they are undertaken (Hodge, 2003). Routines give structure to days and provide the framework that allows individuals to be as productive as possible. Similar to habits, routines are semiautomatic, and they reduce the cognitive processes and decision-making effort required to go about one's everyday life. It has been suggested that up to 90% of everyday behavior is based on habits and routines (Hodge, 2003), so they clearly make a substantial contribution to well-being—both positive and negative. Box 14-1 provides an example of establishing a routine.

Although routines and habits are useful to support optimal occupational performance, they can also hinder occupational performance. It can be difficult to change one's tendency to do things in the same way each time and to develop new habits. This human tendency to resist changing the way one has been doing things can be referred to as **inertia**.

Contrary to popular belief, habits that are unhelpful are not simply "broken." Rather, to change habits, an unhelpful habit should be replaced with a more helpful habit (Hodge, 2003). The most effective way to change an unhelpful habit into a helpful one is to consciously replace the old habit with the new habit and actively practice using the new habit. Through time and with perseverance, the old habit will fade away, and the new habit will replace it and become the new way of doing things. This process can be long and requires concerted effort. Some people say that it takes 21 days to

BOX 14-1 ■ Establishing a Routine

Betty used to regularly attend her local Clubhouse program. She was the lead guide, providing tours to potential new members and interstate and international visitors. She really enjoyed the role because it gave her the opportunity to meet new people and gave her a sense of pride in supporting the functioning of the Clubhouse. She was well liked by others at the Clubhouse, and they were surprised when she stopped attending. When another member reached out with a phone call to check in with Betty, she stated that she stopped attending because she was having "accidents" (urinary incontinence) and was embarrassed by these. She didn't want to use adult incontinence pads, but agreed to talk to one of the staff members about other ideas to manage this issue.

A level II fieldwork student met with Betty to discuss this concern. The student helped Betty manage the issue by establishing a routine. A timer was set on her phone so that Betty was reminded to use the bathroom every hour. At first Betty was reluctant to use the bathroom if she did not feel that she needed to go. However, once convinced that regular trips would reduce the likelihood of accidents, Betty started to follow the routine as established with the timer. Eventually, Betty was able to establish a pattern of using the bathroom more frequently and no longer needed the timer.

replace an old habit with a new one, but in many cases it can be much longer than that (Hodge, 2003).

To support the sustained effort that is required to change a habit, rewards that are focused on the positive outcomes that will be achieved through the change of habit can be very useful (Hodge, 2003). For example, perhaps someone has a habit of checking e-mail and social media on their phone each evening before going to bed, and the OTP suspects that this habit

The Lived Experience

Meghen Mildern

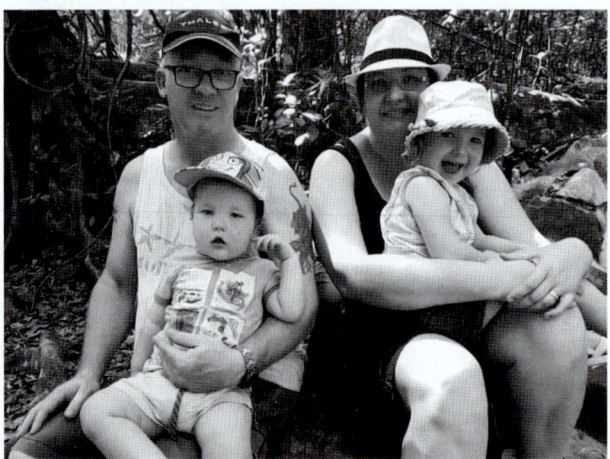

My late teens and early twenties were a very difficult time in my life with regard to my mental health. I was in and out of the hospital with severe depression and thoughts of suicide, and was later diagnosed with bipolar disorder. For a long time, I convinced myself that this was my sentence, and my life was to never get any better. This was my normal.

Despite what I was told by the doctors, I was convinced that I wasn't getting any better because the medication wasn't working properly. I felt I had no control over my illness, and there was nothing I could do to improve my quality of life. As a symptom of my bipolar disorder, I would become obsessed with a topic or interest and buy as many books as I could find.

Ironically, I became obsessed with cognitive therapy and the concept of contributing to your own experience. This led me in the direction of managing my own recovery in terms of the realization that I had control over how I spent my time and the power of having a routine.

I started with little changes, such as making sure I went to bed around the same time and had 8 hours of sleep, reducing my consumption of alcohol, and doing half an hour of exercise. I also came to realize that my recovery was a lot quicker when I was employed in a job meaningful to me. I recognize that I also needed social outlets and to not let myself become isolated, so I also allocated time to leave the house or meet up with friends.

Having a routine gives me comfort and helps me to engage in meaningful activity in my life, which reduces the chances of any relapse. It also provides me the clarity to recognize if I'm not doing so well and when to seek help.

Having children was a concern for me because pregnancy hormones are unpredictable and there was a chance I could suffer from postpartum depression, but I used the same solution that I do for myself and that was to put my children into a routine from the moment they were born. I did have postpartum depression with my first child, but I just kept following the daily routine that I had put together for her and it helped me to focus on the things that needed to be done to keep her happy and healthy. After the first 6 weeks my symptoms had reduced considerably.

I credit my ability to manage my mental health better than most because I recognize the importance of having a routine and engaging in activities both personally and professionally that are meaningful to me. If I had never had that realization I don't know that I would be where I am today.

contributes to difficulty falling asleep. The OTP might make a conscious effort to replace this habit with reading before bedtime and, to make it more likely to happen, have the person place their phone outside their bedroom before going to bed and keep a book on their nightstand. Also see Chapter 11: Motivation for information about how to help people get motivated to change a negative habit. 🤝

Time Use and Mental Health

Several studies have been undertaken to explore the time use of people with psychiatric disabilities (Bejerholm & Eklund, 2004; Eklund et al., 2009; Hayes & Halford, 1996; Krupa et al., 2003; Leufstadius et al., 2006; Minato & Zemke, 2004; Tjörnstrand et al., 2020). Results from these studies, which were conducted in countries as diverse as Australia, Canada, Sweden, and Japan, have generally been very consistent: Compared with the general population, people with psychiatric disability spend less time in productivity or **active leisure** (e.g., sport, hobbies) activities and more time sleeping and in **passive leisure** (sometimes also referred to as "quiet leisure," e.g., using mass media, sitting around) activities. Individuals with psychiatric disability also tend to spend more time alone when compared with the activity patterns of the general population.

In terms of individual experiences, individuals who experience significant amounts of time engaged in these passive leisure activities and large amounts of sleeping (particularly napping during the day) have tended to report lower life satisfaction, quality of life, and other measures of well-being when compared with those who have other patterns of activities (Bejerholm, 2010; Bejerholm & Eklund, 2004; Leufstadius et al., 2006). Although recognizing that occupational balance can only be interpreted via the individuals' subjective experience, this evidence suggests that, for a proportion of people with psychiatric disability (although certainly not all), their days tend to be dominated by activities that have little meaning or purpose, might be completed only to "kill" or "fill" time, might be unsatisfying, and might be associated with poorer well-being.

Interestingly, several research teams have noted the potential similarities in time use between people with psychiatric disability and individuals who are unemployed (Hayes & Halford, 1996; Minato & Zemke, 2004). Although people with psychiatric disability do tend to sleep more than individuals who are unemployed, there are similarities in terms of the significant amounts of time spent in home-based, passive activities (Hayes & Halford, 1996; Minato & Zemke, 2004; Scanlan et al., 2011). Interestingly, this pattern was much less pronounced in individuals with psychiatric disability who were engaged in regular productivity activities (Minato & Zemke, 2004). Considered together, this information suggests that lack of work and other productivity occupations could contribute to the patterns of activity seen in the daily lives of some individuals with psychiatric disability.

Theorists and researchers who have investigated the time use of unemployed individuals have noted that the ability to structure time is often impaired in the context of unemployment (Feather & Bond, 1983; Jahoda, 1982; Wanberg et al., 1997; Waters & Muller, 2003). Without the daily routines afforded by employment (or other social institutions such as education), people often find it challenging to fill their days (Feather & Bond, 1983; Jahoda, 1982; Jahoda & Rush, 1980; Lobo, 1999; Martella & Maass, 2000; Wanberg et al., 1997; Waters & Muller, 2003).

A key theorist in this area, Marie Jahoda, proposed that, in addition to its manifest function of earning a living, employment also provided other latent benefits, including (a) imposed time structure, (b) regular shared experiences and contacts with people outside the immediate family, (c) links to collective goals, (d) personal status and identity, and (e) enforced activity (Jahoda, 1982). Also see Chapter 48: Work and Volunteer Occupations.

The lack of access to certain types of occupational roles (e.g., worker role) clearly can be a significant barrier to optimal time use. Other barriers to optimal time use include lack of financial resources, motivation, social support, and awareness or skills to engage in meaningful and purposeful activities. When finances are limited, individuals can be restricted from participating in certain activities that are costly (e.g., going to restaurants or cinemas) or that are inaccessible by public transport. Individuals with psychiatric disability can also experience difficulties with motivation, which can restrict access to new activities (Bejerholm, 2010; Edgelow & Krupa, 2011).

Similarly, limited social support networks (or a network of social supports that consists of people who spend most of their days working) also restrict individuals' options in terms of activity partners. Finally, lack of awareness of meaningful leisure activities, or limitations in the skills required to find and complete these activities, can also act as a barrier to optimal time use.

At a broader level, the COVID-19 pandemic and the associated lockdowns, quarantine, and social distancing created a great deal of exploration into how time use changed and how this was related to the mental health of individuals and communities. Overall, these changes did appear to have a negative impact on overall mental health, although how people used their time was associated with overall coping. Those individuals who spent more time in outdoor activities and who took up new hobbies were less likely to experience substantial mental health concerns, whereas those who spent more time in the home and engaged in screen-based activities were more likely to experience mental health difficulties (e.g., Bu et al., 2021). Although the overall long-term effects of the pandemic are not yet known, digital communications and more time spent in the home (e.g., through "work from home" activities) certainly will remain. This can make it more challenging to set boundaries around working hours, which can encroach upon other important occupations and potentially diminish mental health. This is especially true for parents and tends to affect working mothers most dramatically (Findley et al., 2022).

To support optimal time use and mental health, OTPs should be encouraged to promote "healthy digital habits" such as limiting screen time, turning off notifications, and reducing the number of apps available on the phone (Pandya & Lodha, 2021). Also see Chapter 11: Motivation, Chapter 49: Connectedness and Belonging, and Chapter 51: Leisure and Creative Occupations.

Mental Health in Culture and Society: The Luddite Club

Catana Brown

During the pandemic, Logan Lane, a high school student in Brooklyn, realized she was consumed by her phone. First, she deleted her Instagram app. Next, she put her phone in a box, but she still was drawn to it. So eventually Logan gave up her iPhone entirely. She now has a flip phone because her parents want to be able to contact her. Without a smartphone, Logan found that her life changed for the better because the way she spent her time changed dramatically. Without her phone she was bored, and boredom led to new interests in reading and drawing. Now, she always has a book with her. Logan also discovered that she was sleeping better, and she was able to wake up earlier and refreshed to start her day. She became interested in school again and looked forward to class and what she might learn.

Logan's own experience caused her to create the Luddite Club. Luddites are people opposed to new things, especially technology. The Luddite Club meets every Sunday, and as of December 2022 the club had 25 members. Because they can't text, they must just show up for the meeting. The members share their experiences during the week, and they discuss the books they are reading. The members of the Luddite Club have to be more intentional about connecting because they can no longer text, but Logan reports that her friendships are closer and more meaningful now.

Logan believes that there is a middle ground, and some people can have a phone but limit their screen time. But for herself, she prefers to go without. She sees parents as a big part of the problem because they encourage phone use by asking their kids to regularly check in, and they tend to be bad role models because parents also spend inordinate amounts of time on their phones. Logan suggests that parents set strict limits as to when phones are allowed, and that they exhibit good digital habits. She suggests that teenagers take a break from their phone so they can see how it can change their life.

Because of their mission the Luddites do not have a social media presence, but readers can find out more about the club by listening to the podcast, which includes an interview with Logan, or read the article about the Luddite Club in the *New York Times*:

https://teenbraintrust.com/podcast-meet-a-teen-who
-gave-up-her-smartphone

https://www.nytimes.com/2022/12/15/style/teens
-social-media.html

Time Use Across the Life Span

The ways in which individuals use their time are also influenced by their stage of life. For example, children tend to spend more time in play and education-related activities than do adults. When compared with adults of working age, older adults often spend more time in leisure activities and less time in formal productivity and work activities. As with the general adult population, there is a complex relationship between time use and well-being in children and older adults.

With children, time spent in structured leisure activities has been associated with lower levels of depression (Desha & Ziviani, 2007), although too much involvement in these activities can create time pressure, which can result in lower levels of well-being (Fredricks, 2012). Over the past 40 years, children's time use has changed. One large study in the United Kingdom exploring school-age children's time use found that there was an increased proportion of time spent at home, more time spent on screen-based activities, and more time engaged in homework (Mullan, 2019). These changes, particularly increased screen time, have prompted concerns that they could have negative implications for mental health.

However, the relationship between screen time and mental health has proved to be quite complex and multifactorial (Atkin et al., 2021; Barthorpe et al., 2020; Kreski et al., 2022; Nagata et al., 2022; Wiciak et al., 2022). One robust finding from a study was that increased time spent in physical activity was associated with better mental health (Atkin et al., 2021).

For adolescents experiencing emerging serious mental illness, supporting good family routines and meaningful time use is particularly important. One small qualitative study from New Zealand suggested that family routines that support a sense of control, occupational balance, and expression of identity were reported to support overall family functioning and well-being (Koome et al., 2012). Other studies have focused on the importance of promoting increased participation in meaningful activities for adolescents with mental illness to ensure they do not experience enduring social disengagement and disconnection in later life (Berry et al., 2022).

Older adulthood is the time when many adults reduce their involvement in some formal productivity roles (e.g., retire from employment, reduce child-related caring activities), but possibly take on other productivity roles (e.g., volunteering or caring for their spouse or partner). Generally older adults report slightly lower levels of well-being than working age adults (Zuzanek, 1998), which may be related to changes in time use associated with retirement from paid employment, involuntary early retirement, or increased time spent caring for a partner (Eagers et al., 2022). Results from one study suggested that those older individuals who maintained their involvement in meaningful roles had higher levels of overall life satisfaction (McKenna et al., 2007), suggesting that support to maintain engagement in important life roles is an important role for OTPs (Eagers et al., 2022).

OTPs are also interested in time use for participants in institutional settings. A case-based research study explored the relationship of time use and quality of life in a long-term care facility for individuals with Alzheimer disease (Wood et al., 2009). Researchers found that, despite retained capacities, participants spent 40% of their daytime dozing or unengaged in activity, and less engagement was associated with lower quality of life.

Environmental factors played a significant role in how participants used their time. The television tended to overwhelm individuals, who were often found sitting still next to the television, but not following what was going on. Meal and snack times were some of the most positive times of day, as participants engaged in activity and interacted with others. Another positive time was when staff engaged participants in brief grooming activities.

This study has important implications for OTPs, who can promote the importance of time use assessments to identify periods when residents are less engaged. The study also suggests that OTPs can mentor and educate direct care staff to design and implement activities that take advantage of the remaining capacities of residents and take an active role in designing living spaces to promote activity engagement (Wood et al., 2009).

Measuring Time Use

Research on time use has a long history in many countries. For many years, various national statistical organizations completed large-scale studies of the ways in which people use time (Hunt & McKay, 2012). These studies explored important measures of the formal and informal economy (e.g., paid and unpaid work, care of children, household division of labor), typically using information from **time diaries** (Fig. 14-1) to examine what the person does, who they do it with, and where the person does it. Data are used to explore the changing nature of time use through time, and data sets are available to researchers across the world to explore specific aspects of time use.

Although these national data sets are valuable in their descriptions of the ways in which people use their time, they do not typically examine the meaning ascribed to activities by individuals. Therefore, researchers (many of them OTPs) have developed several specialized assessment instruments to more consistently gather information about this aspect of time use, some of which are presented in Table 14-1.

Each assessment tool for measuring time use offers advantages and presents disadvantages when used in occupational therapy practice. Each of the advantages and disadvantages should be considered in each individual situation to help to determine which will provide the most useful and meaningful information to guide interventions.

The Occupational Questionnaire (OQ), Modified Occupational Questionnaire (MOQ), and Occupational Experiences Profile (OEP) provide the opportunity to closely explore the ways in which people use their time from a variety of different perspectives. However, simply noting the total scores for the various aspects of time use and proportion of time spent in different types of activity might not highlight the richness of this information. To gain the most complete picture of individuals' time use, the results from these assessments should be further explored in a discussion between the person and OTP to ascertain the meaningfulness of the activities engaged in.

Aldrich and colleagues (2014) suggest that the expanded list of activity types included in the MOQ (also a feature of the OEP) could be advantageous, compared with the more limited categories included in the OQ to support this

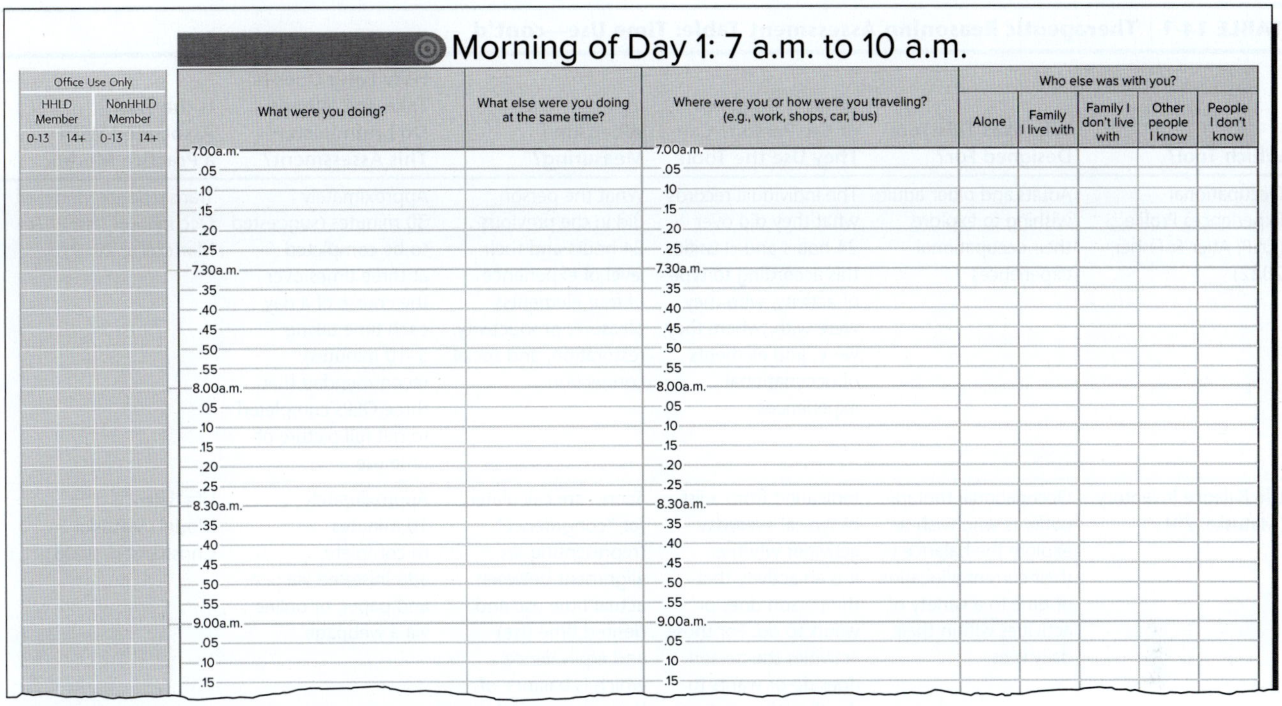

Morning of Day 1: 7 a.m. to 10 a.m.

Office Use Only				What were you doing?	What else were you doing at the same time?	Where were you or how were you traveling? (e.g., work, shops, car, bus)	Who else was with you?				
HHLD Member		NonHHLD Member					Alone	Family I live with	Family I don't live with	Other people I know	People I don't know
0-13	14+	0-13	14+								

7.00a.m.
.05
.10
.15
.20
.25
7.30a.m.
.35
.40
.45
.50
.55
8.00a.m.
.05
.10
.15
.20
.25
8.30a.m.
.35
.40
.45
.50
.55
9.00a.m.
.05
.10
.15

FIGURE 14-1. A sample page from a time diary used by Statistics New Zealand. *Statistics New Zealand and licensed by Statistics NZ for reuse under the Creative Commons Attribution 4.0 International license.*

TABLE 14-1 | Therapeutic Reasoning Assessment Table: Time Use

Which Tool?	Who Was This Tool Designed For?	What Is Required of the Person? Can They Use the Tool?	What Am I Measuring?	How Long Does It Take and Where Do I Administer This Assessment?	Is the Tool Associated With a Practice Model?
Assessment of Time Management Skills (ATMS; White et al., 2013)	Adults with mental illness	Individual answers 30 questions with a Likert scale from none of the time to all of the time.	Use of time management strategies and ability to plan and manage daily life	Takes approximately 10 minutes; can be done anywhere	No
Occupational Questionnaire (OQ; Smith et al., 1986)	Adults wishing to explore their time use (initial research completed with older adults)	The individual records their typical pattern of time use and classifies the activities according to a range of criteria.	What the person does "on a typical day" (in half-hour blocks), classified according to type of activity, competence, importance, and enjoyment	Takes approximately 20–30 minutes; administered via pen and paper, so it can be done anywhere	Model of Human Occupation
Modified Occupational Questionnaire (MOQ; Scanlan & Bundy, 2011)	Adults wishing to explore their time use (initial research completed with young adults who were unemployed)	The individual records what they did the prior day and classifies the activities according to a range of criteria.	What the person did the prior day in 1-hour blocks, classified according to type of activity, reason for doing the activity, value to self, and value to society	Takes approximately 30 minutes; administered via pen and paper, so it can be done anywhere	Not specifically, but based on the OQ, which is based on the Model of Human Occupation
Profiles of Occupational Engagement Among Persons with Severe Mental Illness (POES; Bejerholm et al., 2006)	Adults with psychiatric disability	The individual records what they did in hourly blocks during the past 24 hours and participates in an interview.	Information provided by the individual is used by the therapist to rate nine items that relate to patterns and quality of occupational engagement	Time required is not specifically stated, but estimated to be approximately 30–60 minutes	Not specifically

Continued

TABLE 14-1 | Therapeutic Reasoning Assessment Table: Time Use—cont'd

Which Tool?	Who Was This Tool Designed For?	What Is Required of the Person? Can They Use the Tool?	What Am I Measuring?	How Long Does It Take and Where Do I Administer This Assessment?	Is the Tool Associated With a Practice Model?
Occupational Experiences Profile (OEP; Atler & Fisher, 2022)	Adults and older adults wishing to explore their occupational experiences	The individual records what they did over 24 hours and classifies this according to type of activity, who they were with, where they were, and elements of occupational experiences.	What the person did in the previous 24 hours and their level of experience of four elements: pleasure, productivity, restoration, and social connection	Approximately 30 minutes (suggested to be completed at three times over the course of a day, each time taking 5–10 minutes); recommended that three OEPs completed to get full picture of time use	Transactional Model of Occupation (Fisher & Marterella, 2019)
Life Balance Inventory (Matuska, 2012)	Occupational therapy patients who wish to explore the balance of their current allocation of time to a variety of activities within their daily lives	Indicating from a list of typical everyday activities whether it is an activity that the person does or wants to do. For those activities the person does do or wants to do, they then indicate whether the time they spend on the activity is "too much," "too little," or "about right for me."	Scores are calculated for "congruence" (representing an alignment between actual time use and desired time use) and equivalence, which is balance of time use across the four need-based dimensions of health, social relationships, challenge, and identity.	Approximately 10 minutes to complete, administered via pen and paper, or online via a webpage	Life Balance Model (Matuska & Christiansen, 2008)
Engagement in Meaningful Activity Scale (EMAS; Goldberg et al., 2002)	Adults with disabilities related to psychiatric disability	Responding to a 12-item questionnaire and several open-ended questions	Level of involvement in activities that are personally valuable and meaningful	Takes approximately 10–15 minutes; administered via pen and paper and interview, so it can be done anywhere	Not specifically
Experience Sampling Method (ESM; Csikszentmihalyi & Larson, 1987)	Children and adults	The individual carries a pager or mobile device and then responds to a small set of questions each time when prompted.	What the person was doing, why they were doing it, who the person was doing it with, and how they felt about it	Takes fewer than 5 minutes, seven times per day for 7 days	Csikszentmihalyi's Theory of Flow
Ecological Momentary Assessment (EMA; Stone et al., 1999)	Children and adults	The individual carries a pager or mobile device and then responds to a small set of questions each time when prompted (or in some cases during specific target events or behaviors).	Varies depending on the purpose, but related to what the person was doing, the context of the activity, and how they were feeling	Takes fewer than 5 minutes, several times per day during the course of up to several weeks	Not specifically

discussion and exploration. The Profiles of Occupational Engagement Among Persons with Severe Mental Illness (POES) overcomes some of these limitations by providing a range of coding descriptions to support the administering therapist in analyzing the individual's time use according to several aspects of occupational engagement. However, in doing this, the subjective differences in individuals' experiences might not be fully considered. One disadvantage of all of these "time diary" approaches is that they can be influenced by recall bias

and—if not completed over several days—might not give a full picture of the breadth of activities undertaken by the person.

The brevity and relative ease of interpretation of the Engagement in Meaningful Activities Scale (EMAS) are attractive. However, its format as an "overall" analysis of aspects of meaningfulness does not offer the opportunity to explore specifically what activities the person engages in and how much time they spend doing them. In comparison, the

Lifestyle Balance Questionnaire (LBQ) provides the opportunity to explore a wider range of types of activities and allows the individual to express whether their time use allocation to that activity type is aligned with their desires (i.e., whether it is too much, too little, or just right). This approach can be very useful and helps identify where balances can be adjusted (e.g., reducing time spent in one activity type to focus on another activity type).

However, there are also limitations to this instrument. First, the list of activity types might not be comprehensive, so the questionnaire might not capture all the activities that are important to the person. This is a particular risk for individuals who do not come from Western cultural contexts. Second, for the "equivalence" scores, each activity type is allocated to a predefined "need-based dimension" of occupations (i.e., health, social relationships, challenge, or identity). Given that each individual interprets the purpose and meaning of activities differently, these predefined allocations might not accurately capture the person's overall experiences.

Finally, time sampling approaches (e.g., Experience Sampling Method and Ecological Momentary Assessment) have the advantage of collecting rich information about the person's experience of time use without the risk of recall bias. Although newer technology has made data collection easier (e.g., there are many apps, such as the Participation in Everyday Life app, which can be used on an individual's mobile phone), the time taken for data collection and the need for the person to complete a large number of questionnaires can make this a challenging approach in the practice setting. Collating and "making sense" of the information provided can also be very complex and time consuming for the OTP, which also could affect the feasibility of these approaches in the practice setting.

Interventions to Support Optimal Time Use

There are a variety of interventions available to OTPs to improve individuals' satisfaction with their time use. Some interventions use the core occupational therapy skills of leisure exploration and individually oriented skills training to support engagement in desired activities, whereas others are more specific in their approach. This section describes seven interventions to support optimal time use for individuals living with psychiatric disability. The first of these is a method for integrating new routines and habits into individuals' daily lives, and the following six are focused on developing useful daily rhythms to support optimal well-being. Although evidence for these interventions is still emerging, the range of interventions provides OTPs with a variety of options to address time use.

Being a Psychosocial OT Practitioner

Incorporating Physical Activity into an Already Busy Schedule

Identifying Psychosocial Strengths and Needs

OTPs in general hospital settings frequently work with individuals who have a preexisting mental illness or develop mental health concerns as a secondary consequence of their presenting complaint. Consider the story of Davi, who was admitted to the hospital's cardiac unit after experiencing a myocardial infarction (heart attack). Davi is 48 years old, works as an accountant, and lives with his husband, Dwayne, and their two children, Bradley (12 years old) and Jessica (8 years old), as well as Davi's parents, Eduardo and Manuela.

As part of his rehab, Davi is supposed to participate in regular vigorous exercise. His physician also told Davi that he needed to lose 30 pounds to reach a healthy weight. Davi understands the importance of these lifestyle changes and adheres to the plan while in the hospital. However, when the OTP meets with Davi during his hospital stay, he expresses that he is overwhelmed and cannot comprehend how he will fit vigorous exercise and dietary changes into his daily schedule. The OTP recognizes that individuals are at an increased risk for depression following a heart attack and the importance of addressing these concerns.

Using a Holistic Occupational Therapy Approach

The OTP considers what information they need to gather as part of a semistructured interview. The OTP asks Davi about his primary responsibilities and obligations, what his typical daily and weekly routine consists of, what activities he finds most meaningful, what activities he could spend less time doing, and what actions he could take to address the lifestyle changes recommended by his physician to engage in vigorous exercise and lose weight.

The OTP also decides to use the MOQ to learn about Davi's time use and responsibilities and the Life Balance Inventory to look at his current perspective of satisfactory balance in his time use.

Using this approach, the OTP discovers that:

■ Davi works from home most of the time, which works well for him because it makes caring for the children and his parents easier. He is the primary caregiver in the home, as Dwayne works longer hours.

■ His weekdays are hectic from about 6:30 a.m. until about 9:00 or 10:00 p.m. He works full-time (40 hours per week), but his employer is flexible and allows him to spread those hours over a more extended period of the day. He starts work at 7.30 a.m. after dropping Bradley and Jessica at school and works until about 2:30 p.m., when he goes to pick up the children from school and take them to after-school activities. Then, he prepares dinner for the family and returns to work for another 2 or 3 hours in the evening.

■ His most valued activities involve his family, and he is very unsatisfied with how much time he gets to do meaningful activities with them.

■ His least valued activities are driving in the car and attending work meetings when he feels he doesn't need to be present or contribute to them.

At this point, the OTP focuses on what changes could be made to Davi's and the family's routines to create a better balance and maintain his well-being, while also creating time for additional lifestyle changes, such as vigorous exercise. The OTP brainstorms potential options with Davi and explains the Action Over Inertia and ReDO programs. Together, they identified some opportunities to support better balance, and Davi chose three things he wanted to explore with his family:

1. Making more time in the evenings by "batch cooking" on the weekends rather than cooking every night. He thinks this could be a family event with opportunities for Davi's parents and children to be involved and potentially pass down traditional Brazilian recipes. This change could also support healthier meal preparation to support Davi in losing weight.

2. Trying to multitask during work meetings when he is not contributing information. For example, Davi thinks he could walk on a treadmill or ride an exercise bike during some of the less important meetings to engage in more physical activity during the day.

3. Exploring the idea of riding bikes to school with his children a few days each week instead of driving. Davi thinks this might support more "quality time" with the children and provide another opportunity for more physical activity.

Reflection Questions

1. Davi may have follow-up appointments after discharge, putting more strain on his time. What other strategies might be helpful to ensure his follow-up medical appointments remain manageable and don't overwhelm him?

2. One of the factors related to depression following a heart attack for men is changes in sexual function and satisfaction. How might the OTP discuss changes in satisfaction with sexual activity with Davi? What specific questions could the OTP ask?

3. Reflect on your thoughts about reorganizing time use for someone such as Davi. One of the challenges is that it is impossible to simply add more activities, because to increase time in one activity, time spent in another must be reduced. What strategies or approaches will you use in your practice to help individuals consider this concept and plan for alterations in routines?

Building New Routines and Habits

For some individuals living with psychiatric disability, the presence of cognitive difficulties can make it difficult to solve problems during activities. For these individuals, the development of routines and habits can be especially useful. Once the individual has developed a routine way of doing an activity, they are more likely to be able to complete these activities in a familiar environment where potential problems are minimized or eliminated. This use of routines and habits can support independent performance of activities that can otherwise be difficult for the individual to perform.

The following general principles can be helpful for guiding interventions focused on using routines and habits to promote independent performance:

- Ensure a clear understanding of the individual's strengths and difficulties in planning and problem-solving exists before starting the intervention process. If individuals do not experience difficulties in these areas, the types of interventions described in this section might not be necessary.
- Ensure that skills development focuses on one activity at a time. For example, if the individual wishes to become more independent in travel, laundry, and cooking, they should select which one is most important to focus on first. Once the routine has been established and the person is able to complete the activity without assistance, the intervention can move on to the next most important activity.
- Complete a comprehensive analysis of the activity to be undertaken, with particular attention paid to any decisions that might need to be made or problems that could arise during the activity. Then, devise a series of steps to be undertaken that minimize the need for decision-making and problem-solving during the activity. This will ensure that the individual has the best opportunity to complete the activity independently; for example, simplifying recipes to help the person prepare a meal or devising a public transport plan that minimizes or eliminates the need for changing modes of transport (even if the simpler approach may take somewhat longer).
- Ensure that skills are learned in the environment in which they will be used. Because individuals with cognitive difficulties are likely to have trouble generalizing skills learned in one environment to other environments, skills training should take place in the same environment where activities will be performed (e.g., in the person's home).
- Consider the temporal aspects of the environment. It is optimal to practice skills at the same time of day when the activity would typically be completed. For example, when helping the individual develop a routine of catching the bus to a workplace, training should occur at the time of the day when the person will get on the bus to get to work on time. When supporting an individual to prepare a specific meal, training should occur in the individual's own kitchen at the usual time of day (rather than in a different kitchen at a different time).
- Encourage repetition. Repeated practice supports the development and embedding of new routines and habits. The therapist should support the person to complete the target activity through numerous sessions until they are able to complete the activity without assistance. The number of repetitions required will depend on the complexity of the activity, the person's previous experience with similar activities, and their overall capacity for new learning.
- Take advantage of easily accessible technologies. Smartphone apps such as alarm features, calendars, prompts, and to-do lists can be used as assistive devices to support the development of habits and routines. Although these technologies can be very helpful, it is important to remember that individuals might need support to learn how to use these devices or access the apps. Other devices such as pillboxes can help individuals organize their routines. See Figure 14-2.

Allow support to decrease as the person becomes more independent. As with all occupational therapy interventions, the therapist should provide only as much support as the individual requires. As the person develops these new habits, their need for support will diminish. Once the habit has become a routine, the person will generally be able to continue the activity with minimal support. Because unexpected problems in the environment can interfere with performance, support people should regularly check with the individual to ascertain if they are experiencing any difficulties.

Routines and habits also can be useful in supporting independence by embedding new activities into existing routines. A common example of this is medication use

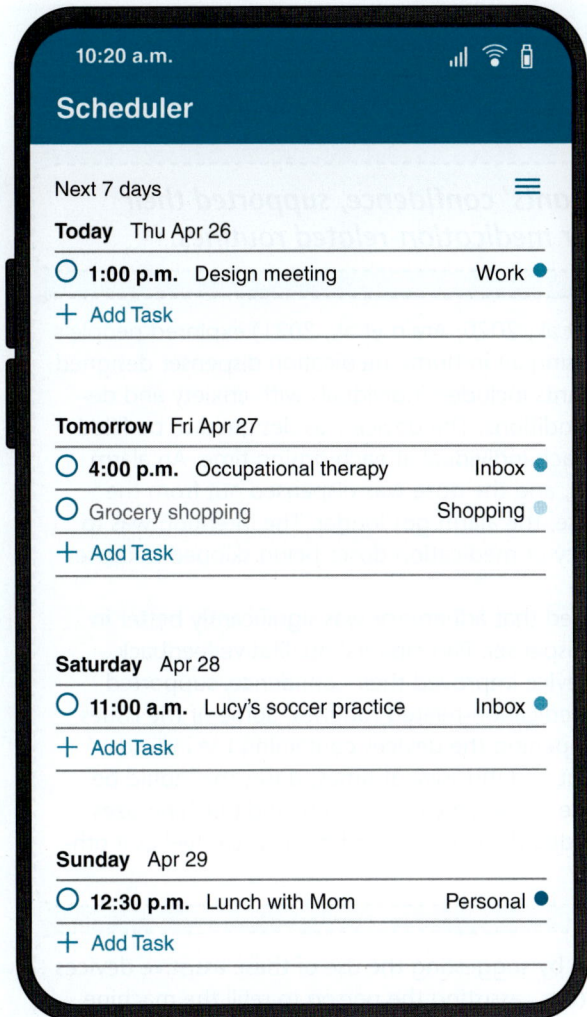

FIGURE 14-2. Example of a smartphone app for scheduling.

(Sanders & Van Oss, 2013). If an individual is required to take medications, embedding this activity into other routines completed at similar times of the day can be helpful. When the practitioner understands what happens in a person's "normal day," they can embed taking medications into the routine by tying the act of taking medications with another routine activity (e.g., drinking morning coffee, brushing teeth, having meals).

Careful attention should be paid to situations in which the medication doses are different at different times of the day. For example, if an individual needs to take one medication in the morning and another in the evening, morning medications could be embedded into the morning routine of making coffee (morning medications are kept close to the coffee pot) and evening medications could be embedded into the routine of having dinner (evening medications are kept on the dinner table).

Action Over Inertia

Action Over Inertia is a specific time use intervention developed by a group of Canadian occupational therapists (Edgelow & Krupa, 2011; Krupa et al., 2021). This intervention approach is designed for individuals living with psychiatric disability whose daily lives are characterized by "pervasive and persistent occupational imbalance and disengagement" (p. 269). Using a workbook (Krupa et al., 2021), the OTP works collaboratively with the individual to reengage with meaningful activities to support optimal health and well-being. The overall process of the intervention is divided into five components:

1. Identifying the need for change and engaging the individual into the change process
2. Exploring current patterns of time use and providing rapid support for engaging in meaningful activities
3. Providing information about the relationship between meaningful activity and well-being
4. Conducting long-term goal planning
5. Monitoring and refining plans on an ongoing basis

An initial randomized controlled trial (RCT) of the Action Over Inertia program demonstrated promising results (Edgelow & Krupa, 2011). Participants were all individuals with psychiatric disability receiving service from Assertive Community Treatment (ACT) teams and were randomized into "control" (routine ACT care) or "treatment" (routine ACT care plus Action Over Inertia) groups. Following 12 weeks of intervention, participants in the treatment group reported an average reduction of 47 minutes per day spent sleeping, and participants in the control group reported an average increase of 22 minutes spent sleeping. Participants in the treatment group all reported that they found the treatment to be useful and would recommend it to other individuals living with psychiatric disability.

Recent studies have evaluated Action Over Inertia in a community-based residential service in Australia (Rees et al., 2021), and the program has been modified to be used with individuals recovering from substance use disorders (Jarrard et al., 2021). Participants in the Australian study reported that Action Over Inertia was helpful in supporting change and recognizing the importance of meaningful activities. In addition, participating in meaningful activities supported the individuals' sense of well-being and recovery (Rees et al., 2021).

Redesigning Daily Occupations

The Redesigning Daily Occupations (ReDO) intervention addresses the importance of developing a balance between restful and reviving occupations (Eklund & Erlandsson, 2014a). It uses the Daily Hassles and Uplift scale to identify negative and positive events experienced by the person in daily life. The intervention works to minimize hassles and increase the experience of uplifts.

This intervention is designed for individuals with stress-related disorders who are working, particularly working women. Working women are particularly prone to difficulties with time management because of challenges associated with managing home and work life, particularly when child care is also involved (Johansson et al., 2012).

ReDO is a 16-week program divided into three phases (Eklund & Erlandsson, 2014a). During Phase I, which takes place during the first 5 weeks, participants analyze their personal patterns of everyday activity. Phase II comprises the next 5 weeks, during which participants work on goal setting and developing strategies to change everyday patterns of time

Evidence-Based Practice

Using Assistive Devices to Develop Habits

> *Assistive devices improved participants' confidence, supported their health, and further developed their medication-related routines.*

RESEARCH FINDINGS

A team of researchers in Canada (Ahmad et al., 2020; Arain et al., 2021) explored people's experiences and outcomes supported by using an in-home medication dispenser designed to support medication adherence. Participants included individuals with anxiety and depression, as well as other chronic health conditions. The device was designed to be filled with the various medications required by each individual at each dosing time. An alarm sounded when it was time to take the dose, and the dose was dispensed out from the machine. If the person did not take the dose, the alarm got louder. The intention was to provide reminders and reduce the frequency of medication doses being skipped because of forgetting.

The RCT (Arain et al., 2021) demonstrated that adherence was significantly better in the group using the in-home medication dispenser. Participants' qualitative feedback (Ahmad et al., 2020) suggested that the device improved their confidence, supported their health, and further developed their medication-related routines. Some of the issues raised by participants included difficulties opening the devices containing the individual doses, reminders that were inconvenient and intrusive at times, doses that could be forgotten if the person was out of the house at the time of the dose, and machine sizes (and the fact that it was in view) that impeded their privacy and made them feel as if others might view them as "sick."

APPLICATIONS

➡ OTPs can support medication adherence by suggesting the use of these assistive devices and supporting increasing independence (e.g., assisting the person to refill the machine by themselves rather than being assisted by others; developing strategies and reminders to take doses out of the machine if the person is leaving the house).

➡ OTPs can support the person to use other, less intrusive, reminder mechanisms (e.g., smartphone reminders) alongside the medication dispenser with the aim of eventually developing the medication routine so that the dispenser is no longer required.

➡ Because this device is only useful when individuals forget to take their medications (rather than deliberately avoid medications), OTPs can provide education and support to individuals to recognize the benefits of adhering to their medications.

REFERENCES

Ahmad, A., Chiu, V., & Arain, M. A. (2020). Users' perceptions of an in-home electronic medication dispensing system: A qualitative study. *Medical Devices: Evidence and Research, 13,* 31–39. https://doi.org/10.2147/MDER.S241062

Arain, M. A., Ahmad, A., Chiu, V., & Kembel, L. (2021). Medication adherence support of an in-home electronic medication dispensing system for individuals living with chronic conditions: A pilot randomized controlled trial. *BMC Geriatrics, 21*(1), 56. https://doi.org/10.1186/s12877-020-01979-w

use. This includes a targeted goal of increasing participation in valued and meaningful occupations. During the final 6 weeks, Phase III, participants implement the identified strategies at work and at home.

In a quasi-experimental study, women with stress-related disorders received ReDO or an intervention with an emphasis on employment counseling (Eklund & Erlandsson, 2014b). At the end of the intervention period, participants receiving ReDO had greater satisfaction and participation in daily occupations, although individuals in the control condition were more likely to return to work.

A shorter, 10-week program (ReDO-10) designed for primary care settings has also been studied in Sweden (Olsson et al., 2020) and Ireland (Fox, Erlandsson,

McSharry, et al., 2022; Fox, Erlandsson, & Shiel, 2022). Initial results are promising, with participants reporting an increased sense of knowledge and confidence, as well as participating in more restorative activities in daily life, although further research is needed to explore how these changes affect broader outcomes.

Balancing Everyday Life

Balancing Everyday Life (BEL; Eklund et al., 2017) was developed based on principles from the ReDO (Eklund & Erlandsson, 2014a) and Lifestyle Redesign (Clark et al., 2012) programs, but it is specifically tailored for individuals with psychiatric disability. It is a group-based program focused on developing a satisfying balance and variety of occupations. It consists of weekly group sessions for 12 weeks and then two additional "booster" sessions in the month following. Topics address activity balance, meaningful activities, strategies to develop and maintain motivation, and exploration of different types of occupations (e.g., work, leisure, and social occupations).

At the completion of the intervention phase of the initial cluster RCT, participants who received BEL reported significantly higher activity engagement, activity balance, and activity value, as well as greater improvement in symptom severity and level of functioning compared with participants who received standard occupational therapy (Eklund et al., 2017). Although some of these between-group differences faded over time, BEL participants maintained a higher activity level and activity value, as well as greater improvements in quality of life, at the 6-month follow-up point compared with the comparison group.

Qualitative studies have also explored participants' perspectives about BEL, including experiencing enhanced sense of value and meaning through feeling connected to others, a sense of belonging through mutual support, and enhanced self-respect and self-worth (Lund et al., 2019). Participants also indicated that one of the key processes that supported these positive outcomes was "breaking a cycle of perceived failure" and experiencing success in making lifestyle changes through applying the strategies learned through BEL.

Interpersonal and Social Rhythm Therapy

Interpersonal and Social Rhythm Therapy (IPSRT) is an intervention designed for individuals with bipolar I mood disorder (Frank et al., 2000, 2007). In addition to providing interventions to support the recognition of early warning signs and other strategies to manage symptoms, IPSRT also focuses on the stabilization of "social rhythms." In the context of this intervention, **social rhythms** refer to the individual's daily routines. In seeking to stabilize social rhythms, individuals are encouraged to maintain regular patterns of meals, social contact, and sleep. This therapy is based on the theory that stable rhythms of daily living support the stability of individuals' mood.

A 2-year outcome study demonstrated that individuals with bipolar I disorder who received IPSRT intervention had significantly longer periods of well-being before experiencing a relapse when compared with individuals who received an alternative intervention (Frank et al., 2005). Outcomes from more recent studies have also suggested that IPSRT can be useful for individuals with major depressive disorder (Crowe, Inder, Douglas, et al., 2020) and may also be adopted into routine clinical practice using a shorter, simplified version called Social Rhythm Therapy (Crowe, Inder, Swartz, et al., 2020).

Meaningful Activities and Recovery

Meaningful Activities and Recovery (MA&R) is a new intervention, designed and delivered by occupational therapists and peer workers, to support individuals with psychiatric disability to increase their participation in activities that are meaningful to them (Bjørkedal et al., 2020). It consists of 11 group-based and 11 individual sessions spread across two manualized courses.

The first course supports participants in exploring and identifying activities that are meaningful to them, and the second course helps participants "anchor" these new activities as habits into their daily lives. An initial qualitative study reported positive experiences from participants often related to their better understanding of meaningful activities, finding enjoyment in everyday activities, and developing a new perspective on their everyday lives (Tepavicharov et al., 2022).

Supported Employment

Although not a specific time use intervention, supporting individuals living with psychiatric disability to engage in employment can also support more effective time use. As previously noted, employment provides support for individuals' time structure. Therefore, if individuals are supported to return to work, their time use is likely to improve. For example, a scoping review found recovery was enhanced when individuals with mental illness spent more of their time in meaningful activities, particularly paid employment and volunteering (Doroud et al., 2015). The approach to **supported employment** with the most substantial evidence base is the Individual Placement and Support (IPS) model (Bond et al., 2012, 2020). Supported employment is described in further detail in Chapter 48: Work and Volunteer Occupations. 🤝

Here's the Point

- The way in which people use their time reflects their roles, routines, and habits and is an important indicator of their overall occupational engagement.
- Having a pattern of time use that is satisfying for the individual is an important aspect of "occupational balance."
- Individuals living with psychiatric disability sometimes experience "occupational imbalance" and a lack of engagement in meaningful activities. People with psychiatric disability spend more time sleeping, napping, and engaged in passive leisure activities than the general population. This may be related to lack of productivity roles such as "worker" or "student," as these roles are often helpful in supporting individuals to structure their time.
- Many assessments of time use patterns use some form of a diary to record what the person does at different points in the day and evaluate how often the individual participates

in meaningful activity. Other assessments evaluate the ability to manage time.

■ Interventions that are focused on supporting individuals with psychiatric disability to develop new routines, engage in more meaningful activities, develop stable daily patterns of activity, or engage in work may be useful in supporting more satisfying patterns of time use. These

satisfying patterns of time use may, in turn, support increased life satisfaction, quality of life, and overall sense of well-being.

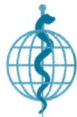 Visit the online resource center at FADavis.com to access the videos.

Apply It Now

1. Analyze Your Time

Analyze your own time use and "occupational balance" using two of the instruments noted in the following list:
■ Modified Occupational Questionnaire (MOQ): available from http://hdl.handle.net/2123/13098
■ Life Balance Inventory: can be completed online at https://minerva.stkate.edu/LBI.nsf
■ Profiles of Occupational Engagement Among Persons with Severe Mental Illness (POES) and Engagement in Meaningful Activities Survey (EMAS): can be downloaded from http://dolivewell.ca/tools-resources/#sthash.UhuUXW5M.dpbs

Use the information gathered to answer the following questions:
■ Does your pattern of time use appropriately reflect your current occupational engagement?
■ What kinds of activities do you spend most of your time doing?
■ From the information collected, what can you say about the "meaningfulness" of the activities you currently undertake?
■ In what ways is your current pattern of time use influenced by existing roles, routines, and habits?
■ Reflect on your own perception of your current "occupational balance." Does the information gathered accurately reflect your current occupational balance? Were there aspects of your occupational engagement or experience that were not effectively captured? Were there aspects of your occupational engagement that you understood more clearly after completing the instruments?

2. Analyze Time Use for an Individual With Mental Health Concerns

Analyze the time use and "occupational balance" of someone who is dealing with mental health concerns. Ask the person to complete one of the instruments listed in Apply It Now Activity #1. Following their completion, have a discussion about the individual's overall sense of "occupational balance." Consider the following questions:
■ Does the information provided reflect the person's subjective sense of "occupational balance"? If not, what additional information did you need to collect to understand the person's current occupational balance?

■ How much of the person's time is spent engaging in meaningful activity? Is this person's experience of time different from or similar to your own?
■ Does this person receive services from a structured program? If so, how does the program affect their time use?
■ What other information did you learn about the person's activities, routines, and habits though the exploration of their time use?
■ How did the person feel about recording their experiences of time use and daily activities?

3. Facilitating Engagement in Meaningful Activity

Although many people today deal with lives that are too full of activity, this chapter indicates that many individuals with mental health issues are experiencing a daily life that lacks meaningful activity. Several of the intervention approaches—Action Over Inertia, ReDO, BEL, and Meaningful Activity and Recovery—were developed by occupational therapists to help individuals with mental health concerns increase their participation. Select two of these approaches and identify (a) what is similar about the two interventions and (b) what is different about the interventions.

4. Video Exercise: Caregiver of Spouse with Alzheimer's on Challenges

Pair up with another student in your class or form a small group of students. Access and watch the "Caregiver of Spouse with Alzheimer's on Challenges" video at the online resource center at FADavis.com. Then, discuss and together answer the following questions:
1. What presents challenges to Nancy in terms of putting her husband on a schedule and filling his time? In what other conditions might caregivers find similar challenges?
2. What strategies would you suggest to Nancy to address the challenges she describes in the video? Can you think of resources that would be helpful to her?
3. Why do you think health-care providers have encouraged Nancy to maintain a consistent schedule with her husband? What message is Nancy sharing with practitioners about person-centered care?
4. Nancy briefly mentions her own needs, but really focuses on Bill's needs. What support/occupational therapy interventions would you recommend for Nancy as caregiver?

Resources

- "Leisure Occupations for Unhoused Individuals" video. In this video, Kailin, an occupational therapist who works in community mental health and homeless services, describes the power of leisure activities to the individuals whom she serves. Kailin talks about the barriers to engaging in leisure that often exist for people who are unhoused. She explains how she integrates the evaluation of leisure in her occupational profile and provides several examples of realistic leisure activities that occupational therapy practitioners can use to support individuals' mental health. Access the video at the online resource center at FADavis.com.
- "Tricks and Techniques from the Mother of an Autistic Son" video. In this video, Laura describes her and her family's creative and adaptive ways of helping their autistic son, Will, succeed. Giving several specific examples of solutions to common problem behaviors and challenges, Laura shares practical wisdom, "tricks and techniques" from 20 years of experience as the mother of a son with autism, with a focus on recognizing and focusing on Will's strengths. Access the video at the online resource center at FADavis.com.
- Action Over Inertia: The Action Over Inertia program supports individuals in overcoming the barriers preventing them from deriving meaning and enjoyment from the wide range of activities that make up their daily life. Krupa, T., Edgelow, M., Chen, S.-P., & Mieras, C. (2021). *Promoting activity and participation in individuals with serious mental illness: The Action Over Inertia approach.* Routledge. https://doi.org/10.4324/9781003111368
- Redesigning Daily Occupations (ReDO): ReDO is an intervention designed to help people develop a balance in their choice of valued and meaningful occupations. The intervention also helps people develop strategies to manage hassles that may occur during occupational engagement. Eklund, M., & Erlandsson, L. K. (2014). Redesigning Daily Occupations (ReDO™): Facilitating return to work among women with stress related disorders. In I. Söderbak (Ed.), *International handbook of occupational therapy interventions* (pp. 553–562). Springer.
- Balancing Everyday Life: BEL is a group program designed to support individuals with psychiatric disability to learn about, self-evaluate, and implement strategies to support their optimal desired level of occupational balance in everyday life. A full manual is not accessible, but more information is available in the original research publication at https://doi.org/10.1186/s12888-017-1524-7.
- Meaningful Activities and Recovery (MA&R): MA&R is group- and individual-based intervention delivered by OTPs and peer workers to support individuals with psychiatric disability to learn about, review, and improve their engagement in activities that are meaningful to them. A full manual is not accessible, but more information about the program can be found in the study protocol at https://doi.org/10.1186/s13063-020-04722-3.
- Interpersonal and Social Rhythm Therapy (IPSRT): IPSRT is designed to help people improve their moods by understanding and working with their biological and social rhythms. The program works in several different kinds of settings, including inpatient and outpatient groups. IPSRT is a compelling adjunctive therapy for people with mood disorders, and it emphasizes techniques to improve medication adherence, manage stressful life events, and reduce disruptions in social rhythms https://www.ipsrt.org.
- PIEL Survey Mobile App: The PIEL Survey app is designed to gather survey data from people in their daily lives. This allows a more complete understanding of a participant's thoughts and feelings than traditional survey methods. The app can be used in an academic research environment or in detailed market research: https://pielsurvey.org. Other information about time sampling apps and approaches can be found at https://www.teamscopeapp.com/blog/6-apps-for-experience-sampling-method-complete-guide and https://psychologicalsciences

.unimelb.edu.au/research/research-initiatives/our-work/feel-research-lab/resources.
- Apps for Time Management: A review of available apps to assist with time management can be found here: https://www.lifehack.org/articles/technology/top-15-time-management-apps-and-tools.html.
- Pill Boxes to Support Medication Adherence: A description of various pill boxes available to support medication adherence can be found at https://www.tabtimer.com.au. This is a commercial website based in Australia, but it provides an overview of the products available, which people might be able to source locally.

References

Ahmad, A., Chiu, V., & Arain, M. A. (2020). Users' perceptions of an in-homer electronic medication dispensing system: A qualitative study. *Medical Devices: Evidence and Research, 13,* 31–39. https://doi.org/10.2147/MDER.S241062

Aldrich, R. M., McCarty, C. H., Boyd, B. A., Bunch, C. E., & Balentine, C. B. (2014). Empirical lessons about occupational categorization from case studies of unemployment. *Canadian Journal of Occupational Therapy, 81*(5), 289–297. https://doi.org/10.1177/0008417414540129

Arain, M. A., Ahmad, A., Chiu, V., & Kembel, L. (2021). Medication adherence support of an in-home electronic medication dispensing system for individuals living with chronic conditions: A pilot randomized controlled trial. *BMC Geriatrics, 21*(1), 56. https://doi.org/10.1186/s12877-020-01979-w

Atkin, A. J., Dainty, J. R., Dumuid, D., Kontostoli, E., Shepstone, L., Tyler, R., Noonan, R., Richardson, C., & Fairclough, S. J. (2021). Adolescent time use and mental health: A cross-sectional, compositional analysis in the Millennium Cohort Study. *BMJ Open, 11*(10), e047189. https://doi.org/10.1136/bmjopen-2020-047189

Atler, K. E., & Fisher, A. G. (2022). Validity and reliability of the Occupational Experience Profile. *Scandinavian Journal of Occupational Therapy, 30*(6), 811–821. https://doi.org/10.1080/11038128.2022.2027009

Barthorpe, A., Winstone, L., Mars, B., & Moran, P. (2020). Is social media screen time really associated with poor adolescent mental health? A time use diary study. *Journal of Affective Disorders, 274,* 864–870. https://doi.org/10.1016/j.jad.2020.05.106

Bejerholm, U. (2010). Occupational balance in people with schizophrenia. *Occupational Therapy in Mental Health, 26,* 1–17. https://doi.org/10.1080/01642120802642197

Bejerholm, U., & Eklund, M. (2004). Time use and occupational performance among persons with schizophrenia. *Occupational Therapy in Mental Health, 20,* 27–47. https://doi.org/10.1300/J004v20n01_02

Bejerholm, U., Hansson, L., & Eklund, M. (2006). Profiles of Occupational Engagement in People with Schizophrenia (POES): The development of a new instrument based on time-use diaries. *British Journal of Occupational Therapy, 69*(2), 58–68. https://doi.org/10.1177/030802260606900203

Berry, C., Hodgekins, J., French, P., Clarke, T., Shepstone, L., Barton, G., Banerjee, R., Byrne, R., Fraser, R., Grant, K., Greenwood, K., Notley, C., Parker, S., Wilson, J., Yung, A. R., & Fowler, D. (2022). Clinical and cost-effectiveness of social recovery therapy for the prevention and treatment of long-term social disability among young people with emerging severe mental illness (PRODIGY): Randomised controlled trial. *The British Journal of Psychiatry, 220*(3), 154–162. https://doi.org/10.1192/bjp.2021.206

Bjørkedal, S. T. B., Bejerholm, U., Eplov, L. F., & Møller, T. (2020). Meaningful Activities and Recovery (MA&R): The effect of a novel rehabilitation intervention among persons with psychiatric disabilities on activity engagement—Study protocol for a randomized controlled trial. *Trials, 21*(1), 789. https://doi.org/10.1186/s13063-020-04722-3

Bond, G. R., Drake, R. E., & Becker, D. R. (2012). Generalizability of the Individual Placement and Support (IPS) model of supported employment outside the US. *World Psychiatry, 11*(1), 32–39. https://doi.org/10.1016/j.wpsyc.2012.01.005

Bond, G. R., Drake, R. E., & Becker, D. R. (2020). An update on Individual Placement and Support. *World Psychiatry, 19*(3), 390–391. https://doi.org/10.1002/wps.20784

Bu, F., Steptoe, A., Mak, H. W., & Fancourt, D. (2021). Time use and mental health in UK adults during an 11-week COVID-19 lockdown: A panel analysis. *The British Journal of Psychiatry, 219*(4), 551–556. https://doi.org/10.1192/bjp.2021.44

Clark, F., Jackson, J., Carlson, M., Chou, C.-P., Cherry, B. J., Jordan-Marsh, M., Knight, B. G., Mandel, D., Blanchard, J., Granger, D. A., Wilcox, R. R., Lai, M. Y., White, B., Hay, J., Lam, C., Marterella, A., & Azen, S. P. (2012). Effectiveness of a lifestyle intervention in promoting the well-being of independently living older people: Results of the Well Elderly 2 Randomised Controlled Trial. *Journal of Epidemiology and Community Health, 66*(9), 782–790. https://doi.org/10.1136/jech.2009.099754

Crowe, M., Inder, M., Douglas, K., Carlyle, D., Wells, H., Jordan, J., Lacey, C., Mulder, R., Beaglehole, B., & Porter, R. (2020). Interpersonal and social Rhythm therapy for Patients with Major depressive disorder. *American Journal of Psychotherapy, 73*(1), 29–34. https://doi.org/10.1176/appi.psychotherapy.20190024

Crowe, M., Inder, M., Swartz, H. A., Murray, G., & Porter, R. (2020). Social rhythm therapy—A potentially translatable psychosocial intervention for bipolar disorder. *Bipolar Disorders, 22*(2), 121–127. https://doi.org/10.1111/bdi.12840

Csikszentmihalyi, M., & Larson, R. (1987). Validity and reliability of the Experience-Sampling Method. *Journal of Nervous and Mental Disease, 175*(9), 526–536. https://doi.org/10.1097/00005053-198709000-00004

Desha, L. N., & Ziviani, J. M. (2007). Use of time in childhood and adolescence: A literature review on the nature of activity participation and depression. *Australian Occupational Therapy Journal, 54*(1), 4–10. https://doi.org/10.1111/j.1440-1630.2006.00649.x

Doroud, N., Fossey, E., & Fortune, T. (2015). Recovery as an occupational journey: A scoping review exploring the links between occupational engagement and recovery for people with enduring mental health issues. *Australian Occupational Therapy Journal, 62*(6), 378–392. https://doi.org/10.1111/1440-1630.12238

Eagers, J., Franklin, R. C., Broome, K., Yau, M. K., & Barnett, F. (2022). Potential occupational therapy scope of practice in the work-to-retirement transition in Australia. *Australian Occupational Therapy Journal, 69*(3), 265–278. https://doi.org/10.1111/1440-1630.12788

Edgelow, M., & Krupa, T. (2011). Randomized controlled pilot study of an occupational time-use intervention for people with serious mental illness. *The American Journal of Occupational Therapy, 65*(3), 267–276. https://doi.org/10.5014/ajot.2011.001313

Eklund, M., & Erlandsson, L. K. (2014a). Redesigning Daily Occupations (ReDO™): Facilitating return to work among women with stress related disorders. In I. Söderbak (Ed.), *International handbook of occupational therapy interventions* (pp. 553–562). Springer.

Eklund, M., & Erlandsson, L. K. (2014b). Women's perceptions of everyday occupations: Outcomes of the Redesigning Daily Occupations (ReDO) programme. *Scandinavian Journal of Occupational Therapy, 21*(5), 359–367. https://doi.org/10.3109/11038128.2014.922611

Eklund, M., Leufstadius, C., & Bejerholm, U. (2009). Time use among people with psychiatric disabilities: Implications for practice. *Psychiatric Rehabilitation Journal, 32*(3), 177–191. https://doi.org/10.2975/32.3.2009.177.191

Eklund, M., Tjörnstrand, C., Sandlund, M., & Argentzell, E. (2017). Effectiveness of Balancing Everyday Life (BEL) versus standard occupational therapy for activity engagement and functioning among people with mental illness—A cluster RCT study. *BMC Psychiatry, 17*(1), 363. https://doi.org/10.1186/s12888-017-1524-7

Feather, N. T., & Bond, M. J. (1983). Time structure and purposeful activity among employed and unemployed university graduates. *Journal of Occupational Psychology, 56*(3), 241–254. https://doi.org/10.1111/j.2044-8325.1983.tb00131.x

Findley, E., LaBrenz, C. A., Childress, S., Vásquez-Schut, G., & Bowman, K. (2022). 'I'm not perfect': Navigating screen time among parents of young children during COVID-19. *Child: Care, Health and Development, 48*(6), 1094–1102. https://doi.org/10.1111/cch.13038

Fisher, A. G., & Marterella, A. (2019). *Powerful practice: A model for authentic occupational therapy.* Center for Innovative OT Solutions.

Fox, J., Erlandsson, L.-K., McSharry, J., & Shiel, A. (2022). How does ReDO®-10 work? Understanding the mechanisms of action of an intervention focused on daily activities and health from the perspective of participants. *Evaluation and Program Planning, 92*, 102092. https://doi.org/10.1016/j.evalprogplan.2022.102092

Fox, J., Erlandsson, L.-K., & Shiel, A. (2022). A feasibility study of the Redesigning Daily Occupations (ReDO™-10) programme in an Irish context. *Scandinavian Journal of Occupational Therapy, 29*(5), 415–429. https://doi.org/10.1080/11038128.2021.1882561

Frank, E., Kupfer, D. J., Thase, M. E., Mallinger, A. G., Swartz, H. A., Fagiolini, A. M., Grochocinski, V., Houck, P., Scott, J., Thompson, W., & Monk, T. (2005). Two-year outcomes for Interpersonal and Social Rhythm Therapy in individuals with bipolar I disorder. *Archives of General Psychiatry, 62*, 996–1004. https://doi.org/10.1001/archpsyc.62.9.996

Frank, E., Swartz, H. A., & Boland, E. (2007). Interpersonal and Social Rhythm Therapy: An intervention addressing rhythm dysregulation in bipolar disorder. *Dialogues in Clinical Neuroscience, 9*(3), 325–332. https://doi.org/10.31887/DCNS.2007.9.3/efrank

Frank, E., Swartz, H. A., & Kupfer, D. J. (2000). Interpersonal and Social Rhythm Therapy: Managing the chaos of bipolar disorder. *Biological Psychiatry, 48*(6), 593–604. https://doi.org/10.1016/S0006-3223(00)00969-0

Fredricks, J. A. (2012). Extracurricular participation and academic outcomes: Testing the over-scheduling hypothesis. *Journal of Youth and Adolescence, 41*, 295–306. https://doi.org/10.1007/s10964-011-9704-0

Goldberg, B., Brintnell, E. S., & Goldberg, J. (2002). The relationship between engagement in meaningful activities and quality of life in persons disabled by mental illness. *Occupational Therapy in Mental Health, 18*(2), 17–44. https://doi.org/10.1300/J004v18n02_03

Hayes, R. L., & Halford, W. K. (1996). Time use of unemployed and employed single male schizophrenia subjects. *Schizophrenia Bulletin, 22*(4), 659–669. https://doi.org/10.1093/schbul/22.4.659

Hodge, J. D. (2003). *The power of habit: Harnessing the power to establish routines that guarantee success in business and in life.* 1st Books.

Hunt, E., & McKay, E. A. (2012). Using population-level time use datasets to advance knowledge of human activity, participation and health. *The British Journal of Occupational Therapy, 75*(10), 478–480. https://doi.org/10.4276/030802212x13496921049789

Jahoda, M. (1982). *Employment and unemployment: A social-psychological analysis.* Cambridge University Press.

Jahoda, M., & Rush, H. (1980). *Work, employment and unemployment: An overview of ideas and research results in the social science literature.* SPRU Occasional Paper Series No. 12. Science Policy Research Unit, University of Sussex.

Jarrard, P., Cunningham, S., Granda, P., Harker, P., Lannan, T., & Price, K. (2021). Who are you without your substance? Transforming occupational time use in recovery. *Modern Applied Science, 15*(6), 19–26. https://doi.org/10.5539/mas.v15n6p19

Johansson, G., Eklund, M., & Erlandsson, L.-K. (2012). Everyday hassles and uplifts among women on long-term sick-leave due to stress-related disorders. *Scandinavian Journal of Occupational Therapy, 19*(3), 239–248. https://doi.org/10.3109/11038128.2011.569942

Koome, F., Hocking, C., & Sutton, D. (2012). Why routines matter: The nature and meaning of family routines in the context of adolescent mental illness. *Journal of Occupational Science, 19*(4), 312–325. https://doi.org/10.1080/14427591.2012.718245

Kreski, N. T., Chen, Q., Olfson, M., Cerdá, M., Hasin, D. S., Martins, S. S., Mauro, P. M., & Keyes, K. M. (2022). Time use and associations with internalizing symptoms from 1991 to 2019 among US adolescents. *SSM-Population Health, 19,* 101181. https://doi.org/10.1016/j.ssmph.2022.101181

Krupa, T., Edgelow, M., Chen, S.-P., & Mieras, C. (2021). *Promoting activity and participation in individuals with serious mental illness: The Action Over Inertia approach.* Routledge. https://doi.org/10.4324/9781003111368

Krupa, T., McLean, H., Eastabrook, S., Bonham, A., & Baksh, L. (2003). Daily time use as a measure of community adjustment for persons served by Assertive Community Treatment teams. *American Journal of Occupational Therapy, 57*(5), 558–565. https://doi.org/10.5014/ajot.57.5.558

Leufstadius, C., Erlandsson, L.-K., & Eklund, M. (2006). Time use and daily activities in people with persistent mental illness. *Occupational Therapy International, 13,* 123–141. https://doi.org/10.1002/oti.207

Liu, Y., Zemke, R., Liang, L., & Gray, J. M. (2021a). Model of Occupational Harmony: A Chinese perspective on occupational balance. *Annals of International Occupational Therapy, 4*(4), e228–e235. https://doi.org/10.3928/24761222-20210601-08

Liu, Y., Zemke, R., Liang, L., & Gray, J. M. (2021b). Occupational harmony: Embracing the complexity of occupational balance. *Journal of Occupational Science,* 1–15. https://doi.org/10.1080/14427591.2021.1881592

Lobo, F. (1999). Young people and unemployment: Does job loss diminish involvement in leisure? *Society and Leisure, 22*(1), 145–170. https://doi.org/10.1080/07053436.1999.10715580

Lund, K., Argentzell, E., Leufstadius, C., Tjörnstrand, C., & Eklund, M. (2019). Joining, belonging, and re-valuing: A process of meaning-making through group participation in a mental health lifestyle intervention. *Scandinavian Journal of Occupational Therapy, 26*(1), 55–68. https://doi.org/10.1080/11038128.2017.1409266

Martella, D., & Maass, A. (2000). Unemployment and life satisfaction: The moderating role of time structure and collectivism. *Journal of Applied Social Psychology, 30*(5), 1095–1108. https://doi.org/10.1111/j.1559-1816.2000.tb02512.x

Matuska, K. (2012). Description and development of the Life Balance Inventory. *OTJR: Occupation, Participation and Health, 32*(1), 220–228. https://doi.org/10.3928/15394492-20110610-01

Matuska, K., & Christiansen, C. H. (2008). A proposed model of lifestyle balance. *Journal of Occupational Science, 15,* 9–19. https://doi.org/10.1080/14427591.2008.9686602

McKenna, K., Broome, K., & Liddle, J. (2007). What older people do: Time use and exploring the link between role participation and life satisfaction in people aged 65 years and older. *Australian Occupational Therapy Journal, 54*(4), 273–284. https://doi.org/10.1111/j.1440-1630.2007.00642.x

Meyer, A. (1922/1983). The philosophy of occupational therapy. *Occupational Therapy in Mental Health, 2*(3), 79–87. https://doi.org/10.1300/J004v02n03_05

Minato, M., & Zemke, R. (2004). Time use of people with schizophrenia living in the community. *Occupational Therapy International, 11*(3), 177–191. https://doi.org/10.1002/oti.205

Mullan, K. (2019). A child's day: Trends in time use in the UK from 1975 to 2015. *The British Journal of Sociology, 70*(3), 997–1024. https://doi.org/10.1111/1468-4446.12369

Nagata, J. M., Cortez, C. A., Cattle, C. J., Ganson, K. T., Iyer, P., Bibbins-Domingo, K., & Baker, F. C. (2022). Screen time use among US adolescents during the COVID-19 pandemic: Findings from the Adolescent Brain Cognitive Development (ABCD) study. *JAMA Pediatrics, 176*(1), 94–96. https://doi.org/10.1001/jamapediatrics.2021.4334

Olsson, A., Erlandsson, L.-K., & Håkansson, C. (2020). The occupation-based intervention REDO™-10: Long-term impact on work ability for women at risk for or on sick leave. *Scandinavian Journal of Occupational Therapy, 27*(1), 47–55. https://doi.org/10.1080/11038128.2019.1614215

Pandya, A., & Lodha, P. (2021). Social connectedness, excessive screen time during COVID-19 and mental health: A review of current evidence. *Frontiers in Human Dynamics, 3,* 684137. https://doi.org/10.3389/fhumd.2021.684137

Rees, E. F., Ennals, P., & Fossey, E. (2021). Implementing an Action Over Inertia group program in community residential rehabilitation services: Group participant and facilitator perspectives. *Frontiers in Psychiatry, 12,* 624803. https://doi.org/10.3389/fpsyt.2021.624803

Sanders, M. J., & Van Oss, T. (2013). Using daily routines to promote medication adherence in older adults. *The American Journal of Occupational Therapy, 67*(1), 91–99. https://doi.org/10.5014/ajot.2013.005033

Scanlan, J. N., & Bundy, A. C. (2011). Development and validation of the Modified Occupational Questionnaire. *American Journal of Occupational Therapy, 65*(1), e11–e19. https://doi.org/10.5014/ajot.2011.09042

Scanlan, J. N., Bundy, A. C., & Matthews, L. R. (2011). Promoting wellbeing in young unemployed adults: The importance of identifying meaningful patterns of time use. *Australian Occupational Therapy Journal, 58*(2), 111–119. https://doi.org/10.1111/j.1440-1630.2010.00879.x

Smith, N. R., Kielhofner, G., & Watts, J. H. (1986). The relationship between volition, activity pattern, and life satisfaction in the elderly. *American Journal of Occupational Therapy, 40*(4), 278–283. https://doi.org/10.5014/ajot.40.4.278

Stone, A., Shiffman, S., & DeVries, M. (1999). Ecological Momentary Assessment. In D. Kahneman, E. Diener, & N. Schwarz (Eds.), *Well-being: The foundations of hedonic psychology* (pp. 26–39). Russel Sage Foundation.

Tepavicharov, N. K., Christensen, J. R., Møller, T., Eplov, L. F., & Bjørkedal, S. T. B. (2022). "Moving on to an Open World": A study of participants' experience in Meaningful Activities and Recovery (MA&R). *Occupational Therapy International, 2022,* 7418667. https://doi.org/10.1155/2022/7418667

Tjörnstrand, C., Eklund, M., Bejerholm, U., Argentzell, E., & Brunt, D. (2020). A day in the life of people with severe mental illness living in supported housing. *BMC Psychiatry, 20*(1), 508. https://doi.org/10.1186/s12888-020-02896-3

Wanberg, C. R., Griffiths, R. F., & Gaving, M. B. (1997). Time structure and unemployment: A longitudinal investigation. *Journal of Occupational and Organizational Psychology, 70*(1), 75–79. https://doi.org/10.1111/j.2044-8325.1997.tb00632.x

Waters, L. E., & Muller, J. (2003). Money or time? Comparing the effects of time structure and financial deprivation on the psychological distress of unemployed adults. *Australian Journal of Psychology, 55*(3), 166–175. https://doi.org/10.1080/00049530042000298632

White, S. M., Riley, A., & Flom, P. (2013). The Assessment of Time Management Skills (ATMS): A practice-based outcome questionnaire. *Occupational Therapy in Mental Health, 29*(3), 215–231. https://doi.org/10.1080/0164212X.2013.819481

Wiciak, M. T., Shazley, O., & Santhosh, D. (2022). An observational report of screen time use among young adults (ages 18–28 years) during the COVID-19 pandemic and correlations with mental health and wellness: International, online, cross-sectional study. *JMIR Formative Research, 6*(8), e38370. https://doi.org/10.2196/38370

Wood, W., Womack, J., & Hooper, B. (2009). Dying of boredom: An exploratory case study of time use, apparent affect, and routine activity situations on two Alzheimer's special care units. *American Journal of Occupational Therapy, 63*(3), 337–350. https://doi.org/10.5014/ajot.63.3.337

Zuzanek, J. (1998). Time use, time pressure, personal stress, mental health, and life satisfaction from a life cycle perspective. *Journal of Occupational Science, 5*(1), 26–39. https://doi.org/10.1080/14427591.1998.9686432

CHAPTER
15
Pain

John V. Rider and Bronwyn Lennox Thompson

Although the experience of pain is universal, the pain experience is unique to each individual. Pain is common and can be experienced at any stage in life. It can be short-lived or persistent and significantly impacts occupational performance and participation.

Regardless of the practice setting or population, occupational therapy practitioners (OTPs) work with people who experience pain; therefore, they need the knowledge and ability to help people develop skills to reduce the impact of pain on occupational performance and participation and improve quality of life. The widespread prevalence of pain and the significant impact on physical, mental, and social health demonstrate a need for comprehensive pain education.

This chapter defines and explores pain, with increased attention to persistent pain; describes the Biopsychosocial Model of Pain; highlights the relationship of pain to all aspects of the occupational therapy domain; provides guidance for assessing pain; summarizes evidence-based occupational therapy interventions; and provides a first-person account of an individual with persistent pain.

Exploring Pain

Persistent or chronic pain affects over 20% (66 million) of adults living in the United States, and of those individuals, over 7% (23 million) report that pain limits their lives or work activities (Zelaya et al., 2020). The prevalence of chronic pain is increasing, with more than one in five adults in the United States experiencing daily chronic pain (Yong et al., 2022). However, this is a conservative estimate, as it does not include data on chronic pain among children and youth, which has been reported to be as high as 30% (Wager et al., 2020).

Pain is the most common reason for seeking medical care in the United States, and it affects the lives of the individuals experiencing pain, their loved ones, and their caregivers (National Center for Complementary and Integrative Health, 2023; Schappert & Burt, 2006). The U.S. Department of Health and Human Services (2019) recognizes pain as a public health problem with significant physical, emotional, and societal costs, estimated between $560 and $635 billion annually. Individuals with chronic pain use primary health-care services five times more often than the general population (Bawa et al., 2015). Beyond medical care, pain costs include the economic costs of disability, lost wages, and decreased productivity.

Acute pain is common and often resolves with healing. However, it can be distressing and directly impacts occupational performance and quality of life. Chronic pain is a global problem that is often misunderstood and undertreated (International Association for the Study of Pain [IASP], 2015). Governing bodies now recognize the obligation to manage pain and relieve suffering as fundamental to health care (IASP, 2015). Furthermore, access to pain management without discrimination is recognized as a basic human right (IASP, 2015).

Risk factors for developing chronic pain include being female; increased age; belonging to a minority group; having lower socioeconomic status; unemployment; lifestyle factors such as smoking, alcohol use, and low physical activity; comorbid health conditions; surgical and medical procedures; sleep disorders; passive coping strategies; negative beliefs about pain; early life adversity; and a history of interpersonal violence or abuse (Mills et al., 2019).

People with chronic pain often experience comorbid psychiatric disorders, particularly mood and anxiety disorders, including posttraumatic stress disorder (PTSD; Arnow et al., 2006; Gatchel et al., 2012; Mills et al., 2019). Evidence suggests a bidirectional relationship between pain and mental health and a bidirectional impact of comorbid chronic pain and mood on functioning (Bondesson et al., 2018; Travaglini et al., 2020). Chronic pain and mental health problems can contribute to and exacerbate each other and affect all aspects of occupational performance and participation.

Definition

The IASP defines "pain" as "an unpleasant sensory and emotional experience associated with, or resembling that associated with, actual or potential tissue damage" (Raja et al., 2020, p. 14). The IASP expands upon this definition with six key notes:

- Pain is always a personal experience that is influenced to varying degrees by biological, psychological, and social factors.
- Pain and nociception (the neural process of encoding noxious stimuli) are different phenomena. Pain cannot be inferred solely from activity in sensory neurons.
- Through their life experiences, individuals learn the concept of pain.
- A person's report of an experience as pain should be respected.

- Although pain usually serves an adaptive role, it may have adverse effects on function and social and psychological well-being.
- Verbal description is only one of several behaviors to express pain; inability to communicate does not negate the possibility that a human or a nonhuman animal experiences pain.

The IASP definition illustrates the physical (sensory) and psychological (emotional) experiences associated with pain. Pain is perceived as both sensory and emotional, and the term is reserved for the experience of pain. The expanded notes convey that pain is a subjective, multifaceted experience. Individual variables, such as age, sex, prior pain experiences, mood, cognitive beliefs (e.g., the meaning of pain), coping style, familial factors, and culture, are known to affect an individual's experience of pain.

Classifications

Classifying pain can help guide evaluation and intervention approaches. Several systems are used to classify pain, including the IASP mechanistic groups (Woolf, 2010), the International Classification of Diseases (ICD) classifications, and the *Diagnostic and Statistical Manual of Mental Disorders (DSM)*.

Pain can also be classified by duration: acute, subacute, and chronic. **Acute pain** is typically associated with tissue damage and inflammation, and subsides as tissue healing occurs. *Subacute pain* typically remains present between 6 weeks and 3 months. **Chronic pain** is not consistently defined but can be considered pain that persists beyond the expected tissue healing time, pain that is present for 3 to 6 months or longer, or pain that serves no evolutionary adaptive function. Definitions of pain based on duration can be problematic because some pain problems can be considered persistent from their onset rather than moving from an acute to a chronic condition (e.g., complex regional pain syndrome). Furthermore, acute pain can last longer than expected (e.g., pain associated with fractures that is present for over 12 months).

Loeser (2018) suggests that pain should no longer be defined by duration but by the location of the main mechanisms involved: peripheral or central, referring to pain caused or maintained by lesions or diseases in the peripheral and/or central nervous systems. This approach is complicated by the difficulty in identifying the mechanisms by which pain persists and because pain often involves multiple processes throughout the peripheral and central nervous systems. OTPs will hear multiple terms and should be aware of their limitations.

The IASP recommends that clinicians classify pain into three mechanistic groups: nociceptive, neuropathic, and nociplastic (IASP, 2012). It is important to recognize that individuals can have a combination of pain types. A basic understanding of nociception and nociceptors is necessary to understand the mechanistic groups. Nociception is the neural process of encoding noxious stimuli. Noxious stimuli can be any stimulus damaging or threatening damage to normal tissues. Encoding noxious stimuli may result in autonomic responses (e.g., elevated blood pressure), behavioral responses (withdrawal reflex), or pain sensations.

However, pain sensation is not necessarily implied, as pain and nociception are different phenomena. Nociceptors are high-threshold sensory receptors of the peripheral somatosensory nervous system capable of transducing and encoding noxious stimuli. The following definitions are based on the IASP pain terminology (2012).

Nociceptive pain arises from actual or threatened damage to nonneural tissue from the activation of nociceptors. Nociceptive pain warns of potential damage. Nociceptor activity is processed at the spinal cord level, often evoking involuntary reflex withdrawal actions before reaching conscious awareness. Once the stimulus is removed, nociceptive activity ceases, and the pain stops. *Inflammatory pain* is nociceptive pain that arises once tissue damage has occurred and is associated with the release of many neurochemicals that both support the removal of necrotic tissue and reduce nociceptive firing thresholds. Once inflammation is resolved, pain also stops. Inflammatory pain can produce **allodynia** (i.e., pain caused by a stimulus that does not normally provoke pain) and **hyperalgesia** (i.e., pain that is experienced as more intense than would usually be expected under typical conditions).

Neuropathic pain arises from an identifiable lesion or disease of the somatosensory system. Neuropathic pain can involve peripheral nerve impingement or a lesion (e.g., diabetic neuropathy, ulnar nerve entrapment), spinal cord lesion (e.g., spinal cord injury, Brown-Sequard syndrome), and lesions or damage in the somatosensory parts of the cortex (e.g., stroke, multiple sclerosis). Similar to inflammatory pain, neuropathic pain can result in allodynia and hyperalgesia, and it is also often accompanied by **dysesthesia** (unpleasant abnormal sensations that can become intense and/or painful), cold or hot sensations, **paresthesias** (numbness, tingling, "pins and needles" sensations), or electric shocklike pain.

Nociplastic pain is the most recent addition to the IASP classifications. Pain in this group is thought to result from alterations in central nervous system processing. It is defined as pain that arises from altered nociception, despite no clear evidence of actual or threatened tissue damage, causing the activation of peripheral nociceptors or evidence of disease or lesion of the somatosensory system causing the pain. Nociplastic pain is the least well-known and most poorly understood classification of pain. Yet, it might account for most persistent pain conditions, such as fibromyalgia, chronic nonspecific low back pain, and migraines (Fitzcharles et al., 2021).

DSM-5 diagnoses may be given to people experiencing chronic pain without identified biological pathology. However, there is no evidence that psychological factors directly *cause* pain. Pain researchers and clinicians recognize that psychological factors such as learning and coping are involved in *all* pain irrespective of etiology or duration, whereas biological changes underpin many psychological phenomena, such as neurophysiological brain changes in perceiving pain (Lena et al., 2022).

Models of Pain

Pain is always a *whole person* experience influenced by biological, psychological, and social factors. Pain can be thought of as emerging from this bio psycho social combination, with pain behavior (i.e., what people do as a response to pain) as the aspect of pain observed by others.

Loeser and Fordyce's Model of Pain

To understand the different aspects of pain that OTPs might treat, readers can consider the "onion ring" model of pain first developed by Loeser and Fordyce (1983), as seen in Figure 15-1.

The inner ring represents biological processes involved in nociception and pain perception. **Nociception** is the neural process of encoding noxious stimuli. More specifically, nociception is encoding high-intensity stimuli from the peripheral nervous system through the spinal cord dorsal horn and up to cortical areas before conscious perception. Modulation occurs at each synapse along the route toward conscious awareness, meaning ascending information may be reduced or enhanced in response to "top-down" processes. Complex networks of cortical activity are involved in determining whether people become aware of nociceptive activity.

Many parts of the brain are involved in processing nociception and related factors, such as emotional responses, sensory qualities (e.g., stinging, sharp, nauseating), the location (e.g., chest, arm, abdomen), and areas dealing with motor preparation. Concurrent activity in brain areas involved in memory, goal-setting, and decision-making contribute to pain perception and appraisal (i.e., interpretation of what the pain means). Nociception is not equivalent to pain.

The next ring represents **pain** or the *sensory and emotional experience* people associate with tissue damage. Pain is a subjective experience people cannot share directly; there is no "pain thermometer." People's experience of pain remains private, and there are no means for determining whether a person's report of pain is a true representation of their experience. Hence, it is also not possible in a health-care setting to determine whether someone is malingering or whether their response is "exaggerated" (Tuck et al., 2019).

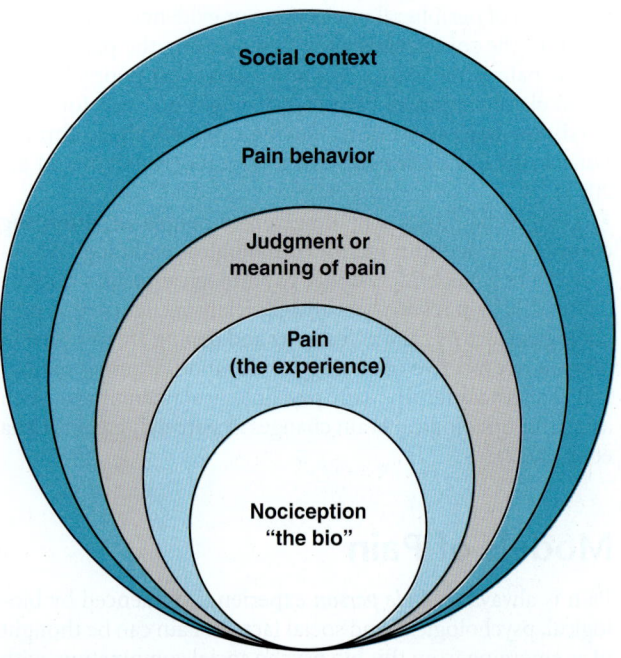

FIGURE 15-1. Loeser and Fordyce's Model of Pain. *Adapted from Loeser, J. D. (1980). Perspectives on pain. In P. Turner (Ed.), Clinical pharmacy and therapeutics (pp. 313–316). Macmillan.*

As pain is perceived, *judgments* are made about current activity and what should be done about it. Judgments are based on an individual's past experiences, observations of others, sociocultural norms and expectations, pain intensity and quality, and influence responses to pain. For example, a person who has previously had migraines will likely notice and interpret the onset of unilateral pain behind the eye, accompanied by nausea, photophobia (light sensitivity), and phonophobia (sound sensitivity), differently from someone having their first episode.

Beliefs and expectations about low back pain are particularly influential because there is a discrepancy between the public understanding of back pain and current evidence. Most low back pain is very uncomfortable; it may settle slowly and reoccur, but it rarely requires imaging or surgery. However, because many people believe the spine is weak and vulnerable to damage, they also think back pain indicates the need for a surgical solution (Ray et al., 2022).

Pain behaviors are the only aspect of pain that can be observed, and depending on the definition of pain behaviors, they may also include thoughts and beliefs (Gross & Fox, 2009). Pain behaviors include involuntary and voluntary actions taken in response to pain. Involuntary actions include the withdrawal reflex, vocalizations (e.g., gasping, groaning, saying "ouch"), muscle guarding, and sympathetic nervous system responses (e.g., increased heart rate, respiration, perspiration). Involuntary responses may have evolutionary utility to protect the person from exposure to noxious stimuli and to communicate with others. Voluntary actions include well-learned behavior, such as gestures and swearing, and complex behaviors, such as taking medication, avoiding activities, or seeking health care. Occupational therapy interventions often target pain behaviors.

The final ring in this model illustrates the influence of **social context** on the pain experience and behavior. Learning influences pain behavior via social learning (Stone et al., 2018) and operant conditioning. Social learning theory shows that the way members of a family group express pain is similar (Stone et al., 2018), whereas operant conditioning processes explain why it is common for someone to utter a curse word after hitting their shin in the privacy of the home but not so much in a very quiet classroom with the professor watching.

Social context also influences a person's judgments of their pain. Young athletes, for example, learn that pain during training is expected, and they can discern the difference between "good pain" and pain from an injury (Tarr & Thomas, 2021). In turn, these socially constructed judgments influence pain behavior, sometimes to the person's detriment if they are focused on an upcoming competition despite having an injury.

Loeser and Fordyce's model helps explain how numerous biopsychosocial factors influence the relationship between nociceptive processes and the eventual pain behaviors clinicians observe. OTPs recognize the complexity involved in understanding an individual's occupational participation. By drawing on the profession's biopsychosocial heritage, OTPs are well placed to understand why people respond differently to what appears to be the same pain problem. This understanding means the profession's approach to helping people enhance their occupational participation does not rely on pain reduction as a prerequisite or primary focus (see Box 15-1).

BOX 15-1 ■ Chronic Pain and Quality of Life

Although the impact of acute pain on emotions and occupational participation is well known, poorly managed chronic pain is associated with significant changes in quality of life (e.g., mood, thoughts, attitudes, lifestyle, and environment; Fine, 2011). As one individual stated: "Every day is a fight. Every morning is a battle to get ready for the day. Every afternoon is a fight to stay awake. Every night is a fight to find sleep. And between every fight is another one: fighting pain, constant pain, day, all night, every single day. The pain hasn't stopped, but it hasn't stopped me.

I am a chronic pain warrior."

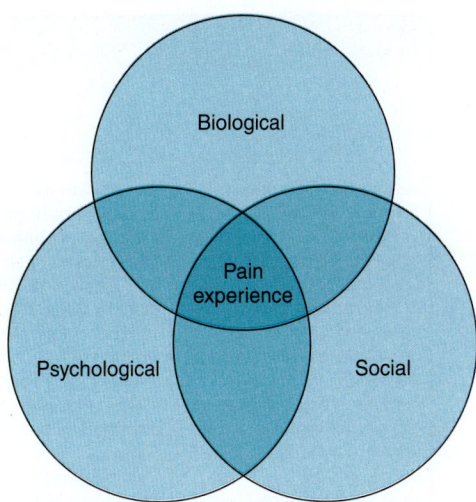

FIGURE 15-2. Biopsychosocial Model of Pain.

Biopsychosocial Model of Pain

Building on Loeser's four dimensions associated with pain, it is important to recognize that to fully understand a person's perception and response to pain, the interrelationships among biological changes, psychological status, and sociocultural context must be considered (Gatchel et al., 2007).

The Biopsychosocial Model of Pain is the most heuristic and widely used approach to understanding and treating pain and "evaluates the integrated whole person, with both the mind and the body together as interconnected entities, recognizing biological, psychological, and social components of pain and illness" (Bevers et al., 2016, p. 99). This model is congruent with occupational therapy's unique perspective on the relationship between a person, their daily activities, and their environment (Fig. 15-2). The Biopsychosocial Model of Pain approach is considered more effective than biomedical approaches in pain management and aligns with commonly used occupational therapy models and frames of reference (American Occupational Therapy Association [AOTA], 2021).

Biological factors include age, genetic factors, nociception, disease, comorbidities, physical health, trauma, tissue injury, immune response, sex differences, nervous system characteristics, sleep participation, the effect of medications, and so on. Psychological factors include coping strategies, stress, thoughts and beliefs about pain, expectations, attitude, anxiety, depression, catastrophizing, past experiences, self-efficacy, and so on. Social factors include cultural beliefs, required activities of daily living (ADLs), economic status, social support, environmental stressors, work situations, relationships, medical care, stigma, social expectations, and so on. The interaction of these factors influences the experience of pain symptoms and disability; therefore, OTPs need to assess and intervene in each area for comprehensive pain management.

Using a biopsychosocial approach, OTPs recognize that pain and the impact of pain on occupational performance and participation is a multidimensional, dynamic interaction among physiological, psychological, and social factors that reciprocally influence one another. OTPs can provide a combination of treatment approaches from the biopsychosocial perspective to meet the unique needs in each area when addressing pain management. Within the Biopsychosocial Model of Pain, OTPs bring a deeper understanding of pain through context and occupation.

Occupational Therapy View of Pain: Context and Occupation

Context refers to the "environmental and personal factors specific to each client that influence engagement and participation in occupations" (AOTA, 2020, p. 9). OTPs consider the contexts of daily life, including environmental factors or aspects of the physical, social, and attitudinal surroundings in which people conduct their lives (AOTA, 2020). Therefore, daily life is where OTPs situate interventions, and participating in daily occupations is the outcome.

In chronic pain practice, occupational therapy aims to help people make sense of and relate to their pain in a way that supports their progress toward optimal occupational participation and performance. Strategies may include demystifying or dethreatening the experience of pain so people can make room for pain and do what matters most to them. It is both necessary and possible for people to live well in the presence of ongoing pain (Lennox Thompson et al., 2020), as pain cannot always be reduced or eliminated, particularly pain arising from neuropathic and nociplastic mechanisms.

Pain may affect occupational engagement through several means. Difficulties with occupational participation and performance arise from:

■ Fear and distress when experiencing pain, and because of efforts to avoid both pain and associated experiences (e.g., reducing participation in daily life to pursue pain treatment, avoiding movements that may cause pain)

■ Unhelpful or "sticky" beliefs about pain that are interpreted literally (e.g., "My disc has slipped, if I move, it will burst," or "My osteoarthritis means my joints are wearing out, so I should stop doing things")

■ Inflexible retaining or adopting a negative sense of self (e.g., "I am a bad parent because I can't play with my children the way I think I should")

■ Remembering past experiences and forecasting future experiences rather than being present with what is (e.g., avoiding an activity because of anticipating a flare-up, remembering a previous occasion when doing an activity hurt, even when pain is not currently present)

Reflective Questions			
Variation	**Selection**	**Retention**	**Context**
Adaptation requires ongoing behavioral variation: What are some different ways the person can engage in their occupations? How can I promote behavioral variation during therapy? How can I explore different ways of engaging in values-based action (occupations) during therapy? How will this intervention support different ways to engage in occupations? If this intervention cannot be used, how else could the person engage in values-based action?	**Adaptation requires selecting options over other possibilities:** Can the person sensitively select how to do what matters, depending on the context and purpose? Do the interventions ensure the person can participate in ways that align with what matters for them in their life contexts? Can the person recognize when ways of doing daily activities are unworkable or limit participation? Does the person know how to distinguish between values-based selection and avoidance-based selection?	**Adaptation involves repeated action over time:** What kinds of support does the person need to develop habits or routine changes? How does the person feel about their ability to change their habits, routines, or rituals? Can the person appreciate the life impact of choice and actions over time? What has worked in the past to help this person develop new habits? Did we explore what this person would like to happen over time?	**Adaptation involves being aware of and responsive to salient contextual features:** Has the person's range of life contexts been explored? Can the person differentiate internal and external parts of their experience? Can the person notice salient features and reflexively adjust their behavior? Does the person have fears, expectations, or beliefs that make them less sensitive to what is actually happening? Does the person know how they can modify occupational participation given contextual changes?

FIGURE 15-3. Reflective questions for adaptation to living with persistent pain. OTPs can use these reflective questions to guide reasoning when developing and integrating pain management coping strategies. *Adapted from Lennox Thompson, B. F., & Ramanauskas, C. (2024). Articulating occupational therapy's unique contribution to pain management.* New Zealand Journal of Occupational Therapy, 71*(1), 26–32.*

- Pursuing strategies that take away from what matters in life (e.g., seeking diagnostic tests and treatments for years after pain onset and diagnosis, refraining from meaningful occupations)
- Being inflexible about actions (e.g., not using activity pacing because it conflicts with current beliefs about laziness)

With direct application to pain management, OTPs' unique and specialized expertise can be described within three key areas:

1. *OTPs know context and meaning.* Occupational therapy clinical reasoning models incorporate the person, their environment, and the occupations the person wants or needs to do (Law et al., 1996).
2. OTPs know occupation is an expression of self-concept (Christiansen, 1999).
3. OTPs know that how individuals adapt to dynamic and changing contexts has implications for health and quality of life (Walder et al., 2021).

When people can no longer engage in preferred occupations, they lose parts of who they are and how they express their sense of self. Maintaining or developing the self-concept involves learning how to adapt everyday activity to enable occupational participation, even if these need to be expressed differently.

OTPs can confidently claim to be "knowledge translation" experts in chronic pain management. Skills and strategies for managing pain must be integrated into daily life, and strategies must become embedded into a person's life while not becoming prescriptive or restrictive. Occupational therapy interventions can bridge the gap between unfamiliar strategies, such as activity pacing, and how people live their lives. OTPs can help individuals develop meta-cognitive skills to

choose the best strategy to suit short- and long-term situations and to identify alternatives when they cannot utilize a preferred strategy. Coping strategies must be well rehearsed, remembered, and contextually used so the individual experiencing pain can still do what matters to them. See also Chapter 10: Coping and Resilience.

An evolutionary lens may be useful to aid clinical reasoning and consider the range of strategies OTPs may explore with individuals experiencing pain. Occupations can be considered adaptive or maladaptive, depending on context and an individual's resources. When a person's resources are constrained by pain, they often alter occupational participation. From an evolutionary perspective, how a person adapts can be evaluated against the principles of *variation, selection, retention,* and *context* sensitivity, focusing on the relevant dimensions and levels within a biopsychosocial framework (Hayes et al., 2020). OTPs can use these principles to evaluate adaptation and to influence action toward an adaptive trajectory.

Figure 15-3 provides reflective questions to guide reasoning when developing and integrating pain management coping strategies. This broad approach to pain management strategies considers a person's capabilities for participating in what matters to them in their daily life contexts, allowing OTPs to support individuals toward increased occupational participation, resilience, and flexibility for the future.

Pain Catastrophizing

As discussed earlier, many biological, social, and psychological factors influence the experience of pain. The state of a person's physical body, the amount and quality of support they get from their family and friends, and their beliefs about pain influence the intensity and quality of all their sensations, including pain. Depression, anxiety, poor self-efficacy, perceived disability, and fear are associated with and considered predictors of pain. However, of all the psychological factors that have been studied and shown to be associated with pain and its impact on people's lives, the single most consistent and strongest factor associated with pain and pain-related outcomes is catastrophizing (Jensen et al., 2011; Pulvers & Hood, 2013; Quartana et al., 2009).

The definition of pain catastrophizing has evolved from its introduction by Albert Ellis (1962) and highlights cognitive beliefs and the thought process surrounding pain. Aaron T. Beck described it as a maladaptive cognitive style initially seen in patients with anxiety and depressive disorders. The early definitions emphasized an irrational negative forecast of future events (Beck et al., 1979; Ellis, 1962). According to Beck and coworkers (1979), patients suffering from pain catastrophizing are maladaptive because they cannot develop additional coping skills that might afford them a more optimistic outlook for the future. More recently, Quartana and colleagues (2009) provided a more comprehensive definition of pain catastrophizing:

> Collectively, pain catastrophizing is characterized by the tendency to magnify the threat value of pain stimulus and to feel helpless in the context of pain, and by a relative inability to inhibit pain-related thoughts in anticipation of, during or following a painful encounter. (p. 2)

Pain catastrophizing is often explored through three constructs or dimensions: magnification, helplessness, and rumination. *Magnification* can be thought of as exaggerating the threat value of pain sensations (e.g., "I am never going to be able to do ___ again because of the pain"). *Helplessness* is perceiving oneself as unable to cope with pain symptoms (e.g., "There is nothing I can do to reduce the intensity of the pain"). *Rumination* refers to an excessive focus on pain sensations (e.g., "I can't stop thinking about how much it hurts") and often interferes with sleep participation and attention.

Pain catastrophizing is an important determinant of pain-related functional outcomes. In general, higher levels of pain catastrophizing are associated with greater pain intensity; increased perceived disability; increased pain-related occupational impairment; greater emotional distress, including depression and anxiety; increased medication use; greater use of medical and mental health-care services; lower rates of returning to work; alterations in social networks; and chronicity of pain (Quartana et al., 2009).

Evidence also suggests that the relationship between catastrophizing and pain emerges early in life and has been observed across a wide range of clinical and experimental pain-eliciting situations, showing a remarkable consistency (Sullivan, 2009). Reductions in catastrophizing prospectively predict reductions in pain and disability (Adams et al., 2007; Sullivan et al., 2006), indicating the potential for catastrophizing as a treatment target for OTPs.

Sensory processing may also affect pain outcomes, as individual sensory processing styles are related to pain coping (Meredith et al., 2015). Meredith and colleagues (2015) found that sensory sensitivity and sensation avoiding were significantly associated with higher levels of catastrophizing, whereas sensation seeking was associated with active coping strategies, such as increasing behavioral activities and using coping self-statements. See also Chapter 9: Sensory Processing and the Lived Sensory Experience. 🤝 Stress is also a significant factor in pain catastrophizing and diverting attention from pain (Meredith et al., 2015). OTPs should consider sensory processing styles when assessing and treating individuals experiencing pain and utilize sensory-informed approaches.

Although pain catastrophizing is predictive of many factors of interest to OTPs when addressing pain, it is important to note that some health-care practitioners and literature have referred to catastrophizing in a derogatory way that is often unhelpful to people living with pain. OTPs need to understand catastrophizing thoughts and their impact on the pain experience. However, OTPs must be cautious about how they refer to catastrophizing. For example, administering the Pain Catastrophizing Scale (PCS; described in the Evaluating Pain section of this chapter) to people and discussing their thoughts and feelings when experiencing pain is often beneficial, but can be done without ever using the word "catastrophizing" or questioning the validity of the person's pain. Assessment, treatment, and education on catastrophizing should never dismiss the person's experience of pain or suggest the pain is their fault. Intervention approaches such as cognitive behavioral therapy (CBT) or Acceptance and Commitment Therapy (ACT) can help people address catastrophizing thoughts and beliefs about pain and increase occupational engagement.

Evaluating Pain

Recognizing the multifaceted and all-encompassing experience of pain often leads to concerns about assessing pain. The American Pain Society has encouraged clinicians to consider pain the "fifth vital sign," hoping that effective pain control would more likely occur if pain were assessed in a similar manner to other vital signs (Morone & Weiner, 2013). Although this has led to more consistent pain intensity ratings, it is not enough for OTPs to only ask, "How intense is your pain on a scale from 1 to 10?" OTPs must carefully assess the multidimensional and biopsychosocial aspects of the pain experience to develop a comprehensive pain management plan in collaboration with the person experiencing pain.

Focusing on pain intensity as a primary measure may inadvertently make pain reduction seem as if it is the only important outcome. Given the complex relationship between pain intensity and disability and the challenge to obtain a minimally clinically important reduction in pain intensity for neuropathic and nociplastic pain, focusing primarily on pain reduction from an intensity perspective may be unhelpful.

Pain is a subjective phenomenon that defies objective measurement. "Pain is always a personal experience that is influenced to varying degrees by biological, psychological, and social factors" (Raja et al., 2020, p. 14). The subjective nature of the pain experience restricts the assessment and interpretation of a person's pain in theoretical, philosophical, diagnostic, and practical terms (Strong & van Griensven, 2014). Too often, the measurement of pain focuses on the magnitude or intensity of pain, overlooking the impact of pain on occupations and physical, emotional, and social health. OTPs must seek to understand the multidimensionality of pain within the context of the person and their daily life.

Furthermore, the impact of pain on a person's daily life needs to be considered in terms of physical limitation and emotional and social influences on health and person-defined well-being (IASP, 2018). Because pain can impact and be influenced by occupations, contexts, performance patterns and skills, and client factors, OTPs should ensure that the evaluation process includes all aspects of the occupational therapy domain (AOTA, 2020). For example, pain often negatively impacts rest, sleep, and health management, necessitating additional targeted assessments. See also Chapter 52: Sleep. 🤝 Pain is often comorbid with mood disorders, and specific assessments for client factors, such as psychosocial functioning, are often warranted.

The evaluation process begins with developing an **occupational profile** and **analysis of occupational performance,** *with specific attention to the impact of pain* (AOTA, 2021). Although factors such as pain intensity, location, type, and frequency should be included, they are only one aspect of the pain assessment. Physical, cognitive, psychosocial, and sensory-perceptual factors related to occupational engagement and the pain experience must also be assessed. OTPs should also consider assessing pain *coping skills, perceptions, cognitive and emotional responses to pain,* and *self-efficacy* (AOTA, 2021).

Another consideration when assessing pain and working with individuals experiencing pain is language. The language used on intake paperwork, during evaluation or treatment, or on discharge instructions can influence people negatively or positively (Manai et al., 2019). For example, the negative, harsh, or stigmatizing language used to describe pain, injury, prognosis, or diagnostic imaging (wear and tear, chronic, degenerative, etc.) can instill fear and hopelessness and enhance pain perception, whereas appropriate language used to educate people throughout their rehabilitation experience can reduce fear, anxiety, pain, and catastrophizing, and foster an environment of healing (Stewart & Loftus, 2018).

Evidence suggests that multiple psychological and environmental factors within a clinical encounter create a context through which people develop negative or positive expectancies about treatments and outcomes (Colloca, 2019; Manai et al., 2019). The **nocebo effect** is the adverse effect that follows an inert treatment, diagnosis, education, or care plan because of negative expectations. Nocebos produce behavioral, functional, and physiological changes leading to increased pain intensity and impact on daily life (Colloca & Finniss, 2012).

For example, using words such as "chronic" and "degenerative" may promote fear of movement, catastrophizing, and distort a person's perception of their body and its ability to adapt, contributing to increased pain intensity and decreased occupational participation. Consider the difference between the following OTP responses to an individual with a new chronic condition: "You are going to have to live with this forever" versus "You may need to make some adjustments moving forward." The **placebo effect** is the opposite phenomenon, where people experience a positive effect because of positive expectations. Verbal and nonverbal clinician language can influence both effects.

Words can heal or harm, and how OTPs interact with persons experiencing pain can significantly impact their pain experience and outcomes in either direction. Expectations about treatment are also shaped by the context in which information is communicated, one's own knowledge, beliefs, past experiences, and dispositional traits. OTPs must recognize personal biases and beliefs about pain and evaluate their verbal and nonverbal behaviors. Klinger and colleagues (2017) suggest practitioners can minimize nocebo effects by reducing negative patient–clinician communication, maintaining a positive therapeutic relationship, addressing people's emotional burdens and cognitive beliefs, and ensuring that education supports positive expectations.

Another critical consideration when assessing pain is the impact of culture, race, ethnicity, religion, and gender on the pain assessment. OTPs must consider cultural aspects relevant to pain expression and the pain experience. Although pain is often a private experience, pain behavior is influenced by social, cultural, and psychological factors (Peacock & Patel, 2008). Cultural expectations and acceptance of pain and whether it is seen as a normal part of life often determine if it is seen as a problem that requires the assistance of healthcare practitioners.

Cultural differences in pain response often result in over- or underestimation of the severity of pain (Givler et al., 2022). For example, decreased pain expression by a person may be viewed as an absence of pain, resulting in the undertreatment of pain and an underrecognition of its impact on occupational performance. To practice cultural humility, OTPs should consider all relevant personal factors (e.g., customs, beliefs, activity patterns, behavioral standards, and expectations of a person's cultural group) when assessing and treating pain and incorporate cultural values when evaluating pain scores.

Before reviewing the types of pain measures, take a moment to complete the reflective activity in Box 15-2, which is adapted from Strong and van Griensven (2014).

After obtaining an *occupational profile* and *observing occupational performance,* the OTP can use a variety of self-report measures and open-ended questions to gather descriptive information about the person's pain experience. OTPs should use open-ended questions that allow for a detailed and emotional expression. Self-report is the "gold standard" of pain measurement because it is consistent with current definitions of pain (Raja et al., 2020). Pain diaries can be used with standardized assessments to understand the impact of pain at specific time points. Information on activity patterns, time use, goal fulfillment, and changes in routines, habits, and roles are also helpful in collaborative goal setting (IASP, 2018). See also Chapter 14: Time Use and Habits. 🤝

Pain measures can be grouped into *self-report, observational,* and *physiological measures.* This chapter provides an overview of all pain measures, emphasizing self-report measures. Self-report measures will be further classified based on the information gained and clinical utilization, as OTPs will commonly use more than one type of assessment with people experiencing pain. The following is not an exhaustive list of all pain assessments but emphasizes self-report measures OTPs can use at no cost and across practice settings.

BOX 15-2 ■ Reflective Activity: Measuring Pain

Take a moment and imagine you are at home and having a severe migraine. You are experiencing significant pain and discomfort, but a big project due for school (or work) tomorrow needs your attention. You choose to make yourself a cup of herbal tea, do some light stretches, lie down with dimmed lights, and listen to some relaxing music to manage the pain so you can work on your project later. Now, imagine you live with someone who has never experienced a migraine, and they are watching you as you go through your pain management routine. Suppose your roommate wants to measure how bad your migraine might be. They could ask you, "How would you rate your migraine on a scale of 0 to 10?"

■ What factors might influence the rating you give when asked this question?

■ How might this apply to other people and their pain ratings?

■ Does this rating provide adequate information about the impact of your migraine on occupational performance and participation?

■ What other questions could your roommate ask to better understand your pain experience?

Now consider if an OTP asked someone living with you to complete an observational pain measure.

■ How accurate do you think their pain measurement would be given their observations of you?

■ How might this scenario apply to people reporting significant pain levels but not demonstrating common pain behaviors?

Another way to measure your pain might be to record your pulse or breathing rate.

■ Do you think these types of measures would tell us anything about the severity of your migraine?

■ What questions could we ask to understand your migraine's impact on things important to you?

■ What questions could we ask to understand how you manage migraines and their impact on your life?

As you complete this activity and read about types of assessments, consider what information you can gain from different pain measures and how this may influence your patient's care plan.

Self-Report Measures

Self-report measures often include questionnaires and can be paired with open-ended questions or additional self-report measures to provide a more in-depth and complete clinical picture (Table 15-1).

General Pain Description

The following scales are unidimensional, as they only measure one factor: the intensity or severity of pain. They are quick and easy to administer and include options for varying levels of communication; however, they oversimplify the pain experience and do not capture the impact of pain on occupational performance or quality of life.

■ *Numerical Rating Scale (NRS):* Individuals indicate which number best represents their pain level using a 0 to 10 scale. Zero represents *no pain,* and 10 represents *extreme pain* (i.e, "worst pain possible"). A reduction of one point in the NRS represents a minimal clinically important difference (MCID) for the person (Salaffi et al., 2004). The MCID is the smallest change in an outcome that a patient would perceive as clinically meaningful (Fig. 15-4).

■ *Visual Analog Scale (VAS):* Individuals indicate their pain level by drawing a vertical mark on a 10-cm horizontal line that represents a continuum between "no pain" and "pain as bad as it could possibly be" (Gift, 1989). The distance measured from the "no pain" anchor to the mark becomes the individual's VAS pain score (Fig. 15-5). Jensen and colleagues (2003) discovered that 100-mm VAS ratings of 0 to 4 mm could be interpreted as no pain, 5 to 44 mm as mild pain, 45 to 74 mm as moderate pain, and 75 to 100 mm as severe pain. A 33% decrease in pain represents a reasonable standard for determining that a change in pain is meaningful for the individual (Jensen et al., 2003).

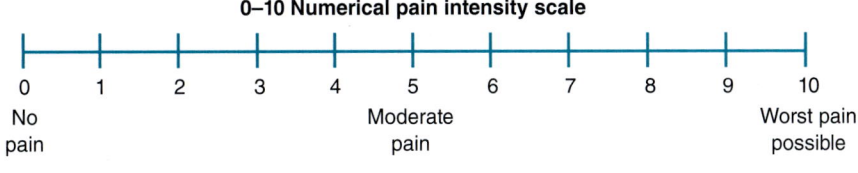

0–10 Numerical pain intensity scale

0　1　2　3　4　5　6　7　8　9　10

No pain　　　　　　Moderate pain　　　　　　Worst pain possible

FIGURE 15-4. Example of a numerical pain intensity scale.

Visual analog scale (VAS)

No pain　　　　　　　　　　　　　Pain as bad as it could possibly be

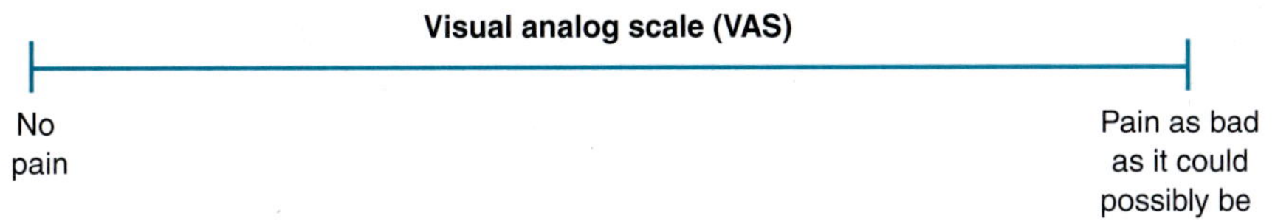

FIGURE 15-5. Example of a Visual Analog Scale.

Evidence-Based Practice

Living Well With Chronic Pain

> *Returning to a sense of self-coherence is key to living well despite chronic pain.*

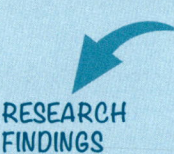

RESEARCH FINDINGS

Using classical grounded theory methodology, Lennox Thompson and colleagues (2020) interviewed 17 individuals living with chronic pain for an average of 13.11 years to understand how and why they believed they were living well despite chronic pain. Findings indicated that the primary concern of people experiencing chronic pain is resolving the problem of disrupted self-coherence (i.e., a belief that personal capabilities, motivations, goals, and ways of engaging in occupations make sense). Returning to a sense of self-coherence consists of three sequential processes of reoccupying self: (1) making sense of pain using an idiographic model; (2) deciding to turn from patient to person, facilitated or hindered by interactions with clinicians and occupational drive; and (3) flexibly persisting, where occupational engaging and coping allow individuals to develop future plans.

APPLICATIONS

➡ Living well with chronic pain involves a process of making sense of the pain experience, deciding to move on with life, and flexibly persisting while pursuing meaningful occupations.

➡ Diagnoses should be accompanied by messages from clinicians that hurt and harm are not equivalent and the need exists for a lifelong approach to managing a chronic problem.

➡ Remaining supportive, demonstrating that the person is unique and being thought of throughout evaluation and treatment, and encouraging engagement in valued occupations allow people experiencing pain to experiment with, and start to engage with, what is important in their lives.

➡ OTPs should help people extend their coping repertoire and encourage flexibility with how these are applied in the pursuit of valued occupations.

REFERENCES

Lennox Thompson, B., Gage, J., & Kirk, R. (2020). Living well with chronic pain: A classical grounded theory. *Disability and Rehabilitation, 42*(8), 1141–1152. https://doi.org/10.1080/09638288.2018.1517195

■ *FACES Pain Rating Scale:* Individuals choose from faces that depict facial expressions ranging from a happy face (0 or no hurt) to a crying face (10 or hurts as if the worst pain imaginable, Fig. 15-6) to indicate pain intensity (Wong & Baker, 1988). These scales are useful for young people and older adults; however, the faces may contain other entities (e.g., depression, anxiety) rather than only pain (Tomlinson et al., 2010).

■ *Verbal Rating Scale (VRS):* Individuals select the words that best describe their pain intensity from 4 to 15 descriptors; corresponding numbers become the pain intensity score (Jensen et al., 1986). Although easy to administer, the VRS assumes equal intervals between the adjectives, and people may not find a descriptor that matches their experience (Fig. 15-7).

Site-Specific Pain Assessments

Site-specific assessments are for pain in specific areas of the body. The following assessments are commonly used in outpatient settings and for outcome measurement, are free to use in clinical practice, and are available in multiple languages.

■ *Disabilities of the Arm, Shoulder, and Hand (DASH):* A widely used questionnaire to measure disability of the upper extremities that asks individuals about symptoms and their ability to perform certain activities. It can measure change over time and has a shorter version called the QuickDASH (Hudak et al., 1996).

■ *Oswestry Pain Disability Index* (ODI; also known as the Oswestry Low Back Disability Questionnaire): A widely used questionnaire to measure how back pain

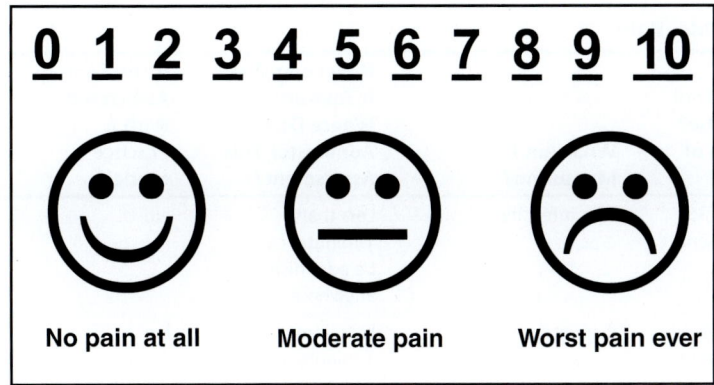

FIGURE 15-6. Example of a FACES Pain Rating Scale.

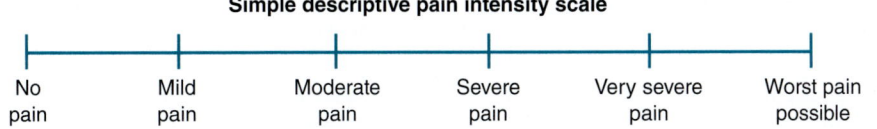

FIGURE 15-7. Example of a simple descriptive pain intensity scale.

has affected an individual's ability to manage everyday life in 10 categories (Fairbank et al., 1980)

■ *Roland & Morris Disability Questionnaire* (RMDQ): A widely used low back pain questionnaire in which individuals indicate whether they agree with 24 statements about how pain impacts different movements and daily activities (Roland & Morris, 1983)

Multidimensional Pain Assessments

Multidimensional assessments cover multiple dimensions of the pain experience, such as pain intensity, frequency, and the degree of interference with daily activities and quality of life, providing more information about the impact of pain on occupational performance. The following measures are free to use in clinical practice and available in multiple languages.

■ *Brief Pain Inventory* (BPI): Assesses the severity of pain, activity interference, and affective interference. Individuals rate on an ordinal scale of 0 (no interference) to 10 (complete interference) how much their pain has interfered with general activity, mood, mobility, work, interpersonal relationships, sleep, and life enjoyment. The BPI is available in short and long forms (Keller et al., 2004; MD Anderson Center, n.d.).

■ *West Haven-Yale Multidimensional Pain Inventory* (WHYMPI): Assesses pain across 12 subscales, three overall domains with 52 total items (Kerns et al., 1985). The three domains assess the pain experience, the responses of others to the individual's communicated pain, and the extent to which the individual participates in daily activities. Each of the 52 items is rated on a scale from 0 (never) to 6 (very often).

■ *McGill Pain Questionnaire* (MPQ): Assesses the quality and intensity of pain with a drawing of the human body and pain descriptors that are classified into 20 categories (Melzack, 1975). Responses are scored to assess the individual's experience of pain across three primary dimensions: sensory (temporal, spatial, pressure, and thermal properties), affective (fear, tension, and autonomic properties), and evaluative (overall intensity of the pain experience). The MPQ also has a short form.

Performance Domains and Client Factors

These assessments provide unique information about the individual's performance patterns or skills and client factors (see Table 15-1). They can help identify additional areas of the occupational therapy domain impacted by pain. The following measures are free to use in clinical practice and available in multiple languages.

■ *Chronic Pain Acceptance Questionnaire–Revised* (CPAQ-R): A 20-item questionnaire that measures acceptance of pain within two factors: activity engagement (pursuit of life activities regardless of pain) and pain willingness (recognition that avoidance and control are often unworkable methods of adapting to chronic pain; McCraken et al., 2004). A short form is also available.

■ *Fear-Avoidance Beliefs Questionnaire* (FABQ): A 16-item questionnaire that measures how an individual's fear-avoidance beliefs about physical activity and work may affect and contribute to their low back pain and resulting disability (Waddell et al., 1993). Modifications for other areas of the body are available.

■ *Pain Catastrophizing Scale* (PCS): A 13-item self-report measure designed to assess catastrophic thinking related to pain within three subscales: rumination, magnification, and helplessness (Sullivan et al., 1995). Adapted versions for children and significant other/proxy responses are available. Scott and colleagues (2014) suggest that a score greater than 24 on the PCS represents a clinically relevant level of catastrophizing and warrants intervention.

TABLE 15-1 | Therapeutic Reasoning Assessment Table: Pain

Which Tool?	Who Was This Tool Designed For?	Is This a Type of Tool the Person Can Use? What Is Required of the Person?	What Am I Measuring?	How Long Does It Take and Where Do I Administer This Assessment?	Is the Tool Associated With a Practice Model?
Numerical Rating Scale (NRS)	Age 6 and older	Person indicates which number best represents their level of pain.	Pain intensity	Less than 1 minute; can be administered anywhere	No
Visual Analog Scale (VAS)	Age 5 and older	Person draws a mark on the line that represents their level of pain.	Pain intensity	Less than 1 minute; can be administered anywhere	No
FACES Pain Rating Scale	Age 3 and older; individuals who have difficulty with written language	Person selects a photograph or drawing of a face that best depicts their level of pain.	Pain intensity	Less than 1 minute; can be administered anywhere	No
Verbal Rating Scale	Age 6 and older	Person selects the word that best describes their pain from a list of descriptors.	Pain intensity	Fewer than 5 minutes; can be administered anywhere	No
Brief Pain Inventory (BPI)	Short form with age 8 and older; long form for adults only	Person indicates how much their pain interferes with different aspects of life (e.g., mood, work, sleep).	Pain intensity and the degree to which pain interferes with life	The short form, which is recommended for clinic use, takes fewer than 5 minutes; can be administered anywhere	No
West Haven-Yale Multidimensional Pain Inventory	Age 18 and older	Person indicates how much their pain has impacted their life and how others have responded.	Pain intensity and the degree to which pain impacts life factors, including participation in daily activities and the responses of others to their communications of pain	Fewer than 15 minutes; can be administered anywhere	Cognitive behavioral models
McGill Pain Questionnaire (MPQ)	Age 13 and older	Person marks areas where they feel pain, selects words that describe pain, and provides information on how pain has changed over time.	Qualitative features of the pain experience	Fewer than 10 minutes; can be administered anywhere	No
Chronic Pain Acceptance Questionnaire–Revised	Age 18 and older	Person indicates their agreement with statements related to their acceptance of chronic pain.	Acceptance of pain within activity engagement and pain willingness	Fewer than 10 minutes; can be administered anywhere	Cognitive behavioral models
Fear-Avoidance Beliefs Questionnaire	Age 18 and older	Person indicates their agreement with statements related to how much physical activities and work affect their back pain.	Beliefs about how work and physical activity affect pain	Fewer than 10 minutes; can be administered anywhere	No
Pain Catastrophizing Scale (PCS)	Age 18 and older; adaptations for children and proxy responses are available	Person indicates the degree to which they have catastrophizing thoughts and feelings when experiencing pain.	Catastrophizing thoughts related to pain	Fewer than 5 minutes; can be administered anywhere	No

TABLE 15-1 | Therapeutic Reasoning Assessment Table: Pain—cont'd

Which Tool?	Who Was This Tool Designed For?	Is This a Type of Tool the Person Can Use? What Is Required of the Person?	What Am I Measuring?	How Long Does It Take and Where Do I Administer This Assessment?	Is the Tool Associated With a Practice Model?
Pain Coping Inventory (PCI) Questionnaire	Age 18 and older; a short version for children is available	Person indicates how often they think or act similar to statements provided when in pain.	Cognitive and behavioral strategies for dealing with chronic pain	Fewer than 15 minutes; can be administered anywhere	Cognitive behavioral models
Pain Self-Efficacy Questionnaire (PSEQ)	Age 18 and older	Person indicates how confident they are in doing activities despite pain.	Confidence in performing activities while in pain	Fewer than 5 minutes; can be administered anywhere	No
Pain Anxiety Symptoms Scale Short Form 20 (PASS-20)	Age 18 and older	Person indicates how frequently they experience pain-related anxiety symptoms.	Pain-related anxiety	Fewer than 10 minutes; can be administered anywhere	No

- *Pain Coping Inventory (PCI) Questionnaire:* A 33-item questionnaire measuring six domains (grouped into active and passive coping dimensions) of cognitive and behavioral strategies for dealing with chronic pain: pain transformation, distraction, reducing demands, retreating, worrying, and resting (Kraaimaat & Evers, 2003)
- *Pain Self-Efficacy Questionnaire (PSEQ):* A 10-item questionnaire that measures the confidence individuals have in performing activities (e.g., household chores, socializing, work, etc.) while experiencing pain (Nicholas, 2007)
- *Self-Compassion Scale (SCS):* A 26-item questionnaire that measures self-compassion through six subscales (self-kindness, self-judgment, common humanity, isolation, mindfulness, and overidentification; Neff, 2003). A short form is also available.
- *Pain Anxiety Symptoms Scale Short Form 20 (PASS-20):* A 20-item questionnaire that measures pain-related anxiety in four subscales: cognitive, escape/avoidance, fear, and physiological anxiety (McCracken et al., 1992). A longer form is also available.

In addition, the *Canadian Occupational Performance Measure (COPM)* and the *Patient-Specific Functional Scale (PSFS)* are frequently utilized within occupational therapy literature and validated for people with pain. The COPM measures an individual's self-perception of performance in everyday living over time and is available in multiple languages (Law et al., 2019). The PSFS is a self-reported, patient-specific measure designed to assess functional change and can be used with individuals of varying levels of independence (Stratford et al., 1995).

Observational Measures

Observational measures refer to what the OTP, other practitioners, or someone close to the person may observe. Observational measures are sometimes referred to as behavioral measures because they are behaviors the person may demonstrate when experiencing pain. These measures can be helpful in combination with self-report measures to identify additional areas of concern, such as environmental or functional performance factors influencing pain.

Observational measures reflect the therapist's pain measurement, failing to account for the person's self-report, and may result in underestimating pain level. OTPs should use self-report when possible.

However, OTPs will encounter people who cannot self-report pain for various reasons, such as impaired cognitive abilities. In these instances, behavioral pain indicators may be the best option to identify and document pain to ensure people receive appropriate pain management (AGS Panel on Persistent Pain in Older Persons, 2002). Behavioral pain indicators are observable behaviors including, but not limited to:

- Facial expressions (e.g., frowning, grimacing, tightly closing eyes, clenching)
- Verbalizations or vocalizations (e.g., moaning, sighing, groaning, grunting, crying)
- Body movements (e.g., rigid/tense posture, guarding, pacing, restricting movement)
- Changes in interpersonal interactions (e.g., aggression, resisting care, withdrawing, disruptive behavior)
- Changes in activity patterns or routines (e.g., appetite changes, changing rest or sleep patterns, sudden cessation of everyday routines)
- Mental status changes (e.g., increased confusion, distress, changes in attentiveness or communication)

Pain behaviors should be observed during functional activities (e.g., transfers, functional mobility, self-care) and at rest. Many standardized pain assessments for individuals with impaired self-report abilities are available online and generally measure aspects of the behavioral pain indicators discussed earlier. These assessments are beyond the scope of this chapter; however, they have been developed for specific populations ranging from children to adults, individuals with intellectual disabilities or in critical care, and adults with dementia.

Physiological Measures

Pain can cause physiological changes such as increased heart rate, respiration, sweating, muscle tension, and other changes associated with stress responses (Middleton, 2003). These changes can be used as an indirect measure of acute pain but are often not beneficial for persistent or chronic pain because the body's responses to acute pain may stabilize over time as the body attempts to maintain homeostasis. However, physiological measures can be useful when self-report or observational measures are not feasible (e.g., in acute care, where individuals may be unconscious and unable to express pain).

OTPs can use pain assessment methods to examine cardiovascular (e.g., heart rate, body temperature, blood pressure), respiratory (e.g., respiratory rate), muscular (e.g., muscle tension), and neurological (e.g., pupils, areas of the brain) changes using various methods such as biometric devices, brain scans, and electrocardiogram monitoring (Korving et al., 2020). Although experimental methods have been utilized in research, they are rarely used in clinical practice. Limitations exist when using physiological measures to identify and quantify pain; however, they may be helpful for specific populations.

The Lived Experience

Hanna Rae Paul

Experiencing chronic pain at the age of 20 left me feeling hopeless and that I would never be able to fulfill the dreams I had at the time. I began to think my life was worthless and that I would never find a significant other who would want to deal with my constant mood swings and angry outbursts. I began to believe I would never have children because I could not care for them. My chronic pain was so persistent that it became the focus of my life, causing me to isolate myself from my friends and stop participating in leisure. I experienced a lot of anxiety when simply going for a walk for fear of the pain I would have later on. I discontinued my workout schedule and began to hate looking at myself in the mirror. I was left unbalanced and eventually had to turn down a job as I could not meet the demands of being on my feet for 8 hours a day.

My initial doctor eventually lost interest in my care, leading me to switch to another pain specialist. After trying two drugs for 6 months and not experiencing any pain relief, my new doctor told me, "You are just going to have to get over it." This angered me greatly and resulted in me taking control of my own health and exploring more holistic approaches to my care. I am now 24 years old and have lived with fibromyalgia for just over 4 years.

The American Pain Society developed a cycle encompassing various stages an individual goes through when experiencing chronic pain. First, my awareness and focus were directed at my pain and physical limitations. This soon became all I could think about, resulting in social isolative behaviors and depression. My depression then increased my fatigue levels, further worsening my pain. There were multiple moments when I took more pills than I was prescribed just to obtain some form of relief.

This cycle resulted in increased emotional distress and disruption in my interpersonal relationships and overall engagement in life. It took 2 long years of suffering both on my end and my family's, as trialing so many drugs left me chemically unbalanced and turned me into someone set off by the smallest things, resulting in angry outbursts. I have been able to live a very rewarding life for the past 2 years as I explored and discovered which interventions work best for me, with the help of an antidepressant, and learning new coping skills from my

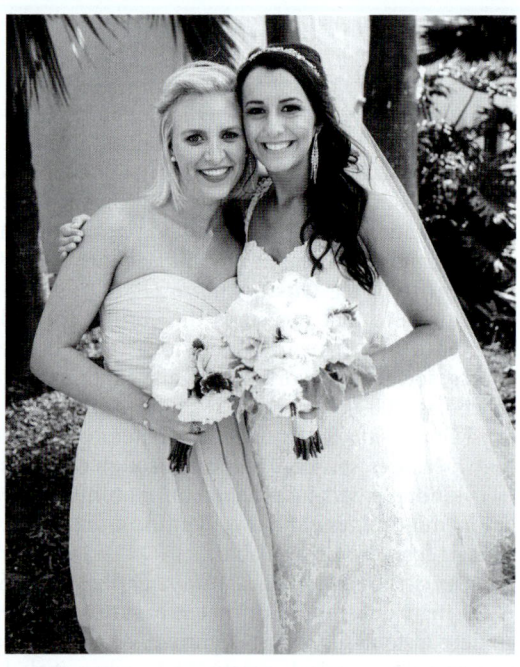

occupational therapist. I had to come to the realization that one day, I would have to listen to my doctors' initial advice that I needed to simply "get over it." The difference is that to "get over it," I would have to go through every stage of the chronic pain cycle.

I would not have made it through this part of my life without the support of my family and friends, who fought for me when I wanted to give up. I also have my parents to thank for firmly saying "No" to my doctors who wanted to put me on narcotics, possibly preventing me from a life of addiction. My pain has not disappeared, but I have learned to manage it by balancing my daily stressors and allowing the pain to become my new "normal." I hope sharing my story gives others suffering from chronic pain a sense of peace and faith that they, too, will overcome the debilitation of pain. I have come to a place in my life where I am thankful for going through this experience, as it has taught me empathy and compassion and brought me closer to my family

Pain Diaries and Time-Use Assessments

Paper and electronic pain diaries provide another means for individuals to communicate their unique pain experiences. Because diaries can record pain triggers and temporal patterns, it is helpful for the person to make regular entries (e.g., each morning/night or after an episode of pain). Typical entries should include a rating of pain intensity, medications or nonpharmacological pain management techniques and their effects, rest time, satisfaction with pain control, activity level, mood, and recurrent thoughts (Pasero & McCaffery, 2011; Turner & Romano, 2001).

OTPs may also ask people to record what they were doing, where they were, and their pain-free activities. For some individuals, however, keeping a diary may exacerbate pain because of the increased attention to pain (Ferrari, 2015). The Occupational Experience Profile (OEP) is an occupation-focused time-use diary where individuals record their daily activities and the personal meanings associated with each activity, helping them become more aware of what they do and experience in everyday life (Atler & Fisher, 2022). The OEP honors the individual's perspective and provides graphics of recorded activities and experience patterns within four occupational experiences: pleasure, productivity, restoration, and social connection (Atler & Fisher, 2022).

The OEP can help people experiencing pain become aware of what they are doing throughout the day and reflect on how those activities impact their feelings, health, and well-being to develop goals for increased occupational engagement (Rider & Tay, 2022).

Measuring Outcomes

OTPs can use many of the assessments listed earlier to measure the efficacy of pain interventions. Clinical improvement can be measured as gains in occupational performance or increased participation in meaningful occupations (e.g., BPI, WHYMPI, PSFS, COPM), reduction in pain intensity (e.g., VAS, NRS, or VRS), changes in beliefs or coping strategies (e.g., PCS, PSEQ, or PCQ), or a reduction of pain behaviors (e.g., measures of observational pain behaviors). Data from pain diaries or the OEP can be used to record increased activity engagement, time use, and social participation. Outcome measures should be clinically meaningful and person-centered.

An effective pain evaluation provides a clear understanding of the person, their problem situation relative to pain, and the physical, psychological, and social contexts influencing or impacted by the person's pain experience. The biopsychosocial model reflects current theories of pain, which argue that pain is not simply the manifestation of an underlying injury or disease process. Contemporary theories of pain are useful for identifying factors that influence pain. For example, low activity levels, poor body mechanics, and inadequate pacing of physical activities can negatively influence the pain experience. Negative thoughts about one's pain experience (e.g., worrying, ruminating on negative aspects of life, focusing on the worst possible outcome) and reactions to pain (e.g., depression, anger, hopelessness) can make self-management of chronic pain more difficult. In contrast, increasing activity tolerance, adjusting beliefs about pain, relaxation training, self-efficacy, a positive attitude and focus on capabilities, and developing proactive strategies to manage one's pain can support self-management.

Intervention

The biopsychosocial model emphasizes the complex and dynamic interaction among physiological (e.g., disease, injury), psychological (e.g., anxiety, fear, catastrophizing), and socio-environmental (e.g., social supports, role obligations, culture) contexts that may perpetuate or even worsen the experience of pain. Because of pain's complex and multidimensional nature, occupational therapy approaches vary widely and must be person-centered. They typically include strategies to alter pain intensity and influence occupational performance. Occupational therapy aims to help people make sense of and relate to their pain in a way that supports their progress toward optimal occupational participation. OTPs assess pain's impact on occupation to establish person-centered interventions and outcomes. OTPs employ occupational modifications so people can participate in what matters to them while undergoing therapy to improve pain and function, using occupations as therapeutic interventions.

Occupations in the pain management context not only mean ADLs but also refer to instrumental ADLs (IADLs), health management, rest and sleep, education, work, play, leisure, and social participation (AOTA, 2020). See the chapters in Part IV: Occupation. OTPs should address all aspects of the occupational therapy domain, as contexts, performance patterns and skills, and client factors are impacted by pain and can influence the pain experience. Pain reduction is intended to enable greater engagement in meaningful occupations; therefore, OTPs must ensure strategies can support occupational participation, preferably through self-management.

Although pain reduction is not always the emphasis, it is often a byproduct of increased occupational participation. OTPs have specialized training in assisting people living with pain to establish life routines and habits to support reliable and consistent participation and explore new occupations as individuals review their lives in light of pain and important values. This section provides several intervention approaches that complement a biopsychosocial model and aim to increase occupational performance through supported self-management. See Being a Psychosocial OT Practitioner at the end of this section for an example of an OTP using a biopsychosocial approach to help a person manage their persistent pain.

Supported Self-Management

Supported self-management is a term used to describe approaches to living with pain that may be employed by the person rather than administered by a health professional. They can be offered one-on-one or in a group setting to capitalize on group interactions (e.g., vicarious learning, encouragement, group problem-solving), and are often based on approaches such as CBT or ACT. Medications, on their own, are not typically considered self-management. However, health literacy, medication management, and self-advocacy may be needed to use medications effectively, report unpleasant side effects, and establish a medication routine.

Along with the strategies discussed in the text that follows, supported self-management includes setting personal goals for areas of life a person may want to focus on, developing plans to achieve these goals, using problem-solving skills, and celebrating successes. Supported self-management may include cognitive restructuring, identifying values-based activities, movement practices including exercise, strategies for managing mood and anxiety, sleep management, effective communication, health literacy, and relapse prevention to help maintain newly formed habits and routines. See also Chapter 45: Self-Care and Well-Being Occupations. 🤝

People living with pain might find it helpful to develop a "personal pain management plan" identifying strategies they have found useful, including details such as what to do, how often to use them, what time of day they are most useful, and options if they cannot use their first choice (Fig. 15-8). A written plan allows people to post it somewhere visible for easy reference, share it with family and other health-care providers, and form the basis of any revised plans over time. Personal pain management plans should be person-centered.

OTPs can incorporate many helpful approaches to pain management; however, it is beyond the scope of this chapter to discuss all available approaches. OTPs can assist people in exploring and incorporating various strategies in their daily lives, such as cognitive behavioral approaches, relaxation, mindfulness, physical agent modalities, exercise or movement-based activity, activity pacing, assistive technology, orthotics, complementary and alternative medicine, adaptive equipment, self-compassion, support groups, environmental and activity modifications, and so on.

A "setback plan" is also integral to a self-management plan. Setbacks may arise from flare-ups in pain or the underlying health condition (e.g., rheumatoid arthritis), changes in daily routines, disruptions from illness, varying emotional states, and so on. A helpful practice is to anticipate setbacks an individual may encounter, asking the person to identify high-risk situations where they have found it challenging to maintain their self-management strategies.

Identifying high-risk situations allows people to be forewarned about times when they may not draw on strategies they know (Fig. 15-9). It can help individuals identify "early warning signs" of lapsing and, together with the OTP, undertake problem-solving to generate practical strategies to resume supported self-management practices. Setback planning and relapse prevention draw on research undertaken in addictions (Larimer et al., 1999) and recognize the influence of the emotional state, social context, and changed routines in triggering reduced use of coping strategies. See also Chapter 12: Emotion Regulation. 🤝

Relapse Prevention

Elbers and colleagues (2020) identify two approaches to relapse prevention. The first is to create an *Insight Card*, in which the person writes down their most meaningful rehabilitation experiences, ideas, and milestones at the top of the card and an environmental cue on the bottom, such as a picture or quote (Fig. 15-10). The second approach is *Values-Based Goal Setting*, in which people identify important personal values and a process to generate goals related to these values. People set calendar reminders, arrange social support, break goals into smaller steps, and identify when,

where, and what they need to do, including obstacles and solutions. By using a systematic approach to this process, people develop skills to sustain behavior change once the immediate support of a therapist is withdrawn, such as after being discharged from therapy services.

Behavioral Approaches

Behavioral approaches in pain management employ mechanisms drawn from learning theory, particularly operant conditioning. They were among the earliest nonmedical approaches for chronic pain, addressing pain behavior so people could do more and reduce medications and health-care use despite continuing to experience pain (Fordyce et al., 1968). Occupational therapy was a vital part of Fordyce's approach to reinforcing "well behavior," using weaving on a loom as one component of supporting the person to remain active.

Unwanted pain behavior is gradually reduced with the person's full informed consent in favor of healthier or adaptive approaches. By ignoring or choosing not to respond to unhelpful behavior, people can gradually resume participating in what matters in their lives. *Fordyce's Behavioral Methods for Chronic Pain and Illness* is the authoritative guide to using behavioral approaches for persistent pain (Main et al., 2014). Occupational therapy interventions commonly incorporate components of operant conditioning. For example, clinicians will give social reinforcement when a person completes between-session tasks or tries a new way of structuring a day. Activity pacing or "quota" strategies to develop a consistent level of daily activity or utilizing biofeedback training employ operant conditioning principles.

A less formal way to use the principles of operant conditioning can be to reduce the number of times a person is asked to rate their pain intensity because this brings the person's attention to their pain rather than what they have been doing. By asking, "What have you been doing?" attention is drawn to occupational participation, and the social responses from the OTP are strongly rewarding. Giving encouragement or praise while remaining neutral and redirecting a conversation away from "pain talk" also employs operant conditioning principles.

Care is needed when utilizing this approach for two important reasons: (1) The person must be fully informed and give consent before using the approach to ensure the person is aware of the rationale for how clinicians and family respond to them; and (2) empathy and compassion for the person, especially when they are distressed or angry, require delicate handling, so the person does not feel rejected when a clinician uses a neutral or redirecting response to illness or pain behavior.

Another behavioral strategy is using an activity "quota" or time period for breaking up activities throughout the day. By reducing the relationship between pain intensity and activity and using time as the guide, people are more consistent, can gradually increase activity duration, and experience fewer pain flare-ups. However, eliminating all flare-ups is unlikely, given that many factors outside an individual's control, such as external stressors and other illnesses, influence pain.

First, a baseline is established, often over a week or two of recordings (e.g., diary, activity tracker, or smartphone). During this time, the person may record the number of steps

My Personal Pain Management Plan	
This plan lists actions you can take to live well even while your pain is still there. Write down WHAT you will do and WHEN you will do it; be specific.	
Strategies:	**My action plan:**
Physical activity Examples: daily stretches, daily exercise, position changes or range of motion, paced & graduated exercise, sitting & standing tolerance, setting a baseline, etc.	*I will do 5 minutes of stretching every morning after having my coffee.* *I will go for a 5-minute walk every afternoon on my break at work. If the weather is bad, I will walk up and down the hallways.*
Managing activities Examples: plan for doing what's important, plan for the day/week using a diary/planner, prioritize, pace, set goals, problem-solve, delegate, notice unhelpful patterns (boom & bust, pain-as-a-guide, avoiding), be flexible, plan time out, reward yourself, etc.	*I will keep a planner and prioritize activities using the "Eisenhower Box" and write "Be flexible" at the top of each week as a reminder.*
Body awareness Examples: breathing, mindfulness, progressive muscle relaxation, distraction, posture changes, stretching, etc.	*I will do a 2-minute progressive muscle relaxation when I notice tension building in my shoulders.*
Sleep Examples: sleep routines (bedtime, morning), sleep environment (devices, temperature, light, noise), medications, sleep log, wind down, etc.	
Thoughts and feelings Examples: notice thoughts and feelings, use positive statements, take time out, plan for fun, monitor mood, CBT/ACT activities, etc.	*I will use a defusion technique (noticing and naming) whenever I get fused with negative thoughts about my pain.* *I will write in my journal each night and allow myself to write positive and negative things without judgment.*
Family and communication Examples: use direct communication, be aware of nonverbal communication, list who can support you, plan time with others, work out family responsibilities, plan date nights, etc.	*I will share this plan with my partner and let them know how they can best support me when I have a flare-up.*
Social and fun Examples: schedule one enjoyable thing a day, fun and social activities, leisure activities inside the home, leisure activities outside the home, have time alone and with others, gratitude journals, etc.	*I will schedule at least one fun activity with friends each weekend and put it on my calendar so I can look forward to it. I will schedule time each week to do things that I enjoy, such as watching a movie, doing calligraphy, and calling my sister.*
Work Examples: identify strengths and skills; identify what you can do reliably and consistently; develop interview or job-seeking skills, effective communication with coworkers/supervisors, "next best steps," household work (household management, caring for others, home/vehicle/yard maintenance), etc.	
Flare-ups Early warning signs, high-risk situations, getting back on track, planning, support, alternatives, etc.	*I will keep my insight card and my setback plan with me at all times.*

FIGURE 15-8. Example of a personal pain management plan. The OTP can list strategies they typically teach during their occupational therapy sessions or identify them with the person. The format is flexible and should be person-centered.

or particular activities, pain intensity, rest periods, and other details that could influence their activity levels. The OTP discusses the sustainability of this routine and identifies features that appear to affect either pain intensity (leading to distress and/or rest) or satisfaction with the current activity pattern.

The OTP then provides modifications or adaptations to break activities into shorter periods, institute more frequent breaks or activity changes, or extend the time or quota for each activity. By gradually increasing (or reducing) the activities according to time rather than pain, the nervous system can

Setback Plan	
Early warning signs of a flare-up (What are my early warning signs and high-risk situations?)	
First steps (What are the first steps [specific actions] I can take immediately?)	
Thinking (What can I tell myself when I am having unhelpful thoughts?)	
Physical (What physical activity can I do [e.g., light stretches, standing, sitting]?)	
Relaxation (What relaxation strategy can I practice [e.g., mindfulness, deep breathing, imagery]?)	
Asking for help (Whom can I ask for help?)	
Distraction (What can I do to refocus my attention?)	
Medication (What medications can I take to help manage pain?)	

FIGURE 15-9. Example of a setback plan template.

Moment: If I am in pain, it does not have to mean that something is broken, injured, or going to get worse.

Memory Cue: HURT ≠ HARM

FIGURE 15-10. Example of an insight card.

adapt, allowing the person to maintain a more consistent and reliable lifestyle of participation in meaningful occupations.

Biofeedback training employs visual or auditory information in response to physiological changes such as skin conductance, surface electromyography (EMG), respiration rate, pulse rate, heart rate variability, and temperature changes. The OTP establishes a baseline and adjusts the biofeedback parameters to provide immediate and ongoing feedback as the individual achieves control over the body response. The approach develops self-regulation over physiological responses to stress, so individuals can better manage their responses to pain fluctuations (Reneau, 2020). Surface EMG can be a training tool to help people adjust their posture and/or monitor muscle fatigue.

Relaxation training offers psychological and physiological benefits, is often used within a multimodal approach, and is commonly a component of biofeedback training, CBT, and ACT. The purpose of relaxation strategies is to decrease the activity of the sympathetic nervous system, leading to multiple detectable physiological effects, ranging from reduced blood pressure, oxygen uptake, respiratory and heart rate, and muscle tension to lower cortisol levels and inhibition of inflammatory processes (Vambheim et al., 2021). Table 15-2 outlines common relaxation strategies.

Graded exposure is based on treatment for phobia and was initially developed for pain-related fear and avoidance (Vlaeyen et al., 2002). Fear avoidance is a common contributor to distress and disability. The Fear-Avoidance Model can explain how pain-related fear is maintained, leading to avoiding activities and reduced participation (Pincus et al., 2010). OTPs can facilitate a process where people undertake previously avoided movements or activities, starting with the least feared (see Vlaeyen et al., 2012, for the definitive guide to graded exposure for pain). People experiencing pain

TABLE 15-2 | Relaxation Strategies for Managing Pain

Strategy	Description
Abdominal or diaphragmatic breathing	Abdominal breathing encourages relaxation and full oxygen exchange and can be incorporated into other relaxation techniques. It involves increasing awareness of breathing patterns, improving breathing efficiency, and slowing down inhalation and exhalation.
Progressive muscle relaxation (PMR)	PMR relieves excess tension that can result in muscle spasms, pain, and fatigue. PMR typically involves (a) focusing attention on a muscle group, (b) systematic tensing and relaxing of major muscle groups for several seconds, (c) focusing attention on how the tensed muscle feels, (d) release of the muscles, and (e) focusing on the sensations of relaxation.
Autogenic training (AT)	AT involves the silent repetition of phrases about homeostasis intended to create calming sensations and relax different body areas. AT includes (a) scanning the mind and body for tension, (b) concentrating on physical and mental states, and (c) concentrating on cues for relaxation. AT also includes practicing controlled breathing.
Guided imagery	Guided imagery techniques employ the purposeful use of mental images to stimulate or recreate sensory perception and can help reduce many symptoms associated with pain.
Mindfulness meditation See also Chapter 12: Emotion Regulation 🤝	Mindfulness meditation is the intentional self-regulation of attention from moment to moment. It involves purposeful and focused attention on the present in a nonjudgmental manner.
Virtual Reality (VR) and Augmented Reality (AR)	VR creates an immersive virtual environment, whereas AR virtually augments a real-world scene. These techniques can distract individuals during painful procedures. They can be used alone and with cognitive behavioral methods and biofeedback to reduce pain and pain interference and encourage increased movement and activity. As technology advances and costs decrease, these techniques may be utilized more heavily in clinical settings.

can use information about an activity's realistic threat (e.g., cognitive restructuring) and self-regulation to reduce physiological arousal and begin doing the activity at a level they can successfully manage. Starting with the least feared activity on a hierarchy, people develop self-efficacy and can return to doing previously avoided activities.

As individuals are gradually exposed to purposeful movements and meaningful activities, OTPs should specifically address pain **self-efficacy** (i.e., beliefs about one's ability to perform a range of tasks despite pain or to cope with pain). Evidence suggests pain self-efficacy is directly related to occupational performance and satisfaction, and OTPs should recognize the importance of engaging people in the experience of "doing" as well as in their belief and ability to "do" (van Huet & Williams, 2007). OTPs can enhance generalization by providing interventions in real-world settings that are variable, unpredictable, and in the context in which people live. Although graded exposure does not directly address pain intensity, this approach targets fears about being overwhelmed by pain, fears of injury or harm, and activity avoidance.

Virtual reality protocols for graded exposure also show promise for delivering therapy to address pain-related fear and disability (Trost & Parsons, 2014; Trost et al., 2021). In general, virtual and augmented reality use in pain management is expanding rapidly with application to acute and chronic pain and benefits to many aspects of the pain experience (Trost et al., 2021).

Self-regulation interventions may include sensory reeducation, desensitization training, and graded exposure. OTPs can use exposure-based interventions causing neuroplastic changes, such as graded motor imagery and mirror therapy, to address complex pain and movement problems.

In contrast with graded exposure, *graded reactivation* does not explicitly address fear. Graded reactivation addresses

physiological changes, including cardiovascular fitness, stamina, and flexibility. The approach is commonly used alongside physical exercise and work-hardening programs, and OTPs may also incorporate other occupations a person needs or wants to do.

Cognitive Behavioral Therapy and Acceptance and Commitment Therapy

CBT and ACT are introduced in Chapter 8: Cognitive Beliefs. 🤝 Readers should refer to this chapter for a more detailed understanding of these approaches. CBT and ACT are evidence-based, practical, hands-on, goal-oriented forms of psychotherapy treatment that OTPs with sufficient training can use across practice settings for pain management. They can be delivered alone or with other evidence-based interventions in group and individual formats and virtually or in person. CBT and ACT encourage people with chronic pain to adopt an active, problem-solving approach to cope with the many challenges associated with chronic pain and involve aspects of cognitive restructuring, behavioral activation, relaxation/mindfulness training, pacing, and graded exposure to physical activity and meaningful occupations.

CBT approaches for chronic pain help individuals identify negative thoughts that influence feelings and behaviors and teach skills to alter or restructure thoughts and behaviors. CBT then works to help individuals understand their thoughts and how they impact behaviors by teaching skills to replace negative or maladaptive thought cycles with more positive or adaptive interpretations and coping skills.

A recent review found CBT to have a positive effect on reducing pain, disability, and distress associated with chronic pain (Williams et al., 2020). The Department of Veterans

Affairs has created a therapist manual for using CBT for chronic pain among veterans, which provides structured sessions covering common CBT topics such as goal setting, exercise and pacing, relaxation training, pleasant activities, cognitive coping, and sleep (Murphy et al., n.d.). This manual is free, available online, and provides an excellent example of CBT interventions for chronic pain (see the Resources section of this chapter).

OTPs can adapt CBT activities or resources for someone experiencing unhelpful or maladaptive thoughts about their chronic pain. For example, helpful interventions can include thought records, the TIC-TOC techniques, self-talk and affirmations, the ABC method, and behavioral experiments. Chapter 8: Cognitive Beliefs features more about these techniques and their application in pain management. 🤝 Figure 15-11 provides an example of a TIC-TOC activity with a person experiencing chronic pain.

Another example of a useful CBT strategy might be developing coping statements to replace unhelpful thoughts. OTPs can help individuals identify helpful thoughts (e.g., The pain flare always passes after a while; I've gotten through this before, and I can get through it again; I don't have to suffer because I have skills I can use to cope; I'm going to focus on what I can do, not what I can't do; or What would I tell a friend who was in pain?) and keep them where they can find them when needed most. Essentially, any technique addressing thoughts or beliefs surrounding chronic pain to alter behavior can be considered a cognitive-belief-oriented approach. Many of the interventions in this chapter fall under the umbrella of CBT. However, because of the wide variety of CBT interventions, this approach is highly individualized and must be person-centered.

ACT extends previous CBT forms and integrates many CBT-related variables into six core therapeutic processes designed to decrease suffering and increase well-being (acceptance, cognitive defusion, contact with the present moment, self-as-context, values, and committed actions; Hayes et al., 1999; Hayes, 2016). ACT aims to help the person with pain develop psychological flexibility and live the life they want. The core processes work together to support this goal.

OTPs can begin with any core process and may not include them all. For example, using an ACT approach, OTPs may help a person develop *acceptance* or willingness to experience pain as only pain and make room for uncomfortable thoughts, feelings, and sensations, rather than fusing (i.e., getting stuck) with unhelpful thoughts such as "pain is horrible," "I shouldn't have any pain," or "I can't do anything with this pain." Being fused with these thoughts often leads to trying to avoid experiences (e.g., thoughts, feelings, and sensations related to pain) by decreasing occupational participation. OTPs can then support individuals in reducing behavioral avoidance and returning to *committed actions* aligned with personal *values* (Thompson, 2013).

ACT is a process-based therapy that fosters openness, awareness, and engagement through a wide range of methods, including exposure-based and experiential methods, metaphors, and values clarification (Feliu-Soler et al., 2018; Hayes et al., 1999). Feliu-Soler and colleagues (2018) summarized evidence from multiple systematic reviews demonstrating positive outcomes in pain intensity, depression, disability, quality of life, anxiety, pain interference, pain acceptance, and functional performance when using ACT for chronic pain. Clinical guidelines have detailed how to use ACT to help people with chronic pain develop greater psychological flexibility and resilience (Moens et al., 2022).

ACT helps individuals experiencing pain see that turning away from pain and distress includes turning away from their values and goals. OTPs help individuals affirm their values and goals and turn toward these by opening up and making room for pain and distress while finding strategies to engage in more meaningful occupations through graded exposure. Readers should refer to The Choice Point in Chapter 8: Cognitive Beliefs 🤝 and consider how an OTP could use this with a person experiencing chronic pain. Consider the examples of ACT interventions presented in Chapter 8: Cognitive Beliefs, 🤝 such as "dropping your anchor" and ACT metaphors available online, to explain and apply the core processes of ACT and how they might help someone experiencing chronic pain develop psychological flexibility and increase occupational engagement.

TIC-TOC ACTIVITY		
Task-Interfering Cognitions (TICs)	**Thought Distortions**	**Task-Oriented Cognitions (TOCs)**
I can't do anything when my pain is really bad.	*Catastrophizing*	*Even when my pain is bad, there are still some things I can do, such as...*
I will only be happy when my pain is completely gone.	*All-or-nothing thinking*	*Even if I have some pain, I can still be happy. There is always something I can do to have a better quality of life.*
I am worthless. I can't help my spouse or my kids. I am so useless.	*Emotional reasoning*	*Even though I can't do everything I used to do, it doesn't mean I can't do anything or that I can't contribute to my family.*

FIGURE 15-11. TIC-TOC example with a person experiencing chronic pain.

Pain Neuroscience Education

Pain Neuroscience Education (PNE) is an educational strategy that OTPs can use that focuses on teaching people more about the biological and physiological processes involved in their pain experience (AOTA, 2021; Louw et al., 2016; Moseley et al., 2004; Rider & Smith, 2023; Rider & Tay, 2022). Evidence suggests that PNE can positively influence pain ratings,

functional performance, psychosocial factors, limitations in movement, pain knowledge, disability, and health-care utilization (Louw et al., 2016).

PNE helps individuals experiencing pain cope and decrease kinesiophobia (fear of movement) and pain catastrophizing (Watson et al., 2019). PNE can be delivered one-on-one or in group settings and utilizes stories, metaphors, examples, pictures, and workbooks to help individuals reconceptualize

---

Being a Psychosocial OT Practitioner

From Pain to Participation: Using a Biopsychosocial Approach to Addressing Chronic Pain

Identifying Psychosocial Strengths and Needs

OTPs in all settings encounter individuals experiencing chronic pain. Consider the story of Jack, who has been living with non-specific low back pain for the last 8 years and is working with an outpatient OTP.

Jack is a 62-year-old veteran and retired plumber. He was referred to occupational therapy by his primary care physician with a chief complaint of low back pain. He lives in a single-story home with his wife and two dogs. His medical history includes lumbar spinal stenosis, degenerative disc disease, osteoarthritis, lumbar spinal fusion (6 years ago), hypertension, PTSD, and depression. Jack uses a front-wheeled walker for short distances and a scooter for long distances. He reports that his back pain caused him to retire early and that his wife assists with most IADLs and lower body dressing. Jack indicates that he tried physical therapy multiple times and eventually had a spinal fusion, resulting in minimal improvements in pain and function.

Jack is distraught while talking about his pain and all it has "taken away" from him over the last 8 years. When asked about hobbies and interests, Jack becomes tearful and focuses on not wanting to burden his wife. When Jack does identify hobbies, he only speaks about them in the past tense and states, "If I could just get rid of the pain, everything else would be fine."

The OTP explains the role of occupational therapy and the biopsychosocial approach in lay terms and asks Jack if he would be willing to consider how pain impacts each area of his life and how addressing these areas might influence his pain. Jack replies, "No one has ever taken the time to talk to me about my pain like this. I don't know if it will help, but I will try anything at this point."

Using a Holistic Occupational Therapy Approach

The OTP obtains a comprehensive occupational profile and gathers more information about Jack's pain experience. He currently uses over-the-counter pain creams, acetaminophen, and heating pads, and avoids movements and activities that he fears will increase his pain. Jack reports minimal relief from his current medications and that pain interferes with his quality of life, general activity levels, walking ability, sleep, mood, and relationships with his family. During functional mobility and lower body dressing, the OTP observes hesitation, guarded movements, and comments demonstrating low pain self-efficacy and catastrophizing.

There are many pain assessments appropriate for Jack. Based on Jack's responses during the occupational profile and interview, the OTP decides to start with the PCS, PCI, and PSEQ to help initiate a discussion on Jack's thoughts and beliefs about pain, beliefs about his capacity to manage his pain, and his current coping mechanisms. The OTP also administers the COPM to capture Jack's self-perception of performance in everyday activities, identify goals, and monitor progress.

Results of the PCS (40/52) indicate high levels of catastrophizing thoughts in all categories. Results of the PCI (102/136) suggest that Jack primarily uses passive coping strategies rather than

active ones. Results of the PSEQ (17/60) indicate Jack is not very confident dealing with pain. The COPM reveals the following meaningful occupations used to develop goals: cooking, lower body bathing/dressing, working on his car, and visiting grandchildren with his wife (average scores are 3.25 for Performance and 2.5 for Satisfaction).

With Jack's permission, the OTP starts by explaining more about the neurophysiology of pain in lay language using metaphors and pictures from PNE. Jack responds well to a commonly used PNE metaphor about how nerves are similar to a home alarm system warning us of danger. The OTP explains how many factors (e.g., fear, failed treatment, family, stress, self-efficacy) can make the alarm more sensitive, causing it to go off when it shouldn't. Using this metaphor, the OTP helps Jack identify what aspects of his life might be causing his alarm system to be too sensitive and what areas he is willing to address to "turn down" the alarm system. He decides to address his worries about burdening his wife and fears that movement and specific activities will worsen his pain.

Through the use of ACT, the OTP helps Jack recognize that he is getting "stuck" on his thoughts about pain and turning away from what he values in life (avoiding things he wants to do for fear of increased pain). After revisiting his values and referring to his COPM results, they explored ACT techniques to make room for unhelpful thoughts about pain and defuse (i.e., get unstuck) from those thoughts so he can be more present and make choices to engage in activities aligned with his values. The OTP provides Jack with specific cognitive defusion techniques to try at home and asks him to begin a pain diary to track his thoughts and progress.

In subsequent sessions, the OTP and Jack review his pain diaries and explore gentle stretches, graded movements, and relaxation strategies, building his capacity to "turn down" the sensitivity of his alarm system. The OTP continues to use PNE and ACT concepts to address Jack's fear-avoidance and catastrophizing thoughts about pain, thereby connecting metaphors to his pain experience. Treatment focuses on occupational participation through graded exposure in the clinic and at home outside of therapy. The OTP slowly grades up cooking and lower body dressing tasks, aligned with operant conditioning principles and building Jack's self-efficacy.

Jack is given homework after each session and continues to keep a pain diary, which progresses to more details about increased occupational participation and less about pain interference. Jack explores multiple pain management approaches (e.g., relaxation, activity pacing, mindfulness, ACT, yoga) as part of occupational therapy and builds his toolbox of strategies. The OTP then guides Jack in creating a written supported self-management plan and a setback plan, drawing on what has helped since starting occupational therapy.

Reflective Questions

1. What other behavioral approaches might be helpful to explore with Jack?
2. How might the OTP specifically address Jack's poor pain self-efficacy?
3. How would the OTP approach the idea of a relapse prevention plan and help Jack develop one as part of a treatment session?

their pain. A growing body of evidence suggests that teaching people experiencing pain more about the neuroscience of pain produces positive immediate and long-term effects (Louw et al., 2016). Guidelines for best practice combine PNE with movement-based therapies or graded exposure (Louw et al., 2011). OTPs can use PNE alongside other evidence-based interventions. More information about learning PNE can be found in the Resources section at the end of this chapter.

Here's the Point

- Pain is a common yet complex experience.
- Pain can impact all aspects of occupational performance and participation.
- Pain is a personal experience influenced by biological, psychological, and social factors.
- Chronic pain and mental health challenges can contribute to and exacerbate each other.

- Evaluation should focus on the impact of pain on occupational performance and participation, physical, emotional, and social health.
- OTPs should seek to understand the multidimensionality of the pain experience within the context of the person and their daily life.
- Intervention approaches should enable occupational performance and participation, preferably through supported self-management.
- OTPs help people make sense of their pain and develop flexible adaptations for the contexts of daily life so they can do what matters most to them.

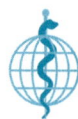 Visit the online resource center at **FADavis.com** to access the video.

Apply It Now

1. Pain Narrative

Individually or with a partner, identify a person experiencing chronic pain or the primary caregiver for someone experiencing chronic pain. Set up a short interview with the specific goal of eliciting the person's pain narrative. You might begin by asking the person to describe the pain and their beliefs about its origins. Ask how the person has dealt with pain and changes in physical activities or occupational participation. Explore positive and negative aspects of the person's interactions and relationships with health-care professionals who treat their pain symptoms. You might also explore the following topics:

- Relationship between their pain experience and self-image
- Impact of their pain experience on relationships with family and friends
- Strategies that they use to cope with pain

Share your interview experiences and stories with your peers. Look for similarities and differences between people's pain experiences.

Reflective Questions
- What did you learn about the pain experience and its impact on daily life?
- What strategies were most helpful in managing pain?
- When comparing your interview with peers, what were common themes among the stories?
- What experiences were unique to your individual?

2. Reflective Activity: Measuring Pain

Review the Reflective Activity on Measuring Pain earlier in the chapter and discuss your thoughts with a peer. Discuss the types of pain assessments and how they might lead to interventions and influence the care plan.

3. Relaxation Techniques

Relaxation techniques can be very helpful in managing pain. The more one practices a technique, the better pain relief is obtained. Rate your tension before and after practicing a relaxation technique (e.g., on a scale of 0 to 10, where 0 equals *completely relaxed* and 10 equals *as tense as possible)*. Go to a quiet, dimly lit room and practice progressive muscle relaxation. You can find many free guided audio clips online.

Reflective Questions
- Were you able to relax? Why or why not?
- How would you teach and practice this technique with a person experiencing pain?
- What other methods or activities provide relaxation for you?

4. Video Exercise: Mental Health and Well-Being During COVID

Pair up with another student in your class or form a small group of students. Access and watch the "Mental Health and Well-Being During COVID" video at the online resource center at FADavis.com. Then, discuss and together answer the following questions.

Reflective Questions
- How did this OTP use a holistic approach to her practice in an outpatient setting while working during the COVID pandemic? Why do you think this was successful?
- The OTP discusses how pain associated with carpal tunnel syndrome can be exacerbated by anxiety and depression. What are other examples of mental health diagnoses/symptoms that might complicate and/or exacerbate physical symptoms? How might OTPs address the interplay of psychosocial and physical conditions?
- Given that mental health challenges can exacerbate pain, physical disabilities, and/or chronic illness, and vice versa,

what might the OTP in this video provide as "homework" to improve the mental health and well-being of people they work with during a pandemic?

■ The practitioner comments that the COVID-19 pandemic "impacted everyone's mental health and well-being." However, the evidence confirms that the pandemic disproportionately affected people with multiple challenges to their social determinants of health. Would the strategies the practitioner in this video used differ if the populations she treated came predominantly from marginalized groups? Explain.

Resources

- American Chronic Pain Association (ACPA): http://theacpa.org. The ACPA offers support and education in pain management to persons with pain, their significant others, and health-care providers.
- American Occupational Therapy Association. (2021). Position statement—Role of occupational therapy in pain management. *American Journal of Occupational Therapy, 75*(Suppl. 3), 7513410010. https://doi.org/10.5014/ajot.2020.75S3001
- International Association for the Study of Pain (IASP): www.iasp-pain.org. The IASP is an international professional forum dedicated to advancing science, practice, and education in the field of pain. The IASP's official journal, *PAIN,* is the premier journal on the subject of pain. IASP has created a curriculum outline on pain for occupational therapy education. The outline is available for free online at https://www.iasp-pain.org/education/curricula/iasp-curriculum-outline-on-pain-for-occupational-therapy.

Textbooks

- Louw, A., Puentedura, E., Schmidt, S., & Zimney, K. (2018). *Pain neuroscience education: Teaching people about pain* (2nd ed.). OPTP.
- Main, C. J., Keepfe, F., Jensen, M., Vlaeyen, J., & Vowles, K. (2014). *Fordyce's behavioral methods for chronic pain and illness: Republished with invited commentaries.* International Association for the Study of Pain.
- Mosely, G. L., & Butler, D. S. (2017). *Explain pain supercharged.* Noigroup Publications.
- Mosely, G. L., Butler, D. S., & Beames T. B. (2019). *The graded motor imagery handbook.* Noigroup Publications.
- Van Griensven, H., & Strong, J. (2023). *Pain: A textbook for health professionals* (3rd ed.). Churchhill Livingstone Elsevier.

Workbooks/Manuals

- Louw, A. (2018). *Why do I hurt? Workbook: Neuroscience education workbook* for *patients with pain.* OPTP.
- Murphy, J., McKellar, J., Raffa, S., Clark, M., Kerns, R., & Karlin, B. (n.d.). *Cognitive behavioral therapy for chronic pain among veterans: Therapist manual.* U.S. Department of Veterans Affairs.
- Otis, J. D. (2007). *Managing chronic pain workbook: A cognitive-behavioral therapy approach.* Oxford University Press, Inc.
- Zoffness, R. (2019). *The chronic pain and illness workbook for teens: CBT and mindfulness-based practices to turn the volume down on pain.* New Harbinger Publications, Inc.
- Zoffness, R. (2020). *The pain management workbook: Powerful CBT and mindfulness skills to take control of pain and reclaim your life.* New Harbinger Publications, Inc.

References

Adams, H., Ellis, T., Stanish, W. D., & Sullivan, M. J. (2007). Psychosocial factors related to return to work following rehabilitation of whiplash injuries. *Journal of Occupational Rehabilitation, 17*(2), 305–315. https://doi.org/10.1007/s10926-007-9082-3

AGS Panel on Persistent Pain in Older Persons. (2002). The management of persistent pain in older persons. *Journal of the American Geriatrics Society, 50*(6 Suppl.), S205–S224. https://doi.org/10.1046/j.1532-5415.50.6s.1.x

American Occupational Therapy Association. (2020). Occupational therapy practice framework: Domain and process—fourth edition. *American Journal of Occupational Therapy, 74*(Suppl. 2), 7412410010p1–7412410010p87. https://doi.org/10.5014/ajot.2020.74S2001

American Occupational Therapy Association. (2021). Role of occupational therapy in pain management. *The American Journal of Occupational Therapy, 75*(Suppl. 3), 7513410010. https://doi.org/10.5014/ajot.2020.75S3001

Arnow, B. A., Enid, M., Hunkeler, M. A., Blasey, C. M., Lee, J., Constantino, M. J., Fireman, B., Kraemer, H. C., Dea, R., Robinson, R., & Hayward, C. (2006). Comorbid depression, chronic pain, and disability in primary care. *Psychosomatic Medicine, 68,* 262–268. https://doi.org/10.1097/01.psy.0000204851.15499.fc

Atler, K. E., & Fisher, A. G. (2022). Validity and reliability of the Occupational Experience Profile. *Scandinavian Journal of Occupational Therapy, 30*(6), 811–821. https://doi.org/10.1080/11038128.2022.2027009

Bawa, F. L., Mercer, S. W., Atherton, R. J., Clague, F., Keen, A., Scott, N. W., & Bond, C. M. (2015). Does mindfulness improve outcomes in patients with chronic pain? Systematic review and meta-analysis. *British Journal of General Practice, 65,* e387–400. https://doi.org/ 10.3399/bjgp15X685297

Beck, A. T., Rush, A. J., Shaw, B. F., & Emery, G. (1979). *Cognitive therapy of depression.* Guilford Press.

Bevers, K., Watts, L., Kishino, N. D., & Gatchel, R. J. (2016). The biopsychosocial model of the assessment, prevention, and treatment of chronic pain. *US Neurology, 12*(2), 98–104. https://doi.org/10.17925/USN.2016.12.02.98

Bondesson, E., Larrosa Pardo, F., Stigmar, K., Ringqvist, Å., Petersson, I. F., Jöud, A., & Schelin, M. E. C. (2018). Comorbidity between pain and mental illness—Evidence of a bidirectional relationship. *European Journal of Pain, 22*(7), 1304–1311. https://doi.org/10.1002/ejp.1218

Christiansen, C. H. (1999). Defining lives: Occupation as identity: An essay on competence, coherence, and the creation of meaning. *American Journal of Occupational Therapy, 53*(6), 547–558. https://doi.org/10.5014/ajot.53.6.547

Colloca, L. (2019). The placebo effect in pain therapies. *Annual Review of Pharmacology and Toxicology, 59,* 191–211. https://doi.org/10.1146/annurev-pharmtox-010818-021542

Colloca, L., & Finniss, D. (2012). Nocebo effects, patient-clinician communication, and therapeutic outcomes. *Journal of the American Medical Association, 307*(6), 567–568. https://doi.org/10.1001/jama.2012.115

Elbers, S., Pool, J., Wittink, H., Köke, A., & Smeets, R. (2020). Exploring the feasibility of relapse prevention strategies in interdisciplinary multimodal pain therapy programs: Qualitative study. *JMIR Human Factors, 7*(4), e21545. https://doi.org/10.2196/21545

Ellis, A. (1962). *Reason and emotion in psychotherapy.* Lyle Stuart.

Fairbank, J. C., Couper, J., Davies, J. B., & O'Brien, J. P. (1980). The Oswestry low back pain disability questionnaire. *Physiotherapy, 66*(8), 271–273.

Feliu-Soler, A., Montesinos, F., Gutiérrez-Martínez, O., Scott, W., McCracken, L. M., & Luciano, J. V. (2018). Current status of Acceptance and Commitment Therapy for chronic pain: A narrative review. *Journal of Pain Research, 11,* 2145–2159. https://doi.org/10.2147/JPR.S144631

Ferrari, R. (2015). Effect of a pain diary use on recovery from acute low back (lumbar) sprain. *Rheumatology International, 35*(1), 55–59. https://doi.org/10.1007/s00296-014-3082-3

Fine, P. G. (2011). Long-term consequences of chronic pain: Mounting evidence for pain as a neurological disease and parallels with other chronic disease states. *Pain Medicine, 12*(7), 996–1004. https://doi.org/10.1111/j.1526-4637.2011.01187.x

Fitzcharles, M., Cohen, S., Clauw, D., Littlejohn, G., Usui, C., & Hauser, W. (2021). Nociplastic pain: Towards an understanding of prevalent pain conditions. *The Lancet, 397,* 2098–2110. https://doi.org/10.1016/S0140-6736(21)00392-5

Fordyce, W. E., Fowler, R. S., & DeLateur, B. (1968). An application of behavior modification technique to a problem of chronic pain. *Behaviour Research and Therapy, 6*(1), 105–107. https://doi.org/10.1016/0005-7967(68)90048-x

Gatchel, R. J., Bo Peng, Y., Peters, M. L., Fuchs, P. N., & Turk, D. C. (2007). The biopsychosocial approach to chronic pain: Scientific advances and future directions. *Psychological Bulletin, 133*(4), 581–624. https://doi.org/10.1037/0033-2909.133.4.581

Gatchel, R. J., Worzer, W. E., Berde, E., Choi, Y., Asih, S., & Hartzell, M. (2012). The comorbidity of chronic pain and mental health disorders: How to manage both. *Practical Pain Management, 12*(2 Pt. 3), 60–80. https://doi.org/10.1037/0003-066X.59.8.795

Gift, A. G. (1989). Visual analogue scales: Measurement of subjective phenomena. *Nursing Research, 38,* 286–287. https://doi.org/10.1097/00006199-198909000-00006

Givler, A., Bhatt, H., & Maani-Fogelman, P. A. (2022). The importance of cultural competence in pain and palliative care. In *StatPearls*. StatPearls Publishing.

Gross, A. C., & Fox, E. J. (2009). Relational frame theory: An overview of the controversy. *The Analysis of Verbal Behavior, 25*(1), 87–98. https://doi.org/10.1007/BF03393073

Hayes S. C. (2016). Acceptance and Commitment Therapy, Relational Frame Theory, and the third wave of behavioral and cognitive therapies—Republished article. *Behavior Therapy, 47*(6), 869–885. https://doi.org/10.1016/j.beth.2016.11.006

Hayes, S. C., Hofmann, S. G., & Ciarrochi, J. (2020). A process-based approach to psychological diagnosis and treatment: The conceptual and treatment utility of an extended evolutionary meta model. *Clinical Psychology Review, 82,* 101908. https://doi.org/10.1016/j.cpr.2020.101908

Hayes, S. C., Strosahl, K. D., & Wilson, K. G. (1999). *Acceptance and Commitment Therapy: An experiential approach to behavior change.* Guilford Press.

Hudak, P. L., Amadio, P. C., & Bombardier, C. (1996). Development of an upper extremity outcome measure: The DASH (disabilities of the arm, shoulder and hand) [corrected]. The Upper Extremity Collaborative Group (UECG). *American Journal of Industrial Medicine, 29*(6), 602–608. https://doi.org/10.1002/(SICI)1097-0274(199606)29:6<602::AID-AJIM4>3.0.CO;2-L

International Association for the Study of Pain. (2012). *IASP taxonomy.* http://www.iasp-pain.org/Taxonomy

International Association for the Study of Pain. (2015). *Access to pain management: Declaration of Montréal.* https://www.iasp-pain.org/advocacy/iasp-statements/access-to-pain-management-declaration-of-montreal

International Association for the Study of Pain. (2018). *IASP curriculum outline on pain for occupational therapy.* https://www.iasp-pain.org/education/curricula/iasp-curriculum-outline-on-pain-for-occupational-therapy

Jensen, M. P., Chen, C., & Brugger, A. M. (2003). Interpretation of Visual Analog Scale ratings and change scores: A reanalysis of two clinical trials of postoperative pain. *Journal of Pain, 4*(7), 407–414. https://doi.org/10.1016/s1526-5900(03)00716-8

Jensen, M. P., Karoly, P., & Braver, S. (1986). The measurement of clinical pain intensity: A comparison of six methods. *Pain, 27*(1), 117–126. https://doi.org/10.1016/0304-3959(86)90228-9

Jensen, M. P., Moore, M. R., Bockow, T. B., Ehde, D. M., & Engel, J. M. (2011). Psychosocial factors and adjustment to chronic pain in persons with physical disabilities: A systematic review. *Archives of Physical Medicine and Rehabilitation, 92*(1), 146–160. https://doi.org/10.1016/j.apmr.2010.09.021

Keller, S., Bann, C. M., Dodd, S. L., Schein, J., Mendoza, T. R., & Cleeland, C. S. (2004). Validity of the Brief Pain Inventory for use in documenting the outcomes of patients with non-cancer pain. *Clinical Journal of Pain, 20,* 309–318. https://doi.org/10.1097/00002508-200409000-00005

Kerns, R. D., Turk, D. C., & Rudy, T. E. (1985). The West Haven-Yale Multidimensional Pain Inventory (WHYMPI). *Pain, 23*(4), 345–356. https://doi.org/10.1016/0304-3959(85)90004-1

Klinger, R., Blasini, M., Schmitz, J., & Colloca, L. (2017). Nocebo effects in clinical studies: Hints for pain therapy. *PAIN Reports, 2*(2), e586. https://doi.org/10.1097/PR9.0000000000000586

Korving, H., Sterkenburg, P. S., Barakova, E. I., & Feijs, L. M. G. (2020). Physiological measures of acute and chronic pain within different subject groups: A systematic review. *Pain Research & Management, 2020,* 9249465. https://doi.org/10.1155/2020/9249465

Kraaimaat, F. W., & Evers, A. W. (2003). Pain-coping strategies in chronic pain patients: Psychometric characteristics of the pain-coping inventory (PCI). *International Journal of Behavioral Medicine, 10*(4), 343–363. https://doi.org/10.1207/s15327558ijbm1004_5

Larimer, M. E., Palmer, R. S., & Marlatt, G. A. (1999). Relapse prevention. An overview of Marlatt's cognitive-behavioral model. *Alcohol Research & Health, 23*(2), 151–160.

Law, M., Baptiste, S., Carswell, A., McColl, M. A., Polatajko, H., & Pollock, N. (2019). *Canadian Occupational Performance Measure* (5th ed.). COPM, Inc.

Law, M., Cooper, B., Strong, S., Stewart, D., Rigby, P., & Letts, L. (1996). The Person-Environment-Occupation Model: A transactive approach to occupational performance. *Canadian Journal of Occupational Therapy, 63*(1), 9–23. https://doi.org/10.1177/000841749606300103

Lena, F., Pappaccogli, M., Santilli, M., Torre, M., Modugno, N., & Perrotta, A. (2022). How does semantic pain and words condition pain perception? A short communication. *Neurological Sciences, 43*(1), 691–696. https://doi.org/10.1007/s10072-021-05577-5

Lennox Thompson, B., Gage, J., & Kirk, R. (2020). Living well with chronic pain: A classical grounded theory. *Disability and Rehabilitation, 42*(8), 1141–1152. https://doi.org/10.1080/09638288.2018.1517195

Lennox Thompson, B. F., & Ramanauskas, C. (2024). Articulating occupational therapy's unique contribution to pain management. *New Zealand Journal of Occupational Therapy, 71*(1), 26–32.

Loeser, J. D. (2018). A new way of thinking about pain. *Pain Management, 9*(1), 5–7. https://doi.org/10.2217/pmt-2018-0061

Loeser, J. D., & Fordyce, W. (1983). Chronic pain. In J. E. Carr & H. A. Dengerink (Eds.), *Behavioral science in the practice of medicine* (pp. 331–345). Elsevier.

Louw, A., Diener, I., Butler, D. S., & Puentedura, E. J. (2011). The effect of neuroscience education on pain, disability, anxiety, and stress in chronic musculoskeletal pain. *Archives of Physical Medicine and Rehabilitation, 92*(12), 2041–2056. https://doi.org/10.1016/j.apmr.2011.07.198

Louw, A., Zimney, K., Puentedura, E. J., & Diener, I. (2016). The efficacy of Pain Neuroscience Education on musculoskeletal pain: A systematic review of the literature. *Physiotherapy Theory and Practice, 32*(5), 332–355. https://doi.org/10.1080/09593985.2016.1194646

Main, C. J., Keepfe, F., Jensen, M., Vlaeyen, J., & Vowles, K. (2014). *Fordyce's behavioral methods for chronic pain and illness: Republished with invited commentaries.* International Association for the Study of Pain.

Manai, M., van Middendorp, H., Veldhuijzen, D. S., Huizinga, T. W. J., & Evers, A. W. M. (2019). How to prevent, minimize, or extinguish nocebo effects in pain: A narrative review on mechanisms, predictors, and interventions. *Pain Reports, 4*(3), e699. https://doi.org/10.1097/PR9.0000000000000699

McCracken, L. M., Vowles, K. E., & Eccleston, C. (2004). Acceptance of chronic pain: Component analysis and a revised assessment method. *Pain, 107*(1-2), 159–166. https://doi.org/10.1016/j.pain.2003.10.012

McCracken, L. M., Zayfert, C., & Gross, R. T. (1992). The Pain Anxiety Symptoms Scale: Development and validation of a scale to measure fear of pain. *Pain, 50*(1), 67–73. https://doi.org/10.1016/0304-3959(92)90113-P

MD Anderson Center. (n.d.). *The Brief Pain Inventory.* https://www.mdanderson.org/research/departments-labs-institutes/departments-divisions/symptom-research/symptom-assessment-tools/brief-pain-inventory.html

Melzack, R. (1975). The McGill Pain Questionnaire: Major properties and scoring methods. *Pain, 1,* 277–299. https://doi.org/10.1016/0304-3959(75)90044-5

Meredith, P. J., Rappel, G., Strong, J., & Bailey, K. J. (2015). Sensory sensitivity and strategies for coping with pain. *American Journal of Occupational Therapy, 69*(4), 6904240010p1–6904240010p10. https://doi.org/10.5014/ajot.2015.014621

Middleton, C. (2003). Understanding the physiological effects of unrelieved pain. *Nursing Times, 99*(37), 28–31.

Mills, S., Nicolson, K., & Smith, B. (2019). Chronic pain: A review of its epidemiology and associated factors in population-based studies. *British Journal of Anaesthesia, 123*(2), e273–e283. https://doi.org/10.1016/j.bja.2019.03.023

Moens, M., Jansen, J., De Smedt, A., Roulaud, M., Billot, M., Laton, J., Rigoard, P., & Goudman, L. (2022). Acceptance and Commitment Therapy to increase resilience in chronic pain patients: A clinical guideline. *Medicina, 58*(4), 499. https://doi.org/10.3390/medicina58040499

Morone, N. E., & Weiner, D. K. (2013). Pain as the fifth vital sign: Exposing the vital need for pain education. *Clinical Therapeutics, 35,* 1728–1732. https://doi.org/doi: 10.1016/j.clinthera.2013.10.001

Moseley, G. L., Nicholas, M. K., & Hodges, P. W. (2004). A randomized controlled trial of intensive neurophysiology education in chronic low back pain. *The Clinical Journal of Pain, 20*(5), 324–330. https://doi.org/10.1097/00002508-200409000-00007

Murphy, J., McKellar, J., Raffa, S., Clark, M., Kerns, R., & Karlin, B. (n.d.). *Cognitive behavioral therapy for chronic pain among veterans: Therapist manual.* U.S. Department of Veterans Affairs. https://www.va.gov/painmanagement/docs/cbt-cp_therapist_manual.pdf

National Center for Complementary and Integrative Health. (2023). *Pain.* https://www.nccih.nih.gov/health/pain

Neff, K. D. (2003). Development and validation of a scale to measure self-compassion. *Self and Identity, 2,* 223–250. https://doi.org/10.1080/15298860390209035

Nicholas, M. K. (2007). The Pain Self-Efficacy Questionnaire: Taking pain into account. *European Journal of Pain, 11*(2), 153–163. https://doi.org/10.1016/j.ejpain.2005.12.008

Pasero, C., & McCaffery, M. (2011). Assessment tools. In C. Pasero & M. McCaffery, *Pain assessment and pharmacologic management* (pp. 49–142). Mosby.

Peacock, S., & Patel, S. (2008). Cultural influences on pain. *Reviews in Pain, 1*(2), 6–9. https://doi.org/10.1177/204946370800100203

Pincus, T., Smeets, R. J., Simmonds, M. J., & Sullivan, M. J. (2010). The fear avoidance model disentangled: Improving the clinical utility of the fear avoidance model. *The Clinical Journal of Pain, 26*(9), 739–746. https://doi.org/10.1097/AJP.0b013e3181f15d45

Pulvers, K., & Hood, A. (2013). The role of positive traits and pain catastrophizing in pain perception. *Current Pain and Headache Reports, 17*(5), 330. https://doi.org/10.1007/s11916-013-0330-2

Quartana, P. J., Campbell, C. M., & Edwards, R. R. (2009). Pain catastrophizing: A critical review. *Expert Review of Neurotherapeutics, 9*(5), 745–758. https://doi.org/10.1586/ERN.09.34

Raja, S. N., Carr, D. B., Cohen, M., Finnerup, N. B., Flor, H., Gibson, S., Keefe, F. J., Mogil, J. S., Ringkamp, M., Sluka, K. A., Song, X. J., Stevens, B., Sullivan, M. D., Tutelman, P. R., Ushida, T., & Vader, K. (2020). The revised International Association for the Study of Pain definition of pain: Concepts, challenges, and compromises. *Pain, 161*(9), 1976–1982. https://doi.org/10.1097/j.pain.0000000000001939

Ray, B. M., Kovaleski, A., Kelleran, K. J., Stilwell, P., Baraki, A., Coninx, S., & Eubanks, J. E. (2022). An exploration of low back pain beliefs in a Northern America based general population. *Musculoskeletal Science & Practice, 61,* 102591. https://doi.org/10.1016/j.msksp.2022.102591

Reneau, M. (2020). Heart rate variability biofeedback to treat fibromyalgia: An integrative literature review. *Pain Management Nursing, 21*(3), 225–232. https://doi.org/10.1016/j.pmn.2019.08.001

Rider, J. V., & Smith, K. (2023). Persistent pain. In S. Dahl-Popolizio, K. Smith, M. Day, S. Muir, & W. Manard (Eds.), *Primary care occupational therapy: A quick reference guide* (pp. 387–400). Springer Publishing Company.

Rider, J. V., & Tay, M. C. (2022). Increasing occupational engagement by addressing psychosocial and occupational factors of chronic pain: A case report. *The Open Journal of Occupational Therapy, 10*(3), 1–12. https://doi.org/10.15453/2168-6408.2027

Roland, M. O., & Morris, R. W. (1983). A study of the natural history of back pain. Part 1: Development of a reliable and sensitive measure of disability in low back pain. *Spine, 8,* 141–144. https://doi.org/10.1097/00007632-198303000-00004

Salaffi, F., Stancati, A., Silvestri, C. A., Ciapetti, A., & Grassi, W. (2004). Minimal clinically important changes in chronic musculoskeletal pain intensity measured on a Numerical Rating Scale. *European Journal of Pain, 8*(4), 283–291. https://doi.org/10.1016/j.ejpain.2003.09.004

Schappert, S. M., & Burt, C. W. (2006). Ambulatory care visits to physician offices, hospital outpatient departments, and emergency departments: United States, 2001-02. Data from the National Health Survey. *Vital and Health Statistics, 13*(159), 1–66.

Scott, W., Wideman, T., & Sullivan, M. (2014). Clinically meaningful scores on pain catastrophizing before and after multidisciplinary rehabilitation: A prospective study of individuals with subacute pain after whiplash injury. *The Clinical Journal of Pain, 30*(3), 183–190. https://doi.org/10.1097/AJP.0b013e31828eee6c

Stewart, M., & Loftus, S. (2018). Sticks and stones: The impact of language in musculoskeletal rehabilitation. *The Journal of Orthopaedic and Sports Physical Therapy, 48*(7), 519–522. https://doi.org/10.2519/jospt.2018.0610

Stone, A. L., Bruehl, S., Smith, C. A., Garber, J., & Walker, L. S. (2018). Social learning pathways in the relation between parental chronic pain and daily pain severity and functional impairment in adolescents with functional abdominal pain. *Pain, 159*(2), 298–305. https://doi.org/10.1097/j.pain.0000000000001085

Stratford, P., Gill, C., Westaway, M., & Binkley, J. (1995). Assessing disability and change on individual patients: A report of a patient specific measure. *Physiotherapy Canada, 47,* 258–263. https://doi.org/10.3138/ptc.47.4.258

Strong, J., & van Griensven, H. (2014). Assessing pain. In H. van Griensven, J. Strong, & A. Unruh (Eds.), *Pain: A textbook for health professionals* (2nd ed., pp. 91–114). Elsevier.

Sullivan, M. J. L. (2009). *The Pain Catastrophizing Scale: User manual.* Departments of Psychology, Medicine, and Neurology, School of Physical and Occupational Therapy, McGill University.

Sullivan, M. J. L., Adams, H., Rhodenizer, T., & Stanish, W. D. (2006). A psychosocial risk factor—Targeted intervention for the prevention of chronic pain and disability following whiplash injury. *Physical Therapy, 86*(1), 8–18. https://doi.org/10.1093/ptj/86.1.8

Sullivan, M. J. L., Bishop, S. R., & Pivik, J. (1995). The Pain Catastrophizing Scale: Development and validation. *Psychological Assessment, 7*(4), 524–532. https://doi.org/10.1037/1040-3590.7.4.524

Tarr, J., & Thomas, H. (2021). Good pain, bad pain: Dancers, injury, and listening to the body. *Dance Research, 39*(1), 53–71. https://doi.org/10.3366/drs.2020.0301

Thompson, B. (2013). Occupational therapy's ACTions: Using ACT within occupational therapy for people with chronic pain. *Ngau Mamae: New Zealand Pain Society,* 4–10.

Tomlinson, D., von Baeyer, C. L., Stinson, J. N., & Sung, L. (2010). A systematic review of FACES scales for the self-report of pain intensity in children. *Pediatrics, 126,* e1168. https://doi.org/10.1542/peds.2010-1609

Travaglini, L. E., Kuykendall, L., Bennett, M. E., Abel, E. A., & Lucksted, A. (2020). Relationships between chronic pain and mood symptoms among veterans with bipolar disorder. *Journal of Affective Disorders, 277,* 765–771. https://doi.org/10.1016/j.jad.2020.08.069

Trost, Z., & Parsons, T. (2014). Beyond distraction: Virtual reality graded exposure therapy for pain-related fear and disability in chronic pain. *Journal of Applied Biobehavioral Research, 19*(2), 106–126. https://doi.org/10.1111/jabr.12021

Trost, Z., France, C., Anam, M., & Shum, C. (2021). Virtual reality approaches to pain: Toward a state of the science. *PAIN, 162*(2), 325–331. https://doi.org/10.1097/j.pain.0000000000002060

Tuck, N. L., Johnson, M. H., & Bean, D. J. (2019). You'd better believe it: The conceptual and practical challenges of assessing malingering in patients with chronic pain. *Journal of Pain, 20*(2), 133–145. https://doi.org/10.1016/j.jpain.2018.07.002

Turner, J. A., & Romano, J. M. (2001). Psychological and psychosocial evaluation. In J. D. Loeser, S. H. Butler, C. R. Chapman, & D. C. Turk (Eds.), *Bonica's management of pain* (3rd ed., pp. 329–341). Lippincott Williams & Wilkins.

U.S. Department of Health and Human Services. (2019). *Pain Management Best Practices Inter-Agency Task Force report: Updates, gaps, inconsistencies, and recommendations.* https://www.hhs.gov/sites/default/files/pmtf-final-report-2019-05-23.pdf

Vambheim, S. M., Kyllo, T. M., Hegland, S., & Bystad, M. (2021). Relaxation techniques as an intervention for chronic pain: A systematic review of randomized controlled trials. *Heliyon, 7*(8), e07837. https://doi.org/10.1016/j.heliyon.2021.e07837

van Huet, H., & Williams, D. (2007). Self-beliefs about pain and occupational performance: A comparison of two measures used in a pain management program. *OTJR: Occupational Therapy Journal of Research, 27*(1), 4–12. https://doi.org/10.1177/153944920702700102

Vlaeyen, J. W., de Jong, J., Sieben, J., & Crombez, G. (2002). Graded exposure in vivo for pain-related fear. In D. Turk & R. Gatchel (Eds.), *Psychological approaches to pain management: A practitioner's handbook* (2nd ed., pp. 210–233). Guilford Press.

Vlaeyen, J. W., Morley, S., Linton, S. J., Boersma, K., & de Jong, J. (2012). *Pain-related fear: Essential guide to treatment.* IASP Press.

Waddell, G., Newton, M., Henderson, I., Somerville, D., & Main, C. J. A. (1993). A Fear-Avoidance Beliefs Questionnaire (FABQ) and the role of fear-avoidance beliefs in chronic low back pain and disability. *Pain, 52,* 157–168. https://doi.org/10.1016/0304-3959(93)90127-B

Wager, J., Brown, D., Kupitz, A., Rosenthal, N., & Zernikow, B. (2020). Prevalence and associated psychosocial and health factors of chronic pain in adolescents: Differences by sex and age. *European Journal of Pain, 24*(4), 761–772. https://doi.org/10.1002/ejp.1526

Walder, K., Molineux, M., Bissett, M., & Whiteford, G. (2021). Occupational adaptation—Analyzing the maturity and understanding of the concept through concept analysis. *Scandinavian Journal of Occupational Therapy, 28*(1), 26–40. https://doi.org/10.1080/11038128.2019.1695931

Watson, J., Ryan, C., Cooper, L., Ellington, D., Whittle, R., Lavender, M., Dixon, J., Atkinson, G., Cooper, K., & Martin, D. (2019). Pain Neuroscience Education for adults with chronic musculoskeletal pain: A mixed-methods systematic review and meta-analysis. *The Journal of Pain, 20*(10), P1140-E1–1140.E22. https://doi.org/10.1016/j.jpain.2019.02.011

Williams, A. C. C., Fisher, E., Hearn, L., & Eccleston, C. (2020). Psychological therapies for the management of chronic pain (excluding headache) in adults. *The Cochrane Database of Systematic Reviews, 8*(8), CD007407. https://doi.org/10.1002/14651858.CD007407.pub4

Wong, D. L., & Baker, C. M. (1988). Pain in children: Comparison of assessment scales. *Pediatric Nursing, 14,* 9–17. PMID: 3344163

Woolf, C. J. (2010). What is this thing called pain? *Journal of Clinical Investigation, 120*(11), 3742–3744. https://doi.org/10.1172/JCI45178

Yong, R. J., Mullins, P. M., & Bhattacharyya, N. (2022). Prevalence of chronic pain among adults in the United States. *Pain, 163*(2), e328–e332. https://doi.org/10.1097/j.pain.0000000000002291

Zelaya, C. E., Dahlhamer, J. M., Lucas, J. W., & Connor, E. M. (2020). Chronic pain and high-impact chronic pain among U.S. adults, 2019. NCHS Data Brief, No. 390. National Center for Health Statistics.

Acquired Physical Disability and Mental Health

CHAPTER 16

Susan Tully

Because of medical advances in recent years, more people are surviving serious injuries than ever before. Improvements in emergency medical care, involving the way patients are stabilized, treated, and transported from the field, as well as lifesaving and limb-saving interventions provided by hospital trauma teams, have helped save countless individuals who decades ago would have succumbed to serious brain, spinal cord, and burn trauma. In addition, the aging of the population and advances in lifesaving therapies that have resulted in reduced mortality rates mean more persons are living with the long-term effects of critical illness and chronic diseases that result in physical disability.

Such progress has contributed to the evolution of a rehabilitation population that can benefit from skilled therapy interventions to help affected individuals both regain lost function and live meaningful lives with the residual challenges left by life-changing injuries, illnesses, and disease. Recovery from a significant injury is a long and complex physical and psychological process that continues long after discharge from a rehabilitation facility (Galvis Arparicio et al., 2021). Successful coping requires the ability to regroup, come to terms with changes in abilities, compensate for deficits, and ultimately find a new way of living that brings satisfaction and fulfillment.

To address the holistic wellbeing of the person with an acquired physical disability the occupational therapy practitioner (OTP) needs to have an understanding of the physical, emotional and psychosocial aspects of recovery. This chapter addresses the complexity of psychosocial adaptation after acquired physical disability and the unique role of OTPs in guiding individuals with newly acquired disabilities to adjust to their new reality, set goals, develop self-efficacy by celebrating and building upon successes, and ultimately achieve a fulfilling life with a different set of skills.

Description of the Condition

The term **acquired physical disability** comprises a wide range of disabilities that can result from trauma or disease, including but not limited to spinal cord injuries (SCIs), traumatic brain injuries (TBIs), stroke, and significant musculoskeletal injuries such as limb amputation, multiple trauma, and burn injuries (Sadiki & Kibirige, 2022). All these conditions are considered severe physical conditions because in most cases they lead to varying degrees of permanent functional loss. Acquired physical disabilities differ from congenital disabilities (disabilities that occur at or around the time of birth) because they occur after a period of typical development (Burnett, 2018).

Although the circumstances surrounding the initial onset and clinical course of a chronic or progressive disease may be substantially different from the sudden nature of a traumatic injury, the onset of symptoms or rapidity of increasing disability can engender similar emotions and ultimately issues of coping and adaptation. Both a malignant brain tumor that declares itself with a grand mal seizure and a progressively deteriorating and ultimately life-limiting disease such as amyotrophic lateral sclerosis (ALS), which leads an individual to seek medical attention to explain extreme fatigue, clumsiness, or frequent falls, can be included in the category of acquired physical disabilities.

Whether the disability is acute or chronic, stable or progressive, the acquisition of a physical disability can result in common stressors, such as feelings of dependence and vulnerability, and it can force an individual to confront the possibility of their own mortality (Liebscher et al., 2022).

Psychological Implications of Physical Disability

Initial reactions to an acquired physical disability typically are characterized by a range of conflicting emotions. Shock, disbelief, anxiety, fear, anger, despair, grief, and mourning are commonly experienced early in the adjustment and recovery process (McDonald et al., 2020). Thoughts such as, "I can't believe this is happening. . . . Is what the doctors are saying really true? What does all this mean?" exemplify this experience.

An individual who sustains a life-changing injury is thrust into an unfamiliar and frightening hospital environment. The medical procedures, personnel, and onslaught of information may seem unrelenting and feel overwhelming. Often heavily medicated, the person struggles to make sense of the unfamiliar medical terms and confusing jargon being spoken by a constant stream of strangers. Pain, noise from beeping monitors, and intrusion from medical staff at all hours keep the patient from getting adequate rest. In the middle of the night, thoughts may drift to the future: "What is going to happen to me? How am I going to live like this? I don't want to be a burden to my family. Am I going to survive? Do I even want to?" Feelings of anxiety and guilt may give way to sadness, despair, and even suicidality. As one's medical condition stabilizes, the focus of care shifts to the rehabilitation process, and new worries and emotions emerge.

Managing daily life with physical problems such as paralysis, spasticity, incoordination, loss of sensation, speech disturbances, vision loss, and pain is an ongoing and demanding process requiring new learning, reacquisition, repetition, and practice of skills. Such efforts are not just a function of physical stamina, but emotional fortitude as well. It is a process that can at times be fraught with feelings of frustration, disappointment, and defeat.

Researchers have rejected a linear or stage-specific model to explain the emotional responses to disability. Instead, they recognize that responses to acquired disability evolve through time relative to the onset of disability as well as across the life span as different developmental stages and challenges are encountered. At different points of time in a person's life, previous issues may resurface, causing individuals to reexperience emotional distress. Individuals face trauma not just in the form of the injury or illness itself, but multiple traumas or losses as a consequence of the condition. Issues such as those in the following list present psychological and emotional challenges to be negotiated.

- Loss of control of basic physical functions
- Changes in ability to participate in previously valued activities
- Changes in relationships with family, friends, and/or sexual partners
- Disruption of cherished roles
- Radically altered body image
- Disruption of self-esteem
- Altered sense of meaning or purpose in life

These *episodic losses* become apparent through time as the individual moves through the rehabilitation process and later attempts to reintegrate back into family roles, participate in the community, and modify life goals (Klonoff, 2010).

Physical recovery is just part of the process for a newly disabled individual; not only does the physical self change, but so too does the psychological self. Several studies that explored the experience of living with a TBI reported that psychosocial factors such as social isolation; health problems such as pain, poor body image, intimacy, and gender role issues; low self-esteem; and cognitive problems were perceived as the most difficult aspects of living with a TBI for the study participants (Khan et al., 2016).

Similar to race, gender, or sexuality, disability is a minority identity with an associated identity development process. Research suggests that establishing a positive relationship to one's minority identity can be protective of physical and mental health (Forber-Pratt et al., 2017). For example, one study that examined disability identity among people with congenital and acquired disabilities found that individuals who had integrated their disability identity into their self-concept reported higher satisfaction with life (Bogart, 2014). Connecting with the community with disabilities and developing disability pride can help people with acquired disabilities combat disability stigma and incorporate their disability into a healthy self-concept (Bogart, 2014). Disability self-concept can include both disability identity (viewing oneself as part of the community with disabilities) and disability self-efficacy (feeling confident in one's ability to manage their disability and achieve their goals; Bogart, 2014).

Although less research exists about disability identity development than racial or sexual identity development, researchers have proposed several different models of disability identity development (Forber-Pratt et al., 2017). One recent model proposes four different statuses of disability identity development: acceptance, relationship, adoption, and engagement (Forber-Pratt & Zape, 2017). The model is framed in terms of statuses and not stages in order to indicate that the development is not linear and people can move back and forth between statuses or even occupy multiple statuses at one time. Table 16-1 provides a brief overview of the statuses. Rehabilitation providers can use this model to identify where people are in their identity development process and connect them to resources that are appropriate for their status.

Isolation

Being in the hospital—particularly for extended periods of time—can leave a person feeling physically and emotionally isolated. While in the hospital, visits and physical contact from friends and family are limited, and the patient is generally cut off from the natural environment, detached from their daily life, surrounded by strangers, and relegated to a type of confinement to the hospital room. As sleep and wake cycles are disrupted, in the absence of orienting cues, the person may even become detached from an accurate sense of the passage of time. Such sensory monotony and/or deprivation have been found to lead to disturbances of thought, cognition, and perception (Senna et al., 2021). Patients who stay in the intensive care unit (ICU) can experience fluctuating states of consciousness, fatigue, distraction, confusion, disorientation, agitation, and depression.

The sometimes dehumanizing aspects of being a patient can be emotionally isolating as well. Upon admission to the hospital, one's self-identifying roles such as "mother," "business owner," or "teacher" are stripped away and subverted to

TABLE 16-1 | Model of Disability Identity Development

Status	Description
Acceptance	The person comes to accept that they are disabled and view themselves as a person with disabilities. Disability becomes a facet of their identity.
Relationship	The person connects with other people with disabilities and forms social relationships. They begin to see themselves as part of the group or community of people with disabilities.
Adoption	The person begins to incorporate some aspects of disability culture or disability community values into their life. For example, they might try on disability humor, take adaptive equipment tips from other people with disabilities, or notice inaccessibility.
Engagement	Having integrated disability into their identity and adopted some values of disability culture, the person begins to act as a role model or leader in/for the community. For example, they might become a peer mentor, speak out about inaccessibility, blog about disability, or engage in disability activism.

Model of Disability Identity Development (Forber-Pratt and Zape, 2017)

that of the role of "patient." An individual may be generically identified via a diagnosis or medical records number; for example, the doctor who states: "I'm headed to see the hip fracture in Bed 2." One's most private moments—disrobing, using the bathroom, bathing—are now conducted in front of strangers. One's body, over which one may or may not have control, is subjected to invasive medical procedures. Patients lose the freedom to spend their time as they wish, come and go as they please, or even to wear their own clothing. This collective stripping away of identity, privacy, and decision-making power can threaten one's self-concept.

For some individuals, a sense of isolation persists long after the person is discharged from the hospital environment. Social isolation can result from activity restriction, architectural barriers that limit access to community resources and accessible transportation, and limited employment opportunities and positive social outlets, as well as the presence of social or attitudinal barriers; for example, the tendency of the public to patronize or ignore persons with disabilities. Even the person with a disability may harbor attitudinal barriers to participation, such as feeling helpless to contribute equally in community-based group activities. Long-term social isolation can result in poor life satisfaction and low self-esteem, and in some people lead to depression and even suicidality (Consortium for Spinal Cord Medicine, 2021).

It is widely held that society at large maintains a range of prejudicial assumptions about people with disabilities, the net effect of which can increase a sense of social isolation in individuals with a disability. Even the perception of social stigma, whether accurate or not, can cause individuals with disabilities to restrict their activity and social participation, leading to an overall poorer psychosocial adjustment. Being an active and engaged community member and learning not to personalize negative biases is considered an adaptive approach for individuals with disabilities (Hitzig et al., 2021). An important role of OTPs is to reinforce and promote a person's personal strengths, individual identity, innate potential, and communication and advocacy skills as they assist with the person's functional reengagement with valued occupations. See Chapter 13: Communication and Social Skills, Chapter 27: Mental Health Stigma and Sanism, and Chapter 49: Connectedness and Belonging. 🤝

Pain

As part of the initial and ongoing occupational therapy evaluation and treatment process, OTPs need to identify the patient's experience of pain and understand how it affects participation in occupation and rehabilitation efforts. Individuals living with disabilities are subject to pain from a variety of sources. Medical procedures such as blood draws and injections are painful and commonplace for someone whose physical condition requires frequent use of the health-care system. Conditions such as spasticity or hypertrophic scarring can require uncomfortable therapy techniques such as range of motion exercises for tight muscles or scar massage on damaged skin.

Through time, the altered movement patterns associated with certain diagnoses may cause mechanical or overuse pain; for example, rotator cuff tears that result from years of using the upper extremities to propel a manual wheelchair. Severe headaches, which are common after TBI, or the burning and shooting (dysesthetic) nerve pain sometimes associated with SCI can be sources of ongoing vexation that prevent an affected individual from being able to fully engage in their meaningful occupations. Complications of weakness or paralysis, such as the development of pressure sores or joint contractures, can themselves not only be extremely painful, but can worsen an individual's disability and extend recovery time.

Studies have shown that ongoing pain has deleterious effects on health, including poor quality sleep, elevated levels of anxiety and depression, and diminished quality of life (Carlozzi et al., 2022). Ongoing pain that negatively affects psychosocial adaptation to disability is problematic for other reasons. The risk for abuse of narcotics or other medications with abuse potential (e.g., diazepam prescribed for spasticity) is high for people with disabilities, as is the potential to "self-medicate" with alcohol (Yuying et al., 2022). The topic of pain is explored in greater detail in Chapter 15: Pain. 🤝

Research has demonstrated that pain can interfere with an individual's emotional adjustment to injury. The sensory loss commonly associated with SCI does not prevent the experience of pain, and chronic pain is a common problem among people with SCI that rates almost as highly as loss of function in terms of impact on quality of life (Ullrich et al., 2013). Severity of pain after SCI was shown to be associated with emotional and cognitive factors more so than physical variables, such as the level of injury, completeness of injury, and the type of surgery for injury.

Catastrophizing or making unrealistic and excessive negative self-statements in response to pain (e.g., "This is unbearable. . . . I cannot function . . .") is related to poorer outcomes including greater pain intensity, greater psychological distress, decreased functional independence, depression, and psychosocial dysfunction (Furrer et al., 2019). Individuals who perceived their injuries as injustices were angrier and less accepting of their disabilities. Such individuals, as well as those who negatively appraised their pain, reported greater pain severity, whereas those who were more accepting of their situation reported lower levels of pain severity (Adams et al., 2019). Pain and feeling helpless or out of control of one's life before discharge from rehabilitation predicted depression in adults with SCI 2 years after injury (Sachdeva et al., 2018).

OTPs can promote the development of self-efficacy and coping skills in patients by encouraging task persistence, distraction, and positive self-talk, which will improve functional outcomes. Occupational therapy interventions designed to increase a person's ability to participate in rewarding occupations, social relationships, physical activity, and functional independence may represent a positive approach to mediating emotional distress and promoting positive adaptation to acquired physical disability.

Body Image

People with acquired physical disability may experience grief related to physical changes and body image concerns, such as loss of a body part, paralysis, spasticity, incoordination, or atrophy. Individuals experiencing a newly acquired disability may also need to integrate unfamiliar and/or unwanted attributes such as scars, contractures, catheters, or feeding tubes into their body schema. Such losses or changes to one's body may symbolize vulnerability or deterioration of one's physical condition, which may be further distressing. Loss of control and mastery over one's physical body can constitute a threat to one's very sense of self and lead a person with a disability to feel as though their place in the world is jeopardized.

Furthermore, for some, a change in physical appearance is akin to a change in identity. *Who am I if I don't even recognize myself in the mirror?* What may seem on the surface to be a person's attempt to come to terms with a perceived loss of attractiveness may actually be an emotional task that runs much deeper. Perhaps a person equates a loss of good looks to a loss of desirability, which can then translate into concerns regarding their acceptability as a partner.

One of the major tasks of psychological adaptation to disability is for individuals to achieve an acceptance of their disability and reintegrate the loss of one's former body image and its effects into a new state of being (De Martino et al., 2021). This requires an individual to make a series of adjustments in their value system with regard to the importance of physical attributes relative to other values. For example, an individual with SCI would come to appreciate personal qualities in themselves other than their physical status (perhaps kindness, creativity, or sense of humor), thus limiting the impact of the disability on other aspects of the self. This shift of focus to one's intrinsic value—rather than one's physical assets or value based on comparisons with others—is necessary for positive adjustment in terms of body image and in other arenas as well (Vázquez-Fariñas & Rodriguez-Martin, 2021).

Relational Intimacy and Gender Role Issues

Sexuality is a vital part of the human experience that is important for self-esteem, self-concept, and quality of life. The expression of sexuality and sensuality is a sign of self-confidence, self-validation, and one's sense of being lovable that reflects a person's emotions, beliefs, values, and hopes for the future (McGrath et al., 2021). The field of occupational therapy recognizes that individuals do not lose their needs and desires for sexual expressiveness and intimacy following the onset of disability (American Occupational Therapy Association [AOTA], 2020: Soler et al., 2018).

Central to one's sexuality is the ability to interact comfortably with others and engage in social relationships and activities that support one's gender identity and allow for expression of gender roles. A person's gender is one of the main ways a person defines their identities; organizes their daily activities, as well as academic, vocational, and leisure pursuits; and informs the way one participates in family, social, and intimate relationships (Mollayeva et al., 2021).

The acquisition of a disability can disrupt a person's ability to perform behaviors that they associated with their gender identity before acquiring a disability (Hanafy et al., 2022). For example, physical gestures (such as opening a door, holding hands, and engaging in intercourse) may be difficult for some to perform after acquiring a physical disability, and changes in ability to perform such tasks may lead the individual to question themselves as a sexual being (McGrath et al., 2019). Therefore, healing the dissonance between preinjury and present life satisfaction is a challenging but necessary process. Redefining self-concept, relinquishing long-held life goals in order to replace them with more realistic but equally meaningful ones, and reconstructing a positive sense of self that accommodates injury-related changes are important aspects of the healing process (Gelech et al., 2019).

Assistance in regaining a sense of sexual identity for a person who becomes disabled as an adult may be a critical component of rehabilitation. In fact, sexual relationships as a measure of supportive interpersonal relationships are positively correlated with good psychosocial adjustment to disability (Barrett et al., 2023). If a health-care practitioner does not raise the issue of sexuality, individuals with disabilities may feel that an essential element of their identity is being ignored. This perceived lack of acceptance may cause a person with a disability to feel as though they are not being regarded as a whole person (Barrett et al., 2023).

Adaptive equipment, environmental modifications, and sexual activity adaptations can help a person engage in sexual activity after changes to their physical abilities. OTPs can play a role in helping a person modify their sexual practices, identify helpful adaptive equipment, or point individuals to educational resources about sex and disability.

Cognition

The process of overcoming many of the physical challenges posed by a disability requires intensive occupational therapy to help the person to learn new information; master compensatory techniques for functional mobility, activities of daily living (ADLs), and community reintegration; and adapt to a new lifestyle. In addition, individuals who successfully adapt to life with a disability must become experts in managing their condition or disease. Successful integration of the vast amount of information one must learn about their disability requires sufficient attention, concentration, memory, problem-solving, abstract reasoning, new learning, and higher-level cognitive skills.

Several diagnoses besides brain injury can cause subtle cognitive dysfunction such as difficulty with attention and concentration and impaired short-term memory and judgment, all of which can affect one's ability to retain, comprehend, and integrate new information. For example, approximately up to 64% of individuals with SCI are now believed to have varying degrees and patterns of cognitive impairment (Sandalic et al., 2022). The causes of the cognitive impairment after SCI may be a mild TBI caused by the same blow to the head and neck that damaged the spinal cord, secondary trauma such as respiratory distress resulting in anoxia, brain damage resulting from a premorbid history of substance abuse, effects of medications, or sleep-disordered breathing that causes hypoxia.

Individuals with depression may exhibit cognitive disturbances in the areas of attention and concentration, speed of information processing, short-term memory, motivation, decision-making, and problem-solving ability (Chakrabarty et al., 2016). Additionally, smoke inhalation in conjunction with a burn injury can cause hypoxic brain injury. As described earlier, the experience of hospitalization in and of itself—including the effects of isolation, pain, and sedating medications—can cause disorientation, confusion, fatigue, and, in extreme cases, delirium, all of which negatively affect cognitive performance. Therefore, regardless of diagnosis, assessment of cognitive abilities is vital to a comprehensive rehabilitation program after acquiring a physical disability. Cognition is discussed in greater detail in Chapter 7: Cognition and Chapter 8: Cognitive Beliefs.

Psychiatric Conditions Associated With Physical Disability

Common psychiatric conditions associated with physical disability include depression and anxiety, posttraumatic stress disorder (PTSD), substance abuse, and suicidal ideation.

Depression and Anxiety

Intense circumstances that expose people to chronic stress for a prolonged period of time increase vulnerability to anxiety and depression. A grieving process should be expected for individuals with a newly acquired disability, and OTPs should be prepared to allow individuals to express their grief. However, individuals with disabilities have a substantially higher risk of experiencing mood disorders (beyond the normal process of grieving and sadness in response to loss) compared with the general population (Wan et al., 2020). Specifically, the loss of role identity, decreased confidence in one's ability to manage effects of disability, declining health status, increased pain, diminished social support system, reduced access to rewarding activities, and unsafe alcohol use are all risk factors for depression in individuals with chronic health conditions (Khan et al., 2016).

For some, depressed mood may peak shortly after diagnosis, whereas for others it may not emerge until the passage of time and the accumulation of many frustrating experiences stemming from physical limitations and/or from encountering social prejudices.

Anxiety may manifest differently whether the disability is chronic or traumatic in nature. When a diagnosis of a chronic illness is involved, anxiety may be future-oriented, taking the form of fear of deteriorating health, fear of an uncertain future, or even fear of death. In contrast, anxiety as a reaction to a traumatic injury may be more past-oriented, and appear as panic regarding the magnitude of the losses and associated grief regarding lost physical or cognitive abilities (Braaf et al., 2019).

When mood disturbance after a serious injury is considered by health-care professionals to be understandable or "normal," it might not be addressed, in which case high levels of negative mood can remain elevated or worsen in the absence of treatment and support (Titman et al., 2019). The presence of negative mood states after the onset of physical disability is associated with additional physical risks and functional implications. For example, in individuals with SCIs, depression increases the risk of undesirable outcomes such as longer hospital stays, fewer improvements during rehabilitation leading to decreased independence in self-care, increased occurrence of preventable medical complications such as pressure sores and urinary tract infections (UTIs, which may be caused by an individual with depression's self-neglect), more time spent in bed, and fewer days spent outside the hospital unit (McDonald et al., 2020).

Even community-dwelling individuals with SCI and high levels of depressive behavior spend more days in bed, have fewer days out of their home, experience more difficulties with transportation, use more paid attendants, and incur increased overall medical expenses (Barclay et al., 2018). The magnifying effect of depression on physical complications has also been noted for other chronic conditions such as type 2 diabetes, multiple sclerosis, and TBI (Leung et al., 2021). When OTPs treat the whole person, they consider emotional as well as physical issues and provide interventions to address emotional concerns. In addition, OTPs who work with individuals with physical illness or acquired disabilities can assist the individual to access additional resources or make appropriate referrals to adjunct therapies (such as psychiatrists, psychologists, social workers, etc.) as needed.

Anxiety and depression may be common reactions to acquired disabilities, but they are not inevitable consequences. Although individuals who sustain traumatic injuries such as TBI and SCI are presented with a traumatic challenge to their physical, psychological, and social well-being, the majority of people living with serious disabilities make a positive psychological adjustment and report a positive quality of life (McDonald et al., 2020). Depression and anxiety are discussed in greater detail in Chapter 18: Anxiety Disorders and Chapter 20: Mood Disorders.

Posttraumatic Stress Disorder

The abrupt and unplanned onset of morbidity and resulting dependence is often a traumatic experience for the individual. The mechanism of injury itself can be a shocking and stressful event, as the majority of physical injuries result from motor vehicle accidents, falls, sports injuries, work-related accidents, interpersonal violence, and disasters (James et al., 2019). The distressing quality of a life-threatening event places those involved at risk for developing PTSD. The characteristic features of PTSD include flashbacks (intrusive memories of the original accident), recurrent nightmares, emotional numbing, persistent symptoms of hyperarousal (increased sympathetic nervous system activity leading to the person being irritable, easily startled, and hypervigilant), and avoidance of stimuli associated with the original trauma (American Psychiatric Association, 2022).

Survivors of physical trauma that leads to disability may experience some of these symptoms. One meta-analysis demonstrated that 23.61% of people with SCI may develop PTSD symptoms, underscoring the need for increased emphasis on treating the psychological aspects of traumatic SCI (Yousefifard et al., 2022). Lodha and colleagues (2020) cited research demonstrating more than 90% of burn victims were found to experience some symptoms of acute stress disorder within the first week of the injury and more than 45% were found to develop signs of chronic stress that could be categorized as PTSD after 1 year. PTSD is discussed in greater detail in Chapter 25: Trauma- and Stressor-Related Disorders. 🤝

Substance Abuse

The issue of substance abuse, as it relates to physical disability, is complex and requires some understanding of premorbid patterns of substance use, how substance use relates to risk-taking behavior and the mechanism of injury, and the effects of postinjury substance use and abuse on rehabilitation and recovery.

It is widely observed that the mechanisms of catastrophic injuries such as SCI and TBI often involve risk-taking behaviors and that the persons most at risk for these injuries are overwhelmingly young males (Ding et al., 2022; National Spinal Cord Injury Statistical Center, 2022). Alcohol and substance use play a significant role in the risk-taking behavior associated with traumatic accidents, including the sorts that commonly account for the majority of brain and spinal cord trauma (Eldridge et al., 2019). Furthermore, the presence of measurable alcohol in the bloodstream at the time of injury is associated with greater severity of both TBI and SCI (El-Menyar et al., 2019).

Preinjury substance abuse is higher in individuals who sustain SCI and TBI as compared with the general population, with more than half of patients admitted for rehabilitation following TBI meeting the diagnostic criteria for alcohol use disorder (AUD; Weil et al., 2018) and up to 80% of adult SCI patients admitted for SCI at one of three trauma centers in the Midwest having used one or more substances (including alcohol, opioids, marijuana, methamphetamines, benzodiazepines, or cocaine) immediately before SCI onset (Eldridge et al., 2019). Such premorbid patterns of substance abuse can worsen after the injury. Vulnerable individuals may turn to drugs or alcohol in an attempt to self-medicate injury-related emotional distress or help them deal with unpleasant emotions such as loss, grief, anger, boredom, or despair.

Other factors that may contribute to an increased risk of abusing substances after acquiring a physical disability include excess unproductive time in one's daily schedule, substance use motivated by a desire for peer acceptance, and use of alcohol representing a return to one's typical preinjury recreational activity (Eldridge et al., 2019).

Substance abuse interferes with rehabilitation and recovery in several ways. Issues related to the personality characteristics associated with substance use such as impaired reasoning, poor impulse control, troubled interpersonal relationships, resistance to authority, and impoverished coping and self-management skills can interfere with an individual's ability to sustain motivation related to rehabilitation efforts (Papamalis, 2020). Substance use has also been shown to increase the incidence of medical complications following injury (Weil et al., 2018). Poor self-care skills and self-neglect may result in an increased incidence of pressure sores, UTIs, and autonomic dysreflexia in persons with SCIs.

Substance use may also interfere with medications prescribed to prevent seizures, control blood pressure, and improve pain and mood postinjury. Substance abuse can also negatively affect sleep, medication compliance, nutritional intake, development of functional skills, and reintegration into family, work, and community roles. Of particular concern is opioid abuse. Opioids are often prescribed for long-term pain control despite recent evidence that opioids appear to have limited benefit for the treatment of chronic pain (Hayes et al., 2018). Prescription opioid use can lead to addiction and unintentional overdose. Overall, substance abuse is correlated with longer lengths of stay, poorer rehabilitation outcomes, decreased life satisfaction, depression, anger, anxiety, and increased risk for reinjury (Wettervik et al., 2021). This topic is discussed in greater detail in Chapter 24: Substance-Related and Addictive Disorders. 🤝

Suicidal Ideation

Physical illness is considered a major risk factor for suicide. Related issues such as chronic stress, dependency, loneliness, grief regarding losses, and setbacks in recovery can lead to feelings of helplessness and hopelessness that lead some people with disabilities to contemplate ending their lives (Stickley et al., 2020). Suggested risk factors for suicide after physical disability include a premorbid history of psychiatric illness that may or may not include past suicide attempts (indeed, some injuries are actually incurred because of suicide attempts) either before injury or during hospitalization, pre- or postmorbid substance abuse, and lack of social support and/or family dysfunction (Lu et al., 2020). Box 16-1 lists risk factors for suicide in the population with disabilities.

Suicide in the population with disabilities can take the form of overt action, self-neglect, or refusal of required care

---

BOX 16-1 ■ Risk Factors for Suicide in the Population With Disabilities

- Male gender
- Depression
- Anger and aggression
- Alcohol and other drug use throughout hospitalization
- Premorbid psychiatric illness
- Prior suicide attempts
- Family disintegration
- Chronic pain
- Multiple medical problems and frequent hospitalizations
- Social isolation

(Choi et al., 2020). Suicide by self-neglect occurs when a person with a disability refuses necessary medical care and stops attending to skin care, hydration, nutrition, and bowel and bladder function (Bombardier et al., 2021). This lack of required care leads to an increase in health problems such as UTIs and other infections, multiple pressure sores, and autonomic dysreflexia, among others, which place the person at increased risk of death from conditions such as sepsis, pneumonia, and stroke. It is important that OTPs take suicidality seriously among persons with acquired disabilities and offer appropriate mental health and suicide prevention interventions. For more about suicide among people with disabilities and suicide in the media, see the Mental Health in Culture and Society feature.

Mental Health in Culture and Society

Aster Harrison

Suicide and Ableism

Suicidality among people with disabilities can sometimes go unnoticed or unquestioned because of ableism. Popular books and movies, such as *Me Before You* and *Million Dollar Baby,* portray suicide of people with acquired disabilities in a romanticized fashion that makes it seem natural and honorable that someone would choose to die rather than to live as disabled. Disability activists critique these ableist portrayals that represent characters as "better dead than disabled" (e.g., Evans, 2016). Disability activists speak out about these films, including protesting at showings of *Me Before You* in 2016 (Quinn, 2016).

Ableist ideas about disability and suicide permeate into the real world and can influence real people into feeling their whole life will be a tragedy when they are disabled. Unfortunately, people with disabilities who want to kill themselves are sometimes provided with help completing their suicides, rather than adequate mental health care and community support to help them see their lives are still worth living.

For example, in 2016, a Black, queer teenager with disabilities, Jerika Bolen, became suicidal. Instead of providing her with mental health care, pain management, and disability community support, her parents threw her a "last dance" presuicide prom and provided her with the means to end her own life. Her condition was not terminal—many people with her disability live well into their 60s. Tragically, she died by suicide with the support of her parents and medical providers at age 14. The media portrayed Jerika's suicide as "inspirational" and "brave" instead of a tragedy as the media tends to portray nondisabled teens' suicides. Disability activists asked, "What might have happened if Jerika's request for a 'last dance' had been met with overwhelming public and media encouragement to live instead of a massive thumb on the scale in support of her death?" (Coleman & Lucas, 2017, para. 12).

It is crucial that people with disabilities who are suicidal are provided with adequate mental and physical health care, including suicide prevention services. For more on suicide, see Chapter 44: Addressing Suicide Across the Continuum 🤝

Effects of Physical Disability on the Family

OTPs need to recognize that the effects of an acquired disability present challenges not only to the person but to their entire family system, as family roles and relationships are drastically altered. Family members undergo significant distress as they experience the trauma of their loved one's unexpected injury or diagnosis and are often unprepared for the emotional and mental demands that accompany learning about their loved one's medical condition. They may cope with multiple losses and changes in family roles as they learn to respond to changes that might result in the physical and/or emotional dependence of their family member.

Some family members may need to adjust to the role of caregiver for their newly disabled family member. Other sources of stress for family members may include role overload, financial strain (related to both loss of income and cost of care), social isolation, an ongoing sense of increased responsibility and upheaval, and decreased quality of life (Klonoff, 2014; Lee et al., 2022).

Common family reactions to a member's disability are depression, anxiety, frustration, guilt, resentment, and a sense of living in perpetual crisis. Family members, particularly those who serve as primary caregivers, may feel isolated or even trapped by the current circumstances (Klonoff, 2010). Along with the individual with a disability, family members experience episodic loss reactions or grief in response to changes in the person's abilities or further realization of limitations. As an example, the family of an elementary school student who sustains a brain injury learns that, because of the severity of his deficits, he will not be able to handle the demands of college life or live independently as an adult, and thus grief reactions are recatalyzed. Over time, some family members themselves report increased chronic health problems and psychosomatic disorders secondary to stress (Eberhard et al., 2019).

On the other hand, many caregivers receive benefits from the act of helping another during times of need. Caregiver burden is reduced when there are reciprocal exchanges, when the relationship is more equitable, and when the caregiver perceives the relationship as satisfying (Hawken et al., 2018).

Marriage and Parenting

Increased physical, emotional, and/or financial dependence on others requires adjustment of relationships. Role changes within the family unit constitute one of the biggest stressors for family members as they are forced to reorganize family routines and redistribute responsibilities in order to assume the long-term role of caregivers. Wives and mothers most often experience the increased responsibilities that come with being the primary caregiver of the disabled family member. This is as opposed to husbands or fathers, who tend to experience more continuity in role performance (January et al., 2019; Wilson et al., 2022).

A spouse or partner serving as caregiver often faces unique challenges and obstacles as compared with a parent serving as caregiver. A spouse or partner who assumes the role of primary caregiver for their mate subsequent to an acquired disability must also adapt to other significant and demanding long-term role changes while continuing to meet the demands of daily family life. In addition to the reallocation of roles or changes in source of income, other challenges may include the ongoing demands of raising children and running a household. Klonoff (2010) suggests that spouses and partners must also manage intangible stressors such as living with a person who is likely to be physically, cognitively, or emotionally very different than they were before the disability, the loss of a reciprocal partnership, and/or the pressure from society not to openly grieve losses or divorce the injured partner.

Siblings and children of a disabled family member also may experience challenging emotional effects of family disruption, including feeling invisible, feeling responsible, having to parent themselves, or becoming secondary caregivers. Therefore, siblings or children may exhibit clinically significant signs of distress such as reports of conflict or family dysfunction or increased anxiety and depression (Haukeland et al., 2021).

Research suggests that family members' adjustment to disability is affected more by the injured person's behavioral, personality, and emotional characteristics than by the severity of physical injury or changes in physical functioning (Jeyathevan et al., 2020). When the disabled family member demonstrates improved control of their emotions, greater self-reliance, enhanced problem-solving abilities, and general optimism, family members tend to report better coping and greater well-being and life satisfaction (Jeyathevan et al., 2020; Klonoff, 2010).

Compassion Fatigue

Compassion fatigue, also known as caregiver burnout, is characterized by a state of physical, emotional, and mental exhaustion in response to the demands of caring for a dependent family member (Klonoff, 2014). Caregivers who are "burned out" may experience fatigue, stress, anxiety, or irritability. These symptoms may be accompanied by a change in attitude or motivation toward providing care—from positive and invested to negative and apathetic. Compassion fatigue intensifies when caregivers do not get respite from the day-to-day physical and emotional demands of caring for a dependent family member.

The lack of respite care can be caused by a lack of resources (e.g., no access to a skilled caregiver, or no money to pay for respite care); the caregiver trying to do too much and not wanting to delegate care; or even a caregiver feeling guilty if they spend time on themself rather than on the family member in need of care. Other sources of caregiver stress include pre- and postinjury factors (such as socioeconomic status and resources) as well as level of vigilance by caregiver (related to the loved one's dependency needs), level of conflict, and loss of sense of self of the caregiver (Klonoff, 2010). If prolonged, such feelings of stress and burnout can lead to depression.

Family members, friends, and others close to the individual are essential to the healing process for a loved one and a valuable resource in recovery. Indeed, rehabilitation outcomes are closely associated with family outcomes (McLeod & Davis, 2023). It is the family's pragmatic adjustment, division of labor, emotional support, and functional assistance that will ultimately empower and enable a person's reacquisition of social roles within the family system and beyond (Klonoff,

2010). Changes in family relationships must be negotiated by all involved in order to establish a new balance.

The challenge for the newly disabled person is to acquire productive and meaningful ways to work, parent, and share responsibilities with their loved ones. The key to sustaining the ability to support and care for a family member with a disability's physical and emotional needs in the long term lies in caregivers addressing their own physical and emotional well-being. OTPs can play an integral role in assisting family members to learn to consider and prioritize their own needs, access available supports, and strive for balance as they endeavor to meet the demands of caring for a loved one. This topic is discussed in greater detail in Chapter 29: Families.

Impact on Occupational Performance

> Occupations are key not just to being a person, but to being a *particular* person, and thus creating and maintaining an identity. Occupations come together within the contexts of relationships with others to provide us with a sense of purpose and structure in our day-to-day activities, as well as over time. When we build our identities through occupations, we provide ourselves with the contexts necessary for creating meaningful lives, and life meaning helps us to be well. (Christiansen, 1999, p. 548)

A key theoretical concept in occupational therapy is that people are what they do; that is, the daily occupations they choose to engage in say something about who they are and how they see themselves. People choose activities that help them fulfill their chosen roles, give them a sense of achievement, connect them with their past, and equip them for their future. But what happens when the ability to engage in daily occupations is changed by illness or injury? In posing a challenge to one's independence in ADLs, the social roles they occupy, the way the individual relates to others, and the person's values, beliefs, and goals for the future, a disability can effect changes to an individual's identity and self-concept.

Role Changes

When people can no longer carry out the tasks they deem essential and valuable to the roles they have chosen to pursue at various stages in their lives, they face having to relinquish those roles and, in so doing, risk relinquishing certain aspects of their identity. A parent may wonder, "If I am no longer able to make my children dinner or give them a bath, what does that say about my role as a parent?" A spouse may feel, "If I cannot return to my job, how can I be a provider for my family and a contributor to my community?"

An acquired physical disability can adversely affect a person's role function in ways that range from minor changes to major upheaval, or even extinction of major life roles. Examples include a worker who loses their job, a spouse who gets divorced, and a parent who can no longer physically care for their children. Such disruption in cherished roles forces one to rethink and ultimately reintegrate constructs such as role identity, family dynamics, and sense of self-worth.

The Past, Present, and Future Selves

Many individuals with acquired disabilities find themselves facing new lives that seem to be missing something that was meaningful to them before the onset of their disability. Loss

The Lived Experience

Pat McBride

For more than 35 years of my life I was a commercial fisherman in Alaska. I started fishing in my early 20's and over time worked my way up to captain and owner of a 100-foot vessel that fished year-round in all the weather and dangerous conditions that the Bering Sea could throw at me and my crew. Commercial fishing is a very high risk occupation that kept me away from home for many months at a time. Living in Alaska means choosing a rugged lifestyle that requires a lot of hard work. My wife and I overcame many challenges to raise our son and build a full life in this beautiful and remote landscape. After so many years of effort and sacrifice, we were ready to enjoy a comfortable retirement.

In February 2011, my wife and I took a trip to visit family in Virginia. While there, we were involved in a motor vehicle accident in which our car rolled over three times and came to rest at the bottom of an embankment. The fact that we were both wearing seatbelts saved our lives. My wife got out of her side of the car and came over to open my door when I realized I could not move my legs. EMTs took her to a hospital via ambulance and a helicopter was called for me. My wife was fortunately only badly bruised, but I soon learned that when the roof of the car caved in on top of me, it had crushed my C-4 and C-5 vertebrae. The doctors diagnosed me with a complete SCI and told me I would never move my limbs again.

I spent the next 3 months in the ICU on a ventilator. I had a feeding tube in my nose, was unable to move or feel anything below my shoulders, and had no bowel, bladder, or sexual function. I became very depressed. I grappled with feelings of not wanting to live this way and felt ready to be with the Lord. The doctors spoke with my wife and family about pulling the plug. Their answer was an emphatic "No." Luckily my wife's twin sister lived close enough to the hospital that they were able to be at my bedside daily. As time went on, I experienced blood clots in my lungs, pneumonia, and breathing difficulties. Still on the ventilator and unable to talk, my depression deepened. When a person suffers a near death injury it usually brings one much closer to a higher power. Without our faith I don't think my wife and I could have survived this whole ordeal.

Since my injury, I have learned that some aspects of having a disability are relative. For instance, I never thought that I would desire to be a paraplegic instead of a quadriplegic. My mindset at the moment is to work hard toward improvement and lessening the burden on my wife and family. I am looking forward to teaching my grandsons many skills that I have developed over the years.

It takes a very knowledgeable person to understand how to care for all the complications of someone with a high-level SCI.

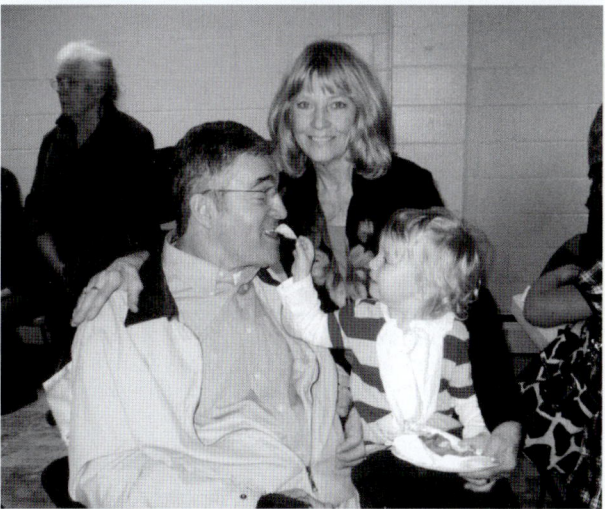

The spouses are often the caregivers, and in many ways they end up living the same life as their injured mate. Often other family members want to give the spouse a break but do not have the know-how or skills to stand in and provide care in order to give the spouse a night off. When you and your spouse take your wedding vows, you say "until death do us part." That takes on new meaning at a time like this when I realize that my wife is now giving her entire life to care for me. It is a very humbling experience. One of the things that has made our marriage more difficult has been living with each other 24-7. Many people have told us we should hire a caregiver because spending some time apart leads to a healthier relationship. That all depends on your financial ability to hire other people.

According to the National Spinal Cord Injury Statistical Center (2022), the average costs associated with an injury such as mine (C4 tetraplegia) is just over $1.1 million the first year, and an average of $202,032 with each subsequent year. A power wheelchair, for example, can cost between $20,000 and $80,000 depending on the severity of the user's injury and the features required. Much of these costs—like attendant care and modifying one's home to be wheelchair accessible—are out of pocket and not covered by insurance. The financial burden, emotional strain, and practical reality of living with a disability can be overwhelming.

I have always been a person that liked the idea of beating the odds; this in itself motivates me to prove that I can rise above this injury and help to motivate other people who have no hope. In the short term I live my life day-to-day. Knowing that I am working hard each day to improve my situation helps me deal with the unforgiving circumstances that go along with this injury.

---

of self encompasses diminished self-knowledge because of cognitive impairments, recognition of postinjury impediments relative to preinjury skills, potential stigmatization by others, and loss of potential opportunities for the "future self." This leads one to grieve their current circumstances and worry about future losses of roles. This incongruity between the preinjury self and the postinjury, unfamiliar, altered self can cause feelings of stress, anxiety, and depression, which threaten psychological well-being (Banerjee et al., 2021). Therefore, an important psychological task of the recovery process is to adequately mourn the past self, learn to cope with the challenges confronting the current self, and develop a new aspired-to future self that is fulfilling and attainable given the changes in one's abilities.

BOX 16-2 ■ Stephanie Nielson—Burn Survivor

In 2008, Stephanie Nielson was a happily married 27-year-old mother of four young children with many hobbies and interests. She wrote a popular blog about motherhood; worked part time as a yoga instructor; enjoyed photography, hiking, and cooking; and was an active member of her church. To celebrate her husband's birthday that year, Stephanie bought him flight lessons, and on August 16 they embarked on a short training flight with his instructor. Shortly after takeoff the plane crashed. Stephanie's husband was injured, the flight instructor was killed, and Stephanie was severely burned over 83% of her body. She was air-evacuated to a burn center and for the next 3 months was kept in a medically induced coma while the medical team fought to keep her alive.

Ultimately Stephanie spent 6 months in the hospital, endured countless skin grafts and surgical procedures, and participated in hundreds of hours of occupational and physical therapy as she struggled to regain her mobility and functional skills. Along the way, Stephanie experienced intense pain, weakness, debilitating deconditioning, and contractures that significantly limited her range of motion. In addition, she had to deal with the emotional turmoil of being severely disfigured. It took her 5 weeks after waking from her coma to finally look at her reflection in a small hand mirror. As she feared, her face was completely transformed. She no longer had eyebrows, or her trademark freckles, or even the full red lips to which she used to love applying lipstick.

"I did it slowly, started with my lips, and went up to my head, and just sort of kind of took it all in piece by, piece by piece," she said. "It was hard, it was so hard . . . but I saw my eyes, and I had eyes, and my eyelashes were there. And so I, I still felt like, you know, I, I was there."

However, for Stephanie, the worst aspect of her circumstance was being separated from her children for many months. The most important part of her recovery consisted of the hard work she undertook to reclaim her role as a mother once she was discharged from the hospital.

As Stephanie resumed writing her blog, she shared her recovery with a readership that, because of the media coverage of her injury, had grown into the millions. She shared stories of what it was like to return home, reintegrate into her family and community, attempt to resume engagement in cherished occupations, and deal with the physical and emotional aftermath of such a life-changing injury.

At the time of the accident, Stephanie's children ranged in age from 6 years to 18 months. While she was in the hospital they were cared for by Stephanie's sisters. When her children were finally allowed to visit her in the hospital, the reunion was bittersweet.

The first to walk into the hospital room was Jane, her younger daughter. The girl was speechless when she saw her mother. "I just will never forget her look that she gave me. . . . And then she put her head down. She wouldn't look at me for the rest of the time. I wanted to die," Stephanie remembered. There was more heartbreak to come. Her youngest child—Nicholas, who was just 18 months old at the time of the crash—didn't know her. Stephanie's sister, Lucy, had been caring for Nicholas and he now cried for her and called her "Mom."

"I was like, 'That's me! You know, but I can't touch you, because my body hurts,'" she remembered. "It was awful."

Stephanie said the rejection by her own children and the limitations imposed by her injuries were almost too much to bear. She said she couldn't do all those little things that mattered so much.

"Just combing my daughter's hair, putting a little bow in her hair, or building blocks with my son, just simple things that mothers take for granted every single day. . . . And I couldn't do it," she said. "So once those little things were taken away, it felt like my life was gone" (ABC News, 2011).

In occupational therapy, an essential goal of rehabilitation and recovery is successful identity reconstruction—putting the pieces of one's self back together in a way that makes sense to the individual, in the context of their life, so as to be satisfying and achieve wholeness. It involves making peace between the self that was, the self that is, and the self one hopes to become. This may involve shifting one's way of thinking about one's life circumstances from a "loss perspective" to an "assets perspective," which reflects a balance of realism and optimism (Klonoff, 2010).

If engagement in certain cherished occupations is no longer possible because of physical or cognitive disability, the person must embark on the process of finding a new valued self. They will need to salvage and strengthen as broad an array of (physical, cognitive, and emotional) skills as possible via their efforts at rehabilitation, and use them to explore and master new occupations and roles (Box 16-2).

Factors Related to Positive Adaptation

Why do some people who acquire a physical disability react with anger or denial, become depressed, withdraw from social and family life, become despondent, and even feel suicidal, whereas others faced with a similar condition find a renewed purpose in life, explore new occupations, acquire new roles, seek ways to engage with and serve their communities, become able to talk about ways their lives have changed for the positive after disability, and thrive despite their circumstances?

Researchers have studied stress and coping in persons who have sustained TBI, SCI, myocardial infarction amputations, and other orthopedic injuries, and have reported that coping style appears to be associated with premorbid personality and social factors and does not appear to be significantly associated with injury-related factors (e.g., severity of neurological symptoms, impairment in ADLs, type of brain pathology). These findings suggest that the inherent coping strategies used had a potentially greater influence on psychological outcome than did severity of injury and degree of functional impairment (Box 16-3; Anson & Ponsford, 2006; Craig et al., 2019; Curran et al., 2000).

Coping

To gain an understanding of individual differences in responding to adversity in the form of an acquired physical disability, it is important for the OTP, individual, and family to understand the importance of an individual's coping style and resilience. Factors that affect an individual's coping strategies include their locus of control, perception of social support, ability to acquire knowledge and communicate about the disability, and generativity.

Whether an individual views their situation as stressful depends on the way the individual appraises the situation

BOX 16-3 ■ "Strong Legs"

Stephanie Nielson

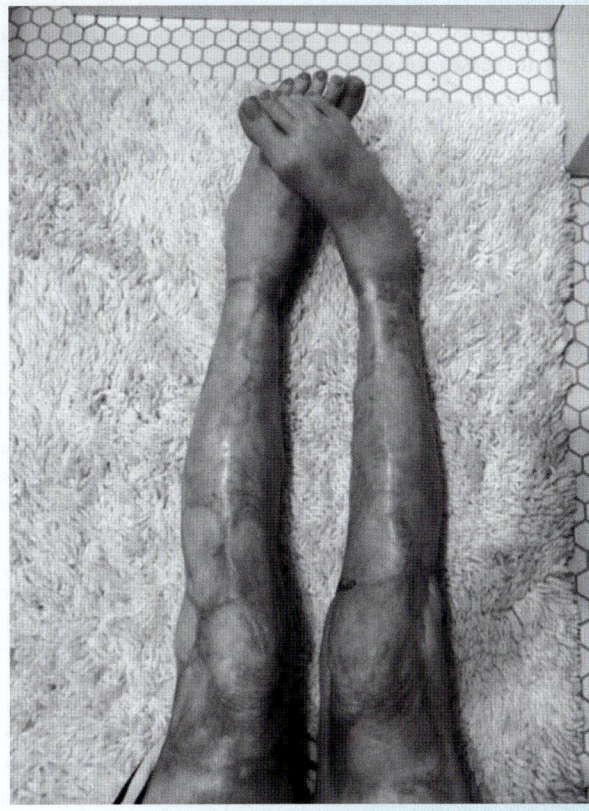

"Finding a new self or coming to terms with the only self one has ever known is reflected in the mirror others place before us." (Fine, 1991, p. 495)

Today while on my daily hike, I waved to a woman who I frequently see on the trail. She is a slower hiker, but always makes it to the top of the trail. I passed her on the way up and smiled (since both of us have earphones in). She smiled back and made her usual facial expression which showed exhaustion, but determination. Several minutes later, after I had made it to the top, I was on my way down and I passed this woman again. This time she waved her hands and gestured to me to take my earphones out. So I did and she said between breaths: "Wow! If I only had your strong legs. . . ."

I appreciated her words of kindness and encouragement probably more than she will ever know. If only she knew that just a few short years ago, I couldn't even stand up or stretch my legs without horrible pain or ripping my skin off. If only she knew the bleeding, the surgeries, and the therapy I endured. If only she knew that most of the skin that covered these babies were (sic) from other parts of my body, and some skin was grown in an incubator in Boston and surgically grafted on. If only she knew the thousands—no, millions—of tears I shed while recovering and pushing myself harder and harder to get better. If only she knew the billions of prayers I offered up to God to sustain and carry me when my legs couldn't.

These sweetheart legs of mine have been through some tough stuff, but without fail they carry me up all kinds of mountains every single day—without a single complaint (mostly). I realize they are not "attractive" or "normal," but they are MY LEGS! And they work just fine. I'd never trade these babies in. They are proof I am a survivor, and can do hard things. And I have the scars to prove it (Nielson, 2015).

PhotoVoice

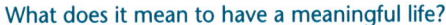

Seven years after the accident, Stephanie has successfully rebuilt a meaningful life. She's achieved independence in all her instrumental activities of daily living (IADLs) and ADLs, resumed many of her cherished occupations, and given birth to a fifth child. Stephanie has added new roles to her life: She's authored a best-selling book about her experiences, become a spokesperson for her church, and travels the country giving speeches and raising money for causes related to recovery from burn injury.

What does it mean to have a meaningful life?

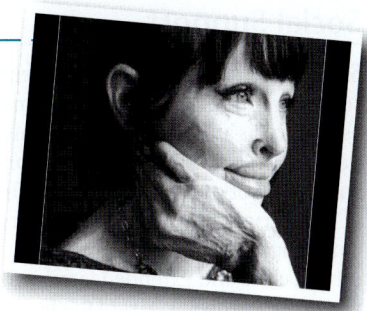

(Lazarus & Folkman, 1984; Shabany et al., 2022). When it comes to a person who is coping with an acquired physical disability, this self-appraisal is based on the person's premorbid personality, including previous successes in handling stressful life situations, problem-solving mentality, locus of control, cultural background, and prior life experience with persons with disabilities (Rogowska et al., 2020). Environmental factors such as perceived level of support, financial status, and opportunities for community and career participation are also integral. The topic of coping is explored in greater detail in Chapter 10: Coping and Resilience. 🤝

Locus of Control

The perception that one has a degree of control regarding a certain life situation (**internal locus of control**) and an active, flexible, problem-focused form of cognitive and behavioral coping style is thought to have a positive impact on rehabilitation outcome, self-care, caregiver coping, psychosocial and emotional adaptation, and self-esteem (Rogowska et al., 2020). **Problem-focused coping** leads individuals to deal directly with a challenging situation either by obtaining more information, acquiring new skills to manage the situation, or by altering the situation or environment (Schoenmakers et al., 2015).

Emotion-focused coping (i.e., managing the feelings provoked by the crisis) does not attempt to change the situation but rather focuses on changing the way the situation is attended to or altering the subjective appraisal of the situation (e.g., positive reappraisal or acceptance of circumstances) and use of calming strategies for aspects of the situation that cannot be controlled (Schoenmakers et al., 2015). OTPs need to understand that coping style extends over a spectrum (i.e., not an either-or concept) and that styles often overlap.

Maladaptive coping is characterized by an external locus of control, worry, magical thinking (i.e., wishing the problem would just go away), denial, blaming oneself or others, use of escape and avoidance strategies (such as overeating, overdrinking, smoking, or medication), and keeping to one's self (Ke & Barlas, 2020). Although some of these coping strategies may be useful temporarily, the exclusive reliance on these styles can be problematic.

Another form of unproductive coping involves passive acceptance of circumstances versus actively adjusting one's lifestyle to make the best of the situation. This ineffective approach involves ongoing efforts to ignore the disability, adoption of a resigned view of the illness, and withdrawal from others (or the reverse, allowing health-care providers such as doctors or therapists to become their sole support network). Though sometimes adaptive early on, when entrenched and chronic, these approaches ultimately render the individual less able to access supportive networks in the community as adjustment problems arise. Such maladaptive coping strategies are associated with significantly higher levels of depression, anxiety, PTSD, psychological dysfunction, and lower self-esteem.

Not surprisingly, maladaptive coping has also been linked to poorer psychological outcome and increased general health problems (including severe pain) following disability (Hoffart et al., 2022).

Social Support

Social support, which involves helping behaviors from a person or group that result in emotional benefits and/or practical assistance, is an important mechanism through which individuals adjust to disability. After the onset of disability, a person's social network tends to contract. Therefore, an important task of recovery is to identify reliable, trustworthy, positive, efficacious "tiers of support" from among one's spouse or significant others, close and extended family members, fictive kin (people who are regarded as part of the family even though they are not related by blood or marriage), friends, a religious community, other social groups, health-care practitioners, and community agencies (Klonoff, 2014).

Social connections help ease emotional burdens through the sharing of experience, advice, and strategies aimed at achieving more realistic and positive appraisals of challenges. Exposure to peers or people with similar injuries is considered beneficial to adjustment to disability through provision of positive role models and emotional support. The ability to meet and talk with others who have similar physical conditions provides several potential benefits to a newly disabled person. If the person with a newly acquired disability has no previous life experience interacting with or knowing persons with disabilities, then peer interaction helps teach them about life with a disability. Being around others with similar physical challenges and seeing them as individuals apart from their disabilities helps foster a sense of normalcy and provides opportunities to learn how others find meaning in life after disability.

Such interactions can also serve to inspire motivation: *If they can have a full life and be happy, then so can I.* Peer interaction offers opportunities to share problems, reduce isolation, increase motivation, see what is possible, inspire hope for the future, and facilitate realistic goal setting. OTPs can play an important role in facilitating positive coping through fostering positive peer role model relationships and community connections (Kannenberg et al., 2016).

It is widely believed that adjustment to disability is strongly correlated with a person's premorbid personality characteristics and coping style, as well as postinjury lifestyle factors such as being married, employed, and socially active, rather than the specific diagnosis or severity of the disability (Wang et al., 2018). OTPs should therefore focus intervention efforts on emphasizing the individual's personal strengths and capitalizing on their personal qualities and life experience beyond one's (changed) physical abilities. This can be achieved by promoting social connections and participation in the community through family and peer relationships, leisure activities, and employment opportunities.

Studies suggest that it is the perceived quality of social support, and not merely the quantity of people providing support, that is positively correlated with psychological well-being and acts as a buffer against psychological distress after injury. Those who believed they had a positive, practical, and reliable support system perceived themselves to be better adjusted to their disabling condition, maintained improved health routines, and ultimately experienced fewer health problems, shorter recovery time, lower blood pressure, less pain, and fewer hospital admissions (Ji et al., 2019). Also see Chapter 28: Social Determinants and Mental Health, Chapter 29: Families, and Chapter 32: The Neighborhood and Community 🤝

Gaining Knowledge and Communicating

An important, ongoing task for OTPs is to assist each individual in adjusting to their disability by gaining a complete understanding of their health condition and its functional implications. This knowledge empowers the individual to cope with the condition in an optimal way. Individuals who feel well informed about their condition and have good communication with their health-care providers perceive themselves as better adjusted to their disability (Kunz et al., 2018; Sadiki & Kibirige, 2022). See the Evidence-Based Practice feature.

One path toward "ownership" of and investment in one's own well-being is for individuals to become "experts" on their disability. Gaining a full understanding of the impact of diagnosis on an individual's health and functional abilities through occupational therapy treatment will equip them with the knowledge and skills needed to be able to adequately solve problems, manage stress, respond to environmental challenges, access community resources, implement adaptations, set realistic goals, and maximize health and independence. This process of increasing self-insight is ongoing; as one navigates different life stages, one continually develops an appreciation of the impact of their disability on various tasks, roles, occupations, and relationships.

It is also important for persons with disabilities to effectively communicate information about their condition.

Evidence-Based Practice

Health Literacy and Acquired Traumatic Brain Injury

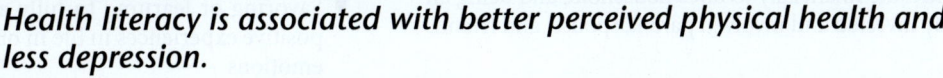

Health literacy is associated with better perceived physical health and less depression.

RESEARCH FINDINGS

A study of 205 individuals with acquired traumatic brain injury found that 69% had adequate health literacy, and 39% had inadequate health literacy (Pappadis et al 2024). When comparing the two groups, people with adequate health literacy were four times more likely to have positive perceived physical health, despite having the same number of physical health conditions as individuals with inadequate health literacy. The researchers concluded that, when individuals were adequately prepared to address health management concerns, they felt better about their physical health. Additionally, people with inadequate health literacy were 3.5 times more likely to be depressed.

APPLICATIONS

➡ OTPs should assess health literacy for people with acquired physical disability.
➡ OTPs should provide health literacy interventions that address health management skills.

REFERENCES

Pappadis, M., Sander, A., Juengst, S., Leon-Novelo, L., Ngan, E., Bell, K., & Lequerica, A. (2024). The relationship of health literacy to health outcomes among individuals with traumatic brain injury: A traumatic brain injury model systems study. *Journal of Head Trauma Rehabilitation, 39,* 103-114. https://doi.org/10.1097/HTR.0000000000000912

This involves developing the assertiveness and social skills to become comfortable talking with others and answering questions about their strengths and limitations. Effective communication skills enable the individual to master the practical realities of day-to-day life with a disability and graciously handle awkward situations (e.g., stares or questions) in a way that educates others and breaks down attitudinal barriers. Also see Chapter 27: Mental Health Stigma and Sanism.

The need to educate others about one's personal strengths and challenges is an important part of occupational therapy treatment, so that the individual can reintegrate back into family and community roles and directly or indirectly aid societal understanding and acceptance of persons with disabilities. As one returns to their home, work, and community environments, they will encounter numerous opportunities to provide information about their specific experience living with a disability. Such scenarios might include the need to educate family members on how to best assist with ADLs without interfering with one's independence, the process of hiring and training a professional caregiver, or the need to educate one's employer on compensations or adaptations that will promote independence in the workplace.

Generativity

In his theory of psychosocial development, Erik Erikson refers to the need of adults to strive to answer the question: "How can I contribute to the world?" **Generativity** refers to the different ways people attempt to "leave their mark" on the world, perhaps by creating or nurturing things that will outlast them, caring for others, or contributing to society in a positive way. The opposite condition, **stagnation**, refers to one's failure to find a way to contribute, which may cause a person to feel unproductive, disconnected, or uninvolved with others, their community, or society in general (Erikson, 1968).

The issue of generativity is one of great salience when an individual is attempting to adapt to life with an acquired physical disability. "The capacity to do something useful for yourself or others is key to personhood, whether it involves the ability to earn a living, cook a meal, put on shoes in the morning, or whatever other skill needs to be mastered at the moment" (Bateson, 1996, as cited in Christiansen, 1999, p. 547). The feeling that one contributes to one's family and community was found to be a positive contributor to adjustment to disability as opposed to the feeling that one contributed little or nothing (Fernandes et al., 2018).

Occupational therapy can help the individual explore and develop opportunities to positively contribute to the lives of others by capitalizing on their personal qualities and life experience in ways beyond one's altered physical abilities. Examples include being interested in others, offering comfort, giving advice, mentoring peers, serving in the community, volunteering, seeking accessible employment opportunities that allow one to contribute financially to one's household, and being an emotionally invested and involved parent, spouse, and friend.

Resilience

Resilience in the rehabilitation setting has been conceptualized as the ability of adults who experience a significant disabling physical injury to be able to positively adapt and adjust in order to maintain relatively stable, healthy levels of psychological and social functioning, and to maintain a positive perception of oneself and the future (Schultz & Brindle, 2022; Yan & Lin, 2022). It has been found that the majority of individuals who acquire physical disabilities are able to reorient themselves and find positive ways to adjust to the many physical and emotional challenges in a way that promotes fulfillment in life (Nalder et al., 2023).

In *Man's Search for Meaning*, Viktor Frankl (1984) explored the idea that choosing one's attitude in any given set of circumstances is a means of having at least the power to determine how you interpret and explain what happens to you and knowing there is more to oneself than current circumstances suggest. After the onset of physical disability, OTPs can help the individual appreciate that although disability may now be a major part of their life, it is not and cannot be the only part.

The ability to find "a silver lining" or something positive in the adverse events of life is a sign of resilience. Viewing hardship and crises as opportunities for learning and growth is associated with maturity and character. Individuals who find something positive—a life lesson or access to a strength or positive quality they didn't realize they had—in an undesirable medical event appear to have a better adjustment to any residual difficulties and survive longer.

For some individuals, occupational therapy can help reframe the injury so that it may serve as an impetus for examining and reorganizing one's priorities in life. This may mean deciding to spend more time on important relationships, looking for ways to serve others, having an enhanced sense of living in the present, seeing a need for more enjoyment in life, seeing life as precious and fragile, and reconsidering one's ideas of productivity and achievement (e.g., becoming less perfectionistic or materialistic) (Klonoff, 2010).

After the onset of disability, individuals find meaning and purpose in different ways:

- Focusing on the positive
- Retaining interests, values, and skills
- Exploring new occupations
- Acquiring new roles
- Expressing gratitude
- Savoring or learning to fully appreciate and enhance positive experiences in life in order to promote positive emotions
- Making new friends
- Seeking ways to engage with and serve their communities
- Becoming able to talk about ways their lives have changed for the positive after disability
- Using intellect and creativity to combat stress and boredom
- Increasing commitment to religion or social causes

The field of positive psychology is concerned with the study of those things that make life worth living. Researchers in this area want to understand what things people do well, and how their efforts influence their well-being, as well as that of their families, friends, and communities. One of the basic themes in positive psychology is defining the "good life" or explaining and promoting the development of traits that contribute to quality of life, a sense of fulfillment and subjective well-being, and happiness (Skarin & Wastlund, 2020).

The following factors can lead to a good life following onset of disability:

- Optimistic attitude
- Healthy behaviors
- Perceived social support
- Positive role adjustment
- Generativity
- Adaptability
- Personal goals
- Financial stability
- Acquisition of knowledge
- Self-efficacy
- Practicing spirituality
- Sense of purpose and meaning

Nalder and colleagues (2023) have identified three elements that promote the good life after acquired physical disability: creating connections to other people, cultivation of positive personal qualities, and development of life regulation qualities, such as autonomy, curiosity, self-control, and the ability to delay gratification and persist in the pursuit of goals. Figure 16-1 shows example actions that can promote the good life following acquired physical disability.

Connections to other people
- Ability to form and maintain relationships
- Socializing with others
- Social comparisons
- Helping others
- Loving others
- Forgiving others

Positive personal qualities
- Finding meaning
- Resilience
- Expressing gratitude
- Humor
- Creativity

Life regulation qualities
- Self-discipline
- Regular physical exercise
- Attending to bodily pleasures
- Finding enjoyment in intrinsically rewarding activities
- Persisting at learning new skills

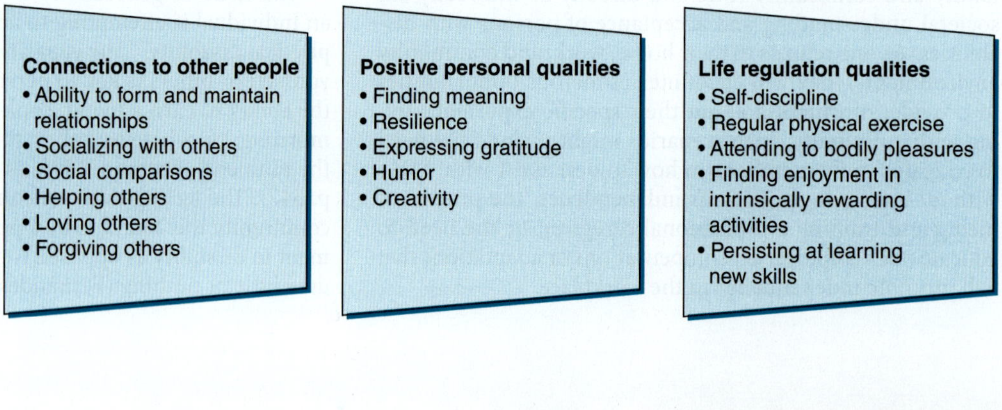

FIGURE 16-1. Promoting the good life following acquired physical disability.

A constructive way for the OTP to help people organize these three elements is by encouraging them to conceptualize the good life after disability as one represented by an appropriate balance of independence (autonomy, choice, motivation to seek or create outcomes that promote well-being and lead to happiness) and interdependence (person's need to relate to and interact with others, especially family, friends, and caregivers). An imbalance in these areas can lead to psychosocial problems (McClure & Leah, 2021). Box 16-4 explores humor as an effective mechanism of dealing with stress and adapting to disability.

Intervention

Table 16-2 outlines common intervention approaches for psychosocial concerns with physical disabilities and identifies the accompanying chapters in this text that provide more detailed information about those approaches. 🤝

BOX 16-4 ■ Humor and Coping

People of all ages and cultures respond to humor. Humor and laughter play an important part in maintaining one's psychological and emotional well-being and are positively correlated with self-concept and vitality in persons with and without disabilities (Papousek, 2018). Sharing humor acts as a means to normalize an abnormal situation, expand one's perspective, and join with others to persevere during trying times. As a learned coping style that focuses on viewing the world from a lighter perspective, it can be an effective mechanism of dealing with stress and adapting to disability.

Humor can have a normalizing effect on abnormal situations by facilitating cognitive restructuring and reframing stressful circumstances. It helps a person expand their perspective and allows them to rise above personal deficiencies by admitting and making light of them. Through the use of humor, individuals can alter their perceptions of stressful circumstances from being overwhelming or insurmountable to being less intimidating, thereby reducing stress and anxiety (Bally & Bernstein, 2019).

Humor tends to draw people closer together, facilitate positive social interactions, and enhance positive emotions (Bally & Bernstein, 2019). People with well-developed senses of humor tend to be flexible thinkers who can make sudden cognitive and perceptual shifts. From a health perspective, having a sense of humor is positively correlated with maturity, stress reduction, improved immune system function, and shorter recuperation times (Papousek, 2018).

John Callahan sustained an SCI at the age of 21 that left him with quadriplegia. After his injury he began drawing by holding a pen between both hands and became a nationally syndicated cartoonist and author of several collections of cartoons.

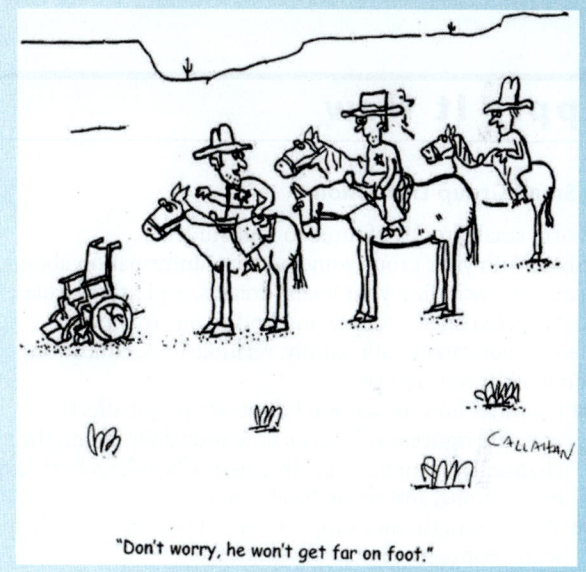

"Don't worry, he won't get far on foot."

TABLE 16-2 | Common Intervention Approaches for Individuals With Physical Disability

Approach	Target(s) of Intervention	Brief Synopsis	Chapters With Additional Information 🤝
Cognitive behavioral approach	Distorted beliefs	Distorted beliefs are identified and then challenged by providing evidence to the contrary.	Chapter 8: Cognitive Beliefs
Therapeutic writing and other creative media	Coping methods, personal understanding, and coming to terms with trauma	Use of writing (e.g., journaling) and other creative media (e.g., painting, dance, and music) to explore losses and sources of resilience	Chapter 10: Coping and Resilience
Mindfulness meditation	Emotional well-being	A form of meditation that focuses awareness nonjudgmentally on the present	Chapter 12: Emotion Regulation
Exercise and other forms of physical activity	Physical conditioning and stress reduction	Promote engagement in preferred physical activities to increase strength and endurance and reduce stress	Chapter 45: Self-Care and Well-Being Occupations
Relaxation strategies	Stress management	Breathing, progressive muscle relaxation, autogenic techniques, and/or guided imagery to promote state of calm	Chapter 15: Pain
Self-advocacy	Reducing stigma and misunderstanding	Developing knowledge of rights and skills to advocate for full inclusion	Chapter 27: Mental Health Stigma and Sanism
Social support	Emotional health, fostering hope, access to resources	Connections to community groups and peer support; working on strengthening established relationships and creating new ones	Chapter 49: Connectedness and Belonging

Here's the Point

■ Adaptation to an acquired physical disability is a complex process that evolves across the life span.

■ In addition to the initial trauma, people with acquired physical disabilities experience episodic losses that become apparent through time as the individual moves through the rehabilitation process and life stages and attempts to reintegrate back into family, social roles, and the community.

■ OTPs need to recognize that the signs and symptoms of conditions such as depression, anxiety, and substance abuse are common but not inevitable consequences of acquired physical disability and provide interventions to address these concerns. They should also make appropriate referrals to additional resources and adjunct members of the health-care team such as psychiatrists, psychologists, and social workers.

■ Family members, friends, and other loved ones are impacted by the disability and may serve in the role of caregivers. OTPs should be aware of the impact on loved ones and provide services to address caregiver needs.

■ OTPs can play an integral role in identifying, facilitating, and promoting personal qualities in their patients that are predictive of favorable psychological outcomes after acquired physical disability. These factors include an internal locus of control, perceived social support, being well informed about one's condition, and a sense of generativity.

■ With proper resources, including occupational therapy interventions, the majority of individuals who live with acquired physical disability make a positive psychological adjustment and report a positive quality of life.

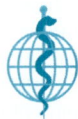 **Visit the online resource center at FADavis.com to access the videos.**

Apply It Now

1. Small Group Discussion

■ Form small groups of three to four students.

■ Share with your group some personal information about yourself, including your goals, dreams, aspirations, roles, habits, cherished occupations, and so on. You may refer to your career path, family, relationships, education, hobbies, travel, and so on.

■ Consider how an acquired disability might affect your life right now. Discuss how your daily life might change. How might your dreams, goals, roles, cherished occupations, and so on, be affected?

■ What strengths and supports would you rely on to help with your recovery?

■ What aspects of an acquired disability might have a positive impact on your life?

2. Reflections on Stephanie Nielson–Burn Survivor (Box 16-2): PEO Analysis

Reread Box 16-2 concerning Stephanie Nielson and complete a Person-Environment-Occupation (PEO) analysis using the template in Appendix A. Consider the following guiding questions:

■ What occupations are important to Stephanie?

■ What personal factors and environmental factors contributed to her recovery and what factors interfered with her recovery?

■ After Stephanie's accident, her appearance dramatically changed. She no longer had a face covered in freckles, no longer resembled her sisters, and even her children didn't recognize her. What challenges did this present to her body image and sense of self?

■ How did Stephanie's inability to carry out the routine tasks of motherhood (braiding her daughter's hair and playing blocks with her son) affect her role identity?

■ How did returning to blogging and sharing her story with a virtual community assist her recovery?

■ Which statuses of disability identity development from the Forber-Pratt and Zape (2017) model (presented in Table 16-1) can you see in Stephanie's story?

3. Identifying Peer Support Resources

The chapter explains that peer support can be very helpful for people in adjusting to acquired physical disabilities. In small groups, work together to identify peer support resources that you could share with people.

■ Where is your nearest Center for Independent Living? Centers for Independent Living often have group meetings, support for training and hiring caregivers, funding for home modifications, and other resources that can be very helpful to people with new disabilities.

■ Are there local support groups for people with specific injuries, such as TBI or SCI?

■ What online peer support resources exist for people with disabilities?

■ Are there local wheelchair or other adaptive sports leagues?

Resources

Books

• Bolte Taylor, J. (2008). *My stroke of insight*. Viking Books.
• Crimmins, C. (2000). *Where is the mango princess? A journey back from brain injury*. Vintage Books.
• Nielson, S. (2013). *Heaven is here*. Hachette Books.
• Purdy, A. (2015). *On my own two feet: From losing my legs to learning the dance of life*. William Morrow Paperbacks.
• Taussig, R. (2020). *Sitting pretty: The view from my ordinary resilient disabled body*. HarperOne, an imprint of HarperCollins Publishers.
• Weiner, J. (2004). *His brother's keeper*. HarperCollins.

Videos

- "Sensory Garden in Geriatric Psychiatric Unit" video. In this video, occupational therapist Callie Ward showcases the sensory garden at an inpatient psychiatric facility. The multisensory garden was designed for occupational therapy groups with a goal of helping participants identify the effects the garden and its related tasks have on their level of arousal. Callie offers specific examples of the many positive effects of the garden on residents, such as collaborating on tasks, problem-solving, encouraging routines, working on cognition, and assisting with self-regulation, among others. She explains how she uses it for active and passive group interventions and in one-to-one sessions. To access the video, visit the online resource center at FADavis.com.
- "Mental Health and Well-Being During COVID" video. Caitlin is an OTP who has worked in outpatient settings with both adults and children. In this video, she talks about how occupational therapy practice during the COVID-19 global pandemic allowed her to see in a new way the effects of stress and anxiety on patient outcomes. She discusses how she incorporates mental health and well-being into her practice and her belief that it promotes successful healing and recovery. To access the video, visit the online resource center at FADavis.com.
- "Any One of Us"—HBO Documentaries: http://www.hbo.com
- "Coma"—HBO Documentaries: http://www.hbo.com
- "Crash Reel"—HBO Documentaries: http://www.hbo.com
- "Gleason"—Amazon Studios
- "Marathon: The Patriots Day Bombing"—HBO Documentaries: http://www.hbo.com
- "Murderball"—MTV Films
- "So Much, So Fast"—PBS: http://www.pbs.org/wgbh/pages/frontline/somuchsofast

Organizations

- Amputee Coalition of America: http://www.amputee-coalition.org
- Brain Injury Association of America: http://www.biausa.org
- Christopher and Dana Reeve Foundation: https://www.christopherreeve.org
- National Stroke Association: http://www.stroke.org
- Parkinson's Foundation: http://www.parkinson.org

Online Resources

- Stephanie Nielson's blog: www.nieniedialogues.com
- https://www.oprah.com/own-relationships/blogger-stephanie-nielsons-daily-struggles-video

References

ABC News. (2011, May 10). *Stephanie Nielson's story: After tragic crash, mom of four nearly lost it all.* http://abcnews.go.com/2020/stephanie-nielsons-story-tragic-crash-mom-lost/story?id=13574901&page=2

Adams, M., Weatherall, M., & Bell, E. (2019). A cohort study of the association between psychosocial factors and pain in patients with spinal cord injury and stroke. *NeuroRehabilitation, 45*(3), 419–427. https://doi.org/10.3233/NRE-192872

American Occupational Therapy Association. (2020). Occupational Therapy Practice Framework: Domain and process—Fourth edition. *American Journal of Occupational Therapy, 74*(Suppl. 2), 7412410010p1–7412410010p87. https://doi.org/10.5014/ajot.2020.74S2001

American Psychiatric Association. (2022). *Diagnostic and statistical manual of mental disorders* (5th ed., text ref.). American Psychiatric Publishing. https://doi.org/10.1176/appi.books.9780890425787

Anson, K., & Ponsford, J. (2006). Evaluation of a coping skills group following traumatic brain injury. *Brain Injury, 20*(2), 167–178. https://doi.org/10.1080/02699050500442956

Bally, S. J., & Bernstein, C. M. (2019). The use of humor to facilitate adaptation to hearing loss: A serious consideration of the potential role of humor in aural rehabilitation Part II. *Journal of the Academy of Rehabilitative Audiology, 52,* 1–13.

Banerjee, M., Hedge, S., Thippeswamy, H., Kulkarni, G. B., & Rao, N. (2021). In search of the 'self': Holistic rehabilitation in restoring cognition and recovering the 'self' following traumatic brain injury: A case report. *NeuroRehabilitation, 48*(2), 231–242. https://doi.org/10.3233/NRE-208017

Barclay, L., Lentin, P., Bourke-Taylor, H., & McDonald, R. (2018). The experiences of social and community participation of people with non-traumatic spinal cord injury. *Australian Occupational Therapy Journal, 66*(1), 61–67. https://doi.org/10.1111/1440-1630.12522

Barrett, O. E. C., Mattacola, E., & Finlay, K. A. (2023). "You feel a bit unsexy sometimes": The psychosocial impact of a spinal cord injury on sexual function and sexual satisfaction. *Spinal Cord, 61,* 52–56. https://doi.org/10.1038/s41393-022-00858-y

Bateson, M. (1996). Enfolded activity and the concept of occupation. In R. Zemke & F. Clark (Eds.), *Occupational science: The evolving discipline* (pp. 5–12). F.A. Davis.

Bogart, K. R. (2014). The role of disability self-concept in adaptation to congenital or acquired disability. *Rehabilitation Psychology, 59,* 107–115. https://doi.org/10.1037/a0035800

Bombardier, C. H., Azuero, C. B., Fann, J. R., Kautz, D. D., Richards, J. S., & Sabharwal, S. (2021). Management of mental health disorders, substance use disorders, and suicide in adults with spinal cord injury: Clinical practice guideline for healthcare providers. *Topics in Spinal Cord Injury Rehabilitation, 27*(2), 152–224. https://doi.org/10.46292/sci2702-152

Braaf, S., Ameratunga, S., Ponsford, J., Cameron, P., Collie, A., Harrison, J., Ekegren, C., Christie, N., Nunn, A., & Gabbe, B. (2019). Traumatic injury survivors' perceptions of their future: A longitudinal qualitative study. *Disability and Rehabilitation, 42*(19), 2707–2717. https://doi.org/10.1080/09638288.2019.1571116

Burnett, S. (2018). Personal and social contexts of disability: Implications for occupational therapists. In H. M. Pendleton & W. Schultz-Krohn (Eds.), *Pedretti's occupational therapy: Practice skills for physical dysfunction* (8th ed., pp. 71–91). Elsevier Mosby.

Carlozzi, N., Freedman, J., Troost, J., Carson, T., Molton, I., Ehde, D., Najarian, K., Miner, J., Boileau, N., & Kratz, A. (2022). Daily variation in sleep quality is associated with health-related quality of life in people with spinal cord injury. *Archives of Physical Medicine and Rehabilitation* 103: 263–273. https://doi.org/10.1016/j.apmr.2021.07.803

Chakrabarty, T., Hadjipavlou, G., & Lam, R. W. (2016). Cognitive dysfunction in major depressive disorder: Assessment, impact and management. *Focus (American Psychiatric Publishing), 14*(2), 194–206. https://doi.org/10.1176/appi.focus.20150043

Choi, J. W., Lee, K. S., & Han, E. (2020). Psychiatric disorders and suicide risk among adults with disabilities: A nationwide retrospective cohort study. *Journal of Affective Disorders, 263,* 9–14. https://doi.org/10.1016/j.jad.2019.11.129

Christiansen, C. H. (1999, November/December). Defining lives: Occupation as identity: An essay on competence, coherence, and the creation of meaning. *American Journal of Occupational Therapy, 53*(6), 547–558. https://doi.org/10.5014/ajot.53.6.547

Coleman, D., & Lucas, C. A. (2017). *Statement on mourning the death of Jerika Bolen.* https://www.notdeadyet.org?statement-on-mourning-the-death-of-jerika-bolen

Consortium for Spinal Cord Medicine. (2021). Management of mental health disorders, substance use disorders, and suicide in adults with spinal cord injury. *Journal of Spinal Cord Medicine, 44*(1), 102–162. https://doi.org/10.1080/10790268.2021.1863738

Craig, A., Tran, Y., Guest, R., & Middleton, J. (2019). Trajectories of self-efficacy and depressed mood and their relationship in the first 12 months following spinal cord injury. *Archives of Physical Medicine and Rehabilitation, 100*(3), 441–447. https://doi.org/10.1016/j.apmr.2018.07.442

Curran, C. A., Ponsford, J. L., & Crowe, S. (2000). Coping strategies and emotional outcome following traumatic brain injury:

A comparison with orthopedic patients. *The Journal of Head Trauma Rehabilitation, 15*(6), 1256–1274. https://doi.org/10.1097/00001199-200012000-00006

De Martino, M. L., De Bartolo, M., Leemhuis, E., & Pazzaglia, M. (2021). Rebuilding body-brain interaction from the vagal network in spinal cord injuries. *Brain Sciences, 11*(8), 1084. https://doi.org/10.3390/brainsci11081084

Ding, W., Hu, S., Wang, P., Kang, H., Peng, R., Dong, Y., & Li, F. (2022). Spinal cord injury: The global incidence, prevalence, and disability from the global burden of disease study 2019. *Spine, 47*(21), 1532–1540. https://doi.org/10.1097/brs.0000000000004417

Eberhard, B., Knüppel Lauener, S., & Mahrer Imhof, R. (2019). Perspectives from family caregivers of persons with spinal cord injury in hospital versus rehabilitation: A pilot study. *Rehabilitation Nursing, 44*(6), 311–318. https://doi.org/10.1097/RNJ.0000000000000143

Eldridge, L. A., Piatt, J. A., Agley, J., & Gerke, S. (2019). Relationship between substance use and the onset of spinal cord injuries: A medical chart review. *Topics in Spinal Cord Injury Rehabilitation, 25*(4), 316–321. https://doi.org/10.1310/sci2504-316

El-Menyar, A., Consunji, R., Asim, M., Mekkodathil, A., Latifi, R., Smith, G., Parchani, A., & Al-Thani, H. (2019). Traumatic brain injury in patients screened for blood alcohol concentration based on the mechanism of injury. *Brain Injury, 33*(4), 419–426. https://doi.org/10.1080/02699052.2018.1553065

Erikson, E. (1968). *Identity: Youth and crisis* (2nd ed.). Norton.

Evans, D. (2016). *Hollywood promotes the idea it is better to be dead than disabled.* https://www.domevansofficial.com/2016/02/11/hollywood-promotes-the-idea-it-is-better-to-be-dead-than-disabled

Fernandes, H. L., Cantrill, S., Shrestha, R. L., Raj, R. B., Allchin, B., Kamal, R., Butcher, N., & Grills, N. (2018). Lived experience of psychosocial disability and social inclusion: A participatory PhotoVoice study in rural India and Nepal. *Disability, CBR & Inclusive Development, 29*(2), 5–23. https://doi.org/10.5463/dcid.v29i2.746

Fine, S. B. (1991). Resilience and human adaptability: Who rises above adversity? *American Journal of Occupational Therapy, 45*(6), 493–503. https://doi.org/10.5014/ajot.45.6.493

Forber-Pratt, A. J., Lyew, D. A., Mueller, C., & Samples, L. B. (2017). Disability identity development: A systematic review of the literature. *Rehabilitation Psychology Journal, 62*(2), 198–207. https://doi.org/10.1037/rep0000134

Forber-Pratt, A. J., & Zape, M. P. (2017). Disability identity development model: Voices from the ADA generation. *Disability and Health, 10*(2), 350–355. https://doi.org/10.1016/j.dhjo.2016.12.013

Frankl, V. (1984). *Man's search for meaning.* Washington Square Press.

Furrer, A., Michel, G., Terrill, A. L., Jensen, M. P., & Müller, R. (2019). Modeling subjective well-being in individuals with chronic pain and a physical disability: The role of pain control and pain catastrophizing. *Disability and Rehabilitation, 41*(5), 498–507. https://doi.org/10.1080/09638288.2017.1390614

Galvis Arparicio, M., Kunz, S., Morselli, D., Post, M., Peter, C., & Carrard, V. (2021). Adaptation during spinal cord injury rehabilitation: The role of appraisal and coping. *Rehabilitation Psychology, 66*(4), 507–519. https://doi.org/10.1037/rep0000410

Gelech, J., Bayly, M., & Desjardins, M. (2019). Constructing robust selves after brain injury: Positive identity work among members of a female self-help group. *Neuropsychological Rehabilitation, 29*(3), 456–476. https://doi.org/10.1080/09602011.2017.1308872

Hanafy, S., Amodio, V., Haag, H., Colquhoun, H., Lewko, J., Quilico, E., Riopelle, R., Archambault, P., Colantonio, A., Lindsay, S., & Mollayeva, T. (2022). Is it prime time for sex and gender considerations in traumatic brain injury? Perspectives of rehabilitation care professionals. *Disability and Rehabilitation, 44*(5), 684–692. https://doi.org/10.1080/09638288.2020.1774670

Haukeland, Y. B., Vatne, T. M., Mossige, S., & Fjermestad, K. W. (2021). Psychosocial functioning in siblings of children with rare disorders compared to controls. *The Yale Journal of Biology and Medicine, 94*(4), 537–544.

Hawken, T., Turner-Cobb, J., & Barnett, J. (2018). Coping and adjustment in caregivers: A systematic review. *Health Psychology Open, 5*(2), 205510291881065. https://doi.org/10.1177/2055102918810659

Hayes, C. J., Payakachat, N., & Li, C. (2018). Evaluation of opioid use among patients with back disorders and arthritis. *Quality of Life Research, 27*(11), 3021–3035. https://doi.org/10.1007/s11136-018-1941-1

Hitzig, S., Cimino, S., Alavinia, M., Basset-Gunter, R., Craven, C., & Guilcher, S. (2021). Examination of the relationships among social networks and loneliness on health and life satisfaction in people with spinal cord injury/dysfunction. *Archives of Physical Medicine and Rehabilitation, 102*(11), 2109–2116. https://doi.org/10.1016/j.apmr.2021.03.030

Hoffart, A., Johnson, S. U., & Ebrahimi, O. V. (2022). Metacognitive beliefs, maladaptive coping strategies, and depressive symptoms: A two-wave network study of the COVID-19 lockdown and reopening. *Journal of Psychiatric Research, 152,* 70–78. https://doi.org/10.1016/j.jpsychires.2022.06.008

James, S. L., Theadom, A., Ellenbogen, R. G., Bannick, M. S., Montjoy-Venning, W., Lucchesi, L. R., Abbasi, N., Abdulkader, R., Abraha, H. N., Adsuar, J. C., Afarideh, M., Agrawal, S., Ahmadi, A., Ahmed, M. B., Aichour, A. N., Aichour, I., Aichour, M. T., Akinyemi, R. O., Akseer, N., . . . Murray, C. J. (2019). Global, regional, and national burden of traumatic brain injury and spinal cord injury, 1990–2016: A systematic analysis for the global burden of disease study 2016. *The Lancet Neurology, 18*(1), 56–87. https://doi.org/10.1016/s1474-4422(18)30415-0

January, A. M., Kelly, E. H., Russell, H. F., Zebracki, K., & Vogel, L. C. (2019). Patterns of coping among caregivers of children with spinal cord injury: Associations with parent and child well-being. *Families, Systems, & Health, 37*(2), 150–161. https://doi.org/10.1037/fsh0000415

Jeyathevan, G., Catharine Craven, B., Cameron, J. I., & Jaglal, S. B. (2020). Facilitators and barriers to supporting individuals with spinal cord injury in the community: Experiences of family caregivers and care recipients. *Disability and Rehabilitation, 42*(13), 1844–1854. https://doi.org/10.1080/09638288.2018.1541102

Ji, Y., Rana, C., Shi, C., & Zhong, Y. (2019). Self-esteem mediates the relationships between social support, subjective well-being, and perceived discrimination in Chinese people with physical disability. *Frontiers in Psychology, 10,* 2230. https://doi.org/10.3389/fpsyg.2019.02230

Kannenberg, K., Amini, D., Hartmann, K., & Delany, J. (2016). Occupational therapy services in the promotion of mental health and well-being. *American Journal of Occupational Therapy, 70*(Suppl. 2), 7012410070p1–7012410070p15. https://doi.org/10.5014/ajot.2016.706S05

Ke, T., & Barlas, J. (2020). Thinking about feeling: Using trait emotional intelligence in understanding the associations between early maladaptive schemas and coping styles. *Psychology and Psychotherapy, 93*(1), 1–20. https://doi.org/10.1111/papt.12202

Khan, F., Amatya, B., Judson, R., Chung, P., Truesdale, M., Elmalik, A., & Galea, M. P. (2016). Factors associated with long term functional and psychological outcomes in persons with moderate to severe traumatic brain injury. *Journal of Rehabilitation Medicine, 48*(5), 442–448. https://doi.org/10.2340/16501977-2084

Klonoff, P. S. (2010). *Psychotherapy after brain injury: Principles and techniques.* Guilford Press.

Klonoff, P. S. (2014). *Psychotherapy for families after brain injury.* Springer.

Kunz, S., Joseph, S., Geyh, S., & Peter, C. (2018). Coping and posttraumatic growth: A longitudinal comparison of two alternative views. *Rehabilitation Psychology, 63,* 240–249. https://doi.org/10.1037/rep0000205

Lazarus, R. S., & Folkman, S. (1984). *Stress, appraisal, and coping.* Springer Publishing Company.

Lee, S.-J., Kim, M.-G., Kim, J. H., Min, Y.-S., Kim, C.-H., Kim, K.-T., & Hwang, J.-M. (2022). Factor analysis affecting degree of depression in family caregivers of patients with spinal cord injury: A cross-sectional pilot study. *International Journal of Environmental Research and Public Health, 19*(17), 10878. https://doi.org/10.3390/ijerph191710878

Leung, J., Gouda, H., Chung, J. Y., & Irmansyah, I. (2021). Comorbidity between depressive symptoms and chronic conditions—Findings from the Indonesia Family Life Survey. *Journal of Affective Disorders, 280,* 236–240. https://doi.org/10.1016/j.jad.2020.11.007

Liebscher, T., Ludwig, J., Lübstorf, T., Kreutzträger M., Auhuber, T., Grittner, U., Schäfer, B., Wüstner, G., Ekkernkamp, A., & Kopp, M. (2022). Cervical spine injuries with acute traumatic spinal cord injury: Spinal surgery adverse events and their association with neurological and functional outcome. *Spine, 47*(1), E16–E26. https://doi.org/10.1097/brs.0000000000004124

Lodha, P., Shah, B., Karia, S., & De Sousa, A. (2020, December 31). Post-traumatic stress disorder (PTSD) following burn injuries: A comprehensive clinical review. *Annals of Burns and Fire Disasters, 33*(4), 276–287.

Lu, Y.-C., Wu, M.-K., Zhang, L., Zhang, C.-L., Lu, Y.-Y., & Wu, C.-H. (2020). Association between suicide risk and traumatic brain injury in adults: A population based cohort study. *Postgraduate Medical Journal, 96*(1142), 747–752. https://doi.org/10.1136/postgradmedj-2019-136860

McClure, J., & Leah, C. (2021). Is independence enough? Rehabilitation should include autonomy and social engagement to achieve quality of life. *Clinical Rehabilitation, 35*(1), 3–12. https://doi.org/10.1177/0269215520954344

McDonald, S., Pugh, M., & Mickens, M. (2020). Resilience after spinal cord injury. *American Journal of Physical Medicine & Rehabilitation, 99*(8), 752–763. https://doi.org/10.1097/PHM.0000000000001371

McGrath, M., Lever, S., McCluskey, A., & Power, E. (2019). How is sexuality after stroke experienced by stroke survivors and partners of stroke survivors? A systematic review of qualitative studies. *Clinical Rehabilitation, 33*(2), 293–303. https://doi.org/10.1177/0269215518793483

McGrath, M., Low, M. A., Power, E., McCluskey, A., & Lever, S. (2021). Addressing sexuality among people living with chronic disease and disability: A systematic mixed methods review of knowledge, attitudes, and practices of health care professionals. *Archives of Physical Medicine and Rehabilitation, 102*(5), 999–1010. https://doi.org/10.1016/j.apmr.2020.09.379

McLeod, J., & Davis, C. G. (2023). Community peer support among individuals living with spinal cord injury. *Journal of Health Psychology, 28*(10), 943–955. https://doi.org/10.1177/13591053231159483

Mollayeva, T., Bordignon, C., Ishtiaq, M., Colquhoun, H., D'Souza, A., Archambault, P., Lewko, J., Quilico, E., & Colantonio, A. (2021). Knowledge of sex and gender and related information needs in patients with traumatic brain injury: In-depth interview study. *Disability and Rehabilitation, 43*(13), 1872–1882. https://doi.org/10.1080/09638288.2019.1683235

Nalder, E., Gillian, K., Hunt, A. W., Hartman, L. R., Szigeti, Z., Drake, E., Shah, R., Shahzad, M., Resnick, M., Pereira, G., & Lenton, E. (2023). Indicators of life success from the perspective of individuals with traumatic brain injury: A scoping review. *Disability and Rehabilitation, 45*(2), 330–343. https://doi.org/10.1080/09638288.2021.2025274

National Spinal Cord Injury Statistical Center. (2022). *Traumatic spinal cord injury facts and figures at a glance.* University of Alabama at Birmingham. https://msktc.org/sites/default/files/SCI-Facts-Figs-2022-Eng-508.pdf

Nielson, S. (2015, March 25). *Strong legs.* http://nieniedialogues.blogspot.com/2015/03/strong-legs.html

Papamalis, F. E. (2020). Examining the relationship of personality functioning and treatment completion in substance misuse treatment. *Substance Abuse: Research and Treatment, 14,* 1–19. https://doi.org/10.1177/1178221820951777

Papousek, I. (2018). Humor and well-being: A little less is quite enough. *Humor, 31*(2), 311–327. https://doi.org/10.1515/humor-2016-0114

Quinn, B. (2016). Disability rights campaigners protest at premiere of Me Before You. *The Guardian.* https://www.theguardian.com/society/2016/may/25/disability-rights-campaigners-protest-at-premiere-of-me-before-you

Rogowska, A. M., Zmaczynska-Witek, B., Mazurkiewicz, M., & Kardasz, Z. (2020). The mediating effect of self-efficacy on the relationship between health locus of control and life satisfaction: A moderator role of movement disability. *Disability and Health Journal, 13*(4), 1–8. https://doi.org/10.1016/j.dhjo.2020.100923

Sachdeva, R., Gao, F., Chan, C. C. H., & Krassioukov, A. (2018). Cognitive function after spinal cord injury: A systemic review. *Neurology, 91*(13), 611–621. https://doi.org/10.1212/wnl.0000000000006244

Sadiki, M. C., & Kibirige, I. (2022). Strategies employed in coping with physical abilities acquired during adulthood in rural South Africa. *African Journal of Disability, 11,* 1–8. https://doi.org/10.4102/ajod.v11i0.907

Sandalic, D., Craig, A., Tran, Y., Arora, M., Pozzato, I., McBain, C., Tonkin, H., Simpson, G., Gopinath, B., Kaur, J., Shetty, S., Weber, G., & Middleton, J. (2022). Cognitive impairment in individuals with spinal cord injury: Findings of a systemic review with robust variance of network meta-analyses. *Neurology, 99*(16), e1779–e1790. https://doi.org/10.1212/wnl.0000000000200957

Schoenmakers, E. C., van Tilburg, T. G., & Fokkema, T. (2015). Problem-focused and emotion-focused coping options and loneliness: How are they related? *European Journal of Ageing, 12*(2), 152–161. https://doi.org/10.1007/s10433-015-0336-1

Schultz, K. R., & Brindle, S. S. (2022). Health care providers' perspectives on resilience and positive adjustment within the spinal cord injury population. *Rehabilitation Psychology, 67*(2), 162–169. https://doi.org/10.1037/rep0000413

Senna, I., Cuturi, L., Gori, M., Ernst, M., & Cappagli, G. (2021). Editorial: Special and temporal perception in sensory deprivation. *Frontiers in Neuroscience, 15,* 671836. https://doi.org/10.3389/fnins.2021.671836

Shabany, M., Ghodsi, S. M., Arejan, R. H., Baigi, V., Ghodsi, Z., Rakhshani, F., Gholami, M., Sharif, P. M., Shool, S., Vaccaro, A. R., & Rahimi-Movaghar, V. (2022). Cognitive appraisals of disability in persons with traumatic spinal cord injury: A scoping review. *Spinal Cord, 60,* 954–962. https://doi.org/10.1038/s41393-022-00756-3

Skarin, F., & Wastlund, E. (2020). Increasing students' long-term well-being by mandatory intervention—A positive psychology field study. *Frontiers in Psychology, 11,* 553764. https://doi.org/10.3389/fpsyg.2020.553764

Soler, M., Navaux, M., & Previnaire, J. (2018). Positive sexuality in men with spinal cord injury. *Spinal Cord, 56,* 1199–1206. https://doi.org/10.1038/s41393-018-0177-9

Stickley, A., Koyanagi, A., Ueda, M., Inoue, Y., Waldman, K., & Oh, H. (2020). Physical multimorbidity and suicidal behavior in the general population in the United States. *Journal of Affective Disorders, 260,* 604–609. https://doi.org/10.1016/j.jad.2019.09.042

Titman, R., Liang, J., & Craven, B. C. (2019). Diagnostic accuracy and feasibility of depression screening in spinal cord injury: A systematic review. *Journal of Spinal Cord Medicine, 42*(Suppl. 1), 99–107. https://doi.org/10.1080/10790268.2019.1606556

Ullrich, P. M., Lincoln, R. K., Tackett, M. J., Miskevics, S., Smith, B. M., & Weaver, F. M. (2013). Pain, depression, and health care utilization over time after spinal cord injury. *Rehabilitation Psychology, 58*(2), 158–165. https://doi.org/10.1037/a0032047

Vázquez-Fariñas, M., & Rodriguez-Martin, B. (2021). "Living with a fragmented body": A qualitative study on perceptions about body changes after a spinal cord injury. *Spinal Cord, 59,* 855–864. https://doi.org/10.1038/s41393-021-00634-4

Wan, F.-J., Chien, W.-C., Chung, C.-H., Yang, Y.-J., & Tzeng, N.-S. (2020). Association between traumatic spinal cord injury and affective and other psychiatric disorders—A nationwide cohort study and effects of rehabilitation therapies. *Journal of Affective Disorders, 265,* 381–388. https://doi.org/10.1016/j.jad.2020.01.063

Wang, Y., Xie, H., & Zhao, X. (2018). Psychological morbidities and positive psychological outcomes in people with traumatic spinal cord injury in Mainland China. *Spinal Cord, 56*(7), 704–711. https://doi.org/10.1038/s41393-017-0044-0

Weil, Z. M., Corrigan, J. D., & Karelina, K. (2018). Alcohol use disorder and traumatic brain injury. *Alcohol Research: Current Reviews, 39*(2), 171–180.

Wettervik, T., Enblad, P., & Lewén, A. (2021). Pre-injury chronic alcohol abuse predicts intracranial hemorrhagic progression, unfavorable clinical outcome, and mortality in severe traumatic brain injury. *Brain Injury, 35*(12–13), 1569–1576. https://doi.org/10.1080/02699052.2021.1975196

Wilson, C. S., DeDios-Stern, S., Bocage, C., Gray, A. A., Crudup, B. M., & Russell, H. F. (2022). A systematic review of how spinal cord injury impacts families. *Rehabilitation Psychology, 67*(3), 273–303. https://doi.org/10.1037/rep0000431

Yan, H., & Lin, H. (2022). Resilience in stroke patients: A concept analysis. *Healthcare, 10*(11), 2281. https://doi.org/10.3390/healthcare10112281

Yousefifard, M., Ramezani, F., Faridaalaee, G., Baikpour, M., Madani Neishaboori, A., Vaccaro, A., Hosseini, M., & Rahimi-Movaghar, V. (2022). Prevalence of posttraumatic stress disorder symptoms following traumatic spinal cord injury: A systematic review and meta-analysis. *Harvard Review of Psychiatry, 30*(5), 271–282. https://doi.org/10.1097/hrp.0000000000000340

Yuying, C., Huacong, W., Navneet, B., & Devivo, M. (2022). Demographic and health profiles of people living with traumatic spinal cord injury in United States during 2015–2019: Findings from the spinal cord injury model systems database. *Archives of Physical Medicine and Rehabilitation, 103*(4), 622–633. https://doi.org/10.1016/j.apmr.2021.11.001

Chronic Health Conditions and Mental Health

Heidi Fischer, Maureen Gecht-Silver, Hilary Marshall, Gina Mulanthara, and Caitlin Smith

Worldwide, people are living longer; however, they are not necessarily living a healthier life absent of chronic conditions. **Chronic diseases** are the number one cause of death and disability worldwide and affect one in three adults (Hajat & Stein, 2018). According to the World Health Organization (WHO), chronic diseases account for 74% of all deaths worldwide (Global Burden of Disease Collaborative Network [GBD], 2019). Four groups of chronic disease account for 80% of all premature death: heart disease, cancer, respiratory diseases (such as chronic obstructive pulmonary disease [COPD]), and diabetes.

In the United States, roughly 60% of adults have at least one chronic condition, and four out of every 10 adults have multiple chronic conditions (Centers for Disease Control and Prevention [CDC], 2023). Furthermore, although life expectancy has increased globally over the last two decades, the COVID-19 pandemic exacerbated the prevalence of chronic disease and created stress on an already burdened health-care system. Long COVID, also known as post-COVID conditions (PCC), has emerged as a chronic health condition that can impact a person's ability to engage in meaningful occupational performance and participation, impacting anywhere from 10% to 35% of people globally (WHO, 2022).

The immense prevalence of chronic disease and the resulting burden on the health-care system has caused a shift toward prevention and management of chronic conditions. The United Nations and WHO have endorsed these efforts by allocating resources and creating goals and strategies to systematically address the burden of chronic disease (Hajat & Stein, 2018). The chronic care model creates a broader system of care with a more collaborative focus that includes the person as an active member of their health-care team. Further, mental health conditions such as depression and anxiety have long been reported to occur concurrently with chronic physical conditions (Bhattacharya et al., 2014). In fact, depression is often linked to the development of chronic diseases such as type 2 diabetes, heart disease, and hypertension (Scott et al., 2016).

Likewise, chronic physical conditions can lead to mental health conditions and have psychosocial implications (Bayliss et al., 2012). Integrating behavioral health into traditional medical care settings can result in a reduction in overall health-care cost, improve individual outcomes, and potentially improve the experience of health care (Thapa et al., 2021).

Occupational therapy practitioners (OTPs) need to understand how chronic health conditions impact the person and their occupations and how the environment interacts with these factors. OTPs work with people who have a chronic health condition, whether it is the primary reason for services or not. In this chapter readers will learn how to effectively work with people experiencing chronic conditions as well as how to promote healthy behaviors to prevent or manage them. Using an occupation-focused lens, the chapter spotlights the unique role OTPs have in supporting people to take an active role in managing their health and occupations to live fully.

This chapter explores the psychosocial impact of living with a chronic health condition by introducing people who experience them on a daily basis. These individuals, as well as their families and care partners, can benefit from collaborating with OTPs in order to take an active role in choosing and implementing strategies to manage symptoms, find ways to carry out valued occupations, and manage emotional changes and psychosocial issues related to their condition(s) on a day-to-day basis.

Although there are common principles and strategies to help people manage their conditions, interventions must be person-centered. Interventions to help people better manage their chronic health conditions are increasingly important as they enable people to participate in valued meaningful occupations and lessen complications associated with their condition(s). Moreover, interventions should not only consider the person and their occupations, but also their environment.

Description of Chronic Health Conditions

Chronic health conditions are disease processes that generally persist over the course of a lifetime and include conditions such as diabetes, heart disease, chronic lung disease, cancer, and arthritis. The CDC defines chronic diseases as conditions that last 1 year or more and require ongoing medical attention, limit activities of daily living (ADLs), or both (CDC, 2023). Others define chronic conditions as those lasting over 3 months, not passed from person to person as in communicable disease, and not likely to go away or be cured (Bernell & Howard, 2016).

Mental Health in Culture and Society

Social Determinants of Health and Systemic Racism

Evidence indicates that social determinants of health (SDOH) or "the conditions in which people are born, grow, work, live, and age" (WHO, n.d.) can impact health outcomes. For example, low household income, food insecurity, racism, and discrimination are linked to higher incidence of chronic disease and serious mental illness (Duong & Bradshaw, 2016; Jones & Neblett, 2017; Paradies et al., 2015; Tarasuk et al., 2013).

Racial and ethnic minority groups experience higher rates of illness and death from chronic conditions such as diabetes, hypertension, and heart disease compared with White populations (CDC, 2021). Black people, once believed to be genetically predisposed to hypertension, are now believed to have higher rates of hypertension because of SDOH (Davis et al., 2014). American Indian and Alaska Native people and Black people are twice as likely as White people to die from diabetes (Hill et al., 2022). In recent years, increased emphasis on holistic approaches and public scrutiny about the inequalities that exist in the health-care system have pushed public health experts and health-care organizations to consider a wider range of factors impacting health (Dean et al., 2013; Knighton et al., 2018).

Rising public consciousness about health equity issues provides a unique opportunity for OTPs to take a leadership role in assessing and addressing SDOH within the context of a person's environment to better understand factors that interact with the person and their occupations and improve health outcomes for individuals with chronic conditions.

Chronic conditions require a different kind of care than acute conditions. Acute conditions are often severe and have a sudden onset such as pneumonia, a broken bone, or an asthma attack. With acute conditions, the causes, treatments, tests, and diagnoses are often clear. The health-care team evaluates and directs treatment over a short period of time. Historically, cancer was treated as an acute condition; however, with the advancements in treatment survivors are now living decades beyond diagnosis. This has shifted cancer into being viewed as a chronic condition as survivors require ongoing monitoring and management of both their original diagnosis and long-term side effects of treatment.

With chronic conditions, the care plan will likely call for a more active role by the person and a long-term shift in the person's sense of life roles, occupations, and daily activities. As such, occupational therapy approaches in the chronic phase shift focus to health management and participation in valued activities.

Despite the type of chronic condition, people can have similar experiences. There are some common ways to manage the condition over time. For example, people with cancer and arthritis often have ongoing long-term appointments with a medical care team. People with hypertension and diabetes are asked to participate in constant monitoring and medication management. People need to manage not only the condition itself, but also the impact of the condition on their daily life. People learn to change the way they perform occupations, such as checking blood sugar before eating a meal.

New occupations often need to be integrated into daily life as well, such as learning how to use a glucometer to measure blood sugar or learning how to check one's blood pressure at

The Lived Experience

Ricardo Nunez

I was born with a visual impairment so I have always been legally blind. When I was younger it was harder for me to accept. In high school, I was told by my mobility teacher to use my cane more, but I refused to. I didn't need it and it didn't work for me. I was constantly bumping into walls and people. Other kids would ask me why I would bump into things and when I told them I was visually impaired, they would ask, "How come you don't use glasses?" I would tell them that glasses don't work for me. They would ask about the cane and I would say that doesn't help me.

When I went to college, I had to realize that no one is looking out for me, but me. I lived in the city and I realized that I had to "look" blind in order to protect myself and get the help that I needed and that's when I started using a cane. The hardest part about it is other people. For example, teachers forget I need accommodations. In the street, people are approaching me with my cane and grabbing me and not asking me if I need help, but just taking me places. The worst is when they are talking about me in front of me. Now that I have a guide dog, people don't approach me or grab me to try to help as much, but they do pay more attention to the dog. She actually gives me emotional support which is more helpful than the guide dog aspect.

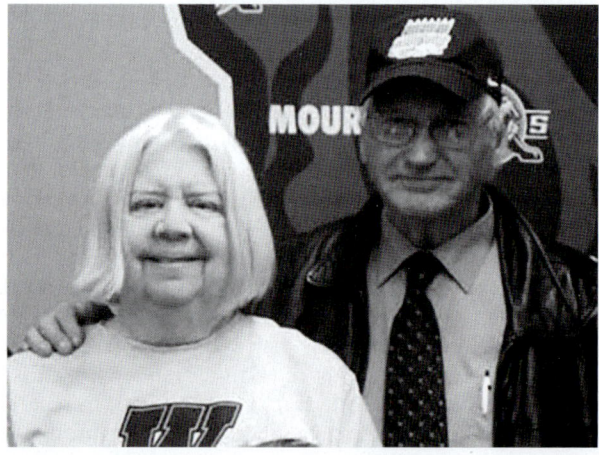

When I was 6 years old, I was diagnosed with type 1 diabetes and when I was 14, I found out I had arthritis. Arthritis affects me the least. With arthritis, it's not as stressful as the blindness and the diabetes. The hardest part about dealing with diabetes is different doctors telling me different things and telling me I'm doing things wrong. I've had diabetes for 23 years. I know my body and my blood sugar enough to know what works for me. I get frustrated when I have to tell

The Lived Experience—cont'd

doctors, "Hey, I already tried that and it doesn't work for me." They put me under the same umbrella as other people, but I also deal with anxiety and what works for them might not work for me. It is really overwhelming at times.

When my blood sugar is up, I have to stop everything that I'm doing to inject insulin, to get some exercise and then it is an ongoing cycle because the stress makes my blood sugar go up, too. Also, when my blood sugar goes up, my body tightens up. When it goes down, I get anxious because if I go outside without anything like insulin or I exercise too much, it might go down. If I go to sleep, I may not wake up again. These are thoughts that I have to work with.

When I'm working with doctors and therapists, I want them to have more compassion. Take the time to understand.

It becomes frustrating when you are being told you are doing something wrong. When you have to explain, "I know what works for me and what doesn't." Instead, listen to my experience and support me to do what I want to do.

Recently, I started a podcast with my cousin and my friend who each have different visual impairments. My brother, who has dyslexia, eventually joined us, too. We choose a topic and talk about it based on our different perspectives and personalities living life. It is called "See It Through My Eyes." It is a way to have everyone talk about their take on a topic. In my 20s, I became comfortable in my own skin and decided that being legally blind is a part of me and it is going to be a part of my life so I need to cope with it and not live in denial and shame.

---

home. Furthermore, there might be a need to modify social roles or work roles. The disease itself can create uncertainty as well as emotional distress. Regardless of how and when the chronic condition began, the experience and management of the condition can have common stressors related to managing a chronic disease. Moreover, many of these stressors can arise from the sociocultural environment. In the preceding Lived Experience feature, Ricardo describes the intersectionality of his identity as a blind person and how the sociocultural environment impacts and sometimes hinders his ability to manage his chronic conditions.

Psychosocial Experience of Chronic Health Conditions

Living with a chronic health condition can elicit various emotional and psychological changes. If the condition is difficult to diagnose, often people can feel frustrated, angry, or disappointed in the health-care team. Some experience anger and grief, whereas others have prolonged distress related to managing the condition. Box 17.1 lists common emotional experiences for people living with chronic health conditions. Some psychological changes are distinct to certain chronic health conditions because of the nature of how they are experienced.

Posttraumatic Stress Symptoms and Posttraumatic Growth

Some chronic conditions, especially those that involve more immediate risk of death or invasive medical procedures such as cancer or cardiac conditions, can result in a person experiencing **posttraumatic stress symptoms** (PTSS). PTSS refer to symptoms similar to those experienced with posttraumatic stress disorder (PTSD), but they do not meet the full criteria for PTSD diagnosis (Pinquart, 2018). Individuals who experience PTSS do not always progress to a clinical diagnosis of PTSD, but they might experience symptoms such as nervousness, fear, intrusive dreams, and anxious thoughts.

> **BOX 17-1 ■ Common Emotions Related to Living With a Chronic Condition**
>
> - Sadness
> - Anger
> - Disbelief
> - Confusion
> - Stress
> - Overwhelm
> - Fear
> - Denial
> - Guilt
> - Loneliness
> - Grief
> - Distress

Although subclinical, PTSS can still greatly impact a person's mental health and ability to participate in daily occupations. In a survey of both hospitalized and nonhospitalized patients following COVID-19 illness, 37.2% reported PTSS 3 months posttreatment (Houben-Wilke et al., 2022).

Posttraumatic growth (PTG) is a more positive psychosocial process experienced by some people with chronic conditions. This term is used to describe the process by which individuals who have encountered a traumatic event reinterpret and find positive meaning in that event (Marziliano et al., 2020). PTG can provide a protective factor against the impact of psychological distress on quality of life (Shand et al., 2015). Growth can be supported by social participation, volunteer work, and physical activity (Connerty & Knott, 2013). See Chapter 5: Trauma-Informed Practice. 🤝

Both PTSS and PTG are frequently found to occur in the cancer population posttreatment. Many individuals experience PTSS and PTG at the same time and can cycle through both while going through the process of coping with their diagnosis and/or treatment (Marziliano et al., 2020). Finding a positive meaning in response to a distressing event can serve as a protective factor. This can have both short-term and long-term impacts on a person's functioning and quality of life.

In the following The Lived Experience feature, Kathy shares the cyclical nature of cancer over the course of her lifetime and dual experience of psychosocial stress and the

The Lived Experience

Kathy Waldinger

First you cry, then you pray. I was having the good life. Two kids in college and only one more at home. I was a healthy, active 46-year-old in the fall of 1993. It was breast cancer awareness month. I never checked my breasts in the shower or otherwise, but all the news and magazines were pushing for check, check, check. So, I was lying on my back on the couch one day and I checked. My heart stopped when I felt a small lump. I told my daughter, "I feel lumpy." She said you need to check it out. So, I called for a doctor appointment. My doctor felt it and said he thought it probably was a benign cyst but just in case will do a mammogram and a needle biopsy. He said it did not have the characteristics of cancer by feeling it. I was relieved and made an appointment for a needle biopsy. That came out okay. Next stop: The mammogram.

Another week later of stress and anxiety, the nurse calls me to tell me good news: The mammogram is clear! I go driving right out into the field where my husband was harvesting corn and jump on the combine, crying and telling my husband the good news.

The doctor said that he knew I was a nervous person and that it was most likely a benign tumor, but I should get it out. He made an appointment for me to see a surgeon. Another week goes by. The waiting is killing me. The surgeon feels it and says the same thing. "It doesn't feel like cancer but let's just take it out anyway." No harm no foul. So, I go in for a lumpectomy. He said it was a 96% chance it would be clear. He later apologized for that statement. I am in the operating room and the whole room gets dead silent. He tells the nurse to take it to lab. He knew.

Another appointment is made for the results. He calmly said to bring my husband along. By this time 4 weeks had passed on the roller coaster ride. I suspected something when I came into the room and the examination bed was propped up. Apparently, they did not want me to pass out. He told us it was cancer and gave us options. This was when the lumpectomy was just becoming popular. My husband asked him what he would do if it was his wife. He said he would treat it like "white on a golf ball" and get a bilateral mastectomy. Being a little bit of a wild person, I told him my breasts were too small anyway just take them both. So that's what we did.

The big topic in all the news and magazines was about lymph nodes. It was conventional wisdom that if it was in your lymph nodes it was a death sentence. Well guess what? It was in my lymph nodes. He took twelve and it was in five. I'm doomed. Depression sets in. You cry and then prayer becomes a priority.

Now I'm meeting my cancer doctor. A real gem. He said not to put too much into the lymph node thing. He said he had patients who had a lumpectomy and no lymph involvement and were gone in 5 years. Others who had lymph node involvement and lived to be in their nineties and died of something else. So, I decided that's going to be me! My neighbor happened to be working as a pathologist in the lab when my breasts came in. She came down to my house a few weeks later with a big pizza to tell me that I had made a good decision. The cancer was also starting in my other breast. WE got it all!

The chemo begins. Once a month for 6 months. They take about 3 hours. They give you chipped ice in a paper cup. I cannot drink out of a paper cup anymore. I wore the same jacket every time. When it was all over, I gave away the jacket. One month after my first chemo, I lost my hair all at once pulling out clumps in the shower. I thought "I better go show my boys as they will have to get used to seeing me that way." One says, "You look like Yoda" and the other says "You look like grandpa." Oh well. A good laugh. Right away I got a wig. I did not want to make others feel uncomfortable seeing my bald head. I tolerated the chemo well and did not miss one time. Yes, it made me feel weirder a week after each one but I looked at it like killing the cancer and decided not to dwell on the side effects.

Stupid things people say to a cancer survivor: I'm in the hospital one day after the surgery and a lady from church calls me and scolds me for not letting her know about my surgery and do I want it in the bulletin? "Kathy Waldinger—cancer." NO! Another lady calls to tell me all about her friend who died of breast cancer. Then she proceeded to tell me how sorry she was, sorry for anything she had said or did to me, only to clear her conscience before I died, I'm sure. "Thanks." Bang! I hung up. I'm at a community dinner and a lady says, "Oh! You are here? Do you eat?" Duh. Yes, and I breathe, talk, and walk. Some people stay away. They are afraid they are going to catch it. If you have not had cancer, you have no idea what it's like. There are many people who are supportive and know just what to say.

In 1993, I told a friend of mine, a fellow mother, that I was afraid I was never going to see my son graduate high school. Four years later at graduation she comes up to me and taps me on the shoulder and says "You made it!" Our preacher said to me, "You know there are worse things than dying." My faith tells me that there are better times to come after we die.

I decided early on that I would try to be positive. While in the hospital, I had a Reach to Recovery volunteer come in to visit and she was very positive. She told me stories about bending over to try on shoes in a shoe store and her boob fell out! She told me when you need to cry, get a sad movie and cry. Get in the shower and cry, cry, cry. Let it all out. And when you need to laugh, really laugh and enjoy every happy thing that comes along. I tried to go to the local breast cancer support group but it was very hard for me emotionally. I felt like it was revisiting the plane wreck every month. Many of the women there were wringing their hands and saying woe is me. There were some who were positive and became role models.

I decided instead to become a Reach to Recovery volunteer. In the training video, they showed a video of a lumpectomy patient. I disliked it and had feelings of jealousy. This patient is still whole. I know why I was assigned to patients who had mastectomies. I wanted to be positive and help people laugh. One of the stories I would tell my patients was how when I ordered my new prostheses, I decided that if I was going to have to pay $500 a piece for each one, I was going to get big

The Lived Experience—cont'd

ones (my real breasts were AA) so I got C's! When I came home sporting my new big breasts, I stuck out my chest to show my husband and his eyes about popped out of his head. Another good laugh.

After chemo, you have to go to the dreaded checkups. First, every 2 months, then they spread out over time for the next 5 long years. Roller coaster ride for sure. Your emotions are all over the place and you hold your breath, get a bunch of tests and wait and wait for the news. Is it coming back? I lived for a long time in denial. I never looked in the mirror. Finally, you get the news—you are cancer free. In 1995, when all the chemo and everything was over, I decided that this would be the first day of the rest of my life. I went back to school and got my Master's degree and got a job teaching. No more cancer. I loved my job and was smiling everyday . . . kids will do that to you!

I went to my first Susan G Komen Race for the Cure. What struck me was that cancer survivors got pink shirts so you *knew* who had it. There were so many young women! Many had a child in a back pack. We were told to gather up and start walking toward the starting line. I had no idea what was coming next. I was not prepared. The crowd on the side lines with white shirts began to cheer and clap. I cried. It was a moment I will never forget. I went back every year as long as I could and soon, I began to become proud of my pink shirt. I began to count the months and the years. I was a survivor.

Fast forward 29 years. I was chatting with a friend of mine from church. She had found a lump under her arm that was cancer. She's a nurse and asked me if I ever checked? God wink. No, why should I? They took it all. I'm a survivor! She told me to check around anyway. So, I did. Remember denial? I found a small lump under my arm! Something told me to mention it at my next wellness check with the doctor. Here we go again. She sent me to the same surgeon. He said 4% chance it is cancer after all these years. I reminded him of his last prediction and he apologized. After 6 weeks of "watching

it" (anxiety) I went back for a final checkup. He was sure that it was not cancer but said just to make sure before I let you go let's do a sonogram.

They rolled in the machine. I watched as it showed upon the screen. Next, we decided to take it out. Indeed, I had blown the odds again. It was cancer. First, I cried but it was different this time. I was going to own it and use it for the good of others. I had been given almost 30 years, so I was grateful. I approached it head on. I had it taken out and agreed to 6 weeks of radiation, 5 days a week. It took me longer to get to the radiation building than it did to get the treatment. A friend of mine from church helped me through it by texting me every day and we counted down the days.

I decided it was going to be an experience I would use to help others with radiation as now I would have that experience. The checkups arrive with the same doctor I had 29 years ago. It was back to a thriller coaster ride; all was going well when 2 years later a tumor marker test came back wacky. They ordered a CT scan. Waiting for the results was agony until I had a talk with myself to be thankful for the testing, be glad for technology to find anything before it turned into something. It was clear. "See you in 3 months!" I realize this is just another bump in the road of life. I continue to take one day at a time and am thankful for every day. I have had other health issues over the years like appendicitis, pancreatitis, gallbladder removal, kidney removal because of stones, diabetes and arthritis.

I try to approach each issue with a positive attitude. I am fortunate to have a supportive family including nine beautiful grandchildren, two daughters-in-law and one son-in-law. I am truly blessed to have a husband who has always treated me with love for 52 years. Two sons who love to laugh with me and my emotional support person, my daughter. As the singer Pink says, "The panic is maybe temporary but when you can't, I will walk you through the turbulence. You are alive, that means you are committed to survive."

positive meaning she was able to find during her journey. Researchers are trying to better understand this complex relationship, but many feel that growth postdiagnosis can help survivors reframe experiences and perceive potential benefits from that experience, which can help moderate symptoms of PTSS (Marziliano et al., 2020; Shand et al., 2015). For practitioners working with these people, it is important to know that each individual will have a unique experience with PTSS and PTG. OTPs should screen for and provide preventive measures for PTSS as well as be aware of and support PTG when it occurs in individuals.

Diabetes Distress

Although the psychosocial impacts of chronic conditions vary widely depending on each individual's unique experiences, some patterns have emerged over time. **Diabetes distress** is one example. This well-documented condition is the emotional response to the stress of managing and living with diabetes, including treatment, symptoms, and the social impact

of chronic illness (Snoek et al., 2015). People with diabetes distress experience an increase in difficult emotions, such as irritability, sadness, fear, anxiety, and depression. These often revolve around the complex self-care routines necessary to manage diabetes, the effects of diabetes on relationships with friends and family, and difficulty finding knowledgeable, trusted health-care providers (Polonsky et al., 2022).

Diabetes distress can have a significant influence on patient outcomes; it has been associated with poor self-management of diabetes and difficulty engaging in management (Aikens, 2012). Therefore, it can also lead to poor glycemic control (Gonzalez et al., 2015; Strandberg et al., 2015). Diabetes distress often presents as a cycle; when patients become overwhelmed, it's more difficult for them to engage in diabetes self-care, which increases their diabetes symptoms and, therefore, their distress. Conversely, decreases in diabetes distress have been associated with decreases in A1c (a biomarker indicating overall control of the disease) through the mechanism of improved self-care (Hessler et al., 2021; Zagarins et al., 2012).

Mental Illness in Culture and Society

Protective Factors

Utilizing a strengths-based approach, OTPs who incorporate protective factors into the occupational therapy process can promote and facilitate positive outcomes with people experiencing chronic conditions. Self-efficacy, social support, and positive emotions such as optimism and gratitude can act as protective factors against disease-related distress and overwhelm for many chronic conditions (American Association of Diabetes Educators, 2020). Furthermore, cultural protective factors can be maximized to tailor interventions; while some societal attitudes emphasize the negative aspects of certain minoritized groups, cultural humility and a strengths-based approach recognize that each culture has inherent strengths that serve as protective factors and can mitigate the impact of chronic conditions.

There is emerging evidence that racial, ethnic, and cultural protective factors are linked to better outcomes for people experiencing chronic conditions (Jones & Neblett, 2016; Koinis-Mitchell et al., 2012; Ramirez et al., 2022). Although there is a need to recognize that each cultural group is heterogeneous, some individuals ascribe to distinct cultural values of the larger group. For example, the Latino ideal of familismo, family connectedness and ideals of collectivism, can serve as protective factors in groups that are experiencing higher rates of chronic conditions such as diabetes and asthma (Koinis-Mitchell et al., 2012; Ramirez et al., 2022). By targeting these positive cultural attributes with humility, OTPs can utilize culturally tailored interventions that may enhance the management of a chronic condition.

Roughly 30% of patients with diabetes experience diabetes distress, and the risks of developing it are believed to be higher among underserved communities, youth, and individuals with more severe diabetes symptoms and additional comorbidities (Snoek et al., 2015). Gariepy and colleagues (2013) found that neighborhood characteristics can also impact diabetes distress rates; residents of safe, well-maintained neighborhoods with sufficient social and material resources reported lower rates of diabetes distress.

Factors such as lack of parks or trails where one can exercise, absence of stores with fresh produce for preparing healthy meals, and limited access to local medical care can profoundly impact health outcomes and raise levels of diabetes distress. The effect of diabetes distress on occupational performance is different for each person. Research suggests that as diabetes distress increases, both work and life productivity decrease (Xu et al., 2020).

As the role of occupational therapy in primary and specialty care increases, the opportunity for OTPs to address diabetes distress is growing. There are several formal programs developed by OTPs and other allied health professionals to address diabetes distress by providing patient education on diabetes management, training patients on goal setting, or strengthening emotional regulation skills.

The Diabetes Distress Scale is a self-report survey evaluating diabetes distress, including subscores for emotional burden, physician-related distress, regimen-related distress, and interpersonal distress. The scale can be used by OTPs as a tool to better understand how distress is impacting a person (Polonsky et al., 2022). Fisher and colleagues (2013) assert that the program methods and structure may be less important than "health care professionals listening to, understanding, acknowledging, and normalizing DD (diabetes distress) so that patients' internal resources can become freer of internal distress–related constraints" (Fisher et al., 2013, p. 2557). These skills are within reach for any OTP, even those without specialized training in diabetes or diabetes distress.

Overwhelm

Living with chronic conditions can result in **overwhelm**, a general term often used in health-care settings when patients have difficulty managing the combined challenges of their **illness burden** (e.g., the impact of symptoms such as pain or fatigue), **treatment burden** (e.g., time, energy, and cognitive load required to adhere to treatment regimens), and environmental or social contexts (e.g., race, socioeconomic status, level of social support, neighborhood characteristics), along with their other valued occupations such as caregiving, work/school, and social participation (Tran et al., 2020).

The cumulative complexity model (Shippee et al., 2012) was developed to describe the experience of people with chronic illness and multimorbidities, in which an individual's capacity is decreased by burden of illness at the same time that workload is increased by burden of treatment (Fig. 17-1). **Workload** encompasses the many tasks related to the patient role, including acquiring, synthesizing, and operationalizing health-related knowledge; making and attending appointments to access information and treatment; establishing and maintaining self-care habits and routines; and monitoring and appraising the effect of this work on health (Leppin et al., 2015).

Often the workload associated with the patient role and the occupation of health management is the time and energy equivalent of a part-time job (Buffel du Vaure et al., 2016). One study of over 2,400 people with chronic conditions found that nearly

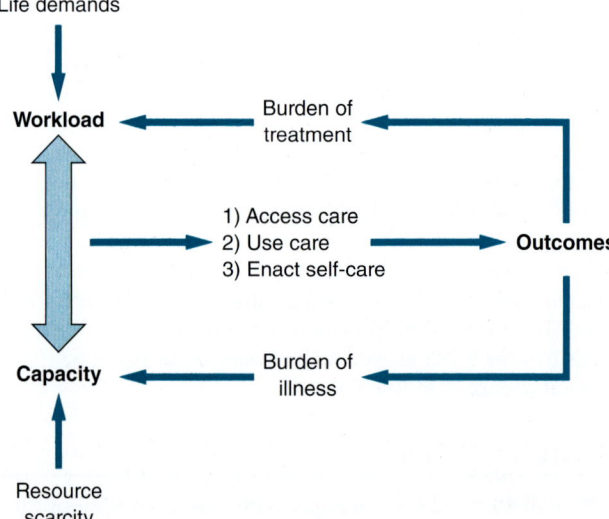

FIGURE 17-1. The Cumulative Complexity Model. *From Leppin, A., Montori, V., & Gionfriddo, M. (2015). Minimally Disruptive Medicine: A pragmatically comprehensive model for delivering care to patients with multiple chronic conditions. Healthcare, 3(1), 50–63. https://doi .org/10.3390/healthcare3010050*

40% of participants rated their treatment burden as unsustainable (Tran et al., 2020). **Capacity** is "the sum total of resources and abilities that a patient can draw on" and includes "physical, mental, social, financial, personal, and environmental domains" (Leppin et al., 2015, p. 52). The relationship between workload and capacity is dynamic, with both aspects fluctuating based on each individual's circumstances at any given time.

When there is workload-capacity imbalance, overwhelm occurs. Patients may disengage from health management, either consciously or unconsciously. They may stop all self-care tasks or continue some aspects of self-care that are most convenient or valuable to them. Therefore, their health-related outcomes typically decline.

Understanding how the balance between workload and capacity affects overwhelm is essential to OTPs working with people with chronic conditions. It's vital that OTPs know both the workload and capacity of their patients in order to appropriately grade and adapt treatment to address individual needs. Minimally Disruptive Medicine (MDM) is an approach to health care that takes into account cumulative complexity and aims to maximize patients' progress toward their own goals (both health related and general) while contributing as little as possible to treatment burden or overwhelm (Leppin et al., 2015).

Therapists can use MDM as a framework to inform their treatment of people with chronic conditions. This means adjusting the intensity of therapy (including home programs) to avoid overwhelming patients. MDM can also be a helpful framework for understanding systems level change needed to better avoid person overwhelm, such as simplified scheduling processes, increased individual access to care coordination services, and streamlined referral to outside resources such as community-based programs that address environmental and social needs such as housing insecurity or lack of child care.

Cognitive Load

Competing priorities, especially for those with multiple chronic conditions, can lead to a sense of diminished resources for all that one must do to manage their health. One may experience impaired cognitive capacity directly related to symptoms of disease or because of cognitive demand exceeding capacity. These challenges might be misidentified by providers as lack of engagement, lack of adherence, or poor ability to problem-solve. More accurately, challenges might be better attributed to difficulty processing and attending to new information because of a naturally limited working memory capacity.

Cognitive load is the amount of information working memory can handle at any given time. When experiencing a chronic condition, the influx of new information can overwhelm natural capacity, outpacing the available cognitive resources. Consequently, it becomes a challenge to process the information presented at the clinic, make decisions regarding course of treatment, or manage all of the tasks that factor into the occupation of disease self-management. People with multiple chronic conditions experience cognitive behavioral challenges that often go unaddressed in standard primary care clinics or traditional medical settings where chronic disease is treated (Winship et al., 2019).

Assessments might consider a person's self-report on the extent to which they are able to engage in their daily health management tasks as well as their valued roles and occupations. Interventions might focus on the environmental level and involve the OTP collaborating with the provider team on strategies to streamline health management tasks and thereby reduce cognitive load. Intervention may also focus inward on the person, with the OTP and person engaging in mindfulness exercises such as meditation.

Habits and routines can be modified or adjusted to decrease cognitive load. For example, the OTP may inquire about a person's daily habits and strategize timing medications with established habits and routines to decrease the cognitive demand of remembering to take a medication. By decreasing the cognitive demand of some of the responsibilities associated with chronic disease management, cognitive abilities can be better redirected to those complex activities and occupations that need them the most. For more information see Chapter 7: Cognition and Chapter 14: Time Use and Habits. 🤝

Psychiatric Conditions Associated With Chronic Health Conditions

Depression and anxiety are the most common mental illnesses associated with chronic disease (Bhattacharya et al., 2014). Depression is connected to diabetes, cardiovascular disease, arthritis, COPD, asthma, and hypertension. Anxiety alone is linked to arthritis, COPD, heart disease, and hypertension. When depression and anxiety co-occur, the associations between chronic health conditions increase.

In a survey of 17 countries exploring the association of chronic illness and mental health conditions, depression and anxiety were associated with 10 chronic physical conditions: asthma, arthritis, back/neck problems, chronic headache, diabetes, heart disease, hypertension, multiple pains, obesity, and ulcer (Scott et al., 2016). PTSD and the mere experience of a traumatic event are related to the development of chronic diseases including type 2 diabetes, cardiovascular disease, hypertension, asthma, arthritis, and respiratory disease (Scott et al., 2013). Anywhere from 5% to 27% of cancer survivors met the clinical diagnosis requirements for PTSD during or posttreatment (Marziliano et al., 2020). Chronic health conditions can lead to mental illness; likewise, the presence of mental health conditions can precipitate chronic disease, resulting in overall poor self-reported quality of life (Bayliss et al., 2012).

When people experience mental illness and a chronic health condition simultaneously, evidence indicates that focusing intervention on the psychiatric condition can impact the physical condition and vice versa (Fig. 17-2). For example, for people who have co-occurring depression and chronic disease, treating the depression can have a cascading impact on the chronic disease. Further, providing tailored care focused on health promotion and disease prevention with people experiencing mental illness can result in improvements in the quality and quantity of their life.

An integrated behavioral health model has been established as an ideal approach for fostering these interventions and has been shown to improve health outcomes, reduce depression, and reduce health-care utilization (Balasubramanian et al., 2017; Dobbins et al., 2016; Miller et al., 2017; Ross et al., 2019). OTPs bring unique expertise to an integrated health-care approach with a focus on how a person's habits, routines, roles, and their environments

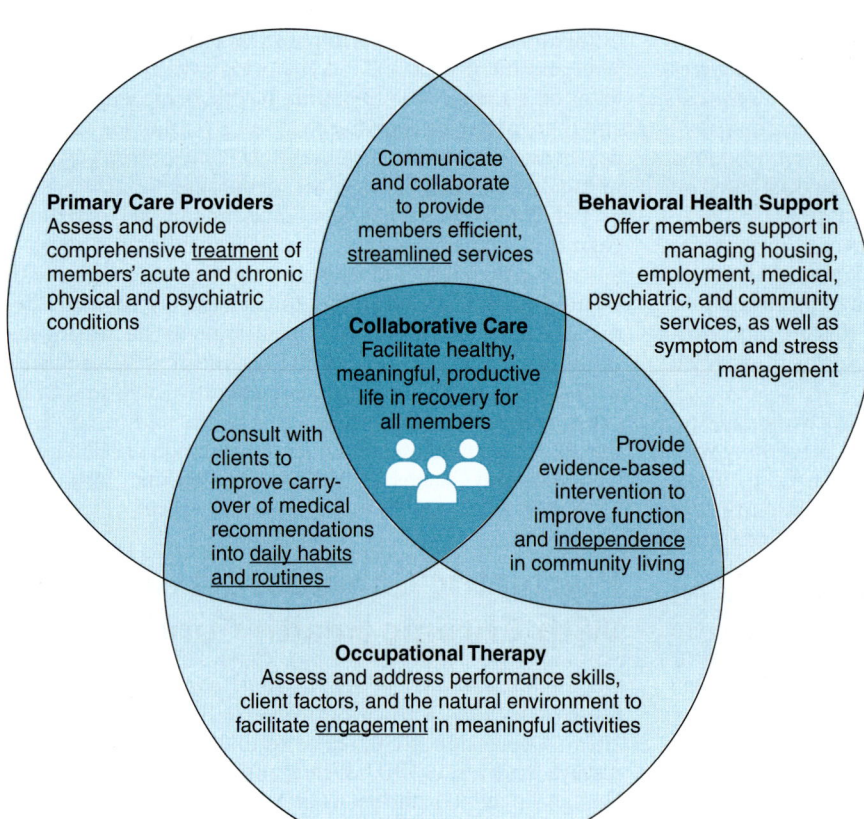

Primary Care Providers
Assess and provide comprehensive <u>treatment</u> of members' acute and chronic physical and psychiatric conditions

Communicate and collaborate to provide members efficient, <u>streamlined</u> services

Behavioral Health Support
Offer members support in managing housing, employment, medical, psychiatric, and community services, as well as symptom and stress management

Collaborative Care
Facilitate healthy, meaningful, productive life in recovery for all members

Consult with clients to improve carry-over of medical recommendations into <u>daily habits and routines</u>

Provide evidence-based intervention to improve function and <u>independence</u> in community living

Occupational Therapy
Assess and address performance skills, client factors, and the natural environment to facilitate <u>engagement</u> in meaningful activities

FIGURE 17-2. Occupational therapy in integrated behavioral healthcare. *Retrieved from Ferlin, A., Fischer, H., Januszewski, C., & Hahn, B. (2019, January). Occupational therapy in integrated behavioral healthcare: A visual service framework. OT Practice, 24(1), 12–17.*

influence their ability to implement health-care recommendations, which can directly impact the management of their chronic condition. Using an occupational lens, practitioners can promote a sense of competency, identity, and well-being and promote healthy lifestyle routines and habits to a wide variety of populations and diagnoses (Dahl-Popolizi et al., 2016; Ferlin et al., 2019; Januszewski & Lukaszewski, 2017; Koverman et al., 2017; Mahaffey, 2009).

Impact of Chronic Health Conditions on Occupational Performance and Participation

Chronic conditions can impact how people perform occupations, as it may require them to learn new occupations and alter participation in daily life. In particular, managing the condition itself can become the central occupation since engaging in the necessary daily routines related to the condition are often required to maintain and promote overall health so that one can participate in all other meaningful occupations. Not only is participation in ADLs impacted by the condition, but living with the condition necessitates new ADLs, instrumental ADLs (IADLs), and occupations.

For example, preparing a meal may be impacted by the symptoms of a chronic condition such as low vision because of diabetes. However, diabetes itself often requires a modification of the occupation of eating as it can directly impact blood glucose levels and alter insulin needs. In this section, self-care, health management, and social participation are highlighted as areas that can be addressed with people who are experiencing chronic conditions.

Self-Care

When considering self-care in the context of chronic illness, it is helpful to think of the symptom-related difficulty of completing ADLs as well as the added challenge of unique self-care tasks that arise because of chronic illness. For someone with a chronic condition, everyday tasks such as bathing, dressing, and eating may take more time and energy to complete. For example, during the survivorship phase of cancer, one might experience cancer-related fatigue and require frequent breaks during grooming. With the onset of a chronic condition, ADL routines may need to change based on physical, emotional, or cognitive changes related to illness.

In addition to challenges completing common ADLs, people with chronic illness also have the additional demand of condition-specific self-care tasks required to maintain their health. In many occupational therapy practice frameworks globally, the self-care tasks related to managing a chronic health condition are included in the occupation of *health management,* which is described in the next section. See Chapter 45: Self-Care and Well-Being Occupations.

Health Management

The World Federation of Occupational Therapy (WFOT) defines occupational therapy as "a client-centered health profession concerned with promoting health and wellbeing through occupation" (WFOT, 2012). The American Occupational Therapy Association (AOTA) recently recognized the centrality of health and wellness by introducing **health management** as an occupation. Health management includes "activities related to developing, managing, and maintaining health and wellness routines, including self-management, with the goal of improving or maintaining health to support participation in other occupations" (AOTA, 2020, p. 32). Engagement in these activities can have a positive impact on achieving wellness with a chronic condition.

Components of health management include (AOTA, 2020):

- Social and emotional health promotion and maintenance
- Symptom and condition management
- Communication with the health system
- Medication management
- Physical activity
- Nutrition management
- Personal care device management

People may work on one or more areas of health management depending on the challenges they face. Although two people may work on the same area of health management, the issues they face may be different and thus the approach will be tailored. For example, one person may need emotional support to engage in positive communication with health-care providers, whereas another may need support to problem-solve the electronic communication system used in their health system.

When considering these unique health management tasks, it is useful to draw on related knowledge from the interdisciplinary team, such as nursing. As alluded to previously, integrated interdisciplinary care of people with chronic disease is considered best practice (Fig. 17-3). Although self-care tasks in the context of chronic disease vary based on condition, they tend to fall into three categories. *Self-care maintenance*

tasks keep health stable and are often informed by guidance from health-care professionals (Riegel et al., 2019). Consistently following a prescribed medication regimen is an example of self-care maintenance.

Self-care monitoring tasks provide information about changes or fluctuations in health (Riegel et al., 2019). They can include objective monitoring, such as recording daily blood pressure readings, and subjective monitoring, such as observing changes in one's own pain or fatigue levels. *Self-care management* tasks use information gathered during monitoring to recognize changes in health and adjust maintenance in response, in an effort to return to a stable state (Riegel et al., 2019). For example, an individual with rheumatoid arthritis may notice increased pain and joint swelling and adjust their diet or medication to address those concerns.

For some conditions, there are well-defined self-care behaviors developed by clinicians and researchers that provide guidance to individuals. In the case of diabetes, the Association of Diabetes Care and Education Specialists (formerly American Association of Diabetes Educators) has identified seven self-care behaviors and focused their education efforts on building patients' skills in those areas. The core behavior is *healthy coping*, which facilitates the other six behaviors and is required for sustainable diabetes management (American Association of Diabetes Educators, 2020).

Healthy coping directly addressed the mental health impact of diabetes by encouraging people to proactively build skills to manage the difficult feelings or situations that may arise from living with a chronic condition. The daily behaviors of *taking medication, healthy eating*, and *being active* make up the second tier of self-care and are often at the core of early treatment planning. *Monitoring* is a parallel to Riegel and colleagues' (2019) *self-care monitoring* and informs the other behaviors. It includes

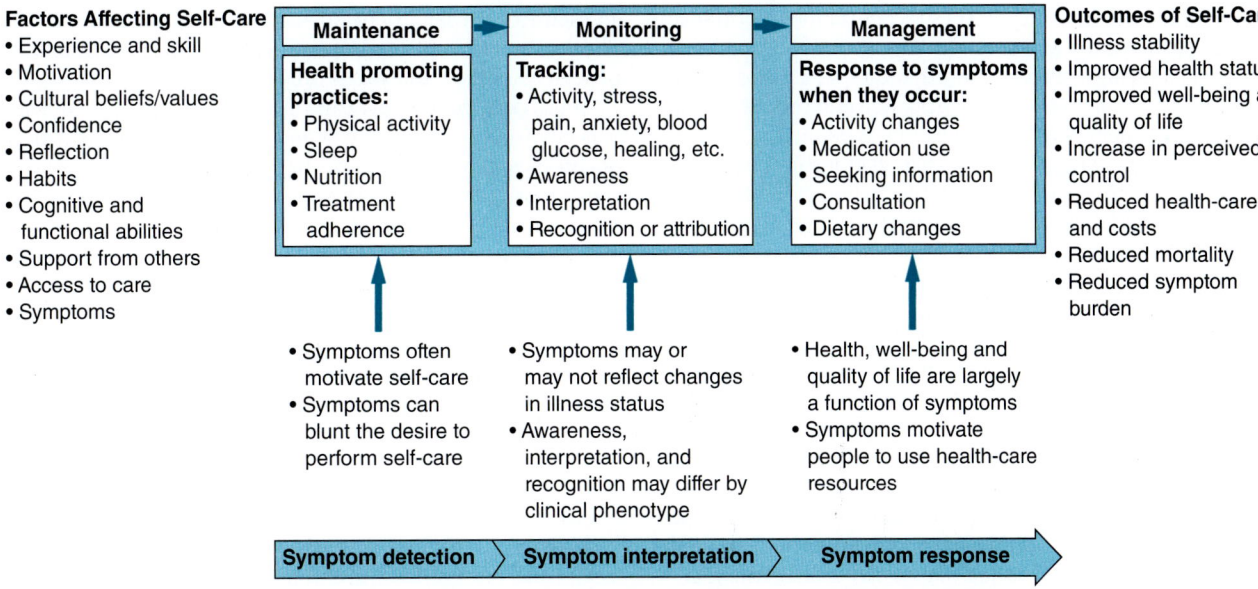

Self-Care of Chronic Illness

Factors Affecting Self-Care	Maintenance	Monitoring	Management	Outcomes of Self-Care
• Experience and skill • Motivation • Cultural beliefs/values • Confidence • Reflection • Habits • Cognitive and functional abilities • Support from others • Access to care • Symptoms	**Health promoting practices:** • Physical activity • Sleep • Nutrition • Treatment adherence	**Tracking:** • Activity, stress, pain, anxiety, blood glucose, healing, etc. • Awareness • Interpretation • Recognition or attribution	**Response to symptoms when they occur:** • Activity changes • Medication use • Seeking information • Consultation • Dietary changes	• Illness stability • Improved health status • Improved well-being and quality of life • Increase in perceived control • Reduced health-care use and costs • Reduced mortality • Reduced symptom burden
	• Symptoms often motivate self-care • Symptoms can blunt the desire to perform self-care	• Symptoms may or may not reflect changes in illness status • Awareness, interpretation, and recognition may differ by clinical phenotype	• Health, well-being and quality of life are largely a function of symptoms • Symptoms motivate people to use health-care resources	

Symptom detection 〉 Symptom interpretation 〉 Symptom response

FIGURE 17-3. Model integrating symptoms with self-care as defined by the Middle-Range Theory of Self-Care of Chronic Illness. Although depicted here as linear, the self-care process features feedback loops. Note that the overlap between the bottom arrows and core self-care model is both theoretical and imperfect and indeed a target of further refinement. *Reprinted with permission from Riegel, B., Jaarsma, T., Lee, C. S., & Strömberg, A. (2019). Integrating symptoms into the Middle-Range Theory of Self-Care of Chronic Illness. Advances in Nursing Science, 42(3), 206–215. https://doi.org/10.1097/ANS.0000000000000237*

not only blood glucose testing, but also documenting blood pressure, activity level, food intake, weight, medication adherence, foot health, oral health, mood, and sleep. *Problem-solving* and *reducing risks* require the highest levels of skill and health literacy; they often drive goal setting and action planning.

For people with chronic conditions, actively engaging in health-related self-care has been linked to improved quality of life (Auld et al., 2018) and fewer hospitalizations (Vellone et al., 2017). For cancer survivors, health-related self-care, such as being active and healthy eating, may help combat long-term side effects of treatment. But although disease-specific self-care behaviors are life sustaining for individuals with chronic conditions, they're also physically, emotionally, and cognitively taxing.

One must learn a host of new skills, ranging from the concrete, such as how to use a blood pressure monitor, to the abstract, such as how to navigate competing concerns of health, relationships, finances, and other major life areas. They require a significant commitment and motivation. It's been estimated that adults with established type 2 diabetes require up to 4 hours *per day* for self-care (Shubrook et al., 2018). That level of demand on patients' finite resources, such as time and energy, can lead to burnout or disengagement from self-care or health care (Fisher et al., 2019). Self-efficacy, social support, and positive emotions such as optimism and gratitude can act as protective factors against disease-related distress and overwhelm for many chronic conditions (American Association of Diabetes Educators, 2020).

Motivational Interviewing can be considered as an approach to increase engagement in health management behaviors. For more information on Motivational Interviewing see Chapter 11: Motivation.

Social Participation

Social participation is defined as activities that involve interaction with others including family, friends, peers, and community members (AOTA, 2020). OTPs recognize the importance of social participation as a crucial component of occupational well-being. Having a chronic condition can put a person at an increased risk for lack of social participation and result in social isolation and loneliness. "Social isolation" is defined as "having infrequent social contact or few social relationships," whereas "loneliness" is defined as "the subjective feeling of being alone, regardless of social interactions" (National Academies of Sciences, Engineering, and Medicine [NASEM], 2020).

Social isolation and loneliness can be risk factors for poor health; they can also arise from the limitations of having a chronic condition (Christiansen et al., 2021). There is a growing body of evidence connecting social isolation and loneliness as risk factors for poor health outcomes (NASEM, 2020). Social connections and support can help people be more able to cope with stress and minimize the impact of stress on their well-being (Christiansen et al., 2021).

Disruption of social participation in people with chronic conditions is common. Social participation may be disrupted because of the time and burden of new self-management activities such as attending physician visits, hospitalizations, and receiving care (Meek et al., 2018). Adults with chronic conditions often report restricting social engagements by skipping social activities, participating less in community engagement or volunteering, and limiting interactions with family and friends (Meek et al., 2018). People may avoid social activities because of fear of judgment or feelings of being a burden to others (Disler et al., 2012; Meek et al., 2018). People who acquire a chronic condition in childhood or as an adolescent may experience social isolation that continues through adulthood. Less time to develop social connections can result in a disruption of social skill developments that result in marked social isolation and decreased quality of life (Howard et al., 2014).

Fostering the development of social skills and the establishment or maintenance of social occupations can be crucial in long-term well-being. Children and adolescents who experience a successful reengagement in social activities were found to perceive themselves as more socially competent and did not report a disruption in social participation later in adulthood (Howard et al., 2014). Similarly, adults who participated in a community reentry program with a focus on social engagement increased their self-efficacy and decreased feelings of loneliness (Kalina et al., 2018). For more information about social engagement see Chapter 13: Communication and Social Skills and Chapter 49: Connectedness and Belonging.

Impact of the Environment on Occupational Performance for People With Chronic Conditions

Environmental factors make up a critical component of assessment and intervention in chronic disease care. An individual's environment is a key player in their capacity to develop routines and habits. Consistent occupational performance requires a certain amount of environmental stability, and the environment also becomes a part of performance (Taylor, 2017). Consider the role of the environment in diabetes care. Family can impact diabetes management and diabetes management in turn can impact the family. Cultural context can influence the value placed on food, the meaning of weight gain or loss, and sense of burden to a health-care system (Youngson, 2019). Physical activity options depend on the climate, time and financial resources, and social influences.

Social determinants of health (SDOH) are part of an individual's environment and context and influence self-management of chronic disease. Among primary care patients with chronic conditions, adverse SDOH are associated with poorer functional capacity (Bonnell et al., 2021). Neighborhood income and stability, perception of neighborhood problems and safety, and walkability influence health outcomes. In individuals with type 2 diabetes, SDOH influence glycemic control, cholesterol, and blood pressure to varying degrees (Walker et al., 2014), and in fact some of these SDOH factors are responsive to intervention (Walker et al., 2015). Perceived discrimination is associated with several negative health outcomes through two mechanisms: (1) compromised ability to fight off disease caused by chronic stress and (2) diminished ability to engage with the health-care system (Cockerham et al., 2017).

OTPs can start to assess for the presence and impact of these factors on a person's life and chronic disease management while completing an occupational profile. Open-ended questions should focus on both the enablers and barriers in a person's environment and can focus specifically on potentially relevant SDOH factors such as the walkability of the person's neighborhood to facilitate outdoor exercises and social experiences when interacting with others in the person's community.

General Considerations When Providing Occupational Therapy Services to People With Chronic Conditions

People with chronic conditions often experience increased burden on their daily lives because of various demands on their time such as attending health-care appointments, managing symptoms of the condition, and learning how to use new technology. OTPs who engage with people who often have more than one chronic condition must rely on their training in person-centeredness, as well as the previously outlined MDM approach. The primary tenet of this approach is moving people toward their own life and health goals while adding to their burden of care as little as possible (Leppin et al., 2015).

Clinicians who adopt an MDM lens see "patients" as whole people with complex lives and finite capacity to take on health-related tasks; these individuals have the right to seek interventions that align with their values and identity. In practice, combining an occupation-focused approach with MDM allows the therapist to tailor interventions that will decrease the burden of care and support the person to manage their health outside a service context.

For people with chronic conditions, self-management includes medication management, emotion regulation, and the organization of life roles. Self-management also includes the confidence to carry out these tasks (Packer, 2013). When a health professional or peer collaborates to teach these skills, it is referred to as **self-management support;** in contrast, when the person uses the skills, it is considered **self-management.** Self-management support refers to interventions that comprise techniques, tools, and programs to help people choose and maintain healthy behaviors through education, building skills, and improving confidence. Self-management skills include self-monitoring, problem-solving, decision-making, action planning, communication with health professionals, and resource utilization. It also refers to a fundamental transformation of the person–caregiver relationship into a collaborative partnership.

Evidence indicates that providing information alone is insufficient to promote self-management (Allegrante et al., 2019; Bodenheimer et al., 2002; Lawn & Schoo, 2010; Lorig & Holman, 2003). The desired outcome for the person, family, or group is:

1. Display knowledge of the condition and its management.
2. Adopt a care plan agreed upon by the person and health professional.
3. Share in decision-making.
4. Monitor and manage signs and symptoms.
5. Manage the impact of the condition on physical, emotional, occupational, and social functioning.
6. Adopt a healthy lifestyle to address risk factors and promote health.
7. Confidently access and use support services.

Many self-management support interventions are held in the community setting (Plow et al., 2011); however, even with limited time in the clinic, therapists can shift to a collaborative approach and engage patients in action planning to individualize their care (Plow et al., 2011). As outlined in the Evidence-Based Practice feature, literature supports the unique role of occupational therapy in supporting health management with people experiencing chronic conditions. Health professionals who support individual self-management will have deeper and more satisfying person relationships and their patients will be more satisfied and have better treatment outcomes related to both their mental health and their chronic condition (see Table 17-1).

TABLE 17-1 | Common Intervention Approaches for Individuals With Chronic Health Conditions

Approach	Target of Intervention	Brief Synopsis	Chapters With Additional Information
Person-Centered Assessment and Intervention	Empower people by focusing on person-identified areas of concern.	Person-centered assessment and intervention allow clinicians to empower people with chronic conditions by focusing on what the person views as a priority and then designing care that is guided by the person's values and goals.	Chapter 2: Recovery and Wraparound Models and Chapter 4: Person-Centered Evaluation
Therapeutic Use of Self	Minimize distress through active listening and empathy.	Tool to build a strong relationship with people and empower them to engage in meaningful occupations	Chapter 13: Communication and Social Skills
Motivational Interviewing	Engagement in health-promoting behaviors	A person-centered manner of interacting that helps the person self-identify reasons for changing	Chapter 11: Motivation
Self-Management Support	ADLs, wellness	Self-management support refers to health professional or peer-facilitated interventions comprising techniques, tools, and programs to help people choose and maintain healthy behaviors through education, building skills and improving confidence.	Chapter 45: Self-Care and Well-Being Occupations

Continued

TABLE 17-1 | Common Intervention Approaches for Individuals With Chronic Health Conditions—cont'd

Approach	Target of Intervention	Brief Synopsis	Chapters With Additional Information
Social Determinants of Health	Sociocultural factors	Remove environmental barriers and promote facilitators; may include policy change	Chapter 45: Self-Care and Well-Being Occupations
Leisure Exploration	Leisure	Identifying and pursuing leisure activities	Chapter 43: Serving Veterans and Service Members Chapter 45: Self-Care and Well-Being Occupations
Lifestyle Redesign	Health and wellness	Creation of habits and routines that are personally meaningful and promote health	Chapter 45: Self-Care and Well-Being Occupations
Lifestyle Physical Activity	Physical health and well-being	Promotion of engagement in active lifestyle to minimize side effects of chronic conditions and reduce stress	Chapter 45: Self-Care and Well-Being Occupations
Social Network Sites	Connection and communication with others	Websites or apps that allow users to communicate	Chapter 33: Virtual Environments
Sleep Hygiene Education	Sleep	Establishing a healthy sleep and rest routine and creating an environment that promotes sleep	Chapter 52: Sleep
Minimally Disruptive Medicine Principles	Move people toward their life and health goals while adding as little as possible to their workload.	These principles are tailored to the person and their context in order to achieve health goals while imposing the least amount of treatment burden possible from the care team.	Chapter 17: Chronic Health Conditions and Mental Health

Evidence-Based Practice

Actively Managing Chronic Conditions

> *People who take an active role in managing their chronic conditions experience better health outcomes.*

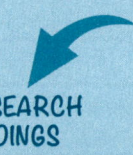

RESEARCH
FINDINGS

Research has demonstrated that people who take an active role in managing their chronic conditions experience better health outcomes. Active self-managers have better control of chronic health conditions, improved physical and emotional health, and more energy to adapt and enjoy life (Allegrante et al., 2019; Lorig & Holman, 2003; Packer, 2013). Self-management support interventions provide benefits when compared with usual care and appear to be as beneficial as cognitive behavioral techniques (Barlow et al., 2002).

OTPs can use an occupation-based approach to self-management support and enhance role management and emotional management, which are not as frequently addressed in traditional programs (Packer, 2013; Plow et al., 2011). OTPs can facilitate an occupation-based, person-centered approach to provide self-management support in community and clinical settings, which is optimal compared with an information only approach that has not been found to be as effective (Lau et al., 2022). A group setting offers opportunities to increase self-efficacy as participants hear about accomplishments and challenges of peer role models that often increase motivation and self-efficacy.

Many people with chronic disease and those with chronic conditions such as stroke leave medical settings uncertain of how to rebuild their lives. Occupation-based self-management groups offer the opportunity to increase participation and life satisfaction (Harel-Katz et al., 2020; Lee et al., 2017; Leland et al., 2017; Stern, 2018; Toole et al., 2013).

Evidence-Based Practice—cont'd

APPLICATIONS

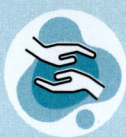

➡ OTPs can use a collaborative approach that goes beyond giving information and includes engaging people in action planning to promote individualized goals and enhanced skill mastery associated with increased self-efficacy (Plow et al., 2011).

➡ OTPs can provide interventions that address role management and emotional management, as well as promote participation, which are not addressed as frequently as medical management (Packer, 2013).

➡ OTPs can implement self-management group interventions that offer opportunities to increase participation and self-efficacy (Harel-Katz et al., 2020; Lee et al., 2017; Toole et al., 2013).

REFERENCES

Allegrante, J. P., Wells, M. T., & Peterson, J. C. (2019). Interventions to support behavioral self-management of chronic diseases. *Annual Review of Public Health, 40,* 127–146. https://doi.org/10.1146/annurev-publhealth-040218-044008

Barlow, J., Wright, C., Sheasby, J., Turner, A., & Hainsworth, J. (2002). Self-management approaches for people with chronic conditions: A review. *Patient Education and Counseling, 48*(2), 177–187. https://doi.org/10.1016/s0738-3991(02)00032-0

Harel-Katz, H., Adar, T., Milman, U., & Carmeli, E. (2020). Examining the feasibility and effectiveness of a culturally adapted participation-focused stroke self-management program in a day-rehabilitation setting: A randomized pilot study. *Topics in Stroke Rehabilitation, 27*(8), 577–589. https://doi.org/10.1080/10749357.2020.1738676

Lau, S. C., Judycki, S., Mix, M., DePaul, O., Tomazin, R., Hardi, A., Wong, A. W. K., & Baum, C. (2022). Theory-based self-management interventions for community-dwelling stroke survivors: A systematic review and meta-analysis. *The American Journal of Occupational Therapy, 76*(4), 7604205010. https://doi.org/10.5014/ajot.2022.049117

Lee, D., Fischer, H., Zera, S., Robertson, R., & Hammel, J. (2017). Examining a participation-focused stroke self-management intervention in a day rehabilitation setting: A quasi-experimental pilot study. *Topics in Stroke Rehabilitation, 24*(8), 601–607. https://doi.org/10.1080/10749357.2017.1375222

Leland, N. E., Fogelberg, D. J., Halle, A. D., & Mroz, T. M. (2017). Occupational therapy and management of multiple chronic conditions in the context of health care reform. *The American Journal of Occupational Therapy, 71*(1), 7101090010p1–7101090010p6. https://doi.org/10.5014/ajot.2017.711001

Lorig, K. R., & Holman, H. (2003). Self-management education: History, definition, outcomes, and mechanisms. *Annals of Behavioral Medicine: A Publication of the Society of Behavioral Medicine, 26*(1), 1–7. https://doi.org/10.1207/S15324796ABM2601_01

Packer, T. L. (2013). Self-management interventions: Using an occupational lens to rethink and refocus. *Australian Occupational Therapy Journal, 60*(1), 1–2. https://doi.org/10.1111/1440-1630.12032

Plow, M. A., Finlayson, M., & Rezac, M. (2011). A scoping review of self-management interventions for adults with multiple sclerosis. *PM&R, 3*(3), 251–262. https://doi.org/10.1016/j.pmrj.2010.11.011

Stern, B. Z. (2018). Critical reflections on self-management support in chronic disease: The value of occupational therapy in health promotion. *The Open Journal of Occupational Therapy, 6*(4), 1–7. https://doi.org/10.15453/2168-6408.1461

Toole, L. O., Connolly, D., & Smith, S. (2013). Impact of an occupation-based self-management programme on chronic disease management. *Australian Occupational Therapy Journal, 60*(1), 30–38. https://doi.org/10.1111/1440-1630.12008

Here's the Point

- Because of the increased prevalence of chronic conditions, there is a shift in health care to focus on management and prevention.
- People with a chronic condition may experience a psychosocial impact both during the diagnosis and the initial medical treatment of the conditions as well as because of the impact of the lifelong self-management of the condition. Some health-care providers may misinterpret emotional reactions as noncompliance or disinterest in health management.
- OTPs should be aware of the association between some psychiatric conditions such as anxiety and depression and certain chronic conditions.

- OTPs should be able to recognize signs and symptoms of posttraumatic stress, PTG, diabetes distress, overwhelm, and impact of chronic conditions on cognitive load. They should also be aware of the impact on self-care, health management, and social participation.
- OTPs can facilitate favorable psychological outcomes by promoting management of a chronic condition, providing person-centered care, evaluating the impact of a person's environment, and promoting engagement in meaningful occupations and activities.

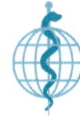

Visit the online resource center at **FADavis.com** to access the videos.

Apply It Now

1. Small Group Discussion

■ Form small groups of three to four students.

■ Share with your group some personal information about yourself, including your roles, meaningful occupations and activities, habits, routines, and goals. You may refer to your career path, family, relationships, education, hobbies, travel, and so on.

■ Consider a time when participation in one role or occupation overtook your ability to participate in other areas of your life; for example, becoming a new caregiver, participating in a sport, or working in a high-demand job. How did this impact your roles, occupations, activities, habits, routines, and goals? Was it more difficult to find time to participate in everything you needed and wanted to do? How did this feel? Now think about people managing a chronic condition: How might this impact their ability to participate in some of the activities you previously discussed?

2. Get Involved in the Community

Volunteer with an organization that serves a specific chronic condition population, such as a local cancer survivor support center or a diabetes support group.

■ What supports and services are provided for the people of this community?

■ What were some of the central issues being discussed by participants?

■ Did anyone discuss any impact on their mental health? If so, what was it?

■ Did you observe any examples of growth or resilience?

Resources

Books

- Miller, T. (2021). *What doesn't kill you: A life with chronic illness—Lessons from a body in revolt.* Macmillan.
- O'Rourke, M. (2023). *The invisible kingdom: Reimagining chronic illness.* Penguin.
- Taylor, J. B. (2009). *My stroke of insight.* Hachette UK.

Videos

- "Playing for Mother Undergoing Cancer Treatment" video. Marylein Serrano is a mother of two children and a speech language therapist who has had several cancer diagnoses. In this video, she discusses how her role as a mother changed during cancer treatment. She describes how playing with her daughter became therapy for herself as well and helped connect her to her role as a mom. She demonstrates her resilience as she describes how she adapted and learned to reconnect with herself, her life, and her children. To access the video, visit the online resource center at FADavis.com.
- "Mental Health and Well-Being During COVID" video. Caitlin is an OTP who has worked in outpatient settings with both adults and children. In this video, she talks about how occupational therapy practice during the COVID-19 global pandemic allowed her to see in a new way the effects of stress and anxiety on patient outcomes. She discusses how she incorporates mental health and well-being into her practice and her belief that it promotes successful healing and recovery. To access the video, visit the online resource center at FADavis.com.
- "Blood Sugar Rising"—PBS Documentary: https://www.pbs.org/wgbh/blood-sugar-rising
- "Dear Jack"—Optic Pictures: https://www.allmovie.com/movie/dear-jack-vm8686194

Online Resources

- The CLEAR (Community Links Evidence to Action Research) Toolkit is a decision aid to support clinicians in assessing SDOH through a four-step process (Treat, Ask, Refer, Advocate): https://www.mcgill.ca/clear/download

Organizations

- Association of Diabetes Education and Care Specialists includes lived experiences, practice tools, and information on how to become a certified diabetes educator: https://www.diabeteseducator.org/practice/practice-tools/app-resources/the-aade7-self-care-behaviors-the-framework-for-optimal-self-management
- The Cancer Support Community/Gilda's Club provides online support to cancer survivors; it also has 175 in-person locations worldwide: https://www.cancersupportcommunity.org
- The American Cancer Society Reach to Recovery website and mobile app provides free peer support for breast cancer survivors: https://reach.cancer.org/p/p1/about
- Susan G. Komen Breast Cancer Foundation funds research endeavors and provides online support and resources for people with breast cancer and their families: https://www.komen.org
- Stupid Cancer provides online support and resources for young adult cancer survivors: https://stupidcancer.org
- The Self-Management Resource Center offers evidence-based 6-week programs across the United States and internationally. These highly structured courses are taught by trained leaders, many with chronic conditions, to promote self-management for people with various chronic conditions: https://selfmanagementresource.com
- The Motivational Interviewing Network of Trainers (MINT) is an international organization of trainers in Motivational Interviewing. The website lists upcoming trainings and contact information for trainers. The library of resources includes books, publications, assessments, videos, and past presentations: https://motivationalinterviewing.org

References

Aikens, J. E. (2012). Prospective associations between emotional distress and poor outcomes in type 2 diabetes. *Diabetes Care, 35*(12), 2472–2478. https://doi.org/10.2337/dc12-0181

Allegrante, J. P., Wells, M. T., & Peterson, J. C. (2019). Interventions to support behavioral self-management of chronic diseases. *Annual Review of Public Health, 40,* 127–146. https://doi.org/10.1146/annurev-publhealth-040218-044008

American Association of Diabetes Educators. (2020). An effective model of diabetes care and education: Revising the AADE7 Self-Care Behaviors®. *The Diabetes Educator, 46*(2), 139–160. https://doi.org/10.1177/0145721719894903

American Occupational Therapy Association. (2020). Occupational therapy practice framework: Domain and process—Fourth edition. *American Journal of Occupational Therapy, 74*(Suppl. 2), 7412410010p1–7412410010p87. https://doi.org/10.5014/ajot.2020.74S2001

Auld, J. P., Mudd, J. O., Gelow, J. M., Hiatt, S. O., & Lee, C. S. (2018). Self-care moderates the relationship between symptoms and health-related quality of life in heart failure. *Journal of Cardiovascular Nursing, 33*(3), 217–224. https://doi.org/10.1097/JCN.0000000000000447

Balasubramanian, B. A., Cohen, D. J., Jetelina, K. K., Dickinson, L. M., Davis, M., Gunn, R., Gowen, K., deGruy, F. V., Miller, B. F., & Green, L. A. (2017). Outcomes of integrated behavioral health with primary care. *Journal of the American Board of Family Medicine, 30*(2), 130–139. https://doi.org/10.3122/jabfm.2017.02.160234

Barlow, J., Wright, C., Sheasby, J., Turner, A., & Hainsworth, J. (2002). Self-management approaches for people with chronic conditions: A review. *Patient Education and Counseling, 48*(2), 177–187. https://doi.org/10.1016/s0738-3991(02)00032-0

Bayliss, M., Rendas-Baum, R., White, M. K., Maruish, M., Bjorner, J., & Tunis, S. L. (2012). Health-related quality of life (HRQL) for individuals with self-reported chronic physical and/or mental health conditions: Panel survey of an adult sample in the United States. *Health Quality of Life Outcomes, 10,* 154. https://doi.org/10.1186/1477-7525-10-154

Bernell, S., & Howard, S. W. (2016, August). Use your words carefully: What is a chronic disease? *Frontiers in Public Health, 4,* 159. https://doi.org/10.3389/fpubh.2016.00159

Bhattacharya, R., Shen, C., & Sambamoorthi, U. (2014). Excess risk of chronic physical conditions associated with depression and anxiety. *BMC Psychiatry, 14,* 10. https://doi.org/10.1186/1471-244X-14-10

Bodenheimer, T., Lorig, K., Holman, H., & Grumbach, K. (2002). Patient self-management of chronic disease in primary care. *Journal of the American Medical Association, 288,* 2469–2475. https://doi.org/10.1001/jama.288.19.2469

Bonnell, L. N., Crocker, A. M., Kemp, K., & Littenberg, B. (2021). The relationship between social determinants of health and functional capacity in adult primary care patients with multiple chronic conditions. *Journal of the American Board of Family Medicine, 34*(4), 688LP–697LP. https://doi.org/10.3122/jabfm.2021.04.210010

Buffel du Vaure, C., Ravaud, P., Baron, G., Barnes, C., Gilberg, S., & Boutron, I. (2016). Potential workload in applying clinical practice guidelines for patients with chronic conditions and multimorbidity: A systematic analysis. *BMJ Open, 6*(3), e010119. https://doi.org/10.1136/bmjopen-2015-010119

Centers for Disease Control and Prevention. (2021, November 24). *Minority health: Racism and health.* https://www.cdc.gov/minorityhealth/racism-disparities/index.html

Centers for Disease Control and Prevention. (2023). *About chronic diseases.* https://www.cdc.gov/chronicdisease/about/index.htm

Christiansen, J., Lund, R., Qualter, P., Andersen, C. M., Pedersen, S. S., & Lasgaard, M. (2021). Loneliness, social isolation, and chronic disease outcomes. *Annals of Behavioral Medicine, 55*(3), 203–215. https://doi.org/10.1093/abm/kaaa044

Cockerham, W. C., Hamby, B. W., & Oates, G. R. (2017). The social determinants of chronic disease. *American Journal of Preventive Medicine, 52*(1), S5–S12. https://doi.org/10.1016/j.amepre.2016.09.010

Connerty, T. J., & Knott, V. (2013). Promoting positive change in the face of adversity: Experiences of cancer and post-traumatic growth. *European Journal of Cancer Care, (22),* 334–344. https://doi.org/10.1111/ecc.12036

Dahl-Popolizio, S., Manson, L., Muir, S., & Rogers, O. (2016). Enhancing the value of integrated primary care: The role of occupational therapy. *Families Systems & Health, 34*(3), 270–280. https://doi.org/10.1037/fsh0000208

Davis, S. K., Gebreab, S., Quarells, R., & Gibbons, G. H. (2014). Social determinants of cardiovascular health among Black and White women residing in Stroke Belt and Buckle regions of the South. *Ethnicity & Disease, 24*(2), 133–143.

Dean, H. D., Williams, K. M., & Fenton, K. A. (2013). From theory to action: Applying social determinants of health to public health

practice. *Public Health Reports, 128*(Suppl. 3), 1–4. https://doi.org/10.1177/00333549131286S301

Disler, R., Gallagher, R., & Davidson, P. (2012). Factors influencing self-management in chronic obstructive pulmonary disease: An integrative review. *International Journal of Nursing Studies, 49*(2), 230–242. https://doi.org/10.1016/j.ijnurstu.2011.11.005

Dobbins, M. I., Thomas, S. A., Melton, S. L. S., & Lee, S. (2016). Integrated care and the evolution of the multidisciplinary team. *Primary Care, 43*(2), 177–190. https://doi.org/10.1016/j.pop.2016.01.003

Duong, J., & Bradshaw. C. P. (2016). Household income level as a moderator of associations between chronic health conditions and serious mental illness. *Journal of Community Psychology, 44*(3), 367–383. https://doi.org/10.1002/jcop.21774

Ferlin, A., Fischer, H., Januszewski, C., & Hahn, B. (2019, January). Occupational therapy in integrated behavioral healthcare: A visual service framework. *OT Practice, 24*(1), 12–17.

Fisher, L., Hessler, D., Glasgow, R. E., Arean, P. A., Masharani, U., Naranjo, D., & Strycker, L. A. (2013). REDEEM: A pragmatic trial to reduce diabetes distress. *Diabetes Care, 36*(9), 2551–2558. https://doi.org/10.2337/dc12-2493

Fisher, L., Hessler, D., Polonsky, W., Strycker, L., Bowyer, V., & Masharani, U. (2019). Toward effective interventions to reduce diabetes distress among adults with type 1 diabetes: Enhancing emotion regulation and cognitive skills. *Patient Education and Counseling, 102*(8), 1499–1505. https://doi.org/10.1016/j.pec.2019.03.021

Gariepy, G., Smith, K. J., & Schmitz, N. (2013). Diabetes distress and neighborhood characteristics in people with type 2 diabetes. *Journal of Psychosomatic Research, 75*(2), 147–152. https://doi.org/10.1016/j.jpsychores.2013.05.009

Global Burden of Disease Collaborative Network. (2019). *Global Burden of Disease study 2019 results.* https://vizhub.healthdata.org/gbd-results

Gonzalez, J. S., Shreck, E., Psaros, C., & Safren, S. A. (2015). Distress and type 2 diabetes-treatment adherence: A mediating role for perceived control. *Health Psychology, 34*(5), 505–513. https://doi.org/10.1037/hea0000131

Hajat, C., & Stein, E. (2018). The global burden of multiple chronic conditions: A narrative review. *Preventative Medicine Reports, 12,* 284–293. https://doi.org/10.1016/j.pmedr.2018.10.008

Harel-Katz, H., Adar, T., Milman, U., & Carmeli, E. (2020). Examining the feasibility and effectiveness of a culturally adapted participation-focused stroke self-management program in a day-rehabilitation setting: A randomized pilot study. *Topics in Stroke Rehabilitation, 27*(8), 577–589. https://doi.org/10.1080/10749357.2020.1738676

Hessler, D., Strycker, L., & Fisher, L. (2021). Reductions in management distress following a randomized distress intervention are associated with improved diabetes behavioral and glycemic outcomes over time. *Diabetes Care, 44*(7), 1472–1479. https://doi.org/10.2337/dc20-2724

Hill, L., Artiga, S., & Haldar, S. (2022). *Key facts on health and health care by race and ethnicity.* Kaiser Family Foundation. https://www.kff.org/racial-equity-and-health-policy/report/key-facts-on-health-and-health-care-by-race-and-ethnicity

Houben-Wilke, S., Goërtz, Y. M., Delbressine, J. M., Vaes, A. W., Meys, R., Machado, F. V., van Herck, M., Burtin, C., Posthuma, R., Franssen, F. M., Vijlbrief, H., Spies, Y., van't Hul, A. J., Spruit, M. A., & Janssen, D. J. (2022). The impact of long COVID-19 on mental health: Observational 6-month follow-up study. *JMIR Mental Health, 9*(2), e33704. https://doi.org/10.2196/33704

Howard, A. F., Tan de Bibiana, J., Smillie, K., Goddard, K., Pritchard, S., Olson, R., & Kazanjian, A. (2014). Trajectories of social isolation in adult survivors of childhood cancer. *Journal of Cancer Survivorship, 8,* 80–93. https://doi.org/10.1007/s11764-013-0321-7

Januszewski, C., & Lukaszewski, K. (2017). Filling the gaps: Occupational therapy services in community mental health. *SIS Quarterly Practice Connections, 2*(1), 13–15.

Jones, S. C., & Neblett, E. W. (2016). Racial–ethnic protective factors and mechanisms in psychosocial prevention and intervention programs for Black youth. *Clinical Child and Family Psychology Review, 19,* 134–161. https://doi.org/10.1007/s10567-016-0201-6

Jones, S. C., & Neblett, E. W. (2017). Future directions in research on racism-related stress and racial-ethnic protective factors for Black youth. *Journal of Clinical Child & Adolescent Psychology, 46*(5), 754–766. https://doi.org/10.1080/15374416.2016.1146991

Kalina, J., Hinojosa, J., Strober, L., Bacon, J., Donnelly, S., & Goverover, Y. (2018). Randomized controlled trial to improve self-efficacy in people with multiple sclerosis: The Community Reintegration for Socially Isolated Patients (CRISP) program. *American Journal of Occupational Therapy, 72*(5), 1–8. https://doi.org/10.5014/ajot.2018.026864

Knighton, A. J., Stephenson, B., & Savitz, L. A. (2018). Measuring the effect of social determinants on patient outcomes: A systematic literature review. *Journal of Health Care for the Poor and Underserved, 29*(1), 81–106. https://doi.org/10.1353/hpu.2018.0009

Koinis-Mitchell, D., McQuaid, E. L., Jandasek, B., Kopel, S. J., Seifer, R., Klein, R. B., Potter, C., & Fritz, G. K. (2012). Identifying individual, cultural and asthma-related risk and protective factors associated with resilient asthma outcomes in urban children and families. *Journal of Pediatric Psychology, 37*(4), 424–437. https://doi.org/10.1093/jpepsy/jss002

Koverman, B., Royeen, L., & Stoykov, M. (2017). Occupational therapy in primary care: Structures and processes that support integration. *The Open Journal of Occupational Therapy, 5*(3), 1–9. https://doi.org/10.15453/2168-6408.1376

Lau, S. C., Judycki, S., Mix, M., DePaul, O., Tomazin, R., Hardi, A., Wong, A. W. K., & Baum, C. (2022). Theory-based self-management interventions for community-dwelling stroke survivors: A systematic review and meta-analysis. *The American Journal of Occupational Therapy, 76*(4), 7604205010. https://doi.org/10.5014/ajot.2022.049117

Lawn, S., & Schoo, A. (2010). Supporting self-management of chronic health conditions: Common approaches. *Patient Education and Counseling, 80,* 205–211. https://doi.org/10.1016/j.pec.2009.10.006

Lee, D., Fischer, H., Zera, S., Robertson, R., & Hammel, J. (2017). Examining a participation-focused stroke self-management intervention in a day rehabilitation setting: A quasi-experimental pilot study. *Topics in Stroke Rehabilitation, 24*(8), 601–607. https://doi.org/10.1080/10749357.2017.1375222

Leland, N. E., Fogelberg, D. J., Halle, A. D., & Mroz, T. M. (2017). Occupational therapy and management of multiple chronic conditions in the context of health care reform. *The American Journal of Occupational Therapy, 71*(1), 7101090010p1–7101090010p6. https://doi.org/10.5014/ajot.2017.711001

Leppin, A., Montori, V., & Gionfriddo, M. (2015). Minimally Disruptive Medicine: A pragmatically comprehensive model for delivering care to patients with multiple chronic conditions. *Healthcare, 3*(1), 50–63. https://doi.org/10.3390/healthcare3010050

Lorig, K. R., & Holman, H. (2003). Self-management education: History, definition, outcomes, and mechanisms. *Annals of Behavioral Medicine: A Publication of the Society of Behavioral Medicine, 26*(1), 1–7. https://doi.org/10.1207/S15324796ABM2601_01

Mahaffey, L. (2009). Incorporating evidence in mental health practice: Articles from the AOTA mental health annotated bibliography project. *American Occupational Therapy Association Special Interest Section Quarterly, 32*(3), 1–4. https://www.aota.org/publications/sis-quarterly/mental-health-sis

Marziliano, A., Tuman, M., & Moyer, A. (2020). The relationship between post-traumatic stress and post-traumatic growth in cancer patients and survivors: A systematic review and meta-analysis. *Psycho-Oncology, 29*(29), 604–616. https://doi.org/10.1002/pon.5314

Meek, K. P., Bergeron, C. D., Towne, S. D., Ahn, S., Ory, M. G., & Smith, M. L. (2018). Restricted social engagement among adults living with chronic conditions. *International Journal of Environmental Research and Public Health, 15*(1), 158–160. https://doi.org/10.17226/25663

Miller, B. F., Ross, K. M., Davis, M. M., Melek, S. P., Kathol, R., & Gordon, P. (2017). Payment reform in the patient-centered medical home: Enabling and sustaining integrated behavioral health care. *American Psychologist, 72*(1), 55–68. https://doi.org/10.1037/a0040448

National Academies of Sciences, Engineering, and Medicine. (2020). *Social isolation and loneliness in older adults: Opportunities for the health care system.* National Academies Press. https://doi.org/10.17226/25663

Packer, T. L. (2013). Self-management interventions: Using an occupational lens to rethink and refocus. *Australian Occupational Therapy Journal, 60*(1), 1–2. https://doi.org/10.1111/1440-1630.12032

Paradies, Y., Ben, J., Denson, N., Elias, A., Priest, N., Pieterse, A., Gupta, A., Kelaher, M., & Gee, G. (2015). Racism as a determinant of health: A systematic review and meta-analysis. *PLoS One, 10*(9), e0138511. https://doi.org/10.1371/journal.pone.0138511

Pinquart, M. (2018). Posttraumatic symptoms and disorders in children and adolescents with chronic physical illnesses: A meta-analysis. *Journal of Child & Adolescent Trauma, 13*(1), 1–10. https://doi.org/10.1007/s40653-018-0222-z

Plow, M. A., Finlayson, M., & Rezac, M. (2011). A scoping review of self-management interventions for adults with multiple sclerosis. *PM&R, 3*(3), 251–262. https://doi.org/10.1016/j.pmrj.2010.11.011

Polonsky, W. H., Fisher, L., Hessler, D., Desai, U., King, S. B., & Perez-Nieves, M. (2022). Toward a more comprehensive understanding of the emotional side of type 2 diabetes: A re-envisioning of the assessment of diabetes distress. *Journal of Diabetes and Its Complications, 36*(1), 108103. https://doi.org/10.1016/j.jdiacomp.2021.108103

Ramirez, R. D., Suarez-Balcazar, Y., Fischer, H. C., & Magasi, S. R. (2022). The occupational participation of Latinx cancer survivors and their family caregivers living in survivorship: A qualitative exploration informed by multiple stakeholders. *Occupational Therapy in Health Care, 36*(2), 116–140. https://doi.org/10.1080/07380577.2021.1907868

Riegel, B., Jaarsma, T., Lee, C. S., & Strömberg, A. (2019). Integrating symptoms into the Middle-Range Theory of Self-Care of Chronic Illness. *Advances in Nursing Science, 42*(3), 206–215. https://doi.org/10.1097/ANS.0000000000000237

Ross, K. M., Klein, B., Ferro, K., McQueeney, D. A., Gernon, R., & Miller, B. F. (2019). The cost effectiveness of embedding a behavioral health clinician into an existing primary care practice to facilitate the integration of care: A prospective, case-control program evaluation. *Journal of Clinical Psychology in Medical Settings, 26*(1), 59–67. https://doi.org/10.1007/s10880-018-9564-9

Scott, K. M., Koenen, K. C., Aguilar-Gaxiola, S., Alonso, J., Angermeyer, M. C., Benjet, C., Bruffaerts, R., Caldas-de-Almeida, J. M., de Girolamo, G., Florescu, S., Iwata, N., Levinson, D., Lim, C. C., Murphy, S., Ormel, J., Posada-Villa, J., & Kessler, R. C. (2013). Associations between lifetime traumatic events and subsequent chronic physical conditions: A cross-national, cross-sectional study. *PLoS One, 8,* e80573. https//doi.org/10.1371/journal.pone.0080573

Scott, K. M., Lim, C., Al-Hamzawi, A., Alonso, J., Bruffaerts, R., Caldas-de-Almeida, J. M., Florescu, S., de Girolamo, G., Hu, C., de Jonge, P., Kawakami, N., Medina-Mora, M. E., Moskalewicz, J., Navarro-Mateu, F., O'Neill, S., Piazza, M., Posada-Villa, J., Torres, Y., & Kessler, R. C. (2016). Association of mental disorders with subsequent chronic physical conditions: World mental health surveys from 17 countries. *JAMA Psychiatry, 73*(2), 150–158. https://doi.org/10.1001/jamapsychiatry.2015.2688

Shand, L., Cowlishaw, S., Brooker, J., Burney, S., & Ricciardelli, L. (2015). Correlates of post-traumatic stress symptoms and growth in cancer patients: A systematic review and meta-analysis. *Psycho-Oncology, 24,* 624– 634. https://doi.org/10.1002/pon.3719

Shippee, N. D., Shah, N. D., May, C. R., Mair, F. S., & Montori, V. M. (2012). Cumulative complexity: A functional, patient-centered model of patient complexity can improve research and practice. *Journal of Clinical Epidemiology, 65*(10), 1041–1051. https://doi.org/10.1016/j.jclinepi.2012.05.005

Shubrook, J. H., Brannan, G. D., Wapner, A., Klein, G., & Schwartz, F. L. (2018). Time needed for diabetes self-care: Nationwide survey of certified diabetes educators. *Diabetes Spectrum, 31*(3), 267–271. https://doi.org/10.2337/ds17-0077

Snoek, F. J., Bremmer, M. A., & Hermanns, N. (2015). Constructs of depression and distress in diabetes: Time for an appraisal. *The Lancet Diabetes & Endocrinology, 3*(6), 450–460. https://doi.org/10.1016/S2213-8587(15)00135-7

Stern, B. Z. (2018). Critical reflections on self-management support in chronic disease: The value of occupational therapy in health promotion. *The Open Journal of Occupational Therapy, 6*(4), 1–7. https://doi.org/10.15453/2168-6408.1461

Strandberg, R. B., Graue, M., Wentzel-Larsen, T., Peyrot, M., Thordarson, H. B., & Rokne, B. (2015). Longitudinal relationship between diabetes-specific emotional distress and follow-up HbA1c in adults with type 1 diabetes mellitus. *Diabetic Medicine, 32*(10), 1304–1310. https://doi.org/10.1111/dme.12781

Tarasuk, V., Mitchell, A., McLaren, L., & McIntyre, L. (2013). Chronic physical and mental health conditions among adults may increase vulnerability to household food insecurity. *The Journal of Nutrition, 143*(11), 1785–1793. https://doi.org/10.3945/jn.113.178483

Taylor, R. (Ed.). (2017). *Kielhofner's Model of Human Occupation* (5th ed.). Wolters Kluwer.

Thapa, B., Laws, M., & Galárraga, O. (2021). Evaluating the impact of integrated behavioral health intervention. *Medicine, 100*(34), e27066. https://doi.org/10.1097/MD.0000000000027066

Toole, L. O., Connolly, D., & Smith, S. (2013). Impact of an occupation-based self-management programme on chronic disease management. *Australian Occupational Therapy Journal, 60*(1), 30–38. https://doi.org/10.1111/1440-1630.12008

Tran, V.-T., Montori, V. M., & Ravaud, P. (2020). Is my patient overwhelmed? *Mayo Clinic Proceedings, 95*(3), 504–512. https://doi.org/10.1016/j.mayocp.2019.09.004

Vellone, E., Fida, R., Ghezzi, V., D'Agostino, F., Biagioli, V., Paturzo, M., Strömberg, A., Alvaro, R., & Jaarsma, T. (2017). Patterns of self-care in adults with heart failure and their associations with sociodemographic and clinical characteristics, quality of life, and hospitalizations: A cluster analysis. *Journal of Cardiovascular Nursing, 32*(2), 180–189. https://doi.org/10.1097/JCN.0000000000000325

Walker, R. J., Smalls, B. L., Campbell, J. A., Strom Williams, J. L., & Egede, L. E. (2014). Impact of social determinants of health on outcomes for type 2 diabetes: A systematic review. *Endocrine, 47*(1), 29–48. https://doi.org/10.1007/s12020-014-0195-0

Walker, R. J., Smalls, B. L., & Egede, L. E. (2015). Social determinants of health in adults with type 2 diabetes—Contribution of mutable and immutable factors. *Diabetes Research and Clinical Practice, 110*(2), 193–201. https://doi.org/10.1016/j.diabres.2015.09.007

Winship, J. M., Ivey, C. K., & Etz, R. S. (2019). Opportunities for occupational therapy on a primary care team. *American Journal of Occupational Therapy, 73*(5), 7305185010p1–7305185010p10. https://doi.org/10.5014/ajot.2019.030841

World Federation of Occupational Therapy. (2012). *About occupational therapy.* https://wfot.org/about/about-occupational-therapy

World Health Organization. (n.d.). *Social determinants of health.* https://www.who.int/health-topics/social-determinants-of-health#tab=tab_1

World Health Organization. (2022, December 7). *Post COVID-19 condition (long COVID).* https://www.who.int/europe/news-room/fact-sheets/item/post-covid-19-condition

Xu, Y., Tong, G. Y. Y., & Lee, J. Y.-C. (2020). Investigation on the association between diabetes distress and productivity among patients with uncontrolled type 2 diabetes mellitus in the primary healthcare institutions. *Primary Care Diabetes, 14*(5), 538–544. https://doi.org/10.1016/j.pcd.2020.04.004

Youngson, B. (2019). Understanding diabetes self-management using the Model of Human Occupation. *British Journal of Occupational Therapy, 82*(5), 296–305. https://doi.org/10.1177/0308022618820010

Zagarins, S. E., Allen, N. A., Garb, J. L., & Welch, G. (2012). Improvement in glycemic control following a diabetes education intervention is associated with change in diabetes distress but not change in depressive symptoms. *Journal of Behavioral Medicine, 35*(3), 299–304. https://doi.org/10.1007/s10865-011-9359-z

CHAPTER
18

Anxiety Disorders

Jackie Fox

It is important to begin an exploration of anxiety disorders with the understanding that anxiety is a natural process within the body and in the human experience. Anxiety and fear were written about in the earliest medical and literary texts and are commonly recognized states across all cultures. Anxiety, as a state, is not in and of itself harmful or even undesirable. It is likely that common anxieties—to social rejection, heights, darkness, strangers, and so on—made clear evolutionary sense in a prehistoric world full of such dangers.

Horwitz and Wakefield (2012) have called anxiety a "living mental fossil," a normal but misplaced expression of humans' biological nature—reflecting a time when acting on such anxieties led to a greater chance of survival. Even today, a person with a complete lack of anxiety or fear would be at very high risk of accidents or social rejection. Nevertheless, for millions of people worldwide, anxiety becomes unmanageable, disproportionate, life limiting, and extremely distressing.

This chapter explores the various ways in which the normal human state of anxiety can become "disordered," describes how anxiety affects occupational performance, and discusses the environmental, cultural, and gender-related factors underlying these common health conditions.

Description of the Condition

People living with anxiety disorders are frequently encountered by occupational therapy practitioners (OTPs) working in all areas of clinical practice. Patients and families with all kinds of health and social challenges will be experiencing reactive anxiety, such as those awaiting surgery, caring for a loved one, or fighting for equal access to housing or services. Anxiety disorders, including generalized anxiety disorder (GAD), phobias, social anxiety, and separation anxiety, are associated with very high rates of health-care usage, particularly in outpatient, primary care, and nonpsychiatric settings (Bandelow & Michaelis, 2022).

People with anxiety disorders may make up 47% of a general practitioner's workload (O'Doherty et al., 2020). Mental health and substance use disorders cause the highest nonfatal burden of disease worldwide, and anxiety disorders are second only to depression on this list. Anxiety disorders lead to considerable loss of quality of life and occupational participation, resulting in approximately 11.2 to 18.4 years of life with a disability (Whiteford et al., 2013).

The diagnoses included in this chapter are based on the diagnostic criteria for anxiety disorders in the newest *Diagnostic and Statistical Manual of Mental Disorders*, 5th Edition, Text Revision (*DSM-5-TR;* American Psychiatric Association [APA], 2022). Although criticized by some authors as being overly reductionistic and pathologizing of some normal reactions (Rodríguez-Testal et al., 2014), the *DSM-5-TR* remains an important diagnostic tool (along with the World Health Organization [WHO] guidelines—the *International Classification of Diseases,* 11th Revision [*ICD-11*; 2022]).

The most significant change in the *DSM-5* involved trauma- and stressor-related disorders (including posttraumatic stress disorder [PTSD] and acute stress disorder) and obsessive-compulsive disorders, which are described separately in their own categories and in different chapters in this textbook. Also of note is that selective mutism and separation anxiety are now considered anxiety disorders (APA, 2022). The following sections outline the separate anxiety disorders.

Anxiety Disorders

Anxiety is an adaptive response resulting in a feeling of apprehensiveness or anticipation of future danger or misfortune. It is accompanied by psychological feelings of worry and distress, along with somatic symptoms of tension (WHO, 2022). The focus of the danger may be internal (such as worry about the self or one's health or abilities), external (worry about other people, circumstances, or threats), or free-floating—when the person cannot describe what they are anxious about. It is important to distinguish between the states of fear and anxiety, although the two may overlap. Fear occurs as an emotional response to a real or imagined imminent threat and usually involves the triggering of the "fight or flight" response and a drive to escape or avoid an impending peril. Anxiety is more future-oriented and involves anticipating a future threat while maintaining bodily tension, vigilance, and caution (APA, 2022).

It is difficult to differentiate between an anxiety disorder and "normal" worry and fear, even for trained psychiatrists or psychologists. For example, most mothers would say, if asked, that they "always" worry about their children, potentially leading to a diagnosis of GAD (Bandelow & Michaelis, 2022). The same is true when considering people with "normal" or culturally valued shyness or modesty as being at risk for social anxiety disorder. As Horwitz and Wakefield (2012) state, "anxiety disorders will generally (but not always) include intense anxiety, but it is not true that intense anxiety generally implies an anxiety disorder, even if in a clinical context it is easy to mistakenly think it does" (p. 111).

For OTPs, who do not take clinical responsibility for medical diagnoses, it is more important to consider ways to help people lower their levels of psychological suffering and try to ameliorate the social, environmental, and occupational factors that are contributing to the anxiety and interfere with participation. The language of "diagnosis" and "symptoms" may not always be helpful and may mask real issues, inequalities, and reactions to daily life challenges (Horwitz & Wakefield, 2012). Nevertheless, for clarity, the following sections describe the diagnostic categories given by the *DSM-5-TR* (APA, 2022)—starting with anxiety disorders diagnosed most commonly in childhood (separation anxiety) and progressing to those more commonly diagnosed in the middle years (GAD).

Separation Anxiety

Of all the anxiety disorders, **separation anxiety disorder** is the earliest diagnosed—most often manifesting in children in their early years of schooling, at approximately 7 years (Bandelow & Michaelis, 2022). The features of separation anxiety include (a) persistent and developmentally excessive worry about being separated from home and attachment figures, usually parents; (b) worry about harm coming to attachment figures or to themselves (such as getting lost, or having an accident); (c) reluctance to be alone or, in older children, to go somewhere without their attachment figure; and (d) clinging and reassurance-seeking behavior, such as school refusal, refusal to sleep alone, and following a parent from room to room (APA, 2022).

Children may have physical symptoms such as headaches, nausea, or stomachache, and the symptoms must be present for at least 4 weeks. Positively, most children with separation anxiety disorder do not go on to have an anxiety disorder in adulthood, and a certain amount of heightened sensitivity to leaving an attachment figure is developmentally normal, particularly at key points such as starting school (APA, 2022).

For some people, separation anxiety can begin in adulthood, without childhood symptoms. However, most adults with the condition also report a history of mood disorders or other emotional difficulties, making this difficult to confirm (Shear et al., 2006). In adults, separation anxiety may manifest as fears about sleeping alone, going on trips away, and worry and panic about serious harm coming to attachment figures (Manicavasaga et al., 1997). Separation anxiety has only recently been identified as a discrete diagnosis in adulthood—with distinct differences between it and other anxiety diagnoses such as agoraphobia or GAD that result in excessive reassurance seeking or fear of leaving home. The lifetime prevalence among adults ages 18 to 64 in the United States is estimated at 6.6%, and among adolescents ages 13 to 17 the rate is 7.7% (Kessler et al., 2012).

Selective Mutism

Selective mutism is a relatively rare condition most often seen in young children (APA, 2022) that is usually also accompanied by another anxiety diagnosis, often social anxiety. It is characterized by consistent failure of the child to speak in certain social situations—usually to teachers, strangers, or those outside the immediate family—despite having the communication skills and language to do so. It is only diagnosed if the disturbance to speech has lasted for more than a month (excluding the first month at school) and where the child can speak at the appropriate developmental level with their immediate family.

Significant disruption to school achievement and social interaction is also part of the diagnostic criteria (WHO, 2022). Clinicians must take care to rule out any other possible reasons for communication difficulties, such as autism spectrum disorder or developmental language disorder.

Specific Phobias

A **phobia** is a marked fear or anxiety about a very specific object or situation. Commonly feared things are blood, flying, heights, certain animals (spiders or snakes), and enclosed places (APA, 2022). Although many phobias reflect evolutionarily understandable fears that likely develop because of humans' natural wariness of wild animals or injury (Horwitz & Wakefield, 2012), in modern society new phobias have developed such as nomophobia—the fear of being without a mobile phone (Rodríguez-García et al., 2020).

People with a specific phobia who do not have other mental health issues rarely seek psychiatric help as most have developed coping strategies to avoid contact with situations they fear (Bandelow & Michaelis, 2022). However, specific phobias are quite common, particularly in children and adolescents. The 12-month community prevalence rate in the United States is approximately 7% to 9% (APA, 2022). The degree to which a phobia affects occupational performance and participation will depend on how easily the feared situation can be avoided.

Social Anxiety Disorder

Social anxiety disorder typically develops in early adolescence, often following a childhood history of shyness or social inhibition. It may develop following a publicly humiliating experience or develop slowly over time. The condition is characterized by marked, intense fear or anxiety of social situations, specifically where the individual fears scrutiny by others. It typically includes intense fear of situations such as speaking in public, being observed, meeting strangers, or having social conversations where the person fears being evaluated negatively by others (APA, 2022). It is only diagnosed if present consistently for 6 months or more.

Social anxiety shows considerable difference in prevalence worldwide. European 12-month prevalence rates are approximately 2.3% compared with 7% in the United States (APA, 2022; Wittchen et al., 2011). Young people account for the majority of cases, and again there are global differences. For example, over 50% of young adults (16–29) in the United States scored above the diagnostic threshold for the condition in 2019, in comparison with 22% of young adults in Indonesia (Jefferies & Ungar, 2020). Social anxiety does not always reach the level of social phobia (where the feared situation is always avoided), but people with social anxiety report an almost constant preoccupation with what people think of them, a sense of "forcing" themselves to function in social situations, and constant cognitive evaluation of social situations, all of which can be exhausting (Clarke & Fox, 2017).

In contrast to those with a phobia, who may be able to cope with their difficulty if certain triggers are avoided, those with social anxiety may hide a high level of psychological distress for many years before seeking help. Shyness, shame, and fear about what others may think are common features of social anxiety, so people may be very reluctant to speak to a health-care provider (Bandelow & Michaelis, 2022). There may also be considerable comorbidity.

The social isolation resulting from social anxiety can lead to the development of depression. Many autistic people also experience social anxiety. Efforts to manage social situations with substances such as alcohol or drugs can themselves become problematic (APA, 2022). Because of these comorbid and risk factors, early intervention for people with social anxiety may prevent future mental health deterioration or loss of functioning (Urish, 2017).

Panic Disorder

A **panic attack**, which is a very intense mental and physical experience, is an abrupt surge of extreme fear or discomfort that can peak in minutes. It includes four or more of the following: palpitations or a racing heart, sweating, trembling, shortness of breath, feeling of choking, chest pain/discomfort, nausea, feeling dizzy or faint, feeling numbness or tingling, feeling unreal or detached from oneself, and fear of losing control, going crazy, or dying (APA, 2022). A person may experience a panic attack from a state of calm or sleep or from a state of anxiety.

Having panic attacks does not necessarily mean that one has panic disorder. Panic attacks can occur in the context of other mental health difficulties or even some medical conditions such as cardiac or respiratory conditions (APA, 2022). People with a specific phobia may experience a panic attack in the presence of the feared stimulus (e.g., heights), and the person can usually identify the trigger of the attack (Roy-Byrne et al., 2006). There are likely to be cultural/societal differences in factors that cause panic attacks, as there are considerable differences in prevalence worldwide. For example, the 12-month prevalence for panic attacks in the United States is 11.2%, but ranges from 2.7% to 3.3% in European countries (APA, 2022). However, most individuals can identify some type of stressor in the months leading up to their first panic attack.

Panic disorder is an experience of recurrent, unexpected panic attacks. Because of the intense physical and emotional distress experienced during a panic attack, those with panic disorder frequently seek help from health-care providers (Bandelow & Michaelis, 2022), sometimes believing that the symptoms represent life-threatening illness such as cardiovascular problems or epilepsy. Panic disorder is diagnosed when panic attacks become recurrent, are accompanied by persistent worry about the attacks or their consequences, avoidance of potential triggers of panic (such as avoiding exercise so as not to experience a raised heart rate), and when the symptoms are not better explained by another medical condition, substance, or mental health condition (such as PTSD; APA, 2022).

People with panic disorder frequently worry about losing control of their feelings and may develop phobias of situations where they perceive there is a possibility of panic attacks (called situational avoidance; Cara, 2013). People with panic disorder may be at increased risk of suicidal ideation and suicide attempts, and early life trauma or mistreatment is a common risk factor for developing the condition (Roy-Byrne et al., 2006).

Agoraphobia

Agoraphobia can develop as a consequence of experiencing panic attacks and can be understood as the person's way of avoiding situations where it might be difficult for them to leave or be embarrassing in the case of another panic attack occurring (APA, 2022). These feared situations are mostly one (or more) of the following five: using public transportation, being in open spaces, being in enclosed spaces, being in a crowded place or standing in line, or being outside of the home alone. Agoraphobia can cause severe occupational performance difficulties for people as these situations are actively avoided or only done in the company of a trusted person.

It is important to clarify that the fear experienced is persistent, lasting more than 6 months, and is out of proportion to the actual danger or threat posed. It can be difficult to differentiate agoraphobia from other anxiety conditions. For example, people with agoraphobia may have a history of panic attacks but now actively avoid the places where panic attacks could occur. One way to differentiate the two experiences is that those with panic disorder are usually more anxious about the panic symptoms themselves, rather than experiencing fear of a specific situation (WHO, 2022).

Agoraphobia peaks in incidence in late adolescence or early adulthood (Bandelow & Michaelis, 2022), and the 12-month prevalence in the U.S. population is 1.7% (Kessler et al., 2012). Long-term agoraphobia, and the accompanying loss of participation in social roles, is associated with other mental health difficulties, particularly substance use problems and secondary depression (APA, 2022).

Generalized Anxiety Disorder

Generalized anxiety disorder (GAD) involves excessive anxiety or worry about multiple situations or everyday life circumstances. To be diagnosed, it must last for at least 6 months (APA, 2022). Other diagnostic criteria of GAD include the symptoms related to sympathetic autonomic overactivity in the body: heart palpitations, nausea, dry mouth, restlessness, fatigue, difficulty concentrating, irritability, muscle tension, and sleep disturbances. The symptoms result in an impaired ability to take part in daily occupations (APA, 2022; WHO, 2022).

GAD is a somewhat controversial diagnosis. Some authors have noted that multiple worries about areas of life such as family, health, finances, or work are not disordered, because the worries may be realistic concerns, or the individual may just be somewhat overly vigilant (Horwitz & Wakefield, 2012). Classifying worry as a disorder leads to a possibility of a large number of potentially false-positive diagnoses, particularly among people who live in circumstances where they face multiple, long-term sources of worry, such as living in long-term poverty. The *ICD-11* does make this distinction, noting that people who live in extremely stressful situations should not be diagnosed as having GAD when their anxiety and worry are appropriate to their circumstances (WHO, 2022).

Twelve-month prevalence rates for GAD are estimated at 2.9% among U.S. adults (APA, 2022) and between 0.2% and 4.3% in European countries. GAD has an older age of onset than the other anxiety disorders, with a median age at onset of 31 (Bandelow & Michaelis, 2022); rates can be as high as 3.4%

in the over-65 age group (Wittchen et al., 2011), although this may reflect population trends (aging population) in the Global North. It is very typical for individuals to have symptoms of both GAD and depression; where GAD is comorbid with depression, people can experience more severe symptoms, lower quality of life, a poorer prognosis, and a higher risk of suicide (Goodwin, 2021). "Anxious depression" is a common presentation of mental health difficulty in primary care.

GAD is a very disabling condition. People can experience disruption to their daily activities in rates similar to those with physical conditions such as diabetes or arthritis. Because of the daily symptoms of tension and the long-term nature of this condition, people with GAD are high users of other medical services, often experiencing manifestations of physical ill health including ulcers, sleep disturbances, chronic pain, and high blood pressure (Hoffman et al., 2008).

The Lived Experience

"Lily"—My Experience of Living with Generalized Anxiety Disorder and Panic Disorder

Where It Began

I can't pinpoint exactly what triggered my anxiety. Looking back now I can recognise that symptoms began around 2019–2020 when I was taking time out to work. By the time I was in my first year of college, I recall every day feeling like a battle between who I knew I was and who the anxiety was making me. I felt I had no control. My emotions were so dysregulated; I began taking everything personally, over analysing and catastrophizing every situation. The physical manifestation of my mental state was something that really impacted my days. My body would be in a constant state of stress leading to continuous trembling throughout the day, heart palpitations and muscle pain. This caused me to miss college, work and affected my ability to socialise.

My sleep and appetite were also affected hugely. Most frustrating was that there were many days where I couldn't pinpoint what was making me feel this way. This later caused panic attacks, which became more and more frequent. I would have up to four panic attacks a week. These were extremely scary and traumatising. I felt like I was going crazy and losing control of myself and sense of reality. The combination of this led to suicidal ideation and extremely low mood that would last weeks. Very important relationships in my life began to suffer as I started to isolate myself with the belief that nothing or no one could ever make this go away.

My Attitude Toward Professional Help

I was reluctant to seek professional help as this felt like confirmation that I was not okay or strong enough to overcome this myself. However, now I know it was my mind frame at the time making me think like this. I was later referred to a psychiatrist from my GP, as my symptoms were progressively getting worse even with medication. The psychiatrist then diagnosed me with GAD with depressive symptoms and panic disorder.

Over the course of 2 years, I struggled with feeling that nothing could ever make this go away. I still had trouble accepting that I needed medication. My symptoms and ways of thinking when in such an anxious state led me to participate in self-destructive behaviours. I felt this was one way to control

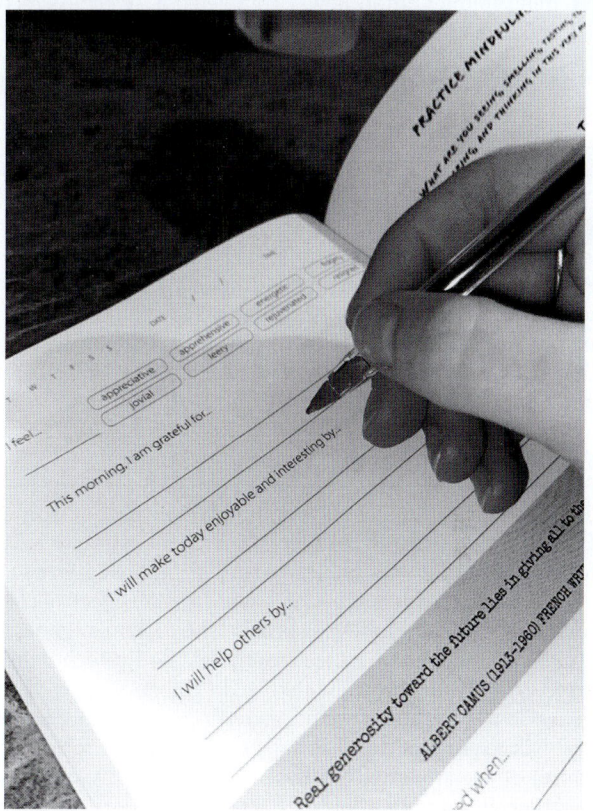

something in my life. I knew if these behaviours made my anxiety worse then I could have something to blame which was easier for me to understand than having no direct cause. These behaviours took me to rock bottom where I was taken to hospital. This rock bottom was the turning point for me. I realised that the way I was living my life was not going to work.

My Recovery and What Worked for Me

My medication dosage was increased, and it was the first time it felt right. I feel it is so important to emphasise that the correct dosage of medication took almost 2 years to find. However, this was what enabled me to make a change along with the realisation following my rock bottom. I decided to try what all of the professionals and my support systems were recommending. It was then that I feel I accepted that I had GAD, and it was okay, I just had to learn how to manage it. I cut out all of the

Continued

The Lived Experience—cont'd

self-destructive behaviours I had been participating in and began developing a daily routine that incorporated healthy occupations such as walking, journaling, and cooking healthy meals.

I also went to counseling, which was a massive fear of mine; however, it provided me with tools I use to this day. It also helped me understand what was going on in my brain and my body, which helped tremendously with my panic attacks. Gratitude was also a huge thing that made a difference, it helped to ground me and put life into perspective. My support systems throughout this whole period were massively important and still are. I still work every day to ensure I stay in the positive mind frame I am in now. I completed a "Wellness recovery action plan" program also which was very beneficial, and I use the strategies I learnt in this every day. I am now excelling in college and in my day-to-day life.

Final Note

Medication is not a bad thing; professional help and management tools provided by counselors did work. Although I hit rock bottom it doesn't mean one has to in order to recover. Had I made use of the available resources earlier I don't think this would have happened. It is a very difficult disorder to live with but for anyone that is struggling with it you can do it, you are not "crazy" and admitting you need help is not a sign of weakness but strength. There is light at the end of the tunnel.

Etiology

As with other mental health conditions, the etiology of anxiety disorders is complex and highly individualized, but it involves an interaction between genetic vulnerability, childhood adversity or stress, precipitating stressors later in life, and temperamental differences (Thibaut, 2017).

Genetics and Heritability

There is a degree of genetic heritability in anxiety disorders. From twin and family studies, researchers estimate a 30% level of heritability for anxiety disorders. There appear to be a large number of genes that, all having a small effect, account for the heritability of these disorders. The particular genes are still being mapped, but the serotonergic and catecholaminergic systems appear to be involved (Thibaut, 2017). These genes do not produce specific anxiety symptoms, but in general will mean a person has a genetic risk factor for one (or more) of the anxiety disorders, and comorbidity of several disorders is common (Shimada-Sugimoto et al., 2015). Panic disorder appears to be particularly heritable.

Precipitating Events and Childhood Experiences

Genetic risk by itself does not fully explain the development of an anxiety disorder. Multiple interactions between genetic risk factors and the environment determine whether children and adults develop an anxiety disorder in childhood. One specific risk factor for an anxiety disorder is having a parent with GAD. Fear and anxiety can be transmitted to infants in verbal and nonverbal ways by a parent with GAD and can put the child at risk for future development of the condition. Even in the first year of life, infants will learn to react with fear and avoidance to stimuli if their parents react in a fearful and anxious way (Aktar et al., 2017).

Infants and young children watch their parents to learn how to react to ambiguous or new situations; in children with an inhibited temperament and a parent with GAD, the child can be at risk of learning an anxious/avoidant method of coping with future situations. Fears can also be transmitted verbally, where parents transmit information about potential threats in everyday situations (e.g., about school) or about future threats (e.g., about failing an examination). Finally, there is evidence that parents with GAD will be excessively cautious and overprotective with their children, potentially limiting their children's exposure to novel situations and the potential to learn from experiences of natural and positive anxiety (Aktar et al., 2017).

A second common risk factor for the development of an anxiety disorder is having **adverse childhood experiences (ACEs)** in early life. ACEs such as exposure to violence, economic hardship, or household dysfunction can lead to permanent neurological changes to the brain structure in developing infants and children because of the prolonged activation of the stress response in such situations (Elmore & Crouch, 2020). Although this is discussed in more detail in Chapter 25: Trauma- and Stressor-Related Disorders, exposure to ACEs is also associated with significantly higher rates of childhood anxiety disorders. Economic hardship is particularly associated with anxiety, and witnessing violence has a stronger association with depression (Elmore & Crouch, 2020).

Anxiety disorders can also develop following a triggering event (or series of events), although people with genetic and childhood risk factors may have lowered resilience and be at greater risk. Specific phobias sometimes (but not always) develop following a traumatic experience with the feared situation (e.g., being trapped in an elevator, or hearing about a feared event such as an aircraft crash on the news; APA, 2022). A frightening experience, such as being separated from a parent or being attacked, is associated with the onset of agoraphobia. People with panic disorder are usually able to identify stressors in the period before their first panic attack (e.g., a death in the family or interpersonal difficulties). Smoking and having negative experiences with drugs are also precipitating factors for panic attacks (APA, 2022).

People in marginalized groups are at heightened risk for developing anxiety disorders as they experience systemic racism directly or vicariously, resulting in an amplified threat response. For example, the rates of suicide are 6.6% higher in men from the Irish Traveller ethnic group than in the general population (All Ireland Traveller Health Study Team, 2010). People of color in the United States or other marginalized groups may experience greater levels of specific phobias (such as blood/injection phobia) because of historical distrust of medical or government services (MacIntyre et al., 2023).

Because of systemic inequalities, marginalized groups in the Global North are also more likely to have childhood experiences of adversity such as living in poverty, having a family member incarcerated, or living in communities where they may witness violence, which present as risk factors for the development of anxiety disorders.

Temperament

Although there might be some variability from situation to situation, people tend to respond to events in a consistent way—showing particular temperament or personality traits. Temperament develops because of interaction between genetic and environmental factors (Rapee, 2002). Having a childhood temperament characterized by shyness, inhibition, withdrawal, and an avoidant style of coping has been linked with the future development of anxiety disorders.

People with an inhibited temperament can be more at risk than other people for developing anxiety in the face of stressors that face the whole community because of how they interpret events. For example, people with an inhibited temperament are more likely to pay selective attention to negative news coverage and so have an increased threat response to current affairs (Urish, 2017). On the other hand, researchers are showing that inhibited temperament can be improved in young children through parental intervention that focuses on reducing overprotectiveness and parental expression of anxiety, as well as encouraging children in exploration and exposure to new situations.

Prevalence

Anxiety disorders are the most prevalent of mental health conditions. Every year across the globe, 10.6% of people will have an anxiety disorder. However, there is substantial variation in geographical spread of these conditions, and accurate prevalence figures for some low-income countries are unknown. The 12-month prevalence of an anxiety disorder is 14% in the European Union countries (Wittchen et al., 2011) and 21.3% in the United States (Bandelow & Michaelis, 2022). Prevalence rates are much lower in Eastern Asian countries (2.8%).

The perception, particularly in Anglophone countries, of a rising prevalence of anxiety disorders needs some clarification (Bandelow & Michaelis, 2022). It is possible that rates of anxiety disorders are prone to what Shorter (2009, p. 427) calls, "cultural shaping," where some diagnoses are more prevalent in particular historical periods based on things such as cultural acceptance, the power of vested interests (such as pharmaceutical companies), cultural movements (such as the self-help movement), and the medicalization of emotional states (Dowbiggin, 2009). The actual prevalence per head of population shows little change from 1990 to 2010

(Baxter et al., 2014), although the COVID-19 outbreak must be considered (see the section that follows). The increase in the numbers of people diagnosed with an anxiety disorder is also because of the longer life spans of people living in most Global North countries, increasing the lifetime prevalence risk (Kessler et al., 2012).

Co-Occurrence of Anxiety Disorders and Neurodiversity

One group of people for whom anxiety disorders are particularly prevalent are those on the autism spectrum. Autistic people may have difficulties initiating and sustaining social communication and interactions, and may have patterns of behavior, interests, or activities that are restricted, rigid, inflexible, and repetitive. Some, but not all, individuals may have some difficulties with intellectual functioning and language (WHO, 2022).

It can be difficult to separate the diagnosis and symptoms of autism and anxiety as there can be some similarities. For example, clarifying whether avoiding social situations is a social anxiety symptom or an autistic coping strategy to avoid social discourse may be challenging. However, there is certainty that the prevalence of anxiety disorders is much higher in autistic people, with an average prevalence rate of about 50%, although some studies report even higher levels (Kent & Simonoff, 2017). Specific phobias are extremely common among autistic children (up to 67%) although this prevalence tends to decrease with age.

Anxiety can be an inherent part of the autistic person's experience. Difficulties with "reading" the emotions of others in social situations, having their own social communication misinterpreted by others, and a strong desire to control everyday life so as to be certain of routines and plans have all been described as highly anxiety provoking by autistic people. Disruptions to everyday life can be perceived as catastrophic, "I need to have everything set in certain order, otherwise it's just not going to get done (and if not adhered to) . . . my life is going to fall apart" (Halim et al., 2018, p. 30).

From a sensory point of view, autistic people can have a very sensitive threat response and may experience terror and fear during sensory experiences (such as loud noises or crowds) that would not trigger the same response in neurotypical individuals. For more information see Chapter 9: Sensory Processing and the Lived Sensory Experience. 🤝 An important clinical feature of anxiety with this population is that there may be very high levels of symptoms and distress without these reaching diagnostic thresholds. However, interventions to improve anxiety can be just as effective for autistic people, with some modifications (Kent & Simonoff, 2017). Key modifications include using social stories to explain complex scenarios, reducing/replacing abstract language, using visual aids and pictures to convey/explain emotions, and focusing more on behavioral modification techniques than metacognitive strategies (Attwood, 2004).

Impact of the COVID-19 Pandemic on Anxiety Disorders

The COVID-19 pandemic was a global stressor, and the societal and health consequences of infection, social isolation, lockdowns, loss/change in employment, and developmental impacts on children may play out over many years to come (Ellyatt, 2022). It may yet be too early to tell (at the time of this writing in 2023) what the long-term effects of the COVID-19 pandemic will be on anxiety disorders. The strict lockdowns imposed in some countries actually helped to reduce the prevalence of anxiety and depressive disorders in the short term, as they led to a feeling of safety and reduced fears of infection. However, in the longer term, the enforced immobility led to an increase in prevalence in anxiety and depression as the loss of social, occupational, and educational opportunities continued.

The COVID-19 lockdown may have worsened anxiety and disability for people who already had difficulties with aspects of daily functioning outside the home (Lokman & Bockting, 2022). Santomauro and colleagues (2021) estimated that globally an additional 76.2 million cases of anxiety disorders could be attributed to the COVID-19 pandemic.

However, some researchers believe that the high prevalence rates of anxiety during 2020 represented an (understandable) acute stress response to a unique and uncertain global situation (Daly & Robinson, 2022) and that coming years will see these additional cases diminish. Population-level rises in anxiety have been seen in many countries in response to crises, such as the Russian invasion of Ukraine in 2022, the cost-of-living crisis in many countries from 2021 onward, and the earlier financial crash of 2008. When surveyed, people may have identified a high number of anxiety symptoms. Yet, this level of perceived threat may be understandable for a person with an underlying vulnerability who was worried about being infected with COVID-19 (Taquet et al., 2021).

The elements of Mental Health First Aid are useful principles for clinicians to apply to the pandemic experience and to future public health crises. Mental health interventions in times of crisis should seek to instill a sense of safety, have a focus on calming activities, emphasize social connectedness, harness/develop self- and community efficacy, and encourage hope (Morganstein, 2022).

Gender Differences

Anxiety disorders are diagnosed in women almost twice as often as in men, and this unequal sex ratio continues across almost all anxiety diagnoses and across the life span. Gender differences are less pronounced in social anxiety, where men have similar prevalence rates. The high rate of diagnosis in women may be because of sociocultural issues and difference in gender presentation (Bekker & van Mens-Verhulst, 2007).

There may be less willingness among men to report symptoms of anxiety, or there may be differences in how anxiety presents for the different genders. For example, social anxiety in women is associated with more internalizing features (e.g., depression or other anxiety disorders), whereas men may use externalizing behaviors, such as using alcohol or drugs to relieve or mask distress (APA, 2022). Alternatively, there may be differences in the diagnostic tool used. In one study, women were twice as likely as men to receive a diagnosis of PTSD when the *ICD-10* was used, compared with no gender difference when the *DSM-IV* was used (Peters et al., 2006).

Nevertheless, there could be some biological reasons why women experience higher rates of anxiety. There is evidence

of gender differences in the brain processes involved in fear and threat (such as hypothalamic-pituitary-adrenal [HPA] axis reactivity) and gonadal hormones that are involved in anxiety (Christiansen, 2015). It appears, however, that what is more important is how these gender differences interact with socialization processes to compound this vulnerability. From early childhood, boys and girls may be socialized differently—with boys being encouraged to face a feared situation more than girls are. This leads to a greater chance for the fear response to be extinguished in boys, whereas girls may be conditioned to avoid a stressful stimulus or to react with anxiety.

In life, women are more likely to be exposed to traumatic events that could precipitate an anxiety disorder, such as sexual trauma, domestic abuse, and relationship stressors (Christiansen, 2015). Women are more likely to experience low pay, unstable employment, and single parenthood (Drapeau et al., 2012) and are vulnerable to stress emanating from the many social roles they play in parenting, caring, and in the community. Gender differences in how social roles are experienced and how domestic work is shared appear to contribute to anxiety. For example, working full time is a protective factor against an anxiety disorder for fathers, but not for mothers (Plaisier et al., 2008).

Rates of anxiety disorders are likely to be even higher in those who do not identify as cisgender. The prevalence of anxiety for people whose sex assigned at birth is different from their current gender identity (nonbinary) was 38%, compared with 14% to 30% of cisgender participants in a study of young U.S. adults (Reisner et al., 2016). Those in treatment for sex reassignment also show higher rates of anxiety than the general population. For nonbinary persons, issues such as parental rejection, childhood victimization, and living with the stress of experiencing incongruence between a person's bodily characteristics and their social expectations are all potential reasons for increased anxiety rates in these communities (Heylens et al., 2014).

Culture-Specific Information

Although guidelines such as the *DSM-5-TR* and the *ICD-11* aim to give objective measurements of what constitutes "normal" and "disordered" mental health, sociocultural differences in shared beliefs, acceptance of "deviance," and the level of importance given to medical diagnoses in different countries will affect how anxiety is perceived (Piko, 2002). This section gives several examples of how anxiety disorders may present differently for people of different cultures around the world.

- People who currently or previously lived in authoritarian regimes such as Russia or Iran may be socialized by the State to mistrust society, to have increased vigilance, an external locus of control, and a sense of learned helplessness. This may be one reason for the increased levels of anxiety disorders among people in Eastern Europe and the former Soviet states (Piko, 2002).
- In collectivist cultures, people may have very high levels of social anxiety but a low prevalence of social anxiety disorder—indicating the importance of social conformity and acceptance in these cultures. One specific example is the syndrome of *"taijin kyofusho"* in Japan and

Korea, which is characterized by fear that the person makes others feel uncomfortable (APA, 2022).

- There are cultural differences in how much independence/interdependence is expected between children and parents, so rates and understanding of separation anxiety will vary widely between individualistic and collectivist cultures. In countries with threats that increase the risk of losing an attachment figure, such as war, displacement, or high crime rates, it is likely that anxiety around separation will understandably be higher (Bögels et al., 2013). The lack of independent exploration encouraged in children in the urbanized Global North has been implicated in a rise in childhood anxiety as children are less self-sufficient (Rapee, 2002).
- The degree to which the somatic symptoms of panic are expressed may also differ among cultures. One example is the syndrome *"ataque de nervios"* ("attack of nerves") among Latin American populations which can manifest as uncontrollable screaming/crying, trembling, depersonalization, and a longer panic attack than is experienced in other populations (APA, 2022). People of Cambodian descent may present with *"khyâl"* attacks that may meet panic attack criteria but the symptoms are attributed to catastrophic fears that *"khyâl"* (a wind-like substance) will rise up in their body and cause serious illness.
- The term *"kufungisisa"* means "thinking too much" in the Shona language of Zimbabwe. Many people in Africa, the Caribbean, and Indigenous communities use the idiom of "thinking too much" to describe rumination or worrying thoughts that could meet the criteria for GAD and are believed to cause distress and somatic problems (APA, 2022).
- In neoliberal societies, there is high pressure, particularly on women, toward individual achievement, unrealistic standards, and harsh self-criticism. Young people in the current generation are more demanding of themselves and of others and believe others are highly demanding of them (Curran & Hill, 2019). This has been linked to a rise in anxiety disorders among young people as they transition to adulthood.

Course

Anxiety disorders tend to start in childhood or early adulthood, peak in the middle years of life, and ease in older age, even without treatment (Bandelow & Michaelis, 2022). Some disorders, such as attachment disorder or selective mutism, are often outgrown, but the individual may always be vulnerable to other anxiety disorders later in life. However, other disorders can be chronic with periods of relapse and remission. Some factors can make anxiety disorders more disabling and worsen the prognosis for individuals. If a person has two or more types of anxiety disorder, chronic physical health complaints, and, particularly, depression as well, the clinical presentation is more difficult and can be chronic.

It is important for people with anxiety disorders to receive treatment and support early, as untreated GAD in particular often leads to major depression and worsening physical health (Wittchen et al., 2003).

Impact on Occupational Performance

This section focuses on how the person, environment, and occupation factors interact for people with different anxiety diagnoses. Anxiety disorders can develop early in childhood and the resulting difficulties in school or academic achievement, social functioning, and quality of life can affect future neurocognitive development, continue into later life, and leave a lasting impact on a person's ability to participate to their satisfaction in daily life (Wittchen et al., 2011).

Person Factors

According to the Person-Environment-Occupation Performance Model (Law et al., 1996), person factors relate to the physical, cognitive, sensory, affective, and spiritual aspects of the person that make them a unique being. Each person has a unique combination of personal factors and life experiences that influences their occupational performance. For people with anxiety disorders, person factors may be affected by symptoms (such as heart palpitations or breathing difficulties) but may also be key to recovery (e.g., spiritual beliefs, psychological flexibility, or motivation).

Physical Factors

The physical symptoms of anxiety occur because of the triggering of the body's threat response symptoms. Although a short-lived adrenaline response because of a threat may actually increase performance, long-term anxiety leads to a large range of symptoms caused by overactivity in the body's sympathetic nervous system. These symptoms may include gastrointestinal discomfort, diarrhea, headaches, dizziness, tremor, restlessness, aching muscles, and insomnia. Cardiac and respiratory symptoms such as tachycardia, feelings of the heart "skipping a beat," constriction in the chest, and hyperventilation can be highly distressing and lead people with anxiety disorders to seek medical help or become anxious about the symptoms themselves, leading to a potential cycle of mounting anxiety (Geddes et al., 2012).

The physical symptoms can be severe but short-lived (as in panic disorder) or more moderate and enduring, but nonetheless distressing (as in generalized anxiety). The long-term impacts of chronic anxiety can be harmful to physical health, and anxiety disorders are associated with concurrent cardiac and gastrointestinal problems, migraines, hypertension, and genitourinary difficulties (Härter et al., 2003).

Because of the sometimes-extreme level of physical discomfort associated with anxiety symptoms, those with anxiety disorders often attempt to reduce their symptoms by avoiding perceived stressors. Those with social anxiety disorder can be more severely disabled than those with GAD—experiencing restrictions in social, home, and work occupations as they avoid potentially anxiety-provoking social situations. Feeling anxious and worried about future symptoms occurring also limits the person's quality of participation in all types of life activities (Hendriks et al., 2014) and reduces the perceived quality and satisfaction in doing daily tasks. Having difficulty sleeping, experiencing pain, and feeling fatigue all impact on a person's ability to maintain employment, and anxiety disorders are associated with a high burden of sick leave (Hoffman et al., 2008).

Cognitive Factors

A distinguishing feature of anxiety disorders is that the individual is highly attentive and responsive to perceived threats in the environment. For example, people with social anxiety report frequent checking of the environment to avoid large groups of people, with constant preoccupation of other people's perceptions of them (Clarke & Fox, 2017). Therefore, people with anxiety may find it more difficult to maintain attention on performing an occupation, particularly in the presence of a perceived threat (Langarita-Llorente & Gracia-Garcia, 2019). They may also have trouble with their short-term memory and have a slower reaction time completing tasks, particularly if there are distractions. However, research in this area is inconsistent, and in several studies people with anxiety disorders have shown no difference when compared to people without anxiety on cognitive tests (Langarita-Llorente & Gracia-Garcia, 2019; Leonard & Abramovitch, 2019).

However, there is evidence to indicate that people with anxiety are more likely to perceive ambiguous situations as anxiety provoking and threatening (Alkozei et al., 2014). This is particularly true of children. A strong basis for cognitive behavioral treatments is exploring and trying to change the patterns of beliefs and thoughts such as catastrophizing (expecting the worst), black-or-white thinking (no tolerance for uncertainty), and stress-inducing beliefs (such as "I must always be liked by others") typically experienced by people with anxiety disorders. See Chapter 7: Cognition and Chapter 8: Cognitive Beliefs.

Sensory Factors

There is a strong relationship between anxiety and sensory processing preferences such that people with anxiety are more likely to respond to the sensory environment with "sensation avoiding" or "sensory sensitivity" patterns—two of Dunn's four proposed sensory processing patterns (Dunn, 1997). Trauma in childhood can lead to disturbances in how the sensory system develops, potentially leading to anxiety disorders in adulthood. People with anxiety disorders may show increased reactivity to sensory stimuli (such as noise), show altered perception of sensory situations (such as in agoraphobia), and will often take steps to limit exposure to stimuli. This is because they may have lower neurological thresholds or hypersensitivity to sensory stimuli (Engel-Yeger & Dunn, 2011).

Avoidance can be a coping strategy for those with this hypersensitivity (or sensory defensiveness). People may avoid crowds or queuing or become resistant/intolerant of change or new experiences. Intimate relationships can be particularly affected as the person may not tolerate being touched or may avoid self-care activities (Abernethy, 2010). See Chapter 9: Sensory Processing and the Lived Sensory Experience.

Affective Factors

Living with an anxiety disorder can be emotionally exhausting. People with GAD report significantly lower satisfaction with life, well-being, vitality, and emotional role functioning than people without GAD. One study indicates that people with GAD report a lower quality of life than people with major depression (Hoffman et al., 2008). The mental and emotional pain of living with anxiety is described as a "whole body" experience that is poorly understood by others and that impacts every aspect of occupational participation by those with lived experience:

> Like everything just shuts down but you just are trying to breathe but you can't, and everything kind of seems just painful and just hard to do, and you just feel so scared. I wish I could just explain it, like, when I just go full on like panic mode I just can't breathe, I can't talk, I just . . . and then I just cry because I can't do anything and it's just very scary . . . I had a full-on blown panic attack at school one time and just, I couldn't do anything. I just sat there and I just couldn't even pick up the phone and call my mom because everything just overwhelms your own body, like the whole feeling. (Woodgate et al., 2020, p. 11)

See Chapter 12: Emotion Regulation.

Environmental Factors

Anxiety as an experience occurs because of an interaction between the person (perhaps with vulnerabilities or other risk factors) and their environment. The person perceives threat or risk in their surroundings or fears that harm will occur in a situation.

For someone with an anxiety disorder, the environment, "the sum total of what surrounds a person," becomes less about a place of "development and growth" but more one with the potential for "danger and damage" (Baptiste, 2017, p. 144). Aspects of the environment, including international threats such as COVID-19, directly provoke anxiety. But anxiety can also occur because of the person–environment interaction—how someone with a vulnerability for anxiety perceives an innocuous environmental situation as threatening. The Mental Health in Society and Culture discusses how technology, specifically doomscrolling, can play a role in anxiety.

Mental Health in Culture and Society

Aster Harrison

Doomscrolling and Anxiety

The environment can have a massive effect on anxiety. According to the *Occupational Therapy Practice Framework,* Fourth Edition (*OTPF-4;* American Occupational Therapy Association [AOTA], 2020), the environment includes products and technology (such as smartphones), attitudes of people around individuals and society, policies and systems, social support and relationships, the natural world, and the human-made built environment.

During the beginning of the COVID-19 pandemic, people were spending a lot of time at home, anxious to know more about the virus and what would happen next. Many people responded to this dramatic change in the political, social, and physical aspects of their environment by using their smartphones to try to access news about the virus and other concerning world events. This desire for information about world events intensified for many Americans in the summer of 2020, as people searched for news about the murder of George Floyd, racial justice protests, and the upcoming American presidential election. Many people found themselves spending long stretches of time—often hours per day—"doomscrolling" on their phone reading discouraging news.

According to Google Trends, the topic of "doomscrolling" was barely discussed before spring of 2020. Online discussion of "doomscrolling" peaked in the fall of 2020 and the winter of 2021, although it still remains a popular topic well into 2023 (Google Trends, n.d.).

Scientific research shows that doomscrolling can worsen anxiety and decrease mental well-being (Satici et al., 2022; Shabahang et al., 2022; Sharma et al., 2022). Doomscrolling can also worsen symptoms of depression and PTSD, especially for those with a history of childhood trauma (Price et al., 2022). Introverts and habitual social media users are more vulnerable to the negative effects of doomscrolling (Satici et al., 2022; Sharma et al., 2022). Researchers hypothesize that doomscrolling can be motivated by anxiety—when a person is anxious about the scary events around them, they may seek news about these negative events on social media (Sharma et al., 2022).

Unfortunately, doomscrolling also seems to worsen anxiety for many, potentially causing a vicious cycle. Doomscrolling can become habitual over time (Sharma et al., 2022), and is related to difficulties with emotional self-regulation (Anand et al., 2022). The negative effects of doomscrolling have been documented in the United States (Price et al., 2022; Sharma et al., 2022), Iran (Shabahang et al., 2022), Turkey (Satici et al., 2022), and other countries.

OTPs can play a role in assisting people who struggle with doomscrolling. OTPs can work with people on emotional self-regulation skills (see Chapter 12: Emotion Regulation 🤝) and managing phone use habits (see Chapter 14: Time Use and Habits 🤝). Approaches such as harm reduction (see Chapter 42: Homelessness and Housing Insecurity 🤝) and Motivational Interviewing (see Chapter 11: Motivation 🤝) could be helpful in assisting people to reduce the time they spend doomscrolling, even as people likely cannot eliminate negative media consumption entirely.

OTPs can also work with people on addressing their anxieties about political or historical events which may spur a desire to doomscroll for information in the first place. OTPs can support people to take values-aligned action in response to historical events through getting involved in occupations such as voting, volunteering, advocacy, or activism. Such occupations can help people connect with similar-minded people and feel satisfaction at taking action to create change (see, for example, Fox & Quinn, 2012).

Physical Factors

The natural environment is inextricably linked to mental health. More frequent visits to green spaces and to coastal areas is associated with lower levels of mental distress. Feeling connected to nature is also strongly associated with positive well-being (White et al., 2021). There are sociocultural differences in how connected to nature different populations feel. People have a higher connectedness to nature in Spain compared with the United Kingdom, for example, and this is linked to mental health differences in these populations (White et al., 2021). However, changes to the natural environment are currently causing a rise in stressors and anxiety disorders for people experiencing the consequences of climate change.

Extreme weather events and changes to local climates are causing disruption to agriculture and the liveability of areas of the planet, but these stressors are disproportionally falling on those already living in poverty. For many others, anxiety about the effects of climate change is rising. However, this anxiety can be adaptive (facilitating people to take action) or maladaptive (causing anxious feelings of helplessness; Taylor, 2020). The changing natural environment is a cause for concern because there is evidence that increased time spent in nature is associated with lower levels of anxiety—at least among those who live predominantly in urban areas. See Chapter 30: Natural Environments. 🤝

Social Factors

Anxiety disorders can severely affect the ability of someone to participate in their social roles to their satisfaction. In social anxiety in particular, job or school performance can be extremely difficult, especially in activities where social judgment is feared, such as giving presentations in college or approaching strangers. People with GAD describe their anxiety as "a grey cloud of worry that follows them everywhere"; this can cause preoccupation, as well as lack of pleasure and full participation in social relationships (Urish, 2017, p. 159).

The work environment can feel alienating, particularly where there may be noise and a busy atmosphere. People with agoraphobia or social anxiety may avoid performing occupations in places where there are many people (e.g., shopping, work meetings, using public transport) or may continue to perform them with considerable emotional effort/distress (Gunnarsson et al., 2021).

Institutional/Public Policy Factors

There is strong evidence that institutional issues such as racism contribute to anxiety disorders for people of color in the United States. Daily exposure to microaggressions, hostile racist contacts on social media, or institutional policies (such as racial profiling) are linked to increased levels of social anxiety, agoraphobia, and trauma-related anxiety and depression (MacIntyre et al., 2023). Because of such experiences, people of color may restrict many areas of occupational participation or experience fear and a threat response in situations where others would not (e.g., when visiting health-care providers).

Political decisions can contribute to stressors or ameliorate them (i.e., through timely health care or social protection policies). Government policies toward things such as health care, employment, and housing can further population-wide stressors. As one Irish professional describes housing policies, "I think about the housing crisis every single day. Some days it's the first sentient thought that enters my head, the vultures claw away at my brain before it's properly woken up . . . the gut-wrenching despair when I see a tent outside . . . the crippling anxiety when I imagine myself in my forties still scrolling Daft (property rental website) for a half decent rental" (Carey, 2022). See Chapter 26: The Public Policy Environment. 🤝

Spiritual Factors

Spiritual or religious beliefs and practices can influence the severity of anxiety disorders. Having positive cognitive or emotional aspects of a spiritual or religious life (such as trusting in God or a higher power) is associated with lower levels of anxiety. However, having negative appraisals (such as fearing a punitive God) is associated with more anxiety. Very strict religious rules can create a context where shame and guilt are common. The cognitive/emotional aspects of spirituality are more important for mental health than just participating in the occupations of religion (attending church or mosque or watching religious media, for example; Rosmarin & Leidl, 2020). Even for those without a formal religion, an attitude of gratitude is associated with lower anxiety, and gratitude practices are now a part of some positive psychology interventions for anxiety disorders. See Chapter 53: Spiritual Occupations.

Virtual Factors

Engaging in the online or virtual world may have some benefits for people with mental health conditions such as anxiety. Social media gives people an opportunity to connect with others experiencing similar difficulties, possibly reducing loneliness for people experiencing social isolation or anxiety. It may also allow people with mental illness to stay in touch with community activities, friends, and family and seek help for their difficulties (Naslund et al., 2020). Digital programs now offer more opportunities for services to offer support for hard-to-reach individuals and can be very acceptable for people who have sufficient agency and technology to use them (Patel et al., 2020).

Nevertheless, a large and growing body of research indicates that social media use and screen time pose an increased risk to mental health in general, and for anxiety and depressive disorders particularly (Naslund et al., 2020). Social media use leads to greater social comparison in young people and can put them at risk for social rejection, "trolling," cyberbullying, and social isolation when online interactions replace real-world social friendships (Rideout & Fox, 2018; Twenge & Campbell, 2018). More time spent on social media is associated with more symptoms of anxiety. Reducing time spent on social media is one clear intervention that OTPs can encourage to reduce anxiety symptoms. Even taking a break for a week from social media can make significant improvements in mental health (Lambert et al., 2022). See Chapter 33: Virtual Environments.

Occupation Factors

It is well recognized that an interrelationship exists between occupation and health and well-being. People organize their occupations into unique patterns, routines, roles, and responsibilities, and they manage varying degrees of different responsibilities and pressures on their occupational engagement over the life span (Baptiste, 2017). For people with anxiety disorders, occupation factors can exacerbate distress (as in someone with social anxiety being required to make a presentation) or relieve it (as in someone with GAD finding relief from tension through a woodland walk).

Occupational Areas and Roles

Some people with anxiety disorders will be greatly disabled in their ability to take part in their occupational roles, whereas others with more specific disorders (such as a specific phobia)

may be able to continue their occupational participation as long as they avoid the feared situation. At a fundamental level, sleep and rest will be particularly affected for someone with an anxiety disorder, particularly in GAD. Individuals will find it difficult to fall asleep, wake frequently, and even experience night terrors (Geddes et al., 2012). The impact of this sleep disturbance feeds into fatigue and loss of performance in daily tasks. GAD can cause difficulties across all occupational areas of life.

People with GAD show the same levels of disruption to life role participation as those with diabetes or arthritis (Hoffman et al., 2008), and it is considered more disabling than the other anxiety disorders. This may be because people with GAD frequently also report physical ill health and somatic symptoms such as headaches or chronic pain. Agoraphobia can exclude a person from occupational areas outside the home in severe cases, or it can mean that the person seeks to be accompanied by a trusted individual (Martin, 2003).

Because children with selective mutism may communicate without difficulty with their parents and siblings, the impact of the diagnosis on occupational performance may not be apparent until the child begins preschool or begins to attend social occasions such as birthday parties. The child may still enjoy leisure or sports occupations that do not require speech such as attending the cinema and be happy to take on nonverbal classroom tasks (APA, 2022).

Occupational Load

Occupational load is "the number of roles, tasks and occupations that an individual undertakes in the course of a specific time span" (Baptiste, 2017, p. 145). Taking an ecological viewpoint, anxiety disorders could be considered as a response to the "intolerably high and relentless demands imposed by modern living conditions," particularly in situations where people feel they do not have control or choices in their daily lives (Piko, 2002, p. 278). However, not all people living with the same demands develop an anxiety disorder, so it is likely that genetic, childhood, or temperamental vulnerabilities interact with these demands in particular ways to produce anxiety for those at risk for it.

Even when people with anxiety disorders can continue to perform their daily occupations, their satisfaction and subjective experience of this participation is lower. There can be a loss of pleasure and, in some cases, occupational imbalance, as distinguished from occupational balance, which is defined as "a relative state, recognizable by a happy or pleasant integration of life activities and demands" (Backman, 2004, p. 208). Amundson described three ways in which occupational life imbalance can affect well-being: where the range of occupations becomes too narrow and risk-averse, where the occupational range is too broad and lacks depth and personal meaning, and "sideline living," when the person is underoccupied, leading to poorer self-efficacy (Amundson, 2001). People with anxiety disorders may present with any of these forms of occupational imbalance at different life stages.

Intervention

With their expertise in adapting and addressing person, occupation, and environment factors, OTPs have the potential to use a range of evidence-based approaches to help

TABLE 18-1 | Common Intervention Approaches for Individuals With Anxiety Disorders

Approach	Target(s) of Intervention	Brief Synopsis	Chapters With Additional Information
Acceptance and Commitment Therapy	Psychological flexibility	Groups and individual programs: Encourage use of self-management tools such as journals, mindfulness, and identifying values.	Chapter 8: Cognitive Beliefs
Cognitive Behavioral Approach	Cognitive scripts and beliefs	Groups and individual programs: Encourage use of self-management tools such as thought diaries.	Chapter 8: Cognitive Beliefs
Building Routines and Time Use That Promotes Meaning and Well-Being	Behavioral regulation–making changes to routines, goals, and intentions	Groups and individual interventions: Explore, set goals, and practice new patterns of time use (e.g., making time for restorative occupations).	Chapter 14: Time Use and Habits
Nature-Based Approaches	Restorative environments and sensory-based mood enhancement	Facilitate group or individual nature-based programs such as forest walking. Encourage and reduce barriers to participation in all groups/populations.	Chapter 30: Natural Environments
Self-Management/Peer-Led Approaches	Peer support and role modeling	Facilitate groups or informal interactions with people with lived experience in recovery to provide hope and peer support. Specific programs include the Wellness Recovery Action Plan.	Chapter 39: Peer-Led Services
Mindfulness	Psychological flexibility	Facilitate mindfulness programs. Encourage mindfulness in everyday occupations (mindful doing).	Chapter 12: Emotion Regulation
Physical Exercise and Lifestyle	Stress response (biological) and reduction (psychological)	Encourage and reduce barriers to participation in active occupations. Facilitate physical activity programs.	Chapter 45 Self-Care and Well-Being Occupations
Sensory Approaches	Promoting sensory self-regulation	Facilitate programs and develop environments (e.g., in hospital settings) that provide opportunities for sensory self-regulation.	Chapter 9: Sensory Processing and the Lived Sensory Experience

improve occupational participation for people with anxiety disorders (Table 18-1).

Medications

Many people with an anxiety disorder are not prescribed (or choose not to take) medication for their symptoms. Rates of health-care utilization vary widely between diagnoses (e.g., those with panic disorder tend to seek help quite quickly, and often from physical health services at first, whereas those with specific phobias may never seek psychological/psychiatric help; Bandelow & Michaelis, 2022).

In general, there are two main groups of medications prescribed for people with anxiety disorders (sometimes called anxiolytics). In the first, oldest group of medications are the benzodiazepines, which target the gamma-aminobutyric acid (GABA) receptors. Use of benzodiazepines is less common today because of fears of dependence, medication abuse, and mortality that can occur with opioids (Bui et al., 2019). In the

second group are the selective serotonin reuptake inhibitors (SSRIs) and serotonin-norepinephrine reuptake inhibitors (SNRIs), which are safer in cases of overdose or misuse and can be used longer without dependence by people with anxiety disorders. However, some authors have questioned the need for lifelong medication use for anxiety disorders, particularly when psychological/rehabilitative approaches can be curative in nature (Bui et al., 2019).

Guidelines for the treatment of people with anxiety disorders recommend using pharmacotherapy and psychosocial treatment approaches together, after self-help/psychoeducation approaches have been tried (Bandelow et al., 2017). SSRIs (such as citalopram, escitalopram, fluoxetine, and sertraline) will be started at a low dose of 10 to 20 mg. There may be some adverse effects, such as restlessness, weight gain, and fatigue, and patients may not see an effect on their anxiety for 4 weeks. SNRIs (such as duloxetine and venlafaxine) are started at higher doses (60–70 mg) and show similar side effects (Bandelow et al., 2017).

Evidence-Based Practice

Acceptance and Commitment Therapy Versus Cognitive Behavioral Therapy

ACT might be more appropriate for use by occupational therapy practitioners than CBT.

RESEARCH FINDINGS

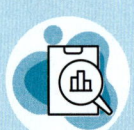

Acceptance and Commitment Therapy (ACT) is one of the so-called new "third wave" psychotherapies. Compared with cognitive behavioral therapy (CBT), the focus in third-wave therapies is on noticing internal experiences, rather than seeing them as "negative" or maladaptive. ACT is as effective as CBT for people with anxiety disorders when compared with treatment-as-usual conditions and in direct comparisons (Twohig & Levin, 2017).

APPLICATIONS

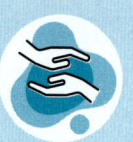

➡ ACT might be more appropriate for use by OTPs than CBT, given that the goal of the former is "promoting functioning and wellbeing" (Gloster et al., 2020, p. 190). However, as both approaches appear equally effective at present, the preferences of the person and the training of the therapist will be important in decision-making.

➡ Using an ACT approach, the OTP would spend time exploring the values of the person and identifying activities and time use that would help them live more closely aligned with those values. In this way, ACT is highly compatible with many existing occupational therapy models and allows the OTP retain their disciplinary focus on occupation.

➡ ACT approaches can be used by OTPs without further certification, although some training and further reading are recommended.

REFERENCES

Gloster, A. T., Walder, N., Levin, M. E., Twohig, M. P., & Karekla, M. (2020). The empirical status of Acceptance and Commitment Therapy: A review of meta-analyses. *Journal of Contextual Behavioral Science, 18,* 181–192. https://doi.org/10.1016/j.jcbs.2020.09.009

Twohig, M. P., & Levin, M. E. (2017). Acceptance and Commitment Therapy as a treatment for anxiety and depression: A review. *Psychiatric Clinics of North America, 40*(4), 751–770. https://doi.org/10.1016/j.psc.2017.08.009

An advantage of the SSRIs and SNRIs is that they also treat the depression symptoms that are commonly experienced by people with anxiety disorders. When stopping treatment, there can be some withdrawal effects, but these are far less severe/frequent when compared with benzodiazepines. However, because of their much quicker effect on anxiety, specific benzodiazepines (lorazepam) may be given in an immediate dose in specific circumstances (e.g., in an acute panic attack; Bandelow et al., 2017).

Here's the Point

■ OTPs are highly likely to work with people with anxiety disorders outside of the psychiatric/mental health services. Most people visit their primary care provider for anxiety concerns and some will present to medical services (e.g., when concerned about panic symptoms). This may not be the reason for referral to occupational therapy, but

co-occurring anxiety should be considered and addressed in all therapy settings.

■ Anxiety disorders are both physically and emotionally distressing. OTPs can provide occupation-focused intervention to increase participation in physical activities, nature-based activities, and activities that promote restoration and sensory self-regulation.

■ OTPs should recognize that anxiety disorders will disproportionally affect people experiencing social inequality and those who have vulnerabilities (genetically or from childhood). Issues such as poverty, poor housing, and racism are structural issues that OTPs can campaign about as a collective (as in AOTA) in order to promote occupational justice.

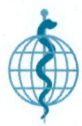

Visit the online resource center at **FADavis.com** to access the videos.

Apply It Now

1. Practicing Psychological Flexibility

In this chapter's The Lived Experience feature, Lily describes using walking and journaling in her recovery from GAD. Over the next week, in your reflective journal, make a note of occupations that are helpful to your mental health and those that are unhelpful. The example in Figure 18-1 will get you started. These should not be special or unusual occupations for you, but rather everyday occupations embedded in your daily life. Just try to notice without judgment the different occupational choices that you make during the day and any impact they have on your stress or anxiety levels.

■ Remember that it is expected that anxiety, as a normal human emotion, will occur and fluctuate during the day. Try to notice without judgment.

■ It is also expected that many meaningful and necessary occupations may cause a rise in anxiety (e.g., sitting for an examination)—this does not make them unhelpful to mental health.

2. Experiencing the Stress Response

When people perceive a threat, their body automatically starts a stress response. Adrenaline triggers the body to be on alert. This week, try something that challenges you (but that you are up for!) and observe (again, without judgment) how your body responds. For example, you could make conversation with a stranger or go out socially on your own. Remember that the human body is designed to experience a certain amount of "normal" anxiety. Try to use the phrase "I'm noticing . . ." as in, "I'm noticing my breathing is shallow" or "I'm noticing that my heart is beating faster." Afterward, do something that naturally diminishes anxiety (e.g., talk to a friend, go for a brisk walk, or sit quietly and take some long deep breaths). Reflect, if you wish, on how it would feel to live long term with ongoing anxiety (as in GAD) or if your experiences escalated to a point where you could not cope with them (as in panic) and how debilitating this would be. Remember that the previous strategies will work for everyday anxiety, but that those with anxiety disorders will need more specialized and ongoing support and help.

3. Video Exercise: Jordon's Lived Experience of Anxiety and Depression

Pair up with another student in your class or form a small group of students. Access and watch the "Jordon's Lived Experience of Anxiety and Depression" video at the online resource center at FADavis.com. Then, discuss and together answer the following questions:

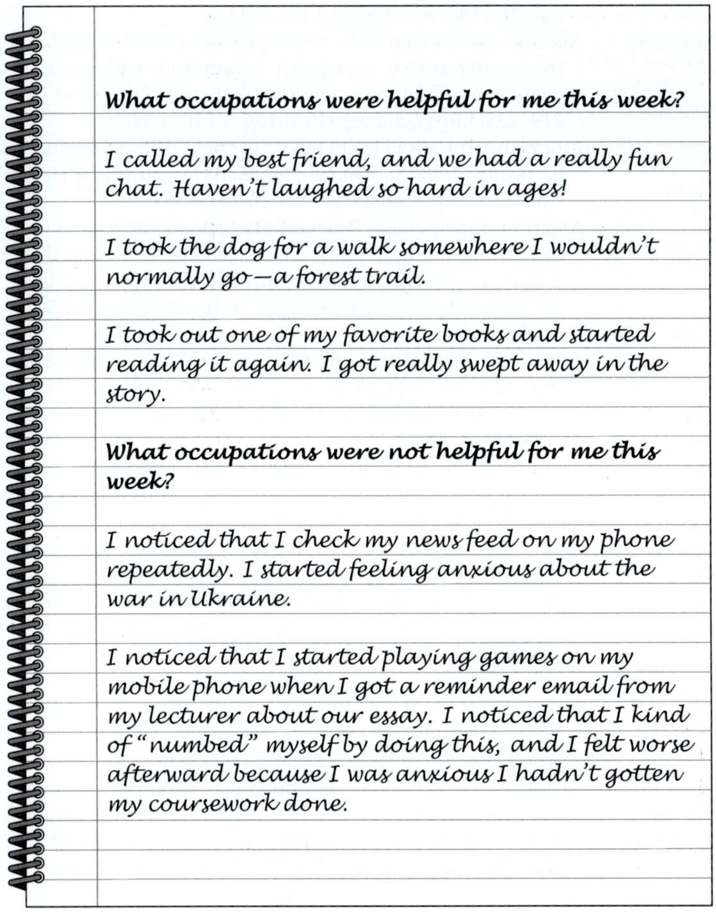

What occupations were helpful for me this week?

I called my best friend, and we had a really fun chat. Haven't laughed so hard in ages!

I took the dog for a walk somewhere I wouldn't normally go—a forest trail.

I took out one of my favorite books and started reading it again. I got really swept away in the story.

What occupations were not helpful for me this week?

I noticed that I check my news feed on my phone repeatedly. I started feeling anxious about the war in Ukraine.

I noticed that I started playing games on my mobile phone when I got a reminder email from my lecturer about our essay. I noticed that I kind of "numbed" myself by doing this, and I felt worse afterward because I was anxious I hadn't gotten my coursework done.

FIGURE 18-1. Reflecting on occupational choices.

Reflection Questions

■ Jordon describes her anxiety in this way: "While I excelled with schoolwork, the taskmaster in my brain wouldn't accept anything less. My internal world was torment. . . . I just did not understand why normal daily activities were such a challenge for me, and it appeared to be a breeze for everyone else." From what you have learned about anxiety, how would you begin working with an individual experiencing these feelings?

■ Jordan learned that her access to mental health treatment as a teen became "a lens that medical providers in the future would view me through," and her mental health label actually misrepresented and invalidated her medical needs. How can OTPs overcome the tendency to view individuals through the lens of their mental health diagnoses? How can we help individuals recognize that their mental health label does not define them?

■ Jordan acknowledges the privileges she had that impacted on her story. How might the story change if Jordan had a minoritized identity, lacked access to mental health care, was unhoused, or if she lacked family and a supportive, caring network? As a practitioner, what steps can you take to recognize and address these social determinants that affect a person's mental health? Through peer support and access to mental health resources, Jordan found connection and the strength to live with her mental health challenges, in part because she discovered the language with which to describe her experience. How can OTPs help individuals find the language to describe their strengths and challenges, and how does providing language around a person's lived experience help them in their overall mental health journey?

Resources

Organizations

- Anxiety and Depression Association of America: http://adaa.org
- National Alliance on Mental Illness: https://www.nami.org/home
- Jigsaw–Youth Mental Health: https://www.jigsaw.ie
- World Health Organization—Global and Developmental Viewpoint on Mental Health: https://www.who.int/health-topics/mental-health#tab+tab_1
- World Federation of Occupational Therapists—Global Occupational Therapy Perspective on Mental Health: https://www.wfot.org/resources/occupational-therapy-and-mental-health

Books

- Bourne, E. (2020). *The anxiety and phobia workbook* (7th ed.). New Harbinger.
- Greenberger, D., & Padesky, C. (2015). *Mind over mood: Change how you feel by changing the way you think* (2nd ed.). Guilford Press.
- Harris, R. (2020). *The happiness trap* (2nd ed.). Psychological Flexibility Pty Ltd.

Videos

- "Jenny's Lived Experience of Sensory Processing Differences" video. Jenny is an occupational therapy doctorate (OTD) student with the lived experience of sensory differences, anxiety, and depression. In this video, she describes how she discovered her diagnosis, how it affects her in the classroom, and what interventions she uses to manage her reactions to stimuli. Importantly, she discusses the need to advocate for herself and for practitioners to help people across the life span to understand their sensory processing needs in order to improve their mental health and overall quality of life. To access the video, visit the online resource center at FADavis.com.
- "Mental Health and Well-Being During COVID" video. Caitlin is an OTP who has worked in outpatient settings with both adults and children. In this video, she talks about how occupational therapy practice during the COVID-19 global pandemic allowed her to see in a new way the effects of stress and anxiety on patient outcomes. She discusses how she incorporates mental health and well-being into her practice and her belief that it promotes successful healing and recovery. To access the video, visit the online resource center at FADavis.com.

References

Abernethy, H. (2010). The assessment and treatment of sensory defensiveness in adult mental health: A literature review. *British Journal of Occupational Therapy, 73*(5), 210–218. https://doi.org/10.4276/030802210X12734991664183

Aktar, E., Nikolić, M., & Bögels, S. M. (2017). Environmental transmission of generalized anxiety disorder from parents to children: Worries, experiential avoidance, and intolerance of uncertainty. *Dialogues in Clinical Neuroscience, 19*(2), 137–147. https://doi.org/10.31887/DCNS.2017.19.2/eaktar

Alkozei, A., Cooper, P. J., & Creswell, C. (2014). Emotional reasoning and anxiety sensitivity: Associations with social anxiety disorder in childhood. *Journal of Affective Disorders, 152–154,* 219–228. https://doi.org /10.1016/j.jad.2013.09.014

All Ireland Traveller Health Study Team. (2010). *All Ireland Traveller Health Study: Summary of findings.* Department of Health and Children. http://hdl.handle.net/10147/111897

American Occupational Therapy Association. (2020). Occupational therapy practice framework: Domain and process—Fourth edition. *American Journal of Occupational Therapy, 74*(Suppl. 2), 7412410010p1–7412410010p87. https://doi.org/10.5014/ajot.2020.74S2001

American Psychiatric Association. (2022). *Diagnostic and statistical manual of mental disorders* (5th ed., text rev.). American Psychiatric Publishing. https://doi.org/10.1176/appi.books.9780890425787

Amundson, N. E. (2001). Three-dimensional living. *Journal of Employment Counseling, 38*(3), 114–127. https://doi.org/10.1002/j.2161-1920.2001.tb00493.x

Anand, N., Sharma, M. K., Thakur, P. C., Mondal, I., Sahu, M., Singh, P., Ajith, S. J., Kande, J. S., Ms, N., & Singh, R. (2022). Doomsurfing and doomscrolling mediate psychological distress in COVID-19 lockdown: Implications for awareness of cognitive biases. *Perspectives in Psychiatric Care, 58*(1), 170–172. https://doi.org/10.1111/ppc.12803

Attwood, T. (2004). Cognitive behaviour therapy for children and adults with Asperger's syndrome. *Behaviour Change, 21*(3), 147–161. https://doi.org/10.1375/bech.21.3.147.55995

Backman, C. L. (2004). Occupational balance: Exploring the relationships among daily occupations and their influence on well-being. *Canadian Journal of Occupational Therapy, 71*(4), 202–209. https://doi.org/10.1177/000841740407100404

Bandelow, B., & Michaelis, S. (2022). Epidemiology of anxiety disorders in the 21st century. *Dialogues in Clinical Neuroscience, 17*(3), 327–335. https://doi.org/10.31887/DCNS.2015.17.3/bbandelow

Bandelow, B., Michaelis, S., & Wedekind, D. (2017). Treatment of anxiety disorders. *Dialogues in Clinical Neuroscience, 19*(2), 93–107. https://doi.org/10.31887/DCNS.2017.19.2/bbandelow

Baptiste, S. (2017). The Person-Environment-Occupation model. In J. Hinojosa, P. Kramer, & C. Brasic Royeen (Eds.), *Perspectives on human occupation: Theories underlying practice* (2nd ed., pp. 137–159). F.A. Davis.

Baxter, A. J., Scott, K. M., Ferrari, A. J., Norman, R. E., Vos, T., & Whiteford, H. A. (2014). Challenging the myth of an "epidemic" of common mental disorders: Trends in the global prevalence of anxiety and depression between 1990 and 2010. *Depression and Anxiety, 31*, 506–516. https://doi.org/10.1002/da.22230

Bekker, M. H. J., & van Mens-Verhulst, J. (2007). Anxiety disorders: Sex differences in prevalence, degree, and background, but gender-neutral treatment. *Gender Medicine, 4*, S178–S193. https://doi.org/10.1016/S1550-8579(07)80057-X

Bögels, S. M., Knappe, S., & Clark, L. A. (2013). Adult separation anxiety disorder in *DSM-5. Clinical Psychology Review, 33*(5), 663–674. https://doi.org/10.1016/j.cpr.2013.03.006

Bui, E., King, F., & Melaragno, A. (2019). Pharmacotherapy of anxiety disorders in the 21st century: A call for novel approaches. *General Psychiatry, 32*, 1–5. https://doi.10.1136/gpsych-2019-100136

Cara, E. (2013). Anxiety disorders. In E. Cara & A. MacRae (Eds.), *Psychosocial occupational therapy: An evolving practice* (3rd ed., pp. 258–307). Delmar Cengage Learning.

Carey, G. (2022, January 5). *Unable to detach—Why I can't stop thinking about the housing crisis.* https://www.alustforlife.com/voice/unable-to-detach-why-i-cant-thinking-about-the-housing-crisis

Christiansen, D. M. (2015). Examining sex and gender differences in anxiety disorders. In F. Durbano (Ed.), *A fresh look at anxiety disorders* (pp. 17–50). InTech. https://doi.org/10.5772/59525

Clarke, J., & Fox, J. (2017). The impact of social anxiety on occupational participation in college life. *Occupational Therapy in Mental Health, 33*(1), 31–46. https://doi.org/10.1080/0164212X.2016.1222323

Curran, T., & Hill, A. P. (2019). Perfectionism is increasing over time: A meta-analysis of birth cohort differences from 1989 to 2016. *Psychological Bulletin, 145*(4), 410–429. https://doi.org/10.1037/bul0000138

Daly, M., & Robinson, E. (2022). Depression and anxiety during COVID-19. *The Lancet, 399*(10324), 518. https://doi.org/10.1016/S0140-6736(22)00187-8

Dowbiggin, I. R. (2009). High anxieties: The social construction of anxiety disorders. *The Canadian Journal of Psychiatry, 54*(7), 429–436. https://doi.org/10.1177/070674370905400703

Drapeau, A., Marchand, A., & Beaulieu-Prevost, D. (2012). Epidemiology of psychological distress. In L. L'Abate (Ed.), *Mental illnesses—Understanding, prediction and control* (pp. 105–134). InTech. https://doi.org/10.5772/30872

Dunn, W. (1997). The impact of sensory processing abilities on the daily lives of young children and their families: A conceptual model. *Infants & Young Children, 9*(4), 23–35. https//doi.org/10.1097/00001163-199704000-0005

Ellyatt, H. (2022, February 10). *Last responders: Mental health damage from Covid could last a generation, professionals say.* https://www.cnbc.com/2022/02/10/covid-pandemic-mental-health-damage-could-last-a-generation.html

Elmore, A. L., & Crouch, E. (2020). The association of adverse childhood experiences with anxiety and depression for children and youth, 8 to 17 years of age. *Academic Pediatrics, 20*(5), 600–608. https://doi.org/10.1016/j.acap.2020.02.012

Engel-Yeger, B., & Dunn, W. (2011). The relationship between sensory processing difficulties and anxiety level of healthy adults.

British Journal of Occupational Therapy, 74(5), 210–216. https://doi.org/10.4276/030802211X13046730116407

Fox, J., & Quinn, S. (2012). The meaning of social activism to older adults in Ireland. *Journal of Occupational Science, 19*(4), 358–370. https://doi.org/10.1080/14427591.2012.701179

Geddes, J., Price, J., & McKnight, R. (2012). *Psychiatry* (4th ed.). Oxford University Press.

Gloster, A. T., Walder, N., Levin, M. E., Twohig, M. P., & Karekla, M. (2020). The empirical status of Acceptance and Commitment Therapy: A review of meta-analyses. *Journal of Contextual Behavioral Science, 18*, 181–192. https://doi.org/10.1016/j.jcbs.2020.09.009

Goodwin, G. M. (2021). Revisiting treatment options for depressed patients with generalised anxiety disorder. *Advances in Therapy, 38*(Suppl. 2), 61–68. https://doi.org/10.1007/s12325-021-01861-0

Google Trends. (n.d.). *Doomscrolling.* https://trends.google.com/trends/explore?date=today%205-y&geo=US&q=doomscrolling&hl=en

Gunnarsson, A. B., Hedberg, A.-K., Håkansson, C., Hedin, K., & Wagman, P. (2021). Occupational performance problems in people with depression and anxiety. *Scandinavian Journal of Occupational Therapy, 30*(2), 148–158. https://doi.org/10.1080/11038128.2021.1882562

Halim, A. T., Richdale, A. L., & Uljarević, M. (2018). Exploring the nature of anxiety in young adults on the autism spectrum: A qualitative study. *Research in Autism Spectrum Disorders, 55*, 25–37. https://doi.org/10.1016/j.rasd.2018.07.006

Härter, M. C., Conway, K. P., & Merikangas, K. R. (2003). Associations between anxiety disorders and physical illness. *European Archives of Psychiatry and Clinical Neuroscience, 253*, 313–320. https://doi.org/10.1007/s00406-003-0449-y

Hendriks, S. M., Spijker, J., Licht, C. M., Beekman, A. T., Hardeveld, F., de Graaf, R., Batlaan, N. M., & Penninx, B. W. (2014). Disability in anxiety disorders. *Journal of Affective Disorders, 166*, 227–233. https://doi.org/10.1016/j.jad.2014.05.006

Heylens, G., Elaut, E., Kreukels, B. P. C., Paap, M. C. S., Cerwenka, S., Richter-Appelt, H., Cohen-Kettenis, P. T., Haraldsen, I. R., & De Cuypere, G. (2014). Psychiatric characteristics in transsexual individuals: Multicentre study in four European countries. *The British Journal of Psychiatry, 204*(2), 151–156. https://doi.org/10.1192/bjp.bp.112.121954

Hoffman, D. L., Dukes, E. M., & Wittchen, H.-U. (2008). Human and economic burden of generalized anxiety disorder. *Depression and Anxiety, 25*(1), 72–90. https://doi.org/10.1002/da.20257

Horwitz, A. V., & Wakefield, J. C. (2012). *All we have to fear: Psychiatry's transformation of natural anxieties into mental disorders.* Oxford University Press.

Jefferies, P., & Ungar, M. (2020). Social anxiety in young people: A prevalence study in seven countries. *PLoS One, 15*(9), e0239133. https://doi.org/10.1371/journal.pone.0239133

Kent, R., & Simonoff, E. (2017). Prevalence of anxiety in autism spectrum disorders. In C. M. Kerns, P. Renno, E. A. Storch, P. C. Kendall, & J. J. Wood (Eds.), *Anxiety in children and adolescents with autism spectrum disorder* (pp. 5–32), Academic Press.

Kessler, R. C., Petukhova, M., Sampson, N. A., Zaslavsky, A. M., & Wittchen, H. U. (2012). Twelve-month and lifetime prevalence and lifetime morbid risk of anxiety and mood disorders in the United States. *International Journal of Methods in Psychiatric Research, 21*(3), 169–184. https://doi.org/10.1002/mpr.1359

Lambert, J., Barnstable, G., Minter, E., Cooper, J., & McEwan, D. (2022). Taking a one-week break from social media improves well-being, depression, and anxiety: A randomized controlled trial. *Cyberpsychology, Behavior, and Social Networking, 25*(5), 287–293. https://doi.org/10.1089/cyber.2021.0324

Langarita-Llorente, R., & Gracia-Garcia, P. (2019). [Neuropsychology of generalized anxiety disorders: A systematic review]. *Revista de Neurologia, 69*(2), 59–67. https://doi.org/10.33588/rn.6902.2018371

Law, M., Cooper, B., Strong, S., Stewart, D., Rigby, P., & Letts, L. (1996). The Person-Environment-Occupation model: A transactive approach to occupational performance. *Canadian Journal of Occupational Therapy, 63*(1), 9–23. https://doi.org/10.1177/000841749606300103

Leonard, K., & Abramovitch, A. (2019). Cognitive functions in young adults with generalized anxiety disorder. *European Psychiatry, 56*(1), 1–7. https://doi.org/10.1016/j.eurpsy.2018.10.008

Lokman, J., & Bockting, C. (2022). Pathways to depressive and anxiety disorders during and after the COVID-19 pandemic. *The Lancet Psychiatry, 9*(7), 531–533. https://doi.org/10.1016/S2215-0366(22)00152-3

MacIntyre, M. M., Zare, M., & Williams, M. T. (2023). Anxiety-related disorders in the context of racism. *Current Psychiatry Reports, 25,* 31–43. https://doi.org/10.1007/s11920-022-01408-2

Manicavasaga, V., Silove, D., & Curtis, J. (1997). Separation anxiety in adulthood: A phenomenological investigation. *Comprehensive Psychiatry, 38*(5), 274–282. https://doi.org/10.1016/S0010-440X(97)90060-2

Martin, P. (2003). The epidemiology of anxiety disorders: A review. *Dialogues in Clinical Neuroscience, 5*(3), 281–298. https://doi.org/10.31887/DCNS.2003.5.3/pmartin

Morganstein, J. C. (2022). Preparing for the next pandemic to protect public mental health: What have we learned from COVID-19? *Psychiatric Clinics, 45*(1), 191–210. https://doi.org/10.1016/j.psc.2021.11.012

Naslund, J. A., Bondre, A., Torous, J., & Aschbrenner, K. A. (2020). Social media and mental health: Benefits, risks, and opportunities for research and practice. *Journal of Technology in Behavioral Science, 5,* 245–257. https://doi.org/10.1007/s41347-020-00134-x

O'Doherty, J., Hannigan, A., Hickey, L., Meagher, D., Cullen, W., O'Connor, R., & O'Regan, A. (2020). The prevalence and treatment of mental health conditions documented in general practice in Ireland. *Irish Journal of Psychological Medicine, 37*(1), 24–31. https://doi.org/10.1017/ipm.2018.48

Patel, S., Akhtar, A., Malins, S., Wright, N., Rowley, E., Young, E., Sampson, S., & Morriss, R. (2020). The acceptability and usability of digital health interventions for adults with depression, anxiety, and somatoform disorders: Qualitative systematic review and meta-synthesis. *Journal of Medical Internet Research, 22*(7), e16228. https://doi.org/10.2196/16228

Peters, L., Issakidis, C., Slade, T. I. M., & Andrews, G. (2006). Gender differences in the prevalence of DSM-IV and ICD-10 PTSD. *Psychological Medicine, 36*(1), 81–89. https://doi.org/10.1017/S003329170500591X

Piko, B. F. (2002). Socio-cultural stress in modern societies and the myth of anxiety in Eastern Europe. *Administration and Policy in Mental Health, 29,* 275–280. https://doi.org/10.1023/a:1015199727651

Plaisier, I., de Bruijn, J. G. M., Smit, J. H., de Graaf, R., ten Have, M., Beekman, A. T. F., van Dyck, R., & Penninx, B. W. J. H. (2008). Work and family roles and the association with depressive and anxiety disorders: Differences between men and women. *Journal of Affective Disorders, 105*(1-3), 63–72. https://doi.org/10.1016/j.jad.2007.04.010

Price, M., Legrand, A. C., Brier, Z. M. F., van Stolk-Cooke, K., Peck, K., Dodds, P. S., Danforth, C. M., & Adams, Z. W. (2022). Doomscrolling during COVID-19: The negative association between daily social and traditional media consumption and mental health symptoms during the COVID-19 pandemic. *Psychological Trauma: Theory, Research, Practice and Policy, 14*(8), 1338–1346. https://doi.org/10.1037/tra0001202

Rapee, R. M. (2002). The development and modification of temperamental risk for anxiety disorders: Prevention of a lifetime of anxiety? *Biological Psychiatry, 52*(10), 947–957. https://doi.org/10.1016/S0006-3223(02)01572-X

Reisner, S. L., Katz-Wise, S. L., Gordon, A. R., Corliss, H. L., & Austin, S. B. (2016). Social epidemiology of depression and anxiety by gender identity. *Journal of Adolescent Health, 59*(2), 203–208. https://doi.org/10.1016/j.jadohealth.2016.04.006

Rideout, V., & Fox, S. (2018). *Digital health practices, social media use, and mental well-being among teens and young adults in the U.S.* Hopelab & Well Being Trust. https://www.hopelab.org/reports/pdf/a-national-survey-by-hopelab-and-well-being-trust-2018.pdf

Rodríguez-García, A.-M., Moreno-Guerrero, A.-J., & Lopez Belmonte, J. (2020). Nomophobia: An individual's growing fear of being without a smartphone—a systematic literature review. *International Journal of Environmental Research and Public Health, 17*(2), 580–599. https://doi.org/10.3390/ijerph17020580

Rodríguez-Testal, J. F., Senín-Calderón, C., & Perona-Garcelán, S. (2014). From *DSM-IV-TR* to *DSM-5*: Analysis of some changes. *International Journal of Clinical and Health Psychology, 14*(3), 221–231. https://doi.org/10.1016/j.ijchp.2014.05.002

Rosmarin, D. H., & Leidl, B. (2020). Spirituality, religion, and anxiety disorders. In D. H. Rosmarin & H. G. Koenig (Eds.), *Handbook of spirituality, religion, and mental health* (pp. 41–60). Academic Press.

Roy-Byrne, P. P., Craske, M. G., & Stein, M. B. (2006). Panic disorder. *The Lancet, 368*(9540), 1023–1032. https://doi.org/10.1016/S0140-6736(06)69418-X

Santomauro, D. F., Mantilla Herrera, A. M., Shadid, J., Zheng, P., Ashbaugh, C., Pigott, D. M., Abbafati, C., Adolph, C., Amlag, J. O., Aravkin, A. Y., Bang-Jensen, B. L., Bertolacci, G. J., Bloom, S. S., Castellano, R., Castro, E., Chakrabarti, S., Chattopadhyay, J., Cogen, R. M., Collins, J. K., & Ferrari, A. J. (2021). Global prevalence and burden of depressive and anxiety disorders in 204 countries and territories in 2020 due to the COVID-19 pandemic. *The Lancet, 398*(10312), 1700–1712. https://doi.org/10.1016/S0140-6736(21)02143-7

Satici, S. A., Gocet Tekin, E., Deniz, M. E., & Satici, B. (2022). Doomscrolling scale: Its association with personality traits, psychological distress, social media use, and wellbeing. *Applied Research in Quality of Life, 18*(2), 833–847. https://doi.org/10.1007/s11482-022-10110-7

Shabahang, R., Kim, S., Hosseinkhanzadeh, A. A., Aruguete, M. S., & Kakabaraee, K. (2022). "Give your thumb a break" from surfing tragic posts: Potential corrosive consequences of social media users' doomscrolling. *Media Psychology, 26*(4), 460–479. https://doi.org/10.1080/15213269.2022.2157287

Sharma, B., Lee, S. S., & Johnson, B. K. (2022). The dark at the end of the tunnel: Doomscrolling on social media newsfeeds. *Technology, Mind, and Behavior, 3*(1), 1–13. https://doi.org/10.1037/tmb0000059

Shear, K., Jin, R., Ruscio, A. M., Walters, E. E., & Kessler, R. C. (2006). Prevalence and correlates of estimated *DSM-IV* child and adult separation anxiety disorder in the National Comorbidity Survey Replication. *American Journal of Psychiatry, 163*(6), 1074–1083. https://doi.org/10.1176/appi.ajp.163.6.1074

Shimada-Sugimoto, M., Otowa, T., & Hettema, J. M. (2015). Genetics of anxiety disorders: Genetic epidemiological and molecular studies in humans. *Psychiatry and Clinical Neurosciences, 69*(7), 388–401. https://doi.org/10.1111/pcn.12291

Shorter, E. (2009). Symposium: Real and unreal in psychiatry. *Canadian Journal of Psychiatry/Revue Canadienne de Psychiatrie, 54*(7), 427–428. https://doi.org/10.1177/070674370905400701

Taquet, M., Holmes, E. A., & Harrison, P. J. (2021). Depression and anxiety disorders during the COVID-19 pandemic: Knowns and unknowns. *The Lancet, 398*(10312), 1665–1666. https://doi.org/10.1016/S0140-6736(21)02221-2

Taylor, S. (2020). Anxiety disorders, climate change, and the challenges ahead: Introduction to the special issue. *Journal of Anxiety Disorders, 76,* 102313. https://doi.org/10.1016/j.janxdis.2020.102313

Thibaut, F. (2017). Anxiety disorders: A review of current literature. *Dialogues in Clinical Neuroscience, 19*(2), 87–88. https://doi.org/10.31887/DCNS.2017.19.2/fthibaut

Twenge, J. M., & Campbell, W. K. (2018). Associations between screen time and lower psychological well-being among children and adolescents: Evidence from a population-based study.

Preventive Medicine Reports, 12, 271–283. https://doi.org /10.1016/j.pmedr.2018.10.003

Twohig, M. P., & Levin, M. E. (2017). Acceptance and Commitment Therapy as a treatment for anxiety and depression: A review. *Psychiatric Clinics of North America, 40*(4), 751–770. https://doi.org /10.1016/j.psc.2017.08.009

Urish, C. (2017). Anxiety disorders. In B. J. Atchison & D. Powers Dirette (Eds.), *Conditions in occupational therapy: Effect on occupational performance* (5th ed., pp. 147–164). Wolters Kluwer.

White, M. P., Elliott, L. R., Grellier, J., Economou, T., Bell, S., Bratman, G. N., Cirach, M., Gascon, M., Lima, M. L., Lõhmus, M., Nieuwenhuijsen, M., Ojala, A., Roiko, A., Wesley Schultz, P., van den Bosch, M., & Fleming, L. E. (2021). Associations between green/blue spaces and mental health across 18 countries. *Scientific Reports, 11*(1), 8903. https://doi.org/10.1038/s41598-021-87675-0

Whiteford, H. A., Degenhardt, L., Rehm, J., Baxter, A. J., Ferrari, A. J., Erskine, H. E., Charlson, F. J., Norman, R. E., Flaxman, A. D., Johns, N., Burstein, R., Murray, C. J. L., & Vos, T. (2013). Global burden of disease attributable to mental and substance use disorders: Findings from the Global Burden of Disease Study 2010. *The Lancet, 382*(9904), 1575–1586. https://doi.org/10.1016/S0140-6736(13)61611-6

Wittchen, H.-U., Jacobi, F., Rehm, J., Gustavsson, A., Svensson, M., Jönsson, B., Olesen, J., Allgulander, C., Alonso, J., Faravelli, C., Fratiglioni, L., Jennum, P., Lieb, R., Maercker, A., van Os, J., Preisig, M., Salvador-Carulla, L., Simon, R., & Steinhausen, H. C. (2011). The size and burden of mental disorders and other disorders of the brain in Europe 2010. *European Neuropsychopharmacology, 21*(9), 655–679. https://doi.org/10.1016/j .euroneuro.2011.07.018

Wittchen, H.-U., Mühlig, S., & Beesdo, K. (2003). Mental disorders in primary care. *Dialogues in Clinical Neuroscience, 5*(2), 115–128. https://doi.org/10.31887/DCNS.2003.5.2/huwittchen

Woodgate, R. L., Tennent, P., Barriage, S., & Legras, N. (2020). The lived experience of anxiety and the many facets of pain: A qualitative, arts-based approach. *Canadian Journal of Pain, 4*(3), 6–18. https://doi.org/10.1080/24740527.2020.1720501

World Health Organization. (2022). *ICD-11: International classification of diseases* (11th rev.). Author. https://icd.who.int/en

Mark E. Hardison and Sofia L. Herrera-Jaureguiberry

The most common eating disorders include anorexia nervosa, bulimia nervosa, binge-eating disorder, and avoidant/restrictive food intake disorder. However, it is common for individuals with one eating disorder to flow through two or more diagnoses across the life span. For example, individuals might transition from anorexia nervosa to bulimia nervosa or from bulimia nervosa to binge-eating disorder (Hilbert et al., 2014). Though the criteria are distinct, each eating disorder diagnosis shares the feature of individuals developing a dysfunctional relationship with food and/or calorie burning and elimination that is rigid and ritualized.

Eating disorders as a group are named for the primary dysfunction with eating. However, as will be discussed, this group of disorders on a deeper level is often about the need to maintain an element of control in life, acting as a harmful coping tool for psychosocial distress, or the expression of traumatic events experienced in childhood or adolescence. Beyond disrupted eating, symptoms may span almost all areas of occupation (e.g., hygiene, social functioning, work, rest) and affect both mental health and physical health (Bradford et al., 2015).

The chapter begins with a personal story of Rudi Pohl, who lives with anorexia nervosa. Hopefully readers will always remember the human struggle involved with any mental health diagnosis: the highs and lows, the strengths, and the striving. Then, the chapter outlines diagnostic criteria for eating disorders. Every individual with an eating disorder has their own unique story; however, understanding the features used to diagnose is helpful in understanding the conditions. This chapter includes a discussion of etiology, prevalence, and course and the impact of the conditions on occupational performance.

Next, the chapter discusses the role of occupational therapy, which aims to help people with eating disorders experience health, wellness, and quality of life through occupational performance and participation in meaningful activities. It highlights challenges inherent in the treatment of individuals with eating disorders, including resistance to change, psychosocial elements, comorbidity, and physical risk factors such as suicide attempts and mortality. Eating disorders are very serious, and often life-threatening conditions. Those struggling with them deserve the best care occupational therapy can provide, along with compassion, patience, and understanding.

Description of Eating Disorders

Eating disorders (EDs) are manifested as disturbances in eating habits or behaviors that stem from an intense fear of being fat and a preoccupation with the perception of one's own weight and shape (American Psychiatric Association [APA], 2022). They are extremely serious and complex mental illnesses that are associated with significant physical, psychological, and social impairments. Evidence indicates that the mortality rate for people with bulimia nervosa is two times that of the general population, and for people with anorexia nervosa the mortality rate is five times as high (van Hoeken & Hoek, 2020). As EDs become more common, the symptom severity for individuals requiring hospitalization is also increasing (Sly & Bamford, 2011). Individuals with more severe forms of EDs tend to be resistant to treatment and susceptible to relapse.

The most recent edition of the *Diagnostic and Statistical Manual of Mental Disorders* (*DSM-5-TR;* APA, 2022) has revised previous diagnostic categories and criteria to better represent the symptoms associated with various EDs. It should be noted that all feeding disorders and EDs described by the *DSM-5-TR* should be considered mutually exclusive. Although EDs may share some similar features, a single diagnosis is given for that point in time that most accurately represents the presentation of any one person's symptoms.

Anorexia Nervosa

Anorexia nervosa (AN) is best characterized by extreme restriction of food intake and/or excessive calorie burning. These behaviors occur because of an intense disturbance of body image and aversion to being perceived by the self or others as fat. AN includes an obsession with food and thinness associated with the refusal to maintain a normal weight for one's age and height (Bulik et al., 2014).

DSM-5-TR Criteria

Because AN develops most often during adolescence, it is sometimes difficult to differentiate between normal growth and developmental changes and the development of the ED. Weight loss is often noted at the time of pubertal menarche, and growing concerns about appearance and body image are common. Therefore, specific diagnostic criteria have

The Lived Experience

Living With Anorexia Nervosa by Rudi Pohl

When did you first realize you might have an ED? How did you know? I think it goes hand in hand, but there was a big difference in timeline as to when I first realized I *might* have an ED, and when I *accepted* I had an ED and decided to ask for help. I can remember being in elementary school when I first started to deal with body image issues. I specifically remember being around 9 years old, trying on clothes in a fitting room and thinking, "I hate how fat my legs are."

As I grew older and the trauma accumulated in my life, the need to control only grew. Later, in undergrad, I was taking an abnormal psychology class which had a unit on EDs. I remember watching a video of a woman who had anorexia and a compulsive exercise addiction. When I saw that girl on the treadmill "running her life away" I saw myself. At this point, I was so weak from my ED that I could hardly twist the cap off of a water bottle or release the parking brake on my car, or even walk up the steps on campus to get to certain classes without feeling like I was going to pass out.

What would you say are some of the things that contributed to developing an ED? I think there was trauma that accumulated throughout my life and within my family system. Some of the trauma included experiences of sexual abuse. I witnessed family members deal with smoking, drug, and alcohol addictions. I watched my father suffer through treatment for hepatitis C and prostate cancer. I was bullied as a child and I think growing up in a "beauty sick society" and being exposed to diet culture, especially within my family, all added to the trauma.

Were there things in the media or society that influenced this? Yes, definitely. Growing up, social media was just evolving so that didn't have an influence on me until later in high school and college. However, women's fashion and health magazines definitely contributed to the way I viewed my body. I remember looking at a woman with washboard abs on the cover of a magazine with the headline "Cameron Diaz' sexy ab workout." I would immediately open the magazine up and rip those pages out so I could do the workout later. Obviously, whichever photoshopped celebrity wearing the unrealistic swimsuit on the cover that month—her body was my goal.

Television also played a big role in introducing the importance of being "pretty," diets, fat-shaming, and unhealthy relationships with exercise. Every summer break, I would spend countless hours watching *America's Next Top Model,* wishing I looked just like girls on the show. Not to mention, in the evenings after school, I watched shows like *The Biggest Loser,* where people lost ridiculous amounts of weight in the most unhealthy ways. I (now regretfully) sat on the bed cheering them on. In more recent years, social media and the internet had an impact on my ED. I found ProAna [anorexia] websites, Thinspiration websites, and Instagram pages, which taught me how to "slowly kill myself," or, in other words, taught me the ins and outs of food restriction, calorie counting, purging, and compulsive exercising.

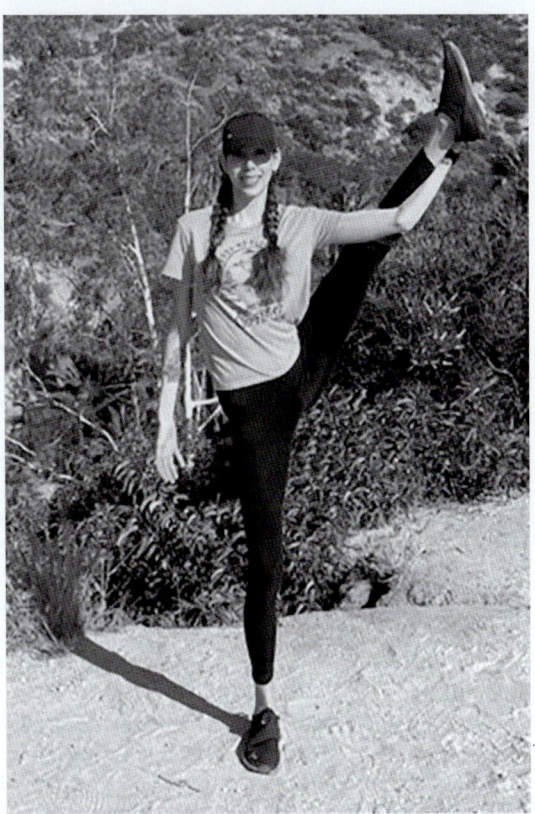

How did family life play a part, if it did? Dieting programs such as Weight Watchers were a big deal in my immediate family. Negative body talk, diets, or weight gain/loss related talk was frequent. It was common to hear unintentional fat-shaming comments amongst family members, "Are you going to eat all of that?" or "Fast food again?" I also had a cousin who was a fitness competitor. I looked up to her and wanted to be just like her, always exercising.

What does having an ED mean for you in day-to-day life? How is it different when you are struggling more versus less? What would you say are the occupations that are most affected by an ED? Bathing/personal hygiene (no motivation, just doing the bare minimum, feeling too weak and tired), eating, sexual activity (not wanting touch, physical contact, hugging), socialization (having conversations, making eye-contact), sleep, working, meal preparation, shopping. My personal warning signs when I am struggling more than usual are an increase in negative body image thoughts, increased body checking, isolating myself from those around me, my hair starting to fall out when I brush it, feeling cold all the time, sleeping more, changes in my mood and energy levels, compulsive exercising, poor sleep, increase in anxiety, and my lower back and knees start to hurt.

In regards to my day-to-day life, I need to maintain an eating schedule. It is usually really rigid, but I am trying to be more flexible. Typically, I *need* to follow my schedule and eat

Continued

The Lived Experience—cont'd

by 7:00 a.m., eat a mid-morning snack at 10:00 a.m., lunch at 12:00 p.m., snack at 3:00 p.m., dinner at 6:00 p.m., snack at 9:00 p.m. I have to do this to keep myself accountable. But, rigidity can interfere. I try to be honest with employers and in relationships about my ED so that I can follow my schedule. I am also a "compulsive exerciser." I walk 3 miles every morning and do an hour of yoga. At night, I do an ab workout. I know it still sounds like a lot, but I really have come a long way.

Are there specific triggers that increase the intensity of your ED? This is the best way I can describe it. In the past, when I was really struggling but didn't know, it was similar to seeing a statue in front of you that was painted blue. But, all the people you love stand beside you and insist the statue is green, but you don't see it. Eventually, you have to learn to trust your loved ones and think, "The statue must be green. They love me and wouldn't lie to me . . . right?" But still, no matter how long you stare at it, the statue is completely blue to you. So your survival depends on trusting their judgment above your own and that is hard to give up. Stress is a big trigger. It can be work stress, fighting with loved ones, comparisons, or experiencing traumas (death). Sometimes, getting sick can be a trigger because it is easier to fall into those maladaptive behaviors like not eating.

What are some ways that the criteria for EDs in psychology don't completely get your experience right? The thought process is that admission to a treatment center will solve everything, but the work continues long after that. Weight restoration or being a specific weight dictates the criteria. There is the belief that being able to eat food at three meals means you don't have an ED. Also, [that EDs are only] experienced by young underweight, White, middle/upper class women. Just because someone is a healthy weight doesn't mean they are not sick.

Let's talk about the term "recovery." Do you consider yourself recovered? What do you think about the word and how do you relate to recovery if you do? No, I do not [consider myself recovered]. For me, recovery looks like having a consistent menstrual cycle. I dream of having kids one day. Recovery for me looks like going through an entire day without thinking how what I eat is going to affect my appearance. Recovery for me looks like not caring what others think about my appearance. I would love to live without those thoughts consuming my mind.

Recovery is not linear. The term "recovery" makes it seem like there is an endpoint, instead it is a process that you continue to change and grow through. Think of recovery like a caterpillar turning into a butterfly. It's a slow process and you do not know what your designs are going to look like, but what you get at the end is a beautiful life. I relate to this because I have relapsed multiple times, but each time I come out of a relapse, I come out stronger and with more life than before.

What were some of the things that helped you work through the hard times? I have spent a lot of time in therapy (in and out of treatment centers). I really feel like yoga saved my life. It taught me how to love my body and

helped me to gain strength. Spending time with family and pets is helpful. Going for walks, doing mindful movement, journaling, and doing art has all been helpful in my recovery. I spent a lot of time reading books about disordered eating and learned about how an ED affects a person long-term. I joined support groups and spent time in intensive outpatient therapy. I wanted to try and manage my ED as holistically as possible, however I had to come to terms with the fact that right now, I need to take medication for anxiety and that has been really helpful.

What would you like OTPs to know about EDs? What role do you see for occupational therapy? As an occupational therapist myself, I do not feel like occupational therapists get enough education about EDs. Even though the field of occupational therapy originated in mental health, I still think practitioners have a hard time figuring out their role and how ED treatment fits into occupational therapy practice. ED treatment in occupational therapy can fit into so many domains. Occupational therapists can help people with EDs learn about coping skills and self-regulation.

There were many times I would become so mad/angry/frustrated and would punch walls or throw things when my meal prep wouldn't go as planned. I felt like if I was going to consume the calories, my food had to be perfect. Occupational therapists can also help with strategies for IADLs like cooking and shopping. There were times when I wouldn't touch butter or use chapstick because I didn't want to gain the calories for touching them. Occupational therapists can address tactile defensiveness, interoception, and socialization. At the height of my ED, I couldn't even look people in the eye or remember how to start a conversation. I lost my social skills because I was so preoccupied by my ED symptoms and exercising. Occupational therapists can teach you how to identify hunger cues and help to identify the signs of relapse such as fatigue and pain.

What were some of the ways that the health-care system did work for you versus didn't work for you? I had a few really bad experiences. For example, at my first therapy session, the therapist called me the wrong name throughout the session. Because of that, I gave up on therapy and went into self-recovery. One intensive-outpatient-therapy program (IOP) I went to was very disorganized, there were a lot of miscommunications and I felt I was treated unfairly. In addition, there are not many facilities in this area that provide ED treatment.

Even though the IOP was not a good experience, it led me to a support group that has been really helpful because it made me feel like I wasn't alone. I also learned about more resources from the support group including a group intervention program for coping skills development led by occupational therapy students. Other things that helped were Art Therapy, individual therapy, and finding the right medication for me with my PCP. There are a lot of problems with our current health-care system and insurance coverage. Above all, it is extremely helpful to have a strong support system when trying to navigate treatment for an ED within this health-care system.

The Lived Experience—cont'd

What is something you want to share that might help others understand what it means to have an ED? Having an ED can make you feel lonely. It is hard to see your peers move on with their lives and you are still learning how to meet your basic needs. It's so hard not to compare yourself to others and when comparing self-criticism is your default. Having an ED is a fight *against* yourself. Recovery is a fight *for* yourself.

What are your hopes for the future for yourself, whether related to ED or not? What would you hope to see in the future in regards to ED treatment? Easier access to treatment, more affordable treatment and early intervention is key. Personally, my hopes are to have a family of my own and raise body-positive children who also have a positive relationship with all foods and exercise. I also hope to help others who are struggling with EDs.

been developed by the APA and recently reviewed in the *DSM-5-TR* (APA, 2022).

In addition to being significantly underweight, individuals with AN also have a strong fear of being fat and the inability to accurately appraise their body. That is, someone with AN may have a persistent and intrusive belief that they have body fat they need to lose while also being emaciated. The body mass index (BMI), calculated as a specific ratio of weight to height (i.e., weight (kg) / height (m)$^2 \times 703$), is the criteria used in the *DSM-5-TR* to determine if someone is underweight.

The BMI range defined as normal by the Centers for Disease Control and Prevention (CDC) is 18.5 to 25 (CDC, n.d.). For context, a woman who is 5 foot, 4 inches, weighing 108 lb, has a BMI of 18.5. Mild anorexia is categorized at a BMI of 17 or higher while still being underweight and meeting the other AN criteria. Moderate anorexia is associated with a BMI between 16 and 16.99 kg/m^2. Severe anorexia is defined as a BMI between 15 and 15.99 kg/m^2, and extreme anorexia is defined as BMI below 15 kg/m^2. A BMI below 13 indicates a life-threatening disorder, but life can also be at risk at higher BMIs, at which precipitous weight loss, unbalanced blood chemistry, and other symptoms are evident.

Subtypes

There are two subtypes of AN: **restricting type** and **binge-eating/purging type**. An individual with the restricting type will decrease their food intake dramatically and continuously, leading to a striking weight loss. Individuals with the binge-eating/purging type of anorexia will go through cycles of eating excessively and compulsively but then negate this by self-induced vomiting, misuse of laxatives, or other means, leading also to striking weight loss. It should be noted that individuals suffering with AN may shift between subtypes (APA, 2022).

Associated Psychological and Physical Conditions

Several psychological and physical comorbidities are observed in individuals with anorexia. The most frequent psychological factors are depression, anxiety, obsessive-compulsive disorders, personality disorders, and mood disorders (APA, 2022). The malnourishment and food restriction observed in anorexia are believed to lead to many physical problems, including the following:

- Hypothermia (a lower-than-normal body temperature)
- Bradycardia (an abnormally slow heart rate) and risk of cardiac failure

- Amenorrhea (absence of a period) or irregular menses
- Edema
- Loss of muscle tone and muscle mass
- Osteoporosis and other skeletal problems
- Hormonal problems
- Skin problems
- Brittle nails and hair, hair loss, and lanugo (a fine, white hair that helps keep the body warm)
- General decrease in bodily functions
- Metabolic, biochemical, renal, and gastrointestinal problems
- Generalized weakness

Most physical problems abate when the individual resumes healthy eating habits, but osteoporosis is irreversible. Finally, deaths from anorexia are most often caused by cardiac arrest secondary to severe food restriction or suicide (APA, 2022).

Bulimia Nervosa

Bulimia nervosa (BN) can also be a life-threatening disorder. Despite an apparently normal weight, those with the disorder share the fear of fatness with those suffering from anorexia. However, an essential distinction in the clinical presentation is the presence of episodes of binging that are associated with different forms of purging and inappropriate compensatory behaviors, such as abuse of laxatives and diuretics.

During a binge-eating episode there is consumption of an abnormally large amount of food along with an intense fear of being unable to stop or control the binge-eating episodes. These episodes are combined with attempts to rid the body of the food by engaging in self-induced vomiting, excessive use of laxatives or diuretics, excessive exercise, or fasting. The binging and purging episodes are typically undertaken in utmost secrecy, and often result in rapid weight gains and losses. Moreover, an overwhelming feeling of guilt and shame follows each episode (APA, 2022).

DSM-5-TR Criteria

Symptomatology of bulimia is characterized by recurrent binge-eating episodes and frenetic compensatory behaviors (APA, 2022). It is important to understand that the amount of food eaten during a binge-eating episode is usually, but not always, larger than what another person would normally eat. For most, it is far more than nibbling during the day or eating between meals. For others, it is the feeling of being "out of control" with food intake that represents a binge. Usually, the person eats very quickly; hence, the duration of the episode is usually short. Severity specifiers for bulimia are based on the number of inappropriate compensatory behaviors per week: Mild bulimia is associated with an average of one to three episodes of inappropriate compensatory behaviors per week, whereas moderate bulimia is associated with four to seven episodes. Severe bulimia is associated with 8 to 13 episodes, whereas extreme cases of bulimia involve 14 or more episodes (APA, 2022).

The *DSM-5-TR* redefined BN and binge-eating disorder, resulting in a decrease in the number of individuals diagnosed with BN to an estimated lifetime prevalence of between 0.85% and 2.8%, with women being two to three times as likely to have the diagnosis (APA, 2022). Peak age of onset is between 15 and 29 years old (van Eeden et al., 2021).

Associated Psychological and Physical Conditions

Several psychological comorbidity factors and other health problems are associated with BN (APA, 2022). The most common psychological factors are mood disorders combined with impulsive actions, such as drug and alcohol abuse, self-harm, sexual disinhibition, and shoplifting. Anxiety and personality disorders are also common.

Problems that occur because of binging, purging, and other weight control strategies are renal problems and electrolytic imbalance (potassium, sodium), leading to headaches, dizziness, loss of balance, and gastrointestinal problems. These problems are mostly because of repeated vomiting. Moreover, the most serious complication related to excessive vomiting is hypokalemia (low blood potassium levels), which can cause cardiac problems. Furthermore, excessive vomiting leads to loss of teeth enamel, dental problems, swelling of salivary glands, chronic sore throat, and irritated vocal cords and deep mouth structures. Excessive use of laxatives can lead to intestinal problems and metabolic imbalance.

Binge-Eating Disorder

Binge eating disorders (BEDs) share the binge-eating characteristic with BN, but do not include purging behaviors.

DSM-5-TR Criteria

In addition to recurrent episodes of binge-eating, the *DSM-5-TR* further describes the binge-eating episode as taking place within a 2-hour time frame, and the amount of food must be clearly larger than what someone else would eat in the same period of time or in the same context (APA, 2022). Also, the binge-eating episode must be accompanied by a feeling of lack of control. Binge-eating episodes involve specific qualities, such as eating more rapidly than usual, eating until the person feels uncomfortably full, eating alone because the person is embarrassed by the amount of food they eat, and/or an overwhelming feeling of guilt and disgust with oneself after the binge-eating episode.

Associated Psychological and Physical Conditions

BED is associated with many psychological and physical conditions (APA, 2022) including an increased risk for obesity and higher health-care utilization. Common comorbid psychological conditions include mood and anxiety disorders.

Avoidant/Restrictive Food Intake Disorder

Avoidant/restrictive food intake disorder (ARFID) is best characterized as a disorder of restricting food intake because of the perception of food as unappetizing, uninteresting, or because of the fear of an aversive consequence of eating. Individuals suffering from ARFID are often described as having a relationship to food that is "choosy," "selective," or "perseverant." This may be because of some sensory elements of the food such as texture, color, taste, or discomfort with feelings of gustatory satiation and fullness. Unlike the other conditions, ARFID is not associated with a disturbance in body image nor with the desire to be thin. This diagnosis was created as the specific extension of eating or feeding disorders developed in infancy or early childhood that have continued into later childhood, adolescence, or beyond (APA, 2022).

DSM-5-TR Criteria

To meet the criteria for ARFID, an individual must show either (a) a sharp decrease in weight or not meeting expected weight gain for developmental stage, (b) a large deficiency in nutrition, (c) being dependent on supplements or a feeding tube to get proper nutrition, and/or (d) a disruption in eating that leads to psychosocial dysfunction. The lack of nutrition from ARFID must not be better described by another medical condition such as physical disruptions in the process of digestion or obsessive-compulsive disorder. Autistic individuals also may show sensory sensitivity to certain foods, but not always in a way that creates a significant deficit in nutrition. That is, autism spectrum disorder is not always comorbid with ARFID, but assigning both diagnoses is appropriate if criteria for both are met (APA, 2022).

OTPs may encounter ARFID as a comorbidity with other developmental disabilities or as an extension of disrupted feeding and eating that began in early childhood. It is important to distinguish ARFID from the other EDs in this chapter as it is the most distinct and there is no evidence of sliding between ARFID and the other EDs as being common. Moreover, the etiology is quite different for ARFID as it does not arise from cultural pressures surrounding body shape nor the use of eating or restricting as a coping mechanism for psychological distress.

Etiology

EDs are pervasive, long-lasting conditions that are exceptionally destructive to well-being and many areas of occupational performance. In the United States, an estimated 29 million individuals will suffer from an ED during their life span (Deloitte Access Economics, 2020). The point prevalence of all EDs combined appears to be on the rise worldwide, increasing from an estimated 4% to 8% of the population starting in the year 2000 through 2018 (Galmiche et al., 2019).

Multiple risk factors can lead to the development of EDs, including genetic predisposition, family disturbance, adverse life events, low self-esteem, high anxiety, identity and self-competence concerns, interpersonal conflicts, and social and cultural pressures to be thin. These factors can influence young women and men to reduce their weight by excessive dieting, exercising, binge/purge routines, and other weight-reducing behavior. Some emerging evidence suggests that the sequence of risk factors develop first from perceived cultural pressure to be thin, then body dissatisfaction, next dieting paired with negative affect, and then the subthreshold onset of ED symptoms (Stice & Van Ryzin, 2019). The highest statistically related risk factors for ED onset are low BMI for anorexia, overeating for bulimia, and body dissatisfaction for BED (Stice & Desjardins, 2018).

There is a cultural perception in the United States that EDs are a White woman's disease; however, recent evidence suggests that the risk factors and prevalence for White women are similar to those for women of other races and ethnicities in the United States (Cheng et al., 2019). It is much more likely that this cultural perception is because of a gap in access to health care, leading to the underdiagnosis of the issue for women of color. Several factors interacting with each other are considered to contribute to the development of EDs.

Figure 19-1 illustrates the multifactorial aspect of these conditions. As shown, predisposing factors are believed to increase the vulnerability of a person to an ED in the presence of precipitating factors. The interaction between predisposing and precipitating factors is believed to lead to the development of an ED. Once the disorder has developed, perpetuating factors keep the person in the cycle of restrictions and compulsions, therefore maintaining the illness.

Early changes from an ED are often satisfying and seen as an improvement by people around the individual, whether family members, peers, or even strangers who might make a comment. It is common to hear someone being complimented on their new figure and weight loss. Unfortunately, comments of that sort reinforce the disordered eating attitudes and behaviors of people who are already vulnerable (Treasure et al., 2008). Consequently, the vulnerable individual will develop strategies to maintain the weight loss and/or increase the restriction and obsessive thoughts about weight and appearances (Pugh & Waller, 2016). Also, the effects of fasting and food restrictions can contribute to the development of cognitive distortions that perpetuate the disorder. For example, the individual thinks of themselves as strong and in control, as demonstrated by the ability to restrict food intake.

Predisposing Factors

Predisposing factors are believed to increase the individual's vulnerability to develop an ED and span biological, social, and cultural realms.

Family Functioning

Interactions within the family system can influence the development of an ED, just as EDs can influence the family's functioning and its dynamic (Barakat et al., 2023; Loeb et al., 2015). However, specific family characteristics can increase an individual's sensitivity to develop an ED, including:

- Alcohol and/or drug abuse in the family
- Family violence
- Sexual abuse
- Overvaluing of appearance and thinness
- Eating habits organized around diets and food restriction

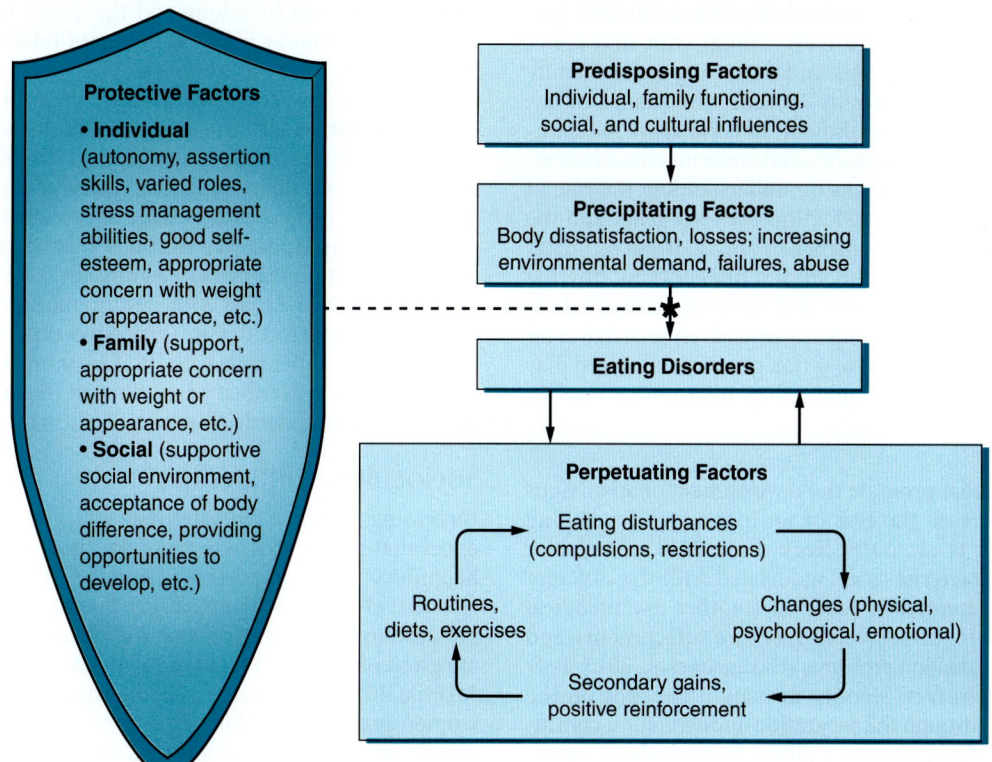

FIGURE 19-1. The development of an eating disorder.

- Lack of opportunity to develop one's independence and autonomy
- Overprotectiveness
- Rigidity
- Excessive or absence of parental control

It is important for occupational therapy practitioners (OTPs) to recognize the impact of caring for someone with an ED on the carer's role, and how the caregiver's reactions may impact their own occupational performance and engagement—as well as that of the person with the ED. Educating and enabling carers to create environments that facilitate adaptive changes for their loved ones is important.

Biology

There is an important body of literature concerning biology and its links to EDs, including strong evidence that serotonin plays a role in the development of EDs. More precisely, on the one hand, serotonin dysregulation (i.e., variability in the concentration levels of serotonin and alteration in its functions) contributes to different signs and symptoms of EDs (Sigurdh et al., 2013). On the other hand, evidence shows that dieting can result in reduced brain serotonin synthesis, leading to more serotonergic dysregulation, which creates a vicious circle in which ED symptomatology is maintained (Gellynck et al., 2013). Increasing evidence links traumatic stress, such as child abuse, to altered serotonin activity (Akkermann et al., 2012). The specific mechanisms of these interactions are still being investigated, but current evidence is strong and suggests promising theoretical and clinical implications for understanding and treating EDs.

Over the past decade, there have been considerable advances in understanding the genetic contribution to EDs (Himmerich et al., 2019; Juli & Juli, 2014; Trace et al., 2013). Genetic and hereditary studies indicate that children of parents who have had EDs and twin siblings with EDs are at higher risk of developing EDs. In fact, having a close family member with AN increases by 10 times the chance of developing anorexia. Yet, it is difficult to tease apart the influence of shared genetics versus shared environmental factors. Ongoing genetic studies focus on understanding the role of genes as well as how the interaction between genes and the environment affects development of an ED. Current estimates of heritability using adoption studies finds that for any ED the heritability is between 59% and 82% (Himmerich et al., 2019). This is an active and ongoing area of research that is far from settled. However, it is clear that genetics do indeed play a significant role in the pathophysiology of disordered eating.

Personality

Characteristics that promote the development of an anxious personality increase the risk of an individual developing an ED (Farstad et al., 2016; Reas et al., 2013). Particular personality characteristics are associated with the different EDs and are presented in Table 19-1. Other psychological factors related to EDs involve insecure attachments and separation-individuation problems (Dakanalis et al., 2015; Ty & Francis, 2013). In fact, identity formation depends on the ability to move through the separation-individuation continuum of normal development. It allows individuals to experiment, learn, identify, evaluate, and compare before deciding what and whom to become (Castellini et al., 2014). Tension

TABLE 19-1 | Overview of Characteristics of Eating Disorders

Disorder	Common Characteristics
Anorexia nervosa (AN)	Compulsivity and perfectionism Desire to conform Lack of initiative and spontaneity Introversion and limited expression of emotions Tendency to avoid risks, danger, and emotions High need for validation from others Excessive self-control Impaired ability to permit self-gratification
Bulimia nervosa (BN)	Impulsivity Seeking sensory stimulations and/or heightened mood states (e.g., substance use, self-harm, sexual relationships) Extroversion Inadequate self-control Impaired ability to cope with delayed or denied self-gratification
Binge-eating disorder (BED)	Low self-esteem Harm avoidance Socially prescribed perfectionism Depressive personality
Avoidant/restrictive food intake disorder (ARFID)	Sensory aversion to food Disinterest in eating Undistorted understanding of body shape and size Possible continuation of feeding concerns from early childhood

between the need to belong and the desire to be independent is influential in ED development (Tabler & Utz, 2015; Wright, 2015).

Moreover, low self-esteem, difficulties in identity formation, negative self-image, and difficulty in establishing fulfilling and meaningful relationships are believed to put people at risk for developing EDs (Doris et al., 2014; Farstad et al., 2016). People with autistic spectrum disorder traits are particularly at risk (Westwood & Tchanturia, 2017); high level of perfectionism is also a significant risk factor (Barakat et al., 2023). Individuals with AN are more likely to have a self-oriented perfectionism (excessive expectations of the self), whereas individuals with BED are more likely to experience a socially prescribed perfectionism (feelings that others demand high standards; Sherry et al., 2014).

Sociocultural Influences

Increasing evidence indicates that social and cultural influences that glorify thinness and associate it with success and happiness play an important role in the development of EDs (Barakat et al., 2023; Wong, 2015). Social reinforcement and cultural norms value people on the basis of physical appearance and place value on obtaining the perfect body (Costa & Melnik, 2016; Pilecki et al., 2016). The image of thin White women promoted in the media influences body image and self-esteem. It sanctions thinness as beauty (Culbert et al., 2015). Despite the fact that most fashion magazine photos are altered to fit certain standards, girls and women still aspire to their images as symbols of beauty and happiness. The message from the media is that to be popular and successful one must be strikingly thin. Also, being overweight is associated with laziness and lack of discipline. People who are overweight can be alienated, rejected by society, and subject to discrimination (Rubino et al., 2020).

Unfortunately, most adolescents are dissatisfied with the way their body looks, and this trend has only increased in the past 10 years. In 2018, an estimated 71% of teens in a large study in Brazil reported they felt too heavy or not thin enough; this spanned both male and female respondents (Gonzaga et al., 2023). Strong evidence supports links between exposure to mass media and low self-esteem and increased body dissatisfaction (Culbert et al., 2015). Earlier studies demonstrated that mass media promoted an ever thinner body type with top models, actresses, and other cultural female icons having become significantly thinner (Dakanalis et al., 2015), whereas more recent trends in body shape have highlighted a desired hourglass shape.

Regardless of momentary trends about being too curvy or not curvy enough, or which parts of the body should be thick or thin, it is all harmful and unachievable standard-setting. Controlling weight and refraining from eating certain foods is perceived as showing strength and determination (Luo et al., 2013; Quick & Byrd-Bredbenner, 2013). To someone with low self-esteem, the pressure to be a certain shape that is promoted by the mass media, in combination with body dissatisfaction, can increase feelings of inadequacy and trigger a cycle of food restriction and dieting.

Technology and, more specifically, social media mean instantaneous and constant contacts with family, friends, worldwide news, celebrities, and even complete strangers. When exploring the impacts of exposure to social media in predominantly White cultures such as Australia, researchers found that exposure to online appearance-related sites is linked to weight dissatisfaction and a drive for thinness (Wilksch et al., 2020), whereas in a more diverse meta-analysis at the multinational level there is a small, if consistent, positive correlation between social media use and body dissatisfaction (Saiphoo & Vahedi, 2019). See Evidence-Based Practice feature.

Protective Factors

Although rarely addressed in the literature, **protective factors** are important when considering the etiology of EDs (Daly, 2015; Gongora, 2014). Moreover, developing protective factors can play an important role in the prevention of EDs, and this can guide families and health-care specialists in the creation of prevention strategies. One important study by Linville and colleagues (2012) involved a qualitative analysis of 22 women who had recovered from an ED. It found that reconnection, close relationships, focusing on overall health and well-being, and compassionate health-care providers were important elements in the recovery process.

Evidence-Based Practice

Media Literacy and Body Image

School-based media literacy interventions have the potential to improve body image.

RESEARCH FINDINGS

A meta-analysis of 17 studies examined the efficacy of media literacy interventions designed to promote positive body image and prevent eating disorders in adolescents (Kurz et al, 2022). All of the interventions helped participants understand how body image is idealized and distorted in the media. Overall, the meta-analysis found positive results for the efficacy of media literacy programs in promoting positive body image. The researchers also found that separate programs for girls and boys were more effective.

APPLICATIONS

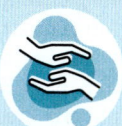

➡ OTPs can help vulnerable individuals develop media literacy.
➡ OTPs can also promote public health messages that promote positive body messaging on social media.

REFERENCES

Kurz, M., Rosendahl, J., Rodeck, J., Muehleck, J. & Berger, U. (2022). School-based interventions improve body image and media literacy in Youth: A systematic review and meta-analysis. *Journal of Primary Prevention, 43,* 5–23. https://doi.org/10.1007/s10935-021-00660-1

The study highlights that getting in touch with feelings of hunger, identifying safe foods, and listening to the body were all safe and helpful ways to discuss eating. On the other hand, hyperfocusing on eating, weight management, and isolation were all hindrances to recovery. The article indicates social relationships and feedback from friends, family, and providers as being very powerful. That is, when relations were patronizing, minimizing, or stigmatizing, it could have a strong negative effect. On the other hand, good social supports were essential and discussion of eating in an intentionally nonstigmatizing way was necessary. Other protective factors identified in quantitative literature include:

- Assertion skills, independence, and autonomy (Bandini et al., 2013; Raykos et al., 2014)
- Opportunity to invest in a variety of roles (e.g., student, friend, club member, worker; Gongora, 2014; van Doornik et al., 2022)
- Ability to use stress management techniques (Berg & Wonderlich, 2013; Kass et al., 2013)
- Positive self-esteem (Frieiro et al., 2022; Obeid et al., 2013)
- Family relationships that allow the person to develop a sense of belonging and individuation (Harrison et al., 2015; Spettigue et al., 2015)
- Social and family environment that is not overly concerned with beauty and thinness (Izydorczyk et al., 2021; Pilecki et al., 2016)
- Spirituality (Goodwin, 2013)

Precipitating Factors

Negative perceptions and thoughts about oneself, one's appearance, the environment, and/or the future can precipitate the development of disordered and unhealthy eating habits, which can eventually result in an ED. A comment on one's body or appearance, a failure, a defeat or a setback, a relationship break-up, or major stress can all precipitate an ED (Cardi et al., 2018; Kjaersdam Telléus et al., 2021). A specific environmental event linked to ED vulnerability is changes in school from one level to another (e.g., moving from primary school to high school, or from high school to college or university) because students must adapt to a new environment with new demands and higher expectations. There is speculation that the stress associated with COVID-19 may have exacerbated or precipitated the onset of EDs in some individuals (Yahya & Khawaja, 2020).

Time spent on social media and number of social media accounts is associated with disordered eating (Wilksch et al., 2020). Social media usage provides opportunities for social comparisons in a context in which thinness and body ideals are regularly presented and revered. Importantly, no single event will lead to an ED; rather, it involves the interactions between multiple factors that significantly increase the risk of developing an ED.

Gender Differences

EDs are more common in women than men, with one review indicating 5.5% to 17.9% of young women and 0.6% to 2.4% of young men have them worldwide (Silén &

Keski-Rahkonen, 2022). However, the perception of EDs as being solely a female concern is often overstated. EDs are not as common in young men, but they appear to be on the rise and may affect as many as 1% of the population. Evidence suggests that up to one in four people with anorexia or bulimia are male, whereas a staggering two-thirds of individuals presenting with ARFID are male (Eddy et al., 2014; Gorrel & Murray, 2019; Hudson et al., 2007).

Very little research even identifies trans and gender diverse identities in their data collection, so the relative rate of incidence and prevalence for these individuals is not widely established. Emerging evidence suggests that trans and gender diverse individuals have unique expressions of EDs as body image concerns are compounded with gender dysphoria and attempts to achieve culturally desirable body shapes (Cusack et al., 2022). The comparison between male and female presentations is more widely researched. Symptom severity, age of presentation, and overall characteristics of EDs comparing males with females are largely similar with certain superficial features of the disorder varying.

Although women and girls seem to report family dynamics as having a larger effect on their ED, for men and boys involvement in sports tends to be a more common precipitating factor (Arnow et al., 2017). Likewise, men and boys have a stronger tendency to use compulsive exercise rather than different purging methods for weight control (Weltzin et al., 2005). The risks of developing anorexia or bulimia are greater when a man or boy's professional and personal recognition is linked to his body (National Eating Disorders Collaboration [NEDC], 2015).

Occupations in which aesthetics and strict dieting practices are directly linked to success increase the risk of developing an ED (Barakat et al., 2023; Crisp, 2006). The same applies in sports in which athletes must maintain a specific weight or those in which low body fat is an advantage. Occupations and sports with a greater risk for EDs in women include ballet, modeling, figure skating, diving, swimming, gymnastics, yoga, and rowing, whereas wrestling and horse racing are particularly associated with male AN (Barakat et al., 2023; Leonkiewicz & Wawrzyniak, 2022). In wrestling, a lower weight allows the individual to participate in a weight class in which he may have a greater advantage. A higher concern with muscularity identified in males combined with distorted perceptions about muscle bulk, eating, and exercise patterns have been associated with increased risk for developing an ED in males (NEDC, 2015).

Mental Illness in Culture and Society

Not All Black Girls Know How to Eat: A Story of Bulimia is an autobiography by Stephanie Covington Armstrong originally published in 2009. The story begins with Stephanie's childhood growing up in Brooklyn, New York, dealing with food insecurity and a cycle of poverty created by racism paired with unhelpful social programs. The author recalls that, "In order to qualify for aid you had to be living well below the poverty line, which we were, but to Uncle Sam we were simply straddling the fence" (p. 4).

Stephanie goes on to describe how her mother had to give up her daughters to foster care for a time in order to make financial ends meet. Stephanie's immediate and extended Black family served as a strong support system during her childhood. Kinship with cousins and sisters helped her explore and play, whereas aunts, uncles, and grandparents helped keep her fed and housed. Stephanie's young, single mother did her best to provide for her daughters, but was also struggling to find security and stability while battling her own mental health issues.

All trust was sadly betrayed by her uncle who initially seemed to be a safe escape from an unstable home life, but then raped her after a night of drinking. This horrific experience affected Stephanie throughout her life, coloring interactions with romantic partners and contributing to her lack of self-esteem: "I refused to hurt, to feel pain, to let anyone close enough to be able to have the power to destroy me again" (p. 52).

Stephanie's teenage years were tumultuous. Her mother found community in political activist and feminist groups, but seemed unaware of Stephanie's emotional suffering and was unable to provide consistent access to food because of her low wages. At this time in her life, Stephanie's relationship with her mother was very challenging. Normal teenage conflicts with parental figures were exacerbated by hunger, poverty, and the building resentment that Stephanie felt for not having been protected from her uncle. "I found myself starving alternately for affection and for food until it became impossible to separate the two" (p. 79).

As soon as Stephanie was old enough, she moved away from her mother and eventually ended up in Los Angeles to attempt starting a career in acting. Pressures to be thin in Hollywood paired with many romantic heart breaks and unstable work had Stephanie at a low point emotionally. Food became the coping mechanism. "[L]ove was the only thing I craved. And so I ate. Instead of admitting to myself how desperately I craved love" (p. 141). Any time a challenge to Stephanie's self-esteem arose, a conflict with friends or lovers built, or pressures of making ends meet loomed, she turned to binging. However, to stay thin, Stephanie also purged by forcing herself to throw up. This pattern was addictive and eventually consumed most of Stephanie's waking hours, interfering with jobs, friendships, romantic partners, and self-care.

The road to recovery for Stephanie was long with many ups and downs. It was challenging to get appropriate treatment because she did not have health-care insurance. Also, "Because I was a Black girl with natural hair who had grown up below the poverty line, no one ever suspected I could be bulimic" (p. 149). She explored the free options of participating in a research project and attending various support groups. The research project was for an experimental medication, but without any other supports in place this option felt unhelpful. Also, Stephanie felt out of place or outright stigmatized in support groups because she was usually the only Black person in those spaces.

Stephanie reflected that she didn't fit the perceived norm of a person with an ED: an upper middle-class, White woman who is thin, in other words, people who seemed to have little in common with Stephanie's experiences and struggles. After persevering through self-doubt, relapse, relocating, and ostracizing from a White support group member, Stephanie was able to find a strong mentor who sponsored her in recovery in the

12-step program. Owing as much to her own tenacity as her mentor's guidance and the support of family and friends, Stephanie was eventually able to build a meaningful life absent of bulimic binging and purging. Now, Stephanie is a successful author and playwright while finding fulfillment in her role as a mother to her daughter.

Stephanie's story is a testament to the complex emotional factors that can contribute to an ED. Surviving sexual trauma, dealing with food insecurity, battling low self-esteem, and seeking comfort from food in the absence of other coping mechanisms are all common themes among people with EDs. This, paired with pressures in her job to stay thin, all compounded on each other. Also, the triggering event for Stephanie's bulimia is a story many share. She came across a magazine article about the concerning rise of bulimia in the United States. More recently, triggering media might come from a TV streaming service, a social media influencer, or an online forum about EDs instead of a magazine article, but the impact is the same. She was feeling particularly vulnerable at the time because of external factors in her life, and Stephanie then used the article as a "how-to" manual for initiating bulimic behaviors.

It is important to recognize that the factors Stephanie faced are common enough and can appear in the lives of many different types of people. Our societal stereotype of the type of person who has an ED is unhelpful, further stigmatizing people who do not fit it and discouraging them from seeking treatment. It's hard enough to deal with an ED, but to have to battle through stereotypes and feel alienated from the community of individuals seeking to heal is especially challenging and unfair.

Impact of Eating Disorders on Occupational Participation/Areas of Occupational Performance

People with EDs experience difficulties participating in self-care, productivity, and leisure occupations, particularly when they involve eating or interactions with others.

Volition

A variety of psychological factors such as perfectionism, cognitive rigidity, and experiential avoidance may impair the individual's volition, or motivation, for action and engagement in occupations. Volition is defined as "a pattern of thoughts and feelings about oneself as an actor in one's world which occur as one anticipates, chooses, experiences and interprets what one does" (Kielhofner, 2008, p. 16). The psychological factors that commonly exist in individuals with EDs combined with an impairment in volition can result in pathologically disabling consequences for these individuals (Kitson, 2012).

Cooper and colleagues (2004) identified five key cognitive concepts commonly affecting motivation, or volition, in persons with EDs that inform the impact of EDs on occupational performance. These concepts are (1) overvaluation of weight, shape, and their control; (2) mood intolerance;

(3) core low self-esteem; (4) perfectionism; and (5) interpersonal problems. Although each individual is unique, there are some common trends in psychological personal factors that might contribute to the development of an ED. The following section explores each of these as well as other commonly affected areas of occupation such as eating, meal preparation, and independent living skills.

Overvaluation of Weight, Shape, and Control

Individuals with EDs are dissatisfied with their body image and preoccupied with their weight and shape (Sharpe et al., 2018). They perceive their bodies and themselves as deserving of criticism, which precipitates avoidance of social interaction, social eating, and body-centric activities (Winecoff et al., 2015). As they attempt to control their food intake, weight, body image, and shape, the EDs take control over their entire occupational being. Ultimately, the person feels controlled by the environment as they get increasingly entrenched in these maladaptive coping behaviors.

Mood Intolerance

People with EDs typically find it difficult to tolerate the negative emotions that are part of the normal experience of adult occupations, roles, responsibilities, and relationships (Henderson et al., 2019). This difficulty is in part linked to a lack of self-acceptance; fear of rejection from others; and impaired emotional, social, and life skills. Participating in maladaptive weight minimization activities allows the person to avoid or alter negative emotions, increases personal control, and reinforces acceptability and self-competence (Cusack, 2013; Nowakowski et al., 2013), which contributes to consolidating disordered eating patterns and beliefs. For example, a person with an ED may avoid dating because of a fear of rejection, or increased food intake restrictions may generate a strengthened sense of competence and being in control.

Dietary restriction or binging/purging and other comorbid behaviors provide distraction from emotionally difficult situations and may provide temporary mood regulation and stress relief. However, people with bulimia and anorexia feel overwhelming shame associated with binging, purging, and restricted eating (Blythin et al., 2020). Furthermore, in some cases, malnutrition (i.e., starvation syndrome) can lead to emotional blunting and a flattened affect, enabling avoidance of intense emotional experience. In other cases, the impact of malnutrition on cognitive functions leads to decreased emotional regulation and emotional expression, increased emotional reactivity, and avoidance or impulsive actions.

Core Low Self-Esteem

Low self-esteem, which has been described as a combination of limited self-liking and self-competence, is a central theme in the development of EDs (Noordenbos et al., 2014) and has a significant impact on occupational performance. The individual's perceived inability to feel acceptable or cope within their social or occupational environment is fueled by distorted beliefs and cognitions about themselves, others, and life in general (MacNeil et al., 2012). This mindset perpetuates low self-esteem and precipitates avoidance of certain adaptive occupations that are perceived as threatening or dissatisfying, such as trying out for a sports team or accepting a promotion (Elliott, 2012).

Perfectionism

Most individuals with EDs have unrealistically high personal standards and believe they are unacceptable and unlovable unless they are perfect (Bills et al., 2023). For people with EDs, eating is frequently linked to greed, fat, and being weak, all of which symbolize unacceptability. The belief that one is unacceptable leads to self-rejection and erroneously expected rejection from others. The individual strives for perfection in daily performance at work and school, at home, and with friends and family. The inability to achieve perfection leads to a sense of failure and shame (Kelly et al., 2014). Feelings of failure and shame are alleviated by weight minimization or other maladaptive coping mechanisms associated with striving for the perfect body (Kelly & Carter, 2013).

Interpersonal Problems

Social anxiety and interpersonal difficulties, which are often linked to insecure early attachments, conflict, or trauma (e.g., neglect, abuse), can lead to impoverished relationships (Sullivan et al., 2020) and social isolation. People with EDs often experience a concern over making mistakes and a general fear in social situations (Delaquis et al., 2023). Furthermore, negative social comparison can contribute to a fear of romantic encounters and physical intimacy (Pinheiro et al., 2010). Impaired interpersonal functioning and social and emotional coping skills of people with EDs (Coombs et al., 2011) often fall short of the demands of diverse social environments.

Interpersonal difficulties and social anxiety are important risk factors for EDs and include excessive shyness, difficulties with trust, managing conflict, and expressing difficult emotions (Harrison et al., 2012; Raykos et al., 2014). As with other areas of occupational performance, body image disturbance and perceived ineffectiveness result in an avoidance of situations in which individuals with EDs could learn and practice interpersonal relationship skills (Zanetti et al., 2013).

Eating Skills and Meal Preparation

Individuals with EDs struggle to eat in a normal, safe, healthy manner and either restrict their food intake to reduce their weight or eat in a dysregulated way (e.g., binging followed by vomiting). They use overcontrolled eating or out of control eating to avoid or alter difficult emotions. These behaviors can lead to emotional dysregulation and increased experiential avoidance of occupations involving eating (Cusack, 2013). People with EDs usually avoid eating with others and public situations involving food, thereby incurring psychosocial harm and occupational deprivation (Morris, 2012).

For people with EDs, eating evokes extreme anxiety, and individuals struggle to identify healthy meals and accurate portion sizes. Food intake is restricted, or digestion of food is avoided, paired with having a very narrow range of foods that they feel safe eating. Foods high in fats and carbohydrates are particularly feared. Eating may be used as a mechanism to manage emotions. Vegetarianism is common, possibly as another means of weight control (Hargreaves et al., 2021). Meals are often eaten excessively slowly or inappropriately fast, sometimes in abnormal, ritualistic, or socially inappropriate ways. Food may be cut into tiny pieces or contaminated with excessive condiments to ensure the experience of eating is self-punitive.

Many individuals have no experience of eating three balanced meals per day in their lifetime. Social situations requiring public eating are either avoided or followed by purging to avoid absorption of calories (Lock et al., 2012). Subsequently, meal preparation is also affected. People with anorexia may avoid and/or obsess about shopping for food, cooking, and eating self-prepared normal-sized meals and snacks (Crouch & Alers, 2014; Lock et al., 2012). Many have very limited cooking skills, whereas others are highly accomplished cooks who enjoy feeding others (Morris, 2012).

Independent Living Skills and Role Functioning

Individuals with EDs may never develop or can lose independent living skills because of impaired self-efficacy, perfectionism, and interpersonal distrust, which leads to an avoidance of participation in these important occupations (Ackard et al., 2014; Wade et al., 2015). Individuals with AN are frequently unable to maintain healthy roles as a worker, friend, leisure participant, and hobbyist (Quiles-Cestari & Ribeiro, 2012). Their lifestyles become significantly imbalanced, often focusing on lengthy eating and disordered or obsessional compulsive routines such as body checking, mirror gazing, cleaning, excessive exercise, and study activities, leading to social isolation (Bulik et al., 2012). These self-reinforcing behaviors may contribute to a maladaptive occupational identity (Elliott, 2012).

The rituals may last many hours a day and become similar to a full-time job, interfering with the development of other adult roles such as worker, leisure participant, and friend (Courty et al., 2015; Robinson, 2014). People with severe and enduring EDs experience a poor quality of life comparable with those of people with other severe and enduring mental illnesses (Rymaszewska & Marurek, 2012).

Intervention

Interventions that may be implemented by OTPs will depend greatly on the level of care at which the encounter occurs. In descending order of severity, treatment for EDs spans medical hospitalization, inpatient/residential treatment, partial hospitalization programs, intensive outpatient programs, individual outpatient mental health services, and self-monitoring including use of support groups. Treatment for EDs can be tricky if an individual does not show outward signs of malnourishment because many of the symptoms are compulsively hidden and carried out in secret.

Moreover, similar to many mental health diagnoses there is a stigma attached to having an ED. One study showed that only a third of individuals interviewed had sought help for their ED over a period of 4 years, and when they did it was often expressed as a desire to lose weight instead of to address ED symptoms (Evans et al., 2011). Barriers included shame and stigma; however, rapport and a nonjudgmental attitude from health-care providers were cited as essential for the women in the study feeling comfortable seeking help. A person's relationship with their ED symptoms can be quite complicated, and typically includes both positive and negative elements (Musolino et al., 2016). That is, acting out ED symptoms sometimes feels similar to self-care, when used as an escape from uncomfortable feelings or processing past traumas.

ED behaviors even help people feel emotionally safe because it allows individuals to feel in control and carry out strongly enforced habits that were in some ways comforting. Symptoms may also be a way to feel productive and a means of gender expression. These are essential tensions that need to be approached with sensitivity and understanding in order to help people move on to more healthy coping strategies. Although ED symptoms blur with an individual's sense of identity, part of the recovery journey is finding ways other than body image to be perceived and valued as a person (Jenkens & Ogden, 2012).

Often people suffering from EDs feel misunderstood by family and medical providers alike who brand them as difficult and cannot understand "why they can't just eat." Caregivers go through their own process of recognizing that their loved one needs help, but sometimes also have negative or harmful appraisals of ED symptoms while blaming themselves for the ED occurring. Caregivers also appeared to feel some desperation in seeking information and help for their loved one. Loss of a sense of control was another theme as caregivers sought to coerce their loved one into gaining weight or eating.

It is clear that caregivers require support in addition to the individual suffering from the ED, and that treatment would benefit from including family in the process when possible. This could include teaching caregivers destigmatization of the ED symptoms and providing accurate information about how to better support their loved one (Fox et al., 2017).

Unfortunately, with current treatments for EDs, the long-term outcomes are poor. Recovery can be a long process, often taking 6 years or more (Franco et al., 2017), but this is likely an underestimate because of the limited length of research follow-up (Arcelus et al., 2011). Estimates of recovery and mortality rates range greatly depending on the source, with as much as half of individuals not recovering fully and up to an astounding 5% of those afflicted with AN dying from the disorder (Franko et al., 2013). Sadly, one in five deaths from AN result from suicide. Predictors of higher mortality rate include alcohol misuse and other comorbid mental health diagnoses (Arcelus et al., 2011).

Multiple systematic reviews report that current interventions have yet to demonstrate strong effect sizes and there is no one specific approach that has emerged as best practice (Kotilahti et al., 2020; Murray et al., 2019; Peat et al., 2017; Zeeck et al., 2018). There is a call to move beyond a simplistic treatment model that overemphasizes weight gain or loss and instead more fully addresses personal and social effects of the disorder, uses harm reduction strategies, and strives to empower people (Hay et al., 2012).

TABLE 19-2 | Common Intervention Approaches for Individuals With Eating Disorders

Approach	Target(s) of Intervention	Brief Synopsis	Chapters With Additional Information 🤝
Cognitive behavioral approach	Distorted beliefs in the context of occupational performance	Distorted beliefs are identified and then challenged by providing evidence to the contrary.	Chapter 8: Cognitive Beliefs
Motivational Interviewing	Promote engagement in change process to adopt healthy lifestyle practices	A form of relationship building that is based on establishing rapport and helping to identify one's own reasons for change	Chapter 11: Motivation
Dialectical behavior therapy	Emotion regulation	Skills training targeting mindfulness meditation, interpersonal effectiveness, emotion regulation, and distress tolerance	Chapter 12: Emotion Regulation
Building health routines and habits	Time use	Learning to reduce engagement in unhealthy routines and adopt healthy routines	Chapter 14: Time Use and Habits
Meditation/mindfulness	Self-care	Focusing on the present in a nonjudgmental manner	Chapter 45: Self-Care and Well-Being Occupations
Meal planning and preparation	Healthy eating	Education and skills training around meal planning, preparation, and healthy eating	Chapter 46: Activities of Daily Living, Instrumental Activities of Daily Living, and Health Management Occupations
Enabling spiritual participation	Providing meaning	Encourage individual to identify spiritual needs and then promote participation in formal religious or informal spiritual activities.	Chapter 53 Spiritual Occupations

Occupational therapy interventions in this setting have yet to be evaluated experimentally. Many of the publications in occupational therapy about ED treatment is older evidence or relies on expert opinion and nonsystematic literature review to describe potential avenues for intervention (e.g., Bradford et al., 2015; Clark & Nayar, 2012; Gardiner & Brown, 2010; Horner, 2006). One other occupational therapy text in mental health (Crouch & Alers, 2014), one survey of OTPs working in mental health settings (Kloczko & Ikiugu, 2006), and a small subjective study that polled participants' opinions about the helpfulness of the intervention (Biddiscombe et al., 2018) demonstrate that occupational therapy self-identifies as having a role in treating EDs.

Key points of interest from these perspectives are that OTPs should work in a collaborative model with other healthcare providers, use a holistic approach to care, and focus on the areas of occupation that are affected by the disorder.

Mealtime support is a foundational practice in inpatient and day treatment programs for individuals with EDs. A survey of intervention settings identified what practices were typically incorporated in mealtime supports (Brockmeyer et al., 2015) and found that most settings provide a kitchen and cooking group, monitor eating and amount of food consumed at mealtimes, and provide role modeling by staff. OTPs are ideally suited to assist with meal planning and cooking interventions; OTPs can model, support, and provide graded exposure for meal planning, shopping, cooking, and eating preplanned meals. They can also assist with modeling by not only eating alongside people but also providing supports and encouraging the use of adaptive coping strategies when feeling distressed during mealtimes. Lastly, OTPs

can help expand the dietary repertoire by providing graded exposures to healthy and avoided foods.

One example of this holistic approach in occupational therapy was a meal preparation group for individuals with EDs developed and led by occupational therapists, which resulted in significant improvements in ability and motivation for meal preparation (Lock et al., 2012). Participants in the group planned a minimum of 10 different meals. Initially, they prepared safe meals and gradually progressed to meals that involved feared foods. Participants received support to eat prescribed portion sizes by eating the meal together in a small group. During the meal, participants were encouraged to use coping strategies when dealing with anxiety or distorted cognitions.

Table 19-2 outlines common intervention approaches for individuals with EDs and identifies the accompanying chapters in this text that provide more detailed information about those approaches.

General Considerations for Occupational Therapy Practitioners When Working With People With Eating Disorders

This section discusses the role of OTPs in working with this population. Consider that ED diagnoses are not a primary diagnosis that would commonly cause a referral for occupational therapy in the United States. However, EDs may be comorbid with a referring diagnosis that would certainly interfere with many areas of occupation and cause occupational therapy services to be indicated.

- This is a developing setting for occupational therapy services. Therefore, no manualized interventions for ED specific to occupational therapy yet exist.
- General principles of occupational therapy services apply to this setting. That is, interventions are indicated that support well-being, manage symptoms, accommodate activities that are challenging, and reduce harm caused by symptoms.
- Specific occupations that should be strongly considered during treatment planning are meal preparation and planning, social engagement, and self-care.
- OTPs should be especially careful to avoid stigmatizing language surrounding weight, body shape and size, food, and meals.
- An autonomy-supportive approach is essential while balancing individual safety. Absolutely no shaming or guilting around food consumption will be helpful. Meet people where they are, be on their side in addressing symptoms, and advocate for their occupational well-being with the health-care team.

Here's the Point

- The diagnoses of AN, BN, BED, and ARFID all involve symptoms around disordered eating but are also characterized by complex psychological impairments and/or cognitive distortions. ARFID is just as serious as BN, AN, and BED but does not share the trait of concern about body shape and size.
- AN, BN, and BED are most often diagnosed in White women, but this disparity is overstated because of underdiagnosis of non-White individuals and differing superficial presentation of these EDs in men. Nonetheless, the severity of EDs and accompanying psychological symptoms appear to be similar for all individuals regardless of gender and sociocultural factors.
- The causes of EDs involve an interaction of biological, psychological, and environmental factors.
- The EDs have a wide-ranging impact on occupational performance beyond eating and include difficulties with many areas of daily living as well as difficulties with social relationships, body image, role development, and independent living skills.

Apply It Now

1. Reflecting on Body Image and Social Media

In the 2020 documentary *Miss Americana,* Taylor Swift reflects, "I've learned over the years it's not good for me to see pictures of myself every day because I have a tendency, and it's only happened a few times, and I'm not in any way proud of it, but I get, I tend to get triggered by something. Whether it's a picture of me where I feel like I looked like my tummy was too big or, or, like someone said that I looked pregnant or something and that'll just trigger me to just starve a little bit. Just stop eating. I thought that I was just like supposed to feel like I was going to pass out at the end of a show or in the middle of it. I thought that was how it was . . . I don't think you know that you're doing that when you're doing it gradually. There's always some standard of beauty that you're not meeting."

The internet has become a vital part of life for many in today's fast-paced world. People use it to stay in contact with others and learn about trends and current events, news, arts, and entertainment. At the same time, exposure to social media can increase body image concerns, body dissatisfaction, and body checking—all potentially leading to the development of an ED. Take a moment to reflect on your own use of social media. Which social media do you use the most? What do you enjoy about using social media? What don't you enjoy about social media? What impact has interacting with social media had on your own body image and mental health, if any?

2. Remembering the Person Behind the Diagnosis

Read Rudi's story of living with AN. Compare and contrast her lived experience with the *DSM-5-TR* criteria for AN. Which elements are present? Which are absent? How does

Rudi's story inform your understanding of the meaning of living with an ED?

3. Stepping Toward Treatment Planning

What are three key strategies that OTPs could use in the treatment of EDs with adolescents? Describe at least one specific occupation that should be strongly considered during occupational therapy intervention planning for individuals with EDs and explain why this may be relevant to clients. Then, using the COAST goal format (Client, Occupation, Assist Level, Specific Condition, Timeline), write a draft of an example goal that might be used in this setting.

4. Acknowledging That Behavior Change Is Hard

Everyone has behaviors they might like to change from time to time. Whether it's going to bed earlier to get better rest, staying hydrated, or remembering to do all of the assigned readings in a class, these can be quite challenging to work toward. Changing the behaviors associated with an ED are only different in that these are more stigmatized and sometimes have more impact on overall health. That does not make them easier to change. In fact, rituals associated with EDs are often very long-standing components of a person's daily routine that they find a lot of comfort in acting out. In order to build empathy for the challenge of changing behavior, identify one health behavior that you are willing to work on this week. Write down each day if you were able to make the change, what barriers you encountered, and how you felt trying to make this change. What insight does this activity give about working with people who have an eating disorder?

Resources

Books for Clinicians

- Brownell, K. D., & Walsh, B. T. (2017). *Eating disorders and obesity: A comprehensive handbook* (3rd ed.). Guilford Press.
- Gaudiani, J. L. (2018). *Sick enough: A guide to the medical complications of eating disorders.* Routledge.
- Lacey, J. H., Bamford, B., & Brown, A. (2010). *Bulimia, binge-eating and their treatment.* Sheldon Press.
- Lask, B., & Bryant-Waugh, R. (2013). *Eating disorders in childhood and adolescence* (4th ed.). Routledge.
- Touyz, S., Le Grange, D., Lacey, H., & Hay, P. (2016). *Managing severe and enduring anorexia nervosa: A clinician's guide.* Routledge.
- Treasure, J., Smith, G., & Crane, A. (2016). *Skills-based caring for a loved one with an eating disorder: The new Maudsley method* (2nd ed.). Routledge.

Clinical Guidelines and Research

- Health Improvement Scotland. (2006). *Recommendations for management and treatment of eating disorders.* http://www.healthcareimprovementscotland.org/previous_resources/best_practice_statement/eating_disorders_in_scotland.aspx
- National Collaborating Centre for Mental Health. (2020). *Eating disorders: Recognition and treatment.* https://www.nice.org.uk/guidance/ng69
- *The Journal of Eating Disorders* (Open Access Journal). http://jeatdisord.biomedcentral.com

More Information About Eating Disorders

- American Psychiatric Association (APA): https://www.psychiatry.org/patients-families/eating-disorders
- Mentalheath.gov: http://www.mentalhealth.gov/what-to-look-for/eating-disorders
- National Health Service (NHS) Choices Advice: https://www.nhs.uk/mental-health/feelings-symptoms-behaviours/behaviours/eating-disorders/overview
- Royal College of Psychiatrists. Eating Disorders for Parents and Carers: http://www.rcpsych.ac.uk/healthadvice/parentsandyouthinfo/parentscarers/eatingdisorders.aspx
- Supportline Problems: Anorexia and Bulimia. Informational page and list of resources: https://www.supportline.org.uk/problems/eating-disorders-anorexia-and-bulimia-support
- National Institute of Mental Health (NIMH). Eating Disorders Informational Page: https://www.nimh.nih.gov/health/topics/eating-disorders

Support Organizations

- Academy of Eating Disorders: https://www.aedweb.org/home
- Australia and New Zealand Academy for Eating Disorders: http://www.anzaed.org.au
- Australian Centre of Excellence in Eating Disorders: http://ceed.org.au
- Beat Eating Disorders: https://www.beateatingdisorders.org.uk
- Butterfly Foundation for Eating Disorders: https://thebutterflyfoundation.org.au
- National Eating Disorders Association (NEDA): https://www.nationaleatingdisorders.org/about-us
- National Eating Disorders Collaboration: http://www.nedc.com.au

Self-Help Websites

- Eating Disorder Recovery: Action Steps: https://www.eatingdisorderrecovery.net/action-steps
- Eating Disorder Treatment: Dialectical Behavioral Therapy Versus Cognitive Behavioral Therapy: http://www.eatingdisorderhope.com/treatment-for-eating-disorders/types-of-treatments/dialectical-behavioral-therapy-dbt
- Help Guide on Eating Disorder Treatment: http://www.helpguide.org/articles/eating-disorders/eating-disorder-treatment-and-recovery.htm
- Recovering From an Eating Disorder: http://au.reachout.com/self-help-tips-for-eating-disorders

Books for Patients and Caregivers

- Bryant-Waugh, R. (2019). *ARFID Avoidant restrictive food intake disorder: A guide for parents and carers.* Routledge.
- Cash, T. F. (2008). *The body image workbook: An 8-step program for learning to like your looks.* New Harbinger.
- Goodman, L. J., & Villapiano, M. (2018). *Eating disorders: The journey to recovery workbook* (2nd ed.). Routledge.
- Graham, P., & Freeman, C. (2019). *Overcoming anorexia nervosa 2nd edition: A self-help guide using cognitive behavioural techniques.* Robinson.
- McKay, M., Wood, J. C., & Brantley, J. (2019). *The Dialectical Behavioral Therapy skills workbook: Practical DBT exercises for learning mindfulness, interpersonal effectiveness, emotion regulation, and distress tolerance* (2nd ed.). New Harbinger Publications.
- Schmidt, U., Treasure, J., & Alexander, J. (2015). *Getting better bite by bite: A survival kit for sufferers of bulimia nervosa and binge eating disorders* (2nd ed.). Routledge.
- Treasure, J., Smith, G., & Crane, A. (2016). *Skills-based caring for a loved one with an eating disorder: The new Maudsley method* (2nd ed.). Routledge.

References

Ackard, D. M., Ritcher, S., Egan, A., & Cronemeyer, C. (2014). Poor outcome and death among youth, young adults and midlife adults with eating disorders: An investigation of the risk factors by age at assessment. *International Journal of Eating Disorders, 47*(7), 825–835. https://doi.org/10.1002/eat.22346

Akkermann, K., Kaasik, K., Kiive, E., Nordquist, N., Oreland, L., & Harro, J. (2012). The impact of adverse life events and the serotonin transporter gene promoter polymorphism on the development of eating disorder symptoms. *Journal of Psychiatric Research, 46*(1), 38–43. https://doi.org/10.1016/j.jpsychires.2011.09.013

American Psychiatric Association. (2022). *Diagnostic and statistical manual of mental disorders* (5th ed., text rev.). American Psychiatric Publishing. https://doi.org/10.1176/appi.books.9780890425787

Arcelus, J., Mitchell, A. J., Wales, J., & Nielsen, S. (2011). Mortality rates in patients with anorexia nervosa and other eating disorders: A meta-analysis of 36 studies. *Archives of General Psychiatry, 68*(7), 724–731. https://doi.org/10.1001/archgenpsychiatry.2011.74

Armstrong, S. C. (2009). *Not all Black girls know how to eat: A story of bulimia.* Lawrence Hill Books.

Arnow, K. D., Feldman, T., Fichtel, E., Lin, I. H., Egan, A., Lock, J., Westerman, M., & Darcy, A. M. (2017). A qualitative analysis of male eating disorder symptoms. *Eating Disorders, 25*(4), 297–309. https://doi.org/10.1080/10640266.2017.1308729

Bandini, L., Sighinolfi, C., Menchetti, M., Morri, M., De Ronchi, D., & Atti, A. R. (2013). Assertiveness and eating disorders: The efficacy of a CBT group training: Preliminary findings. *European Psychiatry, 28*(Suppl. 1), 1. https://doi.org/10.1016/S0924-9338(13)76215-1

Barakat, S., McLean, S. A., Bryant, E., Le, A., Marks, P., National Eating Disorder Research Consortium, Touyz, S., & Maguire, S. (2023). Risk factors for eating disorders: Findings from a rapid review. *Journal of Eating Disorders, 11*(1), 8. https://doi.org/10.1186/s40337-022-00717-4

Berg, K. C., & Wonderlich, S. A. (2013). Emerging psychological treatments in the field of eating disorders. *Current Psychiatry Reports, 15*(11), 1535–1645. https://doi.org/10.1007/s11920-013-0407-y

Biddiscombe, R. J., Scanlan, J. N., Ross, J., Horsfield, S., Aradas, J., & Hart, S. (2018). Exploring the perceived usefulness of practical food groups in day treatment for individuals with eating disorders. *Australian Occupational Therapy Journal, 65*(2), 98–106. https://doi.org/10.1111/1440-1630.12442

Bills, E., Greene, D., Stackpole, R., & Egan, S. J. (2023). Perfectionism and eating disorders in children and adolescents: A systematic review and meta-analysis. *Appetite, 187,* 106586. https://doi.org/10.1016/j.appet.2023.106586

Blythin, S. P. M., Nicholson, H. L., Macintyre, V. G., Dickson, J. M., Fox, J. R. E., & Taylor, P. J. (2020). Experiences of shame and guilt in anorexia and bulimia nervosa: A systematic review. *Psychology and Psychotherapy, 93*(1), 134–159. https://doi.org/10.1111/papt.12198

Bradford, R., Holliday, M., Schultz, A., & Moser, C. (2015). The role of the occupational therapist in the treatment of children with eating disorders. *Journal of Occupational Therapy, Schools, & Early Intervention, 8*(3), 196–210. https://doi.org/10.1080/19411243.2015.1077053

Brockmeyer, T., Friederich, H.-C., Jager, B., Schwab, H. W., Herzog, W., & de Zwaan, M. (2015). [Meal time support for patients with eating disorders: A survey on the clinical practice in German eating disorders centers.] *Psychotherapie, Psychosomatik, Medizinische Psychologie, 65*(3-4), 112–118. https://doi.org/10.1055/s-0034-1389960

Bulik, C. M., Brownley, K. A., Shapiro, J. R., & Berkman, N. D. (2012). Anorexia nervosa. In P. Sturney & M. Hersen (Eds.), *Handbook of evidence-based practice in clinical psychology: Child and adolescent disorders* (Vol. 1, pp. 575–597). John Wiley & Sons.

Bulik, C. M., Trace, S. E., Kleiman, S. C., & Mazzeo, S. E. (2014). Feeding and eating disorders. In D. C. Beidel, B. C. Frueh, & M. Hersen (Eds.), *Adult psychopathology and diagnosis* (7th ed., pp. 473–522). John Wiley & Sons.

Cardi, V., Mallorqui-Bague, N., Albano, G., Monteleone, A. M., Fernandez-Aranda, F., & Treasure, J. (2018). Social difficulties as risk and maintaining factors in anorexia nervosa: A mixed-method investigation. *Frontiers in Psychiatry, 9,* 12. https://doi.org/10.3389/fpsyt.2018.00012

Castellini, G., Trisolini, F., & Ricca, V. (2014). Psychopathology of eating disorders. *Journal of Psychopathology/Giornale di Psicopatologia, 20*(4), 461–470. https://old.jpsychopathol.it/wp-content/uploads/2015/07/14_castellini1.pdf

Centers for Disease Control and Prevention. (n.d.). *About adult BMI.* https://www.cdc.gov/healthyweight/assessing/bmi/adult_bmi/index.html

Cheng, Z. H., Perko, V. L., Fuller-Marashi, L., Gau, J. M., & Stice, E. (2019). Ethnic differences in eating disorder prevalence, risk factors, and predictive effects of risk factors among young women. *Eating Behaviors, 32,* 23–30. https://doi.org/10.1016/j.eatbeh.2018.11.004

Clark, M., & Nayar, S. (2012). Recovery from eating disorders: A role for occupational therapy. *New Zealand Journal of Occupational Therapy, 59*(1), 13–17.

Coombs, E., Brosnan, M., Bryant-Waugh, R., & Skevington, S. M. (2011). An investigation into the relationship between eating disorder psychopathology and autistic symptomatology in a non-clinical sample. *British Journal of Clinical Psychology, 50,* 326–338. https://doi.org/10.1348/014466510X524408

Cooper, M., Whitehead, L., & Boughton, N. (2004). Eating disorders. In J. Bennett-Levy, G. Butler, M. Fennell, A. Hackman, M. Mueller, & D. Westbrook (Eds.), *Cognitive behaviour therapy: Science and practice series, Oxford guide to behavioural experiments in cognitive therapy* (pp. 267–284). Oxford University Press.

Costa, M. B., & Melnik, T. (2016). Effectiveness of psychosocial interventions in eating disorders: An overview of Cochrane systematic reviews. *Einstein (São Paulo, Brazil), 14*(2), 235–277. https://doi.org/10.1590/S1679-45082016RW3120

Courty, A., Godart, N., Lalanne, C., & Berthoz, S. (2015). Alexithymia: A compounding factor for eating and social avoidance symptoms in anorexia nervosa. *Comprehensive Psychiatry, 56,* 217–228. https://doi.org/10.1016/j.comppsych.2014.09.011

Crisp, A. (2006). Anorexia nervosa in males: Similarities and differences to anorexia nervosa in women. *European Eating Disorder Review, 14,* 163–167. https://doi.org/10.1002/erv.703

Crouch, R., & Alers, V. (2014). The treatment of eating disorders in occupational therapy. In R. Crouch & V. Alers (Eds.), *Occupational therapy in psychiatry and mental health* (5th ed., pp. 408–418). John Wiley & Sons. https://doi.org/10.1002/9781118913536

Culbert, K. M., Racine, S., & Klump, K. L. (2015). Research review: What we have learned about the causes of eating disorders—A synthesis of sociocultural, psychological and biological research. *Journal of Child Psychology and Psychiatry and Allied Disciplines, 56*(11), 1141–1164. https://doi.org/10.1111/jcpp.12441

Cusack, A. (2013). *The relationship between acceptance, thought suppression, and eating disordered behavior in an adult eating disorders population.* Chicago School of Professional Psychology.

Cusack, C. E., Iampieri, A. O., & Galupo, M. P. (2022). "I'm still not sure if the eating disorder is a result of gender dysphoria": Trans and nonbinary individuals' descriptions of their eating and body concerns in relation to their gender. *Psychology of Sexual Orientation and Gender Diversity, 9*(4), 422–433. https://doi.org/10.1037/sgd0000515

Dakanalis, A., Carrà, G., Calogero, R., Fida, R., Clerici, M., Zanetti, M., & Riva, G. (2015). The developmental effects of media-ideal internalization and self-objectification processes on adolescents' negative body-feelings, dietary restraint, and binge eating. *European Child & Adolescent Psychiatry, 24*(8), 997–1010. https://doi.org/10.1007/s00787-014-0649-1

Daly, S. B. (2015). Secure body attachment and the prevention of eating disorders: A case application. *Smith College Studies in Social Work (Haworth), 85*(3), 311–329. https://doi.org/10.1080/00377317.2015.1067425

Delaquis, C. P., Godart, N. T., Evhan Group, Fatséas, M., & Berthoz, S. (2023). Cognitive and interpersonal factors in adolescent inpatients with anorexia nervosa: A network analysis. *Children (Basel, Switzerland), 10*(4), 730. https://doi.org/10.3390/children10040730

Deloitte Access Economics. (2020). *The social and economic cost of eating disorders in the United States of America: A report for the strategic training initiative for the prevention of eating disorders and the Academy for Eating Disorders.* https://www.hsph.harvard.edu/striped/report-economic-costs-of-eating-disorders

Doris, E., Westwood, H., Mandy, W., & Tchanturia, K. (2014). A qualitative study of friendship in patients with anorexia nervosa and possible autism spectrum disorder. *Psychology, 5*(11), 1338–1349. https://doi.org/10.4236/psych.2014.511144

Eddy, K. T., Thomas, J. J., Hastings, E., Edkins, K., Lamont, E., Nevins, C. M., Patterson, R. M., Murray, H. B., Bryant-Waugh, R., & Becker, A. E. (2014). Prevalence of *DSM-5* avoidant/restrictive food intake disorder in a pediatric gastroenterology healthcare network. *International Journal of Eating Disorders, 48,* 464–470. https://doi.org/10.1002/eat.22350

Elliott, M. L. (2012). Figured world of eating disorders: Occupations of illness. *Canadian Journal of Occupational Therapy/Revue Canadienne D'Ergotherapie, 79*(1), 15–22. https://doi.org/10.2182/cjot.2012.79.1.3

Evans, E. J., Hay, P. J., Mond, J., Paxton, S. J., Quirk, F., Rodgers, B., Jhajj, A. K., & Sawoniewska, M. A. (2011). Barriers to help-seeking in young women with eating disorders: A qualitative exploration in a longitudinal community survey. *Eating Disorders, 19,* 270–285. https://doi.org/10.1080/10640266.2011.566152

Farstad, S. M., McGeown, L. M., & von Ranson, K. M. (2016). Eating disorders and personality, 2004–2016: A systematic review and meta-analysis. *Clinical Psychology Review, 46,* 91–105. https://doi.org/10.1016/j.cpr.2016.04.005

Fox, J. R., Dean, M., & Whittlesea, A. (2017). The experience of caring for or living with an individual with an eating disorder: A meta-synthesis of qualitative studies. *Clinical Psychology and Psychotherapy, 24,* 103–125. https://doi.org/10.1002/cpp.1984

Franco, K. N., Sieke, E. H., Dickstein, L., & Falcone, T. (2017). *Disease management: Eating disorders.* Cleveland Clinic Center for Continuing Education. https://www.clevelandclinicmeded.

com/medicalpubs/diseasemanagement/psychiatry-psychology/eating-disorders/#bib25

Franko, D. L., Keshaviah, A., Eddy, K. T., Krishna, M., Davis, M. C., Keel, P. K., & Herzog, D. B. (2013). A longitudinal investigation of mortality in anorexia nervosa and bulimia nervosa. *American Journal of Psychiatry, 170*(8), 917–925. https://doi.org/10.1176/appi.ajp.2013.12070868

Frieiro, P., González-Rodríguez, R., & Domínguez-Alonso, J. (2022). Self-esteem and socialisation in social networks as determinants in adolescents' eating disorders. *Health & Social Care in the Community, 30*(6), e4416–e4424. https://doi.org/10.1111/hsc.13843

Galmiche, M., Déchelotte, P., Lambert, G., & Tavolacci, M. P. (2019). Prevalence of eating disorders over the 2000–2018 period: A systematic literature review. *The American Journal of Clinical Nutrition, 109*(5), 1402–1413. https://doi.org/10.1093/ajcn/nqy342

Gardiner, C., & Brown, N. (2010). Is there a role for occupational therapy within a specialist child and adolescent mental health eating disorder service? *British Journal of Occupational Therapy, 73*(1), 38–43. https://doi.org/10.4276/030802210X12629548272745

Gellynck, E., Heyninck, K., Andressen, K. W., Haegeman, G., Levy, F. O., Vanhoenacker, P., & Van Craenenbroeck, K. (2013). The serotonin 5-HT7 receptors: Two decades of research. *Experimental Brain Research, 230*(4), 555–568. https://doi.org/10.1007/s00221-013-3694-y

Gongora, V. C. (2014). Satisfaction with life, well-being and meaning in life as protective factors of eating disorder symptoms and body dissatisfaction in adolescents. *Eating Disorders, 22*(5), 435–449. https://doi.org/10.1080/10640266.2014.931765

Gonzaga, I., Ribovski, M., Claumann, G. S., Folle, A., Beltrame, T. S., Laus, M. F., & Pelegrini, A. (2023). Secular trends in body image dissatisfaction and associated factors among adolescents (2007–2017/2018). *PLoS One, 18*(1), e0280520. https://doi.org/10.1371/journal.pone.0280520

Goodwin, N. P. (2013). Suicide and eating disorders: The role of religiosity, spirituality and religious coping style. *Dissertation Abstracts International: Section B: The Sciences and Engineering, 74*(12-B(E)), 1–100. https://digitalcommons.library.uab.edu/etd-collection/1765

Gorrell, S., & Murray, S. B. (2019). Eating disorders in males. *Child and Adolescent Psychiatric Clinics of North America, 28*(4), 641–651. https://doi.org/10.1016/jchc.2019.05.012

Hargreaves, S. M., Raposo, A., Saraiva, A., & Zandonadi, R. P. (2021). Vegetarian diet: An overview through the perspective of quality of life domains. *International Journal of Environmental Research and Public Health, 18*(8), 4067. https://doi.org/10.3390/ijerph18084067

Harrison, A., Tchanturia, K., Naumann, U., & Treasure, J. (2012). Social emotional functioning and cognitive styles in eating disorders. *British Journal of Clinical Psychology, 51*(3), 261–279. https://doi.org/10.1111/j.2044-8260.2011.02026.x

Harrison, M. E., Norris, M. L., Obeid, N., Fu, M., Weinstangel, H., & Sampson, M. (2015). Systematic review of the effects of family meal frequency on psychosocial outcomes in youth. *Canadian Family Physician, 61*, e96–e106. https://www.cfp.ca/content/cfp/61/2/e96.full.pdf

Hay, P. J., Touyz, S., & Sud, R. (2012). Treatment for severe and enduring anorexia nervosa: A review. *Australian & New Zealand Journal of Psychiatry, 46*(12), 1136–1144. https://doi.org/10.1177/0004867412450469

Henderson, Z. B., Fox, J. R. E., Trayner, P., & Wittkowski, A. (2019). Emotional development in eating disorders: A qualitative metasynthesis. *Clinical Psychology & Psychotherapy, 26*(4), 440–457. https://doi.org/10.1002/cpp.2365

Hilbert, A., Pike, K. M., Goldschmidt, A. B., Wilfley, D. E., Fairburn, C. G., Dohm, F., Walsh, B. T., & Weissman, R. S. (2014). Risk factors across the eating disorders. *Psychiatry Research, 220*, 500–506. https://doi.org/10.1016/j.psychres.2014.05.054

Himmerich, H., Bentley, J., Kan, C., & Treasure, J. (2019). Genetic risk factors for eating disorders: An update and insights into pathophysiology. *Therapeutic Advances in Psychopharmacology, 9*, 1–20. https://doi.org/10.1177/2045125318814734

Horner, R. (2006). Eating disorders: A guide for the occupational therapist. *Occupational Therapy Capstones, 234*, 1–109. https://commons.und.edu/ot-grad/234

Hudson, J., Hiripi, E., Pope, H. G., Jr., & Kessler, R. C. (2007). The prevalence and correlates of eating disorders in the national comorbidity survey replication. *Biological Psychiatry, 61*, 349–358. https://doi.org/10.1016/j.biopsych.2006.03.040

Izydorczyk, B., Sitnik-Warchulska, K., Wajda, Z., Lizińczyk, S., & Ściegienny, A. (2021). Bonding with parents, body image and sociocultural attitudes toward appearance as predictors of eating disorders among young girls. *Frontiers in Psychiatry, 12*, 590542. https://doi.org/10.3389/fpsyt.2021.590542

Jenkins, J., & Ogden, J. (2012). Becoming 'whole' again: A qualitative study of women's views of recovering from anorexia nervosa. *European Eating Disorders Review, 20*, e23–e31. https://doi.org/10.1002/erv.1085

Juli, G., & Juli, L. (2014). The starting point of eating disorders: Role of genetics. *Psychiatria Danubina, 26*, 126–131. https://hrcak.srce.hr/file/385779

Kass, A. E., Kolko, R. P., & Wilfley, D. E. (2013). Psychological treatments for eating disorders. *Current Opinion in Psychiatry, 26*(6), 549–555. https://doi.org/10.1097%2FYCO.0b013e328365a30e

Kelly, A. C., & Carter, J. C. (2013). Why self-critical patients present with more severe eating disorder pathology: The mediating role of shame. *British Journal of Clinical Psychology, 52*(2), 148–161. https://doi.org/10.1111/bjc.12006

Kelly, A. C., Carter, J. C., & Borairi, S. (2014). Are improvements in shame and self-compassion early in eating disorders treatment associated with better patient outcomes? *International Journal of Eating Disorders, 47*(1), 54–64. https://doi.org/10.1002/eat.22196

Kielhofner, G. (2008). *A model of human occupation: Theory and application* (4th ed.). Lippincott Williams & Wilkins.

Kitson, C. (2012). Motivation to change. In J. R. E. Fox & K. P. Goss (Eds.), *Eating and its disorders* (pp. 75–101). John Wiley & Sons. https://doi.org/10.1002/9781118328910

Kjaersdam Telléus, G., Lauritsen, M. B., & Rodrigo-Domingo, M. (2021). Prevalence of various traumatic events including sexual trauma in a clinical sample of patients with an eating disorder. *Frontiers in Psychology, 12*, 687452. https://doi.org/10.3389/fpsyg.2021.687452

Kloczko, E., & Ikiugu, M. N. (2006). The role of occupational therapy in the treatment of adolescents with eating disorders as perceived by mental health therapists. *Occupational Therapy in Mental Health, 22*(1), 63–83. https://doi.org/10.1300/J004v22n01_05

Kotilahti, E., West, M., Isomaa, R., Karhunen, L., Rocks, T., & Ruusunen, A. (2020). Treatment interventions for severe and enduring eating disorders: Systematic review. *International Journal of Eating Disorders, 53*(8), 1280–1302. https://doi.org/10.1002/eat.23322

Leonkiewicz, M., & Wawrzyniak, A. (2022). The relationship between rigorous perception of one's own body and self, unhealthy eating behavior and a high risk of anorexic readiness: A predictor of eating disorders in the group of female ballet dancers and artistic gymnasts at the beginning of their career. *Journal of Eating Disorders, 10*(1), 48. https://doi.org/10.1186/s40337-022-00574-1

Linville, D., Brown, T., Strum, K., & McDougal, T. (2012). Eating disorders and social support: Perspectives of recovered individuals. *Eating Disorders, 20*(3), 216–231. https://doi.org/10.1080/10640266.2012.668480

Lock, L. C., Williams, H. A., Bamford, B., & Lacey, H. (2012). The effectiveness of the St. George's Eating Disorders meal preparation group for inpatients and day patients pursuing full recovery:

A pilot study. *European Eating Disorders Review, 20*(3), 218–224. https://doi.org/10.1002/erv.1134

Loeb, K. L., Le Grange, D., & Lock, J. (2015). Introduction: The role of the family in eating disorders. In K. L. Loeb, D. Le Grange, & J. Lock (Eds.), *Family therapy for adolescent eating and weight disorders: New applications* (pp. 1–5). Routledge.

Luo, J., Forbush, K. T., Williamson, J. A., Markon, K. E., & Pollack, L. O. (2013). How specific are the relationships between eating disorder behaviors and perfectionism? *Eating Behaviors, 14*(3), 291–294. https://doi.org/10.1016/j.eatbeh.2013.04.003

MacNeil, L., Esposito-Smythers, C., Mehlenbeck, R., & Weismoore, J. (2012). The effects of avoidance coping and coping self-efficacy on eating disorder attitudes and behaviors: A stress diathesis model. *Eating Behavior, 13,* 293–296. https://doi.org/10.1016/j.eatbeh.2012.06.005

Morris, R. (2012). Assessment of occupation and social performance. In J. Fox & K. Goss (Eds.), *Eating and its disorders* (pp. 61–73). John Wiley & Sons. https://doi.org/10.1002/9781118328910

Murray, S. B., Quintana, D. S., Loeb, K. L., Griffiths, S., & Le Grange, D. (2019). Treatment outcomes for anorexia nervosa: A systematic review and meta-analysis of randomized controlled trials. *Psychological Medicine, 49*(4), 535–544. https://doi.org/10.1017/S0033291718002088

Musolino, C., Warin, M., Wade, T., & Gilchrist, P. (2016). Developing shared understandings of recovery and care: A qualitative study of women with eating disorders who resist therapeutic care. *Journal of Eating Disorders, 4,* 36. https://doi.org/10.1186/s40337-016-0114-2

National Eating Disorders Collaboration. (2015). *Eating disorders in males.* http://www.nedc.com.au/eating-disorders-in-males

Noordenbos, G., Aliakbari, N., & Campbell, R. (2014). The relationship among critical inner voices, low self-esteem, and self-criticism in eating disorders. *Eating Disorders, 22,* 337–351. https://doi.org/10.1080/10640266.2014.898983

Nowakowski, M. E., McFarlane, T., & Cassin, S. (2013). Alexothymia and eating disorders: A critical review of the literature. *Journal of Eating Disorders, 1,* 21. https://doi.org/10.1186/2050-2974-1-21

Obeid, N., Buchholz, A., Boerner, K. E., Henderson, K. A., & Norris, M. (2013). Self-esteem and social anxiety in an adolescent female eating disorder population: Age and diagnostic effects. *Eating Disorders, 21*(2), 140–153. https://doi.org/10.1080/10640266.2013.761088

Peat, C. M., Berkman, N. D., Lohr, K. N., Brownley, K. A., Bann, C. M., Cullen, K., Quattlebaum, C. M. J., & Bulik, C. M. (2017). Comparative effectiveness of treatments for binge-eating disorder: Systematic review and network meta-analysis. *European Eating Disorders Review, 25*(5), 317–328. https://doi.org/10.1002/erv.2517

Pilecki, M. W., Sałapa, K., & Józefik, B. (2016). Socio-cultural context of eating disorders in Poland. *Journal of Eating Disorders, 4*(11), 2050–2974. https://doi.org/10.1186/s40337-016-0093-3

Pinheiro, A. P., Raney, T. J., Thornton, L. M., Fichter, M. M., Berrettini, W. H., Goldman, D., Halmi, K. A., Kaplan, A. S., Strober, M., Treasure, J., Woodside, B., Kaye, W. H., & Bulik, C. M. (2010). Sexual functioning in women with eating disorders. *International Journal of Eating Disorders, 43*(2), 123–129. https://doi.org/10.1002/eat.20671

Pugh, M., & Waller, G. (2016). The anorexic voice and severity of eating pathology in anorexia nervosa. *International Journal of Eating Disorders, 49*(6), 622–625. https://doi.org/10.1002/eat.22499

Quick, V. M., & Byrd-Bredbenner, C. (2013). Disturbed eating behaviours and associated psychographic characteristics of college students. *Journal of Human Nutrition & Dietetics, 26,* 53–63. https://doi.org/10.1111/jhn.12060

Quiles-Cestari, L. M., & Ribeiro, R. P. P. (2012). The occupational roles of women with anorexia nervosa. *Revista Latino-Americana de Enfermagem, 20*(2), 1–2. https://doi.org/10.1590/s0104-11692012000200004

Raykos, B. C., McEvoy, P. M., Carter, O., Fursland, A., & Nathan, P. (2014). Interpersonal problems across restrictive and binge-purge samples: Data from a community-based eating disorders clinic. *Eating Behaviours, 15*(3), 449–452. https://doi.org/10.1016/j.eatbeh.2014.06.008

Reas, D. L., Ro, O., Karterud, S., Hummelen, B., & Pedersen, G. (2013). Eating disorders in a large clinical sample of men and women with personality disorders. *International Journal of Eating Disorders, 46*(8), 801–809. https://doi.org/10.1002/eat.22176

Robinson, P. (2014). Severe and enduring eating disorders: Recognition and management. *Advances in Psychiatric Treatment, 20*(6), 392–401. https://doi.org/10.1192/apt.bp.113.011841

Rubino, F., Puhl, R. M., Cummings, D. E., Eckel, R. H., Ryan, D. H., Mechanick, J. I., Nadglowski, J., Ramos Salas, X., Schauer, P. R., Twenefour, D., Apovian, C. M., Aronne, L. J., Batterham, R. L., Berthoud, H. R., Boza, C., Busetto, L., Dicker, D., De Groot, M., Eisenberg, D., … Dixon, J. B. (2020). Joint international consensus statement for ending stigma of obesity. *Nature Medicine, 26*(4), 485–497. https://doi.org/10.1038/s41591-020-0803-x

Rymaszewska, J., & Mazurek, J. (2012). The social and occupational functioning of outpatients from mental health services. *Advances in Clinical and Experimental Medicine, 21*(2), 215–223. https://advances.umw.edu.pl/pdf/2012/21/2/215.pdf

Saiphoo, A. N., & Vahedi, Z. (2019). A meta-analytic review of the relationship between social media use and body image disturbance. *Computers in Human Behavior, 101,* 259–275. https://doi.org/10.1016/j.chb.2019.07.028

Sharpe, H., Griffiths, S., Choo, T. H., Eisenberg, M. E., Mitchison, D., Wall, M., & Neumark-Sztainer, D. (2018). The relative importance of dissatisfaction, overvaluation and preoccupation with weight and shape for predicting onset of disordered eating behaviors and depressive symptoms over 15 years. *The International Journal of Eating Disorders, 51*(10), 1168–1175. https://doi.org/10.1002/eat.22936

Sherry, S. B., Sabourin, B. C., Hall, P. A., Hewitt, P. L., Flett, G. L., & Gralnick, T. M. (2014). The perfectionism model of binge eating: Testing unique contributions, mediating mechanisms, and cross-cultural similarities using a daily diary methodology. *Psychology of Addictive Behaviors, 28,* 1230–1239. https://doi.org/10.1037/a0037939

Sigurdh, J., Allard, P., Spigset, O., & Hägglöf, B. (2013). Platelet serotonin transporter and 5-HT2A receptor binding in adolescents with eating disorders. *International Journal of Neuroscience, 123*(5), 333–338. https://doi.org/10.3109/00207454.2012.761215

Silén, Y., & Keski-Rahkonen, A. (2022). Worldwide prevalence of *DSM-5* eating disorders among young people. *Current Opinion in Psychiatry, 35*(6), 362–371. https://doi.org/10.1097/YCO.0000000000000818

Sly, R., & Bamford, B. (2011). Why are we waiting? The relationship between low admission weight and end of treatment weight outcomes. *European Eating Disorders Review, 19*(5), 407–410. https://doi.org/10.1002/erv.1061

Spettigue, W., Maras, D., Obeid, N., Henderson, K. A., Buchholz, A., Gomez, R., & Norris, M. L. (2015). A psycho-education intervention for parents with adolescents with eating disorders: A randomized control trial. *Eating Disorders, 23*(1), 60–75. https://doi.org/10.1080/10640266.2014.940790

Stice, E., & Desjardins, C. D. (2018). Interactions between risk factors in the prediction of onset of eating disorders: Exploratory hypothesis generating analysis. *Behaviour Research and Therapy, 105,* 52–62. https://doi.org/10.1016/j.brat.2018.03.005

Stice, E., & Van Ryzin, M. (2019). A prospective test of the temporal sequencing of risk factor emergence in the dual pathway model of eating disorders. *Journal of Abnormal Psychology, 128*(2), 119–128. https://doi.org/10.1037/abn0000400

Sullivan, J. M., Lawson, D. M., & Akay-Sullivan, S. (2020). Insecure attachment and therapeutic bond as mediators of social, relational, and social distress and interpersonal problems in adult females with childhood sexual abuse history. *Journal of Child Sexual Abuse, 29*(6), 659–676. https://doi.org/10.1080/10538712.2020.1751368

Tabler, J., & Utz, R. L. (2015). The influence of adolescent eating disorders or disordered eating behaviors on socioeconomic achievement in early adulthood. *International Journal of Eating Disorders, 48*(6), 622–632. https://doi.org/10.1002/eat.22395

Trace, S. E., Baker, J. H., Peñas-Lledó, E., & Bulik, C. M. (2013). The genetics of eating disorders. *Annual Review of Clinical Psychology, 9,* 589–620. https://doi.org/10.1146/annurev-clinpsy-050212-185546

Treasure, J. L., Wack, E. R., & Roberts, M. E. (2008). Models as a high-risk group: The health implications of a size zero culture. *British Journal of Psychiatry, 192,* 243–244. https://doi.org/10.1192/bjp.bp.107.044164

Ty, M., & Francis, A. J. (2013). Insecure attachment and disordered eating in women: The mediating processes of social comparison and emotion dysregulation. *Eating Disorders, 21,* 154–174. https://doi.org/10.1080/10640266.2013.761089

van Doornik, S. F. W., Ostafin, B. D., Jonker, N. C., Glashouwer, K. A., & de Jong, P. J. (2022). Satisfaction with normative life domains and the course of anorexia nervosa. *The International Journal of Eating Disorders, 55*(4), 553–563. https://doi.org/10.1002/eat.23691

van Eeden, A. E., van Hoeken, D., & Hoek, H. W. (2021). Incidence, prevalence and mortality of anorexia nervosa and bulimia nervosa. *Current Opinion in Psychiatry, 34*(6), 515–524. https://doi.org/10.1097/YCO.0000000000000739

van Hoeken, D., & Hoek, H. W. (2020). Review of the burden of eating disorders: Mortality, disability, costs, quality of life, and family burden. *Current Opinion in Psychiatry, 33*(6), 521–527. https://doi.org/10.1097/YCO.0000000000000641

Wade, T. D., Wilksch, S. M., Paxton, S. J., Byrne, S. M., & Austin, S. B. (2015). How perfectionism and ineffectiveness influence growth of eating disorder risk in young adolescent girls. *Behaviour Research and Therapy, 66,* 56–63. https://doi.org/10.1016/j.brat.2015.01.007

Weltzin, T. E., Weisensel, N., Franczyk, D., Burnett, K., Klitz, C., & Bean, P. (2005). Eating disorders in men: Update. *Journal of Men's Health and Gender, 2,* 186–193. https://doi.org/10.1016/j.jmhg.2005.04.008

Westwood, H., & Tchanturia, K. (2017). Autism spectrum disorder in anorexia nervosa: An updated literature review. *Current Psychiatry Reports, 19*(7), 41. https://doi.org/10.1007/s11920-017-0791-9

Wilksch, S. M., O'Shea, A., Ho, P., Byrne, S., & Wade, T. D. (2020). The relationship between social media use and disordered eating in young adolescents. *The International Journal of Eating Disorders, 53*(1), 96–106. https://doi.org/10.1002/eat.23198

Winecoff, A. A., Ngo, L., Moskovich, A., Merwin, R., & Zucker, N. (2015). The functional significance of shyness in anorexia nervosa. *European Eating Disorders Review, 23*(4), 327–332. https://doi.org/10.1002/erv.2363

Wong, K.-L. (2015). Social and psychological factors contributing to eating disorders among Caucasian, African American, Asian American, and Hispanic American women. *Dissertation Abstracts International: Section B: The Sciences and Engineering, 76*(2-B(E)), 0419–4217.

Wright, K. M. (2015). Maternalism: A healthy alliance for recovery and transition in eating disorder services. *Journal of Psychiatric & Mental Health Nursing, 22*(6), 431–439. https://doi.org/10.1111/jpm.12198

Yahya, A. S., & Khawaja, S. (2020). The course of eating disorders during COVID-19. *The Primary Care Companion for CNS Disorders, 22*(3), 20com02657. https://doi.org/10.4088/PCC.20com02657

Zanetti, T., Santonastaso, P., Sgaravatti, E., Degortes, D., & Favaro, A. (2013). Clinical and temperamental correlates of body image disturbance in eating disorders. *European Eating Disorders Review, 21*(1), 32–37. https://doi.org/10.1002/erv.2190

Zeeck, A., Herpertz-Dahlmann, B., Friederich, H. C., Brockmeyer, T., Resmark, G., Hagenah, U., Ehrlich, S., Cuntz, U., Zipfel, S., & Hartmann, A. (2018). Psychotherapeutic treatment for anorexia nervosa: A systematic review and network meta-analysis. *Frontiers in Psychiatry, 9,* 158. https://doi.org/10.3389/fpsyt.2018.00158

Mood Disorders

Sara Story and Josh Skuller

Changes in one's emotional state are referred to as mood or sometimes a mood swing. Situations or circumstances can influence one's emotional state or mood. When an individual lives with a mood disorder, the changes or fluctuations in mood may have little to no connection with the current circumstances, experiences, or context. Mood disorders affect people across the life span and cross-culturally. Occupational therapy practitioners (OTPs) know the impact mood disorders can have on an individual's occupational performance and life satisfaction can be detrimental. Mood disorders are among the leading causes of disability globally (United Nations, 2017; World Health Organization [WHO], 2017) and are a significant predictor of suicide across the life span. The connection between mood disorders, such as depression or bipolar disorder, and suicide provides a call to action for OTPs.

OTPs play an important role in mental health promotion and intervention, from aiding in the destigmatization of mood disorders to creating interventions that support engagement in life's meaningful occupations. Mood disorders affect everyone differently, thus suggesting a need for a myriad of treatment options (Box 20-1). This chapter includes information to assist OTPs in learning the different types of mood disorders, the etiology and prevalence of the conditions, their impact on occupational performance, and the most common, evidence-based medical interventions available.

Description of the Condition

Mood disorder is an overarching categorical term that encapsulates conditions where an individual has ongoing feelings of sadness, disengagement, or disinterest in once-valued occupations, or extreme fluctuations from sadness to happiness (U.S. Department of Health & Human Services, 2022). **Unipolar depression** is another categorical term used when referring to low, sad, or unpleasant moods. **Bipolar disorder** is utilized when an individual experiences both ends of the continuum from extreme lows to high levels, such as elation or mania. Often mood disorders occur concurrently with other health conditions, such as anxiety disorders or substance use disorders, as well as medical illnesses such as cardiovascular disease, hypertension, and obesity (Rolin et al., 2020).

Diagnostic and Statistical Manual of Mental Disorders Criteria for Mood Episodes

Diagnostic criteria relating to mood disorders are specified in the *Diagnostic and Statistical Manual of Mental Disorders,* Fifth Edition, Text Revision (*DSM-5-TR;* American Psychiatric Association, 2022). It is important to consider the sociocultural context of individuals with mood disorders to ensure a culturally responsive and holistic approach is taken throughout assessment and treatment. There are three types of mood episodes described in the *DSM-5-TR:* depressive, manic, and hypomanic.

Many associate the term **depression** with moods of sadness, which most have experienced at some point across their life span. Although an individual may experience a moment or brief period of sadness, a diagnosis of depression is frequently classified as a chronic disorder. Warnick and colleagues (2021) suggest depressive disorders are reexperienced with recurrence rates ranging from 50% to 90% after one's first episode. Research indicates the recurrence rate increases with each episode. In addition, depressive disorders are underdiagnosed and undertreated.

A **major depressive episode** occurs when a depressed mood or absence of interest or engagement in all or mostly all activities occurs almost daily for at least 2 weeks. The previously mentioned description is referred to as "Criterion A" (American Psychiatric Association, 2022). "Criterion B" refers to symptoms that interfere with overall engagement and occupational performance or cause clinically significant distress. A **depressive episode** may also be characterized by one's limited capacity to feel pleasure, also known as **anhedonia** (Trøstheim et al., 2020). Depressive episodes may also manifest as feelings of worthlessness and/or recurring thoughts of death, sleep disturbances such as insomnia or hypersomnia, and significant loss or gain in one's appetite patterns and weight.

Manic episodes are classified as a period when one's mood is abnormally and persistently elevated, expansive, or irritable; this abnormal amount of energy lasts at least 1 week (American Psychiatric Association, 2022). To meet the diagnostic criteria, the mood significantly impacts one's social interactions and occupational performance. Other symptoms associated with a manic episode include an inflated

BOX 20-1 ■ David: Medication-Induced Depressive Disorder

David (pseudonym) was recently diagnosed with Crohn disease, an inflammatory bowel disease (IBD). The diagnosis left him feeling "down, with little to no excitement to do meaningful things." In the first few weeks after being diagnosed, he was informed that corticosteroid therapy was going to be the best course of treatment. His health-care provider prescribed a moderate dosage of prednisone, and within a short amount of time David expressed concern for his quick change in moods and overall engagement with the world around him. A side effect of corticosteroid therapy is depression (Brown & Chandler, 2001; Keefer & Kane, 2017). Understanding the chronic nature of IBD, which requires ongoing treatment with corticosteroids, he has great concern for what his new reality may be regarding his emotional state.

After 6 weeks of treatment, David began seeing fewer mood swings but felt a growing concern for his continued lack of desire and engagement in daily life. He decided to address his concern regarding his depressive symptoms with his health-care provider. They decided to stop the corticosteroid therapy to see if the depressive symptoms subsided. Unfortunately, although the depressive symptoms lessened, the IBD symptoms were again becoming unmanageable. David worked closely with his health-care providers to resume corticosteroid therapy for the management of Crohn disease in conjunction with a daily regimen of fluoxetine to manage depressive symptoms, allowing him to resume engagement in his daily life. David's story represents the never-ending battle individuals may experience with navigating life with a mood disorder, in this case, medication-induced depressive disorder.

TABLE 20-1 | Mood Disorder Diagnoses and Episodes

Diagnoses	Episode(s)
Major depressive disorder	Major depressive episode without a manic or hypomanic episode
Bipolar I disorder	Manic episode with or without major depressive episode
Bipolar II disorder	Hypomanic episode with a major depressive episode

Symptomology and one's experience of depression vary based on the individual. The severity and frequency of one's diagnosis may vary from mild to severe, as a single or recurrent episode, and with or without psychotic features. Additionally, specifiers may be added to assist in quantifying the associated features of the depression diagnosis. In accordance with the *DSM-5-TR*, major depression disorder specifiers include anxious distress, mixed features, melancholic, atypical, mood-congruent psychotic, mood-incongruent psychotic, catatonia, peripartum onset, and seasonal pattern features (American Psychiatric Association, 2022).

With the specifier of **anxious distress**, there is a presence of at least two of the following symptoms: feeling tense, unusually restless, concentration challenges because of worry, fear of awful things occurring, and feeling one may lose control of self (American Psychiatric Association, 2022). **Melancholic** features manifest as a loss of pleasure in activities or an inability to react positively to pleasurable stimuli. To meet the criteria for the melancholic specifier, the person must also experience three of the following symptoms: empty mood, psychomotor agitation, inappropriate guilt, significant weight loss, early-morning awakening, and depression that worsens in the morning. Collectively, melancholic features are more frequently seen in inpatient persons who are experiencing a more severe major depressive episode with psychotic features.

Catatonia is associated with mental disorders on the schizophrenia spectrum (see Chapter 23: Schizophrenia Spectrum and Psychotic Disorders 🤝); however, major depressive episodes may incur catatonic features. The specifier for catatonia is applied when the individual experiences marked psychomotor disturbances, exhibiting symptomology such as, but not limited to, stupor, mutism, negativism, or agitation (American Psychiatric Association, 2022). The variability in psychomotor behaviors can manifest in an individual going from waxing to waning motor activity. There is a concern for individuals who experience catatonia in a severe state to be at risk for harming themselves or others.

The **atypical features** specifier is applied to MDD when there is a presence of mood reactivity, weight gain, hypersomnia, leaden paralysis, and/or a pattern of interpersonal rejection sensitivity, which impairs occupational functioning (American Psychiatric Association, 2022). If hallucinations and/or delusions are present during the major depressive episode, the individual is said to have **psychosis**. When psychotic features are present, they are typically categorized as either mood-congruent or mood-incongruent. Mood-congruent would include delusions or hallucinations that follow a typical depressive episode, where the individual might have feelings of inadequacy, guilt, deserved punishment, or even death. In contrast, mood-incongruent features involve

self-esteem, otherwise known as grandiosity; decreased need for sleep; rapid speech; psychomotor agitation; and involvement in high-risk activities such as spending sprees, drug use, or sexual promiscuity.

The same symptoms that were described for a manic episode are present in a **hypomanic episode**, but the symptoms are less severe and do not significantly affect functioning. To meet the criteria for a hypomanic episode, the symptoms need only be present for 4 days. The diagnosis of major depressive disorder (MDD), bipolar I disorder, or bipolar II disorder is based on the combination of episodes. A quick reference for mood disorder diagnoses and episodes is presented in Table 20-1.

Depressive Disorders

Depressive disorders are characterized by sadness, emptiness, or irritable mood that directly impacts the individual's occupational performance or ability to function. To meet the diagnostic criteria for **major depressive disorder (MDD)**, one would experience distinct depressive episodes of at least 2 weeks' duration represented by apparent changes in affect and functioning (American Psychiatric Association, 2022). Because MDD occurs with a depressive episode but with the absence of an episode of mania, hypomania, or mixed features, it is often referred to as **unipolar disorder** (American Psychological Association, 2023; Cuellar et al., 2005). The term "unipolar disorder" or "unipolar depression" is used synonymously with MDD (American Psychological Association, 2023).

delusional or hallucinatory content that is not consistent with depressive themes such as grandiosity.

A **peripartum onset** is characterized by its timing (American Psychiatric Association, 2022). In peripartum onset, the onset of mood symptoms begins during pregnancy or up to 4 weeks after delivery; many refer to mood disorders at this time as postpartum depression. Although the peripartum specifier occurs within 4 weeks of delivery, many women may experience postpartum symptoms through the first 12 months after delivery. Although rare, peripartum episodes can manifest with psychotic features with command hallucinations, such as infanticide.

One's risk of experiencing postpartum mood episodes with psychotic features is elevated if the mother has a history of depressive or bipolar disorder or a family history of bipolar disorders. The severity and frequency of a postpartum episode may vary but exceed the few days or weeks of the "baby blues" (Howland, 2023). Postpartum symptoms may include intense irritability, anhedonia, difficulty bonding with the baby, severe mood swings, and/or functional impairment (Mayo Clinic, 2022c). Nicole's story in Box 20-2 provides an example of postpartum or peripartum onset of depression.

BOX 20-2 ■ Nicole: Peripartum Onset of Major Depressive Disorder

Nicole (pseudonym) was a stay-at-home mother of three boys, with a fourth on the way. She conducted her role as a mother with grace and a giggle. Anyone who knew her was not surprised that she had been blessed with three energetic sons. With the fourth pregnancy, however, things appeared to be a bit different. After approximately 24 to 27 weeks, she appeared more than tired, but also occasionally sad or tearful. Her husband, Braxton (pseudonym), knew something was happening with Nicole during this pregnancy but could not identify exactly what it was.

When asked routine questions at her next prenatal visit, Nicole was more open than usual with her OB-GYN and expressed that she was "not herself." When asked to describe how she was feeling, it was difficult for Nicole to put into words beyond stating, "I feel irritated and like I'm on a hormonal roller coaster, most of the time. My moods feel much different than any I experienced with the past pregnancies." Unsure of what to do, Nicole continued to be open and honest with her care provider and spouse, as well as friends and family.

Once the baby arrived, Nicole became the mother of four handsome boys but still had strong feelings about "not being herself." At her postpartum appointment, Nicole's anger had become extreme, manifesting as near rage. She was often found lying on the floor, crying and even weeping. Braxton identified that even the slightest thing with the new baby could trigger her mood swings. The real concern was for Nicole, the baby, and the other children in the home. Although Braxton worked outside the home, he was unsettled with the idea of leaving Nicole home, given the uncertainty of how her feelings would impact the day. Her moods and actions had become a barrier to her occupational performance relating to herself and her role as a mother.

Nicole's care provider diagnosed postpartum depression, which devastated Nicole as she had associated it with a terrible stigma. Nevertheless, with the support of a care provider, her spouse, and her family, Nicole accepted the recommended treatment of psychotherapy and medication by taking a prescribed selective serotonin reuptake inhibitor (Barbic et al., 2021).

The **seasonal pattern** specifier is utilized in recurrent MDD that occurs at the same time of year, most commonly in winter. Often, the seasonal onset is referred to as **seasonal affective disorder (SAD)**, where a change in one's mood and how one thinks or functions is altered with the changing of the seasons (National Institute of Mental Health [NIMH], 2023b). For an individual to be diagnosed with the seasonal pattern, one must not have exhibited nonseasonal episodes simultaneously with temporal seasonal relational depressive episodes. The specifier of seasonal patterns should not be solely linked to psychosocial stressors. Major depressive episodes with a seasonal pattern may include symptoms of loss of energy, overeating or weight gain, and hypersomnia.

Persistent Depressive Disorder

The chronic form of depression is known as **persistent depressive disorder**, where one experiences depressed moods that consume the majority of one's day and lasts for the majority of 2 years; however, the symptoms are less severe in this form than in MDD (American Psychiatric Association, 2022). In children and/or adolescents, the same symptoms are present for the duration of at least 1 year. If severe symptoms such as suicidal thoughts or psychosis occur, the individual would not receive a diagnosis of persistent depressive disorder.

Depressive episodes may occur in persistent depressive disorder. During periods of severe symptoms when the person meets the criteria for MDD, that would be the diagnosis. However, during periods when the symptoms are less severe, persistent depressive disorder would be the diagnosis. A combination of MDD and persistent depressive disorder is sometimes referred to as **double depression**, and can be particularly debilitating. An individual living with this pattern may describe themselves as constantly feeling "down," and they may struggle to experience day-to-day life without these moods.

Disruptive Mood Dysregulation Disorder

With the publication of the *DSM-5-TR*, a new depressive disorder diagnosis emerged, **disruptive mood dysregulation disorder** (American Psychiatric Association, 2022). Symptoms of the disorder present as persistent irritability and frequent episodes of extreme behavior dysregulation. The irritability may result in temper outbursts, verbal and/or behavioral irritability, as well as ongoing moods of severe irritability or anger. The diagnosis of disruptive mood dysregulation disorder is warranted for children ages 6 through 18, with the onset occurring before age 10. As one reaches adulthood, the individual typically develops unipolar depressive disorder or an anxiety disorder (American Psychiatric Association, 2022).

Bipolar Disorders

Bipolar and cyclothymic disorders are another group of diagnoses categorized under the umbrella of mood disorders. The three types of bipolar disorder are bipolar I, bipolar II, and cyclothymic disorders. Additional bipolar diagnoses may be categorized as substance/medication-induced bipolar disorder.

In order to be diagnosed with **bipolar I disorder**, an individual must experience at least one manic episode. One's manic episode may either be preceded by or follow a hypo-manic or major depressive episode. Hypomanic and depressive episodes are common with bipolar I, but are not required criteria for a diagnosis. In the United States, millions of adults are impacted by the diagnosis of bipolar disorder, often manifesting in their teens or early 20s (Substance Abuse and Mental Health Services Administration [SAMHSA], 2023). Regardless of the age at one's diagnosis, each individual's lived experience with a diagnosis of bipolar I can vary, from mood swings with very high (mania) to extreme lows (depression), with many experiencing life-long impairments in occupational functioning and performance (Koene et al., 2022).

The *DSM-5-TR* suggests that over 90% of those who experience a single manic episode are at an increased likelihood of navigating recurrent mood episodes (American Psychiatric Association, 2022). When an individual experiences a manic episode, euphoria may be present alongside the possibilities of inflated self-esteem and an overcommitment to new projects/tasks. Engagement in behaviors of this magnitude manifests as increased energy levels, ultimately affecting the individual's sleep patterns. Sleep disturbances may be one of the most impactful to one's quality of life (Kraiss et al., 2023).

Because of the increased energy, feelings of euphoria, and sometimes increased productivity, the individual experiencing the symptoms may not see a problem or need for treatment. The change in behaviors often grows in intensity, or can result in drastic changes in routines, behaviors, and preferences (e.g., sudden alteration in one's personal appearance).

The **rapid cycling** specifier is given when four or more episodes occur in 12 months. This specifier may lead to a poorer prognosis including an increased risk for suicide over the span of one's lifetime (American Psychiatric Association, 2022). Suicidal ideation and behavior place one diagnosed with bipolar I at increased risk for a suicide attempt (up to 30 times higher than the general population), with anywhere from 20% to 60% of individuals attempting suicide at least once (Dome et al., 2019).

Bipolar II disorder is distinguished by the presence of a current or past hypomanic episode and a current or past major depressive episode without the presence of a manic episode (American Psychiatric Association, 2022). Within the individual's hypomanic episode, one must exhibit abnormal and persistently elevated or irritable mood and increased energy that is present for the majority of a minimum of 4 days.

Additionally, at least three of the following symptoms must be present: grandiosity, decreased need for sleep, increased talkative behavior, racing thoughts, distractibility, psychomotor agitation, and/or excessive engagement in high-risk activities. Many individuals with bipolar II disorder are diagnosed with MDD, as it is common for the individual not to recognize or acknowledge hypomania. However, bipolar II disorder is not to be considered a lesser form of bipolar disorder. Concern is warranted because of the frequency and duration of depression and the often chronic nature of the diagnosis.

Specifiers may be added to describe the pattern of the mood episode(s) more specifically in bipolar II. Specifiers include anxious distress, rapid cycling, or seasonal pattern (American Psychiatric Association, 2022); these specifiers are the same as those described previously. Although the specifiers may vary based on the type of an episode the individual is experiencing, impulsivity is categorized as a common feature of bipolar II disorder. Impulsive behavior may influence suicidal ideation, behavior, and attempts in individuals with bipolar II disorder, and is often seen during a depressive episode (Zhong et al., 2022).

Additionally, individuals diagnosed with bipolar II disorder experience a high rate of co-occurring mental disorders. For children and adolescents, there is a high rate of co-occurring anxiety disorders (Sala et al., 2010), not drastically different from the adult population, where anxiety and substance use disorders are common (Spoorthy et al., 2019).

When hypomanic and depressive symptoms are recurring and present for at least 2 years in adults, or 1 year for children and adolescents, and do not meet established criteria for hypomanic or major depressive episodes, the diagnosis is **cyclothymic disorder**. Mood disturbances fluctuate between depression and mania, and the symptoms are chronic. Unlike persistent depressive disorder, this diagnosis is often misunderstood or misdiagnosed (American Psychiatric Association, 2022; Bielecki & Gupta, 2022; Medline Plus, 2022). Occupational engagement and performance are disrupted with the onset of symptoms. Although emotional highs and lows occur within cyclothymic disorder, they are less severe than symptoms and moods associated with bipolar I and II disorders (Mayo Clinic, 2022b).

Mental Health in Culture and Society

Aster Harrison

The Icarus Project

The Icarus Project was founded in 2002 by Sascha Altman DuBrul and Jacks McNamara. They created a narrative about mental illnesses as "dangerous gifts." In their original vision statement, they explained their view of bipolar disorder as a "dangerous gift to be cultivated and taken care of rather than as a disease or disorder needing to be 'cured'" (The Icarus Project, 2002, cited in DuBrul, 2014, p. 259). They recognized both how their mental differences could inspire creativity and innovation, and how their bipolar disorder could also lead them to dangerous states of severe isolation or suicidality.

They acknowledged people with bipolar disorder as "members of a group that has been misunderstood and persecuted throughout history, but has also been responsible for some of its most brilliant creations" (The Icarus Project, 2002, cited in DuBrul, 2014, p. 259), and stated that they were "proud" of their identities. Their early goals were for the organization to provide peer support and alternative ways of viewing mental illness beyond the "reductionist framework offered by the current mental health establishment" (The Icarus Project, 2002, cited in DuBrul, 2014, p. 259).

From these beginnings, The Icarus Project expanded into a national group with many local chapters. These local chapters offered support groups for peers with mental illness to gather, help each other, and become friends. The Icarus Project also created a book and a variety of resources—for example, a guide for people who want to come off of psychiatric drugs, a guide about creating community mental health support networks, and a guide to supporting people in crisis. They grew to support people with a variety of different diagnoses and perspectives.

In 2020, The Icarus Project restructured its approach and leadership and renamed itself Fireweed Collective. The intention of the restructuring was to address justice issues that had emerged in the local chapters and take a more explicitly antioppressive and intersectional approach (Fireweed Collective, n.d.-b). The national organization continues to offer educational resources and online support groups. They aim to center "Black, Indigenous, and people of color, disabled and LGBTQIA+ people, immigrants, and low-income people" (Fireweed Collective, n.d.-a, para. 7). They take a Healing Justice (HJ) approach. They define HJ as "a framework rooted in racial justice, disability justice, and economic justice [that] provides us with tools we can use to interrupt the systems of oppression that impact our mental health. Fireweed Collective uses HJ as a guide to help redefine what medicine is, and increase who has access to it" (Fireweed Collective, n.d.-a, para. 1).

The Icarus Project and Fireweed Collective provide examples of approaches to mental illness beyond the mainstream medical and biopsychosocial models.

References

DuBrul, S. A. (2014). The Icarus Project: A counter narrative for psychic diversity. *Journal of Medical Humanities, 35,* 257–271. https://doi.org/10.1007/s10912-014-9293-5

Fireweed Collective. (n.d.-a). *Our framework.* https://fireweed collective.org/our-framework

Fireweed Collective. (n.d.-b). *Our history.* https://fireweedcollective .org/our-history

Etiology

Mood disorders are thought to stem from a combination of biological, environmental, and cognitive/psychosocial factors that combine to form complex issues that are difficult to address with just one simple solution (see Fig. 20-1). Although genetics and biological features are often considered when treating mood disorders, reviewing other related issues such as exposure to stress/trauma, personal history, and the availability of support systems is essential. Other factors that may trigger mood disorders include changes in seasons, childbirth, and substance use.

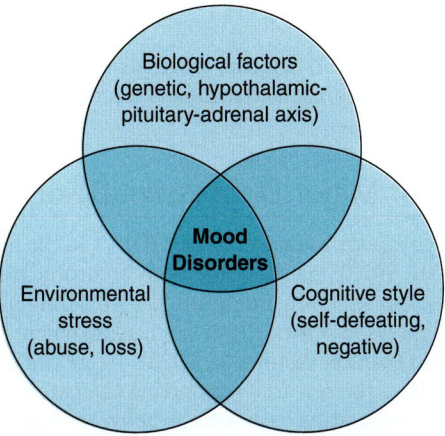

FIGURE 20-1. The etiology of mood disorders involves a complex interaction of biological, environmental, and cognitive factors.

Biological Causes

Depression is related to a lack of norepinephrine and/or serotonin, and mania is associated with an abundance of noradrenaline (Stein et al., 2007). Because of this notion, numerous medications target these neurotransmitters, many of which are quite effective.

Much of the research into the biological causes of mood disorders has focused on the hypothalamic-pituitary-adrenal (HPA) axis. This axis prepares the body for the stress response and works in conjunction with the limbic system, the brain region that controls emotion, to help prepare the body for fight or flight (Wang et al., 2021). It is not known if the biological differences in the brain cause the mood disorder, or if these differences develop because of the disorder. Chronic stress, for example, can release an abundance of cortisol, which can have a lasting effect on the limbic system, including structures such as the amygdala and hippocampus, predisposing an individual to depression.

Repeated exposure to chronic stress is thought to decrease the threshold for depression. Adolescents with MDD show an elevated degree of amygdala activity in response to negative stimuli. They also show a smaller hippocampal volume related to their peers without MDD (Redlich et al., 2018). In addition, changes to the hippocampus are found in individuals with bipolar disorder (Precin, 2023). Because of the limbic system's control of emotions, it can be expected that many episodes of MDD and bipolar disorder are associated with a major stressful event, for example, the death of a loved one, children moving out, or experiencing a near-fatal car collision. Juruena (2014) discussed the term "kindling," which proposes that with each episode, the individual becomes more vulnerable to a future episode.

Circadian rhythm and sleep disturbances are among the major diagnostic criteria for mood disorders and are present in both MDD and bipolar disorder. The "Social Zeitgeber Theory" suggests major stressful events can lead to altered biological rhythms and an increased vulnerability for the development of mood disorders (Ketchesin et al., 2018). In addition to stressful events, circadian rhythm disturbances such as jet lag, shift work, and time changes can lead to mood disorders in some individuals. The previously mentioned HPA axis is also considered to be under circadian rhythm control, and it is thought that disruption to this system can result in the inability to maintain a homeostatic state and can exacerbate a mood disorder (Ketchesin et al., 2018). For more information on sleep, please refer to Chapter 52: Sleep.

Environmental Factors

Adverse childhood experiences (ACEs) are potentially traumatic events that are experienced by children before age 18 (Felitti et al., 1998; King et al., 2022). These can include neglect, physical/emotional/sexual abuse, a family member with mental health issues, or substance use within the household. Children with multiple ACEs are at a greater risk of developing depression related to the constant activation of stress hormones (Felitti et al., 1998). However, there is evidence to support that resilience factors can help children develop coping skills and avoid psychosocial disorders (King et al., 2022). Please refer to Chapter 10: Coping and Resilience and Chapter 25: Trauma- and Stressor-Related Disorders.

Racism and racial trauma are common experiences. Many experience marginalization that can result in stress. For example, Seaton and Iida (2019) found that Black students experienced more depressive symptoms on days when they experienced racial discrimination. This can lead to negative attitudes and biases about the self and the world around them. LGBTQ youth also report similar traumas related to their experiences in school settings.

Kosciw and colleagues (2020) report that LGBTQ youth who experience hostile school environments (homophobic slurs, pronouns disrespected, discouragement from using restrooms and locker rooms aligning with their identity) are more likely to report a lower sense of school belonging, to have lower grade point averages, and to miss school. Many students also report lower levels of self-esteem and consider dropping out of school because of mental health needs such as depression (Kosciw et al., 2020).

Cognitive Styles

Research indicates that cognitive beliefs are influential in developing depression and other psychiatric disorders (Liu et al., 2015: Pössel & Smith, 2020). Stressors caused by trauma and other adverse experiences can lead to negative views and biases of self and the world. This can be especially common in adolescents going through a period of change and development who, therefore, can be more susceptible to depressive symptoms based on past experiences (Pössel & Smith, 2020). Beck's cognitive model of depression and the hopelessness model both contribute to the thought that cognitive vulnerabilities can contribute to stressors caused by daily hassles and life events, which can trigger depressive episodes (Pössel & Smith, 2020).

By continually thinking negative thoughts, individuals tend to develop depressive thinking. The individual eventually assigns negative meaning to relatively benign events; however, to the person with depression, they appear overwhelming and potentially catastrophic. The hopelessness model, similar to Beck's model, focuses on adverse events experienced in life. These events eventually lead to a feeling of hopelessness which in turn causes the individual to develop "hopelessness depression" and quite possibly suicidal ideation (Liu et al., 2015). That said, it is important to point out that not all individuals who experience adverse events develop depression. Refer to Chapter 8: Cognitive Beliefs for a more detailed explanation of this topic.

Prevalence

OTPs, regardless of practice setting, may work with people experiencing some form of depression. There is a growing concern about the prevalence of depressive disorders. In the United States, major depression is considered to be the most common form of mental illness (Mental Health America [MHA], 2023a). Approximately 21% of all American adults are diagnosed and living with a mental illness (MHA, 2023a, 2023b). Within that group, the occurrence of major depression is suggested to account for approximately 8.4% of all U.S. adults and 15.1% of all U.S. youth (ages 12–17; MHA, 2023b).

People with chronic diseases, such as hypertension and diabetes, are noted to have a higher incidence of depression. There is also a strong correlation between depression and cardiovascular issues (Ma et al., 2021). Based on empirical studies, "the estimated prevalence of depression in patients with chronic diseases ranges from 9.3 to 25%" (Ma et al., 2021, p. 2). See Chapter 17: Chronic Health Conditions and Mental Health. People with multimorbid conditions are two times more likely to experience depression than those without multimorbidity (Fortin et al., 2012; Ingle et al., 2017; King et al., 2018). Because of the high prevalence rates of depressive disorders, all practitioners should view themselves as mental health OTPs.

MDD and bipolar disorder are both widespread and make up a considerable percentage of individuals who experience an episode of mental illness, with an estimated 7.8% of adults age 18 and older experiencing a major depressive episode in 2019 (SAMHSA, 2020). For adolescents ages 12 to 17, it is estimated that 15.7% experienced a major depressive episode (SAMHSA, 2020). During the COVID-19 pandemic, an increase in symptoms of depression grew to almost one in six children between 5 and 17 years old, approximately 16.7%, which was up from 14.4% in the prepandemic years (Zablotsky et al., 2022). With the growing number of children and adolescents experiencing depressive symptoms during and postpandemic, there is concern that if left untreated these individuals will continue to experience depression into adulthood (Wang et al., 2022).

It is estimated that 2.8% of U.S. adults experienced bipolar disorder in the past year. Moreover, it is also estimated that 4.4% of U.S. adults experience bipolar disorder at some point in their lives (NIMH, 2023a). Research indicates that Black individuals are more likely to experience depression than white individuals, especially severe depression. Racial tensions are believed to be a risk factor for mental health issues. Discrimination and prejudice are significant risk factors for the onset of depression and can present structural barriers that preclude many Black individuals from obtaining mental health care (Robinson et al., 2022). Additionally, individuals from backgrounds of lower socioeconomic status experience both MDD and bipolar disorder at higher rates than the general population (Shalev et al., 2020; Young et al., 2020).

Course

The course of a mood disorder varies depending on the type of mood. Therefore, each condition is discussed separately in the text that follows.

Course of Major Depressive Disorder

The average age for the onset of an MDD is in the mid to late 20s (Precin, 2023). As someone with a chronic and recurrent illness, an individual diagnosed with MDD may experience a depressive episode that can last anywhere from 6 to 12 months (Bains & Abdijadid, 2023). J. Liu and colleagues (2021) address the research supporting the pathophysiology of MDD by suggesting associations between brain structure alterations and the course of the illness to be a progressive mental disorder evidenced by people in remission who may experience a new depressive episode within a 15-year span of time.

The *DSM-5-TR* reports that comorbid disorders may occur and potentially include substance use, anxiety, and personality disorders (American Psychiatric Association, 2022). Although typically portrayed as a disorder experienced by adults, depression is well documented in both adolescence (Shorey et al., 2022) and childhood (Meister et al., 2020). Children who experience depression carry a much higher risk of continuing the disorder into adolescence and eventually adulthood (American Psychiatric Association, 2022). MDD is also common among older adults, and suicide within this population is a major global public health concern (Obuobi-Donkor et al., 2021).

Course of Bipolar Disorder

Bipolar disorder tends to present and be diagnosed at a younger age than MDD. At least two-thirds of patients diagnosed with this disorder are diagnosed before age 18 (Marangoni, 2018). However, naturalistic and family studies have reported that 50% to 66% of individuals with bipolar disorder developed the condition during their teenage years and that 10% to 20% of this population claim they had experienced symptoms before the age of 10 (Nazeer et al., 2022). An earlier age of onset is associated with a higher prevalence of substance use disorders, higher suicide risk, and more recurrences and relapses.

In addition, pediatric bipolar disorder continues to present consistently into adulthood, with 44% of children displaying manic symptoms into adulthood (Nazeer et al., 2022). Younger onset is associated with a positive family history of mood disorders, comorbidity with anxiety and substance use disorders, rapid cycling course, treatment resistance, more hospitalizations, and suicidal behavior (Marangoni, 2018). Although the symptoms of bipolar disorder may be managed with treatment, the disorder does not truly resolve (NIMH, 2023a). Manic episodes associated with bipolar I typically have at least a 7-day course, with the mean duration estimated at approximately 6 weeks (NIMH, 2023a; Saunders & Goodwin, 2010). The course for depressive episodes may occur for a minimum duration of approximately 2 weeks, with the mean duration being 11 weeks (NIMH, 2023a; Saunders & Goodwin, 2010).

Gender- and Culture-Specific Information

Mood disorders do not discriminate, meaning that this diagnosis can be found in individuals of all ethnicities, genders, and socioeconomic status. That said, there are some populations that tend to experience higher rates of mood disorders. For the Black population, the overall experience of racial trauma can contribute to increased levels of depression (Seaton & Iida, 2019). In addition, many Black individuals live in urban areas associated with higher crime levels, unemployment, pollution, and other poverty-related stressors (Oh et al., 2021), all of which can contribute to the development of mood disorders.

Similar to individuals in the Black community, LGBTQ individuals may also experience higher levels of social stigma, which may cause lower resilience to life stressors (Gmelin et al., 2022). LGBTQ individuals are often victims of bullying and peer rejection, which can lead to decreased mood levels and also suicidal ideation (Pinna et al., 2022).

Suicide Risk

The lows of bipolar disorder and MDD can put some individuals at risk for suicide. Individuals at risk for suicide may express feelings of hopelessness and make statements about no longer wanting to live. It is imperative that OTPs be aware of the signs and symptoms of suicidal ideation so they can quickly make the appropriate recommendation. For more information see Chapter 44: Addressing Suicide Across the Continuum. 🤝 Multiple approaches are required for effective prevention of suicide (Suicide Prevention Resource Center, 2020).

LGBTQ individuals (youth in particular) are especially susceptible to suicidal ideation. In the Trevor Project's inaugural National Survey on LGBTQ Youth Mental Health (2019), 71% of the respondents reported feeling sad or hopeless for at least 2 weeks in the past year. Also of note, 39% of LGBTQ individuals had seriously considered attempting suicide in the past 2 months, whereas more than half of transgender and nonbinary youth had seriously considered suicide. Please refer to the Evidence-Based Practice feature, which briefly discusses suicide and outlines signs of ideation.

OTPs must be aware of the incidence, fatality, and methods of suicide. In 2021, within the United States, over half of all suicides involved a firearm (Gramlich, 2023). When considering the impact by age category, suicide accounted for 32% of gun deaths in children/youth under the age of 18; in contrast, in those older than 18 years of age, suicide accounted for 55% of all gun deaths. There are racial differences in firearm use and suicide in the United States. Considering statistics related to death in children/youth by firearms, 9% of all deaths involving Black children were suicide, whereas 66% of gun deaths involving white children were suicide (Gramlich, 2023). Firearms, the leading means of suicide in the United States, are a public health concern but not the only method of suicide utilized by individuals with mood disorders.

Strangulation/hanging or attempted hanging is another common method of suicide. Ligature risks include anything that is load-bearing and can be used to attach material for hanging or strangulation (e.g., light fixture, bed rail, soap dispenser). Ligature risks can be present in emergency departments where a patient is being evaluated before being admitted to a behavioral health center (Haney, 2018), but can also be present in a behavioral health setting (Patient Safety Authority [PSA], 2018). Many ligature risks can be found throughout health-care settings (see Fig. 20-2), and facilities should utilize a proactive risk assessment process to identify the highest risks to reduce patient harm (PSA, 2018).

Ligature Risks in a
Behavioral Health Room

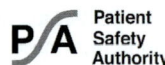

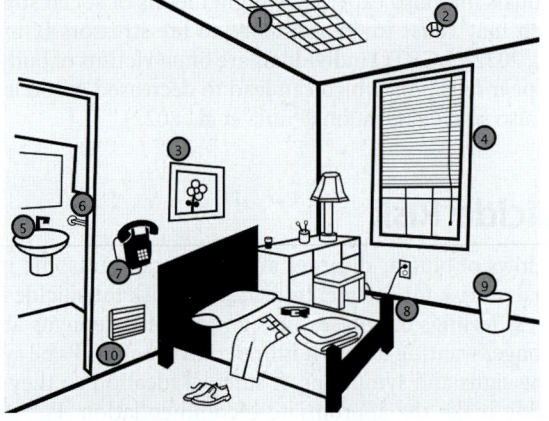

1	Large grill opening for overhead light
2	Fire sprinkler
3	Picture frame
4	Cord for blinds (non-recessed window framing / blind hardware)
5	Exposed plumbing / sink fixture itself
6	Towel bar / grab bar / also a risk if hook
7	Phone (especially if corded)
8	Bed post (only 18" needed for ligature point)
9	Trash can (could also be used as stepping point)
10	Heating grill

©2018 Pennsylvania Patient Safety Authority

FIGURE 20-2. Ligature risks in a behavioral health room. *Image used with permission from the Patient Safety Authority (2018). Risky rooms. https://patientsafety.pa.gov/pst/Pages/Behavioral_Health/risky_rooms.aspx*

Impact on Occupational Performance

The impact mood disorders have on one's occupational performance can vary in severity, but nevertheless they cause a disruption in life satisfaction and one's quality of life. Dissatisfaction with performance or levels of engagement can be devastating to the individual, especially when coinciding with the efforts to manage the symptomology of the mood disorder. Individuals can seek help from various health-care providers in their course of treatment. However, OTPs are uniquely slated to come alongside the individual at any stage in life and at any point in the recovery process. An OTP working with an individual diagnosed with a mood disorder has the ability to understand the individual's roles, habits, and routines and the potential performance problems that may be associated with the individual's diagnosis.

Utilizing the Person-Environment-Occupation (PEO) model (referenced in Chapter 3: Person-Environment-Occupation Model 🤝), the OTP can facilitate evaluations and treatment interventions, regardless of the treatment setting, that focus on the person, the areas of occupation with the most significant impairments, and environmental features that may interfere with or promote engagement and performance.

Specific roles, such as student performance, workplace/job, and parenting, are discussed in the text that follows.

Student Performance

In children and youth, the chemical imbalance and symptoms of depression can have a profound impact on performance in school, as demonstrated by an altered level of energy and impaired concentration, mental ability, outlook, and social interactions. Depressive symptoms may interrupt the acquisition of knowledge that goes beyond academic achievement by impairing performance in life skills. Altered energy levels can have a direct impact on sleep/awake cycles, growth, and age-appropriate physical and psychological development. Additionally, sleep disturbances and altering energy levels can result in emotional outbursts, lability, and even social isolation from family and friends. Low academic achievement can impact future advancement of knowledge, admission and satisfaction with the college experience, learning a vocational skill or trade, ability for future employment, and financial sustainability.

Workplace

Mood disorders may impact occupational performance in work-related tasks. For individuals with depression, apathetic behaviors or prolonged sadness can impact work performance, whereas a worker with a diagnosis of bipolar disorder may display behaviors of mania or agitation (Staglin, 2021).

Whether working on job-related tasks individually or in teams/groups, a disturbance in one's ability to process information, stay focused, and complete tasks directly impacts the dynamics of the work environment. The potential for a decrease in work-related productivity or an inability to interact in social situations changes the work dynamics and may create a tense or hostile work environment between the individual diagnosed with the mood disorder and the employer, direct supervisor, coworkers, and/or other persons or stakeholders. Overall, the individual's occupational performance in the workplace may have effects greater than job performance; it could result in the loss of wages or gainful employment, thereby impacting the livelihood of the individual and others they may support.

Parenting

Another example of depression impacting one's occupational performance can be understood through the role of parenting. The diagnosis of postpartum depression adds an additional barrier to occupational performance. The changes in mood, functional performance, mental stamina, and lability can create challenges for the mother, baby, and other family members. The mother may have a decreased ability to complete self-care tasks, navigate and manage the new responsibilities that come with a newborn/baby, and continue to contribute to the family unit in a way comparable with prediagnosis.

Postpartum depression may create additional barriers, hindering the mother from participating or resuming previous roles, which can generate roles or tasks to other members of the family unit. Taking on these additional tasks may result in additional disruptions when the individual is unfamiliar or inexperienced in carrying out these new roles.

Evidence-Based Practice

Evidence-Based Interventions for People at Risk of Suicide

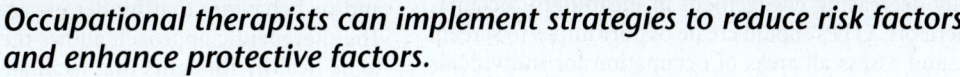

Occupational therapists can implement strategies to reduce risk factors and enhance protective factors.

RESEARCH FINDINGS

Every year, more than 700,000 people commit suicide worldwide. It is suggested that for every suicide, approximately 20 other people may be making an attempt at suicide, with a much larger number potentially experiencing suicidal ideation (WHO, 2022). Although the link between suicide, depression, and alcohol use disorder has been established in high-income countries such as the United States, tragically, a lot of suicides happen out of impulse and an inability to deal with crises related to financial problems (e.g., heavy debts, financial hardship), relationship breakups, or long-term pain or illness.

Suicide is particularly devastating because of the emotional suffering experienced by surviving family members and friends and the disabling effects on people who attempt suicide. Suicide rates vary by age, gender, and ethnic groups, but in general over 70% of global suicides occur in low- and middle-income countries. Additionally, suicide occurs most frequently in males and peaks in adolescence and old age. Suicide was the fourth-leading cause of death among 15- to 29-year-olds globally in 2019 (WHO, 2023).

Several biopsychosocial, environmental, and sociocultural risk factors are associated with suicide, including mental disorders, particularly depression and other mood disorders; job or other financial loss; and social isolation.

Suicide rates are also high among vulnerable groups who experience discrimination, such as refugees and migrants; indigenous peoples; lesbian, gay, bisexual, transgender, intersex (LGBTI) persons; and prisoners. By far, the strongest risk factor for suicide is a previous suicide attempt (WHO, 2023).

In addition, several protective factors for suicide have been identified, including effective behavioral health and clinical care for mental, physical, and substance use disorders, as well as strong connections to individuals, family, community support, and social institutions.

Suicide is complicated and tragic, but it is often preventable. Effective, evidenced-based interventions are available to help people who are at risk for suicide (NIMH, 2022).

APPLICATIONS

➡ OTPs need to understand the biopsychosocial, environmental, and sociocultural risk factors associated with suicide.

➡ OTPs should be familiar with protective factors for suicide and assess their presence in the people they work with.

➡ OTPs can implement strategies to reduce risk factors and enhance protective factors.

REFERENCES

National Institute of Mental Health. (2022). *Suicide prevention.* U.S. Department of Health and Human Services, National Institutes of Health. https://www.nimh.nih.gov/health/topics/suicide-prevention

U.S. Department of Health & Human Services. (2021). *Suicide prevention.* Office on Women's Health in the Office of the Assistant Secretary for Health. https://www.womenshealth.gov/mental-health/get-help-now/suicide-prevention

World Health Organization. (2022). *Creating hope through action.* https://www.who.int/campaigns/world-suicide-prevention-day/2022

World Health Organization. (2023, August 28). *Suicide.* https://www.who.int/news-room/fact-sheets/detail/suicide

Socialization

OTPs should evaluate and monitor the risk for social isolation associated with mood disorder. If social isolation begins to occur, the individual is at risk for worsening symptoms of depression, creating a cycle of withdrawal from others and potentially decreasing engagement in meaningful occupations. Therefore, OTPs should create opportunities to screen, evaluate, and assess all areas of occupation for individuals diagnosed with a mood disorder to ensure a person-centered approach is taken in the treatment planning process.

Intervention

A blend of psychosocial interventions and pharmacological approaches is important in the treatment of individuals with mood disorders. OTPs can provide a variety of psychosocial interventions (see Table 20-2) to assist the individual as they navigate through the recovery continuum and seek to achieve their maximum health status.

Effective treatments may include a variety of psychosocial interventions and approaches, such as cognitive behavior therapy (CBT). CBT is a psychosocial intervention that shifts focus onto acknowledging and changing distorted beliefs and/or behaviors that hinder engagement or performance. The therapeutic approach allows the focus of interventions to be healthy thoughts that facilitate healthy behaviors and feelings supporting one's overall occupational performance.

Another treatment approach could be utilizing Dunn's Model of Sensory Processing, allowing the individual to identify specific sensory needs in order to create an environment or materials that will assist in meeting the individual's sensory processing needs. Upon creation of the materials or even alteration of one's environment to match sensory processing needs, the individual is able to utilize the sensory-focused interventions to enhance occupational engagement and performance.

TABLE 20-2 | **Occupational Therapy Interventions Commonly Used With Individuals Diagnosed With Mood Disorders**

Approach	Target(s) of Intervention	Brief Synopsis	Chapters With Additional Information
Cognitive Behavioral Approach	Distorted beliefs in the context of occupational performance	Distorted beliefs are identified and challenged by providing evidence to the contrary.	Chapter 8: Cognitive Beliefs
Acceptance and Commitment Therapy	Psychological flexibility	Combines acceptance of difficult feelings, thoughts, and circumstances with commitment to constructive activities that address personal goals and values	Chapter 8: Cognitive Beliefs
Dunn's Model of Sensory Processing	Sensory processing needs in the context of occupational performance	Creating environments or materials that meet the individual's sensory processing needs	Chapter 9: Sensory Processing and the Lived Sensory Experience
Interpersonal and Social Rhythm Therapy	Routines	Identifying patterns of activity and restructuring time to create routines	Chapter 14: Time Use and Habits
Family Psychoeducation/ Caring for Yourself	Improving family relationships, support for families and friends	Providing education and support to family members of an individual with a psychiatric condition	Chapter 29: Families
Peer Support Programs	Social connectedness and support	Advocacy, socialization, and education services are provided by persons with lived experience of mental illness.	Chapter 39: Peer-Led Services
Suicide Prevention	Reducing risk of suicide	Reducing risk factors and promoting social connection and engagement in meaningful activity	Chapter 44: Addressing Suicide Across the Continuum
Exercise and Physical Activity	Stress reduction and mood enhancement	Developing physical activity programs or creating ways for engagement in existing programs	Chapter 45: Self-Care and Well-Being Occupations
Supported Education	Goals related to higher education	Individualized support and inclusion to help people succeed in postsecondary education	Chapter 47: Student
Supported Employment	Work	Job placement in sought-after employment positions with follow-along supports	Chapter 48: Work and Volunteer Occupations
Arts and Health Programs	Well-being and health	Creative media utilized to promote self-expression and overall wellness and socialization	Chapter 51: Leisure and Creative Occupations
Sleep Hygiene Education	Restful sleep	Develop and monitor routines and create an environment that promotes sleep	Chapter 52: Sleep

Medications for Depressive Disorders

Many symptoms associated with mood disorders can require pharmacological interventions. Individuals may seek assistance from the OTP to work on medication management, thus increasing one's adherence to the prescribed regimen. When working with individuals on medication management, it is important for the OTP to have working knowledge of drug classifications and commonly prescribed pharmacological interventions. Medication needs will differ based on the mood disorder, severity, and individual medical history.

For individuals diagnosed with depressive disorders, the most common form of pharmacological treatments are selective serotonin reuptake inhibitors (SSRIs), serotonin-norepinephrine reuptake inhibitors (SNRIs), and other antidepressants; see Table 20-3. SSRIs are typically prescribed as a first course of action as they are considered safer with fewer side effects. SNRIs are often utilized when other medication regimens have not produced the desired effect, such as mood regulation or relief from depressive symptoms (Elsevier Mental and Behavioral Health, 2019; Mayo Clinic, 2019). The selection of a pharmacological approach is unique to the individual based upon a myriad of factors, such as diagnosis, medical history and response to other medications, drug interactions, and tolerance (Elsevier Mental and Behavioral Health, 2019).

When SSRIs are prescribed, a common course of action is for the person to be given a small dosage to monitor the medication response (Chu & Wadhwa, 2023). It takes approximately 6 weeks for the medication to take effect. The increase of serotonin has an impact on one's emotions and sleep. Although SSRIs are utilized for the safety and efficacy of treating depression and other psychiatric disorders, they are not without risk or possible side effects. OTPs should be aware of the increased risk for suicidality, especially in the pediatric population who are prescribed SSRIs (Chu & Wadhwa, 2023). Additionally, practitioners should watch for disturbances in sleep, weight changes, anxiety, dizziness, headaches, sexual dysfunction, and gastrointestinal changes as these are common side effects for people taking SSRIs (Chu & Wadhwa, 2023; David & Gourion, 2016; Hu et al., 2004).

As an antidepressant, SNRIs work to regulate one's mood and relieve depression through alleviating feelings of irritability and sadness. The common course of SNRIs takes approximately 8 weeks to observe the medication's full effect (Cleveland Clinic, 2023). Similarly to SSRIs, SNRIs are not without side effects. OTPs should be aware of the increased risk or complications of suicidal thoughts/behaviors, serotonin syndrome, and, when medication regimens are stopped or altered, antidepressant discontinuation syndrome.

Commonly observed side effects may vary by SNRI, but OTPs can monitor for typically occurring ones including nausea/diarrhea, fatigue, drowsiness, dizziness, xerostomia, sexual dysfunction, and diaphoresis (Cleveland Clinic, 2023). Regarding SNRI side effects, OTPs should be concerned and consult with members of the health-care team when the side effects are not mild in severity, do not lessen over time, or significantly impact or impair functional performance. An insufficient response or intolerable side effects to any medication can warrant a change in medication dosage or switching to a new medication.

Medications for Bipolar Disorder

Individuals diagnosed with a bipolar disorder are most commonly treated with mood stabilizers, anticonvulsants, and antipsychotics, as outlined in Table 20-4. An individual's medication regimen should target the type of disorder and symptoms. Medications utilized as a mood stabilizer are often prescribed to assist in controlling either manic or hypomanic episodes. When an individual has symptomology of depression, or if mania exists despite other prescribed medications, an antipsychotic may be added to the medication regimen. Although antidepressants can trigger a manic episode, individuals may be prescribed an antidepressant to help manage depressive symptoms. The antidepressant is likely to be prescribed alongside a mood stabilizer or antipsychotic.

Medications, such as the combination of fluoxetine and olanzapine (Symbyax), work as an antidepressant-antipsychotic (Mayo Clinic, 2022a; Sohel et al., 2022).

TABLE 20-3	Pharmacological Interventions Utilized With Individuals Diagnosed With Depressive Disorders
Drug Class	**Examples**
Selective serotonin reuptake inhibitors (SSRIs)	Citalopram (Celexa) Escitalopram (Lexapro) Fluoxetine (Prozac) Paroxetine (Paxil, Paxil CR, Pexeva) Sertraline (Zoloft) Vilazodone (Viibryd)
Serotonin and norepinephrine reuptake inhibitors (SNRIs)	Duloxetine (Cymbalta) Venlafaxine, extended-release (Effexor XR) Desvenlafaxine (Pristiq, Khedezla) Levomilnacipran (Fetzima)
Other antidepressants (atypical)	Bupropion (Wellbutrin XL, Wellbutrin SR, Aplenzin, Forfivo XL) Mirtazapine (Remeron) Nefazodone Trazodone Vortioxetine (Trintellix)

TABLE 20-4	Pharmacological Interventions Utilized With Individuals Diagnosed With Bipolar Disorders
Drug Class	**Examples**
Mood stabilizers	Lithium carbonate (Eskalith, Lithobid, Lithonate, Lithotabs)
Anticonvulsants	Carbamazepine (Tegretol, Equetro) Divalproex sodium (Depakote, Depakote ER) Gabapentin (Neurontin)
Antipsychotics	Risperidone ER (Risperdal extended-release) Paliperidone ER (extended-release) Quetiapine (Seroquel) Olanzapine (Zyprexa) Aripiprazole (Abilify) Ziprasidone (Geodon) Asenapine (Saphris) Lurasidone (Latuda)

An antidepressant-antipsychotic, such as Symbyax, is used to improve one's mood, help with sleep, improve concentration, and possibly decrease anxiety or nervousness.

In the first few months of treatment with antidepressant medications or if a significant dosage change occurs, OTPs should be aware and observe for signs of a worsening condition, suicidal ideation, or sudden or unusual changes in behavior. Unwanted side effects may appear when taking antidepressants and antipsychotics. With a combination medication such as Symbyax, the antipsychotic portion of the medication may produce a metabolic change such as weight gain or hyperglycemia, placing the person at increased risk for cardiovascular/cerebrovascular issues (National Institutes of Health [NIH], 2021). Practitioners monitoring for potential side effects or efficacy of the prescribed medication can be helpful when collaborating with care team members, such as the psychiatrist, to ensure the pharmacological treatment method and dosage are the best fits for the person.

Other Treatment

The traditional course of treatment for mood disorders includes a pharmacological approach and psychosocial interventions. However, other treatments, such as transcranial magnetic stimulation (TMS) and electroconvulsive therapy (ECT), have been utilized and considered by some as effective treatment methods.

ECT has been utilized for nearly a century in the treatment of mood disorders such as MDD or bipolar disorder when other treatment methods have not been successful (American Psychiatric Association, 2023). The individual is placed under anesthesia in order to receive brief electrical stimulation to the brain. Frequency is based upon the severity of the individual's condition, with typical treatment plans lasting up to three times a week for a total of 6 to 12 treatments. Each treatment involves general anesthesia and a muscle relaxant with electrodes placed on the scalp in specific locations in order to stimulate the brain through controlled electrical pulses. This method causes a seizure that lasts approximately a minute in duration.

TMS is a noninvasive treatment method that may be considered when an individual with a mood disorder has not responded to previous therapies. The treatment includes rapidly alternating magnetic fields that stimulate specific areas of the brain that control mood. Although TMS may not be considered as effective as ECT, it is generally more acceptable because it does not cause a seizure, and the individual remains awake for the duration of the treatment. The typical protocol for TMS includes administration four or five times weekly for up to 4 to 6 weeks (American Psychiatric Association, 2023; National Alliance on Mental Illness [NAMI], 2023).

Another treatment option for individuals with depression is vagus nerve stimulation (VNS). The process involves implanting an electrical pulse generator under the skin of the chest in order to provide intermittent electrical stimulation to the vagus nerve in the neck. The response time to VNS may take months to develop. Because of the time it takes for an individual to respond to VNS, treatment may not be suggested for individuals with acute depression (NAMI, 2023). Additional research studies are needed to assess the overall effectiveness of VNS for treatment-resistant depression.

General Considerations When Providing Occupational Therapy to People With Mood Disorders

Individuals diagnosed with a mood disorder may experience challenges across the recovery continuum such as barriers to medication adherence/management, fluctuation in occupational performance, and variability in life satisfaction.

- OTPs must keep in mind their unique capacity to assist an individual with a mood disorder regardless of age and practice setting.
- Mood disorders are chronic illnesses that impact all areas of occupation, therefore providing a myriad of options regarding selection of appropriate assessments for the focus of occupational therapy interventions to facilitate functional performance and outcomes.
- Considering the progressive or chronic nature of mood disorders as well as the possible side effects from pharmacological treatment approaches, psychosocial interventions may include addressing sleep hygiene, focusing on routines through the use of interpersonal and social rhythm therapy, and suicide prevention.
- OTPs can provide direct services but also have an important role in the consultative process with the healthcare team to ensure a holistic, person-centered approach is taken. The consultative role of the OTP is utilized when observing and collaborating with the psychiatrist regarding the overall effectiveness and potential barriers to the prescribed medication(s).
- Remaining person-centered allows the OTP to consistently consider the environmental context and factors of the individual and assists the person in meeting their highest potential with a focus on function through occupational engagement (Crouch & Alers, 2014; Swarbrick & Noyes, 2018).

Here's the Point

- An individual diagnosed with a mood disorder may have ongoing symptoms of depression or mania, exhibited by feelings of sadness, disengagement or disinterest in once-valued occupations, or extreme fluctuation from sadness to happiness.
- Symptoms may merely meet the diagnostic criteria. Functional performance impacts go beyond basic symptomatology, thus impacting occupational engagement and overall performance.
- Awareness of mood disorders has grown; thus, the prevalence has exponentially grown.

- The risk for suicide/suicidal ideation is higher for individuals affected by some mood disorders in comparison with the general population.
- Mood disorders often impact occupational performance including school, work, parenting, and socialization.
- Treatments must be individualized to ensure a culturally sensitive and holistic approach is taken. Psychosocial and pharmacological interventions may prove beneficial.

- OTPs are skilled in creating psychosocial interventions over all areas of practice for individuals across the life span diagnosed with mood disorders.

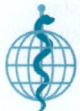 Visit the online resource center at **FADavis.com** to access the videos.

Apply It Now

1. Theory in Practice

Think about an activity that is very important to you. What do you currently do to ensure that you have the optimal fit between person, environment, and occupation (PEO)? Now consider that preferred activity and think about a person who has symptoms of severe depression or a time when you were experiencing sadness. What might impact their overall PEO fit? Do the same for a person diagnosed with bipolar disorder and experiencing a manic episode.

2. Environmental Analysis

Consider the environment in which you work regarding individuals diagnosed with mood disorders and complete a ligature risk assessment to identify the highest risks to reduce patient harm.

3. Examine Political Influence

In a small group identify two to four examples of discrimination in your community as it relates to gender, sexuality, race, or religion. Consider how discrimination might contribute to mood disorders within the stigmatized group.

Resources

- American Academy of Child and Adolescent Psychiatry (AACAP): https://www.aacap.org
- American Psychiatric Association: https://www.psychiatry.org
- Barbic, S., MacKirdy, K., Weiss, R., Barrie, A., Kitchin, V., & Lepin, S. (2021). Scoping review of the role of occupational therapy in the treatment of women with postpartum depression. *Annals of International Occupational Therapy, 4*(4), e249–259. https://doi.org/10.3928/24761222-20210921-02
- Centre for Clinical Interventions: https://www.cci.health .wa.gov.au
- Child Mind Institute: https://childmind.org
- Depression and Bipolar Support Alliance (DBSA): https://www .dbsalliance.org
- Families for Depression Awareness: https://www.family aware.org
- HeretoHelp: https://www.heretohelp.bc.ca
- International Bipolar Foundation: https://ibpf.org
- International Society for Bipolar Disorders (ISBD): https:// www.isbd.org
- Mood Disorders Association of British Columbia (MDABC): https://mdabc.net
- National Alliance on Mental Illness (NAMI): www.nami.org
- National Institute on Mental Health (NIMH): www.nimh .nih.gov
- PanFoundation: https://www.panfoundation.org
- Postpartum Support International: https://www.postpartum.net
- PsychU: https://psychu.org
- Substance Abuse and Mental Health Services Administration (SAMHSA): www.samhsa.gov
- The Mood Disorders Support Group (MDSG): https://mdsg.org
- U.S. Department of Health and Human Services (Mental Health): https://www.mentalhealth.gov

Videos

- "Two Practitioners Discuss Their Work in Suicide Prevention" video. In this video, two occupational therapists, Nadine and Kim, discuss their work in suicide prevention. They share reflections and pearls of wisdom gained in years of practice in this area—both observations about people in crisis and how they have responded as OTPs. They express the role that the occupational lives of these individuals have in their recovery and crisis plans, as well as serving as a springboard for interventions. Nadine and Kim also describe what is rewarding about this work and the crucial need to meet their self-care and well-being needs in order to stay connected to this work. Access the video at the online resource center at FADavis.com.
- "Jordon's Lived Experience of Anxiety and Depression" video. In this video, occupational therapist Jordan describes her lived experience of anxiety and depression. She touches on many issues critical to recovery and occupational therapy practice, including social determinants of health, peer support, and how mental health labels can adversely affect an individual's medical treatment. Importantly, she explains how she has learned to blend her lived experience with her work as an occupational therapist while ensuring she takes care of herself and manages her symptoms. Jordan also offers priceless words of wisdom to OTPs regarding establishing a therapeutic connection with individuals with whom they practice. Access the video at the online resource center at FADavis.com.
- "Jenny's Lived Experience of Sensory Processing Differences" video. Jenny is an occupational therapy doctorate (OTD) student with the lived experience of sensory differences, anxiety, and depression. In this video, she describes how she discovered her diagnosis, how it affects her in the classroom, and what interventions she uses to manage her reactions to stimuli. Importantly, she discusses the need to advocate for herself and for OTPs to help people across the life span to understand their

sensory processing needs in order to improve their mental health and overall quality of life. Access the video at the online resource center at FADavis.com.

- "Civic Engagement Group in an Inpatient Psychiatric Unit" video. In this video, occupational therapist Jennifer speaks about her experience working as an occupational therapy assistant in an inpatient psychiatric unit for individuals with persistent mental illness. She describes a positive experience running civic engagement groups, which proved to do much more than give back to the community. In one project related to voting rights for individuals with felony histories, the group provided opportunities for the residents to practice life skills, feel empowered, and transcend the internalized stigma they faced as people living with mental illness. Access the video at the online resource center at FADavis.com.
- "Mental Health and Well-Being During COVID" video. Caitlin is an OTP who has worked in outpatient settings with both adults and children. In this video, she talks about how occupational therapy practice during the COVID-19 global pandemic allowed her to see in a new way the effects of stress and anxiety on patient outcomes. She discusses how she incorporates mental health and well-being into her practice and her belief that it promotes successful healing and recovery. Access the video at the online resource center at FADavis.com.

References

American Psychiatric Association. (2022). *Diagnostic and statistical manual of mental disorders* (5th ed., text rev.). American Psychiatric Publishing. https://doi.org/10.1176/appi.books.9780890425787

American Psychiatric Association. (2023). *What is electroconvulsive therapy (ECT)?* https://www.psychiatry.org/patients-families/ect

American Psychological Association. (2023). Unipolar disorder. In *APA dictionary of psychology.* https://dictionary.apa.org/unipolar-disorder

Bains, N., & Abdijadid, S. (2023). Major depressive disorder. In *StatPearls.* StatPearls Publishing. https://www.ncbi.nlm.nih.gov/books/NBK559078

Barbic, S., MacKirdy, K., Weiss, R., Barrie, A., Kitchin, V., & Lepin, S. (2021). Scoping review of the role of occupational therapy in the treatment of women with postpartum depression. *Annals of International Occupational Therapy, 4*(4), e249–e259. https://doi.org/10.3928/24761222-20210921-02

Bielecki, J., & Gupta, V. (2022). Cyclothymic disorder. In *StatPearls.* StatPearls Publishing. https://www.ncbi.nlm.nih.gov/books/NBK557877

Brown, E. S., & Chandler, P. A. (2001). Mood and cognitive changes during systemic corticosteroid therapy. *Primary Care Companion to the Journal of Clinical Psychiatry, 3*(1), 17–21. https://doi.org/10.4088/pcc.v03n0104

Chu, A., & Wadhwa, R. (2023). Selective serotonin reuptake inhibitors. In *StatPearls.* StatPearls Publishing. https://www.ncbi.nlm.nih.gov/books/NBK554406

Cleveland Clinic. (2023). *SNRIs (serotonin and norepinephrine reuptake inhibitors).* https://my.clevelandclinic.org/health/treatments/24797-snri

Crouch, R., & Alers, V. (Eds.). (2014). *Occupational therapy in psychiatry and mental health* (5th ed.). Wiley Blackwell.

Cuellar, A., Johnson, S., & Winters, R. (2005). Distinctions between bipolar and unipolar depression. *Clinical Psychology Review, 25*(3), 307–339. https://doi.org/10.1016/j.cpr.2004.12.002

David, D., & Gourion, D. (2016). Antidepressant and tolerance: Determinants and management of major side effects. *Encephale, 42*(6), 553–561. https://doi.org/10.1016/j.encep.2016.05.006

Dome, P., Rihmer, Z., & Gonda, X. (2019). Suicide risk in bipolar disorder: A brief review. *Medicina (Kaunas), 55*(8), 403. https://doi.org/10.3390/medicina55080403

DuBrul, S. A. (2014). The Icarus Project: A counter narrative for psychic diversity. *Journal of Medical Humanities, 35,* 257–271. https://doi.org/10.1007/s10912-014-9293-5

Elsevier Mental and Behavioral Health. (2019, November 14). *Serotonin norepinephrine reuptake inhibitors (SNRIs).* https://elsevier.health/en-US/preview/serotonin-norepinephrine-reuptake-inhibitors-snris

Felitti, V. J., Anda, R. F., Nordenberg, D., Williamson, D. F., Spitz, A. M., Edwards, V., Koss, M. P., & Marks, J. S. (1998). Relationship of childhood abuse and household dysfunction to many of the leading causes of death in adults: The adverse childhood experiences (ACE) study. *American Journal of Preventive Medicine, 14,* 245–258. https://doi.org/10.1016/S0749-3797(98)00017-8

Fireweed Collective. (n.d.-a). *Our framework.* https://fireweedcollective.org/our-framework

Fireweed Collective. (n.d.-b). *Our history.* https://fireweedcollective.org/our-history

Fortin, M., Stewart, M., Poitras, M., Almirall, J., & Maddocks, H. (2012). A systematic review of prevalence studies on multimorbidity: Toward a more uniform methodology. *The Annals of Family Medicine, 10*(2), 142–151. https://doi.org/10.1370/afm.1337

Gmelin, J. H., De Vries, Y. A., Baams, L., Aguilar-Gaxiola, S., Alonso, J., Borges, G., Bunting, B., Cardoso, G., Florescu, S., Gureje, O., Karam, E. G., Kawakami, N., Lee, S., Mneimneh, Z., Navarro-Mateu, F., Posada-Villa, J., Rapsey, C., Slade, T., Stagnaro, J. C., … de Jonge, P. (2022). Increased risks for mental disorders among LGB individuals: Cross-national evidence from the World Mental Health Surveys. *Social Psychiatry and Psychiatric Epidemiology, 57,* 2319–2332. https://doi.org/10.1007/s00127-022-02320-z

Gramlich, J. (2023, April 26). *What the data says about gun deaths in the U.S.* Pew Research Center. https://www.pewresearch.org/short-reads/2023/04/26/what-the-data-says-about-gun-deaths-in-the-u-s

Haney, K. (2018). Keeping psychiatric patients safe in our nation's emergency departments. *The Journal of Legal Nurse Consulting, 30*(2), 20–23.

Howland, J. (2023, February 2). *Mayo Clinic minute: Postpartum depression is more than baby blues.* Mayo Clinic. https://newsnetwork.mayoclinic.org/discussion/2-2-mayo-clinic-minute-postpartum-depression-is-more-than-baby-blues

Hu, X. H., Bull, S. A., Hunkeler, E. M., Ming, E., Lee, J. Y., Fireman, B., & Markson, L. E. (2004). Incidence and duration of side effects and those rated as bothersome with selective serotonin reuptake inhibitor treatment for depression: Patient report versus physician estimate. *The Journal of Clinical Psychiatry, 65*(7), 959–965. https://doi.org/10.4088/jcp.v65n0712

Ingle, V., Pandey, I., Singh, A., Pakhare, A., & Kumar, S. (2017). Screening of patients with chronic medical disorders in the outpatient department for depression using handheld computers as interface and Patient Health Questionnaire-9 as a tool. *International Journal of Applied Basic Medical Research, 7*(2), 129–33. https://doi.org/10.4103/2229-516X.205809

Juruena, M. (2014). Early-life stress and HPA axis trigger recurrent adulthood depression. *Epilepsy & Behavior, 38,* 148–159. https://doi.org/10.1016/j.yebeh.2013.10.020

Keefer, L., & Kane, S. V. (2017). Considering the bidirectional pathways between depression and IBD: Recommendations for comprehensive IBD care. *Gastroenterology & Hepatology, 13*(3), 164–169. https://www.ncbi.nlm.nih.gov/pmc/articles/PMC5439135

Ketchesin, K. D., Becker-Krail, D., & McClung, C. A. (2018). Mood-related central and peripheral clocks. *European Journal of Neuroscience, 51,* 326–345. http://doi.org/10.1111/ejn.14253

King, D., Xiang, J., & Pilkerton, C. (2018). Multimorbidity trends in United States adults, 1988-2014. *Journal of the American Board of Family Medicine, 31*(4), 503–513. https://doi.org/10.3122/jabfm.2018.04.180008

King, L. M., Zori, G., Collins, S. L., Lewis, C., Hack, G., Dixon, B. N., & Hart, M. (2022). What does community resilience mean in the context of trauma informed communities? A scoping review. *Journal of Community Psychology, 50,* 3325–3353. https://doi .org/10.1002/jcop.22839

Koene, J., Zyto, S., van der Stel, J., van Lang, N., Ammeraal, M., Kupka, R., & van Weeghel, J. (2022). The relations between executive functions and occupational functioning in individuals with bipolar disorder: A scoping review. *International Journal of Bipolar Disorder, 10,* 8. https://doi.org/10.1186 /s40345-022-00255-7

Kosciw, J. G., Clark, C. M., Truong, N. L., & Zongrone, A. D. (2020). *The 2019 National School Climate Survey: The experiences of lesbian, gay, bisexual, transgender, and queer youth in our nation's schools.* GLSEN. https://www.glsen.org/sites/default/files/2020-10/NSCS-2019-Full -Report_0.pdf

Kraiss, J., ten Klooster, P., Chrispijn, M., Stevens, A., Doornbos, B., Kupka, R., & Bohlmeijer, E. (2023). A multicomponent positive psychology intervention for euthymic patients with bipolar disorder to improve mental well-being and personal recovery: A pragmatic randomized controlled trial. *Bipolar Disorders, 25*(8), 683–695. https://doi.org/10.1111/bdi.13313

Liu, J., Fan, Y., Zeng, L.-L., Liu, B., Ju, Y., Wang, M., Dong, Q., Lu, X., Sun, J., Zhang, L., Guo, H., Zhao, F., Li, W., Zhang, L., Li, Z., Liao, M., Zhang, Y., Hu, D., & Li, L. (2021). The neuroprogressive nature of major depressive disorder: Evidence from an intrinsic connectome analysis. *Translational Psychiatry, 11,* 102. https://doi .org/10.1038/s41398-021-01227-8

Liu, R. T., Kleinman, E. M., Nestor, B. A., & Cheek, S. M. (2015). The hopelessness theory of depression: A quarter century in review. *Clinical Psychology, 22,* 345–365. https://doi.org/10.1111/cpsp.12125

Ma, Y., Xiang, Q., Yan, C., Liao, H., & Wang, J. (2021). Relationship between chronic diseases and depression: The mediating effect of pain. *BMC Psychiatry, 21*(1), 1–11. https://doi.org/10.1186/s12888 -021-03428-3

Marangoni, C. (2018). ADHD, bipolar disorder, or borderline personality disorder: Getting to the right diagnosis. *Psychiatric Times, 35,* 18–30.

Mayo Clinic. (2019). *Serotonin and norepinephrine reuptake inhibitors (SNRIs).* https://www.mayoclinic.org/diseases-conditions /depression/in-depth/antidepressants/art-20044970

Mayo Clinic. (2022a). *Bipolar disorder.* https://www.mayoclinic .org/diseases-conditions/bipolar-disorder/symptoms-causes /syc-20355955

Mayo Clinic. (2022b). *Cyclothymia (cyclothymic disorder).* https:// www.mayoclinic.org/diseases-conditions/cyclothymia/symptoms -causes/syc-20371275

Mayo Clinic. (2022c). *Postpartum depression.* https://www .mayoclinic.org/diseases-conditions/postpartum-depression /symptoms-causes/syc-20376617

Medline Plus. (2022, July 28). *Cyclothymic disorder.* A.D.A.M. Medical Encyclopedia [Internet]. https://medlineplus.gov/ency /article/001550.htm

Meister, R., Abbas, M., Antel, J., Peters, T., Pan, Y., Bingel, U., Nestoriuc, Y., & Hebebrand, J. (2020). Placebo response rated and potential modifiers in double-blind randomized controlled trials of second and newer generation antidepressants for major depressive disorder in children and adolescents: A systematic review and meta-regression analysis. *European Child & Adolescent Psychiatry, 29,* 253–273. http://doi.org/10.1007/s00787-018-1244-7

Mental Health America. (2023a). *Quick facts and statistics about mental health.* https://mhanational.org/mentalhealthfacts

Mental Health America. (2023b). *The state of mental health in America.* https://mhanational.org/issues/state-mental-health-america

National Alliance on Mental Illness. (2023). *ECT, TMS, and other brain stimulation therapies.* https://www.nami.org /About-Mental-Illness/Treatments/ECT-TMS-and-Other-Brain -Stimulation-Therapies

National Institute of Mental Health. (2022). *Suicide prevention.* U.S. Department of Health and Human Services, National

Institutes of Health. https://www.nimh.nih.gov/health/topics /suicide-prevention

National Institute of Mental Health. (2023a). *Bipolar disorder.* https://www.nimh.nih.gov/health/statistics/bipolar-disorder

National Institute of Mental Health. (2023b). *Seasonal affective disorder.* NIH Publication No. 20-MH-8138. https://www.nimh.nih .gov/health/publications/seasonal-affective-disorder

National Institutes of Health. (2021). *Symbyax.* National Library of Medicine. https://dailymed.nlm.nih.gov/dailymed/drugInfo .cfm?setid=6b28c424-0b7e-4b75-b090-f116b113554e

Nazeer, A., Hashemi, N., Imran, N., Naveed, S., Azeem, M. W., & Skokauskas, N. (2022). Pediatric bipolar disorder. *Journal of Alternative Medicine Research, 14,* 257–266.

Obuobi-Donkor, G., Nkire, N., & Agyapong, V. I. O. (2021). Prevalence of major depressive disorder and correlates of thoughts of death, suicidal behaviour, and death by suicide in the geriatric population—A general review of literature. *Behavioral Sciences, 11,* 142. http://doi.org/10.3390/bs11110142

Oh, H., Nicholson, H. L., Jr., Koyangi, A., Jacob, L., & Glass, J. (2021). Urban upbringing and psychiatric disorders in the United States: A racial comparison. *International Journal of Social Psychiatry, 67,* 307–314. https://doi.org/10.1177/0020764020950781

Patient Safety Authority. (2018). *Risky rooms.* http://patientsafety .pa.gov/pst/Pages/Behavioral_Health/risky_rooms.aspx

Pinna, F., Paribello, P., Somaini, G., Corona, A., Ventriglio, A., Corrias, C., Frau, I., Murgia, R., El Kacemi, E., Galeazzi, G. M., Mirandola, M., Amaddeo, F., Crapanzano, A., Converti, M., Piras, P., Suprani, F., Manchia, M., Fiorillo, A., Carpiniello, B., & The Italian Working Group on LGBTQI Mental Health. (2022). Mental health in transgender individuals: A systematic review. *International Review of Psychiatry, 34,* 292–359. https://doi.org/10.1080/09540261.2022.2093629

Pössel, P., & Smith, E. (2020). Integrating Beck's cognitive theory of depression and the hopelessness model in an adolescent sample. *Journal of Abnormal Child Psychology, 48,* 435–451. http://doi .org/10.1007/s10802-019-00604-8

Precin, P. (2023). Mood disorders. In B. J. Atchison & D. P. Dirette (Eds.), *Conditions in occupational therapy: Effect on occupational performance* (6th ed., pp. 167–180). Wolters Kluwer.

Redlich, R., Opel, N., Bürger, C., Dohm, K., Grotegerd, D., Förster, K., Zaremba, D., Meinert, S., Repple, J., Enneking, V., Leehr, E., Böhnlein, J., Winters, L., Froböse, N., Thrun, S., Emtmann, J., Heindel, W., Kugel, H., Volker, A., … Dannlowski, U. (2018). The limbic system in youth depression: Brain structural and functional alterations in adolescent in-patients with severe depression. *Neuropsychopharmacology, 43,* 546–554. https://doi.org/10.1038 /npp.2017.246

Robinson, M. A., Kim, I., Mowbray, O., & Disney, L. (2022). African Americans, Caribbean blacks and depression: Which biopsychosocial factors should social workers focus on? Results from the National Survey of American Life (NSAL). *Community Mental Health Journal, 58,* 366–375. http://doi.org/10.1007/s10597-021-00833-6

Rolin, D., Whelan, J., & Montano, C. (2020). Is it depression or is it bipolar depression? *Journal of the American Association of Nurse Practitioners, 32*(10), 703–713. https://doi.org/10.1097 /JXX.0000000000000499

Sala, R., Axelson, D. A., Castro-Fornieles, J., Goldstein, T. R., Ha, W., Liao, F., Gill, M. K., Iyengar, S., Strober, M. A., Goldstein, B. I., Yen, S., Hower, H., Hunt, J., Ryan, N. D., Dickstein, D., Keller, M. B., & Birmaher, B. (2010). Comorbid anxiety in children and adolescents with bipolar spectrum disorders: Prevalence and clinical correlates. *The Journal of Clinical Psychiatry, 71*(10), 1344–1350. https://doi.org/10.4088/JCP.09m05845gre

Saunders, K., & Goodwin, G. (2010). The course of bipolar disorder. *Advances in Psychiatric Treatment, 16*(5), 318–328. https:// doi.org/10.1192/apt.bp.107.004903

Seaton, E. K., & Iida, M. (2019). Racial discrimination and racial identity: Daily moderation among black youth. *American Psychologist, 74,* 117–127. http://doi.org/10.1037/amp0000367

Shalev, A., Merranko, J., Gill, M. K., Goldstein, T., Liao, F., Goldstein, B. I., Hower, H., Ryan, N., Strober, M., Iyengar, S., Keller, M., Yen, S., Weinstock, L. M., Axelson, D., & Birmaher, B. (2020). Longitudinal course and risk factors associated with psychosis in bipolar youths. *Bipolar Disorders, 22,* 139–154. http://doi.org/10.1111/bdi.12877

Shorey, S., Ng, E. D., & Wong, C. H. J. (2022). Global prevalence of depression and elevated depressive symptoms among adolescents: A systematic review and meta-analysis. *British Journal of Clinical Psychology, 61,* 287–305. http://doi.org/10.1111/bjc.12333

Sohel, A., Shutter, M., & Molla, M. (2022). Fluoxetine. In *StatPearls.* StatPearls Publishing. https://www.ncbi.nlm.nih.gov/books/NBK459223

Spoorthy, M. S., Chakrabarti, S., & Grover, S. (2019). Comorbidity of bipolar and anxiety disorders: An overview of trends in research. *World Journal of Psychiatry, 9*(1), 7–29. https://doi.org/10.5498/wjp.v9.i1.7

Staglin, G. (2021, April 20). Shedding light on mood disorders in the workplace. *Forbes.* https://www.forbes.com/sites/onemind/2021/04/20/shedding-light-on-mood-disorders-in-the-workplace/?sh=c4b18e93c246

Stein, D. J., Kupfer, D. J., & Schatzberg, A. F. (Eds.). (2007). *American Psychiatric Publishing textbook of mood disorders.* American Psychiatric Publishing.

Substance Abuse and Mental Health Services Administration. (2020). *Key substance use and mental health indicators in the United States: Results from the 2019 national survey on drug use and health.* HHS Publication No. PEP20-07-01-001, NSDUH Series H-55. Author. https://www.samhsa.gov/data.

Substance Abuse and Mental Health Services Administration. (2023). *Living well with serious mental illness.* https://www.samhsa.gov/serious-mental-illness/bipolar

Suicide Prevention Resource Center. (2020). *Effective prevention starts with you.* https://sprc.org

Swarbrick, M., & Noyes, S. (2018). Guest editorial–Effectiveness of occupational therapy services in mental health practice. *American Journal of Occupational Therapy, 72*(5), 7205170010p1–7205170010p4. https://doi.org/10.5014/ajot.2018.725001

The Trevor Project. (2019). *National survey on LGBTQ mental health.* https://www.thetrevorproject.org/wp-content/uploads/2019/06/The-Trevor-Project-National-Survey-Results-2019.pdf

Trøstheim, M., Eikemo, M., Meir, R., Hansen, I., Paul, E., Kroll, S., Garland, E., & Leknes, S. (2020). Assessment of anhedonia in adults with and without mental illness: A systematic review and meta-analysis. *JAMA Network Open, 3*(8), e2013233. https://doi.org/doi:10.1001/jamanetworkopen.2020.13233

United Nations. (2017, February 23). *UN health agency reports depression now 'leading cause of disability worldwide'.* UN News

Global Perspective Human Stories. https://news.un.org/en/story/2017/02/552062

U.S. Department of Health & Human Services. (2021). *Suicide prevention.* Office on Women's Health in the Office of the Assistant Secretary for Health (OASH). https://www.womenshealth.gov/mental-health/get-help-now/suicide-prevention

U.S. Department of Health & Human Services. (2022). *Mood disorders.* https://www.mentalhealth.gov/what-to-look-for/mood-disorders#:~:text=The%20most%20common%20mood%20disorders,Seasonal%20Affective%20Disorder%20(SAD)

Wang, H., van Leeuwen, J. M. C., de Voogd, L. E., Verkes, R., Roozendaal, B, Fernández, G., & Hermans, E. (2021). Mild early life stress exaggerates the impact of acute stress on corticolimbic resting-state functional connectivity. *European Journal of Neuroscience, 55,* 2122–2141. http://doi.org/10.1111/ejn.15538

Wang, S., Chen, L., Ran, H., Che, Y., Fang, D., Sun, H., Peng, J., Liang, X., & Xiao, Y. (2022). Depression and anxiety among children and adolescents pre and post COVID-19: A comparative meta-analysis. *Frontiers in Psychiatry, 13,* 917552. https://doi.org/10.3389/fpsyt.2022.917552

Warnick, S., Van Harrison, R., Parikh, S., Soyster, B., Tremper, A., & Bostwick, J. (2021). *Unipolar depression* [Internet]. Michigan Medicine University of Michigan. https://ncbi.nlm.nih.gov/books/NBK572297

World Health Organization. (2017). *Depression and other common mental disorders: Global health estimates.* Author. https://iris.who.int/bitstream/handle/10665/254610/WHO-MSD-MER-2017.2-eng.pdf?sequence=1.

World Health Organization. (2022). *Creating hope through action.* https://www.who.int/campaigns/world-suicide-prevention-day/2022

World Health Organization. (2023, August 28). *Suicide.* https://www.who.int/news-room/fact-sheets/detail/suicide

Young, C., Zheng, W., Steinwandel, M., Hui, C., Sanderson, M., Blot, W., & Shu, X. (2020). Associations of depressive symptoms with all-cause and cause-specific mortality by race in a population of low socioeconomic status: A report from the southern community cohort study. *American Journal of Epidemiology, 190,* 562–575. http://doi.org/10.1093/aje/kwaa216

Zablotsky, B., Black, L. I., Terlizzi, E. P., Vahratian, A., & Blumberg, S. J. (2022). Anxiety and depression symptoms among children before and during the COVID-19 pandemic. *Annals of Epidemiology, 75,* 53–56. https://doi.org/10.1016/j.annepidem.2022.09.003

Zhong, S., Chen, P., Lai, S., Chen, G., Zhang, Y., Lv, S., He, J., Tang, G., Pan, Y., Wang, Y., & Jia, Y. (2022). Aberrant dynamic functional connectivity in corticostriatal circuitry in depressed bipolar II disorder with recent suicide attempt. *Journal of Affective Disorders, 319,* 538–548. https://doi.org/10.1016/j.jad.2022.09.050

Obsessive Disorders

Susan Noyes

Think about someone who says "I'm so OCD" to describe their need for orderliness or cleanliness. Although many people are concerned with some of the same things that define an obsessive disorder, such as orderliness, germs, or symmetry, the relatively minor annoyance of these things in their lives lies in stark contrast to those whose lives are ruled by their obsessions and associated compulsive behaviors. Although obsessive-compulsive disorder (OCD) is beginning to be conceptualized as a spectrum condition (Vats et al., 2021) similar to other diagnostic categories in the *Diagnostic and Statistical Manual of Mental Disorders,* Fifth Edition *(DSM-5),* significant disruption of daily function because of the symptoms is a requirement for it to become a clinical diagnosis. This is an important distinction for OTPs to know.

This chapter describes the symptoms of the conditions that typically interfere with occupational performance and meaningful daily living, as well as the etiology, course, and prevalence of obsessive disorders. A full appreciation of the impact of OCD symptoms on occupational performance is necessary to inform effective occupational therapy interventions for individuals living with OCD and obsessive-compulsive related disorders (OCRD).

Description of the Condition

Close relationships exist between anxiety disorders (see Chapter 18: Anxiety Disorders 🤝) and many of the obsessive disorders. In the *DSM-IV* (American Psychiatric Association [APA], 1994), the primary symptom of anxiety was thought to be a driving force behind obsessive thoughts and compulsive behaviors. The *DSM-5* (APA, 2013), however, reflects increasing evidence for the distinct diagnostic indicators of OCD and the variety and overlap of OCRD. More complete descriptions of the conditions were deemed necessary to support clinicians in thorough evaluation and accurate diagnosis, and obsessive disorders are now described in a separate chapter from anxiety disorders.

According to the *DSM-5-TR* (APA, 2022), obsessions and/or compulsions must be present for OCD and OCRD to be diagnosed. **Obsessions** are recurrent and persistent thoughts, urges, and/or images that are experienced as intrusive and unwanted; cause marked anxiety and distress; and which the individual attempts to ignore, suppress, or neutralize. Individuals can have a range of obsessive or "worry" thoughts, with content ranging from making a mistake to unintentionally injuring someone while driving.

Typical themes include fear of germs or contamination, taboo thoughts involving sex or religion, and aggressive or violent thoughts toward self or others (National Institute of Mental Health [NIMH], 2022). Other forms of obsessive thinking include *responsibility obsessions* (e.g., fear of harming others because of not being careful); *perfection-related obsessions* such as excessive concern about symmetry or making mistakes; and *scrupulosity* or religious/moral obsessions (International Obsessive Compulsive Disorders Foundation [IOCDF], n.d.).

Compulsions are repetitive behaviors (e.g., hand washing or checking that a door is locked) or mental acts (e.g., counting and praying) that the individual feels driven to perform in response to obsessive thoughts or to comply with perceived rules. These behaviors and mental acts are intended to prevent or reduce the anxiety and distress associated with the obsessive thoughts, but they are excessive and not connected in a realistic way to what they are designed to prevent.

As with all disorders that rise to the level of clinical diagnosis, the symptoms of OCD and OCRD must be excessive, persist beyond developmentally appropriate periods, and significantly impair an individual's ability to function (APA, 2022). This chapter outlines the *DSM-5* criteria for the following disorders: OCD and those categorized as OCRD: body dysmorphic disorder (BDD), hoarding disorder (HD), trichotillomania (TTM), and excoriation disorder. At least two other recently identified public health conditions—online gaming and gambling disorders—have been categorized by the World Health Organization (2015) with the term "Problematic Usage of the Internet" (PUI) and are thought to share genetic risk factors with the OCRD. However, more research is required for a complete understanding of these conditions (Fineberg et al., 2018; Grünblatt, 2021).

Obsessive-Compulsive Disorder

OCD is characterized by obsessions and compulsions that are involuntary and unwanted, cause distress to the individual, and consume more than 1 hour per day (APA, 2022). The obsessive thoughts in OCD are intrusive and unrelenting; stopping them is not simply a matter of "don't think about it." The content of the obsession is specific to each individual, but some common themes in OCD include contamination, symmetry, forbidden or taboo thoughts, and accidentally harming others. The compulsive actions that follow the obsessive thoughts are meant to reduce or eliminate the anxiety associated with the distressing thoughts, for example, washing hands to ease anxiety about contamination, or moving and replacing items on a workspace to achieve a symmetrical arrangement before being able to begin working.

The compulsive actions generally do not work to stop the obsessive thoughts though, and the need to then repeat the actions, hoping for an effect, starts a time-consuming, distressing cycle that the person feels they must engage in. Without treatment, the compulsive actions begin to consume much of the person's time and attention. Habits and routines generated and sustained by these OCD symptoms disrupt the person's ability to engage in meaningful life activities. Understood this way, it is easy for an occupational therapy practitioner (OTP) to see how a person with OCD would struggle with occupational performance in many areas: activities of daily living (ADL), instrumental activities of daily living (IADL), work, school, and social participation.

Further, individuals with OCD and OCRD commonly avoid situations in which their obsessions and/or compulsions are triggered (e.g., public restrooms and social interactions). Consequences impacting occupational performance include avoidance of close relationships because of obsessions about harm, school failure or job loss because of the inability to complete projects in a timely manner, and health issues from avoiding contact with doctors' offices and hospitals.

It is important to distinguish OCD from obsessive-compulsive personality disorder (OCPD), which is categorized separately in the *DSM-5-TR* (APA, 2022). Though the name sounds very similar, OCPD is described as a personality impairment in self-functioning and interpersonal functioning based on an obsessive need for perfection. A person with OCPD finds their identity in their ability to be productive in a work capacity, often leading to overworking. They tend to have obsessively rigid thinking patterns and set unreasonably high goals for themselves and others. People with OCPD demonstrate compulsivity in the persistence of their focus on rigid perfectionism and have difficulty changing their viewpoint.

A primary difference between people with OCD and OCPD is their level of insight; people with OCD generally have an awareness that their obsessions and compulsions are not reasonable or health-supporting, whereas people with OCPD are comfortable with their rigid perfectionism and believe others should be, too (Van Noppen, 2010).

Because of the specificity of symptoms and foci of the obsessions and compulsions involved, the following conditions are categorized as the OCRDs: body dysmorphic disorder, hoarding disorder, trichotillomania, and excoriation disorder.

Body Dysmorphic Disorder

Body dysmorphic disorder (BDD) refers to the preoccupation with perceived flaws or defects in an individual's physical appearance that are not apparent, or appear only slight, to others (APA, 2022). This preoccupation is excessive and leads to repetitive behaviors or mental acts (e.g., comparing oneself with others) that are difficult to control and, on average, consume 3 to 8 hours per day.

One form of BDD that occurs almost exclusively in males is **muscle dysmorphia**. Individuals with this form of the disorder are preoccupied with thoughts that their body is too small or insufficiently muscular, when in fact they have a normal-appearing or even muscular body.

Excessive, repetitive behaviors associated with all forms of BDD include seeking reassurance about appearance, compulsive skin picking, excessive lifting of weights, using anabolic steroids, and having cosmetic surgical procedures. Severe symptoms of BDD result in impaired psychosocial functioning in all areas, but especially in social participation; this ranges from avoiding specific social situations to becoming completely housebound. This also negatively impacts an individual's ability to engage in school or work (APA, 2022). Recent evidence suggests that participation in social networking sites (SNS), either passively or in an appearance-focused manner, can influence body image dissatisfaction. Further, frequent SNS use is indicated as a potential risk factor for developing BDD symptoms (Ryding & Kuss, 2020).

Hoarding Disorder

Formerly considered a rare symptom of OCD, **hoarding disorder** (HD) became a distinct diagnostic category in the *DSM-5* (APA, 2013), and is thought to affect 1.5% to 6% of the general population (Rodriguez & Frost, 2022). Individuals with HD have persistent difficulty discarding or parting with possessions, regardless of their value. In contrast to normative collecting behavior, which is systematic and organized, individuals with HD have long-standing difficulty with organizing their possessions and discarding items, resulting in the accumulation of excessive clutter that interferes with their ability to effectively use the living areas in their homes for their intended purposes.

People who struggle with HD have varying levels of insight into the condition and often do not recognize the excessive acquiring and failure to discard as a problem. For many, the objects become intimately entwined with their identity; as stated by "Marge," a person with HD, "I have all of this; without these things, who am I?" (Spear, 2014, p. 18).

Although the difficulty with cluttering and discarding can present safety risks for individuals with HD and lead to the inability to complete daily living tasks, maintain a safe and sanitary living environment, engage in satisfying family and social relationships, and have good quality of life, attempts to remove or discard possessions by third parties—called *forced clean outs*—typically cause extreme distress to the individual and do not have a positive effect on hoarding behaviors (Clarke, 2019).

Many people with HD have been involved with municipal authorities because of fire hazards, residential code violations, and neighbors' complaints of squalor or pests, often resulting in constant threat of eviction proceedings or losing their housing (APA, 2013). Attempts to mediate these consequences of persistent hoarding behaviors have led cities both in the United States and internationally to develop task forces to address hoarding in their communities. Task force members typically include police and fire personnel, code enforcers, housing and legal agencies, mental healthcare providers and case managers, and, ideally, persons with lived experience of hoarding behaviors (Bratiotis, 2013; Vaingankar et al., 2022).

A subset of individuals with HD hoard animals, referred to as **animal hoarding**. These individuals accumulate large numbers of animals and fail to provide minimal standards of nutrition, sanitation, and veterinary care for the animals. Persons with animal HD experience higher levels of poor sanitation in their living environments (APA, 2013). Although squalor—defined as "the condition of being extremely dirty and unpleasant" (Cambridge Dictionary, n.d.)—occasionally occurs in homes cluttered with objects, it is virtually always present in animal-hoarded homes (Rodriguez & Frost, 2022). Large amounts of animal excrement leading to toxic levels of ammonia in the home environment present health risks to the humans and animals in the home, as well as the potential risk for the home to be condemned (Castrodale et al., 2010; Strong et al., 2019).

People who hoard animals typically demonstrate very poor insight into the problem and this may be because of associated symptoms of delusional thinking and dissociation (APA, 2013; Rodriguez & Frost, 2022).

Trichotillomania and Excoriation Disorder

Both **trichotillomania** (TTM) and excoriation disorder are categorized with OCRD, because they involve recurring repetitive behaviors related to parts of the body, also known as "body-focused repetitive behaviors" (BFRB; Keuthen et al., 2015, p. 10). In both conditions, the behaviors are usually preceded by anxiety or boredom and cause distress and embarrassment. People with BFRB typically report both tension and a sense of urgency before the behavior, and a sense of relief or gratification afterward (APA, 2022).

TTM refers to the repetitive pulling out of one's own hair without intent to cause injury. This results in significant hair loss from any number of body regions, though the most common are the scalp, eyebrows, and eyelashes (APA, 2022). TTM often begins in childhood but can present across the life span, typically in response to stress. Incidence is higher in women than men, but all genders can be affected. Repeated hair pulling over time can result in bald spots, overall thinning of hair, and associated skin injuries. Some individuals ingest the hair they pull, which presents the risk of developing masses in the stomach that can lead to serious gastrointestinal conditions (Houghton & Woods, 2017).

The essential feature of **excoriation disorder** is recurrent skin picking that results in skin lesions (APA, 2022). The persistence of these behaviors, despite repeated attempts to stop and the associated social and medical consequences, defines this as an OCRD (Snorrason et al., 2015). Similar to TTM, excoriation disorder is more common in women, and commonly starts in childhood but can also present later in life. Excoriation disorder causes tissue damage, scarring, and infection (APA, 2022).

TTM and excoriation disorder often occur with each other and also co-occur with depression and anxiety. Both conditions can contribute to social withdrawal and school or work problems caused by absences and stigma (Hallion et al., 2017; Houghton & Woods, 2017).

Etiology

Although research continues to investigate obsessive disorders, their cause is currently unknown. Each condition has unique characteristics; however, common factors have been identified that offer some insight into the basis of OCD and the OCRD. These include genetics; neuroanatomical structure and function; and neurochemical, cognitive and psychological, and environmental factors (NIMH, 2022).

Genetic Factors

As might be expected, many research studies have investigated the possible genetic links in obsessive disorders. OCD in particular demonstrates a strong familial link (Goodman et al., 2014). Close relatives of a person with OCD have a five times higher chance of having OCD; they are also likely to share the same obsessive and compulsive symptoms. Studies of twins have confirmed this, as well as the influence of the environment on the development of OCD (Vaghi, 2021). Genetic risk factors have been found to overlap across all obsessive disorders (Browne et al., 2014; Grünblatt, 2021).

Neuroanatomical Structure and Function Factors

Functional neuroimaging studies have used positron emission tomography (PET) scans and functional magnetic resonance imaging (fMRI) to study OCD and OCRD, thus implicating the prefrontal cortex as the area of the brain most involved with these conditions (Pauls et al., 2014; Vaghi, 2021). Recent studies have identified functional alterations in the nodes of the cortico-striatal-thalamo-cortical circuits, and researchers currently believe that abnormal fronto-striatal neural circuits cause impairment in the executive functions of the brain (Soriano-Mas, 2021; Vaghi, 2021). In OCD and OCRD, hyperactivation of the frontal cortex may play a role in obsessive thoughts because increased activation of the frontal cortex was prominent when obsessive thinking was captured in functional imaging. This hyperactivation may draw additional cortical attention to potential real or imagined threats, resulting in the obsession (Pauls et al., 2014).

Structural imaging using MRI to identify the neuroanatomical underpinnings of OCD and OCRD is ongoing, with a large global study currently underway (Simpson et al., 2020) seeking to identify a "brain signature" (Veltman, 2021, p. 214) for OCD. However, Veltman (2021) also cautions that brain differences in OCD can change over time, so more longitudinal studies are needed to solidify past findings. Findings from such studies can serve to create more targeted therapies and interventions for OCD and OCRD.

Neurochemical Factors

Recent studies suggest there is combined involvement of the serotonergic, dopaminergic, and glutamatergic systems in OCD and OCRD (Grünblatt, 2021). Serotonin is a key neurotransmitter involved with how people manage fear. It affects their ability to process aversive stimuli, develop fear conditioning, and modulate extinction retention. The role of serotonin and another neurotransmitter, gamma-aminobutyric acid (GABA), in anxiety forms the basis for the use of selective serotonin inhibitors and benzodiazepines (which target the GABA system) as medications to treat the anxiety disorders and OCD (Hartley & Casey, 2013).

However, not all individuals with OCD/OCRD experience symptom reduction when the serotonergic system is targeted for treatment, supporting the theory that the neurotransmitters dopamine and glutamate are also implicated in these conditions. More research is needed to determine with certainty the neurochemical system pathways that are involved with OCD and OCRD, which can lead to the development of accurately aligned treatments (Biria et al., 2021).

Cognitive and Psychological Factors

In OCD and OCRD, the behaviors used in attempts to allevi-ate the anxiety of symptoms can be reinforcing. Compulsions in and of themselves are rewarding (Fontenelle et al., 2015) as they lead to at least temporary relief from anxiety. Therefore, when the disturbing thought or anxious feeling recurs, the in-dividual is more likely to engage in the ritual. This pattern is a self-perpetuating cycle (Fig. 21-1). Some compulsions tend to allay a specific concern, such as hand washing performed in conjunction with fears related to contamination. Other com-pulsions, such as symmetry and counting, provide a sense of calm when the individual is anxious. Further, the role of habits in compulsive behaviors is currently being studied to determine both how such uncontrollable habits are formed and how habits might be leveraged as a target for effective intervention in OCD and OCRD (Gillan, 2021).

Environmental Factors

Despite numerous studies of OCD and OCRD, no environ-mental causes have been identified. However, studies do suggest environmental risk factors that may play a part in the development of the condition, including infection and traumatic experiences (Brander et al., 2016; Yang, 2022). For instance, PANDAS, or Pediatric Autoimmune Neuropsychi-atric Disorder Associated with Streptococcal infections, was named by Swedo (2002) as the condition in which OCD was an unexpected result of a child's infection with streptococ-cus. Swedo (2002) postulated that in vulnerable prepubescent children, an abnormal immune response to the streptococ-cus infection affected the basal ganglia, which is known to be involved with OCD symptoms. In contrast to typical OCD onset, PANDAS affects only children and is marked by acute onset of OCD symptoms after streptococcal infection (Brander et al., 2016).

Studies have found relationships between stressful or trau-matic life events and development of OCD. In children, ex-periencing adverse events can lead to OCD, and for adults,

experiencing posttraumatic stress disorder (PTSD) after age 40 significantly increases the likelihood of developing late-onset OCD (Brander et al., 2016; Yang, 2022). Similarly, losses caused by traumatic events may increase the risk for HD (Rodriguez & Frost, 2022).

Prevalence

The lifetime prevalence of OCD has held steady over time at 2% to 3% in the general population around the world (Carmi et al., 2022; Goodman et al., 2014). The cumulative prevalence of all the OCRDs has been estimated at 9.5% (Carmi et al., 2022).

Incidence

The mean age of onset of OCD in the United States is 19.5 years, and onset after age 35 is possible but not typi-cal (APA, 2022). Across the life span, there are two periods when the incidence of OCD increases: during late childhood, known as *early onset,* and in early adulthood, or *late onset.* Early onset OCD is thought to be more heritable than adult late onset OCD (Hauser, 2021).

Gender Differences

Females are affected with OCD at a slightly higher rate in adulthood, with males much more commonly affected in childhood, 25% of them before age 10 (APA, 2013). Male youth with OCD also tend to have related comorbidities, such as tic disorders and attention deficit-hyperactivity dis-order (ADHD; Hauser, 2021).

Culture-Specific Information

OCD and OCRD are known to occur globally, and varying sociocultural elements shape how it presents in individuals (Carmi et al., 2022; Williams, Chapman et al., 2017). Similar-ities exist cross-culturally nonetheless, particularly in symp-toms related to contamination, cleaning, taboo, hoarding, and fear of harm (APA, 2022). Age of onset and gender distribu-tion are also globally similar, with prevalence of the condi-tions evenly distributed around the world (Carmi et al., 2022).

In considering the meaning of culture in a health-care con-text, Nicolini and colleagues (2017) outline four domains to assess—the person's "cultural identity" (p. 286), which includes ethnicity and race, sexual orientation, gender, spiritual beliefs, socioeconomic status (SES), and education; the cultural expla-nation of the disease; the cultural interpretation of stressors and functional level; and cultural elements of the relationship between the health-care provider and patient. For OCD and OCRD, differences in the understanding and presentation of the conditions can vary by specific geographic regions, popu-lations, or religious groups, and overlaps among them.

Williams, Chapman, and colleagues (2017) describe nu-merous examples of this. For instance, *identity OCD,* defined as concerns about undesired change in sexual orientation or gender identity, is a Western-only presentation of OCD; it is not seen in the literature outside the United States. In Kenya,

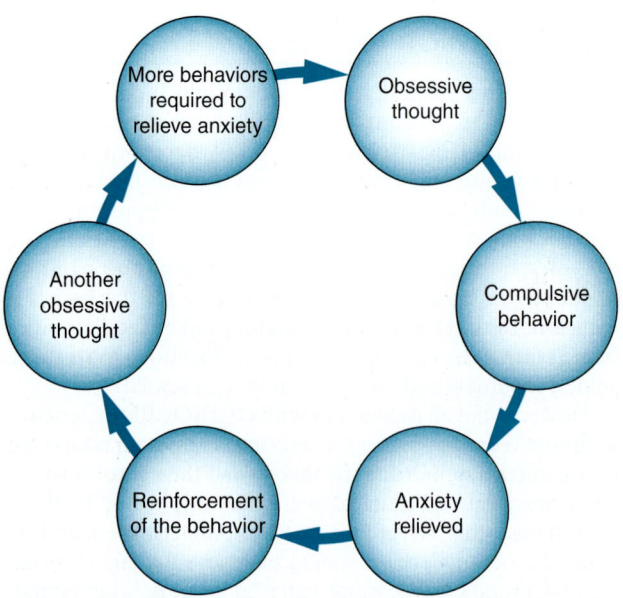

FIGURE 21-1. Cycle of obsessive thoughts and compulsive behaviors.

OCD is thought to be caused by witchcraft, and traditional healers are typically consulted to address symptoms. A large study of African Americans showed that they experienced contamination symptoms at twice the rate of European Americans, and that they tend toward delaying seeking assistance for mental health concerns, or seeking assistance first from healers, friends, elders, or religious leaders (Williams, Taylor et al., 2017).

The collectivist nature of Chinese culture presents unique challenges for OCD, namely, caregiver burden. One study indicated 76 of the 77 households studied reported significant caregiver distress from caring for the individual with OCD, and this involved accommodating or participating in the compulsive behaviors, as well as financial burden—one family had overwhelming water bills because of the patient's cleanliness rituals (Siu et al., 2012).

Studies of some religious communities also reveal a fine line between culturally sanctioned behaviors and what could be considered diagnosable obsessions or compulsions. For instance, higher levels of Christian religiosity also resulted in higher levels of OCD symptoms of washing and controlling thoughts. In the Jewish and Islam cultures, discerning between religious rituals and compulsive behaviors can be difficult because of the emphasis on scrupulosity that focuses on moral or religious issues, and the cleaning rituals that are required in Islam (Williams, Chapman et al., 2017).

Appreciation of the person's full cultural identity offers OTPs the ability to contextually situate their assessment and intervention for OCD and OCRD for best outcomes. See the Mental Health in Culture and Society feature to see an example of how a person's mental health condition may be impacted by discrimination.

Mental Health in Culture and Society

Aster Harrison

Racial Discrimination and Obsessive-Compulsive Disorder

The political and social environment can strongly affect symptoms of OCD. For example, research shows that racial discrimination can worsen symptoms of OCD for African Americans and Black Caribbean Americans (MacIntyre et al., 2023; Williams et al., 2017, 2021). People who experienced more racial discrimination were more likely to report contamination and harm obsessions, as well as washing and repeating compulsions (Williams et al., 2021). Williams (2020) explains that experiences of racism may make Black people hypervigilant about cleanliness in response to racist stereotypes of Black people being less clean.

For some Black people with OCD, experiences of racism can also trigger harm obsessions. Because of societal racism, Black people are often monitored, policed, and treated as threats in public spaces. Individual Black people may become hypervigilant about monitoring their behavior in response to racial discrimination to try to avoid being seen as a threat and harmed or discriminated against again (Williams, 2020).

It is important for OTPs to acknowledge how racial discrimination, trauma, and other environmental factors can influence OCD symptoms. Using a Person-Environment-Occupation (PEO) approach can help practitioners acknowledge that OCD symptoms are not only the result of someone's neurology, but also heavily influenced by environmental stressors and occupational factors. A successful intervention approach can address multiple elements of PEO, and improve PEO fit. OTPs can also play a role in combatting racism in their profession and in society. Because antiblackness has negative health effects, engaging in antiracist advocacy and organizing can be part of their roles in advocating for patient health.

References

MacIntyre, M. M., Zare, M., & Williams, M. T. (2023). Anxiety-related disorders in the context of racism. *Current Psychiatry Reports*, 25(2), 31–43. https://doi.org/10.1007/s11920-022-01408-2

Williams, M. T. (2020). The OCD-racism connection and its impact on people of color. *Psychology Today*. https://www.psychologytoday.com/ca/blog/culturally-speaking/202009/the-ocd-racism-connection-and-impact-people-color

Williams, M. T., Taylor, R. J., George, J. R., Schlaudt, V. A., Ifatunji, M. A., & Chatters, L. M. (2021). Correlates of obsessive-compulsive symptoms among Black Caribbean Americans. *International Journal of Mental Health*, 50(1), 53–77. https://doi.org/10.1080/00207411.2020.1826261

Williams, M. T., Taylor, R. J., Mouzon, D. M., Oshin, L. A., Himle, J. A., & Chatters, L. M. (2017). Discrimination and symptoms of obsessive-compulsive disorder among African Americans. *The American Journal of Orthopsychiatry*, 87(6), 636–645. https://doi.org/10.1037/ort0000285

Course

Individuals may develop OCD in childhood, adolescence, or early adulthood; rarely is the onset after age 40 (Goodman et al., 2014). The course of OCD varies individually, and time of onset influences this. Early onset, or pediatric, OCD tends to present with such cognitive symptoms as intolerance of uncertainty and difficulty with planning and working memory. Challenges with cognitive flexibility and motor inhibition, however, typically present only in late onset OCD (Vaghi, 2021).

In a longitudinal study of OCD, Eisen and colleagues (2013) followed patients with OCD for 5 years and found predictors for remission that included having a primary obsession of overresponsibility for harm, symptoms of lower severity, and shorter length of illness. HD had the least remitting course of any of the OCRDs. This study also found that a longer course of OCD was predicted by the length of time a person had symptoms without intervention, indicating that early identification and intervention for OCD is critical in managing the course of the condition and, by extension, in the person's quality of life.

Impact on Occupational Performance

Regardless of the diagnostic labels a person is given, OTPs are first and foremost concerned with occupational performance. Whether interruptions to daily living occur at home, work, or school, or in social situations, OTPs must be prepared to address the potential impact of a person's obsessions and compulsions on their occupational performance.

OCD and OCRD significantly compromise quality of life and psychosocial functioning. Vats and colleagues (2021) see OCD as a spectrum condition—or obsessive-compulsive spectrum disorders (OCSD). As such, OCD can manifest with varying degrees of impact on occupational performance. For example, Woods and colleagues (2006) calculated that, at a 1% prevalence rate in the working-age population, individuals with TTM alone account for nearly 1 million lost workdays per year because of their symptoms.

Citing recent data, the NIMH reported that adults with OCD scored within a range of impairment from "mild to severe" using the Sheehan Disability Scale. However, in response to questions about the impact of OCD symptoms on work, school, social life, family life, and home responsibilities, the majority had scores in the "serious" and "moderate" levels (NIMH, 2022). These data underscore the need for OTPs to engage people with OCD in a full occupational profile to understand where their symptoms fall on the OCD spectrum so that individualized intervention can be planned accordingly. Two pertinent areas to address for OCD and OCRD are cognitive and psychosocial impairments.

Cognitive Impairments

Farrell and Barrett (2006) reported that, in the case of OCD, disruptive cognitive processes appear to worsen across the developmental trajectory. OCD is often characterized by executive functioning deficits, particularly as they relate to cognitive flexibility and decision-making. Individuals with OCD and OCRD tend to demonstrate patterns of perseverative and inflexible cognition and behavior that are maladaptive in everyday life (Gruner & Pittenger, 2017). Cognitive inflexibility also impacts effective decision-making, and indecisiveness is a common clinical symptom in both children and adults with OCD and OCRD. Increased information-gathering behaviors are frequently noted that are time consuming and can significantly delay decision-making (Hauser, 2021).

OTPs can create interventions that modify the cognitive demands or create adaptations to support successful performance for individuals with OCD and OCRD experiencing cognitive impairments.

Psychosocial Impairments

OCD disrupts engagement in meaningful occupations because individuals, for example, may stop attending social and community activities. Relationships may be disrupted when individuals decline to share in family activities and events involving friends and coworkers. The behaviors associated with OCD can interfere with school, work, and social relationships for two primary reasons (APA, 2013): the time spent engaged in obsessive thinking and the fact that compulsive acts can interfere with completing the tasks necessary for work, school, and home. In addition, many people with OCD avoid situations that are seen as triggers for symptoms.

In his book, *The Man Who Couldn't Stop: OCD and the True Story of a Life Lost in Thought* (2014), author David Adam offers a first-person account of his lived experience with the limitations of his OCD symptoms. He chronicles how he came to obsess over the possibility that he would get AIDS and how that obsession and the resultant compulsive behaviors impacted his daily life for years thereafter. Adam recounts endless hours spent donating blood (because the donation center routinely tested for AIDS) and calling the blood donation center for test results and reassurance, time that he recognized he would otherwise have used to socialize with friends, attend soccer matches, and sleep well.

The tipping point for him in deciding to access treatment was when he realized his baby daughter was becoming part of his OCD. Adam was obsessing over passing HIV to his daughter, and his fear of contaminating her in numerous ways became overwhelming. Consequently, his compulsive behaviors of checking and counting increased, and he also began to have hand-washing compulsions. Recounting his personal experience, David Adam clearly described the psychosocial toll of living a life bound to obsessive thinking and compulsive acts.

Habits, typically understood by OTPs as health-promoting, can nonetheless potentially interrupt occupational performance for people with OCD and OCRD. Instead of efficiency in completing tasks typically afforded by the automatic behaviors that underlie habits, the compulsive behaviors involved in OCD and OCRD represent an extreme form of habit in which automatic behaviors become separated from the person's best intentions not to compulsively repeat them (Gillan, 2021).

OTPs can leverage their knowledge of occupational performance to address the impact of symptoms on the daily lives of individuals who struggle with OCD and OCRD. Assessment and targeted interventions for individuals experiencing occupational performance problems related to obsessive-compulsive symptoms can support the individual to experience successful engagement in meaningful occupations. See this chapter's The Lived Experience feature to better understand the impact of the condition on occupational performance.

Intervention

As for any occupational therapy intervention, good outcomes rely on a thorough assessment. After gathering the occupational profile, assessment tools can be used to extend the understanding of how OCD or OCRD symptoms interrupt the person's occupational performance. This may include assessment of ADL and IADL, cognition, and sensory processing. Using assessment data, occupational therapy intervention for people with OCD and OCRD will be designed to address and improve areas of difficulty in occupational performance.

Table 21-1 outlines common intervention approaches for individuals with OCD and OCRD and identifies the accompanying chapters in this text that provide more detailed information about those approaches.

Digital means of intervention recently have been designed to increase access to and ease of treatment. Vats and colleagues (2021) describe several types of digital intervention for OCD and OCRD, including social media groups for access to both providers and other patients, use of webcams and smartphone cameras for tracking compulsive behaviors as part of a treatment protocol, and smart wearables (watches) to collect and monitor behavioral data and provide clinical support. Also, Roncero and colleagues (2019) found promising results in the

The Lived Experience

Joy Springer

At the time of this writing, Joy Springer was an occupational therapy student. This feature provides many examples of how OCD affects cognition, which in turn affects occupational performance. In addition, Joy provides many examples of strategies that have been useful for her.

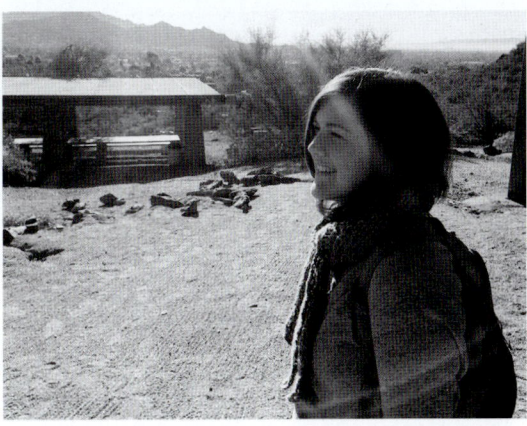

Having OCD means having a brain that sends me mixed messages. For me, OCD is more about the obsessive thoughts than the compulsions that follow. The mixed message from my brain starts with an intrusive/obsessive thought that causes a lot of anxiety. The rational part of my brain tells me that the obsessive thought is completely irrational; the emotional part of my brain makes me feel very anxious. In order to get rid of the anxiety, I perform compulsions. Through time, it takes more compulsions to reduce the anxiety. Rationally, I know that my compulsions aren't helping the situation; emotionally, the compulsions are the only short-term solution to getting rid of the anxiety.

As a child my most pervasive obsessive thought was that I would pull back the shower curtain and be transported to a concentration camp. Even as a child I knew this was impossible. I knew that I could never be transported back in time. But this irrational, impossible thought created the same amount of fear in me *as if* it could come true. Getting in the shower created an immobilizing panic attack. It didn't matter how much my rational brain tried to convince me that I was safe in my own home. My emotional brain was warning me that when I opened that shower curtain I would be transported to my greatest fear.

These fears led to a complex childhood ritual. I started by positioning myself facing the shower curtain and peeking out of the curtain a few times to convince myself I was still in my own home. Then, I would check more and more. Once that compulsion didn't alleviate my anxiety, I added opening and closing the toilet lid to my rituals. Next came turning on every light from the bathroom to my bedroom. If I got out of the shower and realized the hall lights had been turned off, I would be paralyzed by anxiety. I would call for my brothers or parents to turn on the light, giving the excuse that I couldn't find the switches in the dark. On the rare occasions my parents asked about my strange behavior, I was too embarrassed to tell them the truth.

When I entered high school, my intrusive thoughts turned to other fears. Organization became the compulsion that reduced my anxiety. I spent weekends emptying my room and putting my possessions back one item at a time. I would repetitively organize my school notes despite their already pristine organization. Just like with childhood, my time (sometimes an entire day) was filled with anxiety regarding the intrusive thoughts and the compulsions that would keep the anxiety at bay. My shame surrounding my intrusive thoughts was so great that I would tell my friends and family that my stomach hurt and lock myself in the bathroom to perform compulsions. Wherever I was, I would find a way to secretly alleviate my anxiety.

The number of stressors in my life has a huge impact on my OCD. In the 18 months before starting graduate school I had very few symptoms of OCD because I had very few stressors at that time. When I decided to pursue my master's degree in occupational therapy, I entered a career that I love and am very passionate about, but placed myself in a tremendously stressful environment. Going back to school was so stressful that after my first quarter of graduate school my husband and I decided that I needed to go back onto medication to help manage my stress. Unfortunately, I had such a severe reaction to the medication that I was told not to take it any longer.

So far, I have tried six medications from three different drug families, but none of them have worked. Mostly I get the same set of severe physical symptoms: ice pick headaches that don't go away, muscles so tight I can't turn my head, nausea so severe I get sick transitioning from sitting to standing. After this last round of medication, I decided that I couldn't do it anymore. I would have to manage without medications.

The main strategy I use to manage my OCD is called Emotionally Focused Therapy (EFT). This therapeutic approach is actually a couple's therapy method that just happened to help with my OCD. To put it simply, EFT encourages both members of a couple to get in touch with their emotions and share them honestly and openly with their partner. Learning how to connect with my emotions and share them with my husband, Michael, has allowed me to feel safe in discussing my intrusive thoughts and the fears connected with them. Being transparent about my condition has provided the most relief.

In addition to EFT, I use elements of Cognitive Behavioral Therapy (CBT) to help change my internal dialogue. For me, CBT doesn't really help with intrusive thoughts; I know my intrusive thoughts are irrational, so it's better to work on them from an emotional level. I use CBT when I have negative self-talk. Thoughts like "Michael won't love me anymore if I tell him about my latest intrusive thoughts" are best combatted with CBT. In this case, I take the time to tell myself that Michael has never turned away from me, no matter what he's learned about my OCD. Today will be no different.

Most importantly, I've learned to be open about having OCD and to be unashamed in advocating for my needs. The shame and fear surrounding mental illness are potent barriers. I realized that my own silence was perpetuating the shame and fear associated with mental illness. When I had an opportunity to speak to my classmates about my experiences with OCD, I decided to speak up. It was the scariest choice I've ever made. However, my classmates were accepting and some have taken the time to reach out to me to learn more about my experiences or to share their own. Today, I am more open about having OCD than I ever have been before. While I can only share what it's like to have a mental illness from my perspective, I hope that my story leads people to be more open to the experiences of so many others who have a mental illness.

TABLE 21-1 | Common Intervention Approaches for Individuals With Obsessive-Compulsive and Obsessive-Compulsive Related Disorders

Approach	Target(s) of Intervention	Brief Synopsis	Chapters With Additional Information
Cognitive Remediation	Improving executive dysfunction abilities	Graded activities and strategies that target cognitive skill development	Chapter 7: Cognition
Cognitive Adaptation	Changing the environment to compensate for executive dysfunction	Activity analysis and environmental modification to reduce cognitive requirements	Chapter 7: Cognition
Cognitive Behavioral Approach	Distorted beliefs	Distorted beliefs are identified and then challenged by providing evidence to the contrary.	Chapter 8: Cognitive Beliefs
Acceptance and Commitment	Psychological flexibility	Combines acceptance of difficult feelings, thoughts, and circumstances with commitment to constructive activities that address personal goals and values	Chapter 8: Cognitive Beliefs
Dunn's Model of Sensory Processing	Sensory processing needs in the context of occupational performance	Creating environments or materials that meet the individual's sensory processing needs	Chapter 9: Sensory Processing and the Lived Sensory Experience
Mindfulness Meditation	Emotional well-being	A form of meditation practice that focuses awareness nonjudgmentally on the present	Chapter 12: Emotion Regulation
Motivational Interviewing	Enhance motivation for change	Helps individuals identify their values and interests and reasons for change	Chapter 11: Motivation
Building Healthy Routines and Habits	Time use	For individuals with OCD, learning to reduce engagement in unhealthy routines and build supportive habits and routines	Chapter 14: Time Use and Habits
Exercise and Other Forms of Physical Activity	Stress reduction and mood enhancement	Creating physical activity programs or encouraging participation in existing programs	Chapter 45: Self-Care and Well-Being Occupations
Supported Education and Employment	Goals related to higher education and all forms of employment: volunteer, competitive	Individualized, practical support and inclusion to help people succeed in postsecondary education and employment endeavors	Chapter 47: Student; Chapter 48: Work and Volunteer Occupations
Community Clutter and Hoarding Toolkit	Hoarding	Reducing clutter to maintain housing using Motivational Interviewing and goal setting; targets older adults	Chapter 31: The Home Environment: Permanent Supportive Housing

use of a CBT-based mobile app to reduce OCD symptoms in college students. Of course, these treatment options all require the informed consent of the user.

Treatment for OCD and OCRD can include medical interventions (i.e., medications) and several forms of brain stimulation therapies.

Medications

The most commonly used medication for OCD and OCRD is selective serotonin reuptake inhibitors (SSRIs). SSRI medications include fluoxetine (Prozac), paroxetine (Paxil), fluvoxamine (Luvox), sertraline (Zoloft), and citalopram (Celexa). SSRIs have both antiobsessional and antipanic effects; they also have fewer side effects than the older class of antidepressants, but they sometimes produce slight nausea or jitters when people first start to take them. These symptoms fade with time. Some people also experience sexual dysfunction with SSRIs, which may be helped by adjusting the dosage or switching to another SSRI. However, not all people with OCD

or OCRD report relief of their symptoms from using medication, and research on effective pharmacotherapy is ongoing (Pittenger, 2021).

Other Medical Treatments

An increased understanding of the neural pathways associated with mood, thought, and behavior regulation has promoted the use of brain stimulation therapies in the treatment of OCD (Bergfeld et al., 2021). For example, **electroconvulsive therapy (ECT)** is a treatment used for several psychiatric conditions in which seizures are induced with the use of electricity while the person is anesthetized. ECT may be effective in reducing symptoms of OCD in patients with comorbid depression (NIMH, n.d.). **Repetitive transcranial electromagnetic stimulation (rTMS)** is a noninvasive treatment for OCD that is typically used when behavioral and medication interventions have not been effective in reducing symptoms. rTMS involves the external application, via head coil, of variable magnetic fields to excite

Evidence-Based Practice

Exposure and Response Prevention for Obsessive-Compulsive Disorder

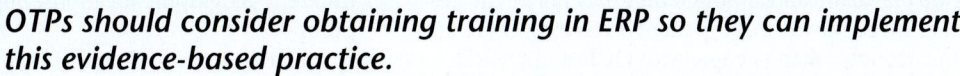

OTPs should consider obtaining training in ERP so they can implement this evidence-based practice.

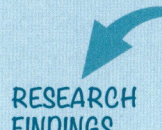

RESEARCH FINDINGS

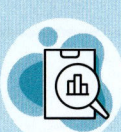

Exposure and response (or ritual) prevention (ERP) is an evidence-based intervention for OCD. It works by slowly and systematically exposing the person to the very objects and situations that trigger their OCD symptoms, while also having the person not engage in the compulsive behavioral response. Current best practice for OCD treatment is CBT that includes ERP combined with SSRI medications. Although recognized as very effective, ERP is often underutilized, for two reasons: Only a limited number of clinicians are adequately trained to provide it, and people with OCD often can't access it or fear that the treatment will be difficult. Innovations currently being studied to improve accessibility and acceptability of ERP treatment include video conferencing, internet-based treatment platforms, and CBT mobile apps (Patel et al., 2021).

APPLICATIONS

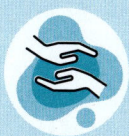

➡ OTPs that provide services to people with OCD should consider obtaining training in ERP so that they have the skills to implement this evidence-based practice.

➡ OTPs should ensure that they are providing ERP within the context of meaningful occupations that have been disrupted by OCD.

REFERENCE

Patel, S. R., Simpson, H. B., & Comer, J. (2021). Innovations in the delivery of exposure and response prevention for obsessive-compulsive disorder. *Current Topics in Behavioral Neuroscience, 49,* 301–329. https://doi.org/10.1007/7854_2020_202

or inhibit areas of the brain. Numerous studies show reduction in OCD symptoms following rTMS. Deep TMS (dTMS) targets deeper cortical regions and has been U.S. Food and Drug Administration (FDA) approved for its effectiveness in hard-to-treat OCD.

Although rTMS and dTMS target cortical areas of the brain for modulation, the use of **deep brain stimulation (DBS)** is directed to subcortical areas (Bergfeld et al., 2021). The most invasive of the brain stimulation therapies, DBS is a neurosurgical form of therapeutic brain stimulation that involves implanting electrodes and subcutaneous pulse generators in the patient's body to provide electrical stimulation to specific brain areas on a programmed schedule (Holtzheimer & Mayberg, 2011). Across numerous studies, DBS has been shown to effect large to very large reductions in OCD symptoms, reduce symptoms of depression and anxiety, and contribute to increased quality of life (Bergfeld et al., 2021).

Many people with OCD utilize a combination of intervention approaches to manage their symptoms, including exposure and response prevention (ERP); see the Evidence-Based Practice feature.

General Considerations When Providing Occupational Therapy to People With Obsessive Disorders

OCD and OCRD co-occur with other mental health conditions, as well as physical conditions and illnesses; therefore, it is very likely that OTPs will encounter people challenged with these symptoms across treatment settings—not just in typical mental health-care facilities. For that reason, all OTPs must be mindful of the symptoms of OCD and OCRD and the ways these can impact occupational performance and engagement with the occupational therapy process:

- Thoughtful therapeutic use of self is critical to establish rapport that allows the person to discuss their OCD or OCRD symptoms as part of occupational therapy assessment and intervention.
- Collaboration with the person's care team, including mental health providers, supports a unified approach to intervention.

■ OTPs can provide advocacy for a person seeking treatment for OCD or OCRD by referring to resources and providers that specialize in these conditions.

Here's the Point

■ OCDs are prevalent, and although they may not be the primary conditions for which the patient is referred, OTPs are likely to encounter many people with OCD and OCRD.

■ Individuals with OCD and OCRD have symptoms that are frequently misunderstood, yet they can cause severe interruption to occupational performance and quality of life.

■ A combination of biological, neurological, psychosocial, and environmental factors contributes to the development of OCD and OCRD.

■ OCD and OCRD are conditions that are seen globally, and cultural factors shape how OCD uniquely presents in different geographic locations, populations, and religious groups.

■ Medical and occupational therapy interventions can reduce symptoms and promote better quality of life and participation in occupations.

Apply It Now

1. PEO Analysis

Read Joy Springer's first-person account of living with OCD ("The Lived Experience") and complete a PEO analysis using the template in Appendix A. Identify factors that support and interfere with occupational performance. Be sure to consider both the personal factors and the environmental factors that might present as facilitators or barriers.

2. Reflect on the First-Person Experience of OCD

Consider the following questions about Joy Springer's narrative:
■ What types of occupations were impaired because of Joy's OCD symptoms?
■ What role could you see for OTPs to support Joy's occupational performance?
■ What personal reaction or feelings did you have after reading Joy's story? How might this affect your work with people with OCD or OCRD?

3. Understanding Intrusive Thoughts

Intrusive thoughts are a key symptom of OCD. Try the following experiment to better understand the process of intrusive thinking.

Set a timer for 5 minutes. For the next 5 minutes, try not to think of white bears.

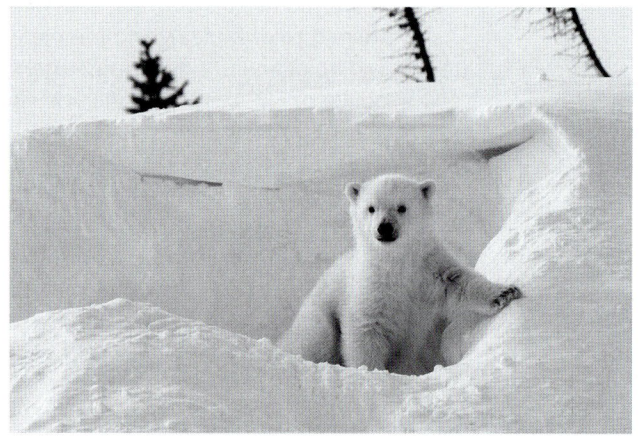

Reflective Questions
■ How many times did you think of white bears? Wegner (1989) first conducted this experiment and described this phenomenon as ironic processes. Attempting to suppress a thought has the opposite effect and causes you to think of it more.
■ Do you ever find yourself stuck with bothersome thoughts that are hard to get rid of? When is this most likely to happen?

Resources

Organizations
- Freedom From Fear: www.freedomfromfear.org
- Hoarding Disorder: www.clutterersanonymous.org
- International OCD Foundation: www.iocdf.org
- National Alliance for the Mentally Ill (NAMI): www.nami.org

Educational Videos
- Public Broadcasting Service (PBS): www.pbs.org
- Stanford Health Library: http://healthlibrary.stanford.edu

Books and Articles
- Chater, C., Shaw, J., & McKay, S. (2013, March). Hoarding in the home: A toolkit for the home healthcare provider. *Home Healthcare Nurse, 31*(3), 144–154. https://doi.org/10.1097/NHH.0b013e3182838847

- Frost, R., & Steketee, G. (2011). *Stuff: Compulsive hoarding and the meaning of things.* Houghton Mifflin Harcourt.
- Grayson, J. (2014). *Freedom from obsessive compulsive disorder: A personalized recovery program for living with uncertainty.* Penguin.
- Hershfield, J., & Corboy, T. (2013). *The mindfulness workbook for OCD: A guide to overcoming obsessions and compulsions using mindfulness and cognitive behavioral therapy.* New Harbinger.
- Sedley, B., & Coyne, L. (2020). *Stuff that's loud: A teen's guide to unspiralling when OCD gets noisy.* Hachette UK.
- Shapiro, L. J. (2015). *Understanding OCD: Skills to control the conscience and outsmart obsessive compulsive disorder.* ABC-CLIO.
- Steketee, G., & Frost, R. (2013). *Treatment for hoarding disorder: Workbook* (2nd ed.). Oxford University Press.

References

Adam, D. (2014). *The man who couldn't stop: OCD and the true story of a life lost in thought*. Picador.

American Psychiatric Association. (1994). *Diagnostic and statistical manual of mental disorders* (4th ed.). American Psychiatric Publishing.

American Psychiatric Association. (2013). *Diagnostic and statistical manual of mental disorders* (5th ed.). American Psychiatric Publishing.

American Psychiatric Association. (2022). *Diagnostic and statistical manual of mental disorders* (5th ed., text rev.). American Psychiatric Publishing. https://doi.org/10.1176/appi.books.9780890425787

Bergfeld, I. O., Dijkstra, E., Graat, I., de Koning, P., van den Boom, B. J., Arbab, T., Vulink, N., Denys, D., Willuhn, I., & Mocking, R. J. (2021). Invasive and non-invasive neurostimulation for OCD. *Current Topics in Behavioral Neurosciences, 49*, 399–436. https://doi.org/10.1007/7854_2020_206

Biria, M., Cantonas, L. M., & Banca, P. (2021). Magnetic resonance spectroscopy (MRS) and positron emission tomography (PET) imaging in obsessive-compulsive disorder. *Current Topics in Behavioral Neurosciences, 49*, 231–268. https://doi.org/10.1007/7854_2020_201

Brander, G., Perez-Vigil, A., Larsson, H., & Mataix-Cols, D. (2016). Systematic review of environmental risk factors for obsessive-compulsive disorder: A proposed roadmap from association to causation. *Neuroscience and Biobehavioral Reviews, 65*, 36–62. https://doi.org/10.1016/j.neubiorev.2016.03.011

Bratiotis, C. (2013). Community hoarding task forces: A comparative case study of five task forces in the United States. *Health and Social Care in the Community, 21*(3), 245–253. https://doi.org/10.1111/hsc.12010

Browne, H. A., Gair, S. L., Scharf, J. M., & Grice, D. E. (2014). Genetics of obsessive-compulsive disorder and related disorders. *Psychiatric Clinics of North America, 37*(3), 319–335. https://doi.org/10.1016/j.psc.2014.06.002

Cambridge Dictionary. (n.d.). Squalor. *In Cambridge online dictionary*. https://dictionary.cambridge.org/us/dictionary/english/squalor

Carmi, L., Brakoulias, V., Arush, O. B., Cohen, H., & Zohar, J. (2022). A prospective clinical cohort-based study of the prevalence of OCD, obsessive compulsive and related disorders, and tics in families of patients with OCD. *BioMed Central Psychiatry, 22*(1), 190. https://doi.org/10.1186/s12888-022-03807-4

Castrodale, L., Bellay, Y. M., Brown, C. M., Cantor, F. L., Gibbins, J. D., Headrick, M. L., Leslie, M. J., MacMahon, K., O'Quin, J. M., Patronek, G. J., Silva, R. A., Wright, J. C., & Yu, D. T. (2010). General public health considerations for responding to animal hoarding cases. *Journal of Environmental Health, 72*(7), 14–19. https://www.jstor.org/stable/26328083

Clarke, C. (2019). Can occupational therapy address the occupational implications of hoarding? *Occupational Therapy International, 2019*, 5347403. https://doi.org/10.1155/2019/5347403

Eisen, J. L., Sibrava, N. J., Boisseau, C. L., Mancebo, M. C., Stout, R. L., Pinto, A., & Rasmussen, S. A. (2013). Five-year course of obsessive-compulsive disorder: Predictors of remission and relapse. *Journal of Clinical Psychiatry, 74*(3), 233–239. https://doi.org/10.4088/JCP.12m07657

Farrell, L., & Barrett, P. (2006). Obsessive-compulsive disorder across developmental trajectory: Cognitive processing of threat in children, adolescents, and adults. *British Journal of Psychology, 97*, 95–114. https://doi.org/10.1348/000712605X58592

Fineberg, N. A., Demetrovics, Z., Stein, D. J., Ioannidis, K., Potenza, M. N., Grunblatt, E., Brand, M., Billieux, J., Carmi, L., King, D. L., & Grant, J. E. (2018). Manifesto for a European research network into problematic usage of the internet. *European Neuropsychopharmacology, 28*(11), 1232–1246. https://doi.org/10.1016/j.euroneuro.2018.08.004

Fontenelle, L. F., Oostermeijer, S., Ferrieira, G. M., Lorenzetti, V., Luiges, J., & Yucel, M. (2015). Anticipatory reward in obsessive compulsive disorder: Are compulsions rewarding? *Journal of Clinical Psychiatry, 76*, e1134–e1135. https://doi.org/10.4088/JCP.14l09499

Gillan, C. M. (2021). Recent developments in the habit hypothesis of OCD and compulsive disorders. *Current Topics in Behavioral Neuroscience, 49*, 147–167. https://doi.org/10.1007/7854_2020_199

Goodman, W. K., Grice, D. E., Lapidus, D. E., & Coffey, B. J. (2014). Obsessive-compulsive disorder. *Psychiatric Clinics of North America, 37*, 257–267. https://doi.org/10.1016/j.psc.2014.06.004

Grünblatt, E. (2021). Genetics of OCD and related disorders: Searching for shared factors. *Current Topics in Behavioral Neuroscience, 49*, 1–16. https://doi.org/10.1007/7854_2020_194

Gruner, P., & Pittenger, C. (2017). Cognitive inflexibility in obsessive-compulsive disorder. *Neuroscience, 345*, 243–255. https://doi.org/10.1016/j.neuroscience.2016.07.030

Hallion, L. S., Tung, E. S., & Keuthen, N. J. (2017). Phenomenology of excoriation (skin picking) disorder. In J. S. Abramowitz, D. McKay, & E. A. Storch (Eds.), *The Wiley handbook of obsessive compulsive disorders* (pp. 806–818). John Wiley & Sons. https://doi.org/10.1002/9781118890233.ch45

Hartley, C., & Casey, B. J. (2013). Risk for anxiety and implications for treatment: Developmental, environmental, and genetic factors governing fear regulation. *Annals of the New York Academy of Sciences, 1304*, 1–13. https://doi.org/10.1111/nyas.12287

Hauser, T. U. (2021). On the development of OCD. *Current Topics in Behavioral Neuroscience, 49*, 17–30. https://doi.org/10.1007/7854_2020_195

Holtzheimer, P., & Mayberg, H. (2011). Deep brain stimulation for psychiatric disorders. *Annual Review of Neuroscience, 34*, 289–307. https://doi.org/10.1146/annurev-neuro-061010-113638

Houghton, D. C., & Woods, D. W. (2017). Phenomenology of trichotillomania. In J. S. Abramowitz, D. McKay, & E. A. Storch (Eds.), *The Wiley handbook of obsessive compulsive disorders* (pp. 817–831). John Wiley & Sons. https://doi.org/10.1002/9781118890233.ch46

International Obsessive Compulsive Disorders Foundation. (n.d.). *What is OCD?* https://iocdf.org/about-ocd

Keuthen, N. J., Tung, E. S., Reese, H. E., Raikes, J., Lee, L., & Mansueto, C. S. (2015). Getting the word out: Cognitive-behavioral therapy for trichotillomania (hair-pulling disorder) and excoriation (skin-picking) disorder. *Annals of Clinical Psychiatry, 27*(1), 10–15.

MacIntyre, M. M., Zare, M., & Williams, M. T. (2023). Anxiety-related disorders in the context of racism. *Current Psychiatry Reports, 25*(2), 31–43. https://doi.org/10.1007/s11920-022-01408-2

National Institute of Mental Health. (n.d.). *Anxiety disorders*. https://www.nimh.nih.gov/health/topics/anxiety-disorders

National Institute of Mental Health. (2022). *Obsessive-compulsive disorder*. https://www.nimh.nih.gov/health/topics/obsessive-compulsive-disorder-ocd

Nicolini, H., Salin-Pascual, R., Cabrera, B., & Lanzagorta, N. (2017). Influence of culture in obsessive-compulsive disorder and its treatment. *Current Psychiatry Reviews, 13*, 285–292. https://doi.org/10.2174/2211556007666180115105935

Patel, S. R., Simpson, H. B., & Comer, J. (2021). Innovations in the delivery of exposure and response prevention for obsessive-compulsive disorder. *Current Topics in Behavioral Neuroscience, 49*, 301–329. https://doi.org/10.1007/7854_2020_202

Pauls, D. L., Abramovitch, A., Rauch, S. L., & Geller, D. A. (2014). Obsessive compulsive disorder: An integrative genetic and neurobiological perspective. *Nature Reviews: Neuroscience, 15*(6), 410–424. https://doi.org/10.1038/nrn3746

Pittenger, C. (2021). Pharmacotherapeutic strategies and new targets in OCD. *Current Topics in Behavioral Neuroscience, 49*, 331–384. https://doi.org/10.1007/7854_2020_204

Rodriguez, C., & Frost, R. O. (2022). *Hoarding disorder: A comprehensive clinical guide*. American Psychiatric Association Publishing.

Roncero, M., Belloch, A., & Doron, G. (2019). Can brief, daily training using a mobile app help change maladaptive beliefs? Crossover randomized controlled trial. *Journal of Medical Internet Research, 7*(2), e11443. https://doi.org/10.2196/11443

Ryding, F., & Kuss, D. (2020). The use of social networking sites, body image dissatisfaction, and body dysmorphic disorder: A systematic review of psychological research. *Psychology of Popular Media, 9*(4), 412–435. https://doi.org/10.1037/ppm0000264

Simpson, H. B., Van Den Heuvel, O. A., Miguel, E. C., Reddy, Y. C., Stein, D. J., Lewis-Fernández, R., Shavitt, R. G., Lochner, C., Pouwels, P. J. W., Narayanawamy, J. C., Venkatasubramanian, G., Hezel, D. M., Vriend, C., Batistuzzo, M. C., Hoexter, M. Q., de Joode, N. T., Costa, D. L., de Mathis, M. A., Sheshachala, K., . . . Wall, M. (2020). Toward identifying reproducible brain signatures of obsessive-compulsive profiles: Rationale and methods for a new global initiative. *BioMed Central Psychiatry, 20*(1), 1–14. https://doi.org/10.1186/s12888-020-2439-2

Siu, B. W. M., Lam, C., & Chan, W. (2012). Pattern and determinants of burden in Chinese families of adults with obsessive-compulsive disorder. *Journal of Anxiety Disorders, 26,* 252–257. https://doi.org/10.1016/j.janxdis.2011.11.008

Snorrason, I., Berlin, G., & Lee, H. (2015). Optimizing psychological interventions for trichotillomania (hair-pulling disorder): An update on current empirical status. *Psychology Research and Behavior Management, 8,* 105–113. https://doi.org/10.2147/PRBM.S53977

Soriano-Mas, C. (2021). Functional brain imaging and OCD. *Current Topics in Behavioral Neuroscience, 49,* 269–300. https://doi.org/10.1007/7854_2020_203

Spear, S. N. (2014). "Friendly Visitor": An occupational therapist's experience of supporting a person with compulsive hoarding disorder. *OT Practice, 19*(4), 16–19.

Strong, S., Federico, J., Banks, R., & Williams, C. (2019). A collaborative model for managing animal hoarding cases. *Journal of Applied Animal Welfare Science, 22*(3), 267–278. https://doi.org/10.1080/10888705.2018.1490183

Swedo, S. E. (2002). Pediatric autoimmune neuropsychiatric disorders associated with streptococcal infections (PANDAS). *Molecular Psychiatry, 7*(2), S24–S25. https://doi.org/10.1038/sj.mp.4001170

Vaghi, M. M. (2021). Neurocognitive endophenotypes of OCD. *Current Topics in Behavioral Neuroscience, 49,* 97–124. https://doi.org/10.1007/7854_2020_197

Vaingankar, J. A., Chang, S., Chong, S. A., Samari, E., Jeyagurunathan, A., Devi, F., Wei, K., Tan, W. M., Chong, R., Ye, P., Lim, L. L., Babjee, R., & Subramaniam, M. (2022). Service providers' perspectives on hoarding management in the community in Singapore. *Singapore Medical Journal, 63*(7), 409–414. https://doi.org/10.11622/smedj.2021005

Van Noppen, B. (2010). *Obsessive compulsive personality disorder (OCPD) fact sheet.* International OCD Foundation. https://iocdf.org/wp-content/uploads/2014/10/OCPD-Fact-Sheet.pdf

Vats, T., Fineberg, N. A., & Hollander, E. (2021). The future of obsessive-compulsive spectrum disorders: A research perspective. *Current Topics in Behavioral Neuroscience, 49,* 461–477. https://doi.org/10.1007/7854_2020_208

Veltman, D. J. (2021). Structural imaging in OCD. *Current Topics in Behavioral Neuroscience, 49,* 201–229. https://doi.org/10.1007/7854_2020_209

Wegner, D. M. (1989). *White bears and other unwanted thoughts: Suppression, obsession, and the psychology of mental control.* Penguin Press.

Williams, M. T. (2020). The OCD-racism connection and its impact on people of color. *Psychology Today.* https://www.psychologytoday.com/ca/blog/culturally-speaking/202009/the-ocd-racism-connection-and-impact-people-color

Williams, M. T., Chapman, L. K., Simms, J. V., & Tellawi, G. (2017). Cross-cultural phenomenology in obsessive-compulsive disorder. In J. S. Abramowitz, D. McKay, & E. A. Storch (Eds.), *The Wiley handbook of obsessive compulsive disorders* (pp. 56–74). John Wiley & Sons. https://doi.org/10.1002/9781118890233.ch4

Williams, M. T., Taylor, R. J., George, J. R., Schlaudt, V. A., Ifatunji, M. A., & Chatters, L. M. (2021). Correlates of obsessive-compulsive symptoms among Black Caribbean Americans. *International Journal of Mental Health, 50*(1), 53–77. https://doi.org/10.1080/00207411.2020.1826261

Williams, M. T., Taylor, R. J., Mouzon, D. M., Oshin, L. A., Himle, J. A., & Chatters, L. M. (2017). Discrimination and symptoms of obsessive-compulsive disorder among African Americans. *The American Journal of Orthopsychiatry, 87*(6), 636–645. https://doi.org/10.1037/ort0000285

Woods, D. W., Flessner, C. A., Franklin, M. E., Keuthen, N. J., Goodwin, R. D., Stein, D. J., & Walther, M. R. (2006). The Trichotillomania Impact Project (TIP): Exploring phenomenology, functional impairment, and treatment utilization. *Journal of Clinical Psychiatry, 67*(12), 1877–1888. https://doi.org/10.4088/jcp.v67n1207

World Health Organization. (2015). *Public health implications of excessive use of the internet, computers, smartphones and similar electronic devices: Meeting report.* Main Meeting Hall, Foundation for Promotion of Cancer Research, National Cancer Research Centre, Tokyo, Japan, 27–29 August 2014. Author.

Yang, S. (2022, June). *Obsessive-compulsive disorder: A general overview.* 8th International Conference on Humanities and Social Science Research (ICHSSR 2022; pp. 2056–2060). Atlantis Press. https://doi.org/10.2991/assehr.k.220504.371

Personality Disorders

Nadine Larivière

In many ways, all people share a common humanity—human body, minds, thoughts, and feelings. In other ways, each person is wholly unique, and no two people can ever have the same experience of life. One's perspectives and interpretations of life events are unique and distinct. Personality is about each person's humanness. Just as people differ in their physical traits, they differ in mental and behavioral traits. There is a wide range of differences in thinking, feeling, and acting. A person's personality reflects their set of enduring dispositions regarding how they think, feel, and act. Personality encompasses nearly every aspect of the human experience: intrapersonal and interpersonal relationships, occupational choices, and modes of functioning. An individual's personality can greatly impact their mental state, self-esteem, general sense of well-being, and overall satisfaction with life (Doughty & Brown, 2019).

This chapter describes current conceptualizations of personality and personality disorders. The specific personality disorders identified in the *Diagnostic and Statistical Manual of Mental Disorders,* Fifth Edition, Text Revision (*DSM-5-TR;* American Psychiatric Association [APA], 2022) are explained, along with the current thinking related to the etiology of these conditions. Also addressed in this chapter, and of particular importance to occupational therapy practitioners (OTPs), is the impact of the personality disorders on occupational participation in different areas of life.

By understanding personality disorders, OTPs are more likely to ensure that persons with personality disorders receive the respect and services they deserve. By understanding the underlying dynamics of personality disorders, OTPs can promote improved treatment outcomes through the building of therapeutic alliances.

Personality

Every person possesses traits and dispositions that they develop from birth, and which will change as life moves onward. The ways in which individuals perceive themselves, their occupations, and the social world are all part of their **personality**.

The American Psychological Association's *Dictionary of Psychology* defines personality as:

> The enduring configuration of characteristics and behaviors that comprises an individual's unique adjustment to life, including major traits, interests, drives, values, self-concept, abilities,

and emotional patterns. Personality is generally viewed as a complex, dynamic integration or totality shaped by many forces, including hereditary and constitutional tendencies; physical maturation; early training; identification with significant individuals and groups; culturally conditioned values and roles; and critical experiences and relationships. (https://dictionary.apa.org/personality)

It is now known that personality traits evident in childhood stabilize throughout life beyond age 30. Such traits are roughly 50% heritable (demonstrated in twin studies), and the remainder can be linked to individuals' unique experiences and how their genetic makeup interacts with the environment. Genetic factors and environmental constancies probably underpin the continuity of personality, whereas changing environmental effects implies plasticity (Newton-Howes et al., 2015). For many years, research examining personality development and studies on personality disorders evolved in parallel, but there is now a growing integrative orientation (Newton-Howes et al., 2015).

An important theory that served as a bridge is the Five-Factor Theory of Personality (big five model) by McCrae and Costa (2008). According to this model, personality is composed of five basic tendencies, endogenous dispositions that are completely uncoupled from environmental influences: (1) neuroticism (negative affectivity, such as anxiety or hostility); (2) extraversion (e.g., assertiveness, excitement seeking); (3) openness to experience (e.g., appreciation of original ideas and adventure); (4) agreeableness (e.g., altruism, compliance); and (5) conscientiousness (e.g., self-discipline, order).

The intrapersonal and interpersonal features that develop over time as expressions of these traits are named characteristic adaptations. They make up the enduring psychological core of the person, which helps the individual adapt and evolve in the environment. For example, the basic tendency of neuroticism would be manifested as low self-esteem, irrational perfectionistic beliefs, and pessimistic attitudes (characteristic adaptations).

Overview of Personality Disorders

Now that personality has been explained, what constitutes a personality disorder? One view suggests a personality disorder exists when personality traits are extreme, and personality development is arrested, delayed, or derailed (Newton-Howes et al., 2015). The classification of personality disorders currently uses a categorical model wherein a person is given a single diagnostic label to describe the associated characteristics of their maladaptive personality traits. This model has existed throughout the various editions of the *DSM*. An alternative model developed by the Personality and Personality Disorder Workgroup for the *DSM-5* was presented in Section III (Emerging Measures and Models) of the manual (APA, 2013), which expands the big five traits described earlier in the chapter.

The alternative model proposes a dimensional perspective such that "personality disorders represent maladaptive variants of personality traits that merge imperceptibly into normality and into one another" (APA, 2013, p. 646). The dimensional model reflects the concept that, rather than compartmentalizing personality traits into discrete diagnoses, an individual's uniqueness is characterized by multiple personality traits of different levels of intensity (APA, 2022).

The current APA definition of a personality disorder in *DSM-5* is "An enduring pattern of inner experience and behavior that deviates markedly from the expectations of the individual's culture, is pervasive and inflexible, has an onset in adolescence or early adulthood, is stable over time, and leads to distress or impairment" (APA, 2013, p. 645).

The enduring pattern manifests in four identified areas: (1) thinking, (2) feeling, (3) interpersonal relationships, and (4) impulse control. Before a diagnosis of a personality disorder can be made, a person must demonstrate significant and persistent difficulties in at least two of these four core areas. These core features combine in various ways to form the 10 specifically identified personality disorders in the *DSM-5*. Each of the 10 personality disorders has its own list of criteria that reflect the observable characteristics associated with that specific condition. By definition, the personality disorders cause functional impairment and subjective distress that can have a strong impact on an individual's occupational participation and performance. Skodol (2005) provides detailed descriptions of these four core areas:

Cognition

Individuals who experience personality disorders demonstrate distortions in the way they think about and interpret their world, and in the way they think about themselves and relationships with others. Table 22-1 outlines examples of interpretations of the self and one's relationship to others.

Affectivity

Each of the specific personality disorders has a specific emotional response pattern associated with it. Some disorders are characterized by a lack of sensitivity or no emotional responsiveness (i.e., constrictive). Other disorders are characterized by a high degree of emotional sensitivity and intensity (i.e., excessively emotional). Others are characteristic of bouncing back and forth between two extremes: from being absolutely overwhelmed with intense feeling at one moment to feeling completely disconnected or "numb" in the next moment (i.e., labile).

For people with personality disorders, there tends to be an extreme degree and persistence of dysregulated affect. The lack of flexibility in the repertoire of emotional responses ultimately leads to problems with chronic anger, irritability, extreme anxiety, and/or lack of empathy.

Impulse-Control Problems

In the same way people with personality disorders tend to have difficulty regulating their emotional responses, they also tend to demonstrate significant difficulties with impulse control. Problems are manifested as extremes on a continuum—the poles being overcontrolled and lack of or undercontrolled impulses. Chronic overcontrol of impulses can manifest as inhibition and significantly limit one's willingness to try new things and lead to overconscientiousness or scrupulousness. Not taking any risks certainly impedes creative self-expression, problem-solving, spontaneity, and fun. In contrast, rigid and persistent undercontrol, or

TABLE 22-1 | Dysfunctional Thinking Patterns

Thinking Pattern	Description	Examples
Black-or-white thinking (also referred to as "all-or-nothing thinking")	The individual demonstrates rigid, polarized thinking. These types of thoughts leave no room for shades of gray. These thoughts do not offer the space for compromising or for considering alternatives or other possible interpretations.	"I never do anything right!" "If he doesn't say he loves me it means he hates me." "If you are right, then I am totally wrong."
Idealizing and then devaluing other people or the self	Seeing others or the self as all good or all bad	"You are the best therapist . . . that other one didn't know what she was doing" to "You have no idea what the hell you're doing—get someone in here who does!"
Distrustful, suspicious thoughts	The motivations of others are questioned, and others are seen as dishonest or harmful.	"She's only saying nice things to me because she wants me to get her a job."
Unusual or odd beliefs	Often in the form of superstitions or worldviews that are extreme	"I can predict where all my friends will go on their next vacation."
Perceptual distortion	Fleeting distortions that the person can usually eventually recognize were not factual	"I thought I heard my name called but I guess I was wrong."

outright lack of control, can manifest itself as recklessness and disregard for the needs and rights of other people.

Interpersonal Problems

Problems with interpersonal relationships are common and considered typical in all personality disorders; in fact, interpersonal problems are the most significant and defining feature shared by the disorders (Hopwood et al., 2013). It is logical that the three defining core features that were previously described (i.e., problems associated with cognition, emotional responses/emotional regulation, and impulse control) cause interpersonal difficulties. Problematic thinking, feeling, and behavior converge to create a negative impact on an individual's capacity to participate in purposeful occupations and their ability to form and maintain healthy and meaningful relationships (Wilson et al., 2017).

However, an interesting peculiarity of personality disorders is that some people with personality disorders will routinely experience difficulties in their relationships, as well as difficulties at work or school, but they do not believe that there is anything wrong. In other words, their personality traits do not appear to be causing *them* any distress; meanwhile, they are causing distress to *everyone around them* (Wilson, et al., 2017). When this is the case, the individual perceives their patterns of thinking, feeling, and behaving as "right" or "normal." It is often the other people in the individual's life who notice the person is frequently difficult to get along with and relate to. It may be clear to others that the individual has a rather narrow view of the world and has great difficulty adapting to life's ordinary challenges.

Evidence-Based Practice

Understanding the Meaning of Self-Harm

> *OTPs can encourage individuals who have engaged in self-harm to share the profound emotions behind their experience.*

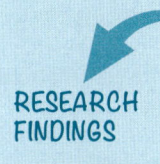

RESEARCH FINDINGS

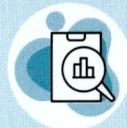

Self-harm is a common way for persons with personality disorders (it is one symptom of borderline personality disorder) to cope with their inner turmoil. It can provoke strong discomfort in health-care professionals. A phenomenological study conducted by Russell and colleagues (2010) in the United Kingdom provided understanding of the possible meanings that self-harm had for a group of four men by giving them a voice to share their experience. They were ages 37 to 58 years old, had been self-harming themselves for at least 5 years, were in heterosexual relationships, and were in regular contact with mental health services. All experienced adverse events in their childhood, such as death of a parent, conflictual relationship between parents, or abuse.

Harming oneself was an escape from reality, bringing oneself into a state resembling a trance (dissociative experience). It was also a way to communicate personal distress. Anticipation of the cutting or burning and its relief was exciting. For some, it was an act of self-punishment after having hurt someone verbally or physically and managing the guilt that followed. Finally, it was a way for them to connect with the notions of vulnerability and invulnerability to pain or death. All viewed this behavior as normal for them. Bringing into the open this intimate experience with oneself can be very moving.

APPLICATIONS

➡ OTPs need to maintain a nonjudgmental attitude.
➡ OTPs need to give space for individuals who have engaged in self-harm to share the profound emotions behind a shocking behavior. The sharing of the experience can be cathartic and therapeutic.

REFERENCE

Russell, G., Moss, D., & Miller, J. (2010). Appalling and appealing: A qualitative study of the character of men's self-harm. *Psychology and Psychotherapy: Theory, Research and Practice, 83,* 91–109. https://doi.org/10.1348/147608309X466826

Specific Personality Disorders

The *DSM-5-TR* groups the 10 separate personality disorders into three "clusters" (APA, 2022). These labeled clusters are NOT diagnoses; rather, they represent a grouping based on descriptive similarities of the disorders in each of the clusters. There is helpful and purposeful utility in doing so because the person can be diagnosed with more than one personality disorder. Research indicates there is a tendency for personality disorders within the same cluster to co-occur (Palomares et al., 2016). Following is a brief discussion of each disorder, including a summary of the core features.

Cluster A

Cluster A is commonly referred to as the "odd or eccentric" cluster and includes paranoid, schizoid, and schizotypal personality disorders. These disorders are dominated by distorted thinking. Common features for individuals with these personality disorders include social awkwardness and social withdrawal. They share links and genetic risks with schizophrenia spectrum disorders (Maass, 2019).

Paranoid Personality Disorder

Paranoid personality disorder is characterized by a pervasive and persistent distrust and suspiciousness of others (APA, 2022). Persons with paranoid personality disorder have great difficulty in establishing close relationships in different contexts. Their excessive suspiciousness and hostility may be experienced in overt arguments and recurrent complaining, or may manifest in quiet, hostile aloofness. Because of a hypervigilance for potential threats, they may act secretively and appear cold and rigid. They can be unforgiving of insults, injuries, or slights. Relationships with authority figures tend to be problematic (Maass, 2019).

In the conceptualization of paranoid personality disorders, there is a discrepancy between the outside that is displayed and the inner world of the individual. Externally, the person can be demanding, mistrustful, driven, moralistic, unromantic, and vigilant. Internally, the person is frightened, timid, self-doubting, and unable to cognitively grasp the totality of events (Maass, 2019).

People with paranoid personality disorder are diagnostically distinguished from individuals with paranoid schizophrenia in that their suspiciousness is plausible rather than psychotic in nature (e.g., their spouse may actually be unfaithful). Although they do not experience ideas of reference nor the delusions (i.e., an entire disconnect from reality) that are associated with schizophrenia, they may experience brief psychotic episodes lasting minutes to hours. Thus, although they are usually unable to acknowledge their negative feelings towards others, they don't lose contact with reality (Maass, 2019).

Schizoid Personality Disorder

Schizoid personality disorder is mainly characterized by a pervasive pattern of social detachment and a restricted range of emotional expression in interpersonal settings (APA, 2022). People with schizoid personality disorder voluntarily choose to be socially isolated. It may be a challenge for them to follow social norms and conventions (Maass, 2019). Although they may not be interested in having sexual experiences and intimate relationships, they may function satisfactorily in the work domain of life, if the type of job doesn't involve a lot of social interactions (APA, 2022). They take little pleasure in activities, although they may participate in mechanical or abstract tasks such as computer or mathematical games (Hoermann et al., 2013).

Schizotypal Personality Disorder

Schizotypal personality disorder is characterized by a pervasive pattern of social and interpersonal deficits marked by acute discomfort, reduced close relationships, and cognitive or perceptual distortions (e.g., paranormal beliefs such as being able to read people's thoughts, or sensing the presence of a person murmuring their name when there is no one in the room; APA, 2022). It is the most impairing of the cluster A personality disorders (Maass, 2019).

The cognitive and perceptual distortions distinguish this disorder from schizoid personality disorder. People with schizotypal personality disorder can express themselves with speech patterns considered vague, circumstantial, or idiosyncratic. These characteristics are distinguishable from a formal thought disorder in that the illusions or misperceptions are of real external stimuli (i.e., they are not hallucinations in which the stimuli are internal) and the conviction around the belief can be challenged through reality testing. Persons with schizotypal personality disorder have similar but less severe cognitive impairments than persons with schizophrenia in areas such as sustained attention, executive functions, or working memory (McClure et al., 2013). Similar to persons with schizoid personality disorder, they may function best in jobs with limited social interactions (McGurk et al., 2013).

Cluster B

Cluster B personality disorders are characterized as dramatic, emotional, or erratic (APA, 2022). This cluster includes antisocial, borderline, histrionic, and narcissistic disorders. Individuals with these disorders share the common feature of problems with impulse control and emotion regulation.

Antisocial Personality Disorder

Antisocial personality disorder is characterized by a pervasive pattern of disregard for, and a violation of the rights of, others, with a lack of empathy or remorse (APA, 2022). People with antisocial personality disorder demonstrate exploitive and manipulative behaviors to gain personal profit or pleasure. They frequently act on impulsive urges without considering the consequences—often placing themselves in risky situations. They are more likely than the general population to die early by suicide, accidents, and homicide. Given the action-oriented nature of persons with antisocial personality disorder, they have an increased likelihood of head injury or neuropsychological impairments (Meloy & Yakeley, 2014).

Individuals with antisocial personality disorder generally have a long history of committing crimes and may spend years in a penal institution. During childhood, deceit and manipulation are central manifestations. They engage in hostile acts such as bullying, intimidation, or hurting animals. They may demonstrate a reckless disregard for property such as setting fires. They may engage in theft and other serious violations of conduct. When this is the case, the child would be diagnosed

The Lived Experience

Alexandre: When a Mental Illness Connects People to Their Humanity

In my life journey, I experienced a major event of betrayal and abuse that generated great anguish and suffering for me, reactivating a previously buried wound. I tried to deal with it on my own for a year, but I found myself in a situational homelessness context, hanging out with people I could drink with to find relief. Then I realized that I needed help. Luckily, my parents accompanied me so that I could be seen by a psychiatrist. After a while of being treated by him, I asked the doctor what my mental illness was. After receiving the information, I learned more about my diagnosis through reading and discussion with other people: schizotypal personality disorder and schizoaffective disorder. I recognized myself so much! I used it as a way to discover and learn about myself, but I didn't want to stick to that, to be seen just through my diagnoses because that's when the stigma can come in.

I have a severe discomfort expressing my feelings with my loved ones. I don't want my emotions to show. Also, it's hard for me to trust, I'm vigilant in a group and so, obviously, it's even harder to integrate into society. I, and others like me, live in the margins. When I'm alone, the specters are there, and I must push myself very hard to reach out to others. However, my role as a peer supporter gives me an accumulation of positive life evidence to counteract rejection and trauma. And . . . I am a person with mystical and spiritual interests. To illustrate, in a book for peer support helpers, there is a representation of cars in a parking lot: a person with schizophrenia is parked in a crooked way; a person with bipolar disorder will not come and park; and the person with schizotypal disorder is in a spaceship!

Living with schizotypal personality disorder has given me a lot of understanding of myself, openness, empathy, and a human understanding that can only be learned in real life. Music has been a constant companion in my life. As Gerry Boulet (a famous French-Canadian singer) would say in his song: today I see life with the eyes of the heart!

---

with **conduct disorder**—considered a *precursor* to an antisocial personality disorder (and would be diagnosed as such when they turn 18). The highest prevalence of this disorder is in males with alcohol use disorder and from substance abuse clinics, prisons, or other forensic settings (APA, 2022).

Antisocial personality disorder has been referred to as sociopathy or psychopathy. It is suggested that sociopathy is the displaying of attitudes and behaviors that are considered antisocial and criminal by society at large but can be considered normal by the subculture or social environment where they developed (e.g., protective survival strategy in low economic rural communities; Maass, 2019). With regard to psychopathy, it includes lack of empathy, grandiosity, and shallow emotions; however, these traits, although often present, are not a requirement for the diagnosis of antisocial personality disorder (Maass, 2019). In addition, psychopathy is not synonymous with histories of criminality (Meloy & Yakeley, 2014).

Borderline Personality Disorder

Of all the personality disorders, **borderline personality disorder** (BPD) has received the most clinical and research attention. Although research has focused on BPD in adulthood, a life span perspective is now suggested to examine the clinical presentation of the features of BPD in adolescence and how it evolves in later years of life (Videler et al., 2019). For persons with BPD, their lifelong vulnerabilities are associated with mentalization, social cognition, impulsivity, emotional lability, and separation insecurity (Videler et al., 2019).

Borderline Personality Disorder in Youth

BPD typically begins in early adolescence and peaks in severity during mid-adolescence (Bornovalova et al., 2009). Teenagers with BPD commonly present with self-harm behaviors, suicidal thoughts and behaviors, affective instability, and inappropriate anger (Thompson et al., 2019). In addition, they are at a higher risk of misusing substances (Scalzo et al., 2018) and many are involved with youth protection services (Chanen et al., 2007). In their daily life, they are most likely struggling at school (Bagge et al., 2004).

Borderline Personality Disorder in Adulthood

The course of BPD from adolescence to adulthood is characterized by a symptomatic switch from a predominance of symptoms related to emotional dysregulation, impulsivity, and suicidality to maladaptive interpersonal functioning and enduring functional impairments, with periods of remission and relapse (Videler et al., 2019).

The essential features are a pervasive pattern of instability in interpersonal relationships, self-image, and affect, along with marked impulsivity in a variety of contexts (APA, 2022). People with BPD suffer from a fear of rejection, separation, or abandonment and have a marked reactivity of mood (e.g., intense anger or sadness) with difficulty regulating emotions. They may act impulsively in potentially self-damaging situations (e.g., reckless driving, gambling) and tend to have recurrent suicidal behaviors, suicidal threats, or self-mutilating behaviors, as well as chronic feelings of emptiness. Sudden changes in interests, goals, and projects reflect an instability in self-identity. Some people with BPD have transient, stress-related paranoid ideation or severe dissociative symptoms (APA, 2022).

For many years, BPD was mistaken for bipolar disorder because of similarities with regard to the presence of mood swings. However, the mood shifts for bipolar disorder change from depression to a manic state, in cycles. In between these episodes, the person will have a more stable mood. With BPD, mood swings are predominantly negative (e.g., anger, intense distress) and occur as part of the person's general

The Lived Experience

Jocelyne (Part 1)

I was diagnosed with borderline personality disorder, officially in 2022, at the age of 52. The portrait of adversity of my childhood can be seen in the 30 or so moves I made in the first 12 years of my life, attendance in eight elementary schools, the rejection of my father in the first 3 years of my life, his departure when I was at the age of 3 and his return 10 months later, the abandonment of my mother three times, and my lodging in a few relatives' homes where I always found security, a real family structure. Starting in 2017, I realized that many of my behaviors and personality traits were dependent on my family upbringing (or experienced as a child):

- my sense of humor (denigrating myself as a joke to avoid the other person doing it);
- my ability to adapt to different types of jobs (e.g., cashier, assistant manager in a restaurant, call center operator, mail clerk, French instructor, secretary, preemployability program facilitator);
- my ability to integrate a group, a team (adopt the rules of the environment);

- my ability to look for solutions (always in "emergency" mode without integrating the tools over a long period of time);
- my ability to spot inconsistencies between the speech of others and their actions (hyper vigilance and hyper mistrust);
- my difficulties to manage conflicts (the little girl inside is afraid that her opinion will be invalidated as it was by her parents);
- self-injury used as self-punishment because I felt misunderstood and angry at myself for failing to be loved and respected (feeling powerless in the face of life and others);
- my suicide attempts (from childhood to adulthood, the last one in 2021) expressed sometimes my need to be taken care of and sometimes my real will to die, because I had lost confidence in the health care system and I was simply exhausted from living.

By 2017, I was hearing the words letting go, caring, boundaries, acceptance. I am just beginning, in 2023, to gradually incorporate them into my habits. (In Part 2 later in the chapter, Jocelyne will share her experience in therapy and with an OTP.)

---

pattern of behaviors rather than in cycles (Maass, 2019). To illustrate BPD in more depth, read about Jocelyne and her life story in this chapter's The Lived Experience feature (part 1).

Borderline Personality Disorder in Older Adults

The prevalence of BPD in community samples tends to decrease with age but it remains high in psychiatric inpatient hospitalization and is growing in residential facilities for older adults (Beatson et al., 2016). There are two main myths with regard to the evolution of BPD over time: (1) Because it is assumed that personality traits remain stable throughout adulthood, BPD features are similar in later years of life (D'Agostino et al., 2022); (2) certain symptoms disappear when aging; thus, BPD is less severe and impairing (Morgan et al., 2013). However, some studies indicate that older adults living with BPD tend to experience a persistence of emotional dysregulation, intense and unstable interpersonal relationships, powerful anger, and attachment insecurity, but that there is a subtler manifestation of impulsivity (Beatson et al., 2016).

A distinctive expression of identity disturbance which is less about shifting interests, projects, and goals and more centered around regrets about life choices is common (Sadavoy, 1996). Finally, there is a heightened presence of depressive-like symptoms, feelings of emptiness, somatic symptoms, and complaints with suicide attempts that tend to be more lethal and deliberate self-harming behaviors, such as misuse of medication (Beatson et al., 2016).

Histrionic Personality Disorder

The essential feature of **histrionic personality disorder** is a pervasive and excessive emotionality as well as attention-seeking behaviors in a variety of contexts (APA, 2022).

Physical appearance is used to draw attention. People with this disorder can spend excessive time, energy, and money on clothes and grooming to impress others. Flamboyant and theatrical actions, with an exaggerated degree of emotional expression and behavior (e.g., embracing casual acquaintances with excessive ardor, sobbing uncontrollably on minor sentimental occasions, flirting openly with their new boss) are common.

People with histrionic personality disorder may use a style of speech that is very impressionistic and strong but lacking in detail and facts. Initially, individuals with a histrionic personality disorder are usually perceived as charming, dynamic, and lively. However, the important drive to get attention can lead to dramatic gestures, such as tantrums or threats, including suicidal gestures. The associated drama easily embarrasses friends and acquaintances and can lead to rejection. They may have difficulty with sincere and deep emotional intimacy. A craving for novelty and stimulation leads to frequent boredom (APA, 2022). Behind these histrionic personality traits, there are high dependency needs.

Narcissistic Personality Disorder

The essential features of persons with **narcissistic personality disorder** include a struggle with grandiosity (expressed overtly or internally); self-esteem fluctuations; intense emotional reactions to perceived threats to their self-experience; fluctuations in empathy; and relational difficulties manifested as self-serving, avoiding, and controlling behaviors (Ronningstam, 2009).

Research proposes two phenotypes of narcissistic personality disorder (Ronningstam, 2010). One profile closer to the *DSM-5* criteria comprises the competitive, arrogant, overt, grandiose, assertive, and aggressive attitudes; these individuals display self-enhancing behaviors in their interactions with others (Ronningstam, 2009). The second profile is more centered around great shyness, insecurity, and shame-ridden characteristics but an equally strong preoccupation with self-enhancing fantasies and strivings. It includes a hyperreactive response to oversights or unfulfilled expectations from others. People with this profile suffer from a strict conscience, harsh self-criticism, and feelings of guilt.

Regardless of the phenotype, persons with a narcissistic personality disorder are at risk for suicide and depression when they face a major wound to their self-esteem (e.g., loss of a job, divorce) or because of repeated disappointments regarding their unfulfilled needs for admiration, approval, and love (Maass, 2019).

Cluster C

Cluster C includes avoidant, dependent, and obsessive-compulsive personality disorders (OCPDs). Referred to as the "anxious and fearful" cluster, individuals with these personality disorders share a high level of anxiety. OCPD is the most prevalent within cluster C personality disorders in the general population and, at the same time, possibly the most disabling (APA, 2022), though OCPD is associated with educational attainment, career success, and wealth (Maass, 2019).

Avoidant Personality Disorder

The essential feature of **avoidant personality disorder** is the demonstration of a pervasive pattern of social inhibition, feelings of inadequacies, and hypersensitivity to any form of criticism (APA, 2022). Although people with avoidant personality disorder desire to make friends, they avoid activities that involve any significant interpersonal contact because of their feelings of insecurity and fears of disappointment or rejection. They feel unwelcome in social situations, regardless of whether such beliefs have any basis (Maass, 2019), and perceive themselves to be socially inept, personally unappealing, or inferior to others.

Additional traits include a withholding of inner feelings and difficulty talking about themselves. They have great difficulty with intimacy and romantic relationships because of low self-esteem. They can be reluctant to take personal risks or engage in new activities because they might cause embarrassment (APA, 2022).

In contrast to the childhood shyness that, in most individuals, tends to gradually dissipate with increasing age, individuals who develop avoidant personality disorder experience increased shyness and avoidance during adolescence and early adulthood, when social relationships with new people and romantic relationships become growingly important. There are several overlaps between avoidant personality disorder and social anxiety disorder. Persons with avoidant personality disorder tend to have more severe problems with self-esteem, mistrust, a vulnerable sense of self, less self-reflexiveness to assist with affect regulation in relational contexts, and more distancing of intimacy (Eikenaes et al., 2013). Their anxiety in social situations may not be as intense as for those with social phobia (APA, 2022).

Dependent Personality Disorder

Dependent personality disorder is characterized by a pervasive and excessive fear of separation and a need to be taken care of that leads to submissive and clinging behaviors. Synthesizing research, Bornstein (2012) suggested dependent personality disorder comprises four dimensions: (1) motivational components (marked need for guidance, help, support, and approval from others); (2) cognitive components (perception of oneself as powerless and ineffectual, coupled with the belief that others are comparatively confident and competent); (3) affective components (tendency to become anxious when required to function autonomously, especially when one's efforts may be evaluated by others); and (4) behavioral components (use of a broad array of self-presentation strategies to strengthen ties to potential caregivers).

The need to maintain important bonds with others often results in unbalanced and distorted relationships. People with these disorders often doubt themselves and self-criticize (APA, 2022). The intense fear of losing support may lead to a vulnerability for manipulation by others (APA, 2022) or, conversely, they become abusive (i.e., domestic violence, child abuse; Bornstein, 2012). Persons with dependent personality disorders face a significant risk of suicide attempts (Chioqueta & Stiles, 2000). Finally, adults with a dependent personality disorder are at increased risk for physical illness and consequent high use of health-care services (Bornstein, 2012) that can lead to an overidentification with the patient role.

Obsessive-Compulsive Personality Disorder

The essential feature of **obsessive-compulsive personality disorder** (OCPD) is a preoccupation with orderliness, perfectionism, and mental and interpersonal control at the expense of flexibility, openness, and efficiency (APA, 2022). Therefore, their self-imposed high standards interfere with task completion and meeting deadlines. Associated with this trait is self-criticism and an intolerance for mistakes. People with OCPD often display an excessive devotion to work and responsibilities at the expense of leisure activities and friendships. Organized activities are preferred when spending time with friends. Relaxing activities can be viewed as a waste of time. They may be perceived by others as rigid, stiff, serious, controlling, and stubborn (APA, 2022). In essence, this is a personality disorder that not only affects interpersonal relationships but also activity performance, occupational engagement, and life balance.

It is important to distinguish OCPD from obsessive-compulsive disorder (OCD). Despite some overlap in characteristics, they are two distinct conditions. Individuals with OCD have insight. They view their thoughts and subsequent behaviors as abnormal, unwanted, and distressing. Individuals with OCPD view their thinking as normal and beneficial. If an individual with an OCPD seeks help from a health-care professional, it would most likely be secondary to interpersonal problems rather than their way of thinking or behaving (Diedrich & Voderholzer, 2015). In addition, the two diagnoses differ in their primary symptoms. The distinguishing characteristic of OCPD is an emphasis on perfectionism and rigid ways of performing an activity.

In OCD, there are clear obsessive thoughts and compulsive behaviors that are associated with anxiety. In contrast, individuals with OCPD find pleasure in carrying out orderly and perfectionistic behaviors. OCD is described in more detail in Chapter 21: Obsessive Disorders.

Prevalence

The World Health Organization (WHO) World Mental Health Surveys is a cross-national study that examined the prevalence of personality disorders in community samples from 13 countries (Colombia, Lebanon, Mexico, Nigeria, China, South Africa, the United States, Belgium, France, Germany, Italy, the Netherlands, and Spain). Overall prevalence rates were reported, as well as rates by clusters. Rates ranged from 2.4% to 7.9% (with the average being 6.1% among the 13 countries). Clusters A, B, and C demonstrated prevalence rates at 3.6%, 1.5%, and 2.7%, respectively (Sansone & Sansone, 2011). Other studies have indicated that international data reflect prevalence rates ranging from 6.1% to 13.4%—with an average of 9.7%.

The most common personality disorder varies from country to country (e.g., OCPD in Australia, avoidant personality disorder in Norway, and schizotypal disorder in Iceland; Sansone & Sansone, 2011). Methodology as well as cultural differences in the recognition and detection of these disorders may offer some explanation as to these differences. Overall, personality disorders affect roughly 9% of the population (Quirk et al., 2016).

The prevalence rates in mental health service users can be quite different. For example, in adults in the general population, BPD has a lifetime prevalence that can range from 1% (Ten Have et al., 2016) to 5.9% (Grant et al., 2008). However, it accounts for 6% of service users in family medicine (Gross et al., 2002), 10% of outpatients in mental health services (Zimmerman et al., 2005), and 20% of inpatients in psychiatric settings (Gunderson, 2011). In the case of persons with schizotypal personality disorder, the opposite pattern is observed. The lifetime prevalence in the general population is estimated at 3.9% (Pulay et al., 2009), whereas it is less than 1.9% in clinical groups (APA, 2022). Finally, as a third example, avoidant personality disorder is prevalent in 2.4% of the general population (Grant et al., 2004) and in 14.7% of outpatients (Zimmerman et al., 2005).

Comorbidity

The presence of other mental disorders concurrently with a personality disorder, including other personality disorders, is very common. The most common comorbid conditions are mostly depressive disorders, anxiety disorders, posttraumatic stress disorder (PTSD), substance use disorders, attention deficit-hyperactivity disorder (ADHD), and eating disorders (David et al., 2016). Moreover, there is growing attention regarding comorbid physical health problems in individuals with personality disorders. A review showed a range of self-reported physical health comorbidities, notably cardiovascular disease and arthritis, from cluster A and B personality disorders (Quirk et al., 2016). Pain-related conditions (e.g., chronic back/neck problems, headache, fibromyalgia, visceral pain) are frequent in persons with BPD (Dixon-Gordon et al., 2018).

Personality Disorders Across the Life Span

Personality disorder characteristics are usually recognized during adolescence or early adult life, although in some cases the traits may be apparent in children and persist into adulthood. For a personality disorder to be diagnosed in an individual younger than 18 years, the features must have been present for at least 1 year. The one exception is antisocial personality disorder, which cannot be diagnosed in individuals under the age of 18 (APA, 2022).

There is very limited research about personality disorders later in life. They may be overlooked or underestimated because they interfere with roles associated with middle adulthood. For example, a limited social network in late life may be caused by death of family members and friends, moving to a residential facility, or transportation challenges to see friends and not because of interpersonal difficulties. A potential minimization bias of personality-related issues in older adults has also been reported (Newton-Howes et al., 2015).

Mental Health in Culture and Society

Aster Harrison

Racial Bias in Diagnosis of Oppositional Defiant Disorder—A Precursor to Antisocial Personality Disorder

Oppositional defiant disorder (ODD) is a childhood disorder defined by "oppositional behaviors," "negativism," and "defiance" (Morrison, 2023, p. 388). These behaviors could include refusing to comply with teacher or parent requests or consistently resisting rules. Although epidemiological research using standardized measures shows that children of different races show approximately equal rates of the oppositional behaviors associated with ODD, clinicians are more likely to assign this diagnosis to Black and Latino children (Ballentine, 2019; Fadus et al., 2020). On the other hand, clinicians are more likely to diagnose white children with similar behaviors with ADHD (Ballentine, 2019; Fadus et al., 2020).

There is a significant stigma associated with an ODD diagnosis and the related diagnosis of conduct disorder (CD) including assumptions that people with these oppositional disorders are dangerous or prone to criminal behaviors. This same stigma is not associated with ADHD (Fadus et al., 2020). Black and Latino children are less likely to receive an ADHD diagnosis overall and are less likely to receive medication when they do receive an ADHD diagnosis (Coker et al., 2016). Because of systemic racism, providers may be more likely to see Black and brown children's oppositional behaviors as threats. Providers might label the same behaviors from white children more empathetically, as hyperactivity or attentional issues. Usually this bias is unconscious and it can occur even for providers who do not hold explicitly racist values.

Once the label of ODD is applied, it can lead to a vicious cycle. Educators and providers may come to expect challenging behaviors from a child labeled with ODD; the child may then feel this bias from the providers and act out against this perceived disrespect. Children with ODD labels are often not assessed for other mental illness diagnoses or given proper access to care. Behaviors that are labeled as defiant may be related to unmet needs associated with other conditions, such as ADHD, PTSD, depression, and anxiety (Fadus et al., 2020). Instead of receiving proper care, children of color may instead receive only punishment for their behaviors associated with mental illness (Marrast et al., 2016).

Autistic scholar and writer Dr. Devon Price explained that "pathological demand avoidance" (an oppositional behavior pattern sometimes associated with autism) can often be logical and powerful in the face of oppressive systems (Price, 2023). This critique could be applicable to ODD as well. For example, North Dakota passed a law that prohibits educators from teaching that racism is embedded into policies, systems, and structures in the United States (Gross, 2022). If you were a Black or Latino child in a classroom taking this teaching approach, you might understandably speak up against the teacher and assert that there are indeed racist policies and histories in the United States. The racial bias associated with ODD is relevant to personality disorders, because many clinicians group ODD with antisocial personality disorder.

The *DSM-5-TR* lists antisocial personality disorder in the chapter on "disruptive, impulse control, and conduct disorders" (alongside ODD) in addition to the chapter on personality disorders (Morrison, 2023). Some clinical guides suggest "some patients may show a progression—for instance from oppositional defiant disorder (ODD) to conduct disorder (CD) to anti social personality disorder (ASPD)" (Morrison, 2023, p. 388). Research indicates racial bias in the diagnosis of conduct disorder as well (Fadus et al., 2020).

Receiving a label of ODD or CD because of racial bias in childhood could increase a clinician's likelihood to view these labeled adults' behavior as associated with ASPD in adulthood. People with ASPD diagnoses are stereotyped as violent and criminal (Sheehan et al., 2016), stereotypes that can compound with racist stereotypes of Black and Latino people. An ASPD diagnosis can make it more difficult to receive needed mental health care rather than punishment and bias (Sheehan et al., 2016).

OTPs can use this information to try to disrupt bias affecting children labeled with ODD and CD. If appropriate, OTPs could advocate for the child to receive assessment for other conditions, such as ADHD, depression, and anxiety. OTPs can advocate for people with ODD, CD, and ASPD diagnoses to receive compassionate mental health care. Moreover, OTPs could educate fellow providers about the potential for bias in diagnosis, and discuss school, clinic, or community education opportunities about racism in health care.

Gender Differences and Possible Bias in Diagnosis

Historically, certain personality disorders were diagnosed more commonly in men (e.g., antisocial and narcissistic personality disorders) and others more frequently in women (e.g., borderline, histrionic, and dependent personality disorders) because of the social representations of certain behaviors. For example, in Western cultures, if a woman brags loudly about her accomplishments, there is a tendency to associate this behavior with histrionic personality disorder, whereas a man displaying that behavior could be seen as narcissistic (Maass, 2019). A literature review conducted by Garb (2021) showed that gender bias in diagnoses was significantly present for antisocial and histrionic personality disorders but not for BPD. Grant and colleagues (2004) reported that there was no gender-specific differences identified in obsessive-compulsive and schizoid personality disorders.

In antisocial personality disorder, there is not only a gender bias but a possible race bias as well. Mikton and Grounds (2007) used vignettes analyzed by forensic psychiatrists. For the near threshold antisocial personality disorder vignette, the percentage of patients who were diagnosed with antisocial personality disorder was 58.4% for white patients and 35.5% for African Caribbean patients.

Although it is thought that these gender differences are reflective of gender-specific patterns, caution is warranted in considering social stereotypes regarding the underdiagnosis or overdiagnosis of specific disorders (APA, 2022).

Culture-Specific Information

Because the diagnostic criteria for personality disorders dictates that the individual's behavior must be outside the social norm for the culture, it is essential to consider the person's ethnic, cultural, and social backgrounds. Personality disorders should not be confused with adaptive problems associated with acculturation following immigration or with the expression of habits, customs, or values stemming from the individual's culture of origin (APA, 2022). An OTP unfamiliar with a person's cultural and religious background may view the person as demonstrating behavior indicative of a personality disorder when, in reality, it is consistent with their cultural norms. For example, religious rituals such as voodoo, evil eye, and shamanism can appear to be schizotypal for some who are uninformed (APA, 2022).

It is especially important that OTPs gain additional information from someone familiar with the person's cultural background and to discuss associated meanings with an individual that they may be seeing in therapy.

Because bias is well documented in health care regarding personality disorders, it is important to discuss stigma that many individuals with personality disorders face.

Stigma

In general, personality disorders are less known and understood by the public than other mental disorders. Typically, because the behaviors associated with personality disorders can be prone to judgment, people with personality disorders are seen as people who misbehave more than persons who suffer and need professional help (Sheehan et al., 2016). In addition, with variable amounts of available information or public speaking peers/role models, it may place a barrier for persons with symptoms to recognize they have a mental health condition and then seek help (Sheehan et al., 2016).

Stigma influences attitudes of health service providers as well. It is documented that stigma can lead to a lack of referral to appropriate services or poor quality of interventions. For example, persons with frequent suicidal threats and attempts are often not taken seriously and are instead viewed as attention-seeking; therefore, they get discharged from emergency services quickly (Sheehan et al., 2016). Finally, stigma can influence stakeholders from the insurance system (e.g., no reimbursement offered as it is not a recognized diagnosis; belief that persons with personality disorders cannot recover) or the employer system (e.g., lack of support and quick dismissal of a person; Juurlink et al., 2019).

Are there differences in the level of experienced stigma between the various personality disorders? One study showed that in treatment-seeking adults with personality problems referred to an intensive psychotherapeutic treatment, there was no impact of a personality disorder diagnosis on the experienced stigma, no effect of the number of personality disorders on experienced stigma, and no difference between different types of personality disorders. Only the paranoid type showed significantly higher stigma scores on the perceived devaluation-discrimination questionnaire (Catthoor et al., 2015).

Etiology

Personality disorders have a biological, psychological, and environmental basis. Events occurring in early childhood exert a powerful influence upon behavior later in life and contribute to the development of personality traits (Raposa et al., 2014). There is also evidence of a genetic predisposition to personality disorders (Carpenter et al., 2013).

An individual's genetics as well as their early life experiences interact in complex ways to influence the development of personality as well as a vulnerability to the development of a personality disorder. Although it may be easier to discuss these two factors (biology/temperament/psychology [e.g., attachment style] and social environment/life experiences) separately, many experts believe that they indeed cannot be totally understood independent of each other (Cloninger et al., 2019).

Genetic Disposition and Biological Factors

Genetic studies involving twins suggest that personality disorders are moderately heritable; however, the specific genes that mediate the risk for personality disorders are unknown (Reichborn-Kjennerud, 2010). Also, certain traits or symptoms, such as emotional lability, can be heritable, much more so than the disorder in its entirety (David et al., 2016). Researchers are studying the genes that regulate neurotransmitters associated with psychopathology such as serotonin, dopamine, and norepinephrine (Ma et al., 2016).

Neuroimaging studies also point to a biological vulnerability for personality disorders.

Although not all personality disorders are well studied using neuroimaging techniques, there are some consistent findings, including abnormalities with the following structures: (a) the amygdala in paranoid personality disorder, (b) the temporal lobe in schizotypal personality disorder, (c) the prefrontal cortex in borderline and antisocial personality disorder, and (d) the fronto-limbic regions in narcissistic disorder and OCPD (Ma et al., 2016).

The influence of biology on behavior is also noted when exploring temperament (i.e., inborn personality disposition). Children are born already possessing primitive personality tendencies. For example, some are born with mild, calm dispositions, whereas others have more anxious/irritable dispositions (e.g., colic). These inborn characteristics are considered genetic factors—similar to the determination of hair and eye color. The connection to genetically determined temperaments is also demonstrated when considering an infant's response to environmental stimuli; some react quickly and sharply to stimuli such as bright lights or loud noises, whereas others react slower and without much attention (Cloninger et al., 2019).

Although research may suggest the genetic relationship of some particular behavioral tendencies, these studies cannot rule out that such behaviors are transmitted through learning mechanisms (i.e., environmental influences). When the difficulties associated with personality disorders can be understood within the context of biological vulnerabilities, it may have an impact on the associated stigma of these disorders. The individual may be viewed as someone who is struggling with challenging emotions and inadequate coping skills, rather than as "intentionally difficult" (Doughty & Brown, 2019).

Psychological Factors

Different theories have been proposed to explain personality development and personality disorders. This section will explore the ones that have led to psychotherapy approaches.

From the psychodynamic perspective, Kernberg (2004) proposed a classification based on the severity of personality organization. **Psychotic personality organization** is characterized by lack of integration of the concept of self and significant others, that is, identity diffusion, a predominance of primitive defensive mechanisms centering on splitting and loss of reality testing. **Borderline personality organization** is characterized by identity diffusion, severe distortions in interpersonal relations, lack of direction in life goals and work, manifestations of primitive defensive mechanisms, lack of anxiety tolerance, difficulties in impulse control, and varying degrees of superego deterioration (antisocial behavior). Borderline, schizoid, schizotypal, paranoid, narcissistic, and antisocial personality disorder compose the borderline personality organization.

Finally, a **neurotic personality organization** includes ego strength reflected in anxiety tolerance, impulse control, effectiveness and creativity in work, and a capacity for intimacy disrupted only by unconscious feelings of guilt manifested in specific pathological patterns of interaction in relation to sexual intimacy. This group is composed of histrionic, obsessive-compulsive, and avoidant personality disorders.

Another perspective to understand personality disorders is through the notion of **mentalization**. It is defined as the act of understanding the experiences and actions of oneself and others, such as assumptions, attitudes, wishes, hopes, intentions, or plans, consciously or unconsciously (Karterud, 2015). In essence, it is "seeing ourselves from the outside and others from the inside" (Bateman & Fonagy, 2016, p. 5). The concept of mentalization is embedded in **attachment theory**. Thus, childhood relationships with parents influence the development of mentalization. When attachment is dysfunctional (e.g., insecure, disorganized, inconsistent), it will result in problems in emotion regulation, attentional control, and self-control, thereby influencing mentalizing skills.

For example, in persons with BPDs, having often lived in family environments where there was neglect of meeting their basic and emotional needs, what is documented and observed clinically is that they can make quick impulse-driven assumptions, express surface judgments based mainly on nonverbal cues, and have a black-or-white type of interpretation (in other theories, this is called splitting). Persons with antisocial personality disorders may read emotions with difficulty although they appear to be very good at reading the minds of others, and they tend to be reluctant to explore their inner world (Bateman & Fonagy, 2016).

A third theory combining notions from the psychodynamic and cognitive behavioral frames of reference is the **schema theory** (Young et al., 2003). In schema theory, individuals with personality disorders have lived toxic childhood experiences where core emotional needs were repeatedly unmet (e.g., secure attachments to others, autonomy, spontaneity, freedom to express one's needs). The child and adolescent living in this context develop early maladaptive schemas comprising memories, emotions, thoughts, and bodily sensations about the self and others.

These pervasive themes are perpetuated (unconsciously or consciously) throughout life during interpersonal experiences. Schema theory applies to persons with borderline and narcissistic personality disorders. In BPD, schemas (self-talk, thoughts, emotional memories), when activated in relationships, will be around the themes of an abandoned, angry, impulsive inner child; a punitive parent; and a detached protector (disconnecting from emotions and others). In narcissistic personality disorders, core schema themes will be about the inner lonely child, the self-aggrandizer, and the detached self-soother. This means that, in essence, they often feel profoundly undeserving of love. Because this is intensely painful, they tend to overcompensate in entitlement, competition, and grandiosity when they are with people and try to distract themselves from their negative feelings when they are alone through overengagement in activities (e.g., work, sports, gaming).

A **biosocial theory of borderline personality disorder** described by Linehan (1993) asserts that this personality disorder is primarily characterized by emotional dysregulation, which emerges from transactions between individuals with biological vulnerabilities (poor impulse control and emotional sensitivity) and specific environmental influences of repeated invalidation experiences associated with expression of emotions. Emotional dysregulation refers to heightened emotional sensitivity, inability to regulate intense emotional responses, and a slow return to emotional baseline. In this state, information processing is distorted or the person freezes. Subsequently, it leads to dysfunctional responses during emotionally challenging events, such as withdrawal or frequent impulsive behaviors and negative thoughts and feelings about self (e.g., shame, hopelessness; Crowell et al., 2009).

Environmental Factors

Biological and genetic factors can predispose an individual to developing a personality disorder, but one cannot underestimate the role of environmental factors and learning mechanisms. Babies are dependent on their caregivers to survive and thrive. The fit between the babies' temperaments and the parents' personalities appears to be particularly crucial in the development of adaptive personality traits (Emami et al., 2024).

Traumatic events occurring early in life in the family or school contexts may have a profound impact on an individual later in life and play an important role in the development of personality disorders (David et al., 2016). Traumatic childhood experiences such as physical, emotional, and sexual abuse and neglect have been identified as risk factors that increase the likelihood of developing personality disorders (Bjorkenstam et al., 2017). In fact, the effects of childhood adversity can persist into old age. One study found older adults who experienced childhood adversity were more than two times more likely to have a diagnosis of personality disorder (Raposa et al., 2014).

Other adverse experiences that may increase the risk of developing a personality disorder include death of a parent in early life, the separation or divorce of parents, the lack of caregiver affection, poor communication within a family, harsh and controlling parenting styles, exposure to extreme bullying, and being in a single parent family (David et al., 2016; Emami et al., 2024). Parental invalidation of a child's emotional experience and sexual assault appears to be particularly predictive of borderline personality traits in individuals who are genetically predisposed to the condition (Carpenter et al., 2013; Hong et al., 2011; Hope & Chapman, 2019).

The relationship between adverse childhood experiences and the development of personality disorders is complex. Although exposure to events does increase the likelihood that a disorder will develop, it is not the case that all abused, neglected, or otherwise stressed children do. This observation suggests that multiple risk factors (both genetic and environmental) combine in a specific way to challenge a child's personality development cognitively (brain's structures and thinking patterns), emotionally, and behaviorally (Crişan et al., 2023). It also suggests that various protective factors (e.g., social support and social involvement) may exist that function to limit the negative effects of trauma and adversity (Johnson et al., 2005).

Finally, the broader social context needs to be considered, although the influence remains to be studied further (David et al., 2016). Evidence for sociocultural factors in certain symptoms indicates changes in prevalence over periods of time. For example, impulsive symptoms in adolescents and young adults (e.g., substance abuse, antisocial behavior, and depression) have increased, both in North America and Europe, since World War II (Paris, 2004). In addition, social scientists have distinguished traditional societies, which have high social cohesion, fixed social roles, and intergenerational continuity, from modern societies, with lower social cohesion, fluid social roles, and less continuity between generations (Paris, 2004). From that perspective, narcissistic personality disorder may be reinforced by the rewarding of individualism and competition in modern societies but buffered in more traditional societies with strong collective values (Paris, 2004).

Impact on Occupational Participation

A few epidemiological studies have compared functioning in everyday life of people with personality disorders, other mental disorders, and the general population. It can be summarized that people with personality disorders, independent of co-occurring mental disorders, display greater impairment in social, occupational, leisure, and global functioning than those with a serious illness such as major depressive disorder (Skodol, 2018). In addition, despite educational and occupational similarities between people with personality disorders and those with other mental disorders, persons with personality disorders have more problems maintaining permanent job positions. They also have more concerns about health (Norén et al., 2007).

Among the different personality disorders, having a diagnosis of avoidant personality disorder, dependent personality disorder, schizoid personality disorder, paranoid personality disorder, and antisocial personality disorder are all significant predictors of social functioning impairment, role emotional impairment, and overall impairment because of mental health problems (Grant et al., 2004). Persons with schizotypal personality disorder and BPD were found to have significantly more impairment at work, in social relationships, and in leisure participation than persons with OCPD.

Functioning in daily life when one has a narcissistic personality disorder is much more variable. On one hand, there are some who can be socially and professionally successful, whereas others who have a concomitant mental disorder, such as an anxiety disorder, can have serious challenges in accomplishing work in a sustainable way (Ronningstam, 2009).

The modes of functioning of persons with personality disorders translate into a subjective feeling of life imbalance, an important occupational outcome. A study comparing life balance between women without mental health issues and women with clusters B and C personality disorders (Larivière et al., 2016) showed that women with a personality disorder felt significantly more imbalanced in their time spent in activities to fulfill physical health needs, have gratifying relationships, and feel competent and engaged. The women with a personality disorder perceived that they were significantly less competent to accomplish work, daily tasks, and rest. Moreover, they felt significantly less interest for all their activities. These findings indicate possible links with boredom in persons with BPD (Masland et al., 2020), narcissistic personality disorder, and antisocial personality disorder (Gunderson et al., 1991).

When boredom is felt in an enduring way and one is intolerant to be in that state, it can have negative consequences on work performance, negligence of home maintenance, physical health (being more sedentary), mental health, emotion regulation, and an increase in risky behaviors to get out of that state or avoid it. Boredom also leads to feelings of lack of meaning, direction, and purpose in life (Martin et al., 2012; Masland et al., 2020). Challenges in specific occupational roles are discussed in greater detail in the text that follows.

Work

Work is an occupation that can be both a source of suffering and a source of success, as it confronts the person with a personality disorder with their interpersonal challenges and emotional vulnerabilities but at the same time offers occupational opportunities to express personal interests, qualities, and competencies, and helps them elevate their self-worth (Dahl et al., 2017; Larivière et al., 2022). Thus, work can be an area of life in which people can overinvest their time, energy, and emotionally as it fulfills several affective needs (e.g., recognition, social affiliation, personal value; Dahl et al., 2017; Potvin et al., 2019).

When comparing overall work functioning between persons with different personality disorders, those with a cluster A personality disorder presented significantly greater degrees of impairment regarding conflicts in the workplace (except schizoid), dismissal, demotions, or unemployment (Hengartner et al., 2014). Participants with cluster B personality disorders all had significant conflicts in the workplace but only those with BPD had significant rates of dismissal, demotions, or unemployment. Finally, for participants with cluster C personality disorders, the profile is more variable. Those with an avoidant personality disorder had significant rates of dismissal or demotion and unemployment; those with a dependent personality disorder had significant conflicts in the workplace, dismissal, or demotion; and those with an OCPD only showed significant conflicts in the workplace.

Work participation has been documented in more depth for persons with BPD. However, clinically, many of the challenges they present are observed in other personality disorders. For example, common difficulties in the work environment include regulating emotions, using ineffective coping strategies to deal with sources of stress or frustration (e.g., avoidance, verbal aggression), and hypersensitivity in interpersonal situations, particularly with the manager, with whom there can be unconscious reactivation of past relations with parents (Dahl et al., 2017; Juurlink et al., 2019). In addition, people with BPD tend to choose a job impulsively, such as following a friend's suggestion (Dahl et al., 2017) and frequently change employment (Sansone & Wiederman, 2013), leading them to have unstable work histories with recurrent or prolonged periods of unemployment.

Larivière and colleagues (2022) have identified six main themes that should be the focus in interventions to support work reintegration of persons with BPD:

1. Personal representations and meaning of work
2. Knowledge about self as a worker (e.g., qualities, preferences, skills, work conditions congruent with current values and needs)
3. Self-management of internal factors (e.g., taking frequent breaks when there are signs of mental fatigue) and

external factors (office arrangement to reduce distractors) that affect cognitive, sensory and mental overload

4. Understanding better "my personal self" versus "my professional self" and the social norms in workplace environments
5. Self-disclosure of mental health conditions at work
6. Work in one's routine and lifestyle: the importance of meaningful activities outside work

In essence, OTPs working on these topics can help persons with personality disorders to consolidate identity, display interpersonal skills that foster good working relationships, empower the person in their choice of employment and ability to self-regulate at work, and support engagement in a variety of activities to function better at work and maintain employment.

Parenthood

Parenting is an important role that is viewed for persons with BPD as being very rewarding and providing a sense of meaning (Bartsch et al., 2016). The challenges that parents with BPD face in assuming their associated responsibilities in that role can be divided into four themes:

1. *Stability in positive discipline with children and in the home environment:* For example, parents may be facing stressors that lead them to cope with emotional dysregulation in inconsistent ways and send mixed messages to their children. They may be rejecting on one occasion or be overly protective. There may also be role reversal where the child takes care of a parent who is suicidal (Bartsch et al., 2016).
2. *Emotional support to their children:* Parents may have difficulty attaching to their child, disengage in child-centered play, or prioritize their needs over the child's (Bartsch et al., 2016).
3. *Communication between parents:* The interpersonal challenges and emotional dysregulation that are core dimensions of BPD affect spousal and parental communication. It may manifest in intense expression of anger both verbally and physically on the part of either parent, and can include threats when one fears abandonment from their partner (Sarkar, 2019).
4. *Negligence or abuse:* As many persons with BPD may have lived in violent environments, they may be more at risk of repeating this pattern (Laulick et al., 2016). Child welfare services are often involved (Laporte et al., 2018).

Parenting has not been extensively researched in persons with other personality disorders, but similar challenges are observed (Johnson et al., 2006). For example, one study found women who experienced some form of violence by their partners obtained higher scores in schizoid, avoidant, self-destructive, schizotypal, borderline, and paranoid personality scales (Pico-Alfonso et al., 2008).

Sleep

Insomnia is more prevalent in persons with cluster C personality disorders (Mahendran et al., 2007). People with obsessive-compulsive personality or avoidant personality features and dependence are those with significantly poorer daytime functioning because of insomnia (Ruiter et al., 2012). They seem to also be more at risk of chronic fatigue syndrome, maybe because of their anxious hyperarousability (Nater et al., 2010; Ruiter et al., 2012).

Persons with BPD also experience insomnia. Studies report that they have a longer latency to fall asleep, more time spent awake during the night, and greater dissatisfaction with sleep quality than persons from the general population (Tisseyre et al., 2022). They may also have unstable routines before sleep and irregular sleeping hours. Understanding insomnia is important as there are links with increased impulsivity and suicidal risk (Tisseyre et al., 2022; Winsper & Tang, 2014). Chronic insomnia is also associated with lower health status, negative work-related consequences (e.g., absenteeism, accidents), and overall lower quality of life (Léger et al., 2002).

Recovery When Living With Personality Disorders

The notion of recovery has been mostly studied with persons with BPD. Findings show that over a 16-year period, 60% met the recovery definition; that is, they had a score of 61 or more on the Global Assessment of Functioning (GAF) scale, worked or attended school full time, and had close relationships for 2 years, with 40% achieving an 8-year recovery (Zanarini, 2019). From a qualitative perspective, the dimensions of life that contribute to recovery are related to the person, their occupations, and the social environment. In a nutshell, when questioned, persons with BPD feel that they are in a process of discovery and learning about the self, others, and activities that resonate and provide new perspectives of life. This contrasts with recovery from a previous well state (Gillard et al., 2015; Larivière et al., 2015). The specific dimensions are presented in Table 22-2.

TABLE 22-2 │ **Lived Experience of Recovery in Borderline Personality Disorder**

Person	Environment	Occupations
• Developing self-acceptance	• Having healthy relationships	• Accomplish activities to take care of
• Becoming self-confident	• Feeling safe and cared for	oneself
• Improving emotional management	• Living in the outside world without having	• Being involved in a meaningful role
• Developing individuation by letting go of	to isolate themselves continually in order	and/or activities
the past and knowing true self: interests and	to feel safe	• Having and maintaining a job
aspirations		• Carrying out a project
• Exploring other ways of seeing life and having		• Taking responsibilities
hope for the future		• Setting short-term and long-term goals

Katsakou & Pistrang, 2018; Larivière et al., 2015; Ng et al., 2019; Shepherd et al., 2016

Treatment

Psychotherapy and medication approaches to treatment for personality disorders are discussed in the text that follows. A table of occupational therapy intervention is included in this section, with references to the chapters which discuss the intervention in detail (Table 22-3).

Psychotherapy

Earlier in this chapter, the etiology of personality disorders was discussed. Various focuses in therapy result from these different frameworks of thought. The evidence-based psychotherapies include dialectical behavioral therapy (Linehan, 1993), mentalization-based treatment (Bateman & Fonagy, 2016), schema-focused therapy (Young et al., 2003), transference-focused psychotherapy (Yeomans et al., 2015), good psychiatric management (Gunderson & Links, 2014), and acceptance and commitment therapy (Zurita Ona, 2020). These therapies all acknowledge that previous experiences (particularly those of early childhood) contribute to the development of personality disorders.

The focus of treatment varies from understanding the reasons or origins of problems to assisting an individual in improving their current level of intrapersonal and interpersonal functioning, which is accomplished by addressing the present-day struggles and difficulties and in developing a more productive life through identifying and meeting specific behavior and skill outcomes. Psychotherapy is often provided through group interventions.

Medication

Medications are available to treat the symptoms associated with personality disorders, but the results of this intervention are limited. It appears that, despite the implementation of evidence-based pharmacotherapy, individuals diagnosed with a personality disorder typically continue to experience symptoms in one or more areas within the identified diagnostic criteria (Triebwasser & Siever, 2007). Medications frequently prescribed as an adjunct to therapy may include (a) anxiolytics (i.e., anti-anxiety medications) to address symptoms of anxiety, agitation, or insomnia; (b) neuroleptics (i.e., antipsychotics) to address episodes of psychosis or, in some cases, extreme anxiety or anger; (c) mood stabilizers to address irritability, impulsivity, and aggression; and/or (d) antidepressants to treat the symptoms of depressed mood, anger, impulsivity, irritability, or the sense of hopelessness that may be associated with personality disorders.

As an OTP, it is important to know the intended purpose of any medications prescribed to assist in education. It is also essential to have an awareness of the potential *side effects* of the medications that individuals are taking as they may have an impact on the person's occupational performance.

Table 22-3 outlines which chapters provide more information on occupational therapy interventions that would be useful for individuals with personality disorders.

TABLE 22-3 │ **Common Intervention Approaches for Individuals With Personality Disorders**

Approach	Target(s) of Intervention	Brief Synopsis	Chapters With Additional Information
Dialectical Behavior Therapy (DBT)	Emotion regulation	Skills training targeting mindfulness meditation, interpersonal effectiveness, emotion regulation, and distress tolerance	Chapter 12: Emotion Regulation
Mindfulness Meditation/ Mindfulness-Based Stress Reduction/Grounding	Enhancing emotional well-being	A form of meditation practice that focuses awareness nonjudgmentally on the present	Chapter 8: Cognitive Beliefs Chapter 10: Coping and Resilience Chapter 12: Emotion Regulation Chapter 43: Serving Veterans and Service Members Chapter 45: Self-Care and Well-Being Occupations Chapter 49: Connectedness and Belonging Chapter 53: Spiritual Occupations
Family Psychoeducation	Improving family relationships	Provides education and support to family members of an individual with a personality disorder	Chapter 29: Families
Peer Support Programs	Social connectedness and support	Education, socialization, and advocacy services provided by persons with a lived experience of mental illness	Chapter 39: Peer-Led Services
Reentry Programs From Criminal Justice System (Antisocial Personality Disorder)	Independent living and adaptive coping	Skills training for independent living and development of coping skills to promote successful reintegration from the criminal justice system to community living	Chapter 40: Criminal Justice Systems

TABLE 22-3 | Common Intervention Approaches for Individuals With Personality Disorders—cont'd

Approach	Target(s) of Intervention	Brief Synopsis	Chapters With Additional Information 🤝
Work Reintegration (Interventions in Early Development)	Support work reintegration process and job tenure	DBT Skills for Employment (Feigenbaum, 2019): support acquisition of the DBT competencies applied to the work domain to tolerate distress, regulate emotions, and problem-solve. Borderline Intervention for Work Intervention (BIWI; Larivière et al., 2022): Activities to improve self-knowledge and self-esteem as a worker; learning strategies applicable at work to better manage emotional dysregulation, sensory and cognitive overload, and physical fatigue; experiences in the community to support mobilization in reintegration in a job that is congruent with current needs and preferences.	Chapter 48: Work and Volunteer Occupations

General Considerations for Occupational Therapy Practitioners When Working With People With Personality Disorders

Even in scholarly literature, people with BPD can be labeled as "difficult" and there is a tendency to caricature the underlying distress and psychologize behaviors in anyone who may be struggling in their context and life situation (Shaw, 2012). In the therapeutic context, it may lead service providers to consciously or unconsciously display invalidating attitudes of increasing impatience, punish the person, or become overcontrolling. Other emotional reactions and perceptions reported by service providers indicate a lack of empathy and poor therapeutic alliance.

For example, persons with dependent personality disorders can be viewed as anxious, clingy, and needy persons, but also compliant, conscientious, eager to please (an authority figure), and with self-awareness of their interpersonal challenges (Bornstein, 2012). With a person with OCD, they can enter therapy with a powerful need to control the situation and the therapist, show a reluctance to trust others (such as peers in group therapy), and have difficulty connecting with their inner vulnerability (Maass, 2019). A third example is with persons with narcissistic personality disorder.

An OTP can fall into several traps influenced by their countertransference (i.e., when an OTP lets past personal experience, thoughts, and feelings [unconscious and conscious] about a person's experience, perceptions, ideas, or emotions shape the way they interact with the person). Because of their attachment and self-esteem issues, persons with narcissistic personality disorder may refrain from self-disclosing, go off-topic to avoid sensitive subjects, be overly critical and blaming of others (including the OTP), and be intolerant to differences in points of view. OTPs can become annoyed, feel as if walking on eggshells, be resentful, get into a competition with the person, or be overly charmed and attracted (Weinberg & Ronningstam, 2020).

A key message is to *look beyond the manifested behaviors and emotions*. Essential professional and relational attitudes and skills include:

- Being sensitive to the life situation of the person and their life/occupational history to connect with underlying affective wounds that are possibly being reactivated. In the here-and-now, there can be a repetition of traumatic memories in the therapeutic relationship. The person's needs will essentially be around care, recognition, security, constancy, autonomy, and respect.
- Being sensitive to cognitive challenges and impairments some persons may have, particularly those with schizotypal personality disorder. Peculiarities of thought and semantic processing make it very difficult for these persons to be understood and/or communicate complex and abstract emotional and psychological states and concepts that are typically required in therapy. Therefore, it is important to tolerate and help the person tolerate these complicated and troubling experiences (Rosell et al., 2014).
- Being sensitive to the attachment challenges that permeate in the therapeutic relationships (e.g., they have rarely had occasions to be consoled when crying or have not been praised often, which may mean defensive reactions when the therapist compliments them on their progress, or they may try to prolong sessions as much as they can).
- Not taking personally negative enactments that the person with a personality disorder might express (mental health professionals tend to unconsciously represent parental figures).
- Being careful not to get into power struggles and arguments (an OTP trying to control their anxiety by becoming authoritarian).
- Being person-centered is essential: having a collaborative approach in goal setting, for example.
- Balancing between validating attitudes (e.g., active listening, reformulation) and moving forward into change

(e.g., problem-solving, exposing in therapeutic activities; Linehan, 1993).
■ Creating therapeutic contracts that clarify mutual expectations regarding engagement in therapy, attitudes, and behaviors in the therapeutic setting and relationship (David et al., 2016; Weinberg & Ronningstam, 2020).

Team discussions and validating support are essential for OTPs to acknowledge their thoughts and feelings and then, to take a step back, self-regulate, make sense of emotionally intense and complex relational situations, understand underlying issues of the person, and link with personal vulnerabilities and experiences.

The Lived Experience

Jocelyne (Part 2)

To conclude this section and the chapter, Jocelyne, who shared earlier her personal story, describes her experience with an OTP and as a peer support:

My therapy with the occupational therapist began in the fall of 2021. Our therapeutic relationship was built on a mutual foundation of listening, respect, trust, and adaptability. The occupational therapist adapted her interventions according to my needs at the time. We could spend a few weeks on the same topic. I had homework to do, for example: fill out a chart of my daily tasks to adopt a balanced routine; do a breathing exercise to welcome and name the emotion; practice confronting my intrusive thoughts by expressing them out loud; make a list of past situations in which I had not asserted myself and role play with the occupational therapist; write mantra phrases to reduce anxiety attacks when they occur, fill out decision grids, etc.

Today, I am learning to use the different tools in my toolbox: mindfulness meditation, breathing exercises, repeating caring and reassuring mantra phrases, introspective or spontaneous writing, puzzles, walking in natural environments. In short, activities that help me regain my calm and that make me feel good. I also use a safety net in which I have identified my triggers, warning signs and people or organizations to contact in case of a crisis. Another thing I have learned in my recovery is that no one is immune to falling into psychological distress. This past year, I have interacted with many peers with different backgrounds. Indeed, before reaching their low point, they had different professions: nurse, social work, teaching, communication, management, event organization, etc.

I have met different service providers in my life as a patient. The therapeutic relationships have not always been harmonious or supportive. At times, I felt ashamed, misunderstood, and especially invalidated in my emotions and my identity. On the other hand, the people who were significant in my recovery showed a benevolent curiosity about my life story, respectfully and patiently welcomed my emotions at the time, reflected my own contradictions with gentleness and humor, pushed my thoughts with their targeted questions, and gave me homework to help me move forward. Some of them showed an amazing capacity to listen and to synthesize, which sometimes disarmed me.

Regardless of the type of therapy, the therapeutic process is both evolutionary and regressive and represents a substantial emotional investment. If I had one word or piece of advice to offer to future occupational therapists, I would say: be curious about the history of each person who comes before you, each one has strengths that they probably forgot about during their psychological distress and have developed new ones that they don't realize. They are in a vulnerable position and the length of their recovery will depend on several factors: their energy, the extent of their support network, their capacity for introspection, the stage they are at in their life (are they ready to receive that message), and especially the attitude and interventions of the therapist.

Today, I wear two hats. I work as a peer support trainer. I lead workshops on service provider-person collaboration with medical and health sciences students. I bring my personal perspective to the clinical cases analyzed by the students. This experience allows me to give back to the next generation by acting as a spokesperson for my peers to our future health care professionals in the hope that the service user will be placed at the center of their care. Through interactions with students, I continue to learn about myself. In 2022, I also took a training course in peer intervention as part of a continuing education program at Laval University (Quebec City). I did my internship within an interdisciplinary team in a psychiatric hospital and then worked as a peer helper/facilitator in a preemployability program with people living with mental health issues.

This work experience was rewarding for my own recovery as well as for regaining my confidence in my abilities and enhancing my self-esteem. I realized that I had certain qualities to practice as a peer counselor: listening, empathy, respect, and curiosity. What distinguishes me as a peer support from professionals is my experiential knowledge and the symbol of hope that I represent, both for the service user and for my professional colleagues. At the time of writing, I have learned that I will soon be starting a new job as a peer support on a pan-Canadian French mental health crisis line.

I am proud of my recovery journey. Who would have thought a few years ago, during my psychotic episodes, that I would become an advocate, that I would be a model of hope and resilience and that I would share my experiential knowledge for educational purposes?

Here's the Point

- Personality traits are characteristics of an individual that persist across situations and contribute to a person's lifelong style of thinking, feeling, behaving, relating, and coping.
- To meet diagnostic requirements for a personality disorder, the identified criteria traits must be inflexible (e.g., repeatedly observed without regard to time, place, and circumstance) and must cause significant functional impairment and/or subjective distress.
- There are three types of personality disorders, described as clusters.
  - Cluster A personality disorders are characterized as odd and eccentric.
- Cluster B personality disorders are characterized as dramatic, emotional, or erratic.
- Cluster C personality disorders are characterized as anxious and fearful.
- Personality disorders are caused by the interaction of vulnerable biology and adverse environmental events.
- Difficulties with self-esteem, mentalization, problematic emotional expression, challenging interpersonal relationships, and impulse-control problems are core features of personality disorders and contribute to challenges with occupational engagement, occupational performance, and life balance in a variety of meaningful activities.

Apply It Now

1. PEO Analysis

Read the lived experiences of Alexandre or Jocelyne and complete a Person-Environment-Occupation (PEO) analysis using the template in Appendix A. Consider the following guiding questions:

- How was receiving a diagnosis helpful and potentially problematic?
- What qualities of service providers, including occupational therapists, contributed to a positive therapeutic relationship.

2. Watch a Movie About a Person With a Personality Disorder

To further assist in integrating the characteristics of personality disorders with occupational performance struggles, the reader is encouraged to choose a movie in which a person with a personality disorder is portrayed. Some movies and characters to consider include:

- *Monster (2003)*—Aileen (antisocial personality disorder)
- *The Glass Menagerie* (1987)—Laura (avoidant personality disorder)
- *Girl, Interrupted (1999)*—Susanna (BPD)
- *Prozac Nation (2001)*—Elizabeth (BPD)
- *Thirteen (2003)*—Evie (BPD)
- *Welcome to Me (2014)* – Alice (BPD)

- *Wall Street (1987)*—Gordon Gekko (narcissistic personality disorder)
- *Lars and the Real Girl (2007)*—Lars (schizoid personality disorder)

Reflective Questions

Reflect on the following questions after watching the movie:

- What pattern of thoughts, feelings, and/or behaviors does the character demonstrate that would indicate the possibility that a personality disorder exists?
- What areas of occupation are negatively affected by the character's pattern of behavior? How are they impacted?
- What performance skills are affected by the movie character's personality disorder?
- What are the occupational roles of the character? Are they impacted by the character's disorder? If so, in what way are they impacted?
- What are the character's routines? Are they impacted by their personality? If so, in what way?
- How does context affect the character throughout the film?
- Are there specific activities that are especially difficult or challenging for the movie character?
- Can you identify any coping strategies the character utilized to manage the perceived difficulties?

Resources

- Emotions Matter: Their mission is to support, educate, and advocate for people impacted by BPD.
  - They have great resources and suggestions to learn more about the lived experience of persons with BPD. https://emotionsmatterbpd.org
- National Education Alliance for Borderline Personality Disorder: Their mission is to provide education, raise public awareness, decrease stigma, and promote research on BPD.
- Disorder: Their mission is to provide education, raise public awareness, decrease stigma, and promote research. It is a great network for families. https://www.borderlinepersonalitydisorder.org
- Mental Health America. *Personality disorders.* https://mhanational.org/conditions/personality-disorder

- Provides accurate and accessible information.
- Centre for Addiction and Mental Health. (2009). *Borderline personality disorder: An information guide for families.* https://camh.ca/-/media/health-info-files/guides-and-publications/borderline-guide-en.pdf

References

American Psychiatric Association (2013). *Diagnostic and statistical manual of mental disorders* (5th ed.). American Psychiatric Publishing. https://doi.org/10.1176/appi.books.9780890425596

American Psychiatric Association. (2022). *Diagnostic and statistical manual of mental disorders* (5th ed., text rev.). American Psychiatric Publishing. https://doi.org/10.1176/appi.books.9780890425787

Bagge, C., Nickell, A., Stepp, S., Durrett, C., Jackson, K., & Trull, T. J. (2004). Borderline personality disorder features predict negative outcomes 2 years later. *Journal of Abnormal Psychology, 113*(2), 279–288. https://doi.org/10.1037/0021-843X.113.2.279

Ballentine, K. L. (2019). Understanding racial differences in diagnosing ODD versus ADHD using critical race theory. *Families in Society, 100*(3), 282–292. https://doi.org/10.1177/1044389419842765

Bartsch, D. R., Roberts, R. M., Davies, M., & Proeve, M. (2016). Understanding the experience of parents with a diagnosis of borderline personality disorder. *Australian Psychologist, 51*(6), 472–480. https://doi.org/10.1111/ap.12174

Bateman, A., & Fonagy, P. (2016). *Mentalization based treatment for personality disorders* (2nd ed.). Oxford University Press.

Beatson, J., Broadbear, J. H., Sivakumaran, H., George, K., Kotler, E., Moss, F., & Rao, S. (2016). Missed diagnosis: The emerging crisis of borderline personality disorder in older people. *Australian and New Zealand Journal of Psychiatry, 50*(12), 1139–1145. https://doi.org/10.1177/0004867416640100

Bjorkenstam, E., Ikselius, L., Burstrom, B., Kosidou, K., & Bjorkenstam, C. (2017). Association between childhood adversity and a diagnosis of personality disorder in young adulthood: A cohort study of 107,287 individuals in Stockhold County. *European Journal of Epidemiology, 32*, 721–731. https://doi.org/10.1007/s10654-017-0264-9

Bornovalova, M. A., Hicks, B., Iacono, W., & McGue, M. (2009). Stability, change, and heritability of borderline personality disorder traits from adolescence to adulthood: A longitudinal twin study. *Development and Psychopathology, 21*, 1335–1353. https://doi.org/10.1017/S0954579409990186

Bornstein, R. F. (2012). Illuminating a neglected clinical issue: Societal costs of interpersonal dependency and dependent personality disorder. *Journal of Clinical Psychology, 68*(7), 766–781. https://doi.org/10.1002/jclp.21870

Carpenter, R. W., Tomko, R. L., & Trull, T. J. (2013). Gene-environment studies and borderline personality disorder: A review. *Current Psychiatry Reports, 15*, 336. https://doi.org/10.1007/s11920-012-0336-1

Catthoor, K., Schrijvers, D., Hutsebaut, J., Feenstra, D., & Sabbe, B. (2015). Psychiatric stigma in treatment-seeking adults with personality problems: Evidence from a sample of 214 patients. *Frontiers in Psychiatry, 6*, 101. https://doi.org/10.3389/fpsyt.2015.00101

Chanen, A. M., Jovev, M., & Jackson, H. J. (2007). Adaptive functioning and psychiatric symptoms in adolescents with borderline personality disorder. *The Journal of Clinical Psychiatry, 68*(2), 297–306. https://doi.org/10.4088/JCP.v68n0217

Chioqueta, A. P., & Stiles, T. C. (2000). Assessing suicide risk in cluster C personality disorders. *Crisis, 25*(3), 128–133. https://doi.org/10.1027/0227-5910.25.3.128

Cloninger, C. R., Cloninger, K. M., Zwir, I., & Keltikangas-Jarvinent, L. (2019). The complex genetics and biology of human temperament: A review of traditional concepts in relation to new molecular findings. *Translational Psychiatry, 9*, 290. https://doi.org/10.1038/s41398-019-0621-4

Coker, T. R., Elliott, M. N., Toomey, S. L., Schwebel, D. C., Cuccaro, P., Tortolero Emery, S., Davies, S. L., Visser, S. N., & Schuster, M. A. (2016). Racial and ethnic disparities in ADHD diagnosis and treatment. *Pediatrics, 138*(3), 1–18. https://doi.org/10.1542/peds.2016-0407

Crişan, Ş., Stoia, M., Predescu, E., Miu, A. C., & Szentágotai-Tătar, A. (2023). The association between adverse childhood events and cluster C personality disorders: A meta-analysis. *Clinical Psychology & Psychotherapy, 30*(6), 1193–1214. https://doi.org/10.1002/cpp.2856

Crowell, S. E., Beauchaine, T. P., & Linehan, M. M. (2009). A biosocial developmental model of borderline personality: Elaborating and extending Linehan's theory. *Psychological Bulletin, 135*(3), 495–510. https://doi.org/10.1037/a0015616

D'Agostino, A., Pepi, R., & Starcevic, V. (2022). Borderline personality disorder and ageing: Myths and realities. *Current Opinion in Psychiatry, 35*(1), 68–72. https://doi.org/10.1097/YCO.0000000000000764

Dahl, K., Larivière, N., & Corbière, M. (2017). Work participation of persons with borderline personality disorders: A multiple case study. *Journal of Vocational Rehabilitation, 46*, 377–388. https://doi.org/10.3233/JVR-170874

David, P., Bertelli, C., & Bérubé, F.-A. (2016). Troubles de la personnalité. In P. Lalonde & G. F. Pinard (Eds.), *Psychiatrie Clinique /Approche bio-psycho-sociale, Tome 1* (4th ed., pp. 926–963). Chenelière Éducation.

Diedrich, A., & Voderholzer, U. (2015). Obsessive compulsive personality disorder: A current review. *Current Psychiatry Reports, 17*, 2. https://doi.org/10.1007/s11920-014-0547-8

Dixon-Gordon, K. L., Conkey, L. C., & Whalen, D. J. (2018). Recent advances in understanding physical health problems in personality disorders. *Current Opinion in Psychology, 21*, 1–5. https://doi.org/10.1016/j.copsyc.2017.08.036

Doughty, K., & Brown, C. (2019). Personality disorders. In C. Brown, V. Stoffel, & J. Muñoz (Eds.), *Occupational therapy in mental health* (2nd ed., pp. 169–181). F.A. Davis.

Eikenaes, I., Hummelen, B., Abrahamsen, G., Andrea, H., & Wilberg, T. (2013). Personality functioning in patients with avoidant personality disorder and social phobia. *Journal of Personality Disorders, 27*(6), 746–763. https://doi.org/10.1521/pedi_2013_27_109

Emami, M., Moghadasin, M., Mastour, H., & Tayebi, A. (2024). Early maladaptive schema, attachment style, and parenting style in a clinical population with personality disorder and normal individuals: a discriminant analysis model. *BMC psychology, 12*(1), 78. https://doi.org/10.1186/s40359-024-01564-5

Fadus, M. C., Ginsburg, K. R., Sobowale, K., Halliday-Boykins, C. A., Bryant, B. E., Gray, K. M., & Squeglia, L. M. (2020). Unconscious bias and the diagnosis of disruptive behavior disorders and ADHD in African American and Hispanic youth. *Academic Psychiatry, 44*(1), 95–102. https://doi.org/10.1007/s40596-019-01127-6

Feigenbaum, J. D. (2019). Dialectical behavioural therapy skills for employment. In M. A. Swales (Ed.), *The Oxford handbook of dialectical behaviour therapy* (pp. 735–768). Oxford University Press.

Garb, H. N. (2021). Race bias and gender bias in the diagnosis of psychological disorders. *Clinical Psychological Review, 90*, 102087. https://doi.org/10.1016/j.cpr.2021.102087

Gillard, S., Turner, K., & Neffgen, M. (2015). Understanding recovery in the context of lived experience of personality disorders: A collaborative, qualitative research study. *BMC Psychiatry, 15*, 1–13. https://doi.org/10.1186/s12888-015-0572-0

Grant, B. F., Chou, S. P., Goldstein, R. B., Huang, B., Stinson, F. S., Saha, T. D., Smith, S. M., Dawson, D. A., Pulay, A. J., Pickering, R. P., & Ruan, W. J. (2008). Prevalence, correlates, disability, and comorbidity of *DSM-IV* borderline personality disorder: Results from the Wave 2 National Epidemiologic Survey on Alcohol and Related Conditions. *The Journal of Clinical Psychiatry, 69*(4), 533–545. https://doi.org/10.4088/jcp.v69n0404

Grant, B. F., Stinson, F. S., Dawson, D. A., Chou, P., Ruan, J., & Pickering, R. P. (2004). Co-occurrence of 12-month alcohol and drug use disorders and personality disorder in the United States: Results from the National Epidemiologic Survey on Alcohol and Related Conditions. *Archives of General Psychiatry, 61*, 361–368. https://doi.org/10.1001/archpsyc.61.4.361

Gross, R., Olfson, M., Gameroff, M., Shea, S., Feder, A., Fuentes, M., Lantigua, R., & Weissman, M. M. (2002). Borderline personality disorder in primary care. *Archives of Internal Medicine, 162*(1), 53–60. https://doi.org/10.1001/archinte.162.1.53

Gross, T. (2022, February 3). *From slavery to socialism, new legislation restricts what teachers can discuss*. NPR. https://www.npr.org/2022/02/03/1077878538/legislation-restricts-what-teachers-can-discuss

Gunderson, J. G. (2011). Clinical practice. Borderline personality disorder. *The New England Journal of Medicine, 364*(21), 2037–2042. https://doi.org/10.1056/NEJMcp1007358

Gunderson, J. G., & Links, P. (2014). *Handbook of good psychiatric management for borderline personality disorder*. American Psychiatric Publishing.

Gunderson, J. G., Zanarini, M. C., & Kisiel, C. L. (1991). Borderline personality disorder: A review of data on *DSM-III–R* descriptions.

Journal of Personality Disorders, 5(4), 340–352. https://doi.org/10.1521/pedi.1991.5.4.340

Hengartner, M. P., Müller, M., Rodgers, S., Rössler, W., & Ajdacic-Gross, V. (2014). Occupational functioning and work impairment in association with personality disorder trait-scores. *Social Psychiatry and Psychiatric Epidemiology, 49,* 327–335. https://doi.org/10.1007/s00127-013-0739-2

Hong, P. Y., Ilardi, S. S., & Lishner, D. A. (2011). The aftermath of trauma: The impact of perceived and anticipated invalidation of childhood sexual abuse on borderline symptomatology. *Psychological Trauma: Theory, Research, Practice, and Policy, 3*(4), 360–368. https://doi.org/10.1037/a0021261

Hope, N. H., & Chapman, A. L. (2019). Difficulties regulating emotions mediates the associations of parental psychological control and emotion invalidation with borderline personality features. *Personality Disorders: Theory, Research, and Treatment, 10*(3), 267–274. https://doi.org/10.1037/per0000316

Hopwood, C. J., Wright, A. G. C., Ansell, E. B., & Pincus, A. L. (2013). The interpersonal core of personality pathology. *Journal of Personality Disorders, 27,* 270–295. https://doi.org/10.1521/pedi.2013.27.3.270

Johnson, J. G., Bromley, E., & McGeoch, P. G. (2005). The role of childhood experiences in the development of adaptive and maladaptive personality traits. In J. M. Oldham, A. E. Skodol, & D. S. Bender (Eds.), *The American Psychiatric Publishing textbook of personality disorders* (pp. 209–223). American Psychiatric Publishing.

Johnson, J. G., Cohen, P., Kasen, S., Ehrensaft, M. K., & Crawford, T. N. (2006). Associations of parental personality disorders and axis I disorders with childrearing behavior. *Psychiatry, 69*(4), 336–350. https://doi.org/10.1521/psyc.2006.69.4.336

Juurlink, T. T., Vukadin, M., Stringer, B., Westerman, M. J., Lamers, F., Anema, J. R., Beekman, A. T. F., & van Marle, H. J. F. (2019). Barriers and facilitators to employment in borderline personality disorder: A qualitative study among patients, mental health practitioners and insurance physicians. *PLoS One, 14*(7), e0220233. https://doi.org/10.1371/journal.pone.0220233

Karterud, S. (2015). *Mentalization-based group therapy (MBT-G). A theoretical, clinical, and research manual.* Oxford University Press.

Katsakou, C., & Pistrang, N. (2018). Clients' experiences of treatment and recovery in borderline personality disorder: A meta-synthesis of qualitative studies. *Psychotherapy Research, 28*(6), 940–957. https://doi.org/10.1080/10503307.2016.1277040

Kernberg, O. F. (2004). Borderline personality disorder and borderline personality organization: Psychopathology and psychotherapy. In J. J. Magnavita (Ed.), *Handbook of personality disorders: Theory and practice* (pp. 92–119). John Wiley & Sons.

Laporte, L., Paris, J., & Zelkowitz, P. (2018). Estimating the prevalence of borderline personality disorder in mothers involved in youth protection services. *Personality and Mental Health, 12*(1), 49–58. https://doi.org/10.1002/pmh.1398

Larivière, N., Couture, É., Blackburn, C., Carbonneau, M., Lacombe, C., Schinck, S. A., David, P., & St-Cyr-Tribble, D. (2015). Recovery, as experienced by women with borderline personality disorder. *Psychiatry Quarterly, 86,* 555–568. https://doi.org/10.1007/s11126-015-9350-x

Larivière, N., Dahl, K., & Corbière, M. (2022). Conception et modèle logique de l'intervention BIWI sur la réinsertion au travail de personnes avec un trouble de personnalité limite [Design and logic model of the BIWI intervention on work reintegration of people with borderline personality disorder]. *Revue Santé Mentale au Québec, 47*(2), 197–220. https://doi.org/10.7202/1098901ar

Larivière, N., Denis, C., Payeur, A., Ferron, A., Levesque, S., & Rivard, G. (2016). Comparison of objective and subjective life balance between women with and without a personality disorder. *Psychiatric Quarterly, 87*(4), 663–673. https://doi.org/10.1007/s11126-016-9417-3

Laulik, S., Allam, J., & Browne, K. (2016). Maternal borderline personality disorder and risk of child maltreatment. *Child Abuse Review, 25,* 300–313. https://doi.org/10.1002/car.2360

Léger, D., Guilleminault, C., Bader, G., Lévy, E., & Paillard, M. (2002). Medical and socioprofessional impact of insomnia. *Sleep, 25*(6), 621–625. https://doi.org/10.1093/sleep/25.6.621

Linehan, M. H. (1993). *Cognitive-behavioral treatment for borderline personality disorder.* Guilford Press.

Ma, G., Fan, H., Shen, C., & Wang, W. (2016). Genetic and neuroimaging features of personality disorders: State of the art. *Neuroscience Bulletin, 32,* 286–306. https://doi.org/10.1007/s12264-016-0027-8

Maass, V. S. (2019). *Personality disorders: Elements, history, examples, and research.* Praeger. https://publisher.abc-clio.com/9781440860461

Mahendran, R., Subramaniam, M., & Chan, Y. H. (2007). Psychiatric morbidity in patients referred to an insomnia clinic. *Singapore Medical Journal, 48,* 163–165.

Marrast, L., Himmelstein, D. U., & Woolhandler, S. (2016). Racial and ethnic disparities in mental health care for children and young adults: A national study. *International Journal of Health Services: Planning, Administration, Evaluation, 46*(4), 810–824. https://doi.org/10.1177/0020731416662736

Martin, M., Sadlo, G., & Stew, G. (2012). Rethinking occupational deprivation and boredom. *Journal of Occupational Science, 19*(1), 54–61. https://doi.org/10.1080/14427591.2011.640210

Masland, S. R., Shah, T. V., & Choi-Kain, L. W. (2020). Boredom in borderline personality disorder: A lost criterion reconsidered. *Psychopathology, 53*(5-6), 239–253. https://doi.org/10.1159/000511312

McClure, M. M., Harvey, P. D., Bowie, C. R., Iacoviello, B., & Siever, L. J. (2013). Functional outcomes, functional capacity, and cognitive impairment in schizotypal personality disorder. *Schizophrenia Research, 144*(1-3), 146–150. https://doi.org/10.1016/j.schres.2012.12.012.

McCrae, R. R., & Costa, P. T. (2008). The Five-Factor Theory of Personality. In O. P. John, R. W. Robins, & L. A. Pervin (Eds.), *Handbook of personality: Theory and research* (3rd ed., pp. 159–181). Guilford Press.

McGurk, S. R., Mueser, K. T., Rebecca Mischel, R., Adams, R., Harvey, P. D., McClure, M. M., Look, A. E., Leung, W. W., & Siever, L. J. (2013). Vocational functioning in schizotypal and paranoid personality disorders. *Psychiatry Research, 210*(2), 498–504. https://doi.org/10.1016/j.psychres.2013.06.019

Meloy, J. R., & Yakeley, J. (2014). Antisocial personality disorder. In G. O. Gabbard (Ed.), *Gabbard's treatments of psychiatric disorders* (5th ed., pp. 1015–1034). American Psychiatric Association Publishing.

Mikton, C., & Grounds, A. (2007). Cross-cultural clinical judgment bias in personality disorder diagnosis by forensic psychiatrists in the UK: A case-vignette study. *Journal of Personality Disorders, 21*(4), 400–417. https://doi.org/10.1521/pedi.2007.21.4.400

Morgan, T. A., Chelminski, I., Young, D., Dalrymple, K., & Zimmerman, M. (2013). Differences between older and younger adults with borderline personality disorder on clinical presentation and impairment. *Journal of Psychiatric Research, 47*(10), 1507–1513. https://doi.org/10.1016/j.jpsychires.2013.06.009

Morrison, J. (2023). DSM-5-TR* made easy: The clinician's guide to diagnosis. Guilford Press.

Nater, U. M., Jones, J. F., Lin, J. M., Maloney, E., Reeves, W. C., & Heim, C. (2010). Personality features and personality disorders in chronic fatigue syndrome: A population-based study. *Psychotherapy and Psychosomatics, 79*(5), 312–318. https://doi.org/10.1159/000319312

Newton-Howes, G., Clark, L. A., & Chanen, A. (2015). Personality disorder across the life course. *Lancet, 385*(9969), 727–734. https://doi.org/10.1016/S0140-6736(14)61283-6

Ng, F. Y. Y., Townsend, M. L., Miller, C. E., Jewell, M., & Grenyer, B. F. S. (2019). The lived experience of recovery in borderline personality disorder: A qualitative study. *Borderline Personality Disorders and Emotional Dysregulation, 6,* 10. https://doi.org/10.1186/s40479-019-0107-2

Norén, K., Lindgren, A., Hällström, T., Thormählen, B., Vinnars, B., Wennberg, P., Weinryb, R. M., & Barber J. P. (2007). Psychological distress and functional impairment in patients with personality disorders. *Nordic Journal of Psychiatry, 61*(4), 260–270. https://doi.org/10.1080/08039480701414973

Palomares, N., McMaster, A., Diaz-Marsa, M., de la Vega, I., Montes, A., & Carrasco, J. L. (2016). Multiple cluster axis II comorbidity and functional outcome in severe patients with borderline personality disorder. *Actas Espanolas de Psiquiatria, 44,* 212–221.

Paris, J. (2004). Sociocultural factors in the treatment of personality disorders. In J. J. Magnavita (Ed.), *Handbook of personality disorders: Theory and practice* (pp. 135–147). John Wiley & Sons.

Pico-Alfonso, M. A., Echeburúa, E., & Martinez, M. (2008). Personality disorder symptoms in women as a result of chronic intimate male partner violence. *Journal of Family Violence, 23,* 577–588. https://doi.org/10.1007/s10896-008-9180-9

Potvin, O., Vallée, C., & Larivière, N. (2019). Meaning and experience of occupations amongst people living with a personality disorder. *Occupational Therapy International, 2019,* 1–11. https://doi.org/10.1155/2019/9030897

Price, D. (2023, March 8). *Devon Price on Instagram: "i diagnose you with anarchist disease."* Instagram. https://www.instagram.com/reel/Cpgmslhuzhb

Pulay, A. J., Stinson, F. S., Dawson, D. A., Goldstein, R. B., Chou, S. P., Huang, B., Saha, T. D., Smith, S. M., Pickering, R. P., Ruan, W. J., Hasin, D. S., & Grant, B. F. (2009). Prevalence, correlates, disability, and comorbidity of *DSM-IV* schizotypal personality disorder: Results from the wave 2 national epidemiologic survey on alcohol and related conditions. *Primary Care Companion to the Journal of Clinical Psychiatry, 11*(2), 53–67. https://doi.org/10.4088/pcc.08m00679

Quirk, S. E., Berk, M., Chanen, A. M., Koivumaa-Honkanen, H., Brennan-Olsen, S. L., Pasco, J. A., & Williams, L. J. (2016). Population prevalence of personality disorder and associations with physical health comorbidities and health care service utilization: A review. *Personality Disorders: Theory, Research, and Treatment, 7*(2), 136–46. https://doi.org/10.1037/per0000148

Raposa, S. M., Mackenzie, C. S., Henriksen, C. A., & Afifi, T. O. (2014). Time does not heal all wounds: Older adults who experienced childhood adversities have higher odds of mood, anxiety and personality disorder. *American Journal of Geriatric Psychiatry, 22,* 1241–1250. https://doi.org/10.1016/j.jagp.2013.04.009

Reichborn-Kjennerud, T. (2010). The genetic epidemiology of personality disorders. *Dialogues in Clinical Neuroscience, 12,* 103–114. https://doi.org/10.31887/DCNS.2010.12.1/trkjennerud

Ronningstam, E. (2009). Narcissistic personality disorder: Facing *DSM-V. Psychiatric Annals, 39*(3), 111–121. https://doi.org/10.3928/00485713-20090301-09

Ronningstam, E. (2010). Narcissistic personality disorder: A current review. *Current Psychiatry Reports,12*(1), 68–75. https://doi.org/10.1007/s11920-009-0084-z

Rosell, D. R., Futterman, S. E., McMaster, A., & Siever, L. J. (2014). Schizotypal personality disorder: A current review. *Current Psychiatry Reports, 16*(7), 452. https://doi.org/10.1007/s11920-014-0452-1

Ruiter, M. E., Lichstein K. L., Nau, S. D., & Geyer J. D. (2012). Personality disorder features and insomnia status amongst hypnotic-dependent adults. *Sleep Medicine, 13*(9), 1122–1129. https://doi.org/10.1016/j.sleep.2012.05.004

Russell, G., Moss, D., & Miller, J. (2010). Appalling and appealing: A qualitative study of the character of men's self-harm. *Psychology and Psychotherapy: Theory, Research and Practice, 83,* 91–109. https://doi.org/10.1348/147608309X466826

Sadavoy, J. (1996). Personality disorder in old age: Symptom expression. *Clinical Gerontologist, 16,* 19–36. https://doi.org/10.1300/J018v16n03_04

Sansone, R., & Sansone, L. (2011). Personality disorders: A nation-based perspective on prevalence. *Innovations in Clinical Neuroscience, 8*(4), 13–18.

Sansone, R. A., & Wiederman, M. W. (2013). Losing a job on purpose: Relationships with borderline personality symptomatology. *Early Intervention in Psychiatry, 7*(2), 210–212. https://doi.org/10.1111/eip.12014

Sarkar, J. (2019). Borderline personality disorder and violence. *Australasian Psychiatry, 27*(6), 578–580. https://doi.org/10.1177/1039856219878644

Scalzo, F., Hulbert, C. A., Betts, J. K., Cotton, S. M., & Chanen, A. M. (2018). Substance use in youth with borderline personality disorder. *Journal of Personality Disorders, 32*(5), 603–617. https://doi.org/10.1521/pedi_2017_31_315

Shaw, P. A. (2012, December). Borderline personality disorder in residential care facilities [Letter to the Editor]. *Annals of Long-Term Care, 20*(12). https://www.hmpgloballearningnetwork.com/site/altc/articles/borderline-personality-disorder-residential-care-facilities.

Sheehan, L., Nieweglowski, K., & Corrigan, P. (2016). The stigma of personality disorders. *Current Opinion in Psychiatry, 18*(11), 1–7. https://doi.org/10.1007/s11920-015-0654-1

Shepherd, A., Sanders, C., Doyle, M., & Shaw, J. (2016). Personal recovery in personality disorder: Systematic review and meta-synthesis of qualitative methods studies. *International Journal of Social Psychiatry, 62*(1), 41–50. https://doi.org/10.1177/0020764015589133

Skodol, A. E. (2005). Manifestations, clinical diagnosis, and comorbidity. In J. M. Oldham, A. E. Skodol, & D. S. Bender (Eds.), *The American Psychiatric Publishing textbook of personality disorders* (pp. 57–89). American Psychiatric Publishing.

Skodol, A. E. (2018). Impact of personality pathology on psychosocial functioning. *Current Opinion in Psychology, 21,* 33–38. https://doi.org/10.1016/j.copsyc.2017.09.006

Ten Have, M., Verheul, R., Kaasenbrood, A., van Dorsselaer, S., Tuithof, M., Kleinjan, M., & de Graaf, R. (2016). Prevalence rates of borderline personality disorder symptoms: A study based on the Netherlands Mental Health Survey and Incidence Study-2. *BMC Psychiatry, 16,* 249. https://doi.org/10.1186/s12888-016-0939-x

Thompson, K. N., Jackson, H., Cavelti, M., Betts, J., McCutcheon, L., Jovev, M., & Chanen, A. M. (2019). The clinical significance of subthreshold borderline personality disorder features in outpatient youth. *Journal of Personality Disorders, 33*(1), 71–81. https://doi.org/10.1521/pedi_2018_32_330

Tisseyre, M., Hudon, A., Giguère, C.-E., Vallières, A., Bastien, C., Bérubé, F. A., & Cailhol, L. (2022). Insomnie et risque suicidaire dans les troubles de la personnalité du groupe B: Une étude comparative transversale [Insomnia and suicide risk in cluster B personality disorder: A comparative cross-sectional study]. *Revue Santé Mentale au Québec, 47*(2), 113–139. https://doi.org/10.7202/1098897ar

Triebwasser, J., & Siever, L. J. (2007). Pharmacotherapy and personality disorders. *Journal of Mental Health, 16*(1), 5–50. https://doi.org/10.1080/09638230601182078

Videler, A. C., Hutsebaut, J., Schulkens, J. E. M., Sobczak, S., & van Alphen, S. P. J. (2019). A life span perspective on borderline personality disorder. *Current Psychiatry Reports, 21*(7), 51. https://doi.org/10.1007/s11920-019-1040-1

Weinberg, I., & Ronningstam, E. (2020). Dos and don'ts in treatments of patients with narcissistic personality disorder. *Journal of Personality Disorders, 34*(Suppl.), 122–142. https://doi.org/10.1521/pedi.2020.34.supp.122

Wilson, S., Stroud, C. B., & Durbin, C. E. (2017). Interpersonal dysfunction in personality disorder: A meta-analytic review. *Psychological Bulletin, 143,* 677–734. https://doi.org/10.1037/bul0000101

Winsper, C., & Tang, N. K. (2014). Linkages between insomnia and suicidality: Prospective associations, high-risk subgroups and possible psychological mechanisms. *International Review of Psychiatry, 26*(2), 189–204. https://doi.org/10.3109/09540261.2014.881330

Yeomans, F. E., Clarkin, J. F., & Kernberg, O. F. (2015). *Transference-focused psychotherapy for borderline personality disorder: A clinical guide.* American Psychiatric Publishing.

Young, J. E., Klosko, J. S., & Weishaar, M. E. (2003). *Schema therapy/A practitioner's guide.* Guilford Press.

Zanarini, M. C. (2019). *In the fullness of time.* Oxford University Press.

Zimmerman, M., Rothschild, L., & Chelminski, I. (2005). The prevalence of *DSM-IV* personality disorders in psychiatric outpatients. *American Journal of Psychiatry, 162*(10), 1911–1918. https://doi.org/10.1176/appi.ajp.162.10.1911

Zurita Ona, P. (2020). *Acceptance & commitment therapy for borderline personality disorder: A flexible treatment plan for clients with emotion dysregulation.* Context Press.

Schizophrenia Spectrum and Psychotic Disorders

Catana Brown and Adam Sakievich

The stigma associated with mental illness can be at least partially attributed to misunderstanding, and of all the diagnoses, schizophrenia may be the most commonly misunderstood. The term "schizophrenia," which is literally translated as "split mind," was coined by Bleuler, who intended to describe a split from reality (Bleuler, 1911, as cited in Heckers, 2011). However, schizophrenia is much more than psychosis. Interestingly, Bleuler was particularly sensitive to the multidimensionality of the condition and the uniqueness of each individual with schizophrenia.

One such unique experience is that of the brilliant mathematician John Nash, made famous in the movie and book *A Beautiful Mind* (Nasar, 1998). John Nash received his PhD from Princeton University in 1950, where he worked on what was to become Nobel Prize–winning contributions to games theory. His theories have gone on to make major contributions to several fields including economics and management. However, after great accomplishments, at the age of 30 Nash was tormented by hallucinations and paranoid delusions, which resulted in divorce, unemployment, and multiple involuntary hospitalizations.

During the most difficult years, Nash received much support from his sister and wife. In the 1970s, although Nash was divorced, his wife Alicia took him into her home, potentially keeping him from homelessness. Alicia believed that living at home within Princeton's mathematical community provided a beneficial environment. At the time he roamed the halls and library and was known on campus as the "Phantom of Fine Hall." He was able to get along in a setting where his eccentricities were accepted.

Eventually, Nash's symptoms abated and he began to reconnect with colleagues and started working on mathematical problems (Kuhn & Nasar, 2002). In 1994 Nash was awarded the Nobel Prize for his work on game theory. He remarried Alicia and was given a position as a senior research mathematician at Princeton University. Nash described the onset of his schizophrenia as caused by intellectual overreaching. During that time period he says his "mind was on strike," explaining that he was not thinking in a socially acceptable manner. Nash and his wife became advocates for community mental health services and were particularly concerned about their son, who also had a diagnosis of schizophrenia (Livio, 2009). Nash and his wife were killed in a tragic car accident in 2015 while riding in a taxi on the New Jersey turnpike.

As remarkable as Nash's life may be, it is not unlike the story of recovery that can be told by many ordinary people who have lived with schizophrenia. Despite the illness and the associated stigma, people with schizophrenia are creating lives characterized by hope and dreams for the future. By better understanding the illness and recognizing the uniqueness of each individual, occupational therapy practitioners (OTPs) can become facilitators of the recovery process.

Description of the Condition

Schizophrenia is a multifaceted and complex condition. Unlike phobias, in which anxiety is the core symptom, or major depression, in which the central symptom is depressed mood, it is difficult to identify specific traits that are shared by all people with schizophrenia. In fact, there is disagreement and controversy as to the cardinal features of schizophrenia and the variability in which symptoms are expressed among individuals with the condition (Tsuang et al., 2000).

Diagnostic and Statistical Manual of Mental Disorders Criteria

To meet the criteria for schizophrenia, an individual must exhibit at least two of the following symptoms for at least 1 month (American Psychiatric Association [APA], 2022): delusions, hallucinations, disorganized speech, disorganized or catatonic behavior, or negative symptoms. At least one of the two symptoms must be delusions, hallucinations, or disorganized speech. Schizophrenia is characterized as a psychotic disorder; hence, the emphasis is on these symptoms. In addition, there must be a marked decline in functioning. Schizoaffective disorder and mood disorders are exclusionary diagnoses.

These symptom criteria represent the acute phase of the illness. The psychotic symptoms of delusions and hallucinations represent one symptom dimension of schizophrenia. **Delusions** are distortions in thought or false beliefs, whereas **hallucinations** are distortions in perception. The two are often related. For example, an individual with schizophrenia can have an auditory hallucination (i.e., "hear voices"). These voices may, for example, tell the individual that they are under surveillance by the FBI, so the individual develops a paranoid delusion that there are "bugs" in the apartment and spies are all around.

According to the *Diagnostic and Statistical Manual of Mental Disorders,* Fifth Edition (*DSM-5*; APA, 2022), the condition must persist for at least 6 months, although it usually lasts for much longer. During residual periods the symptoms may be much less severe, such as odd beliefs instead of actual delusions, or the individual may only experience negative symptoms.

The symptoms of schizophrenia are often classified as positive or negative. **Positive symptoms** represent behavior that is

PhotoVoice

Adam

At my sickest the world was a surreal place where ordinary objects took on ethereal significance. At times it had a bewildering beauty to it, but it was just a phantom in the shadows leading me deeper into darkness. Now lights no longer transport me to heaven, and the earth has stopped trembling where I step. Life is less dramatic, but now I see the beauty of every day creation.

Can the symptoms associated with psychosis possess beauty or provide the individual with other positive experiences?

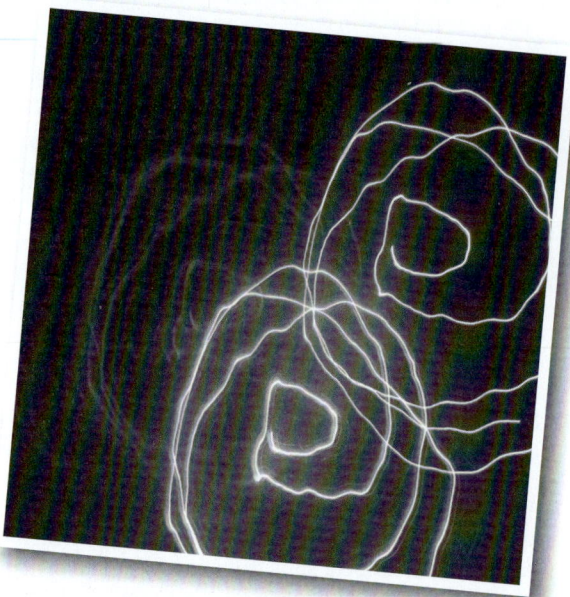

not typically present in other individuals, such as hallucinations, delusions, disorganized thinking, and disorganized behavior. With positive symptoms, perceptions and thoughts assume a richness and idiosyncratic meaning that can be disturbing or scary to the individual who experiences them, or conversely these experiences may be benign or even comforting.

Negative symptoms are the absence of typical function, such as flat affect, social withdrawal, and difficulty initiating activity. Negative symptoms have a greater impact on functioning and are related to early onset, more hospital admissions, poor outcomes, and lower quality of life (Barlati et al., 2022). In summary, the symptoms of schizophrenia include additions to and subtractions from the lived experience. The different symptom clusters are described in greater detail in the text that follows.

Individuals with schizophrenia vary greatly in their expression of symptoms. For example, one person with a diagnosis of schizophrenia may have prominent paranoid delusions, whereas another person with the same diagnosis may have no delusions, but rather a flat affect and speech that is difficult to follow. Some individuals experience significant improvement in symptoms over time, whereas others plateau or get worse. Some individuals with schizophrenia have significant cognitive impairments, and others do not. The heterogeneity of schizophrenia makes the illness equally perplexing and fascinating. Most argue that schizophrenia is not a single disorder but a syndrome or spectrum of psychotic conditions (Barch et al., 2022; Cannon, 2022).

As a syndrome, schizophrenia represents a group of symptoms that tend to cluster together in different combinations but don't have a clear cause or course of treatment. A spectrum suggests that schizophrenia is actually multiple conditions, and with more research people may be able to identify the separate diseases that compose schizophrenia.

Subtypes of Schizophrenia

The heterogeneous nature of schizophrenia has led to numerous attempts to create subtypes; this has been an arduous and frustrating endeavor because there is great variability in symptomatology, course, and outcome among individuals with the condition. The *DSM-IV-TR* listed five subtypes: paranoid, disorganized, catatonic, undifferentiated, and residual (APA, 2000). However, because the reliability and validity of the subtypes was not well established, these were removed in the *DSM-5* (Tandon et al., 2013).

Symptom Clusters

In an effort to better understand the symptoms associated with schizophrenia and to help explain the different manifestations of the condition, many researchers use statistical techniques to identify clusters of symptoms. Different studies indicate different symptom dimensions, but most symptom clusters commonly associated with schizophrenia include psychotic or positive symptoms, negative symptoms (Barlati et al., 2022), and cognitive domains (Sheffield et al., 2018). These symptom clusters suggest that, if an individual has one of the symptoms within a symptom cluster, they are more likely to have other symptoms within that same cluster.

These symptom clusters should not be regarded as subtypes; instead, the prevailing view is that the symptom clusters represent dimensions of schizophrenia (Andreason & Carpenter, 1993). That is, subtypes represent a categorical distinction, and each individual fits into only one subtype. However, from a dimensional perspective, there is overlap among the symptoms, and the emphasis is on the degree to which an individual experiences symptoms in each of the dimensions. Any combination of symptom dimensions is possible. For example, an individual with schizophrenia can have predominant symptoms in just the psychotic dimension, or they can have predominant symptoms in both the negative and cognitive dimensions. Further details about the symptoms in each cluster are provided in Table 23-1.

Psychosis as a symptom cluster is not present only in schizophrenia; it can also manifest in bipolar disorder and more rarely in major depression. Moreover, thinking of psychosis as a continuum means that it may be experienced in nonclinical populations as psychosis proneness or psychotic experiences. Approximately 20% of individuals in the general

TABLE 23-1 | Schizophrenia Symptom Clusters

Cluster	Symptoms
Positive/ Psychotic symptoms	• *Hallucinations:* a disturbance of perception. A perceptual experience that occurs in the absence of a sensory stimulus. Hallucinations can occur in any of the sensory modalities, but auditory hallucinations are the most common in schizophrenia. • *Delusions:* a disturbance in thought that involves a false belief. It is important to take into account a person's cultural and educational background in determining whether a belief is delusional. • *Thought disorder:* a disorganized way of thinking that results in odd ways of speaking, and includes features such as tangential speech (ideas that don't follow a clear train of thought), echolalia (repetition of words or phrases others have said), or neologisms (made-up words).
Negative symptoms	• *Alogia:* speech that is characterized by limited spontaneity, reduced amount, or impoverished content. • *Flat affect:* reduced intensity of emotional expression and response as evidenced through a lack of facial expression, gesturing, and voice inflection. • *Avolition:* difficulty initiating and carrying out goal-directed behavior. • *Anhedonia:* inability to experience pleasure. Individuals no longer enjoy activities that were previously pleasurable. • *Asociality:* withdrawal or avoidance of social contact.
Cognitive impairment	• *Reasoning/problem-solving:* thinking in a logical way and using existing information to choose the best course of action. • *Verbal learning:* acquiring new information through language. • *Visual memory:* ability to recall images. • *Working memory:* manipulation of small amounts of stored information to carry out a cognitive task. • *Attention:* concentrating on a specific aspect of information. • *Processing speed:* time required to attend to and respond to information.

population have some subtle psychotic experiences (van Os et al., 2009). Most people with psychosis proneness have only transitory symptoms; however, environmental factors can increase the risk for someone with psychosis proneness to develop a diagnosable psychotic disorder. Identified

Mental Health in Culture and Society

Aster Harrison

Lessons From "On Radical Empathy and Schizophrenia" by Ben G.

The chapter "On Radical Empathy and Schizophrenia" by Ben G. describes the author's experiences living in a reality that other people did not share. Through a medical lens, these experiences would be labeled as psychosis or symptoms of schizophrenia. Ben G. discusses how profoundly meaningful these states of nonshared reality were, and also the experience of losing access to that world and coming back into experiencing shared reality with others.

Ben G. proposes that people who have never lived through moments of psychosis practice *radical empathy* to connect with those who have had an experience they cannot fully fathom. The author discusses philosopher Thomas Nagel's thought experiment which proposes that a human cannot truly imagine what it is like to be a bat. As one tries to imagine the experience of being a bat, we may think about experiences of being upside down in a human body, or being wrapped in a blanket—but we cannot put ourselves in the position to really envision flying or having wings, having never experienced similar sensations. Similarly, Ben G. proposes that those who have never lived in a reality labeled psychosis cannot truly imagine what these mental states feel like. Lacking the capacity to imagine these states, providers and loved ones often write them off as merely symptoms, rejecting the meaning of the reality experienced during these times.

Ben G. writes, "To say that those years of my life correspond to a brain problem and nothing more, is to view the experience from the outside looking in. It is to reduce my own experience of myself, and at worst, to rob me of the experience altogether" (2014, p. 226).

Radical empathy starts with the practice of acknowledging that we do not fully understand, and that the "experience with psychosis is not to be compared to the experience of someone without it" (Ben G., 2014, p. 225). From this place of humility, we can get curious about the unfamiliar experience and begin to build shared reality with the person. People without psychosis can still trust the meaning and depth of the experience of psychosis, even if it is not within their realm of understanding.

This practice of *radical empathy* with experiences we cannot imagine based on our own life experiences is useful for OTPs. They will never have direct experiences of all of the things their patients have gone through. However, providers do not need to have experienced psychosis to know that that experience of reality is real and meaningful to the patient. Similarly, a provider who has not been forced to flee their home as a refugee, or been homeless, or lived through war can practice *radical empathy* in their work with people who've had these experiences. OTPs can acknowledge that they can't imagine what their bodies and minds would feel like having gone through this, but they can connect with this person, listen to their beliefs and experiences, and trust them anyway.

"On Radical Empathy and Schizophrenia" is part of a book of short stories and chapters about disability called *Criptiques*, which is freely available online.

Reference

Ben G. (2014). On radical empathy and schizophrenia. In C. Wood (Ed.), *Criptiques* (pp. 219–227). May Day. https://criptiques.files.wordpress.com/2014/05/crip-final-2.pdf

environmental risk factors include trauma, cannabis use, and urban living environments. Please read the Mental Health in Culture and Society feature on radical empathy to get a perspective of psychosis from someone who has experienced it.

Negative symptoms are distinguished as an absence of desirable characteristics and include avolition, anhedonia, asociality, flat affect, and alogia (see Table 23-1). Sometimes negative symptoms are divided into primary and secondary symptoms (Galderisi et al., 2021). Primary negative symptoms indicate that they are intrinsic features of schizophrenia. As such, they are persistent and present across the life span. Secondary negative symptoms are caused by other factors such as side effects of medication, depression, or substance use. For example, someone who is depressed may lack motivation (avolition). If treated, secondary symptoms can be ameliorated. Negative symptoms have a greater impact on function than do psychotic symptoms.

Cognitive impairments are not identified as symptoms in the diagnosis of schizophrenia spectrum disorders, but they are recognized as a core feature (Sheffield et al., 2018). Cognitive impairments tend to emerge before the development of schizophrenia and can be useful in targeting individuals who are at high risk of first-episode psychosis. The cognitive impairments in schizophrenia are relatively stable as they are similar for individuals with first-episode psychosis and chronic schizophrenia (Mesholam-Gately et al., 2009; Fatouros-Bergman et al., 2014). Impairments are found in verbal learning, visual memory, working memory, attention, problem-solving, and processing speed and affect long-term outcomes with processing speed and verbal memory particularly predictive of worse outcomes (Cuesta et al., 2022; Sheffield et al., 2018).

Discussions during the development of *DSM-5* included proposals of dimensional approaches in which individuals would be characterized by their most prominent symptoms; however, these changes were not adopted. Although there is empirical support for dimensional diagnoses, there was concern regarding how this method might be used by third-party payers (Carpenter, 2013).

However, there continues to be much interest in dimensional diagnosis for schizophrenia, including a project sponsored by the National Institute of Mental Health (NIMH) called the Research Domain Criteria, which is examining domains of functioning that might be included in a dimensional approach (NIMH, n.d.). There is much overlap in symptoms across disorders. For example, anhedonia is common in both schizophrenia and depression. The Research Domain Criterion improves transdiagnostic understanding of dual

disorders and shows promise with clinical use. Further research is ongoing to better understand the intersectionality of dual disorders (Hakak-Zargar et al., 2022).

Schizoaffective Disorder

Schizoaffective disorder is characterized by a combination of psychotic and mood symptoms. For someone to receive a diagnosis of schizoaffective disorder, criteria must be met for a mood episode (either major depressive or manic) as well as criteria for schizophrenia (APA, 2022). The mood disturbance must be present for the majority of the time in which the individual has experienced the illness. Schizoaffective disorder is now seen as a longitudinal illness and cannot be diagnosed during a single first episode of psychosis.

There is less research examining schizoaffective disorder, but individuals with the condition are generally considered to have better outcomes than individuals with schizophrenia (Jäger et al., 2004). Adam, an occupational therapist and co-author of this chapter, describes his personal experience in this chapter's The Lived Experience feature. His story includes challenges in diagnosing his condition and his own views of recovery.

Etiology

Research into the etiology of schizophrenia explores genetic factors, prenatal factors, structural and functional neuroanatomical differences, dopamine, stress vulnerability, and specific environmental factors. It is likely that biological and environmental factors interact to cause schizophrenia (Fig. 23-1).

Genetic Factors

Family, adoption, and twin studies indicate there is a genetic contribution to schizophrenia. A recent large twin study to date found a heritability estimate of 79% for schizophrenia (Hilker et al., 2018). Yet, these numbers can be misleading because most individuals with schizophrenia do not have a known relative with the condition. Furthermore, the search for specific genetic associations with schizophrenia has been frustrating. There is no biomarker for schizophrenia and what accounts for gene expression for the condition is probably diverse and subtle (Bray, 2008).

Schizophrenia is a polygenetic condition. An important study found 108 genetic risk loci for schizophrenia (Schizophrenia Working Group of the Psychiatric Genomics

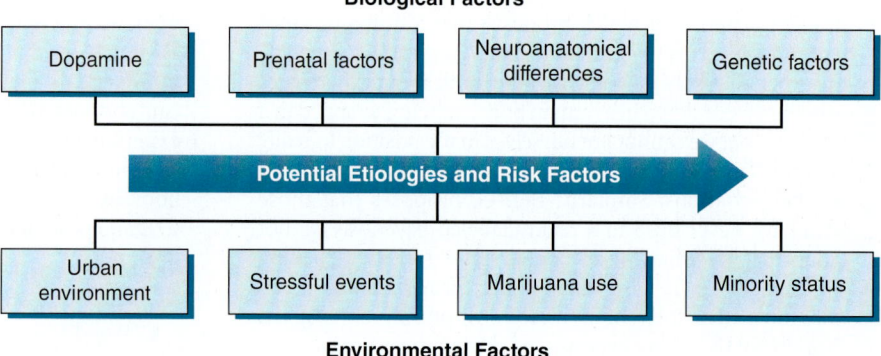

FIGURE 23-1. Research into the etiology of schizophrenia explores genetic factors, prenatal factors, structural and functional neuroanatomical differences, dopamine, stress vulnerability, and specific environmental factors. Biological and environmental factors likely interact to cause schizophrenia.

The Lived Experience

Adam Sakievich

When I'm up, I do everything I set my mind to. For weeks I have endless motivation and energy; every waking hour is spent in productive activity. I don't need to eat. I don't feel like sleeping much. I am a dynamo. People love me when I'm like this. I'm enthusiastic, dedicated, and a lot of fun. I also love *myself* like this. When I am up, I become my ideal self. I don't feel guilty or regretful. I'm good and I always have been good. I'm who I always wanted to be.

Inevitably though, I feel as though I am running forward toward my goals with a large elastic band wrapped around my waist. The other end of the band is mortared into my fears, my guilt, and my past failures. The tension grows greater and greater until everyday activities become increasingly exhausting. I grow irritable, nervous, and anxious. Finally, it snaps me backward and I crash into the dead weight of shame and fear.

All I want is to sleep, to never leave my bed or couch. I put on weight, and the thought of any activity no matter how simple or ordinary is unbearable. I cut myself off from everyone around me. Disappointing people makes me more anxious and guilty. I feel powerless to change my state, like my personal control and will has gone somewhere far away and hidden.

A few times, the elastic band has snapped, so I keep on running, faster, longer, and farther than I have ever gone. The world around me grows unrecognizable, full of strange, secretive truths that only I am privileged to glimpse. I am cut off from reality, alone in a frightening nightmare unable to be shed or awoken from. As with all nightmares, I don't know that I am dreaming. I lose myself in the growing darkness. Who I was has been erased and I don't know if I'll ever find it again. Time dilates and contracts erratically. I cannot tell the past, from the future, from the present. Only when I inexplicably wake up do I realize how very, very far gone I was.

Doctors have struggled to diagnose my illness. Some have said schizoaffective disorder, but some have said it is bipolar disorder with psychotic features. Whatever the name, when I first got sick in high school, it terrified me. It was like my house had been invaded by a large, snarling bear. The bear threatened to destroy everything I hoped for. It was a struggle to finish high school. I had to drop out for much of my sophomore year, but thanks to several teachers who went the extra mile, I was able to return. College was even harder than high school. I would do well for a semester, but the next one always seemed to end in a major crash backwards. Overall, I had to drop out three different times. Because I wasn't comfortable talking about this bear in my mind, I lost many relationships with classmates and professors when I would disappear. I was embarrassed and ashamed. I thought I was a failure, and that everyone else in my life had concluded as much as well.

My doctors helped me find medicine that helps my ups and downs happen less frequently and with much less severity. I also found that by getting enough sleep and eating well I decreased the opportunities for my life to spiral out of control. I learned to recognize internal warning signs, like racing thoughts, as indicators that I needed to slow down. When I am too low, I always try and accomplish a little every day. I've used family and friends as guideposts and supports to help me stay balanced and give me insight when I am lacking it. The bear seemed contained to a comfortably secure pen. He was even a little cuddly, a little loveable.

I was able to graduate from college, and then become an occupational therapist. Most of my career has been on the traditional hospital setting, but I also worked with another colleague to build an occupational therapy program in the behavioral health unit. During my time there, I sympathetically fielded many complaints from my client-peers such as: There is nothing to do. I can't sleep. I want to go outside for just a few minutes. I was frustrated because I had limited ability to help them. Leading a group on improving sleep felt rather futile knowing they would be inspected by flashlights every 15 minutes that night. The heavy hard chairs and thin mattresses, though safe, seemed uncannily well-suited to worsening chronic pain.

We wrote grants and got weighted blankets, rocking chairs, wireless headphones for music, but it still left many problems unsolved. Safety was a frequent barrier to our proposals. I had to live with the dissonance of what I aspired to and the constraints imposed by these restrictions. Over time, it became easier to shrug my shoulders and think, "Well, if it means keeping people safe. . . ."

A few years later I myself was hospitalized again. Now, I felt the sleep deprivation from the thin mattresses and the glaring flashlight. I suffered the boredom of endless sitting. The cameras and locked doors seemed to shout at me, "You are sick. You are broken. You are a wild thing." I could not escape the feeling that, at some level, the staff saw me as dangerous or untrustworthy, bearish even. Perhaps this was why they worried so much about safety. I worry the price of all this overly-restrictive safety comes at the cost of healing and dignity for everyone on those units.

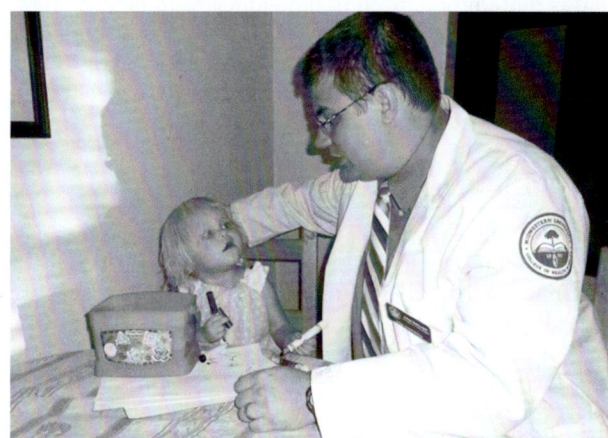

I could relate to the staff's reaction in some sense, because I too initially saw my illness as an unruly disorder, a bear. I too wanted to drive it out or cage it up, to return it to "normal." I used to think returning to normal meant not having to take meds. Then I thought it meant taking meds, but being symptom free. *Now* I understand it isn't about returning to "normal." It is about learning to live and love all aspects of myself, including my schizoaffective or bipolar self. There is no imaginary line between the illness and myself. For good or for ill, it's all just me in here. It's taken me a long time to understand that. Whether I am up or down, staff or hospitalized, no diagnosis can rob me of myself. With all its gifts and curses, strengths and risk, I am the bear.

Consortium, 2014). Furthermore, there is evidence that the genetic risk for schizophrenia, major depression, and bipolar disorder are not discrete, meaning there is no set of genes that distinguishes the different conditions (Cattarinussi et al., 2022). However, the polygenetic risk is associated with widespread cortical anomalies, further supporting the concept of schizophrenia as a neurodevelopmental process. It is likely that several genes act together to increase susceptibility to schizophrenia and that the specific genes that account for the condition may differ among individuals.

Structural and Functional Neuroanatomical Differences

Although there is no definitive neuroanatomical abnormality that is associated with schizophrenia, consistent findings arise when groups of individuals with schizophrenia are studied and compared against individuals without schizophrenia. People with schizophrenia have a reduction of gray matter (cortical thinning) and less surface area of the brain, particularly in the frontal and temporal lobes (Brent et al., 2013; van Erp et al., 2018). It appears that these brain changes occur before the onset of schizophrenia and may begin in adolescence. One theory proposes that during adolescence when normal pruning and specialization of gray matter occurs, individuals with a predisposition toward schizophrenia experience excessive pruning.

In addition to structural abnormalities, individuals with schizophrenia differ from their control counterparts in functional brain activity. One of the most often cited findings in functional brain imaging in schizophrenia is hypofrontality (Townsend et al., 2023). Hypofrontality is indicated by reduced cerebral blood flow or metabolism in the frontal lobe and is more pronounced in individuals with chronic versus first episode of psychosis and in medicated versus nonmedicated individuals. The structural and functional differences in the brains of people with schizophrenia are associated with cognitive impairments and negative symptoms.

Dopamine

The "dopamine hypothesis" of schizophrenia is one of the oldest theories related to the cause of schizophrenia. This theory was initiated in the 1950s, when antipsychotics were first used to treat schizophrenia. Antipsychotic drugs block dopamine activity and reduce psychotic symptoms. Furthermore, drugs that increase dopamine activity, such as amphetamines, can trigger a psychotic episode (Carlsson, 1988). Studies suggest that individuals with schizophrenia have an increase in dopamine synthesis, a greater presynaptic release of dopamine, and higher concentrations of the neurotransmitter at rest (Guillin et al., 2007). The role of dopamine in the symptoms of schizophrenia is unclear, but it has been proposed that dopamine dysregulation plays a role in cognitive processing and the development of delusional thinking and other psychotic symptoms (Howes & Murray, 2014; Howes & Shatalina, 2022).

Stress Vulnerability

The **diathesis stress theory** proposes that exposure to stress is necessary for individuals who are biologically predisposed to schizophrenia to go on to express the condition. There is strong evidence that environmental stressors including daily hassles are associated with the onset of schizophrenia (Tessner et al., 2011) and that impaired stress tolerance or a sensitivity to stress is associated with psychosis and a worsening of symptoms, particularly positive symptoms (Devylder et al., 2013). For individuals with schizophrenia, it is particularly important to take into account the impact of events such as a change in living situation, job interview, and chronic daily concerns such as financial problems and to provide additional supports during these stressful life events.

Environmental Factors

Environmental factors associated with schizophrenia include being part of an underrepresented group, growing up in an urban environment, marijuana use, and prenatal factors. There is a greater incidence of schizophrenia for people of color. However, for individuals who live in a community that is dense with their ethnic/racial group there is a lower risk for schizophrenia, suggesting that it is not ethnicity that increases risk but the degree to which one is underrepresented within a culture (Veling et al., 2008). Living in a community in which one feels a sense of belonging is potentially a protective factor.

Further evidence that social disconnection is a factor in the etiology of schizophrenia comes from studies that show an increased risk of schizophrenia for individuals living in cities. A study that examined urban living as a causal factor sought to determine what it was about the city that led to schizophrenia (Zammit et al., 2010). This study found an increased incidence of schizophrenia in those neighborhoods that experienced greater social fragmentation. Similarly, a longitudinal study of schizophrenia found neighborhood poverty was associated with high risk for psychosis, but social engagement reduced this connection (Ku et al., 2022). These studies suggest that creating connections among individuals at risk for schizophrenia may serve as a preventive measure.

Marijuana use also appears to play a role in the development of schizophrenia. Although the majority of marijuana users do not experience psychosis, for a subgroup of individuals there is an association (Radhakrishnan et al., 2014). Risk increases with earlier age of first use and heavy use. It may be that adolescence presents a critical period of brain vulnerability for those with a genetic predisposition for schizophrenia. In addition, marijuana use is associated with an exacerbation of symptoms, relapse, and a more negative course of the illness. Interestingly, although the tetrahydrocannabinol (THC) component of marijuana is associated with the etiology of schizophrenia, cannabidiol (CBD) appears to have therapeutic effects by improving cognitive and psychotic symptoms (Patel et al., 2020).

During the prenatal and perinatal period there is extreme vulnerability for environmental insults. A large meta-analysis of 152 studies identified 30 risk factors including very young or older maternal or paternal age, maternal or paternal psychiatric conditions, winter birth, famine or nutritional deficiencies during pregnancy, and obstetric complications (Davies et al., 2020). However, all of the risk factors had relatively small odds ratios (OR <2.0), meaning that they increase risk by only a small amount.

Evidence-Based Practice

Social Connection and Schizophrenia

Social connection can play a significant role in recovery for individuals with schizophrenia.

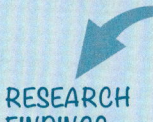

RESEARCH FINDINGS

If social disconnection contributes to the risk of schizophrenia, social connection might provide benefits. One study found that "mattering to other people" played a significant role in recovery (Pernice et al., 2017). Mattering to other people was conceptualized as being valued, being recognized by others, and feeling as though others were concerned about the individual's well-being.

APPLICATIONS

➡ OTPs should recognize the importance of social connection in successful recovery.
➡ OTPs can provide interventions that help individuals with schizophrenia feel as if they matter to other people.

REFERENCE

Pernice, F. M., Biegel, D. E., Kim, J. Y., & Conrad-Garrisi, D. (2017). The mediating role of mattering to others in recovery and stigma. *Psychiatric Rehabilitation Journal, 40,* 395–404. https://doi.org/10.1037/prj0000269

Prevalence and Course

The *DSM-5* reports a prevalence rate of 0.3% to 0.7% of the population (APA, 2013). The prevalence rates are relatively stable across cultures, although the prognosis may vary in different countries, with better outcomes in developing countries. The reason for this difference is unclear but is likely complicated and related to heritable, cultural, and other environmental factors (Jablensky & Sartorius, 2008).

Schizophrenia is typically first diagnosed during the early 20s (Walker et al., 2004). The age of onset can be particularly devastating because this is a time when most people are establishing significant adult relationships and worker roles. However, schizophrenia can develop at any age, although it is rarely diagnosed before adolescence or after age 40. Late-onset schizophrenia is more common in women.

Before meeting the criteria for schizophrenia, most individuals have a prodromal period lasting for weeks or months in which there are nonspecific changes in behavior and experiences. The **prodromal period** is the time between the emergence of early signs of the illness and the point at which the diagnostic criteria for the disorder are met. Identifying the prodrome of schizophrenia may be important for prevention. Some of the most frequently noted early signs of schizophrenia are psychotic-like symptoms, depression, cognitive impairments and a decline in cognition, and social isolation (Keshavan et al., 2011). For example, the individual may report odd perceptual experiences, there may be problems at work or school, or the individual may begin avoiding friends and family.

Efforts at early intervention are receiving increasing attention as long-term disability may be reduced with preventive efforts. For example, because cognitive deficits are significantly related to poor outcomes such as unemployment, early intervention targeting cognition may improve social functioning (Kuo et al., 2022). There is evidence that medication and behavioral interventions such as cognitive behavioral therapy and employment programs provided to high-risk individuals with prodomal symptoms may prevent further decline (Chen, 2019). In addition, there is some evidence that the longer a person with schizophrenia goes without treatment, the poorer the long-term outcome (Penttilä et al., 2014). One of the main problems with preventive treatment of schizophrenia is determining the severity of prodromal symptoms that warrant early intervention.

When Emil Kraepelin first described dementia praecox in 1919 (the disorder that later came to be known as schizophrenia), he depicted the course of the illness as one of progressive decline. This view became so prevalent that the third edition of the *DSM* included the following description: "A complete return to premorbid functioning is unusual—so rare, in fact, that some clinicians would question the diagnosis. However, there is always the possibility of full remission or recovery, although its frequency is unknown.

The most common course is one of acute exacerbations with increasing residual impairment between episodes" (APA, 1981, p. 185). However, research indicates that the long-term outcomes for schizophrenia are much better than indicated by early descriptions (Molstrom et al., 2022). A recent meta-analysis of long-term studies of schizophrenia prognosis found that 24.2% recovered, 35.5% had a good or better outcome, and 40.3% had poor outcomes.

Gender Differences

There is a slightly higher incidence of schizophrenia in males, and schizophrenia is generally less severe for females than it is for males (Hopper et al., 2007). Women experience more depression and are more likely to develop the condition at a later age, whereas men experience more negative symptoms, poorer outcomes, more cognitive impairments, and more substance abuse (Abel et al., 2010).

Culture-Specific Information

Cultural considerations are essential in distinguishing psychotic experiences from commonly held cultural beliefs. For example, in certain religions, it is a typical spiritual experience to hear the voice of God or see visions of people who have died. Schizophrenia is overdiagnosed in some racial groups, with one meta-analysis finding Black Americans to be diagnosed 2.4 times more often than white Americans (Olbert et al., 2018). In addition, immigrants, particularly those who are underrepresented in the areas where they live and those with darker skin, are more likely to be diagnosed with schizophrenia (Bourque et al., 2011).

Social isolation or feeling different from the majority population appears to be linked to a greater risk for psychosis, but other factors include structural racism, discrimination, and racial biases (Nagendra et al., 2023). Additionally, it is important to consider how racism might contribute to the development of psychotic-like symptoms. The term **adaptive paranoia** refers to a healthy suspicion in Black individuals that develops because of police profiling and experiences of racism in everyday environments (Wolny et al., 2023). Experiences of marginalized groups may result in symptoms that lead to the increased diagnosis of psychotic disorders in people of color.

Impact on Occupational Performance

Schizophrenia is recognized as a serious mental illness; as such, the illness can interfere with successful occupational performance. In addition, the social consequences of schizophrenia, such as stigma and poverty, are significant in terms of their impact on daily life.

Cognitive Impairments

Although cognitive impairments are not part of the diagnostic criteria of schizophrenia, impaired cognitive functioning is a core feature of the disorder. Cognitive impairments precede the diagnosis and often persist after psychotic symptoms have remitted (Nuechterlein et al., 2011). In fact, cognitive dysfunction is more strongly associated with functional impairment than symptoms, particularly the positive symptoms of schizophrenia. Cognitive impairments tend to worsen with illness onset, but there does not appear to be a progression of the deficit over time (i.e., the cognitive impairment remains fairly stable). There is a great deal of heterogeneity in the degree to which individuals experience cognitive impairments. Some individuals with schizophrenia have serious cognitive impairments, and some have intact cognitive function, with most individuals falling somewhere in between (Buonocore et al., 2021; Reser et al., 2015).

There has been extensive study of cognition and schizophrenia. A synthesis of systematic reviews on the topic identified five domains of cognition as commonly impaired in people with schizophrenia (Gebreegziabhere et al., 2022). The five domains were processing speed, executive function, memory, verbal fluency, and social cognition.

Processing speed is the amount of time required to perceive information, process that information, and carry out a response. Processing speed appears to be the greatest area of impairment when compared with other cognitive domains in schizophrenia (Knowles et al., 2010) and is a strong predictor of functional outcomes (Nuechterlein et al., 2011). However, a reason for the severity of the impairment is that processing speed impairment is made worse by antipsychotic medications.

Executive function refers to higher-level cognitive processing and includes abilities such as organization, planning, conceptual flexibility, inhibition, and problem-solving. People with schizophrenia often exhibit challenges carrying out tasks because of executive function impairments (Orellana & Slachevsky, 2013). For example, people with schizophrenia are less likely to develop and use scripts or habit patterns when involved in familiar situations such as making an appointment and then going to get a haircut. There are certain steps to follow and social expectations in this situation.

Although many people are unaware of the fact that they are following a script, the person with schizophrenia has more trouble organizing and planning tasks. Individuals with schizophrenia find it particularly difficult to make changes in their behavior and require more feedback and a higher level of certainty before making a change. Obviously, this has important implications for intervention, suggesting that useful and concrete feedback, along with reassurance, should be regularly provided.

Common memory impairments identified in schizophrenia are related to episodic memory and working memory (Palmer et al., 2010). **Episodic memory** pertains to remembering past events or "episodes" that have happened in one's life. **Working memory** is the ability to hold information and manipulate that information for a short period of time to carry out a task. For example, a person might estimate the total cost of items they are planning to purchase to make sure they are staying within their budget. **Verbal fluency** is associated with memory and refers to a person's ability to recall and retrieve verbal information from their memory.

Social cognition refers to the mental processes that are used when relating to other people. Components of social cognition that are impaired in schizophrenia include social cue perception, mentalizing or the ability to take the perspective of others, emotion regulation, and empathy (Green et al., 2015).

Clearly, it is important that cognition be addressed when considering interventions directed toward community living. Skills training and environmental modification should take into account the specific cognitive impairments that are common in schizophrenia. Cognition is explored in greater depth in Chapter 7: Cognition.

Health and Wellness

Individuals with schizophrenia have much higher rates of morbidity and mortality than the general population. For example, people with schizophrenia are four times more likely to die from serious cardiac events than the general population (Enger et al., 2004). An important study found that individuals with schizophrenia have a life expectancy reduced by decades (Colton & Manderscheid, 2006). Obesity is of particular concern, with studies finding obesity associated with greater severity of symptoms and poorer quality of life (Campos-Vazquez & Gonzalez, 2020; Cerimele & Katon, 2013).

In terms of lifestyle practices, individuals with schizophrenia have low levels of physical activity; tend to eat diets rich in calories, fats, and carbohydrates; and are presented with barriers toward accessing primary medical care (Martland et al., 2021; Ringen et al., 2014; Teasdale et al., 2019). Even greater concerns exist today with the increasing evidence that atypical antipsychotics increase the risk for both type 2 diabetes and weight gain in an already vulnerable population. The combination of poor lifestyle behaviors and the side effects of most psychiatric medications (particularly clozapine and olanzapine) contribute to obesity and diabetes in people with schizophrenia (Hirsch et al., 2017).

High rates of smoking present another health risk. It is estimated that people with schizophrenia have rates of cigarette smoking that are at least two times and possibly more than three times greater than the general population (Grant et al., 2004). Several factors contribute to these rates, including the potential for nicotine to reduce negative symptoms, cognitive deficits, and sensory processing abnormalities (George et al., 2000). Smoking-related deaths contribute to the excess mortality rate in schizophrenia.

Severe oral diseases are highly prevalent in this population. Many drugs used to treat schizophrenia have oral side effects. These include severe dry mouth, tardive dyskinesia, and acute dystonic reactions that affect the mouth, tongue, and other head and neck muscle groups. Dry mouth is a particular concern because dryness of the oral tissues increases the rate and severity of periodontal disease and tooth decay. In addition, it can make wearing dentures impossible (King, 1998). Poor oral hygiene directly correlates with the severity of mental illness, which can influence the severity of periodontal disease and cavities (Kang et al., 2022).

One positive finding is that individuals with schizophrenia can benefit from interventions that target lifestyle behaviors (Naslund et al., 2017). Interventions are particularly effective when they are provided over extended periods of time and combine didactic and active learning strategies. OTPs should consider the impact of poor health on occupational performance and contribute to programs that focus on lifestyle changes. The topic of wellness is covered more extensively in Chapter 45: Self-Care and Well-Being Occupations.

Stigma and Poverty

Stigma is possibly the greatest barrier to successful and satisfying community living for people with schizophrenia. One review found that approximately 65% of individuals with serious mental illness experienced stigma, and that stigma was associated with lower quality of life and self-efficacy, as well as feelings of alienation (Gerlinger et al., 2013). Stigma toward schizophrenia can be exacerbated by news stories and social media coverage, especially when the coverage includes content on violence and crime (Battaglia et al., 2022).

It is well established that the term "mental illness" carries a stigma, but schizophrenia appears to be the most stigmatizing of all the mental illnesses (Valery & Prouteau, 2020). Mental illness stigma is associated with negative stereotypes, a belief that individuals will not recover, and a blaming of the individual for their condition. Interestingly, evidence suggests that a greater belief in a biological cause of the disorder is associated with increased stigma. This may be because of the view that a biological disorder is permanent. These findings are important because some antistigma campaigns promote understanding mental illness as a brain disease.

A review examining different methods of changing stigmatizing attitudes found that direct social contact with people with mental illness is more effective than education or indirect social contact. The contact is most effective when there are long-term follow-up strategies. When individuals with mental illness provide antistigma presentations, the message is more effective when there are opportunities for audience discussion and a message that presents positive stories (Corrigan, 2020).

Self-stigma occurs when individuals internalize negative stereotypes. Self-stigma is common in schizophrenia and is associated with poorer functioning, demoralization, and more positive symptoms (Cavelti et al., 2014). However, interventions aimed at reducing self-stigma by improving self-esteem, empowerment, and help-seeking behaviors are effective (Mittal et al., 2012). Additionally, deemphasizing disorder-based models and supporting peer-to-peer groups (such as in the Hearing Voice Movement) has been shown to promote self-esteem and social connection (Beavan et al., 2017).

Most individuals with schizophrenia live in poverty, which presents a major barrier to community living (Zipursky, 2014). Living in impoverished conditions in poor housing situations likely limits opportunities for recovery. For example, people with schizophrenia are less likely to have their own cars and additionally have barriers to using public transportation. Consequently, employment and any other instrumental activity of daily living that takes place outside the home can be challenging. By extension, meeting basic needs for food and shelter is a regular struggle. It is essential to consider the social barriers of stigma and poverty during both the assessment and intervention process of occupational therapy. Also see Chapter 27: Mental Health Stigma and Sanism for more information on this topic.

Intervention

Because of the complexity of schizophrenia and the impact on occupational performance, several chapters in this text provide relevant information regarding assessment and intervention. Table 23-2 outlines common intervention approaches for individuals with schizophrenia and schizoaffective disorder, and identifies the accompanying chapters in this text that provide more detailed information about those approaches. 🤝

Medications

The pharmacological treatment of schizophrenia is based primarily on antipsychotic medications. Antipsychotic medication can be divided into two classes: **first-generation antipsychotics** (also described as conventional) and **second-generation antipsychotics** (sometimes referred to as atypical antipsychotics). The first antipsychotic medication was chlorpromazine (Thorazine; Advokat et al., 2018). Introduced in 1952, it was first noticed that chlorpromazine had a calming effect on people with schizophrenia. Later, psychiatrists recognized that it also reduced hallucinations and delusions. Other common first-generation antipsychotics include haloperidol (Haldol) and fluphenazine (Prolixin). Antipsychotics are dopamine antagonists that work by blocking the dopamine receptors in the brain. The first-generation antipsychotics are most effective in reducing the positive symptoms of schizophrenia; however, they also have many harmful side effects.

The first second-generation antipsychotic was clozapine (Clozaril; Remington, 2003). Clozapine is often effective for individuals who have not responded to other medications.

TABLE 23-2 | Common Intervention Approaches for Individuals With Schizophrenia and Schizoaffective Disorder

Approach	Target(s) of Intervention	Brief Synopsis	Chapters With Additional Information 🤝
Cognitive Remediation	Improving cognitive skills	Graded and repeated practice of cognitive oriented tasks within the context of occupational performance	Chapter 7: Cognition
Cognitive Adaptation	Adapting the environment or task to meet occupational needs	The cognitive demands of an activity are reduced by changing the environment or making the task simpler.	Chapter 7: Cognition
Cognitive Disabilities	Occupations the person "can do," "will do," or "may do"	Identify cognitive level and based on this information maximize strengths and create enabling environment.	Chapter 7: Cognition
Dunn's Model of Sensory Processing	Sensory processing needs in the context of occupational performance	Creating environments or materials that meet the individual's sensory processing needs	Chapter 9: Sensory Processing and the Lived Sensory Experience
Sensory Rooms	Providing sensory input that is calming	In treatment settings a room is created that contains calming sensory input. Individuals can use the room whenever they feel agitated, angry, or anxious.	Chapter 9: Sensory Processing and the Lived Sensory Experience
Social Skills Training	Social skills	Learning and behavioral theories are used with feedback and repeated practice to teach social skills.	Chapter 13: Communication and Social Skills
Permanent Supportive Housing	Independent and stable housing	Individually tailored supports to promote successful living in the person's home of choice	Chapter 31: The Home Environment: Permanent Supportive Housing
Peer Support Programs	Social connectedness and support	Education, socialization, and advocacy services are provided by persons with lived experience of mental illness.	Chapter 39: Peer-Led Services
Activities of Daily Living (ADL) and Instrumental ADL (IADL) Training	ADL and IADL skills	Application of learning and behavioral strategies to promote acquisition of new skills	Chapter 46: Activities of Daily Living, Instrumental Activities of Daily Living, and Health Management Occupations
Supported Education	Goals related to higher education	Individualized, practical support and inclusion to help people succeed in postsecondary education	Chapter 47: Student
Supported Employment	Work	Rapid job placement in competitive employment positions with follow-along supports	Chapter 48: Work and Volunteer Occupations
Creative Arts	Wellness and social participation	Use of creative media to promote wellness and socialization and decrease stigma	Chapter 10: Coping and Resilience Chapter 51: Leisure and Creative Occupations

PhotoVoice

I dread when 8 o'clock comes around because I know I have to take my handful of pills, which practically makes me gag. After I take my pills, they make me shake. I want to talk to my doctor to cut down on the amount of pills I take. I hope to find a doctor that will take the time to listen to me about the side effects and about how the pills are making me feel.

Are there times when you have avoided taking medication as prescribed because of the side effects?

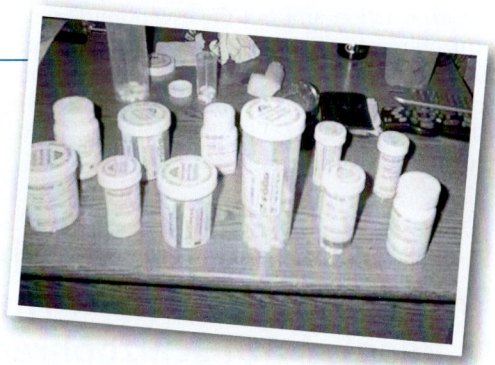

However, it is not used as a first-line drug because of the particularly serious side effect of agranulocytosis (a significant reduction in the number of circulating white blood cells), making the individual highly susceptible to infection. If left untreated, the risk of dying from agranulocytosis is very high. Approximately 1% to 2% of people taking clozapine will develop this condition, so individuals taking this medication must have regular blood monitoring. Other second-generation antipsychotics include risperidone (Risperdal), olanzapine (Zyprexa), quetiapine (Seroquel), ziprasidone (Geodon), and aripiprazole (Abilify).

An important ongoing study titled the U.S. Clinical Antipsychotic Trials of Intervention Effectiveness (CATIE) compared four second-generation psychotics with one another and to a representative first-generation antipsychotic (Revisiting the CATIE Schizophrenia Study, 2008). The findings were surprising and controversial because they indicated that the second-generation antipsychotics were no more effective than the first-generation antipsychotic. Other large studies from England and Europe found similar results. The CATIE study also supported previous work indicating that clozapine was the most effective second-generation drug for individuals who did not respond to a previous medication.

The antipsychotics have many side effects, including sedation, sun sensitivity, anticholinergic effects (dry mouth, constipation, blurred vision), and orthostatic hypertension. Some of the most serious side effects involve movement disorders, which result from the blockage of dopamine in the basal ganglia. Movement disorders include parkinsonlike side effects, akathisia (serious motor restlessness), acute dystonic reaction (a sustained contraction of the muscles of the neck, mouth, and tongue), and tardive dyskinesia. Tardive dyskinesia occurs after long-term treatment with antipsychotic medication and involves involuntary movements, usually of the mouth and tongue. In addition, weight gain and metabolic disturbances are common problems with antipsychotics.

The antipsychotics can have particular side-effect profiles. For example, weight gain is particularly problematic with olanzapine and clozapine, and tardive dyskinesia is much more likely with haloperidol than the second-generation antipsychotics. In some cases, choice of medication may be more based on side effects, and there is evidence to suggest that switching medications to reduce undesirable side effects may not result in a reduction in symptom relief (Newcomer et al., 2013).

Some individuals with schizophrenia do not appear to need antipsychotic treatment throughout their lifetime. One long-term study found that people who discontinued or reduced their medication were more likely to relapse; however, at 7-year follow-up these individuals had a more favorable functional outcome (Harrow et al., 2012; Wunderink et al., 2013). The Common Ground program uses a technology-supported intervention to facilitate a process whereby people with schizophrenia and their physician can share decisions around medication management (MacDonald-Wilson et al., 2021).

The different types of symptoms and impairments that are inherent in schizophrenia (psychosis, negative symptoms, cognitive impairments) make it difficult to find a medication to treat all aspects of the condition. Antipsychotic medications have their greatest impact on psychotic symptoms, and negative symptoms and cognitive impairments often persist or even get worse with medication. In addition, environmental factors such as stigma, medication side effects, and poverty contribute additional difficulties. Clearly, medications provide only partial relief, indicating alternative interventions are essential.

Holistic Perspective

The World Health Organization's (WHO's) Guidance on Community Mental Health Services (2021) argues, "It is critical that mental health systems and services widen their focus beyond the biomedical model to also include a more holistic approach that considers all aspects of a person's life" (p. 21). They cite the need for exploring recovery-based models, peer-to-peer support, and a deemphasis on disorder-based models. One program highlighted by WHO is the Hearing Voices Movement (HVM).

The HVM holds that health is a fundamentally social, cultural, and political process (Corstens et al., 2014). There is a strong emphasis on nonjudgmental perspective and respecting individuals' nonconsensus realities. Groups emphasize peer-to-peer social connection and do not identify as clinically based (Bergner, 2022). HVM has been found to reduce symptoms (Meddings et al., 2004), hospitalizations, and medication usage (Horstein et al., 2020) and to promote self-esteem and social connection (Beavan et al., 2017).

As individuals living with schizophrenia share their stories, they have helped reframe occupational therapy practice such that productive and satisfying community living is now the expectation and not the exception for individuals with schizophrenia. OTPs should seek to implement similar holistic person-led ideals to further stigma reduction, promote social connection, and assist individuals to realize their cherished occupations. OTPs should also advocate for systemic changes wherever possible.

General Considerations When Providing Occupational Therapy to People With Schizophrenia Spectrum and Psychotic Disorders

■ *Person-centered:* The American Occupational Therapy Association (AOTA) emphasizes the importance of creating an occupational profile for each individual person (AOTA, 2017). Because of the high degree of heterogeneity, this is especially true in this population. It is essential to fully appreciate individual strengths, weaknesses, symptomatic presentation, and environmental supports and barriers. Frames of reference that emphasize a comprehensive view of the individual and their environment may include but are not limited to the *Canadian Occupational Performance Model (COPM;* Law et al., 2014) and the *Person-Environment-Occupation Model* (Law et al., 1996).

■ *Appropriate assessment:* OTPs have a wealth of functional assessments at their disposal. Rogers and Holm (2016) listed some of the following functional assessments that may have particular relevance in mental health populations: *The Kohlman Evaluation of Living Skills* (KELS) assesses the ability to complete basic activities of daily living (ADL) and instrumental activities of daily living (IADL) tasks. The *Evaluation of Social Interaction* (ESI) can be used to assess the quality of social interactions. The *Test of Grocery Shopping Skills* (TOGSS) is a cognitive assessment grounded in a functional, routine IADL task. It may be necessary to utilize multiple assessments to fully evaluate a person's needs.

■ *Grade and adapt tasks within environmental contexts:* This population may have several simultaneous barriers to participating in desired occupations across multiple performance skills and contexts including socioeconomic, environmental, cognitive, sensory, and physical conditions. It is essential that OTPs promote function appropriately graded to an individual's capacities and resources. Abaoğlu and colleagues (2020) designed life skills interventions that emphasized increased "independence in daily life and demonstrated positive effects on patient functionality" (p. 57), and they found this showed "improvement in the negative symptoms, general psychopathology and disease severity" (p. 56). For this population as in others, occupation is both the means and the end.

■ *Sensory-based interventions:* Sensory interventions are a rapidly expanding area of growth in mental health populations. High-quality research remains limited but Machingura and colleagues (2018) concluded "that there is preliminary evidence for the existence of sensory modulation disorder in schizophrenia and the effectiveness of sensory modulation interventions for reducing distress" (p. 764). When trying to assist this population, consider a person's overall sensory environment and diet and consider how this may or may not be contributing to their struggle to engage in desired occupations. Consider the use of the *Sensory Processing Measure* or other sensory assessments to provide appropriate data.

■ *Stigma reduction:* Stigma can be difficult to reverse because it has multiple sources, including structural, interpersonal, and internalized self-stigma. OTPs should ensure their own personal biases do not contribute to this problem. Finding opportunities for direct social contact with individuals living with mental illness is an effective way to reduce bias in health-care providers (Carrara et al., 2021). Ensuring mental health literacy and promoting self-advocacy can be useful in reducing self-stigma (National Academies of Sciences, Engineering, and Medicine, 2016). Additionally, peer services, such as the HVM mentioned earlier in the chapter, can be useful in reducing stigma. As a practitioner, remember to accept and understand that the lived experience of mental illness belongs to the individual. Work to support individuals in their journey to understand their mental illness.

Here's the Point

- Schizophrenia and schizoaffective disorder are complex conditions with symptoms from different dimensions including psychosis, disorganized speech and behavior, negative symptoms, and affective symptoms.
- Schizophrenia is a heterogeneous condition with individuals experiencing very different symptom and cognitive profiles. However, efforts to subtype the condition have been unsuccessful.
- Schizophrenia is typically diagnosed in late adolescence and early adulthood and includes a major impact on functioning; however, many individuals experience significant recovery.
- The cause of schizophrenia is unclear but includes a combination of biological and environmental factors.
- Cognitive impairments, differences in sensory processing, and environmental factors can have significant impacts on occupational performance, yet interventions can improve successful engagement in occupations.
- Medications used to treat schizophrenia include first- and second-generation antipsychotics. These medications are most effective in reducing psychosis but have limited impact on negative symptoms and cognition.

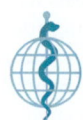 Visit the online resource center at **FADavis.com** to access the videos.

Apply It Now

1. Reflections on John Nash

After reading about John Nash in the introduction to this chapter, complete a Person-Environment-Occupation (PEO) analysis using the template in Appendix A. Feel free to explore other resources that provide additional information about John Nash including the movie, *A Beautiful Mind*. Consider the following guiding questions:

■ What occupations were important to Dr. Nash?
■ What personal factors and environmental factors contributed to his success?
■ What factors interfered with his success?
■ What might have made his recovery easier?

You can also analyze Adam Sakievich's account in this chapter's The Lived Experience feature using the same template and questions. What similarities and differences did you find between the two individuals?

2. Experiencing Environmental Challenges Common for People With Schizophrenia

People with schizophrenia experience many barriers to participation that are separate from the direct effects of the illness. Most people with schizophrenia live in poverty; consequently, many resources that others take for granted can present major obstacles to successful and satisfying community living. For example, many people are unable to afford a car and rely on public transportation or rides from others to get where they need to go. Public transportation in some communities is limited or nonexistent and may be complex or stressful for someone with a serious psychiatric disability. Other issues may include having enough money for essential living expenses such as rent and food. Complete one of the following activities to appreciate external barriers to community living.

a. Public Transportation

If public transportation is available in your community, use it to get to an appointment. Take note of issues such as safety, convenience, schedules, exposure, frustration, and so on during the activity. Consider how the symptoms of schizophrenia along with cognitive impairments and sensory processing impairments would influence the experience. Describe the experience in your Reflective Journal.

b. SNAP Benefits

Go to https//aix-xweb1p.state.or.us/caf_xweb/SNAP_Estimate /frmEstimate.cfm and calculate how much money you would have per day based on your family size. Feed yourself and your family, if applicable, for 1 day on a SNAP budget without using any ingredients you have on hand. Consider your family's satiety, achieving a balanced diet, and providing a variety of food choices when completing this activity.

Reflective Questions

■ What kinds of information did you need to carry out these tasks? How did you go about acquiring this information?
■ What skills did you need to successfully complete the tasks? Did you feel competent when executing the tasks?
■ Did you ask for help from others? If so, were others helpful?
■ What was most challenging?
■ What feelings did you experience?
■ How would it be if you had to rely on public transportation or food stamps all the time?
■ Would the cognitive impairments associated with schizophrenia make these tasks more difficult? In what ways?
■ How might auditory hallucinations affect your experience?
■ If you were feeling paranoid, how would the experience differ?
■ Do you think stigma would play a role in your ability to carry out these tasks if people knew you had schizophrenia?

3. Video Exercise: Nicholas's Lived Experience of Schizophrenia

Pair up with another student in your class or form a small group of students. Access and watch the "Nicholas's Lived Experience of Schizophrenia" video at the online resource center at FADavis.com. Then, discuss and together answer the following questions.

Reflective Questions

■ In the context of Nicholas's story, what was occupational therapy's distinct value for him at the beginning of his mental health journey? How and why did occupational therapy make such a significant impact on his mental wellness/recovery?
■ Nicholas describes that his psychosis caused a breakdown between himself and his community of support. How can OTPs help reduce this type of breakdown, which can occur when individuals experience hallucinations, delusions, paranoia, and a general lack of trust in people and their environment?
■ Nicholas explains that he "exited an inner world and was able to participate in the outside world and . . . what we call . . . shared consensus reality." How would you describe this transformation to a peer or to a patient? How do you think occupational therapy services fostered this connection to his environment and the people in it?
■ In Nicholas's story, we hear a narrative of resilience. From what you learned about him in his video, how does resilience appear to Nicholas? What does resilience mean to you? Are their similarities/differences? How can we maintain an open mind as to how resilience and recovery appear across the spectrum of individuals we work with? Why is this open mindedness about resilience important for their recovery?

Resources

Books/Publications

- Kolker, R. (2020). *Hidden valley road: Inside the mind of an American family.* Anchor Books.
- Nasar, S. (1998). *A beautiful mind.* Simon & Schuster.
- Re-inventing schizophrenia: Updating the construct. (2022). *Schizophrenia Research, 242,* 1–150. A series of essays on the construct of schizophrenia. https://www.sciencedirect.com/journal/schizophrenia-research/vol/242/suppl/C
- Saks, E. R. (2008). *The center cannot hold.* Hyperion.
- Schiller, L., & Bennett, A. (1996). *The quiet room: A journey out of the torment of madness.* Warner Books.
- Spiro, C., & Spiro Wagner, P. (2006). *Divided minds: Twin sisters and their journey through schizophrenia.* St. Martin's Press.
- Wang, E. W. (2019). *The collected schizophrenia.* Graywolf Press.

Educational Videos

- "Schizophrenia: Surviving the World of Normals"—Wellness Reproductions: www.wellness-resources.com
- "Secret Life of the Brain: Part 3: The Teenage Brain"—PBS: http://www.pbs.org/wnet/brain/episode3/index.html
- "West 47th Street"—PBS: http://www.pbs.org/pov/west47thstreet

Organizations

- Hearing Voices Network: www.hearing-voicesorg
- National Alliance for Research on Schizophrenia and Depression (NARSAD): www.narsad.org
- National Alliance on Mental Illness (NAMI): www.nami.org
- National Empowerment Center: www.power2u.org
- Schizophrenia.com: http://schizophrenia.com
- Substance Abuse and Mental Health Services Administration: www.samhsa.gov

Online Resources

- Pat Deegan and Common Ground: www.patdeegan.com
- Elyn R. Saks: A Tale of Mental Illness TED Talk: http://www.ted.com/talks/elyn_saks_seeing_mental_illness
- Eleanor Longden: The Voices in My Head TED Talk: https://www.youtube.com/watch?v=syjEN3peCJw
- Oliver Sacks on Hallucinations—TED Talk: http://www.ted.com/talks/oliver_sacks_what_hallucination_reveals_about_our_mindsPat
- World Health Organization—Guidance on Community Mental Health Services: https://www.who.int/publications/i/item/9789240025707

References

Abaoğlu, H., Mutlu, E., Ak, S., Akı, E., & Anıl Yağcıoğlu, A. E. (2020). The effect of life skills training on functioning in schizophrenia: A randomized controlled trial. *Turk Psikiyatri Dergisi (Turkish Journal of Psychiatry), 31*(1), 50–58. https://doi.org/10.5080/u23723

Abel, K. M., Drake, R., & Goldstein, J. M. (2010). Sex differences in schizophrenia. *International Review of Psychiatry, 22,* 417–428. https://doi.org/10.3109/09540261.2010.515205

Advokat, C. D., Comaty, J. E., & Julien, R. M. (2018). *Julien's primer of drug action* (14th ed.). Worth Publishers.

American Occupational Therapy Association. (2017). AOTA occupational profile template. *The American Journal of Occupational Therapy, 71*(Suppl. 2), 7112420030p1. https://doi.org/10.5014/ajot.2017.716S12

American Psychiatric Association. (1981). *Diagnostic and statistical manual of mental disorders* (3rd ed.). American Psychiatric Publishing.

American Psychiatric Association. (2000). *Diagnostic and statistical manual of mental disorders* (4th ed., text rev.). American Psychiatric Publishing.

American Psychiatric Association. (2013). *Diagnostic and statistical manual of mental disorders* (5th ed.). American Psychiatric Publishing. https://doi.org/10.1176/appi.books.9780890425596.

American Psychiatric Association. (2022). *Diagnostic and statistical manual of mental disorders* (5th ed., text rev.). American Psychiatric Publishing. https://doi.org/10.1176/appi.books.9780890425787

Andreason, N. C., & Carpenter, W. T. (1993). Diagnosis and classification of schizophrenia. *Schizophrenia Bulletin, 19,* 199–214. https://doi.org/10.1093/schbul/19.2.199

Barch, D. M., Karcher, N., & Moran, E. (2022). Reinventing schizophrenia—Embracing complexity and complication. *Schizophrenia Research, 242,* 7–11. https://doi.org/10.1016/j.schres.2021.11.037

Barlati, S., Nibbio, G., Calzavara-Pinton, I., Invernizzi, E., Cadei, L., Lisoni, J., Valsecchi, P., Deste, G., & Vita, A. (2022). Primary and secondary negative symptoms severity and the use of psychiatric care resources in schizophrenia spectrum disorders: A 3-year follow-up longitudinal retrospective study. *Schizophrenia Research, 250,* 31–38. https://doi.org/10.1016/j.schres.2022.10.002

Battaglia, A. M., Mamak, M., & Goldberg, J. O. (2022). The impact of social media coverage on attitudes towards mental illness and violent offending. *Journal of Community Psychology, 50*(7), 2938–2949. https://doi.org/10.1002/jcop.22807

Beavan, V., de Jager, A., & dos Santos, B. (2017). Do peer-support groups for voice-hearers work? A small scale study of Hearing Voices Network support groups in Australia. *Psychosis, 9*(1), 57–66. https://doi.org/10.1080/17522439.2016.1216583

Ben, G. (2014). On radical empathy and schizophrenia. In C. Wood (Ed.), *Criptiques* (pp. 219–227). May Day. https://criptiques.files.wordpress.com/2014/05/crip-final-2.pdf

Bergner, D. (2022, May 17). Doctors gave her antipsychotics. She decided to live with her voices. *The New York Times.* https://www.nytimes.com/2022/05/17/magazine/antipsychotic-medications-mental-health.html?referringSource=articleShare

Bleuler, E. (1911). *Dementia praecox or the group of schizophrenias* (J. Zinkin, Trans.). Deuticke.

Bourque, F., van der Ven, E., & Malla, A. (2011). A meta-analysis of the risk for psychotic disorders among first and second generation immigrants. *Psychological Medicine, 41,* 897–910. https://doi.org/10.1017/S0033291710001406

Bray, N. J. (2008). Gene expression in the etiology of schizophrenia. *Schizophrenia Bulletin, 34,* 412–418. https://doi.org/10.1093/schbul/sbn013

Brent, B. K., Thermenos, H. W., Keshavan, M. S., & Seidman, L. J. (2013). Gray matter alterations in schizophrenia high-risk youth and early-onset schizophrenia: A review of structural MRI findings. *Child and Adolescent Psychiatric Clinics of North America, 22,* 689–714. https://doi.org/10.1016/j.chc.2013.06.003

Buonocore, M., Inguscio, E., Bosinelli, F., Bechi, M., Agostoni, G., Spangaro, M., Martini, F., Bianchi, L., Cocchi, F., Guglielmino, C., Repaci, F., Bosia, M., & Cavallaro, R. (2021). Disentangling cognitive heterogeneity in psychotic spectrum disorders. *Asian Journal of Psychiatry, 60,* 102651. https://doi.org/10.1016/j.ajp.2021.102651

Campos-Vazquez, R. M., & Gonzalez, E. (2020). Obesity and hiring discrimination. *Economics and Human Biology, 37,* 100850. https://doi: 10.1016/j.ehb.2020.100850

Cannon, T. D. (2022). Psychosis, schizophrenia, and states vs. traits. *Schizophrenia Research, 242,* 12–14. https://doi.org/10.1016/j.schres.2021.12.001

Carlsson, A. (1988). The current status of the dopamine hypothesis in schizophrenia. *Neuropsychopharmacology, 1,* 179–186. https://doi.org/10.1016/0893-133X(88)90012-7

Carpenter, W. T. (2013). RDoC and *DSM-5:* What's the fuss? *Schizophrenia Bulletin, 39,* 945–946. https://doi.org/10.1093/schbul/sbt101

Carrara, B. S., Fernandes, R. H. H., Bobbili, S. J., & Ventura, C. A. A. (2021). Health care providers and people with mental illness: An integrative review on anti-stigma interventions. *The International Journal of Social Psychiatry, 67*(7), 840–853. https://doi.org/10.1177/0020764020985891

Cattarinussi, G., Delvecchio, G., Sambataro, F., & Brambilla, P. (2022). The effect of polygenic risk scores for major depressive disorder, bipolar disorder and schizophrenia on morphological brain measures: A systematic review of the evidence. *Journal of Affective Disorders, 310*, 213–222. https://doi.org/10.1016/j.jad.2022.05.007

Cavelti, M., Rusch, N., & Vauth, R. (2014). Is living with psychosis demoralizing? Insight, self-stigma and clinical outcome among people with schizophrenia across 1 year. *Journal of Nervous and Mental Disease, 202*, 521–529. https://doi.org/10.1097/NMD.0000000000000160

Cerimele, J. M., & Katon, W. J. (2013). Associations between health risk behaviors and symptoms of schizophrenia and bipolar disorder: A systematic review. *General Hospital Psychiatry, 35*, 16–22. https://doi.org/10.1016/j.genhosppsych.2012.08.001

Chen, E. Y. H. (2019). Early intervention for psychosis: Current issues and emerging perspectives. *International Review of Psychiatry, 31*(5–6), 411–412. https://doi.org/10.1080/09540261.2019.1667597

Colton, C. W., & Manderscheid, R. W. (2006). Congruencies in increased mortality rates, years of potential life lost, and causes of death among public mental health clients in eight states. *Preventing Chronic Disease, 3*, 1–14.

Corrigan, P. W. (2020). Effect of contact-based interventions on stigma and discrimination. *Psychiatric Services (Washington, D.C.), 71*(12), 1324–1325. https://doi.org/10.1176/appi.ps.711203

Corstens, D., Longden, E., McCarthy-Jones, S., Waddingham, R., & Thomas, N. (2014). Emerging perspectives from the hearing voices movement: Implications for research and practice. *Schizophrenia Bulletin, 40*(Suppl. 4), S285–S294. https://doi.org/10.1093/schbul/sbu007

Cuesta, M. J., Sánchez-Torres, A. M., Moreno-Izco, L., García de Jalón, E., Gil-Berrozpe, G. J., Zarzuela, A., Peralta, V., Ballesteros, A., Fañanás, L., Hernández, R., Janda, L., Lorente, R., Papiol, S., Peralta, D., Ribeiro, M., Rosero, A., & Zandio, M. (2022). Neurocognitive correlates of the varied domains of outcomes at 20 year follow-up of first-episode psychosis. *Psychiatry Research, 318*, 114933. https://doi.org/10.1016/j.psychres.2022.114933

Davies, C., Segre, G., Estradé, A., Radua, J., De Micheli, A., Provenzani, U., Oliver, D., Salazar de Pablo, G., Ramella-Cravaro, V., Besozzi, M., Dazzan, P., Miele, M., Caputo, G., Spallarossa, C., Crossland, G., Ilyas, A., Spada, G., Politi, P., Murray, R. M., . . . Fusar-Poli, P. (2020). Prenatal and perinatal risk and protective factors for psychosis: A systematic review and meta-analysis. *The Lancet. Psychiatry, 7*(5), 399–410. https://doi.org/10.1016/S2215-0366(20)30057-2

Devylder, J. E., Ben-David, S., Schobel, S. A., Kimhy, D., Malaspina, D., & Corcoran, C. M. (2013). Temporal association of stress sensitivity and symptoms in individuals at clinical high risk for psychosis. *Psychological Medicine, 43*, 259–268. https://doi.org/10.1017/S0033291712001262

Enger, C., Weatherby, L., Reynolds, R. F., Glasser, D. B., & Walker, A. M. (2004). Serious cardiovascular events and mortality among patients with schizophrenia. *Journal of Nervous and Mental Disease, 192*, 19–27. https://doi.org/10.1097/01.nmd.0000105996.62105.07

Fatouros-Bergman, H., Cervenka, S., Flyckt, L., Edman, G., & Farde, L. (2014). Meta-analysis of cognitive performance in drug-naïve patients with schizophrenia. *Schizophrenia Research, 158*(1-3), 156–162. https://doi.org/10.1016/j.schres.2014.06.034

Galderisi, S., Mucci, A., Dollfus, S., Nordentoft, M., Falkai, P., Kaiser, S., Giordano, G. M., Vandevelde, A., Nielsen, M. Ø., Glenthøj, L. B., Sabé, M., Pezzella, P., Bitter, I., & Gaebel, W. (2021). EPA guidance on assessment of negative symptoms in schizophrenia. *European Psychiatry, 64*, e23. https://doi.org/10.1192/j.eurpsy.2021.13

Gebreegziabhere, Y., Habatmu, K., Mihretu, A., Cella, M., & Alem, A. (2022). Cognitive impairment in people with schizophrenia: An umbrella review. *European Archives of Psychiatry and Clinical Neuroscience, 272*(7), 1139–1155. https://doi.org/10.1007/s00406-022-01416-6

George, T. P., Ziedonis, D. M., Feingold, A., Pepper, W. T., Satterburg, C. A., Winkel, J., Rounsaville, B. J., & Kosten, T. R. (2000). Nicotine transdermal patch and atypical antipsychotic medications for smoking cessation in schizophrenia. *American Journal of Psychiatry, 157*, 1835–1842. https://doi.org/10.1176/appi.ajp.157.11.1835

Gerlinger, G., Hauser, M., DeHert, M., Lacluyse, K., Wampers, M., & Correll, C. U. (2013). Personal stigma in schizophrenia spectrum disorders: A systematic review of prevalence rates, correlates, impact and interventions. *World Psychiatry, 12*, 155–164. https://doi.org/10.1002/wps.20040

Grant, B. F., Hasin, D. S., Chou, S. P., Stinson, F. S., & Dawson, D. A. (2004). Nicotine dependence and psychiatric disorders in the United States: Results from the National Epidemiological Survey on Alcohol and Related Conditions. *Archives of General Psychiatry, 61*(11), 1107–1115. https://doi.org/10.1001/archpsyc.61.11.1107

Green, M. F., Horan, W. P., & Lee, J. (2015). Social cognition in schizophrenia. *Nature Reviews Neuroscience, 16*, 620–631. https://doi.org/10.1038/nrn4005

Guillin, O., Abi-Dargham, A., & Laruelle, M. (2007). Neurobiology of dopamine in schizophrenia. *International Review of Neurobiology, 78*, 1–39. https://doi.org/10.1016/S0074-7742(06)78001-1

Hakak-Zargar, B., Tamrakar, A., Voth, T., Sheikhi, A., Multani, J., & Schütz, C. G. (2022). The utility of research domain criteria in diagnosis and management of dual disorders: A mini-review. *Frontiers in Psychiatry, 13*, 805163. https://doi.org/10.3389/fpsyt.2022.805163

Harrow, M., Jobe, T. H., & Faull, R. N. (2012). Do all schizophrenia patients need antipsychotic treatment continuously throughout their lifetime? A 20-year longitudinal study. *Psychological Medicine, 42*(10), 2145–2155. https://doi.org/10.1017/S0033291712000220

Heckers, S. (2011). Bleuler and the neurobiology of schizophrenia. *Schizophrenia Bulletin, 37*, 1131–1137. https://doi.org/10.1093/schbul/sbr108

Hilker, R., Helenius, D., Fagerlund, B., Skytthe, A., Christensen, K., Werge, T. M., Nordentoft, M., & Glenthog, B. (2018). Heritability of schizophrenia and schizophrenia spectrum based on the nationwide Danish twin register. *Biological Psychiatry, 83*, 492–498. https://doi.org/10.1016/j.biopsych.2017.08.017

Hirsch, L., Yang, J., Bresee, L., Jette, N., Patten, S., & Pringsheim, T. (2017). Second-generation antipsychotics and metabolic side effects: A systematic review of population-based studies. *Drug Safety, 40*, 771–781. https://doi.org/10.1007/s40264-017-0543-0

Hopper, K., Harrison, G., Janca, A., & Sartorius, N. (Eds.). (2007). *Recovery from schizophrenia: An international perspective. A report from the WHO Collaborative Project, the International Study of Schizophrenia.* Oxford University Press.

Hornstein, G., Putnam, E. R., & Brantisky, A. (2020). How do hearing voices peer-support groups work? A three-phase model of transformation. *Psychosis, 12*(3), 201–211. https://doi.org/10.1080/17522439.2020.1749876

Howes, O. D., & Murray, R. M. (2014). Schizophrenia: An integrated sociodevelopmental-cognitive model. *Lancet, 383*, 1677–1687. https://doi.org/10.1016/S0140-6736(13)62036-X

Howes, O. D., & Shatalina, E. (2022). Integrating the neurodevelopmental and dopamine hypotheses of schizophrenia and the role of cortical excitation-inhibition balance. *Biological Psychiatry, 92*(6), 501–513. https://doi.org/10.1016/j.biopsych.2022.06.017

Jablensky, A., & Sartorius, N. (2008). What did the WHO studies really find? *Schizophrenia Bulletin, 34*, 253–255. https://doi.org/10.1093/schbul/sbm151

Jäger, M., Bottlender, R., Strauss, A., & Möller, H. J. (2004). Fifteen-year follow-up of *ICD-10* schizoaffective disorders compared with schizophrenia and affective disorders. *Acta Psychiatrica Scandinavica, 109,* 30–37. https://doi.org/10.1111/j.0001-690x.2004.00208.x

Kang, J., Palmier-Claus, J., Wu, J., Shiers, D., Larvin, H., Doran, T., & Aggarwal, V. R. (2022). Periodontal disease in people with a history of psychosis: Results from the UK biobank population-based study. *Community Dentistry and Oral Epidemiology, 51*(5), 985–996. https://doi.org/10.1111/cdoe.12798

Keshavan, M. S., DeLisi, L. E., & Seidman, L. J. (2011). Early and broadly defined psychosis risk mental states. *Schizophrenia Research, 126,* 1–10. https;//doi.org/10.1016/j.schres.2010.10.006

King, K. (1998). Dental care of the psychiatric patient. *New Zealand Dental Journal, 94,* 72–82.

Knowles, E. E. M., David, A. S., & Reichenberg, A. (2010). Processing speed deficits in schizophrenia: Reexamining the evidence. *American Journal of Psychiatry, 167*(7), 828–835. https://doi.org/10.1176/appi.ajp.2010.09070937

Kraepelin, E. (1919). *Dementia praecox and paraphrenia.* Chicago Medical Book Co.

Ku, B. S., Aberizk, K., Addington, J., Bearden, C. E., Cadenhead, K. S., Cannon, T. D., Carrión, R. E., Compton, M. T., Cornblatt, B. A., Druss, B. G., Mathalon, D. H., Perkins, D. O., Tsuang, M. T., Woods, S. W., & Walker, E. F. (2022). The association between neighborhood poverty and hippocampal volume among individuals at clinical high-risk for psychosis: The moderating role of social engagement. *Schizophrenia Bulletin, 48*(5), 1032–1042. https://doi.org/10.1093/schbul/sbac055

Kuhn, H. W., & Nasar, S. (Eds.). (2002). *The essential John Nash.* Princeton University Press.

Kuo, S. S., Ventura, J., Forsyth, J. K., Subotnik, K. L., Turner, L. R., & Nuechterlein, K. H. (2022). Developmental trajectories of premorbid functioning predict cognitive remediation treatment response in first-episode schizophrenia. *Psychological Medicine, 53,* 1–10. https://doi.org/10.1017/S0033291722003312

Law, M., Baptiste, S., Carswell, A., McColl, M. A., Polatajko, H., & Pollock, N. (2014). *Canadian Occupational Performance Measure* (5th ed.). CAOT Publications.

Law, M., Cooper, B., Strong, S., Stewart, D., Rigby, P., & Letts, L. (1996). The Person-Environment-Occupation model: A transactive approach to occupational performance. *Canadian Journal of Occupational Therapy, 63*(1), 9–23. https://doi.org/10.1177/000841749606300103

Livio, S. K. (2009, March 14). Mathematician John Nash and family advocate for mental health care. *New Jersey Star-Ledger.* https://www.nj.com/news/2009/03/a_beautiful_challenge_to_help.html

MacDonald-Wilson, K. L., Williams, K., Nikolajski, C. E., McHugo, G., Kang, C., Deegan, P., Carpenter-Song, E., & Kogan, J. N. (2021). Promoting collaborative psychiatric care decision-making in community mental health centers: Insights from a patient-centered comparative effectiveness trial. *Psychiatric Rehabilitation Journal, 44*(1), 11–21. https://doi.org/10.1037/prj0000455

Machingura, T., Shum, D., Molineux, M., & Lloyd, C. (2018). Effectiveness of sensory modulation in treating sensory modulation disorders in adults with schizophrenia: A systematic literature review. *International Journal of Mental Health and Addiction, 16*(3), 764–780. https://doi.org/10.1007/s11469-017-9807-2

Martland, R., Teasdale, S., Murray, R. M., Gardner-Sood, P., Smith, S., Ismail, K., Atakan, Z., Greenwood, K., Stubbs, B., & Gaughran, F. (2021). Dietary intake, physical activity and sedentary behaviour patterns in a sample with established psychosis and associations with mental health symptomatology. *Psychological Medicine, 53*(4), 1–11. https://doi.org/10.1017/S0033291721003147

Meddings, S., Walley, L., Collins, T., Tullet, F., McEwan, B., & Owen, K. (2004). *Are hearing voices groups effective? A preliminary investigation.* The International Hearing Voices Network. https://www.intervoiceonline.org/2678/support/groups/are-hearing-voices-groups-effective.html

Mesholam-Gately, R. I., Giuliano, A. J., Goff, K. P., Faraone, S. V., & Seidman, L. J. (2009). Neurocognition in first-episode schizophrenia: A meta-analytic review. *Neuropsychology, 23*(3), 315–337. https://doi.org/10.1037/a0014708

Mittal, D., Sullivan, G., Chekuri, L., Allee, E., & Corrigan, P. W. (2012). Empirical studies of self-stigma reduction strategies: A critical review of the literature. *Psychiatric Services, 63,* 974–981. https://doi.org/10.1176/appi.ps.201100459

Molstrom, I. M., Nordgaard, J., Urfer-Parnas, A., Handest, R., Berge, J., & Henriksen, M. G. (2022). The prognosis of schizophrenia: A systematic review and meta-analysis with meta-regression of 20-year follow-up studies. *Schizophrenia Research, 250,* 152–163. https://doi.org/10.1016/j.schres.2022.11.010

Nagendra, A., Black, C., & Penn, D. L. (2023). Black Americans and schizophrenia: Racism as a driver of inequities in psychosis diagnosis, assessment, and treatment. *Schizophrenia Research, 253,* 1–4. https://doi.org/10.1016/j.schres.2022.10.007

Nasar, S. (1998). *A beautiful mind.* Simon & Schuster.

Naslund, J. A., Whiteman, K. L., McHugo, G. J., Aschbrenner, K. A., Marsch, L. A., & Bartels, S. J. (2017). Lifestyle interventions for weight loss among overweight and obese adults with serious mental illness: A systematic review and meta-analysis. *General Hospital Psychiatry, 47,* 83–102. https://doi.org/10.1016/j.genhosppsych.2017.04.003

National Academies of Sciences, Engineering, and Medicine. (2016). *Ending discrimination against people with mental and substance use disorders: The evidence for stigma change.* National Academies Press. https://doi.org/10.17226/23442

National Institute of Mental Health. (n.d.). *Research domain criteria (RDoC).* https://www.nimh.nih.gov/research/research-funded-by-nimh/rdoc

Newcomer, J. W., Weiden, P. J., & Buchanan, R. W. (2013). Switching antipsychotic medications to reduce adverse event burden in schizophrenia: Establishing evidence-based practice. *Journal of Clinical Psychiatry, 74,* 1108–1120. https://doi.org/10.4088/JCP.12028ah1

Nuechterlein, K. H., Subotnik, K. L., Green, M. F., Ventura, J., Asarnow, R. F., Gitlin, M. J., Yee, C. M., Gretchen-Doorly, D., & Mintz, J. (2011). Neurocognitive predictors of work outcome in recent-onset schizophrenia. *Schizophrenia Bulletin, 37*(Suppl. 2), S33–S40. https://doi.org/10.1093/schbul/sbr084

Olbert, C. M., Nagendra, A., & Buck, B. (2018). Meta-analysis of Black vs. White racial disparity in schizophrenia diagnosis in the United States: Do structured assessments attenuate racial disparities? *Journal of Abnormal Psychology, 127*(1), 104–115. https://doi.org/10.1037/abn0000309

Orellana, G., & Slachevsky, A. (2013). Executive functioning in schizophrenia. *Frontiers in Psychiatry, 4,* 35. https://doi.org/10.3389/fpsyt.2013.00035

Palmer, B. W., Savla, G. N., Fellows, I. E., Twamley, E. W., Jeste, D. V., & Lacro, J. P. (2010). Do people with schizophrenia have differential impairment in episodic memory and/or working memory relative to other cognitive abilities? *Schizophrenia Research, 116*(2-3), 259–265. https://doi.org/10.1016/j.schres.2009.11.002

Patel, S., Khan, S. M. S., & Hamid, P. (2020). The association between cannabis use and schizophrenia: Causative or curative? A systematic review. *Cureus, 12*(7), e9309. https://doi.org/10.7759/cureus.9309

Penttilä, M., Jääskeläinen, E., Hirvonen, N., Isohanni, M., & Miettunen, J. (2014). Duration of untreated psychosis as predictor of long-term outcome in schizophrenia: Systematic review and meta-analysis. *British Journal of Psychiatry, 205,* 88–94. https://doi.org/10.1192/bjp.bp.113.127753

Pernice, F. M., Biegel, D. E., Kim, J. Y., & Conrad-Garrisi, D. (2017). The mediating role of mattering to others in recovery and stigma. *Psychiatric Rehabilitation Journal, 40,* 395–404. https://doi.org/10.1037/prj0000269

Radhakrishnan, R., Wilkinson, S. T., & D'Souza, D. C. (2014). Gone to pot—A review of the association between cannabis and psychosis. *Frontiers in Psychiatry, 22,* 54. https://doi.org/10.3389/fpsyt.2014.00054

Remington, G. (2003). Understanding antipsychotic "atypicality": A clinical and pharmacological moving target. *Journal of Psychiatry & Neuroscience, 28,* 275–284.

Reser, M. P., Allott, K. A., Killackey, E., Farhall, J., & Cotton, S. M. (2015). Exploring cognitive heterogeneity in first-episode psychosis: What cluster analysis can reveal. *Psychiatry Research, 229*(3), 819–827. https://doi.org/10.1016/j.psychres.2015.07.084

Revisiting the CATIE schizophrenia study. (2008). *Harvard Mental Health Letter, 25,* 1–3.

Ringen, P. A., Engh, J. A., Birkenaes, A. B., Dieset, I., & Andreassen, O. A. (2014). Increased mortality in schizophrenia due to cardiovascular disease—A non-systematic review of epidemiology, possible causes and interventions. *Frontiers in Psychiatry, 5,* 137. https://doi.org/10.3389/fpsyt.2014.00137

Rogers, J. C., & Holm, M. B. (2016, June). Functional assessment in mental health: Lessons from occupational therapy. *Dialogues in Clinical Neuroscience, 18*(2), 145–154. https://doi.org/10.31887/DCNS.2016.18.2/jrogers

Schizophrenia Working Group of the Psychiatric Genomics Consortium. (2014). Biological insights from 108 schizophrenia-associated genetic loci. *Nature, 511,* 421–427. https://doi.org/10.1038/nature13595

Sheffield, J. M., Karcher, N. R., & Barch, D. M. (2018). Cognitive deficits in psychotic disorders: A lifespan perspective. *Neuropsychology Review, 28*(4), 509–533. https://doi.org/10.1007/s11065-018-9388-2

Tandon, R., Gaebel, W., Barch, D. M., Bustillo, J., Gur, R. E., Heckers, S., Malaspina, D., Owen, M. J., Schultz, S., Tsuang, M., Van Os, J., & Carpenter, W. (2013). Definition and description of schizophrenia in *DSM-5. Schizophrenia Research, 150,* 3–10. https://doi.org/10.1016/j.schres.2013.05.028

Teasdale, S. B., Ward, P. B., Samara, K., Firth, J., Stubbs, B., Tripodi, E., & Burrows, T. L. (2019). Dietary intake of people with severe mental illness: Systematic review and meta-analysis. *British Journal of Psychiatry, 214,* 251–259. https://doi.org/10.1192/bjp.2019.20

Tessner, K. D., Mittal, V., & Walker, E. F. (2011). Longitudinal study of stressful life events and daily stressors among adolescents at high risk for psychotic disorders. *Schizophrenia Bulletin, 37,* 432–441. https://doi.org/10.1093/schbul/sbp087

Townsend, L., Pillinger, T., Selvaggi, P., Veronese, M., Turkheimer, F., & Howes, O. (2023). Brain glucose metabolism in schizophrenia: A systematic review and meta-analysis of [18]FDG-PET studies in schizophrenia. *Psychological Medicine, 53*(11), 4880–4897. https://doi.org/10.1017/S003329172200174X

Tsuang, M. T., Stone, W. S., & Faraone, S. V. (2000). Toward reformulating the diagnosis of schizophrenia. *American Journal of Psychiatry, 157,* 1041–1050. https://doi.org/10.1176/appi.ajp.157.7.1041

Valery, K. M., & Prouteau, A. (2020). Schizophrenia stigma in mental health professionals and associated factors: A systematic review. *Psychiatry Research, 290,* 113068. https://doi.org/10.1016/j.psychres.2020.113068

van Erp, T. G. M., Walton, E., Hibar, D. P., Schmaal, L., Jiang, W., Glahn, D. C., Pearlson, G. D., Yao, N., Fukunaga, M., Hashimoto, R., Okada, N., Yamamori, H., Bustillo, J. R., Clark, V. P., Agartz, I., Mueller, B. A., Cahn, W., de Zwarte, S. M. C., Hulshoff Pol, H. E., . . . Turner, J. A. (2018). Cortical brain abnormalities in 4474 individuals with schizophrenia and 5098 control subjects via the Enhancing Neuro Imaging Genetics Through Meta Analysis (ENIGMA) consortium. *Biological Psychiatry, 84*(9), 644–654. https://doi.org/10.1016/j.biopsych.2018.04.023

Van Os, J., Linscott, R., Myin-Germeys, I., Delespaul, P., & Krabbendam, L. (2009). A systematic review and meta-analysis of the psychosis continuum: Evidence for a psychosis proneness–persistence–impairment model of psychotic disorder. *Psychological Medicine, 39*(2), 179–195. https://doi.org/10.1017/S0033291708003814

Veling, W., Susser, E., van Os, J., Mackenbach, J. P., Selten, J. P., & Hoek, H. W. (2008). Ethnic density of neighborhoods and incidence of psychotic disorders among immigrants. *American Journal of Psychiatry, 165,* 66–73. https://doi.org/10.1176/appi.ajp.2007.07030423

Walker, E., Kestler, L., Bollini, A., & Hochman, K. M. (2004). Schizophrenia: Etiology and course. *Annual Review of Psychology, 55,* 401–430. https://doi.org/10.1146/annurev.psych.55.090902.141950

Wolny, J., Moussa-Tooks, A. B., Bailey, A. J., O'Donnell, B. F., & Hetrick, W. P. (2023). Race and self-reported paranoia: Increased item endorsement on subscales of the SPQ. *Schizophrenia Research, 253,* 30–39. https://doi.org/10.1016/j.schres.2021.11.034

World Health Organization. (2021). *Guidance on community mental health services: Promoting person-centred and rights-based approaches.* Author. https://www.who.int/publications/i/item/9789240025707

Wunderink, L., Nieboer, R. M., Wiersma, D., Sytema, S., & Nienhuis, F. J. (2013). Recovery in remitted first-episode psychosis at 7 years of follow-up of an early dose reduction/discontinuation or maintenance treatment strategy: Long-term follow-up of a 2-year randomized clinical trial. *JAMA Psychiatry, 70*(9), 913–920. https://doi.org/10.1001/jamapsychiatry.2013.19

Zammit, S., Lewis, G., Rasbash, J., Dalman, C., Gustafsson, J. E., & Allebeck, P. (2010). Individuals, schools and neighborhood: A multilevel longitudinal study of variation in incidence of psychotic disorder. *Archives of General Psychiatry, 67,* 914–922. https://doi.org/10.1001/archgenpsychiatry.2010.101

Zipursky, R. B. (2014). Why are the outcomes in patients with schizophrenia so poor? *Journal of Clinical Psychiatry, 75*(Suppl. 2), 20–24. https://doi.org/10.4088/JCP.13065su1.05

CHAPTER 24

Substance-Related and Addictive Disorders

Rebecca Knowles

Drinking alcohol, smoking tobacco or marijuana, and taking medications not prescribed or at unsafe levels are examples of what an occupational therapy practitioner (OTP) might identify as risky occupations, because they can lead to unintentional negative health consequences. The potential risk can be further complicated when these substances are consumed while taking psychotropic medications and other medications prescribed for psychiatric conditions or for pain management.

This chapter provides practical information that OTPs can apply to working with individuals, populations, and communities. It highlights the distinct value of mindfully monitoring occupational performance in everyday life as a means of being alerted to the unsafe consequences of mood-altering substances. OTPs impact health, well-being, and quality of life across the health and wellness spectrum, in multiple roles, as members of a health-care team, delivering services in the workplace, homes, schools, and communities, as well as in leadership roles influencing policies and programs. Consequently, regardless of practice area, they need to understand how the use of substances can impact the everyday lives of individuals served; it is a topic deserving of attention, awareness, and, when needed, action.

Description of the Conditions

A common feature of **substance use disorders (SUDs)** is that the individual continues to use the substances, despite significant disruption to meaningful activities across all areas of occupation. Life roles may be compromised: The college student misses classes and eventually drops out; the parent neglects homecare responsibilities, and children suffer; or a person ignores work responsibilities and is fired, causing a loss of financial stability and considerable family upheaval. SUDs do not discriminate by age, gender, race, ethnicity, sexual identity, religious affiliation, geographic location, or socioeconomic status. All segments of society are potentially vulnerable to the consequences of SUDs, which range from fetal alcohol syndrome (FAS) to heroin and opioid addiction, making them among the most serious health problems facing the United States (Substance Abuse and Mental Health Services Administration [SAMHSA], 2022).

According to the *Diagnostic and Statistical Manual of Mental Disorders,* Fifth Edition, Text Revision (American Psychiatric Association [APA], 2022), the diagnosis of SUD involves negative patterns of behaviors involving 11 symptoms across the following four areas:

1. Impaired control (e.g., using more than intended or unable to cut down even when wanting to do so)
2. Social impairment (e.g., unable to meet established roles such as worker or parent)
3. Risky use (e.g., continuing to use despite negative outcomes)
4. Pharmacological criteria (tolerance and withdrawal)

The diagnosis of SUD can range in severity from mild (meets two to three symptoms) or moderate (meets four to five symptoms) to severe (meets six or more symptoms).

The subtypes of drug use disorder are not typically categorized by amount or patterns of use, but they are often delineated by the category of drug (e.g., alcohol, cocaine, nicotine), prescription or nonprescription drugs, age of users, and use by gender. An extensive discussion about subtypes of drug use is beyond the scope of this chapter, but Table 24-1 provides more information on the types of drugs classified in the *DSM-5-TR* (APA, 2022).

Prevalence of Alcohol and Drug Use

According to data from the 2020 National Survey on Drug Use and Health (NSDUH), 40.3 million people (14.5%) age 12 and older had an SUD in the previous year, including 28.3 million with alcohol use disorder and 18.4 million with an illicit drug use disorder (SAMHSA, 2021). Alcohol and tobacco are the most prevalent substances used, with half the population reporting alcohol use (at least one drink) in the previous month, 22.2% reporting binge use, and 6.4% reporting heavy alcohol use. More than 57 million people (20.7%) reported tobacco use in the past month. The category of tobacco expanded in 2020 to include nicotine vaping, with more than 10.4 million reporting use in the past month, and the highest rates among young adults ages 18 to 25 (SAMHSA, 2021).

Illicit drugs include marijuana, cocaine (including crack), hallucinogens (including LSD, PCP, Ecstasy), inhalants, methamphetamine, and prescription psychotherapeutics (including pain relievers, tranquilizers, stimulants, sedatives) when misused (not prescribed or using at a level other than what was prescribed). Illicit drug use over the past year was

TABLE 24-1 | Substance-Related Classes

Class of Substance	Common Forms Available	Mode(s) of Ingestion	Intended Effects	Warning Signs of Use or Overuse	Educational Resources
Alcohol	Beer, wine, hard liquor (i.e., scotch, whiskey, gin, vodka), malt liquor	Drink	Relaxation, lower inhibitions	Intoxication, slurred speech, motor and cognitive slowed responses; injuries caused by automobile accidents, falls, drownings, burns; violence such as homicide, suicide, sexual assault, intimate partner violence; alcohol poisoning; risky sexual practices; fetal alcohol spectrum disorders in pregnant women	http://www.cdc.gov /alcohol/fact-sheets /alcohol-use.htm
Caffeine	Coffee, tea, soda, energy drinks, sweets (chocolate, espresso beans, energy mints), medication (Excedrin, NoDoz)	Drink, eat, or swallow	Energy, alertness	Headaches, restlessness, anxiety	http://www .mayoclinic.org /healthy-lifestyle /nutrition-and -healthy-eating /in-depth/caffeine /art-20049372?pg=1
Tobacco	Cigarettes, cigars, hookah, bidis, kreteks, pipe, smokeless tobacco, e-cigarettes	Smoke, chew, sniff	Relaxation, mild euphoria, decreased appetite	Cardiovascular damage leading to stroke, heart disease; respiratory damage leading to lung cancer, emphysema, chronic bronchitis; worsens asthma; cancers of the body; high-risk pregnancy	http://www.cdc .gov/tobacco /index.htm
Cannabis	Marijuana, THC, THC-rich resins	Smoke joints, blunts, bongs; inhale with use of vaporizers, dabbing resins	"High," altered senses, altered sense of time, mood changes, impaired body movements, difficulty thinking and problem-solving, impaired memory	Long-term effects: brain development, breathing problems, heart rate changes, pregnancy fetal impact; temporary hallucinations and paranoia, worsens symptoms in schizophrenia	http://www .drugabuse.gov /publications /drugfacts /marijuana
Hallucinogens	Lysergic acid diethylamide (LSD, acid, microdots, window panes, blotters), psilocybin (magic mushroom) peyote, DMT, PCP, ketamine	Varied routes: diluted in water, brewed into tea, vaporized, smoked in pipe, snorted	Hallucination: altered sense of reality, intense emotional swings	Anxiety, memory loss, body tremors, numbness; high doses can lead to physical distress (i.e., increased heart rate, body temperature, blood pressure, respiration rate); psychological stress (i.e., extreme panic, fear, anxiety, paranoia, invulnerability, exaggerated strength, and aggression)	https://www.dea .gov/sites/default /files/2020-06 /Hallucinogens -2020.pdf
Inhalants	Volatile solvents (paint thinner, gasoline, glues, felt-tip markers); aerosols (spray paint, deodorant and hair sprays, vegetable oil sprays, fabric protector sprays); gases (nitrous oxide, ether, chloroform); nitrites (amyl or butyl nitrites, poppers, or snappers)	Breathed into the nose or mouth in varied ways: sniffing, snorting, bagging, huffing	Quick-acting euphoria, intoxication-like alcohol effect, slurred speech, incoordinated movements, dizziness	Lightheadedness, hallucinations, delusions; with repeated uses, loss of consciousness and death are possible	http://www .drugabuse.gov /publications /research-reports /inhalants /what-are-inhalants

Continued

TABLE 24-1 | Substance-Related Classes—cont'd

Class of Substance	Common Forms Available	Mode(s) of Ingestion	Intended Effects	Warning Signs of Use or Overuse	Educational Resources
Opioids	Vicodin, Oxycontin, morphine, heroin, codeine	Taken orally, but some can be snorted or injected	Reduce the perception of pain; some experience euphoria	Drowsiness, constipation, mental confusion, nausea, can increase the risk of life-threatening decreased respirations when combined with alcohol and other substances	http://www.drugabuse.gov/publications/research-reports/prescription-drugs/opioids
Central nervous system (CNS) depressants: sedative, hypnotic, or anxiolytics	Valium, Xanax, Ambien, Lunesta, barbituates	Taken orally	Lessen anxiety and sleeplessness by calming and causing drowsiness	Potential for abuse; when stopped, can have rebound effect with seizures or other harmful consequences	https://www.drugabuse.gov/drugs-abuse/commonly-abused-drugs-charts#CNSdepressants
Stimulants: prescription medicines	Dexedrine, Adderall, Ritalin, Concerta	Taken orally	Increase alertness, attention, and energy; elevate blood pressure, heart rate, and respiration	Abuse potential, euphoria, and perceived cognitive enhancers; withdrawal symptoms: fatigue, depression, disturbed sleep patterns, and other hazardous outcomes	https://www.drugabuse.gov/publications/research-reports/prescription-drugs/stimulants
Stimulants: street drugs	Cocaine (coke, C, snow, powder, blow)	Powder might be snorted, injected, used orally on gums, or heated to create crack for inhalation.	Euphoria; talkative; mentally alert; hypersensitive to sight, sound, and touch; temporarily reduces the need to eat and sleep	Potential for toxic amounts to lead to heart attacks, strokes, or seizures, all of which can lead to death	https://www.dea.gov/sites/default/files/2020-06/Cocaine-2020_1.pdf

reported by 59.3 million people (21.4%) age 12 and older (SAMHSA, 2021).

It is noteworthy that caffeine and nicotine misuse commonly occur with other substance-related disorders. Unfortunately, these substances are not typically addressed in substance abuse treatment programs because the acute psychosocial and biological consequences of alcohol and drug abuse and dependence typically take precedence. Substance-related disorders might also involve abuse of multiple substances (e.g., cocaine use coupled with alcohol to reduce the anxiety caused by the cocaine). As part of a health and wellness approach, OTPs need to be prepared to address concerns related to all mood-altering substances to promote awareness of healthy choices and options for harm reduction.

The reader is urged to use Table 24-1 and the additional resources at the end of this chapter to learn more about these and other drugs and their potential effects on individuals receiving occupational therapy intervention across the spectrum of health conditions.

One type of drug use that warrants special consideration is that of opioid use, judged to be at epidemic levels in the United States and causing many unintended overdose deaths. The Centers for Disease Control and Prevention (CDC) in the United States has issued guidelines for health professionals considering epidemic prescription opioid addiction and overdose (Dowell et al., 2022).

In 2021, the CDC estimated there were 107,622 drug overdose deaths in the United States, including 71,238 from synthetic opioids, such as fentanyl (National Center for Health Statistics [NCHS], 2022). Fentanyl is a powerful analgesic, approximately 100 times more potent than morphine (Comer & Cahill, 2019). Even a small amount can be lethal and difficult to detect when mixed with other substances. A 30% increase in overdose deaths was observed between 2019 and 2020, accelerating sharply in March 2020 at the start of the COVID-19 pandemic (Hedegaard et al., 2021). Qualitative findings suggest that unintended consequences of public health mitigation policies, including social isolation, economic stress, decreased access to treatment, and changes in supply of illicit substances, are factors that contributed to this increase (Mattson et al., 2022).

Opioid drugs are powerful. They induce a sense of pleasure and well-being; however, given the stimulation of opioid receptors in deeper regions of the brain, drowsiness and respiratory depression can lead to accidental death. The National Institute on Drug Abuse (NIDA) reports that prescription opioids, including oxycodone, acetaminophen and hydrocodone (Vicodin), morphine, codeine, fentanyl, and methadone, have the same mechanism of action as heroin (NIDA, 2015). When taken for a period, these drugs are associated with increasing levels of tolerance, and more of the drug is needed to produce the same effect.

As individuals take more of the drug, they are at greater risk of overdose. The CDC reports that these powerful pain relievers have been prescribed four times more since 1999, with no concurrent increase in the incidence of pain among

Americans (Dowell et al., 2016). Three populations are identified as being at the highest risk for opioid addiction: (1) adolescents, (2) persons being treated for chronic pain, and (3) persons addicted to another substance (U.S. Department of Health & Human Services, 2016).

Co-Occurring Disorders

SUD and mental health conditions often present together, described as a **co-occurring disorder** (COD; SAMHSA, 2020). Although they influence each other, the relationship is not necessarily causal or directional. Substance use may contribute to the altering of neural processes that predispose an individual to the development of mental health conditions; similarly, mental health conditions can influence the development of an SUD, as individuals may use substances for temporary management of symptoms (Santucci, 2012). Comorbidity can also be attributed to common risk factors, including genetic, epigenetic, and environmental factors; stress; and adverse childhood experiences (Cerdá et al., 2010; He et al., 2022; Nestler, 2014; Santucci, 2012).

According to the 2020 NSDUH survey, 17.0 million adults (18 years or older) in the United States had a COD; of the 14.2 million adults with a serious mental illness (SMI) in 2020, 5.7 million adults also had an SUD (SAMHSA, 2021). In 2020, adults with a COD were more likely to use illicit drugs, smoke marijuana, misuse opioids, binge alcohol, and use tobacco and nicotine products compared with adults without mental illness (SAMHSA, 2021).

Substance abuse by individuals with SMI results in a wide range of adverse consequences, including poorer prognosis, higher costs because of greater use of acute psychiatric services, low compliance with treatment regimens, and overall decreased occupational functioning. Substance use also frequently co-occurs with posttraumatic stress disorder (PTSD), explained in part by individuals using substances to modulate their stress response (Flanagan et al., 2016; Logrip et al., 2012).

Etiology of Substance Use

Substance use is a complex condition, and there are many pathways that contribute to its development. Understanding the neurobiological, psychological, and environmental factors that underlie these conditions also informs OTPs about intervention approaches.

Neurobiological Factors

From a neurobiological perspective, individuals with substance abuse might process the drugs and experience them in ways that lead to compulsive use. For example, individuals with substance abuse disorders tend to have brains that lack inhibitory control and have a dysregulated reward system (Koyama et al., 2017). The cycle of substance use begins with binging/intoxication, is followed by withdrawal, and leads to preoccupation and anticipation of next use (Fig. 24-1). Neurobiological factors contribute to the perpetuation of this cycle (Murnane et al., 2023).

During the initial stage of binge and intoxication, most misused drugs release dopamine and affect other

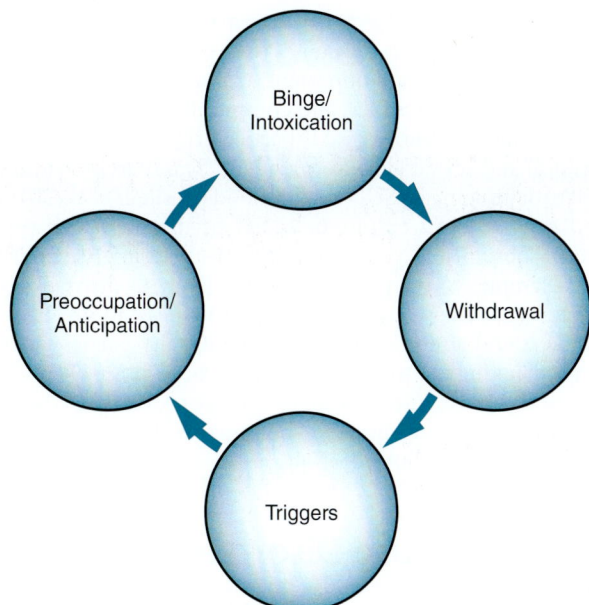

FIGURE 24-1. Cycle of addiction.

neurotransmitter pathways such as the serotonergic and opioid systems. People with substance misuse tend to have an enhanced response to the rewards associated with drugs, which becomes hypersensitized over time and leads to a decreased sensitivity to other types of rewards (Baskin-Sommers & Foti, 2015). A lack of cognitive control or an inability to delay gratification is also associated with a vulnerability for SUDs (Lees et al., 2021).

The discontinuation of substance use leads to the emergence of withdrawal symptoms and cravings. During withdrawal, the individual experiences irritability, pain, and a loss of motivation for natural rewards. Triggers such as drug paraphernalia or a time of day or event associated with drug use leads to cravings. The individual becomes preoccupied with using and this preoccupation/anticipation stage can lead to the release of good feeling neurotransmitters such as cortisol (Kexel et al., 2022). Neuroimaging studies provide support for the cycle of addiction model (Murnane et al., 2023). Pharmacological interventions such as naltrexone and methadone can be useful in addiction recovery programs to decrease positive drug experiences without cessation through a harm-reduction approach (Ma et al., 2019; Qeadan, 2021).

Psychological and Environmental Factors

A biological vulnerability interacts with psychological and environmental factors to create a predisposition to SUDs. Certain personality traits, such as impulsivity and sensation seeking, are associated with a greater likelihood of substance use problems (Hamdan-Mansour et al., 2017). From a behavioral perspective, using drugs and alcohol begins as a goal-directed behavior that is reinforced by dopamine and other reward pathways, which over time becomes habituated. This adaptation is of course influenced by the environment and context (Heinz et al., 2019).

Factors such as poverty, trauma exposure, and social endorsement for substance use speak to sociological considerations that are important to consider when working with individuals, families, and communities. For example, a trauma history before age 11, particularly one that involves physical and sexual violence, greatly increases an individual's risk of developing an SUD in adulthood (Carliner et al., 2016).

Being part of a culture or social environment that promotes substance use can also put individuals at greater risk. For example, young people are more likely to drink excessively when they spend time with friends who are heavy drinkers and attend events such as fraternity parties where binge drinking is a social norm (Kuntsche et al., 2017). From this perspective, interventions aimed at preventing adverse environmental exposure and changing social norms can be useful in reducing substance abuse.

Substance Use Disorder in Specific Populations

Culture-Specific Information and Gender Differences

There are differences in rates of substance use and abuse across cultural and socioeconomic groups. African Americans and Native Americans have higher rates of use than the general population, whereas Asian Americans have lower rates (Khera & Nakamura, 2016). Individuals who tend to use spirituality or religion as a coping mechanism are less likely to have SUDs (Debnam et al., 2017), whereas individuals who are unemployed are at greater risk for substance abuse (McCabe et al., 2017).

Income inequality and health disparity also influence the experience of SUD across populations. After accounting for confounding factors, including local opioid prescription rates, low household income and increased rates of incarceration were both associated with drug-related death (Nosrati et al., 2019).

Overall rates of use and dependency on illicit substances is higher in men in almost all categories, although prescription drug misuse is similar among men and women (CDC, 2016). In the United States in 2020, the most commonly used illicit drug by women was marijuana (16%), followed by psychotherapeutic drugs (6%), including prescription stimulants, tranquilizers, sedatives, and pain relievers (SAMHSA, 2022). The gender gap appears to be narrowing in recent years, as drug overdose deaths have increased dramatically in women (VanHouten et al., 2019).

Women and men have different patterns in substance use from initiation to dependence and recovery. The **telescoping effect** describes how women experience stronger responses to substances and accelerated disease progression, initially using in smaller amounts, but more quickly progressing to addiction (Greenfield et al., 2010). Although treatment outcomes for women and men are largely the same, women tend to experience more significant adverse consequences of SUD because of biological, psychosocial, and environmental factors (McHugh et al., 2018). Approximately 5% of women who are pregnant use substances (Wendell, 2013). Drinking and smoking after the first trimester increases the risk of sudden infant death syndrome (SIDS) by 12-fold (Elliott et al., 2020).

Substance use while pregnant can also lead to neonatal abstinence syndrome (NAS), in which the infant experiences withdrawal at birth. NAS acutely causes dysfunction in the central nervous system of the infant, presenting as a high-pitched cry, sleep difficulties, hypertonicity, tremors, and convulsions, in addition to autonomic and gastrointestinal symptoms (Logan et al., 2013). NAS can lead to long-term effects on neurodevelopment, including cognition, behavior, visual and motor systems, and sleep (Maguire et al., 2016). Historically, women have been excluded from SUD research, which has led to gaps in development of gender-specific treatment. More research is needed to better understand gender differences in substance use.

Substance Use Disorder Across the Life Span

The use of illicit substances has declined among adolescents in the United States, with a dramatic decrease from 2020 to 2021 associated with the COVID-19 pandemic (NIDA, 2022). The Monitoring the Future survey found that only 11% of eighth graders, 21.5% of 10th graders, and 32.6% of 12th graders reported using any illicit drug during the previous year. The most common drugs used were alcohol, nicotine, and cannabis. Ironically, despite the overall decrease in drug use, there has been a dramatic rise in overdose deaths among adolescents because of the increased availability of fentanyl.

Although rates of substance abuse have declined in adolescents and young adults, there is an increase in substance abuse for middle-aged and older adults (Kuerbis, 2020). This increase is associated with the rate of illicit drug use among the baby boomer population, which was higher than previous generations. Cannabis, alcohol, and prescription drugs are the most commonly abused drugs among adults age 50 or older.

There are certain risk factors associated with substance abuse and aging. For example, people who experience chronic pain are often prescribed opioid medication, which has led to an increase in the number of older adults seeking treatment for opioid addiction (NIDA, 2020). In addition, older adults metabolize substances more slowly and may experience heightened sensitivity to alcohol and other drugs, which contributes to falls and motor vehicle accidents.

Impact on Occupational Performance

Having an SUD can affect many occupations identified in the *Occupational Therapy Practice Framework* (*OTPF-4;* American Occupational Therapy Association [AOTA], 2020). These areas include:

- Activities of daily living (ADLs)
- Instrumental activities of daily living (IADLs)
- Rest and sleep
- Education
- Work
- Play
- Leisure
- Social participation

Occupational scientists have proposed that substance use or addiction can be classified as an occupation (Kiepek & Magalhaes, 2011; Wasmuth et al., 2014), meeting the criteria established by Townsend and Polatajko (2013) that occupations give meaning to life; are important to health, well-being, and justice; organize behavior; develop and change during a lifetime; shape and are shaped by environments; and have therapeutic potential. Although the last criterion may be debated, Kiepek and Magalhaes (2011) note the antidepressant effect of smoking tobacco.

Occupations have been understood to have the potential for both positive and negative consequences, gains and harms. For example, some individuals report positive perceptions of cannabis use, including (a) preserving life; (b) navigating the routines of everyday life; (c) understanding the self, identity, and belonging; and (d) expanding the view of the world (Guyonnet et al., 2023).

Canadian occupational therapist Niki Kiepek wrote *Licit, Illicit, Prescribed: Substance Use and Occupational Therapy* (2016), in which she frames use of substances across a continuum and notes not only negative consequences of substance use, but positive and neutral consequences, so as to promote full awareness of how people view their own use and its impact. In addition, Kiepek suggests that substance abuse treatment focuses on reduction of use, but that little attention is directed toward helping people fill the gap with engagement in meaningful activities.

The Lived Experience

Annie

Like a lot of people, I started my relationship with drugs and alcohol when I was a teenager. I went to boarding school in Europe for my last 3 years of high school. In this sheltered, hedonistic world, we were able to buy 2€ bottles of wine and pints of gin. I smoked Moroccan hash. I experimented with harder drugs. I was desperate for connection, and drugs helped me become a different person than who I considered to be myself. I was always quiet and withdrawn, unsure of how I was perceived, since so many girls had hated me in middle school. I knew that my regular way of being bothered a lot of people, so drugs and alcohol were my pass to friends and parties and fun. I came to know myself as a bit of a wild child, but I liked myself better and so did my peers.

When I came home to the states in my early adulthood, I participated in the party culture of my boyfriend and his friends. He and I were the first ones to move out of our parents' houses, so we constantly had people over, and drinking made it fun and bearable for me. We bought weed from friends and acquaintances since it wasn't legal yet. We did other drugs. We felt invincible, and our bodies would bounce back quickly.

My addiction was invisible for a long time since it blended into the background of casual, everyday use by my friends and family. When I got divorced from my husband, my reliance on and relationship with alcohol evolved into a full-blown addiction. Drinking became a part of my personality and my mechanism for dealing with the world. I would get sloppy and do dangerous things, such as unprotected sex, driving under the influence, and generally making a fool of myself. However, I couldn't stop. I didn't have the coping skills or full understanding of my relationship with substances to make a lasting change. Toward the end, I would drink half of a 750 mL bottle of tequila a night. I was miserable and permanently hungover. But nothing helped the anxiety and misery more than the other half of that bottle when I got home.

When COVID first hit and I was alone in my apartment for months, I knew I had to change my relationship with alcohol or I was on the way to death—quickly or slowly, but by my own hand. My social lubricant was no longer necessary to interact with the world, and the real effects of drinking to excess every day were much more apparent in the silence. Two close family friends around my age both lost their lives from complications of alcohol addiction during the early days of the pandemic. I had to confront reality: For almost 20 years, I drank myself into a blackout every night. I tried to quit through my own will power, but it was my only reliable way of falling asleep (passing out) and handling the social and personal demands of my high-stress IT job. The isolation of early COVID helped me separate the way I functioned from the way I was forced to function to conform to societal expectations.

After lots of research, I went into a medical detox facility and then joined an Intensive Outpatient Program (IOP) for women in my city. It was through the IOP that I considered sensory differences as part of my reasons for drinking. IOP helped me learn coping mechanisms and concepts to understand addiction in general. However, I didn't feel I belonged in recovery communities and that I was still missing a piece of the puzzle that explained my personal history of addiction.

While watching Hannah Gadsby's comedy special *Douglas* on Netflix, a line from the show stuck with me, something that people would say to her when suggesting she may be autistic: "I have a piece of information you seem to be missing." Maybe this was my missing piece. I googled "women and autism" and cried for a month while I read about people like me. It took time to fully integrate the idea that my constant feeling of un-belonging since childhood was due to my neurodivergence. Eventually, I sought professional help and received my diagnosis of "Autism Spectrum Disorder Level 1—Social Communication and Restricted, Repetitive Behavior Without Accompanying Intellectual or Language Impairment" or what used to be called Asperger syndrome.

Sensory differences were never discussed during my years of therapy and pharmacological treatments. No one ever suggested that I might be neurodivergent and instead I received treatment for anxiety and depression with no relief. While researching and discussing my experience with other autistic adults, it seems this is a common occurrence. Sensory issues often contribute to our discomfort, and we have less ability to regulate the way these differences affect us. How reassuring it was to know that other people don't like dogs or beaches or

Continued

The Lived Experience—cont'd

parties, not because we're terrible people, but because the sensory experiences can be unbearable! I didn't have the language or context to understand that I experienced things differently than other people.

More than a year after my diagnosis, I am still understanding ways that my sensory differences affected my life and my interactions with people I love. For example, an ex would fall asleep on the couch with the light on, and I would complain about it because it would wake me up. Now I understand I wasn't simply nagging; I was trying to ask for support from my partner for a sensory sensitivity. If I had understood my issue with light, I could have advocated for myself in a more positive and productive way. A friend questioned why I attended

so many concerts when they were painful for me. It never occurred to me that others didn't experience the lights and sounds painfully and that it was just another thing I had to deal with. And I dealt with it by abusing alcohol.

I am learning how to be gentle with myself, learning to give myself space and lots of recovery time if I am in a sensorily overwhelming situation. I say no to a lot more things now. I am living a quieter life than ever before, but I am developing a comfortable, loving relationship with my body for the first time. I spent many years ignoring and repressing my body's signals. It takes time and patience to reconnect with those messages, but it's worth it. I hope others can find this relief and give themselves lots of grace during the process.

Consistent with the Canadian Model of Occupational Performance and Engagement (Townsend & Polatajko, 2013), an analysis of substance use includes an exploration of the interaction between substance use and the environment. Kiepek (2016) helps to draw attention to environmental influences, such as living in communities where substance use is prominent and therefore influences the likelihood that a person uses substances.

Another factor is that use of substances can increase exposure to risky environments; for example, to obtain some substances, the person may enter unsafe neighborhoods. She also emphasizes the influence of healthy environments and suggests that access to adequate housing and social opportunities might decrease substance use, especially if family and peer support is available. Additional environmental features impacting substance use are cultural and religious use for healing and sacred ceremonies, as well as the impact of advertising, law enforcement practices, and substance education in schools.

OTPs work with people and families who may just be becoming aware that the use of substances is impacting their lives, or are already on a path toward recovery. Substance use impacts not only the user's routines but the entire family. The disruption of routines makes it difficult to pursue meaningful occupational roles such as parenting, taking care of a pet, driving a car, maintaining personal finances, eating and exercising in a healthy manner, maintaining a home, and participating with a spiritual community. See Chapter 14: Time Use and Habits. 🤝 For example, a parent using drugs or alcohol might not be able to take their child to an important after-school activity, so the child also misses out on important participation opportunities. Some parents with SUD may have limitations in parenting skills that promote the healthy development of their child, or be challenged to provide a nurturing and safe relationship and home environment.

In addition, a change in substance use or exacerbation of mental health symptoms can affect one's ability to fall or stay asleep, and it can affect the quality of one's rest. Performance in school and work often precipitates outside attention to the negative consequences of an SUD or COD (missed classes or days at work; poor school or work performance; attention from teachers, supervisors, or peers because of performance issues). Chapter 52: Sleep explores this topic in detail. 🤝

Pursuit of playful activities that provide enjoyment, leisure exploration, and participation in environments that are free of substance use can also be early challenges to making healthy changes in occupational routines. Frequently, conscious and deliberate choices about the people and places where one engages in social and community participation need to be considered, as continuing to spend time in using environments with friends who continue to use drugs and alcohol might place the person with an SUD at high risk for relapse. Use of substances is likely woven into the fabric of everyday life and may be used to cope with the symptoms of mental illness. The person seeking recovery and health may need support to rebuild their lifestyle and occupational routines. Also see Chapter 49: Connectedness and Belonging and Chapter 51: Leisure and Creative Occupations. 🤝

Sensory Processing and Substance Use

Sensory processing differences are documented in substance users and may explain some behaviors and their impact on occupational performance. **Sensory processing** describes an individual's experience of perceiving and integrating sensory stimuli from the environment, resulting in a behavioral response (Dunn, 2001).

Individuals with SUDs have demonstrated atypical sensory processing preferences, including stronger patterns of sensory sensitivity, avoidance, and low registration, with gender differences in sensation seeking (Engel-Yeger, 2014; Stols et al., 2013). These differences might be explained by the self-medication hypothesis (Khantzian, 1997), which asserts that individuals with SUD use drugs and alcohol to mediate arousal and affect. Van Gundy and colleagues (2015) identified avoidance as a coping style associated with substance use. Sensory sensitivity and distress are also associated with increased, problematic substance use (Meredith et al., 2020).

Chronic substance use can also change how the brain responds to internal cues (Maracic & Moeller, 2021; Verdejo-Garcia et al., 2012; Wiśniewski et al., 2021).

In addition to sensory processing patterns, OTPs should consider how interoception impacts substance use and occupational participation. For example, patients with SUD can be challenged to respond appropriately to internal cues for hunger,

Evidence-Based Practice

Alternative Habits and Routines

Interventions that provide meaning for a person committed to abstaining from substance use can contribute to treatment retention and lower relapse rates.

RESEARCH FINDINGS

OTPs who address occupational deficits with alternative habits and routines that provide meaning for a person committed to a life of abstaining from substance use can contribute to treatment retention and lower relapse rates (Wasmuth et al., 2014). Social participation and connectedness as a part of building more satisfying relationships can be an important focus of occupational therapy as well as exploring "captivating occupations."

APPLICATIONS

➡ OTPs can use interventions that both "(1) allow individuals to 'lose themselves' in the activity, providing a temporary sense of freedom from anxiety and other concerns, and/or (2) facilitate the development of an increasing sense of mastery and self-efficacy to foster feelings of being 'in control' when desired" (Wasmuth et al., 2014, p. 612).

➡ OTPs can use group activities that promote social interaction with others while engaged in an occupation (Wasmuth et al., 2016).

REFERENCES

Wasmuth, S., Crabtree, J. L., & Scott, P. J. (2014). Exploring addiction-as-occupation. *British Journal of Occupational Therapy, 77*, 605–613. https://doi.org.10.4276/030802214X14176260335264

Wasmuth, S., Pritchard, K., & Kaneshiro, K. (2016). Occupation-based intervention for addictive disorders: A systematic review. *Journal of Substance Abuse Treatment, 62*, 1–9. https://doi.org/10.1016/j.jsat.2015.11.011

---

thirst, fatigue, and hot and cold, which can impact participation in ADLs, including bathing, oral hygiene, feeding, meal preparation, and sleep. For more information see Chapter 9: Sensory Processing and the Lived Sensory Experience. 🤝

Intervention

Interventions for SUD occur in many locations, including hospitals, emergency departments, rehabilitation facilities, mental health centers, private medical or psychology practices, prisons, and community-based self-help groups. SUD treatment is nonlinear; individuals seeking support for SUD may enter and leave treatment anywhere along the continuum of care because of limitations in service access and individual readiness for change. For example, an individual using heroin may be temporarily hospitalized following an accidental overdose, followed by participation in self-help groups upon discharge. Another individual experiencing opioid dependence may access daily support through an outpatient medication-assisted treatment (MAT) program.

There is a discrepancy in the need for substance use treatment with the receipt of services. Of the 41.1 million people 12 years or older who needed substance use treatment in

2020, only 6.5% (2.7 million people) received treatment at a specialty facility (hospital, drug or alcohol rehabilitation facility, or mental health center; SAMHSA, 2020). Adults age 26 or older who needed substance use treatment in the past year were more likely than their counterparts age 12 to 17 or age 18 to 25 to have received substance use treatment at a specialty facility in the past year (SAMHSA, 2020).

Barriers

There are many reasons why a person experiencing an SUD may not be ready for or have access to treatment. A systematic review by Farhoudian and colleagues (2022) identified individual, social, and structural barriers to substance use treatment. These included individual beliefs and perceptions, personality traits, psychiatric comorbidities, stigma, social factors, and legal and policy barriers.

Provider readiness can also be a barrier to treatment. A recent review of OTPs' knowledge and perceptions around SUDS by Mattila et al., 2022 identified limitations in readiness to serve individuals with SUDs. Readers can complete the Self-Assessment: Knowledge and Attitudes About Substance Use in the Apply it Now section of this chapter to better understand their own perceptions and readiness.

Medication-Assisted Treatments

Medication-assisted treatment (MAT) is a developing approach to SUD treatment that uses a harm-reduction approach to support the safety, health, and well-being of individuals in recovery. Providers who are licensed to dispense medications to those seeking treatment for SUDs receive best practice information from the American Society of Addiction Medicine (ASAM). Research on the use of medications to modify substance-related dependence and cravings continues to shape MAT.

Several classifications of drugs are included in most MAT programs: antagonists, agonists, and partial agonists. Three oral medications (naltrexone, acamprosate, and disulfiram) and an injectable form of naltrexone have been approved for treatment of alcohol dependence in the United States. Naltrexone, a narcotics antagonist, binds to receptors in the brain to limit euphoric effects and prevent physical dependence. Naltrexone can be used to mediate the impact of a variety of substance additions, including opioids and alcohol. It is also available in an extended-release formula, sold under the brand name Vivitrol (Swinford-Jackson et al., 2021). Acamprosate (Campral) reduces unpleasant symptoms associated with both craving and withdrawal (Swinford-Jackson et al., 2021).

Considered both a partial agonist and antagonist, the mechanism of action for acamprosate remains unclear, though it may be related to increasing calcium concentration (Schuster et al., 2021). Disulfiram (Antabuse) is an aversive agent that works by inhibiting elimination of acetaldehyde, causing extremely unpleasant gastrointestinal symptoms that mimic an immediate and severe hangover, including nausea, vomiting, jaundice, malaise, and dark urine (Stokes et al., 2024; Swinford-Jackson et al., 2021; Wang et al., 2020).

Methadone is a full agonist used to treat opioid use disorder and chronic pain, which reduces mortality risk (SAMHSA, 2023b; Sordo et al., 2017). In the United States, methadone is most often administered in only opioid treatment programs because of regulatory limits, risk of side effects, and potential for abuse. Global evidence indicates expanded methadone access can be safe and effective (Calcaterra et al., 2019), which is further supported by U.S. findings that suggest office-based administration ("methadone maintenance") to relatively stable and reliable patients has been found to improve treatment retention, satisfaction, employment, and participation in social occupations (McCarty et al., 2021).

Buprenorphine is another medication also used to treat opioid use disorder. It is a partial agonist that can be prescribed in-office and dispensed in sublingual tablets (naloxone, Subutex, Suboxone), as well as other forms (SAMHSA, 2023a). Although buprenorphine is more conveniently accessed, both buprenorphine and methadone treatment are found to be effective at reducing illicit opioid use, craving and withdrawal symptoms, and supporting cessation (Jordan et al., 2019). A systematic review found better neurocognitive functioning in adults receiving buprenorphine and methadone compared with active opioid users, though buprenorphine was associated with better executive functioning, attention, working memory, and learning (Mindt et al., 2022). With advances in the neurosciences and public health research, there is reason to be hopeful that new drugs will be developed and studied.

Mental Health in Culture and Society

Medication-Assisted Treatment: A Harm-Reduction Approach to Motherhood for Women in Recovery

Beyond the known risks and effects of opioids on a woman's body, dependence on opioids can limit participation in meaningful roles and occupations—including motherhood. Through a harm-reduction lens, MAT programs can provide a safe and accessible path through pregnancy, birth, and early infancy for women in recovery. In *The Birth Hour*, a podcast hosted by Bryn Huntpalmer, guest Shannon shares her story of becoming a parent while navigating the challenges and opportunities provided by MAT.

Three years into her recovery, participating in a combination of methadone and therapy services, Shannon reports discovering that she is pregnant. She faces several barriers while navigating her pregnancy, including difficulty accessing health insurance, finding a medical team familiar with methadone treatment, care coordination between providers, changes in employment, discrimination, judgment, and guilt. Shannon demonstrates self-advocacy and proactivity in preparing for her birth, seeking educational resources and developing a support group.

Although it can be medically managed, infants birthed by mothers using methadone have a significant likelihood of experiencing NAS. Shannon's newborn experiences symptoms of opioid withdrawal shortly after the birth and is transferred to the neonatal intensive care unit (NICU). Shannon finds that medical treatment, alongside breastfeeding and support from an experienced and caring nurse, help her son's symptoms resolve and enable her family to return home. Shannon reports that 3 years after birth, her son is healthy and developmentally typical. Though the risk of NAS remains present, MAT programs are one way to make motherhood more accessible to women in recovery.

Integrated Approach

The most effective interventions for substance-related dependence are a combination of psychosocial and pharmaceutical approaches. The psychosocial therapies address the beliefs, coping/stress management techniques, and social skills necessary to function without reliance on substances. Pharmaceutical approaches (i.e., medications) affect the neurochemistry of addiction to reduce the positive effects of the illicit substances and reduce cravings. An integrated treatment approach involves delivering a customized treatment plan combining one or more therapeutic approaches, based on the individual's needs (Colette & Olivier, 2023).

Combining medications with behavioral therapies to treat alcohol use disorder and SUD has been examined in a meta-analysis by Ray and colleagues (2020). The review included a range of pharmacological therapies, including naltrexone, acamprosate, methadone, buprenorphine, and disulfiram, combined with Cognitive Behavioral Therapy (CBT) and other evidence-based modalities. The findings supported the efficacy of an integrated approach, which performed better than usual clinical management or nonspecific counseling services.

TABLE 24-2 | Common Intervention Approaches for Substance Use and Co-Occurring Disorders

Approach	Target(s) of Intervention	Brief Synopsis	Chapters With Additional Information 🤝
Cognitive Behavioral Therapy	Distorted beliefs	Distorted beliefs are identified and then challenged by providing evidence to the contrary.	Chapter 8: Cognitive Beliefs
Motivational Interviewing	Promote engagement in change process to adopt healthy lifestyle practices	A form of relationship building that is based on establishing rapport and helping the individual identify their own reasons for change	Chapter 11: Motivation
Dialectical Behavior Therapy	Emotion regulation	Skills training targeting mindfulness meditation, interpersonal effectiveness, emotion regulation, and distress tolerance	Chapter 12: Emotion Regulation
Mindfulness Meditation	Enhancing emotional well-being	A form of meditation practice that focuses awareness nonjudgmentally on the present	Chapter 12: Emotion Regulation
Permanent Supportive Housing	Independent stable Housing	Individually tailored supports to promote successful living in the person's home of choice	Chapter 31: The Home Environment: Permanent Supportive Housing
Reentry programs from criminal justice system	Independent living and adaptive coping	Skills training for independent living and development of coping skills to promote successful reintegration from the criminal justice system to community living	Chapter 40: Criminal Justice Systems
Enabling Spiritual Participation	Finding meaning	Encourage individual to identify spiritual needs and then promote participation in formal religious or informal spiritual practices	Chapter 53: Spiritual Occupations
Transtheoretical Model of Change	Behavior change	Describes a nonlinear, dynamic progression of health behavior change across six discrete stages.	Chapter 11: Motivation

Other Intervention Approaches

Table 24-2 outlines common intervention approaches for individuals with SUDs and CODs and identifies the accompanying chapters in this text that provide more detailed information about those approaches. 🤝

General Considerations When Providing Occupational Therapy to People With Substance-Related and Addictive Disorders

As a part of the occupational profile, typically conducted as an early step in the evaluation process (AOTA, 2020) while reviewing a person's occupational history, roles, and habits, substance use might be reflected upon as the person shares daily habits and routines. Occupation-based psychoeducation featuring topics such as stress management, lifestyle balance, self-care, leisure, and motivation has been found supportive of recovery and occupational participation (Ryan et al., 2023). Unstructured time can be challenging for individuals in recovery (Kitzinger et al., 2023); OTPs can help individuals better manage time to optimize engagement in meaningful activity.

Regardless of the primary reason the person is being seen by an OTP, inquiring about the use of alcohol, tobacco, caffeine, and other substances is an appropriate part of an overall review of lifestyle habits. The relationship of other health-related routines, such as nutrition, sleep and rest patterns, level of physical activity, and social participation, also can be explored.

When substance use occurs at the level of being a disorder, and the individual's occupational role performance is severely impacted (e.g., problems with self-care, education, parenting, employment, and/or sleep), a referral to comprehensive and integrated physical and behavioral health programs that include OTPs as part of the interprofessional team is indicated.

Consistent with occupational therapy's role in medication management (Siebert & Schwartz, 2017), OTPs should consider the individual's prescription medication use in their evaluation. Because pain is frequently the entry point for addiction, a brief review of prescribed pain medications and reported use can help identify potential for addiction early on. New guidance from the CDC (Dowell et al., 2022) recommends that nonopioid and nonpharmacological pain treatments should be prioritized for most adults experiencing acute pain (less than 1 month); however, there is insufficient evidence to determine the benefits of long-term opioid use to treat subacute (1 to 3 months) or chronic (more than 3 months) pain. OTPs can provide pain management strategies including physical agent modalities, noninvasive and nonpharmacological therapies, and biopsychosocial interventions.

Even when SUD is established, drug and alcohol cessation is not always the primary goal for all individuals. Following a person-centered, occupation-based approach, OTPs can support individuals in identifying strategies to reduce harm and enhance participation in meaningful activities, despite the potential for ongoing substance use. For example, you can support a person with heavy alcohol use to develop a community mobility plan for safe transportation, or implement falls prevention strategies for individuals at higher risk for falls (Shin et al., 2022).

OTPs can also provide referrals for substance-use treatment, including community self-help programs such as Alcoholics Anonymous (AA). Although it is not a wraparound solution, AA can work as well or better than established treatments for alcohol treatment (Kelly et al., 2020). AA can be a powerful entry point for adults with SUD because of its accessibility and low barriers for entry, as groups are available all over the world, remotely and in-person, and there is no cost to join (AA, n.d.).

As with all individuals, OTPs working with people with SUD should emphasize the therapeutic relationship. When people feel stigmatized, judged, or shamed by health-care providers, they are less likely to engage in health services. Be aware of implicit and explicit biases. Use active listening and open-ended questions to build rapport and establish psychological safety with people. The therapeutic mode of empathizing can help form therapeutic alliances and support an individual's motivation to change (Fan & Taylor, 2018).

Here's the Point

- SUDs are complex disorders that can differ in symptoms and impact depending on the substance being abused.
- SUDs are common and OTPs will likely encounter people with SUDs regardless of practice setting.
- SUDs often co-occur with other psychiatric conditions.
- There are differences in the ways that SUDs are manifested across genders and sociocultural groups.
- SUDs are caused by a combination of neurobiological, psychological, and environmental factors.
- SUDs and CODs can be mild, moderate, or severe but can impact all areas of occupational performance.
- SUDs can occur across the life span and impact not only the user but the whole family.
- OTPs should be aware of the advances in MAT, especially for those with opioid addictions; use the stages of change and harm reduction principles to shape their work.

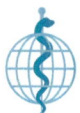 Visit the online resource center at **FADavis.com** to access the video.

Apply It Now

1. Book Review

In *A Common Struggle: A Personal Journey Through the Past and Future of Mental Illness and Addiction* by Patrick Kennedy and Stephen Fried (2016), the former congressman and youngest child of Senator Ted Kennedy describes his personal and political battle with mental illness and addiction, exploring the history of mental health care in the country as well as his and every family's private struggles. In addition to Kennedy's addiction to prescription painkillers, he experienced co-occurring struggles with bipolar disorder and misuse of alcohol. His family history, personal health challenges, and work in the U.S. Congress allow for a unique look at substance-related and addictive disorders.

Reflective Questions
Read the book and answer the following questions:
- How did Kennedy's family history and personal health challenges likely factor into his substance-related and addictive disorders?
- What did you learn from Kennedy's pursuit of personal recovery?
- Describe Kennedy's advocacy for treatment and research of brain diseases.
- What did you learn about policy regarding mental health and substance abuse parity, lack of access to treatment, and receiving different approaches to treatment (medications, psychotherapy, cognitive behavioral approaches)?
- How did you feel about the fact that many aspects of Kennedy's life might be considered privileged? Do you

believe his personal reflections on his lived experiences of healthy and unhealthy occupations are likely to connect with many who have shared those challenges?
- Would you recommend this book to your peers? Why, or why not?

2. PEO Analysis

Reread The Lived Experience feature and complete a Person-Environment-Occupation (PEO) analysis using the template in Appendix A. Consider the following guiding questions:
- Using AOTA's *OTPF-4* (2020), what areas of occupations are negatively affected by substance use?
- What personal and environmental factors acted as supports?
- What personal and environmental factors presented as barriers to recovery?

3. Misconceptions About Substance Use

Misconceptions of SUDs are common. Many people believe that substance abuse is simply a choice. Role-play with a partner how you would help educate a family member about the disease. Access the Rethinking Drinking website at https://www.rethinkingdrinking.niaaa.nih.gov to guide your education, self-awareness, and planning for healthy changes. What information can you present to the family to help them better understand substance use, its etiology, and how it impacts the individual and family?

4. Self-Assessment: Knowledge and Attitudes About Substance Use

Take the Drugs and Drug Users' Problems Perceptions Questionnaire. Here is a link to the questionnaire:
https://portal.ct.gov/-/media/DMHAS/COSIG/drug
seattitudescalepdf.pdf?la=en

Reflective Questions

■ Do you feel as if you are knowledgeable about drugs and drug use?
■ Do you feel comfortable talking to people about their drug use?
■ Do you know where to access resources about working with drug users?
■ Do you think OTPs have a role in addressing drug use in all practice settings?

5. Learn More About Substance Use in Your Community

Consult your own government (country, state, region) reports of prevalence and incidence of SUDs and CODs.

Reflective Questions

■ How do they compare with what is presented in this chapter?
■ Why might some regions have prevalence rates that are higher or lower than others?
■ Why does the use of particular substances vary by region?

■ What do you think contributes to substance use in your area? Are there environmental factors that help mitigate against use?

6. Video Exercise: Aimee's Lived Experience With Substance Use and Autism

Pair up with another student in your class or form a small group of students. Access and watch the "Aimee's Lived Experience With Substance Use and Autism" video at the online resource center at FADavis.com. Then, discuss and together answer the following questions:

Reflective Questions

■ What did Aimee mean when she said using drugs was a way to fill a void, a "god-shaped hole"? Do you think that is a common coping behavior? If so, why?
■ What were the various ways (cognitive, physical/sensory, and behavioral) that Aimee learned to better regulate herself? What relationship did that have to her substance use?
■ How did Aimee come to identify as autistic? What were the behaviors that led her to that conclusion?
■ Aimee describes "scripting" before events—big and small. What does that mean, and what does it potentially signify? When is scripting useful and when might it be a problem for someone with autism?
■ How did Aimee's lived experience impact her role as a student in an occupational therapy program? What were her coping strategies when she felt as though she was "melting down"?

Resources

Information About Specific Drugs

- National Institute on Drug Abuse. To learn more about prescription drugs and other drugs, visit the NIDA website: drugabuse.gov.
- *Substance Abuse and Mental Health Services Administration (SAMHSA).* https://www.samhsa.gov
  This government agency provides many resources including the Office of Recovery at https://www.samhsa.gov/about-us/who-we-are/offices-centers/or and the Providers Clinical Support System (PCSS) at https://www.samhsa.gov/providers-clinical-support-system-pcss
- *Guide to Evidence-Based Practices on the Web:* https://www.samhsa.gov/ebp-web-guide
- *The Rethinking Drinking Website.* This website provides information to the individual who is considering making a change. It includes a free downloadable pamphlet: https://www.rethinkingdrinking.niaaa.nih.gov

References

Alcoholics Anonymous. (n.d.). *Have a problem with alcohol? There is a solution.* https://www.aa.org

American Occupational Therapy Association. (2020). Occupational Therapy Practice Framework: Domain and process—Fourth edition. *American Journal of Occupational Therapy, 74*(Suppl. 2), 7412410010p1–7412410010p87. https://doi.org/10.5014/ajot.2020.74S2001

American Psychiatric Association. (2022). *Diagnostic and statistical manual of mental disorders* (5th ed., text rev.). American Psychiatric Publishing. https://doi.org/10.1176/appi.books.9780890425787

Baskin-Sommers, A. R., & Foti, D. (2015). Abnormal reward functioning across substance use disorders and major depressive disorder: Considering reward as a transdiagnostic mechanism. *International Journal of Psychophysiology, 98*(2 Pt. 2), 227–239. https://doi.org/10.1016/j.ijpsycho.2015.01.011

Calcaterra, S. L., Bach, P., Chadi, A., Chadi, N., Kimmel, S. D., Morford, K. L., Roy, P., & Samet, J. H. (2019). Methadone matters: What the United States can learn from the global effort to treat opioid addiction. *Journal of General Internal Medicine, 34*(6), 1039–1042. https://doi.org/10.1007/s11606-018-4801-3

Carliner, H., Keyes, K. M., McLaughlin, K. A., Meyers, J. L., Dunn, E. C., & Martins, S. S. (2016). Childhood trauma and illicit drug use in adolescence: A population-based national comorbidity survey replication—Adolescent supplement study. *Journal of the American Academy of Child and Adolescent Psychiatry, 55*, 701–708. https://doi.org/10.1016/j.jaac.2016.05.010

Centers for Disease Control and Prevention. (2016). *Drug overdose deaths in the United States hit record numbers in 2014.* https://archive.cdc.gov/#/details?url=https://www.cdc.gov/media/releases/2015/p1218-drug-overdose.html

Cerdá, M., Sagdeo, A., Johnson, J., & Galea, S. (2010). Genetic and environmental influences on psychiatric comorbidity: A systematic review. *Journal of Affective Disorders, 126*(1-2), 14–38. https://doi.org/10.1016/j.jad.2009.11.006

Colette, C., & Olivier, J. (2023). Integrative approaches for the treatment of substance use disorders: A systematic review. *Archives of Clinical Psychiatry, 50*(2), 84–90. https://doi.org/10.15761/0101-60830000000556

Comer, S. D., & Cahill, C. M. (2019). Fentanyl: Receptor pharmacology, abuse potential, and implications for treatment. *Neuroscience and Biobehavioral Reviews, 106,* 49–57. https://doi.org/10.1016/j.neubiorev.2018.12.005

Debnam, K. J., Milam, A. J., Mullen, M. M., Lacey, K., & Bradshaw, C. P. (2017). The moderating role of spirituality in the association between stress and substance use among adolescents: Differences by gender. *Journal of Youth and Adolescence, 47,* 818–828. https://doi.org/10.1007/s10964-017-0687-3

Dowell, D., Haegerich, T. M., & Chou, R. (2016). CDC guideline for prescribing opioids for chronic pain—United States, 2016. *MMWR Morbidity and Mortality Weekly Report Recommendations and Reports, 65*(RR-1), 1–49. https://doi.org/10.15585/mmwr.rr6501e1

Dowell, D., Ragan, K. R., Jones, C. M., Baldwin, G. T., & Chou, R. (2022). CDC clinical practice guideline for prescribing opioids for pain—United States, 2022. *MMWR Morbidity and Mortality Weekly Report Recommendations and Reports, 71*(RR-3), 1–95. http://doi.org/10.15585/mmwr.rr7103a1

Dunn, W. (2001). The sensations of everyday life: Empirical, theoretical, and pragmatic considerations. *American Journal of Occupational Therapy, 55*(6), 608–620. https://doi.org/10.5014/ajot.55.6.608

Elliott, A. J., Kinney, H. C., Haynes, R. L., Dempers, J. D., Wright, C., Fifer, W. P., Angal, J., Boyd, T. K., Burd, L., Burger, E., Folkerth, R. D., Groenewald, C., Hankins, G., Hereld, D., Hoffman, H. J., Holm, I. A., Myers, M. M., Nelsen, L. L., Odendaal, H. J., … Dukes, K. A. (2020). Concurrent prenatal drinking and smoking increases risk for SIDS: Safe Passage Study report. *EclinicalMedicine, 19,* 100247. https://doi.org/10.1016/j.eclinm.2019.100247

Engel-Yeger, B. (2014). Sensory processing disorders among substance dependents. *Cadernos Brasileiros de Terapia Ocupacional (Brazilian Journal of Occupational Therapy), 22*(Especial), 111–118. https://doi.org/10.4322/cto.2014.035

Fan, C. W., & Taylor, R. (2018). Correlation between therapeutic use of self and clients' participation in rehabilitation. *The American Journal of Occupational Therapy, 72*(4_Suppl. 1), 7211500036p1. https://doi.org/10.5014/ajot.2018.72S1-PO5001

Farhoudian, A., Razaghi, E., Hooshyari, Z., Noroozi, A., Pilevari, A., Mokri, A., Mohammadi, M. R., & Malekinejad, M. (2022). Barriers and facilitators to substance use disorder treatment: An overview of systematic reviews. *Substance Abuse: Research and Treatment, 16,* 11782218221118462. https://doi.org/10.1177/11782218221118462

Flanagan, J. C., Korte, K. J., Killeen, T. K., & Back, S. E. (2016). Concurrent treatment of substance use and PTSD. *Current Psychiatry Reports, 18,* 70. https://doi.org/10.1007/s11920-016-0709-y

Greenfield, S. F., Back, S. E., Lawson, K., & Brady, K. T. (2010). Substance abuse in women. *The Psychiatric Clinics of North America, 33*(2), 339–355. https://doi.org/10.1016/j.psc.2010.01.004

Guyonnet, E., Stewart, K. E., & Davis, J. A. (2023). Revealing the meaning of cannabis use as an occupation: A scoping review. *Substance Abuse: Research and Treatment, 17,* 11782218221150113. https://doi.org/10.1177/11782218221150113

Hamdan-Mansour, A. M., Mahmoud, K. F., Al Shibi, A. N., & Arabiat, D. H. (2017). Impulsivity and sensation-seeking personality traits as predictors of substance use among university students. *Journal of Psychosocial Nursing and Mental Health Services, 56*(1), 57–63. https://doi.org/10.3928/02793695-20170905-04

He, J., Yan, X., Wang, R., Zhao, J., Liu, J., Zhou, C., & Zeng, Y. (2022). Does childhood adversity lead to drug addiction in adulthood? A study of serial mediators based on resilience and depression. *Frontiers in Psychiatry, 13,* 871459. https://doi.org/10.3389/fpsyt.2022.871459

Hedegaard, H., Miniño, A. M., Spencer, M. R., & Warner, M. (2021). *Drug overdose deaths in the United States, 1999–2020.* NCHS Data Brief No. 428. National Center for Health Statistics. https://doi.org/10.15620/cdc:112340

Heinz, A., Beck, A., Halil, M. G., Pilhatsch, M., Smolka, M. N., & Liu, S. (2019). Addiction as learned behavior patterns. *Journal of Clinical Medicine, 8*(8), 1086. https://doi.org/10.3390/jcm8081086

Jordan, C. J., Cao, J., Newman, A. H., & Xi, Z. X. (2019). Progress in agonist therapy for substance use disorders: Lessons learned from methadone and buprenorphine. *Neuropharmacology, 158,* 107609. https://doi.org/10.1016/j.neuropharm.2019.04.015

Kelly, J. F., Humphreys, K., & Ferri, M. (2020). Alcoholics Anonymous and other 12-step programs for alcohol use disorder. *Cochrane Database of Systematic Reviews, 3,* CD012880. http://doi.org/10.1002/14651858.CD012880.pub2

Kennedy, P. J., & Fried, S. (2015). *A common struggle: A personal journey through the past and future of mental illness and addiction.* Blue Rider Press.

Kexel, A. K., Kluwe-Schiavon, B., Baumgartner, M. R., Engeli, E. J. E., Visentini, M., Kirschbaum, C., Seifritz, E., Ditzen, B., Soravia, L. M., & Quednow, B. B. (2022). Cue-induced cocaine craving enhances psychosocial stress and vice versa in chronic cocaine users. *Translational Psychiatry, 12*(1), 443. https://doi.org/10.1038/s41398-022-02204-5

Khantzian, E. J. (1997). The self-medication hypothesis of addictive disorders: A reconsideration and recent applications. *Harvard Review of Psychiatry, 4*(5), 231–244. https://doi.org/10.1176/ajp.142.11.1259

Khera, G. S., & Nakamura, N. (2016). Substance use, gender, and generation status among Asian Indians in the United States. *Journal of Ethnicity in Substance Abuse, 17*(3), 291–302. https://doi.org/10.1080/15332640.2016.1201715

Kiepek, N. (2016). *Licit, illicit, prescribed: Substance use and occupational therapy.* CAOT Publications ACE.

Kiepek, N., & Magalhaes, L. (2011). Addictions and impulse-control disorders as occupation: A selected literature review and synthesis. *Journal of Occupational Science, 18,* 254–276. https://doi.org/10.1080/14427591.2011.581628

Kitzinger, R. H., Jr., Gardner, J. A., Moran, M., Celkos, C., Fasano, N., Linares, E., Muthee, J., & Royzner, G. (2023). Habits and routines of adults in early recovery from substance use disorder: Clinical and research implications from a mixed methodology exploratory study. *Substance Abuse: Research and Treatment, 17,* 11782218231153843. https://doi.org/10.1177/11782218231153843

Koyama, M. S., Parvaz, M. A., & Goldstein, R. Z. (2017). The adolescent brain at risk for substance use disorders: A review of functional MRI research on motor response inhibition. *Current Opinion in Behavioral Science, 13,* 186–195. https://doi.org/10.1016/j.cobeha.2016.12.006

Kuerbis, A. (2020). Substance use among older adults: An update on prevalence, etiology, assessment, and intervention. *Gerontology, 66*(3), 249–258. https://doi.org/10.1159/000504363

Kuntsche, E., Kuntsche, S., Thrul, J., & Gmel, G. (2017). Binge drinking: Health impact, prevalence, correlates and interventions. *Psychological Health, 32,* 976–1017. https://doi.org/10.1080/08870446.2017.1325889

Lees, B., Garcia, A. M., Debenham, J., Kirkland, A. E., Bryant, B. E., Mewton, L., & Squeglia, L. M. (2021). Promising vulnerability markers of substance use and misuse: A review of human neurobehavioral studies. *Neuropharmacology, 187,* 108500. https://doi.org/10.1016/j.neuropharm.2021.108500

Logan, B. A., Brown, M. S., & Hayes, M. J. (2013). Neonatal abstinence syndrome: Treatment and pediatric outcomes. *Clinical Obstetrics and Gynecology, 56*(1), 186–192. https://doi.org/10.1097/GRF.0b013e31827feea4

Logrip, M. L., Zorrilla, E. P., & Koob, G. F. (2012). Stress modulation of drug self-administration: Implications for addiction comorbidity with post-traumatic stress disorder. *Neuropharmacology, 62*(2), 552–564. https://doi.org/10.1016/j.neuropharm.2011.07.007

Ma, J., Bao, Y. P., Wang, R. J., Su, M. F., Liu, M. X., Li, J. Q., Degenhardt, L., Farrell, M., Blow, F. C., Ilgen, M., Shi, J., & Lu, L. (2019). Effects of medication-assisted treatment on mortality among opioids users: A systematic review and meta-analysis. *Molecular Psychiatry, 24*(12), 1868–1883. https://doi.org/10.1038/s41380-018-0094-5

Maguire, D. J., Taylor, S., Armstrong, K., Shaffer-Hudkins, E., Germain, A. M., Brooks, S. S., Cline, G. J., & Clark, L. (2016). Long-term outcomes of infants with neonatal abstinence syndrome. *Neonatal Network, 35*(5), 277–286. https://doi.org/10.1891/0730-0832.35.5.277

Maracic, C. E., & Moeller, S. J. (2021). Neural and behavioral correlates of impaired insight and self-awareness in substance use disorder. *Current Behavioral Neuroscience Reports, 8*(4), 113–123. https://doi.org/10.1007/s40473-021-00240-x

Mattila, A. M., Santacecilia, G., & LaCroix, R. (2022). Perceptions and knowledge around substance use disorders and the role of occupational therapy: A survey of clinicians. *Substance Abuse: Research and Treatment, 16,* 11782218221130921. https://doi.org/10.1177/11782218221130921

Mattson, C. L., Kumar, S., Tanz, L. J., Patel, P., & Luo, Q. (2022). Drug overdose deaths in 28 states and the District of Columbia: 2020 data from the State Unintentional Drug Overdose Reporting System (SUDORS). Data Brief, No 1. Centers for Disease Control and Prevention, U.S. Department of Health & Human Services. https://www.cdc.gov/drugoverdose/databriefs/pdf/SUDORS_Data-Brief_Number_1.pdf

McCabe, S. E., West, B. T., Jutkiewicz, E. M., & Boyd, C. J. (2017). Multiple *DSM-5* substance use disorders: A national study of US adults. *Human Psychopharmacology, 32*(5), 1–19. https://doi.org/10.1002/hup.2625

McCarty, D., Bougatsos, C., Chan, B., Hoffman, K. A., Priest, K. C., Grusing, S., & Chou, R. (2021). Office-based methadone treatment for opioid use disorder and pharmacy dispensing: A scoping review. *The American Journal of Psychiatry, 178*(9), 804–817. https://doi.org/10.1176/appi.ajp.2021.20101548

McHugh, R. K., Votaw, V. R., Sugarman, D. E., & Greenfield, S. F. (2018). Sex and gender differences in substance use disorders. *Clinical Psychology Review, 66,* 12–23. https://doi.org/10.1016/j.cpr.2017.10.012

Meredith, P., Moyle, R., & Kerley, L. (2020). Substance use: Links with sensory sensitivity, attachment insecurity, and distress in young adults. *Substance Use & Misuse, 55*(11), 1817–1824. http//doi.org/10.1080/10826084.2020.1766502

Mindt, M. R., Coulehan, K., Aghvinian, M., Scott, T. M., Olsen, J. P., Cunningham, C. O., Arias, F., & Arnsten, J. H. (2022). Underrepresentation of diverse populations and clinical characterization in opioid agonist treatment research: A systematic review of the neurocognitive effects of buprenorphine and methadone treatment. *Journal of Substance Abuse Treatment, 135,* 108644. https://doi.org/10.1016/j.jsat.2021.108644

Murnane, K. S., Edinoff, A. N., Cornett, E. M., & Kaye, A. D. (2023). Updated perspectives on the neurobiology of substance use disorders using neuroimaging. *Substance Abuse and Rehabilitation, 14,* 99–111. https://doi.org/10.2147/SAR.S362861

National Center for Health Statistics. (2022). *Provisional drug overdose death counts.* https://www.cdc.gov/nchs/nvss/vsrr/drug-overdose-data.htm

National Institute on Drug Abuse. (2015). *Prescription opioids and heroin.* https://www.drugabuse.gov/publications/research-reports/relationship-between-prescription-drug-abuse-heroin-use/introduction

National Institute on Drug Abuse. (2020, July 9). *Substance use in older adults. DrugFacts.* https://nida.nih.gov/publications/drugfacts/substance-use-in-older-adults-drugfacts

National Institute on Drug Abuse. (2022). *Most reported substance use among adolescents held steady in 2022.* https://nida.nih.gov/news-events/news-releases/2022/12/most-reported-substance-use-among-adolescents-held-steady-in-2022

Nestler, E. J. (2014). Epigenetic mechanisms of drug addiction. *Neuropharmacology, 76*(Pt. B), 259–268. https://doi.org/10.1016/j.neuropharm.2013.04.004

Nosrati, E., Kang-Brown, J., Ash, M., Mckee, M., Marmot, M., & King, L. (2019). Economic decline, incarceration, and mortality from drug use disorders in the USA between 1983 and 2014: An observational analysis. *The Lancet Public Health, 4,* e326–e333. http://doi.org/10.1016/S2468-2667(19)30104-5

Qeadan, F., Mensah, N. A., Gu, L. Y., Madden, E. F., Venner, K. L., & English, K. (2021). Trends in the use of naltrexone for addiction treatment among alcohol use disorder admissions in U.S. substance use treatment facilities. *International Journal of Environmental Research and Public Health, 18*(16), 8884. https://doi.org/10.3390/ijerph18168884

Ray, L. A., Meredith, L. R., Kiluk, B. D., Walthers, J., Carroll, K. M., & Magill, M. (2020). Combined pharmacotherapy and Cognitive Behavioral Therapy for adults with alcohol or substance use disorders: A systematic review and meta-analysis. *JAMA Network Open, 3*(6), e208279. https://doi.org/10.1001/jamanetworkopen.2020.8279

Ryan, D., Naughton, M., de Faoite, M., Dowd, T., & Morrissey, A. M. (2023). An occupation-based lifestyle lecture intervention as part of inpatient addiction recovery treatment: Exploring occupational performance, balance and personal recovery. *Substance Abuse: Research and Treatment, 17,* 11782218231165123. https://doi.org/10.1177/11782218231165123

Santucci, K. (2012). Psychiatric disease and drug abuse. *Current Opinion in Pediatrics, 24*(2), 233–237. https://doi.org/10.1097/MOP.0b013e3283504fbf

Schuster, R., Winkler, M., Koopmann, A., Bach, P., Hoffmann, S., Reinhard, I., Spanagel, R., Bumb, J. M., Sommer, W. H., & Kiefer, F. (2021). Calcium carbonate attenuates withdrawal and reduces craving: A randomized controlled trial in alcohol-dependent patients. *European Addiction Research, 27*(5), 332–340. https://doi.org/10.1159/000512763

Shin, D., Gill, S. V., Kim, T. W., Magane, K. M., Mason, T., Heeren, T., Winter, M., Helfrich, C., & Saitz, R. (2022). Study protocol for a pilot randomized trial of a virtual occupational therapy fall prevention intervention for people with HIV and alcohol use. *Substance Abuse: Research and Treatment, 16,* 11782218221145548. https://doi.org/10.1177/11782218221145548

Siebert, C., & Schwartz, J. (2017). Occupational therapy's role in medication management. *The American Journal of Occupational Therapy, 71*(Suppl. 2), 7112410025p1–7112410025p20. https://doi.org/10.5014/ajot.2017.716S02

Sordo, L., Barrio, G., Bravo, M. J., Indave, B. I., Degenhardt, L., Wiessing, L., Ferri, M., & Pastor-Barriuso, R. (2017). Mortality risk during and after opioid substitution treatment: Systematic review and meta-analysis of cohort studies. *BMJ (Clinical Research Ed.), 357,* j1550. https://doi.org/10.1136/bmj.j1550

Stokes, M., Patel, P., & Abdijadid, S. (2024). *Disulfiram.* In StatPearls. StatPearls Publishing. https://www.ncbi.nlm.nih.gov/books/NBK459340

Stols, D., Heerden, R. V., Jaarsveld, A., & Nel, R. (2013). Substance abusers' anger behaviour and sensory processing patterns: An occupational therapy investigation. *South African Journal of Occupational Therapy, 43,* 25–34.

Substance Abuse and Mental Health Services Administration. (2020). *TIP 42: Substance use disorder treatment for people with co-occurring disorders.* SAMHSA Publication No. PEP20-02-01-004. https://store.samhsa.gov/sites/default/files/SAMHSA_Digital_Download/PEP20-02-01-004_Final_508.pdf

Substance Abuse and Mental Health Services Administration. (2021). *Key substance use and mental health indicators in the United States: Results from the 2020 National Survey on Drug Use and Health.* HHS Publication No. PEP21-07-01-003, NSDUH Series H-56. Center for Behavioral Health Statistics and Quality. https://www.samhsa.gov/data

Substance Abuse and Mental Health Services Administration. (2022). *2020 National Survey on Drug Use and Health: Women.* https://www.samhsa.gov/data/report/2020-nsduh-women

Substance Abuse and Mental Health Services Administration. (2023a). *Buprenorphine.* https://www.samhsa.gov/medications-substance-use-disorders/medications-counseling-related-conditions/buprenorphine

Substance Abuse and Mental Health Services Administration. (2023b). *Methadone.* https://www.samhsa.gov/medications-substance-use-disorders/medications-counseling-related-conditions/methadone

Swinford-Jackson, S. E., O'Brien, C. P., Kenny, P. J., Vanderschuren, L. J. M. J., Unterwald, E. M., & Pierce, R. C. (2021). The persistent challenge of developing addiction pharmacotherapies. *Cold Spring Harbor Perspectives in Medicine, 11*(11), a040311. https://doi.org/10.1101/cshperspect.a040311

Townsend, E. A., & Polatajko, H. E. (2013). *Enabling occupation II: Advancing an occupational therapy vision for health, well-being, & justice through occupations* (2nd ed.). CAOT Publications ACE.

U.S. Department of Health & Human Services. (2016). *HHS opioid research portfolio brief—Translation science into action.* http://www.hhs.gov/sites/default/files/opioid-report-v4-remediated.pdf

Van Gundy, K. T., Howerton-Orcutt, A., & Mills, M. L. (2015). Race, coping style, and substance use disorder among non-Hispanic African American and White young adults in south Florida. *Substance Use & Misuse, 50*(11), 1459–1469. https://doi.org/10.3109/10826084.2015.1018544

VanHouten, J. P., Rudd, R. A., Ballesteros, M. F., & Mack, K. A. (2019). Drug overdose deaths among women aged 30–64 years—United States, 1999–2017. *MMWR Morbidity and Mortality Weekly Report, 68*(1), 1–5. https://doi.org/10.15585/mmwr.mm6801a1

Verdejo-Garcia, A., Clark, L., & Dunn, B. D. (2012). The role of interoception in addiction: A critical review. *Neuroscience and Biobehavioral Reviews, 36*(8), 1857–1869. https://doi.org/10.1016/j.neubiorev.2012.05.007

Wang, S.-C., Chen, Y.-C., Chen, S.-J., Lee, C.-H., & Cheng, C.-M. (2020). Alcohol addiction, gut microbiota, and alcoholism treatment: A review. *International Journal of Molecular Sciences, 21*(17), 6413. https://doi.org/10.3390/ijms21176413

Wasmuth, S., Crabtree, J. L., & Scott, P. J. (2014). Exploring addiction-as-occupation. *British Journal of Occupational Therapy, 77,* 605–613. https://doi.org/10.4276/030802214X14176260335264

Wasmuth, S., Pritchard, K., & Kaneshiro, K. (2016). Occupation-based intervention for addictive disorders: A systematic review. *Journal of Substance Abuse Treatment, 62,* 1–9. https://doi.org/10.1016/j.jsat.2015.11.011

Wendell, A. D. (2013). Overview and epidemiology of substance abuse in pregnancy. *Clinical Obstetrics Gynecology, 56*(1), 91–96. http://doi.org/10.1097/GRF.0b013e31827feeb9

Wiśniewski, P., Maurage, P., Jakubczyk, A., Trucco, E. M., Suszek, H., & Kopera, M. (2021). Alcohol use and interoception—A narrative review. *Progress in Neuro-psychopharmacology & Biological Psychiatry, 111,* 110397. https://doi.org/10.1016/j.pnpbp.2021.110397

CHAPTER 25

Trauma- and Stressor-Related Disorders

Megan Edgelow

Exposure to trauma is a common experience for both children and adults worldwide. It is estimated that 90% of people will be exposed to trauma over their lifetime, but that only 5% to 15% of the population will go on to develop a related mental health condition (Daskalakis et al., 2018; Oakley et al., 2021). Experts debate the reasons that people are impacted differently by trauma. To date, research shows that some types of trauma are more likely to lead to a diagnosis of posttraumatic stress disorder (PTSD), such as witnessing a death and prolonged trauma exposure, including times of war or social unrest (Daskalakis et al., 2018; Oakley et al., 2021). Globally, rates of PTSD are estimated to be highest in refugees and in survivors of child abuse and domestic abuse; these people would be likely to experience prolonged exposure to trauma (Oakley et al., 2021).

More recently, the global COVID-19 pandemic has exposed humans worldwide to unpredictable situations, restrictions on activities and social interactions, and illness and death (Yunitri et al., 2022). PTSD prevalence has been shown to be high in patients who survived COVID-19 and the health-care professionals who cared for them, demonstrating the fact that the impacts of a disease that is typically thought of as a physical health threat can extend to mental health as well (Yunitri et al., 2022).

Other world events, including racial and political unrest, can also contribute to trauma exposure and resulting emotional impacts. For example, the murder of George Floyd in Minnesota by a police officer in 2020 sparked widespread protests and shone a spotlight on the experiences of African Americans, with more than one third of the American population reporting increased anger and sadness in the aftermath of that event (Eichstaedt et al., 2021). Additionally, researchers have recently pointed to a "dual pandemic" in the United States with the ongoing COVID-19 pandemic and rising rates of gun violence, which have disproportionately impacted racial and ethnic minorities, pointing to the complex impacts of structural racism on the social determinants of health (Schellenberg & Walters, 2022).

With the high probability that people will experience trauma throughout the life course, and the knowledge that racialized and refugee communities have higher rates of trauma exposure and related mental health conditions, it is important that all health care, not just mental health care, be sensitive to this reality. Trauma-informed care (TIC) is increasingly being adopted within health systems to acknowledge that people with a history of trauma exposure may be retraumatized by health-care experiences (Reeves, 2015). For example, someone who has experienced domestic violence and/or sexual assault may find even routine primary care for their physical health to be invasive and may avoid preventive health care and screening.

When health systems adopt a trauma-informed approach, ways to minimize distress and decrease the potential for retraumatization can be considered for intake and assessment processes, the physical design of spaces, and the degree of person choice incorporated into services and programs (Reeves, 2015). This important concept is introduced in Chapter 5: Trauma-Informed Practice and discussed further toward the end of this chapter 🤝.

This chapter describes stress and trauma responses and their connection to physical health, introduces diagnoses in the Trauma- and Stressor-Related Disorders category, explores occupational adaptation and occupational performance, and introduces how occupational therapy practitioners (OTPs) intervene with people who have experienced trauma in order to support their recovery process.

Stress and Trauma

Stressors can be defined as conditions that create demands on a person and may contribute to a stress response, a state of physiological alert or defense that may help achieve a goal or assist with survival (Wheaton et al., 2013). In simpler terms, humans have many activity demands in any given day, including productivity such as work, school, and household activities; self-care such as exercise and medical appointments; and leisure including social engagements and hobbies. Sometimes these demands can be stressful, such as a presentation at work, a test at school, a family member getting sick, or getting stuck in a traffic jam on the way to an important appointment. These types of stressors may be considered ordinary, and people are usually able to adapt and manage the level of stress they experience (Wheaton et al., 2013).

Additionally, some stressors can be thought of as positive life events, such as getting a promotion at work, graduating from college, or buying a new home. Although people may need to manage the stress of these events, chances are they will consider the experience in a positive light. Further, some scholars perceive stress or adversity as an opportunity to persevere and potentially improve psychological health. For example, in the event of a death or a natural disaster, it is common for people to interact with family members, friends, neighbors, or other community members who share their experience and may offer practical and emotional support. Additionally, people may have the opportunity to return this support to others who need it (Mancini, 2019). Social

Mental Health in Culture and Society

Aster Harrison

Lady Gaga's Experiences With Trauma

In 2016, pop star Lady Gaga released a personal letter on the Born this Way Foundation website sharing her diagnosis of PTSD (Gaga, 2016). The letter spoke about how she was overworked and injured on tour, and that continuing to work through the immense pain was traumatizing for her. Some of this experience is detailed in her 2017 documentary, "Five Foot Two" (Moukarbel, 2017).

In the 2016 open letter, Gaga wrote about the neurological processes associated with trauma, including how triggering sights or sounds can send her into dissociation or a fight-or-flight response. She also wrote about how she did psychotherapy and took medication to heal. Later in 2021 in "The Me You Can't See" Apple+ docuseries, she elaborated on her traumatic experiences, which included sexual assault and pregnancy at the age of 19. In this interview, she shared that she was finally able to connect her experience of chronic pain to the psychological trauma she had previously experienced (Jacoby, 2021).

Gaga's goal with coming forward is to spread awareness that PTSD can happen to all types and ages of people, not just to military veterans. She also believes that sharing one's story is therapeutic, and keeping emotions bottled up can worsen emotional and physical pain. The 2016 letter ends with a note from her psychologist, urging others with PTSD symptoms to seek professional help and share their feelings with someone who is supportive.

Gaga's story provides insight into the lived experience of trauma, and is a powerful reminder to fans with PTSD that they are not alone. In the 2021 docuseries she shared that she is "trying to make sure I give back with that experience instead of locking it away and faking it" (Kapadia et al., 2021).

References

Gaga, L. (2016, December 6). *"Head stuck in a cycle I look off and I stare": A personal letter from Gaga.* Born this Way Foundation. https://bornthisway.foundation/personal-letter-gaga

Jacoby, S. (2021, May 21). *Lady Gaga on how her rape, pregnancy, and trauma led to chronic pain.* SELF. https://www.self.com/story/lady-gaga-trauma-chronic-pain

Kapadia, A. (Director), Porter, D. (Director), Kauffman, R. (Segment Director), & Tibbon, T. (Segment Director). (2021, May 21). Say it out loud (Season 1, Episode 1) [TV series episode]. In A. H. Browne, K. Cooperman, C. Cyr, J. Kamen, A. Kapadia, T. Montgomery, D. Porter. P. Harry, D. Sirulnick, O. Winfrey & T. Wood (Executive Producers), *The me you can't see.* Apple+.

Moukarbel, C. (Director). (2017). *Five foot two* [Film]. Live Nation Films, Mermaid Films, & Permanent Wave.

However, sometimes people experience a lot of stressors at once or may experience an unexpected illness or circumstance that leaves them less able to adapt and manage. Further, some events go beyond ordinary stressors to include potentially traumatic events, such as the death of a loved one, experiencing a flood or wildfire near one's home, or being in a car accident (Southwick & Charney, 2004).

Although the acute phase may be distressing or transiently disabling, some people who experience these stressful events will adapt and return to their usual level of function (Shalev, 2002). For others, their distress may seem severe or persist longer than expected, leading people to question what is a normal versus maladaptive response to stress and trauma. This is the subject of ongoing debate in the psychiatric community (Southwick & Charney, 2004), and has even prompted some psychiatrists to wonder if PTSD is overdiagnosed (Tully et al., 2021). However, although a range of experiences and potential symptoms can be considered normal after a stressful or traumatic event, when symptoms persist for months and begin to impact someone's daily activities, they may meet the diagnostic criteria for the mental health conditions that are described further in this chapter.

One type of trauma exposure that it is important to be aware of is **adverse childhood experiences (ACEs)**. ACEs refer to incidents of child abuse, including physical, sexual, and emotional abuse, and child neglect, including physical and emotional neglect, as well as household challenges such as exposure to domestic or substance abuse or the separation or divorce of a parental relationship (Merrick et al., 2017). It is estimated that two-thirds of the population experiences at least one ACE in their childhood, making ACEs very common.

However, although ACEs are common, there is evidence of a graded dose-response relationship, meaning that the more ACEs someone experiences, the more risk they have of heavy drinking, drug use, and suicide attempts as an adult (Merrick et al., 2017). ACEs are also associated with mental and physical illnesses and poor socioeconomic outcomes for adults, making it important to attend to the mental health of people across their life span (Hales et al., 2022).

Impact of Stress, Trauma, and Physical Health

Acute stress can cause short-term adaptation, and stress responses may include increased blood sugar, blood pressure, and heart rate, all of which may be useful if the stressor requires a rapid physical response, such as running away from a predator (Rohleder, 2019). These responses are controlled by the autonomic nervous system (ANS), which includes the **hypothalamic-pituitary-adrenal (HPA) axis** that regulates the fight-flight-freeze response, including levels of the hormone cortisol (Rohleder, 2019).

Chronic exposure to stress may keep provoking the HPA axis, which is not useful if the stressor is not one that requires a physical reaction. Imagine a chief executive officer (CEO) of a publicly traded company who experiences the daily stress of the expectations of shareholders and board members, and who spends much of their day seated in front of a computer. Physical stress responses such as higher blood sugar and blood pressure are not useful adaptations. The chronic

interaction is thought to be a major moderating effect for stress and adversity; in times of shared adversity, this will often spur cooperation, including reports of communities coming together in the face of natural disasters or mass casualties such as the 9/11 disaster in New York City or the Fukushima earthquake and nuclear disaster in Japan (Mancini, 2019).

activation of these stress responses can contribute to physical health issues such as obesity, diabetes, and high blood pressure (Chandola et al., 2006; Rohleder, 2019).

For children who experience ACEs throughout their childhood, research shows that this chronic exposure to stress can increase the risk of physical health issues later in life, and researchers theorize that chronic early life stress may also interfere with the development of the stress response system, creating long-term challenges in coping with stress (Finlay et al., 2022). Obesity, hypertension, chronic illness, and higher mortality rates have all been associated with ACEs (Finlay et al., 2022; Hales et al., 2022).

In line with what is understood about the impact of chronic stress on the body, research has revealed that although PTSD is conceptualized as a mental health condition, it more likely is a whole-body condition that has physical health impacts as well. PTSD is associated with decreased physical functioning and poorer overall health as well as greater health-care utilization and increased mortality (Schnurr, 2022). Research on cardiovascular disease (CVD) shows that PTSD is a significant risk factor for developing and progressing CVD (Krantz et al., 2022; Ryder et al., 2018).

The evidence related to CVD and PTSD has led researchers to theorize that PTSD is a systemic disorder with psychological effects as the "tip of the iceberg" that most often are recognized and receive mental health–oriented treatment (Krantz et al., 2022; Schnurr, 2022). However, the systems affected by PTSD go beyond the cardiovascular system to include the immune, endocrine, and those systems regulating emotional and behavioral responses. Other common comorbidities to PTSD are sleep disorders such as sleep apnea, substance use disorders, and other mental health conditions, such as depression (Krantz et al., 2022). Evidence has also shown that musculoskeletal disorders and chronic pain are associated with PTSD (Lumley et al., 2022; Pacella et al., 2013; Ryder et al., 2018). The connection between trauma and chronic pain is explored further in the Evidence-Based Practice feature that follows.

It is important to keep the physical impacts of stress and trauma in mind when providing health care in settings that

Evidence-Based Practice

Trauma and Chronic Pain

OTPs are ideally positioned to address both physical and mental health conditions such as PTSD and chronic pain.

RESEARCH FINDINGS

Results of a recent meta-analysis demonstrate that PTSD is significantly related to physical health outcomes, including general health, medical conditions, and health-related quality of life (Pacella et al., 2013). Additionally, numerous retrospective studies link trauma or PTSD to chronic pain (Lumley et al., 2022), and the National Center for PTSD (2022) estimates that approximately 15% to 35% of patients with chronic pain also have PTSD.

APPLICATION

➡ It is common for people who experience chronic pain to have also experienced trauma. In fact, earlier trauma is a risk factor for chronic pain.

➡ Centralized pain conditions such as fibromyalgia, migraine headaches, and irritable bowel disease have been most closely linked to trauma and may benefit from emotion-focused therapies.

➡ People who experience chronic pain and have a history of trauma exposure may avoid activity for fear of exacerbating symptoms, but research shows that participating in activity can be an important part of recovery.

➡ OTPs are ideally positioned to address both physical and mental health conditions such as PTSD and chronic pain.

REFERENCES

National Center for PTSD. (2022). *Chronic pain and PTSD: A guide for patients.* U.S. Department of Veterans Affairs. https://www.ptsd.va.gov/understand/related/chronic_pain.asp

Lumley, M. A., Yamin, J. B., Pester, B. D., Krohner, S., & Urbanik, C. P. (2022). Trauma matters: Psychological interventions for comorbid psychosocial trauma and chronic pain. *Pain, 163*(4), 599–603. https://doi.org/10.1097/j.pain.0000000000002425

Pacella, M. L., Hruska, B., & Delahanty, D. L. (2013). The physical health consequences of PTSD and PTSD symptoms: A meta-analytic review. *Journal of Anxiety Disorders, 27*(1), 33–46. https://doi.org/10.1016/j.janxdis.2012.08.004

Ryder, A. L., Azcarate, P. M., & Cohen, B. E. (2018). PTSD and physical health. *Current Psychiatry Reports, 20*(12), 1–8. https://doi.org/10.1007/s11920-018-0977-9

focus on physical health. It is very possible, even likely, that an individual who comes to a cardiac or chronic pain clinic has exposure to chronic stress or has a history of trauma exposure, none of which may be noted in their clinical records. This possibility makes TIC approaches even more important to incorporate outside the mental health system. Additionally, interventions for physical health, such as pain management, physical exercise, improving nutrition, reducing smoking and alcohol consumption, and improving sleep, may all be helpful for people with PTSD (Krantz et al., 2022).

Trauma, Occupational Adaptation, and Resilience

Occupational adaptation is an occupational therapy concept that describes the interaction of the person, occupation, and environment in response to an occupational challenge. People who occupationally adapt to life challenges will experience mastery and competence in their life roles, whereas those who do not may experience occupational disruption or dysfunction (Walder et al., 2021). Walder and colleagues' (2021) concept analysis revealed that the literature conceptualizes occupational adaptation as an internal process, in transaction with the environment, that links to occupational identity, health, and well-being and is a life long and cumulative process.

Research on occupational adaptation has included groups with potential trauma exposure, including brain and hand injuries, forced migrants/asylum seekers, people experiencing homelessness, disaster survivors, and people receiving mental health care (Walder et al., 2021). Lopez (2011) explored occupational adaptation in the context of trauma since trauma exposure impacts both occupational performance and quality of life. Lopez (2011) focused on the protective factors that allow people to overcome distressing circumstances, finding that hope is an important emotional orientation, and that family, peer, social, and community supports are vital for successful occupational adaptation. Additionally, early intervention to support and restore occupational performance, using a person-centered approach that strengthens environmental supports, can help trauma survivors feel more optimistic and effective in daily life (Lopez, 2011).

A concept often associated with successful adaptation in the face of a challenge is **resilience**. Resilience is conceptualized as a return to one's original function after exposure to stress or trauma; it has also been described as a personal trait that enables ongoing positive adaptation to adversity (Tummala-Narra, 2007). Although it has similarities to occupational adaptation, it is not an occupational concept and is used broadly in many disciplines and types of research.

Despite the popularity of the concept of resilience, especially more recently in the COVID-19 pandemic, critiques of resilience have long pointed to its middle class European and North American orientation, with much of its evidence base focused on these populations and on Western values of individuality and independence (Tummala-Narra, 2007). Many scholars point to the role of community in resilience, and that the potential loss of social supports that may come with traumatic experiences is important to attend to (Berry, 2022; Ojukwu et al., 2022; Tummala-Narra, 2007).

Additionally, critiques of resilience push back on a possibly unintentional narrative, that people should just be more resilient in the face of increased stressors, which can neglect the responsibility of social structures and institutions in supporting their citizens (Berry, 2022; Ojukwu et al., 2022; Tummala-Narra, 2007).

Recently, the stressful and traumatic experiences of the COVID-19 pandemic have been explored through healthcare provider narratives, pointing to the burnout, grief, and distress that long preceded the pandemic and has been amplified by the past years of disruption and increased workplace demands in health-care settings (Rosa et al., 2022). There is growing awareness in the health-care system that systemic factors contribute to emotional and mental health, and that there are limits to person-level concepts such as resilience (Rosa et al., 2022). It is important for OTPs to think holistically about a person's personal capacity, social supports, and more broadly their social circumstances when working to support occupational adaptation and resilience. (For more information, see Chapter 10: Coping and Resilience 🤝.)

Description of Trauma- and Stressor-Related Disorders

In 2013, the *Diagnostic and Statistical Manual of Mental Disorders* of the American Psychiatric Association published its fifth edition (*DSM-5),* which made a major change to how disorders of trauma and stress were conceptualized (American Psychiatric Association, 2013).

Previously, reactions to trauma and stress had been categorized along with anxiety disorders, but in this new edition a distinct category was created, called "Trauma- and Stressor-Related Disorders." This moved several diagnoses together in this category, including the common diagnoses of adjustment disorder and PTSD. It created more awareness of the distinct reactions that people have after exposure to trauma, and the category was made more inclusive for a variety of subjective reactions to trauma, as well as lowering the age threshold for children and adolescents (Substance Abuse and Mental Health Services Administration [SAMHSA], 2016). The most recent text revision of the *DSM,* the *DSM-5-TR* (American Psychiatric Association, 2022), maintained the category and the diagnoses within it. The most prevalent mental health conditions in this category are discussed in more detail in this section.

It is important to consider that exposure to stress and trauma can result in diagnoses outside the Trauma- and Stressor-Related Disorders category. With high rates of ACEs in the general population, and a high correlation between ACEs, mental health conditions, and suicide risk, it is possible that many people diagnosed with anxiety disorders, mood disorders, personality disorders, or substance use disorders may all be impacted by stress and trauma (Jiang et al., 2022). Additionally, people may be diagnosed with a Trauma- and Stressor-Related Disorder along with other co-occurring physical and mental health conditions (Fig. 25-1). Relevant information on these diagnoses can be found in Chapter 18: Anxiety Disorders, Chapter 20: Mood Disorders, Chapter 22: Personality Disorders, and Chapter 24: Substance-Related and Addictive Disorders. 🤝

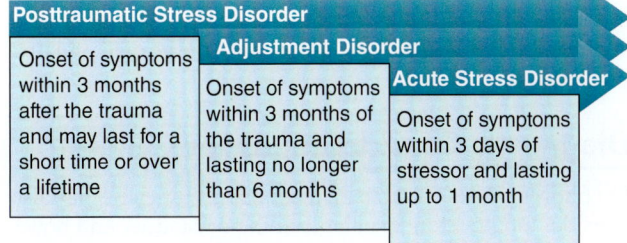

FIGURE 25-1. Comparison of symptom onset and duration for adjustment disorder, acute stress disorder, and PTSD.

Acute Stress Disorder

Acute stress disorder happens when someone develops symptoms following their exposure to a traumatic event, and this reaction lasts between 3 days and 1 month after the event. The traumatic event criteria are similar to the criteria for PTSD, including exposure to actual death or the threat of death, serious injury, or sexual violence, through direct exposure of experiencing or witnessing the event in person, learning the event has happened to a close friend or family member, or being exposed to traumatic details or events through work (e.g., military member, first responder; American Psychiatric Association, 2022).

Diagnostic Features

Reactions to the traumatic event could include extreme or unexpected fear, stress, and pain. Symptoms can include intrusion of thoughts and memories related to the traumatic event, negative mood, dissociative symptoms including the inability to remember parts of the event, avoidance symptoms where efforts are made to avoid reminders of the event, and arousal symptoms including disturbed sleep or heightened startle responses (American Psychiatric Association, 2022).

A diagnosis of acute stress disorder requires symptoms that persist for 3 days to 1 month after the trauma exposure. If symptoms persist longer than this, a diagnosing clinician may consider if adjustment disorder or PTSD is a more appropriate diagnosis. More information on those disorders is provided later in this section.

Prevalence and Course

SAMHSA (2016) estimates that a past year prevalence of the disorder could include 3% of the American population. Some studies have shown that 20% of people who survive accidents may meet the diagnostic criteria, and rates up to 50% have been found for interpersonal events such as rape or assault (American Psychiatric Association, 2022).

Risk and Prognostic Factors

A main risk factor is a prior mental health condition. Avoidant coping styles or catastrophizing are also strong predictors of this disorder. People with prior trauma exposure are at greater risk. This condition is more prevalent in women, which may be attributable to its diagnostic link to abuse, assault, and rape, which more commonly happen to women (American Psychiatric Association, 2022).

Impact on Occupational Performance

The emotional distress and impairment in function of acute stress disorder may interfere with self-care activities, including sleep and maintaining one's health. If a person's reaction includes avoidance and withdrawal, this may interfere with their recovery through missing medical and therapeutic appointments or missing productive activities such as school or work. Because this disorder is a transient condition, the impact on occupational performance is not expected to continue long-term (American Psychiatric Association, 2022).

Adjustment Disorder

Adjustment disorder occurs in response to a stressful life event, or events. The disorder occurs within 3 months of the onset of the stressor(s) and persists for up to 6 months. The symptoms a person experiences, because of the stressor, are generally more severe than would normally be expected for the type of event that occurred (American Psychiatric Association, 2022).

Diagnostic Features

Along with the level of distress experienced being out of proportion to the intensity of the stressor, there must also be impairment in social, occupational, or other areas of function. The diagnosis can be categorized as acute (such as a romantic breakup) or chronic when the disturbance is in response to a chronic stressor (such as a disabling medical condition), and also when the conditions persist longer than 6 months (American Psychiatric Association, 2022).

Prevalence and Course

Adjustment disorders are common, but prevalence data vary widely depending on the group studied and the methods used. Estimates in the United States range from 5% to 20% in outpatient mental health settings, and it was a very common diagnosis in these same settings in Canada, Australia, and Israel in the 1990s, often representing 50% of the patient population (American Psychiatric Association, 2022). By definition, adjustment disorder is a transient disorder, coming on within 3 months of a stressor, and potentially within days in the case of an acute event such as being fired from a job. Acute stressors typically resolve within 6 months, but chronic stressors may be more persistent. If symptoms persist for longer than 6 months, and the stressor or its consequence have ceased, other diagnoses, such as PTSD, might be explored (American Psychiatric Association, 2022).

Risk and Prognostic Factors

People who experience disadvantages or marginalization in life circumstances, such as migrants, refugees, and racialized groups, may be at greater risk of adjustment disorder (American Psychiatric Association, 2022).

Impact on Occupational Performance

The emotional distress and impairment in function from adjustment disorders is often seen in a person's difficulty in productive activities, such as work and school, as well as changes in social relationships. If the disorder is due to a medical condition, such as cancer, the treatment of that condition may decrease occupational performance in usual activities and also impact overall energy and time spent in activities such as self-care. For people with the acute form of the condition, impairment in occupational performance would not be expected past 6 months, as long as the stressor and its consequences have resolved (American Psychiatric Association, 2022).

Posttraumatic Stress Disorder

PTSD is characterized by the development of a pattern of symptoms following a trauma exposure; this includes the symptoms considered with acute stress disorder, with a duration longer than 1 month. The diagnosis requires exposure to actual or threatened death, serious injury, or sexual violence, either directly, by experiencing or witnessing the event in person, or indirectly by learning it happened to a close family member or friend, or experiencing repeated or extreme exposure to the details of traumatic events, such as in the case of first responders or military members (American Psychiatric Association, 2022).

Diagnostic Features

A diagnosis of PTSD requires exposure to an upsetting traumatic event through direct experience, witnessing the event, or learning that it happened to a close family member or friend (American Psychiatric Association, 2022). Symptoms of PTSD fall into the following four categories and can vary in severity:

- *Intrusion:* Having intrusive thoughts such as distressing dreams, involuntary memories, or flashbacks of the event
- *Avoidance:* Avoiding reminders of the traumatic event through avoiding places, people, activities, and situations that may elicit distressing memories
- *Negative alterations in cognitions and mood:* Having an inability to remember aspects of the traumatic event and experiencing negative thoughts and feelings, distorted thoughts, ongoing fear, anger, horror, shame or guilt, decreased interest in activities previously enjoyed, feeling detached from others, or being unable to experience positive emotions
- *Alterations in arousal and reactivity:* Being irritable and having angry outbursts, behaving recklessly or self-destructively, being hypervigilant, being easily startled, or having difficulty concentrating or sleeping (American Psychiatric Association, 2022)

To be diagnosed with PTSD, an adult must have all of the following for 1 month or longer:

- At least one intrusion symptom
- At least one avoidance symptom
- At least two cognition and mood symptoms
- At least two arousal and reactivity symptoms (American Psychiatric Association, 2022)

It is important to note that these symptoms must create distress or impairment in social, occupational, or other important areas of functioning and not be attributable to other medical conditions or the physiological effects of a substance such as a medication or alcohol (American Psychiatric Association, 2022).

Diagnostic Considerations for Children

In children under 6 years old, diagnosing clinicians may also consider a regression in toilet training or bladder and bowel control, regression in motor skills such as walking, acting out the event while playing, and being clingier than normal with caregivers. For older children and teens, symptoms may be similar to adults, but could also include disrespectful, disruptive, or destructive behaviors, as well as guilt about not preventing the traumatic event, or thoughts of revenge (American Psychiatric Association, 2022).

Prevalence and Course

Anyone can develop PTSD at any age, including children; military members, veterans, and first responders; and people who have experienced abuse, a physical or sexual assault, an accident, a disaster, or another serious event (SAMHSA, 2016). The National Center for PTSD (2023) estimates that about 6 in 100 people (8 in 100 women and 4 in 100 men) will experience PTSD at some point in their lives. About 12 million American adults will have PTSD each year, representing only a small proportion of people exposed to trauma (National Center for PTSD, 2023). Symptoms usually begin within 3 months of the trauma but can present earlier or even years after the event (American Psychiatric Association, 2022).

The reactions that individuals have to trauma can be complex and varied, and some populations may have unique levels of exposure and resulting challenges. For example, for refugees who are more likely to be exposed to intentional trauma in addition to displacement from their homes and loss of access to employment and education, rates of PTSD can be much higher than in the general population (Oakley et al., 2021). Other groups also experience greater exposure to trauma through the work they do, including military members, veterans, and first responders, and may have a higher PTSD prevalence than the general population (Carleton et al., 2018). For example, it is estimated that 1.5 million American military members were deployed in the Iraq and Afghanistan Wars from 2001 to 2011 (Baiocchi, 2013), representing significant potential trauma exposure and higher PTSD risk for this population.

Risk and Prognostic Factors

Risk factors for PTSD include childhood adversity, emotional problems and family dysfunction, prior trauma exposure and prior mental health conditions, lower socioeconomic status and education level, and racial discrimination. There is modest evidence for genetic predisposition in the studies of twins, as well as evidence of epigenetic factors from studies of populations exposed to war and conflict (American Psychiatric Association, 2022). Environmental factors can include the severity or "dose" of the trauma and perceived level of threat, as well as the frequency of upsetting reminders and subsequent life challenges including financial stressors (American Psychiatric Association, 2022).

Impact on Occupational Performance

PTSD is associated with high levels of impairment in social, occupational, and physical functioning, potentially leading to reduced quality of life along with physical health problems (American Psychiatric Association, 2022). A scoping review of the occupational therapy literature on PTSD showed that occupational performance impacts are documented across self-care, productivity, and leisure occupational categories (Edgelow et al., 2019). Of the 50 articles included in the review, 29 documented occupational performance issues (OPIs) in self-care, including challenges maintaining health, problems with sleep and rest, community mobility, and meal planning (Edgelow et al., 2019).

The most common self-care OPI was sleep, often caused by increased arousal, flashbacks, and nightmares that may keep the person from falling and staying asleep. Forty of the 50 articles identified issues in productivity, including school performance, safe driving, and working or returning to work, which was the most commonly identified OPI. Leisure OPIs were found in 36 of the 50 articles, including a decrease in interest, pleasure, and meaning experienced in leisure activities, and most commonly issues with friendships and intimate relationships, putting people at risk of social isolation. Regardless of the population, PTSD can have a negative impact on quality of life because of decreased satisfaction with and performance of occupations (Edgelow et al., 2019; Lopez, 2011; Plach & Sells, 2013).

It is important to note that although the most-cited OPIs in the 2019 review were sleep, work, and maintaining social relationships, individual experiences may differ, and the OTP must remain person-centered in their practice and explore any possible occupational challenges (Edgelow et al., 2019).

Prolonged Grief Disorder

Prolonged grief disorder, the newest disorder added to the *DSM* (American Psychiatric Association, 2022), was added to represent a maladaptive grief reaction to the loss of someone who the person had a close relationship with. The severity and duration of the grief reaction must clearly exceed expected social and cultural norms in the individual's context.

Diagnostic Features

The symptoms of prolonged grief disorder include emotional symptoms such as intense pain related to the death, feeling that life is meaningless or emotional numbness, avoidance that can include disbelief about the death or avoidance of reminders of the death, and an impact on function such as difficulty reintegrating with daily life and detachment from others (American Psychiatric Association, 2022).

This disorder can only be diagnosed after 12 months have elapsed since the death for adults and 6 months for children and adolescents. The severity and duration of the grief reaction must clearly exceed expected social and cultural norms in the individual's context (American Psychiatric Association, 2022).

Prevalence and Course

Research shows an approximate prevalence of 10% for those experiencing loss, although there is potential variance across cultures. As the diagnosis is relatively new, prevalence data may change over time (American Psychiatric Association, 2022).

Risk and Prognostic Factors

Risks for developing prolonged grief disorder include a high level of dependency on the deceased person, the death of a child, violent or unexpected deaths, or current economic stressors. There is higher prevalence when the death is related to a spouse/partner or child over other family relationships. Because the grief reaction must clearly exceed expected social and cultural norms in the individual's context to be diagnosed, cultural variation in grief reactions is already considered; however, for cultures that emphasize funerary rituals, the inability to carry out these rituals may put people at greater risk of the disorder (American Psychiatric Association, 2022).

Impact on Occupational Performance

It is likely that someone diagnosed with this disorder will experience challenges with work and social functioning, as well as difficulties coping in daily life. These challenges with coping may manifest in increased use of substances, which may also increase risks of other health consequences. Long-term consequences for children and adolescents can include lower rates of academic attainment (American Psychiatric Association, 2022).

Reactive Attachment Disorder and Disinhibited Social Engagement Disorder

There are two other diagnoses in the Trauma- and Stressor-Related Disorders category that apply only to children: Reactive attachment disorder (RAD) and disinhibited social engagement disorder (DSED). Some children experience early childhood neglect or trauma that can result in insecure attachment and resulting diagnoses. Both of these disorders emerge in childhood and are associated with issues of the child's attachment to caregivers (American Psychiatric Association, 2022). Although there are different classifications and ways of viewing attachment difficulties in the literature, RAD and DSED are included in the category of Trauma- and Stressor-Related Disorders in the *DSM-5-TR* (American Psychiatric Association, 2022).

Diagnostic Features

RAD presents as an inhibited, emotionally withdrawn pattern of behavior (e.g., the child rarely or minimally seeks or responds to comfort when distressed; American Psychiatric Association, 2022). In RAD, there is also a persistent emotional and social disturbance characterized by having at least two of the following:

- Limited expression of positive affect
- Minimal emotional and social responsivity with others
- Episodes of unexplained fearfulness, sadness, or irritability that are evident in nonthreatening interactions with adult caregivers

The behaviors seen in children with RAD are caused by having experienced persistent, extreme patterns of early childhood caregiving in which there was a lack of:

- Meeting basic physical and safety needs
- Comfort and positive emotional bonding experiences
- Developmentally appropriate stimuli and activity opportunities
- Stability in the caregivers
- Opportunities to form selective attachments because of the living situation (e.g., institutions with high child–caregiver ratios)

For a diagnosis of an attachment disorder to be made using the *DSM-5-TR* criteria, it is important to rule out the possibility of the child having a diagnosis of autism (American Psychiatric Association, 2022). In addition, the child must have a developmental age of 9 months or older, and the symptoms and behaviors associated with the attachment must have been evident before age 5. It is important to note that conditions such as language and cognitive delays may co-occur with RAD because of the high degree of neglect experienced during early childhood development.

In children diagnosed with DSED, there is a tendency toward externalizing behaviors, as well as other behaviors that are typically associated with attention deficit/hyperactivity disorder (ADHD). The child will demonstrate at least *two* of the following behaviors:

- Decreased or absent restraint or discretion in approaching or interacting with adults who are unfamiliar
- Overly familiar physical or verbal behavior that is not consistent with age-appropriate boundaries or is not culturally sanctioned
- Willingness to go off with an unfamiliar adult with minimal or no hesitation
- Lack of or absent checking back in after venturing away from adults, even when in unfamiliar settings

The previously noted behaviors are not understood to be driven by issues of impulsivity (as is seen in ADHD); rather, these are socially disinhibited behaviors. Similar to children with RAD, the child must have experienced a pattern of extreme, insufficient early childhood care to receive a diagnosis of DSED; therefore, the caregiving must meet at least one of the previously outlined criteria from RAD (American Psychiatric Association, 2022).

Prevalence and Course

The prevalence of RAD and DESD is unknown and thought to be rare, even in those who have experienced severe early deprivation. RAD is seen more often in young children who have been raised in foster care or institutions, and even in populations with severe neglect, is thought to occur in less than 10% of these children. Research indicates that in low-income community populations in the United Kingdom, prevalence of DESD is up to 2% (American Psychiatric Association, 2022).

Risk and Prognostic Factors

RAD and DSED occur when there has been severe abuse, neglect, and/or deprivation by the primary caregiver(s) for children in early infancy and childhood (usually before age 5).

When a child's basic needs for human affection, comfort, safety, and stimulation are not met by the primary caregiver(s), a pervasive impact on neurodevelopmental, socioemotional, cognitive, and language capacities can be evident (American Psychiatric Association, 2022).

Impact on Occupational Performance

Interpersonal skills can be impacted in both RAD and DESD, which may persist into adolescence and adulthood, putting people at risk of conflict and victimization in interpersonal relationships. Additionally, success in academic and work roles can be impacted because of the ongoing difficulty some people may have in relating to adults and peers (American Psychiatric Association, 2022).

Gender and Cultural Differences

Exposure to stressors and trauma can happen to all people globally, and at any age. However, for trauma- and stressor-related disorders, the prevalence is typically higher in women than in men, which is similar to the prevalence of anxiety disorders and mood disorders (American Psychiatric Association, 2022). The reasons for this gender difference are complex and not fully understood, but they might include unequal exposure to types of traumatic events, higher rates of ACEs in women, and higher rates of help seeking among women (Finlay et al., 2022).

Rates of trauma- and stressor-related disorders are also higher in racialized groups. For example, in the United States, Latinos, African Americans, and Native Americans/Alaska Natives have higher rates of PTSD than non-Latino whites (American Psychiatric Association, 2022). Potential reasons for these differences include differences in risk factors, such as exposure to past trauma, racism, and discrimination; lower quality or availability of treatment; decreased social support and socioeconomic status; and less access to the social resources that facilitate recovery (American Psychiatric Association, 2022).

Intergenerational Trauma

Intergenerational trauma is a term used to describe trauma that is historical and is inherited by or transmitted to future generations. It has been conceptualized as a cycle of trauma, where a parent or grandparent's ACEs may lead to ACEs for the children they go on to parent (Narayan et al., 2021). It has been used to describe the ongoing legacy of slavery for African Americans, the experiences of Holocaust survivors and their families, the impact of trauma for refugee families, and experiences of Indigenous groups in Canada, the United States, and Australia, along with other countries (Graff, 2014; Isobel et al., 2019; Sangalang & Vang, 2017). Often, the trauma is transmitted through parenting relationships, where the parent has experienced trauma and the attachment relationship with their children is impacted, or the family group is not able to provide the support needed in childhood. This can have significant impacts for each generation across their life spans and can predispose future generations to trauma.

PhotoVoice

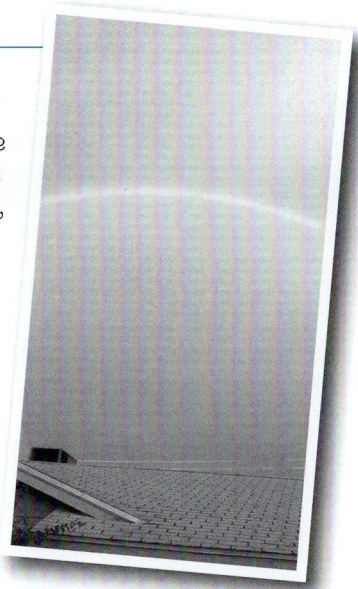

This beautiful rainbow represents the many achievements I have made over the past year. I have overcome trauma, stigma, hatred, and many other obstacles. Throughout the past year I've learned how to make self-care a priority and to accept myself just as I am. It's taken a lot of hard work and determination. But hey, I have that in spades. As anyone who knows me would tell you I've become the best person I can be. I have goals and ambitions. I want to go back to school, make new friends, find a part-time job, etcetera. The possibilities are limitless. For the first time in my life, I am proud of who I've become. I am optimistic, free, compassionate, a peer, sister, aunt, and a friend.

Why are goals and ambitions an indication of recovery?

Emerging research shows that trauma may cause epigenetic changes that are passed on to children, including changes in glucocorticoid and immune-related genes (Daskalakis et al., 2021). Research on intervention for intergenerational trauma shows that the most effective approaches are to help resolve parental trauma through active treatment, and to actively support parent–child attachment through the parenting process (Isobel et al., 2019). However, these interventions can be complicated by the fact that groups vulnerable to intergenerational trauma often experience social disadvantage which can lower access to quality health care and supportive social structures.

Trauma-Informed Care

TIC, a term mentioned in the introduction of this chapter, is incorporated throughout this textbook and addressed specifically in Chapter 5: Trauma-Informed Practice 🤝. TIC has its roots in trauma theory, where psychologists theorized that traumatic memories could be triggered by situations that mimic a past traumatic experience, including sounds, smells, sensations, and verbal and physical interactions (Reeves, 2015). This means that stimuli thought to be noninvasive can cause an unpredictable response for someone with a trauma history.

Health-care settings can be triggering because of the nature of the questioning and physical examination that occurs in these settings. This can be particularly relevant for survivors of physical and/or sexual assault who may have memories tied to physical sensations and may also feel trapped by routine interactions where medical professionals suggest someone relax, or someone is restrained by medical equipment, such as an x-ray or MRI machine (Reeves, 2015). TIC aims to meet the unique needs of trauma survivors and also acknowledges that traumatic experiences and ACEs are so prevalent that it will not be possible to know in advance who may be triggered; as such, all health-care settings should be trauma-informed, including their physical design as well as the health-care services they provide.

Fette and colleagues (2019) recommend that a public health model be adopted to apply TIC at a universal level. OTPs can adopt TIC by using person-centered approaches, telling people what will happen and asking for their permission to proceed as well as inviting them to state their concerns, and giving as much control to people as possible. TIC is highly congruent with a recovery perspective, where people are empowered to ask for what they need and professionals promote the belief that recovery is possible for all (Fette et al., 2019).

Interventions

Because of the short-term nature of acute stress disorder and adjustment disorder, interventions may be focused more on social support or in helping a person to resolve the stressor(s) they are experiencing. When the traumatic experience is longer term and framed as PTSD, more health-care system infrastructure and evidence have been built around intervention.

From a psychology perspective, several types of psychotherapy interventions are recommended for the treatment of PTSD. These include cognitive behavioral therapy (CBT), cognitive processing therapy (CPT), cognitive therapy (CT), and prolonged exposure therapy (American Psychological Association, 2017). Cognitively oriented psychotherapies often examine cognitive beliefs and emotional responses and assist a person in changing the way they interpret and respond to stimuli, where exposure-based psychotherapies work to reduce physiological responses to stimuli and expand the range of places and situations that a person feels confident experiencing (American Psychological Association, 2017). Trauma-focused psychotherapies can be helpful in the recovery process, but have high rates of nonresponse or treatment dropout. They are also not universally accessible, can require significant time to engage in, and have high associated costs (Saeed et al., 2023).

From an occupational therapy perspective, OTPs are interested in supporting occupational adaptation and occupational performance, working from a recovery and trauma-informed perspective to enable people to feel more effective in their daily lives and important life roles (Edgelow & Cramm, 2020; Edgelow et al., 2019). The Occupational Therapy Trauma Intervention Framework (OTTIF; Edgelow & Cramm, 2020) is an evidence-informed clinical reasoning framework that can be used by OTPs to organize their intervention approach by incorporating a person's readiness while remaining occupation-centered.

The intervention framework uses the Canadian Model of Occupational Performance and Engagement (CMOP-E) and occupational therapy enablement skills as key theoretical foundations. This framework directs OTPs to assessment and treatment approaches and includes a core focus on self-regulation in order to acknowledge the emotional and physical responses to trauma that people experience and the role

TABLE 25-1 | Common Intervention Approaches for Trauma- and Stressor-Related Disorders

Approach	Target(s) of Intervention	Brief Synopsis	Chapters With Additional Information
Creative Media	Promoting emotional expression	Person uses writing or other creative media such as painting, dance, or music to tell personal stories.	Chapter 10: Coping and Resilience
Early Intervention for Children	Promoting early access to needed supports	Person recognizes the potential impact of trauma and ACEs on child development and attachment.	Chapter 36: Early Intervention: A Practice Setting for Early Childhood Mental Health Chapter 47: Student
Family Supports	Supporting families and family relationships	Families are part of support networks, and intergenerational trauma is an important consideration in working with families.	Chapter 29: Families
Pain Intervention	Comorbid pain and physical illness	Pain and physical illness can be comorbid with trauma diagnoses. People benefit from interventions for pain management and physical health.	Chapter 15: Pain Chapter 34: Integrated Behavioral Health and Primary Care
Promoting Self-Care	Self-care activities including rest and sleep, and promoting overall wellness	Self-care forms an important foundation for health and recovery.	Chapter 45: Self-Care and Well-Being Occupations Chapter 52: Sleep
Services for Military Members and Veterans	Services tailored to this population with a high prevalence of trauma exposure	People develop coping mechanisms, enhance self-care, and manage stressors while participating in military duties during service and after.	Chapter 43: Serving Veterans and Service Members
Skills Training	Activities of daily living (ADL) and instrumental activities of daily living (IADL) skills	Person applies learning and behavioral strategies to promote acquisition of new skills.	Chapter 46: Activities of Daily Living, Instrumental Activities of Daily Living, and Health Management Occupations Chapter 37: School Mental Health
Supporting Self-Regulation	Emotional and physiological regulation	Skills training involves targeting mindfulness meditation, interpersonal effectiveness, emotion regulation, and distress tolerance.	Chapter 12: Emotion Regulation
Time Use	Time use and participation	Avoidance of activity can occur with trauma exposure. Time use approaches can be helpful for reengaging people in meaningful activities.	Chapter 14: Time Use and Habits
Trauma-Informed Care	Recognizing a person's trauma history and promoting safe health-care experiences	This approach acknowledges the prevalence of trauma, evaluates the potential impact of health-care environments, and promotes the individual's resources and recovery.	Chapter 5: Trauma-Informed Practice

of developing coping skills as a step in the recovery process (Edgelow & Cramm, 2020).

Because of the numerous diagnoses contained within this diagnostic category and their impact on occupational performance and participation, many other chapters in this text provide relevant information. Table 25-1 outlines common intervention approaches for individuals that appear in other chapters.

Medication

Because of the short-term nature of acute stress disorder and adjustment disorder, medications may not be the focus of treatment. For longer-term conditions such as PTSD, the role of medication can be more emphasized. There has been quite a bit of synthesis completed on the efficacy of medications for PTSD. The goals of medication for PTSD include reducing symptoms, reducing avoidance behaviors, treating other comorbid conditions, and improving function (Saeed et al., 2023).

Current American Psychological Association Clinical Practice Guidelines recommend the treatment of PTSD with antidepressants, including sertraline, paroxetine, fluoxetine, and venlafaxine, with insufficient evidence for other types or classes of drugs (American Psychological Association, 2017). Nontraditional treatments including psychedelic medications such as ketamine and MDMA are being investigated with some satisfactory results for efficacy, although their safety and protocols for use are still being studied and they are not part of most treatment guidelines for PTSD (Coquemont et al., 2022). Cannabis has also been studied, with mixed results on its efficacy and some caution remaining on possible negative side effects (Coquemont et al., 2022).

A recent critique of pharmacotherapy for PTSD points out that the efficacy of medications is low, with only 60% of people responding to antidepressants and 20% to 30% of people achieving remission from the disorder (Saeed et al., 2023). Additionally, it may take many months to see a response from medications, and a substantial proportion of people will continue to experience symptoms and difficulties with life function even after taking medications (Saeed et al., 2023). Researchers point to the need for more development of medications, clinical trials, and meta-analysis of the evidence. The lack of a medical "cure" for PTSD also points to the need for person-centered approaches that consider medical, psychological, and occupational approaches to recovery from this complex health condition.

General Considerations When Providing Occupational Therapy to People With Trauma- and Stressor-Related Disorders

The traumatic experiences of people can be invisible to health-care providers, and there can be a lot of shame that goes along with trauma, meaning that many people may not disclose their trauma or have it noted in their health record. However, trauma can be an underlying element to many physical health and pain conditions. It is important to use a trauma-informed approach in all settings to ensure OTPs can understand a person's needs (see Chapter 5: Trauma-Informed Practice 🤝).

The prevalence of traumatic experiences and ACEs is high in the general population and even higher in mental health settings. Considering the presence of traumatic experiences in assessment and intervention approaches in mental health care is important, even when someone's diagnosis is not a trauma- and stressor-related disorder.

Additionally, the complexity of reactions to trauma and its potentially enduring health impacts points to the importance of functional and participatory approaches such as occupational therapy to assist people in coping with the disorder and moving forward toward recovery by increasing personal resources, supports, and efficacy.

Here's the Point

- Everyone will be exposed to stressful events over their life course, and many people will be exposed to a traumatic event. However, not everyone will go on to develop a mental health condition.
- Occupational adaptation is possible in the face of stress and trauma and can be important for OTPs to enable for people.
- TIC is a vital approach across all health-care settings as trauma exposure is associated with increased physical and mental health conditions. People benefit from its person-centered and recovery-focused approach.
- Acute stress disorder and adjustment disorder are shorter-term diagnoses that a person may recover from with or without clinical intervention. Longer-term functional challenges after trauma exposure may lead to a diagnosis of PTSD.
- Current evidence shows that PTSD is a complex, whole-body condition. Current psychotherapy and medication interventions have high rates of person nonresponse and dropout. Many people will retain their PTSD diagnosis even after medical treatment.
- The complexity of reactions to stress and trauma highlights the importance of functional and participatory approaches such as occupational therapy to assist people in coping and moving forward toward recovery.

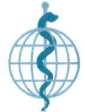

Visit the online resource center at **FADavis.com** to access the videos.

Apply It Now

1. Person-Environment-Occupation (PEO) Analysis

Reread Lady Gaga's experience from earlier in the chapter and complete a PEO analysis using the template in Appendix A. Consider the following guiding questions:
- What occupations are important to her?
- What personal and environmental factors contributed to her recovery process?
- What might have supported an earlier start to her recovery?
- What trauma-informed approaches would be helpful?

2. Experiencing Occupation-Based Challenges

The Edgelow and colleagues (2019) scoping review of occupational therapy and PTSD identified common impacts on occupational performance, including difficulty with sleep, work, and maintaining social relationships.

Reflective Questions
- What feelings come up for you when thinking about stress and trauma?
- How can OTPs be sensitive to the potential trauma histories of people in physical health settings?
- What about in mental health settings?
- What are three strategies you could use to address each of these challenge areas?

Resources

Videos

- "How Do Occupational Therapists Help Individuals Ease Back Into the World After TBI and/or PTSD?" video. https://www.youtube.com/watch?v=M0q_M2S0fvk
- "How This Mental Health Center Is Using Pottery As Therapy" video. https://www.cbc.ca/news/canada/prince-edward-island/pei-pottery-ptsd-mental-health-therapy-serene-view-ranch-1.5726009
- "Joelle Rabow Maletis: The Psychology of PTSD" video. https://www.ted.com/talks/joelle_rabow_maletis_the_psychology_of_post_traumatic_stress_disorder
- "Melissa Walker: Art Can Heal PTSD's Invisible Wounds" video. https://www.ted.com/talks/melissa_walker_art_can_heal_ptsd_s_invisible_wounds?referrer=playlist-what_comes_after_war&autoplay=true
- "Nadine Burke Harris: How Childhood Trauma Affects Health Across a Lifespan" video. https://www.ted.com/talks/nadine_burke_harris_how_childhood_trauma_affects_health_across_a_lifetime?language=en
- "Child in Crisis" video. In this video, occupational therapist Brittany shares her experience working in a psychiatric rehab hospital's adolescent unit with Mikey, an 8-year-old boy presenting with a complex set of challenges. Diagnosed at birth with fetal alcohol syndrome, Mikey has a history of multiple ACEs. On admission, he presented with suicidal and homicidal ideation and symptoms consistent with PTSD. Brittany describes how she did her own research, learned more about Mikey, and developed an intervention that worked well for him and the other children in the group. Access the video at the online resource center at FADavis.com.
- "Managing Challenging Behaviors in Young Children" video. In this video, an occupational therapist and occupational therapy assistant (OTA) discuss the OTA's work in an Operation Breakthrough program within Head Start. The OTA works with young children from at-risk families; together with teachers and other therapists, she helps to catch any developmental delays and intervene as necessary. She describes a particularly challenging behavior in one child and the strategies she uses to help him feel comfortable, safe, and loved, allowing him to better participate in the classroom and individual sessions. Access the video at the online resource center at FADavis.com.
- "Two Practitioners Discuss Their Work in Suicide Prevention" video. In this video, two occupational therapists, Nadine and Kim, discuss their work in suicide prevention. They share reflections and pearls of wisdom gained in years of practice in this area—observations about both people in crisis and how they have responded as practitioners. They express the role that the occupational lives of these individuals have in their recovery and crisis plans, as well as serving as a springboard for interventions. Nadine and Kim also describe what is rewarding about this work and the crucial need to meet their self-care and well-being needs in order to stay connected to this work. Access the video at the online resource center at FADavis.com.
- "Occupational Therapy Approaches in a Shelter for Unaccompanied Refugee Youth" video. In this video, occupational therapist Claudette Fette shares the impactful work she, volunteer students, and staff performed in a massive unaccompanied minor shelter in Texas in 2021. Many of the minors, mostly from Central America, had histories of trauma, and the conditions in the shelter were dismal—lack of meaningful occupations, bullying, untrained staff, and so on. Claudette describes her approach to assessing the environment, training staff, recruiting volunteers, responding to the minors' trauma responses, and creating and supporting occupations and leisure activities. Access the video at the online resource center at FADavis.com.
- "Aimee's Lived Experience With Substance Use and Autism" video. Aimee is an occupational therapist with the lived experience of substance use disorder. In this video, Aimee shares that she was diagnosed with childhood PTSD and that she also realized that she is autistic. She describes the behaviors that led her to that conclusion, her coping strategies, and how her lived experience affected her role as a student in graduate school. Access the video at the online resource center at FADavis.com.

Online Resources

- Adverse Childhood Experiences (ACEs): https://www.cdc.gov/violenceprevention/aces/index.html
- Connected Care Story—Occupational Therapy for Complex Health Concerns: https://www.cbihealth.ca/discover/connected-care-occupational-therapy-ptsd
- Military Family Resiliency: https://www.militaryonesource.mil/parenting/family-life/keeping-your-family-strong-essentials
- Occupational Therapy and PTSD (American Occupational Therapy Association): https://www.aota.org/-/media/corporate/files/aboutot/professionals/whatisot/mh/facts/ptsd%20fact%20sheet.pdf
- Occupational Therapy and PTSD (Canadian Association of Occupational Therapists): https://caot.ca/document/4065/Post%20Traumatic%20Stress%20Disorder%20-%20Fact%20Sheet.pdf

Organizations

- Canadian Institute for Public Safety Research and Treatment (CIPSRT): https://www.cipsrt-icrtsp.ca
- Canadian Institute for Military and Veteran Health Research (CIMVHR): https://cimvhr.ca
- International Society for the Study of Trauma and Dissociative Disorders: http://www.isst-d.org
- National Center for PTSD: http://www.ptsd.va.gov
- SAMHSA Trauma and Violence: https://www.samhsa.gov/trauma-violence

References

American Psychiatric Association. (2013). *Diagnostic and statistical manual of mental disorders* (5th ed.). American Psychiatric Publishing. https://doi.org/10.1176/appi.books.9780890425596

American Psychiatric Association. (2022). *Diagnostic and statistical manual of mental disorders* (5th ed., text rev.). American Psychiatric Publishing. https://doi.org/10.1176/appi.books.9780890425787

American Psychological Association. (2017). *Clinical practice guideline for the treatment of posttraumatic stress disorder (PTSD) in adults.* https://www.apa.org/ptsd-guideline

Baiocchi, D. (2013). *Measuring Army deployments to Iraq and Afghanistan.* Rand.

Berry, M. E. (2022). Radicalising resilience: Mothering, solidarity, and interdependence among women survivors of war. *Journal of International Relations and Development, 25*(4), 946–966. https://doi.org/10.1057/s41268-022-00274-y

Carleton, R., Afifi, T. O., Turner, S., Taillieu, T., Duranceau, S., LeBouthillier, D. M., Sareen, J., Ricciardelli, R., MacPhee, R. S., Groll, D., Hozempa, K., Brunet, A., Weekes, J. R., Griffiths, C. T., Abrams, K. J., Jones, N. A., BeShai, S., Cramm, H. A., Dobson, K. S., … Asmundson, G. J. (2018). Mental disorder symptoms among public safety personnel in Canada. *The Canadian Journal of Psychiatry, 63*(1), 54–64. https://doi.org/10.1177/0706743717723825

Chandola, T., Brunner, E., & Marmot, M. (2006). Chronic stress at work and the metabolic syndrome: Prospective study. *British Medical Journey, 332*(7540), 521–525. https://doi.org/10.1136/bmj.38693.435301.80

Coquemont, C., Georges, C., Massoubre, B., Massoubre, C., & Boulliat, C. (2022). Curative drug treatments for post-traumatic stress disorder: A systematic review of the effectiveness of recent treatments. *American Journal of Internal Medicine, 10*(3), 39–50. https://doi.org/10.11648/j.ajim.20221003.12

Daskalakis, N. P., Rijal, C. M., King, C., Huckins, L. M., & Ressler, K. J. (2018). Recent genetics and epigenetics approaches to PTSD. *Current Psychiatry Reports, 20*, 1–12. https://doi.org/10.1007/s11920-018-0898-7

Daskalakis, N. P., Xu, C., Bader, H. N., Chatzinakos, C., Weber, P., Makotkine, I., Lehrner, A., Bierer, L. M., Binder, E. B., & Yehuda, R. (2021). Intergenerational trauma is associated with expression alterations in glucocorticoid- and immune-related genes. *Neuropsychopharmacology, 46*(4), 763–773. https://doi.org/10.1038/s41386-020-00900-8

Edgelow, M., & Cramm, H. (2020). Developing an occupation-centred framework for trauma intervention. *Occupational Therapy in Mental Health, 36*(3), 270–290. https://doi.org/10.1080/0164212x.2020.1808148

Edgelow, M. M., Macpherson, M. M., Arnaly, F., Tam-Seto, L., & Cramm, H. A. (2019). Occupational therapy and posttraumatic stress disorder: A scoping review. *Canadian Journal of Occupational Therapy, 86*(2), 148–157. https://doi.org/10.1177/0008417419831438

Eichstaedt, J. C., Sherman, G. T., Giorgi, S., Roberts, S. O., Reynolds, M. E., Ungar, L. H., & Guntuku, S. C. (2021). The emotional and mental health impact of the murder of George Floyd on the US population. *Proceedings of the National Academy of Sciences of the United States of America, 118*(39), e2109139118. https://doi.org/10.1073/pnas.2109139118

Fette, C., Lambdin-Pattavina, C., & Weaver, L. L. (2019). Understanding and applying trauma-informed approaches across occupational therapy settings. *OT Practice, 24*(5), 35.

Finlay, S., Roth, C., Zimsen, T., Bridson, T. L., Sarnyai, Z., & McDermott, B. (2022). Adverse childhood experiences and allostatic load: A systematic review. *Neuroscience & Biobehavioral Reviews, 136*, 104605. https://doi.org/10.1016/j.neubiorev.2022.104605

Gaga, L. (2016, December 6). *"Head stuck in a cycle I look off and I stare": A personal letter from Gaga.* Born this Way Foundation. https://bornthisway.foundation/personal-letter-gaga

Graff, G. (2014). The intergenerational trauma of slavery and its aftermath. *The Journal of Psychohistory, 41*(3), 181–197. https://psycnet.apa.org/record/2014-00820-003

Hales, G. K., Saribaz, Z. E., Debowska, A., & Rowe, R. (2022). Links of adversity in childhood with mental and physical health outcomes: A systematic review of longitudinal mediating and moderating mechanisms. *Trauma, Violence, & Abuse, 24*(3), 1465–1482. https://doi.org/10.1177/15248380221075087

Isobel, S., Goodyear, M., Furness, T., & Foster, K. (2019). Preventing intergenerational trauma transmission: A critical interpretive synthesis. *Journal of Clinical Nursing, 28*(7-8), 1100–1113. https://doi.org/10.1111/jocn.14735

Jacoby, S. (2021, May 21). *Lady Gaga on how her rape, pregnancy, and trauma led to chronic pain.* SELF. https://www.self.com/story/lady-gaga-trauma-chronic-pain

Jiang, D. H., Kim, S., Zaidi, A., Cottrell, L., Christopher, M. C., Palacio, T. R., & Rosenfield, P. J. (2022). Insights from expanded adverse childhood experiences screening in a hospital-based outpatient psychiatry service. *The Psychiatric Quarterly, 93*(2), 677–687. https://doi.org/10.1007/s11126-022-09982-7

Kapadia, A. (Director), Porter, D. (Director), Kauffman, R. (Segment Director), & Tibbon, T. (Segment Director). (2021, May 21). Say it out loud (Season 1, Episode 1) [TV series episode]. In A. H. Browne, K. Cooperman, C. Cyr, J. Kamen, A. Kapadia, T. Montgomery, D. Porter. P. Harry, D. Sirulnick, O. Winfrey & T. Wood (Executive Producers), *The me you can't see.* Apple+.

Krantz, D. S., Shank, L. M., & Goodie, J. L. (2022). Post-traumatic stress disorder (PTSD) as a systemic disorder: Pathways to cardiovascular disease. *Health Psychology, 41*(10), 651. https://doi.org/10.1037/hea0001127

Lopez, A. (2011). Posttraumatic stress disorder and occupational performance: Building resilience and fostering occupational adaptation. *Work: Journal of Prevention, Assessment & Rehabilitation, 38*(1), 33–38. https://doi.org/10.3233/wor-2011-1102

Lumley, M. A., Yamin, J. B., Pester, B. D., Krohner, S., & Urbanik, C. P. (2022). Trauma matters: Psychological interventions for comorbid psychosocial trauma and chronic pain. *Pain, 163*(4), 599–603. https://doi.org/10.1097/j.pain.0000000000002425

Mancini, A. D. (2019). When acute adversity improves psychological health: A social–contextual framework. *Psychological Review, 126*(4), 486–505. https://doi.org/10.1037/rev0000144

Merrick, M. T., Ports, K. A., Ford, D. C., Afifi, T. O., Gershoff, E. T., & Grogan-Kaylor, A. (2017). Unpacking the impact of adverse childhood experiences on adult mental health. *Child Abuse & Neglect, 69*, 10–19. https://doi.org/10.1016/j.chiabu.2017.03.016

Moukarbel, C. (Director). (2017). *Five foot two* [Film]. Live Nation Films, Mermaid Films, & Permanent Wave.

Narayan, A. J., Lieberman, A. F., & Masten, A. S. (2021). Intergenerational transmission and prevention of adverse childhood experiences (ACEs). *Clinical Psychology Review, 85*, 101997. https://doi.org/10.1016/j.cpr.2021.101997

National Center for PTSD. (2022). *Chronic pain and PTSD: A guide for patients.* U.S. Department of Veterans Affairs. https://www.ptsd.va.gov/understand/related/chronic_pain.asp

National Center for PTSD. (2023). *How common is PTSD in adults?* U.S. Department of Veterans Affairs. https://www.ptsd.va.gov/understand/common/common_adults.asp

Oakley, L. D., Kuo, W.-C., Kowalkowski, J. A., & Park, W. (2021). Meta-analysis of cultural influences in trauma exposure and PTSD prevalence rates. *Journal of Transcultural Nursing, 32*(4), 412–424. https://doi.org/10.1177/1043659621993909

Ojukwu, E. N., Phillips, J. C., Vance, D. E., & Caine, V. (2022). Thinking with community: A critique of resilience and well-being. *Journal of the Association of Nurses in AIDS Care, 33*(2), 99–102. https://doi.org/10.1097/JNC.0000000000000328

Pacella, M. L., Hruska, B., & Delahanty, D. L. (2013). The physical health consequences of PTSD and PTSD symptoms: A meta-analytic review. *Journal of Anxiety Disorders, 27*(1), 33–46. https://doi.org/10.1016/j.janxdis.2012.08.004

Plach, H. L., & Sells, C. H. (2013). Occupational performance needs of young veterans. *American Journal of Occupational Therapy, 67*(1), 73–81. https://doi.org/10.5014/ajot.2013.003871

Reeves, E. (2015). A synthesis of the literature on trauma-informed care. *Issues in Mental Health Nursing, 36*(9), 698–709. https://doi.org/10.3109/01612840.2015.1025319

Rohleder, N. (2019). Stress and inflammation—The need to address the gap in the transition between acute and chronic stress effects. *Psychoneuroendocrinology, 105*, 164–171. https://doi.org/10.1016/j.psyneuen.2019.02.021

Rosa, W. E., Roberts, K. E., Schlak, A. E., Applebaum, A. J., Breitbart, W. S., Kantoff, E. H., Pessin, H., & Lichtenthal, W. G. (2022). The critical need for a meaning-centered team-level intervention to address healthcare provider distress now. *International Journal of Environmental Research and Public Health, 19*(13), 7801. https://doi.org/10.3390/ijerph19137801

Ryder, A. L., Azcarate, P. M., & Cohen, B. E. (2018). PTSD and physical health. *Current Psychiatry Reports, 20*(12), 1–8. https://doi.org/10.1007/s11920-018-0977-9

Saeed, S. A., Majarwitz, D. J., & Santos, M. G. (2023). Treating PTSD: A review of 8 studies. *Current Psychiatry, 22*(1), 33. https://doi.org/10.12788/cp.0324

Sangalang, C. C., & Vang, C. (2017). Intergenerational trauma in refugee families: A systematic review. *Journal of Immigrant and Minority Health, 19*, 745–754. https://doi.org/10.1007/s10903-016-0499-7

Schellenberg, M., & Walters, A. (2022). The uprise of gun violence in the United States: Consequences of a dual pandemic. *Current*

Opinion in Anesthesiology, 36(2), 132–136. https://doi.org/10.1097/aco.0000000000001218

Schnurr, P. P. (2022). Understanding pathways from traumatic exposure to physical health. In U. Schnyder, & M. Cloitre (Eds.), *Evidence based treatments for trauma-related psychological disorders: A practical guide for clinicians* (2nd ed., pp. 91–108). Springer. https://doi.org/10.1007/978-3-030-97802-0_5

Shalev, A. Y. (2002). Acute stress reactions in adults. *Biological Psychiatry, 51*(7), 532–543. https://doi.org/10.1016/s0006-3223(02)01335-5

Southwick, S. M., & Charney, D. S. (2004). Responses to trauma: Normal reactions or pathological symptoms. *Psychiatry, 67*(2), 170–173. https://doi.org/10.1521/psyc.67.2.170.35960

Substance Abuse and Mental Health Services Administration. (2016). *Impact of the DSM-IV to DSM-5 changes on the National Survey on Drug Use and Health.* https://www-ncbi-nlm-nih-gov.proxy.queensu.ca/books/NBK519697

Tully, J., Bhugra, D., Lewis, S. J., Drennan, G., & Markham, S. (2021). Is PTSD overdiagnosed? *British Medical Journal, 373*, n787. https://doi.org/10.1136/bmj.n787

Tummala-Narra, P. (2007). Conceptualizing trauma and resilience across diverse contexts: A multicultural perspective. *Journal of Aggression, Maltreatment & Trauma, 14*(1-2), 33–53. https://doi.org/10.1300/j146v14n01_03

Walder, K., Molineux, M., Bissett, M., & Whiteford, G. (2021). Occupational adaptation—Analyzing the maturity and understanding of the concept through concept analysis. *Scandinavian Journal of Occupational Therapy, 28*(1), 26–40. https://doi.org/10.1080/11038128.2019.1695931

Wheaton, B., Young, M., Montazer, S., & Stuart-Lahman, K. (2013). Social stress in the twenty-first century. In C. S. Aneshensel, J. C. Phelan, & A. Bierman (Eds.), *Handbook of the Sociology of Mental Health* (2nd ed., pp. 299–323). Springer. https://doi.org/10.1007/978-94-007-4276-5_15

Yunitri, N., Chu, H., Kang, X. L., Jen, H.-J., Pien, L.-C., Tsai, H.-T., Kamil, A. R., & Chou, K.-R. (2022). Global prevalence and associated risk factors of posttraumatic stress disorder during COVID-19 pandemic: A meta-analysis. *International Journal of Nursing Studies, 126*, 104136. https://doi.org/10.1016/j.ijnurstu.2021.104136

The Environment

This part of the text is divided into three sections: Societal Influences, Places, and Mental Health Practice Settings. Although recognized as important by occupational therapy practitioners (OTPs), the environmental component of the Person-Environment-Occupation (PEO) model tends to receive the least attention. This section of the text aims to correct this neglect by providing practitioners with an explicit understanding of the environment and its impact on occupational performance. These chapters also define the frameworks that guide practice, specific environmental assessments, and interventions aimed at creating environments that support meaningful occupational participation. Therapeutic reasoning assessment tables in these chapters provide an easy reference to environmental assessments.

The Societal Influences section focuses on macro elements of the environment that affect participation, such as public policy, stigma, social determinants of health, and the family context. The Places section also takes a broad perspective, and in two new chapters examines the natural and virtual environments. This section also focuses on where people live, love, and work: their neighborhoods, community, and home environments. Finally, the Mental Health Practice Settings section examines the places where OTPs work, particularly settings with either a primary or secondary focus on mental health practice. Some of these settings are emerging areas of practice that have received little attention in other textbooks. Each chapter includes a general description of the setting with information on the needs of the population served. The role of occupational therapy is described, as well as assessments and interventions common to that setting.

PART 3

Societal Influences

SECTION **1**

CHAPTER

26

The Public Policy Environment

Ryan Thomure and Lisa Mahaffey

It is not always obvious in one's day-to-day life, but most people's daily occupations, such as driving, working, and paying household bills, are governed at least in part by policy decisions. For example, a common self-care task is visiting a doctor for an illness or an annual checkup. This simple, everyday task is significantly influenced by local, state, and federal policies. Insurance policy determines which doctors will be paid for under the plan, which services and medications are covered, and possibly even the treatment options available—regardless of best practices.

In fact, one simple change in insurance policy can be powerful. For example, a change in policy that allowed children to remain on their parents' insurance plans to age 26 had incredible ripple effects. This became the law when the Patient Protection and Affordable Care Act (ACA) was passed in 2010 (U.S. Department of Health and Human Services, 2010). Before this policy change, approximately 30% of young adults were uninsured and not likely to seek medical support, despite approximately 50% of young adults having a chronic health condition (Watson et al., 2022).

Many people with disabilities routinely rely on local, state, and federal policies for access to driving and public transportation, the ability to engage in activities to maintain their physical and mental health, assistance in finding a place to live, and opportunities to engage in valued work and leisure. Policy matters!

This chapter describes the policies that affect access to supports for health care and daily living for people across the mental health continuum, particularly those with psychiatric disabilities in the United States. Although policies vary considerably in different countries, there are important similarities in policymaking processes and their effect on occupational participation. Given the fact that participation is the desired outcome of occupational therapy, occupational therapy practitioners (OTPs) must keep current on the local, state, and national policies that influence their practice and the lives of the people they serve. At times it may be necessary

for OTPs to advocate for policies that broaden access and opportunities for occupational participation.

Public Policy, Laws, Regulations, and Politics

Public policies guide action. Public policies regarding mental health reflect the vision that a society has for the mental health of its population and specify frameworks for recognizing, preventing, managing, intervening in, and funding mental health care.

Public Policy

It is valuable to start with a discussion of the different factors that make up what is referred to as *policy*. **Public policy** has been defined as "anything the government chooses to do or not to do" (Dye, 2013; Howlett & Cashore, 2014). Policies typically, though not always, reflect and are significantly informed by the values and objectives of the citizens. They also usually reflect the values and priorities of those in power, such as governing bodies. Political and social discourse drives the formation of policies.

When an influential group of citizens identifies an issue, policymakers can respond by introducing new bills into the legislative process. Policymakers debate the bills both privately and publicly, and competing interest groups vie for their attention. All policies are influenced by the ideology of politicians and community leaders; therefore, changes in leadership can potentially translate to major shifts in policies that affect access to services.

Focusing events can have a powerful effect on the direction of public policy. **Focusing events** are incidents, or a series of incidents, that impact a significant group of people. Lawmakers often respond to focusing events by submitting legislation believed to address the situation, with the goal to mitigate the problems or prevent similar future events. For example, the wars in Iraq and Afghanistan resulted in a high number of returning veterans who experienced symptoms of severe posttraumatic stress disorder (PTSD; Litz & Schlenger, 2009). The needs of these veterans led to implementation of policies meant to improve access to mental health services through the Veterans Administration. Two specific focusing events that affected policy are described in Box 26-1.

BOX 26-1 ■ Focusing Events Impacting Policy

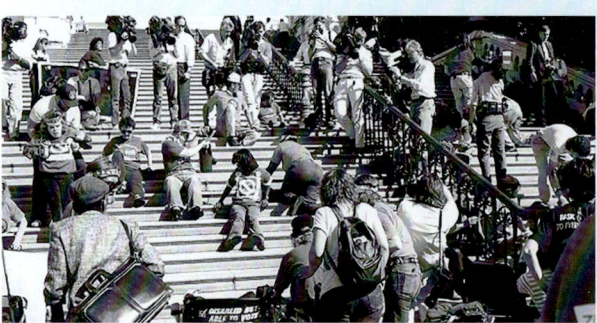

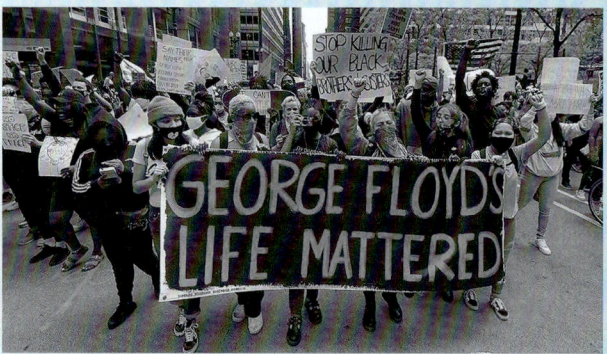

Capitol Crawl: On March 12, 1990, a group of disability activists tossed away their mobility aids and wheelchairs and dragged themselves up the steps of the U.S. Capitol building in Washington, DC. This focusing event came to be known as the Capitol Crawl. The actions of these individuals, during a time Congress was debating civil rights policy for people with disabilities, put a spotlight on the discrimination and life challenges faced by people with disabilities. Four months later, the Americans with Disabilities Act (ADA) was signed into law.

From Elliot, A. (2022, March 29). Capital crawl to access for all. LACDMH Blog. https://dmh.lacounty.gov/blog/2022/03/capitol-crawl-to-access-for-all

Black Lives Matter: The death of George Floyd at the hands of Minneapolis police can be considered a focusing event. His death and the subsequent activism by many individuals and civil rights organizations put the spotlight on racial inequity in the justice system. The George Floyd Justice in Policing Act seeks to address issues such as police accountability, the use of racial profiling, and the use of force. The legislation was approved in the U.S. House of Representatives in 2020 and again in 2021, but since then has failed to garner bipartisan support.

From Daniels, C. M. (2023, May 25). Here's what's changed since George Floyd's murder three years ago. The Hill. https://thehill.com/homenews/race-politics/4020985-heres-whats-changed-since-george-floyds-murder-three-years-ago

---

The Lived Experience

Dawn

As far back as I can remember, I have struggled with depression and self-harm. My earliest memories of this go back to junior high and continue through high school–when I would cut myself with X-ACTO knives and razor blades, carving messages of my sadness and self-loathing. When I entered my twenties, I also began to alternate through periods of extreme highs and out of control behavior. I cycled through relationships, married three times by age 28, and engaged in often heavy daily drinking. Despite these ups and downs, I was highly driven and pushed myself to succeed. I moved through careers in information technology and marketing and eventually settled into a career in insurance and a home life as a wife and mother.

After a traumatic experience at age 30, my depression and anxiety surged, and I developed the need for medication to manage my symptoms. My family doctor worked with me to manage my condition, but 3 months into my fourth marriage, my suicidal thoughts and desires overwhelmed me, and I was forced to admit myself to the psychiatric unit of a local

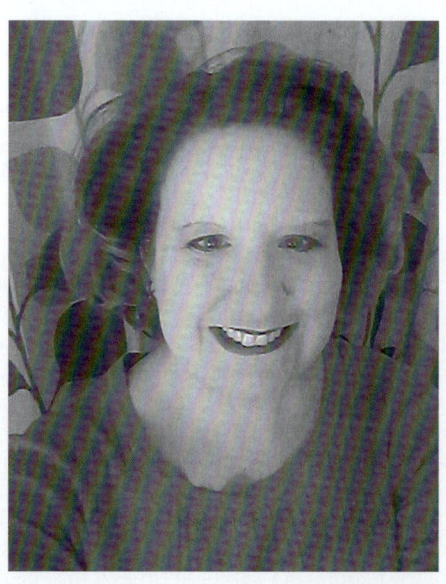

The Lived Experience—cont'd

hospital. I worked with a psychiatrist I met there for nearly a year before a definitive diagnosis was reached: Bipolar II disorder, with anxiety and tendencies of borderline personality disorder. I started on the mood stabilizer lithium, which successfully helped me to manage my ups and downs but with the drawback of a gradual increase in cognitive difficulties and short-term memory loss. These changes to my mental state impaired my self-confidence and increased my anxiety to sometimes debilitating levels.

After more than 3 years as a successful insurance claims analyst and countless 60-hour work weeks I finally succumbed to the difficulties caused by both the disorder and the side effects of my medications, losing both my job and my fourth marriage 3 years later. The following year, and another lost job later, I lost my private health insurance and went on Medicaid. As a person with bipolar disorder, I take multiple medications to manage my symptoms and lessen the "bad" times. At that time, I was taking an antidepressant, thyroid medication, two mood stabilizers, an anxiety medication, and two headache medications (for chronic tension and migraine headaches I had suffered since the traumatic experience 9 years earlier). At the time I went on Medicaid, I had been on these medications for at least 6 months and my antidepressant for 7 years.

When I first encountered my state's four-medication-per-month cap in the public health-care system, the pharmacy explained that my psychiatrist needed only to complete a pre-authorization process and I would be able to get the medication I needed. The reality of the situation was entirely different. The nurses at my doctor's office worked constantly to try to get past the four-script cap for me, and each time I was completely stonewalled by Medicaid. Still unable to work because of my illness, I had used up all my state unemployment and had no income. Paying for medication out of pocket was impossible. Each month, I would end up going anywhere from days to as long as 2 weeks without one or more medications. During those periods I would lie on the floor for hours in tears, feeling hopeless and desperate. Now the single mother of a 12-year-old girl, I had to send my daughter to a friend's house during those days and weeks because I could not care for her. In the end, I would get the medications not because Medicaid authorized them, but because the month started over again. I found I had to bargain with myself over what meds I would take and what I would let slide. Did I want to experience physical pain from the headaches or mental pain from the depression? Should I allow the mania from the bipolar disorder to run out of control or cower under the oppression of rampant anxiety? Every decision was a losing one.

I learned that with some of my meds I could only miss a day or two before beginning an excruciating withdrawal including chills, severe headaches, shaking, nausea, and spiraling depression capped by suicidal thoughts and actions. I ended up in the emergency department (ED) three times in my first year enrolled in Medicaid, all because of the effects of going without my antidepressant and mood-stabilizing medications.

After my second visit, I went through a 6-week partial hospitalization. The third time, unable to face the desperation and withdrawal, I attempted suicide.

After 8 months in the public health-care system, I was able to switch to a Medicaid plan that eliminated the medication cap. Since that time, I have never been turned down for a prescription at the pharmacy. I have not been back to the ED or partial hospitalization. My ongoing instability was 90% caused by having my medications repeatedly withheld. Had the state paid for my medications as prescribed during that period, their cost would have been approximately $3,000. Instead, the state paid approximately $10,200 for medications, ED visits, and partial hospitalization—and I nearly paid with my life. The public health-care system proved to be an expensive game of Russian roulette, forever altering my life. One month before my health-care plan changed, my daughter and I became homeless.

With no family to help us, we had to pack up what we could and move an hour away, the two of us sharing a bedroom in the home of another family. In the new town, case management services for people in my situation were severely lacking compared with what was available before. For 2 years I had relied on assistance from the local mental health center to navigate the complex worlds of Social Security Disability and the state Department of Healthcare Services; this help was now gone. My cognitive difficulties made deciphering these complex systems much more difficult than they may have been for me even 5 years earlier. I inadvertently let my food stamp benefits lapse, which resulted in losing my Medicaid benefits as well. The frustration and helplessness overwhelmed me, throwing me into the worst manic episode I had experienced in 8 years. I descended into out-of-control drinking and rampant sexual activity; I gave up on my medication entirely for more than a month.

In the midst of it all, my Social Security Disability was approved, and I was granted 2 years retroactive benefits. This moved me from the state Medicaid system to the federal Medicare system for my health care, offering a stronger layer of stability in a state with ongoing social services cuts. I was able to replace my car, which had broken down. I purchased a mobile home outright, giving my daughter and me a home of our own once again. Under a state Department of Rehabilitation grant, I am beginning school to learn a new trade that will work better with my challenges. I restarted my medications and my mania gradually subsided, to the amazement of even my own psychiatrist. I have hope and direction, something that I thought I had lost for good. Yet every day, I live under the specter of the public aid and public health-care system. I wonder what will happen next, and will I be strong enough to handle it when it does. At age 40, I don't want to live the rest of my life on disability. I want to have a job again, be independent again. But after all I have experienced, I am left with questions: How do I maintain focus while fighting with the health-care system? How do I get myself out of the system if I can't survive while I am in it?

Laws, Regulations, and Politics

Laws provide the legal and institutional framework with which to implement policy. Policy is a guide for action, and laws function to compel or prohibit behavior. Laws are the rules people live by; they are intended to protect the safety of, and ensure fundamental rights for, the people in a community (Judicial Learning Center, n.d.). For example, the **Americans with Disabilities Act of 1990 (ADA)** represented landmark civil rights legislation written and passed to prohibit discrimination of people with disabilities in all aspects of public life, including employment, education, and transportation. This law also sought to decrease the physical and social barriers in public and private spaces that restricted daily life activities for people with disabilities and sought to decrease discrimination in housing and community organizations as well (ADA, 2010).

The ADA begins by including language that identifies what constitutes a disability to establish whom the law intends to protect; it also defines the environments and circumstances in which the law applies. For example, the ADA specifically prohibits discrimination in transportation, work, and government buildings and in commercial places such as restaurants (ADA.gov, 2020).

Laws outline the processes for enforcement. They are intended to ensure rules are followed and to define consequences for when they are not. Accessibility-related building codes for new construction and reconstruction are one means by which the ADA is implemented. The ADA also includes processes to ensure that the civil rights of people with disabilities are enforced (Box 26-2). This primarily occurs through formal reporting procedures whereby an individual with a disability completes a government claim form indicating, for example, that they were not afforded a necessary accommodation that would allow them to work in a desired position for which they are qualified, or to access a service they need or want (ADA, 2010).

Individuals with psychiatric disabilities may file claims if they have been denied reasonable accommodations such as alternative hours or a change in workspace to support their ability to complete their essential work responsibilities. Because a change in work hours might impact the way the business is conducted, the ADA contains provisions to protect employers and businesses from costs that would cause undue hardship (ADA, 2010).

Regulations are the detailed rules for enforcing laws, including the responsibilities and constraints that constitute what it means to follow laws, and the process for monitoring enforcement. For example, the ADA states that no public entity can discriminate against a qualified person with a disability (ADA, 2010). The regulations define a person with a disability as someone with a physical or mental impairment that limits one or more major life activities.

The ADA law states that no person with a disability shall be excluded from participation in important activities because of architectural, transportation, or social barriers in public spaces. The regulations therefore include language defining what constitutes a public place, identify acceptable ways to remove physical or nonphysical barriers and establish exceptions for when barrier removal is not feasible (ADA, 2010). Regulations can be considered the fine print of the law that specifies how the law should be implemented.

Politics can be defined as activities by individuals or groups that influence the policies of government, including the "debate or conflict" between competing interests (Merriam-Webster, 2015). The political process is characterized by groups of individuals with similar values joining together to influence policy. Because policies are always changing, groups must be vigilant in identifying policy issues that impact their personal lives or work, or, in the case of health-care providers such as OTPs, the people whom they serve.

One role of the American Occupational Therapy Association (AOTA) is to monitor policy efforts and lobby for the interest of their members on the federal level. State associations also perform these functions on behalf of practitioners in their state, including advocating for the profession's state practice act, the law that defines occupational therapy practice and the criteria for obtaining a license in the state. AOTA also has a political action committee (AOTPAC) composed of AOTA members and hired staff members. These people work to further the federal legislative aims of AOTA by supporting the nomination, selection, or election of certain legislators to the federal government. Many state associations also have PACs that support state-level legislators. Box 26-3 describes how OTPs can actively advocate as Qualified Mental Health Providers (QMHPs) and/or Qualified Behavioral Health Providers (QBHPs).

BOX 26-2 ■ The Americans With Disabilities Act Today—The Fight Continues

The passage of the ADA represented a significant win for Americans living with disabilities, but challenges remain. For example:

■ People living with disabilities are approximately half as likely to be employed as their peers without disabilities.

■ People with disabilities continue to experience challenges accessing transportation through inequities such as inaccessible public transit and poor public infrastructure.

■ Aspects of the physical environment can prevent people with disabilities from participating in valued activities.

■ Critical health-care services might be inaccessible because of overly complex patient-facing information or a lack of understanding of people with disabilities on the part of health-care providers.

These are only a few examples of challenges still faced by Americans living with disabilities decades after the passage of the ADA. Many of these challenges can be addressed, at least in part, by policymaking.

Reflective Question: What role can OTPs play in both direct services and partnering with people living with disabilities in advocacy work that addresses these challenges?

From Houtenville, A., & Boege, S. (2019). 2018 annual report on people with disabilities in America. *https://eric.ed.gov/?id=ED595177*

BOX 26-3 ■ Advocacy in Action: Occupational Therapy Practitioners as Qualified Mental Health Providers (QMHPs) and/or Qualified Behavioral Health Providers (QBHPs)

The Issue:

- Despite increasing recognition of the importance of mental health care, there is a shortage of mental health professionals nationwide. OTPs and their allies have advocated for OTPs to be recognized as QMHPs and/or QBHPs in multiple states.

- States that explicitly recognize occupational therapists as QMHPs and/or QBHPs as of 2024 are Illinois, Maine, Massachusetts, Michigan, Missouri, Montana, Oregon, and Virginia.

- Without this recognition, occupational therapists are unable to receive reimbursement for psychosocial occupational therapy services through state payers (e.g., Medicaid).

- Advocacy efforts in other states to recognize occupational therapists as QMHPs and/or QBHPs are ongoing.

The Actions:

- The path to formal recognition of occupational therapists as QMHPs and/or QBHPs has varied by state.

- In ongoing and well-documented advocacy efforts in the state of Indiana, occupational therapists have not yet gained explicit recognition as QBHPs. Because of these advocacy efforts, however, the Indiana Health Coverage Program (Indiana's Medicaid program) has clarified that occupational therapists, despite not yet being recognized as QBHPs, are eligible to receive reimbursement for the provision of psychosocial occupational therapy services (Indiana Health Coverage Program, 2021).

The Impact:

- While efforts to have occupational therapists explicitly recognized as QMHPs and/or QBHPs continue, the advocacy efforts in Indiana demonstrate that there are multiple paths for OTPs to increase their presence in mental health and better serve the needs of individuals, communities, and populations.

- In Indiana, these efforts have resulted in increased access to mental health services for Indianans who are enrolled in Medicaid.

- Wider recognition of occupational therapists as QMHPs and/or QBHPs can play a role in addressing the current and growing discrepancy between the need for and availability of critical mental health services (SAMHSA, 2015).

- All OTPs, whether they are QMPHs/QBHPs or not, have the responsibility to advocate by using their knowledge of occupation to speak to the inadequacies of housing, food security, and insurance policies for people with disabilities.

Evidence-Based Practice

Evidence-Based Policymaking

Creating evidence-based summaries can amplify advocacy efforts.

RESEARCH FINDINGS

The impact of using evidence to inform and develop mental health policy is not yet well established (Williamson et al., 2015). Furthermore, despite an increased focus on using evidence to inform policy in recent years, existing evidence is often misused or underused in the development of policy. In addition, the standard of evidence in mental health policymaking has been found to be, in many cases, significantly less rigorous than clinical research (Hui et al., 2000).

It has been suggested that increasing the level of rigor in policy research and writing could contribute to improved policy outcomes (Oliver & Pearce, 2017). Increased transparency, use of appropriate evidence, and increased levels of collaboration between policymakers and affected parties might play a role in the improvement, development, and implementation of public policy.

At the level of the individual practitioner, common strategies for implementation of evidence-based policymaking include the following.

Continued

Evidence-Based Practice—cont'd

APPLICATIONS

➡ Informing and educating decision-makers by disseminating materials on evidence-based practices and using social marketing approaches to gain the support of key constituencies from leaders to front-line workers (Ward et al., 2012).

➡ Given the lack of rigorous evidence in the field of policymaking, providing educational resources that emphasize cost, quality, or workload reductions can drive behavioral changes that result in the use of evidence-based practices (Cairney & Oliver, 2017; Waters et al., 2011).

➡ A mix of globally relevant and locally relevant or contextualized evidence can be used during deliberations on policy development (Hyde et al., 2016).

➡ OTPs can utilize these strategies to support and influence the use of evidence by decision-makers in mental health policy and planning.

REFERENCES

Cairney, P., & Oliver, K. (2017). Evidence-based policymaking is not like evidence-based medicine, so how far should you go to bridge the divide between evidence and policy? *Health Research Policy and Systems, 15*(1), 1–11. https://doi.org/10.1186/s12961-017-0192-x

Hui, A., Rains, L. S., Todd, A., Boaz, A., & Johnson, S. (2020). The accuracy and accessibility of cited evidence: A study examining mental health policy documents. *Social Psychiatry and Psychiatric Epidemiology, 55*(1), 111–121. https://doi.org/10.1007/s00127-019-01786-8

Hyde, J. K., Mackie, T. I., Palinkas, L. A., Niemi, E., & Leslie, L. K. (2016). Evidence use in mental health policy making for children in foster care. *Administration and Policy in Mental Health and Mental Health Services Research, 43,* 52–66. https://doi.org/10.1007/s10488-015-0633-1

Oliver, K., & Pearce, W. (2017). Three lessons from evidence-based medicine and policy: Increase transparency, balance inputs and understand power. *Palgrave Communications, 3,* 43. https://doi.org/10.1057/s41599-017-0045-9

Ward, V., Smith, S., House, A., & Hammer, S. (2012). Exploring knowledge exchange: A useful framework for practice and policy. *Social Science and Medicine, 74*(3), 297–304. https://doi.org/10.1016/j.socscimed.2011.09.021

Waters, E., Armstrong, R., Swinburn, B., Moore, L., Dobbins, M., Anderson, J., Petticrew, M., Clark, R., Conning, R., Moodie, M., & Carter, R. (2011). An exploratory cluster randomised controlled trial of knowledge translation strategies to support evidence-informed decision-making in local governments (The KT4LG study). *BMC Public Health, 11*(34), 1–8. https://doi.org/10.1186/1471-2458-11-34

Williamson, A., Makkar, S. R., McGrath, C., & Redman, S. (2015). How can the use of evidence in mental health policy be increased? A systematic review. *Psychiatric Services, 66*(8), 783–797. https://doi.org/10.1176/appi.ps.201400329

Policies That Directly Affect Individuals With Psychiatric Disabilities

Policies that influence services and provide funding for people with psychiatric disabilities are influenced by a combination of local, state, and federal programs. The policies in this section have an important role in determining how services are provided and reimbursed. Of significance to OTPs, these policies provide for access to the adaptations and modifications people often need to participate in occupations they value. The laws discussed here can be divided into several policy categories: public assistance programs such as Social Security, Medicaid, and Medicare; private health insurance; civil rights; and policy concerning inpatient commitment. Every OTP should have a working knowledge of these policies that influence the lives of people that receive occupational therapy.

Social Security

The Social Security Act of 1935 was introduced to provide financial assistance to people over 65 who had retired from the labor force. The program was established to be self-supporting and still runs with the expectation that both employers and employees will contribute through payroll taxes. The program is administered by the U.S. Social Security Administration (SSA). The money collected through the Social Security tax was to be used to pay out monetary benefits to people over the age of 65. In this way, current workers would support those who were retired.

In the years since the passing of the original Social Security Act, several amendments have broadened it to provide medical support for older adults, as well as monetary and medical support for specific groups such as veterans, federal employees, those in poverty, and children and adults with physical and psychiatric disabilities (SSA, n.d.-d). Many of the amendments impacting people with psychiatric disabilities are reviewed in this chapter, including additional social insurance programs such as Medicare and means-tested medical assistance programs such as Medicaid.

Social Security Disability Insurance

Social Security Disability Insurance (SSDI) was added as an amendment to the Social Security Act in 1956 to provide a financial safety net for workers who become disabled and are unable to continue working (SSA, n.d.-e). Because this is an insurance program as opposed to a welfare program, both qualification and the monetary amount a person receives monthly are dependent on the Social Security taxes they have paid into the program through employment. Individuals must meet criteria regarding both the length of their work history and the recency of their work. Because it is an insurance program, individuals who acquire a disability after they stopped working or individuals who never or barely worked are not typically eligible.

Applicants must go through a qualification process to determine if they meet the basic requirements. The first step is to determine if a person meets **substantial gainful activity (SGA)**, a monthly earned income amount determined by the federal government to be sufficient for self-support (2023 SGA = $1,470/month; SSA, 2023). A person who cannot maintain an income at or above SGA is then assessed to determine the severity of their disability using two criteria: (1) whether the severity of the disability significantly impacts the individual's ability to obtain or maintain work (e.g., do they have difficulty concentrating or remembering, which interferes with work tasks?) and (2) whether the condition tied to the disability meets the "Listing of Impairments" criteria, SSA's description of conditions that are "severe enough" to warrant benefits.

Each condition has a complicated set of requirements, written in language that is functionally based rather than medical terminology that is symptom based, that must be met to establish "severe enough" for benefits. A health-care provider who is qualified to diagnose mental disorders makes this determination (SSA, n.d.-b). If a person does not have an impairment included on the listing of impairments, they may still qualify for benefits if they can demonstrate that they have limitations in mental functioning that meet the first criteria of significantly impacting work tasks (SSA, n.d.-b).

To apply for SSDI benefits, a physician, or surrogate, must complete a mental residual functional capacity (MRFC) form. This requires the physician to document functional limitations in areas such as activities of daily living (ADLs), instrumental activities of daily living (IADLs), social interaction, or challenges that impact focus, pace, and organization. Many people do not initially qualify for benefits because of the mismatch between medical and Social Security terminology. The MRFC can be completed by OTPs, but forms require a physician's signature endorsing their reports. Substance use disorders cannot be used as a qualifying diagnosis for SSDI, and a person who is diagnosed with such a disorder cannot qualify for SSDI unless they can prove they would still have a disabling mental health condition in the absence of the substance use disorder (SSA, 1995).

Once severity is determined, a decision is made as to whether the person could potentially return to the same work they did before the onset of disability and, if not, whether the person could potentially do any other type of work that will allow them to earn an income above SGA. For example, a person who was teaching before the onset of bipolar disorder will not qualify for SSDI just because they cannot handle tasks related to teaching if it is determined they can handle the tasks for a different job, such as filing in an office, that allows them to meet SGA (SSA, n.d.-a).

This process can represent a significant barrier for many applicants. The supposition that a person can work various positions that are not easily obtained or are no longer common in the United States (e.g., because of automation, outsourcing of many industries) can result in denials for people who cannot realistically obtain work because of their disabilities (Rein, 2022).

The SSA's reliance on the outdated *Dictionary of Occupational Titles* can result in unrealistic assessments of whether jobs that people *could* do are jobs that a person could realistically obtain. This description of eligibility processes can help practitioners reflect on challenges a person may experience navigating this system. Supporting a person to understand SSDI and appropriately self-advocate may be an important therapeutic goal. Discussions of eligibility guidelines may also open the door to other therapeutic goals, such as, for example, supporting the individual to consider realistic employment options that match their values, interests, and functional capacities.

Social Security Disabled Adult Child

Social Security Disabled Adult Child (SSDAC) is a special form of SSDI. To qualify for SSDAC, an individual must be (a) 18 years of age or older; (b) diagnosed with a mental illness that meets the listing of impairment requirements before age 22; (c) the child or dependent of someone who is disabled, retired, or deceased who has worked enough to be eligible for Social Security benefits; (d) unmarried or not married to another person on SSDAC; and (e) earning less than SGA. A person who qualifies for SSDAC receives benefits based on the amount that their parent or legal guardian paid into the Social Security system through Social Security payroll taxes (SSA, n.d.-a).

Medicare

Medicare is one of two government-funded health insurance programs that falls under the umbrella of the Centers for Medicare and Medicaid Services (CMS). In 2020, Medicare covered more than 60 million people (Kaiser Family Foundation, 2020). Medicare provides health insurance for all people eligible for Social Security benefits over the age of 65 and to people under the age of 65 with qualifying disabilities. For a person under 65 with disabilities to qualify for Medicare, they must be eligible for SSDI. Once a person qualifies for SSDI, there is a 24-month waiting period before they are automatically enrolled in Medicare health-care benefits (SSA n.d.-c). Medicare has several parts and options, depending on the recipient's wishes and needs. Table 26-1 summarizes Medicare's parts and options, including what aspects of mental health care are typically covered under various parts of Medicare.

Medicare is a common payer of occupational therapy services, especially for older adults and people with disabilities. As such, OTPs would benefit from developing a basic

TABLE 26-1 | Medicare Parts and Options

Description	Medicare Parts and Options				
	Part A	*Part B*	*Part C*	*Part D*	*Medigap*
Type of coverage	Hospital insurance	Medical insurance	Medicare Advantage	Prescription drug insurance	Supplemental coverage
Description	Inpatient mental health services, skilled nursing, long-term care, hospice, home health, therapy services	Diagnostic and preventive services, outpatient mental health services (e.g., individual psychotherapy, group psychotherapy), partial hospitalization	Includes all services provided in Parts A and B; participant may choose a plan provided through a private health insurance company, which is usually a managed care plan (health maintenance organization [HMO] or preferred provider organization [PPO])	Covers prescription drug costs	Helps to cover out-of-pocket costs and associated Medicare (drug copays, deductibles) costs
Cost	Yearly deductible, coinsurance costs	Yearly deductible, monthly premium; no coverage for prescription drug costs	Administered by private insurers; medical savings accounts include high deductibles	Requires additional premium; includes a penalty for each year not accessed once eligible	Administered by private insurers; available only to those with Medicare Parts A and B, not available to those with Part C

understanding of Medicare and its rules, regulations, and policies as they apply to the people they serve in their setting.

Supplemental Security Income

Supplemental Security Income (SSI), which is administered by the SSA, was amended to the Social Security Act in 1972. SSI is designed to provide monetary income to citizens and qualified noncitizens of the United States who are over age 65, blind, or disabled. Although SSDI is a social insurance program, SSI is a means-tested welfare program (i.e., funds are provided to people who have not been adequately employed and consequently have not paid sufficient Social Security taxes to qualify for SSDI or Social Security Retirement benefits; SSA, n.d.-d). Some states also administer additional supplementary benefits beyond those provided by the federal government.

To qualify for SSI, a person must meet the same criteria as for SSDI: inability to meet SGA and a qualifying condition on the SSA listing of impairments, *and* the individual must have limited resources such as cash, money in the bank, stocks, or other assets. In total, resource limits are $2,000 for an individual and $3,000 for a couple. Most liquid assets can be counted as resources for the purpose of determining eligibility, though a primary residence and vehicle along with several other categories of items are exempted from being considered resources. It is possible for an individual to qualify for both SSI and SSDI, but income received through SSDI will reduce the total amount received through SSI.

In 2023 the maximum federal benefit for SSI was $914 per month for an individual and $1,371 for a married couple in which both persons are eligible for SSI. Because marriage decreases the amount of SSI income received, many people with disabilities feel they must give up their right to marry to maintain their income. The base SSI benefit can also be reduced by other factors, such as other sources of income (including SSDI) or receiving support from a family member.

Medicaid

Medicaid is a means-tested health-care program for people with low income, amended to the SSA in 1965, which aims to aid low-income individuals and families in covering health-care costs. Medicaid is funded through a combination of state and federal funding (Medicaid.gov, n.d.-a) but is administered by individual states. It is considered a means-tested program because to be eligible, a person or a family's assets must fall below a preset threshold (means test).

At its onset, the federal CMS mandated Medicaid coverage for people who qualify for SSI. Because qualification for Medicaid was explicitly tied to qualification for SSI, disincentives to obtain work were inadvertently created. Because these programs are means-tested, income obtained from work may bring an individual's income or assets over the program thresholds, resulting in a loss of benefits. For example, some people may be able to manage a job that would pay them more than the SSI allowance. In the states that have not expanded Medicaid under the ACA, losing SSI could mean losing Medicaid coverage, which could lead to loss of mental health services and potential setbacks to recovery. Although attempts have been made to address these disincentives, rules vary state by state. It is important for people receiving SSI and Medicaid to consult a benefit specialist to understand how work may affect their benefits.

Practitioners working with individuals on Medicaid should understand that there are many ways for an individual to integrate a productive role into their occupational pattern, such as a consistent volunteer role, and that not all people can or wish to work. Furthermore, paid employment is sometimes not the best option for someone as it may jeopardize eligibility for benefits and services that they rely on to maintain their recovery.

Medicaid also covers low-income children and their parents and, in some states, low-income adults without children. The former group is covered through the Children's Health Insurance Program (CHIP) and the latter group is part of the expansion that states could opt into because of the passing of the ACA of 2010 (Kaiser Family Foundation, 2013). Most Medicaid beneficiaries are considered mandatory beneficiaries because they receive SSI. Compared with Medicare, state Medicaid programs often cover a broader set of services. Medicaid covers both community support services and general health-care services, making it possible for people with psychiatric disabilities to improve overall health and avoid institutionalization. This is important, as a high rate of comorbidity exists in people with serious mental illness (SMI), with 87% reporting at least one, 82% two or more, and 69% three or more co-occurring medical conditions.

Furthermore, people with SMI have a life expectancy that is 25 years shorter than the average (Razzano et al., 2015). State Medicaid plans are mandated to include physician, hospital, and nursing home services. States can also opt to include prescription drug; physical, occupational and/or speech therapy; diagnostic screening; and preventive services. Despite these benefits, significant barriers exist for individuals utilizing Medicaid, including a lack of providers who accept Medicaid because of relatively low reimbursement rates compared with private insurance and Medicare (Medicaid and CHIP Payment and Access Commission, 2019).

People who have a significant disability often do not qualify for employer-sponsored health insurance because they cannot meet the minimum hours required for enrollment in benefits. Additionally, if the person was able to get a job, but was unable to keep it, they would be required to reapply for SSI and Medicaid benefits, a time-consuming process during which they would be left without health coverage.

To address these work disincentives, Congress passed the **Medicaid buy-in program** in 1997 and then the **Ticket-to-Work program** in 1999. The Medicaid buy-in program allows people to maintain their Medicaid health insurance by paying a premium or copayments for services. States vary widely in terms of the allowable income threshold for this program. Ticket-to-Work allows people with disabilities to enter work rehabilitation programs and earn an income for a trial period before losing their Medicaid benefits. If they lose their employment because of disability after the trial period, they can be automatically reenrolled without a waiting period (CMS, n.d.-c).

Recently several states have opted to contract out their Medicaid services to private managed care organizations (MCOs). In this contractual agreement, the state's Medicaid authority pays the MCO for each person eligible for Medicaid benefits. In many cases, the MCOs bid for the contract, which opens the door for more competitive rates. Many believe that MCOs will be able to provide more effective care at a reduced cost (Book, 2012). As of 2022, two thirds of all Medicaid recipients are enrolled in MCOs.

Reports on the quality measures remain mixed for people with disabilities using these plans. That said, there is an effort by the government to leverage the big contracts with the large insurance companies that manage these plans to start addressing social determinants of health. For example, over half of the MCO states have put requirements in place for behavioral health screenings and some require community reinvestment (Hinton & Raphael, 2023).

Many OTPs will not find it necessary to develop an "in depth" understanding of the programs just described. However, being able to describe and differentiate the basic tenets of the various programs that people they work with may be enrolled in or be eligible for is critical. It can help OTPs understand, for example, opportunities and challenges that may be brought about by a person's insurance coverage. Having this basic understanding can enhance an OTP's ability to better understand the context of the people they serve. Practitioners may find that some of the individuals they work with have in-depth understandings of the programs and lived experiences related to eligibility, as well as the challenges of enrollment, loss of coverage, or impact of coverage changes. Learning to respectfully ask about these experiences can improve one's understanding of the programs.

Food Security and Housing Policies

Many people in the United States and other countries struggle to afford food, housing, and basic living expenses. Some U.S. policies are focused on providing goods and services to these segments of the population that are struggling with meeting basic needs. These policies are financed by all taxpayers, but they are not linked to SSA. This section describes social policies that target hunger and housing.

Food Security Policies

The presence of one household member with a psychiatric disability predicts a 300% increase in the risk of poverty (Vick et al., 2012). Food and nutrition programs can offer the assistance needed to stretch grocery dollars or provide food in times of need. Federal programs administered through the U.S. Department of Agriculture (USDA) include the Supplemental Nutrition Assistance Program (SNAP), The Emergency Food Assistance Program (TEFAP), and programs specifically designed to assist mothers and children (USDA, n.d.-a).

In 1939, the USDA initiated the Food Stamp Program (FSP), and 25 years later Congress passed the Food Stamp Act of 1964 to increase the ability of low-income people to purchase nutritious food. Building upon this foundation, the Food and Nutrition Act of 2008 solidified the federal commitment to food assistance programs and renamed the program SNAP. The income eligibility for SNAP is determined by individual states on an annual basis and is updated based on changes in the cost of living. In 2022, over 42 million individuals in over 22 million households participated in SNAP. The average monthly benefit per person was approximately $257 (USDA, n.d.-b).

Issues of food security may have a significant impact on mental health. For example, during the COVID-19 pandemic, food insecurity was associated with over a 250% higher risk of anxiety and/or depression (Fang et al., 2021). OTPs must understand the full context in which individuals live, and consistent access to nutritious food is a critical part of that context. In the Being a Psychosocial OT Practitioner feature, readers will learn how an occupational therapy team worked together to support an individual as he became more food secure.

Being a Psychosocial OT Practitioner

Advocacy to Address Food Insecurity

Identifying Psychosocial Strengths and Needs

Juan and Carla are an occupational therapy team working in community mental health in a state that is under a consent decree with the Department of Justice. The state has traditionally used its long-term care mental health dollars to pay for institutionalization in nursing homes rather than building and supporting community-based programs. Because of this, the state was sued by the Department of Justice for violation of Title II of the ADA, which stated that people have a right to receive their services in the communities of their choice. The state entered a consent decree agreeing to build community support programs. Juan, along with a group of OTPs working in community mental health, advocated to get the state to require occupational therapy services as part of the consent decree.

Using a Holistic Occupational Therapy Approach

Juan is part of an occupational therapy team with occupational therapy assistant (OTA) Carla. Together, they have been assigned to a building that is part of a cluster housing program, a form of permanent supportive housing. In this program, most residents have transitioned out of nursing homes and are learning how to live successfully in the community. Juan and Carla support people as they learn to clean, shop, cook, and connect to community resources, creating routines that support participation in the roles and social activities they desire. All the people they work with are either on Medicaid or are dually eligible for Medicaid and Medicare. They also qualify for housing vouchers through the Department of Housing and Urban Development (HUD), SNAP benefits, and reductions on utilities. Few can afford internet access, though the building does offer a computer space, with access to the internet as a service with their rent.

However, many people are forced to use the library or support services if they want to communicate with others via email, search for housing, or even apply for a job. One of the biggest challenges is the fact that many people leaving the nursing homes have developed multiple health problems because of inactivity and poor access to healthy foods. Juan and Carla have been instrumental in helping the housing staff locate and secure apartments that are accessible given the shortage of affordable housing and the limited number of landlords that accept HUD housing vouchers. They have had to teach people how to advocate for access to accessible transportation and are often the

discipline supporting people as they also learn to manage their health conditions on a limited disability income, as well as SNAP benefits that are often insufficient.

Today Carla is working with Duane, who receives only $37 a month in SNAP benefits. Duane's budget identifies additional money from his SSI income totaling about $135 a month for food. He has a medical diagnosis of diabetes and there is some question about an autoimmune disorder, but no one has been able to identify what it is. Carla and Duane are working on developing strategies to get a week's worth of groceries given Duane's limited income. With Carla's help, Duane has learned to go to the food pantry and get any meat and staples he can get before the two of them sit down to plan the meals and grocery list using what Duane was able to get at the pantry. They work together to plan meals that meet the recommendations of Duane's dietitian. This is a challenge, as nutritious food is often unaffordable.

Duane relies on public transportation, so Carla helps him find coupons and stores with deals on the bus routes. Unfortunately, that means that Duane can spend a large part of a day just getting groceries every week. Carla is also teaching Duane to cook more meals for himself so that he can avoid costly fast food that is not on his recommended diet. Carla, Juan, and Duane, along with several other members of the community mental health center, have decided to get involved in an advocacy movement to increase SNAP benefits, and to increase access to better quality foods for SNAP participants, such as getting the local farmers market to accept the SNAP benefit card.

Reflective Questions

1. What do you view as a unique role that occupational therapy can play in helping people understand and utilize benefits compared with what is already being done by other professionals such as social workers and case managers?
2. Regarding Duane's dietary needs, in what way does occupational therapy provide support that is not provided by the registered dietitian that Duane is already working with? How can he benefit from occupational therapy intervention in this area?
3. With this case in mind, do you think it is appropriate for OTPs to act as advocates for policy and political change within the context of their paid positions as health-care providers? Why or why not?

Low-Income Housing Policies

On any given night in the United States, more than half a million people will be unhoused (U.S. Department of Housing and Urban Development [HUD], 2022). In addition to the significantly increased risk of experiencing homelessness for people with psychiatric disabilities (Elbogen et al., 2021), being unhoused can significantly impact the degree to which individuals with psychiatric disabilities are able to manage their health and well-being (Coe et al., 2015).

The increasingly widely utilized **Housing First** model posits that having the security of a place to call home can be a prime factor in the path to recovery and has been shown to be a motivating factor to engage in treatment (Padgett et al., 2016). While the evidence for the impact of the Housing First model continues to develop, there is reason to believe it may have a significant impact on the ability of individuals with psychiatric disabilities and substance use disorders to live as

safely and independently as possible (Woodhall-Melnik & Dunn, 2016).

Despite this widening recognition of the critical role that housing can play in supporting the well-being of people with and without disabilities, there continue to be significant challenges related to housing availability, accessibility, affordability, and security (Anacker, 2019). The National Low Income Housing Coalition (NLIHC) found that there are only 37 affordable and available housing units for every 100 low-income renters (NLIHC, 2022), meaning that many low-income renters, including those with disabilities, will not have access to housing that they can afford.

The **Section 8 housing voucher system** is designed to play a role in assisting low-income individuals and families in obtaining housing. With Section 8 vouchers, renters typically pay no more than 30% of their income toward rent. Vouchers work in two ways: (1) Through the Housing Choice Voucher

Program, a tenant-based voucher allows the tenant to use the Section 8 housing subsidy for their choice of housing, which remains with the tenant when they move; and (2) a project-based voucher remains with the housing to be used by the next tenant (HUD, 2022). In the latter program, property owners typically reserve a certain number of units for low-income renters in exchange for a government subsidy.

Because the program is applicable only to rental housing and because property owners are not required only to accept Section 8 vouchers, voucher holders may have trouble finding housing that meets their preferences regarding quality, location, or both. People with disabilities may also experience difficulties in finding housing that is accessible, both in terms of the physical environment of the unit but also in the opportunities it provides for access to engagement in valued occupation, connection to needed medical services, proximity to support systems, and so on.

This section is intended to provide only a brief overview of low-income housing policies. Because of occupational therapy's focus on engagement and participation within the person's natural environment, a basic understanding of housing policy and the effect it may have on the individuals the policy serves may benefit OTPs regardless of setting. See Chapter 31: The Home Environment: Permanent Supportive Housing and Chapter 42: Homelessness and Housing Insecurity. 🤝

Private Health Insurance

Approximately 36% of people experiencing mental health challenges are covered by employer-sponsored private health insurance. Most of these health insurance policies are run by for-profit organizations, but there has been an increase in not-for-profit insurers because of financial support through the ACA (National Alliance on Mental Illness [NAMI], n.d.). Although there are no federal mandates for what is covered by employers or individually purchased insurance policies obtained outside the health insurance marketplace, there are mandated services at the state level. Understanding the state mandates for insurance may be particularly helpful for practitioners who are involved in nontraditional areas of practice (e.g., community behavioral health centers, homeless shelters).

Two key pieces of legislation specifically address health-care services for mental health challenges: the Mental Health Parity and Addiction Equity Act (MHPAEA) and the ACA. In 2008, Congress passed the MHPAEA (U.S. Department of Labor, 2010). The MHPAEA addresses the fact that, before its passage, many insurance plans covered mental health services at a different rate than physical health services, and such services often came with higher out-of-pocket expenses. The MHPAEA mandates that out-of-pocket costs and access to treatment be equal for mental health, substance abuse, and physical health. See Chapter 34: Integrated Behavioral Health and Primary Care. 🤝

Multiple provisions of the ACA are important to people with psychiatric disabilities; these provisions are summarized in Box 26-4. The passage of the ACA was related to a framework called the **Triple Aim** put forth by the Institute for Healthcare Improvement (IHI), an independent not-for-profit organization. The Triple Aim strives to improve the personal experience of health-care services, improve the health of the population, and reduce the per capita expense

---

> **BOX 26-4 ■ Provisions of the Affordable Care Act That Affect Individuals With Psychiatric Disabilities**
>
> - Coverage of mental health and substance abuse services is federally mandated for insurance companies that wish to be included in state insurance exchanges.
> - The preexisting conditions clause is eliminated for all insurance plans, which allows people with long-standing psychiatric needs to qualify for plans both from the insurance exchanges and employer-provided plans.
> - Children are allowed to be covered under their parents' insurance until age 26, addressing the need for access to services such as the early identification and treatment for first-time psychosis.
> - The Medicaid expansion option, which raises allowable income limits and eases restrictions for adults without children, has resulted in more people with psychiatric disabilities gaining access to health care under the Medicaid program.
> - Provisions were made for the creation of primary care services through medical homes, providing integrated behavioral and physical health care for individuals with psychiatric diagnoses.

(IHI, 2015). This initiative addresses the fact that the U.S. health-care system is the most expensive in the world yet underperforms relative to other developed nations in terms of health outcomes, access, efficiency, and equity (Davis et al., 2014). Many of the provisions of the ACA align with the Triple Aim framework.

Civil Rights Policy

The 1960s brought about a major paradigm shift in disability policy, essentially moving disability services from a medical model focused on cure or containment to a civil rights model in which support in the community was considered a basic human right (Longmore & Umansky, 2001). This paradigm shift came about because of grassroots activism by people with disabilities, including advocates for the rights of people with psychiatric disabilities (Longmore & Umansky, 2001). Although there are still many people with psychiatric disabilities who, for a variety of reasons, are not receiving the support promised through these acts of Congress, there is hope that through time people can advocate for the supports promised in the laws.

The Rehabilitation Act of 1973 was enacted primarily to provide government funding to states, by way of grants, for the purpose of providing vocational training, and to expand federal funding for researching and developing work training programs, specifically for people with significant disabilities. It is this law that provides funding for the vocational rehabilitation programs and the Ticket to Work Program discussed earlier. The Rehabilitation Act requires affirmative action in hiring people with disabilities by agencies and contractors that receive any form of federal funding, which includes schools, universities, and public transportation. The act also establishes requirements for dissemination of any information by federal agencies or contractors for electronic and information technology (ADA.gov, 2020).

However, because of a small section in the act, Section 504, that was added during the legislative process, it became the first law to formally ban discrimination based on disability. *Section 504 of the Rehabilitation Act* is the section most credited for changing the disability landscape. Section 504 states,

> No otherwise qualified individual with a disability in the United States, as defined in section 705(20) of this title, shall, solely by reason of her or his disability, be excluded from the participation in, be denied the benefits of, or be subjected to discrimination under any program or activity receiving federal financial assistance or under any program or activity conducted by any Executive agency or by the United States Postal Service. (ADA.gov, 2020)

The inclusion of Section 504 marked the first time any legislation recognized that lack of accommodation for full participation in the community was a form of discrimination. The passing of the act set off a legislative shift that began to favor access to civil and human rights for disabled people. Passing the law was, however, only a critical first step; it was only with continued advocacy by disability rights advocates demanding enforcement of the law that positive changes developed for people with disabilities. See Box 26-5 to learn more about the 504 sit-in, a response to the government's refusal to enact rules to enforce Section 504.

The ADA, inspired by the passing of Section 504, is the first civil rights law passed specifically to address the basic human rights of people living with disabilities. The law is meant to protect people from discrimination based on disability in employment, state and federal government services, commercial facilities, telecommunications, and transportation. The ADA has four titles that detail the specific provisions, but Title II is the provision most relevant for people with psychiatric disabilities. Title II "prohibits discrimination against qualified individuals with disabilities in all programs, activities, and services of public entities" (ADA National Network, n.d., p. 1). Public entities include any federal, state, or local organization providing services using public money such as transportation, housing support, employment support, and other long-term care services.

Title II of the ADA is the basis for the current shift to community-based mental health care. The regulations under Title II require any organization providing services to people with disabilities to do so in the most integrated setting possible. Medicare and Medicaid dollars have not traditionally been earmarked for home- and community-based services. Their benefits were, and in the case of Medicare still are, earmarked for hospital care and nursing facilities, an unintended consequence referred to as the *institutional bias*. This stems from policies that favor the provision of care in institutional as opposed to community settings.

Without a payment structure for these services, there was little incentive for states to spend dollars to create community-based services. That started to change after a 1999 Supreme Court ruling referred to as the **Olmstead Decision**. This decision ruled that the plaintiffs, two women with disabilities who were institutionalized in a Georgia nursing facility, had the right to live and receive all services in the community of their choice.

BOX 26-5 ■ Section 504 and the Disability Civil Rights Movement

Shortly after the 1973 Rehabilitation Act was signed into law, the Nixon Administration recognized the far-reaching consequences of Section 504. The language was broad and covered any organization receiving government funds. Schools, libraries, transportation systems, postal services, and civic buildings where the government or publicly supported education programs intersected with civilians would all be required to be made accessible.

When attempts to roll back the legislation didn't work, the administration opted to neglect to enforce the law by simply not writing the regulatory rules for that section. Without regulatory rules, it was impossible to determine basic provisions such as who was disabled or what the term "otherwise qualified" meant.

The Department of Health, Education and Welfare (HEW) was tasked to write the rules in 1973, but 4 years later no regulations were in place, even though the Office of Civil Rights provided HEW with a draft. When the Carter Administration came into power, they set up a task force to "study" the proposed rules. In response to the lack of action, disability advocates formed a cross disability organization called the American Coalition of Citizens with Disabilities (ACCD).

ACCD began to organize individuals with disabilities, including people with psychiatric disabilities, to protest the lack of action. The film *Crip Camp* (available on Amazon Prime) tells the story of the leaders and the grassroots effort that had its roots in a camp for kids with disabilities in New York. ACCD eventually gave HEW an

ultimatum. If regulations were not handed down by April 4, 1977, the disability community would participate in demonstrations in the form of sit-ins at the eight regional HEW headquarters around the United States. On April 5, those sit-ins began.

It is important to remember that organizing people with physical disabilities at a time when there was little accessible transit and little in the way of support services was challenging. Most of the sit-ins ended within a few days, but the sit-in at the HEW headquarters in San Francisco became a focal point and lasted 26 days. Food, medications, and other needs were brought into the headquarters with help from the Glide Community Church and the Black Panther Party. The ACCD leaders orchestrated the news coverage, eventually pushing the HEW director, Califano, to call a hearing with ACCD leaders in Washington, DC.

A private businessman agreed to provide a plane to fly leaders to Washington, DC given airflight was still largely not accessible. After days of hearings, HEW and other leaders agreed to move forward with the regulations. Section 504 wasn't strongly enforced but it was the first time that a law recognized the civil rights of people with disabilities and identified inaccessibility as a form of discrimination. The sit-in and the work that followed would lead to the passing of the Americans with Disabilities Act some 20 years later. See footage from the Section 504 sit-ins and the hearings at: https://dredf.org/web-log/2015/07/26/translating-the-power-of-504.

From Cone, K. (n.d.). A short history of the 504 sit-in. Disability Education and Defense Fund. https://dredf.org/504-sit-in-20th-anniversary/short-history-of-the-504-sit-in

Because of this decision several things happened. The U.S. Justice Department filed several lawsuits in states with high numbers of people in nursing homes. These states entered consent decrees in which they agreed to expand community-based services to avoid going to court. To support the states in this process, the federal government created the **Money Follows the Person (MFP) demonstration project** (Medicaid n.d.-b). State participation in MFP is voluntary so not all states have these grants. An MFP grant provides funding specifically for costs associated with transitioning to the community from an institution. When people move into a nursing home, they lose most of their possessions.

The stipend covers expenses such as the security deposit, a cell phone, cooking tools, towels, furniture, and any other things a person needs to live safely in an apartment. MFP funding will end in 2024, but bills to fund it permanently are regularly submitted in Congress. Aside from supporting states to meet people's civil rights, there is a push to shift long-term care dollars away from expensive institutions to cheaper and more desirable home- and community-based services. As of 2021, MFP dollars have helped to successfully transition over 100,000 people, reducing long-term care costs for this group by nearly two thirds (Göttlich, 2022).

OTPs can search the website of the Department of Human Services in their state to see if there is a consent decree related to institutionalization of people with disabilities. These consent decrees offer an opportunity for OTPs to be paid competitively for work in home- and community-based mental health and intellectual and developmental disabilities (IDD) service organizations. When people move from institutions to their own apartments, they may struggle with decision-making, and they are often unfamiliar with disability rights, new technology, and public transportation (Chow & Priebe, 2013). Occupational therapy's focus on assessing performance skills, and on supporting problem-solving and self-determination through occupation, is unique and valuable to the organizations tasked with this responsibility.

See Chapter 31: The Home Environment: Permanent Supportive Housing and Chapter 35: Practice Across the Continuum of Service Needs. 🤝

Policy Concerning Inpatient Commitment

Occasionally a person with a psychiatric disability has experiences that are so severe they are unable to acknowledge the reality of their situation. If the person meets the state's legal criteria for commitment, the person can be involuntarily admitted to an inpatient facility for a short period (typically 72 hours) for an emergency psychiatric evaluation. A judge's order is required for the person to be committed beyond the initial emergency period.

Civil commitment standards exist in every state, but the legal criterion for commitment varies by state. According to the Treatment Advocacy Center (n.d.), most states adhere to either the "grave disability" standard (inability to care for self, leading to possible physical danger) or the "need for treatment" standard (the person is unable to seek help because they are experiencing symptoms that may lead to deterioration of their physical or psychiatric state).

Committing an individual to treatment against their will creates a dilemma between the ethical principles of beneficence and autonomy. Advocates for people with mental health challenges have diverse opinions on the issue. Mental Health of America (2015) takes a strong stand for the autonomy of the individual, agreeing with the Bazelon Center for Mental Health Law (n.d.) that civil commitment should be "in response to an emergency, and then only when based on a standard of imminent danger of significant physical harm to self or others and when there is no less restrictive alternative" (p. X). On the other hand, NAMI favors broader, more flexible standards for civil commitment, given that "proof of dangerousness often produces(s) unsatisfactory outcomes because individuals are allowed to deteriorate needlessly before involuntary commitment and/or court-ordered treatment can be instituted" (NAMI, 2016, p. 64).

In recent years, there have been attempts to develop alternatives to inpatient hospitalization that allow individuals experiencing a mental health crisis to remain in the community. An example of such an initiative is the peer respite center. According to the National Empowerment Center (NEC), a **peer respite center** is a "voluntary, short term, overnight program that provides community-based, nonclinical support to help people find new understanding and ways to move forward" (NEC, n.d., para. 1).

Peer respite centers provide safe spaces for individuals experiencing a mental health crisis. The care is primarily provided by trained peer support specialists who identify as having lived experience of mental health challenges. The centers also have professional staff such as social workers who are trained to assess and triage people to higher levels of care if it is determined they need more support. Many such spaces are open access and can provide a valuable alternative to the emergency room (Fuller, 2020). Programs such as the peer respite centers and other noninstitutional community resources can play a vital role in reducing the incidence of inpatient psychiatric hospitalization and promoting increased autonomy for individuals living with psychiatric disabilities because they can help individuals develop the skills and support network they need to manage their mental health crisis.

In July 2022, the federal government launched the 988 Suicide & Crisis Lifeline (988 Suicide & Crisis Lifeline, n.d.). This is a national effort to replace the complicated network of suicide hotlines with a single, easily remembered talk and text line for people experiencing a mental health crisis, similar to how 911 works for a physical health crisis. Similar to 911, when someone calls 988 it will route the call to mental health–related resources in the local area. Unlike 911, though, the calls are routed to the organizations that run the original Lifeline. Many local suicide hotlines have someone trained to respond to these calls to assess the needs of the caller and connect them to the mental health supports that they need.

The support structure for community-based mental health has varied widely across states; therefore, the rollout of 988 has been far more successful in states with strong crisis-based mental health services. In states with strong crisis-based mental health services, approximately 3% of calls are routed to the police and those are typically calls in which the mental health assessor cannot determine the person's safety (Saunders, 2023). In other states, where mental health support networks are not as strong, the numbers of calls routed to police remain higher. See Chapter 41: State Hospitals. 🤝

The 988 service remains a relatively new development and there are ongoing efforts to increase the public's awareness and use of the service. After launching in July 2022, the 988 service received a 43% increase in call, text, and chat volume compared with its predecessor service (Lifeline) through December 2022 (Saunders, 2023). This increase in utilization represents many more individuals getting services they need to stay safe in the community during a mental health crisis.

Mental Health and Education Policy

According to the National Education Association, the mental health needs of students have significantly increased since 2016. Between 2016 and 2019, before the pandemic, the number of children diagnosed with anxiety rose by 27% and the number of children diagnosed with depression rose by 24%. Between 2020 and 2021, 15% of teens experienced a major depressive episode, over 300,000 more teens than the year before (Flannery, 2022). University students have also experienced an increase in mental health needs in recent years (Lipson et al., 2022).

Education policies do identify provisions for providing mental health supports in the schools, and OTPs can have a role. Children spend about one sixth of their waking hours in schools, so school-based mental health services allow for early intervention and access to care, especially for low-income students (Ed100, n.d.; Panchal et al., 2022). The U.S. Department of Education (DOE) recognizes that school-based mental health services result in decreased absenteeism and better outcomes for the mental health and school participation for all children (Panchal et al., 2022). Educators have observed that when children are anxious, depressed, or struggling with other mental health challenges, their learning is impacted (Flannery, 2022).

The **Every Student Succeeds Act** (ESSA; DOE, 2015) is the overarching education law in the United States. The intent of the law is to support innovation in education as well as provide funding for high-quality, evidence-based education programs and preschools (DOE, 2015). ESSA sets standards for accountability for schools and districts based on several factors. The primary method is periodic milestone testing; however, ESSA also requires schools to monitor and report on at least one other quality measure such as college readiness, advanced coursework, school safety, or any number of other standards identified in the law. When lawmakers approved ESSA, they specifically worked to put in provisions that increase support for identifying and implementing unique interventions for struggling schools and districts, rather than pulling funding as happened with previous laws (DOE, 2015).

There are several provisions written into ESSA that offer opportunities to create mental health supports in the nation's elementary and secondary schools. ESSA articulates a connection between the mental health of students and overall student achievement, school climate, and graduation rates. The law does not specify a particular approach to mental health; instead, they authorize various funding streams, especially for schools targeted for additional support. Funding can be used for any number of different efforts such as universal screening for mental and behavioral health, implementation of a multitiered system of support for positive behavior interventions, mental health and wellness promotion services, and efforts to engage families around mental health support.

There is also a provision to train staff to identify mental health challenges early, participate in suicide prevention programs, improve culturally sensitive education practices, and improve school climate through curbing violence and bullying (National Association of School Psychologists, n.d.).

One of the key provisions of ESSA is the recognition that states control how they implement the requirements of the law. To ensure compliance, every state is required to file an ESSA plan with the DOE. These plans must be updated periodically and are publicly available. Practitioners working with school-age children and youth can search for their state's ESSA plan to see how the mental health provisions are being implemented in their states.

Because of OTPs' mental health training and recognition as mental health providers nationally and in many states, OTPs are recognized in ESSA as qualified to fill the role of Specialized Instructional Support Personnel (SISP). In this role, OTPs can contribute not only to the services for children and youth with mental health issues, but also to supporting school-wide efforts to improve social and emotional learning and healthy participation in all the social environments in school such as the classroom, cafeteria, and recess (Bazyk et al., 2022).

The **Individuals with Disabilities Act** (IDEA; DOE, n.d.) is the primary federal education legislation that governs education for children with disabilities. The law has four purposes: (1) to provide access to a free and "appropriate" education for children with disabilities addressing their unique needs, (2) to protect the education rights of children and their parents, (3) to aid state and local education authorities so they can provide the needed educational services, and (4) to provide funding and oversight to determine the effectiveness of special education services (DOE, n.d.). A 2008 amendment, passed with the implementation of ESSA, added this clarification to the original law:

> Disability is a natural part of the human experience and in no way diminishes the rights of individuals to participate in or contribute to society. Improving educational results for children with disabilities is an essential element of our national policy of ensuring equality of opportunity, full participation, independent living and economic self-sufficiency for individuals with disabilities.

This language is important because it identifies education as a civil right and situates the necessity of education for full inclusion in society. In addition to requiring a free and appropriate education for children with disabilities, IDEA sets the minimum standards and requirements for educating children with disabilities starting in early intervention and going through high school. It also governs how the law will be enforced. Similar to many policies, IDEA provides a specific definition of disability:

> A child with intellectual disabilities, hearing impairments (including deafness), speech or language impairments, visual impairments (including blindness), serious emotional disturbance, orthopedic impairments, autism, traumatic brain injury, or other health impairments, or specific learning disabilities; and who, by reason thereof, needs special education and related services. (IDEA, 2004)

IDEA consists of four parts covering (1) general provisions; (2) the scope of disability services, including children with emotional disturbance; (3) services for early intervention and preschool; and (4) funding opportunities for training and implementation. IDEA is funded by Congress every year through appropriations that are used to provide money to schools in the form of grants and to researchers and higher education for education research and to develop training programs targeted at specific needs (DOE, n.d.).

Section 504 is another disability policy in the schools that requires accommodation for qualifying children with mental health challenges. Section 504 requires that school districts provide a free appropriate public education (FAPE) to qualified students who have a physical or mental impairment that substantially limits one or more major life activities (DOE, Office for Civil Rights, n.d.). If a child has a 504 plan in school, it is because they did not qualify for services under the narrower requirements of IDEA. Section 504 is not an education law. It is a civil rights law that guarantees a person's rights throughout their lifetime, but there is no funding for children with 504 plans through this law as there was with IDEA.

Compliance with Section 504 is enforced through a complaint process, similar to the ADA. If someone files a complaint stating that their child is not receiving services they are entitled to, and this complaint is found to be legitimate, the school could lose some of their federal funding. Although Section 504 does not provide any financial support to schools for the services, schools may be able to get reimbursed for qualifying services rendered to children covered by Medicaid. This, similar to all other Medicaid funding, is dependent on the state. According to the DOE, to be protected under Section 504, a student must be determined to (a) have a physical or mental impairment that substantially limits one or more major life activities, or (b) have a record of such an impairment, or (c) be regarded as having such an impairment (DOE, Office for Civil Rights, n.d.).

Both Section 504 and IDEA identify mental health diagnoses in their list of qualifying conditions. However, having a psychiatric diagnosis doesn't guarantee that a student will be able to gain access to accommodations and other services. Children only qualify for accommodations and supports when the challenges associated with the condition "adversely affect" their academic performance. Proving that a child is struggling specifically because of a psychiatric disability, as opposed to other factors, can be a challenge. This is especially true given that many psychiatric disabilities could be considered "invisible" disabilities, especially compared with physical disabilities.

IDEA explicitly defines emotional disturbance for the purposes of deciding if a child meets criteria. However, some argue that the parameters are relatively unclear. For example, terms such as "extended period" and "inappropriate feelings" are not explicitly defined and may be interpreted differently by different people. OTPs can recognize the many barriers to participation, not just in the classroom but in the cafeteria, at recess, in physical education, or in classrooms and school spaces that require management of multiple sensory inputs (Bazyk et al., 2022). See Chapter 37: School Mental Health and Chapter 47: Student.

In 2021, the Office of Special Education and Rehabilitation Services, part of the DOE, released a report called "Supporting Child and Student Social, Emotional, Behavioral, and Mental Health Needs" (DOE, 2021). This report contains seven recommendations for addressing the mental health needs of children in schools.

School-based OTPs can bring a unique contribution to the implementation of several of the recommendations. For example, in occupational therapy literature there is growing evidence that supports the relationship between a sense of mental well-being and positive and satisfying experiences in valued activities, at school, and with friends (Tokolahi et al., 2018), addressing the first and third recommendations related to promoting well-being and providing evidence-based interventions to children in schools. Box 26-6 lists the seven DOE recommendations for addressing mental health and lists some specific action steps OTPs can take to support these recommendations.

BOX 26-6 ■ Addressing Department of Education Recommendations for Supporting Child and Student Social, Emotional, Behavioral, and Mental Health Needs

DOE Recommendation	Action Steps for Practitioners
1. Prioritize Wellness	• Acknowledge one's mental health training and address the multidimensional aspects of wellness in their interventions. • Recognize that children with disabilities have a right to balance the different dimensions of wellness and consider occupational therapy interventions that recognize social, occupational, intellectual, and other forms of wellness. • Emphasize that routine self-care activities are a key to wellness, not just for children, but in support of teachers and staff as well.
2. Enhance Mental Health Literacy and Reduce Stigma	• Embrace one's training to use occupation to develop positive mental health. • Talk to children, parents, and employees about how occupational engagement builds resilience, affords dignity of risk, and supports a positive sense of self. • Be trained or become certified trainers for Youth Mental Health First Aid to support broader discussions of mental health challenges and how to respond.

Continued

BOX 26-6 ■ Addressing Department of Education Recommendations for Supporting Child and Student Social, Emotional, Behavioral, and Mental Health Needs—cont'd

DOE Recommendation	Action Steps for Practitioners
3. Implement Evidence-Based Practices	• Become familiar with the Multi-Tiered Systems of Support for mental health needs, and the evidence for occupation-focused interventions that fall under Tier 1 and Tier 2. • Support and lead Tier 1 programs such as the ones highlighted in Every Moment Counts (Bazyk, 2022), or interventions around bullying. • Support and lead Tier 2 programs with programs such as Coping Cat (Kendall & Hedtke, 2006); Check In, Check Out (Hawken et al., 2006); or by using an occupational focus group process to support mental health needs (Egan et al., 2023).
4. Establish an Integrated Framework of Supports	• Advocate by articulating the roots of the profession and acknowledging the occupational therapy training positions OTPs contribute to school-wide mental health programs. • Advocate for, support, and lead efforts to bring together all disciplines to look at mental health from a systems perspective instead of ad-hoc, reactive approaches to addressing mental health. • Use one's background in human occupation and occupational balance and engagement to be integral contributors to school-wide mental health teams.
5. Leverage Policy and Funding	• Advocate for inclusion on mental health school-wide teams and connect to resources that will support a greater understanding of the policies that govern access to funding sources for mental health supports. • Participate in advocacy efforts aimed at recognizing OTPs as mental health providers as a first step to increasing needed mental health services in school settings. • Connect with children's mental health lobbying organizations to help support inclusion of occupational therapy in policy and regulation documents.
6. Enhance Workforce Capacity	• Advocate for occupational therapy, which is ensconced in the school systems and included on individualized education plans (IEPs), to be recognized by the U.S. Department of Education and have OTPs recognized as mental health providers. • Learn to articulate occupational therapy's role in mental health and the evidence to support this to administrators and those who are currently recognized as mental health providers. • Reconsider any practice focused on reductionistic practices, which often results in "othering" children with disabilities; as such, this can be a source of frustration and poor mental health (Bazyk, 2022).
7. Use Data for Decision-Making	• Become adept with data-based decision-making processes focused on outcomes driven by children as well as parents. • Recognize that data collection on mental health outcomes could include data on the development of roles and role tasks, task analyses to identify efficient ways for children to complete their work, monitoring outcomes of self-advocacy efforts, or observations of effective recess play skills. • Infuse occupational perspectives in school-wide screenings by examining volitional components such as belief in capacity, sense of self-control, development of interests and values, and a student's overall sense of efficacy.

Specific Policies That Affect Occupational Therapy Practice

The Primary and Behavioral Healthcare Integration grant program was established in 2009 by the Substance Abuse and Mental Health Services Administration (SAMHSA) to address the myriad health issues of individuals with high support needs (SAMHSA, 2014a). Integrated behavioral and physical care for individuals with psychiatric disabilities is supported by evidence of their medical vulnerability, which is well documented in studies of mortality and morbidity (Delaney et al., 2013). This orientation to holistic care is a good fit for OTPs who understand both the physical and psychological aspects of a person, having long recognized the "mind-body interrelationship" (Mosey, 1996, cited in AOTA, 2010, p. 80). See Chapter 34: Integrated Behavioral Health and Primary Care. 🤝

The Excellence in Mental Health Act was signed in 2013 to expand funding for services to community mental health (National Council for Community Behavioral Health, 2013).

Subsequently, Congress passed the Protecting Access to Medicare Act of 2014 (Medicaid.gov, n.d.-c). Section 223 of this act established a demonstration project to create Certified Community Behavioral Health Clinics (CCBHCs) in eight states to improve health care for people with high support needs through delivery of evidence-based services. In November 2014, SAMHSA held a listening session to help determine the criteria for the CCBHCs. An unprecedented number of OTPs contributed to the listening session, introducing policymakers to the role that occupational therapy plays in integrated care and making a strong case for recognizing the benefit of occupational therapy in improving the lives of people with SMI.

In May 2015, occupational therapy achieved a "great victory" when SAMHSA listed occupational therapy as part of the suggested staffing of the CCBHCs (AOTA, 2015, para. 1). Former AOTA President Virginia Stoffel remarked, "This is a huge opportunity for the profession to return to our mental health roots and provide needed services to those who can most benefit from occupational therapy. Because the new CCBHCs will be required to provide integrated care, this is a chance for us to show how our broad understanding of both physical health and behavioral health helps bridge these different worlds of service provision" (AOTA, 2015, para. 4).

Several attempts have been made to expand the role of occupational therapy in mental health services through federal legislative efforts. Most recently, the bipartisan Occupational Therapy Mental Health Parity Act (S. 4712) sought to increase recognition of occupational therapy as a profession that can address mental and behavioral health disorders. Introduced in 2022, the bill has not yet been voted on as of this writing (Parsons, 2022).

In 2014 Congress increased funding through State Mental Health Block Grants by 5% to specifically address early diagnosis and treatment for people with psychiatric disabilities (SAMHSA, 2014b), which can open the door for increasing occupational therapy services in this area. Evidence-based programs to address first-episode psychosis, such as Oregon's Early Assessment and Support Alliance (EASA), have occupational therapy written into the guidelines. At EASA, OTPs bring their distinct knowledge of the person-occupation-environment (PEO) interaction to their work as group leaders, and identify motor, visual-spatial, social interaction, cognitive, and sensory issues that may be interfering with performance (Waite, 2014).

The Portland Identification and Early Referral Program (PIER), a pilot program codeveloped by an occupational therapist in Portland, Maine, also has integrated occupational therapy into its services. PIER was the basis of the national Early Detection and Intervention for the Prevention of Psychosis Program (EDIPPP), which was funded to establish the PIER program in several sites across the United States. Data from the EDIPPP trial indicates that occupational therapy has had positive outcomes (Waite, 2014).

OTPs are well suited to collaborate with individuals with high support needs who are transitioning from nursing homes to the community because of the enforcement of the Olmstead Decision. The nursing home environment can prevent residents from practicing many ADLs (e.g., medication management, self-care) and IADLs (e.g., money management, cooking, shopping, community mobility). Practitioners work with residents to relearn everyday skills, manage their health conditions, and achieve full participation in community life.

Here's the Point

- Given that participation is the desired outcome of occupational therapy, OTPs must keep current on the local, state, and national policies that influence their practice and the lives of the people they serve, and at times may advocate for policies that broaden opportunities for occupational participation.
- Federal and state policies determine how health-care services are reimbursed, providing or restricting access to the supports, adaptations, and modifications people need to participate in occupation.
- The ADA, the Olmstead Decision, and recent state legislative efforts open the door for OTPs to increase their presence in behavioral health. By collaborating with those with psychiatric disabilities, they help them to lead the life they want (and deserve) to live.

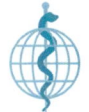 Visit the online resource center at **FADavis.com** to access the videos.

Acknowledgments

The authors would like to acknowledge Dr. Celeste Januszewski, who contributed to this chapter in the last edition of this text.

Apply It Now

1. Applying for Services

Explore the process of applying for a specific program such as SNAP or Medicaid. Gain an appreciation of the application process from start to finish and consider how you as an OTP might assist an individual with mental health challenges in applying for such programs. Then, consider how you might support this individual in developing strategies for obtaining a month's worth of healthy food using the limited monetary support provided by SNAP.

2. Local Resources

Identify your local center for independent living (e.g., the center for independent living that serves Chicago is Access Living [accessliving.org]). Explore the resources they offer and consider how people you work with might benefit from their services.

3. Advocacy

Explore AOTA's advocacy webpage (https://www.aota.org /advocacy). Using AOTA's legislative action center, write a letter to your elected representatives about an issue that matters to you and your profession.

4. Education

The ESSA requires every state to file a plan explaining how they intend to comply with the law. Research your state's ESSA compliance plan (e.g., Kentucky's can be found at https://education.ky.gov/comm/Documents/Kentucky%20 Consolidated%20State%20Plan.pdf). Based on what is in your state's act, make a list of the opportunities that exist for OTPs to support the mental health of students.

5. Video Exercise: "Occupational Therapy Approaches in a Shelter for Unaccompanied Refugee Youth"

Pair up with another student in your class or form a small group of students. Access and watch the "Occupational Therapy Approaches in a Shelter for Unaccompanied Refugee Youth" video at the online resource center at FADavis. com. Then, discuss and together answer the following questions.

Reflective Questions
- Many of the youth at this shelter were engaged strictly in survival occupations; some were bullied by staff, and they all lacked control and autonomy over their day-to-day life. How do you think the OTPs' introduction of opportunities for engagement in leisure and creative occupations affected the minors' mental health during their short-term stay at the shelter? How did the OTPs use occupational engagement to form meaningful connections with the youth?
- Claudette spoke about creating trauma-informed training for the staff at the shelter to help increase their understanding of trauma, what trauma responses can look like, and how to avoid further traumatizing the youth. Why was it important for Claudette and the students she recruited to work with not only the youth but also the staff who interacted directly with the youth daily? How did this training likely support directly the mental health and well-being of the staff, as well as the youth?
- Claudette explained that, "Our big strategy was to be part of the environment and learn how things were operating there and embed ourselves in the operations with our knowledge of occupation and just support both the faculty, the staff, and the youth in being able to engage." How did this approach lead to planning and decision-making that reflected cultural humility and trauma-sensitive interventions?
- In what ways did Claudette and her students demonstrate cultural humility in their daily interactions as well as in the interventions they created for the youth at the shelter?

6. Video Exercise: "Civic Engagement Group in an Inpatient Psychiatric Unit"

Pair up with another student in your class or form a small group of students. Access and watch the "Civic Engagement Group in an Inpatient Psychiatric Unit" video at the online resource center at FADavis.com. Then, discuss and together answer the following questions.

Reflective Questions
- What do you believe made this civic engagement group successful? How did Jennifer ensure the group focused on a topic that was meaningful and relevant to the individuals participating in the group? Why is collaboration and choice so important in all therapeutic interactions?
- In what ways did this OTP go "the extra mile" and turn the group into more than just civic engagement? How did she provide for individuals to feel a sense of empowerment?
- Jennifer describes starting a group that was "looking at what's happening outside of the clinical experience and outside of the residents themselves." Why do you think that was important, and how did she accomplish it?

Resources

- AOTA Advocacy: https://www.aota.org/advocacy
  Current news and resource links on AOTA's congressional, regulatory, and state policy work; includes how you can become involved in advocacy work and how you can contact your elected representatives.
- AOTA Advocacy Events: https://www.aota.org/advocacy/hill-day
  Contains information on opportunities for advocacy, including Hill Day, an annual event where occupational therapy students and OTPs are encouraged to go to Washington DC to advocate for the profession.
- AOTA Legislative Action Center: https://www.aota.org/takeaction
  Information on federal issues that AOTA is actively engaged in; includes members of Congress and where they stand on these issues, plus a link to send a message directly from your smartphone to your senator and representative.
- AOTA Political Action Committee (AOTPAC): https://www.aota.org/advocacy/political-action-committee
  AOTPAC is a committee of AOTA members that works to influence the outcome of federal elections to advance the legislative aims of AOTA.
- Bazelon Center for Mental Health Law: http://www.bazelon.org
  Legal advocacy organization that advocates for full inclusion of people with disabilities.
- Centers for Independent Living: http://www.ilru.org/projects/cil-net/cil-center-and-association-directory
  Resource to connect with your local center for independent living, which are consumer-controlled, cross-disability agencies that often sponsor advocacy events.
- Kaiser Family Foundation: KFF.org
  A nonprofit organization focused on health care in the United States and the role of the United States in global health policy. Includes thoughtful balanced analysis of health-care policy.
- Mental Health of America: https://mhanational.org
  Mental health advocacy organization.
- National Alliance on Mental Illness (NAMI): http://www.nami.org
  Mental health advocacy organization.
- National Coalition for Mental Health Recovery (NCMHR): http://www.ncmhr.org
  Advocacy organization that strives to keep the consumer voice in health-care policy issues.
- Olmstead Enforcement: http://www.ada.gov/olmstead
  Information on the Olmstead Decision and the Department of Justice's efforts to enforce it.
- "Veteran's Caregiver on Advocacy and VA Support" video. Nancy is the spouse and caregiver of a veteran with early onset Alzheimer disease. In this video, she shares about his diagnosis and the arduous process of applying for VA benefits. In her case, the application was successful, and she describes how critical those resources have been for her and her husband. Nancy urges OTPs to work with social workers to ensure families of veterans receive the benefits they have earned. Access the video at the online resource center at FADavis.com.

Publications

- *American Journal of Occupational Therapy*: Health Policy Perspectives is an opinion column written by OTPs that addresses the link between current policy issues and the impact on practice.
- *OT Practice* Magazine: The Capital Briefing column provides updates on federal, state, and regulatory issues impacting the profession.

References

988 Suicide & Crisis Lifeline. (n.d.). *988 Suicide and Crisis Lifeline homepage.* https://988lifeline.org

ADA.gov. (2020). *A guide to disability rights laws.* https://www.ada.gov/resources/disability-rights-guide

ADA National Network. (n.d.). *What is the Americans with Disabilities Act (ADA)?* https://adata.org/learn-about-ada

American Occupational Therapy Association. (2010). Occupational therapy services in the promotion of psychological and social aspects of mental health. *American Journal of Occupational Therapy, 64*(6 Suppl.), S78–S91. https://doi.org/10.5014/ajot.2010.64S78

American Occupational Therapy Association. (2015, May 21). *New community behavioral health centers: Occupational therapy listed in final criteria.* http://www.aota.org/Advocacy-Policy/Congressional-Affairs/Legislative-Issues-Update/2015/community-behavioral-health-occupational-therapy-criteria.aspx#sthash.iN8DlyJF.dpuf

Americans with Disabilities Act of 1990. Pub. L. No. 101–336, 104 Stat 327 (1990). https://www.govinfo.gov/content/pkg/STATUTE-104/pdf/STATUTE-104-Pg327.pdf

Americans with Disabilities Act Title III Regulations. (2010). *Part 36: Nondiscrimination on the basis of disability by public accommodations and in commercial facilities.* https://www.ada.gov/law-and-regs/regulations/title-iii-regulations

Anacker, K. B. (2019). Introduction: Housing affordability and affordable housing. *International Journal of Housing Policy, 19*(1), 1–16. https://doi.org/10.1080/19491247.2018.1560544

Bazelon Center for Mental Health Law. (n.d.). *Position statement on involuntary commitment.* http://www.bazelon.org/wp-content/uploads/2017/04/Position-Statement-on-Involuntary-Commitment.pdf

Bazyk, S. (2022). *Occupational therapy: Promoting participation in occupation.* Every Moment Counts. https://everymomentcounts.org/about/about-occupational-therapy

Bazyk, S., Myers, S., Romaniw, A., Virone, M., Greene, S., Fette, C., Thomas, L., Test, L., Thorman, J., & Rupp, T. (2022). *Occupational therapy's role as SISPs under ESSA.* https://s3.us-east-2.amazonaws.com/s3.everymomentcounts.com/wp-content/uploads/2022/05/03202516/FINAL_OT-ESSA-Admin_4-25-22.pdf

Book, R. (2012, October 18). Benefits and challenges of Medicaid managed care. *Forbes.* https://www.forbes.com/sites/aroy/2012/10/18/benefits-and-challenges-of-medicaid-managed-care/#5bfaea8e720f

Cairney, P., & Oliver, K. (2017). Evidence-based policymaking is not like evidence-based medicine, so how far should you go to bridge the divide between evidence and policy? *Health Research Policy and Systems, 15*(1), 1–11. https://doi.org/10.1186/s12961-017-0192-x

Chow, W. S., & Priebe, S. (2013). Understanding psychiatric institutionalization: A conceptual review. *BMC Psychiatry, 13,* Article 169. https://doi.org/10.1186/1471-244X-13-169

Coe, A. B., Moczygemba, L. R., Gatewood, S. B. S., Osborn, R. D., Matzke, G. R., & Goode, J.-V. R. (2015). Medication adherence challenges among patients experiencing homelessness in a behavioral health clinic. *Research in Social and Administrative Pharmacy, 11*(3), e110–e120. https://doi.org/10.1016/j.sapharm.2012.11.004

Cone, K. (n.d.). *A short history of the 504 sit-in.* Disability Education and Defense Fund. https://dredf.org/504-sit-in-20th-anniversary/short-history-of-the-504-sit-in

Davis, K., Stremikis, K., Squires, D., & Schoen, C. (2014). *Mirror, mirror on the wall. How the performance of the US health care system compares internationally.* The Commonwealth Fund. http://www.resbr.net.br/wp-content/uploads/historico/Espelhoespelhomeu.pdf

Delaney, K., Robinson, K., & Chafetz, L. (2013). Development of integrated mental health care: Critical workforce competencies.

Nursing Outlook, 61(6), 384–391. https://doi.org/10.1016/j.outlook.2013.03.005

Dye, T. R. (2013). *Understanding public policy.* Pearson.

Ed100. (n.d.). *School hours: Is there enough time to learn?* https://ed100.org/lessons/schoolhours#:~:text=Each%20year%20consists%20of%20about,1%2C000%20of%20them%20in%20school

Egan, B. E., Sears, C., & Keener, A. (2023). *Occupational therapy groups for addressing mental health challenges in school-aged populations: A tier II resource.* Slack, Inc.

Elbogen, E. B., Lanier, M., Wagner, H. R., & Tsai, J. (2021). Financial strain, mental illness, and homelessness: Results from a national longitudinal study. *Medical Care, 59*(Suppl. 2), S132–S138. https://doi.org/10.1097/MLR.0000000000001453

Fang, D., Thomsen, M. R., & Nayga, R. M. (2021). The association between food insecurity and mental health during the COVID-19 pandemic. *BMC Public Health, 21*(1), 607. https://doi.org/10.1186/s12889-021-10631-0

Flannery, M. E. (2022). *Mental health in schools: The kids are not all right.* National Education Association. https://www.nea.org/advocating-for-change/new-from-nea/mental-health-schools-kids-are-not-all-right

Fuller, K. (2020). *Responding to crisis: The crisis living room.* https://www.nami.org/Blogs/NAMI-Blog/September-2020/Responding-to-Crisis-The-Crisis-Living-Room

Göttlich, V. (2022). *Policy note: Important changes to Money Follows the Person (MFP).* Administration for Community Living. https://acl.gov/news-and-events/acl-blog/policy-note-important-changes-money-follows-person-mfp

Hawken, L. S., Pettersson, H., Mootz, J., & Anderson, C. (2006). *The behavior education program: A check-in, check-out intervention for students at risk.* Guilford Press.

Hinton, E., & Raphael, J. (2023). *10 things to know about Medicaid managed care.* Kaiser Family Foundation. https://www.kff.org/medicaid/issue-brief/10-things-to-know-about-medicaid-managed-care

Houtenville, A., & Boege, S. (2019). *2018 annual report on people with disabilities in America.* https://eric.ed.gov/?id=ED595177

Howlett, M., & Cashore, B. (2014). Conceptualizing public policy. In I. Engeli & C. R. Allison (Eds.), *Comparative policy studies: Conceptual and methodological challenges* (pp. 17–33). Palgrave Macmillan UK. https://doi.org/10.1057/9781137314154_2

Hui, A., Rains, L. S., Todd, A., Boaz, A., & Johnson, S. (2020). The accuracy and accessibility of cited evidence: A study examining mental health policy documents. *Social Psychiatry and Psychiatric Epidemiology, 55*(1), 111–121. https://doi.org/10.1007/s00127-019-01786-8

Hyde, J. K., Mackie, T. I., Palinkas, L. A., Niemi, E., & Leslie, L. K. (2016). Evidence use in mental health policy making for children in foster care. *Administration and Policy in Mental Health and Mental Health Services Research, 43,* 52–66. https://doi.org/10.1007/s10488-015-0633-1

Indiana Health Coverage Program. (2021). *IHCP clarifies that scope of occupational therapy practice may include behavioral health services.* https://provider.indianamedicaid.com/ihcp/Banners/BR202137.pdf

Individuals with Disabilities Education Act, 20 U.S.C. § 1401 (2004). https://sites.ed.gov/idea/statute-chapter-33/subchapter-i/1401

Institute for Healthcare Improvement. (2015). *The IHI Triple Aim initiative.* http://www.ihi.org/Engage/Initiatives/TripleAim/pages/default.aspx

Judicial Learning Center. (n.d.). *What is a law?* http://judiciallearningcenter.org/law-and-the-rule-of-law

Kaiser Family Foundation. (2013). *Summary of the Affordable Care Act.* https://www.kff.org/health-reform/fact-sheet/summary-of-the-affordable-care-act

Kaiser Family Foundation. (2020). *Total number of Medicare beneficiaries.* https://www.kff.org/medicare/state-indicator/total-medicare-beneficiaries/?currentTimeframe=0&sortModel=%7B%22colId%22:%22Location%22,%22sort%22:%22asc%22%7D

Kendall, P. C., & Hedtke, K. A. (2006). *Coping cat workbook* (2nd ed.). Workbook Publishing.

Lipson, S. K., Zhou, S., Abelson, S., Heinze, J., Jirsa, M., Morigney, J., Patterson, A., Singh, M., & Eisenberg, D. (2022). Trends in college student mental health and help-seeking by race/ethnicity: Findings from the National Healthy Minds Study, 2013–2021. *Journal of Affective Disorders, 306,* 138–147. https://doi.org/10.1016/j.jad.2022.03.038

Litz, B. T., & Schlenger, W. E. (2009). PTSD in service members and new veterans of the Iraq and Afghanistan Wars: A bibliography and critique. *PTSD Research Quarterly, 20,* 1–8. https://www.ptsd.va.gov/publications/rq_docs/V20N1.pdf

Longmore, P., & Umansky, L. (2001). *The new disability history.* New York University Press.

Medicaid and CHIP Payment and Access Commission. (2019). *Physician acceptance of new Medicaid patients.* http://www.macpac.gov/wp-content/uploads/2019/01/Physician-Acceptance-of-New-Medicaid-Patients.pdf

Medicaid.gov. (n.d.-a). *Financial management.* https://www.medicaid.gov/medicaid/financial-management/index.html

Medicaid.gov. (n.d.-b). *Money follows the person.* https://www.medicaid.gov/medicaid/ltss/money-follows-the-person/index.html

Medicaid.gov (n.d.-c). *Section 223 demonstration program to improve community mental health services.* https://www.medicaid.gov/medicaid/finance/223-demonstration/index.html

Mental Health of America. (2015, March 7). *Position statement 22: Involuntary mental health treatment.* http://www.mentalhealthamerica.net/positions/involuntary-treatment#_edn1

Merriam-Webster. (2015). Politics. In *Merriam-Webster Online Dictionary.* http://www.merriam-webster.com/dictionary/politics

National Alliance on Mental Illness. (n.d.). *Types of health insurance.* https://www.nami.org/Learn-More/Health-Insurance/Types-of-Insurance

National Alliance on Mental Illness. (2016). *Public policy platform* (12th ed.). https://www.nami.org/wp-content/uploads/2023/10/Public-Policy-Platform-up-to-12-09-16.pdf

National Association of School Psychologists. (n.d.). *ESSA mental and behavioral health services for decision-makers.* https://www.nasponline.org/research-and-policy/policy-priorities/relevant-law/the-every-student-succeeds-act/essa-implementation-resources/essa-mental-and-behavioral-health-services-for-decision-makers

National Council for Community Behavioral Health. (2013, March). *Excellence in Mental Health Act.* https://www.thenationalcouncil.org/resources/excellence-in-mental-health-and-addiction-treatment-act/

National Empowerment Center. (n.d.). *Directory of peer respites.* https://power2u.org/directory-of-peer-respites

National Low Income Housing Coalition. (2022). *The gap—A shortage of affordable homes.* https://nlihc.org/sites/default/files/gap/Gap-Report_2022.pdf

Oliver, K., & Pearce, W. (2017). Three lessons from evidence-based medicine and policy: Increase transparency, balance inputs and understand power. *Palgrave Communications, 3,* 43. https://doi.org/10.1057/s41599-017-0045-9

Olmstead v. L. C. 527 U.S. 581 (1999).

Padgett, D., Henwood, B. F., & Tsemberis, S. J. (2016). *Housing first: Ending homelessness, transforming systems, and changing lives.* Oxford University Press.

Panchal, N., Cox, C., & Rudowitz, R. (2022). *The landscape of school-based mental health services.* Kaiser Family Foundation. https://www.kff.org/other/issue-brief/the-landscape-of-school-based-mental-health-services

Parsons, H. (2022). *Occupational Therapy Mental Health Parity Act introduced in Senate.* American Occupational Therapy Association. https://www.aota.org/advocacy/advocacy-news/2022/ot-mental-health-parity-act

Razzano, L. A., Cook, J. A., Yost, C., Jonikas, J. A., Swarbrick, M. A., Carter, T. M., & Santos, A. (2015). Factors associated with co-occurring medical conditions among adults with serious mental disorders. *Schizophrenia Research, 161*(2–3), 458–464. https://doi.org/10.1016/j.schres.2014.11.021

Rein, L. (2022, December 27). Social Security denies disability benefits based on list with jobs from 1977. *The Washington Post.* https://www.washingtonpost.com/politics/2022/12/27/social-security-job-titles-disabled-applicants-obsolete

Saunders, H. (2023). *Taking a look at 988 Suicide & Crisis Lifeline implementation one year after launch.* Kaiser Family Foundation. https://www.kff.org/other/issue-brief/taking-a-look-at-988-suicide-crisis-lifeline-implementation/#:~:text=On%20July%2016%2C%202022%2C%20the,and%20state%20funded%20crisis%20centers

Social Security Administration. (n.d.-a). *Disability benefits—How you qualify.* https://www.ssa.gov/benefits/disability/qualify.html#anchor2

Social Security Administration. (n.d.-b). *Disability evaluations under Social Security—Mental disorders.* https://www.ssa.gov/disability/professionals/bluebook/AdultListings.htm

Social Security Administration. (n.d.-c). *General information.* https://www.ssa.gov/disabilityresearch/wi/medicare.htm

Social Security Administration. (n.d.-d). *Historical background and development of Social Security.* https://www.ssa.gov/history

Social Security Administration. (n.d.-e). *1956 Social Security amendments.* https://www.ssa.gov/history/tally56.html

Social Security Administration. (1995). *Drug addiction and alcoholism.* https://www.ssa.gov/OP_Home/cfr20/416/416-0935.htm

Social Security Administration. (2023). *Substantial gainful activity.* https://www.ssa.gov/OACT/COLA/sga.html

Substance Abuse and Mental Health Services Administration. (2014a). *Primary and behavioral healthcare integration.* http://www.samhsa.gov/grants/grant-announcements/sm-15-005

Substance Abuse and Mental Health Services Administration. (2014b). *Serious mental illness: A new block grant priority.* http://www.samhsa.gov/samhsaNewsLetter/Volume_22_Number_4/serious_mental_illness_block_grant_priority

Substance Abuse and Mental Health Services Administration. (2015). *Planning grants for Certified Community Behavioral Health Clinics.* https://www.samhsa.gov/grants/grant-announcements/sm-16-001

Tokolahi, E., Vandal, A. C., Kersten, P., Pearson, J., & Hocking, C. (2018). Cluster-randomized controlled trial of an occupational therapy intervention for children aged 11–13 years, designed to increase participation to prevent symptoms of mental illness. *Child and Adolescent Mental Health, 23*(4), 313–327. https://doi.org/10.1111/camh.12270

Treatment Advocacy Center. (n.d.). *Map of state SMI resources.* https://www.treatmentadvocacycenter.org/look-up-your-state/

U.S. Department of Agriculture. (n.d.-a). *Child nutrition programs.* https://www.ers.usda.gov/topics/food-nutrition-assistance/child-nutrition-programs

U.S. Department of Agriculture. (n.d.-b). *Supplemental Nutrition Assistance Program (SNAP).* http://www.fns.usda.gov/snap

U.S. Department of Education. (n.d.). *About IDEA.* https://sites.ed.gov/idea/about-idea/#IDEA-History

U.S. Department of Education. (2015). Every Student Succeeds Act of 2015, Pub. L. No. 114-95, § 1177 Stat. 1806. U.S. Government Publishing Office. https://www.congress.gov/114/plaws/publ95/PLAW-114publ95.pdf

U.S. Department of Education. (2021). *Supporting child and student social, emotional, behavioral, and mental health needs.* http://:www2.ed.gov/documents/students/supporting-child-student-social-emotional-behavioral-mental-health.pdf

U.S. Department of Education, Office for Civil Rights (n.d.). *Protecting students with disabilities: Frequently asked questions about*

Section 504 and the education of children with disabilities. https://www2.ed.gov/about/offices/list/ocr/504faq.html

U.S. Department of Health and Human Services. (2010). *About the Affordable Care Act.* https://www.hhs.gov/healthcare/about-the-aca/index.html

U.S. Department of Housing and Urban Development. (2022). *The 2022 Annual Homelessness Assessment Report (AHAR) to Congress. Part 1: Point-in-time estimates of homelessness.* Author. https://www.huduser.gov/portal/sites/default/files/pdf/2022-ahar-part-1.pdf

U.S. Department of Justice: Civil Rights Division. (2009). *A guide to disability rights laws.* http://www.ada.gov/cguide.htm#anchor65610

U.S. Department of Labor. (2010). *Fact sheet: The Mental Health Parity and Addiction Equity Act of 2008 (MHPAEA).* https://www.dol.gov/sites/dolgov/files/ebsa/about-ebsa/our-activities/resource-center/fact-sheets/mhpaea.pdf

Vick, B., Jones, K., & Mitra, S. (2012). Poverty and severe psychiatric disorder in the U.S.: Evidence from the medical expenditure panel. *Journal of Mental Health Policy and Economics, 15,* 83–96.

Waite, A. (2014). On the brink: Occupational therapy program helps address early psychosis. *OT Practice, 19*(11), 9–12. http://www.aota.org/Publications-News/otp/Archive/2014/6-30-14/on-the-brink.aspx#sthash.S0v2L7ls.dpuf

Ward, V., Smith, S., House, A., & Hammer, S. (2012). Exploring knowledge exchange: A useful framework for practice and policy. *Social Science and Medicine, 74*(3), 297–304. https://doi.org/10.1016/j.socscimed.2011.09.021

Waters, E., Armstrong, R., Swinburn, B., Moore, L., Dobbins, M., Anderson, J., Petticrew, M., Clark, R., Conning, R., Moodie, M., & Carter, R. (2011). An exploratory cluster randomised controlled trial of knowledge translation strategies to support evidence-informed decision-making in local governments (The KT4LG study). *BMC Public Health, 11*(34), 1–8. https://doi.org/10.1186/1471-2458-11-34

Watson, K. B., Carlson, S. A., Loustalot, F., Town, M., Eke, P. I., Thomas, C. W., & Greenlund, K. J. (2022). Chronic conditions among adults aged 18–34 years—United States, 2019. *MMWR Morbidity and Mortality Weekly Report, 71*(30), 964–970. https://doi.org/10.15585/mmwr.mm7130a3

Williamson, A., Makkar, S. R., McGrath, C., & Redman, S. (2015). How can the use of evidence in mental health policy be increased? A systematic review. *Psychiatric Services, 66*(8), 783–797. https://doi.org/10.1176/appi.ps.201400329

Woodhall-Melnik, J. R., & Dunn, J. R. (2016). A systematic review of outcomes associated with participation in Housing First programs. *Housing Studies, 31*(3), 287–304. https://doi.org/10.1080/02673037.2015.1080816

Mental Health Stigma and Sanism

Aster Harrison and Jaime Phillip Muñoz

Stigma is an all-too-common feature of the social environment. Individuals diagnosed with mental illnesses, regardless of country or culture, experience feeling devalued and treated as less acceptable than others in their communities (Parcesepe & Cabassa, 2013; Thornicroft, 2006). They are also confronted with **sanism**, which is defined by Vermont Psychiatric Survivors as "a form of systemic and systematic discrimination and oppression of people who have been diagnosed with psychiatric disorders, or who have or are perceived to have mental differences or emotional distress" (2018, para 1). As they attempt to manage their illness and resume daily life, they often are confronted with challenging decisions such as whether or how much to disclose about their illness to family, friends, employers, teachers, and landlords. Stigma can worsen mental health symptoms, including suicidality (Oexle et al., 2017; Oexle et al., 2018). Discrimination based on mental illness can also worsen self-stigma, mental health symptoms, well-being, and life satisfaction (Chan & Tsui, 2023).

This chapter explores the impact of stigma and sanism in the social environment and explores frameworks for understanding stigma and sanism and the processes by which they impact individuals with mental illnesses and their families. It describes ways of measuring stigma and conducting anti-stigma interventions. Finally, it defines the role of occupational therapy in addressing stigma and sanism from an occupational justice perspective.

Stigma in the Social Environment

One of the earliest definitions of stigma was offered by Goffman, who described it as an "attribute which is deeply discrediting" and as "an undesired differentness" (1963, p. 3). Social psychologists have defined "stigma" as comprising cognitive, emotional, and behavioral aspects known as stereotypes, prejudice, and discrimination (Werner et al., 2012). **Stigma** can be defined as negative attitudes and a behavioral chain that begins by applying a stigmatizing mark to a person, progresses through the attitude structures, and results in discrimination. Ascribing a mark of shame or dishonor begins by labeling a person with a mental illness with some negative stereotype such as the belief that such individuals are lazy, unclean, or dangerous. These prejudicial attitudes can then lead to stigmatizing actions and discrimination that can be more covert (e.g., avoiding eye contact or interaction) or more overt (e.g., excluding behaviors, bias, dehumanization, aggression; Bos et al., 2013).

It is widely recognized that stigma occurs at multiple levels, which can be categorized most simply as public stigma (i.e., interpersonal, or societal-level conditions) and self-stigma (i.e., intrapersonal appraisals; Hatzenbuehler et al., 2014). **Public stigma** refers to endorsement of negative stereotypes of individuals with the specific condition by others, such as family members and the general population. Public stigma can include prejudice (i.e., a hostile attitude toward a person simply because they belong to a group judged to have objectionable qualities) and can lead to discriminatory behaviors (St. Louis & Roberts, 2013). **Self-stigma** occurs when stigmatized individuals agree with and internalize negative stereotypes; the person believes that they are deviant or shamefully different (Kleinman, 1988; Tsang et al., 2016). Both public and self-stigma are detrimental to recovery and full community participation for people with mental illness.

Definitions of stigma not only emphasize a difference that devalues the person but also specify that stigma occurs within social interactions, or within the social environment (Bos et al., 2013). This is an important point because it affirms that stigma is not an attribute of the person but an attribute of the social context. The World Health Organization's (WHO) *International Classification of Functioning, Disability, and Health (ICF)* reinforces this view by recognizing a variety of problems specifically related to the social environment (e.g., social exclusion and rejection, discrimination, and persecution) that can negatively impact health and a person's full participation in community life (WHO, 2001).

Stigma in the social environment may increase the risk for negative mental and physical health outcomes for individuals in multiple groups, including racial and ethnic minorities; lesbian, gay, bisexual, transgender, and queer (LGBTQ) people; fat people; and individuals with physical or mental illnesses (Hatzenbuehler et al., 2014; St. Louis & Roberts, 2013). Stigmatized individuals may experience poor self-esteem, negative emotions, and behavioral withdrawal, and they may often conceal their stigmatized status from others. Furthermore, the individuals may use secrecy and withdrawal to cope with stigma, thus restricting access and willingness to seek health care (Morrison et al., 2013; Silverman, 2013).

The negative consequences of social stigma may include marginalization, segregation, and restricted personal freedoms (Miller Polgar & Landry, 2004). An example is a person whose social invitations or opportunities at work are reduced following hospitalization for major depressive disorder. The potential negative social environment for recovery that is created by negative public perceptions and stigmatization of people with mental illness is important for occupational therapy

PhotoVoice

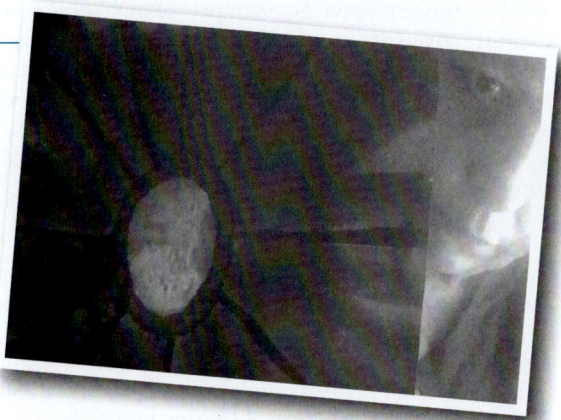

L

Depression is similar to a dark cloud that falls on you. Trauma puts you in situations that our mind cannot comprehend and can cause us to feel things that tear us apart. But everyone experiences the same human emotions, those with a "diagnosis" just endure them deeper and longer. "Diagnosed people" have the same traits as the rest of society . . . we are just "more." There is a fine line between CREATIVITY and INSANITY, or "insight." I did my college thesis on that. Many, if not all, of the great artists, musicians, scientists, inventors, and visionaries have had "more." As humans on this Earth, we are all the same, some of us are just "more" of certain parts than others . . . both painful and creative. Sometimes, to see less is to see more. But that depends on how YOU want to look at it.

Self-stigma is defined and discussed in this chapter. How does this concept apply here? How does this PhotoVoice relate to the concept of Mad Pride? How does Mad Pride relate to stigma? What strategies might OTPs use to "see less" so we can "see more"?

BOX 27-1 ■ Seeking a Life With Dignity

Zhìháo was diagnosed with schizophrenia when he was 24. He grew up in a typical family household in Taiwan and was an excellent student, graduating near the top of his class. While in college, he began to have difficulties relating to others. He spent a lot of time alone, both inside and outside of class, and didn't participate in extracurricular activities or clubs. He often chose to stay in his dorm room or to study alone at the library when his peers engaged in social activities. This was not hard to do because classmates did not often initiate meaningful conversations with Zhìháo.

In contrast to his high school performances, Zhìháo only earned average marks in his college courses and struggled to keep up in many classes. When he came home for breaks his family was confused and frustrated by his drop in performance and limited their interactions outside the home to save face (i.e., not be embarrassed) with extended family and friends who were similarly confused by the changes in Zhìháo.

Zhìháo never really felt that he fit in with his college peers socially and was often suspicious of the motives of others. Some peers bullied him, and others criticized his interaction style. He rarely felt genuine kindness from most college peers. He did not date, even though he desperately wanted a relationship. Despite these challenges, he graduated with an engineering degree.

After graduation, he had difficulty finding a suitable job with adequate salary. Eventually, he found work at a milling company, but was fired soon after he revealed his illness to his colleagues. Even though he has found other jobs, he has difficulty maintaining

continuous employment. When he does find a job, Zhìháo often feels that he receives lower wages than others. He has a strong desire to earn his own living and to be a productive member of society.

Outside of work, he has tried participating in social and service groups, but he has not found a place where he feels accepted as he is. He is often lonely and finds it hard to make friends. He is thankful that the welfare system in Taiwan supports his living but also feels being labeled a schizophrenic makes it hard for others to accept him. Sometimes he tells others that he is depressed rather than revealing that he has schizophrenia. When he does this, he feels others seem less fearful or uncomfortable around him and some even try to empathize. Overall, Zhìháo accepts himself as he is and often feels exhausted by the effort he spends just trying to fit in and from dealing with stigma. He desperately wants to live a life with dignity and productivity.

Reflection Questions

- Create a list of experiences described in the story that reflect clear evidence of Zhìháo's stigmatization.
- What do you think the consequences of stigma in the social environment were for Zhìháo? Explain your responses to a peer.
- Apply a person-environment-occupation (PEO) framework to understand Zhìháo's experiences.
- What clues from the story help you determine occupations that Zhìháo finds meaningful and important?

---

practitioners (OTPs) to consider. Practitioners will encounter these challenges directly when working with people with serious mental illness in the community, where obtaining affordable, safe housing and having adequate financial resources for the necessities of daily life are common challenges. In Box 27-1, Zhìháo's story provides examples of some of his lived experiences with various types and levels of stigma.

Theories of Stigma and Sanism

Goffman (1963) was one of the first to extensively discuss the negative effects of stigma on individuals with serious mental illnesses. Initially, labeling theory and normalization were

predominant social science theories used to study stigma. These theories continue to be relevant to the understanding of stigma, and recent modifications and critiques of these frameworks are presented in the text that follows. Many disciplines, including medicine, criminology, and psychology, continue to examine stigma and its consequences. This research has led to other theories that OTPs may use to understand and address stigma.

Labeling Theory

Labeling theory grew out of the sociological study of deviance (Becker, 1963). According to labeling theorists, certain groups have sanctioned power to define or "label" what is and is not socially deviant. Examples of such groups in power include government officials and medical professionals (Jones, 1998). For example, police officers label certain behaviors deviant and may detain or punish someone behaving outside the norm.

Similarly, mental health professionals determine if a person's self-report and observed behavior meet criteria for a *Diagnostic and Statistical Manual of Mental Disorders (DSM)* diagnosis and proceed according to their socially sanctioned role to "label" someone with a mental illness and recommend intervention. The writers of the *DSM,* too, play a major role in labeling which behaviors are considered normal and which are considered deviant (Crowe, 2020). Therefore, the basis of labeling theory is that a judgment occurs, particularly by individuals with power and authority, to decide that the behavior deviates from the norm (Becker, 1963).

Normalization Theory

Normalization theory is based on the work of labeling theorists, yet it provides an alternative view that people who are typically disenfranchised in society are excluded; in other words, it has become normal in society to stigmatize and exclude (Jones, 1998; Wolfensberger, 1972, 1984). Normalization theorists posit that a label forces an individual into a deviant role, and an individual's subsequent behavior and response to others are determined by expectations surrounding the label. For example, youth labeled as juvenile delinquents may demonstrate behaviors associated with this label when they are faced with lowered expectations or lowered opportunities from the adults around them after a criminal conviction. Normalization theory reasons that, because labeling and stigmatization can have a negative impact, intervention should focus on reducing elements that emphasize difference and create opportunities for social participation in naturally occurring groups and settings within the broader community.

Application of normalization theory is apparent in the design of inclusive environments in which program and environmental designs that emphasize difference (e.g., "special" buses, camps, and congregate housing) are replaced with supporting interventions that emphasize opportunities for social role development. That is, the focus is not solely on skill development, but creating opportunities for the person with a disability to engage in roles such as friend, neighbor, student, and coworker more naturally. A family-centered intervention aligned with the "normalization" approach could be encouraging the parents of a child with attention difficulties and social challenges to join noncompetitive, age-appropriate social activities, such as Girl Scouts, rather than enrolling the child in a therapeutic social skills group composed only of children with similar limitations. In the Girl Scout setting, the child becomes part of a normally occurring community group that offers opportunities to develop skills with peers.

Other Stigma Theories

In addition to labeling and normalization theories, there are other theories that may help practitioners better understand the phenomenon of stigma (Martin et al., 2008). These include Minority Group Perspective (Susman, 1994), Rite of Passage Theory (Turner, 1969), and the Modified Labeling

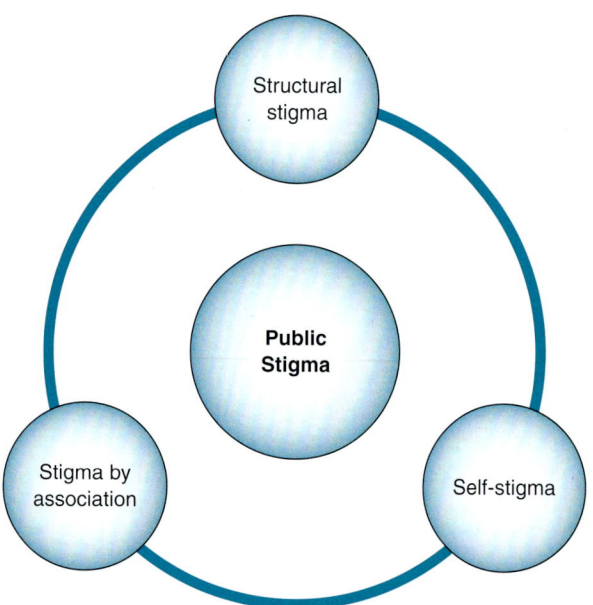

FIGURE 27-1. Pryor and Reeder's Model of Stigma.

Theory (Link et al., 1989). Collectively, these approaches provide ways of examining stigma from a variety of vantage points. Pryor and Reeder (2011) analyzed the diverse stigma literature and proposed a model of stigma that attempts to provide an evidence-based, organizational framework for understanding the processes and impact of stigmatization. Their dynamic model defines four interrelated types of stigmas that operate at societal, interpersonal, and individual levels (Fig. 27-1).

Public stigma is at the core of Pryor and Reeder's (2011) model. Public stigma is manifest in the way people react cognitively, affectively, and behaviorally to a person who is believed to have a stigmatized condition. For example, meeting a person diagnosed with schizophrenia may trigger reactions that include negative beliefs that the person is the product of poor parenting (cognitive), that the person is dangerous and should be feared (affective), and that the person should be avoided (behavioral).

Persons who possess these stigmatized conditions are often acutely aware of the public stigma and therefore may demonstrate self-stigma when they anticipate the stigma or internalize the negative stigmatizing beliefs. For example, a person living with bipolar disorder may begin to limit their social participation because they anticipate being devalued or treated negatively by others. This person may also begin to agree with the stigma and believe in a whole range of negative and self-stigmatizing statements such as, "People are right to expect less of me because of my illness." "I won't be able to accomplish much because of my bipolar disorder, so why should I even try?" This consequence of self-stigmatization has been referred to as the "why try" effect because this attitude reflects the negative impact on a person's motivation to achieve life goals (Corrigan et al., 2009).

People who have internalized such negative beliefs about themselves and their condition are likely to experience psychological distress, have a sense of reduced self-worth, and may engage in maladaptive behaviors such as being reluctant to advance their status through work or education (Corrigan et al., 2014).

Family members and friends of the person with the stigmatized condition may also feel the devaluation of being stigmatized. Pryor and Reeder (2011) refer to this as **stigma by association**. For example, suppose a father whose son comes home from college after his first psychotic break notices that his once friendly and supportive neighbors never come around anymore and the frequent invitations to cookouts and parties that were part of the neighborhood norm in the past are no longer extended to their family. Last week, while out in his yard, his son was arguing loudly with a voice in his head. A neighbor who was walking by told the father he needed to learn to control his son. Thus, individuals experiencing stigma by association can be subject to decreased social support, feelings of isolation, a loss of status and respect, and disrupted family relationships (Pryor & Reeder, 2011).

On a broader socioenvironmental level, **structural stigma** occurs when society and societal institutions operate in ways that weave inequities and injustices into their laws, policies, or practices. Therefore, structural stigma may intentionally restrict opportunities for people with mental illnesses or create unintentional consequences that limit opportunities for participation (Corrigan et al., 2014). For example, when people believe that individuals with substance abuse disorders are dangerous, they may be disinclined to be supportive or to befriend that individual and they may advocate and support policy initiatives that restrict the freedoms and rights of the person with such conditions.

Since Goffman's (1963) influential work more than 60 years ago, researchers have continued to explore how stigma is manifest both in the broader context of society and in more intimate day-to-day social interactions. As health-care providers, OTPs can use theories of stigma to better understand the processes of stigmatization and guard against becoming a source of that stigma in their personal and professional lives. In the case of structural stigma, it may be useful to consider that it took decades of disability activism to force Congress to pass the Americans with Disabilities Act (ADA) and the Mental Health Parity and Addiction Equity Act to address the clear inequities in opportunities for education, employment, and health care that exist for people with physical and psychiatric disabilities.

Furthermore, people with mental illness had to fight for enforcement of the ADA after its passage; for example, through the case that Lois Wilson and Elaine Curtis took to the Supreme Court (Olmstead Decision) to assert their right to live in the community when they were being involuntarily institutionalized (Equip for Equality, 2019). The need for these laws is evidence that structural inequities exist in U.S. society. The passage of these laws does not mean that these structural challenges do not continue to persist.

In most U.S. states, restrictions are placed on the civil rights of people with mental illness and/or people deemed mentally incompetent (a subjective term that could be interpreted differently in each case; Walker et al., 2016). These restrictions include laws limiting the rights of people with mental illness and/or intellectual disability to vote, hold an elective office, maintain custody of their children or adopt children, get married or divorced, or serve on a jury (Walker et al., 2016). For example, 43 U.S. states have laws on the books that can prevent people with intellectual disabilities and/or mental illness from voting (Kopel, 2017). Inaccessibility and other structural barriers can also reduce the ability of people with mental illness to vote, even in states without

these laws (Harrison, 2018). Research has shown that laws restricting the rights of people with mental illnesses have increased since 1989 (Walker et al., 2016).

Internationally, a review of the laws in 193 countries found that 71 countries restrict the rights of people with mental illness to marry (Bhugra et al., 2016). Considering the right to employment, within health-care fields, many states ask questions on the licensure application that may exclude people with mental illnesses or other disabilities from becoming licensed health-care professionals. Most of the state medical licensure applications for future physicians and 46% of occupational therapy licensure applications contain questions that conflict with the ADA (Groth & Scoby, 2019; Jones et al., 2018). Taken together, these policies represent widespread structural stigma, discrimination, and occupational injustices that harm people with mental illnesses. OTPs can use their skills in advocacy to partner with people with mental illness and their families and other allies to help deconstruct structural stigma. See Chapter 26: The Public Policy Environment and Chapter 28: Social Determinants and Mental Health.

Mad Studies and Theories of Sanism

Another way to think about bias and discrimination that affects people labeled as mentally ill is through the concept of sanism. Sanism is one of many common, toxic -isms that are prevalent in societies throughout the world, all of which reinforce oppression, injustice, and inequity (see Fig. 27-2). The Mad movement and the academic field of Mad Studies explain that sanism is a form of structural oppression whereby people who are—or who are perceived to be—mentally ill are treated as inferior to people who are perceived to be "sane" (Vermont Psychiatric Survivors, 2018; Wolframe, 2013).

The Mad movement is an umbrella term used in this chapter to encompass a variety of historical and modern movements for the liberation of people who are labeled as "mentally ill." The word "Mad" is a reclaimed slur that comes from the British English word for "crazy." This word has been reclaimed within the movement as an identity and often a

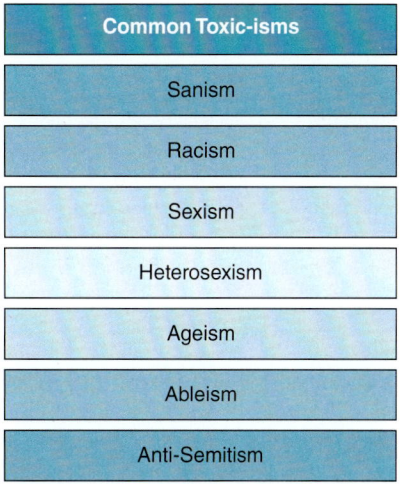

Common Toxic-isms
Sanism
Racism
Sexism
Heterosexism
Ageism
Ableism
Anti-Semitism

FIGURE 27-2. Common toxic-isms.

point of pride. One of the earliest iterations of the Mad movement was the "mental patients' liberation movement," in which current and former patients of mental institutions came together to protest their treatment in those institutions and in society. These patients pointed out many of the inhumane conditions at mental institutions, as well as bias in the mental health-care system.

Later iterations of the movement included the "consumer/survivor/ex-patient movement (c/s/x movement)." The c/s/x movement continued to critique the mental health-care system and protest for the rights of people who have been psychiatrized (labeled with psychiatric diagnoses and/or treated with psychiatric treatments). This movement prioritizes the leadership and wisdom of people who have experienced psychiatric treatment (Menzies et al., 2013; Starkman, 2013).

Another important contingency of the movement is the antipsychiatry movement (Diamond, 2013). This group of activists and scholars heavily critiques psychiatry and other "psy-disciplines" (psychology, clinical social work, mental health occupational therapy, mental health nursing, etc.) and in some cases calls for abolition of the current mental health-care system. The antipsychiatry contingent points out injustices in psychiatric treatment, including how women, LGBTQ people, and people of color are more likely to be institutionalized or medicated as a form of social control.

Some in the antipsychiatry contingent wholly reject biomedical models of mental illness and believe that there is no biological basis for mental illness (Burstow, 2015). Rather, they emphasize the role of trauma and oppression in creating mental distress (for examples of Mad approaches to trauma and oppression creating mental distress, see Filson, 2016 and The Icarus Project, 2015). Another important contingent of the movement is Mad Pride (Diamond, 2013). Those in the Mad Pride contingent view their mental differences as natural and desirable forms of human diversity.

Mad Studies is an academic discipline associated with the Mad movement (Menzies et al., 2013). Mad Studies scholars critique sanism and psychiatry. They also explore Mad people as a minority group, including the "history, culture, and language of madness and Mad people" (Menzies et al., 2013, p. xi).

In this way, Mad Studies has much in common with other minority studies disciplines such as Women's Studies and African American Studies. One thing that all contingents of the Mad movement and Mad Studies have in common is their acknowledgment of Mad people as a minority group that experiences oppression.

One of the strengths of thinking about sanism and how it affects Mad people is that it turns OTPs' focus from what is wrong with Mad people to what is wrong with the environment and society around Mad people. Stigma is not a natural feature of mental illness. Rather, sanism embedded in society imbues mental illness with stigma and leads Mad people to experience discrimination once they are labeled as "mentally ill." Analyzing sanism can allow people to focus less on how Mad people need to change to recover from their mental illness symptoms, and more on how society needs to change to better affirm and support people with mental illnesses.

Another benefit of acknowledging sanism as a structural oppression is that it allows people to better view how sanism interlocks with other forms of structural oppression, such as racism and sexism (Wolframe, 2013). For example, Black people with mental illnesses experience both sanism and racism simultaneously. This intersection of racism and sanism is too often deadly in the case of police brutality (Shadravan et al., 2021). At least 25% of people murdered by police have documented mental illnesses (DeGue et al., 2016). Black people are nearly three times more likely than white people to be killed by police, even though they are less likely than white people to be armed during such encounters with police (DeGue et al., 2016).

People with mental illness face sanist stereotypes that they are dangerous. However, people with mental illness are far more likely to be victims of violent crimes than to be perpetrators (Ghiasi et al., 2023). Black people are also wrongly stereotyped as more dangerous than white people. In encounters with the police, these sanist and racist stereotypes can intersect and compound. Examples of sanism are illustrated in Table 27-1, which defines the Four I's of oppression. The application of the Four I's of oppression (Chinook Fund, n.d.) to sanism is inspired by the work of Elliot Fukui (2020).

TABLE 27-1 | How Sanism Perpetuates Oppression

Type of Oppression	Definition	Example
Ideological oppression	Societal beliefs that people with mental illness are inferior to people without mental illness	People commonly use sanist language that associates mental illness with negative traits; for example, calling someone they disagree with "insane" or "nuts," or calling violent or racist actions "crazy."
Institutional oppression	Discrimination against people with mental illness is codified into laws, policies, and organizations.	Laws in many states make it possible for people to lose the right to vote or to hold public office because of a mental illness diagnosis (Walker et al., 2016). The case of Britney Spears's guardianship fight is a well-known example of someone losing their rights to self-determination because of a mental illness diagnosis (Spears, 2023).
Interpersonal oppression	Bias against people with mental illness shows up in personal social relationships.	People may choose not to date or be friends with someone with schizophrenia, or they may make fun of classmates with unusual speech or behaviors.
Internalized oppression	People with mental illness believe negative societal views about mental illness themselves.	A person may belittle themselves for their diagnosis and tell themselves that they just need to "snap out of it," rather than approaching themselves with acceptance, patience, and care.

Stigma and Mental Health Care

The global financial costs, morbidity, and mortality of mental illness clearly outpace any other health condition (Vigo et al., 2016), yet many individuals with mental illness do not receive mental health care. In the United States and Australia, for example, fewer than one-half of the adults experiencing a mental illness receive care (Substance Abuse and Mental Health Services Administration [SAMHSA], 2015; Whiteford et al., 2013). The 2021 National Survey on Drug Use and Health found that 27.6% of people with any mental illness and 65.1% of people with serious mental illness reported an unmet need for mental health services (they wanted mental health care and did not receive it; SAMHSA, 2021). The unmet need was highest among young adults, with 43.9% of those ages 18 to 25 with any mental illness and 65.1% of those with severe mental illness reporting an unmet care need.

The following section describes several specific stigma processes and their impact on help-seeking.

The Lived Experience

Grady Newton

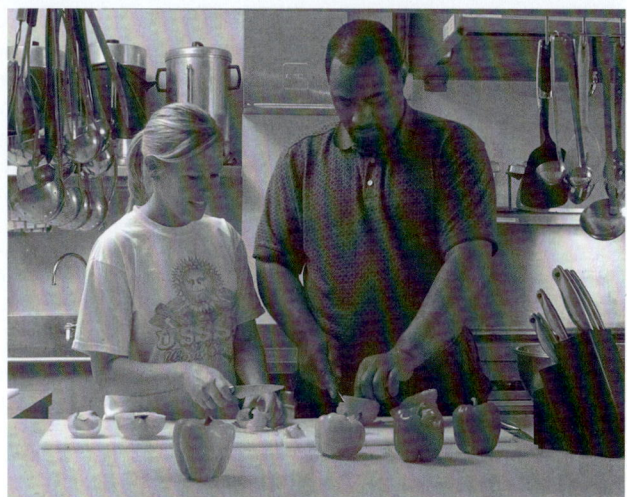

Years ago, I went through a 2-hour psychodiagnostic test and verbal consultation with a psychiatrist, and he said I was sane. I then went for a second opinion with a different psychiatrist. Without any testing this psychiatrist called me a name, that I had a mental illness, and told me to go to the drop-in center. That was the last time I saw that psychiatrist. I've seen four psychiatrists altogether. Once you get diagnosed with mental illness, it's tough to get back into society without that name.

Writing this is one way for me to speak on my own behalf. When you are looked upon as mentally ill, you lose your voice. I want to give a general statement about what I live like. This is my viewpoint.

Wyandot Center is a place I attend that has a foundation, doctors, nurses, case management, and staff. I respect the Wyandot Center with a good group of people that hear me. I feel like I've lost something in life by being called mentally ill; it is a personal loss. There are groups to attend, and I show up for my share of the program. When they have the groups and classes, I take in the information and enjoy it fully. In my everyday life, I know I am not alone or at least hope not. A goal of mine is persevering through this so-called mental illness. I don't believe the psychiatrist; I think I've been misjudged. My attitude and my behavior must remain to the best of my ability even when relaxing.

I believe education is important. It helps you in the long run. I went to Kansas State University. I have 250 credits and a C average with a major in Social Sciences, with an emphasis in Criminology. I had a full football scholarship, and I was a fifth-year senior. I redshirted myself, so I played for 4 of the 5 years. I was an outside linebacker, the most athletic position on the field. I was honorable mention, All-American even though I was on the losingest team in college football. I was team captain for the whole season. I was a free agent for the Washington Commanders. I signed the contract, I reported to training camp, but then I left. I looked at the situation and decided instead of seeking money I sought God. I got to keep the signing bonus.

I left the Commanders, and then I got a job as a detention officer in a correctional facility the same year. I worked there for 2 years. They terminated the whole job. Because I had this job, I now get an SSDI check—it is like workman's compensation. It shows that I have worked, but I'm disabled. I used to get the check myself in the mail, but I decided I wanted to have a payee. A payee is someone that takes the check, pays the rent, and then gives me a disbursement check once a week. I get a little more than $100 a week. But once you have a payee it's hard to get it back. I must decide what to do with the check, decide how to budget and what to eat.

When I must see the psychiatrist, the nurse, or occupational therapy students, or take my medication, I feel like my life is the subject. I get fired up and empowered. I question why this is happening to me. So, I go to the library to get books that help me learn. Checking those books out is my answer and antidote. I take my medication, but I must find a way to heal myself, to be as healthy as I can. My reading consists of the Holy Bible King James Version, *Introduction to Criminology, Psychological Theories of Motivation, The 26 Letters, Evil the Shadow Side of Reality,* and many more. These books help me gain strength during my lifelong trial. Reading is like eating healthy food.

I watch what I say, and I watch what I do for myself and the Wyandot Center Staff and business associates because sometimes people jump to conclusions or say things against me because of the stigma of this mental illness. For instance, one early mid-afternoon eating was on my mind. I decided to go to the cafeteria at KU Medical Center. I usually go there without incident. I was a few steps past the cafeteria when a policeman was standing in a doorway on a cell phone talking to someone. I noticed him talking on the cell phone. He said "Hi" to me. I felt uncomfortable. I responded by saying, "Why are you saying hi to me?" He said "Hi" again, and I turned in the direction

Continued

The Lived Experience—cont'd

of peace toward him and repeated, "Why are you saying hi to me?" while he was still talking on his cell phone.

The police officer then went screaming into hysterics. He disappeared through a door and alarmed the whole unit. They arrested me and handcuffed me from head to toe and gave me a ticket for resisting arrest. I believe this is associated with Wyandot Mental Health Center calling me mentally ill. I don't mean they know each other, but being called mentally ill and having this incident with the police officer reminds me of the same sort of stigma.

I didn't show up for my court date, but I turned myself in. They were not able to verify the arresting incident but set another court date. I wrote a citizen's report explaining what had happened. I showed this to the prosecuting attorney and the attorney said the story coincides with the police report and dismissed the charges. This is unheard of. I have to say I won, and I got my $100 back. I think the law should be respected because the law is there for a reason. Trying to figure out the problem personally on my own is my true nature. This is what I do to protect myself and my world. I have people telling me I'm mentally ill, but I tell myself I'm sane because that is my own interpretation of my past, present, and future. Hopefully, the interpretation of your own life story is protected, so you won't have to go through what I'm going through.

I've developed a model to help me interpret my life. There are different elements that interact that form a variety of patterns that give the illusion of greater differences than really exist. When you are in a situation, this model helps explain how you look at the characters in the room, what is said, and how to pay attention to your surroundings. I call the model my PK matrix, which can be viewed on the right.

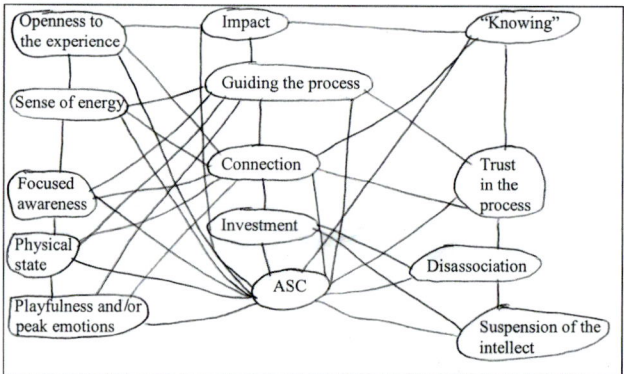

The Asbury Café is a place where I work. The café is held in a church every Wednesday. We fit into the church's schedule. The people that come to eat may go to the church but anybody who wants to get a meal can come to eat. I try to work harder when I'm there. I like the job. I've been there for 7 years, and I've never had a job that long. I cook a little, I do clean up, take the money, and am nice to the patrons that eat there, and they are nice to me. I compare it with other restaurants in the area, and it is one of the best places that I've been to eat. I gave a speech during the church services to get more patrons to come to eat at the Asbury Café. I hoped that I could say something that would make them come and eat with us. Lately we have had new people coming to eat at the café, and we get compliments. They say the food is good every time. There is an incredible hospitality and respect that is shared at the Asbury Café.

Public Perceptions of People With Mental Illnesses

In a systematic review of 36 articles evaluating public stigma toward individuals with mental illness, Parcesepe and Cabassa (2013) concluded many hold beliefs that people with mental illness are more likely to be a danger to themselves or others, are incompetent, or are more likely to engage in criminal behavior than the public. In their analysis, these researchers also reported that blaming, shaming, or punishing such individuals was a typical stigmatizing response.

In her study of public opinions about disclosing a mental illness, Donnelly (2017) demonstrated that the public clearly perceives the negative stigma attributed to people with mental illness. Most respondents in Donnelly's study indicated that if they had a mental illness, they would be unwilling to disclose this disability in employment, academic, and vocational counseling situations and would only be inclined to disclose such information when seeking health care.

Stigmatizing Responses

Negative attitudes and beliefs about people with mental illness often lead to overt, negative stigmatizing responses including discrimination. For example, stigma can be demonstrated through **social distance**; that is, a measure of how willing a person is to exclude those with mental illness in various social situations (e.g., not wanting the person to be a neighbor or marry into one's family, or not wanting to work closely with someone with such an illness; Boyd et al., 2010). Studies that have examined social distance found the public was most likely to want to keep their distance from individuals who had substance use disorders, those abusing alcohol, and those with psychotic and depressive disorders (Parcesepe & Cabassa, 2013).

Some stigmatizing perceptions differ based on the sociodemographic characteristics. For example, in their systematic review of studies of stigma and perceived violence and dangerousness, Parcesepe and Cabassa (2013) reported that children with depression were considered more likely to be violent and dangerous than adults with depression; ethnic minorities (Blacks Hispanics, Asians) were believed to be more dangerous than whites; and people with less education were believed to be more dangerous than those with more education.

Compared with people without mental illnesses, people with mental illness are more likely to experience housing discrimination, unemployment, and homelessness (Corbiere et al., 2011; Corrigan & Shapiro, 2010). See Chapter 28: Social Determinants and Mental Health and Chapter 32: The Neighborhood and Community. 🤝

Coping and Disclosure

When people with mental illnesses perceive and internalize stigma, it has a negative impact on their coping behaviors, sense of dignity, and general pursuit of meaning and happiness (Corrigan et al., 2014). Most individuals with severe psychiatric illnesses report that they experience discrimination or anticipate discrimination (Mestdagh & Hansen, 2014; Ye et al., 2016). This expectation of negative consequences extends to college students as well. In their meta-analysis, Li and colleagues (2014) concluded that clear evidence existed that the more college students anticipated negative stigmatizing effects of help-seeking, the less likely they were to seek mental health care. Similarly, students with mental illnesses participating in a recent focus group study reported that stigma is a major problem on college campuses (Turosak & Siwierka, 2021). See Chapter 10: Coping and Resilience. 🤝

In a systematic review of 144 studies examining stigma and help-seeking behavior, Clement and colleagues (2014) reported that stigma is a highly ranked barrier to help-seeking and that concerns regarding disclosure were the most common. These included believing that disclosure would lead to shame and embarrassment, concerns about social judgment and labeling, and fears of discrimination in employment and education. These researchers also reported concerns about stigma related to disclosure disproportionately impacting the health-seeking behavior for individuals in the military, males, minority ethnic groups, and young people (Clement et al., 2014). A clear trend in their analysis of nearly 150 studies was that these groups were least likely to disclose a mental illness.

Stigma and Culture

Stigma is a phenomenon that is present in every culture; however, there is diversity in the ways that stigma is exhibited and experienced across different cultures and contexts (Abdullah & Brown, 2011). A systematic review examining mental health stigma in the United States found that Asian American, Latinx American, and Black American groups tended to report higher levels of public and/or self-stigma surrounding mental illness as compared with white American groups (Misra et al., 2021). Yu and colleagues (2021) found that individuals residing in countries with more collectivist cultural traditions reported higher levels of self-stigma after experiences of public stigma. This may be because individuals in more interdependent cultures tend to greatly value community members' opinions of them, and more actively prioritize maintaining the reputation of their family and community than individuals from individualistic cultural backgrounds (Yu et al., 2021).

Yang and colleagues (2014) completed a systematic review of stigma literature that intentionally considered the impact of culture on stigma by examining how stigma interfered with the person's ability to do those activities that "mattered most" within their specific cultural context. In Chinese American communities, for example, cultural aspects of what matters most include "saving face" (avoiding humiliation) and preserving the family lineage. A person whose mental illness threatened their ability to effectively engage in interactions that could lead to marriage proposals to ensure the family lineage could be perpetuated would experience increased stigma because of this perceived deficit (Abdullah & Brown, 2011; Yang et al., 2007; Yang et al., 2013). A recent systematic review that considered self-stigma in different geographic areas found the highest rates of self-stigma of mental illness in participants from Southeast Asia and the Middle East (Dubreucq et al., 2021).

In Yang and colleagues' (2014) review of studies examining stigma in immigrant Latinx communities, stigma was considered most harmful when a person's mental illness negatively impacted their ability to work hard and to overcome problems. These aspects of Latinx culture may also negatively impact adherence to medication regimens because someone needing psychiatric medications might be more likely to be seen by others in the community as weak and incapable of working hard to overcome their problems (Yang et al., 2014). Further, a Latina whose capacity to be a mother and good caregiver was limited by her psychiatric illness was prone to stigmatization because these maternal expectations are also very strong cultural values in Latinx communities (Collins et al., 2008).

Some of the cultural themes that impacted stigma revolved around hesitancy in some African American communities to disclose private thoughts or "family business," stigma, and distrust of mental health service providers (Alang, 2019; Joo et al., 2011). In African American communities, some psychiatric symptomology was viewed through a cultural frame that attributed these symptoms to a weakness of spirituality and faith (Johnson et al., 2009). Many Black Americans have experienced racism during health-care encounters or anticipate potential racism during health-care encounters, which can also serve as a barrier to care. A mixed methods study of unmet need for mental health care among Black Americans found that "racism causes mistrust in mental health service systems" (Alang, 2019, p. 346) and addressing racism must be a priority to improve access to care.

OTPs can be culturally responsive by acknowledging possible differences in mental health stigma across cultures and opening a dialogue for individuals to share about their cultural beliefs surrounding mental health. Furthermore, it is important to acknowledge that people may be experiencing stigma based on more than one identity. For example, in addition to experiencing stigma related to mental illness, people may experience public and self-stigma associated with race, ethnicity, socioeconomic status, gender, sexual orientation, religion, or disability. An intersectional, mixed methods study of discrimination based on mental illness, race, and sexuality found that people of color and lesbian, gay, or bisexual (LGB) people with mental illness face multiple kinds of discrimination simultaneously (Holley et al., 2016). See Chapter 28: Social Determinants and Mental Health. 🤝

Family Stigma

Many of the consequences of stigma (e.g., self-stigmatization, devaluing the self, isolation, and the reluctance to seek personal care) that are experienced by the person with a mental illness are also experienced by that person's family, spouse, partner, and network of friends (Werner et al., 2011). Stigma by association can cause distress to those closest to the person with mental illness.

Family members may manifest their distress in multiple ways. Many experience psychological distress related to caring for the family member with a mental illness as they attempt to regulate a multitude of feelings that may arise during caregiving, such as guilt, empathy, anger, sympathy, regret, love, frustration, hope, anxiety, hopelessness, and depression (Larson & Corrigan, 2008). Depending on how these feelings are managed, they can contribute to internalized stigma for the person with mental illness themself who may fear that they are seen as a "burden." Families can also hold stigmatizing attitudes about their loved ones' mental illness themselves (Sousa et al., 2012).

Family members may experience stigma when they believe others blame them for their family member's mental illness, such as when others suggest that the family's poor parenting resulted in the person's illness (Larson & Corrigan, 2008). Children of parents with mental illness also experience significant stigma by association and structural stigma.

In addition to directly experiencing stigma, these individuals can also be distressed by anticipating potential future stigma (Dobener et al., 2022). The consequences of family stigma may be emotional (e.g., feeling disrespected, desperate, anxious, embarrassed), social (e.g., having a poor reputation, experiencing discrimination), and interpersonal (e.g., isolating the family or being shunned, avoiding relationships, efforts to hide the family member's mental illness, bullying; Dalky, 2012; Muralidharan et al., 2014; Park & Park, 2014; Pirutinsky et al., 2010; Reupert et al., 2021). Similar to other forms of stigma, family stigma can also discourage people from seeking help (Reupert et al., 2021). Therefore, families require support, education, and their own interventions to address the impact of stigma (Drapalski et al., 2008).

OTPs working with family members of persons with mental illness should make asking about family members' experiences with stigma a routine component of their evaluation processes and engage in family education and support in both professional and peer-run groups. Practitioners can draw on their training in cognitive and problem-solving strategies and their person-environment-occupation (PEO) practice framework to engage families in strengths-based strategies that build resiliency and reduce the negative impact of stigma.

Measurement of Stigma

Reliable and valid assessments exist to measure self-stigma, family stigma, public stigma, and stigmatizing beliefs held by health-care providers. Measuring the degree of internalized stigmatization or the level of impact of stigma on an individual's life can help both the stigmatized person and the OTP better understand the impact of stigma and the individual's response to stigma. These data can inform intervention planning and support advocacy that strengthens policies to combat stigma.

Two valid and reliable options for measuring self-stigma are the Self-Stigma of Mental Illness Scale (SSMIS; Corrigan et al., 2006) and the Internalized Stigma of Mental Illness (ISMI) Scale (Ritsher et al., 2003). Both forms also have reliable and valid shortened versions (Boyd et al., 2014; Corrigan et al., 2012). Both instruments can be used to understand the level to which a person self-stigmatizes. Table 27-2 shows sample items from the ISMI Scale.

Measuring the level of stigma experienced by family members of people with mental illness may also be useful for the OTP working with these families. The Stigma Assessment Tool for Family Member Caregivers of Patients with Mental Illness (SAT-FAM) is a scale designed to measure stigma experienced by family members. The SAT-FAM demonstrated good content validity, face validity, internal consistency, and test-retest reliability in preliminary research (Shamsaei & Holtforth, 2020).

The OTP intervening in the social and cultural environment may also wish to measure public stigma, or specifically measure stigma among health-care providers. Two measures for assessing public stigma are the Attribution Questionnaire (AQ; Corrigan, 2008) and the Attitudes to Mental Illness Questionnaire (AMIQ; Luty et al., 2006). The AQ measures stigma by presenting a short vignette (fictional case story) about a person with a mental illness and then asking questions about this fictional person. The vignette in the 27-item version of the AQ reads, "Harry is a 30-year-old single man with schizophrenia. Sometimes he hears voices and becomes upset. He lives alone in an apartment and works as a clerk at

TABLE 27-2 | Sample Items From the Internalized Stigma of Mental Illness (ISMI) Scale by Subscale

Subscale	Sample Items
Alienation	• I feel out of place in the world because I have a mental illness. • People without mental illness could not possibly understand me. • I feel inferior to others who don't have a mental illness.
Stereotype endorsement	• People can tell that I have a mental illness by the way I look. • Mentally ill people tend to be violent. • I can't contribute anything to society because I have a mental illness.
Discrimination experience	• Others think that I can't achieve much in life because I have a mental illness. • People often patronize me, or treat me as if I am a child, just because I have a mental illness. • Nobody would be interested in getting close to me because I have a mental illness.
Social withdrawal	• I don't talk about myself much because I don't want to burden others with my mental illness. • I don't socialize as much as I used to because my mental illness might make me look or behave "weird." • I avoid getting close to people who don't have a mental illness to avoid rejection.
Stigma resistance (reverse-coded questions)	• I feel comfortable being seen in public with someone who is obviously a person with mental illness. • People with mental illness make important contributions to society. • Living with mental illness has made me a tough survivor.

Excerpted from Ritsher, J. B., Otilingam, P. G., & Grajales, M. (2003). Internalized Stigma of Mental Illness: Psychometric properties of a new measure. Psychiatry Research, 121, 31–49. https://doi.org/10.1016/j.psychres.2003.08.008

a large law firm. He had been hospitalized six times because of his illness" (Corrigan, 2008, p. 10).

Then, the person taking the assessment must rate their level of agreement (from 1 = "not at all" to 9 = "very much") with statements about Harry. The statements reflect stigmatizing beliefs, ranging from, "I would feel aggravated by Harry," to "Harry would terrify me," to "If I were an employer, I would interview Harry for a job" (Corrigan, 2008, pp. 10–11). The AMIQ also uses fictional vignettes to measure stigma. The AMIQ vignettes are about five people with stigmatizing life circumstances: substance use disorders, depression, schizophrenia, and a criminal conviction. The AMIQ also includes two vignettes of life circumstances that are less typically stigmatized in the United Kingdom: being a Christian and having diabetes (Luty et al., 2006). The AMIQ allows for comparison of the level of stigmatizing attitudes people express about the characters with the different conditions.

The Opening Minds Stigma Scale for Health Care Providers (OMS-HC) is specifically designed to measure stigma among health-care providers. It can also be used to evaluate the effectiveness of an anti-stigma intervention (Modgill et al., 2014). An OTP who is delivering an anti-stigma intervention at their workplace for their colleagues could administer this assessment pre- and posttraining to see if their training was effective in reducing stigmatizing attitudes toward patients with mental illness. An OTP might also want to take this assessment themselves and use it as a tool for self-reflection. Table 27-3 contains sample items from the OMS-HC.

Table 27-4 outlines key information about common evaluation tools to help guide the OTP's therapeutic reasoning during the evaluation processes. An OTP who therapeutically incorporates discussion of the results of these assessment tools can help a person to understand the impact of the stigma, evaluate their personal responses to it, and help identify adequate strategies to cope with it. Practitioners should be cautious and remember that a therapeutic discussion of stigma never situates the problem within the person; rather, stigma is a failing of society and a social injustice (Corrigan et al., 2011).

Anti-Stigma Interventions

In his early work, Goffman (1963) defined stigma as a social process that is manifest in interpersonal interaction and relationships and that sociocultural structures of society impact these processes. Referencing Goffman's work, Pescosolido

(2013) reminds readers that, "if stigma emanates from social relationships, the solution to understanding and changing must similarly be embedded in changing social relationships and the structures that shape them" (p. 15).

There are multiple pathways through which stigma leads to discrimination and other negative outcomes. However, OTPs have the knowledge and skills to both prevent and address the negative impact of stigma. Practitioners can do this by orchestrating opportunities that encourage the public, including people with mental illness, to routinely participate in social occupations together. Practitioners can also support people with mental illness to develop their own capacities to create and sustain social relationships. Practitioners can also play an advocacy role in speaking out against negative public perceptions of mental illness.

A variety of interventions have been developed to combat stigma. In a meta-analysis of 27 randomized controlled trials assessing anti-stigma programs, Griffiths, and colleagues (2014) reported that programs designed to address social distance produced small but significant reductions in stigma across a variety of mental illnesses. Even more promising results were reported for programs that used educational interventions and those that emphasized personal contact with people with mental illnesses as a strategy to reduce stigma (Griffiths et al., 2014).

There are various ways to categorize anti-stigma interventions. Michaels and colleagues (2014) suggested that interventions can be categorized as education, social contact, and advocacy. Educational interventions focus on educating individuals about mental illness, whereas social contact interventions are built around the concept that personal contact with someone with mental illness can reduce stigma. Advocacy interventions include approaches that raise consciousness about mental illness, efforts to decrease negative attitudes and stigmatizing representations of people with mental illness, policy-focused strategies, and protests. In practice, these categories are not absolute, that is, an educational intervention can include an advocacy component. Various examples of anti-stigma interventions are described in the text that follows. Table 27-5 summarizes the consequences of stigma and strategies to reduce their effect.

Interventions to Reduce Public Stigma

Shahwan and colleagues (2022) conducted focus groups with people with lived experience of mental illness and caregivers about stigma. The participants identified four main suggestions for strategies to address stigma: "(1) raising

---

TABLE 27-3 | Sample Items From the Opening Minds Stigma Scale for Health Care Providers (OMS-HC)

Factor	Sample Items
Attitudes of health-care providers toward people with mental illness	• I am more comfortable helping a person who has a physical illness than I am helping a person who has a mental illness. • More than half of people with mental illness don't try hard enough to get better. • Health-care providers do not need to be advocates for people with mental illness.
Disclosure/Help-seeking	• If I were under treatment for a mental illness, I would not disclose this to any of my colleagues. • I would see myself as weak if I had a mental illness and could not fix it myself.
Social distance	• I would still go to a physician if I knew that the physician had been treated for a mental illness (reverse scored). • I would not want a person with mental illness, even if it were appropriately managed, to work with children.

Excerpted from Modgill, G., Patten, S. B., Knaak, S., Kassam, A., & Szeto, A. C. (2014). Opening Minds Stigma Scale for Health Care Providers (OMS-HC): Examination of psychometric properties and responsiveness. BMC Psychiatry, 14(120), 1–10. https://doi.org/10.1186/1471-244X-14-120

TABLE 27-4 | **Therapeutic Reasoning Assessment Table: Stigma**

Which Tool?	Who Was This Tool Designed For?	What Am I Measuring?	How Long Does It Take and How Do I Administer This Assessment?	Is the Tool Reliable and Valid?	Are There Additional Versions Available?
Internalized Stigma of Mental Illness (ISMI) Scale (Ritsher et al., 2003)	Persons with various types of stigmatizing conditions, such as psychiatric disabilities or HIV/AIDS	Subjective experience of stigma in subscale areas of naming alienation, social withdrawal, stereotype endorsement, discrimination experience, and stigma resistance	A 29-item self-report checklist that can be self-administered; typically takes 20–30 minutes	Good internal consistency; retest reliability; and concurrent, convergent, and discriminant validity (Corrigan et al., 2006) Subset scales have good internal consistency and good test-retest reliability (Corrigan et al., 2013; Ritsher & Phelan, 2004)	Short form is available with 10 items (Boyd et al., 2014; Corrigan et al., 2012). Consistency and reliability in short version reflect that of the full version (Boyd et al., 2014).
Self-Stigma of Mental Illness Scale (SSMIS; Corrigan et al., 2012)	Ethnic and racial minorities and immigrants, persons diagnosed with a psychiatric disability, and people with concealable diagnoses such as those with HIV/AIDS	Assesses perceived levels of internalized stigma including awareness and agreement of stereotypes, self-concurrence, and self-esteem decrement	A 40-item self-report checklist that can be self-administered; Typically takes 20–30 minutes	Satisfactory internal consistency and test-retest reliability (Corrigan et al., 2006)	Short version has 20 items and demonstrates good reliability and validity (Corrigan et al., 2013).
Stigma Assessment Tool for Family Members and Caregivers of Patients with Mental Illness (SAT-FAM; Shamsaei & Holtforth, 2020)	Family member caregivers (Shamsaei & Holtforth, 2020)	Items target perceived and experienced stigma that families and caregivers of people with mental illnesses experience.	Can be self-administered and has 30 items	Demonstrates good content validity, face validity, internal consistency, and test-retest reliability (Shamsaei & Holtforth, 2020)	N/A
Attribution Questionnaire (AQ)	Assesses individuals' attributes toward their family member regarding their mental health. (Sousa et al., 2012)	The items reflect the family's feelings of responsibility, pity, anger, dangerousness, fear, help, coercion, segregation, and avoidance (Sousa et al., 2012).	Can be self-administered and has 27 questions	Demonstrates good convergent validity, construct validity, and internal and test-retest reliabilities (Brown, 2008; Corrigan et al., 2004; Link et al., 2004)	Short version AQ-9 (Corrigan et al., 2002) Revised Attribution Questionnaire—nine items that can be used for adolescents (Pinto et al., 2012; Watson et al., 2004) Children's Attribution Questionnaire (AQ-8-C)—eight items for children 10–18 (Corrigan et al., 2005; Pinto et al., 2012; Watson et al., 2004) Available in Persian (Atashi et al., 2022), Spanish (Muñoz et al., 2015), Italian (Pingani et al., 2012), Swedish (McAllister et al., 2021), and Turkish versions (Akyurek et al., 2019)

TABLE 27-4 | Therapeutic Reasoning Assessment Table: Stigma—cont'd

Which Tool?	Who Was This Tool Designed For?	What Am I Measuring?	How Long Does It Take and How Do I Administer This Assessment?	Is the Tool Reliable and Valid?	Are There Additional Versions Available?
Attitudes to Mental Illness Questionnaire (AMIQ; Luty et al., 2006)	Assesses the attitudes of members of the public. The test can be used to assess the effectiveness of anti-stigma methods (Luty et al., 2006).	Assesses people's attitudes toward patients with mental illnesses (Luty et al., 2006)	Can be self-administered and has five items (Luty et al., 2006)	Has good content validity; face validity, construct, and criterion validity; test-retest reliability; alternative test reliability (Luty et al., 2006)	N/A
Opening Minds Stigma Scale for Health Care Providers (OMS-HC; Kassam et al., 2012)	Health-care providers; for use in educational realms to evaluate health-care courses and as part of quality assurance initiatives within health-care systems (Kassam et al., 2012)	Assesses attitudes and behaviors of health-care providers regarding individuals with mental illness (Modgill et al., 2014)	Can be self-administered and is a 20-item self-report questionnaire (Modgill et al., 2014)	Demonstrates good internal consistency, satisfactory test-retest reliability, and sensitivity to change (Kassam et al., 2012; Modgill et al., 2014)	Available in Hungarian (O˝ri et al., 2020), German (Zuaboni et al., 2021), and Brazilian versions (Carrara et al., 2023) Chilean version includes cultural adaptation and Spanish language translation (Sapag et al., 2019). The 15-item and 12-item versions are available with psychometric analysis best supporting the 15-item version (Modgill et al., 2014).

TABLE 27-5 | Stigma and Oppression: Strategies to Reduce Their Effect

Type of Stigma or Oppression	Strategies to Reduce the Effect
Public stigma and ideological oppression	• Education • Social contact • Advocacy • Positive media representation
Self-stigma and internalized oppression	• Cognitive skill-based approach (e.g., cognitive behavioral therapy) and coping skills • Peer support • Exposure to positive media • Participation in mental health advocacy organizations
Stigma by association and interpersonal oppression	• Skill-based approach and coping skills • Assertive communication to address bias in the moment with loved ones • Mediation • Exposure to positive representation • Workshops and courses about unlearning bias
Structural stigma and institutional oppression	• Advocate for the passage of the laws to address the issues • Spread awareness of occupational injustices

mental health awareness, (2) social contact, (3) advocacy by influential figures or groups, and (4) the legislation of anti-discriminatory laws" (Shahwan et al., 2022, p. 1). These priorities align with many of the anti-stigma interventions that have been designed to date and can also serve as guidelines for future anti-stigma interventions.

Several teams of researchers have developed effective methods of addressing mental health stigma through theatre and storytelling. Wasmuth and colleagues (2022) have used the Identity Development Evolution and Sharing

(IDEAS) program to effectively reduce negative attitudes about several different stigmatized populations. When conducting IDEAS, the team initially conducts interviews with individuals with lived experience of stigma. For the 2022 study, the team interviewed Black women, transgender and gender nonconforming people, and people with substance use disorders. Then, the team worked with a playwright and professional actors to transform the information from the interviews into a play. Finally, the play was performed in front of audiences of health-care providers. After viewing

PhotoVoice

Al

Social stigma affects the mentally ill and is seen as a mark of disgrace or dishonor. People can behave badly by exposing others to nerve agents and radiation, which causes mental illness, and long-term exposure causes multiple sclerosis. People target healthy people who want to take advantage of them for their own financial gain. The mentally ill have been mistreated throughout history. One victory is in recognizing the bad treatment. Collaboration of peers can change our future and overcome the trauma of bad treatment. Community awareness and recognizing all as equals can help overcome stigma. Every hand in the picture represents coming together to fight stigma for a new start.

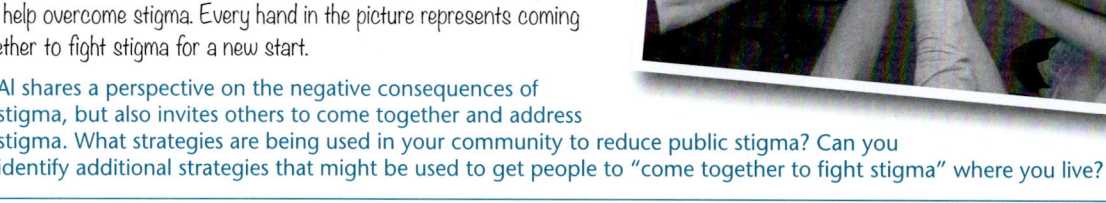

Al shares a perspective on the negative consequences of stigma, but also invites others to come together and address stigma. What strategies are being used in your community to reduce public stigma? Can you identify additional strategies that might be used to get people to "come together to fight stigma" where you live?

the play, the audience showed significant decreases in stigmatizing attitudes about these groups, as measured by the Acceptance and Action Questionnaire-Stigma (AAQ-S; Wasmuth et al., 2022).

Another stigma reduction program is called This Is My Brave (TIMB). TIMB is a live, onstage storytelling performance wherein people with lived experience of mental illness share their stories in a creative format, such as through poetry, comedy, or a musical performance. Preliminary research showed that the in-person version of TIMB contributed to a reduction in stigmatizing attitudes among audience members (Kosyluk et al., 2018). A later study conducted a randomized controlled trial of the effectiveness of a video recording of TIMB performances in reducing audience stigma (Kosyluk et al., 2021). The study showed the TIMB recording contributed to a reduction in perceived difference from people with mental illness and desire for social distance from people with mental illness among the TIMB viewers (Kosyluk et al., 2021).

In one intervention, Magliano (2022) tested whether distance education featuring personal experiences and scientific evidence could be used to reduce students' prejudices toward people with schizophrenia. This intervention included two 3-hour educational lessons that provided definitions of stigma, shared first-person accounts of stigma and its effects, and shared scientific evidence about stigma and mental health with particular focus on schizophrenia. The master's level students in this study were majoring in psychology, and the interventions supported positive changes in their attitudes toward persons with schizophrenia. Patten and colleagues (2012) designed a randomized controlled study to investigate the efficacy of contact-based education to reduce stigma in pharmacy students. Students who attended the 2-hour educational session were better able to interact with persons with mental illness than those who did not attend the session. The results reflected a small effect but showed that even brief contact-based education could reduce stigma.

In keeping with the occupational therapy value of person-centeredness, the best practice for conducting interventions to reduce public stigma is to have individuals with lived experience of mental illness involved at every stage of the development and implementation of the program. One study testing the effectiveness of a 3-hour anti-stigma workshop led by people with lived experience of mental illness ("experts by experience" [Świtaj et al., 2019, p. 1219]) found that the workshops significantly reduced stigmatizing attitudes among attendees. The positive effect on attendees' desire for "social distance, stigmatizing attributions, and beliefs about self-determination for people with mental illness" (Świtaj et al., 2019, p. 1219) persisted 6 months after the workshop.

The Time to Change (TTC) social marketing campaign in England focused on reducing stigma toward individuals with mental illnesses through increased social media contact. This education and advocacy program used social media to reach the public and encourage positive changes in attitudes and behavior toward persons with mental illness throughout England (Evans-Lacko et al., 2013). An investigation of the effectiveness of the mass media component of TTC found that the campaign facilitated moderate levels of public awareness. However, there was no significant longitudinal improvement in the public's overall knowledge or behavior over the entire campaign period.

Such interventions to reduce public stigma could be an excellent role for OTPs. These interventions could be considered "education" or "advocacy" type interventions according to the *Occupational Therapy Practice Framework: Domain and Process,* Fourth Edition *(OTPF-4).* The *OTPF-4* also highlights the practitioner's role in addressing occupational injustice (American Occupational Therapy Association [AOTA], 2020).

Addressing structural stigma embedded into laws and policies is also a key area where OTPs can intervene. Here, OTPs can follow the lead of established organizations that support people with mental illness, especially those working from a Mad Pride or Recovery perspective. A few such organizations include Fireweed Collective, Institute for the Development of Human Arts (IDHA), Project LETS, and the Hearing Voices Network. These organizations are linked in the Resources section of this chapter.

Critiquing and protesting discriminatory policies is one way to address structural stigma and sanism. IDHA and other

Evidence-Based Practice

Addressing Self-Stigma and Stigma by Association

Internalized stigma exacerbates negative lived experiences of stigma for individuals with mental illness.

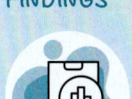

RESEARCH FINDINGS

The self-efficacy of people with mental illnesses is negatively impacted when they internalize stigma and accept the negative stereotypes about their condition held by others. These individuals are also less likely to seek help or adhere to treatment if they do (Dubreucq et al., 2021). Further, though country- and culture-related variations exist, the experience of self-stigma occurs in all peoples and all cultures worldwide (Dubreucq et al., 2021).

Individual- and group-based interventions aimed at reducing self-stigma typically encourage discussion of a person's lived experiences with various forms of stigma, often employ a psychoeducational approach, and frequently intentionally discuss the pros and cons of disclosure (Rüsch & Kösters, 2021). Mental health service providers need to be vigilant in their own practices to avoid adding to a person's negative lived experiences of stigma (Mills et al., 2020). Providers must also practice self-care as they are often subject to diminished job satisfaction and burnout when they face stigma by association (Yanos et al., 2020).

APPLICATIONS

➡ All campaigns directed toward reduction of stigma should be recovery-oriented and intentionally consider cultural factors.

➡ People experiencing mental illness should not be left to deal with stigma on their own. OTPs can support and model strategic disclosure, can advocate for peer-supported stigma self-management interventions, and can help individuals build skills for disclosure that tell the right story, to the right people, at the right time.

➡ OTPs can play an essential role in dispelling stigma, in all its forms, by highlighting and celebrating occupational therapy's role in addressing function across the mental health continuum.

➡ Practitioners in mental health can address stigma by association by collaborating with interdisciplinary colleagues to create programs that enhance practitioner well-being, and which focus on and share coping strategies for dealing with stigma by association among mental health professionals.

REFERENCES

Dubreucq, J., Plasse, J., & Franck, N. (2021). Self-stigma in serious mental illness: A systematic review of frequency, correlates and consequences. *Schizophrenia Bulletin, 47*(5), 1261–1287. https://doi.org/10.1093/schbul/sbaa181

Mills, H., Mulfinger, N., Raeder, S., Rüsch, N., Clements, H., & Scior, K. (2020). Self-help interventions to reduce self-stigma in people with mental health problems: A systematic literature review. *Psychiatry Research, 284,* 112702. https://doi.org/10.1016/j.psychres.2019.112702

Rüsch, N., & Kösters, M. (2021). Honest, open, proud to support disclosure decisions and to decrease stigma's impact among people with mental illness: Conceptual review and meta-analysis of program efficacy. *Social Psychiatry and Psychiatric Epidemiology, 56,* 1513–1526. https://doi.org/10.1007/s00127-021-02076-y

Yanos, P.T., DeLuca, J. S., Salyers, M. P., Fischer, M. W., Song, J., & Caro, J. (2020). Cross-sectional and prospective correlates of associative stigma among mental health service providers. *Psychiatric Rehabilitation Journal, 43*(2), 85–90. https://doi.org/10.1037/prj0000378

organizations have been speaking out against the involuntary commitment policies in New York City and other places (IDHA, n.d.). In November 2022, New York City Mayor Eric Adams issued a directive declaring that people with mental illness seen in public in New York could be detained by police and involuntarily hospitalized, even if they were not threatening the safety of others (Newman & Fitzsimmons, 2022). This policy stems from intersecting sanist and classist beliefs that people with mental illness and unhoused people are dangerous and violent. This directive encourages police and other city officials to judge the behavior of people in public and violate their rights to self-determination by detaining them if they behave in an unusual manner. This policy represents an occupational justice issue and would be an appropriate subject of advocacy by OTPs.

Interventions to Reduce Self-Stigma

Two studies investigated whether a structured, group-based intervention called **narrative enhancement and cognitive therapy (NECT)** could effectively reduce self-stigma. NECT programs include elements of psychoeducation, cognitive restructuring, and building narratives with positive identities (Yanos et al., 2012). Results showed that individuals in the NECT group had less self-stigma and better insight than those in the control group. In a later quasi-experimental study examining the effect of NECT (Roe et al., 2014), participants showed significant reductions in self-stigma and an increase in self-esteem and quality of life when compared with the control group after 20 NECT sessions (1 hour/week).

Two additional evidence-based programs for self-stigma reduction are the "Coping Internalized Stigma Program" (PAREI) and the "Ending Self-Stigma" (ESS) program. PAREI is an eight-session group intervention that includes "psychoeducation, cognitive behavioral therapy, and mutual support" (Díaz-Mandado & Periáñez, 2021, p. 1). One study found that after completing PAREI, the people with mental illness in the intervention group experienced a significant decrease in self-stigma as compared with the control group (Díaz-Mandado & Periáñez, 2021). Similar to NECT and PAREI, ESS is a group intervention that involves psychoeducation and cognitive behavioral approaches (Lucksted et al., 2017).

ESS also directly educates participants about stigma. A randomized controlled trial of the effectiveness of ESS found that people who went through the 9-week ESS program experienced significant short-term decreases in self-stigma as measured by the SSMIS and the ISMI measure (Lucksted et al., 2017). An adapted version of the ESS designed specifically for people with posttraumatic stress disorder (PTSD) also exists (ESS-P). A preliminary randomized trial showed that veterans with PTSD who participated in the ESS-P experienced decreased self-stigma and depression symptoms. Participants also showed increases in self-efficacy and feelings of belonging (Drapalski et al., 2021).

Sibitz and colleagues (2013) investigated the efficacy of an empowerment and recovery-oriented program in a day clinic on internalized stigma for people with schizophrenia spectrum disorders. The study included group and individualized sessions using a psychoeducation format. In addition to psychoeducation for people with mental illness, health-care team members were educated in the recovery model and better identifying strengths of people with mental illness. The results showed that the psychoeducation participants had a reduction in internalized stigma, whereas the wait-list control group had a minimal increase in internalized stigma.

Another model that shows promise in the reduction of both public stigma and self-stigma is the Recovery College model. Recovery Colleges are educational programs in which people with and without mental illness learn about mental illness and well-being alongside each other. The educational programming is codeveloped and cofacilitated by mental health-care providers ("experts by training") and people with mental illness ("experts by experience"; Thériault et al., 2020, p. 928). The college operates under an adult education model and participation is open to people with mental illness, health-care providers, caregivers, and members of the public. This model allows for education about mental illness as well as social contact between people with different relationships to mental illness. Recovery Colleges take an empowerment-focused and strengths-based approach, in keeping with the tenets of the recovery model. Some evidence from the United Kingdom suggests that attending a Recovery College can reduce self-stigma of mental illness (Nurser et al., 2017) as well as improve public and health-care provider attitudes about mental illness (Crowther et al., 2019).

This brief review of the evidence demonstrates that anti-stigma interventions can be effective in reducing stigma, just as Griffiths and colleagues (2014) reported in their meta-analysis. Practitioners can be assured that growing research does support using educational interventions, skill-based interventions, and social contact approaches (filmed or lived) as effective ways to encourage reductions in negative attitudes of the general population and health-care professionals. Although changing attitudes may be achieved by short-term courses or workshops, changing behaviors toward stigmatized individuals may require social-contact interventions.

In a similar vein, OTPs should recognize that the evidence supports using interventions with cognitive and skill training components and that these can be effective in reducing self-stigma. Psychoeducational approaches, which are often employed by OTPs, have been found to be effective in reducing self-stigma and improving positive coping skills. Interventions that target the broader social, cultural, and legal environment—such as advocacy—may often be needed to transform institutional sanism and structural stigma. See Chapter 39: Peer-Led Services.

Stigma and Occupational Justice

Occupational justice, a derivative of social justice, refers to the right of every individual to have access to, and the ability to engage in, the variety of occupations necessary to support health and wellness (Wilcock & Hocking, 2015). Research indicates there are negative consequences to social stigma that can impede occupational justice (Østerud, 2023). Because one of the goals of the recovery movement is consumer-driven care and social participation in communities of choice, anything that impedes an individual from exercising self-determination is of concern to OTPs.

OTPs, who are advocating for occupational justice, are calling for support of individual mental well-being by addressing social strategies beyond traditional occupational therapy interventions, particularly for individuals whose self-determination is impacted by poverty, unemployment, or unstable housing (Duncan, 2004; Durocher et al., 2014; Farias et al., 2016). Such occupational therapy intervention includes occupational empowerment, enablement, and

Being a Psychosocial OT Practitioner

Deana Muñoz, MS, OTR/L

Framing Coping as Positive Self-Management

Identifying Psychosocial Strengths and Needs

OTPs often work with people who qualify for Medicaid or low-cost public health-care plans designed for those who earn too much to qualify for Medicaid but not enough to afford private health insurance. Stephen is 8 years old and qualifies for Medicaid. He was referred by his pediatrician to a private, multidisciplinary pediatric outpatient practice that commonly sees children for fine motor and visual motor delays, regulation difficulties, and "sensory challenges." Because there is a shortage of behavioral health facilities, many children referred to occupational therapy for functional skill deficits also present with anxiety and depression that is not being addressed by any other health-care providers.

Stephen's functional skill referral specified "visual motor integration deficits." In addition to his visual motor integration challenges, Stephen had also been diagnosed with a moderate intellectual disability, dyslexia, and attention deficit-hyperactivity disorder combined type. Reports of "multiple meltdowns each day" suggested Stephen had difficulty self-regulating. Stephen's mother, Bree, admitted that she used alcohol and stimulants during her pregnancy with Stephen.

Stephen and his mother had recently moved to the area. Bree shared that they had fled their home and moved to a new state to escape physical abuse from Stephen's biological father. Just before their move, Stephen's father left their home with his younger brother and did not return. Bree and Stephen have had no contact with them since fleeing. Her social support in the community consists of a cousin who occasionally provides child care. Stephen and Bree's housing situation is fluid, and they have spent some nights sleeping in their vehicle. Despite these challenges, Stephen and Bree have a very strong bond.

At a recent parent-teacher conference, Stephen's teacher noted his difficulty with reading and writing and expressed concern about his frequent physical and verbal outbursts in class. Stephen receives school-based occupational therapy services, but school officials suggested that Bree seek additional services to address his mental health challenges and ensure he does not fall further behind his peers. Bree is resistant to suggestions that Stephen has mental health challenges. She pulled Stephen from speech and counseling because of perceived disrespect from the therapists, who also suggested that further assistance and/or medication may be necessary.

Using a Holistic Occupational Therapy Approach

Using a combination of assessments designed to identify a range of motor skill difficulties in addition to adaptive and social-emotional skill challenges, the OTP and Bree created an occupational profile. This profile presented Stephen's handwriting and behavioral challenges as part of a larger picture, including difficulties with visual motor, auditory, and oral processing, which sometimes impacted his attention, cognition, and communication.

During occupational therapy sessions, it became clear that challenges with self-esteem and emotional regulation impacted Stephen's ability to participate in scholastic and social activities just as much as his difficulties with visual motor integration. He struggled to persist with tasks and frequently gave up when he experienced a problem, often hiding under the table or becoming tearful. Stephen used words such as "stupid" and "bad" to describe himself and often hit his head when upset. He reported that some kids at school called him "crazy" and put rocks in his food. Sensory sensitivities to tactile, auditory, and oral input distressed Stephen. In the school environment, these sensitivities overwhelmed him, making engaging in social and scholastic activities difficult.

Bree notes that she and Stephen have not had stable housing or been able to set a routine schedule. After school, Stephen struggles to calm down, to eat meals in one sitting, to complete his homework, and can't settle down for bed. Each time they move to another place, Stephen sleeps poorly, and he frequently asks to join Bree in her bed.

The OTP works with Stephen to identify sensory preferences and trial sensorimotor strategies and activities to address daily regulation and attention. Using the Goal Attainment Scale (GAS) system, they created a personalized way to track Stephen's progress that did not compare him to his peers but showed his own individual growth in handwriting legibility, letter formation, and behaviors. Framing coping skill use in a way that related to practical skills improved Bree's buy-in to the home program, and the OTP was careful not to mention words that might be perceived as related to mental illness.

Level of EXPECTED OUTCOME— 3 months	Rating	Expected Outcome (Effectively utilize coping skills to decrease daily meltdowns with minimal support for coregulation)
MUCH MORE than expected	+2	1–2 meltdowns per week, 10–15 minutes
MORE than expected	+1	1 meltdown per day, 15–20 minutes
EXPECTED outcome	0	Currently, 2–3 meltdowns per day, 20–30 minutes
LESS than expected	-1	2–3 meltdowns per day, 30–40 minutes
MUCH LESS than expected	-2	15+ meltdowns per week, 30–40 minutes

Using the GAS system helped Bree and Stephen see that it was possible to make progress while allowing for mistakes to be made. The OTP and Stephen engaged in coping skills exploration and involved Bree in each session to allow Stephen to teach her the skills he had learned, improve his own mastery, provide Bree with a chance to participate in a positive therapy experience, and build her trust in the therapeutic process. The OTP collaborated with Stephen's school counselor and school OTP to implement successful strategies at home, school, and the clinic.

Reflection Questions

1. How might the OTP address Stephen's self-stigmatization and negative self-talk using strategies that accommodate his cognitive and communicative challenges?
2. The OTP in this story was careful to present the idea of using coping skills and practical skills to manage Stephen's behavioral challenges and avoided using terms that Stephen or his mother might identify with mental illness. Role-play a conversation with Stephen's mother and use your own words to describe the focus of occupational therapy using nonstigmatizing language.
3. What are some ways you could help Stephen develop self-advocacy skills to combat stigmatization from peers and request assistance from adults when experiencing bullying behaviors?

enrichment to address occupational risks associated with deprivation, alienation, and imbalance. These interventions occur not only at the individual level but also at the community and policymaking systems levels.

Here's the Point

- Stigma and sanism are consistent features in the social environment and can have a profound, negative impact on people with mental illness, their families, and significant others.
- There are various theories of stigma and sanism that can help OTPs understand the processes of stigma and how to intervene.
- Individuals with mental illness, their families, and health-care providers all need to be educated on the processes and impacts of stigmatization and sanism.
- Stigma can be understood in terms of public stigma, self-stigma, stigma by association, and structural stigma. Each type of stigma warrants a different intervention approach.

- Assessment of level of stigmatization is possible and can help OTPs address the impact of stigma through interventions.
- Evidence shows there are effective ways to reduce stigma. Anti-stigma and anti-sanism efforts are consistent with OTPs' emphasis on occupational justice.

Acknowledgments

Dr. Harrison would like to thank research assistants Jordan Crisci, Katie McLaughlin, and Janna Rus for their valuable assistance with literature searches to update the evidence in this chapter. The authors would also like to acknowledge Dr. Ay-Woan Pan, who contributed to this chapter in the last edition of this text.

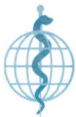

Visit the online resource center at **FADavis.com** to access the videos.

Apply It Now

1. Reflections on Grady's Lived Experience Story

Reread this chapter's The Lived Experience feature that shares Grady's story.

Reflective Activities
- Create a list of experiences that are described in the story that reflect clear evidence of stigmatization.
- Create a table with two columns. Label one column "Public Stigma" and the other column "Self-Stigma." Sort everything in your initial list into these two columns.
- Discuss your analysis with a peer to describe and defend your thinking.
- Return to the story and apply a PEO framework to understand Grady's experiences. What do you know about Grady that helps you develop an occupational profile? What clues from the story help you determine occupations that Grady finds meaningful and important?
- Identify personal and environmental factors that support or detract from Grady's participation in occupations in a variety of environments. Consider how they may have changed or whether they have remained the same over time.
- Imagine what might make it easier for Grady to engage in the occupations he enjoys. What steps can OTPs take to make it easier for Grady to engage in a dignified and productive life?

2. First-Person Accounts in Popular Media, Blogs, and Online Sources

Read some of the lived experiences of people with mental illness collected in one of the following sources. Create a bulleted list of those and look for common themes. What do you notice about these stories? What are consistent themes? Discuss your analysis with some peers.

- "Personal Stories" feature in the MindFreedom.org website (2006): http://www.mindfreedom.org/personal-stories/personal-stories
- "Share Your Story" feature in the National Alliance on Mental Illness website (NAMI, n.d.-a.): http://www.nami.org/Get-Involved/Share-Your-Story
- "Disability Visibility": disabled narratives in podcasts, stories, and art on this website: https://disabilityvisibilityproject.com/podcast-2

3. Representation of Mental Illness in the Media

Get together in a group with four or five of your classmates. Have each person search the internet for items that depict mental illness in popular culture (TV, movies, video games, advertisements, etc.) and choose a clip that is 2 to 5 minutes long. Share your clips within your group or with the rest of your class and discuss them.

Reflective Questions
- What messages do these clips portray to the public regarding people with mental illness? How about to the individual with a diagnosis of a mental illness?
- How do these clips contribute to stigma?
- What other conditions do people live with that are portrayed in this way?
- Do these clips contribute to stereotypes?
- How often are people exposed to messages such as those portrayed in the clips?

4. Self-Reflection on Stigma

Take the OMS-HC yourself. It is available through the Mental Health Commission of Canada at https://www.mentalhealthcommission.ca/English/initiatives/11874/opening-minds

After taking the questionnaire, reflect on your answers.

Reflective Questions

- Do your answers indicate some stigma about mental illness?
- If so, what could you do to address this stigma?

5. Stigma Reduction Programs

Participate in a stigma reduction initiative. Two options that are available free and online are:

- Manic Monologues interactive website (Burton & Hofmeister, 2021): https://manicmonologues.mccarter .org
- Amazing Adventure Against Stigma game (Carrot Salmon, 2021): https://antistigma.psy.cuhk.edu.hk

There are also in-person programs in some cities, such as TIMB (This Is My Brave, n.d.) and Erasing the Distance (Erasing the Distance, n.d.). After participating in the activity, ask yourself the following.

Reflective Questions

- Did this activity affect your attitudes about mental illness? If so, how did this activity affect your attitudes about mental illness?
- What evidence-based strategies for stigma interventions did this activity use?
- Who else might benefit from participating in this activity? How could you share it with them?

6. Video Exercise: Student Panel Discusses Running Groups in Mental Health Settings

Pair up with another student in your class or form a small group of students. Access and watch the "Student Panel Discusses Running Groups in Mental Health Settings" video at the online resource center at FADavis.com. Then, discuss and together answer the following questions.

Reflective Questions

- The students stated they were surprised by the welcome they experienced from individuals in this mental health setting. Is it possible that stigma and stereotypes about people with mental illness influenced their expectations about working with individuals in a psychiatric day program? Explain.
- How do you think the students were able to connect with and learn from the individuals they served with the lived experience of mental illness?
- Several students mentioned that they felt very welcomed by staff and participants and that the participants were especially receptive to the groups they offered. What about

the students and participants might have come together to make things work so well?

- Why do you think the team approach was emphasized by the students as helping them be successful in running the groups?
- How does it make you feel to hear these students recognize that part of the learning is feeling anxious about independently running groups in a mental health setting? What strategies can you use to manage anxiety and give yourself the best opportunity to succeed when running groups?

7. Video Exercise: Student Perceptions of Bias and Stigma

Pair up with another student in your class or form a small group of students. Access and watch the "Student Perceptions of Bias and Stigma" video at the online resource center at FADavis.com. Then, discuss and together answer the following questions

Reflective Questions

- What did it take for these students to recognize and honestly reflect on their personal biases and assumptions about unhoused individuals? How did connecting and working with unhoused individuals shape their current perspectives, and how can they use this new perception in their future practice regardless of the setting they work in?
- What shared lived experiences, desires, and life goals helped these students humanize the unhoused individuals they saw in clinic? What effect do you think that had on their work with the individuals?
- One student mentioned that, from this experience, he realized how mental health challenges were a common experience in unhoused populations. He commented that, although mental health conditions are becoming more widely acknowledged and discussed in society, unhoused individuals often are excluded from that conversation. Why do you suppose that occurs? How can OTPs help ensure that the mental health needs of unhoused individuals are considered at a societal level?
- Students having their own lived experiences with people who are unhoused at the occupational therapy clinic were surprised at the significant heterogeneity in the population and how stereotypes that usually are attributed to people who are unhoused often did not apply. What strategies did the students use that helped them to understand the lived experiences of people at the clinic and to dismantle their own biases and stigmatizing behaviors?

Resources

- Criptiques—This free e-book, edited by Caitlin Wood, is a collection of essays from writers with lived experiences of disability. The essays are intended to be generative and to spark discussion and debate about disability: https://criptiques.files .wordpress.com/2014/05/crip-final-2.pdf

- Fireweed Collective—A healing justice organization that offers many resources about mental health, crisis, and addressing sanism (Fireweed Collective, n.d.): https://fireweedcollective.org
- Hearing Voices Network—An organization that offers peer support and other affirming alternatives to conventional mental health treatment for people who hear voices or have visions. One of their missions is to reduce stigma associated with

hearing voices and having visions (Hearing Voices Network, n.d.): https://www.hearing-voices.org
- Initiatives: Opening Minds From Mental Health Commissions of Canada—This Canadian website develops and disseminates resources that specifically focus on improving the lives and experiences of people with mental illness and their families (Mental Health Commission of Canada, n.d.): https://www.mentalhealthcommission.ca/English/initiatives/11874/opening-minds
- Institute for the Development of Human Arts (IDHA)—An organization working toward "a new paradigm of Transformative Mental Health" which centers "systemic change," "experiential knowledge," and "holistic care" (IDHA, n.d.). They offer many trainings and resources: https://www.idha-nyc.org
- National Alliance on Mental Illness (NAMI): I Am Stigma Free—This website, based in the United States, provides information and resources for individuals and companies to use in combating mental health stigma (NAMI, n.d.-b). https://www.nami.org/stigmafree
- NAMI Queens/Nassau—This website is hosted by the Queens/Nassau, New York branch of the NAMI and offers lesson plans (for a small fee) on mental illness for children and adolescents as a part of NAMI's Campaign to End Discrimination: http://www.btslessonplans.org/about_began.html
- Project LETS—An organization specializing in "building just, responsive, and transformative peer support collectives and community mental health care structures that do not depend on state-sanctioned systems that trap out folks in the medical/prison-industrial complex" (Project LETS, 2021, para. 1). They offer workshops for health-care providers and community members, peer support groups, and more: https://projectlets.org
- SAMHSA's Resource Center to Promote Acceptance, Dignity and Social Inclusion Associated with Mental Health (ADS Center)—This SAMHSA site links to multiple resources for addressing stigma: https://www.samhsa.gov/sites/default/files/overcoming-stigma-ending-discrimination-resource-guide.pdf
- TOOLKIT for Evaluating Programs Meant to Erase the Stigma of Mental Illness, Patrick Corrigan Illinois Institute of Technology—This toolkit provides several tools that can be used to measure the impact of anti-stigma programs. The copyright holder of all tools grants permission to use these measures freely (Corrigan, 2008): https://www.montefiore.org/documents/Evaluating-Programs-Meant-to-Erase-the-Stigma-of-Mental-Illness.pdf
- World Health Organization, Stigma and Discrimination—This website, based in Denmark, describes the WHO European Mental Health Action Plan to end mental health discrimination and stigma (WHO, 2023): http://www.euro.who.int/en/health-topics/noncommunicable-diseases/mental-health/priority-areas/stigma-and-discrimination
- "Nicholas' Lived Experience of Schizophrenia" video. Nicholas is an occupational therapist living with the lived experience of schizophrenia. In this video, he describes his first episode of psychosis and the crucial role that occupational therapy played in his recovery. Nicholas emphasizes the importance of engaging with other people during rehabilitation and how, through occupational engagement, he discovered reconnection, felt loved, and found a sense of meaning and purpose. Access the video at the online resource center at FADavis.com.
- "First Fieldwork Experience in Inpatient Mental Health" video. In this video, Casey describes her first fieldwork experience in occupational therapy, which took place in an inpatient mental health setting. Casey shares what she was nervous about before her fieldwork coleading a group and then how things actually turned out. She emphasizes the benefit of creating detailed activity proposals before each group and learning to modify activities as needed on the spot. Access the video at the online resource center at FADavis.com.
- "Aster's Lived Experience of Suicidality" video. Aster is an occupational therapist, educator, and disability researcher who shares their experience with major depression and suicidality. In this video, Aster openly and courageously describes an episode of suicidality that resulted in taking a leave of absence from work. Aster discusses the actions and resources that helped them get through the crisis, including creating a psychiatric advanced directive, planning for their safety, and stopping an asthma medication that was worsening their symptoms. Aster's video also addresses the topics of social connectedness, stigma, and trauma recovery following a mental health crisis. To access the video, visit the online resource center at FADavis.com.

References

Abdullah, T., & Brown, T. L. (2011). Mental illness stigma and ethnocultural beliefs, values, and norms: An integrative review. *Clinical Psychology Review, 31,* 934–948. https://doi.org/10.1016/j.cpr.2011.05.003

Akyurek, G., Efe, A., & Kayihan, H. (2019). Stigma and discrimination towards mental illness: Translation and validation of the Turkish version of the Attribution Questionnaire-27 (AQ-27-T). *Community Mental Health Journal, 55*(8), 1369–1376. https://doi.org/10.1007/s10597-019-00438-0

Alang, S. M. (2019). Mental health care among Blacks in America: Confronting racism and constructing solutions. *Health Services Research, 54*(2), 346–355. https://doi.org/10.1111/1475-6773.13115

American Occupational Therapy Association. (2020). Occupational therapy practice framework: Domain and process—Fourth edition. *The American Journal of Occupational Therapy, 74*(Suppl. 2), 7412410010p1–7412410010p87. https://doi.org/10.5014/ajot.2020.74S2001

Atashi, A., Corrigan, P., Shakiba, S., Pourshahbaz, A., & Al-khouja, M. (2022). Mental illness stigma: The psychometric properties of the Persian version of the Attribution Questionnaire (AQ-27-P). *Journal of Psychosocial Rehabilitation and Mental Health, 9,* 189–196. https://doi.org/10.1007/s40737-021-00251-7

Becker, H. S. (1963). *Outsiders: Studies in the sociology of deviance.* Free Press.

Bhugra, D., Pathare, S., Nardodkar, R., Gosavi, C., Ng, R., Torales, J., & Ventriglio, A. (2016). Legislative provisions related to marriage and divorce of persons with mental health problems: A global review. *International Review of Psychiatry, 28*(4), 386–392. https://doi.org/10.1080/09540261.2016.1210577

Bos, A. E., Pryor, J. B., Reeder, G. D., & Stutterheim, S. E. (2013). Stigma: Advances in theory and research. *Basic and Applied Social Psychology, 35*(1), 1–9. https://doi.org/10.1080/01973533.2012.746147

Boyd, J. E., Katz, E. P., Link, B. G., & Phelan, J. C. (2010). The relationship of multiple aspects of stigma and personal contact with someone hospitalized for mental illness, in a nationally representative sample. *Social Psychiatry and Psychiatric Epidemiology, 45*(11), 1063–1070. https://doi.org/10.1007/s00127-009-0147-9

Boyd, J. E., Otilingam, P. G., & Deforge, B. R. (2014). Brief version of the Internalized Stigma of Mental Illness (ISMI) scale: Psychometric properties and relationship to depression, self-esteem, recovery orientation, empowerment and perceived devaluation and discrimination. *Psychiatric Rehabilitation Journal, 3,* 17–23. https://doi.org/10.1037/prj0000035

Brown, S. A. (2008). Factors and measurement of mental illness stigma: A psychometric examination of the Attribution Questionnaire. *Psychiatric Rehabilitation Journal, 32*(2), 89–94. https://doi.org/10.2975/32.2.2008.89.94

Burstow, B. (2015). *Psychiatry and the business of madness: An ethical and epistemological accounting.* Palgrave Macmillan.

Burton, Z., & Hofmeister, E. (Creators). (2021). *The manic monologues* [Interactive Online Studio]. McCarter Theatre Center.

Carrara, B. S., Sanches, M., Bobbili, S. J., de Godoy Costa, S., de Sousa, Á. F. L., de Souza, J., & Ventura, C. A. A. (2023).

Validation of the Opening Minds Scale for Health Care Providers (OMS-HC): Factor structure and psychometric properties of the Brazilian version. *Healthcare, 11*(7), 1–14. https://doi.org/10.3390/healthcare11071049

Carrot Salmon. (2021). *Amazing adventure against stigma* [Web-based Video Game]. https://www.carrotsalmon.com/projects/antistigma

Chan, K. K. S., & Tsui, J. K. C. (2023). Longitudinal impact of experienced discrimination on mental health among people with mental disorders. *Psychiatry Research, 322,* 115099. https://doi.org/10.1016/j.psychres.2023.115099

Chinook Fund. (n.d.). *4 I's of oppression.* https://chinookfund.org/wp-content/uploads/2015/10/Supplemental-Information-for-Funding-Guidelines.pdf

Clement, S., Schauman, O., Graham, T., Maggioni, F., Evans-Lacko, S., Bezborodovs, N., Morgan, C., Rüsch, J., Brown, S. L., & Thornicroft, G. (2014). What is the impact of mental health-related stigma on help-seeking? A systematic review of quantitative and qualitative studies. *Psychological Medicine, 45*(1), 11–27. https://doi.org/10.1017/S0033291714000129

Collins, P. Y., Von Unger, H., & Armbrister, A. (2008). Church ladies, good girls, and locas: Stigma and the intersection of gender, ethnicity, mental illness, and sexuality in relation to HIV risk. *Social Science Medicine, 67,* 389–397. https://doi.org/10.1016/j.socscimed.2008.03.013

Corbiere, M., Zaniboni, S., Lecomte, T., Bond, G., Gilles, P. Y., & Lesage, A. (2011). Job acquisition for people with severe mental illness enrolled in supported employment programs: A theoretically grounded empirical study. *Journal of Occupational Rehabilitation, 21*(3), 342–354. https://doi.org/10.1007/s10926-011-9315-3

Corrigan, P. (2008). *A toolkit for evaluating programs meant to erase the stigma of mental illness.* https://www.montefiore.org/documents/Evaluating-Programs-Meant-to-Erase-the-Stigma-of-Mental-Illness.pdf

Corrigan, P. W., Druss, B. G., & Perlick, D. A. (2014). The impact of mental illness stigma on seeking and participating in mental health care. *Psychological Science in the Public Interest, 15*(2), 37–70. https://doi.org/10.1177/1529100614531398

Corrigan, P. W., Larson, J., & Rusch, N. (2009). Self-stigma and the "why try" effect: Impact on life goals and evidence-based practices. *World Psychiatry, 8,* 75–81. https://doi.org/10.1002/j.2051-5545.2009.tb00218.x

Corrigan, P. W., Lurie, B. D., Goldman, H. H., Slopen, N., Medasani, K., & Phelan, S. (2005). How adolescents perceive the stigma of mental illness and alcohol abuse. *Psychiatric Services, 56*(5), 544–550. https://doi.org/10.1176/appi.ps.56.5.544

Corrigan, P. W., Michaels, P. J., Vega, E., Gause, M., Watson, A. C., & Rusch, N. (2012). Self-Stigma of Mental Illness Scale—Short form: Reliability and validity. *Psychiatric Research, 199*(1), 65–69. https://doi.org/10.1016/j.psychres.2012.04.009

Corrigan, P. W., Roe, D., & Tsang, W. (2011). *Challenging the stigma of mental illness: Lessons for therapists and advocates.* John Wiley and Sons. https://doi.org/10.1002/9780470977507

Corrigan, P. W., Rowan, D., Green, A., Lundin, R., River, P., Uphoff-Wasowski, K., White, K., & Kubiak, M. A. (2002). Challenging two mental illness stigmas: Personal responsibility and dangerousness. *Schizophrenia Bulletin, 28*(2), 293–309. https://doi.org/10.1093/oxfordjournals.schbul.a006939

Corrigan, P. W., & Shapiro, J. R. (2010). Measuring the impact of programs that challenge the public stigma of mental illness. *Clinical Psychology Review, 30*(8), 907–922. https://doi.org/10.1016/j.cpr.2010.06.004

Corrigan, P. W., Sokol, K. A., & Rusch, N. (2013). The impact of self-stigma and mutual help programs on the quality of life of people with serious mental illnesses. *Community Mental Health Journal, 49*(1), 1–6. https://doi.org/10.1007/s10597-011-9445-2

Corrigan, P. W., Watson, A. C., & Barr, L. (2006). The self-stigma of mental illness: Implications for self-esteem and self-efficacy. *Journal of Social and Clinical Psychology, 25*(8), 875–884. https://doi.org/10.1521/jscp.2006.25.8.875

Corrigan, P. W., Watson, A. C., Warpinski, A. C., & Gracia, G. (2004). Stigmatizing attitudes about mental illness and allocation of resources to mental health services. *Community Mental Health Journal, 40*(4), 297–307. https://doi.org/10.1023/B:COMH.0000035226.19939.76

Crowe, M. (2020). Constructing normality: A discourse analysis of the *DSM-IV. Journal of Psychiatric and Mental Health Nursing, 7*(1), 69–77. https://doi.org/10.1046/j.1365-2850.2000.00261.x

Crowther, A., Taylor, A., Toney, R., Meddings, S., Whale, T., Jennings, H., Pollock, K., Bates, P., Henderson, C., Waring, J., & Slade, M. (2019). The impact of Recovery Colleges on mental health staff, services and society. *Epidemiology and Psychiatric Sciences, 28*(5), 481–488. https://doi.org/10.1017/S204579601800063X

Dalky, H. F. (2012). Perception and coping with stigma of mental illness: Arab families' perspectives. *Issues in Mental Health Nursing, 33*(7), 486e491. https://doi.org/10.3109/01612840.2012.676720

DeGue, S., Fowler, K. A., & Calkins, C. (2016). Deaths due to use of lethal force by law enforcement: Findings from the National Death Reporting System, 17 U.S. States, 2009–2012. *American Journal of Preventative Medicine, 51*(5), S173–S187. https://doi.org/10.1016/j.amepre.2016.08.027

Diamond, S. (2013). What makes us a community? Reflections on building solidarity in anti-sanist praxis. In B. A. LeFrançois, R. J. Menzies, & G. Reaume (Eds.), *Mad matters: A critical reader in Canadian mad studies* (pp. 64–77). Canadian Scholars' Press Inc.

Díaz-Mandado, O., & Periáñez, J. A. (2021). An effective psychological intervention in reducing internalized stigma and improving recovery outcomes in people with severe mental illness. *Psychiatry Research, 295,* 113635. https://doi.org/10.1016/j.psychres.2020.113635

Dobener, L. M., Fahrer, J., Purtscheller, D., Bauer, A., Paul, J. L., & Christiansen, H. (2022). How do children of parents with mental illness experience stigma? A systematic mixed studies review. *Frontiers in Psychiatry, 13,* 813519. https://doi.org/10.3389/fpsyt.2022.813519

Donnelly, C. (2017). Public attitudes toward disclosing mental health conditions. *Social Work in Mental Health, 15*(3), 588–599. https://doi.org/10.1080/15332985.2017.1302039

Drapalski, A. L., Aakre, J., Brown, C. H., Romero, E., & Lucksted, A. (2021). The Ending Self-Stigma for Posttraumatic Stress Disorder (ESS-P) program: Results of a pilot randomized trial. *Journal of Traumatic Stress, 34*(1), 69–80. https://doi.org/10.1002/jts.22593

Drapalski, A. L., Marshall, T., Seybolt, D., Medoff, D., Peer, J., Leith, J., & Dixon, L. B. (2008). Unmet needs of families of adults with mental illness and preferences regarding family services. *Psychiatric Services, 59*(6), 655–662. https://doi.org/10.1176/ps.2008.59.6.655

Dubreucq, J., Plasse, J., & Franck, N. (2021). Self-stigma in serious mental illness: A systematic review of frequency, correlates, and consequences. *Schizophrenia Bulletin, 47*(5), 1261–1287. https://doi.org/10.1093/schbul/sbaa181

Duncan, M. (2004). Promoting mental health through occupation. In R. Watson & L. Swartz (Eds.), *Transformation through occupation* (pp. 198–218). Whurr Publishers.

Durocher, E., Rappolt, S., & Gibson, B. E. (2014). Occupational justice: Future directions. *Journal of Occupational Science, 21*(4), 431–442. https//doi.org/10.1080/14427591.2013.775693

Equip for Equality. (2019). *Olmstead—20 years of community integration.* https://www.equipforequality.org/olmstead-20-years-of-community-integration

Erasing the Distance. (n.d.). *Home: What is mental illness?* https://www.erasingthedistance.org

Evans-Lacko, S., Malcolm, E., West, K., Rose, D., London, J., Rusch, N., Little, K., Henderson, C., & Thornicroft, G. (2013). Influence of Time to Change's social marketing interventions on stigma in England 2009–2011. *The British Journal of Psychiatry, 202*(Suppl. 55), S77–S88. https//doi.org/10.1192/bjp.bp.113.126672

Farias, L., Laliberte Rudman, D., & Magalhães, L. (2016). Illustrating the importance of critical epistemology to realize the promise of occupational justice. *OTJR: Occupation, Participation and Health, 36*(4), 234–243. https://doi.org/10.1177/1539449216665561

Filson, B. (2016). The haunting can end: Trauma-informed approaches in healing from abuse and adversity. In J. Russo & A. Sweeney, *Searching for a rose garden: Challenging psychiatry, fostering Mad studies* (pp. 20–24). PCCS Books.

Fireweed Collective. (n.d.). *Homepage.* https://fireweedcollective.org

Fukui, E. (2020, August 2). *Education for the people: Best practices in facilitation.* [Online Workshop] Crip Camp: The Official Virtual Experience.

Ghiasi, N., Azhar, Y., & Singh, J. (2023). Psychiatric illness and criminality. In *StatPearls*. StatPearls Publishing. https://www.ncbi.nlm.nih.gov/books/NBK537064

Goffman, E. (1963). *Stigma: Notes on the management of spoiled identity.* Prentice-Hall.

Griffiths, K. M., Carron-Arthur, B., Parsons, A., & Reid, R. (2014). Effectiveness of programs for reducing the stigma associated with mental disorders. A meta-analysis of randomized controlled trials. *World Psychiatry, 13,* 161–175. https://doi.org/10.1002/wps.20129

Groth, M., & Scoby, M. (2019). Access to occupational therapy practice: A review of current licensing processes in the United States. *Occupational Therapy Capstones,* 421. https://commons.und.edu/ot-grad/421

Harrison, E. A. (2018). Voting rights. In T. Heller, S. Parker Harris, C. Gill, & R. P. Gould (Eds.), *Disability in American life: An encyclopedia of concepts, policies, and controversies,* (pp. 698–701). Bloomsbury Publishing.

Hatzenbuehler, M. L., Bellatorre, A., Lee, Y., Finch, B. K., Muennig, P., & Fiscella, K. (2014). Structural stigma and all-cause mortality in sexual minority populations. *Social Science & Medicine, 103,* 33–41. https://doi.org/10.1016/j.socscimed.2013.06.005

Hearing Voices Network. (n.d.). *Welcome.* https://www.hearing-voices.org

Holley, L. C., Mendoza, N. S, Del-Colle, M. M., & Lynette Bernard, M. (2016). Heterosexism, racism, and mental illness discrimination: Experiences of people with mental health conditions and their families. *Journal of Gay and Lesbian Social Services, 28*(2), 93–116. https://doi.org/10.1080/10538720.2016.1155520

Institute for the Development of Human Arts. (n.d.). *Community care, not coercion.* https://www.idha-nyc.org/community-care

Johnson, M., Mills, T. L., DeLeon, J. M., Hartzema, A. G., & Haddad, J. (2009). Lives in isolation: Stories and struggles of low-income African American women with panic disorder. *CNS Neuroscience Therapy, 15,* 210–219. https://doi.org/10.1111/j.1755-5949.2009.00079.x

Jones, D. (1998). Deviance. In D. Jones, S. Blair, T. Hartery, & R. K. Jones (Eds.), *Sociology and occupational therapy: An integrated approach* (pp. 93–104). Churchill Livingstone.

Jones, J. T. R., North, C. S., Vogel-Scibilia, S., Myers, M. F., & Owen, R. R. (2018). Medical licensure questions about mental illness and compliance with the Americans with Disabilities Act. *The Journal of the American Academy of Psychiatry and the Law, 46*(4), 458–471. https://doi.org/10.29158/JAAPL.003789-18

Joo, J. H., Wittink, M., & Dahlberg, B. (2011). Shared conceptualizations and divergent experiences of counseling among African American and white older adults. *Qualitative Health Research, 21,* 1065–1074. https://doi.org/10.1177/1049732311404247

Kassam, A., Papish, A., Modgill, G., & Patten, S. (2012). The development and psychometric properties of a new scale to measure mental illness related stigma by health care providers: The Opening Minds Scale for Health Care Providers (OMS-HC). *BMC Psychiatry, 12*(1), 1–12. https://doi.org/10.1186/1471-244X-12-62

Kleinman, A. (1988). *The illness narratives: Suffering, healing and the human condition.* Basic Books.

Kopel, C. (2017). Suffrage for people with intellectual disabilities and mental illness: Observations on a civic controversy. *Yale Journal of Health Policy, Law, and Ethics, 17*(1), 209–250. https://pubmed.ncbi.nlm.nih.gov/29756757

Kosyluk, K., Marshall, J., Conner, K., Macias, D. R., Macias, S., Michelle Beekman, B., & Her, J. (2021). Challenging the stigma of mental illness through creative storytelling: A randomized controlled trial of This Is My Brave. *Community Mental Health Journal, 57*(1), 144–152. https://doi.org/10.1007/s10597-020-00625-4

Kosyluk, K., Marshall, J., Diana, R. M., Andrus, D., Guerra, D., Robinson, M., Ostos, A., & Chapman, S. (2018). Examining the impact of This Is My Brave on mental illness stigma and willingness to seek help: A pilot study. *Community Mental Health Journal, 54*(3), 276–281. https://doi.org/10.1007/s10597-018-0238-8

Larson, J. E., & Corrigan, P. (2008). The stigma of families with mental illness. *Academic Psychiatry, 32*(2), 87e91. https://doi.org/10.1176/appi.ap.32.2.87

Li, W., Dorstyn, D. S., & Denson, L. A. (2014). Psychosocial correlates of college students' help-seeking intention: A meta-analysis. *Professional Psychology: Research and Practice, 45*(3), 163–170. https://doi.org/10.1037/a0037118

Link, B. G., Cullen, F. T., Struening, E. L., Shrout, P. E., & Dohrenwend, B. P. (1989). A modified labeling theory approach to mental disorders: An empirical assessment. *American Sociological Review, 54*(3), 400–423. https://doi.org/10.2307/2095613

Link, B. G., Yang, L. H., Phelan, J. C., & Collins, P. Y. (2004). Measuring mental illness stigma. *Schizophrenia Bulletin, 30*(3), 511–541. https://doi.org/10.1093/oxfordjournals.schbul.a007098

Lucksted, A., Drapalski, A. L., Brown, C. H., Wilson, C., Charlotte, M., Mullane, A., & Fang, L. J. (2017). Outcomes of a psychoeducational intervention to reduce internalized stigma among psychosocial rehabilitation clients. *Psychiatric Services (Washington, D.C.), 68*(4), 360–367. https://doi.org/10.1176/appi.ps.201600037

Luty, J., Fekadu, D., Umoh, O., & Gallagher, J. (2006). Validation of a short instrument to measure stigmatised attitudes towards mental illness. *Psychiatric Bulletin, 30*(7), 257–260. https://doi.org/10.1192/pb.30.7.257

Magliano L. (2023). Bringing psychology students closer to people with schizophrenia at pandemic time: A study of a distance anti-stigma intervention with in-presence opportunistic control group. *Journal of Psychosocial Rehabilitation and Mental Health, 10,* 287–299. https://doi.org/10.1007/s40737-022-00308-1

Martin, J. K., Lang, A., & Olafsdottir, S. (2008). Rethinking theoretical approaches to stigma: Framework Integrating Normative Influences on Stigma (FINIS). *Social Science Medicine, 67*(3), 431–440. https://doi.org/10.1016/j.socscimed.2008.03.018

McAllister, A., Burström, B., & Corrigan, P. (2021). Cultural adaptation and validation of the Attribution Questionnaire for stigma towards disability pension applicants for use among psychiatrists and general practitioners in Sweden. *BMC Psychology, 9*(1), 27. https://doi.org/10.1186/s40359-021-00523-8

Mental Health Commission of Canada. (n.d.). *Opening minds.* https://www.mentalhealthcommission.ca/English/initiatives/11874/opening-minds

Menzies, R., LeFrançois, B., & Reaume, G. (2013). Introducing Mad studies. In B. A. LeFrançois, R. J. Menzies, & G. Reaume (Eds.), *Mad matters: A critical reader in Canadian Mad studies* (pp. 1–22). Canadian Scholars' Press Inc.

Mestdagh, A., & Hansen, B. (2014). Stigma in patients with schizophrenia receiving community mental health care: A review of qualitative studies. *Social Psychiatry and Psychiatric Epidemiology, 49*(1), 79–87. https://doi.org/10.1007/s00127-013-0729-4

Michaels, P. J., Corrigan, P. W., Buchholz, B., Brown, J., Arthur, T., Netter, C., & MacDonald-Wilson, K. L. (2014). Changing stigma through a consumer-based stigma reduction program. *Community Mental Health Journal, 50*(4), 395–401. https://doi.org/10.1007/s10597-013-9628-0

Miller Polgar, J., & Landry, J. E. (2004). Occupations as a means for individual and group participation in life. In C. H. Christiansen

& E. Townsend (Eds.), *Introduction to occupation: The art and science of living* (pp. 197–220). Prentice Hall.

Mills, H., Mulfinger, N., Raeder, S., Rüsch, N., Clements, H., & Scior, K. (2020). Self-help interventions to reduce self-stigma in people with mental health problems: A systematic literature review. *Psychiatry Research, 284,* 112702. https://doi.org/10.1016/j.psychres.2019.112702

MindFreedom International. (2006, August 28). *Personal stories.* https://mindfreedom.org/front-page/personal-stories

Misra, S., Jackson, V. W., Chong, J., Choe, K., Tay, C., Wong, J., & Yang, L. H. (2021). Systematic review of cultural aspects of stigma and mental illness among racial and ethnic minority groups in the United States: Implications for interventions. *American Journal of Community Psychology, 68*(3-4), 486–512. https://doi.org/10.1002/ajcp.12516

Modgill, G., Patten, S. B., Knaak, S., Kassam, A., & Szeto, A. C. (2014). Opening Minds Stigma Scale for Health Care Providers (OMS-HC): Examination of psychometric properties and responsiveness. *BMC Psychiatry, 14*(120), 1–10. https://doi.org/10.1186/1471-244X-14-120

Morrison, A. P., Birchwood, M., Pyle, M., Flach, C., Stewart, S. L., Byrne, R., Patterson, P., Jones, P. B., Fowler, D., Gumley, A. I., & French, P. (2013). Impact of cognitive therapy on internalised stigma in people with at-risk mental states. *British Journal of Psychiatry, 203*(2), 140–145. https://doi.org/10.1192/bjp.bp.112.123703

Muñoz, M., Guillén, A. I., Pérez-Santos, E., & Corrigan, P. W. (2015). A structural equation modeling study of the Spanish Mental Illness Stigma Attribution Questionnaire (AQ-27-E). *American Journal of Orthopsychiatry, 85*(3), 243–249. https://doi.org/10.1037/ort0000059

Muralidharan, A., Lucksted, A., Medoff, D., Fang, L. J., & Dixon, L. (2014). Stigma: A unique source of distress for family members of individuals with mental illness. *Journal of Behavioral Health Services & Research, 43*(3), 484–493. https://doi.org/10.1007/s11414-014-9437-4

National Alliance on Mental Illness. (n.d.-a). *Share your story.* https://www.nami.org/Get-Involved/Share-Your-Story

National Alliance on Mental Illness. (n.d.-b). *Stigma free.* https://www.nami.org/Get-Involved/Pledge-to-Be-StigmaFree

Newman, A., & Fitzsimmons, E. G. (2022, December 14). New York City to involuntarily remove mentally ill people from streets. *The New York Times.* https://www.nytimes.com/2022/11/29/nyregion/nyc-mentally-ill-involuntary-custody.html

Nurser, K., Hunt, D., & Bartlett, T. (2017). Do Recovery College courses help to improve recovery outcomes and reduce self-stigma for individuals who attend? *Clinical Psychology, 300,* 32–37. https://doi.org/10.53841/bpscpf.2017.1.300.32

Oexle, N., Ajdacic-Gross, V., Kilian, R., Müller, M., Rodgers, S., Xu, Z., Rössler, W., & Rüsch, N. (2017). Mental illness stigma, secrecy and suicidal ideation. *Epidemiology and Psychiatric Sciences, 26*(1), 53–60. https://doi.org/10.1017/S2045796015001018

Oexle, N., Waldmann, T., Staiger, T., Xu, Z., & Rüsch, N. (2018). Mental illness stigma and suicidality: The role of public and individual stigma. *Epidemiology and Psychiatric Sciences, 27*(2), 169–175. https://doi.org/10.1017/S2045796016000949

Öri, D., Rózsa, S., Szocsics, P., Simon, L., Purebl, G., & Győrffy, Z. (2020). Factor structure of the Opening Minds Stigma Scale for Health Care Providers and psychometric properties of its Hungarian version. *BMC Psychiatry, 20,* 1–9. https://doi.org/10.1186/s12888-020-02902-8

Østerud, K. L. (2023). Mental illness stigma and employer evaluation in hiring: Stereotypes, discrimination and the role of experience. *Sociology of Health & Illness, 45*(1), 90–108. https://doi.org/10.1111/1467-9566.13544

Parcesepe, A. M., & Cabassa, L. J. (2013). Public stigma of mental illness in the United States: A systematic literature review. *Administration and Policy in Mental Health and Mental Health*

Services Research, 40(5), 384–399. https://doi.org/10.1007/s10488-012-0430-z

Park, S., & Park, K. S. (2014). Family stigma: A concept analysis. *Asian Nursing Research, 8,* 165–171. https://doi.org/10.1016/j.anr.2014.02.006

Patten, S. B., Remillard, A., Phillips, L., Modgill, G., Szeto, A., Kassam, A., & Gardner, D. M. (2012). Effectiveness of contact-based education for reducing mental illness-related stigma in pharmacy students. *BMC Medical Education, 12,* 120. https://doi.org/10.1186/1472-6920-12-120

Pescosolido, B. A. (2013). The public stigma of mental illness: What do we think; What do we know; What can we prove? *Journal of Health and Social Behavior, 54*(1), 1–21. https://doi.org/10.1177/0022146512471197

Pingani, L., Forghieri, M., Ferrari, S., Ben-Zeev, D., Artoni, P., Mazzi, F., Palmieri, G., Rigatelli, M., & Corrigan, P. W. (2012). Stigma and discrimination toward mental illness: Translation and validation of the Italian version of the Attribution Questionnaire-27 (AQ-27-I). *Social Psychiatry and Psychiatric Epidemiology, 47*(6), 993–999. https://doi.org/10.1007/s00127-011-0407-3

Pinto, M. D., Hickman, R., Logsdon, M. C., & Burant, C. (2012). Psychometric evaluation of the revised Attribution Questionnaire (r-AQ) to measure mental illness stigma in adolescents. *Journal of Nursing Measurement, 20*(1), 47–58. https://doi.org/10.1891/1061-3749.20.1.47

Pirutinsky, S., Rosen, D. D., Shapiro Safran, R., & Rosmarin, D. H. (2010). Do medical models of mental illness relate to increased or decreased stigmatization of mental illness among orthodox Jews? *The Journal of Nervous and Mental Disease, 198*(7), 508–512. https://doi.org/10.1097/NMD.0b013e3181e07d99

Project LETS. (2021). *Our mission.* https://projectlets.org/mission

Pryor, J. B., & Reeder, G. D. (2011). HIV-related stigma. In J. C. Hall, B. J. Hall, & C. J. Cockerell (Eds.), *HIV/AIDS in the post-HAART era: Manifestations, treatment, and epidemiology* (pp. 790–806). PMPH-USA.

Reupert, A., Gladstone, B., Helena Hine, R., Yates, S., McGaw, V., Charles, G., Drost, L., & Foster, K. (2021). Stigma in relation to families living with parental mental illness: An integrative review. *International Journal of Mental Health Nursing, 30*(1), 6–26. https://doi.org/10.1111/inm.12820

Ritsher, J. B., Otilingam, P. G., & Grajales, M. (2003). Internalized Stigma of Mental Illness: Psychometric properties of a new measure. *Psychiatry Research, 121*(1), 31–49. https://doi.org/10.1016/j.psychres.2003.08.008

Ritsher, J. B., & Phelan, J. C. (2004). Internalized stigma predicts erosion of morale among psychiatric outpatients. *Psychiatry Research, 129*(3), 257–265. https://doi.org/10.1016/j.psychres.2004.08.003

Roe, D., Hasson-Ohayon, I., Mashiach-Eizenberg, M., Derhy, O., Lysaker, P. H., & Yanos, P. T. (2014). Narrative Enhancement and Cognitive Therapy (NECT) effectiveness: A quasi experimental study. *Journal of Clinical Psychology, 70*(4), 303–312. https://doi.org/10.1002/jclp.22050

Rüsch, N., & Kösters, M. (2021). Honest, open, proud to support disclosure decisions and to decrease stigma's impact among people with mental illness: Conceptual review and meta-analysis of program efficacy. *Social Psychiatry and Psychiatric Epidemiology, 56,* 1513–1526. https://doi.org/10.1007/s00127-021-02076-y

Sapag, J. C., Klabunde, R., Villarroel, L., Velasco, P. R., Álvarez, C., Parra, C., Bobbili, S. J., Mascayano, F., Bustamante, I., Alvarado, R., & Corrigan, P. (2019). Validation of the Opening Minds Scale and patterns of stigma in Chilean primary health care. *PLoS One, 14*(9), 1–14. https://doi.org/10.1371/journal.pone.0221825

Shadravan, S. M., Matthew, L. E., & Vinson, S. Y. (2021). Dying at the intersections: Police-involved killings of Black people with mental illness. *Psychiatric Services, 72*(6), 623–625. https://doi.org/10.1176/appi.ps.202000942

Shahwan, S., Goh, C. M. J., Tan, G. T. H., Ong, W. J., Chong, S. A., & Subramaniam, M. (2022). Strategies to reduce mental illness stigma: Perspectives of people with lived experience and caregivers. *International Journal of Environmental Research and Public Health, 19*(3), 1632. https://doi.org/10.3390/ijerph19031632

Shamsaei, F., & Holtforth, M. G. (2020). Development and psychometric testing of the Stigma Assessment Tool for Family Caregivers of People with Mental Illness. *East Asian Archives of Psychiatry, 30*(3), 73–78. https://doi.org/10.12809/eaap1938

Sibitz, I., Provaznikova, K., Lipp, M., Lakeman, R., & Amering, M. (2013). The impact of recovery-oriented day clinic treatment on internalized stigma: Preliminary report. *Psychiatry Research, 209*(3), 326–332. https://doi.org/10.1016/j.psychres.2013.02.001

Silverman, M. J. (2013). Effects of music therapy on self- and experienced stigma in patients on an acute care psychiatric unit: A randomized three group effectiveness study. *Archives of Psychiatric Nursing, 27*(5), 223–230. https://doi.org/10.1016/j.apnu.2013.06.003

Sousa, S. D., Marques, A., Rosário, C., & Queirós, C. (2012). Stigmatizing attitudes in relatives of people with schizophrenia: A study using the Attribution Questionnaire AQ-27. *Trends in Psychiatry and Psychotherapy, 34*(4), 186–197. https://doi.org/10.1590/s2237-60892012000400004

Spears, B. (2023). *The woman in me.* Galaxy Books.

Starkman, M. (2013). The movement. In B. A. LeFrançois, R. J. Menzies, & G. Reaume (Eds.), *Mad matters: A critical reader in Canadian Mad studies* (pp. 27–37). Canadian Scholars' Press Inc.

St. Louis, K. O., & Roberts, P. M. (2013). Public attitudes toward mental illness in Africa and North America. *African Journal of Psychiatry, 16*(2), 123–133. https://doi.org/10.4314/ajpsy.v16i2.16

Substance Abuse and Mental Health Services Administration. (2015). *More Americans continue to receive mental health services, but substance use treatments remain low.* https://www.samhsa.gov/newsroom/press-announcements/201509170900

Substance Abuse and Mental Health Services Administration. (2021). *Results for the 2021 national survey on drug use and health: Graphics from the key findings report.* https://www.samhsa.gov/data/sites/default/files/reports/rpt39443/2021_NNR_figure_slides.pdf

Susman, J. (1994). Disability, stigma and deviance. *Social Science Medicine, 38*(1), 15–22. https://doi.org/10.1016/0277-9536(94)90295-X

Świtaj, P., Grygiel, P., Krzyżanowska-Zbucka, J., Sonik, J., Chrostek, A., Jahołkowski, P., Wciórka, J., & Anczewska, M. (2019). The evaluation of the impact of anti-stigma training led by "experts by experience" on participants' attitudes towards persons with mental illness. *Psychiatria Polska, 53*(6), 1219–1236. https://doi.org/10.12740/PP/109818

The Icarus Project. (2015). *Madness and oppression: Paths to personal transformation and collective liberation.* Creative Commons. https://fireweedcollective.org/wp-content/uploads/2018/11/MadnessAndOppressionGuide.pdf

Thériault, J., Lord, M. M., Briand, C., Piat, M., & Meddings, S. (2020). Recovery Colleges after a decade of research: A literature review. *Psychiatric Services, 71*(9), 928–940. https://doi.org/10.1176/appi.ps.201900352

This Is My Brave. (n.d.). *Homepage.* https://thisismybrave.org

Thornicroft, G. (2006). *Shunned: Discrimination against people with mental illness.* Oxford University Press.

Tsang, H. W. W., Ching, S. C., Tang, K. H., Lam, H. T., Law, P. Y. Y., & Wan, C. N. (2016). Therapeutic intervention for internalized stigma of severe mental illness: A systematic review and meta-analysis. *Schizophrenia Research, 173*, 45–53. https://doi.org/10.1016/j.schres.2016.02.013

Turner, V. W. (1969). *The ritual process: Structure and anti-structure.* Cornell University Press.

Turosak, A., & Siwierka, J. (2021). Mental health and stigma on campus: Insights from students' lived experience. *Journal of Prevention & Intervention in the Community, 49*(3), 266–281. https://doi.org/10.1080/10852352.2019.1654264

Vermont Psychiatric Survivors, Inc. (2018, May 7). *What is sanism?* [Feed Post]. Facebook. https://www.facebook.com/VermontPsychiatricSurvivors/photos/a.1861132230617777/1890353577695642

Vigo, D., Thornicroft, G., & Altun, R. (2016). Estimating the true global burden of mental illness. *The Lancet Psychiatry, 3*(2), 171–178. https://doi.org/10.1016/S2215-0366(15)00505-2

Walker, A. M., Klein, M. S., Hemmens, C., Stohr, M. K., & Burton, V. S., Jr. (2016). The consequences of official labels: An examination of the rights lost by the mentally ill and mentally incompetent since 1989. *Community Mental Health Journal, 52*(3), 272–280. https://doi.org/10.1007/s10597-015-9941-x

Wasmuth, S., Pritchard, K. T., & Belkiewitz, J. (2022). Bridging the humanities and health care with theatre: Theory and outcomes of a theatre-based model for enhancing psychiatric care via stigma reduction. *Psychiatric Rehabilitation Journal, 46*(4), 285–292. https://doi.org/10.1037/prj0000551

Watson, A. C., Otey, E., Westbrook, A. L., Gardner, A. L., Lamb, T. A., Corrigan, P. W., & Fenton, W. S. (2004). Changing middle schoolers' attitudes about mental illness through education. *Schizophrenia Bulletin, 30*(3), 563–572. https://doi.org/10.1093/oxfordjournals.schbul.a007100

Werner, P., Goldstein, D., & Heinik, J. (2011). Development and validity of the family stigma in Alzheimer's disease scale (FS-ADS). *Alzheimer Disease and Associated Disorders, 25*(1), 42–48. https://doi.org/10.1097/WAD.0b013e3181f32594

Werner, S., Corrigan, P., Ditchman, N., & Sokol, K. (2012). Stigma and intellectual disability: A review of related measures and future directions. *Research in Developmental Disabilities, 33*(2), 748–765. https://doi.org/10.1016/j.ridd.2011.10.009

Whiteford, H. A., Buckingham, W. J., Harris, M. G., Burgess, P. M., Pirkis, J. E., Barendregt, J. J., & Hall, W. D. (2013). Estimating treatment rates for mental disorders in Australia. *Australian Health Review, 38*(1), 80–85. https://doi.org/10.1071/AH13142

Wilcock, A. A., & Hocking, C. (2015). An occupational justice perspective of health. In A. A. Wilcock & C. Hocking (Eds.), *An occupational perspective of health* (pp. 390–419). Thorofare, NJ: Slack, Inc.

Wolfensberger, W. (1972). *The principle of normalisation in human services.* National Institute on Mental Retardation.

Wolfensberger, W. (1984). A reconceptualisation of normalisation as social role valorisation. *Mental Retardation, 34*, 22–25.

Wolframe, P. M. (2013). The madwoman in the academy, or, revealing the invisible straightjacket: Theorizing and teaching saneism and sane privilege. *Disability Studies Quarterly (Disability and Madness), 33*(1). https://doi.org/10.18061/dsq.v33i1.3425

World Health Organization. (2001). *International classification of functioning, disability, and health.* Author.

World Health Organization. (2023). *Mental health.* https://www.who.int/europe/health-topics/mental-health#tab=tab_1

Yang, L. H., Kleinman, A., Link, B. G., Phelan, J. C., Lee, S., & Good, B. (2007). Culture and stigma: Adding moral experience to stigma theory. *Social Science Medicine, 64*, 1524–1535. https://doi.org/10.1016/j.socscimed.2006.11.013

Yang, L. H., Purdie-Vaughns, V., Kotabe, H., Link, B. G., Saw, A., Wong, G., & Phelan, J. C. (2013). Culture, threat, and mental illness stigma: Identifying culture-specific threat among Chinese American groups. *Social Science Medicine, 88*, 56–67. https://doi.org/10.1016/j.socscimed.2013.03.036

Yang, L. H., Thornicroft, G., Alvarado, R., Vega, E., & George, B. (2014). Recent advances in cross-cultural measurement in psychiatric epidemiology: Utilizing "what matters most" to identify culture-specific aspects of stigma. *International Journal of Epidemiology, 43*(2), 494–510. https://doi.org/10.1093/ije/dyu039

Yanos, P. T., DeLuca, J. S., Salyers, M. P., Fischer, M. W., Song, J., & Caro, J. (2020). Cross-sectional and prospective correlates of associative stigma among mental health service providers. *Psychiatric Rehabilitation Journal, 43*(2), 85–90. https://doi.org/10.1037/prj0000378

Yanos, P. T., Roe, D., West, M. L., Smith, S. M., & Lysaker, P. H. (2012). Group-based treatment for internalized stigma among persons with severe mental illness: Findings from a randomized controlled trial. *Psychological Services, 9*(3), 248–258. https://doi .org/10.1037/a0028048

Ye, J., Chen, T. F., Paul, D., McCahon, R., Shankar, S., Rosen, A., & O'Reily, C. L. (2016). Stigma and discrimination experienced by people living with severe and persistent mental illness in assertive community treatment settings. *International Journal of Social Psychiatry, 62*(6), 532–541. https://doi.org/10.1177 /0020764016651459

Yu, B. C. L., Chio, F. H. N., Mak, W. W. S., Corrigan, P. W., & Chan, K. K. Y. (2021). Internalization process of stigma of people with mental illness across cultures: A meta-analytic structural equation modeling approach. *Clinical Psychology Review, 87,* 102029. https://doi.org/10.1016/j.cpr.2021.102029

Zuaboni, G., Elmer, T., Rabenschlag, F., Heumann, K., Jaeger, S., Kozel, B., Mahlke, C. I., Theodoridou, A., Jaeger, M., & Rüsch, N. (2021). Psychometric evaluation of the German version of the Opening Minds Stigma Scale for Health Care Providers (OMS-HC). *BMC Psychology, 9*(86), 1–7. https://doi.org/10.1186 /s40359-021-00592-9

28 Social Determinants and Mental Health

Jaime Phillip Muñoz and Meghan Blaskowitz

A significant proportion of occupational therapy education and training, particularly in the United States and other Global North countries, is dedicated to addressing occupational performance challenges at the person level. This is essential learning. It is undeniable that occupational therapy interventions directed at an individual level are critically important, but Person-Environment-Occupation (PEO) and other practice models in occupational therapy emphasize the dynamic interaction of the person with their environment through their occupations (Baum et al., 2015; Law et al., 1996; Townsend & Polatajko, 2007). Practice frameworks in the United States (American Occupational Therapy Association [AOTA], 2020b), Canada (Polatajko et al., 2013), and Australia (Australian Health Practitioner Regulation Agency, 2018), as well as the World Federation of Occupational Therapists (WFOT) educational standards (WFOT, 2016), all include social context as a critical occupational therapy domain that affects occupation, health, and well-being. The research evidence that social factors impact health and wellness and create and sustain health inequities is plentiful and irrefutable (Lucyk & McLaren, 2017; Islam, 2019; World Health Organization [WHO], 2023).

This chapter focuses on social context. It examines how social determinants of health (SDOH)—the conditions in which people are born, grow, live, learn, love, work, and age—can shape health and mental health outcomes, and how social forces and systemic and structural injustices shape these conditions and limit opportunities for occupation. In this chapter, the terminology "social drivers of health" is used; a bit later, the chapter provides explanations about how this terminology shifts one's perspective on one's ability to control these factors. The chapter explores the impact of these social drivers on mental health and provides examples of how these drivers influence the transactional processes between person, environment, and occupation. From this point on, to avoid any confusion between determinants and drivers, the acronym SDOH is used to refer to social drivers of health. The chapter then presents theoretical constructs and frameworks that support establishment of a therapeutic alliance and guide therapeutic reasoning and practices related to health equity and addressing SDOH. The chapter closes by proposing actions and processes OTPs can take part in to advance diversity, justice, equity, inclusion, and accessibility.

Socioenvironmental Factors Impacting Health

In this textbook, mental health is discussed as existing on a continuum. Mental health anchors one end of this continuum and mental illness the other. An individual can be at any point on this continuum and one's position can shift as one's circumstances improve or deteriorate. Markers on the continuum in Figure 28-1 primarily identify person-oriented indicators such as a person's mood, sleep, physical and social activity, behavior, and cognitive functioning. However, a person's mental health cannot be fully understood or influenced if it is isolated from the socioenvironmental forces and contexts that shape and sustain mental health. Practitioners must absolutely consider diagnosis and medical conditions in their practice, but if social, economic, and political factors of the environments where a person lives, loves, learns, and works are not considered, then an OTP's ability to maintain a holistic perspective of the person and understand the relationship between occupation, justice, inclusion, and health will be limited (AOTA, 2023b; Bailliard, 2023; Hammell, 2021; Lysack et al., 2023).

In the United States, and internationally, framing how to prevent, understand, and address ill health has long been dominated by a focus on individual behavior and biology. For example, the *Diagnostic and Statistical Manual of Mental Disorders,* Fifth Edition, Text Revision (*DSM-5-TR;* American Psychiatric Association [APA], 2022) and the *International Classification of Diseases,* 11th Edition (*ICD-11;* WHO, 2019) both use symptomatology to classify the immense diversity of human emotion, behavior, and relationships to create discrete categories of mental illness. These medicalized systems of diagnostic labeling routinely locate the causes of psychological conditions in the brain, underlying organic pathologies, genetics, and biochemical processes of the individual; at the same time, they focus less attention on symbolic systems of the mind or the socioenvironmental conditions that impact mental health and well-being (Fisher, 2022; Johnstone et al., 2018; Kotov et al., 2021). Certainly, behaviors such as smoking, using alcohol and drugs, diet, and exercise are important individual behaviors to address, but concentrating the gaze on individual behaviors limits a health professional's ability to question and understand behavior in context. Context matters!

Continuum of Care in Mental Health

Crisis	Struggling	Surviving	Thriving	Excelling
• Very anxious • Severely depressed • Detached from reality • Safety concerns • Poor sleep • Decreased ADLs • Getting through the day-to-day is taxing • Disengaged • Numb	• Anxious • Depressed • Tired • Safety risks still may be present • Poor sleep and low appetite • Decreased ADLs • Slow • Engagement is a struggle	• Worried/nervous • Sad • Irritable • Distracted • Withdrawn • Difficulty engaging in ADLs, IADLs, and meaningful occupations • Barriers with lifestyle balance	• Positive • Calm • Sleeping and eating well • Acceptance • Meaning in narrative, roles, and occupations • Purpose • Commitment to recovery • Social connections	• Cheerful • Connected to self, others, and environments of choice • Focused attention • Meaning in doing • Balance between enjoyment and mundane stressors • Enjoyment in everyday life

FIGURE 28-1. Continuum of care in mental health. *Adapted and informed by the following sources: Delphis. (2020, June 30). The mental health continuum is a better model for mental health. https://delphis.org.uk/ mental-health/continuum-mental-health; Merryman, M. B., & Riegel, S. K. (2007). The recovery process and people with serious mental illness living in the community: An occupational therapy perspective.* Occupational Therapy in Mental Health, 23(2), 51–73. https://doi.org/10.1300/J004v23n02_03; Spaniol, L., & Wewiorski, N. J. (2012). *Phases of the recovery process from psychiatric disabilities.* International Journal of Psychosocial Rehabilitation, 17(1), 116–133. Sutton, D. J., Hocking, C. S., & Smythe, L. A. (2012). *A phenomenological study of occupational engagement in recovery from mental illness.* Canadian Journal of Occupational Therapy, 79(3), 142–150. https:// doi.org/10.2182/cjot.2012.79.3.3

A 2008 WHO final report titled *Health Equity Through Action on the Social Determinants of Health* provided early impetus to consider the impact of context on health. This report defined **social determinants of health (SDOH)** as nonmedical factors impacting health outcomes, examined evidence for the relationships between these factors and health, and defined initial strategies to promote **health equity** (WHO, 2008). In this WHO report, factors such as nutrition, education, employment, and living environment were identified as social determinants and were believed to apply to nearly everyone. Since this initial 2008 WHO report, research on social determinants has grown exponentially (Islam, 2019; Lucyk & McLaren, 2017). In addition, researchers have identified factors related to health equity for specific populations (Kim, 2019) or conditions (Jeste et al., 2022; WHO, 2023) including social determinants specifically impacting mental health (Alegría et al., 2018; Kallivayalil & Enara, 2022). This broader set of SDOH and the forces that sustain health inequity are presented in Figure 28-2. Notably, occupation is not listed as an SDOH; however, OTPs would agree that one's ability to participate in meaningful activities affects one's ability to thrive.

A holistic PEO approach requires OTPs to consider that each person they encounter in therapy is embedded in a set of complex social, political, economic, and cultural systems that influence every aspect of that individual's social identities, health, and well-being (Hammell, 2017b). An OTP must consider whether the person referred for service is someone who has experienced trauma, poverty, racism, homophobia, domestic violence, or adverse childhood experiences (ACEs), or is someone who lives in an area with high concentrations of crime, pollution, unemployment, political oppression, or which lacks any green spaces (Galvaan, 2015; Hammell & Beagan, 2017; Martín et al., 2015). Each of these contextual features is increasingly recognized as a factor that can contribute to psychological distress that ultimately impacts a person's opportunity for occupation and ability to achieve desired occupational performance outcomes (Fisher, 2022; Kotov et al., 2021; Office of Disease Prevention and Health Promotion, n.d.).

Social Drivers (Determinants) of Health

Public health researchers have increasingly recognized that a person's risk for physical and/or psychiatric disability is less associated with individual factors and much more likely caused by a person's exposure to social and economic inequities and a unique set of SDOH present from birth (Artiga, 2020; Froehlich-Grobe et al., 2021; Schillinger, 2020). As displayed in Figure 28-2, the list of socioenvironmental factors impacting health has grown to include factors such as socioeconomic status (SES), housing, education, health services/ insurance, the physical environment, food security, and systemic and structural inequities such as racism, sexism, and homophobia.

Although many of these factors are out of a person's control, they have enormous impact on an individual's physical and mental health. These factors significantly influence individual and group differences in health status, and a lifetime of poor SDOH can lead to a myriad of physical and mental health disparities. Multiple studies find that SDOH are the main "drivers" of health status, accounting for 45% to 60%

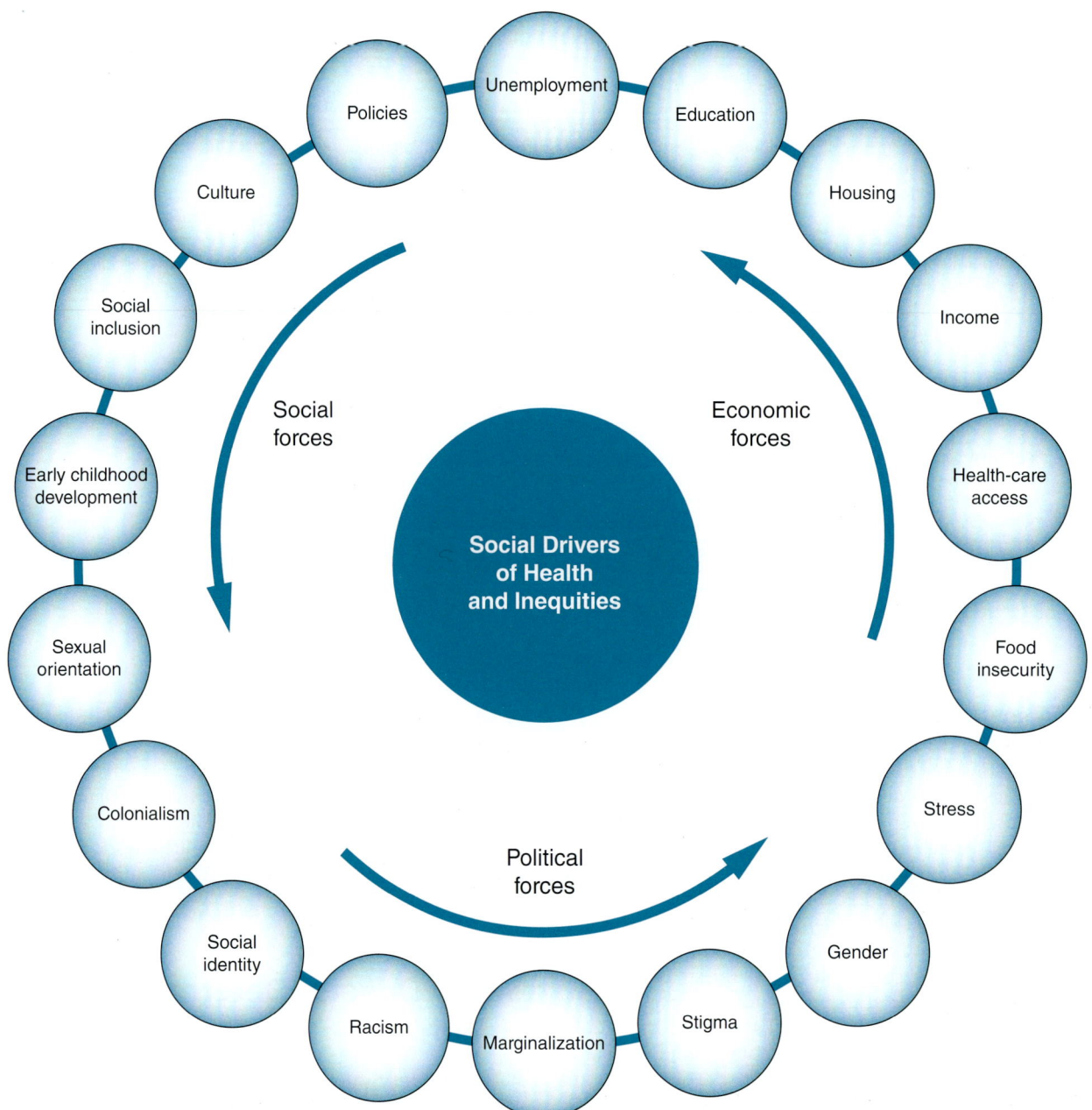

FIGURE 28-2. Social drivers (determinants) of health and inequities.

of a person's risk for illness or disability (Centers for Disease Control and Prevention [CDC], 2022; Drake & Rudowitz, 2022; Froehlich-Grobe et al., 2021; Schillinger, 2020; U.S. Department of Health & Human Services [USDHHS], 2023; Whitman et al., 2022).

The USDHHS recently proposed that social and environmental conditions be referred to as **social drivers of health** (Sheingold et al., 2022; USDHHS, 2024). The term "determinants" can lead to a perception that nothing can be done to change one's trajectory; poor health is fate. Using the term "drivers" helps to reframe perspectives to underscore that people, communities, and indeed whole societies have control and can implement systemic changes to address these SDOH (AOTA, 2023b; Office of the Assistant Secretary

for Planning and Evaluation [ASPE], 2023; Elevance Health, 2022). Table 28-1 identifies many SDOH and uses the five domains defined by the U.S. Office of Disease Prevention and Health Promotion to organize these factors. The examples presented in this table are frequently listed across these key domains, but some diversity exists related to specific contexts in different countries (USDHHS, 2024). For example, SDOH defined by the Canadian government also list factors within the person, their environment, and in and outside the health-care system, and specifically include racism (Public Health Agency of Canada, 2023). In India, demographic factors such as gender identity and inequality, racism, sexual orientation, and immigration status are specifically identified as SDOH (Chelak & Chakole, 2023).

TABLE 28-1 | Social Drivers of Health

Neighborhood and Built Environment	Health-Care Access and Quality	Social and Community Context	Education Access and Quality	Economic Stability
• Quality and stability of housing • Transportation options and traffic • Public safety, including crime rate and violence levels • Walkability • Green space accessibility, including parks and playgrounds • Air and environmental quality and conditions • Access to clean drinking water and healthy food options	• Health insurance coverage • Provider availability • Access to primary and preventive care • Quality of care • Provision of culturally and linguistically responsive care • Health promotion initiatives • Health and mental health literacy levels	• Social integration and civic participation • Political activity and advocacy • Universal accessibility for people of all abilities • Community engagement • Levels of gender inequality, racism, ableism, stigma, and discrimination • Incarceration levels • Access to legal services • Social service availability	• High school graduation levels • Literacy and language levels • Access to preschools and early childhood education • Adult education opportunities • Workforce development and vocational training availability • Access to quality schools and vocational training • Attainment of higher education	• Employment and job security • Income and debt levels • Quality of jobs and working conditions • Food security levels • Financial strain and poverty levels • Housing costs

From Agency for Healthcare Research and Quality. (2020). About SDOH in health care. *Author. https://www.ahrq.gov/sdoh/about.html; U.S. Department of Health & Human Services. (2023).* Health equity in Healthy People 2030. *Office of Disease Prevention and Health Promotion. https://health.gov/healthypeople/priority-areas/health-equity-healthy-people-2030; World Health Organization. (2024, January).* Health equity. *https://www.who.int/health-topics/health-equity#tab=tab_1*

Social Drivers and Mental Health Disparities

Some social drivers are more strongly linked to mental health outcomes than others (Kivimäki et al., 2020; Reiss et al., 2019), particularly racism and socioeconomic status (Lopez et al., 2021; Schouler-Ocak et al., 2021). Other drivers that increase the risk of mental illness include poor access to health-care services, systemic and structural racism, stigma and discrimination, ACEs, poverty and income inequity, housing instability, and unemployment (APA, 2023; Pester et al., 2023; Shim & Starks, 2021). Globally, populations that are poor and disadvantaged experience stressors impacting their physical and mental health; these impacts are cumulative and can

persist across the life span and for generations (Alegría et al., 2018, Morgan et al., 2020).

In early seminal research on the connection between social drivers and mental health, Allen and colleagues (2014) applied a multilevel framework that considered life course from prenatal to old age, community context including the environment and health-care systems, country level political and economic factors, cultural factors, and policies influencing mental health care to analyze the impact of social drivers. These researchers found those who were poor and marginalized in society were most affected by these social drivers (Allen et al., 2014). This cumulative and interactive effect of SDOH on the risk of health and mental health inequities is well established in the research literature (Lund et al., 2018; Mao & Agyapong, 2021; Pester et al., 2023). Figure 28-3 presents an image designed to

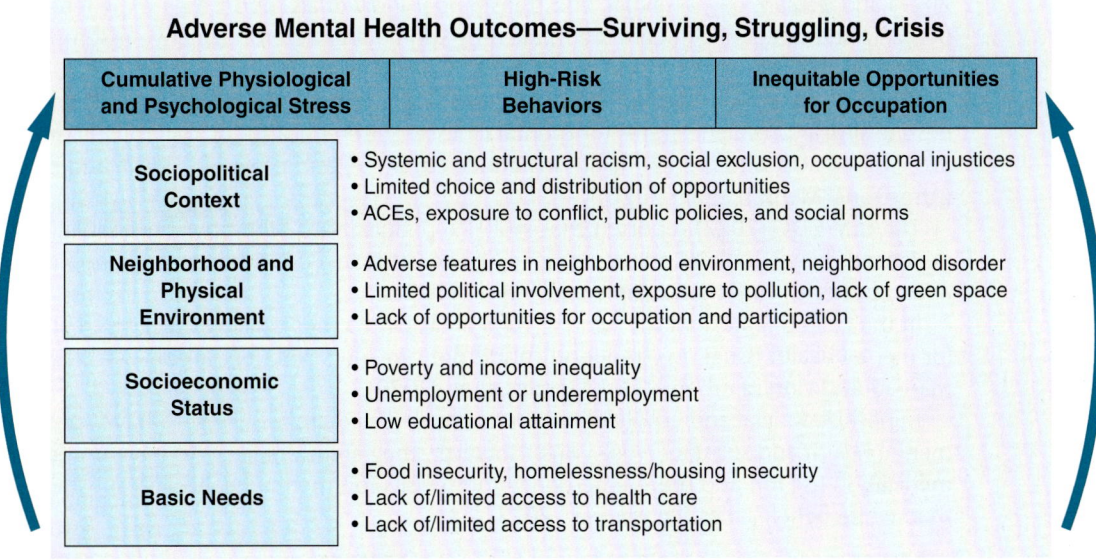

FIGURE 28-3. Social drivers of mental health.

help learners identify and visualize SDOH that research has shown negatively impacts mental health and sustains unequal distribution of opportunities for many individuals (APA, 2023; Lund et al., 2018; Pester et al., 2023; Shim & Starks, 2021).

In terms of mental health care, diverse and minoritized populations are oppressed. They are more likely to be overdiagnosed, underdiagnosed, and misdiagnosed with mental illness; have poorer access to mental health care, and have limited access to culturally responsive and linguistically appropriate mental health services. They are also less likely to receive evidence-based treatments and are often overinstitutionalized in inpatient mental health facilities, correctional institutions, and child welfare and juvenile justice systems (Londono Tobon et al., 2021; Priester et al., 2016, Teplin et al., 2023; USDHHS, 2023). For many people with minoritized social identities, the decision to seek mental health care is based on a complex interaction among individual and family variables, cultural beliefs and practices, and issues of access to and trust of the mental health-care delivery system (APA, 2023; WHO, 2023). For example, immigrant and refugee populations have distinct mental health needs that vary across this heterogeneous group. Factors such as race, ethnicity, age, developmental stage, immigration status, and place of residence within the United States can all impact one's mental health needs, but disparities in access to mental health care exist for all immigrant and refugee populations (Rodriguez et al., 2021). Punitive laws impacting immigration, education, and employment exert a compounding negative impact on the health and well-being of immigrant populations and their communities (Rodriguez & Rodriguez, 2020; Vargas & Ybarra, 2017). See Chapter 27: Mental Health Stigma and Sanism.

The Evidence-Based Practice feature accompanying this section summarizes findings from several recent studies reflecting mental health disparities in minoritized populations and inequities in mental health services. OTPs can aid in overcoming these barriers and closing health disparity gaps by intentionally informing themselves about the social, cultural, and environmental characteristics that can influence a person's perception of mental health, their health-seeking behaviors, their experience and expression of psychiatric symptoms, and the ease or difficulty of accessing and participating fully in mental health care.

Health Equity

WHO (2024) defines "equity" as "the absence of unfair, avoidable, or remediable differences among groups of people, whether those groups are defined socially, economically,

---

Evidence-Based Practice

Mental Health Disparities

Using a lens of health equity supports cultural humility and helps OTPs ask difficult questions with compassion and respect.

RESEARCH FINDINGS

Transgender adults, regardless of race or ethnicity, exhibit mental distress and report life-long depression diagnoses at a higher rate than white cisgender adults (Robertson et al., 2021) and lesbian, gay, bisexual, and transgender individuals report their experiences of receiving mental health care are marked by stigma and heteronormative assumptions (Rees et al., 2021).

African Americans in the United States have worse mental health outcomes than whites despite similar prevalence rates for mental illnesses, often because of systemic racism, poor SES, limited access to mental health insurance coverage, and provider stigma and bias (Armstrong-Mensah et al., 2020).

The U.S. CDC (2022) reported that in 2019, people living with physical disabilities experienced depression and anxiety, smoked more, were less physically active, and had less access to health care than people without disabilities

In the United States, adults living in rural areas with a mental illness receive treatment for mental health issues less frequently and from providers with less specialized training than adults living in urban areas (Morales et al., 2020).

Minoritized racial and ethnic older adults on Medicaid are less likely to have specialty mental health and substance use visits. However, they are more likely to have unmonitored medication use for, and more emergency room visits for, mental health and substance use than white beneficiaries (Fung et al., 2023).

Evidence-Based Practice—cont'd

APPLICATIONS

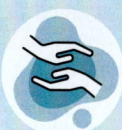

➡ OTPs can consciously and consistently build their knowledge and skills for delivering culturally responsive care and practice reflective cultural humility to demonstrate self-awareness of personal and societal biases, prejudices, and stigma.

➡ OTPs can employ a health equity lens when creating an occupational profile, learn to ask about issues related to social drivers in kind and compassionate ways, and document data about social challenges to ensure the team considers these issues in planning.

➡ OTPs can advocate for individuals and families (e.g., write letters on a person's behalf related to housing, immigration, courts, or educational institutions) and help individuals learn about and practice the skills for accessing benefits or programs that they may be eligible for (e.g., child benefits, classes, low-cost day care, food security programs).

REFERENCES

Armstrong-Mensah, E., Patel, H., Parekh, P., & Lee, C. (2020). Mental health inequities and disparities among African American adults in the United States: The role of race. *Research in Health Science, 5*(3), 23–32. https://doi.org/10.22158/rhs.v5n3p23

Centers for Disease Control and Prevention. (2022). *Health equity for people with disabilities.* Author. https://www.cdc.gov/ncbddd/humandevelopment/health-equity.html#ref

Fung, V., Price, M., McDowell, A., Nierenberg, A. A., Hsu, J., Newhouse, J. P., & Cook, B. L. (2023). Coverage parity and racial and ethnic disparities in mental health and substance use care among Medicare beneficiaries. *Health Affairs, 42*(1), 83–93. https://doi.org/10.1377/hlthaff.2022.00624

Morales, D. A., Barksdale, C. L., & Beckel-Mitchener, A. C. (2020). A call to action to address rural mental health disparities. *Journal of Clinical and Translational Science, 4*(5), 463–467. https://doi.org/10.1017/cts.2020.42

Rees, S. N., Crowe, M., & Harris, S. (2021). The lesbian, gay, bisexual, and transgender communities' mental health care needs and experiences of mental health services: An integrative review of qualitative studies. *Journal of Psychiatric Mental Health Nursing, 28,* 578–589. https://doi.org/10.1111/jpm.12720

Robertson, L., Akré, E.-R., & Gonzalez, G. (2021). Mental health disparities at the intersections of gender, identity, race, and ethnicity. *LGBT Health, 8*(8), 526–535. https://doi.org/10.1089/lgbt.2020.0429

demographically, or geographically or by other dimensions of inequality (e.g., sex, gender, ethnicity, disability, or sexual orientation)" (para. 1). Health equity exists when everyone has opportunities to live a healthy life and achieve well-being. In a society where health equity existed, everyone would have equal access to high-quality health care and be valued irrespective of their social identities (CDC, 2019; Office of Disease Prevention and Health promotion, n.d.).

OTPs are routinely confronted with the impact of health inequities on the lives of people they serve (Johnson & Lavalley, 2021; Restall et al., 2018; Synovec & Aceituno, 2020). They see firsthand that when society does not value all people and resources are not distributed equally (e.g., economic resources, access to health/mental health care), the result is often higher rates of health and mental health disparities in certain communities and populations (Hammell, 2020a, 2021). For example, people with housing, transportation, and robust social supports are more likely to have better health and mental health outcomes than those who are unhoused, are subject to systemic racism, and/or lack social supports (Synovec & Aceituno, 2020). Achieving health equity requires that health OTPs use a multitiered socioecological or public health approach to intervention. Practitioners using a PEO approach informed by lenses of equity and ecological systems theory can wield a powerful tool that helps them recognize and address SDOH and health inequities (Hammell, 2021; Johnson et al., 2022; Restall et al., 2018).

Decades ago, Bronfenbrenner (1979) proposed an **ecological systems theory** that emphasized the dynamic and reciprocal interplay between the individual, biological and psychological factors, society, and multiple levels of the environment. Bronfenbrenner's approach has been refined and applied to a variety of mental health challenges and to address SDOH and issues of health equity (Finan & Yap, 2021; Golden & Wendel, 2020; Hill, 2021; McLeroy et al., 1988; Tebb & Brindis, 2021). A socioecological framework adapted from Bronfenbrenner's seminal work and informed by additional public health researchers is presented in Figure 28-4. This framework identifies five levels of influence impacting human behavior: (1) intrapersonal; (2) interpersonal; (3) community, organizational, and institutional; (4) policy; and (5) socioenvironmental (Golden & Wendel, 2020; McLeroy et al., 1988). These levels are described in the text that follows.

Intrapersonal Level

The intrapersonal level is focused on factors within the individual; this person level is at the core of the image in Figure 28-4. Practitioners applying PEO models are well versed at evaluating and intervening at this level and typically consider factors such as the person's physical, mental, and interpersonal abilities; self-concept; personality; and ability to plan and self-regulate when planning interventions. An approach informed by SDOH intentionally considers the impact of chronic oppression-based lived experiences

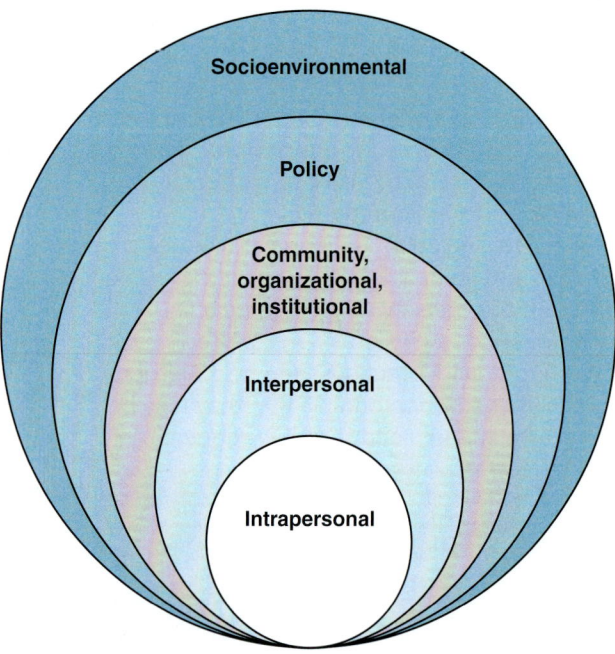

FIGURE 28-4. Socioecological framework for addressing health equity.

on a person's functioning. Chronic racism, sexism, ableism, homophobia, and stigma can all negatively affect function (Williams et al., 2023).

Interpersonal Level

The second level focuses on interpersonal processes. When OTPs evaluate a person's social environment, they consider the people and contexts a person interacts with most often. This can include formal and informal social networks such as family members, caregivers, friends, shopkeepers, clergy, neighbors, or coworkers. Practitioners intervening at this level focus on interpersonal interactions within these networks. For example, an OTP working with an individual focused on recovery may combine skills training with arranging a conversation between the individual and their employer to discuss workplace accommodations that could be mutually beneficial.

Community, Organizational, and Institutional Level

Community and organizational factors may include formal and informal networks within a defined area; for example, the local neighborhood and different health, education, and social service organizations within the neighborhood. An OTP applying a socioecological framework and seeking to address social drivers and health equity at this level may focus on spaces where the individuals they are working with interact in face-to-face ways. An OTP might create opportunities for occupation by strengthening relationships between local organizations. For example, they may work with contacts at the local library to make space for art activities for teenagers in the neighborhood who may be at risk, and then arrange for the library to collaborate with a local art studio to schedule a show featuring the youths' art. The OTP's focus here is building ties for coordination and collaboration

between organizations so that these connections promote health and provide opportunities for occupation. An ultimate health-promoting goal would be to have these connections become prominent and habitual parts of the community's norms and values (Finan & Yap, 2021; McLeroy et al., 1988).

Organizational and institutional elements included in this level of the socioecological framework have their own rules and social norms. OTPs should consider whether these operational rules and regulations create inequities. For example, consider the OTP who is working with Rachel, a person who is unhoused, unemployed, diagnosed with an anxiety disorder, and has a history of trauma. Program staff at the shelter, unaware of the impact of Rachel's anxiety and past traumas, are frustrated that she does not use communal shower facilities at assigned times and that her morning routine of arranging and rearranging her limited personal space at the shelter results in her always being late when leaving the sleeping area in the morning. Staff interpret these behaviors as Rachel's intentional disregard for agency rules. The OTP could work with program staff to use a labeling system so all of Rachel's personal items have a designated space, advocate that she be allowed to complete hygiene routines before bedtime instead of in the morning, and could provide staff education on complex traumas. These approaches might fit Rachel's needs and also benefit other people who need similar accommodations in this setting. See Chapter 32: The Neighborhood and Community. 🤝

Policy Level

This level includes local, state, and national laws and policies. OTPs must have good working knowledge of how policies, procedures, regulations, and laws that impact the health of communities are developed, advocated for, and analyzed. These policies impact health and health equity. For example, in the United States, people cannot smoke in public buildings; there are rules for workplace safety; food items people buy in stores are required to provide nutrition labeling; and individuals expect clean, safe drinking water from a water fountain. They also expect to be treated fairly in schools, in health-care facilities, and by law enforcement officials. Practitioners seeking to address change at this level can advocate for greater funding and/or policies that close structural gaps in health and mental health care and which address SDOH for individuals, communities, and populations (Flaubert et al., 2021; Golden & Wendel, 2020; Hammell, 2017a, 2017b; Hammell & Beagan, 2017). Every OTP who becomes knowledgeable about policy development must in turn make efforts to increase public awareness on specific health and mental health issues a routine part of their practice. Advocacy can be a form of occupation when OTPs create environments where they participate and encourage others to participate in the political processes of policy development. See Chapter 26: The Public Policy Environment. 🤝

Socioenvironmental Level

This outermost level of the socioenvironmental framework in Figure 28-4 encompasses all the other levels to represent the pervasive nature of systemic racism, structural violence, and other intersecting forms of oppression in education and health-care processes and systems that perpetuate unequal treatment of minoritized populations (Berger & Miller, 2021;

Braveman et al., 2022; Hammell, 2021; Sharif et al., 2021). A few examples of systemic oppression include inequitable access to and quality of health care, discrimination in employment, injustices in the education system, and environmental injustices and inequities in law enforcement and the criminal justice system (Braveman et al., 2022; Sharif et al., 2021; Sexton et al., 2020). These inequities are systemic because they are deeply embedded in attitudes and beliefs, as well as in laws, written and unwritten policies, and standard practices (Melton-Fant, 2022). OTPs need to employ multiple and varied strategies at the local, state, and national level to affect the kind of changes that dismantle the structures perpetuating disadvantage. Some strategies for addressing systemic racism and other forms of oppression are provided later in this chapter, but one effective approach may be framing the challenges through a lens of occupation. Showing up, speaking up, gathering friends and coworkers, organizing the neighborhood, voting, or leading organizations that are working for change are all purposeful occupations addressing health equity. This chapter's Being a Psychosocial OT Practitioner feature shares Jonathon's story and illustrates how socioenvironmental factors at various levels affect participation and how these factors can be addressed. See Chapter 32: The Neighborhood and Community.

Being a Psychosocial OT Practitioner

Meghan Blaskowitz, DrPH, OTR/L

Addressing Participation in Community Context

Identifying Psychosocial Strengths and Needs

To be truly person-centered, OTPs must intentionally consider how SDOH impact a person across their lifetime. Jonathon is in his late 50s and lives in an intermediate care facility (ICF, or group home) in Forest Hills, Queens, with seven other men who are blind and/or have intellectual and developmental disabilities (IDDs). Jonathon is blind, has a mild intellectual disability (ID), and has schizophrenia. He's taken risperidone (Risperdal) since his teens; because of this, he has tardive dyskinesia and holds his neck in constant extension, consistently smacks his lips, and engages in facial grimacing. Many people he interacts with have significant difficulty seeing past these behaviors.

When stressed, Jonathon occasionally yells, "Leave me alone, nurse!" Staff believe this is a result of living most of his childhood and young adulthood in Willowbrook State School. Willowbrook was New York's largest state institution, housing more than 6,000 individuals with psychiatric and intellectual disabilities until it closed in the late 1980s. When Jonathon was born, it was commonplace for physicians to advise families to institutionalize their child born with IDD, often soon after birth. Families that ignored this advice found few public supports or services.

Jonathon is known to be a "gentle giant." Standing 6'5", he's extremely kind, chatty, and agreeable with his roommates, group home staff, and his OTP and mental health professionals who visit him weekly. He's lived at his group home for nearly 12 years and is close with more senior peers, especially Arthur and Bobby. The group home is located between two neighborhoods—one more affluent neighborhood and another neighborhood of low to middle socioeconomic status—and is at least 8 to 10 blocks from resources like grocery stores, gyms, and green spaces. Food access in Jonathon's walkable neighborhood is via a Chinese restaurant and various bodegas, which are small, independently owned corner stores located throughout New York City; they sell coffee, soda, chips, candy—mostly unhealthy snacks.

Jonathon is unemployed and subsists financially on Medicaid Home & Community Based Services (HCBS) waiver funding. He receives additional state funding as a result of a combined family lawsuit that forces Willowbrook to fund services that promote community inclusion for its residents. These funding sources pay for housing and long-term support services including around-the-clock direct support professionals, medications, and transportation. He also receives monthly Supplemental Security Income (SSI) payments.

Jonathon's only living relative is his mom. She is elderly but visits him every Shabbos. She also occasionally takes Jonathon out to lunch or to synagogue on major Jewish holidays. Jonathon was referred to occupational therapy to help support his social participation and instrumental activities of daily living (IADLs).

Using a Holistic Occupational Therapy Approach

The OTP completed a standard occupational therapy evaluation, interview, and performance-based observation and concluded that Jonathon has good insight and can do most of his basic activities of daily living (ADLs) independently, although he eats with his hands. Jonathon requires moderate-maximal assistance for all IADLs (e.g., laundry, meal preparation, money/financial management, community mobility). He is respectful of his roommates but has little interaction with peers and few leisure interests. He spends most of his time alone in his room, listening to old radio programs and the news.

Jonathon ambulates independently within his own home but requires assistance from a sighted guide to get around his community. In the past, he's received services to support his mobility, train his direct support personnel (DSPs) in how to be a sighted guide, and obtain a walking cane and regular eye care/examinations. Although there are several subway stops within 5 to 10 blocks of his home, Jonathon has never engaged in subway travel training. He relies solely on Access paratransit service, or his staff/the residential van for transportation. Staff express concern about Jonathon going into the community alone and worry that he'll be taken advantage of. He never learned how to identify bills, so he doesn't know when he's handing bodega staff a $5 versus a $20 bill.

The OTP works with Jonathon to elicit his goals for participation. He expresses a desire to make friends in and outside his home, participate in his community of Forest Hills to a greater degree, and to become more politically active so he can vote regularly. Despite his desire to keep up with current events and politics, he has never participated in an election.

Reflective Questions

1. Considering strategies for understanding and addressing SDOH and social needs, how can the OTP support Jonathon at intrapersonal, interpersonal, community, and policy levels?
2. How might oppression, occupational rights, occupational possibilities, and occupational apartheid be applied to Jonathon's story?
3. How could you help Jonathon address his self-defined goals and develop self-advocacy skills to combat stigmatization he may experience from others when venturing outside his group home to participate more in his community?

Social Identity, Intersectionality, and Mental Health Care

Humans have multiple, intersecting, social identities that make up who they are. Each person is born into a biological sex, race, SES, culture, or place that was entirely out of their control; nonetheless, they make up one's original core identity. Over time, one's social identities shift and change in response to the experiences gathered over a lifetime. Sometimes, with increased experiences and exposure to alternate identities, a person may choose to deny aspects of their original identities when they no longer match how they feel inside, the lifestyle that they lead, or their value system.

Some dimensions of one's identity (e.g., race, physical and [dis]ability status) are primary and central to one's core identity. These identities inform how a person moves about the world and interacts with those around them, including interactions with the health-care system. Unfortunately, throughout history and still today, a person's social identities have been used as vehicles of oppression by people and systems from the "in group" harnessed against individuals labeled as part of the "out group" (Horner-Johnson, 2021). Many individuals who hold minoritized identities have been subject to systemic and personally mediated racism and ableism across their life span (Young et al., 2020), including by OTPs (Beagan et al., 2023; Hammell, 2020a, 2021; Johnson et al.,

2022). Although one's social identities can be a protective factor for some and support one's mental health, all too often a lifetime of oppression can be a causative factor of mental illness for individuals, communities, and populations.

In Figure 28-5, some of the myriad social identities a person can hold are presented. Some can be considered primary and others secondary dimensions of social identity. When an OTP is creating an occupational profile and considering PEO interactions, applying a lens of intersectionality can help OTPs to intentionally consider a person's social identities and may help them better understand the individual's occupational performance and choices. While examining Figure 28-5, readers are invited to reflect on their own primary and secondary social identities and consider how their identities may interact to position them in a place of power and privilege, or as potentially vulnerable to discrimination. During self-reflection, it may be useful to think about interactions and experiences with others in different contexts, such as among family and friends, as an OTP working with individuals from various walks of life, or out in the community.

Intersectionality is a concept introduced by Kimberlé Crenshaw in the late 1980s to describe the interconnected nature of social categorizations such as race, class, and gender, creating overlapping systems of discrimination or disadvantage (Crenshaw, 1989). A person with one or more of these

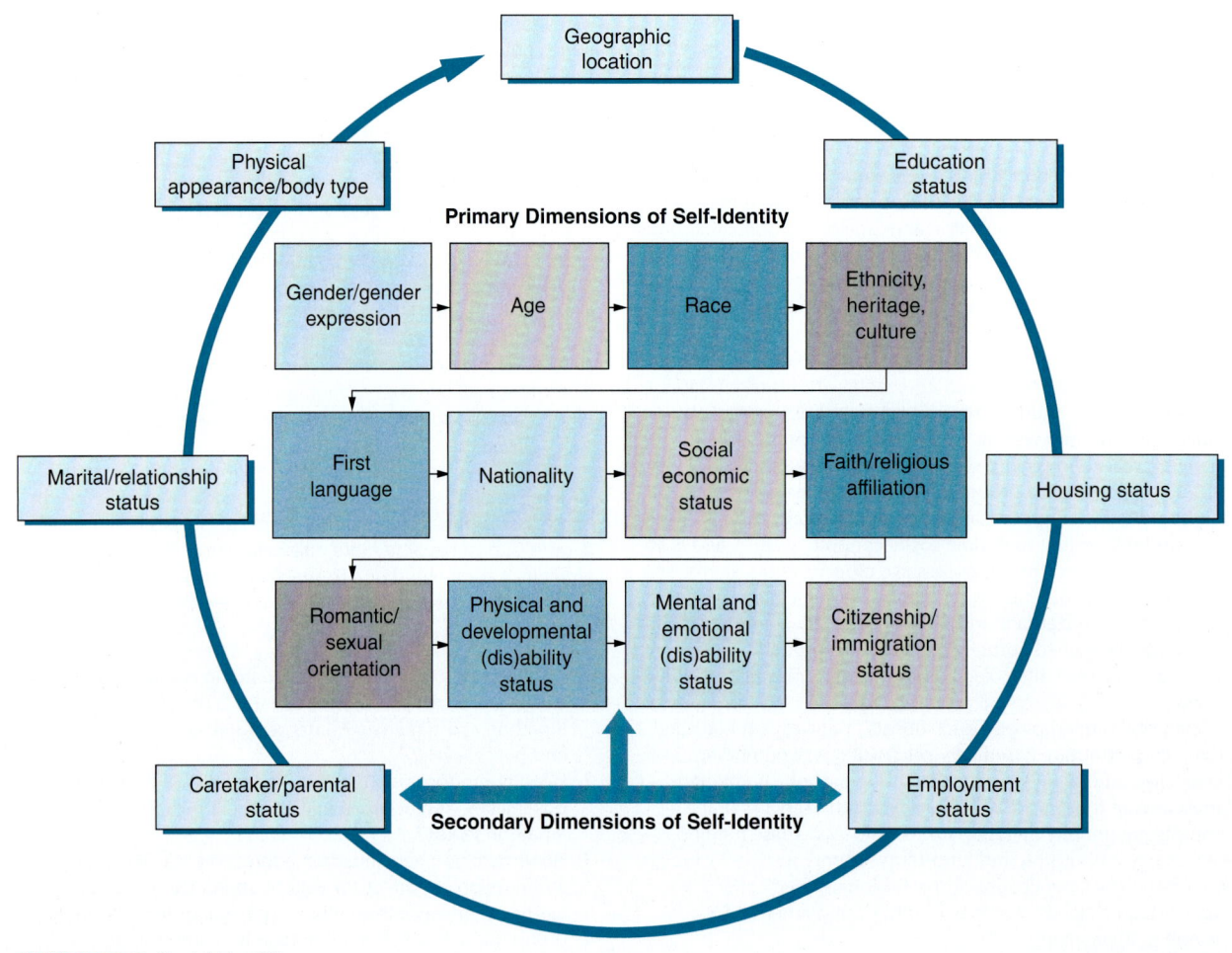

FIGURE 28-5. Social identities.

identities likely has a wide-ranging set of lived experiences that have both enhanced and challenged their development over their life course (Horner-Johnson, 2021). Intersectionality theory posits that discrimination and oppression multiplies for those with multiple minoritized social identities. For instance, a Black transgender woman with a disability likely experiences greater stigmatization than a Black cisgender able-bodied woman because she holds additional gender and disability status identities that society negatively stereotypes. Mental health challenges disproportionately impact individuals who hold minoritized social identities, especially those with multiple minoritized identities (Khanolkar et al., 2022; Oexle & Corrigan, 2018). The following description of intersectionality may help OTPs thoughtfully reflect on how identity, SDOH, oppression, and health equity are interconnected.

> Intersectionality is a way of understanding and analyzing complexity in the world, in people, and in human experiences. The events and conditions of social and political life and the self can seldom be understood as shaped by one factor. They are shaped by many factors in diverse and mutually influencing ways. When it comes to social inequality, people's lives, and the organization of power in a given society are better understood as being shaped not by a single axis of social division, be it race or gender or class, but by many axes that work together and influence each other. (Collins & Bilge, 2016, p. 2)

An OTP who applies a health equity lens informed by an understanding of social identity and intersectionality is one who

The Lived Experience

Cynthia's Story—What's My Purpose?

Editor's Note: Many stories could have been told for this feature. Often these stories include a main character who is someone whose social identities seem exotic, strange, or different. When asked how she describes herself, Cynthia replies she is "an African American woman in my mid-40s" who is "just a plain American."

I was diagnosed with depression way back in 1980. But I've been depressed all my life. I can remember when I was in preschool. The teacher told my mother that I was "antisocial" cause I didn't socialize with the other children. I had one friend, and if she wasn't there, then I had no friends. I kept to myself. I wasn't mean. I was just in my own head and doing my own thing.

I was always real shy to where I was even scared to talk to my own mother. I'm just now getting out of that within the last couple years. I've always been off by myself. I don't think of myself as an antisocial person, but I function better by myself. Most of my friends have a mental illness. My closest friend has a few diagnoses. I think sometimes that I can relate more to a person who has a mental illness because if people don't understand mental illness, like if you tell them that you have a mental illness, they'll think that you're crazy. That's their automatic thought. It jumps to something like, well you must be off balance, dangerous or crazy! That's the way they explain you. It gives them an excuse not to even try to get to know you.

Sometimes *I AM OFF BALANCE!!* At those times, I can relate to my friend because when I'm feeling down or some other kind of way, then I can talk to her because she can understand what I'm feeling because she's been there too. Most times, other people don't get it; even my own sister. When I tell my sister, she's like, she says, "It's a mind thing and you can get out of it." My son's father is like that too, he's like, "It's just a will thing." That might be a general feeling within Black communities; just be stronger, get faith. It's something in you; a weakness thing—something that you should be able to overcome if you just try harder. They don't think it is something that requires medication and stuff like that. It's not a disease. It's just something that you can overcome if you really want to overcome it. If you don't overcome it, well that's on you—you ain't trying hard enough. My sister is slowly

coming around more to understand that I do have a mental illness and it's not something that I can just turn on and turn off. It's not something that I control, but it is something I can manage better sometimes. So, she's coming around to that perspective.

I don't tell certain people about my mental illness because, to me, I think people gonna judge you if you say you have a mental illness. I think it will hinder you in a lot of different things. Like I couldn't go to a job and share, "Oh by the way I have a mental illness." You know, I won't get that job because I told them. That is society in general. When people see homeless people on the street, they try to avoid them. They think that they are crazy, but that's not the case a lot of times. It's just that certain circumstances happen. Things happen and you can't afford to live in a house—you are not crazy; you just don't have resources. That's how I think people think about mental illness too. I think that if people knew you had a mental illness, they would walk around you or step to the other side of the street to avoid you.

I was in a welfare office applying for housing once, and I decided I'm not going to tell them that I am mentally ill because it's a judging thing. In the welfare office they make it so hard for you to get benefits, and sometimes the workers act like they are paying you out of their own pocket. I feel like, OK, I have worked in my life too and I'm not planning on being on welfare all my life. It is supposed to be there for people who need it when they need it. Just admitting I need it is hard enough, but they judge you. They judge you and they make you go through some pain. Especially when you get workers who think that they are better than you are because you aren't working, and they are. So, you learn little tricks through experience and word of mouth. I'm not going to say that I work the system, but I've learned that there are certain things you have to do with the system because if you don't, you're not going to get any benefit. People with mental illness or who are homeless tell each other what we need to know, because the workers won't tell you nothing. You share information.

I graduated from the occupational therapy employment program and my intentions were to get a job. I did get a job last October, but I didn't keep it very long, and after a while I decided I should apply for Social Security Disability. That's

Continued

The Lived Experience—cont'd

my record; after a while I can't keep a job. I thought that a job would keep me sane, but it didn't. I felt that if I had a job, I would feel like I had a purpose in life because I felt useless when I wasn't working. I like to work, but I don't tend to stay on a job for a long time. I felt like I was getting worse instead of getting better, and I stopped taking my meds. So, my depression came back. I was trying to change with the occupational therapy employment program, but it didn't work out. I'm to the point right now where I really want to work. I honestly do want to work, but with Social Security, you can only work so many hours before you lose your benefits. It's risky for me.

If I were to describe myself culturally, I would say I am middle-aged, but I'm still young. I'm a person with a mental illness. I have been an addict. I consider myself a mother; a mother of three. I'm not going to say lower class, but I live in poverty. I think I struggle a lot with identifying myself or who I am or my purpose, that's what I struggle a lot with. What is my purpose?

Reflective Questions

- Using Figure 28-5, what are some primary and secondary identities you might ascribe to Cynthia? Explain your reasons for choosing these identities.
- Apply the concept of intersectionality to the identities you assigned to Cynthia. Hypothesize how these intersecting identities may support Cynthia's occupational functioning. How might they impede her functioning?
- Based on specific content in Cynthia's story, what lived experiences that she shares do you think might influence her own sense of social identity or how others may perceive her? Explain.

intentionally engages in deep reflection to consider the ways race, gender, social class, ableness, sexual orientation, and other identities may constitute and operate as intersecting systems of oppression for many individuals (Young et al., 2020). Readers are encouraged to use this chapter's The Lived Experience feature about Cynthia to apply concepts from this discussion of social identity, intersectionality, and mental health.

Concepts and Frameworks

This chapter frames health equity as a broad public health issue. The COVID-19 pandemic and disproportionate response to this crisis was a catalyst for many to refocus on SDOH and to recognize just how unequal health-care access and resources are in the United States and other parts of the world (Campo-Arias & De Mendieta, 2021; Gibson et al., 2021; Maffly-Kipp et al., 2021). The evidence that an unequal burden is placed on marginalized, minoritized, and oppressed communities and how health is stratified by various features of identity such as race, socioeconomic class, gender, (dis)ability, geographic location, and sexuality is irrefutable (APA, 2023; CDC, 2023; Thurston et al., 2023). This section shares some concepts and frameworks that OTPs can use to better understand and take actions in their practice to address health equity and SDOH. If OTPs want to embrace anti racism and begin to dismantle systemic inequities, they must integrate these concepts into the language they use when discussing inequities in occupation, study frameworks that address oppression, and adopt frameworks that intentionally address occupational justice (Emery-Whittington et al., 2024; Johnson et al., 2024).

Cultural Humility

Health-care professionals have identified the need to shift from a focus on acquiring cultural competence to practicing with **cultural humility** (Agner, 2020; Campinha-Bacote, 2019; Grenier, 2020; Lekas et al., 2020). Approaches focused on cultural competency emphasize acquiring knowledge of multiple and diverse cultures, often without creating opportunities for experiential learning or interaction with minoritized individuals or groups (AOTA, 2020a; Grenier et al., 2020). Knowledge and self-awareness alone will not mitigate oppression and racism. Practitioners must critically reflect on their own biases and seek to examine the lived experiences of minoritized individuals through a lens of intersectionality. It is essential to identify the power dynamics operating in health-care interactions and recognize the social drivers that affect the health behaviors and occupational choices of minoritized populations (Anderson, 2022; Irvine-Brown et al., 2020).

An OTP who works to develop cultural humility can be a better ally to marginalized and minoritized populations. An *ally* is a person who fights for the rights of marginalized groups that they are not a part of. Acquiring cultural humility is a lifelong learning process requiring commitment to constant self-reflection and self-critique to identify individual assumptions and biases (Tervalon & Murray-Garcia, 1998). Practitioners who do not engage in deep and regular self-reflection risk proposing interventions that align with their own cultural values and biases and that may be inconsistent with the needs of the person they are treating. Practicing with cultural humility requires OTPs to recognize that power imbalances exist within health-care interactions and systems; these power dynamics must be acknowledged and addressed. Cultural humility is fostered when OTPs reach out and affiliate with individuals and advocacy groups addressing barriers to health equity (Anderson, 2022; Ginsberg & Mayfield-Clarke, 2021; Grenier et al., 2020).

Occupational Consciousness

The concept of **occupational consciousness** emerged in the work of Dr. Elelwani Ramugondo (2012, 2015, 2024). It is a useful construct for OTPs, specifically because it addresses one's capacity to pause and intentionally question the dynamics of cultural hegemony in everyday life and occupations. **Cultural hegemony** refers to the idea that in a culturally diverse society, the ruling class dominates and shapes culture and ideology through social structures, systems, and institutions to ensure that their worldview (e.g., beliefs, perceptions, values, mores) is the accepted cultural norm (Gramsci, 1975). An OTP with occupational consciousness recognizes that racism is systemic and normalized in laws and rules; social structures and practices designed to maintain inequities in health care; education; economics; and the criminal justice system. If racism is to be dismantled, it must be recognized. That seems a simple thing, but public consent for the status quo is believed to be provided in unconscious and uncritical ways that can limit human agency and which typically work against the public's own interests (Gachon, 2021). Ramugondo (2024) highlighted this point when positing that in everyday doing, everyone, at some level, is complicit in perpetuating the structural aspects of their socioenvironmental context that oppress opportunities for some and provide advantages for others. Just as using a lens of health equity encourages OTPs to consider the SDOH that impact health status and health-related behavior, a lens of occupational consciousness demands that OTPs intentionally probe the dynamics of power, dominance, and oppression and to question what opportunities do and do not exist for people to participate in occupation. Practitioners can become more occupationally conscious when they attend to the power dynamics impacting day-to-day life in an intentional way that disrupts the status quo and questions hegemonic dynamics influencing their own lives and the lives of people they work with (Ramugondo, 2015, 2024).

Occupational Choice

Many OTPs are familiar with Mary Reilly's quote espousing the perspective of occupational choice: "Man, through the use of his hands, as they are energized by mind and will, can influence the state of his own health" (Reilly, 1962, p. 2). Occupational therapy has long held that people make autonomous choices to engage in meaningful occupations that ultimately impact their mental health and well-being (Kielhofner, 2008; Yerxa, 2000). Practitioners are encouraged to interrogate the opposite. Does everyone have the same opportunities to engage in doing, being, becoming, and belonging? **Occupational choice** is a concept amplified within occupational science scholarship and used to challenge the perspective that the locus of control for one's choices always lies entirely within the individual (Brennan & Gallagher, 2017; Galvaan, 2012; Hammell, 2020b).

When choice is considered through a lens of occupational justice, one may understand that choice is often contextually situated; opportunities for occupation are not equally distributed, and choice is influenced by the lifestyles, expectations, resources, and dominant values of social groups in social contexts (Gallagher et al., 2015; Hammell, 2020a, 2020b). Conceptualizing occupational choice this way may help ensure that individual services and programs that OTPs developed are not a poor match or even oppressive to individuals or communities who lack the opportunity to make these occupational choices. Multiple studies have already demonstrated that when applying the concept of occupational choice through a lens of occupational justice, OTPs are provided a way to more deeply and broadly consider how context influences one's autonomy to make choices, particularly for oppressed and minoritized populations (Brennan & Gallagher, 2017; Dowers et al., 2019; Galvaan, 2015; Hammell, 2020b; Murthi & Hammell, 2021). Cultural humility, occupational consciousness, and occupational choice are all concepts that can help an OTP prepare themselves to address SDOH and health equity. Additional conceptual lenses to support practice grounded in occupational justice and help promote antiracist practices appear in Table 28-2.

TABLE 28-2 | Conceptual Lenses for Health Equity

Conceptual Lens	Description
Occupational apartheid	Highlights the fact that different groups of people experience "restriction or denial of access to dignified and meaningful participation in occupations of daily life based on race, colour, disability, national origin, age, gender, sexual preference, religion, political beliefs, status in society, or other characteristics. Occasioned by political forces, its systematic and pervasive social, cultural, and economic consequences jeopardize health and well-being as experienced by individuals, communities, and societies" (Kronenberg & Pollard, 2005, p. 67).
Occupational possibilities	Practitioners applying this concept intentionally consider the way that possibilities for occupation are grounded in power structures; that is, occupations are made available or not by systems and structures operating in and impacting the lives of people where they live. This concept encourages one to question the range of occupational possibilities available for individuals who, for example, live in poverty, have multiple intersecting and minoritized identities, are elderly, or are disabled (Laliberte Rudman, 2010).
Occupational rights	Viewing occupation as a human right requires OTPs to focus on what people can do, aggressively assess environmental barriers impacting access, build their capacity to recognize structural inequalities, and take action and aspire to practice in a manner that prioritizes addressing access and structural inequities to occupational participation (Hammell, 2015; Pollard et al., 2009).
Oppression	This lens encourages OTPs to consider how oppression operates through power. When individuals in one social group experience harm while individuals in another group receive corresponding benefits, that is oppression. Identifying and naming oppression in one's practice and in the daily life experiences of others encourages OTPs to call out systemic injustices in the power relationships in education, housing, economic, legal, and health-care systems (Freire, 1970; Pooley & Beagan, 2021).

From Freire, P. (1970). Pedagogy of the oppressed. Bloomsbury Academic; Hammell, K. W. (2015). Occupational rights and critical occupational therapy: Rising to the challenge. Australian Occupational Therapy Journal, 62, 449–451. https://doi.org/10.1111/1440-1630.12195; Kronenberg, F., & Pollard, N. (2005). Overcoming occupational apartheid: A preliminary exploration of the political nature of occupational therapy. In F. Kronenberg, S. S. Algado, & N. Pollard (Eds.), Occupational therapy without borders: Learning from the spirit of survivors (pp. 58–86). Elsevier; Laliberte Rudman, D. (2010). Occupational terminology: Occupational possibilities. Journal of Occupational Science, 17(1), 55–59. https://doi.org/10.1080/14427591.2010.9686673; Pollard, N., Sakellariou, D., & Kronenberg, F. (2009). A political practice of occupational therapy. Churchill Livingstone Elsevier; Pooley, E. A., & Beagan, B. L. (2021). The concept of oppression and occupational therapy: A critical interpretive synthesis. Canadian Journal of Occupational Therapy, 88(4), 407–417. https://doi .org/10.1177/00084174211051168

Capabilities, Opportunities, Resources, and Environments (CORE) Approach

Key points in a WFOT position statement on occupation and human rights state that every person has the right to "participate in a range of occupations that support survival, health and well-being," . . . [to] choose occupations without pressure, force, coercion or threats . . . [and to] freely engage in necessary and chosen occupations without risk to safety, human dignity or equity (WFOT, 2019, p. 1). Framing occupational participation as a human right obligates OTPs to use occupation-centered practices and frameworks to address systemic and structural issues that enable or restrict participation (Doll et al., 2023; Pereira et al., 2020). The CORE approach is a framework that guides this type of therapeutic reasoning and targets occupational participation and social inclusion (Pereira, 2017; Pereira et al., 2020; Pereira & Whiteford, 2018). CORE structures practice by identifying four critical aspects impacting inclusion and participation: capabilities, opportunities, resources, and environments (Pereira, 2017).

Addressing capabilities requires OTPs to understand what individuals want to do and who they want to be, as well as identify and address barriers that may interfere with these goals. Practitioners often consider the term "capabilities" from a person-oriented perspective; that is, what does the person have the ability to do? In the CORE framework, the OTP still asks about what the person wants to do, needs to do, and can do, but they also consider what opportunities the person has to engage in that doing and the enablement strategies that can be used to build opportunities. An OTP using the capabilities perspective asks whether the person is afforded opportunities to engage in personally valuable, meaningful occupation (Pereira et al., 2020).

When building opportunities, an OTP plans and creates prospects for occupations that can support doing, being, and belonging. In the CORE approach, an OTP seeks to identify circumstances that limit participation and advocate to generate opportunities for occupation. Doing and becoming require resources. When addressing the resource component in the CORE approach, OTPs must consider the personal, social, physical, material, technological, emotional, and financial resources available that support a person's full realization of capabilities. Intervention may require mobilizing resources.

Addressing environments, the final component of CORE, requires OTPs to critically examine sociocultural environments with a particular intent to design, enhance, and/or modify these in ways that support the person's social inclusion, personal growth, and overall health and well-being (Pereira, 2017; Pereira et al., 2020). It is critical for the OTP to consider how environments support a person's individual occupations and support collective occupations that promote equity and social inclusion (Ramugondo & Kronenberg, 2015). *Collective occupations* are "occupations that are engaged in by individuals, groups, communities, and/or societies in everyday contexts; these may reflect an intention toward social cohesion or dysfunction, and/or advancement of or aversion to a common good" (Ramugondo & Kronenberg, 2015, p. 10). The CORE framework "provides a platform for occupational possibilities and creative exploration, where the goal is for the person seeking occupational outcomes to have agency, choice and be in control over the enablement process" (Pereira, 2017, p. 433).

Occupation-Based Community Development (OBCD) Framework

OTPs and scholars from around the world have proposed context-specific frameworks to address oppression and build health equity at a community level. Some examples include the Social Occupational Therapy approach originating in Brazil (Malfitano, 2021), the Community Development Framework (CDF) from Germany (Melville et al., 2023), the Community Centered Practice Framework from Australia (Hyett et al., 2019), and the OBCD framework from South Africa (Galvaan & Peters, 2017), which is the focus of this next section of this chapter.

In the OBCD framework, occupation is both a means and an ends for creating collaborative partnerships that build both individual and collective agency and which are directed at addressing SDOH (Galvaan & Peters, 2017; Mthembu, 2021). OTPs using the OBCD framework engage in iterative discourse, listen, and solicit indigenous ideas and solutions that involve the community and population in action-oriented problem-solving to address structural inequities. They build collaborative partnerships with communities to create opportunities for participation that fit the context, are socially inclusive, and improve quality of life for members of the community (Albuquerque & Farias, 2022; Galvaan et al., 2024; Mthembu, 2021). Four iterative processes in the OBCD framework guide practice: (1) initiating intervention; (2) designing; (3) implementation; and (4) monitoring, reflection, and evaluation.

Initiating Intervention

Initiating intervention requires OTPs to identify stakeholders, build relationships, and develop a deep understanding of context. During this stage, OTPs use concepts such as SDOH, occupational justice, and health equity to identify the broad range of social and occupational identities operating within the community. In collaboration with the community, an OTP creates a mutual understanding of context, of groups and subgroups in the community, and of other interprofessional colleagues working in the community, and identifies key community leaders. It is important to identify common occupations in the community; how people think about participating in these occupations; and the cultural, economic, social, and other structural factors that shape doing, being, becoming, and belonging in the community. Useful tools in this stage include therapeutic use of self, participant observation, interviewing, PhotoVoice techniques, and occupational and context analysis. Key goals are to build collaborative relationships and establish a mutual understanding of the focus for intervention. Therapeutic use of self is critical, and the strategies OTPs employ to understand the community's perspectives and priorities set the tone for how opportunities for occupational engagement are framed (Galvaan & Peters, 2017; Galvaan et al., 2024).

Designing

Designing is a dynamic, iterative process. Effective design requires OTPs to identify the kinds of occupations that are typically engaged in, barriers and supports to participation, structural inequities impacting opportunities for engagement in occupations, and what local resources support engagement. Mutuality in the design phase is enhanced by iterative discussions with key stakeholders about possibilities for occupational engagement. Encouraging community members to use their words to frame problem situations, define solutions, and choose strategies that are culturally relevant to their context is key.

Another critical step of design is testing out **occupational possibilities** (Laliberte Rudman, 2010). That is, by understanding that occupation is contextually situated, the OTP identifies the ways and types of doing that are realistically available for individuals within the socioenvironmental context of the community. Designing offers multiple opportunities to build and/or strengthen connections between networks that can provide the resources (e.g., time, human, financial) to facilitate access to opportunities and other resources.

Implementation

In the implementation phase, the OTP and community allies collaboratively use occupation as the mechanism for change. An OTP routinely engaging in active reflection to learn from experiences can maximize success in this stage. Kolb's reflective cycle is one framework that supports active reflection (Kolb, 1984). The reflective cycle begins with the OTP paying attention to their internal reactions and what is going on around them during concrete experiences that occur during implementation. Reflective observation comes next. This processing stage of the cycle requires OTPs to reflect deeply on their concrete experiences, attend to nuance, and focus on surprising or unexpected observations. In the abstract conceptualization phase, the OTP connects their observations to concepts and frameworks that help them understand and explain the experiences. For example, specific concepts such as occupational justice, collective occupations (Núñez et al., 2022), social and environmental determinants of health (Smith, 2023), occupational choice (Galvaan, 2012; Hammell, 2020b), occupational imagination (Laliberte Rudman, 2014), occupational consciousness (Ramugondo, 2012), intersectionality, or occupational possibilities (Laliberte Rudman, 2015) can extend an OTP's analysis of their observations. The next step in this reflective learning cycle is active experimentation. Here the OTP puts conceptual understanding into action by testing hypotheses, checking their thinking, and planning their next moves. This of course leads the OTP back to new concrete experiences that support continuous reflection on action. Active experimentation in the OBCD approach should test how occupations chosen in the implementation phase effectively stimulate occupation engagement.

Monitoring, Reflection, and Evaluation

At the monitoring, reflection, and evaluation stage, OTPs must collaborate on decisions such as:

- What aspects of the intervention are a priority to monitor and evaluate?
- What strategies for data collection best fit the context?
- Who are the best choices for collecting the data?
- How will evaluation tools reflect community involvement?
- What are the best ways to collaboratively analyze data and disseminate results to the community?

Processes consistent with **participatory action research** approaches, which include methods emphasizing participation and action by members of communities affected by the research, can be especially useful at this stage (Vaughn & Jacquez, 2020). Continued use of an active reflection cycle informs ongoing adjustments in this phase. An OTP must effectively utilize strategies that elicit the expectations, perceptions, and lived experiences of all community participants, as this can result in useful data. Some useful strategies include developing short questionnaires or surveys and using focus groups to gather data. These strategies to assess intervention outcomes and solicit feedback from the community regarding the degree to which interventions are effectively addressing the priorities of the community are culturally relevant, and are creating relevant opportunities for community members to exert their own agency in ways that improve social inclusion, participation, and the quality of life in their community. They are all recommended strategies. When done well, this phase of monitoring, reflection, and evaluation leads to invigorated, productive dialogue between all partners on the next iteration of design.

Occupational therapy models of practice that address racism and health equity, as well as target community development, do exist. Although most are relatively recent, they show strong signs of future potential. Some additional occupational therapy frameworks are presented in Table 28-3. Practitioners are also encouraged to research established public health frameworks designed to support individuals in developing healthy routines and behaviors. Some of these include the Health Belief Model (Glanz et al., 2015), the Theory of Reasoned Action (Ajzen & Fishbein, 1980), and the Transtheoretical "Stages of Change" Model (Prochaska & Velicer, 1997). The Transtheoretical "Stages of Change" Model is frequently used in community mental health practice to support people with substance use disorder (SUD) address health behaviors. Using this model, the individual and the OTP work in concert to assess their level of readiness for change and take stage-appropriate steps to incrementally incorporate healthy behavioral changes (Witkiewitz et al., 2022).

Addressing Social Determinants and Health Equity

This section begins with a story about addressing problem situations and taking action. Three OTPs were having a picnic on the bank of a large stream, enjoying the day. Suddenly they notice a person flailing in the current of the stream trying desperately to get to shore. The three immediately form a human chain, reach into the water, and pull the person out. Almost immediately, another person flails by and they pull that person out, too. This situation repeats itself again and again and the three dutifully pull each person from the stream. After a bit, one of the OTPs unexpectedly bolts from the bank and begins to run upstream. The others yell frantically that they need help, but the OTP yells back, "I am going to go stop whoever is throwing these people in!"

Allow the stream in this story to represent SDOH that disproportionately impact health and opportunities for occupational participation. This imagery of a stream is presented in Figure 28-6 and is often used in public health literature (Castrucci & Auerbach, 2019; Flaubert et al., 2021). It helps to

TABLE 28-3 | Frameworks for Health Equity

Framework	Description
Do-Live-Well Framework	The framework encourages critical reflexivity, community advocacy, and dialogue at a systems level about how day-to-day occupations impact health and well-being. The framework defines eight dimensions of experience (activating the physical body, connecting with others, taking care of oneself, etc.) and five concepts related to activity patterns (engagement, meaning, balance, control/choice, routine) that assist an OTP to take a deep dive into links between doing and health outcomes. Outcomes for health and wellness, social factors, and contextual forces impacting what people can do on a day-to-day basis are also included in this framework (Hamilton et al., 2023; Moll et al., 2015).
Equity Lens for Occupational Therapy	This framework is based on the Canadian Practice Process Framework (CPPF) and layers on a logic model to support development and evaluation of programs and a health equity lens to sharpen the focus on SDOH. The authors propose a four-step model that involves (1) considering the context, (2) creating a logic model for each step of the CPPF, (3) applying an equity lens, and (4) identifying actions (Restall et al., 2018).
PAIRE: Recognize Privilege, Acknowledge Injustice, and Reframe Perspective to Reach Equity Model	This practice model provides a guided focus on three "inner" factors in the health-care process: (1) the individual or community receiving services, (2) the person/team providing services, and (3) prioritized occupations. Practitioners are also directed to focus on three "outer" factors: (1) access and availability of services; (2) justice, including how systems and policies impact an individual's ability to access health care and the need to potentially change harmful policies; and (3) context including the culture and sociopolitical systems that support or stymie a person's ability to engage in prioritized occupations (Hoyt et al., 2023).

From Hamilton, K. A., Letts, L. J., Larivière, N., & Moll, S. E. (2023). Revisiting the Do-Live-Well Health Promotion Framework: A citation content analysis. Canadian Journal of Occupational Therapy, 90(3), 297–302. https://doi.org/10.1177/00084174221149268; Hoyt, C. R., Clifton, M., Smith, C. R., Woods, L., & Taff, S. D. (2023). Transforming occupational therapy for the 21st century PAIRE: Recognize Privilege, Acknowledge Injustice, and Reframe Perspective to Reach Equity. Occupational Therapy in Health Care, 1–24. https://doi.org/10.1080/07380577.2023.2265479; Moll, S. E., Gewurtz, R. E., Krupa, T. M., Law, M. C., Larivière, N., & Levasseur, M. (2015). "Do-Live-Well": A Canadian framework for promoting occupation, health, and well-being. Canadian Journal of Occupational Therapy, 82(1), 9–23. https://doi.org/10.1177/0008417414545981; Restall, G. J., MacLeod Schroeder, N. J., & Dubé, C. D. (2018). The Equity Lens for Occupational Therapy: A program development and evaluation tool. Canadian Journal of Occupational Therapy, 85(3), 185–195. https://doi.org/10.1177/0008417418756421

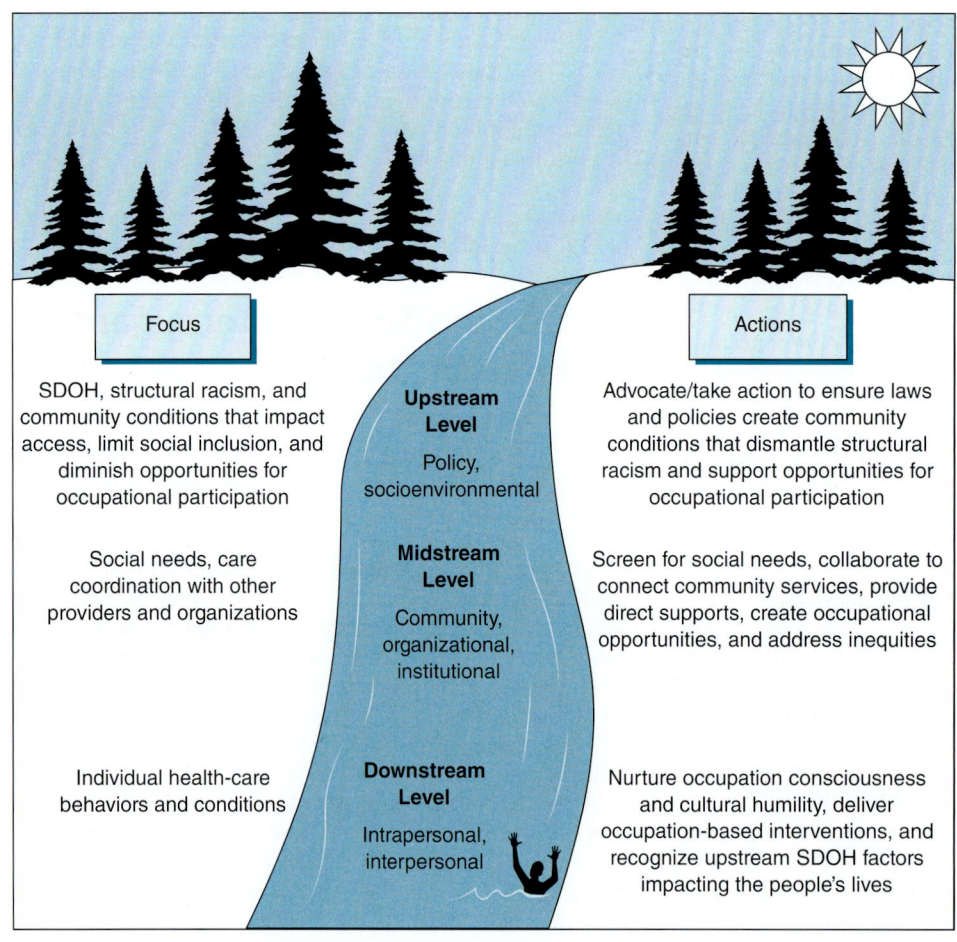

FIGURE 28-6. Addressing SDOH and social needs.

reinforce the use of a socioecological model and reflects that the downstream health behaviors and conditions at an individual level are significantly impacted by upstream factors—oppression, systemic racism, and SDOH—that operate at a socioenvironmental level. This image can help an OTP visualize where and how they might act on SDOH. Most OTPs work downstream, addressing health conditions and behaviors at the individual level, usually in clinics, hospitals, schools, and people's homes. If occupational therapy is to support efforts to dismantle racist systems and structures that perpetuate health disparities, OTPs will need to work across all levels of the socioecological model (CDC, 2022; Hammell, 2021). The following sections present approaches that can help OTPs address SDOH. They are organized across the levels of the socioecological model discussed earlier (see Fig. 28-4). This is not an exhaustive list, but it provides resources and tactics that can be useful for addressing health disparities.

Intrapersonal Level

A holistic OTP committed to developing their own cultural humility and occupational consciousness and dedicated to joining efforts to dismantle racism and SDOH that lead to health inequities must begin within, at an intrapersonal level. Action steps at this level include personal efforts to engage in critical reflection to allow deep consideration of the upstream SDOH factors impacting the lives of people they treat. Pitonyak and her colleagues (2015) have argued that OTPs who are truly person-centered in their practice attend to societal factors that impact a person's ability to participate in occupation. Further, they argue that failure to apply a socioecological lens leads to continued health disparities and occupational deprivation/imbalance for individuals receiving occupational therapy. Practitioners are encouraged to hone their community observation skills by using windshield or walking surveys. Such tools can structure one's observations and note-taking while walking or driving through a community and encourage one to pay close attention to elements such as housing, accessibility, the streetscape, public transportation, schools, political activity, and community organizations that often go unnoticed (Center for Community Health and Development, 2023). Using lenses of occupational choice and occupational possibilities while completing such observations and surveys may further increase one's awareness of SDOH impacting community health.

Embracing social and occupational justice and inclusion as core tenets of the occupational therapy profession obligates OTPs to commit to being antiracist and antiableist in their ideology and therapeutic practice. Throughout their careers, OTPs will engage with individuals who hold a multitude of intersecting social identities. However, the occupational therapy workforce remains predominantly white and female, whereas minoritized populations are overrepresented in disability communities (AOTA, 2023a; Ross & Bateman, 2019). Committing to **anti racism** means that an OTP is actively working to dismantle and eliminate racism nationally, locally, and in all personal interactions. Providing antiracist and inclusive health interventions that address SDOH reflects one's effort to dismantle health disparities for all communities and populations (Ahmed-Landeryou, 2024; Emery-Whittington et al., 2024; Lerner & Kim, 2024).

Johnson and colleagues (2022) have recommended a variety of approaches OTPs can employ to practice anti racism in their own lives and in therapeutic practices. A first step is embracing cultural humility, acknowledging that cultural learning often entails unlearning prejudices that people have been enculturated with from an early age, and relearning new ways of thinking, being, and moving through the world. It can be personally challenging to acknowledge biases, prejudice, and stigma and work toward dispelling them. It may be unsettling for individuals who have chosen to enter occupational therapy, a social justice–oriented profession, to think that they hold biases. However, an initial step to dispelling racism is admitting that all people hold racist and ableist ideologies (Lavalley & Johnson, 2020). The Harvard University's Implicit Association Tests (IAT) are a suite of open-access tools that can serve as a starting point for initiating some of this personal work (Harvard University Office for Equity, Diversity, Inclusion, and Belonging [OEDIB], 2024). A series of studies have been conducted to understand OTPs' bias toward people who hold various social identities using Harvard's IAT tools. The results of these studies reflected the gender, anti-fat, and ableist bias that exist among occupational therapy students and OTPs (Friedman et al., 2022; Friedman & VanPuymbrouck, 2021; VanPuymbrouck & Friedman, 2023). Practitioners may also find that the Attitudes Towards People with Disabilities Scale (Myong et al., 2021) can be a useful instrument for deeply examining attitudes and perceptions of community integration, discomfort in interactions, and feeling a sense of burden or charitability toward individuals with disabilities.

Each new therapeutic encounter offers an opportunity to critically reflect on one's biases and social identities. Using lenses of power and privilege to guide this reflection on one's own identities and those of individuals that one treats may help one attend to systemic and structural forces that impact lived experiences. It may be useful to revisit the Social Identity concepts included in Figure 28-5 to reinforce reflection on primary and secondary social identities. Table 28-4 presents a Therapeutic Reasoning Assessment that includes brief descriptions of tools that an OTP might consider using to support the development of cultural humility, uncover biases, and practice critical reflection skills. An essential caveat to note here is that tests of bias and self-awareness are useful for critical reflection and building one's knowledge, but knowledge alone does not mitigate racism. An antiracist OTP is one who actively opposes racism and inequities.

Interpersonal Level

Proficient OTPs are master interviewers. Experience talking about and closely observing an individual's occupational performances makes most OTPs very competent ethnographers as well. It is critical, however, that OTPs hone their skills to glean information about social needs and contextual opportunities and barriers in addition to individual-level factors and performance skills. Reflective OTPs consider questions such as: Does this person have access to transportation to support their attendance and compliance with occupational therapy and mental health appointments? Do they have access to technology, Wi-Fi, and health/technological literacy skills to be able to access these

TABLE 28-4 | Therapeutic Reasoning Assessment Table

Which Tool?	Who Was This Tool Designed For?	What Is Required of the Person Being Assessed?	What Am I Measuring?	How Long Does It Take and Where Do I Administer This Assessment?	Is the Tool Associated With a Practice Model?
Attitudes and Perspectives toward Persons with Disabilities (Myong et al., 2021)	Designed for health-care professionals; can be used with adults 18 or older	Objective self-reflection on 32 items examining attitudes and perspectives	Self-perceived attitudes and perspectives toward people with disabilities	Complete in a quiet space supporting private reflection in 20 minutes	Not identified
Cultural Humility Self-Reflection Tool for School Mental Health Professionals (School Mental Health Ontario, 2024)	Designed for health-care professionals working in schools, but the items are applicable to a variety of practice settings	Objective self-reflection to rate self on 32 items focused on cultural humility to document strengths and to set goals for growth	Self-perceived cultural humility that explores awareness, knowledge, and skills related to cultural humility	Complete checklist in a quiet space supporting private reflection in 20 minutes; goal setting may take an additional 20 minutes	Cultural Humility Model
Implicit Association Tests (OEDIB, 2024)	Any adult 18 or older	Objective self-reflection to sort words reflecting attitudes or beliefs on a range of sociocultural topics	Self-understanding of attitudes and beliefs that a person is unable or unwilling to report or is not consciously aware of	Complete any one of 18 different tests in a quiet space supporting 15–20 minutes of private reflection	Cognitive and implicit bias
Inventory for Assessing the Process of Cultural Competence Among Health-Care Professionals–Revised (Campinha-Bacote, 2002)	Health-care professionals with a high level of health literacy; available in many languages	Objective self-reflection; respondent rates self on 20 items focused on cultural competency	Self-perceived cultural competence focused on cultural desire, cultural awareness, cultural knowledge, cultural skills, and cultural encounters	Administer in a quiet space that supports 10–15 minutes of private reflection	Process of Cultural Competence Model
Upstream Risks Screening Tool & Guide	Health-care professionals with a high level of health literacy	Objective self-reflection; subject responds to 28 interview questions focused on SDOH domains	Assesses a person's social needs and concerns in five SDOH domains: economic stability, education, social/community context, neighborhood and physical environment, and food	Administer in a quiet space that supports 20–25 minutes of private conversation	SDOH
WellRx Questionnaire (Page-Reeves et al., 2016)	Health-care professionals with a high level of health literacy	Objective self-reflection; tool includes 11 items requiring yes/no response and focusing on various socioeconomic challenges	Tool is intended to be a quick screening of social needs (e.g., food and housing security, employment, safety)	Administer in a quiet space that supports 10 minutes of private conversation	SDOH

therapies remotely? Does this person have safe housing? Are they food secure? Does the community where they live provide them with safe access to green space? Are there affordable community health programs they can access if they choose to do so? Practitioners who can consider such questions are more likely to create an occupational profile that considers social needs and the impact of SDOH on occupational performance and health behaviors.

At an intrapersonal level, an OTP who critically reflects and knows to ask about social needs has laid a good foundation. Knowing and doing are different abilities. Being able to respectfully ask potentially sensitive questions is an interpersonal skill that takes practice. An OTP must develop an interviewing approach where creating a relationship is more important than gathering data. Motivational Interviewing (MI) is one good method (Frey et al., 2021). When done well, the OTP is an empathic listener who empowers a person and helps them understand and articulate their own goals and motivations; the OTP also helps a person speak clearly about what may be getting in the way of their recovery (Frey & Hall, 2021). **Empathic inquiry** is another effective approach. Empathic inquiry is grounded in MI and trauma-informed care; OTPs use interpersonal skills to engage, empathize with, support, summarize, action plan, and collaborate with the person (Oregon Primary Care Association, 2023). This approach has been found to be effective when interviewing individuals about SDOH (Thornton & Persaud, 2018). Using an empathic inquiry approach requires the OTP to prioritize human connection as the goal of the interview and to understand the person's lived experiences, concerns, and perspectives. Finally, an OTP who is adept at using the Intentional Relationship Model (Taylor, 2020) may find that the therapeutic modes of advocating, collaborating, empathizing, encouraging, instructing, and problem-solving in this model may also be an effective approach to developing SDOH inquiry skills. Questions an OTP may use to prompt dialogue around some SDOH topics are presented in the text that follows. These are followed by prompts that can support critical reflection on one's interviewing skills and the context of service delivery where one practices.

Dialogue Prompts

- When I asked you to describe yourself, you said [insert gender, race, ethnicity, sexuality, etc.]. What does that identity mean to you?
- Do you feel as if your identity as [insert gender, race, ethnicity, sexuality, etc.] makes it harder or easier to deal with things?
- What are some of your biggest challenges in the community? What do you feel might be causing these challenges?
- What are some of the things you do in your community that you enjoy the most? What activities make you feel most supported in the neighborhood?
- Are there people or places in the community that make these problems better? Worse?
- What are some things I can do that could make talking about this more comfortable?

Reflection Prompts

- What could make my approach more openly welcoming and hospitable?
- Do the practices intentionally or unintentionally reflect a middle-class perspective and value system that elicits resistance from people accessing services?
- Is the person's ability to access health care impacted by availability?
- What opportunities truly exist for community members to take a direct role in health-care access?
- Does poverty or economic insecurity impact a person's capacity to adhere to treatment interventions?
- Does the availability or cost of transportation impact the person's ability to access services?

In public health, a variety of screening tools are being developed and tested to help OTPs identify health-related social needs. For example, the Centers for Medicare & Medicaid Services' (CMS) *Health-Related Social Needs Screening Tool* (CMS, 2021) is a 26-item screening tool that can help an OTP attend to social needs in several areas such as housing stability, food insecurity, interpersonal safety, financial strain, mental health, and disabilities. Items such as, "Do you speak a language other than English at home?" or "Because of a physical, mental, or emotional condition, do you have serious difficulty concentrating, remembering, or making decisions?" can be answered yes or no, whereas others such as, "How often do you feel lonely or isolated from those around you?" ask for a frequency with a range such as never to always (CMS, 2021, pp. 6–10). The Therapeutic Reasoning Assessment in Table 28-4 shares additional tools that an OTP might consider using to screen and interview around social needs.

Community, Organizational, and Institutional Level

When OTPs work midstream, often in community-based settings or with individuals and populations who may be unhoused, are food insecure, have histories of trauma, or have poor access to employment and education, they attend to individual needs, but also focus more intentionally on social needs. If an OTP has intentionally screened for social needs (housing, food security, access, etc.) when completing their occupational profiles, these data combined with an occupational perspective can inform their collaboration with others in the community. Using an occupational perspective to inform decision-making on how best to provide direct supports and ensure services target social needs, as well as build access and social inclusion, can improve options for occupation that benefit the health of the community.

SES is identified as a powerful predictor of social determinants; therefore, it's important that OTPs make the time to understand how to support a person's access to community health and mental health resources. This sometimes requires a role shift from direct intervention to care coordinator, which is a health-care professional who can link individuals with important resources addressing SDOH. These may include transportation (e.g., access reduced passes for Uber or Lyft); access to housing, food, and utilities (e.g., temporary housing, food stamps, free and reduced-cost school lunch for children, *Low Income Home Energy Assistance Program* [*LIHEAP*]); or access to community programs (e.g., Alcoholics Anonymous/Narcotics Anonymous, trauma-informed care, free yoga or exercise classes). This means that OTPs must do their homework! It is important to know what is available, to make connections with key leaders in the community and key individuals in organizations, and to be ready to share knowledge of resources that fit the health and social needs of those they work with.

OTPs making a difference at this level should expect to collaborate with multidisciplinary team members and seek out social workers, case managers, medical doctors, and mental health professionals to collectively work to address social determinants for the individuals they treat. The CORE and OBCD frameworks discussed earlier both emphasized partnering with critical stakeholders such as community members and leaders as well as directors of social, religious, political, and environmental organizations. Both models provide some guidelines for approaching these tasks.

OTPs providing community- or center-based mental health services can work to ensure day-to-day practices at these facilities are welcoming and intentionally address social determinants and systemic discrimination impacting their workforce and the people using their services. Practical examples of actionable steps might include reviewing organizational practices on the use of pronouns, using a person's preferred name in electronic health records/charts, or offering gender-neutral bathrooms in a setting with an LGBTQ population in the community. Evaluate educational materials, handouts, and pamphlets to ensure they meet National Institutes of Health recommendations to be written at a sixth- to seventh-grade reading level. Work with or lead the team to create a system for reporting microaggressions in the workplace for service users and OTPs who are victims of racism. A final point here is the importance of documentation. Practitioners must use the language of SDOH in their documentation and specify the social needs they uncover when creating occupational profiles. When OTPs specifically include content regarding SDOH factors such as housing or food insecurity, racism, stigma and discrimination, unsafe neighborhood environments, limited employment opportunities, and/or access issues related to education and health care, they are building data that can help identify the most pressing needs for a population and communities (AOTA, 2022; Haggans, 2023).

Policy and Socioenvironmental Level

Working even further upstream requires OTPs to concentrate on improving community conditions and access to occupations. The focus of efforts at this level involves changes to laws, regulations, and policies that address SDOH and health equity, and create conditions in the community that support health, social inclusion, and occupational participation for everyone. Practitioners address upstream factors when they advocate, use their expertise and collaborate with key stakeholders to bring an occupational opportunity and participation lens to government policies at the local, state, and federal levels. OTPs can support policies that close mental health disparity gaps for communities and populations by familiarizing themselves with public health policies aimed at addressing racism, structural inequities, and SDOH. For example, OTPs might advocate that services in their community for people with intellectual and developmental disabilities (IDDs) and mental health needs utilize a Systemic, Therapeutic, Assessment, Resources, and Treatment (START) model approach (National Center for START Services, 2024). This evidence-based model is consistent with community-built and community-informed

practices that address SDOH. AOTA's Legislative Advocacy Center maintains an advocacy issues page that can help OTPs gain understanding of current bills proposed or under review by the Senate and House of Representatives, some of which would close disparity gaps for individuals with mental health diagnoses (AOTA, 2024).

The authors of this chapter argue that OTPs can and do work downstream, midstream, and upstream (see Fig. 28-6), can do so simultaneously, and that it is every OTP's responsibility to work to dismantle racism, as well as systemic and structural inequities that drive poor health outcomes for oppressed and minoritized populations.

Here's the Point

- A holistic PEO approach requires OTPs to consider that each person they encounter in therapy is embedded in a set of complex social, political, economic, and cultural systems that influence every aspect of that individual's social identities, health, and well-being.
- Multiple social drivers increase the risks of mental illness, including poor access to health care, systemic and structural racism, stigma, ACE, income inequity, housing instability, and unemployment. Racism and SES are strongly linked to mental health outcomes.
- Working toward health equity, so that everyone has a fair and just opportunity to attain health and well-being, is enhanced when OTPs use a PEO approach informed by lenses of equity and ecological systems.
- By understanding that humans have multiple, intersecting social identities, OTPs can use a lens of intersectionality to intentionally consider a person's social identities and help them better understand the individual's occupational opportunities and choices.
- OTPs and scholars are creating concept and practice frameworks that OTPs can use to better understand and take actions that address racism, health equity, and SDOH.
- Racism is a powerful structural inequity operating in health-care systems. Practitioners must address this and other inequities at multiple levels including individual, interpersonal, community and policy levels.

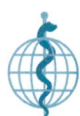 Visit the online resource center at **FADavis.com** to access the videos.

Apply It Now

1. Exploring Social Identities in My Community

Scan your community and identify an event to participate in or a setting to visit. Your choice should be an event or place that is just outside your comfort zone and not a group, population, or setting that is routine for you. Choose something that will present a new experience. Events or places might include a Pride weekend parade or festival, an ethnic festival such as Polish-Fest or Dia de los Muertos celebrations, a drag show, a political or consciousness-raising

event such as a protest or a Hearing Voices Network event, or any number of events that may exist in your area. Do your homework and research the event online as much as you can. Before you attend the event, think about what you expect to see, hear, smell, feel, and so on. It is best if you write some of these assumptions down or create a brief audio note on your phone that documents your preattendance expectations. Attend the event and then answer the following reflective questions.

Reflective Questions
- What did you notice? Consider the experience in terms of all your senses. What sights, sounds, smells, and feelings did you most notice?
- Read or listen to your preattendance notes/audio message. Reflect on the experience. How did the actual experience of the event compare with your expectations?
- Consider the people you interacted with, met, or observed while at this event. How might their primary social identities overlap with your own? How might they differ?

2. Social Identity and Behavior

In this exercise, use a lens of social identity to understand and situate behavior. Read and reflect on the following questions and write brief answers to each of them. These questions are designed to help you examine how you have come to think about what constitutes normal and abnormal behavior and to consider the impact of identity on behavior. For each question, try to provide an example that helps explain your response. When you have responded to each question, pair up with a peer and compare your responses with the following reflective questions.

Reflective Questions
- What are my own boundaries for what I think constitutes normal and abnormal behavior? How did I learn to define what constitutes normality? Have my boundaries changed over time?
- Reexamine Figure 28-1, which is a visualization of a mental health continuum including Excelling-Thriving-Surviving-Struggling-Crisis. What assumptions underlie your own conceptual models about mental illness and about how you think about and understand the behavior of others?
- This chapter has defined multiple ways that social drivers influence human experience and behavior, health, and mental health. Create one example, your own example, of how factors such as racism, poverty, homophobia, ableism, or violence influence human experience and behavior.
- How might a person's social identity influence the kinds of challenges to health and mental health that they report or the meaning the person attaches to these problems?

3. Social Identity Collage

Reexamine Figure 28-5. Create a collage that represents you and your primary and secondary identities. At a basic level, you can draw a medium-sized circle in the middle of a page representing you surrounded by layers of additional smaller circles, each labeled with characteristics from Figure 28-5 that you feel apply to you or that are important to you. You can also be more creative and use images and words that you draw, download, or find in printed materials to represent characteristics of your identity. Use the following reflective questions to consider what you have created.

Reflective Questions
- What was your first or most automatic thought when you started this task?
- How did you experience the task?
- What characteristics of your identity did you automatically include in your description and which did you reflect a bit more on before adding or leaving out?
- In what way are the characteristics of your identity the same or different from those of your peers?
- Do you think any of these characteristics might impact your approaches to evaluation and intervention with others? Explain.

4. Social Determinants of My Mental Health

Consider the neighborhood where you grew up or live in now. On a piece of paper or your device, answer these following questions with "yes" or "no."
- Is there an adequate food supply and easy access to fresh foods?
- Is most of the housing in this neighborhood good to high quality with consistent upkeep?
- Is the area you are thinking about economically stable and vibrant?
- Do people in this area have strong social relationships and are they civically and politically involved at various levels?
- Is there good transportation available?
- Is there adequate green space?
- Can people in this neighborhood easily access high-quality educational and health services?

Reflective Questions
- If all or most of your answers to these questions are "yes," try to articulate how each of the "yes" characteristics in your neighborhood may have supported your health and mental health.
- If all or most of your answers to these questions are "no," try to articulate how each of the "no" characteristics in your neighborhood may present challenges to your health and mental health.
- With a colleague, discuss your analysis of your neighborhood through lenses of SDOH and health equity.

5. *Healthy People 2030* SDOH Infographics

Follow the URL displayed at the end of this activity. You will find easy to read SDOH infographics. These are well done illustrations providing concise examples of how social drivers influence health and mental health across various domains of the socioecological environment including economics, education, health-care access, the neighborhood environment, and school and community contexts. Download an infographic that most interests you and prepare to share and discuss the content with a peer who does the same: https://health.gov/healthypeople/priority-areas/social-determinants-health/literature-summaries#block-sdohinfographics

Resources

Videos

- "Positive Mindset Creative Arts Festival" video. This video showcases the Positive Mindset Creative Arts Festival, held at the Queensland Children's Hospital in Australia. This annual children's festival promotes positive thinking about mental health and increases help-seeking behaviors with a creative arts focus. It is a notable example of how OTPs can contribute to community health efforts. The emphasis is on art as an occupation and creating space in the community to encourage and celebrate mental health. In addition, the event promotes the idea of social connection and belonging centered around self-expression of feelings across the mental health continuum and how that ultimately encourages the sense of connection and belonging with people and communities. Access the video at the online resource center at FADavis.com.
- "Managing Challenging Behaviors in Young Children" video. In this video, an occupational therapist and occupational therapy assistant (OTA) discuss the OTA's work in an Operation Breakthrough program within Head Start. The OTA works with young children from at-risk families; together with teachers and other therapists, she helps to catch any developmental delays and intervene as necessary. She describes a particularly challenging behavior in one child and the strategies she uses to help him feel comfortable, safe, and loved, allowing him to better participate in the classroom and individual sessions. Access the video at the online resource center at FADavis.com.
- "Jordon's Lived Experience of Anxiety and Depression" video. In this video, occupational therapist Jordan describes her lived experience of anxiety and depression. She touches on many issues critical to recovery and occupational therapy practice, including SDOH, peer support, and how mental health labels can adversely affect an individual's medical treatment. Importantly, she explains how she has learned to blend her lived experience with her work as an occupational therapist, while ensuring she takes care of herself and manages her symptoms. Jordan also offers priceless words of wisdom to OTPs regarding establishing a therapeutic connection with individuals with whom they practice. Access the video at the online resource center at FADavis.com.
- "Occupational Therapy Approaches in a Shelter for Unaccompanied Refugee Youth" video. In this video, occupational therapist Claudette Fette shares the impactful work she, volunteer students, and staff performed in a massive unaccompanied minor shelter in Texas in 2021. Many of the minors, mostly from Central America, had histories of trauma, and the conditions in the shelter were dismal—lack of meaningful occupations, bullying, untrained staff, and so on. Claudette describes her approach to assessing the environment, training staff, recruiting volunteers, responding to the minors' trauma responses, and creating and supporting occupations and leisure activities. Access the video at the online resource center at FADavis.com.
- "Student Perceptions of Bias and Stigma" video. In this video, four occupational therapy students reflect on how they came to recognize and work through their own biases against people who are unhoused. Each describes meeting and working in a student-run occupational therapy clinic with individuals who were unhoused and/or experiencing mental illness. They explain how engaging with these individuals and learning their stories became the impetus for transformative learning. Access the video at the online resource center at FADavis.com.
- "Cooking Group in a State Mental Hospital" video. In this video, occupational therapist Samuel Gentile describes an extremely meaningful therapeutic group he runs in a state mental hospital. Samuel's weekly cooking group allows him to assess individuals' occupational performance and physical health, as well as help them develop functional skills. He shares why the experience is so powerful for the hospital residents and what it has taught him as an OTP. Access the video at the online resource center at FADavis.com.

Books

- Dsouza, S. A., Galvaan, R., & Ramugondo, E. (2017). *Concepts in occupational therapy: Understanding southern perspectives.* Manipal University Press. Various authors, mostly from India and South Africa, provide examples of occupational therapy practice addressing socioeconomic, cultural, and political factors. Application of occupational therapy and occupational science concepts to practice in Global South countries provides a global perspective that can inform practice.
- Ivlev, S. R. (2023). *Occupational therapy disruptors: What global OT practice can teach us about innovation, culture, and community.* Jessica Kinsley Publishers. The editor of this collection has gathered perspectives from OTPs around the globe. Their stories of culturally relevant practice provide a global lens on occupational therapy in a range of cultural and political contexts that can broaden and inform one's reflexivity and practice.
- Lopes, R. E., & Malfitano, A. P. S. (2020). *Social Occupational Therapy: Theoretical and practical designs.* Elsevier. This book offers both theoretical and practical chapters regarding occupational therapy's role in addressing the social needs of vulnerable populations. The text emphasizes occupation as a human right, examines occupational therapy's role as a social profession, and shares examples of OTPs responding to social issues.
- Musharrat, J. A.-L. (2023). *Anti-racist occupational therapy: Unsettling the status quo.* Jessica Kinsley Publishers. The editor of this collection has gathered perspectives from minoritized OTPs spanning a variety of practice and academic settings. Readers will expand their knowledge of antiracist practices that are accessible and sustainable.

Websites

- The Office of Minority Health Resource Center: https://minorityhealth.hhs.gov/office-minority-health-resource-center. This website is maintained by the USDHHS and includes a wealth of information that can be applied to minoritized populations. Consumers, professionals, and researchers are provided free online resources from a substantial document collection. This site also allows one to ask for a customized request of information on funding opportunities that may match your needs.
- The National Center for Cultural Competence: https://nccc.georgetown.edu. This website provides a wealth of information about cultural and linguistic competence. Among other things, you will find information about conceptual frameworks for cultural competency, tools for assessing your own cultural competence, and practical resources to support cross-cultural care for children, adults, and families.
- Trying Together—Anti-Racism Tools: https://tryingtogether.org/community-resources/anti-racism-tools. Trying Together is a community-based organization operating in southwestern Pennsylvania. Their focus is on early childhood care and education for professionals, families, and caregivers. They have multiple resources loaded on their website and an entire page dedicated to anti-racism where OTPs will find hundreds of tools, videos, short articles, and other resources focused on anti-racism.
- World Health Organization—Social Determinants of Health: https://www.who.int/health-topics/social-determinants-of-health#tab=tab_1. This page on the WHO's website provides solid descriptions of SDOH and health equity and defines both key challenges and critical actions to take to address health inequities. Multiple resources that help OTPs gain a global perspectives of SDOH are found on this site.

References

Agency for Healthcare Research and Quality. (2020). *About SDOH in health care*. Author. https://www.ahrq.gov/sdoh/about.html

Agner, J. (2020). Moving from cultural competence to cultural humility in occupational therapy: A paradigm shift. *American Journal of Occupational Therapy, 74*(4), 7404347010p1–7404347010p7. https://doi.org/10.5014/ajot.2020.038067

Ahmed-Landeryou, M. J. (2024). *Antiracist occupational therapy: Unsettling the status quo.* Jessica Kingsley Publishers.

Ajzen, I., & Fishbein, M. (1980). *Understanding attitudes and predicting social behavior.* Prentice Hall.

Albuquerque, S., & Farias, L. (2022). Occupational therapists' perceptions of the need to enact health promotion in community development through occupational justice. *Cadernos de Terapia Ocupacional, 30,* 1–17. https://doi.org/10.1590/2526-8910.ctoAO23253070

Alegría, M., NeMoyer, A., Falgàs Bagué, I., Wang, Y., & Alvarez, K. (2018). Social determinants of mental health: Where we are and where we need to go. *Current Psychiatry Reports, 20*(11), 95. https://doi.org/10.1007/s11920-018-0969-9

Allen, J., Balfour, R., Bell, R., & Marmot, M. (2014). Social determinants of mental health. *International Review of Psychiatry, 26*(4), 392–407. https://doi.org/10.3109/09540261.2014.928270

American Occupational Therapy Association. (2020a). Educator's guide for addressing cultural awareness, humility, and dexterity in occupational therapy curricula. *The American Journal of Occupational Therapy, 74*(3), 7413420003p1–7413420003p19 https://doi.org/10.5014/ajot.2020.74S3005

American Occupational Therapy Association. (2020b). Occupational therapy practice framework: Domain and process—Fourth edition. *The American Journal of Occupational Therapy, 74*(Suppl._2), 7412410010p1–7412410010p87. https://doi.org/10.5014/ajot.2020.74S2001

American Occupational Therapy Association. (2022). *AOTA occupational profile community mental health–Homelessness example.* Author. https://www.aota.org/-/media/corporate/files/practice/manage/documentation/community-mental-health-occupational-profile-example.pdf

American Occupational Therapy Association. (2023a). *AOTA 2023 compensation and workforce survey.* AOTA Press. https://library.aota.org/AOTA-Workforce-Salary-Survey-2023-members

American Occupational Therapy Association. (2023b). *Evolving OT in response to societal needs.* https://www.aota.org/-/media/corporate/files/practice/practice-essentials/practice-engagement-and-capacity-building/evolving-ot-in-response-to-society-needs.pdf

American Occupational Therapy Association. (2024). *Advocacy issues.* AOTA's Legislative Advocacy Center. https://www.aota.org/advocacy/issues

American Psychiatric Association. (2022). *Diagnostic and statistical manual of mental disorders* (5th ed., text rev.). https://doi.org/10.1176/appi.books.9780890425787

American Psychiatric Association. (2023, February). *Report of the presidential task force on the social determinants of mental health.* American Psychiatric Publishing. https://www.psychiatry.org/getmedia/b73d3f7b-94dd-4a52-9267-e83328247325/2022-APA-TFSDMH-Board-of-Trustees-December-Report.pdf

Anderson, S. H. (2022). Cultivating cultural humility in occupational therapy through experiential strategies and modeling. *The Open Journal of Occupational Therapy, 10*(4), 1–7. https://doi.org/10.15453/2168-6408.1962

Armstrong-Mensah, E., Patel, H., Parekh, P., & Lee, C. (2020). Mental health inequities and disparities among African American adults in the United States: The role of race. *Research in Health Science, 5*(3), 23–32. https://doi.org/10.22158/rhs.v5n3p23

Artiga, S. (2020). *Health disparities are a symptom of broader social and economic inequities.* Kaiser Family Foundation. https://www.kff.org/policy-watch/health-disparities-symptom-broader-social-economic-inequities

Australian Health Practitioner Regulation Agency. (2018). *Australian occupational therapy competency standards.* https://www.occupationaltherapyboard.gov.au/Codes-Guidelines/Competencies.aspx

Bailliard, A. (2023). Occupational justice. In G. Gillen & C. Brown (Eds.), *Willard and Spackman's occupational therapy* (14th ed., pp. 139–160). Wolters Kluwer.

Baum, C. M., Christiansen, C. H., & Bass, J. D. (2015). The Person-Environment-Occupation-Performance (PEOP) model. In C. H. Christiansen, C. M. Baum, & J. D. Bass (Eds.), *Occupational therapy: Performance, participation, and well-being* (4th ed., pp. 49–56). Slack, Inc.

Beagan, B. L., Bizzeth, S. R., Pride, T. M., & Sibbald, K. R. (2023). Racism in occupational therapy: "It's part of who we are . . . ." *British Journal of Occupational Therapy, 86*(3), 171–175. https://doi.org/10.1177/03080226231153345

Berger, J. T., & Miller, D. R. (2021). Health disparities, systemic racism, and failures of cultural competence. *The American Journal of Bioethics, 21*(9), 4–10. https://doi.org/10.1080/15265161.2021.1915411

Braveman, P. A., Arkin, E., Proctor, D., Kauh, T., & Holm, N. (2022). Systemic and structural racism: Definitions, examples, health damages and approaches to dismantling. *Health Affairs, 41*(2), 171–178. https://doi.org/10.1377/hlthaff.2021.01394

Brennan, G. J., & Gallagher, M. B. (2017). Expectations of choice: An exploration of how social context informs gendered occupation. *Irish Journal of Occupational Therapy, 45*(1), 15–27. https://doi.org/10.1108/IJOT-01-2017-0003

Bronfenbrenner, U. (1979). *The ecology of human development: Experiments by nature and design.* Harvard University Press.

Campinha-Bacote, J. (2002). *The process of cultural competence in the delivery of healthcare services: A culturally competent model* (4th ed.). Transcultural C.A.R.E. Associates.

Campinha-Bacote, J. (2019). Cultural competemility: A paradigm shift in the cultural competence versus cultural humility debate—Part 1. *The Online Journal of Issues in Nursing, 24*(1). https://www.doi.org/10.3912/OJIN.Vol24No01PPT20

Campo-Arias, A., & De Mendieta, C. T. (2021). Social determinants of mental health and the COVID-19 pandemic in low-income and middle-income countries. *Lancet Global Health, 9*(8), e1029–e1030. https://doi.org/10.1016/S2214-109X(21)00253-9

Castrucci, B. C., & Auerbach, J. (2019, January 16). Meeting individual social needs falls short of addressing social determinants of health. *Health Affairs Blog.* https://doi.org/10.1377/hblog20190115.234942

Center for Community Health and Development. (2023). *Windshield and walking surveys.* Center for Community Health and Development at the University of Kansas. https://ctb.ku.edu/en/table-of-contents/assessment/assessing-community-needs-and-resources/windshield-walking-surveys/main

Centers for Disease Control and Prevention. (2019). *Social determinants of health: Frequently asked questions.* https://www.cdc.gov/nchhstp/socialdeterminants/faq.html

Centers for Disease Control and Prevention. (2022, September). *Health equity for people with disabilities.* https://www.cdc.gov/ncbddd/humandevelopment/health-equity.html#ref

Centers for Disease Control and Prevention. (2023). *Disability and Health Data System (DHDS).* National Center on Birth Defects and Developmental Disabilities, Division of Human Development and Disability.

Centers for Medicare & Medicaid Services. (2021). *Health-Related Social Needs Screening Tool.* Author. https://www.cms.gov/priorities/innovation/files/worksheets/ahcm-screeningtool.pdf

Chelak, K., & Chakole, S. (2023). The role of social determinants of health in promoting health equality: A narrative review. *Cureus, 15*(1), e33425. https://doi.org/10.7759/cureus.33425

Collins, P. H., & Blige. S. (2016). *Intersectionality.* Polity Press.

Crenshaw, K. (1989). Demarginalizing the intersection of race and sex: A Black feminist critique of antidiscrimination doctrine, feminist theory, and antiracist politics. *University of Chicago Legal Forum, 1,* 8. http://chicagounbound.uchicago.edu/uclf/vol1989/iss1/8

Delphis. (2020, June 30). *The mental health continuum is a better model for mental health.* https://delphis.org.uk/mental-health/continuum-mental-health

Doll, J., Malloy, J., & Gonzales, R. (2023). Social determinants of health: Opportunity for occupational therapy. *American Journal of Occupational Therapy, 77*(4), 7704090010. https://doi.org/10.5014/ajot.2023.050360

Dowers, E., White, C., Kingsley, J., & Sewnson, R. (2019). Transgender experiences of occupation and the environment: A scoping review. *Journal of Occupational Science, 26,* 496–510. https://doi.org/10.1080/14427591.2018.1561382

Drake, P., & Rudowitz, R. (2022). *Tracking social determinants of health during the COVID-19 pandemic.* Kaiser Family Foundation. https://www.kff.org/coronavirus-covid-19/issue-brief/tracking-social-determinants-of-health-during-the-covid-19-pandemic

Elevance Health. (2022, February 25). *Social drivers vs. social determinants of health: Unstacking the deck.* https://www.elevancehealth.com/our-approach-to-health/whole-health/social-drivers-vs-social-determinants-of-health-unstacking-the-deck

Emery-Whittington, I., Leite, J., & Ivlev, S. (2024). Antiracism as means and ends. In M. J. Ahmed-Landeryou (Ed.), *Antiracist occupational therapy: Unsettling the status quo* (pp. 119–136). Jessica Kingsley Publishers

Finan, S. J., & Yap, M. B. (2021). Engaging parents in preventive programs for adolescent mental health: A socio-ecological framework. *Journal of Family Theory and Review, 13*(4), 515–527. https://doi.org/10.1111/jftr.12440

Fisher, M. (2022). Moving social policy from mental illness to public wellbeing. *Journal of Social Policy, 51*(3), 567–581. https://doi.org/10.1017/S0047279421000866

Flaubert, J. L., Le Menestrel, S., Williams, D. R., & Wakefield, M. K. (Eds.). (2021). *The future of nursing 2020–2030: Charting a path to achieve health equity.* National Academies Press. https://doi.org/10.17226/25982

Freire, P. (1970). *Pedagogy of the oppressed.* Bloomsbury Academic.

Frey, A. J., & Hall, A. (2021). *Motivational Interviewing for mental health clinicians: A toolkit for skills enhancement.* PESI Publishing.

Frey, A. J., Lee, J., Small, J. W., Sibley, M., Owens, J. S., Skidmore, B., Johnson, L., Bradshaw, C. P., & Moyers, T. B. (2021). Mechanisms of Motivational Interviewing: A conceptual framework to guide practice and research. *Prevention Science, 22,* 689–700. https://doi.org/10.1007/s11121-020-01139-x

Friedman, C., Feldner, H., & VanPuymbrouck, L. (2022). Anti-fat biases of occupational and physical therapy assistants. *Occupational Therapy in Health Care, 36*(1), 63–83. https://doi.org/10.1080/07380577.2021.1972380

Friedman, C., & VanPuymbrouck, L. (2021). Impact of occupational therapy education on students' disability attitudes: A longitudinal study. *The American Journal of Occupational Therapy, 75*(4), 7504180090. https://doi.org/10.5014/ajot.2021.047423

Froehlich-Grobe, K., Douglas, M., Ochoa, C., & Betts, A. (2021). Social determinants of health and disability. In D.J. Lollar, W. Horner-Johnson, & K. Froehlich-Grobe (Eds.), *Public health perspectives on disability* (2nd ed., pp. 53–90). Springer. https://doi.org/10.1007/978-1-0716-0888-3_3

Fung, V., Price, M., McDowell, A., Nierenberg, A. A., Hsu, J., Newhouse, J. P., & Cook, B. L. (2023). Coverage parity and racial and ethnic disparities in mental health and substance use care among Medicare beneficiaries. *Health Affairs, 42*(1), 83–93. https://doi.org/10.1377/hlthaff.2022.00624

Gachon, N. (2021). Hegemony. In N. Gachon (Ed.), *Bernie Sanders's democratic socialism: Holding utopia accountable* (pp. 122–141). Palgrave Macmillan.

Gallagher, M., Pettigrew, J., & Muldoon, O. (2015). Occupational choice of youth in a disadvantaged community. *British Journal of Occupational Therapy, 78,* 622–629. https://doi.org/10.1177/0308022615583065

Galvaan, R. (2012). Occupational choice: The significance of socio-economic and political factors. In G. E. Whiteford & C. Hocking (Eds.), *Occupational science: Society, inclusion and participation* (pp. 152–162). Wiley-Blackwell.

Galvaan, R. (2015). The contextually situated nature of occupational choice: Marginalised young adolescents' experiences in South Africa. *Journal of Occupational Science, 22,* 39–53. https://doi.org/10.1080/14427591.2014.912124

Galvaan, R., & Peters, L. (2017). Occupation-based community development: A critical approach to occupational therapy. In S. Dsouza, R. Galvaan, & E. Ramugondo (Eds.), *Concepts in occupational therapy: Understanding Southern perspectives* (pp. 172–182). Manupal University Press.

Galvaan, R., Peters, L., Cornelius, C., & Richards, L. (2024, January). *Occupation-based community development: Strategies for promoting potential.* https://mandelainitiative.org.za/wp-content/uploads/2021/09/87_Galvaan_Occupation%20based%20community%20development_strategies%20for%20promoting%20potential.pdf

Gibson, B., Schneider, J., Talamonti, D., & Forshaw, M. (2021). The impact of inequality on mental health outcomes during the COVID-19 pandemic: A systematic review. *Canadian Psychology, 62*(1), 101–126. https://doi.org/10.1037/cap0000272

Ginsberg, S. M., & Mayfield-Clarke, B. (2021). Applying concepts of cultural humility in CSD education. *Teaching and Learning in Communication Sciences & Disorders, 5*(3), 1–10. https://doi.org/10.30707/tlcsd5.3.1649037688.632982

Glanz, K., Rimer, B. K., & Viswanath, K. (2015). *Health behavior: Theory, research, and practice* (5th ed.). Jossey-Bass.

Golden, T., & Wendel, M. L. (2020). Public health's next step in advancing equity: Re-evaluating epistemological assumptions to move social determinants from theory to practice. *Frontiers in Public Health, 8,* Article 131. https://doi.org/10.3389/fpubh.2020.00131

Gramsci, A. (1975). *Prison notebooks.* Columbia University Press.

Grenier, M.-L. (2020). Cultural competency and the reproduction of white supremacy in occupational therapy education. *Health Education Journal, 79*(6), 633–644. https://doi.org/10.1177/0017896920902515

Grenier, M.-L., Zafran, H., & Roy, L. (2020). Current landscape of teaching diversity in occupational therapy education: A scoping review. *The American Journal of Occupational Therapy, 74*(6), 7406205100p1–7406205100p15. https://doi.org/10.5014/ajot.2020.044214

Haggans, J. (2023). Identifying social determinants (drivers) of health using AOTA's occupational profile template. *OT Practice, 28*(11), 42–43. https://www.aota.org/publications/ot-practice/ot-practice-issues/2023/practice-improvement-perk-identifying-social-determinants?utm_campaign=2023_OTI_Lead%20Nurture%20Emails

Hamilton, K. A., Letts, L. J., Larivière, N., & Moll, S. E. (2023). Revisiting the Do-Live-Well health promotion framework: A citation content analysis. *Canadian Journal of Occupational Therapy, 90*(3), 297–302. https://doi.org/10.1177/00084174221149268

Hammell, K. W. (2015). Occupational rights and critical occupational therapy: Rising to the challenge. *Australian Occupational Therapy Journal, 62,* 449–451. https://doi.org/10.1111/1440-1630.12195

Hammell, K. W. (2017a). Critical reflections on occupational justice: Toward a rights-based approach to occupational opportunities. *Canadian Journal of Occupational Therapy, 84*(1), 47–57. https://doi.org/10.1177/0008417416654501

Hammell, K. W. (2017b). Opportunities for well-being: The right to occupational engagement. *Canadian Journal of Occupational Therapy, 84*(4-5), 209–222. https://doi.org/10.1177/0008417417734831

Hammell, K. W. (2020a). Action on the social determinants of health: Advancing occupational equity and occupational rights.

Cadernos Brasileiros de Terapia Ocupacional, 28(1), 378–400. https://doi.org/10.4322/2526-8910.ctoARF2052

Hammell, K. W. (2020b). Making choices from the choices we have: The contextual-embeddedness of occupational choice. *Canadian Journal of Occupational Therapy, 87*(5), 400–411. https://doi.org/10.1177/0008417420965741

Hammell, K. W. (2021). Social and structural determinants of health: Exploring occupational therapy's structural (in)competence. *Canadian Journal of Occupational Therapy, 88*(4), 365–374. https://doi.org/10.1177/00084174211046797

Hammell, K. W., & Beagan, B. (2017). Occupational injustice: A critique. *Canadian Journal of Occupational Therapy, 84*(1), 58–68. https://doi.org/10.1177/0008417416638858

Harvard University Office for Equity, Diversity, Inclusion, and Belonging. (2024). *Implicit Association Test (IAT).* Author. https://edib.harvard.edu/implicit-association-test-iat

Hill, B. (2021). Expanding our understanding and use of the Ecological Systems Theory Model for the prevention of maternal obesity: A new socioecological framework. *Obesity Reviews, 22,* e13147. https://doi.org/10.1111/obr.13147

Horner-Johnson, W. (2021). Disability, intersectionality, and inequity: Life at the margins. In D. J. Lollar, W. Horner-Johnson, & K. Froehlich-Grobe (Eds.), *Public health perspectives on disability* (2nd ed., pp. 91–106). Springer. https://doi.org/10.1007/978-1-0716-0888-3_4

Hoyt, C. R., Clifton, M., Smith, C. R., Woods, L., & Taff, S. D. (2023). Transforming occupational therapy for the 21st century PAIRE: Recognize Privilege, Acknowledge Injustice, and Reframe Perspective to Reach Equity. *Occupational Therapy in Health Care,* 1–24. https://doi.org/10.1080/07380577.2023.2265479

Hyett, N., Kenny, A., & Dickson-Swift, V. (2019). Re-imagining occupational therapy clients as communities: Presenting the community-centred practice framework. *Scandinavian Journal of Occupational Therapy, 26*(4), 246–260. https://doi.org/10.1080/11038128.2017.1423374

Irvine-Brown, L., Tommaso, A. D., Malfitano, A. P., & Molineux, M. (2020). Experiences of occupational therapy education: Contexts, communities, and Social Occupational Therapy. *Cadernos Brasileiros de Terapia Ocupacional, 28*(1), 330–342. https://doi.org/10.4322/2526-8910.ctoARF1931

Islam, M. M. (2019). Social determinants of health and related inequalities: Confusion and implications. *Frontiers in Public Health, 7,* 11. https://doi.org/10.3389/fpubh.2019.00011

Jeste, D. V., Koh, S., & Pender, V. B. (2022). Perspective: Social determinants of mental health for the new decade of healthy aging. *American Journal of Geriatric Psychiatry, 30*(6), 733–736. https://doi.org/10.1016/j.jagp.2022.01.006

Johnson, K., Kirby, A., Washington, S., Lavalley, R., & Faison, T. (2022). Linking antiracist action from the classroom to practice. *American Journal of Occupational Therapy, 76*(5), 7605347010. https://doi.org/10.5014/ajot.2022.050054

Johnson, K. R., & Lavalley, R. (2021). From racialized think-pieces toward anti-racist praxis in our science, education, and practice. *Journal of Occupational Science, 28*(3), 404–409. https://doi.org/10.1080/14427591.2020.1847598

Johnson, K. R., Washington, S., Opuku, E. N., & Adomako, E. S. (2024). Antiracist occupational therapy education: Perspectives from Ghana, the United Kingdom, and the United States of America. In M. J. Ahmed-Landeryou (Ed.), *Antiracist occupational therapy: Unsettling the status quo* (pp. 68–83). Jessica Kingsley Publishers.

Johnstone, L., & Boyle, M., with Cromby, J., Dillon, J., Harper, D., Kinderman, P., Longden, E., Pilgrim, D., & Read, J. (2018). *The Power Threat Meaning Framework: Towards the identification of patterns in emotional distress, unusual experiences and troubled or troubling behaviour, as an alternative to functional psychiatric diagnosis.* British Psychological Society. https://www.madinamerica.com/wp-content/uploads/2020/12/The-Power-Threat-Meaning-Framework.pdf

Kallivayalil, R. A., & Enara, A. (2022). Mental health in an unequal world: The role of social determinants. *Indian Journal of Social Psychiatry, 38*(1), 3–6. https://doi.org/10.4103/ijsp.ijsp_48_22

Khanolkar, A., Bolster, A., Tabor, E., Frost, D. M., Patalay, P., & Redcliff, V. (2022). *Lived experiences and their consequences for health in sexual and ethnic minority young adults in the UK—A qualitative study.* University College London. https://www.ucl.ac.uk/cardiovascular/sites/cardiovascular/files/mmi_health_-_br_feb_2022_web.pdf

Kielhofner, G. (2008). *A Model of Human Occupation: Theory and application* (4th ed.). Williams & Wilkins.

Kim, P. J. (2019). Social determinants of health inequities in indigenous Canadians through a life course approach to colonialism and the residential school system. *Health Equity, 3*(1), 378–381. https://doi.org/10.1089/heq.2019.0041

Kivimäki, M., Batty, G. D., Pentti, J., Shipley, M. J., Sipilä, P. N., Nyberg, S. T., Suominen, S. B., Oksanen, T., Stenholm, S., Virtanen, M., Marmot, M. G., Singh-Manoux, A., Brunner, E. J., Lindbohm, J. V., Ferrie, J. E., & Vahtera, J. (2020). Association between socioeconomic status and the development of mental and physical health conditions in adulthood: A multi-cohort study. *Lancet Public Health, 5*(3), e140–e149. https://doi.org/10.1016/S2468-2667(19)30248-8

Kolb, D. A. (1984). *Experiential learning: Experience as the source of learning and development.* Prentice-Hall.

Kotov, R., Krueger, R. F., Watson, D., Cicero, D. C., Conway, C. C., DeYoung, C. G., Eaton, N. R., Forbes, M. K., Hallquist, M. N., Latzman, R. D., Mullins-Sweatt, S. N., Ruggero, C. J., Simms, L. J., Waldman, I. D., Waszczuk, M. A., & Wright, A. G. C. (2021). The hierarchical taxonomy of psychopathology: A quantitative nosology based on consensus of evidence. *Annual Review of Clinical Psychology, 17*(1), 83–108. https://doi.org/10.1146/annurev-clinpsy-081219-093304

Kronenberg, F., & Pollard, N. (2005). Overcoming occupational apartheid: A preliminary exploration of the political nature of occupational therapy. In F. Kronenberg, S. S. Algado, & N. Pollard (Eds.), *Occupational therapy without borders: Learning from the spirit of survivors* (pp. 58–86). Elsevier.

Laliberte Rudman, D. (2010). Occupational terminology: Occupational possibilities. *Journal of Occupational Science, 17,* 1, 55–59. https://doi.org/10.1080/14427591.2010.9686673

Laliberte Rudman, D. (2014). Embracing and enacting an 'occupational imagination': Occupational science as transformative. *Journal of Occupational Science, 21*(4), 373–388. https://doi.org/10.1080/14427591.2014.888970

Laliberte Rudman, D. (2015). Situating occupation in social relations of power: Occupational possibilities, ageism and the retirement 'choice'. *South African Journal of Occupational Therapy, 45*(1), 27–33. https://doi.org/10.17159/2310-3833/2015/v45no1a5

Lavalley, R., & Johnson, K. R. (2022). Occupation, injustice, and anti-black racism in the United States of America. *Journal of Occupational Science, 29*(4), 487–499. https://doi.org/10.1080/14427591.2020.1810111

Law, M., Cooper, B., Strong, S., Stewart, D., Rigby, P., & Letts, L. (1996). Person–Environment–Occupation Model: A transactive approach to occupational performance. *Canadian Journal of Occupational Therapy, 63,* 9–23. https://doi.org/10.1177/000841749606300103

Lekas, H. M., Pahl, K., & Lewis, C. F. (2020). Rethinking cultural competence: Shifting to cultural humility. *Health Services Insights, 13,* 1–4. https://doi.org/10.1177/1178632920970580

Lerner, J. E., & Kim, A. (2024). "This is about heart knowledge": The disconnect between anti-racist knowledge and practice among white students in social work education. *Social Work Education,* 1–19. https://doi.org/10.1080/02615479.2024.2324901

Londono Tobon, A., Flores, J. M., Taylor, J. H., Johnson, I., Landeros-Weisenberger, A., Aboiraloi, O., Avila-Quintero, V. J., & Bloch, M. H. (2021). Racial implicit associations in psychiatric diagnosis, treatment, and compliance expectations. *Academic Psychiatry, 45*(1), 23–33. https://doi.org/10.1007/s40596-020-01370-2

Lopez, L., Hart, L. H., & Katz, M. H. (2021). Racial and ethnic health disparities related to COVID-19. *Journal of the American Medical Association, 325*(8), 719–720. https://doi.org/10.1001/jama.2020.26443

Lucyk, K., & McLaren, L. (2017). Taking stock of the social determinants of health: A scoping review. *PLoS One, 12,* e0177306. https://doi.org/10.1371/journal.pone.0177306

Lund, C., Brooke-Sumner, C., Baingana, F., Baron, E. C., Breuer, E., Chandra, P., Haushofer, J., Herrman, H., Jordans, M., Kieling, C., Medina-Mora, M. E., Morgan, E., Omigbodun, O., Tol, W., Patel, V., & Saxena, S. (2018). Social determinants of mental disorders and the sustainable development goals: A systematic review of reviews. *The Lancet Psychiatry, 5*(4), 357–369. https://doi.org/10.1016/S2215-0366(18)30060-9

Lysack, C. L., Adamo, D. E., & Galvaan, R. (2023). Social economic and political factors that influence occupational performance. In G. Gillen & C. Brown (Eds.), *Willard and Spackman's occupational therapy* (14th ed., pp. 224–242). Wolters Kluwer.

Maffly-Kipp, J., Eisenbeck, N., Carreno, D. F., & Hicks, J. (2021). Mental health inequalities increase as a function of COVID-19 pandemic severity levels. *Social Science & Medicine (1982), 285,* 114275. https://doi.org/10.1016/j.socscimed.2021.114275

Mafitano, A. P. S. (2021). Social context and social action. In R. Lopes & A. P. S. Malfitano (Eds.), *Social Occupational Therapy: Theoretical and practical designs* (pp. 48–56). Elsevier.

Mao, W., & Agyapong, V. I. O. (2021). The role of social determinants in mental health and resilience after disasters: Implications for public health policy and practice. *Frontiers in Public Health, 9,* 658528. https://doi.org/10.3389/fpubh.2021.658528

Martín, I. Z., Flores Martos, J. A., Millares, P. M., & Björklund, A. (2015). Occupational therapy culture seen through the multifocal lens of fieldwork in diverse rural areas. *Scandinavian Journal of Occupational Therapy, 22*(2), 82–94. https://doi.org/10.3109/11038128.2014.965197

McLeroy, K. R., Bibeau, D., Steckler, A., & Glanz, K. (1988). An ecological perspective on health promotion programs. *Health Education Quarterly, 15,* 351–377. https://doi.org/10.1177/109019818801500401

Melton-Fant, C. (2022). Health equity and the dynamism of structural racism and public policy. *The Milbank Quarterly, 100*(3), 628–649. https://doi.org/10.1111/1468-0009.12581

Melville, A., Schiller, S., Engelen, A.-M., & Kramer-Roy, D. (2023). Perceptions of occupational therapists in the United Kingdom on the applicability of the reflective framework for community development in occupational therapy. *British Journal of Occupational Therapy, 86*(2), 158–168. https://doi.org/10.1177/03080226221121744

Merryman, M. B., & Riegel, S. K. (2007). The recovery process and people with serious mental illness living in the community: An occupational therapy perspective. *Occupational Therapy in Mental Health, 23*(2), 51–73. https://doi.org/10.1300/J004v23n02_03

Mthembu, T. G. (2021). A commentary of occupational justice and occupation-based community development frameworks for social transformation: The Marikana event. *South African Journal of Occupational Therapy, 51*(1), 72–75. https://doi.org/10.17159/2310-3833/2021a10

Moll, S. E., Gewurtz, R. E., Krupa, T. M., Law, M. C., Larivière, N., & Levasseur, M. (2015). "Do-Live-Well": A Canadian framework for promoting occupation, health, and well-being. *Canadian Journal of Occupational Therapy, 82*(1), 9–23. https://doi.org/10.1177/0008417414545981

Morales, D. A., Barksdale, C. L., & Beckel-Mitchener, A. C. (2020). A call to action to address rural mental health disparities. *Journal of Clinical and Translational Science, 4*(5), 463–467. https://doi.org/10.1017/cts.2020.42

Morgan, C., Gayer-Anderson, C., Beards, S., Hubbard, K., Mondelli, V., Di Forti, M., Murray, R. M., Pariante, C., Dazzan, P., Craig, T. J., Reininghaus, U., & Fisher, H. L. (2020). Threat, hostility and violence in childhood and later psychotic disorder: Population-based case-control study. *The British Journal of Psychiatry, 217*(4), 575–582. https://doi.org/10.1192/bjp.2020.133

Murthi, K., & Hammell, K. W. (2021). 'Choice' in occupational therapy theory: A critique from the situation of patriarchy in India. *Scandinavian Journal of Occupational Therapy, 28*(1), 1–12. https://doi.org/10.1080/11038128.2020.1769182

Myong, Y., Shin, H. I., Lee, J. E., Cho, W., & Yi, Y. G. (2021). Development and validation of a new scale to assess attitudes and perspectives toward persons with disabilities. *Annals of Rehabilitation Medicine, 45*(4), 331–340. https://doi.org/10.5535/arm.21046

National Center for START Services. (2024). *START Model.* https://centerforstartservices.org/START-Model

Núñez, C. M. V., Hernández, S. S., & Alarcón, A. H. (2022). Collective occupations and nature: Impacts of the coloniality of nature on rural and fishing communities in Chile. *Journal of Occupational Science, 29*(2), 252–262. https://doi.org/10.1080/14427591.2021.1880264

Oexle, N., & Corrigan, P. W. (2018). Understanding mental illness stigma toward persons with multiple stigmatized conditions: Implications of intersectionality theory. *Psychiatric Services, 69*(5), 587–589. https://doi.org/10.1176/appi.ps.201700312

Office of Disease Prevention and Health Promotion. (n.d.). *Healthy People 2030: Building a healthier future for all.* U.S. Department of Health and Human Services. https://health.gov/healthypeople

Office of the Assistant Secretary for Planning and Evaluation. (2023). *Social determinants of health.* https://aspe.hhs.gov/topics/health-health-care/social-determinants-health

Oregon Primary Care Association. (2023). *Empathic inquiry.* https://orpca.org/empathic-inquiry

Page-Reeves, J., Kaufman, W., Bleeker, M., Norris, J., McCalmont, K., Ianakieva, V., Ianakieva, D. I., & Kaufman, A. (2016). Addressing social determinants of health in a clinical setting. The WellRx Pilot in Albuquerque, New Mexico. *The Journal of the American Board of Family Medicine, 29*(3), 414–418. https://doi.org/10.3122/jabfm.2016.03.150272

Pereira, R. B. (2017). Towards inclusive occupational therapy: Introducing the CORE approach for inclusive and occupation-focused practice. *Australian Occupational Therapy Journal, 64*(6), 429–435. https://doi.org/10.1111/1440-1630.12394

Pereira, R. B., & Whiteford, G. (2018). Advancing understandings of inclusion and participation through situated research. In N. Pollard, H. van Bruggen, & S. Kantartzis (Eds.), *Occupation based social inclusion* (pp. 129–145). Whiting & Birch.

Pereira, R. B., Whiteford, G., Hyett, N., Weekes, G., Di Tommaso, A., & Naismith, J. (2020). Capabilities, Opportunities, Resources and Environments (CORE): Using the CORE approach for inclusive, occupation-centred practice. *Australian Occupational Therapy Journal, 67*(2), 162–171. https://doi.org/10.1111/1440-1630.12642

Pester, D. A., Jones, L. K., & Talib, Z. (2023). Social determinants of mental health: Informing counseling practice and professional identity. *Journal of Counseling & Development, 101,* 392–401. https://doi.org/10.1002/jcad.12473

Pitonyak, J. S., Mroz, T. M., & Fogelberg, D. (2015). Expanding client-centred thinking to include social determinants: A practical scenario based on the occupation of breastfeeding. *Scandinavian Journal of Occupational Therapy, 22*(4), 277–282. https://doi.org/10.3109/11038128.2015.1020865

Polatajko, H. J., Craik, J., Davis, J., & Townsend, E. A. (2013). Canadian Practice Process Framework. In E. A. Townsend &

H. J. Polatajko, *Enabling occupation II: Advancing an occupational therapy vision for health, well-being, and justice through occupation* (2nd ed., p. 233). CAOT Publications ACE.

Pollard, N., Sakellariou, D., & Kronenberg, F. (2009). *A political practice of occupational therapy.* Churchill Livingstone Elsevier.

Pooley, E. A., & Beagan, B. L. (2021). The concept of oppression and occupational therapy: A critical interpretive synthesis. *Canadian Journal of Occupational Therapy, 88*(4), 407–417. https://doi.org/10.1177/00084174211051168

Priester, M. A., Browne, T., Iachini, A., Clone, S., DeHart, D., & Seay, K. D. (2016). Treatment access barriers and disparities among individuals with co-occurring mental health and substance use disorders: An integrative literature review. *Journal of Substance Abuse Treatment, 61,* 47–59. https://doi.org/10.1016/j.jsat.2015.09.006

Prochaska, J. O., & Velicer, W. F. (1997). The Transtheoretical Model of Health Behavior Change. *American Journal of Health Promotion, 12*(1), 38–48. https://doi.org/10.4278/0890-1171-12.1.38

Public Health Agency of Canada. (2023). *Social determinants of health and health inequalities.* https://www.canada.ca/en/public-health/services/health-promotion/population-health/what-determines-health.html

Ramugondo, E. (2012). Intergenerational play within family: The case for occupational consciousness. *Journal of Occupational Science, 19*(4), 326–340. https://doi.org/10.1080/14427591.2012.710166

Ramugondo, E. (2015). Occupational consciousness. *Journal of Occupational Science, 22*(4), 488–501. https://doi.org/10.1080/14427591.2015.1042516

Ramugondo, E., & Kronenberg, F. (2015). Explaining collective occupations from a human relations perspective: Bridging the individual-collective dichotomy. *Journal of Occupational Science, 22*(1), 3–16. https://doi.org/10.1080/14427591.2013.781920

Ramugondo, E. (2024). Occupational consciousness. In G. Gillen & C. Brown (Eds.), *Willard and Spackman's occupational therapy* (14th ed., pp. 161–177). Wolters Kluwer.

Rees, S. N., Crowe, M., & Harris, S. (2021). The lesbian, gay, bisexual, and transgender communities' mental health care needs and experiences of mental health services: An integrative review of qualitative studies. *Journal of Psychiatric Mental Health Nursing, 28,* 578–589. https://doi.org/10.1111/jpm.12720

Reilly, M. (1962). Occupational therapy can be one of the greatest ideas of 20th century medicine. *American Journal of Occupational Therapy, 16,* 1–9. https://doi.org/10.1177/000841746303000102

Reiss, F., Meyrose, A. K., Otto, C., Lampert, T., Klasen, F., & Ravens-Sieberer, U. (2019). Socioeconomic status, stressful life situations and mental health problems in children and adolescents: Results of the German BELLA cohort-study. *PLoS One, 14*(3), e0213700. https://doi.org/10.1371/journal.pone.0213700

Restall, G. J., MacLeod Schroeder, N. J., & Dubé, C. D. (2018). The Equity Lens for Occupational Therapy: A program development and evaluation tool. *Canadian Journal of Occupational Therapy, 85*(3), 185–195. https://doi.org/10.1177/0008417418756421

Robertson, L., Akré, E.-R., & Gonzalez, G. (2021). Mental health disparities at the intersections of gender, identity, race, and ethnicity. *LGBT Health, 8*(8), 526–535. https://doi.org/10.1089/lgbt.2020.0429

Rodriguez, D. X., Hill, J., & McDaniel, P. N. (2021). A scoping review of literature about mental health and well-being among immigrant communities in the United States. *Health Promotion Practice, 22*(2), 181–192. https://doi.org/10.1177/1524839920942511

Rodriguez, S. C., & Rodriguez, D. X. (2020). *Hay que tener fe*: The challenge of being a Latina DACA college student. *Peace and Conflict: Journal of Peace Psychology, 26*(4), 390–402. https://doi.org/10.1037/pac0000445

Ross, M., & Bateman, N. (2019). *Meet the low wage workforce.* Brookings Institute. https://vtechworks.lib.vt.edu/items/5aa41ff5-6518-4969-b802-75ca1446616c

Schillinger, D. (2020). The intersections between social determinants of health, health literacy, and health disparities. *Studies in Health Technology and Informatics, 269,* 22–41. https://doi.org/10.3233/SHTI200020

School Mental Health Ontario. (2024, January). *Cultural Humility Self-Reflection Tool for School Mental Health Professionals.* Author. https://smho-smso.ca/wp-content/uploads/2022/10/Cultural-humility-self-reflection-tool-for-school-mental-health-professionals.pdf

Schouler-Ocak, M., Bhugra, D., Kastrup, M., Dom, G., Heinz, A., Küey, L., & Gorwood, P. (2021). Racism and mental health and the role of mental health professionals. *European Psychiatry, 64*(1), E42. https://doi.org/10.1192/j.eurpsy.2021.2216

Sexton, S. M., Richardson, C. R., Schrager, S. B., Bowman, M. A., Hickner, J., Morley, C. P. Mott, T. F., Pimlott, N., Saultz, J. W., & Weiss, B. D. (2020). Systemic racism and health disparities: A statement from editors of family medicine journals. *Evidence-Based Practice, 23*(10), 3–4. https://doi.org/10.1097/EBP.0000000000001113

Sharif, M. Z., García, J. J., Mitchell, U., Dellor, E. D., Bradford, N. J., & Truong, M. (2021). Racism and structural violence: Interconnected threats to health equity. *Frontiers in Public Health, 9, 676783.* https://doi.org/10.3389/fpubh.2021.676783

Sheingold, S., Zuckerman, R., Alberto, C., Samson, L., Lee, E., & Aysola, V. (2022, September). *Reflections accompanying a report on addressing social drivers of health: Evaluating area-level indices* (Issue Brief No. HP-202226). Office of the Assistant Secretary for Planning and Evaluation, U.S. Department of Health & Human Services. https://aspe.hhs.gov/sites/default/files/documents/7814e2c613d6004f419b357ed85b8d7d/Area-level-Indices-ASPE-Reflections.pdf

Shim, R. S., & Starks, S. M. (2021). COVID-19, structural racism, and mental health inequities: Policy implications for an emerging syndemic. *Psychiatric Services, 72*(10), 1193–1198. https://doi.org/10.1176/appi.ps.202000725

Smith, D. L. (2023). Social and environmental determinants of occupation: An intersectional concept focused on occupational justice and participation. *Journal of Occupational Science,* 1–7. https://doi.org/10.1080/14427591.2023.2212676

Spaniol, L., & Wewiorski, N. J. (2012). Phases of the recovery process from psychiatric disabilities. *International Journal of Psychosocial Rehabilitation, 17*(1), 116–133.

Sutton, D. J., Hocking, C. S., & Smythe, L. A. (2012). A phenomenological study of occupational engagement in recovery from mental illness. *Canadian Journal of Occupational Therapy, 79*(3), 142–150. https://doi.org/10.2182/cjot.2012.79.3.3

Synovec, C. E., & Aceituno, L. (2020, January 1). Social justice considerations for occupational therapy: The role of addressing social determinants of health in unstably housed populations. *Work, 65*(2), 235–246. https://doi.org/10.3233/WOR-203074

Taylor, R. R. (2020). *The intentional relationship: Occupational therapy and use of self.* F.A. Davis.

Tebb, K. P., & Brindis, C. D. (2021). Understanding the psychological impacts of teen pregnancy through a socio-ecological framework and life course approach. *Seminars in Reproductive Medicine, 40*(01/02), 107–115. https://doi.org/10.1055/s-0041-1741518

Teplin, L. A., Abram, K. M., & Luna, M. (2023). Racial and ethnic biases and psychiatric misdiagnoses: Toward more equitable diagnosis and treatment. *American Journal of Psychiatry, 180*(6), 402–403. https://doi.org/10.1176/appi.ajp.20230294

Tervalon, M., & Murray-Garcia, J. (1998). Cultural humility versus cultural competence: A critical distinction in defining physician training outcomes in multicultural education. *Journal of Health Care for the Poor and Underserved, 9*(2), 117–125. https://doi.org/10.1353/hpu.2010.0233

Thornton, M., & Persaud, S. (2018, September 30). Preparing today's nurses: Social determinants of health and nursing education.

OJIN: The Online Journal of Issues in Nursing, 23(3), Manuscript 5. https://doi.org/10.3912/OJIN.Vol23No03Man05

Thurston, I. B., Alegría, M., Hood, K. B., Miller, G. E., Wilton, L., & Holden, K. (2023). How psychologists can help achieve equity in health care—Advancing innovative partnerships and models of care delivery: Introduction to the special issue. *American Psychologist, 78*(2), 73–81. https://doi.org/10.1037/amp0001153

Townsend, E., & Polatajko, H. (2007). *Enabling occupation II: Advancing an occupational therapy vision for health, well-being & justice through occupation.* Canadian Association of Occupational Therapists Publications.

U.S. Department of Health & Human Services. (2023). *Health equity in Healthy People 2030.* Office of Disease Prevention and Health Promotion. https://health.gov/healthypeople/priority-areas /health-equity-healthy-people-2030

U.S. Department of Health & Human Services. (2024, January). *Social determinants of health. Healthy People 2030.* Office of Disease Prevention and Health Promotion. https://health.gov/healthypeople /priority-areas/social-determinants-health

VanPuymbrouck, L., & Friedman, C. (2023). Early career occupational therapists' experiences during the COVID-19 pandemic. *Occupational Therapy in Health Care,* 1–20. Advance online publication. https://doi.org/10.1080/07380577.2023.2175291

Vargas, E. D., & Ybarra, V. (2017). U.S. citizen children of undocumented parents: The link between state immigration policy and the health of Latino children. *Journal of Immigrant and Minority Health, 19*(4), 913–920. https://doi.org/10.1007/s10903-016 -0463-6

Vaughn, L. M., & Jacquez, F. (2020). Participatory research methods: Choice points in the research process. *Journal of Participatory Research Methods, 1*(1), 1–13. https://doi.org/10.35844/001c .13244

Whitman, A., De Lew, N., Chappel, A., Aysola, V., Zuckerman, R., & Sommers, B. D. (April 2022). *Addressing social determinants of health: Examples of successful evidence-based strategies and current federal efforts* (Issue Brief No. HP-202212). Office of the Assistant Secretary for Planning and Evaluation, U.S. Department of Health & Human Services.

Williams, M., Osman, M., & Hyon, C. (2023). Understanding the psychological impact of oppression using the Trauma Symptoms of Discrimination Scale. *Chronic Stress, 7,* 24705470221149511. https://doi.org/10.1177/24705470221149511

Witkiewitz, K., Pfund, R. A., & Tucker, J. A. (2022). Mechanisms of behavior change in substance use disorder with and without formal treatment. *Annual Review of Clinical Psychology, 18*(1), 497–525. https://doi.org/10.1146/annurev-clinpsy-072720-014802

World Federation of Occupational Therapists. (2016). *Minimum standards for the education of occupational therapists.* Author. https://wfot.org/resources/new-minimum-standards -for-the-education-of-occupational-therapists-2016-e-copy

World Federation of Occupational Therapists. (2019). *Occupational therapy and human rights.* https://www.wfot.org/resources/ occupational-therapy-and-human-rights

World Health Organization. (2008). *Closing the gap in a generation: Health equity through action on the social determinants of health.* Commission on Social Determinants of Health, Final Report. https://www.who.int/publications/i/item/WHO-IER-CSDH-08.1

World Health Organization. (2019). *International statistical classification of diseases and related health problems* (11th ed.). Author. https://icd.who.int

World Health Organization. (2023). *Social determinants of health.* Author. https://www.who.int/health-topics/social -determinants-of-health#tab=tab_

World Health Organization. (2024, January). *Health equity.* Author. https://www.who.int/health-topics/health-equity#tab=tab_1

Yerxa, E. J. (2000). Occupational science: A renaissance of service to humankind through knowledge. *Occupational Therapy International, 7,* 87–98. https://doi.org/10.1002/oti.109

Young, R., Ayiasi, R. M., Shung-King, M., & Morgan, R. (2020). Health systems of oppression: Applying intersectionality in health systems to expose hidden inequities. *Health Policy and Planning, 35*(9), 1228–1230. https://doi.org/10.1093/heapol/czaa111

Becca Allchin and Claudette Fette

Mental health needs occur in the context of families. Families can be a pivotal support for recovery; they are resilient and experience a variety of states and associated tasks as they seek to adapt to challenges along the mental health continuum. Many report areas of growth including increased compassion, better communication skills, and stronger relationships. Occupational therapy practitioners (OTPs) can provide effective support by seeking to work with whole families through strengths-based, culturally responsive, family-focused practice and by taking on an occupational justice lens that acknowledges and advocates for families impacted by societal and environmental discrimination and injustice. Occupational therapy's ethos aligns well with these collaborative and person-driven approaches that seek to help identify strengths and build capacity for health and wellness. Furthermore, there are many resources within and beyond occupational therapy to provide a firm foundation for this work. This chapter describes and provides examples of how OTPs can partner with families using approaches that understand a family's needs relative to life span, role demands, and the conditions and needs of varied states of adaptation. The focus of these approaches is working with families to build relationships in support of family recovery.

Overview of the Family

Having supportive relationships is a critical component of recovery across the life span, and so it is important to think about support for families as a target of intervention, as well as how therapists champion families at the level of population. The Substance Abuse and Mental Health Services Administration (SAMHSA, 2017) describes *family* as those people who consider themselves a family because of their interaction, situation, psychological attachment, and satisfaction of mutual social needs and support. Families are diverse and not limited to one specific family structure. For instance, a family might include relatives such as parents, grandparents, and siblings; spouses or partners; children; people in cohabitation or friends; those with kinship responsibilities and extended family; foster parents; and others not necessarily directly related to a person (Hillebregt et al., 2019). Families may be headed by single parents, by grandparents, or by LGBTQ (lesbian, gay, bisexual, transgender, or questioning) adults (Jaffe & Cospar, 2014). Today, family is any social group whose members care about each other, and are committed to each other regardless of whether they are related or live in the same household (Smith et al., 2020).

When working with families, OTPs need to consider the family as a whole and look at the interrelated nature of their occupations, rather than merely viewing other family members as part of one individual's social context. At the core of occupational therapy is the belief that occupations are pivotal for well-being and are embedded in the everyday life of individuals, families, groups, communities, organizations, and populations (Whiteford & Townsend, 2011). The social political context of everyday life provides inequitable opportunities to engage in occupations that promote well-being, requiring the OTP to consider the context clues, as well as social and system structures, that shape occupational choice (Hammell, 2020). The context and the people around the individual influence the person's choice, engagement, and participation in the occupations they need as well as those that are required and those they want to do. Practitioners can take this perspective by considering the following factors: systemic policies and community support for families, family occupations, performance patterns and responses, culture, and life span development. **Family-focused care** sees the family and individual as a whole unit and directs intervention across both practice areas and conditions, especially around long-term conditions in both physical and mental health (Hackett & Cook, 2016; Hillebregt et al., 2019; Smith et al., 2020). Evidence-informed family-focused practices are highlighted in this chapter's Evidence-Based Practice feature.

Family Adaptation

Family resilience is the ability for families to cope and rebound during life transitions, stress, or adversity (Walsh, 2021). Mental health challenges, with their associated demands and losses, have the potential to disrupt family relationships and well-being, or conversely to strengthen the family when they respond with unified action and commitment. Families can use internal and/or external resources to problem-solve, develop new solutions, and institute effective changes, which allow the family to positively adapt and move forward; at other times, a family may become overwhelmed by increased stressors and shift into survival mode. Thus, the development of resilience is a dynamic process that is context dependent and changes over time (Walsh, 2016).

In keeping with Emily Perl Kingsley's (1987) Italy-Holland analogy for raising a child with a disability, being in a family in which someone experiences mental health challenges is similar to someone landing in Holland when they thought they were traveling to Italy. When planning a trip to Italy,

Evidence-Based Practice

Family-Focused Practice

In family-focused practice, occupational therapy evaluation and intervention are focused on the family's occupations, habits, and routines.

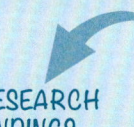
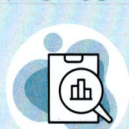

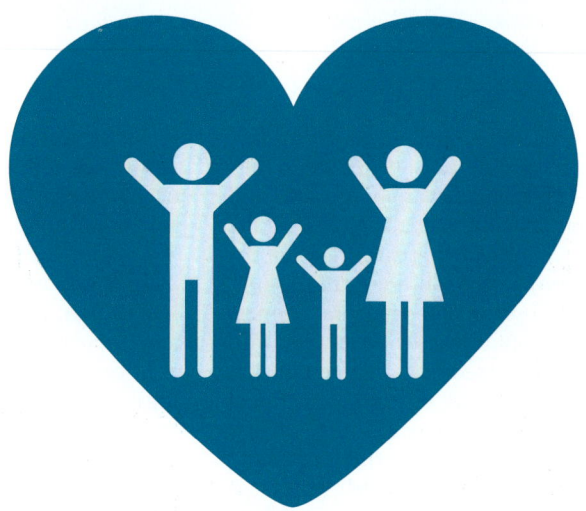

Family-focused practice views the whole family as a unit rather than a collection of individuals. This means, as an OTP, your evaluation and intervention are focused on the family's occupations, habits, and routines. This avoids the danger of pitting members against each other in allocation of resources, perspective taking, and so on. It supports your identification and utilization of family strengths in support of goals that benefit everyone in the family. Tompson and colleagues (2017) found that family-focused practice was more effective than individual supportive therapy. Using a structured approach with a focus on supporting family strengths and coping was particularly effective for youth between 7 and 14 years old with mood disorders.

APPLICATIONS

➡ In family-focused practice, OTPs need to keep these four principles in mind (Trowse et al., 2013):

1. The family is the central unit of attention.
2. Maximize the families' options and choices.
3. Prioritize strengths-focused perspectives.
4. Emphasize culturally and spiritually sensitive approaches.

REFERENCES

Tompson, M. C., Sugar, C. A., Langer, D. A., &.Asarnow, J. R. (2017). A randomized clinical trial comparing family-focused treatment and individual supportive therapy for depression in childhood and early adolescence. *Journal of the American Academy of Child & Adolescent Psychiatry, 56*(6), 515–523. https://doi.org/10.1016/j.jaac.2017.03.018

Trowse, L., Hawkins, K., & Clark, J. (2013). *Putting families at the centre of recovery.* COPMI GEMS edition 14. https://www.copmi.net.au/professionals-organisations/copmi-what-works/research-summaries-gems/gems-edition14

this person bought summer clothing and got maps and tour guides for all the Italian sites they expected to see. The person boarded the plane, excited; however, when the plane landed they found themself in Holland. It's cold, they don't have appropriate clothing, and their maps don't work. But eventually, the person gets sweaters and a coat, along with some sensible shoes, and begins to learn their way around. They begin to see that Holland has windmills; lovely, colorful tulips; and even Rembrandts. As the person's friends tell them all about their time in Italy, the individual experiences a sense of loss, but then grows to love Holland, too. Families frequently don't start with the specialized knowledge and skills required to manage mental ill health, but instead start with whatever tools their families passed on to them, and those are frequently Italian at best. There are adjustments to living in Holland.

Families and even individual family members are unique in the ways that they respond to a family member's mental ill health. Family members do not necessarily move through their responses in predictable sequences. Figure 29-1 provides a graphic representation of common responses in managing mental illness in the family, with blue circles representing states that family members and/or families often experience, each with a white text box with frequent areas of focus for that state. Given the stigma surrounding mental illness, families often start their journey with a fair amount of fear and confusion as they begin in *survival* mode, where they may struggle between reacting (with denial, anger, shame) or coping (Miller, 1997). The journey toward a diagnosis can be long and difficult, with family members trying to make sense of what is happening and get support. Products of this experience may include grieving the loss of what they expected for their loved one, learning to hold compassion for each other, and/or learning appreciation of small moments as they move into *seeking* (Bourke-Taylor, 2022; Miller, 1997), which often features longing for meaning and wellness. For some families, a diagnosis may offer relief by providing an explanation for changes in a family member's behavior. They may have expectations that obtaining a label will result in treatment that will "fix" their family member so that they can reconnect back to the life they had before their loved one's illness.

As families acquire knowledge, new perspectives, and an appreciation for their strengths and those of their loved ones, families may move into **acceptance**; with this, they may begin work toward *occupational justice*. Here, wraparound and recovery models with their focus on strengths and building capacity for participation begin to make sense as families strive to educate and advocate. Some family members may take on professional advocacy and peer support roles with other families (resources and programs developed by families for families are discussed later in this chapter). They may begin to embrace neurodiversity and advocate for others to see differences, not deficits. As they hit their stride, often finding new opportunities, and perhaps even experiencing **posttraumatic growth**, families may look to find a *balance* (Bourke-Taylor, 2022) that is health promoting and sustainable across roles, routines, self-care, productivity, leisure, and their environments (Mynard, 2020). Families may move through the balance, acceptance, justice, seeking, and survival states in a nonlinear way; for example, grief may loop back to survival rather than into seeking, or balance may give way to advocacy/justice or seeking in response to external stigma.

In addition to working through their own states as they adapt to caregiving for someone with mental health needs, families also must navigate their context. Matthews and colleagues (2021) listened to parents raising children with a range of developmental disabilities and created a model that reflects their interactions within systems, their families, and themselves. Those contexts are represented by gray ovals around the outer portion of Figure 29-1, and families' interactions with them are featured in black type within the

---

BOX 29-1 ■ Framing and Language Matter

There is a shift away from presenting mental ill health through a deficit-saturated medical model that viewed the person by their incapacities, the ill health as something to be fixed, and the person and family members as needing services provided by expert OTPs.

Additionally, the individualized framing of mental ill health can lead to separating its effect on different family members. For example, when a parent experiences mental ill health, children have been viewed as at risk. This has had the unfortunate result of promoting a "pity the child" view for workers, activating a rescue or fix response, limiting the scope of children's agency, and promoting a false choice between their parent's needs versus their own, and with parents feeling shamed and blamed for an illness they didn't choose.

In the context of families in which a member experiences mental ill health, everyone experiences shifts in their individual and collective occupations. The well-being of all family members is best supported by promoting/enabling/equipping families to be a resource to each other to promote everyone's well-being.

---

ovals. Family interactions with **systems** include managing impressions, employing savvy, influencing, sacrificing, and advocating for change. Within the context of family, families construct spaces of care, adjust their lives and homes, anticipate disruption, and expand boundaries of care. Family members adapt, celebrate strengths, reframe their experiences to construct a sense of growth, and configure new expectations within themselves (Matthews et al., 2021).

It is important for OTPs to appreciate that family experiences and responses to mental illness differ for parents, spouses or partners, siblings, and children in families, so OTPs must respond effectively to the family members' differing needs while, at the same time, holding them together. Whole-of-family well-being is more than just attending to each individual member's needs (Foster et al., 2016). Families can be the best resource to their members when the well-being outcomes for one can promote well-being outcomes for another. An individually focused medical framework can invite OTPs to be drawn into pitting one member's outcomes against another's. Families are better served when OTPs are intentional about the language they use and understand that the disruption has impacted each member of the family in an individual way (see Box 29-1). Practitioners should act as facilitators to build shared understanding of those impacts and pathways to meet the needs of different family members.

A strengths-based perspective may counter the deluge of negative messages from systems and the community that people living with mental health needs and their families face. Helping families to maintain an overall family balance can foster resilience through time. Hence, Walsh (2016) suggests key processes in building family resilience: (a) making meaning out of adversity, whereby a family comes to make sense of mental illness and to discover what it means for their family's sense of identity; (b) developing a hopeful outlook by focusing on strengths and potential; then (c) finding a pathway for rising above adversity.

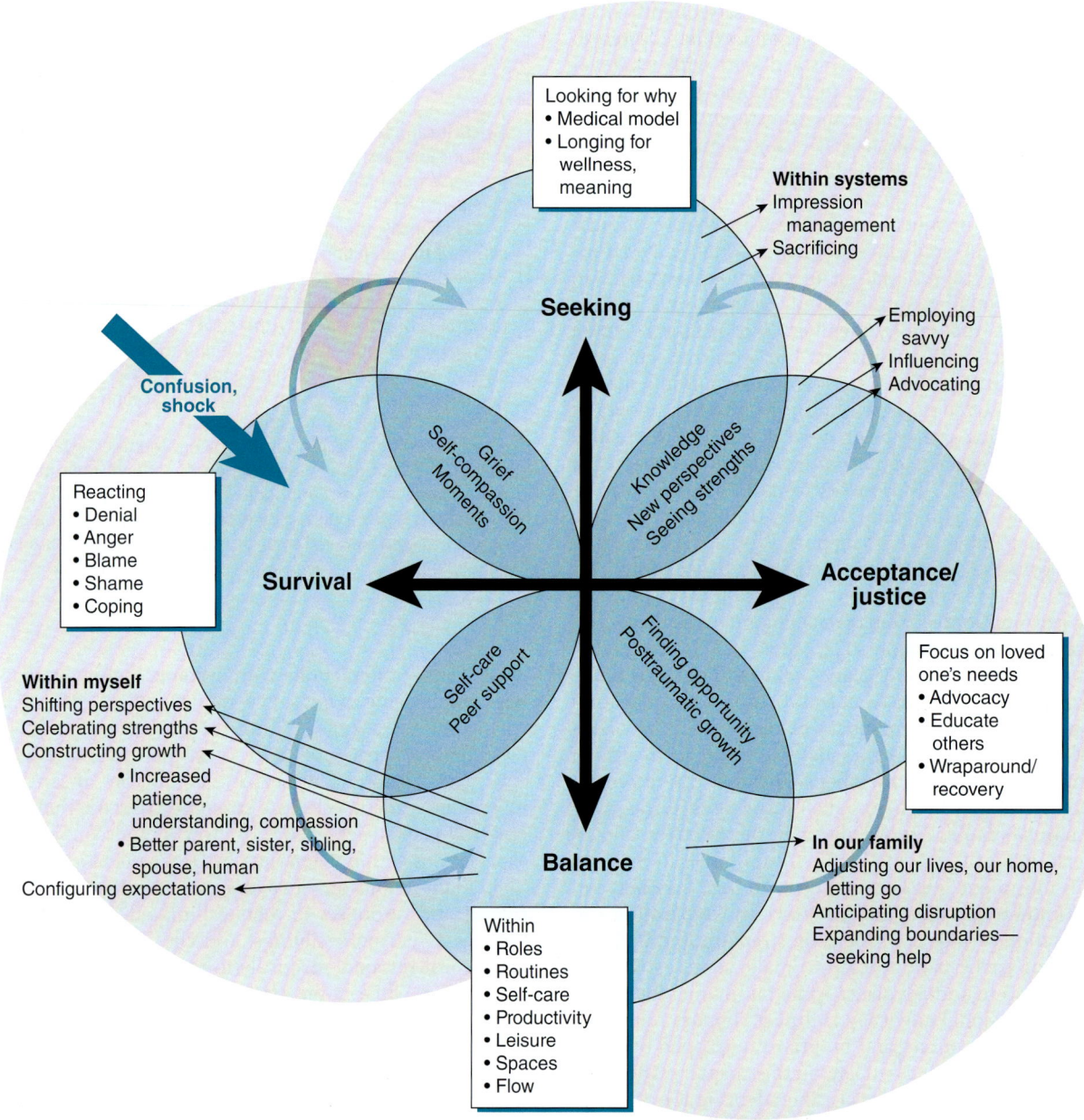

FIGURE 29-1. Fette's synthesis of models reflecting states, tasks, and transitions around family adaptation from Bourke-Taylor (2022), Kübler-Ross & Kessler (2014), Miller (1997), and Mynard (2020) in blue circles and text, superimposed on Matthews and colleagues' (2021) family context outputs at the level of systems, family, and self. *Used with permission from Claudette Fette.*

Family Culture as Context

A particular family's culture provides an overarching context for understanding the family's responses, roles, communication styles, problem-solving, decision-making, conflict resolution, mental health-seeking attitudes, and behaviors. Practitioners are encouraged to view each family as a unique culture shaped by forces operating within and external to the family (Jaffe & Cospar, 2014; Nicholson et al., 2014). The principle of *family voice and choice* from wraparound (community-based guiding principles and practices that serve as an alternative to residential placement for young

people) speaks to the special value placed on distinct cultural traditions that families hold, whether those are aligned with race, ethnicity, or other differences or are just specific to a particular family. For example, some families may use language that another might find offensive. As OTPs, it is important for OTPs to reflect on their own cultures to assure that they are not pushing their own bias and cultural norms onto others. See Chapter 2: Recovery and Wraparound Models.

Some populations have a history of cumulative trauma and barriers to participation in dominant economic and cultural systems (Hankerson et al., 2022; Western Australian

Health, 2020), which has resulted in generations of people of color experiencing systemic abuse, discrimination, and consequently, difficulty trusting helpers who are often members of dominant and privileged classes. Because most OTPs are still members of these dominant cultures and often don't accurately reflect the diversity of those whom they serve, they must strive for cultural humility. Families need providers to show increased capacity to effectively work and communicate with them, and provide still more culturally responsive services, wherein providers resemble them and treat them with respect (Jain et al., 2019). Disparities in prevalence of mental health needs and mental health outcomes for minoritized children and/or those who live in poverty are made worse by housing instability, food insecurity, increased stress, economic hardship, lack of access to mental health care or quality schools, and safe play spaces (Jain et al., 2019; Stenersen et al., 2022). Transgender and gender diverse people with strong family support demonstrate less drug and alcohol use, report less victimization, and claim better mental health, so Trinh and colleagues (2022) assert the need to provide family support to families of choice and to educate regarding the needs of gender diverse people.

Barriers to seeking help and obtaining adequate care also include the ways that people think about mental illness, its causes, and its treatment. In some cultures, physical and psychological problems are not viewed as separate, so emotional information may be reported as bodily symptoms (e.g., fatigue may mean despair in Chinese culture), with families viewing the causes of illness as related to spiritual, social, interpersonal, and psychological problems (Leong & Kalibatseva, 2011; Subu et al., 2022). Within this cultural context, the family may be seen as morally and socially responsible for the person's behavior; therefore, mental illness can be seen to bring stigma to the whole family, not just the individual (Fernandes et al., 2018; Subu et al., 2022).

In other cultures, a frank discussion of mental health issues may be considered inappropriate and insensitive, and dealing with such issues outside the family is not the cultural norm. In many Hispanic and Asian families, for example, family unity is highly valued, and the network of social relationships often extends beyond marital or biological ties (Leong & Kalibatseva, 2011; Subu et al., 2022). This can also mean a family-focused approach may be more relevant than individually oriented mental health care (Price-Robertson et al., 2017). See Chapter 27: Mental Health Stigma and Sanism and Chapter 28: Social Determinants and Mental Health. 🤝

Life Span and Occupations of Families: A Developmental Perspective

Families are systems that evolve and change across the life course and generations. Adaptation is required as relationships within the members change and boundaries shift through losses and additions (Hetherington, 2003; Walsh, 2016). A developmental perspective is a useful framework for understanding the life stage of each family member and the family as a unit within society (Keeble-Devlin, 2012). Using a life span or developmental perspective enables the OTP to consider the various occupational roles of different family members and see how these roles and activity patterns change as people age and circumstances change over their lifetimes. Families are more than their individual members, however, so there is a need to consider occupations families do together or apart. Kantartzis (2017) describes family occupations as the "day-to-day network of doing and connectedness . . . [built on] embodied memories and shared skills and knowledge" (p. 21). Family occupations include family members in planning, discussing, and doing, thus shaping routines, identity, and culture. "Family" is experienced and expressed through family occupations such as shared holidays, celebrations, and traditions. Considering the family occupations and how they shift to meet the changing needs of the family members enables the OTP to identify a family's strengths, challenges, and resources to manage these transitions (Jaffe & Cospar, 2014; Jakobsen et al., 2021; Kantartzis, 2017). Appreciating that disequilibrium is often a normal aspect of family transitions can also help the OTP to support a family to anticipate challenges and proactively plan how to address them. Every family is unique in its membership, how it develops, and its individual and collective occupations, requiring the OTP to provide a curious, nonjudgmental approach to inquiry (Jaffe & Cospar, 2014). Some common roles and occupations seen in family members are presented in the text that follows.

Children

Occupations of young children are mostly carried out with another person in an interactive routine in which both actors play an active part, such as feeding and eating (Olson, 2004). These co-occupations in families are reciprocal tasks with shared emotionality, intentionality, and physicality (Aubuchon-Endsley et al., 2020). Play and self-care occupations such as eating, dressing, and toileting are the primary occupations of preschool children; they start as co-occupations and gradually become occupations that can be done individually. School-age children extend their range of occupations as they participate in new roles, including student, friend, and hobbyist (Jaffe & Cospar, 2014). Within family life, children take on occupations that support and maintain the household, such as cleaning or preparing meals, with expectations and appropriate responsibilities determined by culture and society. Siblings often participate in occupations together, such as playing, doing daily living tasks, and going to school, with their individual interests and activity pursuits becoming more differentiated as they get older. Family life, in its broadest sense, is the environment in which children grow and develop, providing just right challenges and possibly also demands that don't meet children's needs. Through listening to families in early childhood systems, Jain and colleagues (2019) found families focused on children's positive social and emotional development, as well as hopes for their child's education, communication skills, independence, happiness, and career success.

Adults

Adults participate in varied roles that serve their individual and family needs, including worker, care provider, home maintainer, friend, community member, and parent (Jaffe & Cospar, 2014). Occupations may be gendered, with women having a greater percentage of their time engaged in occupations related to household management and child rearing, or they may be more egalitarian. Many roles are held simultaneously, requiring complex organizational and emotional processing, and adults commonly need to prioritize some occupations over others or combine outcomes into one occupation. Occupations adults are required to do are commonly enfolded within parenting occupations such as combining play with household work.

Parenting occupations are multilayered with a focus on both monitoring a child's needs and environments to fulfill basic, developmental, and social needs, and on building parenting capacity (Lim et al., 2022). Parenting occupations go on through the lifetime, changing to fit the life stage of the parent–child relationship (Francis-Connolly, 2004) and remain in the background even while carrying out other occupations.

The sociopolitical environment of the family, as well as individual dispositions, shape role priorities. The emphasis an adult family member places on a particular role fluctuates as they transition through life. For example, employment, leisure, and community engagement occupations might have greater priority in early adult life. Parenting occupations may have greater focus in the middle of life, which might shift again to employment and community engagement as their children move into adulthood themselves. Providing care for older family members may also take predominance in this period. In later adult life, members might place less emphasis on employment occupations and have more resources for leisure occupations. This time of life might also create opportunities for taking a different role in child-raising occupations.

Impact of Mental Ill Health and Needs for Particular Groups

The mental ill health of a family member impacts the family, its members, and their occupations in different ways. Negative outcomes cannot be assumed; the ways a family and its members respond to the adversities they face and the support and resources they have access to are pivotal in determining outcomes. Family members identify increased mental health literacy, empathy, and resilience in the context of their experiences (Abraham & Stein, 2015) alongside the losses, grief, and adjustment noted previously. Although the focus of OTPs is often on the person with the mental ill health, all family members are impacted by the disruptions that result from the symptoms, the side effects of treatment, and the social consequences of mental ill health.

Symptoms of mental ill health such as mood changes, disordered thinking, sensory sensitivity, and disturbed perception can impact a person's ability to function in their usual or expected occupations. These symptoms may also result in changed behavior such as social withdrawal, lowered motivation, poor self-care, irritability, and unusual actions. These

changes can be difficult for the person and those around them to fully comprehend and can lead to complicated communications, greater potential for misunderstandings, and relational disengagement (Reupert & Maybery, 2016). A person's limited capacity for their self-care, education, employment, household, or parenting occupations may require accommodation by other family members, creating temporary or more permanent shifts in roles and occupations, such as shopping, cooking, banking, general household chores, and child and/or pet care (Chaffey & Fossey, 2004).

Treatment, its side effects, and the recovery process can also interfere with establishing and maintaining family occupations. The absences created by hospital admissions interrupt parent–child attachment and disrupt everyday family life (Reupert & Maybery, 2016). The focus on one's own recovery needs can shift the focus from family or community occupations to individual occupations (Awram et al., 2017). Common side effects of medications, such as morning drowsiness, can make it more challenging to get to school or work or to facilitate children's routines. These in turn can disrupt the occupations and relationships within families, shown in loss of usual routines, celebrations, and traditions. In these cases, others often step into care providing or parenting roles. These changes within families can also limit everyone's contact and engagement with people and occupations outside the family.

Interrupted or loss of employment and education exposes families to poverty and social isolation (Pohlan, 2019). Negative community attitudes about the value and capability of people with mental ill health can shrink their and their family's social networks and lead to discrimination, self-isolation, or other's withdrawal (Allan et al., 2018; Koschorke et al., 2014; Larson & Corrigan, 2008; Reupert & Maybery, 2015). Added to this, the self-stigma people also experience can lessen their willingness to seek help and silence communication within the family (Koschorke et al., 2014; Weimand et al., 2013). These social consequences of poor mental health can expose families to intergenerational disadvantage and poorer quality of life (Bland & Foster, 2012; Hayes et al., 2015; Weimand et al., 2013).

Let's look further at the needs of specific family members.

Needs of Children Whose Parents Have Mental Ill Health

Children growing up in families where a parent has mental ill health are a diverse group with a range of needs depending on their experiences and circumstances (Australian Infant, Child, Adolescent and Family Mental Health Association [AICAFMHA], 2004). Support for the child is best done in partnership with parents to support the strengthening of the parent–child relationship and family well-being. With their egocentric view of the world, children can be fearful of the changes in family members and family life and see themselves as responsible. OTPs can promote well-being to children by being curious about their experience of family life and the parents' mental ill health, enabling them to have age-appropriate explanations and messages that underscore the parent's mental ill health is not their fault and facilitating the building of a shared understanding in the family. Children can pick up the social cues and negative attitudes that can silence communication in families. Practitioners can facilitate parents to invite ongoing conversations with their children about their experiences and assist in the building of networks of support around the child to help them know they are not alone. Peer connections with others in the same situation can support understanding and lessen the impact of stigma (Shalaby & Agyapong, 2020). Reflecting with the child about their experiences can help the parent and the OTP understand how the adjusted roles and responsibilities in family life are impacting on the child's daily routines and valued occupations. The OTP can work with the network of formal support such as child care and schools, as well as informal supports such as neighbors, friends, and family, to promote problem-solving to cocreate balance.

Needs of Siblings

OTPs should ask about, acknowledge, and validate the experiences of siblings. Siblings can be a significant influence throughout life providing connection, enabling participation, and providing strength through life's ups and downs. These relationships are commonly the first in which children learn to resolve conflict and work together with others. Each family's experience of the disruption to sibling co-occupations and relationships will depend on their age and sibling order as well as their sibling's level of disability. Shifts in care arrangements and doing less together can in turn mean siblings lose emotional connections with each other (Ewertzon et al., 2012). Facilitating connection, shared enjoyment, and positive interactions can help to alleviate the challenges faced within family relationships (Olson, 2006). Practitioners can help families to identify and facilitate sibling co-occupations such as shared activities (Pierce, 2009) and invite siblings to codevelop family events (van der Sanden et al., 2014). As children and adolescents are still developing emotional resources and strategies for coping with challenges (Purcell et al., 2012; van der Sanden et al., 2014), developmentally appropriate support for their personal needs and emotions will be needed. Using a curious approach, OTPs can enable exploration of each family member's experience of family life and their siblings' mental ill health, facilitating parents to provide age-appropriate explanations that emphasize it's not the child's fault. This will support building a shared understanding to promote collective and individual mental well-being.

Needs of Parents of Children With Emotional Disturbances

Developmentally, parenting has inherent expectations about the responsibility to protect children and provide them with what they need to become fully functioning people who contribute to the family group and to their community and who eventually form their own families and live independently. Parents may struggle with a sense of responsibility for their child having developed mental ill health. They may feel guilt or shame and may struggle through the states of adaptation to this new normal, similar to Kingsley's (1987) adjustment to Holland example used

in the earlier analogy. They may struggle with not knowing how to best help and almost certainly get lots of often misguided advice from others living in Italy. Additionally, in childhood, families often must navigate between several, often contradictory, models. Behavioral models confer one set of diagnoses and often see causation as some facet of a child's environment, reinforcing negative behaviors. In this model, families may be asked to set up reinforcement schedules and follow routines intended to address behaviors to be extinguished. Trauma-informed practices would instead see many of these behaviors as needs, but the extent to which trauma is understood in child-serving systems varies broadly. Behavioral models are reflected in a common cultural understanding of undesired behaviors; they may be embraced by one family but be a source of conflict for another. In U.S. schools, educational systems often incorporate behavioral strategies, but rather than specific diagnoses, children may fall under the larger umbrella term "serious emotional disturbance" (SED).

Psychiatric models may confer a completely different set of diagnoses for the same symptoms. Therapy in this paradigm might include medication, perhaps play therapy, or if a child is old enough to employ metacognition, cognitive behavioral or other evidence-informed, language-based therapies. Children with histories of trauma may have still other interventions. Families have the challenge of working their way through these competing explanations for their child's behavior and figuring out how to best support their child as well as the whole family system. As therapists, it is helpful first to listen and validate people's experience, connecting them to peer supports who have already faced negotiating these competing understandings and systems. Practitioners can provide parents with education regarding the often-confusing labels, symptoms, and needs around their child. They can also enable practical accommodations to address the child's sensory, psychosocial, and cognitive needs, as well as identify strengths and participation in occupations around those.

Needs of Spouses and Partners

Although intimate relationships can take extra work to maintain when one or both partners have mental health issues, some partners described experiencing increased closeness when their choice to remain with a partner was grounded in a sense of love rather than obligation (Gurayah, 2016; Lewis, 2016). The impact of illness on the relationship and the experience of partners and spouses varies depending on the severity of disability, the familiarity of the illness, and the internal and external resources available (Jungbauer et al., 2004). If they haven't had previous experience of their partner's illness, they may be surprised by the impact that the illness has on themselves and the relationship, causing them to experience stress and shock (Jungbauer et al., 2004; Lewis, 2016; Mizuno et al., 2011). Companionship and intimate relationships may be affected because of medications, exhaustion, or lack of sexual attraction following symptoms, and in turn may disrupt major life decisions such as starting a family (Mizuno et al., 2011; Östman & Björkman, 2013). An OTP can equip the person with mental health needs and their partner to communicate openly about their experiences to help limit misunderstandings. It may also be

The Lived Experience

Claudette Fette

My oldest son, Aaron, heard voices from early childhood, but we did not understand what was happening. He was kicked out of several day cares and was seeing a psychologist by age 5. Because his pediatrician and all the therapists we saw framed his issues as behavioral, we lived by all manner of charts and reinforcement systems that were a source of frustration and repeated failure for us all. He also had lots of difficulty learning, which started about the same time as the hallucinations. Unfortunately, with the best of intentions, we focused a lot on remediating his deficits, which meant that he rarely got to experience himself as competent. He was brilliant but that was not his experience.

At 12, we exhausted his lifetime maximum for mental health insurance and were told to relinquish custody to the state to access care. Instead, we found a program where he was supposed to go to treatment in the day and come home at night, but it turned out to be a horribly abusive, tough love style "troubled teen industry" (TTI) program. He did not come home for nearly a year and when he did, he had both severe mental illness and trauma. By age 15, he had learned to hop trains, going to whatever city the train stopped in, staying maybe 2 weeks until his delusions became too much, then getting onto another train to another city. He lived mostly on the streets across the United States and Canada for the next 25 years.

At first, we tried forcing him to stay home, but that only drove him farther away. We began to realize that if we wanted to have a relationship with Aaron, it would be on his terms, and we came to embrace a sort of radical acceptance. Before cell phones, we got an 800 number so he could call whenever he wanted. He would sometimes call five or six times a day and we would work through reality testing which threats were real and which were not. Soon many other traveling homeless youth called that line; to check in, let each other know where they were, or just to talk to a mom. Aaron started coming through town a couple of times a year and bringing other youth. One of the first years, several came for Christmas. We fed and loved them and relished in the house full of laughing youth laying all over the living room floor watching videos. They left behind an entrenched lice infestation, and we learned to keep Rid Lice Treatment and clean clothes of all sizes so that when they came, we could treat them and their clothes. I would bring whoever wanted to go with me to church, but we cleared the pews. Soon, other parishioners would move when I sat down whether the kids were with me or not. They lived in Italy, and we chose to stay in Holland.

Some strategies that we found helpful along the way have since been incorporated into several interventions. Our whole

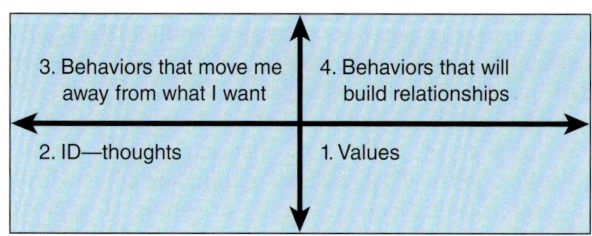

| 3. Behaviors that move me away from what I want | 4. Behaviors that will build relationships |
| 2. ID—thoughts | 1. Values |

family experienced trauma. Aaron was not safe. Dialectical behavioral therapy (DBT; Linehan & Wilks, 2015) has a focus on distress tolerance, and we certainly experienced distress. DBT divides distress tolerance skills into three categories: (1) sensory body awareness—which falls in line with most trauma practice as it starts with self-regulation strategies, (2) crisis survival techniques—which is about stepping back, taking a deep breath; not responding impulsively, and (3) reality acceptance. Another useful contemporary framework is Acceptance and Commitment Therapy (ACT; Hayes, 2019). The figure shown above walks through an ACT exercise in Gordon and Borushok's (2017) workbook. It starts with (1) identifying the values we wanted to live, (2) identifying thoughts that interfere with those values, (3) identifying behaviors that those thoughts were driving that were not helping us live our values, and (4) behaviors that would help us live our values. We wanted a relationship with Aaron (1). Our belief that his choices were unacceptable and that he had to fit our expectations (2) were driving us to do things that were pushing him away, such as engaging law enforcement to attempt to make him stay home (3). We had to instead choose behaviors that would prioritize rebuilding and sustaining our relationship with Aaron (4), which brought us to *radical acceptance*.

Other strategies that helped were finding other families with our experience, finding meaning, and staying occupied. I channeled energy into learning, advocacy, and creating resources for other families. I became an occupational therapist in that quest. I garden, write, and create. Aaron and I have just finished a book that is intended to advocate for better supports for individuals and families. Our family has realized posttraumatic growth. We learned how to better support Aaron's brothers. We are all more compassionate and more fully formed human beings because we are part of our family.

Image Source: The ACT exercise is derived from Gordon and Borushok's (2017) workbook. Below the horizontal line are internal processes; above are behaviors. Thoughts and behaviors left of the vertical line are driving away from what is desired, whereas those to the right move toward desired outcomes.

---

appropriate to see the partner separately to enable expression of issues they may be initially hesitant to voice in front of their partner such as grief at unexpected changes in the relationship. Partners may lose practical assistance with day-to-day family life, including financial security, and must adapt or

take on additional roles within the relationship. An OTP can support the couple to collaboratively problem-solve strategies for organizing and managing day-to-day home and family life and facilitate both parties to access support to meet their needs as individuals and partners.

Needs of Parents With Mental Ill Health

In addition to the everyday demands faced by all parents, parents with mental ill health face unique challenges as they meet the needs of their own mental and physical health and the needs of children and other family members (Awram et al., 2017; Nicholson, 2010). Parents with mental ill health need OTPs to actively value the parenting role, parent–child relationships, and family life to enable open, trusting conversations that are protective of everyone in the family unit's well-being (Goodyear et al., 2022). Many adults with mental ill health are parents and have described the role as rewarding, enabling personal growth, and supporting their recovery (Hackett & Cook, 2016; Maybery et al., 2015). Parents with mental ill health, however, also often worry about the impact of their ill health on their children; they feel a heightened responsibility for their child's problems and experience guilt and self-doubt (Goodyear et al., 2022). With the isolating impact of stigma, parents with mental ill health may lack the normalizing social network of other parents that gives perspective and helps them not feel alone. Parents at times struggle to find ways to talk to and help their children understand about mental ill health, sometimes thinking it's protective for them to not know. Using a nonjudgmental approach, OTPs can create safe reflective spaces to explore how their parenting role, the parent–child relationship, and family life are impacted by their ill health and promote parenting self-awareness, self-management, and parental agency (Goodyear et al., 2022). Practitioners can further support whole-of-family well-being by supporting social inclusion of parents and families, supporting parents to problem-solve everyday family-life challenges, and encourage family occupations that promote family well-being (Hackett & Cook, 2016). In the Being a Psychosocial OT Practitioner feature, an OTP provides examples of working with a family to identify strengths and resources in the family and creating a family care plan that integrates the parents' shared vision of occupations that support child rearing.

Being a Psychosocial OT Practitioner

Using Family-Focused Practice

Identifying Psychosocial Strengths and Needs

OTPs working in community adult mental health settings commonly work with people who are parents. However, the systems and models of care often result in the psychosocial needs of their parenting and family occupations being obscured and the opportunity to promote the mental health and well-being of the whole family lost.

Sue is a new mother with a lived experience of hearing voices. She and her husband, Marco, have been together for 5 years and had planned to start a family for a year or two. Family is important to Marco, who grew up in a bustling extended Italian family that lives close by and provides social connection and support to Sue and Marco. Sue has little contact with her own family, with whom she shares a history of family violence and estranged relationships. Sue appreciates the support Marco's family provides but can find them too much at times.

After birth, she and her son Harry returned home with Marco's extended family providing meals and dropping in to provide support. The visiting maternal-child health nurse noted that she had a good connection with Harry and could provide for his needs, but that she appeared to become overwhelmed and distressed quickly, especially when there were others in the house. On their next community mental health service visit, the physician referred Sue to see an OTP at the clinic to support her transition to parenthood.

Using a Holistic Occupational Therapy Approach

In the initial meeting, the OTP and Sue drew up a three-generation genogram charting the strengths and resources of her and Marco's family. The OTP asked Sue about the daily living patterns and the family occupations she and Marco had established before Harry was born and how they had changed since his birth. Sue related that she and Marco loved nature and would take walks together before Marco went to work and when he got home in the evening. During this time, they would take note of the flowering plants and talk about their days. She indicated that since Harry was born, their walks were sporadic, and although Marco appeared to love to show Harry the world, she found them less enjoyable as she was worried about Harry needing a diaper change or feed.

With Sue's permission, the OTP met with Sue and Marco together to explore what was important to them both about being parents and how they supported Harry. Sue and Marco identified that being parents was fulfilling a dream, and they had shared visions of helping Harry grow up caring for the world and being connected to family. Sue reflected that she was feeling very stressed about getting things right, and she couldn't use her usual strategies to self-regulate, resulting in feeling overwhelmed more frequently. Marco said that he'd found the changes to daily routines difficult and was thankful for the rhythms of his work and his family's frequent visits to support running things around the home. Marco was surprised to find that Sue wondered if the extra visits from Marco's family were to check on her and catch her doing something wrong. He also didn't know that Sue worried about being a good enough mother because of hearing voices and that things might not go well for Harry.

The OTP works with Sue to better understand her sensory preferences and find new self-regulation strategies to help manage her distress. Together, Sue, Marco, and the OTP develop a family care plan to work toward establishing new family occupations and explore how the extended family could be seen as a support for Sue and Harry when Marco is at work.

Reflective Questions

1. What other Family Models could be used with Sue, Marco, and Harry to promote family well-being?
2. What assessments could help gain a greater understanding of Sue's parenting occupations?
3. How could you design a treatment to build Sue's confidence in her parenting occupations?

Collaboration and Partnering With Families: Family-Focused Practice

Family-focused practice broadens perspectives from a narrow focus on the mental health consumer to one that includes their family and caregivers (see this chapter's Evidence-Based

Practice feature). Strengths of a person (even when unwell), and the well-being and strengths of all family members, along with their vulnerabilities and needs in keeping with trauma-informed care, are included (Falkov et al., 2020). Partnering with family is important even when service delivery is individually focused.

Practitioners partner with families for two purposes: (1) to reduce distress and build resilience and well-being for family members, and (2) to improve outcomes for the identified person using the service (Dixon et al., 2001; Mottaghipour & Bickerton, 2005; Wyder & Bland, 2014). As relationships are central to the recovery and well-being for all family members, a pivotal role of the OTP is to work with families to facilitate understanding of mental health needs, support healing in relationships, and build the networks of support needed by all family members. Critical practices to partnering with families and carers have been defined as (a) identifying and acknowledging, (b) engaging and communicating, (c) involving in the assessment and planning/collaboration in a person's treatment, (d) exploring the family members' or carer's own needs, (e) providing or offering them ongoing support, (f) providing psychoeducation, and (g) providing or recommending referrals to address their own needs (Lakeman, 2008; Maybery et al., 2021). Mottaghipour and Bickerton (2005), in their pyramid of family care, advocate that all OTPs can meet families' needs for information, communication, and education on coping skills and dealing with crises. Box 29-2 lists standards for partnering with family/carers that all OTPs should integrate into their practice routines and advocate for in places where they work.

Practitioners use open and reciprocal communication to create and maintain trusting environments that emphasize the strengths of the family and facilitate families feeling respected and validated. The collaborative approach assumes that families have capacity as well as family recovery as their main goal. Family participation in care and treatment of people with mental illness across the life span provides strong evidence for better outcomes for the person with the mental ill health and their family members (Lakeman, 2008). There is greater acceptance of family participation in child-focused

systems than those serving adolescents and adults. These services have noted barriers related to the organization (funding, staffing, models of care), OTP (attitudes, skills, confidence, perception of confidentiality), family (time, previous negative experience, location), and the person with mental ill health (relationship, confidentiality, perception of family willingness) that can limit engagement with families (Wonders et al., 2019). Wonders and colleagues (2019) advocate that OTPs need to actively enable positive family inclusion by working collaboratively with the person with mental ill health to facilitate choice, build understanding, and overcome the barriers.

Practitioners should deliberately invite family to take part in care and attend to family support needs related to both information and emotional support (Aass et al., 2021). Menear and colleagues (2022) suggest that adolescents and adults identify desired family members to be invited to initial sessions. Families may share information and receive education even if OTPs do not have permission to share specific information with them; they can facilitate discussion, assist with development of care plans, and state where they can provide support (Menear et al., 2022). Moen and colleagues (2021) proposed a Family-Centered Support Conversation (FCSC) intervention that included (a) conversations to assess and establish a relationship; (b) focus on strengths across cognitive, affective, and behavioral domains; (c) data regarding family daily life experiences; and (d) strategies for the future. Professionals implementing FCSC reported that it gave them a new tool to include families, helped them build skills for facilitating a safe space, and enabled working through confidentiality concerns by letting the person lead. Although they reported the shift to a strengths focus was hard, they learned more about daily life from families and came to realize that a person's recovery cannot be separated from their surroundings and everyday life.

Family-Sensitive Organizational Cultures

At the level of universal or tier 1 interventions (see Chapter 2: Recovery and Wraparound Models 🤝), OTPs can advocate for systemic practices that better support families. Fette and colleagues (2009) asserted that systems set the tone for relationships with families, and can be negatively impacted by stigma, attitudes, and administrative barriers. Families also bring their own barriers: isolation, a history of negative experiences, fear, and mistrust. Mental health professionals can participate in the creation of environments where families feel respected and included in care, and where family caregiver needs are addressed (Aass et al., 2021; Allchin et al., 2022; Moen et al., 2021).

In child-focused services in the United States, family-led support and advocacy organizations began to push for the shift in language from family-centered to family-driven alongside the development of the Systems of Care (SOC) movement, insisting on not only being in the driver's seat for their child's care, but also in building systems that elevate the role of families, recalling the disability rights slogan, "Nothing About Us Without Us" (del Vecchio et al., 2023; National Federation of Families [NFF], 2008). The family-led component of the National Community of Practice on Collaborative School Behavioral Health surveyed families across the United States to craft a family-driven definition of family

---

BOX 29-2 ■ Six Partnership Standards

A guide developed by Mental Health Carers Australia has six partnership standards for working with family/carers that OTPs can use to self-assess their practice (Mind Australia and Helping Minds, 2016):

1. Carers and the essential role they play are identified at first contact, or as soon as possible thereafter.
2. Staff are carer aware and trained in carer engagement strategies.
3. Policy and practice protocols regarding confidentiality and sharing of information are in place.
4. Defined staff positions are allocated for carers in all service settings.
5. A carer introduction to the service and staff is available, with a relevant range of information across the care settings.
6. A range of carer support services is available.

engagement in child-focused systems (Fette et al., 2009). They defined family engagement as:

> An active and ongoing process that facilitates opportunities for all family members to meaningfully participate and contribute to all decision making for their children, and in meaningful involvement with specific programs and with each other. (p. 8)

They modeled family engagement as a process along a continuum that may move toward increased engagement, but that also sometimes slides backward away from that goal. Systems increase engagement, beginning with developing respect, then engaging in effective communication, taking initiative to find solutions, embracing strengths, building family capacity as experts, and finally including families as equals. Conversely, activities that decrease engagement are a lack of respect and resources, negative communication, inflexibility, fragmented systems, increased barriers to family leadership, and finally actively threatening families (Fette et al., 2009). Working within family-sensitive organizational cultures and with a critical mass of other therapists committed to families strengthens OTPs who are striving to build family supports (Moen et al., 2021). The next section presents frameworks from outside and within the occupational therapy profession that can be used for family-focused practice.

The Family Model: Two-Generation Mental Health Needs

The Family Model is a two-generation health-promoting conversation for families in which a parent has mental health challenges. The model, presented in Figure 29-2, provides a framework for working collaboratively with parents and children in building the family's capacity to have ongoing conversations. The semistructured conversation aims to create change in family life through developing a care plan and shared understanding within the family and between the family and the OTP. The conversation focuses on the two most important things for each person and utilizes a visual Family Model diagram to draw attention to each of the domains and their relationships (arrows).

Its six domains are: (1) parent's mental health needs; (2) child's mental health and development; (3) parent and child relationships; (4) protective factors, resilience, and resources/risk factors and stressors; (5) adult and child services; and (6) culture and community (Falkov et al., 2020).

This intervention can be used in both adult- and child-focused service settings: In *adult-focused service settings* it is used as a parent/OTP conversation that acknowledges the parental role, explores how their children are doing, develops a family care plan, and incorporates actions into recovery care planning (Falkov et al., 2020). In *child-focused service settings,* the structured conversation is with the whole family working through each domain and relationship and developing a shared care plan (Hoadley et al., 2017, 2019).

Recovery Frameworks With Adults

In adult mental health practices, SAMHSA describes recovery as a "process of change through which individuals improve their health and wellness, live a self-directed life, and strive to reach their full potential" (SAMHSA, 2012, p. 3). Individuals experiencing mental ill health and their families can have

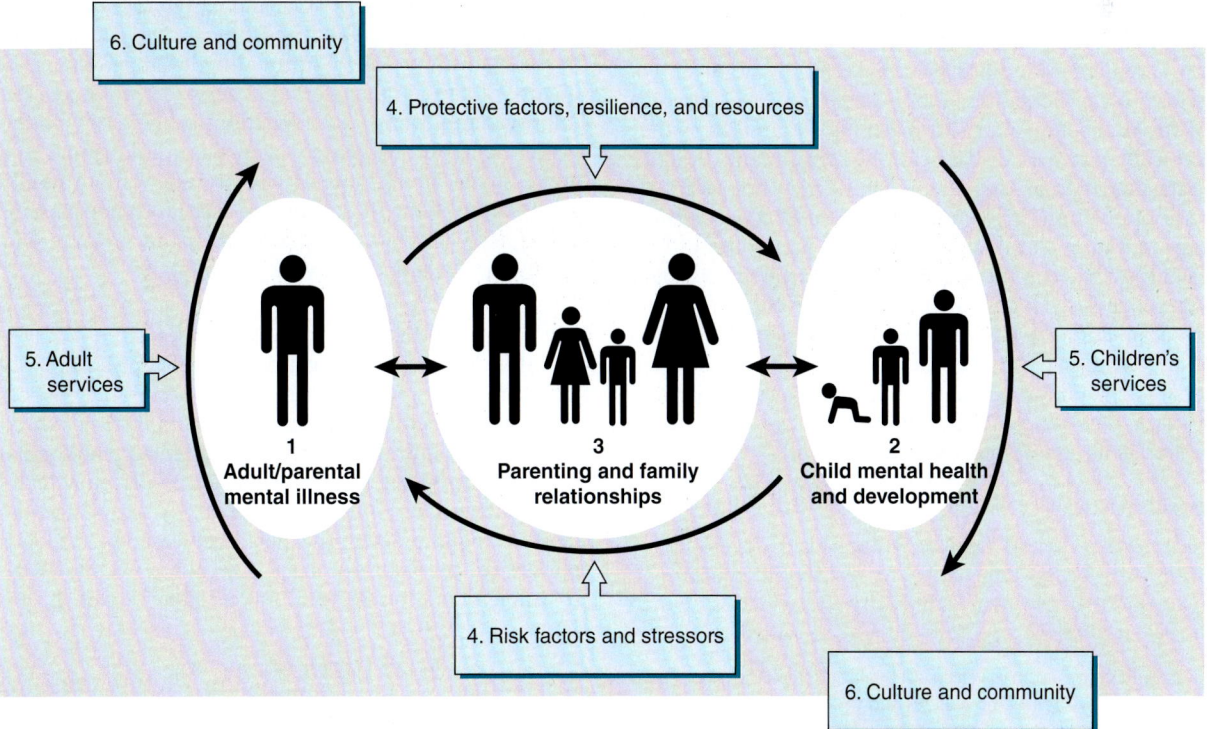

FIGURE 29-2. Family Model diagram. *Adapted from* The Family Model Handbook: An Integrated Approach to Supporting Mentally Ill Parents and Their Children. *Pavilion Publishing and Media Ltd, July 2013. https://pavpub .com/children-mental-health/the-family-model-handbook?srsltid=AfmBOorEjbBdF1zMPUTAGCjZJpO-iLsyvYECQ0d DUh2Ze3ZqN3dOZEcO*

> **BOX 29-3** ■ **Strategies to Promote Family Recovery**
>
> Linking the concepts of family resilience and recovery, Price-Robertson and colleagues (2016) proposed six strategies that OTPs can use to promote family recovery:
> 1. Understand that recovery occurs in a family context.
> 2. Focus on strengthening parent–child relationships.
> 3. Support families to identify what recovery means to them.
> 4. Acknowledge and build on family strengths, while recognizing vulnerabilities.
> 5. Assist family members to better understand and communicate about mental illness.
> 6. Link families into their communities and other resources that support parents and children.

> **BOX 29-4** ■ **Guiding Principles of Family-Driven Support**
>
> 1. Shared decision-making and responsibility for outcomes occur across providers and families.
> 2. Families and youth are given needed information to make informed decisions.
> 3. All children, youth, and families have advocates, family of choice, or families with lived experience to ensure their voices are heard.
> 4. Families and family-run organizations provide peer support and knowledge.
> 5. Families and family-run organizations provide direction for funding services and supports, and advocate for choice.
> 6. Providers actively shift from provider to family driven.
> 7. Administrators allocate resources to make family-driven methods work at the point of service and be sustainable.
> 8. Effort is made to change attitudes in the community by removing barriers and discrimination.
> 9. Communities and providers embrace and celebrate diversity and work to decrease disparities.
> 10. All who work with children, youth, and families continually advance their own cultural and linguistic responsiveness.
>
> *From National Federation of Families. (2008).* Working definition of family-driven care. *https://www.ffcmh.org/resources-familydriven*

---

differing ideas about what constitutes recovery; therefore, a family recovery perspective focuses on supporting the family to explore, direct, and shape changes in their lives, not solely focus on what families might do to support an individual's personal recovery. The topic of recovery and the four dimensions that support recovery are covered in more detail in Chapter 2: Recovery and Wraparound Models. 🤝 Family recovery is about all family members being able to make sense of their experiences and move forward with their lives. Effective strategies to promote family recovery are listed in Box 29-3.

Frameworks for Children and Youth

Practices for children and youth may naturally include families because children live in the context of family. However, in traditional mental health systems, treatment focused on the child and/or youth also persists in practice. Pragmatic features of practice settings may make family involvement easier or more difficult. In school-based practice, OTPs must make very deliberate efforts to reach out to families as they are typically not part of the school environment. Practice in acute hospitals or outpatient clinics may not routinely provide opportunities for family-focused practices. These settings require intentional planning and preparation to include family that may go beyond what is covered by typical billing processes. Historically, early childhood and home health practices have partnered with families in developing goals and creating opportunities for follow through in occupational participation between sessions, but even those may not include the strengths and needs of other family members as deliberate targets of intervention.

Wraparound

In community mental health, wraparound developed as a community-based alternative to residential placement. Wraparound uses the term "family driven," which is defined by the NFF (2008) as:

> Families have a primary decision-making role in the care of their own children as well as the policies and procedures governing care for all children in their community, state, tribe, territory and nation. This includes: [1] Choosing culturally and linguistically competent supports, services, and providers; [2] Setting goals; [3] Designing, implementing, and evaluating programs; [4] Monitoring outcomes; and [5] Partnering in funding decisions. (p. 1)

The NFF definition also lays out 10 principles of **family-driven** support. Principles are tools for accountability for individual OTPs as well as agencies and systems. The American Academy of Child and Adolescent Psychiatry (AACAP, 2022) states the importance of SOC and family-driven practices in providing access to mental health care for youth with SED in the community and as providing leverage for increasing quality of care. They assert that active family participation improves family and youth functioning, increases family empowerment, and decreases reliance on professional support and systems. Identifying areas of competence in families is a key component in strengths-based assessment. Guiding principles OTPs can use that help ensure they are offering family-driven supports are shared in Box 29-4.

Family Group Decision Making

Family Group Decision Making (FGDM) is another family-focused practice with roots in restorative justice that is practiced in child and adult welfare. FGDM has three key elements: (1) It draws up an action-oriented plan for clarifying and monitoring goals; (2) it is family-driven, which here means the person in need and the family set the agenda and develop and implement the plan together; and (3) it has three phases: (a) preparation phase, (b) conference meeting, and (c) implementation and evaluation (Hillebregt et al., 2019).

Occupational Justice

An occupational justice framework calls all OTPs to advocate for inclusive practices and to attend to the impact of social drivers of health and systemic racism. Using this framework, OTPs can support families by advocating for their needs at systems or population levels. Michels and colleagues (2022) assert the importance of family networks in mitigating poverty and food insecurity for people living with severe mental ill health and states that supporting families is an important component of intervention. Tyo and McCurry (2023) affirm caregiver resilience and effective coping as products of good physical and mental health, characteristics of both the caregiver and recipient of care, access to adequate support, and decreased stigma. Brock-Baca and colleagues (2022) identified substantial impacts on family time, finances, employment status secondary to raising a child with severe mental health needs, and suggested use of two-generation strategies to simultaneously address child and family mental health, including job training, employment supports and behavioral health services, high fidelity wraparound, and support from families with lived experience.

Many people living with mental ill health end up in the criminal justice system because of social and economic burdens and the fragmented and inadequate systems charged with supporting them in the community. There is a call for systemic change that would recognize the cultural, economic, and resource needs of families but also go beyond and embrace families as potential drivers of solutions regarding what is a crisis in access to mental health care (Isobel et al., 2019; Jain et al., 2019). The National Alliance on Mental Illness (NAMI) has successfully launched anti-stigma campaigns that seek to eliminate the negative social status and secondary consequences of vilifying families living with mental illnesses (https://www.nami.org/blogs/nami-blog/october-2017/9-ways-to-fight-mental-health-stigma). SAMHSA has initiated the National Family Support Technical Assistance Center (https://www.nfstac.org) to both extend their focus on families across the life span (from its origin in children's mental health) and link family advocates across mental health and substance use recovery. The NFF (https://www.ffcmh.org) has initiated a campaign to shift advocacy language from mental health *awareness* to *acceptance* to feature more active language. Their current slogan is *Accept - Advocate - Act!*

Matching Advocacy to Family Needs

Practitioners should be familiar with local and regional family support organizations and connect families to organizations that might best meet their needs. For example, NAMI has historically embraced a medical or biopsychosocial understanding of mental illness and may be a better fit for families in the Seeking phase of adapting to mental health needs (Fig. 29-1) and/or those who are at ease with a more medical orientation that seeks to label and understand the illness itself. In contrast, a family in the Acceptance/Justice or Balance states may be a better match with NFF, which is closely aligned with wraparound, or some of the MAD Pride–aligned peer-to-peer psychiatric survivor groups who focus on recovery and justice and embrace a focus on enabling meaning and participation. Recovery-oriented practices are more likely to embrace ideas of neurodivergence and compensatory strategies whose aim is *living a life anyway* instead of remediating illness. Likewise, families experiencing alcohol and/or substance use disorder may align more with traditional Al-Anon support groups, newer SMART Recovery family meetings, or even harm reduction movement organizations. These are often volunteer, peer-to-peer support networks and represent

diverse perspectives requiring the OTP to be familiar with both their nuances and what is available in the area and online. See Chapter 27: Mental Health Stigma and Sanism. 🤝

It is also important for OTPs to be aware of predatory groups with potentially harmful practices. These align with prevailing cultural mores in the United States that have a history of seeing families as more part of the problem than the solution. An example is tough love, which advocates showing love by holding rigid boundaries and insisting upon desired behaviors even if that means rejecting the person whose behavior they want to change. There are also some common support groups who may veer from family support into extreme practices that ostracize. At their worst, these have spawned so called "treatment" programs collectively known as the "troubled teen industry (TTI)." See this chapter's The Lived Experience for an example. Other examples may include extremist groups who may prey on individuals who are socially isolated and estranged from family yet are seeking to belong somewhere.

Occupational Therapy Frameworks

Occupational therapy practice frameworks help guide OTPs to identify their role in the provision of family-focused services. Several occupational therapy frameworks see human occupation as an interaction between person (family), the environment, and their occupations. Examples include the Canadian Model of Occupational Performance and Engagement (Polatajko et al., 2007), the Kawa Model (Iwama, 2006; Iwama et al., 2009), Kielhofner's Model of Human Occupation (MOHO; Taylor, 2017), and Occupational Adaptation (OA; Schultz, 2013).

Occupational Adaptation

Working from an OA framework, the OTP is the agent of the environment, and the person and family are the agents of change. This approach aligns well with recovery and wraparound's emphasis on individuals as drivers of change. In OA, the mechanisms of change are persons' three-part internal adaptive response mechanisms: adaptive response modes, adaptation energy, and adaptive response behaviors. **Adaptive response modes** are (a) the extent to which responses are habitual and routine (existing modes), (b) an adaptation of habituated behaviors (modified modes), or (c) a novel way of doing something (new modes) by a person or group. For a family, an existing mode is something they have been doing that is automatic; for example, in this chapter's The Lived Experience account, Fette's family had been trained in behavioral techniques when Aaron was very young and that was how they understood change (existing mode). As that failed, they learned tough love strategies, which were easily incorporated into their existing behavioral strategies (modified). Finally, when those were still not working, they shifted into radical acceptance, which was a completely new mode.

Adaptation energy compares the easy use of secondary energy in habituated behaviors to the high primary energy costs of change. New behaviors come with a cost (primary energy) and are not as efficient as automatic behaviors (secondary energy). The Fettes did not have to use any primary energy to implement the behavioral strategies that they knew, but learning a whole new paradigm required effort to implement. The primary energy demanded for change also meant they had decreased energy reserves or tolerance left over.

They had a finite amount of energy that was tied up in the need to develop new behaviors that would enable a relationship with Aaron.

Adaptive response behaviors (ARBs) are the third and final piece of the adaptive response generation subprocess. These are classified as primitive, transitional, or mature. **Primitive** or hyperstable ARBs are experienced as being stuck, often repeating behaviors that are clearly not working. With the Fettes, this was demonstrated in failed efforts to force Aaron to stay home. Primitive behaviors are the least effective ARBs, but they are what is initially resorted to when people feel overwhelmed. **Transitional** ARBs are common coming out of primitive states and they often serve to knock people off balance a bit to get unstuck. Schultz (2013) initially referred to these as hypermobile because they often include trial-and-error responses; they are more adaptive than primitive ARBs because one might accidentally try something that works. When Aaron was failing out of middle school, the Fettes tried more counselors, supplements, medications, new psychiatrists, and sadly that TTI program. Finally, after Aaron was on the streets, they developed **mature** ARBs, which resulted in more effectively appraising the potential for outcomes from their efforts and building capacity to rebuild and sustain a relationship with their oldest son.

Kawa Model

Kawa (Iwama, 2006; Iwama et al., 2009) uses the metaphor of a river to emphasize the interrelatedness of the whole system rather than the independent self, making it a good fit for partnering with families. The model provides an opportunity to explore a family's experience through a narrative, looking at their collective life as a river. It looks at both the length of the river, examining its past, present, and future, and a cross section of the river, exploring their current experience.

From the source to the ocean, a river's quality and character will alter, widening in parts to an easy flow and narrowing in parts with rapids and a fast pace. Working in partnership with a family, the length of the river can be used to understand the family's perspective on their context, identifying family identity, strengths, and challenges, and hearing their hopes for the future.

A cross section of a river reveals the *riverbanks, rocks, driftwood,* and the *river* flowing in the spaces between. Using these interrelated constructs, the OTP and the family can explore the family's current experience. The *river* represents the life flow of the family and their overall occupations and can be explored by asking families to describe the flow of their life, what they enjoy doing together, and their everyday activities. The *riverbanks* represent their social and physical environments that contain and control their life flow. These might be explored through asking about formal and informal networks of support, their living arrangements, and where their occupations are carried out. The circumstances that block their life flow and cause difficulties or disruption are represented by *rocks*. Asking about, and having families name, the difficulties they are facing, what they want to do but are unable to do, or things they want to change can help to identify what gets in the way of the family's occupations. The *driftwood* represents the family's personal resources that influence their life flow positively (pushing rocks out of the way) or negatively (getting stuck between the rocks). These resources can be family characteristics; beliefs; values and principles; skills, abilities, and experiences; and their material and social capital.

The process of developing the picture of their river can create opportunities for the family to see their situation differently through identifying strengths and resources and promoting their family identity. It can also facilitate them to explore ways to utilize their resources to enable family life flow that can promote family well-being.

Model of Human Occupation

MOHO is an occupation-based conceptual framework and practice model that aims to understand how people select (volition), organize (habituation), and undertake (performance capacity) their occupations, and the environmental contexts that influence all aspects of these occupations, such as constraining or enabling them (Kielhofner, 2008; Taylor, 2017). As people engage in an activity, they interpret the experience through the lens of their values, beliefs, and previous experiences (Did I enjoy it? Was I successful? Did it meet my expectations?). This interpretation shapes how they see themselves in relation to that activity (occupational identity), which affects how they might anticipate participating in that activity, thereby affecting their future choices (Kielhofner, 2008; Kramer & Bowyer, 2007). MOHO understands human occupation as dynamic with change occurring in response to shifts in skills, values, roles, habits, routines, and environment.

There is a collection of tools to find information about values, interests, competencies, roles, and routines from both the subjective lived experience and objective observational perspective. Information gathered is drawn together into a narrative to understand the person's OA (in MOHO, this is the outcome rather than the internal adaptive process explained earlier in the practice theory OA) through the alignment of occupational identity and occupational capacity (Parkinson & Brooks, 2021).

When using a MOHO lens, the OTP and the family build an understanding of fit between their occupational identity and occupational capacity. Asking about what is important to them individually and collectively (beliefs/values/culture/interests) and their perception of their capacity and efficacy to act in their own world can help the OTP to understand how their views on mental ill health may impact engagement in previous or new occupations. Exploring how family life is organized through their roles, patterns, habits, and routines can help to understand how these may have been disrupted or reorganized in the context of a family member's mental ill health. Exploring the family's capacity to engage in their family occupations by exploring both the objective observed view and their subjective lived experience provides insight into how the experience of having a family member with mental ill health impacts family functioning. Armed with this information, the family and OTP can collaboratively develop new responses to the new activity, role, and routine demands to promote everyone's well-being, improve family functioning, and gain a greater sense of competence.

Evaluation and Intervention

The *Occupational Therapy Practice Framework* (*OTPF;* American Occupational Therapy Association [AOTA], 2020) guides evaluation focused on individual, caregiver,

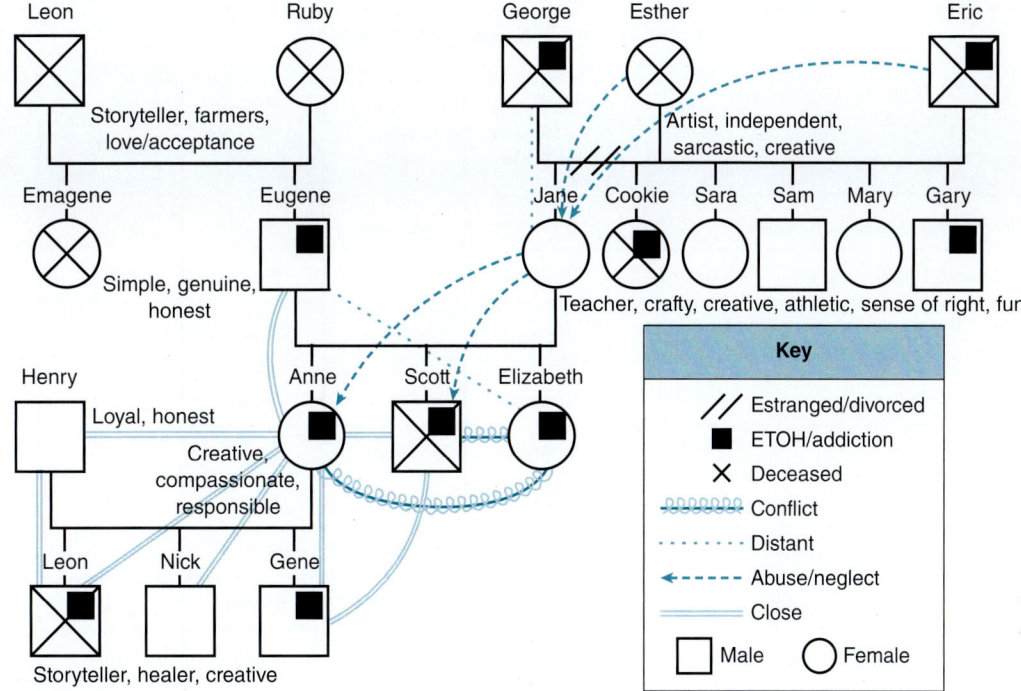

FIGURE 29-3. When creating a family genogram, include at least three generations. Graphics can be used to depict strengths of family that are passed down; these serve as both a legacy and a way to identify assets. They can additionally identify how close or strained relationships are and intergenerational abuse and conflict.

group, or population levels. Evaluation includes the occupational profile and the analysis of occupational performance. In family-focused practice, an occupational profile may be generated for the family. The focus of data gathering is on the family's occupational history, their collective experiences, daily living patterns, what they want and need to do as a family unit, and supports and barriers for their health and well-being (AOTA, 2020). While completing a family occupational profile, the OTP must be sensitive to the family's values, culture, environment, and contextual factors. Practitioners must also acknowledge the strengths, resources, and expertise of families. Families experience a variety of challenges, and family members are usually doing the best they can. Promoting the family's sense of control and acknowledging their strengths can assist families in developing the necessary skills to cope with mental illness and address the specific needs identified by the family.

At the end of the occupational profile, the OTP reviews the information and forms a working hypothesis for what occupations and contexts need to be addressed (AOTA, 2020). Most importantly, OTPs listen to the family and analyze the occupations and performance patterns they have identified. If needed, the OTP may use tools, such as a family genogram to gather history (Fig. 29-3); self-report tools such as the Role Checklist (Oakley et al., 1986) to identify current roles and their value; or ParentingWell® Strengths & Goals, which are used to self-identify capacity in parenting occupations (Fig. 29-4). These tools are a starting point for partnering with families to develop goals and plans. Once the Analysis of Occupational Performance is complete, OTPs generate an interpretive summary and work with families to identify desired goals and objectives.

Family Interventions

The *OTPF* lists occupational therapy interventions as (a) establish/restore, (b) modify, (c) maintain, (4) prevent, and (5) create (AOTA, 2020). In practice with families, OTPs may work alongside families to help them establish or restore occupations that they identify as valuable, as well as performance patterns that enable those. Practitioners use a modification approach when they facilitate compensatory strategies in the environment to enable effective performance of tasks such as medication management, self-care, or organization. They may support maintaining roles and routines that are important to families and enabling participation in valued occupations to prevent deterioration of those roles and routines. A whole-of-family approach helps to prevent the cascade effects of mental ill health that can lead to intergenerational challenges, deteriorated family functioning, loss of custody of children, and/or isolation. Often adjustments within the family to accommodate mental health challenges lead to increased capacity within family members; OTPs may help identify these and create new opportunities.

Occupational perspectives support family-focused practice by offering a positive focus on a family's strengths and enabling positive joint activities rather than focusing on problems in family dynamics (Hackett & Cook, 2016). The concepts of family-focused recovery and family resilience have a natural alignment with the principles of occupational therapy, particularly those focused on strengths and success-oriented goals (Merryman & Riegal, 2007). Family members need access to strengths-based care that offers support, education, and practical strategies to both support each other and attend to their own mental health (Aass et al., 2021; Moen et al., 2021).

ParentingWell® Strengths & Goals					
Here is a list of things you may need to do as a parent. For each one that applies to you, *circle* the answer that describes you best.	**This is a strength of mine.**	**I do this okay.**	**I'd like to do this better.**	**Does not apply.**	**Check items to work on.**
1. Manage everyday household tasks	Strength	Okay	Better	DNA	
2. Plan and make healthy meals	Strength	Okay	Better	DNA	
3. Understand the relationship between my feelings and my actions	Strength	Okay	Better	DNA	
4. Manage my family's money	Strength	Okay	Better	DNA	
5. Set limits with my child	Strength	Okay	Better	DNA	
6. Have positive interactions/visits with my child	Strength	Okay	Better	DNA	
7. Have a pleasant routine with my child	Strength	Okay	Better	DNA	
8. Find fun things to do with my child	Strength	Okay	Better	DNA	
9. Get adequate child care for my child	Strength	Okay	Better	DNA	
10. Balance work or school, and parenting	Strength	Okay	Better	DNA	
11. Know what to do when my child has problems	Strength	Okay	Better	DNA	
12. Identify my child's strengths	Strength	Okay	Better	DNA	
13. Have positive "family time"	Strength	Okay	Better	DNA	
14. Know my legal options as a parent	Strength	Okay	Better	DNA	
15. Get help for myself, if I need it	Strength	Okay	Better	DNA	
16. Talk with my child about my situation or worries	Strength	Okay	Better	DNA	
17. Keep in touch with my child who is not living with me	Strength	Okay	Better	DNA	
18. Live a substance-free lifestyle	Strength	Okay	Better	DNA	
19. Communicate well with my child	Strength	Okay	Better	DNA	
20. Have good relationships with my child's caregivers/helpers	Strength	Okay	Better	DNA	
21. Express anger without hurting anyone	Strength	Okay	Better	DNA	
22. Keep my child and myself safe	Strength	Okay	Better	DNA	
23. Make time to take care of myself	Strength	Okay	Better	DNA	
24. Manage stress and worries in healthy ways	Strength	Okay	Better	DNA	
25. Cope with bad things that have happened to me in my life	Strength	Okay	Better	DNA	
26. Get special services and supports for my child	Strength	Okay	Better	DNA	
27. Other:	Strength	Okay	Better	DNA	

FIGURE 29-4. ParentingWell® strengths & goals self-assessment form. *Courtesy U.S. Department of Health and Human Services, Substance Abuse and Mental Health Services Administration, Center for Mental Health Services.*

Family psychoeducation based on partnership with consumers and families, information sharing, building social support, problem-solving, and skills development is within the scope of occupational therapy practice. Family members may be coteachers in a multifamily group approach. Core elements of family psychoeducation programs include establishing respectful relationships; offering education about mental illness, mental health, and recovery; managing difficult situations and challenges; creating a strengths-based environment; and fostering mutual support and participation in family support groups. This approach also emphasizes communication skills and problem-solving, two areas in which OTPs have knowledge and skills, particularly as they apply to everyday life (see the Resources section). Practitioners may access online materials such as those discussed later in the self-help resources, promote family access, and use them to develop and facilitate multifamily groups and create activities centered on family occupational participation.

Support, Resources, and Programs

OTPs can draw on a wide range of resources and programs available to assist families affected by mental illness. Emotional and practical support is essential in helping families to cope successfully with life changes. This support can come from peer and/or professionally led support groups. Family-led mutual support groups offer family members the opportunity to connect with others with shared experience, build hope, and learn from one another. One side benefit to COVID-19 was that it has increased web-based resources and support available to isolated families.

A population with specific needs is military families. Occupational performance difficulties in relationships, school, physical health, sleep, and driving were identified among military service personnel after combat duty (Plach & Sells, 2013). Occupational therapy should be a key component of programs supporting military families to address issues and optimize their health and well-being (Cogan, 2014). Understanding military culture (the Veterans Administration [VA] has provider toolkits) and the resources in the area is important, as military families move frequently and may not be familiar with local and state regulations or resources. There are websites with information, resources, and programs specifically for military service personnel and their families, which can assist OTPs to guide and support them (see Resources). See Chapter 43: Serving Veterans and Service Members. 🤝

Family Peer Supports

Family or carer peer workers are trained family members who have their own experience of family with mental illness. There is a growing workforce of family peer workers/professionals internationally who work directly with families and/or at a system level. They provide support to families through courses/programs, resources, and individual consultations. Many are limited to work with families within the system they are employed in. Family peer support offers the unique opportunity for participants to build hope from others who have been where they are; learn from the experiences of other family members, friends, and carers; and find mutual support among peers (Bourke et al., 2015).

Family support and educational courses or programs led by trained and accredited peer facilitators have evidence showing a reduction in worry, tension, and distress of families (Stephens et al., 2011). An example of this is the NAMI Family to Family (FTF) program, which is a 12-week education course for family and friends of people living with mental illness in the United States. It offers information and support through presentations, discussions, and group activities (see Resources). NAMI groups frequently embrace a more medical or biopsychosocial perspective, often with a focus on mental illnesses rather than recovery. Families who need support with advocacy and navigating complex systems (schools, justice, etc.) may benefit from family peers associated with the NFF, who are more closely aligned with wraparound or recovery models.

A mix of volunteer and paid family support providers is available within family-run organizations, but these vary broadly, sometimes serving individuals in a specific program, or being specific to a diagnosis or group of families. Several states in the United States have SAMHSA-funded statewide family networks, which could be allied with NAMI and/or NFF. Practitioners should get to know local and state organizations and see what specific resources they offer. Since COVID, many support groups have created online options, which may eliminate geographic barriers for many families. See Chapter 39: Peer-Led Services. 🤝

Self-Help Tools for Families, Friends, and Communities

Rethink Mental Illness is a UK-based organization that aims to promote a better life for people affected by mental illness. It provides several resources for families, friends, and carers, which are accessible from their website (see Resources). *Caring for Yourself,* a self-help workbook for family and friends supporting people with mental illness, created by Rethink Mental Illness and the Meriden Family Programme in the United Kingdom is downloadable from their website. This workbook is designed for use either by family members and friends to work through independently, or in education programs and support groups for families and carers that could also be supported by OTPs (Fadden et al., 2012). The workbook covers a range of topics, including carer support, recovery and hope, information and resources, communication skills, problem-solving, goal setting, and relapse management (see Resources).

In addition to group support for other family members, siblings and children of people with mental health needs also benefit from their own groups to meet other families coping with the same challenges as well as to develop effective strategies for resilience (Feriante et al., 2022). Rethink Mental Illness has developed a Siblings Network to provide information and support resources for anyone whose brother or sister has experienced mental health issues. The Sibling Toolkit, developed by the Siblings Network, also provides web-based tools to help siblings look after their own well-being, and to support a brother or sister experiencing mental health issues. It features personal stories and videos of siblings sharing their experiences and what they have learned (see Resources). COPMI (Children Of Parents with Mental Illness) is an Australian initiative that provides web-based resources, including booklets, videos for children, and resources for families when a family member has mental health issues (https://www.copmi.net.au).

The NAMI Parents and Teachers as Allies program is designed to create supportive school communities by raising awareness among educators of mental health issues and early warning signs and building their skills to partner effectively with families affected by mental illness and local support services (see Resources). The locally delivered Parents and Teachers as Allies program is led by a young adult with lived experience of mental health issues, a parent, and a teacher (Burland & Nemec, 2007). In addition, a program aimed at middle and high school students called NAMI Ending the Silence has been developed to raise awareness and change perceptions and understanding of mental illness (Burland & Nemec, 2007). NAMI Ending the Silence involves presentations by a young adult living with mental illness and a family member telling their stories (see Resources).

Here's the Point

- Families are best supported as a whole unit rather than a collection of individuals.
- OTPs may serve as direct care providers, consultants, advocates, and social systems change agents to promote family-focused mental health care.
- Practitioners, because of their occupational perspective, understanding of roles and performance patterns, and collaborative approach, are well suited to support families.
- Well-developed practice frameworks for family-focused practice exist and are compatible with *OTPFs*.
- Practitioners should advocate for families within their service delivery setting.

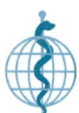 Visit the online resource center at **FADavis.com** to access the videos.

Apply It Now

1. Reflexivity

It is important that OTPs check their own bias and refrain from imposing their values onto the families they work with. As norms change across societies, it is recommended that OTPs use supervision to work through ethical dilemmas. For example, discipline using corporal punishment—a norm in past generations—has shifted with knowledge of more effective forms of parenting practices. What were the norms from your childhood? How could you support families whose norms include practices that people have come to see as potentially harmful? With a peer, discuss how you might approach this topic of discipline or another ethical dilemma with a family you may work with.

2. Family Occupations

What are the occupations that are valued and enjoyed in your family? Reflect on how they were chosen, how they have shaped your family identity and who plays what roles in them. Consider how they might be able to continue if a family member couldn't contribute as they had previously. Consider how family occupations differ in other families.

3. Finding Local Resources

- Explore what specific resources exist for families in your community to support their mental health and well-being (e.g., support groups specifically for parents, mothers, or fathers; after-school activities).
- Develop your own list of local family resources, including family support groups, family education programs, and current web resources or reading materials appropriate for families.

4. Using Frameworks for Family Involvement

Reflect on the organizational characteristics within a fieldwork placement or workplace you have experienced. Use the following questions to guide your thinking about family-focused practices at this setting. If you find apparent gaps in services, consider how these might be addressed to create family-sensitive or family-inclusive services.

Reflective Questions

- When a family first encounters this setting, what information (e.g., culturally relevant information leaflets, education resources, support groups) do they receive about the service?
- How does the service routinely consider the experiences and needs of the whole family?
- What family-focused interventions does the service offer? What, if any, gaps in services are apparent?

5. Education Using First-Person Accounts

Explore resources in your community that offer first-person accounts of individuals' lived experiences that can give you and your peers the opportunity to learn about mental illness and its impact on families.

- Deveson, A. (1991). *Tell me I'm here.* Penguin.
- Hinshaw, S. P. (2004). Parental mental disorder and children's functioning: Silence and communication, stigma and resilience. *Journal of Clinical Child and Adolescent Psychology, 33*(2), 400–411. https://doi.org/10.1207/s15374424jccp3302_22
- Mom's Blog on Aaron–Voices website: https://aaron-voices.com/moms-blog
- Sane website: *People like us*—lived experience stories: https://www.sane.org/spotlight-on/families-carers

6. Relative Mastery: Applying the Occupational Adaptation Model

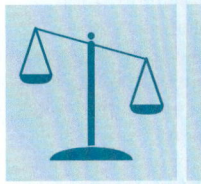  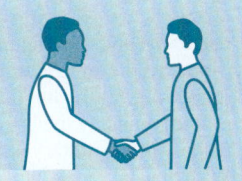

Efficiency   Effectiveness   Satisfaction (self, others)

Observable outcomes in OA are framed as **relative mastery**, which includes efficiency, effectiveness, satisfaction to self, and satisfaction to others. Using this chapter's The Lived Experience *radical acceptance* story, identify when you believe the Fettes' responses were *efficient* in terms of their use of time, money, energy, and other resources. At what point did they successfully build a relationship with Aaron (*effectiveness*)? What was their level of *satisfaction* at various points in their story? What was the level of satisfaction of others in their environment? Explain/discuss your responses with a peer.

7. Video Exercise: Prioritizing Family During a Mother's Cancer Treatment

Pair up with another student in your class or form a small group of students. Access and watch the "Prioritizing Family During a Mother's Cancer Treatment" video at the online resource center at FADavis.com. Then, discuss and together answer the following questions.

Reflective Questions
■ How did Marylein work to prioritize her family during cancer treatments?
■ Marylein focuses on the invaluable support she received from her family, an outward focus. Would you also encourage Marylein to consider self-care strategies? If so, how might you introduce these?

■ What was the role of social connectedness and belonging in Marylein's story?

8. Video Exercise: Tricks and Techniques From the Mother of an Autistic Son

Pair up with another student in your class or form a small group of students. Access and watch the "Tricks and Techniques From the Mother of an Autistic Son" video at the online resource center at FADavis.com. Then, discuss and together answer the following questions.

Reflective Questions
■ Laura and her husband were creative, adaptive, and person-centered when it came to understanding Will's diagnosis and learning how to help him. How can OTPs intentionally listen and learn from families to elicit and build on their solutions?
■ Think about Laura's story about anticipating that Will would be deluged with broad questions when the family returned from a trip to Sweden and how she created a strategy to help him respond. How did the use of visuals help Will address events in his life and learn to regulate his emotions? In what ways was this helpful to his family as well as Will himself?
■ Laura describes using the technique of social stories—both spoken and visual—to prepare Will for his daily routine, transitions, changes, and choices. In what ways did that help Will and his family? What other types of individuals might benefit from the use of social stories? How might you include them in your occupational therapy practice?
■ Watching this video, you might feel exhausted just listening to Laura's stories and thinking of her and her husband's efforts. Describe the time and emotional commitment it took for them to participate with Will in intensive therapy at school and at home, as well as maintain full-time jobs. What supports would have been helpful to the family? What self-care methods would you recommend to a mother like Laura?

Resources

U.S.-Based Mental Health Support Organizations
• Family Run Executive Director Leadership Association (FREDLA): https://www.fredla.org/helpful-websites. FREDLA includes many family run organizations in the United States. They have an extensive list of organization websites that provide valuable resources for families.
• National Federation of Families: https://www.ffcmh.org/resources. Find Family Advocacy & Support Resources on multiple topics such as Crisis Resources, Mental Wellness and Self-Care, Learning Disabilities, Suicide Prevention, and multiple other topics. Scroll down to the "Mental Wellness and Self-Care" link under Resources and look at the self-care infographics. Or go to the top navigation bar, select the

Advocacy Toolkit, and scroll down to the links under "Help Me Learn to Advocate."
• Family Education & Support—The National Alliance on Mental Illness (NAMI) Family-to-Family (FTF) Program: https://www.nami.org/Find-Support/NAMI-Programs/NAMI-Family-to-Family. Follow this link to find out more about NAMI's free 8-week course for families.
• Mental Health America: https://mhanational.org. This website shares a wide variety of resources including advocacy tools. Excellent national statistics/information can be found in their annual *State of Mental Health in America* report (https://mhanational.org/issues/state-mental-health-america).
• Youth MOVE National: Voices of Youth With Lived Experience: https://youthmovenational.org. Here you can connect youth to chapters with other young people in their area or click on

the provider tab and check out their training on how to better advocate for youth-driven infrastructure and how to support youth as leaders in systems change.

Videos

- "Occupational Therapy Collaboration in Early Head Start" video. In this video, an occupational therapist and occupational therapy assistant describe their partnership while working collaboratively at an Early Head Start program. They explain the importance of a team approach to tiered intervention services and how they work together to support children, parents, and staff. This includes strategizing on how to implement creative intervention ideas and address challenges with individual children, some of whom have experienced trauma. Access the video at the online resource center at FADavis.com.
- "Veteran's Caregiver on Advocacy and VA Support" video. Nancy is the spouse and caregiver of a veteran with early-onset Alzheimer disease. In this video, she shares about his diagnosis and the arduous process of applying for VA benefits. In her case, the application was successful, and she describes how critical those resources have been for her and her husband. Nancy urges OTPs to work with social workers to ensure families of veterans receive the benefits they have earned. Access the video at the online resource center at FADavis.com.
- "Caregiver of Spouse With Alzheimer Disease on Challenges" video. Nancy is the wife and caregiver of a man with early-onset Alzheimer disease. Her husband, Bill, had an exciting civilian career, as well as a U.S. Navy career. In this video, she describes the challenges they face now that he is unable to work, particularly because he has few hobbies or friends. Nancy shares her struggle maintaining a schedule and filling his time, and describes how she encourages occupations that are meaningful to him. Access the video at the online resource center at FADavis.com.
- "Laura's Experience as a Mother of an Autistic Son" video. Laura is the mother of an adult son, Will, who was diagnosed with autism at age 3. In this video, she describes what Will was like as a baby and what signs she and day-care teachers first noticed. She explains what the evaluation process was like and how it felt when she learned that her loving, talkative, playful child had autism. Occupational therapy, social skills therapy, speech therapy, and other services—as well as intensely involved parents—laid the groundwork for Will to succeed in school and go on to fulfill his occupational dream as a young adult. Access the video at the online resource center at FADavis.com.
- "Aster's Lived Experience of Suicidality" video. Aster is an occupational therapist, educator, and disability researcher who shares their experience with major depression and suicidality. In this video, Aster openly and courageously describes an episode of suicidality that resulted in taking a leave of absence from work. They discuss the actions and resources that helped them get through the crisis, including creating a psychiatric advance directive, planning for their safety, and stopping an asthma medication that was worsening their symptoms. Aster's video also addresses the topics of social connectedness, stigma, and trauma recovery following a mental health crisis. To access the video, visit the online resource center at FADavis.com.

Military Family Resources

- VA Provider Toolkit for Co-Occurring Disorders: https://www.mentalhealth.va.gov/communityproviders. This website provides OTPs with evidence-based strategies to support veterans with co-occurring disorders such as posttraumatic stress disorder (PTSD), head injuries, mood disorders, and substance abuse.
- FREDLA—Resources for Military Families: https://www.fredla.org/resources-for-military-families. This website has links to

access resources to support military families. On this site, go to the "Best Military Family Resources" link to access a military wife and mom's informed list of essential resources.
- Mental Health America: http://www.mentalhealthamerica.net/military-mental-health. This website includes information, resources, and programs specifically for military service personnel and their families.
- Military One Source: https://www.militaryonesource.mil/parenting/family-life/family-resilience. This one-stop website is maintained by the U.S. Department of Defense with lots of resources for military families. Go to the "Support for Families With Special Needs" link for information on resources, benefits, and other programs for families with children with special needs.

International Resources

- Emerging Minds : https://emergingminds.com.au/families/Minds. This website develops free resources to help OTPs and families support children's mental health and well-being.
  - Go to the "Professionals" tab to find online training resources: https://emergingminds.com.au/practitioners
  - Go to the "Families" tab for free resources for all families: https://emergingminds.com.au/families
- Emerging Minds Children of Parents With Mental Illness (COPMI; Australia; www.copmi.net.au) provides resources for parents with mental ill health, their children, and family and friends.
- Rethink Mental Illness (UK): https://www.rethink.org/help-in-your-area/about-services-and-groups. This website has resources for people living in the United Kingdom. However, anyone can access their Carers Hub with easy segments on a range of topics from supporting someone with suicidal thoughts to guidance in understanding mental health conditions and how to help.
- Meriden—*Caring for Yourself* online workbook: http://meridenfamilyprogramme.com/recovery/what-carers-families-and-friends-can-do-to-help-themselves/caring-for-yourself. This free workbook is intended to support carers and covers everything from self-care and communication to relapse management.
- The Children's Society (UK): https://www.childrenssociety.org.uk/information/young-people/young-carers. This website provides a wealth of information for young people caring for family members, ranging from accessing financial resources for kids in the United Kingdom to how to cope with living with an alcohol-dependent adult.
- ParentingWell (United States): https://www.cbhknowledge.center/parentingwell-resources. This site includes resources and a workbook to support OTPs' skill development in working with parents with mental illness and their family.
- SANE Family/Carers: https://www.sane.org/spotlight-on/families-carers. This website provides support for caregivers from others with lived experience and features a blog, fact sheets, and personal stories.

References

Aass, L. K., Moen, O. L., Skundberg-Kletthagen, H., Lundqvist, L. O., & Schröder, A. (2021). Family support and quality of community mental health care: Perspectives from families living with mental illness. *Journal of Clinical Nursing, 31*(7-8), 935–948. https://doi.org/10.1111/jocn.15948

Abraham, K. M., & Stein, C. H. (2015). Stress-related personal growth among emerging adults whose mothers have been diagnosed with mental illness. *Psychiatric Rehabilitation Journal, 38*(3), 227. https://doi.org/10.1037/prj0000128

Allan, E., Najm, A., Fernandes, H., & Allchin, B. (2018). Participatory lived experience research: Barriers and enablers for social inclusion for people with psychosocial disability in Afghanistan. *Journal of Mental Health and Psychosocial Support in Conflict Affected Areas, 16*(3), 222–230. https://doi.org/10.4103/INTV.INTV_39_18

Allchin, B., Weimand, B. M., O'Hanlon, B., & Goodyear, M. (2022). A sustainability model for family-focused practice in adult mental health services. *Frontiers in Psychiatry, 12,* 2578. https://doi.org/10.3389/fpsyt.2021.761889

American Academy of Child and Adolescent Psychiatry (AACAP) Committee on Community-Based Systems of Care and AACAP Committee on Quality Issues. (2022). Clinical update: Child and adolescent behavioral health care in community systems of care. *Journal of the American Academy of Child & Adolescent Psychiatry, 62*(4), 367–384. https://doi.org/10.1016/j.jaac.2022.06.001

American Occupational Therapy Association. (2020). Occupational therapy practice framework: Domain and process—Fourth edition. *The American Journal of Occupational Therapy, 74*(Suppl. 2), 7412410010p1–7412410010p87. https://doi.org/10.5014/ajot.2020.74S2001

Aubuchon-Endsley, N. L., Gee, B. M., Devine, N., Ramsdell-Hudock, H. L., Swann-Thomsen, H., & Brumley, M. R. (2020). A cohort study of relations among caregiver–infant co-occupation and reciprocity. *OTJR: Occupational Therapy Journal of Research, 40*(4), 261–269. https://doi.org/10.1177/1539449220905791

Australian Infant, Child, Adolescent and Family Mental Health Association. (2004). *Principles and actions for services and people working with children of parents with a mental illness.* Author.

Awram, R., Hancock, N., & Honey, A. (2017). Balancing mothering and mental health recovery: The voices of mothers living with mental illness. *Advances in Mental Health, 15*(2), 147–160. https://doi.org/10.1080/18387357.2016.1255149

Bland, R., & Foster, M. (2012). Families and mental illness: Contested perspectives and implications for practice and policy. *Australian Social Work, 65*(4), 517–534. https://doi.org/10.1080/0312407X.2011.646281

Bourke, C., Sanders, B., Allchin, B., Lentin, P., & Lang, S. (2015). Occupational therapy influence on a carer peer support model in a clinical mental health service. *Australian Occupational Therapy Journal, 62,* 299–305. https://doi.org/10.1111/1440-1630.12235

Bourke-Taylor, H. (2022). *The journey of mothers fact sheet.* https://healthymothers-healthyfamilies.com/assets/main/PDFs/1.-Journey-fact-sheet.pdf

Brock-Baca, A. H., Zundel, C., Fox, D., & Nagel, N. J. (2022). Partnering with family advocates to understand the impact on families caring for a child with a serious mental health challenge. *The Journal of Behavioral Health Services & Research, 50,* 315–332. https://doi.org/10.1007/s11414-022-09821-4

Burland, J., & Nemec, P. (2007). NAMI training programs. *Psychiatric Rehabilitation Journal, 31*(1), 80–82. https://doi.org/10.2975/31.1.2007.80.82

Chaffey, L., & Fossey, E. (2004). Caring and daily life: Occupational experiences of women living with sons diagnosed with schizophrenia. *Australian Occupational Therapy Journal, 51,* 199–207. https://doi.org/10.1111/j.1440-1630.2004.00460.x

Cogan, A. M. (2014). Supporting our military families: A case for a larger role for occupational therapy in prevention and mental health care. *American Journal of Occupational Therapy, 68,* 478–483. https://doi.org/10.5014/ajot.2014.009712

del Vecchio, P., Dmitrovic, D., & Sweet, E. (2023). *The role of families in SAMHSA's Office of Recovery* [Webinar]. Administration for Community Living. https://acl.gov/news-and-events/announcements/samhsa-webinar-role-families-samhsas-office-recovery

Dixon, L., McFarlane, W. R., Lefley, H., Lucksted, A., Cohen, M., Falloon, I., Miklowitz, D., Solomon P., & Sondheimer, D. (2001).

Evidence-based practices for services to families of people with psychiatric disabilities. *Psychiatric Services, 52*(7), 903–910. https://doi.org/10.1176/appi.ps.52.7.903

Ewertzon, M., Cronqvist, A., Lutzen, K., & Andershed, B. (2012). A lonely life journey bordered with struggle: Being a sibling of an individual with psychosis. *Issues in Mental Health Nursing, 33,* 157–164. https://doi.org/10.3109/01612840.2011.633735

Fadden, G., James, C., & Pinfold, V. (2012). *Caring for yourself—Self-help for families and friends supporting people with mental health problems.* Rethink Mental Illness and Meriden Family Programme. https://meridenfamilyprogramme.com/recovery/what-carers-families-and-friends-can-do-to-help-themselves/caring-for-yourself

Falkov, A., Grant, A., Hoadley, B., Donaghy, M., & Weimand, B. M. (2020). The Family Model: A brief intervention for clinicians in adult mental health services working with parents experiencing mental health problems. *Australian & New Zealand Journal of Psychiatry, 54*(5), 449–452. https://doi.org/10.1177/0004867420913614

Feriante, J., Shayani, A., Lauer, E., Pressman, A., & Rubin, E. (2022). Sibling support program: A novel peer support intervention for parents, caregivers and siblings of youth experiencing mental illness. *Healthcare, 10,* 908. https://doi.org/10.3390/healthcare10050908

Fernandes, H. L., Cantrill, S., Shrestha, R. L., Raj, R. B., Allchin, B., Kamal, R., Butcher, N., & Grills, N. (2018). Lived experience of psychosocial disability and social inclusion: A participatory PhotoVoice study in rural India and Nepal. *Disability, CBR & Inclusive Development, 29*(2), 5–23. https://doi.org/10.5463/dcid.v29i2.746

Fette, C. V., Glimpse, C. R., Rodarmel, S. L., Carter, A., Derr, P., Fallon, H., & Miller, K. (2009). Spatiotemporal Model of Family Engagement: A qualitative study of family-driven perspectives on family engagement. *Advances in School Mental Health Promotion, 2*(4), 4–18. https://doi.org/10.1080/1754730X.2009.9715712

Foster, K., Maybery, D., Reupert, A., Gladstone, B., Grant, A., Ruud, T., Falkov, A., & Kowalenko, N. (2016). Family-focused practice in mental health care: An integrative review. *Child & Youth Services, 37*(2), 129–155. https://doi.org/10.1080/0145935X.2016.1104048

Francis-Connolly, E. (2004). Mothering across the lifecourse. In S. A. Esdaile & J. A. Olson (Eds.), *Mothering occupations: Challenge, agency, and participation* (pp. 28–51). F.A. Davis.

Goodyear, M. J., Allchin, B., Burn, M., von Doussa, H., Reupert, A., Tchernegovski, P., Sheen, J., Cuff, R., Obradovic, A., Solantaus, T., & Maybery, D. (2022). Promoting self-determination in parents with mental illness in adult mental health settings. *Journal of Family Nursing, 28*(2), 129–141. https://doi.org/10.1177/10748407211067308

Gordon, T., & Borushok, J. (2017). *The ACT approach.* Pesi Publishers.

Gurayah, T., Govender, P., Naidoo, D., Fewster, D. L., & Lingah, T. (2016). Faces of caregiving in a South African context. In D. Sakellariou & N. Pollard (Eds.), *Occupational therapies without borders: Integrating justice with practice* (2nd ed., 373–380). Elsevier.

Hackett, E., & Cook, S. (2016). Occupational therapists' perspectives of how they support the parenting role of mental health service users who have children. *Occupational Therapy in Mental Health, 32*(1), 32–49. https://doi.org/10.1080/0164212X.2015.1091280

Hammell, K. W. (2020). Making choices from the choices we have: The contextual embeddedness of occupational choice. *Canadian Journal of Occupational Therapy, 87*(5), 400–411. https://doi.org/10.1177/0008417420965741

Hankerson, S. H., Moise, N., Wilson, D., Waller, B. Y., Arnold, K. T., Duarte, C., Lugo-Candelas, C., Weissman, M. M., Wainberg, M., Yehuda, R., & Shim, R. (2022). The intergenerational impact of structural racism and cumulative trauma on depression. *American*

Journal of Psychiatry, 179, 434–440. https://doi.org/10.1176/appi.ajp.21101000

Hayes, L., Hawthorne, G., Farhall, J., O'Hanlon, B., & Harvey, C. (2015). Quality of life and social isolation among caregivers of adults with schizophrenia: Policy and outcomes. *Community Mental Health Journal, 51*(5), 591–597. https://doi.org/10.1007/s10597-015-9848-6

Hayes, S. C. (2019). *A liberated mind: How to pivot toward what matters.* Avery.

Hetherington, E. M. (2003). Social support and the adjustment of children in divorced and remarried families. *Childhood, 10*(2), 217–236. https://doi.org/10.1177/0907568203010002007

Hillebregt, C. F., Scholten, E. W. M., Post, M. W. M., Visser-Meily, J. M. A., & Ketelaar, M. (2019). Family group decision-making interventions in adult healthcare and welfare: A systematic literature review of its key elements and effectiveness. *BMJ Open, 9,* e026768. https://doi.org/10.1136/bmjopen-2018-026768

Hoadley, B., Falkov, A., & Agalawatta, N. (2019). The acceptability of a single session family focused approach for children/young people and their parents attending a child and youth mental health service. *Advances in Mental Health, 17*(1), 44–54. https://doi.org/10.1080/18387357.2018.1480398

Hoadley, B., Smith, F., Wan, C., & Falkov, A. (2017). Incorporating children and young people's voices in child and adolescent mental health services using the Family Model. *Social Inclusion, 5*(3), 183–194. https://doi.org/10.17645/si.v5i3.951

Isobel, S., Allchin, B., Goodyear, M., & Gladstone, B. M. (2019). A narrative inquiry into global systems change to support families when a parent has a mental illness. *Frontiers in Psychiatry, 10,* 421006. https://doi.org/10.3389/fpsyt.2019.00310

Iwama, M. (2006). *The Kawa Model: Culturally relevant occupational therapy.* Churchill Livingstone/Elsevier.

Iwama, M. K., Thomson, N. A., & Macdonald, R. M. (2009). The Kawa Model: The power of culturally responsive occupational therapy. *Disability and Rehabilitation, 31,* 1125–1135. https://doi.org/10.1080/09638280902773711

Jaffe, L., & Cospar, S. (2014). Working with families. In J. Case-Smith & J. C. O'Brien (Eds.), *Occupational therapy for children and adolescents* (7th ed., pp. 129–162). Elsevier.

Jain, S., Reno, R., Cohen, A. K., Bassey, H., & Master, M. (2019). Building a culturally responsive, family-driven early childhood system of care: Understanding the needs and strengths of ethnically diverse families of children with social-emotional and behavioral concerns. *Children and Youth Services Review, 100,* 31–38. https://doi.org/10.1016/j.childyouth.2019.02.034

Jakobsen, F. A., Ytterhus, B., & Vik, K. (2021). Adult children's experiences of family occupations following aging parents' functional decline. *Journal of Occupational Science, 28*(4), 525–536. https://doi.org/10.1080/14427591.2020.1818611

Jungbauer, J., Wittmund, B., Dietrich, S., & Angermeyer, M. C. (2004). The disregarded caregivers: Subjective burden in spouses of schizophrenia patients. *Schizophrenia Bulletin, 30*(3), 665–675. https://doi.org/10.1093/oxfordjournals.schbul.a007114

Kantartzis, S. (2017). Exploring occupation beyond the individual: Family and collective occupation. In D. Sakellariou & N. Pollard (Eds.), *Occupational therapies without borders: Integrating justice with practice* (2nd ed., pp. 19–28). Elsevier.

Keeble-Devlin, B. (2012). Disorders of childhood: A developmental and family perspective. In G. Meadows, J. Farhall, E. Fossey, M. Grigg, F. McDermott, & B. Singh (Eds.), *Mental health in Australia: Collaborative community practice* (3rd ed., pp. 578–602). Oxford University Press.

Kielhofner, G. (2008). *Model of Human Occupation: Theory and application* (4th ed.). Lippincott, Williams & Wilkins.

Kingsley, E. P. (1987). *Welcome to Holland.* https://www.emilyperlkingsley.com/welcome-to-holland

Koschorke, M., Padmavati, R., Kumar, S., Cohen, A., Weiss, H. A., Chatterjee, S., Pereira, J., Naik, S., John, S., Dabholkar, H., &

Balaji, M. (2014). Experiences of stigma and discrimination of people with schizophrenia in India. *Social Science & Medicine, 123,* 149–159. https://doi.org/10.1016/j.socscimed.2014.10.035

Kramer, J., & Bowyer, P. (2007). Application of the Model of Human Occupation to children and family interventions. In S. B. Dunbar (Ed.), *Occupational therapy models for intervention with children and families.*

Kübler-Ross, E., & Kessler, D. (2014). *On grief and grieving: Finding the meaning of grief through the five stages of loss.* Simon & Schuster.

Lakeman, R. (2008). Practice standards to improve the quality of family and career participation in adult mental health care: An overview. *International Journal of Mental Health Nursing, 17,* 44–56. https://doi.org/10.1111/j.1447-0349.2007.00510.x

Larson, J. E., & Corrigan, P. (2008). The stigma of families with mental illness. *Academic Psychiatry, 32,* 87–91. https://doi.org/10.1176/appi.ap.32.2.87

Leong, F. T. L., & Kalibatseva, Z. (2011). Cross-cultural barriers to mental health services in the United States. *Cerebrum, 2011*(5), 1–13. https://www.ncbi.nlm.nih.gov/pmc/articles/PMC3574791

Lewis, L. (2016). Meta-ethnography of qualitative research on the experience of being a partner to an individual with schizophrenia spectrum disorder. *Issues in Mental Health Nursing, 38*(3), 219–232. https://doi.org/10.1080/01612840.2016.1259699

Lim, Y. Z. G., Honey, A., & McGrath, M. (2022). The parenting occupations and purposes conceptual framework: A scoping review of 'doing' parenting. *Australian Occupational Therapy Journal, 69*(1), 98–111. https://doi.org/10.1111/1440-1630.12778

Linehan, M., & Wilks, C. R. (2015). The course and evolution of dialectical behavior therapy. *American Journal of Psychotherapy, 69*(2), 97–110. https://doi.org/10.1176/appi.psychotherapy.2015.69.2.97

Matthews, E. J., Puplampu, V., & Gelech, J. M. (2021). Tactics and strategies of family adaptation among parents caring for children and youth with developmental disabilities. *Global Qualitative Nursing Research, 8,* 1–18. https://doi.org/10.1177/23333936211028184

Maybery, D., Jaffe, I. C., Cuff, R., Duncan, Z., Grant, A., Kennelly, M., Ruud, T., Skogoy, B. E., Weimand, B., & Reupert, A. (2021). Mental health service engagement with family and carers: What practices are fundamental? *BMC Health Services Research, 21,* 1–11. https://doi.org/10.1186/s12913-021-07104-w

Maybery, D., Reupert, A., & Goodyear, M. (2015). Goal setting in recovery: Families where a parent has a mental illness or a dual diagnosis. *Child and Family Social Work, 20*(3), 354–363. https://doi.org/10.1111/cfs.12084

Menear, M., Girard, A., Dugas, M., Gervais, M., Gilbert, M., & Gagnon, M. P. (2022). Personalized care planning and shared decision making in collaborative care programs for depression and anxiety disorders: A systematic review. *PLoS One, 17*(6), e0268649. https://doi.org/10.1371/journal.pone.0268649

Merryman, M. B., & Riegal, S. K. (2007). The recovery process and people with serious mental illness living in the community: An occupational therapy perspective. *Occupational Therapy in Mental Health, 23,* 51–73. https://doi.org/10.1300/J004v23n02_03

Michels, C., Hallgren, K. A., Cole, A., Chwastiak, L., & Cheng, S. C. (2022). The relationship among social support, food insecurity and mental health for adults with severe mental illness and type 2 diabetes: A survey study. *Psychiatric Rehabilitation Journal, 45*(3), 212–218. https://doi.org/10.1037/prj0000525

Miller, N. B. (1997). *Nobody's perfect: Living and growing with children who have special needs.* Paul Brookes Publishing.

Mind Australia and Helping Minds. (2016). *A practical guide for working with carers of people with a mental illness.* Mind Australia, Helping Minds, Private Mental Health Consumer Carer Network (Australia), Mental Health Carers Arafmi Australia and Mental Health Australia. https://www.mindaustralia.org.au/sites/default/files/publications/A_practical_guide_for_working_with_people_with_a_mental_illness.pdf

Mizuno, E., Iwasaki, M., & Sakai, I. (2011). Subjective experiences of husbands of spouses with schizophrenia: An analysis of the husbands' descriptions of their experiences. *Archives of Psychiatric Nursing, 25*(5), 366–375. https://doi.org/10.1016/j.apnu.2011.03.001

Moen, O. L., Aass, L. K., Schröder, A., & Skundberg-Kletthagen, H. (2021). Young adults suffering from mental illness: Evaluation of the family-centred support conversation intervention from the perspective of mental healthcare professionals. *Journal of Clinical Nursing, 30,* 2886–2896. https://doi.org/10.1111/jocn.15795

Mottaghipour, Y., & Bickerton, A. (2005). The Pyramid of Family Care: A framework for family involvement with adult mental health services. *Australian e-Journal for the Advancement of Mental Health, 4*(3), 210–217. https://doi.org/10.5172/jamh.4.3.210

Mynard, L. (2020, July). *The new normal: Navigating everyday life during COVID-19.* Occupational Therapy Australia. https://otaus.com.au/publicassets/97c2319e-0bc0-ea11-9434-005056be13b5/The%20New%20Normal_ebook_Final.pdf

National Federation of Families. (2008). *Working definition of family driven care.* https://www.ffcmh.org/resources-familydriven

Nicholson, J. (2010). Parenting and recovery for mothers with mental disorders. In B. Levin & M. Becker (Eds.), *A public health perspective of women's mental health* (pp. 359–372). Springer.

Nicholson, J., Wolf, T., Wilder, C., & Biebel, K. (2014). *Creating options for family recovery: A provider's guide to promoting parental mental health.* Employment Options, Inc.

Oakley, F., Kielhofner, G., Barris, R., & Reichler, R. K. (1986). The Role Checklist: Development and empirical assessment of reliability. *Occupational Therapy Journal of Research, 6,* 157–170. https://doi.org/10.1177/153944928600600303

Olson, J. A. (2004). Mothering co-occupations in caring for infants and young children. In S. A. Esdaile & J. A. Olson (Eds.), *Mothering occupations: Challenge, agency, and participation* (pp. 28–51). F.A. Davis.

Olson, L. (2006). What do we know about the daily interactions between children with mental illness and their parents? *Occupational Therapy in Mental Health, 22*(3/4), 11–22. https://doi.org/10.1300/J004v22n03_02

Östman, M., & Björkman, A. (2013). Schizophrenia and relationships: The effect of mental illness on sexuality. *Clinical Schizophrenia & Related Psychoses, 7*(1), 20–24. https://doi.org/10.3371/CSRP.OSBJ.012513

Parkinson, S., & Brooks, R. (2021). *A guide to the formulation of plans and goals in occupational therapy.* Routledge.

Pierce, D. (2009). Co-occupation: The challenges of defining concepts original to occupational science. *Journal of Occupational Science, 16*(3), 203–207. https://doi.org/10.1080/14427591.2009.9686663

Plach, H. L., & Sells, C. H. (2013). Occupational performance needs of young veterans. *American Journal of Occupational Therapy, 67,* 73–81. https://doi.org/10.5014/ajot.2013.003871

Pohlan, L. (2019). Unemployment and social exclusion. *Journal of Economic Behavior & Organization, 164,* 273–299. https://doi.org/10.1016/j.jebo.2019.06.006

Polatajko, H. J., Townsend, E. A., & Craik, J. (2007). Canadian Model of Occupational Performance and Engagement (CMOP-E). In E. A. Townsend & H. J. Polatajko (Eds.), *Enabling Occupation II: Advancing an occupational therapy vision of health, well-being, & justice through occupation* (pp. 22–36). CAOT Publications ACE.

Price-Robertson, R., Obradovic, A., & Morgan, B. (2017). Relational recovery: Beyond individualism in the recovery approach. *Advances in Mental Health, 15*(2), 108–120. https://doi.org/10.1080/18387357.2016.1243014

Price-Robertson, R., Olsen, G., Francis, H., Obradovic, A., & Morgan, B. (2016). *Supporting recovery in families affected by parental mental illness.* Child Family Community Australia, Australian Institute of Family Studies. https://aifs.gov.au/cfca/publications/supporting-recovery-families-affected-parental-mental-illness

Purcell, R., Parker, A., Goldstone, S., & McGorry, P. (2012). Youth mental health: A new stream of mental health care for adolescents and young adults. In G. Meadows, J. Farhall, E. Fossey, M. Grigg, F. McDermott, & B. Singh (Eds.), *Mental health in Australia: Collaborative community practice* (3rd ed., pp. 603–614). Oxford University Press.

Reupert, A. E., & Maybery, D. J. (2015). Stigma and families where a parent has a mental illness. In A. E. Reupert, D. J. Maybery, J. Nicholson, M. Gopfert, & M. V. Seeman (Eds.), *Parental psychiatric disorder: Distressed parents and their families* (3rd ed., pp. 51–60). Cambridge University Press.

Reupert, A. E., & Maybery, D. J. (2016). What do we know about families where parents have a mental illness? A systematic review. *Child & Youth Services, 37*(2), 98–111. https://doi.org/10.1080/0145935X.2016.1104037

Schultz, S. (2013). Theory of Occupational Adaptation. In B. A. Schell, G. Gillen, M. Scaffa, & E. S. Cohn (Eds.), *Willard and Spackman's occupational therapy* (12th ed., pp. 527–540). Lippincott, Williams & Wilkins.

Shalaby, R. A. H., & Agyapong, V. I. (2020). Peer support in mental health: Literature review. *JMIR Mental Health, 7*(6), e15572. https://doi.org/10.2196/15572

Smith, J., Ali, P., Birks, Y., Curtis, P., Fairbrother, H., Kirk, S., Saltiel, D., Thompson, J., & Swallow, V. (2020). Umbrella review of family-focused care interventions supporting families where a family member has a long-term condition. *Journal of Advanced Nursing, 76,* 1911–1923. https://doi.org/10.1111/jan.14367

Stenersen, M. R., Kelly, A., Bracey, J., Marshall, T., Cummins, M., Clark, K., & Kaufman, J. S. (2022). Understanding racial-ethnic disparities in wraparound care for youths with emotional and behavioral disorders. *Psychiatric Services, 73*(5), 526–532. https://doi.org/10.1176/appi.ps.202100086.

Stephens, J. R., Farhall, J., Farnan, S., & Ratcliff, K. M. (2011). An evaluation of Well Ways, a family education programme for carers of people with a mental illness. *Australian & New Zealand Journal of Psychiatry, 45,* 45–53. https://doi.org/10.3109/00048674.2010.522170

Substance Abuse and Mental Health Services Administration. (2012). *SAMHSA's working definition of recovery: 10 guiding principles of recovery.* https://store.samhsa.gov/sites/default/files/pep12-recdef.pdf

Substance Abuse and Mental Health Services Administration. (2017). *Substance Abuse and Mental Health Services Administration website.* https://www.samhsa.gov

Subu, M. A., Holmes, D., Arumugam, A., Al-Yateem, N., Dias, J. M., Rahman, S. A., Waluyo, I., Ahmed, F. R., & Abraham, M. S. (2022). Traditional, religious, and cultural perspectives on mental illness: A qualitative study on causal beliefs and treatment use. *International Journal of Qualitative Studies on Health and Wellbeing, 17*(1), 2123090. https://doi.org/10.1080/17482631.2022.2123090

Taylor, R. (Ed.). (2017). *Kielhofner's Model of Human Occupation: Theory and application* (5th ed.). William and Wilkins.

Tompson, M. C., Sugar, C. A., Langer, D. A., & Asarnow, J. R. (2017). A randomized clinical trial comparing family-focused treatment and individual supportive therapy for depression in childhood and early adolescence. *Journal of the American Academy of Child & Adolescent Psychiatry, 56*(6), 515–523. https://doi.org/10.1016/j.jaac.2017.03.018

Trinh, M. H., Aguayo-Romero, R., & Reisner, S. L. (2022). Mental health and substance use risks and resiliencies in a U.S. sample of transgender and gender diverse adults. *Social Psychiatry and Psychiatric Epidemiology, 57,* 2305–2318. https://doi.org/10.1007/s00127-022-02359-y

Trowse, L., Hawkins, K., & Clark, J. (2013). *Putting families at the centre of recovery.* COPMI GEMS edition 14. https://www.copmi.net.au/professionals-organisations/copmi-what-works/research-summaries-gems/gems-edition14

Tyo, M. B., & McCurry, M. K. (2023). Model of family caregiver resilience and burden in opioid use disorder: A theoretical framework. *Advances in Nursing Science, 46*(2), 147–157. https://doi.org/10.1097/ANS.0000000000000448

van der Sanden, R., Stutterheim, S., Pryor, J., Kok, G., & Bos, A. (2014). Coping with stigma by association and family burden among family members of people with mental illness. *The Journal of Nervous and Mental Disease, 202*(10), 710–717. https://doi.org/10.1097/NMD.0000000000000189

Walsh, F. (2016). *Strengthening family resilience* (3rd ed.). Guilford Press.

Walsh, F. (2021). Family resilience: A dynamic systemic framework. In M. Ungar (Ed.), *Multisystemic resilience: Adaptation and transformation in contexts of change* (pp. 255–270). Oxford Academic. https://doi.org/10.1093/oso/9780190095888.003.0015

Weimand, B. M., Hall-Lord, M. L., Sällström, C., & Hedelin, B. (2013). Life-sharing experiences of relatives of persons with severe mental illness—A phenomenographic study. *Scandinavian Journal of Caring Sciences, 27*(1), 99–107. https://doi.org/10.1111/j.1471-6712.2012.01007.x

Western Australian Health. (2020). *Journey of health and wellbeing.* https://www.youtube.com/watch?v=cDYGjkcjUdg

Whiteford, G., & Townsend, E. (2011). Participatory occupational justice framework (POJF 2010): Enabling occupational participation and inclusion. In F. Kronenberg, N. Pollard, & D. Sakellariou (Eds.), *Occupational therapies without borders-Volume 2: Towards an ecology of occupation-based practices* (pp. 65–84). Churchill Livingstone.

Wonders, L., Honey, A., & Hancock, N. (2019). Family inclusion in mental health service planning and delivery: Consumers' perspectives. *Community Mental Health Journal, 55,* 318–330. https://doi.org/10.1007/s10597-018-0292-2

Wyder, M., & Bland, R. (2014). The recovery framework as a way of understanding families' responses to mental illness: Balancing different needs and recovery journeys. *Australian Social Work, 67*(2), 179–196. https://doi.org/10.1080/0312407X.2013.875580

Places

SECTION 2

CHAPTER

30

Natural Environments

Amy Wagenfeld

This chapter begins with an historical accounting of the evolution of the human connection with nature. It describes how and when the relationship between nature and health in humans transformed from survival and subsistence into a more pleasurable experience that forebearers recognized as health promoting. This nature and health connection includes a long-standing relationship in which occupational therapy has deep roots, which are fascinating and well worth exploring.

This chapter presents a review of the literature, beginning with theories that support the nature and health relationship. It examines evidence that nature positively influences physical and mental health and facilitates learning. The chapter also provides case studies of therapeutic garden design projects that the author contributed to, vignettes about practitioners worldwide who are engaged in nature-related endeavors, and strategies for occupational therapy practitioners (OTPs) to incorporate nature into therapeutic practice.

Nature and Health

Before reading any further, please consider this question: What is **nature**? Although complex to quantify, nature represents the physical world as compared with human-made creations (Hartig et al., 2014). Some people may think of nature as a body of water, weather, wind, mountain ranges, forests, rain, snow, plants, trees, and/or animals; none of these things are made or caused by people. This list excludes gardens because they are a human creation; however, they certainly do include nature. In this chapter gardens are included as another part of nature, particularly when thinking about nature-based experiences and their therapeutic application. Collectively, research finds that engagement with nature and its human-derived counterpart, gardens, can be health promoting, which is the essence of occupational therapy.

Research shows that layering on the experiential components of nature is another story worth exploring. One person might equate nature with a positive personal experience they had while strolling in a park. For another, it is the joy and satisfaction that comes from harvesting a basket of luscious ripe tomatoes that they have tended from tender seedlings, the wonder of watching a storm roll across the mountains, the act of photographing flowers in bloom, or the fun of kicking up a pile of crunchy fall leaves or inhaling the heady fragrance of roses in bloom. Some people experience a profound sense of awe and contentment while hiking in the woods or walking on a quiet beach. Experiences with nature may be restorative, calming, exhilarating, or frightening. The ways in which humans experience nature are intensely personal.

As OTPs tasked to improve occupational engagement and performance, bringing nature into therapeutic intervention can be meaningful and satisfying for both OTPs and the people they work with. Using nature as a foundation of occupational therapy intervention is as old as the profession, but often overlooked or underrepresented as a viable occupation-based intervention. Incorporating nature into occupational therapy practice can start as an aspirational goal in which the OTP is the steward of nature-based intervention in their workplace. Ultimately, using nature as a therapeutic tool is an achievable goal in many practice settings.

Why Nature Matters in Daily Life

The World Health Organization (WHO) defines health as "a state of complete well-being and not merely the absence of disease or infirmity" (WHO, 2024, p. 1). Connecting humans with nature can lead to health. This fact is recognized in one of the United Nations' sustainable development goals, which states, "By 2030, [to] provide universal access to safe, inclusive and accessible, green and public spaces, in particular for women and children, older persons and persons with disabilities" (United Nations, 2016, Target 11.7). Nature occurs in varying degrees, from wilderness to a tended garden, and includes plants and nonhuman animals in various grades and scales with myriad opportunities for human interaction

(Bratman et al., 2012). For many, nature is a source of pleasure, comfort, and interest. Ancient scholars, philosophers, and physicians exhorted the value of nature. Throughout history, the landscape has been equated with its therapeutic value and health-promoting qualities (Ward-Thompson, 2011). Nature experiences can occur inside (e.g., tending house plants and looking out a window) or outside; both are health promoting (Kondo et al., 2020; Korpela et al., 2016; Soga et al., 2021; Swank et al., 2020). Contemporary research has demonstrated that when people are engaged with nature, their physiology changes for the better, as does mental health (Bratman et al., 2019; Jimenez et al., 2021; Ross & Mason, 2017). Quite simply, nature matters because experiencing it improves mental health, physical health, and the capacity to learn, to socialize, and to live to the fullest (Choe et al., 2020; Hall & Knuth, 2019; Meidenbauer et al., 2020; White et al., 2019).

Historical Foundations

Humans' earliest connections with nature were predicated around survival, as it was relied upon as a source of food, shelter, clothing, and medicine (Beil, 2021; Keniger et al., 2013). By the second century BCE, Greco-Roman scholars and physicians began to identify a positive relationship between nature and health (Baker, 2018), considering them to be the "'non-natural' factors, understood to influence the course of health and sickness" (Ward-Thompson, 2011, p. 189). Greek scholars identified ideal landscapes as being places that provided opportunities for engagement in many activities that might be prescribed for healthy living (Ward-Thompson, 2011). Interestingly, the ancient Persian word *pairi-daeza* is the origin of the modern word "paradise," which is the heavenly or ideal landscape (Hobhouse, 2004). During the Middle Ages, gardens began to be considered therapeutic spaces (Stigsdotter et al., 2011). These early explanations of the importance of nature were prescient, as contemporary research now validates what was viewed as truth in ancient societies throughout the world.

Farms and gardens located adjacent to or on the campuses of hospitals and other care and correctional facilities have long provided the environment and context for meaningful engagement in occupation, production, and socialization (Sempik, 2010). In the latter part of the 19th century, Benjamin Rush, the father of American psychiatry, recognized the value of nature as therapeutic intervention, and under his tenure at the Philadelphia Hospital he saw to it that the campus was heavily greened and patients were given opportunities to garden and stroll along pathways on the campus as part of their rehabilitation. Under Rush's influence, other public and private hospitals followed suit (Detweiler et al., 2012; Gunderman, 2020; Penn Medicine, n.d.). During and following World War I, returning wounded veterans to U.S. hospitals precipitated the start of using horticulture in clinical settings, most notably by occupational therapists, as part of psychiatric and physical rehabilitation. More recently, and setting the stage for all future nature and health studies, Ulrich (1984) published a seminal paper on the impact of nature on healing that has been guiding modern health-care experts and designers ever since. Over a period of 8 years, Ulrich reviewed the medical records of two groups of patients recovering from gallbladder surgery. One group had windows with a view of trees, the other a view of a brick wall. Ulrich (1984) found that patients who had a view of trees spent a shorter time in the hospital, had fewer prescribed painkillers, and made fewer negative notes about staff. Today, there is overwhelming evidence in support of the value of nature-based interventions to improve physical and emotional health, well-being, and learning. This evidence is shared throughout this chapter.

Contributions by Occupational Therapy

Occupational therapy has a long-standing history of using gardening as intervention (Wagenfeld & Atchison, 2014). Dating back to 1932, the positive effects of gardening and interacting with plants have been acknowledged in occupational therapy literature (e.g., Clarke, 1950; Hartwell, 1932; Southcott, 1951). Archival photographs in the American Occupational Therapy Association's (AOTA's) Wilma West Library portray individuals engaged in these activities. Early in the profession's history, gardening was used as therapy, particularly with veterans and individuals with psychiatric diagnoses. No formal research evidence was available to support the impact of early nature-based therapy; the evidence was grounded in practitioners' lived experiences. For example, in her article "Gardening as a Therapeutic Experience," published in the 1950 issue of the *American Journal of Occupational Therapy*, Elizabeth Clarke shared,

> There are many types of activities in which patients may become interested, perhaps one of the most profitable, yet relaxing and enjoyable to all those requiring physical exercise is that of gardening. The values derived from gardening, whether the participation is passive or very strenuous are far reaching, and give each person a chance to re-create and express himself. (p. 109)

Contemporary practice demands that interventions be evidence-based. The profession is generating evidence that gardening as an occupational therapy intervention is sustainable and supports healthy eating, exercise, elevation of mood, and social engagement (Adevi & Mårtensson, 2013; Wagenfeld & Atchison, 2014). One early qualitative inquiry found that people with neurological damage who received occupational therapy that included working in a training garden reported beneficial and productive outcomes (Jonasson et al., 2007). More recently, OTPs surveyed about their rationales for using gardening as an intervention reported that the activity is meaningful, purposeful, motivating, fun, and person-centered. When these OTPs were involved in designing the garden, it was interpreted as being more useful as a therapeutic environment (Wagenfeld & Atchison, 2014). These researchers concluded that environmental context supports occupational engagement and heightens the meaningfulness and purposefulness of gardening (Wagenfeld & Atchison, 2014). In another qualitative study of a group gardening intervention for adults with mental health diagnoses, the OTPs who facilitated the group reported it facilitated positive growth, skill building, and coping (Joyce & Warren, 2016). Similar to the Wagenfeld and Atchison study, Joyce and Warren (2016) also found that the setting mattered in terms of providing the environment in which there was an opportunity to make lifestyle changes. A recent scoping review on the use of outdoor environments for individuals with dementia found that occupations facilitated outdoors were beneficial in terms of increased participation in activities and social connectivity, reduced agitation, and improved sleep quality (Ng et al., 2022). The evidence supporting the use of nature-based interventions in occupational therapy practice remains limited; however, with an established connection between gardening and wellness, OTPs can effectively provide such intervention on an individual or group level (Ng et al., 2022; Persson & Erlandsson, 2014; York & Wiseman, 2012).

Ecosocial Occupational Therapy

Algado and Townsend (2015) consider the intersection between occupation, occupational justice, and ecology to be a concept called **ecosocial occupational therapy**. This concept not only has meaning for the profession but is also a way for it to contribute to planetary health. Environmental health is critical to human health, recognizing at the same time the increasing impact of humans on environmental health. Notably, biodiversity, one indicator of health, is decreasing because of pollution, unsustainable development practices, and destruction of the natural environment (Clark et al., 2014). Engaging in social justice–based ecological efforts, such as cleaning up trash-ridden parks or recycling plastic bottles, is inherently occupation-based, as suggested by Algado and Townsend (2015). In the realm of nature-based occupational intervention, ecosocial occupational therapy could mean maintaining an active composting system in the therapy garden. Raised beds could be constructed from sustainably harvested woods or recycled plastic "boards." Drying flowers and saving the seeds to plant the following season could be a meaningful sensory and fine motor activity. Planting a garden with native plants could reduce the water consumption needed to sustain the garden. The occupational therapy discipline has unique opportunities to address climate change, as discussed in Box 30-1.

Nature and Human Health Theories

Several theories and hypotheses inform the health and nature context and the impact of nature and the environment on human health and well-being. The hypothesis of biophilia posits that people's affiliation with nature is innate and both biological and emotional. **Biophilia** explains why people keep pets and have plants in and around their homes: because they make people content and happy (Wilson, 1984). A recent meta-analysis of experimental studies examining the emotional impact of human exposure to natural environments concluded there was a significant effect; exposure increased positive emotions and decreased negative affect (Gaekwad et al., 2022).

Stress Reduction Theory posits physiological stress is relieved through contact with nature (Ulrich et al., 1991). Conversely, complex environments such as modern urban cities require more brain power to navigate and to evaluate the safety of these built environments, which can increase stress and anxiety, particularly for individuals who are already unwell or under pressure (Memari et al., 2021). Stress can accentuate other health conditions and thereby prevent or slow

---

BOX 30-1 ■ Occupational Therapy's Opportunities to Address Climate Change

According to Occupational Therapists for Environmental Action (OTEA), "Human occupation is directly linked to climate change as its cause and the root of all solutions" (OTEA, n.d., para. 11). Climate change is, in fact, a global issue impacting all facets of human life, including physical and mental health and economic well-being (AOTA, 2022). Professional understanding of how the physical environment impacts engagement in daily life makes OTPs well suited to advocate for engagement in sustainable and health-promoting occupations on an individual and community level (Garcia Diaz & Richardson, 2021). The AOTA 2022 policy paper, *Policy E.16, Occupational Therapy's Commitment to Sustainability and Climate Change,* identifies 12 outcomes that OTPs and students are encouraged to take action for as a means to mitigate the serious implications of climate change both now and for the future of global planetary health.

American Occupational Therapy Association. (2022). *Policy E.16, occupational therapy's commitment to sustainability and climate change.* https://www.aota.org/-/media/corporate/files/aboutaota/officialdocs/policies/policy-e16-20220908.pdf
Garcia Diaz, L. V., & Richardson, J. (2021). Occupational therapy's contributions to combating climate change and lifestyle diseases. *Scandinavian Journal of Occupational Therapy, 30*(7), 992–999. https://doi.org/10.1080/11038128.2021.1989484
Occupational Therapists for Environmental Action. (n.d.). *Occupational therapy and climate change.* https://www.otenvironmentalaction.com/ot-climate

---

healing (O'Connor et al., 2021). Being in nature reduces the impact of sympathetic nervous system activation that stress and anxiety cause; muscles become less tense, blood pressure lowers, and brain activity slows down. At the same time, being in nature triggers positive emotional, physiological, and psychological-neurological responses in humans (Lim et al., 2021; Scott et al., 2021).

The **Attention Restoration Theory** explains the ability of the brain to relax in nature and thereby reduce stress and anxiety. Every time a person pulls their car over at a scenic overlook to quietly gaze at an expanse of nature, stops along a walk fascinated by the rays of the sun slanting through the clouds, or feels the comfort of a light breeze gently caress their face, they have experienced the effect of attention restoration. This theory suggests that being in a natural environment is restorative; it helps people recover from mental fatigue and improves brain function worn down by everyday stress and anxiety (Kaplan, 1995; Kaplan & Kaplan, 1989). Being in nature restores the ability of the brain to intensely focus, pay attention, and think more clearly. There is evidence that stress reduction and attention restoration occur concurrently and thereby improve cognition (Kaplan, 1995; Kaplan & Kaplan, 1989).

Cognitive neuroscience supports the argument that the quality and type of environment affect human health and well-being, can reduce stress and anxiety, and can impact human behavior and performance (Williams Goldhagen, 2017). It is well established with these many theories and an increased body of research that the environment and being in nature are important to human health and well-being

Evidence-Based Practice

Nature in the Workspace

> *Occupation-based nature interventions improve emotional well-being.*

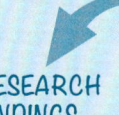

RESEARCH FINDINGS

A weekly exposure of 120 minutes of time spent in nature, including gardening, is associated with improved physical and mental health and well-being (White et al., 2019). The purpose of this research was to understand the impact of a one-time, short-term plant-based intervention on the emotional state of employees at an urban office building (Wagenfeld et al., 2019). A pre-/posttest design study used a visual analog emoticon assessment tool, the *Interaction with Nature* scale, to measure differences in emotional state before and after participating in a planting activity. As a group, 22 participants potted up a succulent plant to display in their workspace. Statistically significant findings suggest that a short-term occupations-centered nature intervention can improve emotional state.

APPLICATIONS

➡ Practitioners can introduce gardening as a group mental health intervention to support improved emotional state.
➡ Practitioners may benefit from engaging in gardening activities as part of staff meetings to improve mental health and sense of restoration and camaraderie.

REFERENCES

Wagenfeld, A., Schefkind, S., & Hock, N. (2019). Measuring emotional response to a planting activity for staff at an urban office setting. *Open Journal of Occupational Therapy, 7*(2), Article 5. https://doi.org/10.15453/2168-6408.1532

White, M. P., Alcock, I., Grellier, J., Wheeler, B. W., Hartig, T., Warber, S. L., Bone, A., Depledge, M. H., & Fleming, L. E. (2019). Spending at least 120 minutes a week in nature is associated with good health and wellbeing. *Scientific Reports, 9*(1), 1–11. https://doi.org/10.1038/s41598-019-44097-3

(Frumkin et al., 2017). **Nature prescribing** is becoming widely accepted as a valid form of drug-free health care and is improving users' experiences and therapy environments in health-care settings and on college campuses (Cornell Health, n.d.; Kondo et al., 2020; Wagenfeld & Marder, 2024). In the context of increasing health-care costs and serious environmental challenges, it is critical to make use of the therapeutic qualities of nature to support health and well-being in the built environment and health-care settings. Table 30-1 outlines these theoretical approaches and their implications for occupational therapy practice.

Linking Evidence to Nature and Health

The amount of green space in the living environment has encouraging health associations and is therefore critical in urban planning (Maas et al., 2006). People who live in a neighborhood with more trees feel healthier and report a reduced impact of their chronic conditions (Brown et al., 2016; Holland et al., 2021; Kardan et al., 2015). Research also suggests that regular visits to green spaces could reduce the prevalence of depression and high blood pressure in urban populations while achieving greater social cohesion in the neighborhood (Coventry et al., 2021; White et al., 2021). Access to green space has the potential for substantial medical cost savings considering the vast amounts of money spent on treating depression alone (Shanahan et al., 2016). Additional positive outcomes from being in nature include improved environmental conditions, such as air quality by trees filtering pollutants, improved stormwater runoff, reduced temperature and heat island effect, diminished energy demand, the provision of pollination and wildlife habitats, and carbon sequestration and storage (Hartig et al., 2014). The amount of green space in the living environment has encouraging health associations and is therefore critical in urban planning (Maas et al., 2006).

Contact with nature offers many opportunities for health improvements such as reduced physiological stress (Ulrich et al., 1991, 2020), better sleep (Gladwell et al., 2016; Mancus et al., 2021), attention restoration (Crossan & Salmoni, 2021; Qui et al., 2021), enhanced immune function (Pryor et al., 2021), improved mental capacity (Weerasuriya et al., 2019), increased physical activity (Christiana et al., 2021), and social connectedness (McNeil et al., 2022). Research shows reduced stress levels and reduced blood pressure to be an outcome of being immersed in nature (Jones et al., 2021).

Personal perception, purpose, and meaning of life are often reconsidered when one is in nature. For example, people may draw personal symbolism from a garden experience that helps them to make sense of personal life circumstances

TABLE 30-1 | Applying Nature and Health Theories in Occupational Therapy

Theory	Key Principle	Implication for Practice
Biophilia Theory	Humans' connection to nature is innate and includes an emotional connection to living things.	Connecting people with nature can support therapeutic interventions by boosting a person's immune system, supporting psychosocial health, creating social connectedness, and facilitating physical recovery.
Stress Reduction Theory	Nature calms and can help humans recover from both psychological and physiological stress.	When provided with opportunities to engage with nature on their own terms, people may experience improvement in physiological and psychological capacity, thus enhancing the quality of their therapeutic intervention.
Attention Restoration Theory	Time spent in nature, or even looking at or listening to nature, improves humans' capacity to concentrate and combats mental fatigue.	Inviting people to engage with outdoor and indoor nature-enriched places of respite and refuge can be restorative and reduce stress; in turn, these experiences enhance therapeutic intervention.
Cognitive Neuroscience	The quality and type of environment affects human health and well-being, can reduce stress and anxiety, and impacts human behavior and performance.	With increasing health-care costs and burgeoning environmental challenges, it is imperative to make use of the therapeutic qualities of nature to support health and well-being in the built environment and health-care settings, such as through nature prescriptions.

and illness (Blaschke et al., 2017). Access to nature promotes well-being and can positively impact the health of older people in disadvantaged areas, most likely because of more time being spent outdoors exercising or because of the stress-reducing quality of nature (Brown et al., 2016). Other benefits from passive contact with nature can include reduced hospital stay, less pain medication, quicker patient recovery (Ulrich, 1984), and contribution to a happier workforce (Cordoza et al., 2018). Nature-based solutions are good for people and the environment (Vujcic et al., 2017).

Mental Health and Nature

The World Bank predicts that 7 of 10 people will live in cities by 2050 (World Bank, 2022). In this context and with increasing environmental challenges, social isolation and increased loneliness are causing a mental health crisis. Medical services are struggling with increasing requests for mental health services, and contact with nature can be a tool to improve mental health in urban health-care settings. The COVID-19 pandemic highlighted the importance of access to nature for mental health with increased visitation rates to parks and nature reserves during restrictions and lockdowns (Jackson et al., 2021; Lõhmus et al., 2021; Ribeiro et al., 2021).

Scientific interest in the health benefits of nature has increased in recent years. Improved mood, life fulfillment, greater happiness, boosted well-being, and increased self-esteem and confidence have been reported when humans are in contact with nature (Wendelboe-Nelson, et al., 2019). Being in nature can alleviate mental health conditions and support mental health interventions. For example, research shows the benefits of community gardens and public open space for increased prosocial behavior and social connectedness (Lampert et al., 2021).

Evidence-based health benefits of nature contact for improved mental health include reduced depression (Balanzá-Martínez, & Cervera-Martínez, 2022) and reduced anxiety (Coventry et al., 2021). A narrative review by Ray and Jakubec (2014) found that access to nature in the form of therapeutic landscapes may reduce anxiety and thereby

may improve the health of individuals with cancer. Similarly, a systematic review and meta-synthesis by Blaschke (2017) found access to nature offers benefits to individuals with cancer by enabling interaction with nature and thereby offering the experience of nature as a "secure base" while dealing with their life challenges and outlook for the future. Blaschke (2017) argues that nature is supportive of individuals' needs in work through clinical and personal difficulties. In this chapter's The Lived Experience that follows, Roger shares his own experiences of how nature-based activities, specifically gardening, have been a key part of his physical and psychological recovery.

With regard to environmental context, there are interesting findings that support the role of nature in buffering mental health. The correlation between green space and reduced aggressive behavior in residential neighborhoods can be demonstrated (Bogar & Beyer, 2016; Kuo & Sullivan, 2001; Senel, 2020; Younan et al., 2016) and alludes to the health benefits of conducting behavioral or rehabilitation therapy in a natural setting. Additionally, reduced symptoms of inattention and aggression have been reported for children who regularly play in natural environments (Faber Taylor & Kuo, 2009, 2011).

Physical Health and Nature

There are many physical health benefits when people interact with nature including improved health in general, increased immune function, better eyesight, superior children's motor skills and balance, reduced stress and anxiety, and a diminished risk of obesity and cardiovascular disease (Coventry et al., 2021; Lampert et al., 2021). Recent technological advances have improved living and working conditions, with menial and heavy tasks being performed by machines, thus impacting physical health by making people less physically active. A sedentary lifestyle is clearly linked to obesity and a reduction in physical activities (Silveira et al., 2022). A study showed an association of neighborhood green spaces and body mass index (BMI) in children (Jia et al., 2021); thus, it is important to encourage children to spend time outside to increase physical activity and thereby reduce weight

The Lived Experience

Roger: The Transformative Nature of Gardening

Gardening. For me in many ways it has been transformative. There are some things that I've discovered in gardening that have added so much to a very difficult life. I suppose I'm getting ahead of myself, so please let me explain. My name is Roger (pseudonym). I'm a 57-year-old accountant from the Midwest region of the U.S. Throughout my life I have had to deal with many chronic illnesses and disabilities, both physical and mental. Much of my life has been spent watching things being taken away from me, but with gardening, I found something that gave me so much back.

It is hard to explain how much gardening has given back to me without explaining a little bit about me and my disabilities. I have multiple sclerosis and have been living with it for about 26 years. Over time it continues to rob me of my flexibility, my coordination, and at times my emotional resiliency. I also have significant back issues which compound these problems. I have significant spinal stenosis as well as spondylosis, both of which can cause substantial pain. In terms of mental health, I have treatment-resistant C-PTSD, as well as having to deal with multiple occurrences of major depressive disorder. For me the world can be a very bleak place; that is, until I discovered the little ray of sunshine that is gardening. I'm not claiming that gardening has cured me; what I am saying is gardening has provided me with something where I can get relief. It has done so much more than any therapy session or pharmaceutical, and it is something that is literally life-giving for me.

I really didn't get into gardening until I was in my 30s. My wife, who grew up on a farm, always had a green thumb and needed to be outside in nature and wanted to start large gardens. We set about getting some raised beds built in our backyard. While I helped with it, most of it was stuff that my wife worked on. I was always a little bit hesitant, because I didn't feel like I knew what I was doing, but I enjoyed being outside with her and our young daughter, working on the vegetables and flowers that we planted. More recently, we obtained some raised planters which have opened up new avenues to gardening for me. As I am extremely tall at 6' 5," I can no longer bend to work on things in a standard raised bed without pain. What we work

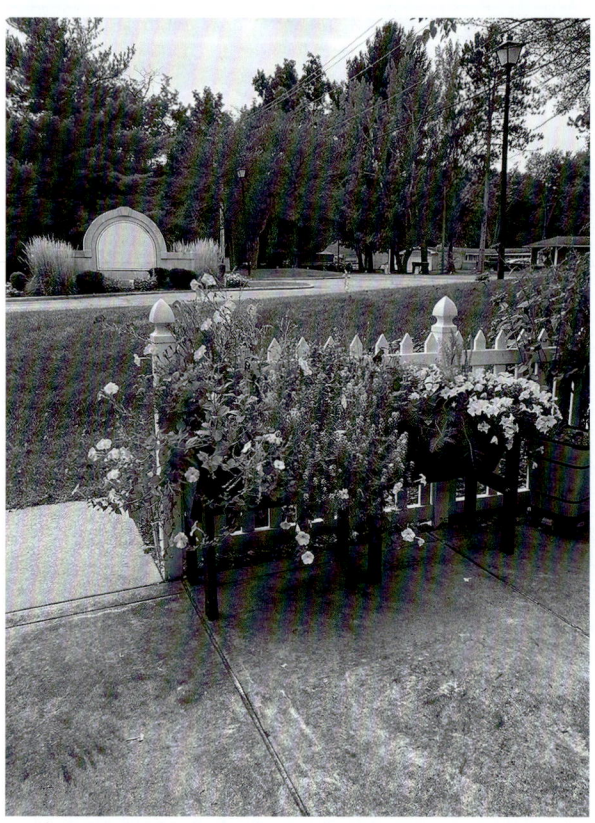

with now stands about 3½ to 4 feet tall and it is extremely easy for me to plant and tend our small little patio garden. I find myself going outside multiple times a day to "check on the garden." I get great joy, watching them sprout, grow, and either bloom or fruit. I find peace in the garden, I feel connected to nature, and I feel responsible in helping the plants grow. As I write this I look outside and it is lightly snowing, and the raised beds are covered with tarps, and it is all a rather depressing scene. However, I smile when I think about plans for planting in just a few months. That's one of the things about gardening, all you have to do is be present with nature and do your work, and you get exponentially more back than you ever put out.

(Kim et al., 2016). While the association of physical activity, availability of green space, and risk of obesity is established, more research is required to define what type of nature in the green space has the ability to reduce obesity (Teixeira et al., 2021) across the life course. Neighborhoods in residential areas with large and small parks and good park maintenance were associated with a lower BMI (Stark et al., 2014). It is suggested that longitudinal studies tracking changes in BMI through childhood in relation to levels of green space are needed to support cross-sectional study results (Sanders et al., 2015). The risk of type 2 diabetes is also significantly lower in green neighborhoods; therefore, developing, advocating, and maintaining green spaces in residential areas is critical in fighting the type 2 diabetes epidemic (Khan et al., 2021; Thiering et al., 2016).

People have been walking in forests, an experience called forest bathing or shinrin-yoku, a term coined in 1982 by the Japanese Ministry of Agriculture, Forestry, & Fisheries, for personal enjoyment and health benefits for millennia. Forest bathing is a contemplative process where in one is totally immersed in nature and uses all their senses to see, smell, feel, and listen to the forest. It is an ancient eastern Asian practice steeped in culture and tradition. Research has demonstrated that forest bathing enhances the human immune system and is beneficial to human health (Antonelli et al., 2022; Doimo et al., 2020; Furuyashiki et al., 2019; Yu et al., 2017). Older adults with chronic heart failure who engage in forest bathing demonstrated improved antioxidant function and improved mood. These health outcomes show the potential of nature as an effective tool to improve cardiovascular syndromes (Mao et al., 2017). Further, participants with chronic pain benefited from a 2-day forest therapy trip; these individuals showed physiological improvements in their heart rate variability, immune function, and life circumstances (Han et al., 2016). Although being in nature encourages physical activity, the phenomena of physical activities in nature leading to health outcomes is yet to be fully understood. Evidence notwithstanding, when appropriate, bringing individuals outside for therapy may be a complementary approach that supports therapeutic outcomes (Wagenfeld & Marder, 2024).

When people cannot be immersed in nature, health and healing can be enhanced by facilitating a different form of nature experience, specifically, bringing pictures and incorporating sounds of nature into health-care practices. These practices distract patients during flexible bronchoscopy and serve as an effective, low-cost and noninvasive tool in addition to standard pain medication (Diette et al., 2003). Similarly, a study found that viewing scenes of nature and listening to the sounds of nature during a painful bone marrow aspiration and biopsy, performed under local anesthetic, may reduce pain and therefore be a safe and cost effective way to reduce pain during the procedure (Lechtzin et al., 2010). Even the presence of potted plants in hospitals has been found to have therapeutic postoperative effects, resulting in less pain medication and positive physiological reactions evident in lower blood pressure and heart rate and fewer complaints about pain, anxiety, and weariness (Yeo, 2021). The health benefits from potted plants in hospitals suggest they could be a low-cost, drug-free and noninvasive treatment tool that needs to be considered in the health-care environment (Raanaas et al., 2016). In accordance with health-care facility guidelines, plants may be a healthful addition to clinics, as are photographs of nature. Introducing recorded nature sounds or opening windows, as tolerated, may also be considered. Refer to Box 30-2, regarding the Fisher House VA Puget Sound Healing Garden, as an example of the benefits of nature on physical health.

BOX 30-2 ■ Fisher House VA Puget Sound Healing Garden

Fisher House is a nonprofit organization dedicated to providing a no cost "home away from home" for families of veterans receiving medical care at major military and VA medical centers. The Therapeutic Garden is an outdoor environment conducive for residents displaced from their homes and experiencing a traumatic medical situation and, often, associated grief and loss. These personal issues are exacerbated by environmental conditions such as lack of natural lighting or ventilation and imposing waiting rooms, corridors, and treatment rooms that offer little in the way of environmental comfort or respite. Applying the Attention Restoration Theory, the goal was to create a verdant oasis within the institutional environment to support physical, emotional, and spiritual healing for veterans and their families.

To understand the physical and emotional needs of veterans and their families, students collaborated throughout the design-build with an occupational therapist (Amy Wagenfeld) and a veteran combat medic currently receiving services at the VA. Collaborations included site visits to Fisher House and a series of participatory design community meetings. Participants provided valuable insight and compiled a wish list of amenities and functions for the garden.

The final design included several distinct elements that are unified through planting materials and Americans with Disabilities Act (ADA) and universal design guidelines. Access to the garden is through a patio containing raised vegetable planters. The various heights and configurations of the planters enable all who care to garden the ability to do so in an ergonomically safe manner. An 8-foot wide gravel path winds throughout the site and links all of the elements by creating a contiguous 0.1 mile walking loop of the property. The wide paths enable people walking or wheeling to experience the garden side by side. A bench swing looks out over a small lawn area, providing a relaxing place for caregivers to watch their children play or to rest and reflect. A water feature embraced by a flowing bench wall and steel-framed gazebo provides visual interest and soothing sounds. Both the gazebo and bench wall incorporate principles of universal design so those using wheelchairs can comfortably and equitably sit with their ambulatory peers.

A final feature is a small level bridge with kick rails, spanning a rain garden. Here the path links a more secluded part of the garden with features such as a private retreat area, a raised yoga deck with low-effort access via a gently sloped ramp, an outdoor living room with gliding benches and a sculptural element evoking a sense of water and movement, and raised container gardens for vegetables and herbs. It also contains berry trees for increased wildlife habitat and aromatic plantings to enrich the senses. This project was a collaborative design process that provided an

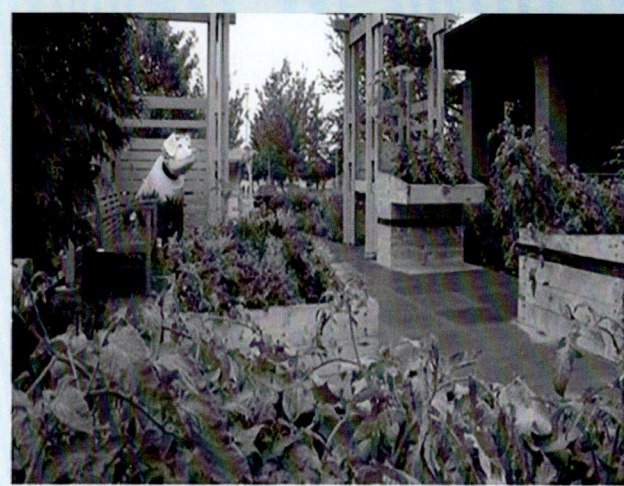

Universally designed planting beds.

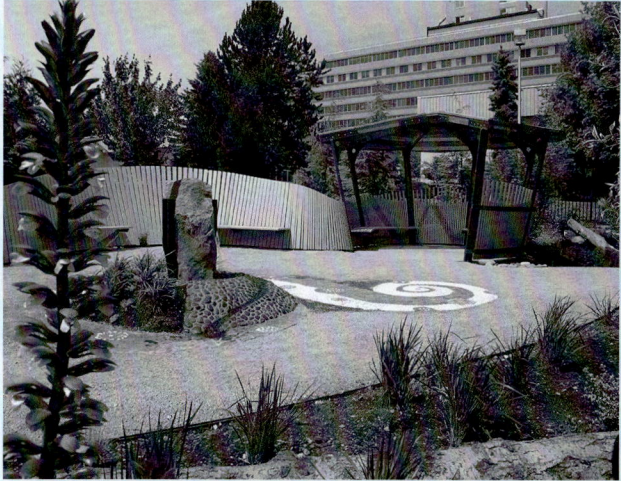

Seating configuration welcomes all visitors. *Photos courtesy of Amy Wagenfeld and Daniel Winterbottom.*

amenity for a deserving community in need. Response to the garden remains overwhelmingly positive. The garden has won a national award.

Cognition and Nature

There are cognitive benefits of engaging with nature, both inside and outside. These benefits can occur across the life course and for people in various life situations (Jimenez et al., 2021). Children who engage in at least 10 to 90 minutes of outdoor recreation during the school day demonstrate increased attention restoration, preparing them to be better able to learn (Mason et al., 2021). Providing university students with opportunities to engage in outdoor recreation is also associated with cognitive rejuvenation (Puhakka, 2021). In the workplace, when attention is given to greening the indoor environment, employees are more productive, energized, and focused (Klotz & Bolino, 2021). For veterans receiving treatment for posttraumatic stress disorder, using nature-based therapy as an adjunct to traditional mental health intervention demonstrated reduced symptomology, leading to better focus and capacity to process (Bettmann et al., 2021). Providing nature-based activities for older adults with dementia has been associated not only with improved sleep and reduced stress, but also in some circumstances improved cognition (Evans et al., 2021).

Being in nature has demonstrated physical and emotional health; led to cognitive, environmental, and societal benefits; and offers an immersive experience that visually, acoustically, and emotionally takes people away from the often highly emotional, disorienting, and unfamiliar experience of the health-care system. The health and wellness benefits of nature are evident and should be used to support healing and recovery after illness or surgery where possible. Nature is good for human health and well-being; regardless of their practice setting, people should intentionally seek ways to integrate nature to support therapeutic goals. This intentionality could take on the form of facilitating therapy outdoors, including nature-focused art in the clinic and ambient nature sounds (Wagenfeld & Marder, 2024). Refer to Box 30-3, which discusses the Kline Galland Home Marty Bender Unfold/Unfurl Family Garden, as an example of the benefits of nature on cognition.

Loss and Lack of Nature

This chapter presents several theories explaining the relationship between nature and health. Research provides evidence that supports this positive relationship. Practitioners can be confident that building opportunities for individuals to connect with nature can provide holistic benefits to people's physical and mental health, as well as support learning. The positive relationship between humans and nature was evident during the COVID-19 pandemic. Many people turned to nature for exercise, comfort, and solace, and children often learned outside (Bustamante et al., 2022; Jackson et al., 2021; Kang et al., 2022). Although these benefits are universal, not everyone has equitable access to experience the health-promoting qualities of nature. Recall that biophilia posits that humans' affinity for nature is innate. Arguably, then, a lack of equitable access to nature is an occupational injustice (Pizarro, 2018; Wilson, 1984). This section explores elements such as personal factors, environment-related factors, the built environment, and safety, and how they can and often do lead to exclusion from a much needed daily infusion of nature

Personal Factors

The *Occupational Therapy Practice Framework*, Fourth Edition *(OTPF-4)* describes personal factors as:

BOX 30-3 ■ Kline Galland Home Marty Bender Unfold/Unfurl Family Garden

Kline Galland Home is a skilled nursing long-term senior care facility in the heart of Seattle, Washington. Its mission and values are, "A living commitment, inspired by Jewish values, to provide exceptional senior care by exceptional people . . . every day, in every way, for everyone." The previous courtyard garden was rarely utilized because of unsafe, failing paving; minimal shade or shelter; and an abundance of invasive ivy. In a two quarter academic design and build studio cotaught by Professor Daniel Winterbottom and Amy Wagenfeld, University of Washington landscape architecture students worked closely with residents, families, and staff to create the 3,500 square foot Unfold/Unfurl Garden, inspired by the way a scroll or book unfolds to reveal its stories.

As the ultimate users of the site, residents and staff commented on ideas generated by students while articulating their needs and preferences, which were reflected in the final design. Their input was essential in designing the garden and to its success, because while the students used their skills and knowledge gained through studio lectures on the aging process and nature and health theories to execute the design, Kline Galland residents and staff relied on the students to understand their vision for the garden and to create a space that truly met the needs and wishes of their community. The Unfold/Unfurl Garden is now an intergenerational gathering space, where people of all ages can come together to share their own stories, histories, and memories with loved ones, as well as enjoy the sensorial phenomena, sounds, smells, and seasonality

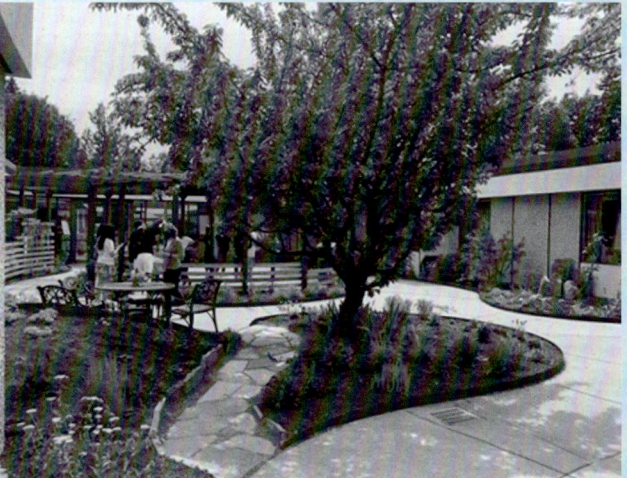

Seating nooks provide spaces for conversation and viewing. *Photo courtesy of Amy Wagenfeld.*

of nature. Similar to an unfolding book, each person has a story to tell, and this garden contains a variety of spaces where the exchange of these stories can occur and residents can experience the powerful healing and therapeutic benefits of nature.

the unique features of a person that are not part of a health condition or health state and that constitute the particular background of the person's life and living . . . [and are the neutral] . . . internal influences affecting functioning and disability . . . [that] . . . reflect the essence of the person—who they are. (AOTA, 2020, p. 10)

Personal factors may include, but are not limited to, "sexual orientation, gender identity, race, ethnicity, socio-economic status, lifestyle, and health conditions and fitness status that might impact an individual's occupations but are not the main concern of occupational therapy" (AOTA, 2020, p. 10). Outdoor environments can and do influence personal factors in myriad ways, both positively and negatively. In this chapter's Being a Psychosocial OT Practitioner feature, the practitioner in the story, Jamil, identifies personal factors that help Violet reengage in doing using nature-based activities.

Terms such as **JEDI** (justice, equity, diversity, and inclusion) or **DEI** (diversity, equity, and inclusion) are commonly used to present visions of social change that address historical and ongoing systemic injustices. They also create a society where all can participate, differences are respected and celebrated, and everyone is included. These terms are linked to experiencing the natural environment. Justice in its broadest sense is having fair access to opportunities, which in the built or natural environment can be thought of as environmental justice (Hammell, 2021). In nature, this means that people living in underserved neighborhoods have the same quality and quantity of well-maintained and safe parks that a more affluent neighborhood might have. Equity focuses on how some people and groups receive privileges and some do not (Warner & Dillenschneider, 2019). Equity occurs when people get the support that they need. Taking the park analogy further, it means that where there are benches, the benches have armrests to make getting up and down from seating easier, and that there is ample space next to the bench for a wheelchair user to sit. Diversity considers people's varying

Being a Psychosocial OT Practitioner

A Spot of Tea to Help Rediscover Direction

Identifying Psychosocial Strengths and Needs

Practitioners in all practice areas work with individuals with psychosocial needs such as depression and anxiety that can affect occupational performance and lead to a decline in function. Violet is an 18-year-old college freshman at a local community college. She has always loved cooking and is an avid consumer of food podcasts and food-related social media. Violet's long-term goal is to have a salad-focused food truck; she knows the journey to becoming a successful food entrepreneur is a long one, but she is determined to see it happen. Violet is planning to take business courses at community college and then transfer to a culinary school to complete her undergraduate degree.

One day, while experimenting with a new recipe for a salad pizza, the knife slipped while Violet was dicing tomatoes for the pizza, and she severely lacerated the median nerve of her left hand. Violet required extensive surgical repair and is currently being treated by an occupational therapist (Jamil) with a certified hand therapist (CHT) designation. Therapy is progressing well, and Violet is gaining range of motion and strength in her left hand. Despite her gains, functional performance is not improving as expected and Violet has expressed fear of returning to cooking, particularly using a knife. She is questioning whether she even wants to pursue a culinary career and has withdrawn from her business classes for the rest of the year. Although she was never considered outgoing, being somewhat reserved in her social interactions, Violet now spends most of her days in her bedroom listening to music and sleeping.

Violet's occupational therapist is concerned that her fear avoidance of returning to the kitchen cooking and withdrawal from all social engagements puts Violet at risk for further long-range functional decline and social withdrawal.

Using a Holistic Occupational Therapy Approach

Violet has shared with Jamil that she was bullied as a child. She dealt with weight issues and was teased for wanting to share recipes with her friends' parents rather than to play with her friends. During the initial evaluation, Violet told Jamil that she has experienced transient episodes of depression and ongoing anxiety since early adolescence and has had multiple courses of medication, which she is currently not taking. She told Jamil that she is has felt glum and, in her words, "directionless" since the accident.

Jamil is a gardener and has recently taken a couple of plant-related courses through his local cooperative extension service. He noticed that after the last course he took on herbal wreath making he felt very calm and restored, which was especially noteworthy because his workday had been particularly taxing. This transformative experience got him thinking that perhaps trying to incorporate nature-based activities into Violet's intervention plan could be beneficial. A brief evidence-based research search confirmed his hunch that interacting with nature can promote elevated mood and decreased stress and anxiety.

At Violet's next session, Jamil brings up the idea of working with dried herbs to make teas. The activity is purposeful, sequential, bilateral, and social, and although not cooking, it is a culinary related task. Skeptical, but an avid tea drinker, Violet reluctantly agrees. Together, Violet and Jamil discuss what will be needed to make tea bags and plan the activity. All materials are purchased and ready to go. At the beginning of the next session, Jamil introduces a temperature scale (visual analog) and asks Violet to use her left index finger to point to where on the scale her perceived level of anxiety is. On a scale of 1 to 10, with 1 none and 10 maximal, Violet points to the number 9. After using physical agent modalities (PAMs) and other manipulative and strengthening tasks, Violet and Jamil begin the teabag-making activity. He observes that Violet is more verbal and is initiating conversation. She is making eye contact and even laughed a few times at his bad jokes. She used her left hand to hold the tea ingredients' mixing bowl and to stabilize the tea bags and ready them for the herbs without prompting. The session ends with five tea bags to take home and a recheck on the temperature scale. Using her left ring finger, Violet points to the number 2. Violet tells Jamil that she had fun and wants to try other activities that involve herbs. She suggested making herbal vinegar. He affirms her request, and the session concludes.

Reflective Questions

1. What nature and health theories align with incorporating nature-based activities into Violet's intervention plan?
2. How might the practitioner use plants and plant materials as a metaphor for Violet's sense of anxiety and social withdrawal?
3. How would you incorporate a culinary activity that involves fresh herbs and produce into the intervention session with the goal of increasing social interaction and reducing anxiety?

BOX 30-4 ■ Edgerley Family Horizons for Homeless Children Play Garden

The Edgerley Family Horizons for Homeless Children Play Garden is a place that facilitates high-quality early education, provides opportunities for developmentally appropriate play, and ensures comprehensive support services are available for children and their families experiencing homelessness. It also establishes a landmark physical presence for the organization in Boston's diverse Roxbury neighborhood.

Designed by StudioMLA in collaboration with Amy Wagenfeld, the entire 45,000 square foot project included renovating the existing building as well as designing and installing a play garden. The design team worked very closely with Horizon's administration and staff. The intensity of this collaborative process enabled the design team to better understand what the garden needed to be. Completed in 2020, the 5,000 square foot outdoor play space, which Dr. Wagenfeld focused much of her work on, incorporates trauma-responsive design strategies as well as graded challenge, choice, and balanced sensory enrichment to better support the children and families that Horizons for Homeless Children serves. The play space is built on top of a parking garage and provides a broad range of opportunities for infants, young and older toddlers, preschool-age children, and all children to play on their terms, in

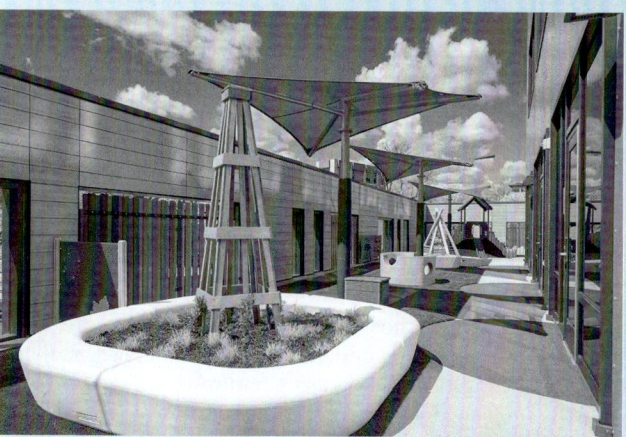

An axial view of the play garden. *Photo courtesy of Rosemary Fletcher.*

a natural, welcoming environment. This was an incredibly rewarding experience, and the renovated garden and interior spaces are working spectacularly for children, their families, and staff.

---

identities, perspectives, and backgrounds. In a park, restrooms could be designated all gender, and plantings and public art could be representative of local community culture (Chen et al., 2021). Inclusion is feeling welcomed. In this JEDI-focused park there are no steps, and pathways are wide and smooth enough for two wheelchairs or two caregivers pushing strollers to move in tandem. Any signage uses only simple and universally understandable icons and Braille. Refer to Box 30-4, regarding the Edgerley Family Horizons for Homeless Children Play Garden, as an example of supporting personal and environmental factors.

Environment-Related Factors

The *OTPF-4* identifies environmental factors as "aspects of the physical, social, and attitudinal surroundings in which people live and conduct their lives . . . [and encompass] natural environment and human-made changes to the environment" (AOTA, 2020, p. 36). The component most germane to a discussion about occupational therapy and natural environments is the physical geography. One example of the physical geography shared in Table 4 of the *OTPF-4* is "raised flower beds in a backyard garden" (AOTA, 2020, p. 36). What if this raised bed does not meet the needs of the intended users, or for that matter any users? Or more generally speaking, what if there is a mismatch between the physical geography and the person wanting and needing to use it?

Practitioners might consider the concept of **environmental press** to examine the person–environment fit. Specifically, it would involve examining the match or mismatch between person variables, such as physical health, functional skills, cognition, quality of life, and sense of efficacy, and environmental variables such as the home, neighborhood, and community (Lawton & Nahemow, 1973). Does the environment press for the just right level of adaptive function? Regarding equity, specifically access to outdoor environments, environmental press factors into an individual's ability to experience

the health-promoting capacities of nature. When environmental press overwhelms personal factors—for example, a child with a disabling condition cannot participate equitably on a community playground because the equipment limits participation—this is an unjust situation.

Practitioners are trained to understand the important relationship between a person's environment and their capacity to participate in meaningful occupation. This is the essence of the Person-Environment-Occupation-Performance (PEO-P) model (Baum et al., 2015). Think about this: Raised flower beds that lack access for individuals who want or need to sit to garden and to do so in an ergonomically correct way with their front body directly facing the garden disrupts the PEO-P relationship and can cause harm to the physical body and one's mental health. To help to overcome environmental barriers to participation and reduce or eliminate environmental press, OTPs do indeed have a role in creating outdoor environments that support, rather than impede, participation. Refer to Box 30-5, regarding The Healing Gardens of Queensland Children's Hospital (QCH), for an example of such environmental factors.

Built Environment

Nature can support the physical and social-emotional health and well-being, as well as cognitive capacities, of individuals and practitioners in health-care, educational, and community settings.

User needs depend on the individual and their personal circumstances, on their life situation, and on their mental and physical capacity to deal with individual requirements for physical, psychosocial, and mobility adjustments after serious illness (Blaschke et al., 2020). Therapeutic outdoor environments must be purposefully designed, which means suiting both user and practitioner needs, and be well-integrated into treatment programs to support intervention. In this way, they enable emotional, mental, and physical health benefits for individuals, their caregivers, staff, and volunteers.

BOX 30-5 ■ The Healing Gardens of Queensland Children's Hospital (QCH)

Contributed by Katharina Nieberler-Walker

The QCH opened in 2014, having taken 8 years to design, construct. and commission. The Community Plaza and 11 healing gardens at the QCH are purposefully designed and well-integrated into the hospital program for the benefits of patients, their families, staff, and the broader community. Located on a highly built out inner-city site in Brisbane, 75% of the QCH site area is allocated to public open space and healing gardens, with only 25% of the site area covered by conventional roof.

The design of the healing gardens draws on stress reduction and supportive design, salutogenesis, and biophilia and biophilic design theories. The building design allows natural light to penetrate deeply into the building and affords views to the gardens and surrounding landscape. The healing gardens cater to a variety of user needs, such as time out from the clinical hospital environment and the need for social interaction, relaxation, recreation, physical exercise, and nature-based therapy in an environment that feels familiar and normal.

The gardens appeal to all the senses. Nature is presented in innovative ways including six 30-year-old fig trees, a children's playground that invites exploration at the Community Plaza, and green monoliths, epiphyte columns, and tropical plants that create Jungle Gardens. A Secret Garden offers respite from the clinical hospital environment. It is designed as a green haven for mindfulness and conversation and is located next to the parent's retreat and stay space. An Adventure Garden supports fundraising events and therapy programs and is accessible to staff, patients, and invited visitors only. Here, gardens are colocated with the physiotherapy department and gymnasium for easy access and outdoor rehabilitation therapy. The Adventure Garden is designed with a wheelchair training run and training ramp, a basketball hoop, a horizontal climbing wall, a universally accessible swing, and an herb garden. Dedicated Mental Health Gardens gently enrich the senses and a Staff Garden enables staff to relax and recuperate for the next shift. Many of these gardens are accessible to the general public and offer sheltered seating areas, a picnic lawn protected by green monoliths, and spectacular views to the river. Please see https://www.youtube.com/watch?v=PlkW2ENG2Yw.

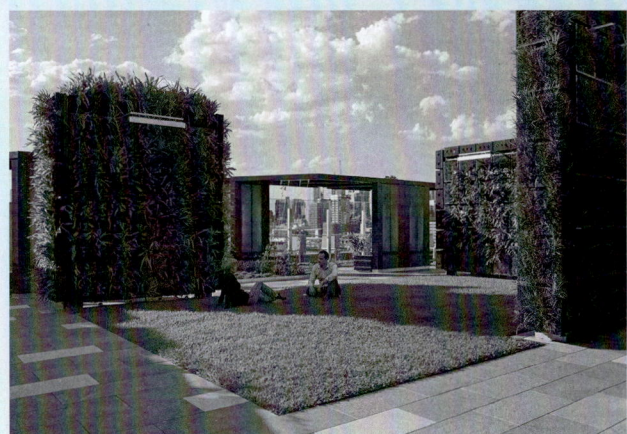

The garden green.

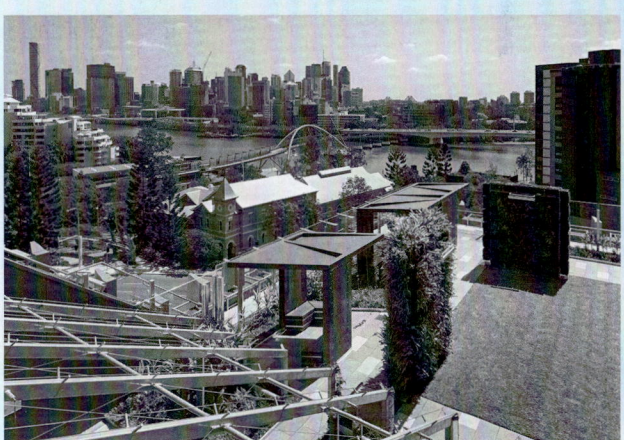

A bird's eye view. *Photos courtesy of Christopher Fredrick Jones.*

Safety

Environmental safety is paramount for nature-based treatment and goes beyond physical safety. Pollen, soil, fungi, and other allergens associated with plants can in some cases worsen asthma and thereby affect nature-based therapy (Fuertes et al., 2014, 2016). It is important for OTPs to be aware of an individual's general health conditions, as well as their personal experiences with nature, phobias, and negative nature experiences before introducing nature-based interventions.

Utilizing outdoor spaces and gardens for mental health may be difficult in some situations where there are physical safety considerations related to self-harm. Although safety is paramount, it is also important to consider the purpose of such spaces and the impact on users. It is important for OTPs to understand risks but to emphasize benefits with designers and stakeholders. Talking points that focus on optimizing performance instead of dwelling on risk can shift perspectives and enable the design of spaces that support the mental capacity of individuals, leading to safe, suitable, and dignified environments for recovery. Refer to Box 30-6, regarding the Els for Autism Sensory Arts Garden, for an example of supporting safety.

Nature-Based Occupations

This section focuses on translating the evidence that nature-based occupations can support an individual's health, mental health, and well-being. Application scenarios present examples where nature is the main focus of occupational therapy intervention. Each has been used in some capacity by the author Amy Wagenfeld in her clinical and design practice. The scenarios start with quiet contemplation, then gardening, followed by a more physical activity–focused example, and then conclude with the most important occupation of childhood: play.

Quiet Contemplation in Nature

Exposure to nature, whether it occurs inside or outside, can positively influence a person's mental health. In nature, many find peace and contentment, well-being, reduced stress, and the opportunity to engage in personal reflection

BOX 30-6 ■ The Els for Autism Sensory Arts Garden

Located on a 26-acre campus in Jupiter, Florida, the Els Center of Excellence offers multiple, innovative programs designed to meet the needs of autistic individuals and their caregivers. Completed in 2016, The Els for Autism Sensory Arts Garden is a nearly 14,000 square foot garden. Working very closely and collaboratively, the landscape architecture firm, DirtWorks, PC, Amy Wagenfeld | Design, and staff at Els for Autism created a garden that nurtures all eight sensory systems; provides alerting and calming experiences; is predictable and has repeating elements, yet is very fun; and contains multiple universal design principles including perceptible information, tolerance for error, and equity.

The evidence-based design process sought to create a garden space where everyone could thrive. Theories such as Sensory Integration, the Attention Restoration Theory, and Prospect and Refuge were applied to the garden design and are reflected in the final product. There are learning spaces and social gathering spaces where yoga, storytelling, music, and tabletop activities are facilitated. There are spaces for retreat, and for engagement. The children are outside in the garden for at least 20 minutes a day and the completely enclosed garden eliminates risk of elopement. Because the garden was deliberately designed with safety and surveillance in mind, no matter where they are in the garden, staff

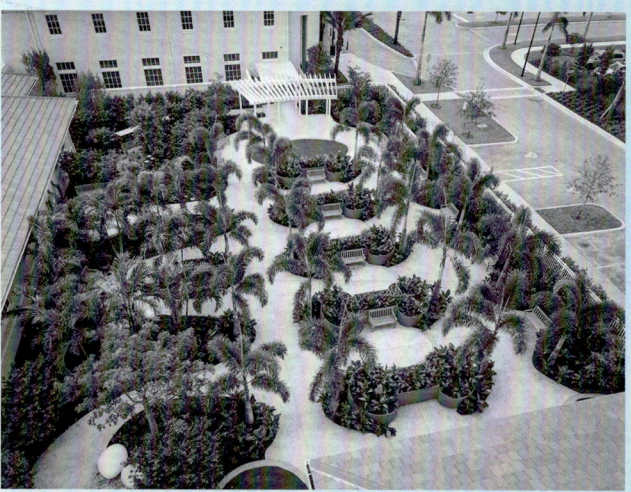

An overview of the garden. *Photograph courtesy of DirtWorks.*

can see the entire expanse, so children are free to do what they want and need to do. The garden has won multiple national and international awards.

TABLE 30-2 | Cozy Plant Refuge

Intervention Goals	Materials	Simplified Instructions

• Logan will self-initiate use of the cozy refuge and practice one anxiety management technique for at least 10 minutes each workday.	• Identify a quiet area in a clinic or other facility, such as the terminus of a hallway, a small room, or a closet.
	• If using the terminus of a hallway, obtain a privacy screen, preferably one made of natural materials.
	• Include potted and/or hanging plants arranged in the space and ensure the capacity for rearranging them as needed and desired by the person using the space.
	• Other materials/features:
	  • A small water feature
	  • Dimmable lights
	  • Wooden table and wooden chairs (no more than two)
	  • Beanbag or other body hugging seat
	  • Journaling and drawing materials
	  • Aromatherapy diffuser and oils
	  • Audio system with nature sounds
		1. Invite participant into the space.
		2. If using a hall end terminus, move privacy screen into place and dim lights to tolerance of the user.
		3. If using a closet or small room, also dim lights to tolerance of the user.
		4. Invite user to select an essential oil of their choice (only a suggestion) and add a few drops to the diffuser.
		5. Invite the person to listen to nature sounds of their choice (only a suggestion).
		6. Invite the person to journal, draw, and/or simply be quiet.
		7. Duration: 5–20 minutes as tolerated.
		8. Adapt as needed to meet the user's needs and consider how this intervention could be carried over to a person's workplace.

(Berger et al., 2022; Puhakka, 2021). Exposure to nature is easily graded from cultivating and tending to indoor plants, to participating in a weekly mindfulness-based stress reduction intervention outdoors, to immersion in a forest therapy program. Each of these approaches has proved effective in supporting positive mental health outcomes such as reducing self-isolation, depression, and stress, as well as buffering the impact of trauma (Bettmann et al., 2021; Choe & Sheffield, 2022; Park et al., 2021; Yan et al., 2022). The following application scenario capitalizes on providing an opportunity for quiet contemplation in nature (also see Chapter 10: Coping and Resilience 🤝):

Logan, a 49-year-old Asian American man, receives weekly outpatient services at a local mental health treatment center. He was diagnosed with posttraumatic stress disorder (PTSD) after witnessing his best friend being murdered in a racially focused hate crime. He cannot sleep or eat and is unable to return to his office job. His employer allows him to work remotely for now, but ultimately wants him to return to the office, 3 days per week. Logan loves his job and wants to one day return to the office, but first knows that he must heal as best he can.

Logan's occupational therapist, Winston, is aware of the evidence connecting nature-based interventions and reduced anxiety. When constructing Logan's occupational profile, Winston recorded Logan's interest in plants. Logan reported that his mother always had a lot of plants in their home, and he always enjoyed watering them. Winston thinks nature-based interventions may help Logan now and support his integration back to the office. He and Logan talk about it and Logan is willing to give it a try. Although the center has no outdoor space except for a parking lot, Logan has learned that indoor nature is also health promoting. With encouragement from his supervisor, Winston creates a cozy plant refuge area that Logan is the first to use. Table 30-2 outlines what he did.

Gardening

Gardening offers myriad opportunities for individuals to experience occupational engagement through the sensory rich, motoric, and cognitive acts of planting, tending, harvesting, and making use of the harvest (Matuska, 2013). Many people consider gardening to be a meaningful, participatory, purposeful, and goal-oriented activity (Hewitt et al., 2013). Gardening is surprising. The surprise comes from a flower that goes from bud to full opening overnight or a seedling pushing through the earth on its way to growing into a plant. Gardening is also repetitive. The repetition of gardening are the chores, such as weeding and watering. For many, these tasks are meditative and focusing (Franck et al., 2021; O'Nuallain, 2021; Veldheer et al., 2020).

Consider the following application scenario concerning gardening and physical rehabilitation:

Alberta is a home health practitioner and an avid gardener whose specialty is growing heirloom tomatoes. During an initial assessment she met Maurizio, an 82-year-old man of Italian descent who has early-stage dementia, depression, and is recovering from a right-sided cerebrovascular accident. Maurizio also loves to garden. He is ambulatory with stand by assist and has mild left side neglect. Before his stroke, Maurizio took great pleasure in growing herbs that his wife lovingly used to make sauces, salads, and sweet treats. Maurice and his wife are living with their daughter and her family. The home has a 1/8-acre lot with a patio that is accessed directly from the kitchen. Maurizio's daughter is open to having Alberta use the yard as a therapeutic environment for him. Collaboratively, Maurizio and Alberta decide to use the next therapy session to work outside and create a container garden. As part of the person-centered process and to address cognitive issues, Alberta and Maurizio plan the container garden to determine what it should contain. Alberta encourages Maurizio to page through seed catalogs using his left hand and arm to address motor skills. To address mental health skills, they also discuss how each plant that Maurizio wants to choose makes him feel. They both determine that the session was productive and look forward to planting. Fortunately, Alberta's partner owns a garden store and willingly provides her with all the materials she needs to facilitate this outdoor nature activity. Table 30-3 outlines the materials needed and simplified instructions to create an herbal container garden.

Wilderness Program for Mental Health

Most of the research conducted on the influence of nature on adolescents centers on engagement in outdoor wilderness programs and finds that experiences such as hiking, biking, running, and outdoor exercise improve cognition, attention, and self-awareness (Mayer et al., 2009). Group-based outdoor adventure interventions such as rock climbing and hiking experiences are understood to enhance coping skills, self-confidence, and autonomy because they are goal directed and challenge each participant and also encourage a prosocial group mentality (Rosenberg et al., 2014). For example, results of one study found that young adults with cancer who participated in a weeklong outdoor adventure program reported decreased levels of stress and improved self-efficacy and experienced a greater sense of social support (Zebrack et al., 2017). This chapter's Practitioner Profile feature describes the efforts of an occupational therapist Mubangizi Benedicto, who includes activities in a wildlife nature preserve at the Serenity Centre (SC), a Ugandan treatment and rehabilitation facility for individuals diagnosed with substance use disorders and co-occurring mental illnesses.

In the application scenario that follows, the occupational therapist advocates for outdoor-based therapeutic activities targeting socioemotional health: *William, an occupational therapist, has received permission from his supervisor to*

TABLE 30-3 | Herbal Container Gardening

Intervention Goals	Materials	Simplified Instructions
• Maurizio will actively engage in the plant selection process for the container garden and choose three plants from a selection of 10 images. • Maurizio will use his left arm to turn the pages in a plant catalog 50% of the time. • Maurizio will use one verb to describe how each of the three plants he selected makes him feel.	• 12"–16" diameter pot or container with a drainage hole and drain tray • Potting soil (do not use topsoil as it is too dense for container gardens) • 1 thriller, showy plant (e.g., lemon verbena) • 1–2 spiller, cascading plants (e.g., dittany) • 1–2 filler plants, one that will spread and fill the pot (e.g., thyme) • Garden gloves • Trowels • Scoop for potting soil • Paper or table cover for worktable • Water	1. Cover work surface. 2. Place herb seedling plants, pot, and drainer tray on work surface. 3. Open bag or container of potting soil. 4. Scoop potting soil into the pot until about two-thirds full. 5. To visualize the final product, arrange herb plants (still in their seedling pots) in larger pot with thriller upright in the middle, fillers upright around the thriller, and spillers angled about 30–45 degrees at the edge of the pot. 6. Gently depress the plant seedling pots into the potting soil. 7. Gently remove the plants from their seedling pots and gently massage the roots. 8. Place the seedlings on the worktable. 9. Gently remove the seedling pots from the larger pot. 10. Place the seedlings into the larger pot, taking care to gently spread the roots, remembering where each needs to be and how they should be oriented. 11. Use the trowel or scoop to carefully fill in the areas around the herb seedlings with additional potting soil until the pot is full (to the top of the planting line). 12. Place the pot on the drain tray. 13. Gently water the plants. 14. Adapt the activity as needed to address motor, cognitive, and/or mental health issues.

develop daylong therapeutic wilderness programs for the adolescents he works with in a juvenile correctional facility. William, accompanied by two staff workers, will be taking three people at a time to a nature preserve. There are many safety and security issues to overcome in the planning, but William is undaunted as he firmly believes that providing this type of therapeutic programming for the youth he works with will benefit their mental health and promote prosocial behaviors. In his research, William determines that identifying one specific place to facilitate the programs is a good idea because it sets forth a level of predictability and comfort for the youth, but in reality, there is nothing predictable about nature. So, although

the site remains constant, there is always something different to experience. After looking around the community, William finds an appropriate site for the program in a nearby forest preserve that has a small clearing. William determines that the first session should focus on a team building activity. He has presented the plan to his supervisor and discussed the logistics and responsibilities that each staff worker will be tasked with doing. As a warmup activity intended to address social-emotional and problem-solving skills, William planned the first activity of the day to be web making (Table 30-4). Please note that safety precautions regarding the use of sharps and string must be taken when facilitating this activity.

TABLE 30-4 | Web Making

Intervention Goals	Materials	Simplified Instructions
• Individuals will actively initiate their part of the activity 75% of the time. • Individuals will share one reflection of their group experience and constructively respond to another person's experience with no more than one prompt 90% of the time.	• Scissors • String	1. Group facilitators will serve as needed as active assistants, not as participants. 2. In advance of facilitating the activity, cut 10′ long lengths of string, enough for each adolescent to have one piece. 3. Gather adolescents into a large 20′ diameter circle with at least arms' width length between each of them. 4. Give each adolescent a piece of string, then ask them to place one end on the ground and slowly walk out the string so that they all meet in the center of the circle, holding the other end of their string. 5. With one end of the string in their hands, meet at the center and tie all the ends of the string together in a knot, so all pieces are connected. 6. Drop the knotted end of the string onto the ground. 7. Walk backwards out to the other end of the string. 8. Pick up the end of the string and, while holding it, begin to weave in and out between the other participants until there is no more string left. 9. Slowly and carefully unwind until everyone is back at the edge of the circle, holding the end of their fully extended string. 10. After the activity, gather the group members and invite them to share how the experience made them feel, both as an individual and as a group member. 11. Invite each person to constructively respond to another's comment.

Note: Scissors may be needed to untangle some participants.
Adapt the activity as needed to address motor, cognitive, and/or mental health issues.

Practitioner Profile

Mubangizi Benedicto, OTR, Head of the Occupational Therapy Department at Serenity Centre: www.Serenitycentre.org

Serenity Centre (SC) is a Ugandan treatment and rehabilitation facility for individuals diagnosed with substance use disorders and co-occurring mental illnesses. SC envisions a healthy world society free from substance dependencies through prevention and treatment. For over 21 years, SC has supported over 20,000 individuals recovering from alcoholism and drug abuse to regain occupations and live purposeful and sober lives. Referrals come from public and private health facilities, religious and Christian community nonprofits, self-referrals, and family and friends of individuals struggling with substance abuse and mental illness. Most receiving services at SC are men (86%) varying in age from 18 to 75, but the vast majority are young. Nearly all (90%) report a diagnosis of depression, bipolar disorder, attention deficit-hyperactivity disorder (ADHD), PTSD, anxiety, or schizophrenia.

OTPs use the Canadian Model of Occupational Performance to guide person-centered evaluation. A person's medical, psychiatric, forensic, and occupational histories; functional, cognitive, motor, and neuromusculoskeletal performances; and strengths and weaknesses are documented using a locally developed tool. The OTP and multidisciplinary team assess each individual to determine if they can benefit from a nature-based occupational therapy. We administer checklists of nature activities distributed in occupational domains of work, leisure, and self-care to assess the level of interest in these activities. Primary challenges include poor self-care, lack of routines, unemployment, anhedonia, difficulty setting goals, and poor time and self-management. Individual and group occupational therapy services are provided in residential, community, and family settings. Specific nature-aided activities are prepared and adapted to meet each person's occupational performance issues while providing a therapeutic, sensory rich environment where individuals learn and regain a variety of skills.

Practitioner Profile—cont'd

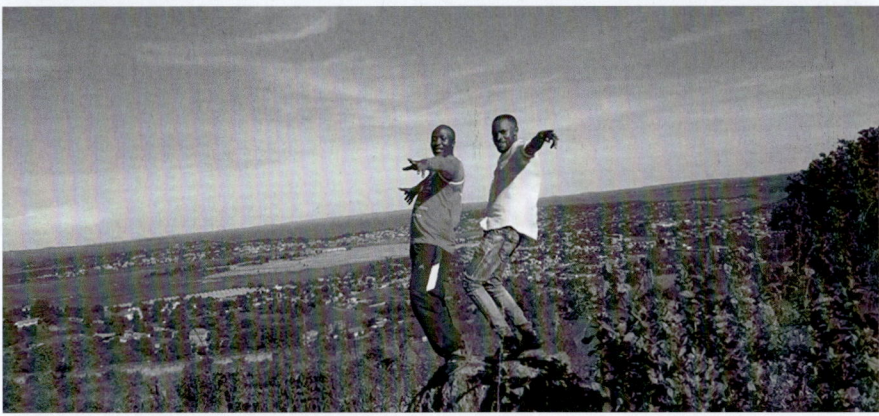

Joy after completing a 20-minute hike and rock climbing for site seeing.

Nature-aided therapeutic activities can be structured and unstructured and are designed to address each person's occupational performance issues. Activities include the following:

- A (visual) "big five" hunt for lions, leopards, rhinos, elephants, and African buffalo in the park challenges emotional regulation, attention, organization, flexibility, critical thinking, motor and perceptual skills, and sensory processing, and provides diversion from negative stimuli and thoughts.

- Creating a nature swing out of creeping stems challenges bilateral coordination, motor planning, tremors secondary to medication and drug abuse, visual motor skills, sensory processing, concentration, problem-solving, and emotion regulation.

- Completing a 20-minute hike to zipline for 5 minutes across a lake serves as a behavioral substitution for substance use and addresses hyperactivity secondary to excessive energy, which along with poor social skills, and negative thought diversion is often observed in individuals with manic symptoms.

Supporting individuals to interact with nature is a means to support sensory and emotional regulation. Team building activities completed in nature often require the integration of multiple cognitive, performance, and perceptual skills and interpersonal negotiation skills. Occupational therapy practitioners can design and lead nature-based activities that provide participants engaging opportunities to strengthen impulse controls, to learn to take safe risks, to communicate effectively with others, to be flexible, to practice mindfulness and coping, and to build greater self-awareness.

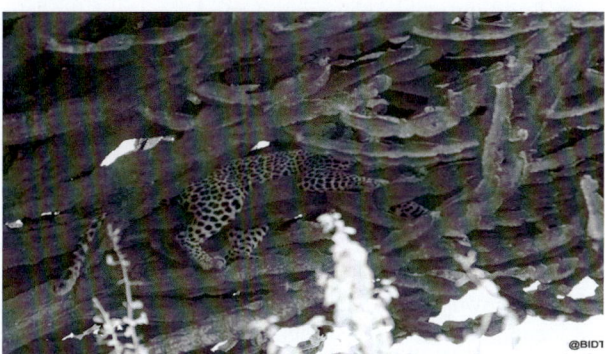

Spotting a leopard while completing a (visual) big five hunt for lion leopards, rhinos, elephants, and African buffalo in the park.

Play

Play is the primary occupation of childhood. One of many definitions of play is "an imaginative private reality, contains elements of make-believe, and is nonliteral" (Yogman et al., 2018, p. 2). While engaged in play, children can learn to take risks, be creative, and test the limits of their physical, social, and emotional skills on their own terms. Outdoor play in childhood is so important that a landmark 2007 American Academy of Pediatrics paper recommended between 30 and 60 minutes of daily outdoor play or exercise to maintain health and well-being. It cannot be stressed enough that every child, regardless of skill or ability, deserves to participate in play. In fact, the seminal 1959 *UN Declaration on the Rights of the Child* documented play as a right of every child. The occupation of play is described in more detail in Chapter 50: Play.

Consider the following application scenario concerning creative ways to facilitate understanding what features are desired in the play space:

Miranda is a school-based practitioner working in an urban school district. Recently, she learned that hard work and diligence pay off. Working closely with a team of parents, teachers, school administrators, and one of the district's physical therapists, they wrote a grant that was funded to design and install a nature-based play space in the small outdoor space on the elementary school grounds. They have retained a landscape design firm to work with the team pro bono to help design and install the play space. Right now, Miranda is thinking about the type of features the play space needs to first and foremost support the children who she works with. As a person-centered and evidence-driven practitioner, she wants to create and facilitate hands-on learning and listening sessions so that the team can understand what the play space needs to be. After reading

TABLE 30-5 | Edible Model Making

Intervention Goals	Materials	Simplified Instructions
• Individuals will initiate and actively engage in the activity 75% of the time with no prompts from the OTP. • Individuals will interact with others in the groups 50% of the time, sharing at least one positive comment about another's work during the session.	Food items such as small crackers, cookies, frosting, woven and stick pretzels, cereal rings, small marshmallows, pillow mints or other small candies, raisins, broccoli, and so on Markers and/or crayons	Draw the outline of a space to be designed on mat board or posterboard. If this activity is group-based, use a larger board. If the intention is for each individual to create their own vision board, use smaller pieces of mat or poster board. Place all food items into bowls or trays. Invite participants to gather building materials and place them in their work space and use them to design and/or draw elements that represent what they want to see included in the space.

about **participatory design workshopping**, she developed these group activities to facilitate with children, parents, and school personnel. The goals for these activities are to authentically understand what children, parents, and school personnel envision as being important and meaningful elements to be included in the play space and why they are important to each person. Once the workshopping is completed, she will compile the information and share with the team to guide the design process.

Examples of participatory design strategies for children:

- Chalk drawing on sidewalks or asphalt surfaces on the school grounds
- Building edible playground models out of food (see Table 30-5 and Fig. 30-1)
- Collaging
- Recording video and audio "interviews"

Examples of participatory design strategies for adults:

- *Card sorts:* Create a deck of at least 15 cards that contain images of playground equipment that adults sort in rank order from 1 to 15, with their most favored element being 1 and least favorite 15.
- *Image preference boards:* Adhere images of playground equipment to large sheets of poster board that are displayed on easel walls. Provide adults with green and red stickers; green stickers represent favored items, and red are not favored.
- *Video and audio "interviews":* This strategy provides opportunities for adults to verbally share their views.

Here's the Point

- There is a long history of the health-promoting value of participation in natural environments and nature-based intervention.
- A theoretical foundation has been established that supports a positive nature and health relationship.

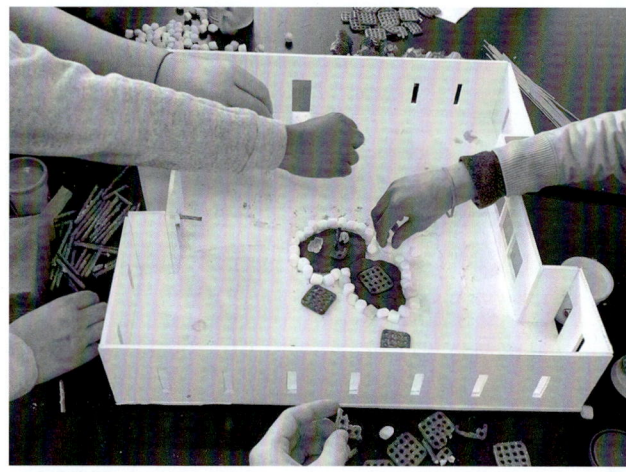

FIGURE 30-1. Edible model making. *Photo courtesy of Julie Stevens.*

- An ever-expanding body of research supports nature as a means to improve mental and physical health, cognition, and social-emotional status.
- Connecting nature with occupation is highly therapeutic, and for many people and OTPs is a gratifying, meaningful, and purposeful activity.
- Practitioners have long used nature, particularly gardening, as a therapeutic intervention, though limited research has been published by OTPs on its effects on individuals and groups.

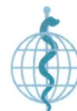

Visit the online resource center at **FADavis.com** to access the video.

Apply It Now

1. Reflective Walk Exercise

If climate and space permit, on 2 separate days, take a 15- to 20-minute walk in a favorite park and a 15- to 20-minute walk in a busy urban area. Note to yourself how you feel before you leave and then when the walk concludes. In class, share the impact of the experience with classmates. How might this activity be carried out in a mental health facility? Besides verbalizing the impact of the experience, how else might you invite individuals to share how they feel?

2. Addressing Climate Change

Review the AOTA policy on climate change (https://www .aota.org/-/media/corporate/files/aboutaota/officialdocs/ policies/policy-e16-20220908.pdf). Working in small groups, select one of the 12 stated outcomes and identify how you as an emerging OTP will address the selected outcome on an individual and community level.

3. Planning a Therapeutic Gardening Program

You want to start a therapeutic gardening program with the individuals you work with at a Veterans Administration facility providing services for individuals with PTSD. What reasons and evidence would you, as a new OTP, share with a supervisor to move the program forward?

4. Biophilia in the Workspace

With biophilia in mind, how might you enhance your workplace setting while still adhering to any infection control or other facility guidelines?

5. Video Exercise: Sensory Garden in Geriatric Psychiatric Unit

Pair up with another student in your class or form a small group of students. Access and watch the "Sensory Garden in Geriatric Psychiatric Unit" video at the online resource center at FADavis.com. Then, discuss and together answer the following questions.

Reflective Questions

■ Why are participation and engagement so important for residents of inpatient psychiatric facilities? What specific examples of the effect of the multisensory garden on residents' mental health and well-being does Callie describe?

■ What are the specific benefits of sensory stimulation for aging adults, and why is it so important for this population's mental health and well-being? What other populations might benefit from similar nature-based interventions?

■ Callie must consider the physical needs and abilities of everyone she works with in the geriatric psych unit, as well as evaluate performance challenges to ensure the garden is universally accessible and meets the diverse needs of all individuals (e.g., sensory, physical, social, emotional, leisure). What other specific design or therapeutic activity considerations might you implement in the sensory garden for this population?

■ In what ways is Callie using her rehabilitation, disability, and participation lens and skills to support the residents' mental health and well-being?

■ Although Callie is framing her work in a geriatric psychiatric unit, how might she help facilitate gardening as a leisure activity that a person could pursue after discharge and when living in their home or a community setting?

Resources

- Greener Allied Health Professional Hub: https://www.england .nhs.uk/ahp/greener-ahp-hub. Throughout the world, OTPs are taking action, becoming stewards of the land, and working toward environmental sustainability. For example, under the leadership of occupational therapist Ben Whitaker of the National Health Service in the UK, there is an active group of OTPs who participate in the Greener Allied Health Professional Hub. This site shares many links on sustainability and examples of recent efforts by the Greener Allied Health Professional Hub.

- Occupational Therapists for Environmental Action (OTEA): https://www.otenvironmentalaction.com. In the United States, a group that is making waves is OTEA. Their mission—"We're transforming occupational therapy in the United States to improve individual, community, and planetary health. We want your help"—sums it up well. The group is inclusionary and welcomes new members who have a passion for the planet, occupational therapy, and ways in which OTPs can improve not only the health of populations they serve, but the health of the planet.

- Social and Therapeutic Horticulture for Palliative Care (STH4PC): https://sth4pc.wordpress.com. Located in the United Kingdom, this group called STH4PC maintains a website with years of resources and postings. The group's goal

is to promote the use of social horticulture as a therapeutic intervention, particularly in hospice and other palliative care settings. Many of its members are OTPs whose practice incorporates nature-based interventions. They meet regularly and share ideas for practice.

- NatureOT: www.natureot.com.au. Bronwyn Paynter, BAppSc(OccTh)*UniSA,* PostgradDip(OT)*La Trobe,* GradCertPermDesign *CQU,* Dip PM, DipGov(OHS), is an occupational therapist from Adelaide, South Australia. She is the director of NatureOT and recognizes that connecting people with nature supports both human AND planetary well-being. Her website shares evidence about nature's connection to well-being and reflects her innovative coaching and consulting nature-based practice designed to help OTPs across the globe include more nature in their own lives, work, and all areas of occupational therapy practice.

- *Nature-Based Allied Health Practice: Creative and Evidence-Based Strategies.* Written by Amy Wagenfeld and Shannon Marder and published by Jessica Kingsley Publishers, this evidence-based and accessible book demonstrates easily workable, creative, tried-and-tested strategies for bringing nature into therapy. Resources are included to help assess a program's readiness to incorporate nature, create plans to take therapy outdoors (or bring the outside in), and evaluate the impact it could have for individuals and groups.

References

Adevi, A. A., & Mårtensson, F. (2013). Stress rehabilitation through garden therapy: The garden as a place in the recovery from stress. *Urban Forestry & Urban Greening, 12*(2), 230–237. https://doi.org/10.1016/j.ufug.2013.01.007

Algado, S. S., & Townsend, A. E. (2015). Eco-social occupational therapy. *British Journal of Occupational Therapy, 78*(3), 182–186. https://doi.org/10.1177/0308022614561239

American Academy of Pediatrics. (2007). *Active healthy living: Prevention of childhood obesity through increased physical activity.* http://pediatrics.aappublications.org/content/117/5/1834.full.pdf

American Occupational Therapy Association. (2020). Occupational therapy practice framework: Domain and process—Fourth edition. *American Journal of Occupational Therapy, 74*(Suppl. 2), 7412410010p1–7412410010p87. https://doi.org/10.5014/ajot.2020.74S2001

American Occupational Therapy Association. (2022). *Policy E.16, Occupational therapy's commitment to sustainability and climate change.* https://www.aota.org/-/media/corporate/files/aboutaota/officialdocs/policies/policy-e16-20220908.pdf

Antonelli, M., Donelli, D., Carlone, L., Maggini, V., Firenzuoli, F., & Bedeschi, E. (2022). Effects of forest bathing (shinrin-yoku) on individual well-being: An umbrella review. *International Journal of Environmental Health Research, 32*(8), 1842–1867. https://doi.org/10.1080/09603123.2021.1919293

Baker, P. (2018). Identifying the connection between Roman conceptions of 'Pure Air' and physical and mental health in Pompeian gardens (*c*.150 BC–AD 79): A multi-sensory approach to ancient medicine. *World Archaeology, 50*(3), 404–417. https://doi.org/10.1080/00438243.2018.1487332

Balanzá-Martínez, V., & Cervera-Martínez, J. (2022). Lifestyle prescription for depression with a focus on nature exposure and screen time: A narrative review. *International Journal of Environmental Research and Public Health, 19*(9), 5094. https://doi.org/10.3390/ijerph19095094

Baum, C. M., Christiansen, C. H., & Bass, J. D. (2015). The Person-Environment-Occupation- Performance (PEOP) model. In C. H. Christiansen, C. M. Baum, & J. D. Bass (Eds.), *Occupational therapy: Performance, participation, and well-being* (4th ed., pp. 49–56). Slack, Inc.

Beil, K. (2021). Nature therapy: Part one: Evidence for the healing power of contact with nature. *Journal of Restorative Medicine, 11*(1), 1–7. https://doi.org/10.14200/jrm.2021.0101

Berger, J., Essah, E., Blanusa, T., & Beaman, C. P. (2022). The appearance of indoor plants and their effect on people's perceptions of indoor air quality and subjective well-being. *Building and Environment, 219*, 109151. https://doi.org/10.1016/j.buildenv.2022.109151

Bettmann, J. E., Prince, K. C., Ganesh, K., Rugo, K. F., Bryan, A. O., Bryan, C. J., Rozek, D. C., & Leifker, F. R. (2021). The effect of time outdoors on veterans receiving treatment for PTSD. *Journal of Clinical Psychology, 77*(9), 2041–2056. https://doi.org/10.1002/jclp.23139

Blaschke, S. (2017). The role of nature in cancer patients' lives: A systematic review and qualitative meta-synthesis. *BMC Cancer, 17*(1), Article 370. https://doi.org/10.1186/s12885-017-3366-6

Blaschke, S., O'Callaghan, C. C., & Schofield, P. (2020). Nature-based supportive care opportunities: A conceptual framework. *BMJ Supportive and Palliative Care, 10*(1), 36–44. https://doi.org/10.1136/bmjspcare-2017-001465

Blaschke, S., O'Callaghan, C. C., Schofield, P., & Salander, P. (2017). Cancer patients' experiences with nature: Normalizing dichotomous realities. *Social Science and Medicine, 172*, 107–114. https://doi.org/10.1016/j.socscimed.2016.10.024

Bogar, S., & Beyer, K. M. (2016). Green space, violence, and crime: A systematic review. *Trauma, Violence & Abuse, 17*(2), 160–171. https://doi.org/10.1177/1524838015576412

Bratman, G. N., Anderson, C. B., Berman, M. G., Cochran, B., De Vries, S., Flanders, J., Folke, C., Frumkin, H., Gross, J. J., Hartig, T., Kahn, P. H., Jr., Kuo, M., Lawler, J. J., Levin, P. S., Lindahl, T., Meyer-Lindenberg, A., Mitchell, R., Ouyang, Z., Roe, J., . . . Daily, G. C. (2019). Nature and mental health: An ecosystem service perspective. *Science Advances, 5*(7), eaax0903. https://doi.org/10.1126/sciadv.aax0903

Bratman, G. N., Hamilton, J. P., & Daily, G. C. (2012). The impacts of nature experience on human cognitive function and mental health. *Annals of the New York Academy of Sciences, 1249*(1), 118–136. https://doi.org/10.1111/j.1749-6632.2011.06400.x

Brown, S. C., Lombard, J., Wang, K., Byrne, M. M., Toro, M., Plater-Zyberk, E., Feaster, D. J., Kardys, J., Nardi, M. I., Perez-Gomez, G., Pantin, H. M., & Szapocznik, J. (2016). Neighborhood greenness and chronic health conditions in Medicare beneficiaries. *American Journal of Preventative Medicine, 51*(1), 78–89. https://doi.org/10.1016/j.amepre.2016.02.008

Bustamante, G., Guzman, V., Kobayashi, L. C., & Finlay, J. (2022). Mental health and well-being in times of COVID-19: A mixed-methods study of the role of neighborhood parks, outdoor spaces, and nature among US older adults. *Health & Place, 76*, 102813. https://doi.org/10.1016/j.healthplace.2022.102813

Chen, K., Zhang, T., Liu, F., Zhang, Y., & Song, Y. (2021). How does urban green space impact residents' mental health: A literature review of mediators. *International Journal of Environmental Research and Public Health, 18*(22), 11746. https://doi.org/10.3390/ijerph182211746

Choe, E. Y., Jorgensen, A., & Sheffield, D. (2020). Does a natural environment enhance the effectiveness of Mindfulness-Based Stress Reduction (MBSR)? Examining the mental health and wellbeing, and nature connectedness benefits. *Landscape and Urban Planning, 202*, 103886. https://doi.org/10.1016/j.landurbplan.2020.103886

Choe, E. Y., & Sheffield, D. (2022). The role of natural environments in the effectiveness of brief Mindfulness-Based Stress Reduction (brief MBSR): Depression, anxiety, stress and hair cortisol from a randomized trial. *Journal of Public Health and Emergency*, 1–14. https://doi.org/10.21037/jphe-22-13

Christiana, R. W., Besenyi, G. M., Gustat, J., Horton, T. H., Penbrooke, T. L., & Schultz, C. L. (2021). A scoping review of the health benefits of nature-based physical activity. *Journal of Healthy Eating and Active Living, 1*(3), 154–172. https://doi.org/10.51250/jheal.v1i3.25

Clark, N. E., Lovell, R., Wheeler, B. W., Higgins, S. L., Depledge, M. H., & Norris, K. (2014). Biodiversity, cultural pathways, and human health: A framework. *Trends in Ecology & Evolution, 29*(4), 198–204. https://doi.org/10.1016/j.tree.2014.01.009

Clarke, E. (1950). Gardening as a therapeutic experience. *American Journal of Occupational Therapy, 4*(3), 109–110, 116.

Cordoza, M., Ulrich, R. S., Manulik, B. J., Gardiner, S. K., Fitzpatrick, P. S., Hazen, T. M., Mirka, A., & Perkins, R. S. (2018). Impact of nurses taking daily work breaks in a hospital garden on burnout. *American Journal of Critical Care, 27*(6), 508–512. https://doi.org/10.4037/ajcc2018131

Cornell Health. (n.d.). *Nature Rx.* https://health.cornell.edu/resources/health-topics/nature-rx

Coventry, P. A., Brown, J. E., Pervin, J., Brabyn, S., Pateman, R., Breedvelt, J., Gilbody, S., Stancliffe, R., McEachan, R., & White, P. L. (2021). Nature-based outdoor activities for mental and physical health: Systematic review and meta-analysis. *SSM-Population Health, 16*, 100934. https://doi.org/10.1016/j.ssmph.2021.100934

Crossan, C., & Salmoni, A. (2021). A simulated walk in nature: Testing predictions from the Attention Restoration Theory. *Environment and Behavior, 53*(3), 277–295. https://doi.org/10.1177/0013916519882775

Detweiler, M. B., Sharma, T., Detweiler, J. G., Murphy, P. F., Lane, S., Carman, J., Chudhary, A. S., Halling, M. H., & Kim, K. Y. (2012). What is the evidence to support the use of therapeutic gardens for the elderly? *Psychiatry Investigation, 9*(2), 100–110. https://doi.org/10.4306/pi.2012.9.2.100

Diette, G. B., Lechtzin, N., Haponik, E., Devrotes, A., & Rubin, H. R. (2003). Distraction therapy with nature sights and sounds reduces pain during flexible bronchoscopy: A complementary approach to routine analgesia. *Chest, 123*(3), 941–948. https://doi.org/10.1378/chest.123.3.941

Doimo, I., Masiero, M., & Gatto, P. (2020). Forest and wellbeing: Bridging medical and forest research for effective forest-based initiatives. *Forests, 11*(8), 791. https://doi.org/10.3390/f11080791

Evans, S. C., Atkinson, T., Rogerson, M., & Bray, J. (2021). Nature-based activities for people living with dementia: A nice day out or a matter of human rights? *Working With Older People, 26*(1), 64–75. https://doi.org/10.1108/WWOP-08-2021-0040

Faber Taylor, A., & Kuo, F. E. (2009). Children with attention deficits concentrate better after walk in the park. *Journal of Attention Disorders, 12*(5), 402–409. https://doi.org/10.1177/1087054708323000

Faber Taylor, A., & Kuo, F. E. (2011). Could exposure to everyday green spaces help treat ADHD? Evidence from children's play settings. *Applied Psychology: Health and Well-Being, 3*(3), 281–303. https://doi.org/10.1111/j.1758-0854.2011.01052.x

Franck, E., Haegdorens, F., Goossens, E., Van Gils, Y., Portzky, M., Somville, F., Abuawad, M., Slootmans, S., & Van Bogaert, P. (2021). The role of coping behavior in healthcare workers' distress and somatization during the COVID-19 pandemic. *Frontiers in Psychology, 12*, 684618. https://doi.org/10.3389/fpsyg.2021.684618

Frumkin, H., Bratman, G. N., Breslow, S. J., Cochran, B., Kahn, P. H., Jr., Lawler, J. J., Levin, P. S., Tandon, P. S., Varanasi, U., Wolf, K. L., & Wood, S. A (2017). Nature contact and human health: A research agenda. *Environmental Health Perspectives, 125*(7), 075001. https://doi.org/10.1289/EHP1663

Fuertes, E., Markevych, I., Bowatte, G., Gruzieva, O., Gehring, U., Becker, A., Berdel, D., von Berg, A., Bergström, A., Brauer, M., Brunekreef, B., Brüske, I., Carlsten, C., Chan-Yeung, M., Dharmage, S. C., Hoffmann, B., Klümper, C., Koppelman, G. H., Kozyrskyj, A., . . . Heinrich, J. (2016). Residential greenness is differentially associated with childhood allergic rhinitis and aeroallergen sensitization in seven birth cohorts. *Allergy, 71*(10), 1461–1471. https://doi.org/10.1111/all.12915

Fuertes, E., Markevych, I., von Berg, A., Bauer, C.-P., Berdel, D., Koletzko, S., Sugiri, D., & Heinrich, J. (2014). Greenness and allergies: Evidence of differential associations in two areas in Germany. *Journal of Epidemiology and Community Health, 68*(8), 787–790. https://doi.org/10.1136/jech-2014-203903

Furuyashiki, A., Tabuchi, K., Norikoshi, K., Kobayashi, T., & Oriyama, S. (2019). A comparative study of the physiological and psychological effects of forest bathing (shinrin-yoku) on working age people with and without depressive tendencies. *Environmental Health and Preventive Medicine, 24*, 1–11. https://doi.org/10.1186/s12199-019-0800-1

Gaekwad, J. S., Moslehian A. S., Roös, P. B., & Walker, A. (2022). A meta-analysis of emotional evidence for the biophilia hypothesis and implications for biophilic design. *Frontiers in Psychology, 13*, 750245. https://doi.org/10.3389/fpsyg.2022.750245

Garcia Diaz, L. V., & Richardson, J. (2021). Occupational therapy's contributions to combating climate change and lifestyle diseases. *Scandinavian Journal of Occupational Therapy, 30*(7), 992–999. https://doi.org/10.1080/11038128.2021.1989484

Gladwell, V. F., Kuoppa, P., Tarvainen, M. P., & Rogerson, M. (2016). A lunchtime walk in nature enhances restoration of autonomic control during night-time sleep: Results from a preliminary study. *International Journal of Environmental Research and Public Health, 13*(3), 280. https://doi.org/10.3390/ijerph13030280

Gunderman, R. B. (2020). Medical valor in plague time: Dr. Benjamin Rush. *Perspective, 27*(6), 889–891. https://doi.org/10.1016/j.acra.2020.04.014

Hall, C. R., & Knuth, M. J. (2019). An update of the literature supporting the well-being benefits of plants: Part 2. Physiological health benefits. *Journal of Environmental Horticulture, 37*(2), 63–73. https://doi.org/10.24266/0738-2898-37.2.63

Hammell, K. W. (2021). Occupation in natural environments; health equity and environmental justice. *Canadian Journal of Occupational Therapy, 88*(4), 319–328. https://doi.org/10.1177/00084174211040000

Han, J.-W., Choi, H., Jeon, Y.-H., Yoon, C.-H., Woo, J.-M., & Kim, W. (2016). The effects of forest therapy on coping with chronic widespread pain: Physiological and psychological differences between participants in a forest therapy program and a control group. *International Journal of Environmental Research and Public Health, 13*(3), 255. https://doi.org/10.3390/ijerph13030255

Hartig, T., Mitchell, R., De Vries, S., & Frumkin, H. (2014). Nature and health. *Annual Review of Public Health, 35*, 207–228. https://doi.org/10.1146/annurev-publhealth-032013-182443

Hartwell, D. M. (1932). *Landscape gardening and floriculture as occupational therapy treatment.* Presented at the sixteenth annual meeting of the American Occupational Therapy Association, Detroit, Michigan, September 12–14, 1932.

Hewitt, P., Watts, C., Hussey, J., Power, K., & Williams, P. (2013). Does a structured gardening programme improve well-being in young onset dementia? A preliminary study. *British Journal of Occupational Therapy, 76*(8), 355–361. https://doi.org/10.4276/030802213X13757040168270

Hobhouse, P. (2004). *Gardens of Persia.* Kales Press.

Holland, I., DeVille, N. V., Browning, M. H., Buehler, R. M., Hart, J. E., Hipp, J. A., Mitchell, R., Rakow, D. A., Schiff, J. E., White, M. P., Yin, J., & James, P. (2021). Measuring nature contact: A narrative review. *International Journal of Environmental Research and Public Health, 18*(8), 4092. https://doi.org/10.3390/ijerph18084092

Jackson, S. B., Stevenson, K. T., Larson, L. R., Peterson, M. N., & Seekamp, E. (2021). Outdoor activity participation improves adolescents' mental health and well-being during the COVID-19 pandemic. *International Journal of Environmental Research and Public Health, 18*(5), 2506. https://doi.org/10.3390/ijerph18052506

Jia, P., Dai, S., Rohli, K. E., Rohli, R. V., Ma, Y., Yu, C., Pan, X., & Zhou, W. (2021). Natural environment and childhood obesity: A systematic review. *Obesity Reviews, 22*, e13097. https://doi.org/10.1111/obr.13097

Jimenez, M. P., DeVille, N. V., Elliott, E. G., Schiff, J. E., Wilt, G. E., Hart, J. E., & James, P. (2021). Associations between nature exposure and health: A review of the evidence. *International Journal of Environmental Research and Public Health, 18*(9), 4790. https://doi.org/10.3390/ijerph18094790

Jonasson, I., Marklund, B., & Hildingh, C. (2007). Working in a training garden: Experiences of patients with neurological damage. *Australian Occupational Therapy Journal, 54*(4), 266–272. https://doi.org/10.1111/j.1440-1630.2007.00634.x

Jones, R., Tarter, R., & Ross, A. M. (2021). Greenspace interventions, stress and cortisol: A scoping review. *International Journal of Environmental Research and Public Health, 18*(6), 2802. https://doi.org/10.3390/ijerph18062802

Joyce, J., & Warren, A. (2016). A case study exploring the influence of a gardening therapy group on well-being. *Occupational Therapy in Mental Health, 32*(2), 203–215. https://doi.org/10.1080/0164212X.2015.1111184

Kang, N., Bell, S., Ward Thompson, C., Zheng, M., Xu, Z., & Sun, Z. (2022). Use of urban residential community parks for stress management during the COVID-19 lockdown period in China. *Frontiers in Psychology, 13*, 816417. https://doi.org/10.3389/fpsyg.2022.816417

Kaplan, R., & Kaplan, S. (1989). *The experience of nature: A psychological perspective.* Cambridge University Press.

Kaplan, S. (1995). The restorative benefits of nature: Toward an integrative framework. *Journal of Environmental Psychology, 15*(3), 169–182. https://doi.org/10.1016/0272-4944(95)90001-2

Kardan, O., Gozdyra, P., Misic, B., Moola, F., Palmer, L. J., Paus, T., & Berman, M. G. (2015). Neighborhood greenspace and health in a large urban center. *Scientific Reports, 5,* 11610. https://doi.org/10.1038/srep11610

Keniger, L. E., Gaston, K. J., Irvine, K. N., & Fuller, R. A. (2013). What are the benefits of interacting with nature? *International Journal of Environmental Research and Public Health, 10,* 913–935. https://doi.org/10.3390/ijerph10030913

Khan, J. R., Sultana, A., Islam, M., & Biswas, R. K. (2021). A negative association between prevalence of diabetes and urban residential area greenness detected in nationwide assessment of urban Bangladesh. *Scientific Reports, 11*(1), 1–9. https://doi.org/10.1038/s41598-021-98585-6

Kim, J.-H., Lee, C., & Sohn, W. (2016). Urban natural environments, obesity, and health-related quality of life among Hispanic children living in inner-city neighborhoods. *International Journal of Environmental Research and Public Health, 13*(1), 121. https://doi.org/10.3390/ijerph13010121

Klotz, A. C., & Bolino, M. C. (2021). Bringing the great outdoors into the workplace: The energizing effect of biophilic work design. *Academy of Management Review, 46*(2), 231–251. https://doi.org/10.5465/amr.2017.0177

Kondo, M. C., Oyekanmi, K. O., Gibson, A., South, E. C., Bocarro, J., & Hipp, J. A. (2020). Nature prescriptions for health: A review of evidence and research opportunities. *International Journal of Environmental Research and Public Health, 17*(12), 4213. https://doi.org/10.3390/ijerph17124213

Korpela, K. M., Stengård, E., & Jussila, P. (2016). Nature walks as a part of therapeutic intervention for depression. *Ecopsychology, 8*(1), 8–15. https://doi.org/10.1089/eco.2015.0070

Kuo, F. E., & Sullivan, W. C. (2001). Environment and crime in the inner city: Does vegetation reduce crime? *Environment and Behavior, 33*(3), 343–367. https://doi.org/10.1177/0013916501333002

Lampert, T., Costa, J., Santos, O., Sousa, J., Ribeiro, T., & Freire, E. (2021). Evidence on the contribution of community gardens to promote physical and mental health and well-being of non-institutionalized individuals: A systematic review. *PLoS One, 16*(8), e0255621. https://doi.org/10.1371/journal.pone.0255621

Lawton, M. P., & Nahemow, L. (1973). Ecology and the aging process. In C. Eisdorfer & M. P. Lawton (Eds.), *Psychology of adult development and aging* (pp. 619–674). American Psychological Association.

Lechtzin, N., Busse, A. M., Smith, M. T., Grossman, S., Nesbit, S., & Diette, G. B. (2010). A randomized trial of nature scenery and sounds versus urban scenery and sounds to reduce pain in adults undergoing bone marrow aspirate and biopsy. *Journal of Alternative and Complementary Medicine, 16*(9), 965–972. https://doi.org/10.1089/acm.2009.0531

Lim, Y. S., Kim, J., Khil, T., Yi, J., & Kim, D. J. (2021). Effects of the forest healing program on depression, cognition, and the autonomic nervous system in the elderly with cognitive decline. *Journal of People, Plants, and Environment, 24*(1), 107–117. https://doi.org/10.11628/ksppe.2021.24.1.107

Lõhmus, M., Stenfors, C. U., Lind, T., Lauber, A., & Georgelis, A. (2021). Mental health, greenness, and nature related behaviors in the adult population of Stockholm County during COVID-19-related restrictions. *International Journal of Environmental Research and Public Health, 18*(6), 3303. https://doi.org/10.3390/ijerph18063303

Maas, J., Verheij, R. A., Groenewegen, P. P., de Vries, S., & Spreeuwenberg, P. (2006). Green space, urbanity, and health: How strong is the relation? *Journal of Epidemiology and Community Health, 60*(7), 587–592. https://doi.org/10.1136/jech.2005.043125

Mancus, G., Hill, S. V., Carter, P., Payne-Foster, P., Krishnamurthy, M., Kazembe, A., & Cody, S. L. (2021). Nature-based therapies for sleep disorders in people living with human immunodeficiency virus. *Nursing Clinics, 56*(2), 189–202. https://doi.org/10.1016/j.cnur.2021.02.002

Mao, G., Cao, Y., Wang, B., Wang, S., Chen, Z., Wang, J., Xing, W., Ren, X., Lv, X., Dong, J., Chen, S., Chen, X., Wang, G., & Yan, J. (2017). The salutary influence of forest bathing on elderly patients with chronic heart failure. *International Journal of Environmental Research and Public Health, 14*(4), 368. https://doi.org/10.3390/ijerph14040368

Mason, L., Ronconi, A., Scrimin, S., & Pazzaglia, F. (2021). Short-term exposure to nature and benefits for students' cognitive performance: A review. *Educational Psychology Review, 34,* 1–39. https://doi.org/10.1007/s10648-021-09631-8

Matuska, K. (2013). The healthy harvest. *Occupational Therapy Journal of Research, 33*(4), 179. https://doi.org/10.3928/15394492-20130827-01

Mayer, F. S., Frantz, C. M., Bruehlman-Senecal, E., & Dolliver, K. (2009). Why is nature beneficial? The role of connectedness to nature. *Environment and Behavior, 41*(5), 617–643. https://doi.org/10.1177/0013916508319745

McNeil, D. G., Singh, A., & Chambers, T. (2022). Exploring nature and social-connectedness as mediators of the relationship between nature-based exercise and subjective wellbeing. *Ecopsychology, 14*(4), 226–234. https://doi.org/10.1089/eco.2022.0013

Meidenbauer, K. L., Stenfors, C. U. D., Bratman, G. N., Gross, J. J., Schertz, K. E., Choe, K. W., & Berman, M. G. (2020). The affective benefits of nature exposure: What's nature got to do with it? *Journal of Environmental Psychology, 72,* 101498. https://doi.org/10.1016/j.jenvp.2020.101498

Memari, S., Pazhouhanfar, M., & Grahn, P. (2021). Perceived sensory dimensions of green areas: An experimental study on stress recovery. *Sustainability, 13*(10), 5419. https://doi.org/10.3390/su13105419

Ng, L., Oliver, E., & Laver, K. (2022). Beyond garden design: A review of outdoor occupation in hospital and residential care settings for people with dementia. *Australian Occupational Therapy Journal, 70*(1), 97–118. https://doi.org/10.1111/1440-1630.12826

Occupational Therapists for Environmental Action. (n.d.). *Occupational therapy and climate change.* https://www.otenvironmentalaction.com/ot-climate

O'Connor, D. B., Thayer, J. F., & Vedhara, K. (2021). Stress and health: A review of psychobiological processes. *Annual Review of Psychology, 72,* 663–688. https://doi.org/10.1146/annurev-psych-062520-122331

O'Nuallain, F. (2021). *Seeds of mindfulness: 101 mindful moments in the garden.* Dover Publications.

Park, C. H., Chun, J., Hahm, Y., Kang, D. H., & Park, B. J. (2021). Effects of a forest therapy program on reducing PTSD and depression and improving mood states in fire officers. *Journal of People, Plants, and Environment, 24*(6), 693–705. https://doi.org/10.11628/ksppe.2021.24.6.693

Penn Medicine. (n.d.). *Dr. Benjamin Rush.* https://www.uphs.upenn.edu/paharc/features/brush.html

Persson, D., & Erlandsson, L.-K. (2014). Ecopation: Connecting sustainability, glocalisation and well-being. *Journal of Occupational Science, 21*(1), 12–24. https://doi.org/10.1080/14427591.2013.867561

Pizarro, E., Estrella, S., Figueroa, F., Helmke, F., Pontigo, C., & Whiteford, G. (2018). Understanding occupational justice from the concept of territory: A proposal for occupational science. *Journal of Occupational Science, 25*(4), 463–473. https://doi.org/10.1080/14427591.2018.1487261

Pryor, A., Harper, N., & Carpenter, C. (2021). Outdoor therapy: Benefits, mechanisms and principles for activating health, wellbeing, and healing in nature. In G. Thomas, J. Dyment, & H. Prince (Eds.), *Outdoor environmental education in higher education* (pp. 123–134). Springer.

Puhakka, R. (2021). University students' participation in outdoor recreation and the perceived well-being effects of nature. *Journal of Outdoor Recreation and Tourism, 36,* 100425. https://doi.org/10.1016/j.jort.2021.100425

Qiu, L., Chen, Q., & Gao, T. (2021). The effects of urban natural environments on preference and self-reported psychological restoration of the elderly. *International Journal of Environmental Research and Public Health, 18*(2), 509. https://doi.org/10.3390/ijerph18020509

Raanaas, R. K., Patil, G., & Alve, G. (2016). Patients' recovery experiences of indoor plants and views of nature in a rehabilitation center. *Work, 53*(1), 45–55. https://doi.org/10.3233/WOR-152214

Ray, H., & Jakubec, S. L. (2014). Nature-based experiences and health of cancer survivors. *Complementary Therapies in Clinical Practice, 20*(4), 188–192. https://doi.org/10.1016/j.ctcp.2014.07.005

Ribeiro, A. I., Triguero-Mas, M., Santos, C. J., Gómez-Nieto, A., Cole, H., Anguelovski, I., Silva, F. M., & Baró, F. (2021). Exposure to nature and mental health outcomes during COVID-19 lockdown. A comparison between Portugal and Spain. *Environment International, 154,* 106664. https://doi.org/10.1016/j.envint.2021.106664

Rosenberg, R. S., Lange, W., Zebrack, B., Moulton, S., & Kosslyn, S. M. (2014). An outdoor adventure program for young adults with cancer: Positive effects on body image and psychosocial functioning. *Journal of Psychosocial Oncology, 32*(5), 622–636. https://doi.org/10.1080/07347332.2014.936652

Ross, M., & Mason, G. J. (2017). The effects of preferred natural stimuli on humans' affective states, physiological stress and mental health, and the potential implications for well-being in captive animals. *Neuroscience & Biobehavioral Reviews, 83,* 46–62. https://doi.org/10.1016/j.neubiorev.2017.09.012

Sanders, T., Feng, X., Fahey, P. P., Lonsdale, C., & Astell-Burt, T. (2015). Greener neighbourhoods, slimmer children? Evidence from 4423 participants aged 6 to 13 years in the longitudinal study of Australian children. *International Journal of Obesity, 39*(8), 1224–1229. https://doi.org/10.1038/ijo.2015.69

Scott, E. E., LoTemplio, S. B., McDonnell, A. S., McNay, G. D., Greenberg, K., McKinney, T., Uchino, B. N., & Strayer, D. L. (2021). The autonomic nervous system in its natural environment: Immersion in nature is associated with changes in heart rate and heart rate variability. *Psychophysiology, 58*(4), e13698. https://doi.org/10.1111/psyp.13698

Sempik, J. (2010). Green care and mental health: Gardening and farming as health and social care. *Mental Health and Social Inclusion, 14*(3), 15–22. https://doi.org/ 10.5042/mhsi.2010.0440

Senel, B. (2020). Fuzzy Dematel analysis on the examination of physical characteristics emergency room affecting the efficiency of doctors. *Mathematics in Engineering, Science and Aerospace, 11*(1), 77–90. http://nonlinearstudies.com/index.php/mesa/article/view/2150

Shanahan, D. F., Bush, R., Gaston, K. J., Lin, B. B., Dean, J., Barber, E., & Fuller, R. A. (2016). Health benefits from nature experiences depend on dose. *Scientific Reports, 6*(1), 28551. https://doi.org/10.1038/srep28551

Silveira, E. A., Mendonça, C. R., Delpino, F. M., Souza, G. V. E., de Souza Rosa, L. P., de Oliveira, C., & Noll, M. (2022). Sedentary behavior, physical inactivity, abdominal obesity and obesity in adults and older adults: A systematic review and meta-analysis. *Clinical Nutrition ESPEN, 50,* 63–73. https://doi.org/10.1016/j.clnesp.2022.06.001

Soga, M., Evans, M. J., Tsuchiya, K., & Fukano, Y. (2021). A room with a green view: The importance of nearby nature for mental health during the COVID-19 pandemic. *Ecological Applications, 31*(2), e2248. https://doi.org/10.1002/eap.2248

Southcott, B. (1951). Gardening for the rehabilitation of the injured workman. *Canadian Journal of Occupational Therapy, 18,* 27–30. https://doi.org/10.1177/000841745101800106

Stark, J. H., Neckerman, K., Lovasi, G. S., Quinn, J., Weiss, C. C., Bader, M. D. M., Konty, K., Harris, T. G., & Rundle, A. (2014). The impact of neighborhood park access and quality on body mass index among adults in New York City.

Preventive Medicine, 64, 63–68. https://doi.org/10.1016/j.ypmed.2014.03.026

Stigsdotter, U. K., Palsdottir, A. M., Burls, A., Chermaz, A., Ferrini, F., & Grahn, P. (2011). Nature-based therapeutic interventions. In K. Nilsson, M. Sangster, C. Gallis, T. Hartig, S. de Vries, K. Seeland, & J. Schipperijin (Eds.), *Forests, trees and human health* (pp. 309–342). Springer. https://doi.org/10.1007/978-90-481-9806-1_11

Swank, J. M., Walker, K. L., & Shin, S. M. (2020). Indoor nature-based play therapy: Taking the natural world inside the playroom. *International Journal of Play Therapy, 29*(3), 155–162. https://doi.org/10.1037/pla0000123

Teixeira, A., Gabriel, R., Quaresma, L., Alencoão, A., Martinho, J., & Moreira, H. (2021). Obesity and natural spaces in adults and older people: A systematic review. *Journal of Physical Activity and Health, 18*(6), 714–727. https://doi.org/10.1123/jpah.2020-0589

Thiering, E., Markevych, I., Brüske, I., Fuertes, E., Kratzsch, J., Sugiri, D., Hoffmann, B., von Berg, A., Bauer, C.-P., Koletzko, S., Berdel, D., & Heinrich, J. (2016). Associations of residential long-term air pollution exposures and satellite-derived greenness with insulin resistance in German adolescents. *Environmental Health Perspectives, 124*(8), 1291–1298. https://doi.org/doi:10.1289/ehp.1509967

Ulrich, R. S. (1984). View through a window may influence recovery from surgery. *Science, 224*(4647), 420–421. https://doi.org/10.1126/science.6143402

Ulrich, R. S., Cordoza, M., Gardiner, S., Manulik, B., Fitzpatrick, P., Hazen, T. M., & Perkins, R. (2020). ICU patient family stress recovery during breaks in a hospital garden and indoor environments. *Health Environments Research & Design Journal, 13*(2), 810–812. https://doi.org/10.1177/1937586719867157

Ulrich, R. S., Simons, R. F., Losito, B. D., Fiorito, E., Miles, M. A., & Zelson, M. (1991). Stress recovery during exposure to natural and urban environments. *Journal of Environmental Psychology, 11*(3), 201–230. https://doi.org/10.1016/S0272-4944(05)80184-7

United Nations. (2016). *The sustainable development goals report.* UN DESA. https://desapublications.un.org/publications/global-sustainable-development-report-2016

Veldheer, S., Winkels, R. M., Cooper, J., Groff, C., Lepley, J., Bordner, C., Wagner, A., George, D. R., & Sciamanna, C. (2020). Growing healthy hearts: Gardening program feasibility in a hospital-based community garden. *Journal of Nutrition Education and Behavior, 52*(10), 958–963. https://doi.org/10.1016/j.jneb.2020.07.006

Vujcic, M., Tomicevic-Dubljevic, J., Grbic, M., Lecic-Tosevski, D., Vukovic, O., & Toskovic, O. (2017). Nature based solution for improving mental health and well-being in urban areas. *Environmental Research, 158,* 385–392. https://doi.org/10.1016/j.envres.2017.06.030

Wagenfeld, A., & Atchison, B. (2014). "Putting the occupation back in occupational therapy:" A survey of occupational therapy practitioners' use of gardening as an intervention. *The Open Journal of Occupational Therapy, 2*(4), Article 4. https://doi.org/10.15453/2168-6408.1128

Wagenfeld, A., & Marder, S. (2024). *Nature-based allied health practice: Creative and evidence-based strategies.* Jessica Kingsley Publishers.

Wagenfeld, A., Schefkind, S., & Hock, N. (2019). Measuring emotional response to a planting activity for staff at an urban office setting. *Open Journal of Occupational Therapy, 7*(2), Article 5. https://doi.org/10.15453/2168-6408.1532

Ward-Thompson, C. (2011). Linking landscape and health: The recurring theme. *Landscape and Urban Planning, 99*(3-4), 187–195. https://doi.org/10.1016/j.landurbplan.2010.10.006

Warner, R. P., & Dillenschneider, C. (2019). Universal design of instruction and social justice education: Enhancing equity in outdoor adventure education. *Journal of Outdoor Recreation, Education, and Leadership, 11*(4), 320–334. https://doi.org/10.18666/JOREL-2019-V11-I4-9543

Weerasuriya, R., Henderson-Wilson, C., & Townsend, M. (2019). A systematic review of access to green spaces in healthcare facilities. *Urban Forestry & Urban Greening, 40,* 125–132. https://doi.org/10.1016/j.ufug.2018.06.019

Wendelboe-Nelson, C., Kelly, S., Kennedy, M., & Cherrie, J. W. (2019). A scoping review mapping research on green space and associated mental health benefits. *International Journal of Environmental Research and Public Health, 16*(12), 2081. https://doi.org/10.3390/ijerph16122081

White, M. P., Alcock, I., Grellier, J., Wheeler, B. W., Hartig, T., Warber, S. L., Bone, A., Depledge, M. H., & Fleming, L. E. (2019). Spending at least 120 minutes a week in nature is associated with good health and wellbeing. *Scientific Reports, 9*(1), 1–11. https://doi.org/10.1038/s41598-019-44097-3

White, M. P., Elliott, L. R., Grellier, J., Economou, T., Bell, S., Bratman, G. N., Cirach, M., Gascon, M., Lima, M. L., Lõhmus, M., Nieuwenhuijsen, M., Ojala, A., Roiko, A., Schultz, P. W., van den Bosch, M., & Fleming, L. E. (2021). Associations between green/blue spaces and mental health across 18 countries. *Scientific Reports, 11*(1), 1–12. https://doi.org/10.1038/s41598-021-87675-0

Williams Goldhagen, S. (2017). *Welcome to your world: How the built environment shapes our lives.* Harper.

Wilson, E. O. (1984). *Biophilia.* Harvard University Press.

World Bank. (2022). *Urban development.* https://www.worldbank.org/en/topic/urbandevelopment/overview

World Health Organization. (2024). *Constitution.* https://www.who.int/about/accountability/governance/constitution

Yan, L., Liu, F., & Meng, X. (2022). Questionnaires assessing the anxiety alleviation benefits of indoor plants for self-isolated population during COVID-19. *International Journal of Low-Carbon Technologies, 17,* 300–307. https://doi.org/10.1093/ijlct/ctab102

Yeo, L. B. (2021). Psychological and physiological benefits of plants in the indoor environment: A mini and in-depth review. *International Journal of Built Environment and Sustainability, 8*(1), 57–67. https://doi.org/10.11113/ijbes.v8.n1.597

Yogman, M., Garner, A., Hutchinson, J., Hirsh-Pasek, K., Golinkoff, R. M.; Committee on Psychosocial Aspects of Child and Family Health; Council on Communications and Media. (2018). The power of play: A pediatric role in enhancing development in young children. *Pediatrics, 142*(3), e20182058. https://doi.org/10.1542/peds.2018-2058

York, M., & Wiseman, T. (2012). Gardening as an occupation: A critical review. *British Journal of Occupational Therapy, 75*(2), 76–84. https://doi.org/10.4276/030802212X13286281651072

Younan, D., Tuvblad, C., Li, L., Wu, J., Lurmann, F., Franklin, M., Berhane, K., McConnell, R., Wu, A. H., Baker, L. A., & Chen, J.-C. (2016). Environmental determinants of aggression in adolescents: Role of urban neighborhood greenspace. *Journal of the American Academy of Child & Adolescent Psychiatry, 55*(7), 591–601. https://doi.org/10.1016/j.jaac.2016.05.002

Yu, C. P., Lin, C. M., Tsai, M. J., Tsai, Y. C., & Chen, C. Y. (2017). Effects of short forest bathing program on autonomic nervous system activity and mood states in middle-aged and elderly individuals. *International Journal of Environmental Research and Public Health, 14*(8), 897. https://doi.org/10.3390/ijerph14080897

Zebrack, B., Kwak, M., & Sundstrom, L. (2017). First Descents, an adventure program for young adults with cancer: Who benefits? *Supportive Care in Cancer, 25*(12), 3665–3673. https://doi.org/10.1007/s00520-017-3792-7

The Home Environment: Permanent Supportive Housing

Deborah B. Pitts

Recovery for persons labeled with psychiatric disabilities involves a "reclaiming of the self" (Davidson & Strauss, 1992; Sells et al., 2004, p. 334; Sutton et al., 2012), a self that is often compromised by disruptions in engagement in occupational roles and the social stigma attached to mental illness (Milbourn et al., 2015). This reclaiming of the self is best accomplished through "role recovery" processes that include access to opportunities for engagement in occupations within supportive contexts (Leamy et al., 2011; Sutton et al., 2012).

Permanent supportive housing is one type of supportive context that has been developed and disseminated internationally to promote recovery by providing persons labeled with psychiatric disabilities access to the role of tenant. For persons seeking recovery, having a sense of home as a safe, supportive place to live, sleep, and carry out meaningful occupational roles can make the difference between full and limited participation in everyday life (Borg & Davidson, 2007; Padgett, 2007; Polvere et al., 2013).

This chapter describes the philosophical and operational elements of permanent supportive housing, including ways in which occupational therapy contributes to this service model. In particular, this chapter addresses how opportunities for choice, autonomy, privacy, and freedom are operationalized in the delivery of permanent supportive housing services and supported by public policy initiatives. It also illustrates occupational therapy's role in facilitating the transition from homelessness to housing and the provision of flexible supports to ensure successful housing tenure.

Home as Facilitating Context for Recovery

Experiencing a "sense of home" in one's living environment is said to promote a sense of well-being and contribute to overall quality of life (Seamon, 2015; Tuan, 2012). Philosophy, geography, and environmental psychology distinguish a sense of place from the spatial dimensions of a specific environmental context and emphasize the deep meaning and value that particular places can have for humans (Tuan, 1977), including the presence of personal objects (Borg et al., 2005; Csikszentmihalyi & Halton, 1981). A sense of home is particularly important for individuals with psychiatric disabilities, especially given the disruptions to stable housing that they have often experienced (Padgett, 2007; Piat et al., 2017).

This may be particularly important for persons experiencing homelessness as they transition into being housed (Boland et al., 2021; Chan, 2020; Marshall, Boland, et al., 2021; Marshall, Cooke, et al., 2021).

Recovery involves self-changes that include an individual's effort at "rebuilding/redefining [a] positive sense of identity" (Leamy et al., 2011, p. 448). Securing housing can lay a foundation upon which persons labeled with psychiatric disabilities who were formerly homeless "get back on track" and "explore new avenues" (Polvere et al., 2013, p. 111). Padgett (2007) describes "ontological security" as "the feeling of well-being that arises from a sense of constancy in one's social and material environment which, in turn, provides a secure platform for identity development and self-actualization" (p. 1926). In the accompanying PhotoVoice feature, Glen shares the powerful impact that having a consistent place to call home makes on his life.

Despite the potential for a sense of home to provide a place for recovery, permanent supportive housing contexts have been found to be somewhat contested places for experiencing a sense of home. For example, Alaazi et al. (2015) found in their exploration of Indigenous people's experience that a "sense of home remained disconnected for their housing experience, in the sense of being connected to land, family, and community" (p. 36). The same researchers noted that being in scattered versus community and family living situations in permanent supportive housing, as well as the restrictive guest practices (i.e., limited number of guests at a time, limited length of overnight stays) left residents feeling isolated. Further, they emphasize that for Indigenous people, "home is a blend of domestic, ceremonial, and spiritual spaces that allow for construction of a sense of belonging and health" (p. 36).

Permanent supportive housing settings did not afford or provide space or opportunities for residents to engage in such practices (e.g., sweat lodge, pipe ceremony). In addition, for persons labeled with psychiatric disabilities, their experience of being "at home" can be significantly impacted by specific features of the built environment (Fossey et al., 2020; Friesinger et al., 2019).

A Place for Control and Self-Determination

Empowerment has been identified as a key component of the recovery experience; it represents the experience of taking "personal responsibility" and "control over [one's

PhotoVoice

Glen

My house is a safe haven where I find peace and serenity. Not only is my house a home to me, but a place the squirrels call home as well. I enjoy watching the squirrels. Their interactions and movements relax me. I feel a sense of responsibility to the squirrels. I feed them corn, sunflower seeds, and bread daily. Every day I know when I get home, they will be waiting for me to feed them. While I am taking care of the squirrels, I am also taking care of myself because I feel peaceful and relaxed. It gives me a sense of recovery.

Can you analyze Glen's comments about his house and its impact on his recovery using the person-environment-occupation (PEO) perspective? Be sure to consider routines, meaning, impact on identity, and the physical and social environments.

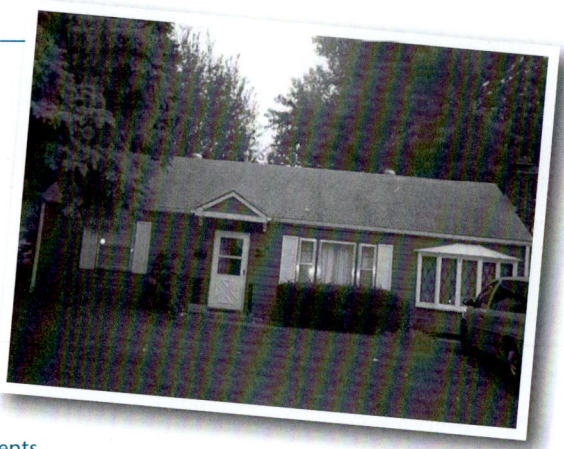

life" (Leamy et al., 2011). Having or being in one's own place seems to uniquely provide for such experiences (Borg et al., 2005; Kirst et al., 2014; Padgett, 2007; Polvere et al., 2013). Making even mundane choices about one's everyday life in one's own home comes to be experienced as personally meaningful and empowering—particularly when considered in stark contrast with previous experiences in psychiatric hospitals and/or residential treatment programs, where decisions about one's daily life were made by staff and/or driven by program rules (Farnworth & Muñoz, 2009; Fenton et al., 2014).

However, such opportunities aren't experienced without their tensions. As one transitions from homelessness or institutional life, they need time for "trying out and experimenting" how to make wise choices and feel confident about doing it on one's own (Lindstrom et al., 2009). Borg and colleagues (2005) provide some sense of how a person labeled with psychiatric disability describes the opportunities that home provides for establishing a sense of control and self-determination.

> The fact that I've been allowed to kind of just wander along. Allowed to make all the decisions without being put in place so much. That has been important to me . . . because when you're allowed to make mistakes as you go along, without being corrected all the time, then you realize that what you are doing might not be such a good idea. Like "sleeping in" in the mornings. (Borg et al., 2005, p. 249)

Building policies adopted by permanent supportive housing entities were also experienced as problematic. For example, tenants viewed surveillance practices such as the use of cameras and on-site staff as enhancing safety and security. However, building policies that limited access to the building communal spaces and amenities and regulated guests were seen as limiting autonomy and choice (Burgess et al., 2021).

A Place for Privacy and Freedom

The right to privacy is considered an important human right, and most democracies include legal and regulatory processes to protect privacy. Freedom to engage in certain types of personal actions within one's home is linked to this right to privacy. For persons labeled with psychiatric disability,

having one's own home may offer them privacy and freedom from the surveillance that comes with being placed—some consumers would say incarcerated—in psychiatric hospitals or long-term institutional settings (e.g., skilled nursing homes or residential care homes; Lindstrom et al., 2009; Padgett, 2007).

Having privacy also means that home can serve as a place of retreat, "as [a] haven[s] from the noise and stress of urban life" (Padgett, 2007, p. 1931), particularly from the social demands of daily life (Brown, 1996; Raphael-Greenfield & Gutman, 2015). This perspective is consistent with Corin and Lauzon's (1991) foundational work on "positive withdrawal" as an intentional, recovery-oriented strategy engaged in by persons labeled with schizophrenia as a way to mediate their interaction with the social world (Davidson, 2003; Sells et al., 2004).

Yet, having privacy and freedom also has its risks. Persons labeled with psychiatric disabilities must "balance privacy and social life" (Borg et al., 2005, p. 249) when living in their own place (Fossey et al., 2020; Raphael-Greenfield & Gutman, 2015). Studies exploring the experience of loneliness for persons labeled with psychiatric disabilities in supportive housing have been mixed (Weiner et al., 2010). Borg and colleagues (2005) again provide readers with a sense of how important privacy and freedom can be:

> I don't know. It's my private place. I don't want people to see me—that there are lots of dust balls around, dishes not done . . . whatever. I live my social life outside my home. At home I'm myself. (p. 250)

A Place for Engaging in Daily Life

Some of the earliest contemporary studies exploring recovery for persons labeled with psychiatric disability emphasized how being able to again engage in the everyday, mundane activities—such as making coffee or listening to the radio in one's own home—was experienced as important (Davidson & Strauss, 1992; Young & Ensing, 1999). Opportunities to engage in self-care practices, be active, and to connect with others were reported as particularly important (Young & Ensing, 1999). This perspective resonates with well-known mental health consumer researcher and advocate Patricia Deegan's findings on what she calls "personal medicine," which she defines as "non-pharmaceutical activities and strategies that serve to decrease symptoms and increase personal wellness" (Deegan, 2005, p. 32).

Qualitative studies exploring the experience of individuals who have transitioned from homelessness or long-term residential treatment settings into permanent supportive housing have found that being housed offers a "place" from which this reengagement can happen (Borg et al., 2005; Padgett, 2007; Raphael-Greenfield & Gutman, 2015).

> . . . you get your own room, you mind your business, you live by yourself, you know. You go down to the park, you look at the birds. Look at the dogs. What the hell. You say hello to normal people. (Padgett, 2007, p. 1931)

The importance of healthy routines is further explored in Chapter 14: Time Use and Habits.

Need for and Barriers to Access to Housing

The need for and barriers to securing housing for persons labeled with psychiatric disabilities include the limitations and problems associated with historical and institutional approaches to providing housing, as well as homelessness and poverty. Stigma and discrimination are other issues to consider.

Limitation of the Linear Continuum Approach

Early models of housing for persons labeled with psychiatric disabilities provided sequential and graded reintroduction into community life, primarily from institutions. The idea underlying this approach, referred to as the **linear continuum paradigm** (Ridgway & Zipple, 1990), was to match the needs of the person with the level of housing. The person then moved from one level of care to another as their level of support needs changed and living skills improved. Understood as a transitional approach, proponents of the linear continuum argued that people discharged from psychiatric hospitals needed a place to develop the skills for community living before "going it alone."

It was believed that skill development was especially needed because lengthy institutional stays of the time may have atrophied what independent living skills existed before the hospital admission or limited the individual's ability to develop such skills if they had not had any tenure in independent living before that admission (Glasscote et al., 1971; Raush & Raush, 1968; Rothwell & Doniger, 1966). One of the earliest examples of one level of care in the linear continuum paradigm, the **halfway house**, was Woodley House. Located in Washington, DC, Woodley House was developed and staffed by occupational therapists Joan Doniger and Edith Maeda. The initial halfway house established in 1958 housed 10 residents and was expanded in the mid-1970s to include an apartment program as well (Doniger et al., 1963; Kresky et al., 1976; Rothwell & Doniger, 1966).

Paul Carling (Hogan & Carling, 1992) is credited with first challenging this approach. One criticism of this approach was that, for persons labeled with psychiatric disabilities, moving from one level of care to the next disrupted the formation of interpersonal relationships that were critical for success and satisfaction, and the need to adjust to each new context was seen as stressful (Forchuk et al., 2006). Tsemberis and Asmussen (1999) identified additional risks, including:

- Skills learned for successful functioning in a structured congregate setting are not necessarily transferable to an independent living situation.
- Residents of such settings lack choices and freedoms; residential treatments offer standardized levels of care to which the person must adapt.
- Placement into a level of supervised housing is based on the decision of clinical staff, and people are afforded little privacy or control. (p. 116)

Problems With Custodial Housing

Custodial housing settings include congregate-living environments that are most often operated for profit by private landlords, including residential care homes, boarding homes, and board and care homes. The term **board and care home** describes living arrangements that provide shelter, food, and 24-hour supervision or protective oversight and personal care services to residents. Other terms for board and care homes include *homes for the aged, residential care homes, adult foster care, domiciliary care,* and *assisted-living facilities.* These might best be understood as sites of profound occupational deprivation (Farnworth & Muñoz, 2009; Hammell & Iwama, 2012; Suto & Frank, 1994).

Although regulations in some states may require such settings to have an activity program, this may depend on the size of the home (i.e., number of residents) and is often limited. Seldom are such programs individually tailored or based on personal preferences consistent with a recovery-orientation, unless that resident has outreach support from other mental health services. In addition to having limited site-based activity programs and/or physical plants that support a range of activity opportunities (e.g., outside spaces), few of these settings assist residents in accessing recreational and cultural activities in the community (Substance Abuse and Mental Health Services Administration [SAMHSA], 2006).

Risk and Impact of Homelessness

Persons labeled with psychiatric disabilities have been identified as having a greater risk of experiencing homelessness, particularly those receiving or having received services from the public mental health system (Folsom et al., 2005; Kuno et al., 2000; Roos et al., 2014; Viron et al., 2014). In addition, homelessness is understood to have serious consequences for one's recovery, including increased long-term psychological, social emotional, and health risks, as well as increased risk of trauma and assault (Castellow et al., 2015; Padgett et al., 2012; Tsai & Rosenheck, 2015). The topic of homelessness is covered in more detail in Chapter 42: Homelessness and Housing Insecurity.

Impact of Poverty

Poverty has been linked to increased morbidity and mortality (Boyer et al., 2014). Given that persons labeled with psychiatric disabilities are less likely to be employed and receiving federal disability payments, they are also more likely to be living in poverty (National Alliance on Mental Illness [NAMI], 2014; Sylvestre et al., 2018). Poverty limits access to the basics needed for everyday life, seriously restricts full participation in meaningful roles, and constrains a person's ability to secure access to safe, affordable housing. In 2023, the average income for a person receiving federal disability support through Supplemental Security Income (SSI) in the United States was more than $4,000 below the federal poverty guidelines.

- The U.S. Department of Health & Human Services (USDHHS) for 2024 defines poverty in one-person households as an annual income of $15,000.
- The U.S. Social Security Administration (SSA) identified the annual SSI federal payments for 2024 for an individual as $11,321.49 ($943.00 monthly).

Individuals receiving federal disability support through the Social Security Disability Insurance (SSDI) program are slightly more advantaged, but still hover near the federal poverty level. There are some efforts to reduce the impact of poverty associated with SSDI and SSI. For example, in some states persons receiving such benefits may also be eligible for the U.S. Department of Agriculture (USDA) Food and Nutrition Service's Supplemental Nutrition Assistance Program (SNAP), more commonly known as "food stamps." In addition, the SSA also has special rules that make it possible for persons receiving Social Security or SSI to work and still receive benefits.

Stigma and Discrimination

Stigma and discrimination are significant barriers to recovery in general and access to safe and affordable housing in particular (Pescosolido et al., 2010), and both have been found to negatively impact the stability of housing for persons who have experienced homelessness (Mejia-Lancheros et al., 2021). Discrimination in housing may occur when individuals document that they are unemployed and/or receiving SSDI or SSI as their main income source. In addition, multiple or extended periods of psychiatric hospitalization and/or homelessness mean that an individual may not have well-established tenancy histories.

Community resistance, often referred to as "not in my back yard," or NIMBYism, to locating housing for different disability groups has been documented, and the reactions of communities toward integration of persons labeled with psychiatric disabilities have been particularly harmful (Piat, 2000; Zippay & Lee, 2008). This may impact strategies utilized by supportive housing developers and local governmental authorities to site new housing projects for persons labeled with psychiatric disabilities (Fjellfeldt et al., 2021). See Chapter 27: Mental Health Stigma and Sanism, Chapter 28: Social Determinants and Mental Health, and Chapter 32: The Neighborhood and Community. 🤝

Public Policy Initiatives to Address Barriers to Housing

Both nationally and internationally, public policy efforts have been leveraged to address the previously identified barriers and to increase access for persons labeled with psychiatric

disabilities to safe, affordable housing. In the United States, the New Freedom Commission on Mental Health (USDHHS, 2003) and the SAMHSA's Transformation Action Agenda (USDHHS, 2005) promoted the adoption of permanent supportive housing by state and local mental health authorities.

Although there were efforts by some institutions during the mid-1800s "moral treatment" and the early 1900s "mental hygiene" eras in the United States to help those individuals being discharged to resettle into the community following an extended hospitalization experience (Goldstein & Godemont, 2003; Meyer, 1915/1952; Tuntiya, 2006), these programs were never widespread. More recent public policy efforts have focused on homelessness, which has been identified as a national crisis (National Law Center on Homelessness & Poverty, 2017; United States Interagency Council on Homelessness. A significant number of persons experiencing homelessness are also experiencing mental illness and/or substance abuse (SAMHSA, 2023). See Chapter 26: The Public Policy Environment. 🤝

The Right to Live in the Community

The right to live in the community is seen as a key civil rights protection for persons labeled with psychiatric disabilities (Dorvil et al., 2005). The U.S. 1990 *Americans with Disabilities Act* (ADA) extended protections established by Section 504 of the Rehabilitation Act of 1973, requiring that persons living with disabilities be provided services in the most integrated setting and appropriate to their needs.

The **Olmstead Integration Mandate** ensured these protections. *Olmstead* was the 1999 U.S. Supreme Court decision in response to a case presented to the court on behalf of Lois Curtis and Elaine Wilson. Both women remained in a state long-term psychiatric hospital despite their treatment team having recommended discharge to a community program. The treatment team had been unable to find a community resource that met their needs. Considered a landmark decision, the Supreme Court found that institutional confinement deprives people of most of what is valued in life: family relations, social contacts, work, educational advancement and cultural enrichment (*Olmstead v. L.C.*, 1999).

The Supreme Court's decision included the requirement that public entities "administer services, programs, and activities in the most integrated setting appropriate to the needs of the qualified individuals with disabilities" (28 C.F.R. 35.130(d)). Each state is now required to submit an *Olmstead* plan to the Centers for Medicare and Medicaid Services (CMS) that addresses how they will meet the integration mandate as part of their long-term care systems. In addition, there have been efforts on the part of advocates to utilize the Olmstead Integration Mandate to reduce the use of institutional settings, in particular Institutions for Mental Disease (IMD) and nursing homes as long-term placement options for persons labeled with psychiatric disability.

For example, two ADA/*Olmstead*-related court consent decrees in the State of Illinois—*Williams v. Quinn* (2010; IMD residents specifically) and *Colbert v. Quinn* (2011; nursing home residents specifically)—have required the state to evaluate and assist persons labeled with psychiatric disability residing in such institutions to be given the opportunity to live in the community. Illinois is noted here specifically, because Illinois occupational therapy practitioners (OTPs) succeeded in leveraging these legal actions to secure an expanded role for occupational therapy in mental health services (Mahaffey et al., 2015). Despite these efforts, in recent reviews of *Olmstead* given its 20th anniversary, advocates argued that it has not resulted in the hoped for full integration for persons labeled with psychiatric disabilities (Luken, 2022). Indeed, there have been some calls to "bring back the asylum" (Sisti, 2015, p. 243).

The Right to Fair Housing and Equal Access

Federal protections from discrimination because of disability are critical for access to permanent supportive housing for persons labeled with psychiatric disabilities. In the United States, the **Fair Housing Act (Title VIII of the Civil Rights Act of 1968)** prohibits discrimination in the sale, rental, and financing of dwellings based on race, color, religion, sex, or national origin. The Fair Housing Act was amended in 1988 to include persons with disabilities. It is illegal to deny housing, make housing otherwise unavailable, threaten, or intimidate. Equal access allows people opportunities to live where they want to live.

Along with **Section 504 of the Rehabilitation Act** and Title II of the ADA, the Fair Housing Act obligates landlords, property managers, and other housing providers to make reasonable accommodations and ensure that their housing practices are accessible and nondiscriminatory. Reasonable accommodations may include allowing a service animal despite "no pet" policies, reserving a parking space, allowing a live-in aide, allowing a nontenant to use laundry facilities, moving from one unit to another without a fee, changing the rent due date, and accepting a reference from a mental health provider if an applicant has no recent rental history.

The Right to Affordable Housing

Access to affordable and safe housing has been identified as a basic human right (Hartman, 1998; King, 2003; Thiele, 2002). Whereas previously identified public policy initiatives addressed the discrimination protections, the cost of housing can also be prohibitive, especially in urban areas. Although some states may provide financial resources for the development of supported housing (e.g., the California Mental Health Services Act–supported housing initiative), the primary source of public funds for financing new housing construction and rehabilitation of existing properties that provide rental assistance in the United States is the federal-level **Department of Housing and Urban Development** (HUD; see Table 31-1).

A key benefit of having HUD housing rental assistance is that the individual tenant is obligated to pay only 30% of their income for rent, despite the market value of the unit they are renting. This can make housing much more affordable when one's primary source of income is SSDI, SSI, and/or low-wage employment. In many parts of the United States, an affordable housing crisis has been documented further, especially for renters and low-income individuals and families (Ault et al., 2015), because of the scarceness of basic affordable housing options.

Permanent Supportive Housing

Permanent supportive housing has been described as "independent housing coupled with the provision of community-based mental health services" (Wong & Solomon, 2002, p. 13). Supportive housing emerged as a response to the limitations of the linear continuum paradigm described earlier, and as a way to facilitate transition from homelessness (Tsemberis & Eisenberg, 2000). It is an approach informed by the belief that:

> Every person with a psychiatric disability deserves a range of housing choices and *to live in a home of his or her own* (emphasis added). That includes the full rights of tenancy, including a lease, a key, privacy, and the choice of roommate, where relevant. (National Council on Disability, 2008)

The "Supported Life" Approach

Supported housing has evolved, along with other "supported life" approaches (e.g., supported employment and supported education), as a natural environment strategy to facilitate community integration for persons labeled with psychiatric disabilities (Salzer & Baron, 2006). Supported life approaches are founded on the belief that people with disabilities should have access to the same living, learning, and working environments as those individuals without disabilities. Persons with disabilities should not be segregated in "specialized" settings such as congregate living, or group homes, and/or sheltered work situations (Salzer & Baron, 2006).

Supported life approaches acknowledge that persons with disabilities *may* need certain types and levels of intensity of support beyond that typically accessed by persons without disabilities. However, supported life advocates emphasize the interdependent nature of human existence and emphasize that everyone, even people without disabilities, need ongoing support to sustain participation in living, learning, and working environments of choice. Whatever the nature of supports, the supported life perspective emphasizes that the support should be provided in real-world contexts and only at a level preferred by the person with the disability to ensure that they can sustain successful and satisfying participation in that environment (Kirsh et al., 2009).

Supported life approaches argue that the best way to learn to do "something" is to *do* that something. This is most commonly referred to in the community-integration literature as a paradigm shift from a "train-place" to a "place-train" perspective in psychiatric rehabilitation philosophy (Corrigan & McCracken, 2005).

The **place-train perspective** acknowledges the contextualized nature of learning and habit formation, particularly for major life roles, and eschews assumptions regarding the need for preparatory or transitional experiences (hence questioning the programs that train first in simulated environments) for persons with disabilities. Advocates of this approach acknowledge the developmental nature of skill building and habit formation across the life span. They emphasize that self-care, domestic care, and work-related habits and routines are learned and established by practicing them in those contexts in which they would be used with the specialized support of more skilled others and with the socioemotional support needed to take risks.

The Lived Experience

Peace of Mind

Marilyn Davis, in collaboration with her OTP Tessa Milman

I've lived here for a year now. I applied to live in this apartment about 10 years ago, and I had been on the waiting list ever since then. I was living with a boyfriend in Covina, and when my boyfriend put me out, I went and lived with one of my girlfriends in Fullerton. So I was totally homeless at that time. Garden Villa (the apartments) had called me while I was staying with him to come in for the interview. But I guess God just didn't feel like helping me out at that time and made it very difficult for me. So it took me like 3 months to get in here after they called me.

When I first moved in, it was wonderful. It was exhilarating to have my own place, you know with no rules, nobody telling me what I can and cannot do. That was the greatest joy of it all, having my own place. I made me some tacos—which is my favorite. You know money was scarce for me at that time. Food was really tight. I went hungry there for a few days, but God provided for me. You know from my church, I got a little help from my church. They gave me a check to get some food because I was without for about a month when I first moved in.

What do I like about being here? My peace of mind. My solitude. That I can be in here and think and plan the rest of my life out. It was hard to do that when I didn't have my own place. The pressures of being in somebody else's house, where you got to do what they want you to do—it was very hard. Even though I was paying my money to be there, I didn't have control of my own life.

There are some things about this place that bother me. The constant wantin' to come in and see this and do that and always knocking on my door with notices for this, that, and the other. I mean these inspections—I don't think they are warranted like they should be. They come in, I mean every 2 or 3 months there is somebody wanting to come into my house and see something or do something. It doesn't make me feel comfortable. Because a lot of times I don't feel good—I don't feel like getting up because of my physical ailments. You know . . . And having to jump up and down for them is not good for me. Sometimes, when I know the manager is coming, I light up a cigarette real quick and start smoking. The manager doesn't like cigarette smoke, so when he opens the door and smells it, he tells me he will just come back another time. I have to do those kinds of things to keep my privacy. I'd really just rather relax. But other than that it's a quiet building. You know people are not running up and down the hallways and that's a good thing.

Since I've lived here, I'm not as stressed out as I was before. I don't have to take as many medications just to have some peace of mind. Before, I was taking everything the doctor was giving me just to have some peace of mind. Even though it left me out of it, I'd rather feel out of it than be in it because then I would have been arguing with people. So I just stayed out of it. Now that I have an environment that gives me peace of mind, I don't have to take the medication as often. Every now and then I get depressed, of course, you know, this is my first time ever living alone. You know the first time I really ever lived alone was back in 1979 when I divorced my husband, but I wasn't alone for long. You know . . . But you know this is the first time I've ever really lived alone—no children, no nothing. It's a big difference. Of course I get lonely in here; I want some company. But I think about it—I'm like, "Do I really need company? No." I can watch TV all night if I want to. And not having anybody telling me to "turn the TV down or off or cut the lights or clean this up"—it's a big weight off my shoulders, a big weight.

Core Elements of Permanent Supportive Housing

The core elements of permanent supportive housing include choice of housing; functional separation of housing and services; decent, safe, and affordable housing; housing integration; access to housing; and flexible, voluntary, and recovery-focused services (SAMHSA, 2010b, p. 1).

Choice of housing distinguishes permanent supportive housing from other approaches by its fundamental commitment to providing consumers with "choice/control over where they live, how they live, and the professional support that they receive" (Nelson & Peddle, 2005, p. 1573). Paul Carling (1993, 1995) and Ridgway & Zipple (1990) are credited with defining this key characteristic of supported housing, noting the philosophical perspective of the independent living movement for persons with physical disabilities as a key influence. This feature of permanent supportive housing challenges what is often described as the coercive nature of discharge placement decisions (SAMHSA, 2010b; see Box 31-1). Research suggests that what is most important about choice in housing is its impact on the tenant's psychological well-being and subjective quality of life (Friesinger et al., 2019; Tsai & Rosenheck, 2012).

Functional separation of housing and services is considered a critical operational element in permanent supportive housing. This feature ensures that the tenant with psychiatric disabilities is the primary lessee or mortgage holder, not a mental health or social service agency. It is important that the housing provided as part of permanent supportive housing be a "home for life . . . [not a] treatment way-station" (Bigelow, 1998, p. 403). Access to the housing is based solely on the person meeting their tenancy obligations, not on the individual's compliance with treatment or willingness to accept the support services offered. Therefore, it is recommended that the mental health agency providing the support services *not* serve as the landlord.

Many mental health agencies providing housing services partner or contract with a property management company to handle property management issues, whereas the mental health agency continues to focus on the provision of the support services. When a single agency performs both the property management and support services, it is important to institute procedures that establish a "firewall" between these

TABLE 31-1 | U.S. Public Policy Initiatives Providing Funding for Permanent Support Housing

Federal Program	Who Is Eligible?	What Is Provided?
Housing and Urban Development (HUD) Housing Choice Voucher Program	Very low income families, older adults, and those who are disabled	Assists very low income families, older adults, and those who are disabled to afford decent, safe, and sanitary housing in the private market. The participant is free to choose any housing that meets the requirements of the program and is not limited to units located in subsidized housing projects. Housing choice vouchers are administered locally by public housing agencies (PHAs). The PHAs receive federal funds from HUD to administer the voucher program. A housing subsidy is paid to the landlord directly by the PHA on behalf of the participant. The participant then pays the difference between the actual rent charged by the landlord and the amount subsidized by the program.
Housing and Urban Development (HUD) Section 811 Supportive Housing Program for Persons With Disabilities	Nonprofit agencies	Provides funding to develop and subsidize rental housing with the availability of supportive services for very low and extremely low income adults with disabilities. Authorized to operate in two ways: (1) the traditional way, by providing interest-free capital advances and operating subsidies to nonprofit developers of affordable housing for persons with disabilities; and (2) providing project rental assistance to state housing agencies.
Housing and Urban Development (HUD) Continuum of Care (CoC) Program	Individuals who are homeless with disabilities, primarily psychiatric disabilities and addiction	Designed to promote a community-wide commitment to the goal of ending homelessness; to provide funding for efforts by nonprofit providers, states, Indian Tribes or tribally designated housing entities (TDHEs; as defined in section 4 of the Native American Housing Assistance and Self-Determination Act of 1996 [25 U.S.C. 4103]), and local governments to quickly rehouse homeless individuals, families, persons fleeing domestic violence, dating violence, sexual assault, and stalking, and youth while minimizing the trauma and dislocation caused by homelessness; to promote access to and effective utilization of mainstream programs by homeless individuals and families; and to optimize self-sufficiency among those experiencing homelessness.
Money Follows the Person (MFP)	Persons who reside in a hospital, a nursing home, an intermediate care facility for people with intellectual disabilities, or an institution for people with a mental illness who could be served in a home- or community-based setting	Federal grant Medicaid program that was established to make home- and community-based services (HCBS) more accessible to seniors and persons with disabilities, while simultaneously decreasing the need for Medicaid-funded nursing home care

two functions. As noted by SAMHSA (2010b), "vigilance is needed to ensure that confidentiality is maintained and that coercion does not occur" (p. 2).

Decent, safe, and affordable housing addresses the critical importance of the quality of the living environment to recovery, as well as how the common experience of poverty can make this element of support housing so challenging to achieve (Henwood et al., 2015; Padgett, 2007; Raphael-Greenfield & Gutman, 2015; Ridgway et al., 1994; Whitley & Henwood, 2014). A key strategy for increasing the quality and affordability of housing for persons labeled with psychiatric disabilities has been to ensure access to housing subsidies. In the United States, HUD is responsible for ensuring access to affordable housing, and some of the initiatives outlined in Table 31-1 are available to persons labeled with psychiatric disabilities and addiction.

Although affordability is a key concern, safety is also an important component of permanent supportive housing. The experience or need for safety is partly influenced by past experiences of trauma, as well as the "unpredictability of street and shelter life" (Raphael-Greenfield & Gutman, 2015).

The concept of **housing integration**, ensuring that people with psychiatric disabilities live alongside individuals without psychiatric disabilities, rather than clustered in predominantly psychiatric communities, relates directly to the *Olmstead* decision described earlier, specifically that the expressed preferences of persons labeled with psychiatric disabilities and addiction must be considered in housing programs (Tsai et al., 2010; Tsai & Rosenheck, 2012). Although there are different configurations of permanent supportive housing, advocates argue that **scattered-site housing** or mixed-use buildings are more likely to achieve this objective (SAMHSA, 2010b). In scattered-site housing, persons in need of permanent supportive housing reside in apartment buildings in which the majority of tenants are not people with psychiatric disabilities. This housing configuration is more aligned with a key criterion for integration.

A common criticism of community integration efforts is that persons labeled with psychiatric disabilities may be living in the community but are not fully engaged in the life of the local community (Whitley & Henwood, 2014; Yanos et al., 2012).

BOX 31-1 ■ Housing and Coercion: Why Coercion Is Not Part of Evidence-Based Practice

Coercion undermines the helping alliance and the ethical relationship between helpers and consumers.

Coercing people to accept a particular residential setting and prebundled set of services rarely meets people's unique needs.

Coercing people to live in a particular place or accept a particular service package may violate federal law and policies, which prohibits discrimination or social segregation based on disability.

Coercion often denies consumers the right to live as others do, including the right to take an active role in their home and community.

Coercive programs often engender and maintain social stigma.

Coercion can be especially counterproductive in helping people who have experienced trauma.

From Substance Abuse and Mental Health Services Administration. (2010). Permanent supportive housing: Training frontline staff (Module 3, p. 7). HHS Pub. No. SMA-10-4509. Center for Mental Health Services, U.S. Department of Health and Human Services.

Therefore, attention to facilitating daily routines and rituals that engage the person in the local community must be included in any supported housing context (Marshall & Rosenberg, 2014; Marshall, Boland, et al., 2021; Raphael-Greenfield & Gutman, 2015; Stergiopoulos et al., 2014). This could include, for example, participating in local organizations, attending local social and recreational events, and voting.

Access to housing is intended to address both the discriminatory protections that have been established (*Olmstead v. L.C.* 1999), and the readiness perspective argued by the linear continuum model described earlier. **Housing First** is an approach to permanent supportive housing intended to target persons labeled with psychiatric disabilities and addiction who are also experiencing homelessness (Tsemberis, 2010; Tsemberis & Asmussen, 1999; Tsemberis & Eisenberg, 2000; Tsemberis et al., 2004).

Key elements of this approach include rapid placement in housing, low barrier admission policies, and few to no programmatic prerequisites (e.g., sobriety or other readiness criteria). Housing First combines scattered-site housing with what is known as intensive case management and/or Assertive Community Treatment (ACT). Housing First providers do "whatever it takes" to support the tenant.

Whatever it takes means finding the methods and means to engage a client, determine his or her needs for recovery, and create collaborative services and support to meet those needs. This concept may include innovative approaches to "no-fail" services in which service provision and continuation are not dependent upon amount or timeliness of progress, or on the client's compliance with treatment expectations, but rather on individual needs and individual progress and/or pace on their path to recovery. Clients are not withdrawn from services based

on pre-determined expectations of response. (California Institute for Mental Health [CIMH], 2011, p. 12)

The Housing First model has been widely disseminated both nationally and internationally, and research has demonstrated its effectiveness (Aubry et al., 2014; Kirst et al., 2015; O'Shaughnessy et al., 2020). In addition to the United States, Canada (Gaetz et al., 2013) and Australia (Johnson et al., 2012), in particular, have prioritized the Housing First approach and contributed substantially to the research regarding this approach, particularly the portability of innovative programs across borders. Also see Chapter 35: Practice Across the Continuum of Service Needs.

When paired with access to housing, **flexible, voluntary, and recovery-focused services** serve the critical "support" function. A hallmark of these services is that they are provided at an intensity directed by the tenant—not by the tenant's mental health services provider. As such, the level and nature of the supports change as the person's needs or wants change. Common support services used by people labeled with psychiatric disabilities include financial support to pay for rent, professional support to assist with obtaining and maintaining the apartment, choices for safe and comfortable housing, and opportunities for social contact and community integration (SAMHSA, 2010a). Varying configurations for support service exist across permanent supportive housing contexts.

Because some HUD programs finance supportive services, as well as housing subsidies, organizations that provide housing may have residential service coordinators (RSCs) or case managers on their staff to provide support services. RSCs or case managers are most typically nonlicensed mental health providers who might have lived experience in recovery and/or homelessness. They serve as the primary support person in permanent supportive housing settings and are the primary provider with whom OTPs working in permanent supportive housing will collaborate.

In addition to RSCs or case managers, mental health and/or substance abuse providers may also be available depending on the configuration and funding in a particular jurisdiction. In addition to HUD, the U.S. publicly funded health plan for low-income individuals known as Medicaid has also been leveraged to fund supportive services, in particular services that target the mental health and general health needs of tenants (Burt et al., 2014).

When scattered-site approaches are used, the tenant is more likely to be supported by mental health providers from an ACT or intensive services community mental health team. Internationally, OTPs are part of such teams (Arbesman et al., 2011; Fossey et al., 2006; Marshall & Rosenberg, 2014; Nolan & Swarbrick, 2002).

Occupational Therapy in Permanent Supportive Housing

OTPs can make meaningful contributions and play important roles in facilitating the transition to and sustained success for persons with mental illness in permanent supportive housing. Internationally, OTPs have demonstrated these contributions in both practice and research

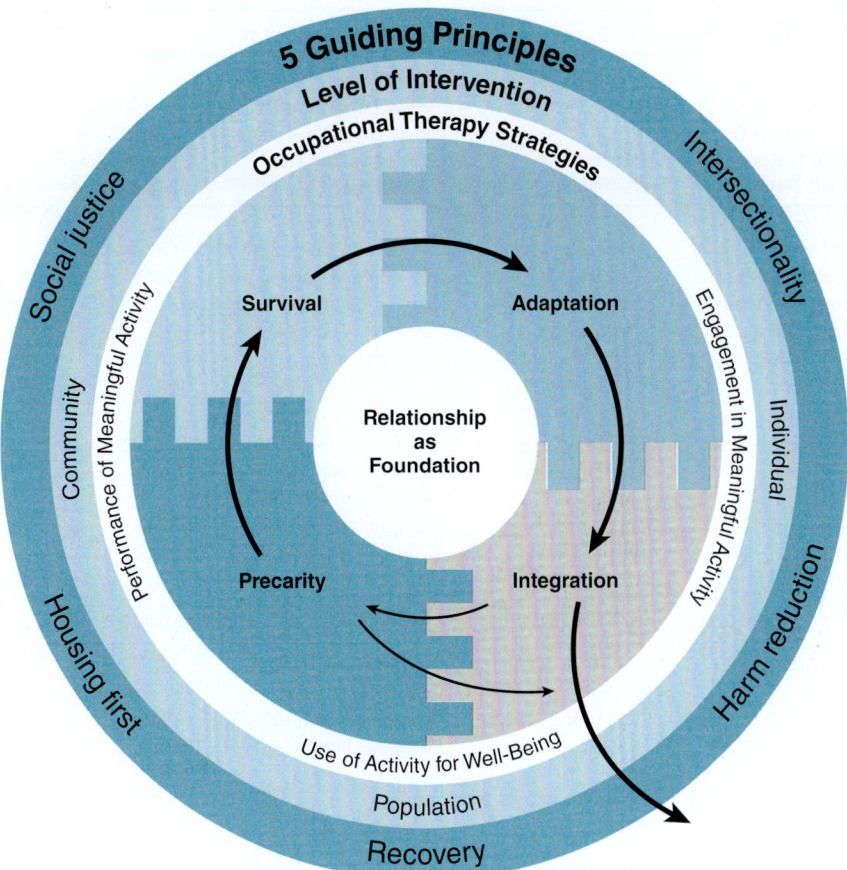

FIGURE 31-1. Bridging the Transition From Homeless to Housed Framework. *From Marshall, C. A., Barbic, S., Gewurtz, R., Roy, L., Lysaght, R., Ross, C., Becker, A., Cooke, A., & Kirsh, B. (2020).* Bridging the transition from homeless to housed: A social justice framework to guide the practice of occupational therapists *(p. 7).* Ontario Society of Occupational Therapists.

(Fossey et al., 2006; Kirsh et al., 2009; Kirsh et al., 2011; Marshall, Boland, et al., 2021; Nolan & Swarbrick, 2002; Raphael-Greenfield & Gutman, 2015) and are making contributions to the theoretical perspectives (see Fig. 31-1) regarding the transition to housing as well (Marshall, Boland et al., 2020; Marshall, Cooke et al., 2021; Marshall & Rosenberg, 2014).

OTPs in permanent supportive housing may serve as direct service providers and/or consultants to other team members. As a **direct service provider**, the OTP will meet with individual tenants, utilizing the findings from their own assessment as well as information from other team members. When the OTP is serving as a **consultant** to other team members, they will utilize the findings from their assessment to give the team guidance regarding the design of individually tailored supports to meet the tenant's needs. Whether a direct service provider or consultant, the OTP brings their unique perspective on humans as occupational beings, along with occupational therapy values, knowledge, and skill sets related to occupation, participation, and psychiatric disability.

Practitioners in the permanent supportive housing context are most likely to be members of an intensive community mental health team (i.e., ACT team) or be directly employed by the housing organization itself. When the OTP is a member of an ACT team, providing housing supports will be only one part of their "generalist" role within a transdisciplinary team. That is, the OTPs will address all areas of occupational needs, and not simply focus on housing. Practitioners

directly employed by the housing organization are more likely to function as specialists with a particular focus on the individual's successful tenancy.

Table 31-2 outlines key information about common evaluation tools to help guide the OTP's therapeutic reasoning during the evaluation process. These tools are likely to be familiar to OTPs, as they are not designed to specifically address housing issues. However, reflective OTPs applying culturally responsive approaches will use these tools to elicit evaluative data that supports their understanding of and interventions for the persons' housing issues.

Facilitating the Transition

Persons with psychiatric disabilities are most often transitioning to permanent supportive housing either from the streets after extended periods of homelessness or from long-term institutional settings, such as board and care homes, residential treatment settings, skilled nursing facilities, and/or state hospitals.

The process of transition is best understood as complex and fraught with risks and challenges (Raphael-Greenfield & Gutman, 2015), particularly in the early days of transitioning to housing from the streets for persons experiencing homelessness (Stergiopoulos et al., 2014). Marshall (2016) explicitly frames this move from the street to housing as an

TABLE 31-2 | Therapeutic Reasoning Assessment Table: The Person in the Home Environment

Which Tool?	Who Was This Tool Designed For?	Is This a Type of Tool the Person Can Do? What Is Required of the Person?	What Am I Measuring?	How Long Does It Take and Where Do I Administer This Assessment?	Is the Tool Associated With a Practice Model?
Occupational Performance History Interview-II (OPHI-II; Kielhofner et al., 2004)	Adolescents and adults with cognitive capacity sufficient to engage in reflection	Semistructured interview format requires person to be able to reflect and verbally communicate	Person's occupational identity, occupational competence, and occupational behavior settings (e.g., home, work)	Approximately 45 minutes, plus time for documentation, and can be conducted in any context conducive to conversation	Model of Human Occupation (MOHO)
Occupational Self-Assessment (OSA), Version 2.2 (Baron et al., 2006)	Adolescents and adults with cognitive capacity sufficient to engage in reflection	Self-report format	Person's perception of occupational competence and importance for specific set of everyday activities	Administrative time varies depending on person, typically completed within 30 minutes, with additional time for review and goal setting	MOHO
Residential Environment Impact Scale (Fisher et al., 2014)	Primarily intended for community-dwelling adults with disabilities residing in group homes, supportive housing, or independent housing	Semistructured interview of resident and staff, if present, informed by specific interview; therapist observation of engagement in activities within residence and "walk-through"	Impact of environment (i.e., space, objects, relationships, activities) on person–occupation engagement	Administration time varies on components completed; estimated time is 3 hours	MOHO
Test of Grocery Shopping Skills (TOGSS; Brown et al., 2009)	Individuals labeled with psychiatric disabilities experiencing functional difficulties	Standardized assessment in which person is required to find 10 specific grocery items in a grocery store	Evaluating person's *executive functioning* ability, as measured by accuracy and efficiency in locating specific grocery items	Administration time varies depending on individual; usually fewer than 30 minutes	Not associated with a specific conceptual practice model
Allen Cognitive Level Screen 5 (ACLS-5; Allen et al., 1992; Earhart et al., 2022)	Individuals who have, or are suspected to have, impairments in cognition that affect their *global* ability to function	Standardized assessment that requires person to follow verbal/visual directions and to problem-solve in order to complete three different leather lacing tasks	*Functional cognition,* including the complex and dynamic interactions between a person's cognitive abilities and their context that produce observable task behavior	Administration time depends on a person's cognitive capacity and fatigue level; results of screening should never be used alone, but must be verified with other tools (e.g., ADM, RTI-E)	Cognitive Disabilities Model
Allen Diagnostic Modules (ADM; Earhart, 2006)	Individuals who have, or are suspected to have, impairments in cognition that affect their *global* ability to function	Standardized assessment that requires person to manipulate tools and materials to replicate various craft activities from a sample (e.g., placemat)	*Functional cognition,* including the complex and dynamic interactions between a person's cognitive abilities and their context that produce observable task behavior	Administration time depends on a person's cognitive capacity and fatigue level; it can be conducted in any setting that has a table top; often conducted in group format with up to four persons	Cognitive Disabilities Model

TABLE 31-2 | Therapeutic Reasoning Assessment Table: The Person in the Home Environment—cont'd

Which Tool?	Who Was This Tool Designed For?	Is This a Type of Tool the Person Can Do? What Is Required of the Person?	What Am I Measuring?	How Long Does It Take and Where Do I Administer This Assessment?	Is the Tool Associated With a Practice Model?
Routine Task Inventory-Expanded (RTI-E; Katz, 2006)	Individuals who have, or are suspected to have, impairments in cognition that affect their *global* ability to function	Interview of person and caregiver based on routine task checklist, and therapist observation of person's performance of routine tasks	*Routine task behavior,* including self-care, instrumental activities of daily living (IADL) at home and in community, social communication, readiness for work	Administration time varies depending on areas assessed, as well as communicative ability of person and caregiver	Cognitive Disabilities Model
Adolescent/Adult Sensory Profile (AASP; Brown & Dunn, 2002)	Adolescents and/or adults experiencing functional difficulties	Self-report questionnaire; can also be administered by reading questions and recording person's responses	Person's perception of everyday sensory experiences in comparison with population	Administration time 10–15 minutes, with additional time to score and interpret findings	Dunn's Sensory Processing Model

"**occupational transition**," drawing on the work of Crider and colleagues (2014, as cited in Marshall, 2016) who note "the importance of meaningful engagement, how occupations are disrupted and impacted, the use of occupation to regain control, and that a new occupational balance emerges as a result of the transition" (p. 12). Drawing on research exploring self and narrative theories of housing transitions for persons who were formerly homeless, Marshall and Rosenberg (2014) make a case for a focus on helping the person in permanent supportive housing to develop a **housed identity** (Marshall & Rosenberg, 2014, p. 330). They emphasize that:

> Enhancing a person's opportunity to engage in occupations associated with those performed during a housed state may be a way of fortifying a positive sense of self and may contribute to the development of a new identity as a "housed person." Engaging in occupations required to function independently as a person who is housed may also lead to decreased marginalization and increased social inclusion. By facilitating the transition from homeless to housed in a way that promotes the development of a housed identity and increases opportunities to engage in occupations, the likelihood of future relapse into homelessness may also be decreased. (Marshall & Rosenberg, 2014, p. 334)

OTPs in their role as direct service providers can facilitate the person's development of a housed identity by supporting the development of new daily routines that offer structure and are tied to their role as tenant. Further, the OTPs in their role as consultants can help the housing team be patient as the person moves away from temporal rhythms associated with street-based "survival occupations" to set and meet new goals once housed (Marshall et al., 2018, p. 42).

Although a significant amount of effort in permanent supportive housing has been focused on facilitating the transition of persons from homelessness to housing, facilitating the transition of persons from long-term institutional settings to housing is also of critical importance (SAMHSA, 2006).

Given that few institutional settings afford an individual the opportunity to engage in home care routines in particular, there have been efforts to address this population's transitional needs while still institutionalized (Leedahl et al., 2015). From a recovery-oriented perspective, this is particularly important given the evidence in the United States, and potentially other countries, that there has been an increase in the use of long-stay residential care centers (Knable et al., 2015) and, as noted earlier, calls to "bring back the asylum" (Sisti et al., 2015).

Housing options are always limited by the available housing in any particular community. Despite this limitation, the person's choice of housing must be guided by their personal preferences and unique support needs. It is the role of the housing team to facilitate this process in such a way that the housing that is secured meets the person's preferences and needs. OTPs are well suited for engaging in this process given their deep understanding of person-in-context, as well as the functional consequences of psychiatric disorders.

In addition, the occupational therapy profession uses assessment tools and intervention approaches that can help the person and the housing team identify support needs and design individually tailored support strategies, thus providing the team with valuable information to support their efforts in facilitating the transition process and help match the person to available housing options. One example of an OTP's interventions with transition to housing is provided in Box 31-2.

There is an important caveat that must be taken into account given the critical place that choice has in permanent supportive housing: The person's preferences take precedence over the assessed support needs. This means that the housing team is expected to support the choice of housing made by the person, even if they have concerns about its fit with the person's support needs. Although this may be challenging, in permanent supportive housing the team does "whatever it takes"

BOX 31-2 ■ A Story of Freedom

Contributed by Julian Prado, OTD, OTR/L

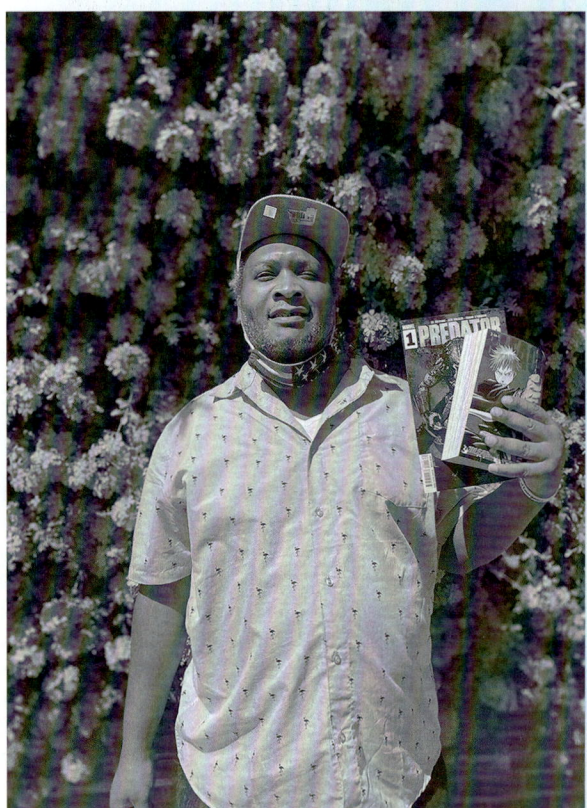

"Freedom. I don't have to share my space with anyone. I finally have my own place that I can take care of and I can do what I want. I feel free."—Kahwan

Kahwan is a 43-year-old Black man who loves comic books, enjoys listening to music, and hopes to return to school. He has a small community of friends that he's been in mental health programs with and many reside in the same building. Outside these friends and the staff, he has limited social supports. Kahwan received his label of mental illness, unspecified psychotic disorder, in his early 20s and reports feeling stigmatized. He was connected to a forensic mental health agency after being charged with a felony and being deemed unfit to stand trial.

Kahwan was placed in the FIST (Felony Incompetent to Stand Trial) community-based restoration program. He receives case management, psychotherapy, occupational therapy, and engages in a court competencies curriculum. After completing the FIST program, he was placed in an interim housing site to await permanent housing. He transitioned to the agency's Intensive Case Management Services (ICMS), which provides intensive wraparound services to high-need/high-barrier behavioral health populations in the LA County jail. ICMS includes case management, psychotherapy, substance use support, medication management, and occupational therapy. The program provides interim and permanent supportive housing for some of the most underserved, or highest utilizers, in the LA County system. Kahwan was referred to occupational therapy by an ICMS program manager to support preparations for living in his own apartment. Julian, Kahwan's occupational therapist completed an occupational profile and utilized the Occupational Self-Assessment to create person-centered goals.

Kahwan expressed interest in building home care skills and participating in leisure activities. While at interim housing, he is responsible for laundry and daily housekeeping. Kahwan experiences chronic low back pain and self-reports consistent symptoms of anxiety.

Some activities in his daily routine exacerbate his low back pain and limit his engagement in interim housing programming. Julian provided education around pacing and ergonomic positioning to use during activities of daily living and instrumental activities of daily living (ADLs/IADLs) to reduce back pain and to allow for engagement in activities beyond chores. Julian also supported Kahwan to explore leisure activities. Wait time for permanent housing is long and Kahwan worried excessively, impacting his mood and interactions with peers and housing staff. Julian taught Kahwan sensory strategies to support self-regulation and self-soothing when he felt overwhelmed by worrisome thoughts and anxiety.

After a year in interim housing, Kahwan moved into his own studio apartment in a metropolitan neighborhood of Los Angeles. He had access to onsite support staff including his OTP. Once settled, Kahwan asked for modified ergonomic strategies that fit his new living space and he continued to practice sensory strategies. Kahwan had difficulty adjusting to his new identity as a housed person and creating routines in his new home. He kept clothes in a large duffle bag and there was clutter throughout his home. Julian supported Kahwan in establishing home care routines around de-cluttering and laundry through the use of a visual chore schedule. The OTP also supported Kahwan to explore art-based leisure activities and to reengage in reading comic books.

Just over a year later, Kahwan is now a student at a local college studying business administration. He shares his studio apartment with his beloved cat, "Star." He meets regularly with his OTP, who supports his efforts to manage student responsibilities, maintain his apartment, and complete pet care routines. When reflecting on his work with Julian, his OTP, Kahwan noted, "I like how you approach situations and help me do things I wasn't sure I could."

Reflective Question

1. Reread Kahwan's story paying specific attention to Julian's use of self as Kahwan's OTP. Using examples from the story and Figure 31-2, define where you think Julian's approach exists on this continuum. Explain your response.

to meet the support needs within whatever housing the person chooses. Because OTPs highly value person-centered services, they may struggle with supporting the person's choice, and feel morally and legally obligated to be protective (American Occupational Therapy Association [AOTA], 2020).

Deegan (2005) drew on perspectives regarding self-determination for persons with disabilities to argue for what she calls the "recovery zone" (see Fig. 31-2). The recovery zone is that place on the continuum between doing nothing in response to a person's actions, despite concern, versus pushing the person to do what is wanted regardless of their point of view. Deegan, in her work on intentional care, calls this the "neglect over protect continuum," and emphasizes that OTPs can neither abandon nor control the person with whom they are working; rather, OTPs need to stay engaged, remain supportive, and explore options.

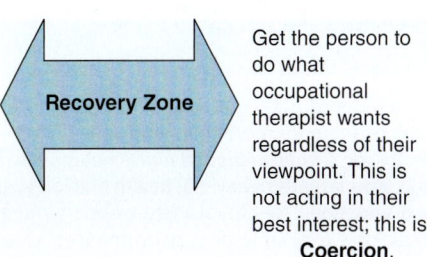

FIGURE 31-2. The recovery zone is that place on the continuum between doing nothing in response to a person's actions, despite concern, versus pushing the person to do something regardless of their point of view.

Helping the person to identify their preferences can be facilitated in many ways. The SAMHSA *Permanent Supportive Housing Evidence-Based Practices* toolkit (2010a) provides a housing preference checklist in its Tools for Tenants section. This checklist invites the person to rate the importance of certain aspects of their living environment; neighborhood; access to support, security, and visitors; and activities and pets.

Facilitating Sustained Tenancy

Once housing has been secured, the housing team must shift its focus to providing the supports needed to facilitate the person's housing tenure and success. This includes explicit strategies to facilitate effective tenancy behaviors and to promote community integration. Providing flexible supports within a supported-life approach means that the supports are enhanced or faded as needed and/or preferred by the tenant. A key aspect of supported-life approaches is the notion of providing the just-right supports, not more or less than is needed to ensure successful tenancy and community integration. The SAMHSA *Permanent Supportive Housing Evidence-Based Practices* toolkit emphasizes that "no cookie-cutter rules or approaches will work in every situation" (2010a, p. 5-2), noting that flexible supports include providing practical assistance, offering emotional support, teaching life skills, encouraging engagement in meaningful activity, supporting wellness, expanding social support networks, and so on.

Research indicates that departures from permanent supportive housing are more likely to be the result of problems rather than personal choice and often result in transitions back to higher levels of care (Wong & Solomon, 2002). Persons with problematic departures were more likely to be identified by housing providers as less likely to perform life skill tasks and to require more intensive supports (Wong & Solomon, 2002). Research exploring the early support needs of tenants in Housing First programs found that addressing social isolation, substance misuse, and life skills training were considered important by tenants and housing team members (Polvere et al., 2013; Stergiopoulos et al., 2014).

The need for explicit *life skills training*, in particular home management skills, may be related to periods of homelessness during which the person developed street-dwelling habits and routines, rather than those needed for being housed. In addition, periods of institutional living also limited the person's opportunity to engage in home care management routines. Practitioners in permanent supported housing can address each of these identified concerns, in particular life skills that may be impacted by neurocognitive deficits and sensory processing disruptions (Fossey et al., 2006).

OTPs are adept at determining whether the person has the **functional cognition** needed for successful enactment of home care routines, especially the more complex tasks that require judgments or the need to anticipate risks (e.g., cooking and budgeting). Practitioners can help housing teams identify and design individually tailored environmental supports when uptake of skills training is limited. In occupational therapy, cognition and process skills are most typically assessed through performance-based measures.

During the past decades, research regarding assessment practices in mental health has called for ecologically valid tools (Fossey et al., 2006; McKibbin et al., 2004), as well as tools that mediate what has been called the "competence/performance" distinction (Bromley & Brekke, 2010). This distinction represents what is well understood in occupational therapy: The ability to perform a skill does not mean that it will be performed in life when needed. Allen and colleagues (1992) clarified this in their articulation of the cognitive disabilities conceptual practice model's functional cognition—"can do, will do, may do"—guidance (McCraith et al., 2011). Such a view supports the need for assessment tools that help OTPs to better understand performance.

Various practice models can be applied to guide the OTP's therapeutic reasoning to address functional cognition. One example is the Cognitive Disabilities Model (Allen et al., 1992; McCraith et al., 2011; www.allencognitive.com), which identifies markers for when a person is most likely to be able to safely live without supports. Practitioners utilizing this conceptual practice model can provide guidance regarding what types of cognitive and/or environmental cues are needed to ensure successful performance of each home care management routine that the person must perform.

In addition, OTPs can advocate for housing organizations to conduct routine assessment of functional cognition given that many people experiencing psychiatric disability, substance abuse, and extended periods of homelessness may have residual cognitive deficits that can help explain their difficulties in independent living (Green et al., 2015; Rempfer, et al., 2003). If the housing organization takes this view, then OTPs can take the lead on educating both the property management and residential support services staff regarding how cognition impacts function. Having this understanding may allow these staff members to be less frustrated and more supportive as tenants make efforts to manage their day-to-day lives. Box 31-3 provides an example of the therapeutic reasoning an OTP might use to explore how addressing functional cognition can support success in staying housed for some individuals. Also see Chapter 7: Cognition and Chapter 8: Cognitive Beliefs.

In addition to neurocognitive impairments, persons labeled with psychiatric disabilities may also experience *sensory processing disruptions* (Bailliard & Whigham, 2017; Brown et al., 2002, 2020), in particular hypersensitivity (Kinnealey et al., 1995). Sensory processing disruptions impact quality of life (Pfeiffer et al., 2014; Sanchis-Asensi et al., 2022; Serafini et al., 2016) and mediating sensory defensiveness through

BOX 31-3   ■   Cognition and Housing

Jasper, a permanent supportive housing tenant, is a veteran presenting with posttraumatic stress syndrome (PTSD). He has a history of substance use and lived on the street for over two decades before moving into permanent supportive housing. Jasper spends most of his time in his unit and doesn't go out much. He has an in-home support worker who helps with home maintenance, and he welcomes and is responsive to support he receives from an ACT team and the on-site housing case manager. A Level II fieldwork occupational therapy student is at the housing site every day. The ACT team case manager is considering reducing support because their sense is that Jasper is doing well. The occupational therapy student works with Jasper almost daily, with visits varying from just a hello and check-in to longer visits. Recent check-ins with Jasper and the housing case manager note the following:

■ Jasper reported to the housing case manager that his toilet was not working right. The housing case manager helped Jasper submit a work order. Several days later the maintenance team worker arrived; however, during exchanges with this worker, Jasper stated the toilet was working fine. Maintenance left without checking the toilet.

■ The ACT team provides Jasper with money management and an in-home support worker does Jasper's shopping. Jasper reported to the housing case manager that he has no money to give his support worker. In exploring the situation with Jasper, the housing case manager learned that the ACT team case manager is on vacation.

■ Jasper also reported to the housing case manager that he is out of night medications. The housing case manager knows that the ACT team nurse had been doing home medication management visits, including setting up Jasper's pill case. Jasper reports that he has not seen the ACT team nurse for a while.

■ Jasper enjoys drinking soda daily. During an in-unit visit, the occupational therapy student notices many empty soda cans on the kitchen counter. The occupational therapy student has never noticed this before. Exploring further, Jasper shares that one of his neighbors collects cans and that neighbor recycles them for extra cash. The occupational therapy student knows, but it appears that Jasper does not, that this neighbor recently

entered a substance use residential rehabilitation program and will be there for more than a month.

Therapeutic reasoning around functional cognition: What's happening? Given Jasper's behavioral health and long-term homelessness, the occupational therapy student wonders whether cognitive deficits possibly explain Jasper's performances. Would providing individually tailored cognitive supports be of value? If so, what might they be?

■ *Would Jasper benefit from cognitive supports to track and prepare for future events?* The work order was put in, but Jasper didn't know when service would happen. The maintenance team schedules based on their availability and just "stops by" rather than prescheduling appointments. Jasper likely relied on a "brittle" verbal memory here. Since, the case manager likely did most of the actions to submit the work order, Jasper didn't have procedural memory to rely on as a future prompt. Jasper may not have a place in his unit to note such things (refrigerator, etc.). Further, Jasper may have adjusted to the problem with his toilet, which is often what happens, or the problem with the toilet could have resolved itself.

■ *Would Jasper benefit from cognitive supports to notice changes and initiate some action to avoid future problems?* Jasper didn't notice the amount of cans building up as a concern. This visual cue wasn't sufficient to prompt him to become aware that his neighbor hadn't visited and to find out why. He may have noticed the ACT team nurse hadn't visited, but this was not sufficient to cue him that this might impact his medication supply/practice. Only when his medication ran out did he notice the change. He connected this to his nurse visits only when the case manager initiated exploration of the situation. Jasper may have known the community mental health team case manager was on vacation, but prior planning may not have occurred regarding his need for money management. Reliance on the ACT team for two very important activities may warrant them not reducing their support yet or at all unless alternative supports, possibly natural supports, can replace the support—"serving as a cognitive exoskeleton"—the ACT team is providing. This may be especially important because the support from the occupational therapy student is time limited as well.

environmental adaptations may contribute to housing success (Brown, 2001). Tenants with sensory processing disruptions may experience very modest levels of noise coming from neighboring apartments as highly toxic and uncomfortable. They may initiate complaints to the apartment manager or directly to the tenant who is making the noise. This can result in problematic neighbor relations when the neighbor does not understand how everyday activities are experienced so loudly. In such cases, conflict resolution assistance may be required to help facilitate communications between the two tenants.

With assistance from the OTP, the tenant experiencing the noise levels can better understand the sensory experiences and initiate strategies that will help to mediate their discomforts (Brown, 2001). The OTP can also educate the mental health provider, apartment manager, and possibly other tenants about how sensory disruptions can impact function; this can help promote a community of support within the supported housing setting. See Chapter 9: Sensory Processing and the Lived Sensory Experience. 🤝

Hoarding has been previously identified as a concern in permanent supportive housing. Its identification as a disorder

in the recently updated *Diagnostic and Statistical Manual of Mental Disorders* (5th ed., text revision [*DSM-5-TR*], American Psychiatric Association [APA], 2022; Bratiotis & Steketee, 2015) has focused attention on this disorder. People with hoarding disorder have persistent difficulty getting rid of or parting with possessions because of a perceived need to save the items. Attempts to part with possessions create considerable distress and lead to decisions to save them. The resulting clutter disrupts the ability to use living spaces (APA, 2022). In the United States, hoarding has been identified as a disability for which reasonable accommodations in housing can be secured under the ADA and the Fair Housing Laws (Ligatti, 2013).

Assessments beyond the initial diagnosis of hoarding have been developed to facilitate intervention planning (Frost & Hristova, 2011). For example, the Clutter Image Scale (Frost et al., 2008) can be used to match the person's current level of clutter or hoarding to pictures of rooms within the home at various degrees of clutter. Approaches to hoarding include the use of community-level hoarding task forces made up of public safety, mental health, and social service organizations

(Bratiotis, 2013), cognitive behavioral therapy (Steketee et al., 2010), and peer support (Frost et al., 2012).

Clarke (2019) framed hoarding from an occupational perspective, partly as a challenge to a medical model frame. In framing "hoarding as an activity" (p. 7), Clarke goes on to consider how the "doing" . . . "being" . . . "belonging" . . . "becoming within hoarding" offers the OTP ways to see hoarding as having purpose and meaning to the individual, but with profound impact on the person's health (pp. 7–8). Clarke emphasizes that:

> An understanding of hoarding as a daily occupation can also support consideration of alternative interventions to what are currently offered, appreciating that the removal of items, such as in a decluttering process, will not specifically stop a person hoarding if this is the person's daily occupation and constructs daily tasks, roles, and routines. (p. 10)

Toolkits providing guidance on how to respond to hoarding practices have been authored and/or developed by OTPs; here are two examples:

- *The Community Clutter & Hoarding Toolkit* (Chater & Levitt, 2011) focuses mostly on addressing the needs of the older adult and hoarding.
- *Compulsive Hoarding: Frontline Worker's Toolkit* (Simmons & Richardson, 2013) specifically addresses the needs of persons labeled with psychiatric disabilities.

Although OTPs engaged in mediating hoarding practices have most typically assessed safety and/or directly assisted persons in their home, they can also use their knowledge and skill sets to support other providers in their work with persons who hoard. Reducing hoarding practices and working with persons who hoard is understood to be challenging, slow going, and best grounded in team-based meaningful therapeutic relationships (Koenig et al., 2012).

Optimizing Health and Condition Management

Concern regarding the health and wellness of persons with psychiatric disability was put front and center when research demonstrated higher mortality rates for persons with psychiatric disability (Lutterman et al., 2003), a finding that persists in the United States and internationally (Fiorillo et al., 2019; Firth et al., 2019; Plana-Ripoll et al., 2020). People experiencing long periods of homelessness who transition from the street to being housed often present with multiple comorbid medical conditions that have not been well managed (Rider et al., 2021), despite the availability of street medicine and/or clinic-based primary care clinics for persons experiencing homelessness.

When the complexity of these health comorbidities is combined with the previously noted functional cognition deficits, persons who have transitioned into housing require substantial levels of support beyond case management to schedule, get to, and communicate with the primary care provider (PCP), as well as to engage in the self-care management practices for conditions such as diabetes (e.g., skin and insulin level checks).

In the United States, integration of behavioral health and primary care services has been promoted for the past two decades (Koyangi & Carty, 2004), and is a key part of the Affordable Care Act in the United States. Permanent supportive housing providers are exploring differing configurations to address the comorbid health conditions that tenants and/or residents present (Larimer et al., 2009). For example, partnerships between permanent supportive housing providers and PCPs have been established (Burt et al., 2014; Wilkins, 2015). Such initiatives colocate primary care clinics within permanent supportive housing and has been referred to as "housing for health."

These partnerships are leveraging opportunities within Medicaid, the U.S. health insurance for low-income individuals, and the Affordable Care Act's expansion of Federally Qualified Health Centers (FQHCs), health centers serving low-income communities to deliver not only mental health services but primary care services as well (Corporation for Supportive Housing [CSH], 2011; Post, 2008).

OTPs internationally have already established their presence in primary care, and efforts are underway to do the same in the United States (AOTA, 2020). OTPs' expertise in addressing habits and routines, developing cognitive supports, and understanding the impact of medical conditions on function can target these concerns (Synovec et al., 2020). Practitioners working in the permanent supportive housing field can bring critical information to the housing team as unique professionals who address both mental and physical health together in the context of their impact on function. See Chapter 34: Integrated Behavioral Health and Primary Care. 🤝

Facilitating Occupational Engagement and Community Participation

Although it seems obvious that a focus for OTPs in permanent supported housing should be facilitating occupational engagement, there are particular reasons to highlight this point. Occupational deprivation is one of the key problems associated with institutional residential settings (Farnworth & Muñoz, 2009). Persons labeled with psychiatric disabilities are often transitioning from these settings into permanent supportive housing and experience residual disability associated with long stays in such settings. This is distinct from the disability associated with the illness itself; rather, this disability and disempowerment results from the lack of opportunities for personally relevant and meaningful activity or occupation (Blank et al., 2014; Sutton et al., 2012). In addition, boredom has been implicated in the misuse of substances and increase in psychiatric symptoms (Corvinelli, 2008; Hoxmark et al., 2012).

Persons who have experienced homelessness often report experiencing boredom and social isolation once they transition into housing (Borg et al., 2005; Marshall et al., 2019; Marshall, Keogh-Lim, et al., 2020; Raphael-Greenfield & Gutman, 2015), especially those who experience comorbid behavioral health conditions. In a systematic review, Marshall, Boland, and colleagues (2020) found that the supportive services provided in permanent supportive housing settings, including those informed by a Housing First approach, failed to consistently address community integration. In addition, the nature of the built environment or the policies of the permanent supportive housing setting may limit access to meaningful activity, for example, when communal areas of the housing site are limited, ill-configured, and/or nonexistent (Friesinger et al., 2019) and/or the policies established by the housing provider limit access to common areas and/or restrict guest visitation.

Given the previously noted research regarding the problematic departures, what is already known about the low employment rates for persons with psychiatric disabilities, and the clear evidence that engagement in occupation facilitates recovery (Mee & Sumsion, 2001; Mee et al., 2004; Strong, 1998; Sutton et al., 2012), access to occupational engagement and community participation must be addressed (Marshall & Rosenberg, 2014; Marshall, Boland, et al., 2020).

OTPs can strongly advocate to address this area of need when working in permanent supportive housing and/or ACT

teams that support persons with psychiatric disability in housing (Krupa et al., 2002; Townsend, 1998). Manualized interventions developed by OTPs can be utilized within permanent supportive housing and include Krupa and colleagues' (2010) *Action Over Inertia: Addressing the Activity-Health Needs of Individuals With Serious Mental Illness* and Parkinson's (2014) *Recovery Through Activity: Increasing Participation in Everyday Life.*

An example of occupational therapy's distinct role in supported housing settings is provided in Box 31-4. The setting

---

BOX 31-4 ■ RC's Story–Coming Inside: PEO Frames Transition to Housing

Contributed by Silvia Hernandez Cuellar, OTD, OTR/L

RC, now 66 years old, had been living her life outside for 28 years before deciding "to come inside." She made this decision after considering her personal health status and the well-being of her beloved pets. Explaining her decision, she said, "I came inside because of [my cat and my dog]. Professor is going to be 15, he can't be outside like that anymore." Living outside brought RC a healing freedom she craved, one that allowed her to escape her troubles and worries. Her escape included traveling that took her across state lines and into the mountains where she would yell into the wilderness, bringing about a catharsis that transformed into a coping mechanism she embraced.

Since transitioning to being housed, RC has been processing her life inside and adjusting to her new role as a housed person. For the first few months, RC refused to touch anything in her unit, explaining, "I kept thinking in the back of my mind 'mhm, yeah right . . . someone is going to come and tell me it was a joke.'" Assimilating has been challenging for RC. She had to learn to re-engage in new or modified occupations different from those she performed when unhoused. Financial management (i.e., allocating money for food, rent, utilities, and household items), home management (i.e., risk and fears around failing inspection), shopping, getting groceries, meal preparation, clean up, and even using the appliances in her unit were all new challenges. Figure 31-3 visualizes some of RC's challenges through the PEO model.

RC identified goals to decorate her apartment so it created a homey feel while still passing unit inspections and to complete grocery shopping and more meal preparation at home. These goals directly impact housing retention, which is the ICMS ultimate goal. RC's strengths and supports include having a stable

income (SSI), living close to retail and grocery stores, having an *In-Home Support Service (IHSS)* worker, being tech savvy with her cell phone (downloading apps, making online purchases, managing online banking, etc.), her creative vision for decorating and making up recipes, and her openness to work with service providers including occupational therapy. Barriers and limitations include her physical health (i.e., visual impairments, history of multiple sclerosis), having a fixed income, aspects of her social/cultural environment (i.e., property management judgmental attitudes), and her physical environment (i.e., unit layout and kitchen appliances in her unit).

Misfit between the person, environment, and occupation does not support RC's optimal occupational performance. RC spends most of her fixed income on DoorDash for meals and Amazon/Wish for apartment decor, sometimes going over budget. This impacts her ability to pay rent because RC does not always consider the implications of her expenses and spending patterns. Despite having a fully functioning kitchen, money for groceries, and a grocery store nearby, personal and environmental factors inhibited RC's access and ability to maximize use of the resources at hand. For example, RC's chronic health conditions (visual impairments and multiple sclerosis) and layout of her unit's kitchen and the appliances in her unit made grocery shopping and meal preparation more challenging and less enjoyable, posed potential safety risks, and depleted RC's energy. Other PEO misfits were identified. Although RC has a creative eye for decorating her apartment, her ideas, such as wanting to bring the outside into her home by having a tent in the unit and laying synthetic grass carpet, clashed with the housing management rules and cultural norms. Addressing the disconnects in RC's PEO through an occupational therapy informed lens involved the following.

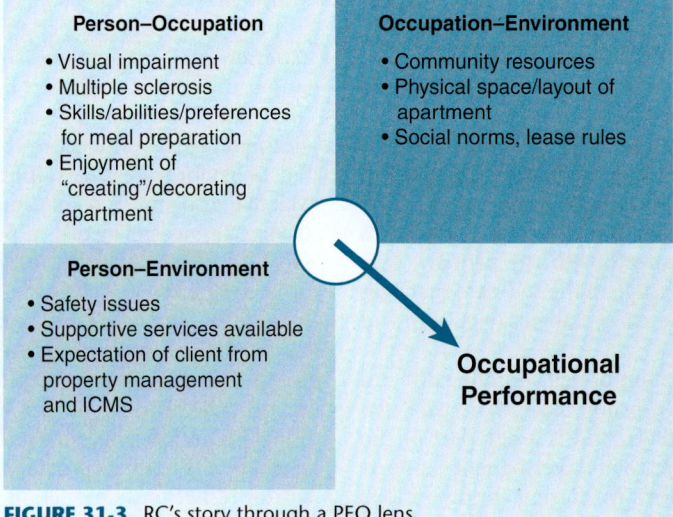

Person–Occupation

- Visual impairment
- Multiple sclerosis
- Skills/abilities/preferences for meal preparation
- Enjoyment of "creating"/decorating apartment

Occupation–Environment

- Community resources
- Physical space/layout of apartment
- Social norms, lease rules

Person–Environment

- Safety issues
- Supportive services available
- Expectation of client from property management and ICMS

Occupational Performance

FIGURE 31-3. RC's story through a PEO lens.

Education:

- Focused on health management and recognizing cause and effect (e.g., impact of symptoms [headaches, blurred vision, body aches, fatigue]) on occupational engagement.
- Teaching energy conservation as a strategy for maintaining engagement in valued occupational activities.
- Sharing the PEO model with SJC staff to highlight the interaction of factors impacting RC's behavior and to inform the plan of care and service referral and delivery.
- Using knowledge on disability and understanding the evidence on how health conditions and social factors impact function and participation to advocate for RC and to prevent occupational performance issues from affecting tenancy.

Doing With:

- Accompanying RC to the grocery store and the bank. Using rideshare together to facilitate self-efficacy and address her safety concerns. This also allows for further evaluation of key competencies (functional community mobility, functional cognition, etc.) through naturalistic observations.

Modifying Occupation and/or Environment:

- Using activity analysis to identify characteristics of the occupations or environments that could be modified or reasonably accommodated for; for example, lowering kitchen furniture to allow RC to sit during meal prep and using a hot plate/electric griddle/crock pot for cooking instead of the stove.

Evidence-Based Practice

Need for Occupational Engagement and Community in Supportive Housing

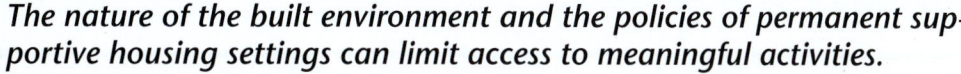

The nature of the built environment and the policies of permanent supportive housing settings can limit access to meaningful activities.

RESEARCH FINDINGS

Persons who have experienced homelessness often report experiencing boredom and social isolation once they transition into housing (Marshall & Rosenberg, 2014: Marshall et al., 2018, 2019, 2020), especially those who experience comorbid behavioral health conditions. In a systematic review, Marshall and colleagues (2020) found that the supportive services provided in permanent supportive housing settings, including those informed by a Housing First approach, failed to consistently address community integration. In addition, the nature of the built environment or the policies of the permanent supportive housing setting can limit access to meaningful activity; for example, when communal areas of the housing site are limited, ill-configured, and/or nonexistent (Friesinger et al., 2019), and/or the policies established by the housing provider limit access to common areas and/or restrict guest visitation.

APPLICATIONS

➡ OTPs in permanent supportive housing must address the risk of boredom and isolation by targeting their services to occupational engagement and community participation.

➡ OTPs in permanent supportive housing settings can work with housing providers to develop policies and practices to support occupational engagement and community.

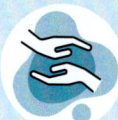

REFERENCES

Friesinger, J. G., Topor, A., Boe, T. D., & Larsen, I. B. (2019). Studies regardng supported housing and the built environment for people with mental health problems: A mixed-methods literature review. *Health Place, 57,* 44–53. https://doi.org/10.1016/j.healthplace.2019.03.006

Marshall, C. A., Boland, L., Westover, L. A., Marcellus, B., Weil, S., & Wickett, S. (2020). Effectiveness of interventions targeting community integration among individuals with lived experiences of homelessness: A systematic review. *Health and Social Care, 28*(6), 1843–1862. https://doi.org/10.1111/hsc.13030

Marshall, C. A., Davidson, L., Li, A., Gewurtz, R., Roy, L., Barbic, S., Kirsh, B., & Lysaght, R. (2019). Boredom and meaningful activity in adults experiencing homelessness: A mixed-methods study. *Canadian Journal of Occupational Therapy, 86*(5), 1–14. https://doi.org/10.1177/0008417419833402

Marshall, C. A., Lysaght, R., & Krupa, T. (2018). Occupational transition in the process of becoming housed following chronic homelessness. *Canadian Journal of Occupational Therapy, 85*(1), 33–45. https://doi.org/10.1177/0008417417723351

Marshall, C. A., & Rosenberg, M. W. (2014). Occupation and the process of transition from homelessness: L'occupation et le processus de transition de l'itinérance au logement. *Canadian Journal of Occupational Therapy, 81*(5), 330–338. https://doi.org/10.1177/0008417414548573

is St. Joseph Center (SJC), a comprehensive mental health and homeless service organization providing permanent supportive housing in Greater Los Angeles. Silvia Hernandez Cuellar, OTD, OTR/L, completed a postprofessional occupational therapy doctorate residency in one of SJC's permanent supportive housing sites. Over the year of her residency, Dr. Cuellar worked with RC. In Box 31-4, RC's story unfolds and elucidates how occupational therapy, and in particular the Person-Environment-Occupation (PEO) model, is used to understand RC's lived experience and support her sustained tenancy.

RC's story reinforces what OTPs understand, that "behavior is influenced and cannot be separated from contextual influences, temporal factors, and physical and psychological characteristics" (Law et al., 1996, p. 10). A distinct value of occupational therapy is that OTPs routinely consider the congruence of the person, environment, and occupation and tailor interventions to address the interaction of these components (Cramm, 2009; Law et al., 1996). This approach refocuses the attention to the notion that adapting to a housed identity comes with the demands of new occupation(s) in new/different environments and shifts away from perpetuating stereotypes and labeling of individuals as irresponsible or noncompliant.

Here's the Point

- Most persons labeled with psychiatric disabilities prefer living in their own place, rather than in congregate housing.
- Permanent supportive housing rather than custodial and/or congregate living arrangements facilitates recovery for persons labeled with psychiatric disabilities, by providing opportunities for choice, autonomy, privacy, and freedom.
- Providing housing alone is not sufficient to facilitate recovery; supportive services are essential in optimizing recovery outcomes.
- Public policy initiatives that promote the right to live in the community, the right to fair housing and equal access, and the right to affordable housing are essential to making permanent supportive housing available and successful.
- Occupational therapy has a role to play in permanent supportive housing by facilitating transition to housing and providing flexible supports for persons labeled with psychiatric disabilities.

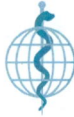 Visit the online resource center at **FADavis.com** to access the video.

Apply It Now

1. Self-Reflection on Living Independently

If you have lived independently or are currently living independently, reflect on your experience with meeting the day-to-day obligations of being a tenant.

Reflective Questions
- Have you consistently met all of your rental, mortgage, or utility payment deadlines?
- Have you ever been evicted or had your utilities turned off because of late or failed payments?
- How well are you maintaining the upkeep of your living environment?
- What emotional and physical resources do you need to call upon regularly to maintain the habits and routines related to maintaining your environment in a way that is satisfying to you?
- What supports have you needed or called upon to maintain your living situation?
- What interpersonal and other problem-solving strategies do you use to meet daily challenges?
- Did you feel a sense of home? If so, how did you make that happen?

2. Supported Housing Services

Contact a local community mental health agency that provides supported housing services to persons with psychiatric disabilities. Learn as much as you can about the services they offer. For example, how many supported housing units do they have available? How many do they need to meet the needs of people with psychiatric disability in your community? If there are not enough housing units to meet those needs, what other types of housing options (e.g., residential care) are available? Talk with the agency representatives about the challenges they have had in locating and establishing housing in your local community. Have they had any experiences with NIMBY-type responses to their efforts? What strategies did they employ, and how effective were they in countering negative reactions?

Resources

Web-Based Resources
- Bazelon Center for Mental Health Law: http://www.bazelon.org. The mission of the Judge David L. Bazelon Center for Mental Health Law is to protect and advance the rights of adults and children who have mental disabilities. The Bazelon Center envisions an America where people who have psychiatric disabilities or developmental disabilities exercise their own life choices and have access to the resources that enable them to participate fully in their communities.
- Pathways Housing First Institute: https://www.pathwayshousingfirst.org. This site provides training and consultation for the Housing First Model, and is directed by Sam Tsemberis, PhD, founder of this model.

- Corporation for Supportive Housing: http://www.csh.org. The mission of CSH is to advance solutions that use housing as a platform for services to improve the lives of the most vulnerable people, maximize public resources, and build healthy communities. CSH has provided consultation and training to sites around the United States in their efforts to develop permanent supportive housing.
- Department of Housing and Urban Development (HUD): http://www.hud.gov. HUD administers federal aid to local housing agencies (HAs) that manage the housing for low-income residents at rents they can afford.
- SAMHSA Homelessness and Housing: https://www.samhsa.gov/homelessness-programs-resources. SAMHSA supports programs that address homelessness and increase access to permanent housing for people with mental and/or substance use disorders.

Books and Other Resources

- Padgett, D. K., Henwook, B. F., & Tsemberis, S. J. (2016). *Housing First: Ending homelessness, transforming systems, and changing lives.* Oxford University Press.
- Schutt, R. K. (2011). *Homelessness, housing, and mental illness.* Harvard University Press.
- Sylvestrie, J., Nelson, G., & Aubry, T. (2017). *Housing, citizenship, and communities for people with serious mental illness.* Oxford University Press.
- Tsemberis, S. (2015). *Housing First manual: The Pathways Model to End Homelessness for People With Mental Illness and Addiction.* Hazelden.

Video

- "Student Perceptions of Bias and Stigma" video. In this video, four occupational therapy students reflect on how they came to recognize and work through their own biases against people who are unhoused. Each describes meeting and working in a student-run occupational therapy clinic with individuals who were unhoused and/or experiencing mental illness. They explain how engaging with these individuals and learning their stories became the impetus for transformative learning. Access the video at the online resource center at FADavis.com.

References

Alaazi, D. A., Masuda, J. R., Evans, J., & Distasio, J. (2015). Therapeutic landscapes of home: Exploring Indigenous people's experiences of Housing First intervention in Winnipeg. *Social Science and Medicine, 147,* 30–37. https://doi.org/10.1016/j.socscimed.2015.10.057

Allen, C., Earhart, C., & Blue, T. (1992). *Occupational therapy treatment goals for physically and cognitively disabled.* American Occupational Therapy Association.

American Occupational Therapy Association. (2020). Role of occupational therapy in primary care. *American Journal of Occupational Therapy, 74*(Suppl. 3), 7413410040p1–7413410040p16. https://doi.org/10.5014/ajot.2020.74S3001

American Psychiatric Association. (2022). *Diagnostic and statistical manual of mental disorders* (5th ed., text rev.). American Psychiatric Publishing. https://doi.org/10.1176/appi.books.9780890425787

Arbesman, M., D'Amico, M., Gibson, R. W., & Jaffe, L. (2011). Occupational therapy interventions for recovery in the areas of community integration and normative life roles for adults with serious mental illness: A systematic review. *AJOT: American Journal of Occupational Therapy, 65*(3), 247–256. https://doi.org/10.5014/ajot.2011.001297

Aubry, T., Tsemberis, S., Adair, C. E., Veldhuizen, S., Streiner, D., Latimer, E., Sareen, J., Patterson, M., McGarvey, K., Kopp, B., Hume, C., & Goering, P. (2014). One-year outcomes of a randomized controlled trial of Housing First with ACT in five Canadian cities. *Psychiatric Services, 66*(5), 463–469. https://doi.org/10.1176/appi.ps.201400167

Ault, M., Sturtevant, L., & Viveiros, J. (2015, March). *Housing landscape 2015.* Center for Housing Policy.

Bailliard, A. L., & Whigham, S. C. (2017). Linking neuroscience, function, and intervention: A scoping review of sensory processing and mental illness. *American Journal of Occupational Therapy, 71*(5), 7105100040p1–7105100040p18. https://doi.org/10.5014/ajot.2017.024497

Baron, K., Kielhofner, G., Lyenger, A., Goldhammer, V., & Wolenski, J. (2006). *Occupational Self Assessment (OSA).* Version 2.2. Model of Human Occupation Clearinghouse, University of Illinois at Chicago.

Bigelow, D. A. (1998). Supportive homes for life versus treatment way-stations: An introduction to TAPS Project 41. *Community Mental Health Journal, 34*(4), 403–405. https://doi.org/10.1023/A:1018740124488

Blank, A. A., Harries, P., & Reynolds, F. (2014). 'Without occupation you don't exist': Occupational engagement and mental illness. *Journal of Occupational Science, 22*(2), 197–209. https://doi.org/10.1080/14427591.2014.882250

Boland, L., Yarwood, R., & Bannigan, K. (2021). 'Making a home': An occupational perspective on sustaining tenancies following homelessness. *Housing Studies, 38*(7), 1239–1259. https://doi.org/10.1080/02673037.2021.1935757

Borg, M., & Davidson, L. (2007). The nature of recovery as lived in everyday experience. *Journal of Mental Health, 17*(2), 129–140. https://doi.org/10.1080/09638230701498382

Borg, M., Sells, D., Topor, A., Mezzina, R., Marin, I., & Davidson, L. (2005). What makes a house a home: The role of material resources in recovery from severe mental illness. *American Journal of Psychiatric Rehabilitation, 8*(3), 243–256. https://doi.org/10.1080/15487760500339394

Boyer, L., Baumstarck, K., Iordanova, T., Fernandez, J., Jean, P., & Auquier, P. (2014). A poverty-related quality of life questionnaire can help to detect health inequalities in emergency departments. *Journal of Clinical Epidemiology, 67*(3), 285–295. https://doi.org/10.1016/j.jclinepi.2013.07.021

Bratiotis, C. (2013). Community hoarding task forces: A comparative case study of five task forces in the United States. *Health & Social Care in the Community, 21*(3), 245–253. https://doi.org/10.1111/hsc.12010

Bratiotis, C., & Steketee, G. (2015). Hoarding disorders: Models, interventions, and efficacy. *Focus, 13*(2), 175–183. https://doi.org/10.1176/appi.focus.130202

Bromley, E., & Brekke, J. S. (2010). Assessing function and functional outcome in schizophrenia. *Current Topics in Behavioral Neuroscience, 4,* 3–21. https://doi.org/10.1007/7854_2010_40

Brown, C. (1996). A comparison of living situation and loneliness for people with mental illness. *Psychiatric Rehabilitation Journal, 20*(2), 59–63. https://doi.org/10.1037/h0095383

Brown, C. (2001). What is the best environment for me? A sensory processing perspective. *Occupational Therapy in Mental Health, 17*(3/4), 115–125. https://doi.org/10.1300/J004v17n03_08

Brown, C., Cromwell, R. L., Filion, D., Dunn, W., & Tollefson, N. (2002). Sensory processing in schizophrenia: Missing and avoiding information. *Schizophrenia Research, 55*(1–2), 187–195. https://doi.org/10.1016/s0920-9964(01)00255-9

Brown, C., & Dunn, W. (2002). *Adolescent/Adult Sensory Profile.* Psychological Corporation.

Brown, C., Karim, R., & Steuler, M. (2020). Retrospective analysis of studies examining sensory processing preferences in people with a psychiatric condition. *American Journal of Occupational Therapy, 74*(4), 7404205130p1–7404205130p11. https://doi.org/10.5014/ajot.2020.038463

Brown, C., Rempfer, M., & Hamera, E. (2009). *The Test of Grocery Shopping Skills.* AOTA Press.

Brown, C., Tollefson, N., Dunn, W., Cromwell, R., & Filion, D. (2001). The adult sensory profile: Measuring patterns of sensory processing. *American Journal of Occupational Therapy, 55*(1), 75–82. https://doi.org/10.5014/ajot.55.1.75

Burgess, H., Vorobyova, A., Marziali, M., Loeh, K., Jongbloed, K., Von Bischoffshausen, O., Salters, K. A., Hogg, R. S., & Parashar, S. (2021). Supportive housing building policies and resident psychological needs: A qualitative analysis using self-determination theory. *Housing Studies, 38*(4), 642–660. https://doi.org/10.1080/02673037.2021.1900548

Burt, M., Wilkins, C., & Locke, G. (2014). *Medicaid and permanent supportive housing for chronically homeless individuals: Emerging practices from the field.* U.S. Department of Health and Human Services.

California Institute for Mental Health. (2011). *Adult 2011: Full service partnership tool kit. California Department of Mental Health.* https://bhcsproviders.acgov.org/providers/qi/docs/full_service_partnership_toolkit.pdf

Carling, P. J. (1993). Housing and supports for persons with mental illness: Emerging approaches to research and practice. *Hospital & Community Psychiatry, 44,* 439–449. https://doi.org/10.1176/ps.44.5.439

Carling, P. J. (1995). *Return to community: Building supports systems for people with psychiatric disabilities.* Guilford Press.

Castellow, J., Kloos, B., & Townley, G. (2015). Previous homelessness as a risk factor for recovery from serious mental illnesses. *Community Mental Health Journal, 51,* 1–11. https://doi.org/10.1007/s10597-014-9805-9

Chan, D. V. (2020). Safe spaces, agency, and connections to "regular stuff": What makes permanent supportive housing feel like "home." *Rehabilitation Counseling Bulletin, 63*(2), 102–114. https://doi.org/10.1177/0034355218814927

Chater, C., & Levitt, E. (2011). *The community clutter & hoarding toolkit.* VHA Home Healthcare.

Clarke, C. (2019). Can occupational therapy address the occupational implications of hoarding? *Occupational Therapy International, 2019,* 1–13. https://doi.org/10.1155/2019/5347403

Colbert v. Quinn, No. 7-C-4737 (N.D. Ill 2011).

Corin, E., & Lauzon, G. (1991). Positive withdrawal and the quest for meaning: The reconstruction of experience among schizophrenics. *Psychiatry, 55*(3), 279–281. https://doi.org/10.1080/00332747.1992.11024600

Corporation for Supportive Housing. (2011). *Integrating FQHC health care services with permanent supportive housing in Los Angeles.* Corporation for Supportive Housing and United Homeless Healthcare Partners.

Corrigan, P. W., & McCracken, S. G. (2005). Place first, then train: An alternative to the Medical Model of Psychiatric Rehabilitation. *Social Work, 50*(1), 31–39. https://doi.org/10.1093/sw/50.1.31

Corvinelli, A. (2008). Alleviating boredom in adult males recovering from substance use disorder. *Occupational Therapy in Mental Health, 21*(2), 1–11. https://doi.org/10.1300/J004v21n02_01

Cramm, H. (2009). The Person-Environment-Occupation circle tool: A simple way to bridge theory into practice. *Occupational Therapy Now, 11*(3), 19–21.

Crider, C., Calder, R., Bunting, K. L., & Forwell, S. (2014). An integrative review of occupational science and theoretical literature exploring transition. *Journal of Occupational Science, 22*(3), 304–319. https://doi.org/10.1080/14427591.2014.922913

Csikszentmihalyi, M., & Halton, E. (1981). *The meaning of things: Domestic symbols and the self.* Cambridge University Press.

Davidson, L. (2003). *Living outside mental illness: Qualitative studies of recovery in schizophrenia.* New York University Press.

Davidson, L., & Strauss, J. (1992). Sense of self in recovery from severe mental illness. *Psychology and Psychotherapy, 65*(2), 131–145. https://doi.org/10.1111/j.2044-8341.1992.tb01693.x

Deegan, P. (2005). The importance of personal medicine: A qualitative study of resilience in people with psychiatric disabilities. *Scandinavian Journal of Public Health, 33,* 29–35. https://doi.org/10.1080/14034950510033345

Doniger, J., Rothwell, N. D., & Cohen. R. (1963). Case study of a halfway house. *Psychiatric Services, 14*(3), 191–199. https://doi.org/10.1176/ps.14.4.191

Dorvil, H., Morin, P., Beaulieu, A., & Robert, D. (2005). Housing as a social integration factor for people classified as mentally ill. *Housing Studies, 20*(3), 497. https://doi.org/10.1080/02673030500062525

Earhart, C. A. (2006). *Using Allen diagnostic module-2nd edition assessments.* S&S Worldwide.

Earhart, C. A., McCraith, D. B., & Riska-Williams, L. (2022). *Manual for the version 5 of the Allen Cognitive Level Screen, second edition.* https://allencognitive.com

Farnworth, L., & Muñoz, J. P. (2009). An occupational and rehabilitation perspective for institutional practice. *Psychiatric Rehabilitation Journal, 32*(3), 192–198. https://doi.org/10.2975/32.3.2009.192.198

Fenton, K., Larkin, M., Boden, Z. V. R., Thompson, J., Hickman, G., & Newton, E. (2014). The experiential impact of hospitalisation in early psychosis: Service-user accounts of inpatient environments. *Health & Place, 30,* 234–241. https://doi.org/10.1016/j.healthplace.2014.09.013

Fiorillo, A., Luciano, M., Pompili, M., & Sartorius, N. (2019). Editorial: Reducing the mortality gap in people with severe mental disorders: The role of lifestyle psychosocial interventions. *Frontiers in Psychiatry, 10,* 434. https://doi.org/10.3389/fpsyt.2019.00434

Firth, J., Siddiqi, N., Koyanagi, A., Siskind, D., Rosenbaum, S., Galletly, C., Allan, S., Caneo, C., Carney, R., Carvalho, A. F., Chatterton, M. L., Correll, C. U. Curtis, J., Gaughran, F. Heald, A., Hoare, E., Jackson, S. E., Kisely, S., Lovell, K., . . . Stubbs, B. (2019). The Lancet Psychiatric Commission: A blueprint for protecting physical health in people with mental illness. *The Lancet Psychiatry, 6*(8), 675–712. https://doi.org/10.1016/S2215-0366(19)30132-4

Fisher, G., Forsyth, K., Harrison, M., Angarola, R., Kayhan, E., Noga, P. L., Johnson, C., & Irvine, L. (2014). *User's Manual Residential Environment Impact Scale* (Version 4.0). Model of Human Occupation Clearinghouse, Department of Occupational Therapy, University of Illinois at Chicago.

Fjellfeldt, M., Hogstrom, E., Berglund-Snodgrass, L., & Markstrom, U. (2021). Fringe or not fringe? Strategies for localizing supported accommodation in a post-deinstitutional era. *Social Inclusion, 9*(3), 201–213. https://doi.org/10.17645/si.v9i3.4319

Folsom, D. P., Hawthorne, W., Lindamer, L., Gilmer, T., Bailey, A., Golshan, S., Garcia, P., Unützer, J., Hough, R., & Jeste, D. V. (2005). Prevalence and risk factors for homelessness and utilization of mental health services among 10,340 patients with serious mental illness in a large public mental health system. *American Journal of Psychiatry, 162*(2), 370–376. https://doi.org/10.1176/appi.ajp.162.2.370

Forchuk, C., Nelson, G., & Hall, G. B. (2006). "It's important to be proud of the place you live in": Housing problems and preferences of psychiatric survivors. *Perspectives in Psychiatric Care, 42*(1), 42–52. https://doi.org/10.1111/j.1744-6163.2006.00054.x

Fossey, E., Harvey, D., & McDermott, F. (2020). Housing and support narratives of people experiencing mental health issues: Making my place, my home. *Frontiers in Psychiatry: Social Psychiatry and Psychiatric Rehabilitation, 10,* 939. https://doi.org/10.3389/fpsyt.2019.00939

Fossey, E., Harvey, C., Plant, G., & Pantelis, C. (2006). Occupational performance of people diagnosed with schizophrenia in supported housing and outreach programmes in Australia. *The British Journal of Occupational Therapy, 69,* 409–419. https://doi.org/10.1177/030802260606900904

Friesinger, J. G., Topor, A., Boe, T. D., & Larsen, I. B. (2019). Studies regarding supported housing and the built environment for people with mental health problems: A mixed-methods literature review. *Health Place, 57,* 44–53. https://doi.org/10.1016/j.healthplace.2019.03.006

Frost, R., & Hristova, V. (2011). Assessment of hoarding. *Journal of Clinical Psychology, 67*(5), 456–466. https://doi.org/10.1002/jclp.20790

Frost, R., Ruby, D., & Shuer, L. (2012). The buried in treasures workshop: Waitlist control trial of facilitated support groups for hoarding. *Behaviour Research and Therapy, 50*(11), 661–667. https://doi.org/10.1016/j.brat.2012.08.004

Frost, R., Steketee, G., Tolin, D., & Renaud, S. (2008). Development and validation of the clutter image rating. *Journal of Psychopathology and Behavioral Assessment, 30*(3), 193–203. https://doi.org/10.1007/s10862-007-9068-7

Gaetz, S., Scott, F., & Gulliver, T. (2013). *Housing First in Canada: Supporting communities to end homelessness.* Canadian Homelessness Research Network Press.

Glasscote, R. M., Gudeman, J. E., & Elpers, R. (1971). *Halfway houses for the mentally ill.* American Psychiatric Association.

Goldstein, J. L., & Godemont, M. L. (2003). The legend and lessons of Geel, Belgium: A 1500-year-old legend, a 21st century model. *Community Mental Health Journal, 39,* 441–458. https://doi.org/10.1023/A:1025813003347

Green, M., Llerena, K., & Kern, R. (2015, July). The "right stuff" revisited: What have we learned about the determinants of daily functioning in schizophrenia? *Schizophrenia Bulletin, 41*(4), 781–785. https://doi.org/10.1093/schbul/sbv018

Hammell, K. R. W., & Iwama, M. K. (2012). Well-being and occupational rights: An imperative for critical occupational therapy. *Scandinavian Journal of Occupational Therapy, 19*(5), 385–394. https://doi.org/10.3109/11038128.2011.611821

Hartman, C. (1998). The case for a right to housing. *Housing Policy Debate, 9*(2), 223–246. https://doi.org/10.1080/10511482.1998.9521292

Henwood, B., Derejko, K. S., Couture, J., & Padgett, D. (2015). Maslow and mental health recovery: A comparative study of homeless programs for adults with serious mental illness. *Administration and Policy in Mental Health and Mental Health Services Research, 42*(2), 220–228. https://doi.org/10.1007/s10488-014-0542-8

Hogan, M. F., & Carling, P. J. (1992). Normal housing: A key element of a supported housing approach for people with psychiatric disabilities. *Community Mental Health Journal, 28*(3), 215–226. https://doi.org/10.1007/BF00756818

Hoxmark, E., Wynn, T. N., & Wynn, R. (2012). Loss of activities and its effect on the well-being of substance abusers. *Scandinavian Journal of Occupational Therapy, 19,* 78–83. https://doi.org/10.3109/11038128.2011.552120

Johnson, G., Parkinson, S., & Parsell, C. (2012). *Policy shift or program drift? Implementing Housing First in Australia.* AHURI Final Report No. 184. Australian Housing and Urban Research Institute.

Katz, N. (2006). *Routine Task Inventory-Expanded.* Allen Cognitive Network. https://www.allen-cognitive-network.org/index.php/allen-cognitive-model/routine-task-inventory-expanded-rti-e

Kielhofner, G., Mallinson, T., Crawford, C., Nowak, M., Rigby, M., Henry, A., & Walens, D. (2004). *The Occupational Performance History Interview-II (OPHI-II). Version 2.1.* University of Illinois. https://moho-irm.uic.edu/productDetails.aspx?aid=31

King, P. (2003). Housing as a freedom right. *Housing Studies, 18*(5), 661–672. https://doi.org/10.1080/02673030304259

Kinnealey, M., Oliver, B., & Wilbarger, P. (1995). A phenomenological study of sensory defensiveness in adults. *American Journal of Occupational Therapy, 49,* 444–451. https://doi.org/10.5014/ajot.49.5.444

Kirsh, B., Gewurtz, R., & Bakewell, R. (2011). Critical characteristics of supported housing: Resident and service provider perspectives. *Canadian Journal of Community Mental Health, 30*(1), 15–30. https://doi.org/10.7870/cjcmh-2011-0002

Kirsh, B., Gewurtz, R., Bakewell, R., Singer, B., Badsha, M., & Giles, N. (2009). *Critical characteristics of supported housing:*

Findings from the literature, residents and service providers. Wellesley Institute: Advancing Urban Health.

Kirst, M., Zerger, S., Misir, V., Hwang, S., & Stergiopoulos, V. (2015). The impact of a Housing First randomized controlled trial on substance use problems among homeless individuals with mental illness. *Drug and Alcohol Dependence, 146*(1), 24–29. https://doi.org/10.1016/j.drugalcdep.2014.10.019

Kirst, M., Zerger, S., Wise Harris, D., Plenert, E., & Stergiopoulos, V. (2014). The promise of recovery: Narratives of hope among homeless individuals with mental illness participating in a Housing First randomised controlled trial in Toronto, Canada. *BMJ Open, 4,* e004379. https://doi.org/10.1136/bmjopen-2013-004379

Knable, M. B., Cantrell, C., Meer, A. V., & Levine, E. (2015). The availability and effectiveness of residential treatment for persistent mental illness. *Psychiatric Annals, 45*(3), 109–113. https://doi.org/10.3928/00485713-20150304-04

Koenig, T. L., Leiste, M. R., Spano, R., & Chapin, R. K. (2012). Multidisciplinary team perspectives on older adult hoarding and mental illness. *Journal of Elder Abuse & Neglect, 25*(1), 56–75. https://doi.org/10.1080/08946566.2012.712856

Koyangi, C., & Carty, L. (2004). *Get it together: How to integrate physical and mental health care for people with serious mental disorders.* Bazelon Center for Mental Health Law.

Kresky, M., Maeda, E. M., & Rothwell, N. D. (1976). The apartment program: A community-living option for halfway house residents. *Psychiatric Services, 27*(3), 153–154. https://doi.org/10.1176/ps.27.3.153

Krupa, T., Edgelow, M., Chen, S., Mieras, C., Almas, A., Perry, A., Radloff-Gabriel, D., Jackson, J., & Bransfield, M. (2010). *Action Over Inertia: Addressing the activity-health needs of individuals with serious mental illness.* Canadian Occupational Therapy Association.

Krupa, T., Radloff-Gabriel, D., Whippey, E., & Kirsh, B. (2002). Reflections on . . . occupational therapy and Assertive Community Treatment. *Canadian Journal of Occupational Therapy, 69*(3), 153–157. https://doi.org/10.1177/000841740206900305

Kuno, E., Rothbard, A. B., Averyt, J., & Culhane, D. (2000). Homelessness among persons with serious mental illness in an enhanced community-based mental health system. *Psychiatric Services, 51*(8), 1012–1016. https://doi.org/10.1176/appi.ps.51.8.1012

Larimer, M., Malone, D., Garner, M., Atkins, D., Burlingham, B., Lonczak, H., Tanzer, K., Ginzler, J., Clifasefi, S. L., Hobson, W. G., & Marlatt, G. (2009). Health care and public service use and costs before and after provision of housing for chronically homeless persons with severe alcohol problems. *Journal of the American Medical Association, 301,* 1349–1357. https://doi.org/10.1001/jama.2009.414

Law, M., Cooper, B., Strong, S., Stewart, D., Rigby, P., & Letts, L. (1996). The Person-Environment-Occupation model: A transactive approach to occupational performance. *The Canadian Journal of Occupational Therapy, 63*(1), 9–23. https://doi.org/10.1177/000841749606300103

Leamy, M., Bird, V., Le Boutillier, C., Williams, J., & Slade, M. (2011). Conceptual framework for personal recovery in mental health: Systematic review and narrative synthesis. *The British Journal of Psychiatry, 199*(6), 445–452. https://doi.org/10.1192/bjp.bp.110.083733

Leedahl, S. N., Chapin, R. K., Wendel, C., Anne Baca, B., Hasche, L. K., & Townley, G. W. (2015). Successful strategies for discharging Medicaid nursing home residents with mental health diagnoses to the community. *Journal of Social Service Research, 41*(2), 172–192. https://doi.org/10.1080/01488376.2014.972012

Ligatti, C. C. (2013). Cluttered apartments and complicated tenancies: A collaborative intervention approach to tenant "hoarding" under the Fair Housing Act. *Suffolk University Law Review, 46*(1), 79–109.

Lindstrom, M., Lindberg, M., & Sjostrom, S. (2009). Home bittersweet home: The significance of home for occupational transformations. *International Journal of Social Psychiatry, 57*(3), 284–299. https://doi.org/10.1177/0020764009354834

Luken, S. (2022). Policy recommendations to address housing shortages for people with severe mental illness. *Psychiatric Services, 73*(3), 329–334. https://doi.org/10.1176/appi.ps.202100158

Lutterman, T., Ganju, V., Schacht, L., Shaw, R., Monihan, K., & Huddle, M. (2003). *Sixteen state study on mental health performance measures.* Center for Mental Health Services, Substance Abuse and Mental Health Services Administration.

Mahaffey, L., Burson, K. A., Januscewski, C., Pitts, D., & Preissner, K. (2015). Role for occupational therapy in community mental health: Using policy to advance scholarship of practice. *Occupational Therapy in Health Care, 29*(4), 397–410. https://doi.org/10.3109/07380577.2015.1051689

Marshall, C. A. (2016). *Occupation, homelessness, and the transition to becoming housed among chronically homeless persons.* Queens University, Kingston.

Marshall, C. A., Boland, L., Westover, L. A., Isard, R., & Gutman, S. A. (2021). A systematic review of occupational therapy interventions in the transition from homelessness. *Scandinavian Journal of Occupational Therapy, 28*(3), 171–187. https://doi.org/10.1080/11038128.2020.1764094

Marshall, C. A., Boland, L., Westover, L. A., Marcellus, B., Weil, S., & Wickett, S. (2020). Effectiveness of interventions targeting community integration among individuals with lived experiences of homelessness: A systematic review. *Health and Social Care in the Community, 28*(6), 1843–1862. https://doi.org/10.1111/hsc.13030

Marshall, C. A., Cooke, A., Gewurtz, R., Barbic, S., Roy, L., Ross, C., Becker, A., Lysaght, R., & Kirsh, B. (2021). Bridging the transition from homelessness: Developing an occupational therapy framework. *Scandinavian Journal of Occupational Therapy, 30*(7), 953–969. https://doi.org/10.1080/11038128.2021.1962970

Marshall, C. A., Davidson, L., Li, A., Gewurtz, R., Roy, L., Barbic, S., Kirsh, B., & Lysaght, R. (2019). Boredom and meaningful activity in adults experiencing homelessness: A mixed-methods study. *Canadian Journal of Occupational Therapy, 86*(5), 1–14. https://doi.org/10.1177/0008417419833402

Marshall, C. A., Keogh-Lim, D., Koop, M., Barbic, S., & Gewurtz, R. (2020). Meaningful activity and boredom in the transition from homelessness: Two narratives. *Canadian Journal of Occupational Therapy, 87*(4), 253–264. https://doi.org/10.1177/0008417420941782

Marshall, C. A., Lysaght, R., & Krupa, T. (2018). Occupational transition in the process of becoming housed following chronic homelessness. *Canadian Journal of Occupational Therapy, 85*(1), 33–45. https://doi.org/10.1177/0008417417723351

Marshall, C. A., & Rosenberg, M. W. (2014). Occupation and the process of transition from homelessness: L'occupation et le processus de transition de l'itinérance au logement. *Canadian Journal of Occupational Therapy, 81*(5), 330–338. https://doi.org/10.1177/0008417414548573

McCraith, D., Austin, S., & Earhart, C. (2011). The Cognitive Disabilities Model in 2011. In N. Katz (Ed.), *Cognition, occupation, and participation across the life span: Neuroscience, neurorehabilitation, and models of intervention in occupational therapy* (3rd ed., pp. 383–406). AOTA Press.

McKibbin, C. L., Brekke, J. S., Sires, D., Jeste, D. V., & Patterson, T. L. (2004). Direct assessment of functional abilities: Relevance to persons with schizophrenia. *Schizophrenia Research, 72*(1), 53–67. https://doi.org/10.1016/j.schres.2004.09.011

Mee, J., & Sumsion, T. (2001). Mental health clients confirm the motivating power of occupation. *The British Journal of Occupational Therapy, 64,* 121–128. https://doi.org/10.1177/030802260106400303

Mee, J., Sumsion, T., & Craik, C. (2004). Mental health clients confirm the value of occupation in building competence and self-identity. *The British Journal of Occupational Therapy, 67,* 225–233. https://doi.org/10.1177/030802260406700506

Mejia-Lancheros, C., Lachaud, J., Woodhall-Melnik, J., O'Campo, P., Hwang, S. W., & Stergiopoulos, V. (2021). Longitudinal inter-relationships of mental health discrimination and stigma with housing and well-being outcomes in adults with mental illness and recent experience of homelessness. *Social Science & Medicine, 268,* 113463. https://doi.org/10.1016/j.socscimed.2020.113463

Meyer, A. (1915/1952). The extra-institutional responsibilities of state hospitals for mental disease. In E. Winters (Ed.), *The collected papers of Adolf Meyer: Mental hygiene* (Vol. IV, pp. 229–236). Johns Hopkins University Press.

Milbourn, B., McNamara, B., & Buchanan, A. (2015). The lived experience of everyday activity for individuals with serious mental illness. *Health Sociology Review, 24*(3), 270–282. https://doi.org/10.1080/14461242.2015.1034747

National Alliance on Mental Illness. (2014). *Road to recovery: Employment and mental illness.* Author.

National Council on Disability. (2008). *Inclusive livable communities for people with psychiatric disabilities.* Author.

National Law Center on Homelessness & Poverty. (2017). *Don't count on it: How the HUD point-in-time count underestimates the homelessness crisis in America.* https://homelesslaw.org/wp-content/uploads/2018/10/HUD-PIT-report2017.pdf

Nelson, G., & Peddle, S. (2005). *Housing and support for people who have experienced serious mental illness: Value base and research evidence.* Wilfrid Laurier University.

Nolan, C., & Swarbrick, M. (2002). Supportive housing occupational therapy home management program. *AOTA Mental Health Special Interest Section Quarterly, 25*(2), 1–3.

Olmstead v. L.C. 527 U.S. 581 (1999).

O'Shaughnessy, B., Manning, R. M., Greenwood, R. M., Vargas-Moniz, M., Loubiere, S., Spinnewijn, F., Gaboardi, M., Wolf, J. R., Bokszczanin, A., Bernad, R., Blid, M., Ornelas, J., & The HOME-EU Consortium Study. (2020). Home as base for a well-lived life: Comparing the capabilities of homeless service users in Housing First and the Staircase of Transition in Europe. *Housing, Theory and Society, 38*(3), 343–364. https://doi.org/10.1080/14036096.2020.1762725

Padgett, D. K. (2007). There's no place like (a) home: Ontological security among persons with serious mental illness in the United States. *Social Science & Medicine, 64,* 1925–1936. https://doi.org/10.1016/j.socscimed.2007.02.011

Padgett, D. K., Smith, B. T., Henwood, B. F., & Tiderington, E. (2012). Life course adversity in the lives of formerly homeless persons with serious mental illness: Context and meaning. *American Journal of Orthopsychiatry, 82*(3), 421–430. https://doi.org/10.1111/j.1939-0025.2012.01159.x

Parkinson, S. (2014). *Recovery through activity: Increasing participation in everyday life.* Speechmark.

Pescosolido, B. A., Martin, J. K., Long, J. S., Medina, T. R., Phelan, J. C., & Link, B. G. (2010). "A disease like any other"? A decade of change in public reactions to schizophrenia, depression, and alcohol dependence. *American Journal of Psychiatry, 167*(11), 1321–1330. https://doi.org/10.1176/appi.ajp.2010.09121743

Pfeiffer, B., Brusilovskiy, E., Bauer, J., & Saltzer, M. S. (2014). Sensory processing, participation, and recovery in adults with serious mental illness. *Psychiatric Rehabilitation Journal, 37*(4), 289–296. https://doi.org/10.1037/prj0000099

Piat, M. (2000). The NIMBY phenomenon: Community residents' concerns about housing for deinstiutionalized people. *Health & Social Work, 25*(2), 127–138. https://doi.org/10.1093/hsw/25.2.127

Piat, M., Seida, K., Sabetti, J., & Padgett, D. (2017). (Em)placing recovery: Sites of health and wellness for individuals with serious mental illness in supported housing. *Health & Place, 47,* 71–79. https://doi.org/10.1016/j.healthplace.2017.07.006

Plana-Ripoll, O., Musliner, K. L., Dalsgaard, S., Momen, N. C., Weye, N., Christensen, M. K., Agerbo, E., Iburg, K. M., Laursen, T. M., Mortensen, P. B., Pedersen, C. B., Petersen, L. V., Santomauro, D. F., Vilhjálmsson, B. J., Whiteford, H. A., & McGrath, J. J. (2020). Nature and prevalence of combinations of mental disorders and their association with excess mortality in a population-based cohort study. *World Psychiatry, 19*(3), 339–349. https://doi.org/10.1002/wps.20802

Polvere, L., Macnaughton, E., & Piat, M. (2013). Participant perspectives on housing first and recovery: Early findings from the At Home/Chez Soi project. *Psychiatric Rehabilitation Journal, 36*(2), 110–112. https://doi.org/10.1037/h0094979

Post, P. A. (2008). *Defining and funding the support in permanent supportive housing: Recommendations of health centers service homeless people.* National Health Care for Homeless Council, Corporation for Supportive Housing.

Raphael-Greenfield, E. I., & Gutman, S. A. (2015). Understanding the lived experience of formerly homeless adults as they transition to supportive housing. *Occupational Therapy in Mental Health, 31*(1), 35–49. https://doi.org/10.1080/0164212x.2014.1001011

Raush, H. L., & Raush, C. L. (1968). *The Halfway House Movement: A search for sanity.* Appleton-Century-Crofts.

Rempfer, M. V., Hamera, E. K., Brown, C. E., & Cromwell, R. L. (2003). The relations between cognition and the independent living skill of shopping in people with schizophrenia. *Psychiatry Research, 117*(2), 103–112. https://doi.org/10.1016/S0165-1781(02)00318-9

Rider, J. V., Selim, J., & Garcia, A. (2021). Assessing functional disability among persons experiencing homelessness. *American Journal of Occupational Therapy, 75*(Suppl. 2), 7512505192p1. https://doi.org/10.5014/ajot.2021.75S2-RP192

Ridgway, P., Simpson, A., Wittman, F. D., & Wheeler, G. (1994). Home making and community building: Notes on empowerment and place. *The Journal of Mental Health Administration, 21*(4), 407–417. https://doi.org/10.1007/BF02521359

Ridgway, P., & Zipple, A. M. (1990). The paradigm shift in residential services: From the linear continuum to supported housing approaches. *Psychosocial Rehabilitation Journal, 13*(4), 11–31. https://doi.org/10.1037/h0099479

Roos, L. E., Distasio, J., Bolton, S.-L., Katz, L. Y., Afifi, T. O., Isaak, C., Goering, P., Bruce, L., & Sareen, J. (2014). A history in-care predicts unique characteristics in a homeless population with mental illness. *Child Abuse & Neglect, 38*(10), 1618–1627. https://doi.org//10.1016/j.chiabu.2013.08.018

Rothwell, N. D., & Doniger, J. M. (1966). *The Psychiatric Halfway House.* Charles C. Thomas.

Salzer, M. S., & Baron, R. C. (2006). *Community integration and measuring participation.* University of Pennsylvania Collaborative on Community Integration.

Sanchis-Asensi, A., Trivino-Juarrez, J. M., Sanchis-Alminana, H., & Romero-Ayuso, D. (2022). Relationship between sensory profile and self-perceived quality of life in people with schizophrenia: An exploratory study. *Occupational Therapy in Mental Health, 39*(3), 295–313. https://doi.org/10.1080/0164212X.2022.2125925

Seamon, D. (2015). *A geography of the lifeworld: Movement, rest and encounter.* Routledge Taylor & Francis Group.

Sells, D., Stayner, D., & Davidson, L. (2004). Recovering the self in schizophrenia: An integrative review of qualitative studies. *Psychiatric Quarterly, 75*(1), 87–97. https://doi.org/10.1023/b:psaq.0000007563.17236.97

Serafini, G., Gonda, X., Pompili, M., Rihmer, Z., Amkore, M., & Engel-Yeger, B. (2016). The relationship between sensory processing patterns, alexithymia, traumatic childhood experiences, and quality of life among patients with unipolar and bipolar disorders. *Child Abuse & Neglect, 62,* 39–50. https://doi.org/10.1016/j.chiabu.2016.09.013

Simmons, R., & Richardson, S. (2013). *Compulsive hoardings: Frontline workers' toolkit.* Orbit Group Limited.

Sisti, D. A., Segal, A. G., & Emanuel, E. J. (2015). Improving long-term psychiatric care: Bring back the asylum. *Journal of the American Medical Association, 313*(3), 243–244. https://doi.org/10.1001/jama.2014.16088

Steketee, G., Frost, R. O., Tolin, D. F., Rasmussen, J., & Brown, T. A. (2010). Waitlist-controlled trial of cognitive behavior therapy for hoarding disorder. *Depression and Anxiety, 27*(5), 476–484. https://doi.org/10.1002/da.20673

Stergiopoulos, V., Gozdzik, A., O'Campo, P., Holtby, A., Jeyaratnam, J., & Tsemberis, S. (2014). Housing First: Exploring participants' early support needs. *BMC Health Services Research, 14*(1), 167. https://doi.org/10.1186/1472-6963-14-167

Strong, S. (1998). Meaningful work in supportive environments: Experiences with the recovery process. *American Journal of Occupational Therapy, 52*(1), 31–38. https://doi.org/10.5014/ajot.52.1.31

Substance Abuse and Mental Health Services Administration. (2006). *Transforming housing for people with psychiatric disabilities report.* (2006). Center for Mental Health Services.

Substance Abuse and Mental Health Services Administration. (2010a). *Permanent supportive housing evidence-based practices.* Center for Mental Health Services, U.S. Department of Health and Human Services.

Substance Abuse and Mental Health Services Administration. (2010b). *Permanent supportive housing: Training frontline staff.* Center for Mental Health Services, U.S. Department of Health and Human Services.

Substance Abuse and Mental Health Services Administration. (2023). *Expanding access to and use of behavioral health services for people experiencing homelessness.* Center for Mental Health Services, U.S. Department of Health and Human Services.

Suto, M., & Frank, G. (1994). Future time perspective and daily occupations of persons with chronic schizophrenia in a board and care home. *American Journal of Occupational Therapy, 48*(1), 7–18. https://doi.org/10.5014/ajot.48.1.7

Sutton, D. J., Hocking, C. S., & Smythe, L. A. (2012). A phenomenological study of occupational engagement in recovery from mental illness. *Canadian Journal of Occupational Therapy, 79*(3), 143–150. https://doi.org/10.2182/cjot.2012.79.3.3

Sylvestre, J., Notten, G., Kerman, N., Polillo, A., & Czechowki, K. (2018). Poverty and serious mental illness: Toward action on a seemingly intractable problem. *American Journal of Community Psychology, 61*(2), 153–165. https://doi.org/10.1002/ajcp.12211

Synovec, C. E., Merryman, M., & Brusca, J. (2020). Occupational therapy in integrated primary care: Addressing the needs of individuals experiencing homelessness. *The Open Journal of Occupational Therapy, 8*(4), 1–14. https://doi.org/10.15453/2168-6408.1699

Thiele, B. (2002). The human right to adequate housing: A tool for promoting and protecting individual and community health. *American Journal of Public Health, 92*(5), 712–715. https://doi.org/10.2105/ajph.92.5.712

Townsend, E. (1998). *Good intentions overruled: A critique of empowerment in routine organization of mental health services.* University of Toronto Press.

Tsai, J., Bond, G., Salyers, M., Godfrey, J., & Davis, K. (2010). Housing preferences and choices among adults with mental illness and substance use disorders: A qualitative study. *Community Mental Health Journal, 46,* 381–388. https://doi.org/10.1007/s10597-009-9268-6

Tsai, J., & Rosenheck, R. A. (2012). Consumer choice over living environment, case management and mental health treatment in its relation to outcomes. *Journal of Health Care for the Poor and Underserved, 23*(4), 1671–1677. https://doi.org/10.1353/hpu.2012.0180

Tsai, J., & Rosenheck, R. A. (2015). Risk factors for homelessness among US veterans. *Epidemiologic Reviews.* https://doi.org/10.1093/epirev/mxu004

Tsemberis, S. (2010). *Housing First: The pathways model to end homelessness for people with mental illness and addiction.* Hazelden.

Tsemberis, S., & Asmussen, S. (1999). From streets to homes: The pathways to housing consumer preference supported housing model. In K. J. Conrad (Ed.), *Homelessness prevention in treatment of substance abuse and mental illness: Logic models and implementation of eight American projects* (pp. 113–131). Haworth Press.

Tsemberis, S., & Eisenberg, R. F. (2000). Pathways to housing: Supported housing for street-dwelling homeless individuals with psychiatric disabilities. *Psychiatric Services, 51*(4), 487–493. https://doi.org/10.1176/appi.ps.51.4.487

Tsemberis, S., Gulcur, L., & Nakae, M. (2004). Housing First, consumer choice, and harm reduction for homeless individuals with a dual diagnosis. *American Journal of Public Health, 94*(4), 651–656. https://doi.org/10.2105/ajph.94.4.651

Tuan, Y. F. (1977). *Space and place: The perspective of experience.* University of Minnesota Press.

Tuan, Y. F. (2012). *Humanist geography: An individual's search for meaning.* George F. Thompson Publishing.

Tuntiya, N. (2006). Making a case for the Geel model: The American experience with family care for mental patients. *Community Mental Health Journal, 42,* 319–330. https://doi.org/10.1007/s10597-005-9029-0

U.S. Department of Health and Human Services. (2003). *The President's New Freedom Commission on Mental Health achieving the promise: Transforming mental health care in America.* Author.

U.S. Department of Health and Human Services. (2005). *Transforming mental health care in America—The federal action agenda: First steps.* Author.

Viron, M., Bello, I., Freudenreich, O., & Shtasel, D. (2014). Characteristics of homeless adults with serious mental illness served by a state mental health transitional shelter. *Community Mental Health Journal, 50*(5), 560–565. https://doi.org/10.1007/s10597-013-9607-5

Weiner, A., Roe, D., Mashiach-Eizenberg, M., Baloush-Kleinman, V., Maoz, H., & Yanos, P. (2010). Housing model for persons with serious mental illness moderates the relation between loneliness and quality of life. *Community Mental Health Journal, 46*(4), 389–397. https://doi.org/10.1007/s10597-009-9279-3

Whitley, R., & Henwood, B. F. (2014). Life, liberty, and the pursuit of happiness: Reframing inequities experienced by people with severe mental illness. *Psychiatric Rehabilitation Journal, 37*(1), 68–70. https://doi.org/10.1037/prj0000053

Wilkins, C. (2015). Connecting permanent supportive housing to health care delivery and payment systems: Opportunities and challenges. *American Journal of Psychiatric Rehabilitation, 18*(1), 65–86. https://doi.org/10.1080/15487768.2015.1001690

Williams v. Quinn, 748 F. Supp. 2d 892 (N.D. Ill. 2010).

Wong, Y. I., & Solomon, P. L. (2002). Community integration of persons with psychiatric disabilities in supporting independent housing: A conceptual model and methodological considerations. *Mental Health Services Research, 4*(1), 13–28. https://doi.org/10.1023/a:1014093008857

Yanos, P. T., Stefancic, A., & Tsemberis, S. (2012). Objective community integration of mental health consumers living in supported housing and of others in the community. *Psychiatric Services, 63*(5), 438–444. https://doi.org/10.1176/appi.ps.201100397

Young, S. L., & Ensing, D. S. (1999). Exploring recovery from the perspective of people with psychiatric disabilities. *Psychiatric Rehabilitation Journal, 22*(3), 219–232. https://doi.org/10.1037/h0095240

Zippay, N., & Lee, S. K. (2008). Neighbors' perceptions of community-based psychiatric housing. *Social Services Review, 82*(3), 395–417. https://doi.org/10.1086/592857

The Neighborhood and Community

Carrie Anne Marshall and Terry Krupa

In recent years, increased attention has been dedicated to the role of environments, including neighborhoods and communities, in supporting or detracting from mental well-being (Mahmoudi Farahani, 2016). This evidence has led to increased research, policy, and practice efforts directed toward realizing the capacity of neighborhoods and communities to influence the mental health and well-being of all citizens. This growing interest in neighborhoods and communities within the mental health field is good news for occupational therapy practitioners (OTPs).

The profession is defined by its focus on participation and function in meaningful activities, which naturally occur in neighborhood and community environments (Egan & Restall, 2022). After all, people come to build their social networks through the activities they spend time doing, as they typically engage in activities with others in the physical spaces of their neighborhoods and within the communities to which they belong (Ramugondo & Kronenberg, 2015).

This chapter focuses on an often neglected but important environment—the neighborhood and the communities in which people occupy their time. People live, socialize, recreate, and conduct many instrumental activities of daily living (IADLs) within their neighborhoods and communities. One of the most meaningful ways that people spend their time is with individuals who compose communities within their neighborhoods and beyond. All too often, individuals who live with mental illness face exclusion from their neighborhoods and communities. This is an unfortunate reality given the essential role that neighborhoods and communities play in promoting recovery. By experiencing belonging within their neighborhoods and communities, people can grow, heal, and develop as individuals irrespective of whether they live with mental illness.

In the following sections, the text provides definitions for "neighborhood" and "community" and discusses their associations with occupational performance, engagement, and experience. The text also explores specific challenges and opportunities that neighborhoods pose for individuals who live with mental illness. Further, the chapter discusses ways in which neighborhoods and communities may influence the mental well-being of all persons, whether diagnosed with a mental illness or not. To guide practice, the chapter provides an overview of assessment and intervention approaches that can be used at the neighborhood and community levels.

Defining Neighborhoods and Communities

The terms "neighborhood" and "community" are often used to refer to geographic locations. Although the terms are typically used interchangeably, there are differences. **Neighborhoods** can be conceptualized as the loosely bound physical space that surrounds the area in close proximity to an individual's place of residence. Neighbors are people who share space around where one lives. They can become friends, but even when they do not, they are often considered to be a potential source of informal support. Neighbors might, for example, lend out tools, help out with picking up groceries, or send their children to help look after someone's home when the owners are away. At the very least, neighbors are people whom one might expect to share an interest in maintaining the neighborhood as a welcoming and safe place to live as well as a potential place to build a sense of community.

Community, on the other hand, is oriented to people and relationships. The people and relationships that make up a community may be in one's neighborhood, but may also be located in other neighborhoods, regions, or beyond. For example, people may have relationships with their neighbors, which is one type of community, but they can also belong to communities with individuals from other neighborhoods. These communities are often centered around an activity such as activism, employment, a person's profession, sports, or other leisure activities. Increasingly, it is common to be a member of an online community through social media or online gaming. See Chapter 33: Virtual Environments.

Interdependence and Mental Health

Occupational therapy is a profession that emphasizes the importance of promoting the "independence" of individuals living with a range of health and social conditions. Independence is defined in occupational therapy as having choice over one's activities and the ability to perform them in chosen ways without the support of others (Collins, 2017). Interdependence, on the other hand, involves relying on relationships to engage in and perform desired activities (Collins, 2017). The latter has less often been a focus of occupational therapy; consequently, the profession has historically emphasized individuality and "doing" alone.

Scholars are increasingly questioning the extent to which occupational therapy has embraced a Westernized, individualistic view of disability and occupation, and the extent to which a focus on independence reflects the neoliberal values of the cultures in which the profession originated. As such, these scholars have called for a greater focus on interdependence as a way of acknowledging the interconnectedness of all living things, to recognize that independence and interdependence necessarily coexist, and to reduce a Westernized and ableist focus within the profession (Hammell, 2023; Kirby, 2015).

By promoting both interdependence and independence together, occupational therapy has the potential to help individuals living with mental illness to construct lives that enable them to function and participate in activities both independently and also with the support of others when needed or desired. Approaches directed at the levels of neighborhoods and communities have the potential to promote interdependence, which has been historically undervalued in the occupational therapy profession.

Current Interest in Neighborhoods and Communities

There is a growing recognition that OTPs' understanding of mental health and mental illness has been overly focused on individual risk and that a more balanced view that integrates social and ecological perspectives is needed (World Health Organization [WHO], 2014). For example, research conducted in the past several years indicates that individuals living with serious mental illness in high-income countries die 10 to 20 years sooner than individuals in the general population, often because of the inadequate social conditions in which they are situated (Vigo et al., 2016). These social conditions include living in poverty, having insufficient access to food and housing, and experiencing the negative impacts of social exclusion resulting from stigma and discrimination. Research indicates that stigma and discrimination are disproportionately experienced by persons living with mental illness and substance use disorders (Hack et al., 2020; Murney et al., 2020).

Symptoms of stigma and discrimination are evident in the fact that persons living with mental illness are more likely to live in poverty, experience homelessness (Hossain et al., 2020), live in food insecure households, and have insufficient access to meaningful activities and relationships that are protective of mental health (Doroud et al., 2015). As wealth inequality grows in high-income countries, this discrimination is felt stronger than ever before. Although many individuals who live with mental illness are able to find inroads into community and remain in the neighborhoods of their choosing, a disturbing number of persons who live with mental illness are thrust into precarious living situations and are often denied the right to live free of discrimination within their neighborhoods and communities (Marshall et al., 2023). Such conditions make it challenging for anyone to attain mental well-being and are especially detrimental for individuals living with mental illness. See Chapter 27: Mental Health Stigma and Sanism and Chapter 28: Social Determinants and Mental Health.

Knowledge of these realities has led to the proliferation of scholarship focused on social determinants of mental health (WHO, 2014). Social determinants of mental health include social factors that influence mental health for better or worse, including housing and living conditions, employment and work conditions, transportation, income, and access to services. These associations have been researched from a broad range of perspectives. For example:

- In a systematic review of 63 studies, researchers identified that neighborhood crime was strongly associated with the mental health of residents (Baranyi et al., 2021). Higher rates of crime were specifically associated with increased depression, psychological distress, anxiety, and psychosis. The authors argued that there is a need for community-level approaches aimed at reducing crime as a mental health promotion strategy.
- Researchers studying youth mental health have identified that depression, anxiety, suicide ideation, aggression, conduct disorder, and property offenses were lower among young people residing in neighborhoods with greater social cohesion (Kingsbury et al., 2020).
- Fong and colleagues (2019) found that having a sense of neighborhood identity moderates the effects of socioeconomic disadvantage. Further, the authors found that individuals who had a sense of identity as a member of their neighborhood reported better mental health.
- In research with individuals who experience homelessness and mental illness, studies have identified that individuals often struggle to integrate into their communities during and following homelessness (Marshall et al., 2023). In related research, community integration has been demonstrated to be poorly targeted by many existing interventions designed to support persons living with mental illness who are leaving homelessness; however, interventions that included engagement in meaningful activity and peer support demonstrated effectiveness (Marshall et al., 2020).
- Research conducted during the COVID-19 pandemic in the United Kingdom indicated that the solidarity resulting from participating in collaborative community initiatives aimed at supporting fellow citizens through the pandemic predicted psychological bonding that was associated with improved mental well-being (Bowe et al., 2022).

These studies represent only a small fraction of a broad and growing area of interdisciplinary research that helps OTPs to understand how neighborhoods and communities influence the mental well-being of their members as well as inform the development of policy and other intervention approaches.

Trends Drawing Attention to Neighborhood and Community Approaches

Changes in how people support persons living with mental illness in the present day, coupled with structural changes in high-income countries internationally in recent years, have resulted in increased interest in scholarship and the development and evaluation of solutions aimed at neighborhoods and communities. These changes include deinstitutionalization and growing wealth inequality.

Deinstitutionalization

Until the 1980s, persons living with mental illness often received support for mental illness within institutional settings. Although institutions were viewed as providing individuals living with mental illness "asylum" from the pressures of daily life in the community, they also had the unintended effect of excluding individuals from their communities, as many individuals were admitted to inpatient settings for decades of their lives, and these institutions were seen as costly and inhumane (Erickson, 2021). This, coupled with the fact that psychiatric institutions were frequently overcrowded, resulting in an erosion in the standard of care, led to a growing wave of criticism from academics and advocates alike, who increased pressure for community-based solutions to support individuals living with mental illness (Ben-Moshe, 2020; Goffman, 1961; Szasz, 1970). This resulted in a process of **deinstitutionalization** in which psychiatric institutions were gradually closed and replaced with community-based approaches that supported persons living with mental illness in regular neighborhoods and communities.

Although the original intent of deinstitutionalization was to promote the community reintegration of people who experienced long stays in institutions, such as psychiatric hospitals, it has evolved to have a larger focus on the prevention of institutionalization of people living with mental illness in the community.

As the process of deinstitutionalization has unfolded over several years, with large psychiatric institutions still closing in high-income countries within the last two decades, reception to this approach has been mixed. In the present day, access to mental health care in the community is severely underfunded, resulting in a dire shortage of inpatient mental health beds and growing waitlists for community-based mental health services.

As a consequence, many individuals living with mental illness are left floundering in their communities without adequate support or receiving care through systems that inappropriately serve their needs such as shelters and criminal justice systems (Brown, 2022; Lamb & Weinberger, 2020). This unfortunate reality has left researchers, policymakers, practitioners, and persons with lived experiences and their families advocating for the development and evaluation of innovative solutions to more effectively support individuals living with mental illness in their communities—not a return to institutionalization, but rather a more effective and appropriate system of supports.

Persons living with mental illness, particularly those with serious and persistent forms of illness, require careful attention to the stabilization of their mental illness, including active involvement in illness self-management and careful consideration of their housing situations in community settings. Finding ways of integrating in their communities and helping them to build active social networks within their neighborhoods and beyond is an essential approach to promoting good community-based mental health care. Individuals living with mental illness require a range of complex skills of community living and access to the resources, supports, and opportunities that all citizens need to establish themselves in their communities. Occupational therapy is a critical part of helping individuals to develop these skills at individual, community, and population levels. See Chapter 27: Mental Health Stigma and Sanism.

Growing Wealth Inequality

It is an unfortunate reality that wealth inequality is growing internationally, and this has disproportionately affected individuals living with mental illness in various communities. Mental illness and poverty are deeply intertwined, with a range of research studies indicating that poverty is both a cause and a consequence of mental illness (Ridley et al., 2020). Ridley and colleagues (2020) report that across studies, persons living with mental illness have fewer opportunities for employment and are therefore more likely to live in low-income housing. Further, studies included in this review provide evidence that mental illness among persons living in poverty is caused by experiences of trauma, low social status, violence and crime in their neighborhoods, and constant worry associated with living on an insufficient income with little savings to draw upon (Ridley et al., 2020).

Growing wealth inequality, coupled with a housing market that continues to increase in value and a lack of government investment in public and supportive housing, has resulted in a growing homelessness crisis in most countries internationally. This crisis has disproportionately affected individuals living with mental illness in various communities, with up to 98% of persons experiencing homelessness being people who also live with mental illness (Hossain et al., 2020). Having inadequate access to housing not only presents barriers to accessing services for persons living with mental illness, but frequently results in increased exposure to trauma, traumatic brain injury, and substance use that only further complicates mental illness.

In addition to rising rates of homelessness, growing wealth inequality means that persons living with mental illness are also experiencing increases in food insecurity, placing them at risk of developing other chronic diseases (Teasdale et al., 2020). In one study conducted with 19 women living in social housing in Canada, all but two reported that they had been diagnosed with mental illness, despite the fact that mental illness was not an inclusion criterion. Further, more than half indicated that food security was a problem, with nearly 32% indicating that they experienced moderate to high levels of food insecurity (Marshall et al., 2021). These studies and others highlight the intersectional nature of mental illness for persons living in various communities.

Occupying a range of social locations such as being a person living with psychiatric disability, being a woman, and living in poverty can intersect to create a situation where persons with mental illness are profoundly excluded from their neighborhoods and mainstream communities such that even their basic needs for housing and food are unmet. See Chapter 28: Social Determinants and Mental Health.

Social Capital in Neighborhoods and Communities

Social capital theory was introduced by a range of theorists including Bourdieu, Coleman, and Putnam (Field, 2016). It can be thought of as the power that individuals hold in society that is gained or lost through the relationships that they build and the social positions that they occupy. This power can be conceptualized as a form of currency that can determine the influence that one has in their community as well as the opportunities afforded to them by others in that community. The influence that a person has in their neighborhood and community is often determined by the social capital that they have accumulated, which is typically developed through civic participation and informal relationship-building.

Social capital can be held by individuals, neighborhoods, and communities. High social capital neighborhoods and communities are characterized by increased levels of trust and reciprocity where neighbors and community members take care of one another and actively advocate for better living conditions and resources for individual members as well as the collective (Ehsan et al., 2019).

A range of factors determine the social capital that an individual, neighborhood, or community may have and how each may be associated with mental health, mental illness, and occupation. These can be conceptualized using a framework for understanding how neighborhoods and communities enable or constrain the occupational lives of people and ultimately influence mental health and mental illness. These dimensions include the following (represented in Fig. 32-1):

- Organization and activism
- Neighborhood socioeconomic status (SES)
- Neighborhood safety
- Resident mobility
- Diversity
- Community attitudes

Neighborhood Organization and Activism

Neighborhood social structures and interactions can be characterized by the extent to which they reflect civic participation, a sense of identity, equality among members, and community responsibility and reciprocity. Social capital

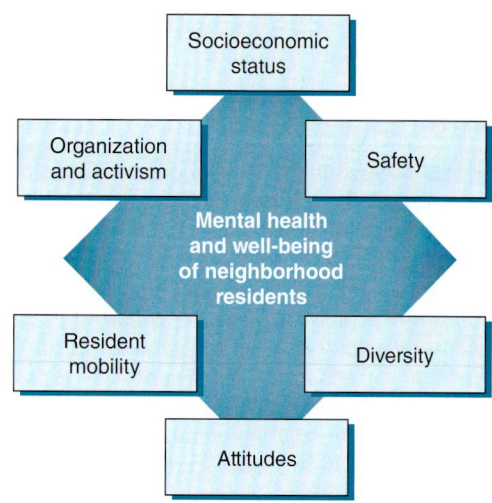

FIGURE 32-1. Dimensions of mental health and well-being in neighborhood communities. This framework can help OTPs understand how neighborhoods and communities enable or constrain the occupational lives of people and ultimately influence mental health and mental illness.

represents these characteristics, which engender cooperation and trust among community members. Although more research is needed, studies have demonstrated relationships between social capital and mental health, including the effectiveness of social capital interventions for improving mental well-being (Flores et al., 2018).

The mechanisms by which social capital influences the mental health of individuals are complex. A review of research across the life span conducted by Almedom and Glandon (2008) indicated that social capital offers its positive effects through at least four pathways: (1) the ability of social norms to influence positive health-related behaviors; (2) the ability of social networks to enhance positive psychological processes such as self-esteem, confidence, and control; (3) social networks, which increase access to health and social resources and amenities; and (4) a reduction in illicit and criminal activities.

PhotoVoice–For Students Only

I had the biggest struggle with just finding a place. Or even getting showings . . . when you would go to a showing, they would ask "Are you a student?" and if you said no, they would shut off . . . there was a lot of discrimination because I'm on [disability-related social assistance]. I would either be immediately rejected, or people would tell me about their bad experience with a [disability-related social assistance] person, which apparently gave them the stigma that every person on [disability-related social assistance] is bad . . . or I would be asked really uncomfortable questions about my disability. [Gavin, a person with lived experiences of mental illness and homelessness]

Are there characteristics or symbols that, if present in a neighborhood, may communicate to a person that they are unwelcome?

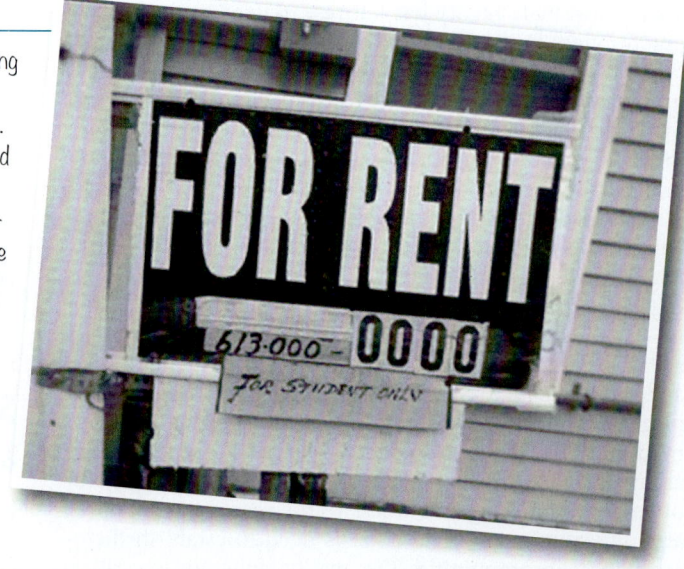

Neighborhood Socioeconomic Status

Neighborhoods constitute an important external condition for recovery by offering access to a range of work, education, self-care, social, and recreational opportunities that are consistent with basic human rights. These opportunities can create a positive culture of hope that can enable a full occupational life beyond the limits of mental illness. Persons who live with mental illness and experience poverty, however, are more likely to live in poorer neighborhoods characterized by a range of social disadvantages, and this can have a serious impact on occupational performance, engagement, and experience. For example, children living in neighborhoods characterized by poverty experience academic and behavioral difficulties more often than children from wealthier areas (Morrissey & Vinopal, 2018).

Persons living in poorer neighborhoods also have fewer opportunities for high-quality employment characterized by higher wages, benefits, and opportunities for professional advancement. Instead, persons living in socially disadvantaged neighborhoods are more likely to obtain precarious employment with few benefits that only sustains their poverty over time. This is highly problematic as precarious employment is more likely to expose individuals who are residents of low-income neighborhoods to hazardous work environments that place them at risk of further disability and thereby compound social disadvantage further (Bonney et al., 2022).

Socioeconomic disadvantage is also reflected in conditions that are uninviting to, or constrain, involvement in meaningful activity. In a study exploring transitions from homelessness to housing, researchers identified that a lack of material resources was a primary barrier to engagement in meaningful activity, and that living in environments such as shelters in disadvantaged neighborhoods limited these options further (Marshall, Gewurtz, et al., 2024).

Factors that prevent engagement in meaningful activity for persons who experience homelessness include the need to follow the rules established formally in shelters, permanent supportive housing programs, and law enforcement, or informally on the street or in urban encampments. These formal and informal rules often dictate which activities persons with experiences of homelessness can or cannot participate in beyond the influence of material resources in their neighborhoods. See Chapter 42: Homelessness and Housing Insecurity.

Neighborhood Safety

The relative prevalence of crime and violence is of particular concern in disadvantaged neighborhoods. Feeling safe in one's own neighborhood is important for positive occupational performance, yet existing research indicates the persons living with serious mental illness are more likely to be victims of violence in their neighborhoods (Bhavsar et al., 2020). Concerns about personal security and the presence of antisocial behaviors, such as substance use and the presence of an open market for illicit substances, have been associated with psychological distress and poorer mental health. In one study, single women living with mental illness in social housing described how a perceived lack of safety in their apartment building led to social isolation in their apartments, which severely restricted the activities in which they could participate

in their daily lives and consequently led to further difficulties with attaining mental well-being (Marshall et al., 2020).

For persons living with mental illness, having fewer opportunities to participate in meaningful activity, coupled with the presence of an active market for illicit substances in the neighborhood, may lead to increased participation in activities involving the use of substances (Marshall, Easton, et al., 2024). This can result in worsening mental health by creating co-occurring disorders of mental illness and substance use, which also may lead to increasing vulnerability and victimization. In a scoping review focusing on the use of methamphetamine among persons who experience homelessness, for example, participants in the included studies who used methamphetamine were more likely to experience violence and victimization in their neighborhoods (Carrillo Beck et al., 2022).

Resident Mobility

Resident mobility is the movement of residents in and out of a neighborhood through time (Silver et al., 2002). In a neighborhood with high resident mobility, people do not stay very long and there is a high rate of "turnover" in homes. High levels of resident mobility are believed to compromise mental health by negatively impacting the development of strong social networks that can allay the risks associated with vulnerability to symptoms of mental illness.

Individuals living with mental illness who are at risk of homelessness experience high levels of residential mobility, as well as the inability to create meaningful community connections that support meaningful activity engagement. This can pose risks to the mental health of the person who is forced to move because of the loss of a tenancy, and can also pose risks to other residents in the neighborhood. For example, the extent to which people move beyond the boundaries of their own neighborhood in the typical course of their daily activities is a concept referred to as "activity space" (Vallée et al., 2011).

Research has suggested that residents in disadvantaged neighborhoods have higher rates of depression when their activity space limits them to their immediate neighborhood, but that limited activity space does not appear to have the same impact within more advantaged neighborhoods. This is likely because of the fact that persons living in low-income neighborhoods are less likely to have reliable access to transportation options to engage in activities that occur further afield.

One example of how residential mobility influences meaningful activity engagement and mental well-being is revealed through the many persons with mental illness who are forced to live in urban encampments because of a lack of deeply affordable housing and appropriate shelter spaces. This problem continues to increase in many high- and middle-income countries, and became especially visible during the COVID-19 pandemic (Boucher et al., 2022).

Persons living with mental illness in urban encampments are frequently forced to relocate from neighborhoods by municipal governments. These municipal governments are driven by the desire to preserve the availability of public spaces such as parks and the belief that there is a need to control the proliferation of crime and violence that is attributed to the presence of urban encampments. As there is no other place to go, persons who experience homelessness are forced to find other places in the community that are further from view and the services that are designed to support them. This leads to a worsening of mental health because of disconnection from communities of mutual support provided by other encampment residents and outreach services that provide support there.

The ongoing precarity that results from being denied the right to adequate housing, coupled with being constantly driven away from encampments with no other place to go, can severely impair one's ability to engage in activities that are meaningful. This is because one is forced to engage in survival activities with little opportunity to explore other activities that support self-actualization. Further, the ability of encampment residents to take on meaningful community roles is impaired by the constant precariousness of housing that, in some cases, continues for several years of their lives.

Neighborhood Diversity

Neighborhood diversity can contribute in positive and negative ways to mental health. Persons who occupy social conditions such as oppressed races, genders, or sexual orientations or who live with disabilities may be particularly vulnerable to exclusion in neighborhoods that are more heterogeneous, in their demographic makeup and that exclude these groups. Conversely, when neighborhoods are more heterogeneous, individuals who occupy similar social locations, such as being a member of the 2SLGBTQ+ community or identifying with a particular race or religion, may engender a feeling of safety, acceptance, and mutual support.

In one Australian study, increases in ethnic diversity in neighborhoods resulted in poorer mental health of residents, leading the authors to conclude that there is a need for neighborhood interventions that promote trust and belonging across ethnic groups to engender more positive mental health (Awaworyi Churchill et al., 2019). Historically, persons living with mental illness have been excluded from their communities, which is largely linked to a history of excluding persons with mental illness through institutionalization. The legacy of this approach to mental health care has resulted in a culture of "Not In My BackYardism" (NIMBYism), wherein community members who identify the behaviors of persons with mental illness as problematic may seek to eradicate such individuals from neighborhood spaces. See Chapter 28: Social Determinants and Mental Health.

Community Attitudes

Public stigma and the discrimination of people who experience mental illness is a well-known issue. It is of particular importance when considering one's neighborhood, because social proximity and social interactions characterize community environments. Stigma can enforce exclusion from relationships, activities, and physical spaces and places that constitute the neighborhood. See Chapter 27: Mental Health Stigma and Sanism.

The neighborhood environment may be an important context in which to change stigmatizing attitudes and their associated discriminatory behaviors. Interpersonal contact between individuals living with mental illness and members of the public has gained prominence as an effective way to reduce stigma, particularly when the nature of the contact can disconfirm negative beliefs and attitudes. Such approaches can mitigate the stigma of mental illness and the potential for the

emergence of NIMBYism in neighborhoods, as well as the need to be incorporated into strategies that aim to create inclusive neighborhoods for all (Shearer et al., 2021). By definition, neighborhoods bring people into contexts that allow for a range of social exchanges. Therefore, neighborhood residents may become more likely to accept their neighbors with mental illnesses through time, with multiple contacts, and through the opportunity to interact collaboratively and as equals.

Stigma or the perception of stigma in the neighborhood may affect an individual's willingness to accept treatment or rehabilitation. In some cases, the ways in which mental health services are delivered in community settings may promote stigma by compromising one's perception or actual status as neighbors. In one study, participants living with mental illness described mental health professionals contributing to their experience of stigma by openly carrying medications into their homes and by arriving for home appointments in cars that they felt could easily be connected to mental health services (Krupa et al., 2005). This has led scholars to advocate for education for health professionals that encourages the acknowledgement of the stigma that professionals hold and encourages behaviors that reduce stigma in practice (Ungar et al., 2016).

Intervening to Develop Supportive Neighborhood Communities

Most mental health services are primarily directed at attending to the needs, limitations, and strengths of individuals with mental illness, with a view to enabling person-level changes that will lead to community integration. Historically, occupational therapy practices have largely focused on the skills that people need to "fit in" and successfully participate in meaningful neighborhood and community activities.

Within inpatient and day program settings, OTPs are challenged in their efforts to address the occupational issues of the people they treat because they practice at a distance from the neighborhood and community contexts within which these occupations occur. Today, people who are admitted to inpatient mental health settings are typically experiencing acute illness or their mental health has destabilized in the midst of a crisis in community life.

It can be difficult for the OTPs working in inpatient settings to envision the individual making the transition back to neighborhood life, especially if the person's inpatient stay has been long. However, the OTP's role in the inpatient context still includes integrating a return to the neighborhood and community context into short- and long-term goals and collaborating alongside interdisciplinary teams to do the same. Efforts to improve the recovery orientation of inpatient services have resulted in the development of a recovery competency framework for inpatient providers (Chen et al., 2013). This framework includes specific competencies related to enabling the transition to community life, such as:

- Connecting people who are inpatients and their significant others to community services and resources
- Connecting people who are inpatients to their most significant healing relationships and supports in the community

The Lived Experience

Niq

Shared experience brings us together as humans, whether that is bonding through long hikes with our dogs or discussing our histories and the places where our experiences dovetail, or working on a garden together, or sharing a worldview, or being the person who they call for advice or a sober outlook when they are "drunk" and upset. The decision to choose positive connection does not mean leaving behind the folks we know who are struggling but finding new paths through that struggle and new ways of being together. Sometimes folks won't be along for the ride, and that comes with its own sense of grief and loss. Choosing community, joy, and recovery does not mean abandoning those we are connected to who are having a more difficult time, even with that person is ourselves.

I am so lucky to have become friends with the wonderful people who I count as my community. Community is so key to a well lived life in recovery from housing instability, substance dependence, and both the trauma that contributed to it and that was a product of it. We are there for each other through rough patches and share and celebrate "the good" together. The communities that form around positive activities and that help us through the rough times are so important. For me, the folks who I have worked with or for, whether that is through tattooing or farming or cooking, have my back in a way that so many of the folks I met strictly through a community of "activism" or "faith" do not. For me, my community included the folks who I do life affirming activities with. This can be walking our dogs together, or sharing food, talking about our excitements or fears, or attending online meditation sessions. It is often helping each other out when we are able in the ways we can offer outside of guilt or compulsion. Celebrating important moments with these people has shown me what community can truly mean.

Connection to others outside of ourselves is so critical for humans in our development and recovery. When these things are broken, it leads to a deep sense of destabilization, shame, and grief that, often, substances are the obvious substitute for. But the use of these substances can also act as a barrier to connection.

Finding folks who understand, and finding, uplifting, and celebrating the ways that our lived experiences are similar even when it is not apparent on the surface, really helps us feel less alone and more connected. When we connect through lived experience, we learn from each other, support each other, and grow together in ways that can generate healing not only for ourselves, but for others. Even when they are drawing their own conclusions, whether that is around substance use, or political identity, or relationship structures, or faith, or priorities, we mutually respect each other and offer what balance and comfort and help we can. These are the folks who I have found who deeply enrich my life and who make my recovery from trauma and trauma-reactions possible.

I've recently moved to a new city, and am excited about the opportunity that it presents, away from the triggers of old-time bad experiences and connections that were formed during years of active substance dependence. Some of these people I still count as my closest people, regardless of their own sobriety, but I am missing the folks who have been solid in my life, and I am lucky enough to have a car so that I can go back and visit them. We are still finding time for each other, even as we grow and connect with new people as well. Honestly, at the end of the day, I feel like I'm finally building an understanding of what a healthy and supportive family can look like and am grateful to have found my people. Community is something that acts less like a fortress and more like a welcome shore you can always return to and that grows and changes with the tide. I can honestly say that these folks who mutually choose to walk with me have changed and saved my life.

■ Anticipating potential problems or issues in making community connections and strategizing accordingly
■ Helping people to plan and solve problems related to the transition to community life
■ Integrating community resources in the work of the inpatient setting
■ Strengthening partnerships with local community services and helping with transition processes such as referral and follow-up (adapted from Chen et al., 2013)

In community-based services, OTPs have the opportunity to practice directly in the individual's neighborhood and community environment. They can develop community-based services that offer individuals access to a range of self-care, productivity, and leisure interventions to enhance occupations experienced in daily life and to reduce their experiences of marginalization. If these programs are truly part of the neighborhood, they will be sensitive to the types and range of knowledge and skills that are expected of all community residents, including those with mental illness.

These programs capitalize on the individual's personal abilities and potential within communities. When the community is viewed as a resource and interventions are designed to assist individuals with mental illness to truly become members of their communities, the result can be a feeling of belonging instead of isolation. The Being a Psychosocial OT Practitioner feature provides a great example of an occupational therapist supporting an individual to reengage in their community.

The information provided in this chapter thus far has highlighted the profound influence that the neighborhood and community have on the occupational lives of people with mental illness. It suggests that, in addition to individual-level service approaches, adequate attention must be given to approaches directed to the level of the neighborhood and community. These approaches focus on identifying the needs, limits, and capacities of the neighborhood and community, with a view to facilitating the capacity of the neighborhood to enhance, and be enhanced by, the occupations of all their residents. These approaches can be conceptualized as a form

Being a Psychosocial OT Practitioner

Reengaging in the Community

Contributed by Paula M. Cook, OTD, OTR/L

Identifying Psychosocial Strengths and Needs

OTPs routinely work with individuals experiencing exclusion from their neighborhoods and communities because of physical and mental illnesses that negatively impact their recovery and quality of life. Consider the story of Evelyn and how OTPs can support participation at the neighborhood and community levels.

Evelyn is a 65-year-old woman who lives with her husband, Arnold, in a one-story bungalow in a large city. They live in a middle-class, historical neighborhood. Evelyn had a stroke 2 years ago, which resulted in left hemiparesis. Before her stroke, she worked as a guard in an art museum, which required a bus ride and long hours of standing. She and Arnold were avid travelers.

Evelyn attended inpatient rehabilitation and outpatient therapy, then received home health therapies for several months after her stroke. Although she no longer attends therapy, she continues with the home exercise program she learned during her home health visits. She performs these as part of her daily morning routine. Once a month, she attends a stroke support group led by an OTP at the community hospital outpatient clinic.

Evelyn uses a cane around her home and a manual wheelchair for longer outings. Since her stroke, she has used paratransit services for community mobility. She likes the door-to-door service of paratransit but is increasingly frustrated at the tardiness and unreliability. She is interested in riding the bus again, but not doing so alone.

Although she loves her stroke support group, Evelyn feels her physical health is all she talks about anymore. When she leaves her home, it is mainly for health management reasons. She misses going out for other reasons, like working and grocery shopping, and wishes she was more confident about going places without her husband. Evelyn feels lonely and bored in her home and is experiencing symptoms of depression.

Using a Holistic Occupational Therapy Approach

The OTP is the stroke support leader at the community hospital outpatient clinic. At the end of a support group session, Evelyn mentions how boring it is at home. The other group members nod knowingly and share their experiences of feeling stuck, too. One member asks her why she doesn't go to other places, and Evelyn replies there is nowhere to go. She laments her days feel so long, and before she knows it, she is back here the next month, and not much has changed. The OTP closes out the session and makes a note to discuss community participation in the next session.

While Evelyn waits for her ride, the OTP continues the conversation with Evelyn and uses the Activity Card Sort to understand what activities Evelyn currently does, what she has stopped doing since her stroke, and what she wishes to do. She currently reads a lot on her phone and does simple cooking and cleaning. She misses seeing artwork, earning money, and helping people. She stopped using the bus for fear of falling and missing her stop. She misses seeing the same bus driver daily and making small talk with him. While her long-term goal would be to ride the bus again, Evelyn does not feel ready for that yet. She wishes she could do more than come to these meetings.

The OTP and Evelyn brainstorm ways to get her out of her house more. The OTP works with several other individuals in Evelyn's neighborhood and knows that the local library is a valuable resource. Evelyn knew there was a branch in her neighborhood, though she wasn't too familiar with it because she was so busy working before. Evelyn made a plan to go there next Friday with Arnold. It's close enough that Arnold can walk and push her in her wheelchair. The OTP asks Evelyn to note what supports and barriers she encounters during that outing and report to the stroke support group next month. The OTP follows up with a phone call to confirm the outing is still on her schedule and troubleshoot any planning or accessibility concerns.

At the next month's stroke support group, Evelyn shares her outing experience. They decided to go on a Friday morning as Arnold was off work. They noticed the sidewalks were somewhat uneven in places, but overall Evelyn thought she could walk there with Arnold and her cane the next time. When they arrived at the library, Evelyn needed to use the restroom and had difficulty locating it. The restroom was in the back of the library, but once there, Evelyn appreciated that the accessible stall was closest to the sinks. She expected it to be quiet, being that it was a library on a weekday morning; however, the library had a soft buzz of toddlers and parents who just finished a storytime playgroup. The staff was very helpful as she updated her information to get a library card. She enjoyed choosing the artwork for the card and was surprised she could customize it. The last time she was there, all the cards had the same green and white design. Evelyn became a bit overwhelmed when she saw all the books on display. The librarian offered a few recommendations, which Evelyn chose to borrow.

Arnold quietly followed her around the library. He showed her a small space with local art on exhibit and many free programs like book clubs, holiday crafts, and a puzzle exchange. Evelyn noticed a sign for an upcoming neighborhood garage sale and considered selling some things cluttering her hallway.

She said the main barriers were the restroom location, unexpected noise, and the number of books. The main support was the social support from Arnold and the helpful staff. Overall, she was pleasantly surprised by all the different offerings. She expected it to be "a whole lot of books and not much else."

The other members of the stroke support group listen with encouragement. One mentions that the library has museum passes, so she can go for free. Another member offers to meet her at the library next time because she lives across the street. Someone else asks what days and times they were open. Evelyn shares what she knows and thanks the group for their support. She exchanges contact information with two members and stays after to discuss plans for future library visits.

Reflective Questions

1. List different ways the support group might be structured to better support peer-led activities that foster community participation.
2. What opportunities for advocacy do you notice in Evelyn's story? How might the OTP support Evelyn and other group members in pursuing advocacy that addresses some of these issues?
3. What opportunities for maximizing peer support and community participation might exist in this community-based support group compared with other more traditional settings (e.g., rehabilitation hospitals, outpatient settings)?

of **community development**, a process of building local communities to support the well-being of both individual community members and the community as a whole.

Although there are many definitions of community development, the definition proposed by Gibbon, Gibbon et al. (2002) is one that aligns well with the focus of this chapter: Community development is "a process that increases the assets and attributes which a community is able to draw upon in order to improve their lives" (p. 485). This definition integrates notions of community development, community empowerment, and capacity building to address health and well-being concerns in the community's population.

It is critical that occupational therapy values remain fundamental to community development approaches; that is, occupational therapy practice focused at the level of the neighborhood and community must reflect the fundamental values of personal choice, empowerment, respect for basic human dignities, and respect for individual knowledge and experience. A community development approach includes the values of equal access to meaningful occupations within the community and to the resources and supports that facilitate these occupations.

The implementation of these values in practice will increase the likelihood of sustainability of positive change. Indeed, the notion of community development practice that is espoused in this chapter is consistent with the philosophy and values of occupational justice, a community situation in which "each person and community could meet their own and others' survival, physical, mental and social development needs through occupation that recognised and encouraged individual and communal strengths" (Wilcock & Townsend, 2014, p. 542).

Mental health and public health experts have proposed the development of integrated approaches to address common mental health and well-being problems in local communities. This integrated approach would see the systematic integration of evidence-informed health service practice and community development approaches with a view to optimizing and broadening the scope of outcomes.

For example, in such an integrated approach, evidence-based models, such as strengths-based case management (Fukui et al., 2012), might be explicitly and formally connected to established community development practices such as grassroots organization, participatory needs assessments, coalition building, asset mapping, and capacity building. Such an integrated approach would have the potential to expand the resource base for mental health-related care, engage the commitment of local communities and neighborhoods, and empower people with mental illness to participate directly with community members and to be recognized as important stakeholders, potentially strengthening the positive outcomes already achieved by the model.

With their focus on supporting occupations in the natural community context, OTPs could serve as leaders in building and sustaining such an integrated approach. For example, Lauckner et al. (2011) conducted a case study of three different OTPs working as community developers to develop a conceptual framework for occupation-focused community development practice.

Assessing Neighborhoods and Developing a Neighborhood Profile

Neighborhoods are complex entities with multiple structural and relational components. The dimensions of neighborhood communities described earlier provide a basic framework for community assessment and understanding the complex associations between occupation and the neighborhood environment. These dimensions can be used by OTPs to work collaboratively with persons with mental illness to create a neighborhood profile. The profile can include both a description of important neighborhood characteristics and a visual map locating important resources and activities.

The neighborhood profile has meaning when it leads to a process of exploration and evaluation in relation to the individual's occupational performance and experience. For example, a neighborhood profile can identify specific resources in the community to support leisure interests. It can also lead to a discussion of neighborhood barriers that interfere with active participation in community supports, such as encountering places or people that make an individual feel unsafe. The profile can also help identify difficulties accessing needed resources (e.g., limited transportation options). In this way, the neighborhood profile becomes personalized—that is, a vehicle for raising the individual's awareness of the context of their daily life and reflecting on themself as a member of a community. Figure 32-2 shows a sample template for a neighborhood profile.

The neighborhood profile can lead to discussions about other potentially supportive neighborhoods. Individuals, for example, may continue to maintain social and occupational connections with their previous neighborhoods, and these may serve to counterbalance challenges arising in the present neighborhood. Similarly, extending the boundaries of the neighborhood can reveal opportunities that are aligned with the individual's values and interests while still being readily accessible. Community colleges, for example, often offer a wide range of courses and educational schedules that are accessible to the larger community.

Practitioners who work in programs that serve a large number of individuals from one, or only a few, neighborhood communities will benefit from developing formal neighborhood profiles. Formal neighborhood profiles create an accurate representation of a neighborhood community with regard to information about the population, employment rates, business and industry, land use, educational opportunities, housing, recreational resources, and health services. These profiles are developed both by spending time in and being immersed in the community, and also from existing databases that can be accessed through internet and library services.

Beyond collaboration with people with mental illnesses, this type of neighborhood profile is essential for larger initiatives focused on assisting individuals with mental illness as a collective to establish themselves in their communities. For example, OTPs who are interested in developing employment, occupational, and leadership opportunities for people living with mental illness in a particular neighborhood can initiate and support the development of a work integration social

Neighborhood Profile	
Considerations	
1. Demographics of individuals living in the neighborhood—age, family structure (single, couples, families with young children), ethnic/cultural groups, socioeconomic status	1. _____ _____ _____

2. Housing
  a. Types of housing—single family, apartments, condos
  b. Availability
  c. Cost
	2. _____
	  a. _____
	  b. _____
	  c. _____

3. Safety
  a. Crime rates, types of crime
  b. Policing, neighborhood watch organizations
  c. Dangerous/safe areas
	3. _____
	  a. _____
	  b. _____
	  c. _____

4. Businesses
  a. Shopping (grocery stores, pharmacy, clothing, thrift stores)
  b. Banks and other financial services (money orders)
	4. _____
	  a. _____
	  b. _____

5. Leisure and recreational resources—parks, movie theaters, walking paths, coffee shops, museums	5. _____ _____

6. Employment
  a. Types of employment in the neighborhood
  b. Unemployment rates
	6. _____
	  a. _____
	  b. _____

7. Public transportation
  a. Cost, availability of passes for people with mental illness
  b. Routes, access to important locations
	7. _____
	  a. _____
	  b. _____

8. Social services—health services, food banks, housing assistance	8. _____
9. Educational resources—libraries, schools (K–12), community colleges	9. _____
10. Day care (child and elder); after-school programs	10. _____
11. Religious organizations	11. _____
12. Community clubs and organizations (e.g., scouting, recreational sports, political organizations, social clubs)	12. _____
13. Neighborhood newspapers/newsletters, online resources	13. _____
14. Aesthetics—architecture, cleanliness, art, natural spaces, pollution	14. _____
15. Intangibles—friendliness, openness to outsiders, acceptance of nonconformity	15. _____

FIGURE 32-2. Sample template for a neighborhood profile. Profiles can help raise an individual's awareness of the context of their daily life and reflect on what it means to be a member of a community.

enterprise (WISE). WISEs are social enterprises that provide job opportunities for individuals who are facing exclusion from traditional forms of employment and have demonstrated effectiveness for positively addressing the stigma of mental illness in previous research (Krupa et al., 2019).

Practitioners may also support the development of a WISE that is completely consumer-run. This type of community economic development effort will depend on the resources and services available and the economic needs of the community to ensure viability of the business. The neighborhood profile will also help reveal the potential for the credibility and recognition of the business, and subsequently the employees, in the community.

Dynamic Assessment of Neighborhood and Community Capacity

A second approach to neighborhood community assessment focuses on revealing the potential assets and capacities of communities. Community researchers Kretzmann and McKnight (1993) argued that the traditional path to community development, overcome by the overwhelmingly negative influences that exist in neighborhoods in trouble (unemployment, high crime rates, lack of resources, low social capital, etc.), has centered on identifying needs, problems, and limitations. The result is that the interventions that follow are based on the view that the neighborhood is deficient and requires external resources to diagnose and correct the problems. This deficit-based approach can leave the community reliant on external expertise and fail to capitalize on community strengths and capacities.

Kretzmann and McKnight (1993) argued that all communities have the inherent capacity for sustained regeneration. To release this capacity, they highlight the importance of approaches that serve to identify and build on the community's own capacities. This community-building perspective has gained respect as the preferable approach to guide the development of occupational therapy practice in the area of community development (Lauckner et al., 2011).

Practitioners who assess a neighborhood from a capacity-building approach focus their efforts on understanding how to release the assets of the community to successfully engage persons with mental illness in the occupations of the neighborhood. Using the framework proposed by Kretzmann and McKnight (1993) and Kretzmann et al. (2005), the assessment would include the following steps:

1. Identify the skills and resources (e.g., time, skills from past education and work experiences, knowledge of music, family and friends with a range of skills and resources, computer experience, and previous experience in organizing or participating in communities) that people living with mental illness can contribute to their communities.

2. Identify community assets (e.g., local associations, community groups, churches, and public institutions such as schools, libraries, and local businesses) that could serve as potential partners for people with mental illness.

3. Determine how reciprocal and productive connections can be formed using the capacities of people with mental illness and the assets of the community. (For example, members of the local senior center may wish to hire individuals to assist with looking after their homes when they are away; local public schools may be interested in developing opportunities for students to learn about diversity and acceptance, including gaining an understanding of mental illness; or a local committee focusing on accessibility issues may benefit from members who can help broaden their view beyond physical accessibility.)

Practices to Support Change

Considering the neighborhood as the target of intervention requires practices that may be unfamiliar or even uncomfortable to some OTPs. However, the profession has developed the knowledge base and continues to build practice expertise in the area of environmental modifications. When applied to the neighborhood and community, OTPs can address the occupational needs of people served within community environments. As OTPs advance their understanding of the modifiable aspects of neighborhoods and communities that can be strategically addressed to improve mental health and well-being, innovative and effective practice strategies are likely to follow. The following are suggestions for ways in which practitioners can become more involved in neighborhoods and creating environments that support community living for people with mental illness.

Promoting Neighborhood Regeneration

Practitioners who work in community mental health can make significant contributions by promoting initiatives to overcome the dimensions of neighborhood environments that are barriers to occupation for people living with mental illness. Typically, efforts to change the community include advocacy directed at municipal or state governments to influence these structures to change community conditions. Although advocacy efforts will always be an integral part of community development, it is possible for OTPs, together with the individuals they serve, to identify and collaborate with local community networks to participate in the process of neighborhood regeneration, which involves eliminating barriers and creating supports that promote satisfying and productive daily life for people in that community.

For example, OTPs working in community regeneration can address community safety issues by working with community leaders, agencies, and stakeholders, including persons living with mental illnesses, to increase the patrol of parks and play areas, increase lighting at night, develop Neighborhood Watch programs, and improve affordable public transportation. OTPs are capable of linking these initiatives explicitly to positive changes in occupation for all residents, but specifically for vulnerable individuals including persons living with mental illness.

For example, positive changes in affordable transportation can be linked explicitly to improving opportunities for people living with mental illness to contribute meaningfully to their communities, and neighborhood patrols and lighting could enable their ability to access opportunities for leisure and recreation (McKibbin et al., 2014). Practitioners can work with individuals and their families to develop strategies for increasing feelings of personal safety, such as providing information about where and when to travel outside the home, identifying others to walk with, and increasing social connections with neighbors. In addition, OTPs can work with community organizations whose efforts impact the physical environment to create opportunities for socialization, such as organizations that are planting trees, developing accessible community gardens, managing rainwater retrieval projects, maintaining green spaces, or cleaning blighted lots. See Chapter 30: Natural Environments.

Supporting Neighborhood Partnerships

Building partnerships that connect the occupation-related assets of neighborhood communities and residents can require considerable attention and support. Practitioners will

Evidence-Based Practice

At-Risk Youth

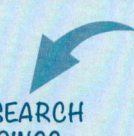

> *OTPs can engage at-risk youth in programs that bring about community change and support positive development.*

RESEARCH FINDINGS

In community neighborhood environments where levels of poverty are high and there is limited development of both public and private sector organizations, neighborhood youth are at risk for experiencing lifelong physical, mental health, and social inequities. Contemporary frameworks for positive youth development under such circumstances include attention to building the capacity of youth, but also strengthening community resources and opportunities and engaging youth directly in the processes and activities that bring about community change (Edberg et al., 2017).

APPLICATIONS

➡ OTPs can engage youth in programs that help increase their awareness of environmental issues that can impact their lives and support them to develop activities and organizations that encourage positive development (Edberg et al., 2017).

➡ Youth living with mental illness and their families can collaborate with OTPs, other mental health practitioners, and policymakers to transform mental health services using community-based participatory research approaches that draw on their unique knowledge of what supports are effective and relevant in their lives (Malla et al., 2018).

REFERENCES

Edberg, M. C., Cleary, S. D., Andrade, E. L., Evans, W. D., Simmons, L. K., & Cubilla-Batista, I. (2017). Applying ecological positive youth development theory to address co-occurring health disparities among immigrant Latino youth. *Health Promotion Practice, 18*(4), 488–496. https://doi.org/10.1177/1524839916638302

Malla, A., Shah, J., Iyer, S., Boksa, P., Joober, R., Andersson, N., Lal, S., & Fuhrer, R. (2018). Youth mental health should be a top priority for health care in Canada. *The Canadian Journal of Psychiatry, 63*(4), 216–222. https://doi.org/10.1177/0706743718758968

need to apply their broad base of knowledge and critical reasoning skills to enable the growth of these partnerships.

Consider the example of a senior center that partners with individuals with mental illness to develop employment opportunities. The OTP may find that an individual expresses a desire for employment and a genuine interest in this employment opportunity, but still experiences difficulty in carrying out the work. In this case, the OTP must work with the individual to identify and address the barriers to this partnership. Perhaps it is a person-level issue, such as physical conditioning or the lack of a specific task or social skill that is the issue. Perhaps the barrier is the occupation itself, such as a lack of adequate equipment to carry out the job. Or perhaps the problem rests in the environment, such as a disability pension system that presents the individual with a financial disincentive for paid work.

An important consideration in supporting neighborhood partnerships is the need to avoid the tendency to automatically explain partnership struggles as evidence of limitations and functional difficulties associated with mental illness. Building partnerships to enable occupation is a strategy based on developing new types of relations and interactions. In a situation in which there is limited experience with this type of partnership, and therefore few concrete examples to draw on, the automatic response can be to define the current struggles based on the old and familiar social relationships and labels.

Empowering Peer Support

There is a high rate of people living with mental illness in communities, yet communities and service systems have historically been constructed in a way that isolates them from the supportive structures of their neighborhood communities and the support and experiences of their peers. Engagement in peer support is not for everyone, but for many individuals with mental illness, their experiences with peer support can be transformative. The outcomes of studies on peer supports report mixed results, although there is evidence that peer support can influence important aspects of neighborhood living such as housing stability and use of community resources (Chinman et al., 2014).

In one systematic review exploring the effectiveness of peer support interventions for persons living with mental illness, across studies researchers identified a moderate positive effect of peer support on self-reported recovery and

TABLE 32-1 | Examples of Neighborhood Interventions

Category of Intervention	Examples
Neighborhood regeneration	• Establish Neighborhood Watch programs. • Promote affordable child care. • Work with local law enforcement on mental illness awareness. • Start monthly neighborhood clean-up activities. • Initiate block parties or community fairs. • Create a safe walking path. • Develop an afterschool program. • Establish reduced-cost bus passes for people with disabilities.
Neighborhood partnerships	• Public library provides meeting space; people with mental illness create art displays. • Senior center members have opportunities for employment (e.g., house sitting, helping out around the home); people with mental illness have time and services to volunteer or provide for pay. • Public schools and community colleges are interested in disability awareness; people with mental illness can provide educational programs. • Accessibility committees need information to improve neighborhood accessibility; people with mental illness have real-life experiences.
Peer support	• Develop a consumer-run organization. • Create a consumer business. • Connect consumers who live in the same apartment complex. • Establish a mentorship program (e.g., one peer teaches others how to use public transportation).

self-empowerment but found that it was not effective for improving clinical symptoms or service use (White et al., 2020). Despite these moderate effects, for many persons who live with mental illness, peer support is a critical intervention in supporting their recovery that has been instrumental in supporting resilience and well-being.

In addition to the enormous potential for benefits to the individual, peer initiatives are vehicles for individuals with mental illness, as a collective, to develop a shared legacy of support, skills, and experience. Whitley and Campbell (2014), for example, demonstrated that even informal forms of peer support could provide the support that people with serious mental illness require to engage actively in their neighborhoods and communities.

Supporting the development of peer partnerships in neighborhood communities can be a distinct intervention of occupational therapy practice. This may include initiatives such as facilitating the development of self-help groups (Roush, 2008) and peer-led programming. One such approach, "recovery colleges," involves the delivery of curricula developed and codelivered with persons living with mental illness to individuals in the community who may benefit from the curricula (Thériault et al., 2020).

In recovery colleges, program participants are called "students" and do not have to have received a diagnosis to register for "courses" delivered through the recovery college. The courses offered are aimed at supporting mental health promotion and recovery for all citizens in a community, thereby recognizing the ubiquity of mental illness in many communities. This is a distinctly community-based approach. Empowering peer support can also be an important underlying element of all occupational therapy intervention in neighborhoods.

Emerging from the previous examples, people might see developing the employment opportunity through the senior center into a registered business, owned and operated by individuals with mental illness; evolving the partnership with the accessibility committee into a participatory research project that engages individuals in hosting focus groups to involve others in the community who live with mental illness;

and displaying artwork at the public library as a vehicle for establishing an artist's cooperative. Table 32-1 summarizes three potential areas of neighborhood intervention. See Chapter 39: Peer-Led Services.

Here's the Point

- Neighborhoods can present both opportunities and barriers to the occupational experiences and occupational performance for citizens.
- People living with mental illness can be particularly vulnerable to the barriers to occupation presented in neighborhoods.
- Although community-based mental health services are now widespread, most services continue to be delivered at the individual level despite the need for neighborhood and community-level intervention.
- A growing body of research has identified important structures and elements within communities that are associated with mental health and well-being. Many of these are amenable to change.
- Person-environment-occupation models have guided OTPs to attend directly to the context of occupations. As OTPs advance their understanding of the modifiable aspects of neighborhoods and communities that can be strategically addressed to enable occupation and ultimately improve mental health and well-being, innovative and effective practices are likely to follow.
- OTPs can use established community development approaches to build community capacities so that individuals with mental illness can access and benefit from a broad range of meaningful occupational opportunities.

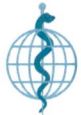 Visit the online resource center at FADavis.com to access the videos.

Apply It Now

1. Applying the Lived Experience

Consider Niq's story from this chapter's The Lived Experience feature regarding how community was pivotal in his recovery. Imagine how you might support someone with similar experiences to develop community using an occupational lens. For example, how might you help him to engage in occupation with others so that he could feel as if he belongs in his community?

2. Your Neighborhood

Think about your current neighborhood. Make a list of neighborhood characteristics that enable or restrict mental health and well-being. Identify specific resources in the neighborhood that you feel support your physical or mental health. Identify any characteristics of the neighborhood that make you anxious, frustrated, unhappy, or lonely. Do you feel at home and connected in your neighborhood? Why or why not?

Now imagine that you are working as an OTP with an individual with mental illness who has just moved into your neighborhood. How do the same resources that support or hinder you as a student apply to this individual? How do they help or hinder the individual with mental illness to feel connected and supported within your neighborhood? Explain your answer and give examples.

3. Comparing and Contrasting Neighborhood Profiles

Think about your neighborhood. Use the guidelines in this chapter (Fig. 32-2) to create a comprehensive neighborhood profile of your neighborhood. Select another neighborhood that you are less familiar with. Consider selecting a neighborhood that you have a sense is quite different from your own. Create a comprehensive neighborhood profile for this new community context. Compare these neighborhoods with respect to the opportunities and barriers they pose for occupation. Explain your thinking.

Alternatively, get together with classmates who live in different neighborhoods and compare and contrast the different neighborhoods. Consider how the neighborhoods would impact the lived experience of a person living with a mental illness.

4. Barriers to Activities

Choose an activity in which you regularly engage in within your neighborhood. While you are participating in this activity, think about how a person experiencing mental illness might be included or excluded from participating. Consider how the activity might be changed to make it more inclusive. What barriers would you expect, and how might they be overcome?

5. Video Exercise: Positive Mindset Creative Arts Festival

Pair up with another student in your class or form a small group of students. Access and watch the "Positive Mindset Creative Arts Festival" video at the online resource center at FADavis.com. Then, discuss and together answer the following questions.

Reflective Questions

■ Why are community events and initiatives like this so important? What barriers might limit participation in such occupations for people with mental health challenges?

■ How do events like this promote positive mental health in the general population?

■ What are some examples of other spaces in which OTPs can get involved and take action to universally promote positive mental health and increase social belonging and connection?

■ The video shares one example of the impact of generating opportunities for participation for individuals who might not have access to creative occupations. What knowledge and skills would you need to design similar opportunities in your own community?

Resources

Websites

- Asset-Based Community Development Institute. DePaul University's Irwin W. Steans Center for Community-Based Service Learning & Community Service Studies: https://resources.depaul.edu/abcd-institute/resources/Pages/tool-kit.aspx. This website contains multiple resources regarding asset-based community development that are free to download and use.
- Ontario Healthy Communities Coalition. Tool: Mapping your community assets: http://www.ohcc-ccso.ca/en/courses/community-development-for-health-promoters/module-two-process-strategies-and-roles/tool-mapp. This Canadian website provides access to online trainings about community asset mapping.
- Beaulieu, L. J. (2002). *Mapping the assets of your community: A key component for building local capacity.* Southern Rural

Development Center, Mississippi State: http://srdc.msstate.edu/trainings/educurricula/asset_mapping/asset_mapping.pdf. This website contains a pdf resource that describes how to go about mapping the assets of a community in order to build local capacity.
- Community Tool Box: http://ctb.ku.edu/en. This website is developed and maintained by the Center for Community Health and Development at the University of Kansas. It has a multitude of free resources specifically designed to help people build healthy neighborhoods and facilitate social change.
- Northern Initiative for Social Action: http://nisa.on.ca. This organization is an example of a mental health consumer-run organization that helps members build and maintain their own skills and well-being and contribute in meaningful ways in their community through active social recovery.

Videos

- "It's in Our Hands: Asset-Based Community and Economic Development in Practice" by Jenny Cameron:
  - Part 1: https://www.youtube.com/watch?v=I1r_h9GeV2Q
  - Part 2: https://www.youtube.com/watch?v=ptLjXNECrFs
- "Leisure Occupations for Unhoused Individuals" video. In this video, Kailin, an occupational therapist who works in community mental health and homeless services, describes the power of leisure activities to the individuals whom she serves. Kailin talks about the barriers to engaging in leisure that often exist for people who are unhoused. She explains how she integrates the evaluation of leisure in her occupational profile and provides several examples of realistic leisure activities that OTPs can use to support individuals' mental health. Access the video at the online resource center at FADavis.com.
- "Civic Engagement Group in an Inpatient Psychiatric Unit" video. In this video, occupational therapist Jennifer speaks about her experience working as an occupational therapy assistant in an inpatient psychiatric unit for individuals with persistent mental illness. She describes a positive experience running civic engagement groups, which proved to do much more than give back to the community. In one project related to voting rights for individuals with felony histories, the group provided opportunities for the residents to practice life skills, feel empowered, and transcend the internalized stigma they faced as people living with mental illness. Access the video at the online resource center at FADavis.com.
- "Principles and Practices of Asset-Based Community Development" with Howard Lawrence, Cormac Russell, and John McKnight: https://youtu.be/uWUsnnHbjS0

Articles

- Guillory, J. D., Everson, J. M., & Ivester, J. G. (2006). Community development: Lessons learned about coalition building and community connections for stakeholders with disabilities. *Community Development, 37*(3), 83–96. https://doi.org/10.1080/15575330.2006.10383110
- Hyett, N., Kenny, A., & Dickson-Swift, V. (2019). Re-imagining occupational therapy clients as communities: Presenting the community-centred practice framework. *Scandinavian Journal of Occupational Therapy, 26*(4), 246–260. https://doi.org/10.1080/11038128.2017.1423374
- Richardson Bruna, K., McNelly, C. A., Greder, K., & Rongerude, J. (2020). Youth dialogue and design for educational possibility: Eliciting youth voice in community development. *Journal of Community Practice, 28*(2), 121–131. https://doi.org/10.1080/10705422.2020.1757006

Essential Books

- Born, P. (2012). *Community conversations: Mobilizing the ideas, skills, and passion of community organizations, governments, businesses, and people.* BPS Books.
- Born, P. (2014). *Deepening community: Finding joy together in chaotic times.* Berrett-Koehler.
- Kretzmann, J. P., & McKnight, J. L. (1993). *Building communities from the inside out: A path toward finding and mobilizing a community's assets.* Institute for Policy Research.
- Ledwith, M. (2015). *Community development in action: Putting Freire into practice.* Policy Press.
- Ledwith, M. (2020). *Community development: A critical approach.* Policy Press.
- McKnight, J. (1995). *The careless society: Community and its counterfeits.* Basic Books.
- McKnight, J., & Block, P. (2011). *The abundant community: Awakening the power of families and neighborhoods.* Berrett-Koehler.
- Russell, C., & McKnight, J. (2022). *The connected community: Discovering the health, wealth, and power of neighborhoods.* Berrett-Koehler.

References

Almedom, A. M., & Glandon, D. (2008). Social capital and mental health: An updated interdisciplinary review of primary evidence. In I. Kawachi, S. V. Subramanian, & D. Kim (Eds.), *Social capital and health* (pp. 191–214). Springer.

Awaworyi Churchill, S., Farrell, L., & Smyth, R. (2019). Neighbourhood ethnic diversity and mental health in Australia. *Health Economics, 28*(9), 1075–1087. https://doi.org/10.1002/hec.3928

Baranyi, G., Di Marco, M. H., Russ, T. C., Dibben, C., & Pearce, J. (2021). The impact of neighbourhood crime on mental health: A systematic review and meta-analysis. *Social Science & Medicine, 282,* 114106. https://doi.org/10.1016/j.socscimed.2021.114106

Ben-Moshe, L. (2020). *Decarcerating disability: Deinstitutionalization and prison abolition.* University of Minnesota Press.

Bhavsar, V., Sanyal, J., Patel, R., Shetty, H., Velupillai, S., Stewart, R., Broadbent, M., MacCabe, J. H., Das-Munshi, J., & Howard, L. M. (2020). The association between neighbourhood characteristics and physical victimisation in men and women with mental disorders. *British Journal of Psychiatry Open, 6*(4), e73. https://doi.org/10.1192/bjo.2020.52

Bonney, T., Rospenda, K. M., Forst, L., Conroy, L. M., Castañeda, D., Avelar, S., Castañeda, Y., Holloway, A., & Hebert-Beirne, J. (2022). Employment precarity and increased risk of hazardous occupational exposures among residents of high socioeconomic hardship neighborhoods. *Annals of Work Exposures and Health, 66*(9), 1122–1135. https://doi.org/10.1093/annweh/wxac062

Boucher, L. M., Dodd, Z., Young, S., Shahid, A., Bayoumi, A., Firestone, M., & Kendall, C. E. (2022). "They have their security, we have our community": Mutual support among people experiencing homelessness in encampments in Toronto during the COVID-19 pandemic. *SSM-Qualitative Research in Health, 2,* 100163. https://doi.org/10.1016/j.ssmqr.2022.100163

Bowe, M., Wakefield, J. R., Kellezi, B., Stevenson, C., McNamara, N., Jones, B. A., Sumich, A., & Heym, N. (2022). The mental health benefits of community helping during crisis: Coordinated helping, community identification and sense of unity during the COVID-19 pandemic. *Journal of Community & Applied Social Psychology, 32*(3), 521–535. https://doi.org/10.1002/casp.2520

Brown, P. (Ed.). (2022). *The transfer of care: Psychiatric deinstitutionalization and its aftermath* (Vol. 7). Routledge.

Carrillo Beck, R., Szlapinski, J., Pacheco, N., Sabri Laghaei, S., Isard, R., Oudshoorn, A., & Marshall, C. A. (2022). Violence and victimisation in the lives of persons experiencing homelessness who use methamphetamine: A scoping review. *Health & Social Care in the Community, 30*(5), 1619–1636. https://doi.org/10.1111/hsc.13716

Chen, S., Krupa, T., Lysaght, R., McCay, E., & Piat, M. (2013). The development of recovery competencies for in-patient mental health providers working with people with serious mental illness. *Administration and Policy in Mental Health, 40*(2), 96–116. https://doi.org/10.1007/s10488-011-0380-x

Chinman, M., George, P., Dougherty, R. H., Daniels, A. S., Ghose, S. S., Swift, A., & Delphin-Rittmon, M. E. (2014). Peer support services for individuals with serious mental illnesses: Assessing the evidence. *Psychiatric Services, 65,* 429–441. https://doi.org/10.1176/appi.ps.201300244

Collins, B. (2017). Independence: Proposing an initial framework for occupational therapy. *Scandinavian Journal of Occupational Therapy, 24*(6), 398–409. https://doi.org/10.1080/11038128.2016.1271011

Doroud, N., Fossey, E., & Fortune, T. (2015). Recovery as an occupational journey: A scoping review exploring the links between occupational engagement and recovery for people with enduring mental health issues. *Australian Occupational Therapy Journal, 62*(6), 378–392. https://doi.org/10.1111/1440-1630.12238

Edberg, M. C., Cleary, S. D., Andrade, E. L., Evans, W. D., Simmons, L. K., & Cubilla-Batista, I. (2017). Applying ecological positive youth development theory to address co-occurring health disparities among immigrant Latino youth. *Health Promotion Practice, 18*(4), 488–496. https://doi.org/10.1177/1524839916638302

Egan, M., & Restall, G. (Eds.). (2022). *Promoting occupational participation: Collaborative relationship-focused occupational therapy: 10th Canadian occupational therapy guidelines.* Canadian Association of Occupational Therapists. CAOT Press.

Ehsan, A., Klaas, H. S., Bastianen, A., & Spini, D. (2019). Social capital and health: A systematic review of systematic reviews. *SSM-Population Health, 8,* 100425. https://doi.org/ 10.1016/j.ssmph .2019.100425

Erickson, B. (2021). Deinstitutionalization through optimism: The Community Mental Health Act of 1963. *American Journal of Psychiatry Residents' Journal, 16*(4), 6–7. https://doi.org/10.1176 /appi.ajp-rj.2021.160404

Field, J. (2016). *Social capital.* Routledge.

Flores, E. C., Fuhr, D. C., Bayer, A. M., Lescano, A. G., Thorogood, N., & Simms, V. (2018). Mental health impact of social capital interventions: A systematic review. *Social Psychiatry & Psychiatric Epidemiology, 53*(2), 107–119. https://doi.org/10.1007/s00127-017-1469-7

Fong, P., Cruwys, T., Haslam, C., & Haslam, S. A. (2019). Neighbourhood identification and mental health: How social identification moderates the relationship between socioeconomic disadvantage and health. *Journal of Environmental Psychology, 61,* 101–114. https://doi.org/10.1016/j.jenvp.2018.12.006

Fukui, S., Goscha, R., Rapp, C. A., Mabry, A., Liddy, P., & Marty, D. (2012). Strengths model case management fidelity scores and client outcomes. *Psychiatric Services, 63,* 708–710. https://doi .org/10.1176/appi.ps.201100373

Gibbon, M., Labonte, R., & Laverack, G. (2002). Evaluating community capacity. *Health and Social Care in the Community, 10,* 485–491. https://doi.org/10.1046/j.1365-2524.2002.00388.x

Goffman, E. (1961). *Asylums: Essays on the social situation of mental patients and other inmates.* Anchor Press.

Hack, S. M., Muralidharan, A., Brown, C. H., Drapalski, A. L., & Lucksted, A. A. (2020). Stigma and discrimination as correlates of mental health treatment engagement among adults with serious mental illness. *Psychiatric Rehabilitation Journal, 43*(2), 106. https://doi.org/10.1080/17482631.2020.1744926

Hammell, K. W. (2023). A call to resist occupational therapy's promotion of ableism. *Scandinavian Journal of Occupational Therapy, 30*(6), 745–757. https://doi.org/10.1080/11038128.2022.21308211

Hossain, M. M., Sultana, A., Tasnim, S., Fan, Q., Ma, P., McKyer, E. L. J., & Purohit, N. (2020). Prevalence of mental disorders among people who are homeless: An umbrella review. *International Journal of Social Psychiatry, 66*(6), 528–541. https://doi .org/10.1177/0020764020924689

Kingsbury, M., Clayborne, Z., Colman, I., & Kirkbride, J. (2020). The protective effect of neighbourhood social cohesion on adolescent mental health following stressful life events. *Psychological Medicine, 50*(8), 1292–1299. https://doi.org/10.1017 /S0033291719001235

Kirby, A. V. (2015). Beyond independence: Introducing Deweyan philosophy to the dialogue on occupation and independence. *Journal of Occupational Science, 22*(1), 17–25. https://doi.org /10.1080/14427591.2013.803297

Kretzmann, J. P., & McKnight, J. L. (1993). *Building communities from the inside out: A path toward finding and mobilizing a community's assets.* ACTA Publications.

Kretzmann, J. P., McKnight, J. L., Dobrowolski, S., & Puntenney, D. (2005). *Discovering community power: A guide to mobilizing local assets and your organization's capacity.* School of Education and Social Policy Northwestern University. https://resources.depaul.edu/ abcd-institute/publications/publications-by-topic/Documents /kelloggabcd.pdf

Krupa, T., Eastabrook, S., Hern, L., Lee, D., North, R., Percy, K., Von Briesen, B., & Wing, G. (2005). How do people who receive Assertive Community Treatment experience this service? *Psychiatric Rehabilitation Journal, 29*(1), 18–24. https://doi .org/10.2975/29.2005.18.24

Krupa, T., Sabetti, J., & Lysaght, R. (2019). How work integration social enterprises impact the stigma of mental illness: Negotiating perceptions of legitimacy, value and competence. *Social Enterprise Journal, 15*(4), 475–494. https://doi.org/10.1108 /SEJ-12-2018-0075

Lamb, H. R., & Weinberger, L. E. (2020). Deinstitutionalization and other factors in the criminalization of persons with serious mental illness and how it is being addressed. *CNS Spectrums, 25*(2), 173–180. https://doi.org/10.1017/S1092852919001524

Lauckner, H. M., Krupa, T. M., & Paterson, M. L. (2011). Conceptualizing community development: Occupational therapy practice at the intersection of health services and community. *Canadian Journal of Occupational Therapy, 78*(4), 260–268. https://doi .org/10.2182/cjot.2011.78.4.8

Mahmoudi Farahani, L. (2016). The value of the sense of community and neighbouring. *Housing, Theory and Society, 33*(3), 357–376. https://doi.org/10.1080/14036096.2016.1155480

Malla, A., Shah, J., Iyer, S., Boksa, P., Joober, R., Andersson, N., Lal, S., & Fuhrer, R. (2018). Youth mental health should be a top priority for health care in Canada. *The Canadian Journal of Psychiatry, 63*(4), 216–222. https://doi.org/10.1177/0706743718758968

Marshall, C. A., Boland, L., Westover, L. A., Marcellus, B., Weil, S., & Wickett, S. (2020). Effectiveness of interventions targeting community integration among individuals with lived experiences of homelessness: A systematic review. *Health & Social Care in the Community, 28*(6), 1843–1862. https://doi.org/10.1111/hsc.13030

Marshall, C. A., Easton, C., George, C., Oudshoorn, A., Wathen, N., & Forchuk, C. (2024). *Methamphetamine and homelessness: A mixed-methods study in two urban centres in Ontario, Canada.* Manuscript in development.

Marshall, C. A., Gewurtz, R., Ross, C., Becker, A., Cooke, A., Roy, L., Lysaght, R., & Kirsh, B. (2024). Beyond securing a tenancy: Using the capabilities approach to identify the daily living needs of individuals during and following homelessness. *Journal of Social Distress and Homelessness, 33*(1), 81–95. https://doi.org/10.1080 /10530789.2022.2070098

Marshall, C. A., Phillips, B., Holmes, J., Todd, E., Hill, R., Panter, G., Easton, C., Landry, T., Collins, S., Greening, T., O'Brien, A., Jastak, M., Ridge, R., Goldszmidt, R., Shanoff, C., Rudman, D., Carlsson, A., Aryobi, S., Szlapinski, J., . . . Oudshoorn, A. (2023). "I can't remember the last time I was comfortable about being home": Lived experience perspectives on thriving following homelessness. *International Journal of Qualitative Studies on Health and Well-Being, 18*(1), 1–15. https://doi.org/10.1080/17482631.2023.2176979

Marshall, C. A., Tjörnstrand, C., Downs, E., Devries, R., & Drake, F. (2021). "Nobody cares about you as a group of people": A mixed methods study of women living in congregate social housing in Ontario, Canada. *Housing and Society, 48*(1), 21–42. https://doi .org/10.1080/08882746.2020.1793285

McKibbin, C. L., Kitchen, K. A., Wykes, T. L., & Lee, A. A. (2014). Barriers and facilitators of a healthy lifestyle among persons with serious and persistent mental illness: Perspectives of community mental health providers. *Community Mental Health Journal, 50,* 566–576. https://doi.org/10.1007/s10597-013-9650-2

Morrissey, T. W., & Vinopal, K. M. (2018). Neighborhood poverty and children's academic skills and behavior in early elementary school. *Journal of Marriage and Family, 80*(1), 182–197. https:// doi.org/10.1111/jomf.12430

Murney, M. A., Sapag, J. C., Bobbili, S. J., & Khenti, A. (2020). Stigma and discrimination related to mental health and substance use issues in primary health care in Toronto, Canada: A qualitative study. *International Journal of Qualitative Studies on Health and Well-Being, 15*(1), 1744926. https://doi.org/10.1080/17482631 .2020.1744926

Ramugondo, E. L., & Kronenberg, F. (2015). Explaining collective occupations from a human relations perspective: Bridging the individual-collective dichotomy. *Journal of Occupational Science, 22*(1), 3–16. https://doi.org/10.1080/14427591.2013.781920

Ridley, M., Rao, G., Schilbach, F., & Patel, V. (2020). Poverty, depression, and anxiety: Causal evidence and mechanisms. *Science, 370*(6522), eaay0214. https://doi.org/10.1126/science.aay0214

Roush, S. (2008). Starting a dual diagnosis anonymous meeting: The role of the clinician. *Journal of Dual Diagnosis, 4*(2), 158–169. https://doi.org/10.1080/15504260802066992

Shearer, A. L., Roth, E., Cefalu, M. S., Breslau, J., McBain, R. K., Wong, E. C., Burnam, M. A., & Collins, R. L. (2021). Contact with persons with mental illness and willingness to live next door to them: Two waves of a California survey of adults. *Psychiatric Services, 72*(1), 23–30. https://doi.org/10.1176/appi.ps.202000064

Silver, E., Mulvey, E. P., & Swanson, J. W. (2002). Neighborhood structural characteristics and mental disorder: Faris and Dunham revisited. *Social Science and Medicine, 55,* 1457–1470. https://doi.org/10.1016/s0277-9536(01)00266-0

Szasz, T. (1970). *The manufacture of madness.* Harper & Row.

Teasdale, S. B., Morell, R., Lappin, J. M., Curtis, J., Watkins, A., & Ward, P. B. (2020). Prevalence and correlates of food insecurity in community-based individuals with severe mental illness receiving long-acting injectable antipsychotic treatment. *British Journal of Nutrition, 124*(4), 470–477. https://doi.org/10.1017/S0007114520001191

Thériault, J., Lord, M. M., Briand, C., Piat, M., & Meddings, S. (2020). Recovery colleges after a decade of research: A literature review. *Psychiatric Services, 71*(9), 928–940. https://doi.org/10.1176/appi.ps.201900352

Ungar, T., Knaak, S., & Szeto, A. C. (2016). Theoretical and practical considerations for combating mental illness stigma in health care. *Community Mental Health Journal, 52,* 262–271. https://doi.org/10.1007/s10597-015-9910-4

Vallée, J., Cadot, E., Roustit, C., Parizot, I., & Chauvin, P. (2011). The role of daily mobility in mental health inequalities: The interactive influence of activity space and neighbourhood of residence on depression. *Social Science & Medicine, 73,* 1133–1144. https://doi.org/10.1016/j.socscimed.2011.08.009

Vigo, D., Thornicroft, G., & Atun, R. (2016). Estimating the true global burden of mental illness. *The Lancet Psychiatry, 3*(2), 171–178. https://doi.org/10.1016/S2215-0366(15)00505-2

White, S., Foster, R., Marks, J., Morshead, R., Goldsmith, L., Barlow, S., Sin, J., & Gillard, S. (2020). The effectiveness of one-to-one peer support in mental health services: A systematic review and meta-analysis. *BMC Psychiatry, 20*(1), 1–20. https://doi.org/10.1186/s12888-020-02923-3

Whitley, R., & Campbell, R. D. (2014). Stigma, agency and recovery amongst people with severe mental illness. *Social Science & Medicine, 107,* 1–8. https://doi.org/10.1016/j.socscimed.2014.02.010

Wilcock, A., & Townsend, E. (2014). Occupational justice. In B. A. B. Schell, M. Scaffa, G. Gillen, & E. S. Cohn (Eds.), *Willard and Spackman's occupational therapy* (12th ed., pp. 541–552). Lippincott Williams & Wilkins.

World Health Organization. (2014). *Social determinants of mental health.* https://iris.who.int/bitstream/handle/10665/112828/9789241506809_eng.pdf?sequence=1

Josh Skuller and Sara Story

Judy utilizes a smartphone app to engage in video calls with her children and grandchildren who live across the country. Davion has a diagnosis of attention deficit-hyperactivity disorder (ADHD) and finds the flexibility of online college courses helps to meet his academic needs. Malia utilizes social media to keep up with friends but also receives support through an online LGBTQIA+ network. Individuals engage in occupations throughout their day in both physical (i.e., brick and mortar) and virtual (cyber) environments.

It is important for occupational therapy practitioners (OTPs) to recognize the choices individuals make pertaining to when, why, and how they choose virtual participation versus physical participation so they can support individuals in exercising their choices and accessing the virtual environment. The Person-Environment-Occupation (PEO) model (Law et al., 1996) can help OTPs consider the fit between an individual, their preferred occupations, and participation within virtual environments.

This chapter explores the virtual realm of occupations, how and why individuals choose to engage in them, and how OTPs can create interventions within the virtual context to help support a person's goals. These interventions may involve connecting an individual with a social media group, working within the parameters of telehealth or other assistive technology (AT) devices (apps), and using this technology to support participation. See Chapter 3: Person-Environment-Occupation Model. 🤝

Defining the Virtual Environment

Effective practitioners always consider context when providing occupational therapy services. The *Occupational Therapy Practice Framework: Domain and Process,* Fourth Edition (*OTPF-4*; American Occupational Therapy Association [AOTA], 2020) defines context as "a broad construct defined as the environmental and personal factors specific to each client (person, group, population) that influence engagement and participation in occupations" (p. 9). The *OTPF-4* exemplifies the fact that occupational therapy literature often uses the terms "context" and "environment" interchangeably, but also delineates personal and environmental factors. The *OTPF-4* environmental factors include nature, social supports, attitudes of society and others, systems and policies, and the focus of this chapter, products and technology.

Environmental factors encompass "physical, social, and attitudinal surroundings" (AOTA, 2020, p. 9), which take on a whole different meaning when referring to virtual environments. Within the field of occupational therapy, engagement in the cyber world regarding evaluative and treatment methodologies has grown to the extent that telemedicine and virtual care are becoming mainstream aspects of practice.

The concept of "telehealth" has grown exponentially since the COVID-19 pandemic. In *Occupational Therapy and Telehealth,* the World Federation of Occupational Therapists (WFOT, 2021) defines **telehealth** as "the use of information and communication technologies to deliver health-related services when the provider and client are in different physical locations" (p. 1). Therefore, in occupational therapy practice, the cyber world provides a new context in which people, groups, and populations can find comfort in virtual surroundings, identity through social meaning, and expanded opportunities for learning, play, support, community, and services.

Use of Assistive Technology in Mental Health

Over the years, technology use has evolved from large computers that filled an entire room to individuals engaging with smartphones (Table 33-1 and Fig. 33-1). Roger O. Smith, in his Eleanor Clarke Slagle Lecture (2017), pointed out that technology will continue to integrate into daily life at an increasingly fast pace; therefore, it is crucial that occupational therapy professionals increase their technology knowledge and skills. When considering the virtual environment, it is important to recognize the umbrella of AT services, which covers the technology required to make engagement within the virtual environment possible.

So, what is **assistive technology** (AT)? Two formal definitions are commonly used. In the United States, the Assistive Technology Act of 1998 (amended in 2004 and known as the "Tech Act") defines AT as, "Any item, piece of equipment, or product system whether acquired commercially off the shelf, modified, or customized that is used to increase, maintain, or improve functional capabilities of individuals with disabilities."

The Tech Act defines **assistive technology service** as "any service that directly assists an individual with a disability in the selection, acquisition or use of an assistive technology device" (Assistive Technology Act of 1998). The World Health Organization (WHO) defines AT and products as "any product, instrument, equipment, or technology adapted or specially designed for improving the functioning of a disabled person" (WHO, 2001, p. 180). This international definition is congruent with the Tech Act statement.

TABLE 33-1 | Computer Technology Timeline

1940s	Several computing systems were introduced including the Atanasoff-Berry Computer and the ENIAC, both of which utilized vacuum tubes and took up a lot of space.
1950	UNIVAC 1101 was the first computer to store and run a program from memory.
1968	Hewlett Packard created the HP9100A, considered to be the first mass-marketed computer.
1970	The world's first video call took place.
1974	The Micral, the first microcomputer, was created.
1975	The IBM 5100, the first portable computer, was created; it weighed 55 pounds.
1976	Apple I, the first Apple computer, was created.
1981	The first IBM pc (home computer) was created.
1986	IBM introduced the first laptop computer (the PC convertible). It weighed 12 pounds.
1992	Tandy, by Radio Shack, created the first multimedia computer.
1992	AT&T launched the video phone, which worked over standard phone lines and had a $1,600 price tag.
2003	Apple introduced the iSight, an external webcam which could be used with iChat and Skype, which were also introduced in 2003.
2007	Apple introduced the iPhone, the first smartphone. Several companies also created smartphones shortly after.
2010	Apple introduced the iPad, the beginning of tablet computers.
2010	Apple introduced FaceTime, the much-anticipated ability to communicate through video.
2012	Oculus Rift was introduced, igniting the incorporation of virtual reality into daily life.
2020	The COVID-19 pandemic forced everyone to utilize the virtual environment (i.e., Zoom, FaceTime, and other virtual methods) to conduct daily life.
After 2020	Since 2020, technology has become more sophisticated. What will be next?

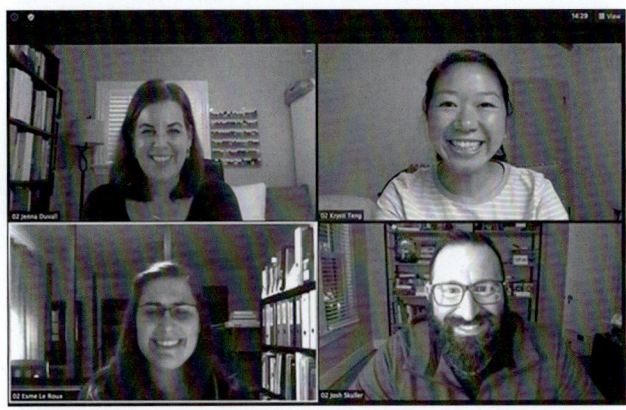

FIGURE 33-1. The use of computer technology is routine and pervasive in many parts of the world. These OTPs from Australia, California, and Kentucky are engaged in an online learning continuing education course through Zoom.

- Education: equal access to education is provided
- Participation in cultural life, recreation, leisure, and sports

Consideration must be given to how social determinants of health impact accessibility of virtual environments. Individuals living in rural areas, minoritized populations, and/or those who are socioeconomically disadvantaged have an added barrier to accessing the physical and psychosocial health benefits the virtual environment can provide (Benda et al., 2020; Yoon et al., 2020). The lack of access to the internet is an issue of equity when it limits accessibility to information and services, diminishes an individual's freedom of expression, limits equal access to educational pursuits, and directly interferes with occupational engagement in leisure pursuits involving the virtual environment.

Application of the Virtual Environment for Occupational Therapy Practitioners

Practitioners must intentionally engage in therapeutic reasoning when determining the appropriate AT interventions for an individual. The use of AT to support occupations (AOTA, 2020) and participation in the virtual environments is considered a virtual intervention, which per the *OTPF-4* (AOTA, 2020) includes videoconferencing, teleconferencing, or mobile telephone application (app) technology. A reflective OTP is one that is intentional when choosing a framework to back their therapeutic reasoning behind their recommendations for use of AT.

This textbook utilizes the PEO framework; however, in the field of AT, there are additional frameworks to consider. One particular framework, the Human Activity Assistive Technology (HAAT) model (Cook et al., 2020), very closely aligns with the PEO model because it explores what the human being is doing in relation to AT. The overall emphasis of this model is based on the person being engaged in activities within their preferred environments and the use of AT to support this engagement (Cook et al., 2020). The HAAT model also puts the human and activity first, meaning that they should always

AT is one of many strategies used to lessen the disabling influence of many environments (Cook et al., 2020). For many individuals across the mental health continuum, participation within a virtual environment can help to remove barriers to completing daily tasks within physical environments; as such, the virtual environment becomes an AT. It is important that OTPs recognize the potential of assistive technologies when planning interventions for people with mental illness and across the mental health continuum.

For nearly 20 years, the United Nations (UN) in their Convention on the Rights of Persons with Disabilities (2006) has posited that disability occurs at the intersection of the person and the context in which they live and that the extent of disability is different for individuals living in different contexts (UN, 2006). Examples in this document that support the use of the virtual environment to enable participation include:

- Accessibility: providing equitable access to information and services
- Freedom of expression and opinion and access to information: the use of the internet

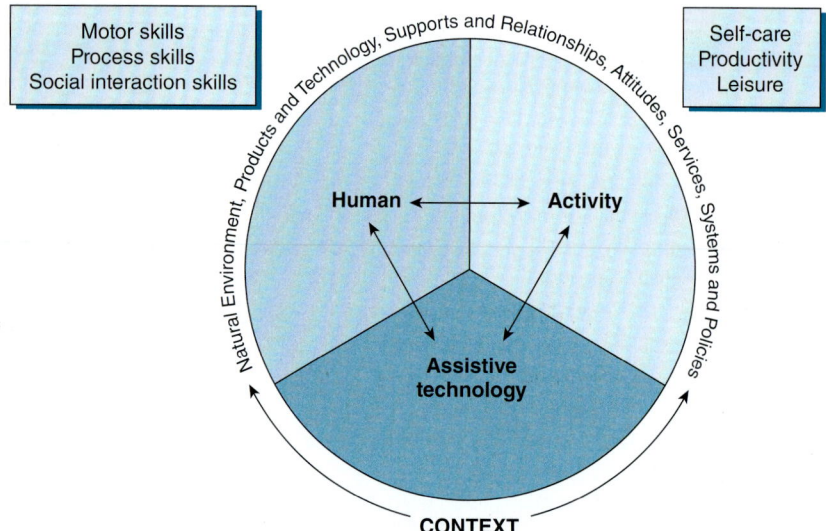

Motor skills
Process skills
Social interaction skills

Self-care
Productivity
Leisure

Natural Environment, Products and Technology, Supports and Relationships, Attitudes, Services, Systems and Policies

Human ← → Activity

Assistive
technology

CONTEXT

FIGURE 33-2. The HAAT model adapted from Cook, Polgar, and Encarnação (2020) is consistent with a PEO approach in that it emphasizes the transactional relationship between the person, the activity, and their context while using AT.

TABLE 33-2 | Hierarchy of Assistive Technology

Category	Description	Examples
High tech assistive technology	Items often have sophisticated computer systems and typically need to be plugged into an electrical outlet.	• Smartphone • Tablet • Home PC and accessories (i.e., webcam) • Video gaming system • Apps
Low tech assistive technology	Any item that can be purchased off the shelf at a commercial market. These items are typically nonelectronic or do not have sophisticated electronics.	• Daily schedule board • Pill minder • Fidget spinner • Worry stone • Planner • Wellness Recovery Action Plan (WRAP) Binder
No tech assistive technology	AT solutions that are made with whatever the individual has lying around. These can be utilized as a temporary solution until something more permanent can be purchased; however, if it works well for the individual, this might be a permanent solution.	• Using electric tape and a whiteboard to create a wall schedule/calendar • Using bathroom cups with day and time written on them to create a pill minder

be considered first. AT is then added in to support these two components within their environments (Cook et al., 2020).

Figure 33-2 presents a visual representation of the HAAT model that integrates elements of occupational therapy's PEO approach. Using the HAAT model can help frame decision-making, allowing OTPs to determine the appropriate equipment suggestions to support a person to engage in the virtual environment.

Technology Hierarchy

When considering AT, it is important to understand the continuum of AT that is available to the consumer. AT categories are high tech, low tech, and no tech (Table 33-2). High tech devices typically involve a computer system and include smartphones/tablets with accompanying apps, desktop computers, web

cameras, meeting software (e.g., Zoom), and so on. Low tech devices can include schedule boards, pill minders, and reading strips. Low tech solutions are typically purchased off the shelf.

Lastly, no tech solutions consist of utilizing whatever is available at the moment to create an assistive device; for example, using a 3-inch classroom binder as a slant board for a student who requires a slanted surface when working. The no tech solution may be either temporary or, for some individuals, it may work very well for them and will become a permanent device. In this chapter, AT focuses on high tech devices and solutions, because they are most common in the virtual environment.

High tech devices such as computer systems, smartphones, and tablets have all become a part of mainstream technology, meaning that they are available to most consumers and can be purchased from many general stores (Cook et al., 2020). With the advancement of these technologies and apps, individuals are able to participate in the virtual environment for a variety of reasons throughout the life span. OTPs need to understand the devices people will utilize and how they will choose to engage with these devices in order to participate in their preferred occupations. These topics will be explored further throughout the chapter.

Use of Apps

For many people, apps have become an integral part of life, allowing individuals to participate in the virtual environment. Many grocery store chains have created an app that can be used on a smart device. For example, with the touch of an app on a smartphone, an individual can access their grocery store, use previous shopping lists, decide what they need, and then order their groceries for delivery, should shopping in a grocery store be too stressful for them. Individuals can utilize apps for guided meditations, to encourage and track weight loss, for better sleep, and to track workouts. Apps can help individuals develop coping skills and experience calm throughout their day.

Some apps can be used as an accessory to behavioral health treatment. For example, Virtual Hope Box (National Center for Telehealth and Technology) provides coping strategies for individuals who are experiencing distress by providing distracting activities, breathing exercises, and coping

cards, among other strategies. In addition, a phone icon on the app allows quick access by telephone to the individual's behavioral health team, should they be in an acute crisis. By having knowledge of apps, OTPs can help individuals select what might be a good fit to help them function in their daily occupations between sessions and after discharge from therapy. Table 33-3 provides some examples of apps OTPs might recommend and shares some of the therapeutic goals and reasoning behind these recommendations.

Technology Innovation Centers

Health care is a dynamic environment where new knowledge is learned and applied and new processes are constantly being considered. In health care and in education technology, innovation centers are being created as spaces to create and explore digital health-care solutions. For example, OTPs seeking to identify new virtual experiences for the older adult population could utilize an innovation technology center, such as the Thrive Center, located in Louisville, Kentucky. Established to promote healthy aging and put the spotlight on innovation in health care, the Thrive Center is designed to immerse seniors in technology to help increase their quality of life. Because technology can often be overwhelming for

TABLE 33-3 | Examples of Apps to Help Engage in Daily Occupations

Type of App	Why Recommend It?	Expected Outcomes
Mindfulness • Headspace • Calm • Fabulous: Daily Habit Tracker • Day One Journal • Finch: Self Care Widget Pet	Offers individuals the opportunity to bring their coping strategies with them for whenever they would need them. Virtual strategies can also help to replace a pencil-and-paper system.	Improved ability to utilize coping strategies to participate in daily tasks. When using activities on a personal device, the individual "fits in" with those around them who are also engaging with their devices.
ADL/IADL • Shipt: Same Day Delivery • Amazon Prime • Timers: Already on phone/tablet • Reminders: Already on phone/tablet • Mint: Budget & Expense Manager • Many grocery stores have apps for shopping and grocery delivery	Many individuals with mental health issues may find that using reminders on their devices and using premade grocery lists can help their daily productivity. Budget apps can help to show expenses in real time.	Improved medication adherence and ability to participate independently in ADL/IADL activities.
Cognition • Calendar: Already on phone/tablet • Google Calendar • Structured-Daily Planner • Evernote Notes Organizer • Elevate • Luminosity • Duolingo	Rather than using a pencil-and-paper planner, apps can offer infinite reminders, provide timers, and keep notes all together rather than relying on a binder or notebook. Apps can also be used to help develop cognitive skills (Elevate, Luminosity, Duolingo).	Improved organization and executive function skills. Cognition apps can also help with thinking through complex situations.
Leisure • Yoga Studio: Beginner Classes • TikTok • Hidden Objects: Puzzle Games • YouTube • There are many puzzle/game options in the various app stores	Provides individuals with the opportunity to be distracted from their symptoms. May also be able to engage with others through social media features on apps (TikTok).	Distraction from symptoms and can potentially help the individual to develop new interests.
Social Connectedness • FaceTime • Zoom • Facebook • Instagram • WhatsApp Messenger	Gives individuals the opportunity to participate in a community and feel a sense of belonging. Also allows those who may be homebound to engage with family, friends, and so on.	Provides a feeling of support and connectedness. Can help individuals build a supportive community of similar-minded peers.

BOX 33-1 ■ jDome BikeAround at Thrive Louisville

This technology allows an individual to get exercise on a stationary bike, but it also allows the rider to engage in exploring neighborhoods, reminisce on their older neighborhoods, and so on. Many newer exercise bikes such as Peloton utilize similar technology.

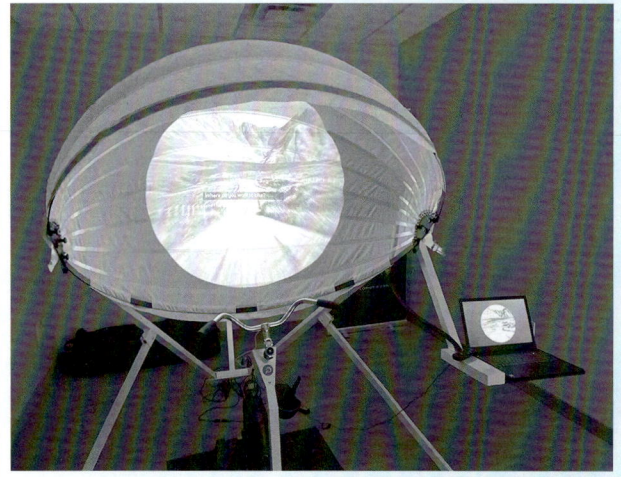
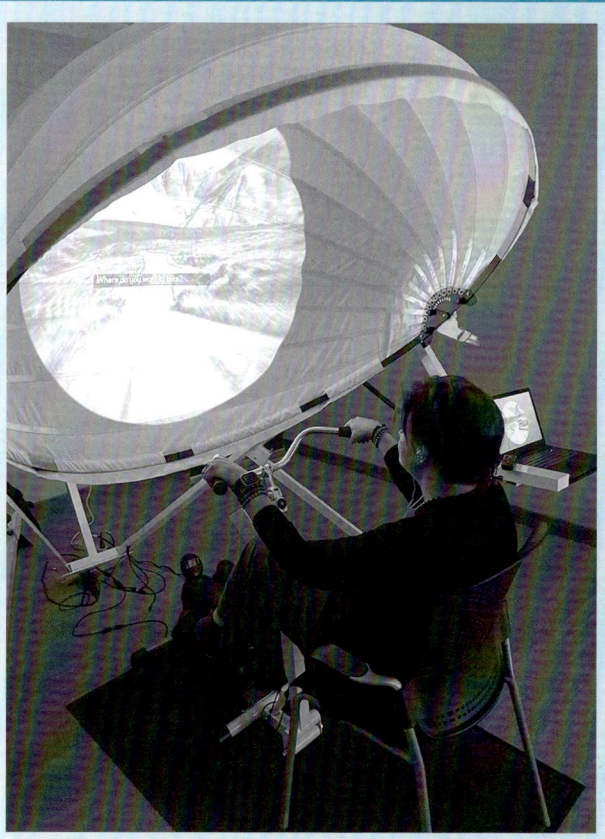

this population, the Thrive Center is designed to help make this technology accessible.

Equipment utilized at the Thrive Center includes the jDome BikeAround (Box 33-1). This bicycle, created in Sweden, is an example of innovative technology focusing on virtual engagement to assist the aging population and those diagnosed with dementia. The primary focus of the jDome BikeAround experience is to provide the individual with an opportunity to engage in physical exercise through stationary cycling while immersing themselves in sensory stimulation for reminiscence.

In addition to technology innovation centers, the Tech Act requires each state to have an **assistive technology resource center** (ATRC). ATRCs may be a part of a university campus or another agency (such as Thrive) or they may be a free-standing center. ATRCs, similar to technology innovation centers, are available to demonstrate AT and advise consumers on the best devices to fit their unique needs. In addition, ATRCs have a loan closet so consumers can try out equipment to determine what will fit their needs. Table 33-4 includes examples of some prominent technology innovation centers around the United States.

Virtual Environments Throughout the Life Span

Much of the world is experiencing a paradigm shift to a much higher engagement in the cyber world. For many, the use of technology is growing across the life span. Although some individuals may not have the means to have technology at their homes, it is common to see this technology in use at libraries, community centers, and within school settings, increasing the accessibility to everyone. Because technology has become so accessible, many children begin interacting with it at a very young age and it quickly becomes a part of their world at home and at school. Many adolescents and adults use technology on a daily basis for communication, scheduling, and networking. Older adults are becoming more technologically savvy, and many elderly individuals use technology to help keep up with their grown children and grandchildren, providing inclusivity in the family, especially if they are far away from one another.

Participation in virtual environments can be considered in several different categories of use, including learning, managing physical and mental health, socializing, playing/gaming, and seeking and providing support. While engagement within a virtual environment across the life span is growing, a digital divide continues to exist. Practitioners must be cognizant of the clear evidence that exists linking socioeconomic variables to access and participation in virtual environments (Mubarak et al., 2020; Vassilakopoulou & Hustad, 2023).

Learning

The *OTPF-4* defines education as an occupation; it refers to activities needed for learning and participating in the educational environment (AOTA, 2020). People may participate in education as occupation in formal, informal, and virtual

TABLE 33-4 | Examples of Technology Innovation Centers

Innovation centers work with a variety of people with a range of conditions. In addition to these centers, the Tech Act requires every state to operate ATRCs. These may be free-standing agencies or they may be a part of another agency such as a university.

Technology Innovation Center	Description
Ingles House: https://www.inglis.org/about-us	Located in Pennsylvania (Pittsburgh and Philadelphia), they have free-standing innovation centers that allow individuals with disabilities the opportunity to engage in technology to improve overall quality of life.
Colorado State University Assistive Technology Resource Center: https://www.chhs.colostate.edu/atrc	An example of an ATRC on a university campus within the department of occupational therapy. Offers AT services to members of the campus community (student and employee) to promote inclusion and accessibility.
The Center for Discovery: https://thecenterfordiscovery.org/our-services/medical-clinical-services/assistive-technology-innovation	Located in New York, this organization hosts the Innovation Labs, which is designed to engage the services of engineers, artists, designers, and so on, to help problem-solve and create solutions to improve the lives of individuals with disabilities.
World Health Organization Collaborating Centre for Research on Assistive Technology: https://www.ucl.ac.uk/who-cc-assistive-technology/world-health-organization-who-collaborating-centre-research-assistive-technology	The WHO collaborates with the Global Disability Innovation Hub to drive research, practice research, and accelerate innovation that improves access to assistive technology for a more fair and just world.

contexts across the life span, including preschool, high school, trade school, higher education, and through adulthood and old age. Educational technology can be a key aspect of making education accessible and supporting a learner's goals.

Formal Education

Education can be classified as formal when an individual participates in academic coursework, nonacademic areas of the educational environment (lunch/recess), extracurricular activities (sports/clubs), technological education (online/distance learning), and vocational education. Formal education is often considered to happen Monday to Friday during school hours; however, individuals can also participate in formal education during other times as well. As an example, a Jewish child may participate in religious school on Sunday mornings and Hebrew school one to two afternoons a week after school hours.

Education can be considered informal when it involves participating in classes for fun or self-enrichment outside of a regular academic curriculum (AOTA, 2020). For example, an adult could take a bonsai class in hopes of developing a new leisure activity. The educational component is important. Using the bonsai example, the individual needs to learn how to handle and prune the tree, learn to use wire to bend a branch, and get comfortable using tools required in this art form. However, the outcome of this class is the skills learned versus test taking and earning an academic grade.

It's important to consider how individuals access their education. Within formal education, it is becoming more commonplace for people to have options to engage in online education or schooling provided outside of brick-and-mortar buildings. Some private/charter schools, as well as some public schools, have created virtual school or virtual classroom options, a trend that increased substantially because of the COVID-19 pandemic.

Occupational, physical, and speech therapy services can also be delivered virtually within the school setting. For example, the Breakfast Club (Friedman, 2022) initially began because of the COVID-19 pandemic. This program was put into place to help create structure/routine for students who were learning from home because of school closure. It is an interprofessional collaboration between an occupational therapist, physical therapist, and speech language pathologist and was provided through a virtual platform first thing in the morning to help children develop social/emotional skills, self-regulation, and motor skills; it also gave them the opportunity to have a positive start to their day. The Breakfast Club is currently being continued in this particular school district as a virtual offering.

By doing so, multiple classrooms can engage with the occupational, physical, and speech therapists at the same time, allowing multiple students to work on needed skills through an interprofessional collaboration—something that can be very challenging within the confines of a traditional classroom setting.

For many OTPs, the process of delivering services through the virtual environment can be classified as telehealth. Telehealth, being a service delivery model, can be utilized in all major areas of occupational therapy and can fit very well into educational activities (Zylstra, 2013). OTPs can, for example, group several students in different schools for a therapy session through telehealth, which can be more efficient than driving to individual schools to treat students.

In the educational setting, OTPs may work with students who have not been identified for special education services through the Multi-Tiered System of Support (MTSS). MTSS provides support to students based on three tiers, each one providing more intensive services. Practitioners can use the virtual environment as a part of MTSS to help support students who are identified as being at risk either academically or with mental health concerns (Rortvedt & Jacobs, 2019). Mental health issues are often identified in school-aged children, and MTSS can help support them in the educational environment.

Practitioners can work at Tier-1 providing supports, such as the Breakfast Club, to all students within a school setting to help support the classrooms. At Tier-2 of MTSS, prevention services are provided to students who are considered to be at risk. A practitioner might meet with a small group of students to discuss hobbies and help the students to develop leisure interests. Tier-3 is designed to be intensive and individualized for students identified with a mental illness. The OTP can meet with the student in Tier-3 to help teach stress reduction and coping techniques to increase time spent in class (Bazyk, 2019). Students at each tier of MTSS can receive services through the virtual environment. See Chapter 37: School Mental Health and Chapter 47: Student.

Virtual Learning in Higher Education

Students who decide to attend college can also participate in virtual learning. It is becoming more commonplace for students to choose to take online courses to help complete their degree requirements (Zhang et al., 2023). Some students do so to help round out their schedules and allow for more flexibility in how they complete their coursework. For example, a student can take in-person classes on Monday, Wednesday, and Friday and synchronous online classes on Tuesday and Thursday, which reduces commuting time to campus should they live further away from the school. Synchronous online classes have a dedicated class meeting time and tend to feel similar to a seated class on a campus; however, the student will use computer technology such as Zoom to attend their class virtually.

Other students may work full time and may choose to take online courses that are more asynchronous in nature, allowing them time to work and the flexibility of when they can complete their assignments.

Asynchronous classes typically consist of preloaded assignments and lectures and a weekly schedule. Students can work on their assignments at their own pace on their own schedule and upload them by a predetermined due date. Because the lectures are prerecorded, students participating in asynchronous classes can listen to them as many times as needed to help learn the material. Virtual university courses can also be beneficial to students who experience health or mental health issues. For example, a student who is a veteran with posttraumatic stress disorder (PTSD) might be challenged by a crowded college campus. This person may elect to take some courses in the evening when the college campus is not as busy, as well as online offerings to help fill in the gaps for classes that can't be taken at night. This may assist with reducing the stress of navigating the crowded college campus during prime hours.

Massive Open Online Courses (MOOCs) are another way to help people who want to increase their academic skills but who cannot access a traditional college campus either geographically or financially. Through the use of these courses, individuals can build their academic repertoire, which may help to fill in learning gaps and can also demonstrate knowledge needed for a career. Most MOOCs are offered for free; however, some are also offered at cost if the individual is receiving college credit for the course (https://www.mooc.org).

OTPs need to recognize the value of online course offerings, especially when working with individuals who are interested in attending or returning to college. The virtual environment can help to break down barriers that traditionally might interfere with college attendance for many students.

Informal Education

Informal education involves education outside of a traditional graded/outcomes-based manner (AOTA, 2020). Individuals may engage in informal learning to help develop new skills, such as learning a new language or cooking different foods, or to develop new leisure activities, such as drawing or knitting. The virtual environment is an excellent approach for individuals pursuing informal learning opportunities.

Informal learning in the virtual environment can be structured or unstructured and can be offered through online platforms or through an app. For example, an individual may be interested in learning a new language such as Spanish either for fun or to help increase their job skills. Rather than enrolling in a college Spanish course, the individual may choose to utilize an app such as Duolingo to help develop their language skills. Another person may decide they want to learn how to cook Thai food. YouTube is an excellent place to start. YouTube allows individuals to peruse different cooking offerings, and they can choose to subscribe (for free) and follow different instructors so they can develop their cooking skills and cook different dishes.

When looking to learn a new skill, some individuals may choose to enroll in more formal online offerings. Khan Academy is a free service offering online academic courses. It is important for an OTP to be aware of what is offered in their local communities. For example, in Louisville, Kentucky (where one of the chapter authors resides), Jefferson County Public Schools along with Louisville Learns/Ed2go has a variety of adult learning activities ranging from the arts to science to financial literacy. While these courses have a cost associated with them, they are all offered virtually. Some courses are self-paced, so that the participant learns as they go, and others may have specific online meeting times to teach a skill and support the participants to practice skills.

In addition, people may also choose to utilize MOOCs as mentioned in the formal education section. These courses can also help to build skills and start new leisure pursuits. See Box 33-2 for examples of virtual offerings through Louisville Learns and worldwide offerings through Mooc.org. Many public libraries also have opportunities for virtual engagement through the use of streaming services for book discussions or podcasts for author interviews. It is important for OTPs to be familiar with offerings for informal learning to help individuals they treat be aware of their options. This is an effective way to support informed decision-making, support individuals to create their own educational goals, and help people pursue and monitor their goal attainment.

Managing Physical and Mental Health

The concept of virtual health is one that has emerged in the last few decades and exponentially grown since the COVID-19 pandemic. As the use of the internet grew during the .com era, it created opportunities for new models of virtual health-care delivery to emerge. **Virtual health** or virtual health care occurs when products or services are delivered in a technology-based format influenced by the use of virtual platforms, such as telemedicine (Harrop, 2001) and digital communications, such as patient portals (Jung & Padman, 2014). Often, terms such as "telemedicine" or "telehealth" may be used when referring to the context of virtual health (Majerowicz & Tracy, 2010). Although some may attempt to use it interchangeably, the two terms are not the same.

BOX 33-2 ■ Examples of Virtual Course Offerings

Louisville Learns: Example menu for online adult learning opportunities

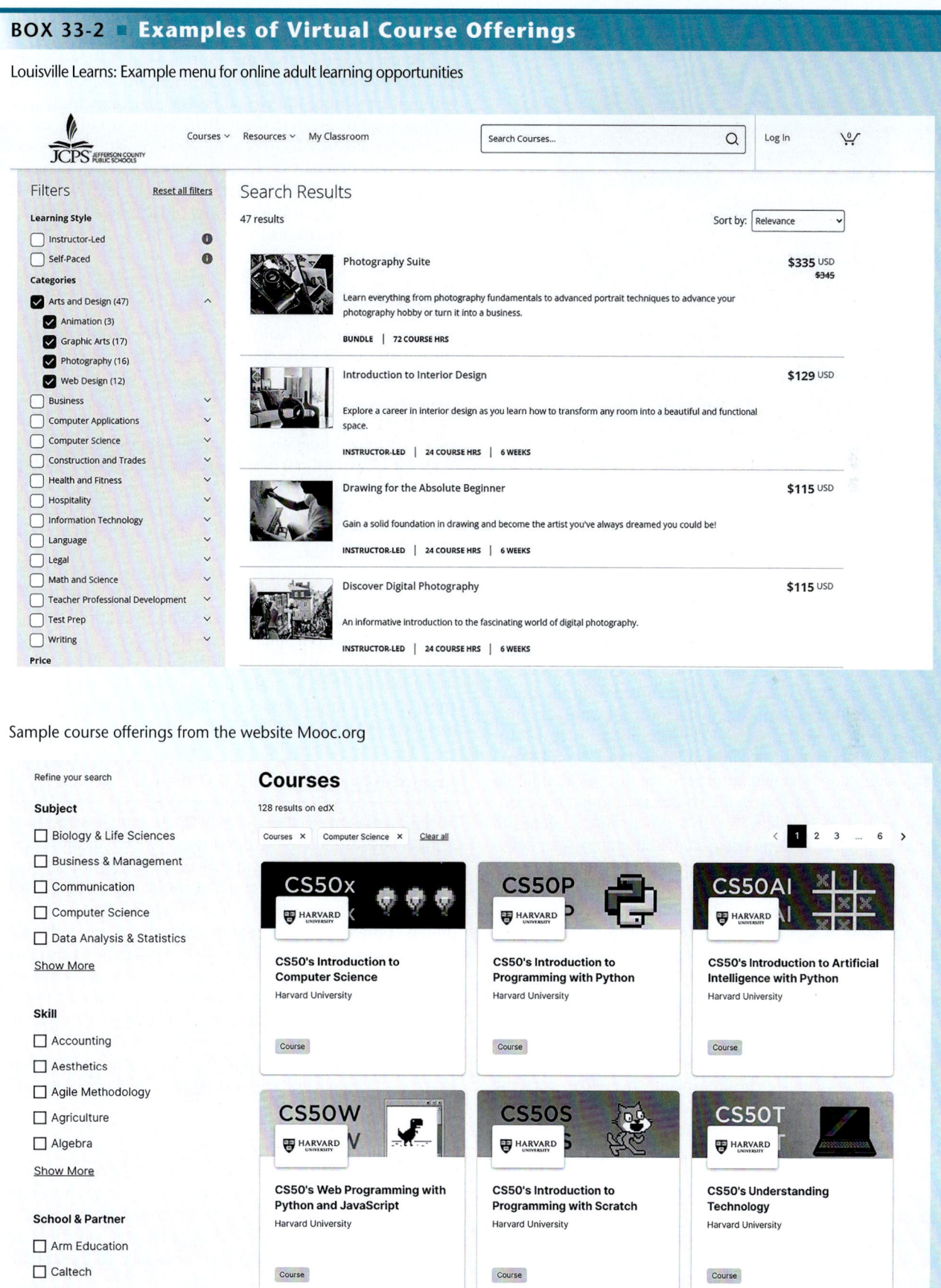

Sample course offerings from the website Mooc.org

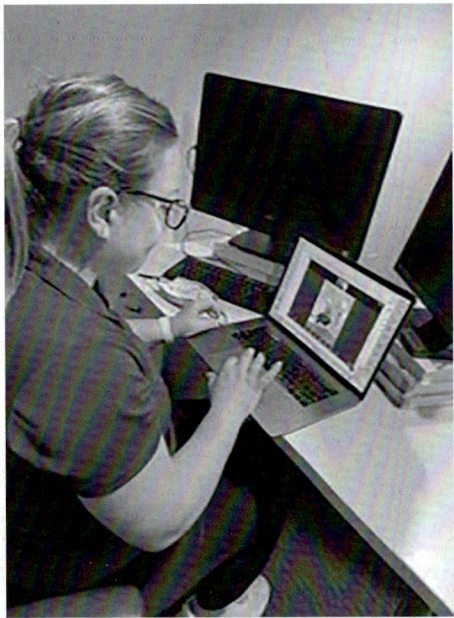

FIGURE 33-3. Telehealth can support the occupational therapy process in a variety of engaging and innovative ways. Dr. McBride used it to access needs and evaluate a person's home for accessibility and fall risks.

The Office of the National Coordinator for Health Information Technology (ONC) offers a definition guide, stating, "telemedicine refers specifically to remote clinical services" (HealthIT.gov, 2019, para. 1). When considering the realm of virtual health, OTPs often gravitate toward what is known as telehealth. For example, an OTP can utilize a Health Insurance Portability and Accountability Act of 1996 (HIPAA) compliant, secure virtual platform to conduct an evaluation and assessment that shapes the intervention plan and continuation of services delivered in a synchronous telehealth format. In Figure 33-3, an occupational therapist seen delivering telehealth services by way of completing a virtual home assessment for a person living in a rural community.

Occupational therapy via telehealth creates a pathway for the provision of services to people living in rural communities and the delivery of services and/or consultations for home-bound people or their caregivers. It also provides access to specialists from across the country or cross-nationally. In this chapter's Practitioner Profile feature, Quiana Long discusses her practice and illustrates how an OTP can even deliver telehealth across continents.

Practitioners using telehealth not only need to understand the terminology, but also need to understand and adhere to practice guidelines. When using telehealth, the OTP is expected to continue to uphold privacy, security, and confidentiality laws and regulations such as HIPAA and the Family Educational Rights and Privacy Act (FERPA) while also ensuring consumers have a clear understanding of their rights and responsibilities when accessing telehealth services. Guidance as it relates to telehealth broadly and occupational therapy specifically can be found in multiple sources. Some key

documents providing frameworks for delivering telehealth are listed and described in Table 33-5.

The use of a telemedicine approach can foster opportunities for practitioners to utilize telehealth when working within the realm of the virtual health environment. Consideration must be given to the individual's means of access and technology literacy for receiving services within the virtual health environment. Community support services along with occupational therapy interventions may be beneficial in the health, well-being, and/or recovery process of the individual, groups, and populations.

Socializing

The virtual learning realm creates opportunities for social participation and multiple occasions for individuals to build and strengthen social interaction skills. Virtual interactions, whether focused on learning or leisure activities, take place in a unique social environment. Social interactions are a vital aspect of occupation and practitioners should creatively consider how they can best support social participation and social interdependence in virtual environments (*OTPF-4*, AOTA, 2020). Virtual social environments can provide individuals across the life span with a broad array of choices for engaging with others.

For example, a student in school has options for social participation when working in virtual school activities, while a young adult may seek to engage with peers through interactive online gaming, and an older adult may connect with family members across the globe through the use of apps or social media. Thus, an individual's level of participation and engagement will vary based on the context and personal factors (AOTA, 2020; Smallfield et al., 2014).

Social Media

Social media emerged in the early 2000s, and its exponential growth has resulted in the development of what can be identified as social environments. One's participation in social media may have originated from the desire to be virtually connected to someone they previously met in-person. As digital connections continue to grow, many see daily interactions occurring through the use of social environments. In many experiences, the social environment has manifested into providing one with a sense of connection and belonging, eliminating barriers and borders that once occurred when only brick-and-mortar environments existed. Although social media provides a myriad of opportunities for occupational engagement and connection, it is not without potential negative repercussions.

Though many individuals seek to find community and belonging in the virtual environment using social media platforms, there are legitimate concerns about the rise in negative engagement. Parents and practitioners alike must be vigilant to ensure virtual interactions do not foster paths for cyberbullying, online predation, or suicidality, especially in young adolescents (Gu et al., 2022; Pellegrino et al., 2022; Schonfeld et al., 2023).

Practitioner Profile

Quiana Long, MS, OTR/L, HCPC Reg.

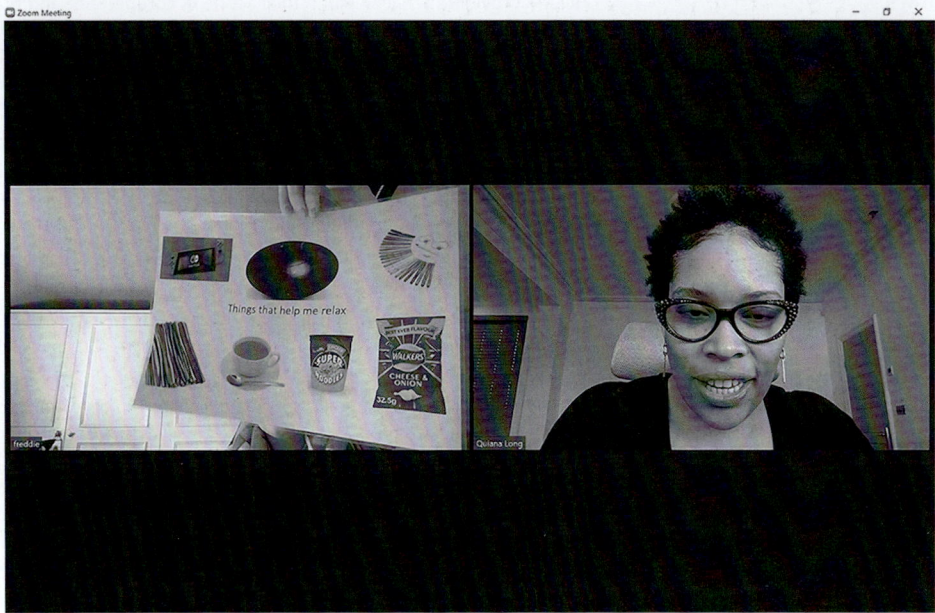

Bright Skies Therapy & Consulting is a small, dynamic practice I founded during the height of COVID. My goal was to reach as many families as possible while achieving a life-long goal of birthing my own business. I think of myself as #thereallifeOT because I've been both the professional and the parent/carer. My lived experiences include raising a child with a heart condition that resulted in various additional diagnoses (e.g., developmental delay, vision problems, failure to thrive) and caring for my mother who lost her battle with multiple sclerosis in 2013. These experiences presented challenges, kept me humble, and molded me into the dynamic practitioner I am today. These adversities taught me to approach each child and their family with empathy and understanding.

I am a skilled practitioner with the same drive and passion for occupational therapy today that I had when I graduated. I've continued my education by completing SI training, becoming a licensed Zumbini instructor, and earning the National Board for Certification in Occupational Therapy (NBCOT) Pediatrics Practice Area Emphasis badge. I am NBCOT certified and HCPC registered (a UK qualification), and hold membership in AOTA and RCOT (Royal College of Occupational Therapists).

I have dedicated my career to helping children and their families/support circles, from all walks of life, to achieve a sense of accomplishment, happiness, and lasting quality of life. I have worked with children living with various diagnoses and strive to support the whole child. I've been told I'm personable, engaging, and compassionate; a practitioner who believes "it takes a village" to help nurture a child. I understand the importance of teamwork, collaboration, caregiver involvement, and the family unit.

I learned about telehealth during employee orientation at my very first therapy job. I was immediately intrigued. I saw the benefits of reaching those without access to face-to-face health care, of delivering convenient care that realistically fit in these families' lives, and saw I could support more families. My passion to be a teletherapist was realized during the pandemic. During COVID, I used my occupational therapy skills to support children and their families learning to navigate an unfamiliar online world. My practice included students attending a special needs school in the United Kingdom. Helping these children navigate learning along with their sensory processing, executive functioning, attention, motor, and social-emotional challenges in an unstructured, comfortable setting called home proved to be a beautiful challenge. I also found myself as a key support for parents.

Crossing country borders virtually has been a great personal experience. I live in the United States now, but also provide telehealth services to families in the UK. In my telehealth practice, I place key importance on family routines, culture, age, home environment, and the family's access to material. Maintaining engagement and addressing functional limitations and goals requires a lot of preparation, planning, and organization. These are all outcomes I try to encourage in the children and their families. It truly becomes a joint effort.

The most difficult aspect of working within the virtual environment is keeping the person I am working with engaged. It takes a great deal of flexibility, quick thinking, and preparation. I find joy in the dynamic nature of telehealth and love the challenge of navigating time differences and experiencing two different cultures simultaneously. A constant for me is the familiar feeling of brightening a child/family's world through occupational therapy.

TABLE 33-5 | Key Documents and Practice Guidelines for Telehealth

Document	Key Practice Guidelines
AOTA Position Paper *Telehealth in Occupational Therapy* (AOTA, 2018)	Emphasizes that an OTP must meet standards for minimum qualifications; these include providing services within their scope of competence and practice; complying with federal and state regulations; adhering to the AOTA Code of Ethics, as well as HIPAA and FERPA regulations; delivering safe and effective services; and demonstrating working knowledge of technology used for the delivery of services while being able to troubleshoot with the person should issues arise.
Code of Ethics (WFOT, 2016)	Outlines key factors an OTP must consider before engaging in telehealth practices, including professional licensure or registration requirements, the occupational therapy community at large, and personal factors such as the reason for the referral, evaluation and assessment measures, and intervention(s) that may be employed.
Global Standard for Accessibility of Telehealth Services (WHO, 2022)	Guides health-care providers with a set of technical requirements as a checklist to ensure equitable services are being provided.
Principles in Delivering Telerehabilitation Services (American Telemedicine Association, 2020)	Outlines guidelines or standards associated with the use of telehealth and guiding principles for the administration and delivery of clinical services (Richmond et al., 2017).
Position Statement: *Occupational Therapy and Telehealth* (WFOT, 2021)	Defines professional regulations for OTPs and outlines telehealth services as follows: "may be synchronous (real-time) interactions with the client (e.g. videoconference, telephone, remote monitoring applications ['apps'] and gaming technologies); and/or asynchronous (i.e., "store-and-forward") transmission of data (e.g. video, photos, electronic mail) between the provider and the client" (WFOT, 2021, p. 1).
State licensure laws and practice acts	Practitioners are responsible to be informed and adhere to national/federal or state laws and regulations, as well as practice guidelines and standards set forth by governing organizations, regulatory bodies, and licensing and credentialing agencies.

Many youths participate in social media to keep in touch with their friends and to promote self-expression. It can also make them a target for cyberbullying. Cyberbullying is bullying that occurs through online platforms or technology; it may be worse than traditional bullying because of the anonymous course it can take (i.e., there is no face-to-face confrontation; Schonfeld et al., 2023). Unfortunately, for some individuals, cyberbullying can become pervasive enough that they may choose to take their own lives, thus creating the term "cyberbullicide" (Schonfeld et al., 2023). For more information about suicide, please refer to Chapter 20: Mood Disorders and Chapter 44: Addressing Suicide Across the Continuum.

Human Behavior in Social Environments

Human behavior in virtual social environments, specifically how interactions have changed with one another, has been studied since the rise of **social network sites** (**SNS**; Pantic, 2014). In a seminal work, Kraut and colleagues (1998) suggested engagement in the cyber world would affect human behavior, specifically aspects of social participation and occupational engagement (AOTA, 2020). For adolescents and teens, social interaction is critical for the development of social skills.

OTPs know that social skills support participation in occupation and often take a more global or public health approach when focusing on social skills programming with these groups regardless of the presence of mental health concerns. Arbesman et al. (2013), for example, discovered that occupational therapists "believed that children who were able to interact in peer and social environments . . . were more likely to successfully participate in school and in the home and community environments" (p. e121).

The virtual environment is now easier for many across the globe to access. Practitioners can use their activity and occupational analysis skills to consider the unique manner in which virtual social contexts can impact participation. For example, a student located in the United States may feel more at ease discussing barriers to occupational performance with a peer in an online community who resides across the globe, rather than openly sharing the concerns with a friend who attends the same brick-and-mortar school.

An individual may demonstrate an increase in openness when interacting with others in virtual rather than physical social environments; this can be witnessed across the life span. For example, an older adult who resides in a senior community might not feel comfortable sharing intimate thoughts or feelings with someone they engage with on a daily basis. However, this same older adult's behavior may change when they are provided the opportunity to connect and dialogue with someone in a virtual environment, such as an online chat or videoconferencing support group, in which others are experiencing a similar situation related to health or well-being (Smallfield et al., 2014).

Interpersonal interactions, communication skills, and an individual's social environment can be directly impacted by the culture and practices of the social networks they interact with. The impact of participation in varied SNS on the individual's mental health can be negative or positive

(Kreski et al., 2021). The research regarding social media has mixed outcomes with some studies capturing some degree of both positive and negative effects on the mental health of children, teens (Orben & Przybylski, 2019), or adults. Practitioners may find the use of the PEO model beneficial when examining the option of a social environment where SNS engagement fulfills the category of meaningful occupation.

SNS can create social environments that create emotional and psychological burdens that challenge an individual's mental health. Cyberbullying and the online disinhibition effect (Suler, 2004), which is a tendency to show less constraint in communication online than one would normally show in person, are two examples of how people can experience harm or personal attacks from a myriad of social media platforms (Cimke & Cerit, 2021). Instances of cyberbullying could include creating a disparaging profile of a peer to rate their appearance or popularity or sending mean or even threatening statements to an individual through instant text or video messages.

In addition to the potential for verbal aggression to manifest from the use of social media, another growing concern from the use of SNS is the direct effect on communication skills. With a growth in online communication, the ways in which children, adolescents, teens, and young adults engage

Evidence-Based Practice

Social Media and Mental Health

OTPs need to be aware of both the negative effects and benefits of social media on people.

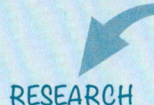

RESEARCH FINDINGS

Research continues to focus on the effects social media has on the mental health of children, teens, and young adults. One's use of social media/SNS has evidence to support both positive and negative effects with regard to mental health outcomes. Negative effects of social media/SNS can directly impact one's perception of self, potentially influence self-harming behaviors or engagement in the emotional harm of others. On the contrary, the positive effects of social media/SNS can generate a sense of community, create opportunities for affirmation of self or others, and foster an outlet for positivity beliefs and behaviors.

APPLICATIONS

➡ Practitioners should be aware of and alert so they can identify and respond to the negative effects social media/SNS can have on children and teens (Abi-Jaoude et al., 2020; Chou & Edge, 2012; Stiglic & Viner, 2019). These can include:
- Depressive symptoms and changes to and/or challenges with self-esteem (Barry et al., 2017; Boers et al., 2019; George et al., 2018)
- Suicidal ideation and/or self-harm behaviors (Cohen & Biddle, 2022; John et al., 2018; Sedgwick et al., 2019)
- Evidence of being targeted by cyberbullying as a victim (Hamm et al., 2015; Kowalski et al., 2014)

➡ Practitioners should be aware of and look to capitalize on the positive effects social media/SNS can have on children and teens. Social media/SNS activities can:
- Support community building (Anderson et al., 2022; George et al., 2018)
- Foster self-affirming behaviors and practices (Cingel et al., 2022)
- Be a positive outlet for self-expression (Anderson et al., 2022; Austin-McCain, 2017)

REFERENCES

Abi-Jaoude, E., Naylor, K., & Pignatiello, A. (2020). Smartphones, social media use and youth mental health. *Canadian Medical Association Journal, 192*(6), E136–E141. https://doi.org/10.1503/cmaj.190434

Anderson, M., Vogels, E., Perrin, A., & Rainie, L. (2022, November 16). *Connection, creativity, and drama: Teen life on social media in 2022.* Pew Research Center. https://www.pewresearch.org/internet/2022/11/16/connection-creativity-and-drama-teen-life-on-social-media-in-2022

Austin-McCain, M. (2017). An examination of the association of social media use with the satisfaction with daily routines and healthy lifestyle habits for undergraduate and graduate students. *The Open Journal of Occupational Therapy, 5*(4), Article 6. https://doi.org/10.15453/2168-6408.1327

Continued

Evidence-Based Practice—cont'd

Social Media and Mental Health

Barry, C., Sidoti, C., Briggs, S., Reiter, S., & Lindsey, R. (2017). Adolescent social media use and mental health from adolescent and parent perspectives. *Journal of Adolescence, 61,* 1–11. https://doi.org/10.1016/j.adolescence.2017.08.005

Boers, E., Afzali, M., Newton, N., & Conrod, P. (2019). Association of screen time and depression in adolescence. *JAMA Pediatrics, 173,* 853–859. doi:10.1001/jamapediatrics.2019.1759

Chou, H. T., & Edge, N. (2012). "They are happier and having better lives than I am": The impact of using Facebook on perceptions of others' lives. *Cyberpsychology, Behavior & Social Networking, 15,* 117–121. https://doi.org/10.1089/cyber.2011.0324

Cingel, D., Carter, M., & Krause, H. (2022). Social media and self-esteem. *Current Opinion in Psychology, 45,* 101304. https://doi.org/10.1016/j.copsyc.2022.101304

Cohen, R., & Biddle, L. (2022). The influence of social media on suicidal behaviour among students. In S. Mallon & J. Smith (Eds.), *Preventing and responding to student suicide: A practical guide for FE and HE settings* (pp. 94–107). Jessica Kingsley Publishers.

George, M., Russell, M., Piontak, J., & Odgers, C. (2018). Concurrent and subsequent associations between daily digital technology use and high-risk adolescents' mental health symptoms. *Child Development, 89,* 78–88. http://doi.org/10.1111/cdev.12819

Hamm, M., Newton, A., Chisholm, A., Shulhan, J., Milne, A., Sundar, P., Ennis, H., Scott, S., & Hartling, L. (2015). Prevalence and effect of cyberbullying on children and young people: A scoping review of social media studies. *JAMA Pediatrics, 169*(8), 770–777. https://doi.org/10.1001/jamapediatrics.2015.0944

John, A., Glendenning, A., Marchant, A., Montgomery, P., Stewart, A., Wood, S., Lloyd, K., & Hawton, K. (2018). Self-harm, suicidal behaviours, and cyberbullying in children and young people: Systematic review. *Journal of Medical Internet Research, 20*(4), e129. https://doi.org/10.2196/jmir.9044

Kowalski, R., Giumetti, G., & Schroeder, A. (2014). Bullying in the digital age: A critical review and meta-analysis of cyberbullying research among youth. *Psychology Bulletin, 140,* 1073–1137. https://doi.org/10.1037/a0035618

Sedgwick, R., Epstein, S., Dutta, R., & Ougrin, D. (2019). Social media, internet use and suicide attempts in adolescents. *Current Opinion in Psychiatry, 32*(6), 534–541. https://doi.org/10.1097/YCO.0000000000000547

Stiglic, N., & Viner, R. (2019). Effects of screen time on the health and well-being of children and adolescents: A systematic review of reviews. *BMJ Open, 9*(1), e023191. https://doi.org/10.1136/bmjopen-2018-023191

or interact is changing (American Academy of Pediatrics, 2018; Kreski et al., 2021). Changes are observed in the frequency of face-to-face interactions, the quality of social interactions that impact interpersonal relationships, and the possibility that one may lack some social skills (Larson, 2021). The notion that an individual's way of communication and interacting with others is changing can be attributed to a generational shift where many current youths, particularly in more economically developed countries, cannot understand day-to-day life without instant internet access, social media, or SNS (Abi-Jaoude et al., 2020).

Social Skill Development

An individual's interaction with and use of the virtual environment experienced an exponential growth during the height of the COVID-19 pandemic and has continued. The social aspect of the virtual environment fostered a sense of belonging cross-culturally, allowing individuals of all ages to connect during the uncertainty of the pandemic. Skills required for communication and social connection in virtual social environments differ from those of in-person interactions. For example, virtual communication, although not limited to written form, creates opportunities for inference and open interpretation of the intended message.

It is likely most people have received an email where the message was questioned, the intent seemed unclear, and there was a feeling that one should or should not read into the sender's use of a message in ALL CAPS. The point here is that

OTPs may find that some people they work with need to learn and practice the skill sets needed for engaging in communication with a new peer or group in virtual contexts. Practitioners should consider context and personal factors (AOTA, 2020) as the virtual environment can provide opportunities for interaction with individuals from a myriad of backgrounds. Skills that may have been present with in-person communication, such as reading nonverbal communication, using clarifying questions, or asking someone to repeat themselves when the listener did not initially grasp the communication, are less likely to occur in the virtual environment.

The virtual social environment can provide an individual with an opportunity to be bold or open in sharing information from behind a screen. Although openness may be needed to foster growth and/or healing of the individual, it is imperative one understands the skills may differ from virtual to in-person communication. Most skills of effective in-person communication still apply in the virtual social environment, but additional skills such as learning to seek clarification, how to move in and out of conversations, and the ability to avoid misinterpretation of messages or misinformation can be critical.

Video and Gaming Systems

Video game systems are common in many households; these range from PC consoles to entertainment systems such as the PlayStation to handheld systems such as the Nintendo Switch. Many of these systems are now integrated with the home internet to allow individuals to go online and interact with others. For example, on the Nintendo Switch, the game Animal Crossing: New Horizons allows players to visit each other's islands and interact with each other as well as the island inhabitants. On the PlayStation, players can participate in games such as World of Warcraft, Elder Scrolls Online, and Final Fantasy, all of which are classified as **massively multiplayer online (MMO) gaming**.

OTPs may choose to incorporate video gaming, **role-playing games (RPGs), virtual reality (VR)** experiences, and **multi-user virtual environments (MUVE)** into their treatment to help people build social interaction skills and develop leisure skills. These activities allow individuals to create a character and become whoever they want within the gaming world, which can ultimately be very empowering in the recovery process.

Massively Multiplayer Online/ Role-Playing Games

MMOs are online video games with a large number of players on the same server. MMOs can allow individuals to cooperate and compete with each other and sometimes create meaningful relationships with individuals from around the world. Practitioners should consider whether encouraging the use of MMO-type games or RPGs could help encourage social interaction for people they work with. Based on the concept of "gamification," a term conceptualized as utilizing game-based designs, elements, and principles to target mental health, digital gaming has been showing promise in psychiatric practice (Banerjee et al., 2021).

Through the use of MMO gaming and RPGs, many individuals are able to find a community of similar-minded individuals. Specific social skills to practice could include setting up times to engage in game play and maintaining reciprocal communication with other players through the video game system either with voice through a headset or by typing in a communication box on the screen. For individuals who have conditions such as PTSD, anxiety, or depression, which may make it difficult to leave the house, video gaming can provide an outlet for social interaction and can also help distract the individual from their symptoms, allowing them to feel a sense of calm while playing but also a sense of success as they work through the many requirements of the game.

For many individuals, online gaming can help to create a source of community. In addition, games also provide a "playful" experience and the user is not necessarily aware of the fact that they may be participating in mental health intervention, a fact that can make this treatment modality more acceptable in naturalistic settings (Banerjee et al., 2021).

Role-Playing Games

Dungeons & Dragons (D&D) is a popular RPG. D&D has a large following with individuals from the middle grades through adulthood participating in gaming sessions that can take place in many forms. In a practice setting, role-playing games can be utilized as a therapeutic tool because its narrative structures about overcoming adversity and exploring alternative identities mirror some aspects of mental health recovery (Baker et al., 2023).

While many individuals create their characters and engage in this activity in person, the COVID-19 pandemic saw individuals stretch their role-playing skills to engage in D&D through Zoom or another online platform. D&D itself has traditionally been a very inclusive game and many individuals with a variety of diverse needs have found comfort and a sense of belonging through participation in this activity. By adding Zoom to D&D, the game is now more portable and individuals can still engage should they need to travel for some reason, or they are unable to leave their home. Through Zoom, players can share a screen to help show the game board to all players (usually by the dungeon master, the person running the game). Google Dice Roller can also be utilized to simulate a dice roll, so each participant does not have to keep up with the multiple dice required for this activity.

Because of the inclusivity of the virtual environment, individuals can use this game to help develop their leisure activities, social skills, and ultimately help to create a community of similar-minded individuals for themselves. OTPs may choose to incorporate RPGs such as D&D into a treatment plan because they can help aid friendship and relationship maintenance, mitigate social anxiety, improve social skills, reduce stress, and provide connection with others (Baker et al., 2023). D&D may also eventually move from a treatment modality to a developed leisure activity, which the person may continue to engage in outside of occupational therapy intervention.

AVATAR Training

Audio Visual Assisted Therapy Aid for Refractory (AVATAR) therapy is a therapist-assisted computerized treatment program designed to target distressing auditory verbal hallucinations (voices) in participants whose symptoms have typically been resistant to medication (Garety et al., 2021). In the Garety and colleagues study, participants with a diagnosis of schizophrenia participated in this therapy for nine 60-minute sessions, which were done through a VR type setting. Therapists create an "avatar" of the perpetrator or distressing voice and, over each session, the participant works to address their voice.

During the initial three sessions, the avatar is quite dominant; however, as the individual learns how to cope with, and develops, power and control, the avatar eventually becomes less hostile. The use of AVATAR therapy has provided positive results among individuals diagnosed with schizophrenia, including the reduction of distressing voices (Garety et al., 2021). While the individuals conducting this research are not OTPs, practitioners who are working in psychiatric settings should be aware of this technology to help people manage their symptoms. AVATAR training is also emerging as a treatment methodology in the United Kingdom for people in community prisons (van Rijn et al., 2015). The pilot program was avatar-based, VR therapy to "improve mental health outcomes and mental well-being of prisoners" (van Rijn et al., 2015, p. 1).

Virtual Reality

VR technology has moved from a gaming system to gathering traction as a potential treatment option in the rehabilitation world. VR has been defined as computer-produced

BOX 33-3 ■ Use of Virtual Reality Within an Orthopedic Setting

Juliet Steffe, OTD, OTR/L, CHT

I've always been interested in technology. Before using VR in practice, I used VR programs to improve my public speaking skills and to learn to control my anxiety when giving presentations. I was familiar with the technology and kept abreast of the evidence on the use of VR in health care, so I was excited when our orthopedic practice acquired a VR unit. The unit used technology to address chronic pain and contained programs for meditation and games to encourage a person's physical and mental engagement to provide distraction from pain.

Just after getting the unit, I evaluated a man presenting 2 months after a wrist laceration at work. He had soft tissue and nerve involvement affecting the use of his dominant hand, particularly his thumb. During evaluation, he avoided moving his wrist and hand and reported pain of 8/10. His hand was swollen and stiff. He had developed a fear of moving his hand and voiced anxiety about being touched on the hand. Whenever I attempted to assess motion, he would pull his hand away. On his initial visit, he didn't tolerate manual soft tissue mobilization or modalities. I wasn't sure how to get him moving to break his pain cycle. On the next visit, even though he'd never experienced VR, he agreed to try the VR program for pain reduction.

We selected a program for distraction where he could interact within a virtual environment. I explained I would provide gentle range of motion (ROM) to his injured hand in this session. While he was engaged with the VR, I initiated gentle effleurage and joint mobilization without him resisting or reporting any increase in his pain. We continued to use VR in subsequent visits. Therapy was graded by incorporating active wrist and hand motions and having him squeeze a stress ball or perform wrist active range of motion (AROM) while using the VR. Eventually, he participated in therapy without the VR distraction. Realizing he could use his hand with less pain, he accepted typical manual treatments and exercises to regain hand function.

We've also used VR technology to manage pain in a woman diagnosed with chronic regional pain syndrome (CRPS). She reported difficulty managing anxiety because of her ongoing pain. We used a VR program to learn meditation and relaxation. Her treating therapist successfully integrated VR into her care plan during heat and electrical stimulation to help her relax during treatment. Allowing this woman to have just a 20-minute break from her pain helped her understand how to manage her pain.

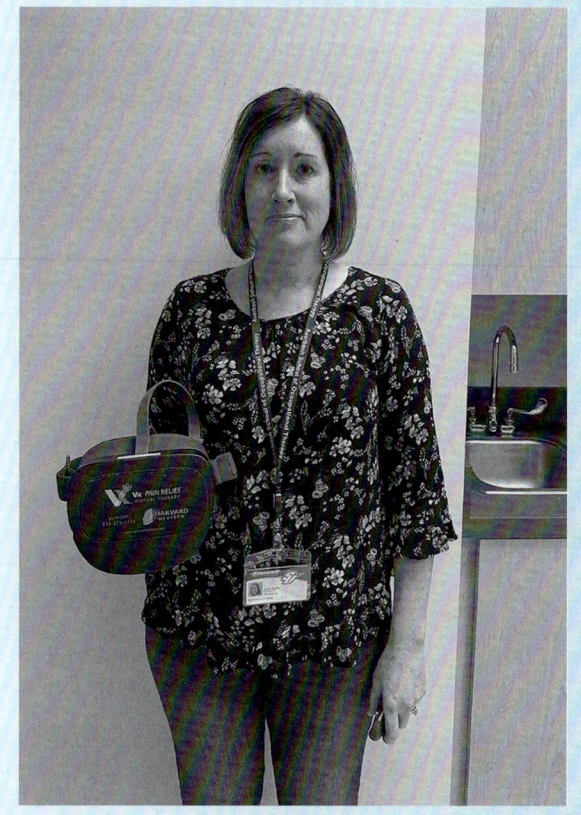

VR technology is also useful for patient education. We have used a program provided by a psychologist who is present in the VR environment. This mental health and pain expert addresses the VR user directly, explains the mind–body connection, and teaches how to control pain through mental exercises and an understanding of the pain cycle. This technology is not for everyone, but in my experience, VR provides another avenue for addressing mental health issues often accompanying physical conditions.

---

images and sounds representing a place or situation in which one can engage (Cote et al., 2023). The *OTPF-4* lists VR as an environmental factor for OTPs to consider (AOTA, 2020). Practitioners may choose to utilize VR in the clinic setting to help distract an individual from symptoms that can help to ease anxiety, promote healing, and support function. In Box 33-3, Dr. Steffe shares one story of using VR as part of her holistic interventions.

The use of VR can be quite helpful to teach a variety of life skills to individuals with intellectual and developmental disabilities in a controlled/safe setting before practicing these skills in the real world (Panerai et al., 2018).

These simulated activities can be great for the practitioner who can then review the VR session with the individual, discuss what happened and what changes they may want to make, and allow them to engage in the VR session again to build up their skill set. For example, a person may want

to walk to the grocery store to make purchases, but they have difficulty with wayfinding. VR can be utilized to teach adults with intellectual disabilities various routes (in the safety of the practice setting) and can also be utilized to simulate a grocery store setting so they can work on making purchases without getting overwhelmed in an actual community setting. In addition, VR has been utilized to teach individuals with intellectual disabilities how to safely cross the street (Oakes, 2022). Figure 33-4 shows occupational therapy students trying out VR equipment to better understand the experience of using this equipment.

In addition to teaching life skills, VR can also be utilized to teach job interviewing skills. Virtual Interactive Training Agents (ViTA) has been shown to improve the efficacy for job interviewing skills in individuals with autism and other developmental disorders. Job interviews can be very anxiety inducing for many individuals; for those on the autism

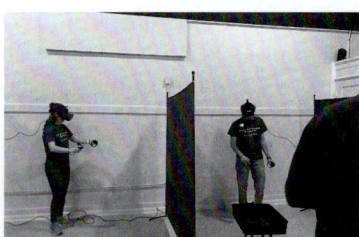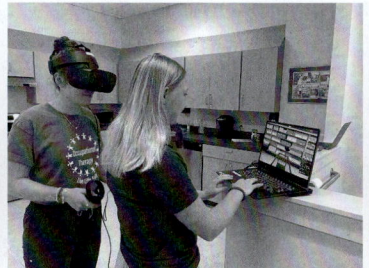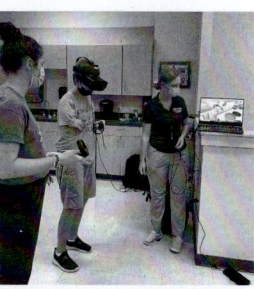

FIGURE 33-4. Occupational therapy students engage in VR life skills activities during Life Skills: Enabling Technology (LSET), a student-run program out of Spalding University's Auerbach School of Occupational Therapy. Students are paired with an adolescent from the community and engage them in prevocational and life skills using technology. Here, you can see the student working with an LSET participant to use VR to learn self-help skills, similar to ViTA.

spectrum, this can be especially difficult. ViTA is a curriculum that allows individuals with autism and developmental disabilities to learn effective interviewing skills and other hidden aspects of the interview process such as greetings, appropriate small talk, and leaving the interview (Burke et al., 2021).

The use of intelligent virtual agents has allowed this intervention to remove the human bias from the interview process and allows the participants to practice interviewing in a nonthreatening environment before their actual job interviews. ViTA has shown to be an effective tool to enhance interview skills and self-efficacy for this population (Burke et al., 2021), and it could also be effective when working with individuals with other diagnoses as well (Fig. 33-4).

Virtual Reality With English Language Learners

When considering the use of VR, associations are made that the functionality is focused on leisure, play, or social skill development. For learners where English is a foreign language (EFL), VR can be applied as a feasible learning tool. Tai and Chen (2021) summarized the effectiveness of utilizing VR through mobile-rendered head-mounted displays (MVR) with adolescent EFL learners. The benefits of VR for EFL learners included an increase in the learner's level of engagement, mediated cognitive processing issues, decreased potential anxiety levels, and supported information retention (Tai & Chen, 2021).

Additional literature is emerging in the area of EFL learners utilizing VR for learning in the virtual environment. Yeh, Tseng, and Heng (2022) discuss the benefits of VR for Taiwanese EFL college students when focusing on intracultural learning. Findings of the study suggest additional benefits may exist across the age continuum of the learner, with the college students demonstrating a stronger intracultural awareness. Overall, the emerging practice of utilizing VR for skill building in a social context to assist EFL learners may translate to the usability in occupational therapy interventions both internationally and cross-culturally.

The virtual environment provides the individual with opportunities for skill building in a safe, controlled setting where emphasis can be placed on an inter- or intracultural awareness and learning. Practitioners may consider the use of VR with EFL learners when focusing treatment interventions on skill development, whether social or educational skills.

Multi-User Virtual Environments

MUVEs are virtual platforms where individuals are able to create a virtual self (similar to an avatar) and then explore virtual environments and worlds. MUVEs pair nicely with VR technology, but they differ in the aspect that multiple individuals are able to participate in an environment, hence the term "multi-user" (Fokides, 2017). MUVEs essentially allow the simulation of real or imaginary environments that fool the human senses and trick individuals into believing that they are in a real world.

The most common MUVE is Second Life (2024). In Second Life, individuals are able to engage with music clubs, role-playing communities, virtual cinemas, and so on. Second Life also claims to be an inclusive haven of self-expression and allows individuals to connect with others who share similar stories and interests (https://secondlife.com). Although the platform for MUVEs is different, an OTP may consider utilizing MUVEs in a similar manner as MMOs and RPGs. Thus, individuals can develop social interaction skills and learn to problem-solve as they develop and sustain friendships and participate in leisure activities. Overall, these skills can be generalized into meaningful social interactions within a physical environment as well.

Virtual Mental Health Communities

The virtual environment can be utilized in a way that creates a sense of community or support for individuals. Individuals are now able to schedule virtual appointments that range from medical evaluations and needs to mental health counseling. Although the COVID-19 pandemic required these virtual visits, many individuals have found the convenience to be enticing. Rapid growth in the online support communities was evident during and after the onset of the COVID-19 pandemic (Bauer & Ngondo, 2022). Traditional, brick-and-mortar environments for support communities previously placed an additional barrier, such as transportation or access, to those needing a support group. Individuals now can routinely access a wide range of support services in a virtual capacity, allowing them to build or strengthen their support community.

Virtual Mental Health Communities (VMHCs) are communities that meet through a virtual platform (such as Zoom) and are virtual spaces where individuals with similar interests can connect and discuss issues and offer mutual support to each other. VMHCs often offer more immediate access to support and can be very beneficial. For example, if a person lives in a rural area, does not have reliable transportation, or is afraid of attending a physical meeting for their own safety, VMHCs can provide a sense of community and belonging. The levels of support can vary, and might be checking in with a sponsor or attending a virtual Alcoholics Anonymous (AA) meeting.

During the global COVID-19 pandemic, the shutdown provided many who needed to speak to a counselor or peer support specialist with an alternative of interacting virtually using options such as texting or phone calls, virtual conferencing using apps, or web-based programming. Many support group environments switched to online meetings and virtual gatherings during the pandemic, but continuing to offer this format for participation may decrease attendance challenges.

Support groups are a source of social connection, offering aid through the use of sharing lived experiences and challenges, as well as offering methods for accountability. Traditional 12-step recovery programs, such as AA or Narcotics Anonymous (NA), have provided a foundation for healing and growth through the use of peer support. To be clear, across the globe groups such as AA and NA have been offering some forms of web-based support since the mid-1990s. However, the COVID-19 pandemic accelerated the evolution of online service delivery models for support groups such as AA and NA.

The evolution of their service delivery models was reflected in an expansion of the previously existing web-based supports, allowing for programs to increase online availability and access beyond face-to-face options. Several 12-step recovery programs' online presence were highlighted during the initial months of the global pandemic shutdown. Since then, access to support groups has become readily available for many across the globe, in multiple languages. Virtual support groups can vary in offerings; examples range from a one-on-one support, such as Project LETS, to a group format such as that offered by the Fireweed Collective.

Project LETS and the Fireweed Collective are VMHCs that aim to create peer support for those with mental illness, disability, trauma, and neurodivergence. Project LETS provides a good example of the benefits a VMHC can bring by using an inclusive international, culturally and socially responsive support group including adolescents and adults. All of the peer mental health advocates through Project LETS have lived experience with mental illness, disability, trauma, and/or neurodivergence, allowing individuals the opportunity to have a one-on-one meeting with someone with a similar lived experience who can see the individual for themself and not as a category or diagnosis. OTPs may find virtual communities such as Project LETS and Fireweed Collective helpful when working with people who may feel isolated and need someone who they can share their lived experiences with.

The use of virtual support may come in various forms of technology advancements, such as Wisdo, which is best understood as a social health platform. Wisdo is an app-based resource that allows the individual to create their profile and level of connection in the VMHC through the selection of community, peer support, and skill-building support groups. Practitioners may help individuals choose the supports they feel they want and need, navigate the use of these virtual communities, and support people as they consider how they want to create their profile for app resources such as Wisdo. Practitioners are also encouraged to become knowledgeable about virtual mental health resources offered by organizations such as the National Alliance of Mental Illness (NAMI) or the Anxiety and Depression Association of America (ADAA).

When an OTP considers social participation and engagement for an individual in the virtual setting, previously mentioned options may use AT whether through online education, social environments (SNS), virtual play, or even VMHC. These myriads of options are not all-inclusive, as technology advancements allow occupational therapy interventions to continuously evolve.

As occupational therapy continues to propel into technological advances, many disparities continue to exist that may prevent some individuals from being able to fully access all aspects of the virtual environment (funding, environment, etc.). OTPs should consider whether social determinants of health may impact a person's access to and participation in virtual environments and, when advocating for the most useful pieces of technology, help support their participation and promote a better quality of life.

Here's the Point

- Individuals across the life span are engaging in the use of technology to participate in their daily occupations; this includes participation within the virtual environment.
- The virtual environment and its associated technology fall under the umbrella of AT.
- OTPs need to be knowledgeable of apps that can help individuals participate in daily living.
- The virtual environment has become a space where individuals across the life span, and their caregivers, can find meaning and a sense of belonging that can foster a sense of well-being, recovery, safety, and support.
- Individuals are engaging in virtual learning activities either formally or informally at an increasing rate across the life span. OTPs can provide services to students in K–12 settings identified for special education, but can also recommend participation virtually for informal learning.
- Occupational therapy services can be delivered through telehealth via HIPAA-compliant platforms to people who may be homebound, reside in rural areas, or live outside the United States.
- OTPs can help individuals build skills such as job interviewing through the use of VR.
- Individuals engage in play/leisure through online gaming. OTPs can assist in leisure exploration through these platforms.
- OTPs can help individuals connect with virtual social networks to help join communities and receive support through a variety of outlets.

Apply It Now

1. Accessibility Features

On one of your devices (laptop, phone, or tablet), please locate the accessibility features. Select a few of these features to try out on your device. Which features did you like the most/least? Can you see yourself continuing to utilize these features as a part of your daily life? Why or why not? Imagine you are working with a person with an intellectual disability attending high school who is struggling with visual perceptual skills. What features would be useful to them to complete academic tasks?

2. Social Media Networking

Take a few minutes to evaluate your social media accounts (please don't get lost in the scroll!). Take some time to categorize the groups that you may be involved with on social media (AOTA, NBCOT, your school page, etc.). Why are you particularly interested in these groups? How have these groups helped to shape who you are today? How would you describe your typical social interaction patterns within these groups? Are there other categories that you want to add to your social media groups or are there groups that you no longer utilize and may want to consider deleting?

3. Virtual Participation

Consider the following scenarios. How would you respond to the individual's request?

- Janet, a 33-year-old female, has severe depression and lacks initiation. However, she is interested in art and wants to learn how to draw. She shares that she is afraid to attend an in-person art class. Identify specific virtual tools and processes that an OTP might suggest to Janet to pursue her leisure interest.
- Geo, a 19-year-old nonbinary college student, recently moved into an apartment and has no communication with their family because of differences in values. They were bullied in middle and high school and feel very isolated. How can an OTP help Geo find a supportive community? Identify aspects of the community that might be important to Geo.
- Peter, a 35-year-old military veteran, served two tours of duty overseas and was injured in combat. Since returning home and leaving the service, he has labored to adjust to civilian life. He struggles with PTSD and gets very anxious when he is out in the community, particularly when he anticipates crowded situations. He desperately wants to routinely complete his instrumental activities of daily living (IADL) activities, such as shopping, managing his finances, and monitoring his health care. Identify three to five specific strategies a practitioner could suggest to help Peter become successful with IADL activities.
- Susan, a 75-year-old grandma, loves her grandchildren; however, they recently moved across the country and she misses them. Susan has little experience with computers. How might a practitioner help Susan keep in contact with her children and grandchildren while she successfully ages in place? What features would be most important to Susan?

Resources

- Rehabilitation Engineering and Assistive Technology Society of North America (RESNA): https://www.resna.org. This site is dedicated to educating the public about AT, which includes the virtual environment (similar to AOTA, but for AT!).
- Thrive Center: https://www.thrivecenterky.org. This is an innovation hub where innovators can showcase products that may enhance the lives of the older adult through the use of technology.
- Project LETS: https://projectlets.org. This is a national grassroots organization and movement led by and for folks with lived experience of mental illness/madness, disability, trauma, and neurodivergence.
- Fireweed Collective: https://fireweedcollective.org. This site offers mental health education and mutual aid through a healing justice lens.
- AOTA Telehealth Resources: https://www.aota.org/practice/practice-essentials/telehealth-resources. This page offers information to occupational therapy students and practitioners interested in using telehealth as a part of their practice.

References

Abi-Jaoude, E., Naylor, K., & Pignatiello, A. (2020). Smartphones, social media use and youth mental health. *Canadian Medical Association Journal, 192*(6), E136–E141. https://doi.org/10.1503/cmaj.190434

American Academy of Pediatrics. (2018). *Children and media tips from the American Academy of Pediatrics.* https://www.aap.org/en/patient-care/media-and-children

American Occupational Therapy Association. (2018). Telehealth in occupational therapy. *American Journal of Occupational Therapy, 72*(Suppl. 2), 7212410059p1–7212410059p18. https://doi.org/10.5014/ajot.2018.72S219

American Occupational Therapy Association. (2020). Occupational therapy practice framework: Domain and process—Fourth edition. *American Journal of Occupational Therapy, 74*(Suppl. 2), 7412410010p1–7412410010p87. https://doi.org/10.5014/ajot.2020.74S2001

American Telemedicine Association. (2020). *Telehealth: Defining 21st-century care.* Telehealth Taxonomy. https://marketing.americantelemed.org/hubfs/Files/Resources/ATA_Telehealth_Taxonomy_9-11-20.pdf

Anderson, M., Vogels, E., Perrin, A., & Rainie, L. (2022, November 16). *Connection, creativity, and drama: Teen life on social media in 2022.* Pew Research Center. https://www.pewresearch.org/internet/2022/11/16/connection-creativity-and-drama-teen-life-on-social-media-in-2022

Arbesman, M., Bazyk, S., & Nochajski, S. M. (2013). Systematic review of occupational therapy and mental health promotion, prevention, and intervention for children and youth. *American Journal of Occupational Therapy, 67*, e120–e130. https://doi.org/10.5014/ajot.2013.008359

Assistive Technology Act of 1998, as amended. Pub. L. No. 108-364, § 3, 118 Stat. 1707 (2004). https://www.govinfo.gov/content/pkg/PLAW-108publ364/html/PLAW-108publ364.htm

Austin-McCain, M. (2017). An examination of the association of so-cial media use with the satisfaction with daily routines and healthy lifestyle habits for undergraduate and graduate students. *The Open Journal of Occupational Therapy, 5*(4), Article 6. https://doi .org/10.15453/2168-6408.1327

Baker, I. S., Turner, I. J., & Koteram, Y. (2023, May). Role-play games for mental health (why not?): Role for initiative. *International Journal of Mental Health and Addiction, 21,* 3901–3909. https:// doi.org/10.1007/s11469-022-00832-y

Banerjee, D., Vajawat, B., & Varshey, P. (2021). Digital gaming inter-ventions: A novel paradigm in mental health? Perspectives from India. *International Review of Psychiatry, 33,* 435–441. https://doi .org/10.1080/09540261.2020.1839392

Barry, C., Sidoti, C., Briggs, S., Reiter, S., & Lindsey, R. (2017). Adolescent social media use and mental health from adolescent and parent perspectives. *Journal of Adolescence, 61,* 1–11. https:// doi.org/10.1016/j.adolescence.2017.08.005

Bauer, J. C., & Ngonda, P. S. (2022). Moms, memes, and mitigating pandemic stress: Exploring themes and implications in an aca-demic mamas' Facebook group. *Women's Studies in Communica-tion, 45,* 45–69. https://doi.org/10.1080/07491409.2022.2030607

Bazyk, S. (2019). Occupational therapy's role in school mental health. In C. Brown, V. C. Stoffel, & J. P. Muñoz (Eds.), *Occupa-tional therapy in mental health: A vision for participation* (2nd ed., pp. 809–837). F.A. Davis.

Benda, N. C., Veinot, T. C., Sieck, C. J., & Ancker, J. S. (2020). Broad-band internet access is a social determinant of health! *American Journal of Public Health, 110,* 1123–1125. https://doi.org/10.2105 /AJPH.2020.305784

Boers, E., Afzali, M., Newton, N., & Conrod, P. (2019). Association of screen time and depression in adolescence. *JAMA Pediatrics, 173,* 853–859. https://doi.org/10.1001/jamapediatrics.2019.1759

Burke, S. L., Li, T., Grudzien, A., & Garcia, S. (2021). Brief report: Improving employment interview self-efficacy among adults with autism and other developmental disabilities using Vir-tual Interactive Training Agents (ViTA). *Journal of Autism and Developmental Disorders, 51,* 741–748. https://doi.org/10.1007 /s10803-020-04571-8

Chou, H. T., & Edge, N. (2012). "They are happier and having better lives than I am": The impact of using Facebook on perceptions of others' lives. *Cyberpsychology, Behavior & Social Networking, 15,* 117–121. https://doi.org/10.1089/cyber.2011.0324

Cimke, S., & Cerit, E. (2021). Social media addiction, cyberbully-ing and cyber victimization of university students. *Archives of Psychiatric Nursing, 35,* 499–503. https://doi.org/10.1016/j.apnu .2021.07.004

Cingel, D., Carter, M., & Krause, H. (2022). Social media and self-esteem. *Current Opinion in Psychology, 45,* 101304. https:// doi.org/10.1016/j.copsyc.2022.101304

Cohen, R., & Biddle, L. (2022). The influence of social media on suicidal behaviour among students. In S. Mallon & J. Smith (Eds.), *Preventing and responding to student suicide: A practical guide for FE and HE settings* (pp. 94–107). Jessica Kingsley Publishers.

Cook, A. M., Polgar, J. M., & Encarnação, P. (2020). *Assistive tech-nologies: Principles and practice* (5th ed.). Elsevier.

Cote, D., Ryan, M., Stevens, L., & Simmons, C. D. (2023, June). Integrating virtual reality gaming into OT interventions. *OT Practice, 28*(6), 22–26.

Family Educational Rights and Privacy Act. 20 U.S.C. § 1232g; 34 C.F.R. Part 99 (1974).

Fokides, E. (2017). Pre-service teachers' intention to use MUVEs as practitioners—A structural equation modeling approach. *Journal of Information Technology: Research, 16,* 47–68. https:// doi.org/10.28945/3645

Friedman, Z. L. (2022, July). The Breakfast Club: Enduring lessons for stronger school-based relationships. *OT Practice,* 12–16.

Garety, P., Edwards, C. J., Ward, T., Emsley, R., Huckvale, M., McCrone, P., Rus-Calafell, M., Fornells-Ambrojo, M., Gumley, A.,

Haddock, G., Bucci, S., McLeod, H., Hardy, A., Peters, E., Myin-Germeys, I., & Craig, T. (2021). Optimising AVATAR ther-apy for people who hear distressing voices: Study protocol for the AVATAR2 multi-centre randomised controlled trial. *Trials, 22*(3), 66. https://doi.org/10.1186/s13063-021-05301-w

George, M., Russell, M., Piontak, J., & Odgers, C. (2018). Concur-rent and subsequent associations between daily digital technol-ogy use and high-risk adolescents' mental health symptoms. *Child Development, 89,* 78–88. https://doi.org/10.1111/cdev.12819

Gu, C., Liu, S., & Chen, S. (2022). Fight or flight? Curvilinear rela-tions between previous cyberbullying victimization experiences and continuous use of social media: Social media rumination and distress as chain mediators. *Behavioral Sciences, 12,* 421. https:// doi.org/10.3390/bs12110421

Hamm, M., Newton, A., Chisholm, A., Shulhan, J., Milne, A., Sundar, P., Ennis, H., Scott, S., & Hartling, L. (2015). Prevalence and effect of cyberbullying on children and young people: A scoping review of social media studies. *JAMA Pediatrics, 169*(8), 770–777. https://doi.org/10.1001/jamapediatrics.2015.0944

Harrop, V. M. (2001). Virtual healthcare delivery: Defined, modeled, and predictive barriers to implementation identified. *Proceedings AMIA Symposium,* 244–248.

Health Insurance Portability and Accountability Act. Pub. L. No. 104-191, 110 Stat. 1936 (1996). https://www.govinfo.gov/content /pkg/PLAW-104publ191/pdf/PLAW-104publ191.pdf

HealthIT.gov. (2019). *Frequently asked questions: What is telehealth?* The Office of the National Coordinator for Health Information Technology. https://www.healthit.gov/faq/what-telehealth -how-telehealth-different-telemedicine

John, A., Glendenning, A., Marchant, A., Montgomery, P., Stewart, A., Wood, S., Lloyd, K., & Hawton, K. (2018). Self-harm, suicidal behaviours, and cyberbullying in children and young people: Systematic review. *Journal of Medical Internet Research, 20*(4), e129. https://doi.org/10.2196/jmir.9044

Jung, C., & Padman, R. (2014). Virtualized healthcare delivery: Understanding users and their usage patterns of online medi-cal consultations. *International Journal of Medical Informatics, 83*(12), 901–914. https://doi.org/10.1016/j.ijmedinf.2014.08.004

Kowalski, R., Giumetti, G., & Schroeder, A. (2014). Bullying in the digital age: A critical review and meta-analysis of cyberbully-ing research among youth. *Psychology Bulletin, 140,* 1073–1137. https://doi.org/10.1037/a0035618

Kraut, R., Patterson, M., Lundmark, V., Kiesler, S., Mukophadhyay, T., & Scherlis, W. (1998). Internet paradox: A social technology that reduces social involvement and psychological well-being? *American Psychologist, 53*(9), 1017–1031. https://doi.org/10.1037 /0003-066X.53.9.1017

Kreski, N., Platt, J., Rutherford, C., Olfson, M., Odgers, C., Schulenberg, J., & Keyes, K. (2021). Social media use and de-pressive symptoms among United States adolescents. *Journal of Adolescent Health, 68,* 572–579. https://doi.org/10.1016 /j.jadohealth.2020.07.006

Larson, L. (2021). Social media use in emerging adults: Investigating the relationship with social media addiction and social behavior. *Psi Chi Journal of Psychological Research, 26*(2), 228–237. https:// doi.org/10.24839/2325-7342.JN26.2.228

Law, M., Cooper, B., Strong S., Stewart, D., Rigby P., & Letts, L. (1996). The Person-Environment-Occupation model: A trans-active approach to occupational performance. *Canadian Jour-nal of Occupational Therapy, 63,* 9–23. https://doi.org/10.1177 /000841749606300103

Majerowicz, A., & Tracy, S. (2010). Telemedicine: Bridging gaps in healthcare delivery. *Journal of AHIMA, 81*(5), 52–58.

Mubarak, F., Suomi, R., & Kantola, S. P. (2020). Confirming the links between socio-economic variables and digitalization worldwide: The unsettled debate on digital divide. *Journal of Information, Communication and Ethics in Society, 18*(3), 415–430. https://doi .org/10.1108/JICES-02-2019-0021

Oakes, L. R. (2022). Virtual reality among individuals with intellectual and/or developmental disabilities: A systematic literature review. *Therapeutic Recreation Journal, 56*, 281–299. https://doi.org/10.18666/TRJ-2022-V56-I3-11184

Orben, A., & Przybylski, A. (2019). Screens, teens, and psychological well-being: Evidence from three time-use-diary studies. *Psychological Science, 30*, 682–696. https://doi.org/10.1177/0956797619830329

Panerai, S., Catania, V., Rundo, F., & Ferri, R. (2018). Remote home-based virtual training of functional skills for adolescents and young adults with intellectual disability: Feasibility and preliminary results. *Frontiers in Psychology, 9* (Article 1730), 1–6. https://doi.org/10.3389/fpsyg.2018.01730

Pantic, I. (2014). Online social networking and mental health. *Cyberpsychology, Behavior and Social Networking, 17*, 652–657. https://doi.org/10.1089/cyber.2014.0070

Pellegrino, A., Abe, M., & Shannon, R. (2022). The dark side of social media: Content effects on the relationship between materialism and consumption behaviors. *Frontiers in Psychology, 13*, 870614. https://doi.org/10.3389/fpsyg.2022.870614

Richmond, T., Peterson, C., Cason, J., Billings, M., Terrell, E. A., Lee, A. C. W., Towey, M., Parmanto, B., Saptono, A., Cohn, E. R., & Brennan, D. (2017). American Telemedicine Association's principles for delivering telerehabilitation services. *International Journal of Telerehabilitation, 9*(2), 63–68. https://doi.org/10.5195/ijt.2017.6232

Rortvedt, D., & Jacobs, K. (2019). Perspectives on the use of a telehealth service-delivery model as a component of school-based occupational therapy practice: Designing a user-experience. *Work, 62*, 125–131. https://doi.org/10.3233/WOR-182847

Schonfeld, A., McNiel, D., Toyoshima, T., & Binder, R. (2023). Cyberbullying and adolescent suicide. *The Journal of the American Academy of Psychiatry and the Law, 51*(1), 112–119. https://doi.org/10.29158/JAAPL.220078-22

Second Life. (2024). *Explore. Discover. Create.* (online video game). Retrieved May 14, 2024, from https://secondlife.com

Sedgwick, R., Epstein, S., Dutta, R., & Ougrin, D. (2019). Social media, internet use and suicide attempts in adolescents. *Current Opinion in Psychiatry, 32*(6), 534–541. https://doi.org/10.1097/YCO.0000000000000547

Smallfield, S., Haag, B., Poston, A., Giger, J. T., & Anderson, W. D. (2014). Promoting social participation: Teaching technology to older adults. *OT Practice, 19*(14), 13–16.

Smith, R. O. (2017). Technology and occupation: Past, present, and the next 100 years of theory and practice (Eleanor Clarke Slagle Lecture). *American Journal of Occupational Therapy, 71*, 7106150010p1–7106150010p15. https://doi.org/10.5014/ajot.2017.716003

Stiglic, N., & Viner, R. (2019). Effects of screen time on the health and well-being of children and adolescents: A systematic review of reviews. *BMJ Open, 9*(1), e023191. https://doi.org/10.1136/bmjopen-2018-023191

Suler, J. (2004). The online disinhibition effect. *Cyberpsychology & Behavior, 7*(3), 321–326. https://doi.org/10.1089/1094931041291295

Tai, T.-Y., & Chen, H. H.-J. (2021). The impact of immersive virtual reality on EFL learners' listening comprehension. *Journal of Educational Computing Research, 59*(7), 1272–1293. https://doi.org/10.1177/0735633121994291

United Nations. (2006). Convention on the Rights of Persons with Disabilities. *Treaty Series, 2515,* 3.

van Rijn, B., Cooper. M., Jackson, A., & Wild, C. (2015). Avatar-based therapy within prison settings: Pilot evaluation. *British Journal of Guidance & Counselling, 45*(3), 268–283. https://doi.org/10.1080/03069885.2015.1068273

Vassilakopoulou, P., & Hustad, E. (2023). Bridging digital divides: a literature review and research agenda for information systems research. *Information Systems Frontiers, 25*, 955–969. https://doi.org/10.1007/s10796-020-10096-3

World Federation of Occupational Therapists. (2016). *Code of ethics.* http://wfot.org/resources/code-of-ethics

World Federation of Occupational Therapists. (2021). *Occupational therapy and telehealth.* https://wfot.org/resources/occupational-therapy-and-telehealth

World Health Organization. (2001). *International classification of functioning, disability, and health.* Author.

World Health Organization. (2022). *WHO-ITU global standard for accessibility of telehealth services.* World Health Organization and International Telecommunication Union. https://www.who.int/publications/i/item/9789240050464

Yeh, H.-C., Tseng, S.-S., & Heng, L. (2022). Enhancing EFL students' intracultural learning through virtual reality. *Interactive Learning Environments, 30*(9), 1609–1618. https://doi.org/10.1080/10494820.2020.1734625

Yoon, H., Jang, Y., Vaughan, P. W., & Garcia, M. (2020). Older adults' internet use for health information: Digital divide by race/ethnicity and socioeconomic status. *Journal of Applied Gerontology, 39*, 105–110. https://doi.org/10.1177/0733464818770772

Zhang, R., Bi, N. C., & Mercado, T. (2023). Do Zoom meetings really help? A comparative analysis of synchronous and asynchronous online learning during COVID-19 pandemic. *Journal of Computer Assisted Learning, 39*, 210–217. https://doi.org/10.1111/jcal.12740

Zylstra, S. E. (2013). Evidence for use of telehealth in pediatric occupational therapy. *Journal of Occupational Therapy, Schools & Early Intervention, 6*, 326–355. https://doi.org/10.1080/19411243.2013.860765

Deborah Pitts and Brent Braveman

ontemporary perspectives on health care emphasize the integration of behavioral health and primary care services, with the goals of improving health outcomes and reducing health-care costs. Although the concept of integration is not new, the enactment of the Patient Protection and Affordable Care Act (ACA) of 2010, with its emphasis on prevention, wellness, and primary care, has significantly shifted the landscape for such efforts in the United States. In addition, concern over the segregation of health services into "silos" of physical health and behavioral health have long been identified as contributing to poorer health and mental health outcomes (Kathol et al., 2015).

New emphasis on integrated care for service settings in the United States, including Federally Qualified Health Centers (FQHCs), Certified Community Behavioral Health Clinics (CCBHCs), and **patient-centered medical homes (PCMHs),** has provided the opportunity for occupational therapy practitioners (OTPs) to play a more central role as part of an interprofessional behavioral health and primary care team and for providing intervention within these settings and in the evolving health-care system.

This chapter provides an overview of the integration of behavioral health and primary care, describes key policies, presents approaches to the design and delivery of integrated behavioral health services, and describes ways in which OTPs can engage in this emerging practice context.

Understanding Integration

A helpful way of understanding integration in the mental health practice context is to consider two ways in which integration has evolved in the mental health service system: first, the integration of mental health and substance abuse services into what has become known as "behavioral health,"

and second, the integration of primary care and behavioral health services. Although the focus of this chapter is on the latter, understanding integration in both ways is useful for all OTPs.

Integration of Mental Health and Substance Abuse Services into Behavioral Health

Historically, mental health and substance use recovery services were seen as distinct and separate. This separation occurred at all levels—the level of the individual provider, the program, the organization, and the regulatory and policy levels. This has been the case for both private and publicly funded substance use and mental health recovery services. Early efforts at integration occurred because of the understanding that persons with serious mental illness (SMI) were also increasingly presenting with substance-related disorders (Drake et al., 2004). An example of these efforts includes development and dissemination of the Substance Abuse and Mental Health Services Administration's (SAMHSA) Evidence-Based Toolkit on Integrated Treatment for Co-Occurring Disorders (SAMHSA, 2010). Updates on co-occurring disorders can be found on the SAMHSA website (https://www.samhsa.gov/co-occurring-disorders).

Despite the development of evidence-based practice approaches, barriers to addressing co-occurring disorders continued, including differing perspectives on how to treat, billing restrictions, and the challenges of communicating between the two types of providers (Padwa et al., 2014). Over the last decade, efforts at integration have resulted in the consolidation of state and local government departments of mental health and substance abuse services into "behavioral health" departments. These new initiatives brought mental health and substance use recovery providers together in new ways and challenged the traditional views about substance use and mental health disorders. Researchers, policymakers, and advocates in the United States acknowledge that "even with great advances in behavioral health policy in the last decade, the problems of mental illness and addiction persist in the United States—so more needs to be done" (Alegria et al., 2021, p. 226).

Integration of Primary Care and Behavioral Health

The integration of behavioral health and primary care services means that both settings consider all health conditions at the same time (National Council for Mental Wellbeing, 2023; SAMHSA, 2012). The actual services provided can occur in various models and settings, such as community mental health centers, primary care clinics, FQHCs, and CCBHCs (both described later in this chapter). **Integrated behavioral health care (IBHC)** therefore is the consideration of mental health and substance use conditions, along with any other health conditions within the same episode of care, as well as across the person's life span (Commonwealth Fund, 2022).

The Agency for Healthcare Research and Quality (AHRQ, 2015), in defining integrated behavioral health care, notes that "care may address mental health and substance abuse conditions, health behaviors (including their contribution to chronic medical illnesses), life stressors and crises, stress-related physical symptoms, and ineffective patterns of health care utilization." A key element of this integration is that it is *bidirectional* (Mauer & Jarvis, 2010). This means that behavioral health moves into the primary care setting, *and* primary care moves into the behavioral health setting. Without

bidirectionality, integration is incomplete and health risks ensue (Gerrity et al., 2014).

The move toward integration of behavioral health and primary care has been influenced by various factors, including the well-acknowledged perspective that there is "no health without mental health" (Prince et al., 2007, p. 859), promoted by the World Health Organization (WHO). Research findings show the profound difference in mortality rates for persons with mental illness (Manderscheid et al., 2008; Walker et al., 2015). For decades, WHO's constitution has stated that "health is state of complete physical, mental and social well-being and not merely the absence of disease or infirmity" (WHO, 1948, p. 1).

The WHO *World Mental Health Report: Transforming Mental Health for All* (2022) recommits to the view that "mental health is an integral part of our general health and well-being and a basic human right" (p. xiv). Further, noting the importance of integrated behavioral health, the American Medical Association and leading medical associations established the Behavioral Health Integration (BHI) Collaborative in 2020 to serve as a resource for physician practices to move toward full integration. Box 34-1 shares an example of how the integration of primary and behavioral health care can support a person's recovery.

Impact of Behavioral Health on Overall Health

To examine the impact of behavioral health on overall health, this section addresses disease burden, prevalence data, and mortality and health disparities for individuals with serious psychiatric disabilities.

BOX 34-1 ■ My Health—Making Sense of Integrated Care

This feature shares John's lived experience of receiving IBHC. John works part time for a local mental health center as a peer provider. He was diagnosed with schizophrenia his first year of college. He left college then and for several years his symptoms made it difficult for him to function. He's been hospitalized over 25 times, most recently 4 years ago. It was a brief hospitalization, and he was discharged quickly.

John, now 45, hopes to become a certified peer support specialist and is taking classes to earn a human services worker certificate at a community college. He's much older than most of the other students. He was assisted to reenter college about 2 years ago and is now finishing up his last semester and an internship. After he earns his certificate, he hopes to move into a full-time position with the mental health agency he works for now.

John spent several years being treated by this same mental health agency's Assertive Community Treatment (ACT) team. The ACT team encourages each person's recovery and full participation in daily life by focusing on the whole person. Just as he entered school 2 years ago, he and his team decided to help him transition to a lower level of support. Where before he was receiving multiple visits per week from the ACT team for support, now he would be seen once or twice per month. At first, John was worried about transitioning to less intense support services, but once he made the move, he found it worked out. He likes being less reliant on the ACT team and has more confidence about being able to take care of himself.

John has been taking olanzapine (Zyprexa) for several years. However, he and his psychiatrist discussed changing his medications out of concern he may develop diabetes. John had gained weight after starting this medication, but the symptom relief was substantial, and he didn't want to risk going backward with his psychiatric symptoms. John feels medications made the difference in his being able to go to school. He has not developed diabetes, but it is something that he, his primary care physician, and his psychiatrist monitor.

John is committed to finishing his certificate program, managing his medications to control his symptoms, and monitoring his health in general and the onset of symptoms of diabetes specifically. He is concerned about arranging stable health care that addresses all his needs and integrates care for his mental and physical health at one setting. As he makes progress toward completion of a certificate program and the potential of working full time, he wonders what type of resources are available in his community to meet his primary care needs over the long term.

Reflective Questions

1. ACT teams practice from a transdisciplinary perspective. How might this approach support integrated care?

2. Psychiatric medication can contribute to what is referred to as the metabolic syndrome. Where might John learn more about this interaction?

Disease Burden and Prevalence

The impact of a health problem can be discussed in terms of disease burden, in which the impact is measured by factors such as cost, mortality and morbidity, years lost because of disease (YLDs), quality of adjusted life years (QALYs), and disability-adjusted life years. "Mental and substance disorders were one of the leading causes of disease burden in 2010. They were responsible for 7.4% of global disability adjusted life years (DALYs) and 22.9% of global years living with a disability (YLDs), making them the fifth leading cause of DALYs and the leading cause of YLDs" (Whiteford et al., 2015, p. 3). It was estimated that mental disorders in 2019 resulted in 418 million DALYs, or 16% of global DALYs (Arias et al., 2022). Insel, Collins, and Hyman (2015) calculated that the global impact of spending on mental health care and lost productivity was $2.5 trillion a year and would rise to $6 trillion by 2030. Comparatively, this is "more than heart disease and more than cancer, diabetes, and respiratory diseases combined" (Insel et al., 2015, p. 128).

The prevalence of mental health issues and their impact on primary care needs is significant. In 2014, the Centers for Disease Control and Prevention's National Ambulatory Medical Care Survey reported the following for primary care office visits:

- Mental disorders accounted for just over 7% of the primary diagnoses made.
- Depression was present in 10.3% of patients making office visits, and alcohol misuse, abuse, or dependence and substance abuse or dependence was noted at almost 4% of visits. Depression screening was ordered at just over 4% of visits.
- Psychotherapy, mental health counseling, stress management, and substance abuse or alcohol abuse counseling were ordered at almost 5% of office visits.
- Antidepressants were the third most frequently mentioned drugs at office visits.

The same survey reported that in 2020 there were over 2.4 million visits to emergency departments (EDs) that were attributed to psychological and mental disorders (National Center for Health Statistics, 2021). Influences on mental health issues and primary care needs are constantly evolving. For example, according to the American Psychological Association (2020), "Despite several months of acclimating to a new reality and societal upheaval spurred by the COVID-19 pandemic, Americans are struggling to cope with the disruptions it has caused. Nearly 8 in 10 adults (78%) say the coronavirus pandemic is a significant source of stress in their life. And, 2 in 3 adults (67%) say they have experienced increased stress over the course of the pandemic."

Mortality and Health Disparities for Persons With Serious Mental Illness

In the United States, evidence that persons with serious psychiatric disabilities were dying 25 years earlier than other Americans, largely because of treatable medical conditions (Firth et al., 2019; Manderscheid et al., 2008; WHO & UNICEF, 2018), significantly influenced the push to incorporate wellness-oriented services within the public mental health system. Physical health in people with mental illness leads to significantly poorer overall health outcomes. People with mental illness have an increased risk of physical disease as well as reduced access to adequate health care. Therefore, physical health disparities are observed across the entire spectrum of mental illnesses in low-income, middle-income, and high-income countries. The high rate of physical comorbidity, which often has poor clinical management, drastically reduces life expectancy for people with mental illness, and also increases the personal, social, and economic burden of mental illness across the life span (Firth et al., 2019).

Specific vulnerability factors for this population that contribute to poorer health outcomes include "much higher rates of cardiovascular disease, diabetes, respiratory disease, and infectious disease (such as HIV/AIDS) than the general population" (Firth et al., 2019, p. 675). More specifically:

- Higher rates of modifiable risk factors, including smoking, alcohol consumption, poor nutrition/obesity, lack of exercise, unsafe sexual behavior, intravenous drug use, and residence in group care facilities and homeless shelters
- Poverty, homelessness, unemployment, victimization, trauma, and incarceration
- Social isolation/stigma and discrimination
- Side effects from psychiatric medications, including weight gain, diabetes, high cholesterol and abnormal triglyceride levels, insulin resistance, and metabolic syndrome
- Impact of mental illness–related symptoms that can mask the symptoms of medical/somatic illnesses
- Lack of coordination between mental health systems and primary care
- Polypharmacy—use of multiple medications with harmful drug interactions (Center for Mental Health Services [CMHS], 2007, pp. 1–2).

Concerns regarding the impact of psychiatric status on overall health have been identified over the decades, and concerted efforts have been made to identify and intervene against the health risk factors for persons with mental illness in the last 20 years (Bagalman et al., 2022; Firth et al., 2019; U.S. Department of Health and Human Services [DHHS], 1999, 2003, 2005; WHO & UNICEF, 2018). For example, SAMHSA's Wellness Initiative is used to raise awareness of health disparities and increased mortality rate for people with SMI and/or substance-related disorders, which includes the National Wellness Week hosted each fall in the United States (SAMHSA, 2016). Occupational therapist Margaret (Peggy) Swarbrick's Eight Dimensions of Wellness has come to serve as a guide for wellness initiatives within the U.S. public mental health system.

A key element of the efforts to improve the overall health status of persons with mental illness has been to leverage the recent growth in the commitment to the integration of behavioral health and primary care services (WHO, 2021, 2022). This has included the development and evaluation of evidence-based interventions that target key health risks for persons with SMI, in particular the obesity that is often secondary to psychiatric medications and sedentary lifestyles, and smoking cessation (Bartels & Desilets, 2012). For example, the Nutrition and Exercise for Wellness and Recovery (NEW-R) is an intervention developed because of collaboration between an occupational therapy researcher Catana Brown and her colleagues Jeannine Goetz, a registered dietitian, and Cherie Bledsoe, a consumer advisor (Brown et al., 2006, 2011a, 2011b, 2015).

A recent randomized controlled trial demonstrated the effectiveness of the NEW-R in a community mental health population (Brown et al., 2023). This intervention manual and other resources are currently available from the University of Illinois Center on Psychiatric Disability and Co-Occurring Medical Conditions, Center on Integrated Health Care & Self-Directed Recovery (https://www.center4healthandsdc .org/new-r.html).

Challenges of Nonintegrated Care

Nonintegrated care results in several significant disadvantages, including poorer health outcomes and increased health-care costs, especially for individuals with high levels of need (Cheung et al., 2019; Hoff et al., 2020; Reiss-Brennan et al., 2010). SAMHSA (2022) reported that in 2021, 15.5 million adults age 18 or older perceived an unmet need for mental health care at some point in that year. Among adults who reported a need for mental health care, 7.1 million adults did not receive any mental health services in the past year. Individuals whose health-care services are not integrated specifically suffer with regard to treatment of depression (Butler et al., 2011; Gilbody et al., 2006).

Major depression among patients with chronic medical illnesses increases the burden of physical symptoms and can result in functional impairment, poorer outcomes, and increased medical costs (Ramanuj et al., 2019). Depression also impairs self-care, decreases adherence to treatments for chronic medical illnesses, and causes increased mortality (Unutzer et al., 2009; Zikos & Afolayan-Oloye, 2021). The relationship between improved treatment adherence and lowered costs is well documented (Cutler et al., 2018; Sokol et al., 2005).

IBHC can be more expensive than usual care in the short term, but it yields better outcomes and may offset costs in the long run (Gilbody et al., 2006; Levin & Chisholm, 2016; Ross et al., 2019). Estimates of cost savings vary, but literature on the cost offset of integrating behavioral health services suggests that savings may be as much as 20% to 40% for well-designed programs. Melek (2012) stated in a report prepared for Milliman (a large actuarial firm) that, "The evidence for medical cost offsets that can be achieved through effective management of behavioral conditions remains elusive and in need of additional study. It should be noted, however, that in the case when total healthcare costs were compared, up to a 50% decrease in healthcare costs was observed" (p. 9).

Fewer than 50% of all those referred for mental or behavioral health (MH/BH) treatment by a primary care provider (PCP) in nonintegrated systems ever follow through with the referral or initiate MH/BH treatment (Auxier et al., 2012; Kessler, 2012; Wittchen et al., 2022). Reasons for this include the self-stigma against MH/BH services; the "trust gap" where individuals are often more willing to disclose BH concerns to those they trust, especially for people with trauma histories; experience of long wait lists for specialty services such as MH/BH care; and the financial burdens of copays/coinsurance. Social determinants of health challenges (e.g., lost work time, transportation to/from new medical provider, arrangement of child care, and so on) and/or additional burden on the person (related to calling and scheduling appointments, figuring out how to attend appointments, etc.) places additional motivation, volition, and executive functioning/cognitive demands on people who may already be struggling.

Public Policy Supports for Integrated Behavioral Health and Primary Care

IBHC has been supported through significant public policy initiatives over the last few decades. A brief summary of U.S.-based initiatives is provided in the next section of this chapter.

Mental Health Parity and Addiction Equity Act

During the past several decades, U.S. legislation has addressed expansion of insurance coverage for behavioral health. In 1996, Congress passed the Mental Health Parity Act. The law prohibited large, employer-sponsored group health plans (i.e., those with more than 50 employees) from setting lower annual lifetime dollar limits on mental health benefits than those applied to medical benefits (Goodell, 2014). In 2008, Congress passed the Mental Health Parity and Addiction Equity Act (MHPAEA), which "prevents group health plans and health insurance issuers that provide mental health or substance use disorder (MH/SUD) benefits from imposing less favorable benefit limitations on those benefits than on medical/surgical benefits" (Centers for Medicare & Medicaid Services, 2023, Introduction, para. 1).

The MHPAEA also applied to large group health plans and health insurance issuers that chose to include MH/SUD benefits in their benefit packages; it did not mandate MH/SUD coverage. Approximately one-third of individuals who were covered in the individual market had no coverage for substance use disorder services, and nearly 20% had no coverage for mental health services, including outpatient therapy visits and inpatient crisis intervention and stabilization (Office of the Assistant Secretary for Planning and Evaluation, 2011). In 2014, the ACA extended the directives of the MHPAEA and required insurance coverage of MH/SUD services as 1 of 10 essential health benefits (EHB) categories.

Evidence of low parity compliance has been a concern of mental health and substance use services advocates for years and was demonstrated in a 2022 report from the U.S. Department of Labor, Department of the Treasury, and the DHHS. Therefore, enforcement enhancements have been recommended (Pestaina, 2022). Further efforts to improve the MHPAEA include simplifying the standards, taking a closer look at medical management criteria, assessing how parity can address network adequacy challenges, and evaluating enforcement tools. See Chapter 26: The Public Policy Environment.

Affordable Care Act: Impact on Primary Care in the United States

The passage of the ACA in 2010 emphasized the role of primary care in the U.S. health-care system and, more importantly, required mental health and substance use services to be a covered benefit in all health plans. Under the ACA, all new small group and individual market plans are required to cover the EHB categories, including MH/SUD services, and are required to cover them at parity with medical and surgical benefits. The ACA essentially expanded insurance coverage, including coverage of MH/SUD to millions of previously uninsured Americans through access to private health insurance in the individual and small group markets, the health insurance marketplaces (i.e., state or federally facilitated health insurance exchanges), and Medicaid (Congressional Budget Office, 2013). The ACA defined primary care as:

> Health services that cover a range of prevention, wellness, and treatment for common illnesses. Primary care providers include doctors, nurses, nurse practitioners, and physician assistants. They often maintain long-term relationships with you and advise and treat you on a range of health-related issues. They may also coordinate your care with specialists. (Healthcare.gov, 2014, para. 1)

Patient-Centered Medical Home

The ACA not only increased health insurance coverage and delineated essential primary health-care benefits, but it also defined primary care models and intervention settings. For example, a key component of the ACA is the PCMH, a primary care model based on patient-centered, coordinated, team-driven care and supported by strong health information technology (American Occupational Therapy Association [AOTA], 2012).

The PCMH is accountable for meeting the large majority of each patient's physical and mental health-care needs, and coordinates care across all elements of the broader health-care system. The medical home model promotes an interdisciplinary team-based approach to care of a patient through a spectrum of disease states, including behavioral health challenges, and across the various stages of life. The AHRQ emphasizes the PCMH's specific functions and attributes—comprehensive care; patient-centered, coordinated care; accessible services (i.e., shorter wait times when urgent care needed); and quality and safety. More information regarding PCMHs is available from the ARHQ website: https://www.ahrq.gov/ncepcr/research/care-coordination/pcmh/index.html.

Federally Qualified Health Centers

FQHCs, often referred to as "safety net" clinics for underserved populations, focus on integrating care across the full range of services, not just medical but oral health, vision, behavioral health, and pharmacy. They are locally based nonprofit organizations governed by a board of directors. FQHCs include all organizations receiving grants under Section 330 of the U.S. Public Health Service Act (PHSA). FQHCs qualify for enhanced reimbursement from Medicare and Medicaid, as well as other benefits. They must serve an underserved area or population, offer a sliding fee scale, provide comprehensive services, have an ongoing quality assurance program, and have a governing board of directors (Health Resources and Services Administration [HRSA], 2016). FQHCs may be community health centers, migrant health centers, health care for homeless centers and/or health centers for residents of public housing.

New funding provided through the ACA expanded services offered through health centers, with funds targeted specifically to (a) support ongoing health center operations; (b) create new health center sites in medically underserved areas; and (c) expand preventive and primary health-care services, including oral health, behavioral health, pharmacy, and/or enabling services at existing health center sites. In particular, health centers emphasize coordinated primary and preventive services or a "medical home" that promotes reductions in health disparities for low-income individuals, racial and ethnic minorities, rural communities, and other underserved populations.

Health centers place emphasis on the coordination and comprehensiveness of care, the ability to manage individuals with multiple health-care needs, and the use of key quality improvement practices, including health information technology (HRSA, 2014, p. 2). In 2014, funding was targeted to establish or expand behavioral health services, including adding new personnel, developing mental health and substance use disorder service, and expanding integrated models of primary care.

Occupational therapy has had a limited presence in FQHCs to date; however, there is an opportunity for expanded involvement. AOTA has strongly promoted occupational therapy's inclusion in primary care and integrated behavioral health settings including FQHCs. "Occupational therapy practitioners make a distinct contribution in primary care by recognizing and addressing the impact of roles, habits and routines on management of chronic illness and development of health lifestyles" (AOTA, 2020b, p. 3). Because FQHCs focus on comprehensive, whole person services, OTPs are seen as a natural fit. People served by FQHCs face multiple barriers to accessing appropriate health services. According to AOTA (2020b), "integration of occupational therapy into FQHC primary care settings reduces these barriers and can increase access to occupational therapy services through integrated and co-located care for individuals who might not otherwise have the ability to receive occupational therapy interventions" (p. 7).

Certified Community Behavioral Health Clinics

CCBHCs were authorized in 2014 under the Protecting Access to Medicare Act (PAMA) and were designed to address challenges experienced by community mental health centers. This included "pressure to provide an increasingly broad array of mental health, substance use, and primary care services for individuals with comorbid conditions" and their reliance on "a patchwork of federal and state funds and philanthropy to supplement the cost of care for Medicaid beneficiaries and the uninsured" (Brown et al., 2021).

The CCBHC model is designed to ensure access to coordinated comprehensive behavioral health care. CCBHCs are required to serve anyone who requests care for mental health or substance use, regardless of their ability to pay, place of residence, or age—including developmentally appropriate care for children and youth. CCBHCs must meet standards for the range of services they provide and they are required to get people into care quickly. An important feature of the

CCBHC model is that it requires crisis services that are available 24 hours a day, 7 days a week.

CCBHCs are required to provide a comprehensive array of behavioral health services so that people who need care are not caught trying to piece together the behavioral health support they need across multiple providers. In addition, CCBHCs must provide care coordination to help people navigate behavioral health care, physical health care, social services, and the other systems in which they are involved. CCBHCs are required to provide nine core services, which they can provide directly or via formal relationships with designated collaborating organizations (DCOs):

1. Crisis Services
2. Treatment Planning
3. Screening, Assessment, Diagnosis, and Risk Assessment
4. Outpatient Mental Health and Substance Use Services
5. Targeted Case Management
6. Outpatient Primary Care Screening and Monitoring
7. Community-Based Mental Health Care for Veterans
8. Peer, Family Support, and Counselor Services
9. Psychiatric Rehabilitation Services

OTPs are included in the staffing suggestions for CCBHCs. According to AOTA as of 2021, OTPs are working in several CCBHCs. For example, Monarch (https://monarchnc.org) is a North Carolina statewide provider of services for persons with mental illness or substance use disorders. Its CEO is an OTP. Monarch began its efforts to integrate occupational therapy to specifically support mental health and substance use disorder treatment into its CCBHC in 2020. For more information about CCBHCs, check with the National Council for Mental Wellbeing's CCBHC Success Center at https://www.thenationalcouncil.org/program/ccbhc-success-center.

Frameworks for Integrating Behavioral Health and Primary Care

Over the past two decades, frameworks have been developed to define *levels* or *models* of integration. Each of these frameworks offer different ways to understand how integration can occur, including identifying which providers are involved and which individuals might be best served by which level or component of a given model. These models have emphasized a distinction between collaborative and integrated care. In **collaborative care**, a person will "perceive they are getting a separate service from a specialist [i.e., behavioral health specialist], albeit one who collaborates closely with their physician," as opposed to **integrated care** where the person will "perceive [behavioral health] to be a routine part of their health care" (Collins et al., 2010, p. 6).

SAMHSA-HRSA's Center for Integrated Health Solutions standard framework for *levels of integration* (Table 34-1)

TABLE 34-1 | SAMHSA's Six Levels of Collaboration/Integration

Coordinated Key Element: Communication		Colocated Key Element: Physical Proximity		Integrated Key Element: Practice Change	
Level 1 *Minimal Collaboration*	*Level 2* *Basic Collaboration at a Distance*	*Level 3* *Basic Collaboration Onsite*	*Level 4* *Close Collaboration Onsite With Some System Integration*	*Level 5* *Close Collaboration Approaching an Integrated Practice*	*Level 6* *Full Collaboration in a Transformed Merged Integrated Practice*
Separate facilities and separate systems Rare communication about cases Communication typically based on a particular provider's need for specific information about a mutual patient	Separate facilities and separate systems Providers view each other as resources Periodic communication about shared patients Specific issues typically drive these communications Behavioral health typically viewed as specialty care	Colocation in same facility May or may not share the same practice space Separate systems, but communication becomes more regular Occasional meeting to discuss shared patients Referral process between practice areas Team and how it operates are not clearly defined Most decisions about patient care to be done independently by individual providers	Colocation in the same practice space Closer collaboration among providers Beginning of integration in care through some shared systems May share some medical records Consultation on complex patients with multiple health-care issues Personal communication among providers Providers have a better basic understanding of each other's roles	High levels of collaboration and integration between providers Function as a true team Frequent personal communication Actively seek system solutions to barriers to care integration for a broader range of patients Some issues, such as the availability of an integrated medical record, may not be readily resolved Understanding of the different roles team members need to play Some change in practice and structure to better achieve goals	Highest level of integration, involving the greatest amount of change Single transformed or merged practice Providers and patients view the operation as a single health system treating the whole person Principle of treating the whole person is applied to all patients, not just targeted groups

From Heath, B., Wise Romero, P., & Reynolds, K. (2013, March). A review and proposed standard framework for levels of integrated healthcare. SAMHSA-HRSA Center for Integrated Health Solutions.

TABLE 34-2 | **Four Quadrant Clinical Integration Model**

	Quadrant II	Quadrant IV
HIGH ← BEHAVIORAL HEALTH RISK/COMPLEXITY → **LOW**	Individuals with high behavioral health and low physical health needs Served in primary care and specialty mental health settings (Example: Individuals with bipolar disorder and chronic pain) Note: When mental health needs are stable, often mental health care can be transitioned back to primary care.	Individuals with high behavioral health and high physical health needs Served in primary care and specialty mental health settings (Example: Individuals with schizophrenia and metabolic syndrome or hepatitis C)
	Quadrant I	**Quadrant III**
	Individuals with low behavioral health and low physical health needs Served in primary care setting (Example: Individuals with moderate alcohol abuse and fibromyalgia)	Individuals with low behavioral health and high physical health needs Served in primary care setting (Example: Individuals with moderate depression and uncontrolled diabetes)

LOW ◄——— PHYSICAL HEALTH RISK/COMPLEXITY ———► HIGH

From Collins, C., Hewson, D. L., Munger, R., & Wade, T. (2010). Evolving models for behavioral health integration in primary care (p. 8). Milbank Memorial Fund.

has been a useful way to understand how well integration between primary care and behavioral health services has been achieved in a particular practice context (Heath et al., 2013).

Another framework for understanding IBHC is the Four Quadrant Clinical Integration Model (Table 34-2). This framework was developed by the U.S.-based National Council for Mental Wellbeing (formerly National Council for Community Behavioral Health). The Four Quadrant Clinical Integration Model describes potential scenarios for ways to meet the person's medical and psychiatric needs and has been a useful approach to understanding the person's needs in IBHC (Collins et al., 2010). In this framework, the risk and complexity of an individual's behavioral health *and* physical health needs inform the development and planning of health-care services. Quadrant I patients have low behavioral and physical health risks and needs, and Quadrant IV patients have the most complex risks and needs. The story in Box 34-2 introduces Grace, a woman with a complex set of behavioral and physical health needs.

Although these frameworks serve as useful guides for integrating care, challenges exist for successful implementation of integrated behavioral health and primary care. For the U.S. health-care system, these challenges were identified over approximately two decades ago by the Bazelon Center for Mental Health Law and remain problematic:

- Patterns of financing, lack of time to collaborate, and lack of reimbursement for collaborative work even if time is found
- Cultural barriers between primary care and mental health delivery systems and practitioners
- Lack of practitioner training in the other areas of health care
- Information-sharing issues, including system differences and confidentiality practices

BOX 34-2 ■ Street Medicine for Grace

Grace has been living on the street for the last year. A homeless outreach service practicing integrated care—sometimes referred to as "street medicine"—has been visiting her regularly for the last 2 years or so. The outreach team has included a nurse practitioner, social worker, psychiatrist, and an OTP. On occasion, she has been willing to take psychiatric medications, but not on a regular basis. She is suspicious of medication because for several years before she became homeless, she had been taking psychiatric medications and experienced severe akathisia. She also refuses offers of housing, although the team has registered her with a housing registry hosted by the local housing authority and health department.

Grace refuses to eat anything but food scraps that she gets from a dumpster outside a McDonald's near where she spends much of her time. The homeless outreach team has brought her fresh fruit and other healthier foods, but she just throws it away when they leave. The last time that Grace was visited by the team, she was found wandering and appeared very delirious. She allowed them to transport her to the nearest ED and it was found that her blood sugar was very high. The medical team also did a full physical and found that Grace also appears to be hypertensive, and when they removed her shoe they found that she had a wound that wasn't healing.

Reflective Question

1. Apply the Four Quadrant Clinical Integration Model using the details of Grace's behavioral and physical health risks and needs. Which quadrant would you place Grace in? Explain.

- Access problems to either mental health or primary care, which discourage or block referral and collaboration
- Consumer issues and concerns (Grazier et al., 2016; Koyangi, 2004, p. 10)

Since the publication of this report, there have been efforts to address these barriers, in particular reimbursement (Kathol et al., 2014), information technology, and workforce development (Hoge et al., 2014). As described earlier, the ACA addressed some of these barriers as well, such as improving access through full implementation of mental health parity. However, there remains significant room for improvement as barriers in the workforce, training, and technology remain (Commonwealth Fund, 2022).

Health Navigators: A Role for the Mental Health Peer Support Specialist

As efforts to promote integration have evolved, particularly in underserved populations with significant health disparities, the use of **health navigators** has become more common (Lemak et al., 2004; Wells et al., 2018). Lemak and colleagues (2004) described health navigators as functioning as community health workers (CHWs). The American Public Health Association defines a CHW as, "a frontline public health worker who is a trusted member of and/or has an unusually close understanding of the community served. This trusting relationship enables the worker to serve as a liaison/link/intermediary between health/social services and the community to facilitate access to services and improve the quality and cultural competence of service delivery" (American Public Health Association, 2017).

The training of health professionals such as OTPs focuses on advanced clinical knowledge and skills, whereas the CHW is expected to exhibit a variety of nonclinical skills, in particular, the ability to develop trust and rapport (American Public Health Association, 2014; Wells et al., 2018). A systematic review demonstrated that CHWs practicing as health-care navigators in primary care improved chronic disease management outcomes (Mistry et al., 2021).

Overall, the training and credentialing of CHWs are very uneven in the United States. Currently, 13 states operate certification programs (AZ, CT, IN, KY, MA, MD, NJ, NM, NV, MY, OH, OR, and TX), four states' programs are privately run by independent credentialing boards (FL, MO, PA, VA), and four states (AR, KS, MI, SC) run their program through CHW association or CHW association-led committee (Association of State and Territorial Health Officials [ASTHO], 2022). Although the Bureau of Labor Statistics estimates that there are over 58,000 CHWs nationwide, there is no national consensus on appropriate competencies, training, and certification (Coffinbargar et al., 2022). The CHW Core Consensus Project "primary aims are to expand cohesion in the field and to contribute to the visibility and greater understanding of the full potential of CHWs to improve health, community development, and access to systems of care" (Rosenthal et al., 2022, p. 13).

Brekke and colleagues (2013; Kelly et al., 2014) drew on the CHW approach and the well-implemented peer support specialist role in community mental health programs to carve out a role for these providers as health navigators. The Peer Health Navigation initiative is informed by Gelberg, Andersen, and Leake's Behavioral Model of Health Service Use for Vulnerable Populations (Brekke et al., 2013), which contends that the use of health services is influenced by an individual's predisposing characteristics, enabling resources, need for care, and personal health-care habits.

Peer health navigators are trained to help people with an SMI self-manage their physical health-care and wellness needs. Brekke and colleagues modified the original model to include the impact of psychiatric status and barriers to access related to the division or separation of mental health and primary care services. The peer health navigator serves as a "bridge," mediating the impact of the person's health behavior on their utilization of health services to improve overall health outcomes. Health navigation in this context is a comprehensive health-care engagement and self-management intervention provided by individuals with lived experience (peers) to individuals with severe mental health challenges.

Peer health navigators receive training, which includes explicit guidance in assessment and planning, coordinated linkages, consumer education, and cognitive behavioral strategies. Table 34-3 identifies the tasks and focus of the peer health navigators intended to improve health outcomes for persons with SMI. Research has demonstrated the effectiveness of the Bridge Peer Health Navigation intervention in improving the health status of persons with SMI (Brekke et al., 2019; Kelly et al., 2017). See Chapter 39: Peer-Led Services. 🤝

TABLE 34-3 | Tasks and Focus of Peer Health Navigators

Health and Wellness Needs	Consumer Awareness	Scanning Environmental Resources	Initial Provider Contact	Getting the Appointment	Waiting Room Experience	Examination Room Experience	Treatment Plan and Follow-Up
Work with service coordinators and mental health providers to assess a person's need for navigation Conduct health-care service screening with individuals Help with insurance benefits as necessary	Conduct health and wellness assessments with individuals Work with person to set health and wellness goals and the means to achieve those goals Provide health education tailored to a person's goals	Find providers and/or health clinics Develop relationships with providers and clinics Find insurance and/or benefits information	Assist with making appointments (role-play and in vivo) Coach individuals in making appointments	Provide appointment reminders Assist with and coach regarding transportation needs	Help with provider forms Model interactions with staff and other individuals (role-play and in vivo) Coach interactions with staff and others (in vivo) Act as stigma buffer	Model interactions with medical personnel (role-play and in vivo) Coach interactions with medical personnel (in vivo) Help individuals communicate needs Act as stigma buffer	Assist with treatment compliance, treatment plan, follow-up or specialty care, prescriptions

From Brekke, J. S., Siantz, E., Pahwa, R., Kelly, E., Tallne, L., & Fulginiti, A. (2013). Reducing health disparities for people with serious mental illness: Development and feasibility of a Peer Health Navigation intervention. Best Practices in Mental Health, *9*(1), 72.

The Lived Experience

Catherine

Catherine Clay is a mother, a wife, a friend, a notable advocate, and a health navigator. She has been living with a diagnosis for more than 20 years and has been actively engaged in her recovery since 2011.

Health navigators, according to Catherine, are "life bridgers," bridging the gap between mental health and physical health. As a health navigator, Catherine is able to provide support for individuals with SMI, helping them to seek out and receive quality health services. She connects members of her community with public services—such as the NAMI, UMMA Clinic, YWCA, the Villages—and private health services. "I help my community by modeling healthy behavior. I support them when they need it, but I teach them that they can do it alone," Catherine says. Catherine remembers an eye-opening experience as a health navigator:

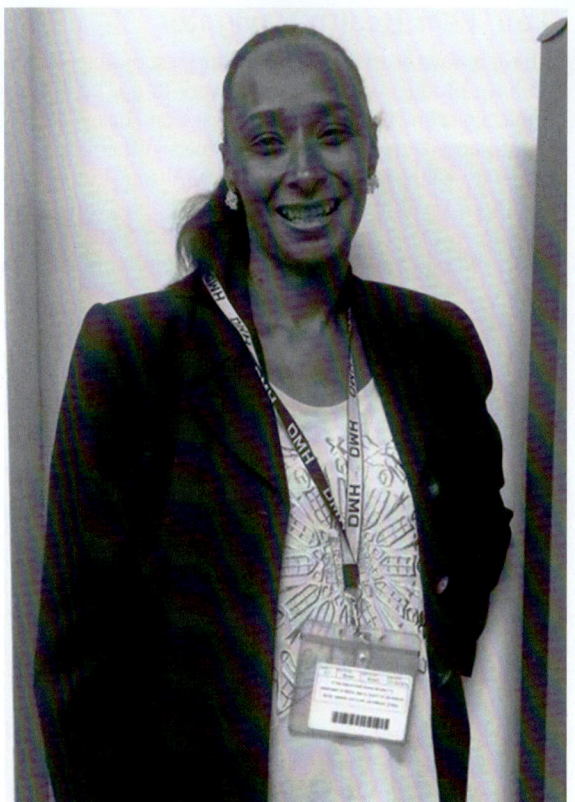

A friend was pregnant. She had no insurance. The clinic she went to, it was really bad. They told her she had an STD, that's what she thought. They never gave her meds, I couldn't believe it. I told her she needed to see the doctor—she needed to find out what was wrong and get medication. She asked me to go, she said "I'm afraid to talk to them, can you come?" I sat down with her and did an Ask Me Three. That's something I learned as a navigator. I helped her to write three questions that she wanted to ask the doctor. The doctor fills out the bottom part with instructions and then I sit down and go over it—in words they understand, not the complicated doctor language. So we made one and went to the clinic. It turned out she didn't have an STD, they only wanted to check the baby— to make sure it didn't have Down syndrome or anything. She was nervous, thinking the whole time that she was pregnant and had an STD. That's the thing about being a health navigator. I got to help her.

Peer advocates such as Catherine fill a unique role as health navigators, providing guidance and support through the lens of an experienced peer. "Health navigators need to be peer advocates," Catherine explains, "Someone with lived experience. We can give help without judgment. It comes from the community. We provide resources that we used ourselves. It's important."

Through her training as a health navigator, Catherine has learned to model healthy behaviors for her community and is currently working on a proposal to implement the peer health navigator program at the Women's Community Reintegration Services and Education Center. "Individuals with mental illness forget about their physical health, they shorten their life span." Catherine identifies the most prominent barriers to the receipt of medical care as people's misunderstanding of health practitioners, inconvenience of care, lack of understanding about coverage, and fear of denial. "They're afraid to be told no. They don't realize they can just ask—ask for more, ask for a different doctor, ask about their care. I help them ask and help them understand the answer," Catherine says.

Catherine believes strongly in her work as a health navigator. Being a health navigator motivates her to maintain her own health and promotes her own recovery by giving her a forum to speak about her own experiences. Catherine has received myriad awards from the Los Angeles County Department of Mental Health for her advocacy, including their highest honor, the "profile of hope," in 2013. As a health navigator—or life bridger, as she calls it—Catherine is working to educate her community, connect them to health resources, and support their improved quality of life. "I believe I help give a voice to the voiceless, and hope to the hopeless." (Catherine Clay as told to Leah Goodman, OTS, 2015)

The Lived Experience

Lou, Peer Health Navigator

I have always been an organized and responsible person. I like to have productive and creative work to do, be it in my personal life or my work life. I like to take on challenges and I am most happy working with people to help them improve their life and health. I graduated with a BA from the University of Southern California majoring in philosophy with a minor in psychology. I had a 20-year career at USC School of Medicine from 1977 to 1997 working with patients with Parkinson disease in the Department of Neurology.

Since 2011, I have had a career at Pacific Clinics as a health navigator, and starting in 2013, lead health navigator for the agency. I supervise 30 health navigators and am a member of the health navigation training team. I love my job providing health navigation services, training new health navigators, and serving as the unofficial "ambassador" for the program. Health navigation is a short-term intervention that pairs a consumer living with mental illness with a health navigator in order to help the consumer learn how to navigate the medical system on their own.

Just meeting me or being around me, you might not guess that I have been living with depression for the last 22 years. Through the years I have learned my depression triggers. I learned that loss is a trigger for me. Changing jobs, a death in the family, the end of a relationship, moving to a new home, or a combination of significant stressors could plunge me back into depression. I learned that I have several physical feelings at the onset of depression: I feel a heavy, dark weight descending upon me coupled with a feeling of doom and extreme fatigue. I learned that there are significant red flags to be aware of. If I start to have trouble getting to sleep, or staying asleep for more than 2 weeks, depression might be a factor. I learned that having difficulty reading or getting out of the house in my free time were other significant red flags. I have had three episodes of depression in the last 22 years and all have been triggered by a combination of significant loss and stressful life events, either on the job or in my personal life.

I have learned to be very aware of my physical and mental health and have included massage, aromatherapy, meditation, and creative activities such as singing, painting, and playing the ukulele to enhance my life going forward. Today, I am truly grateful that I am living my life in recovery.

My story has enabled me to work more effectively with my health navigation consumers and also other health navigators. I can relate to the challenges consumers have because I have been in their shoes. I am better able to hold hope for them as we work together because I know what it is like to lose hope. I have found that appropriately sharing a bit of my lived experience allows consumers to open up and trust me more readily. The consumers I have worked with have run the gamut between a 21-year-old young man with bipolar disorder to a 60-year-old woman with schizophrenia. The young man had never been to a primary care doctor in his life, thinking that he was supposed to go to the ED for care because that is what

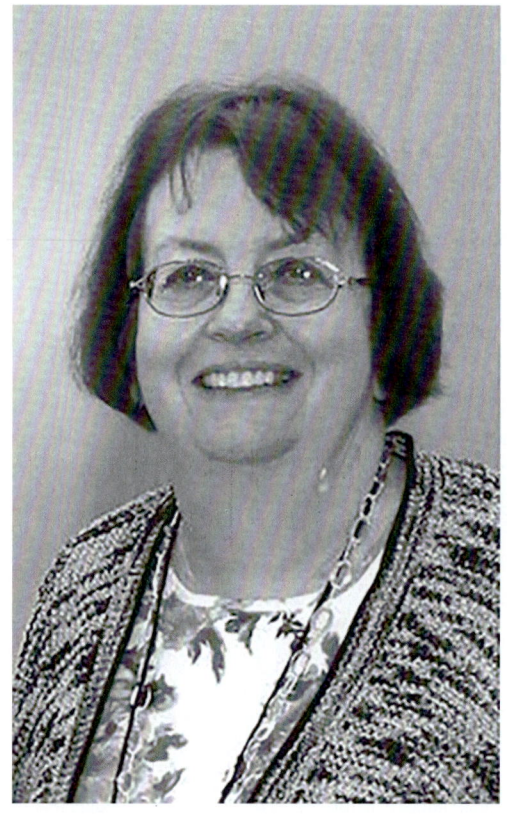

his mother did. The older adult woman was very proud and resilient—she was used to doing things for herself but now faced stage 4 pancreatic and liver cancer.

As a health navigator I have the opportunity to help consumers learn to make doctor's appointments, communicate effectively with their primary care physician and medical office staff, fill out necessary forms at the medical office, find a new doctor or specialist, organize their schedule with a calendar, and organize their medical paperwork for easy access while at the doctor's office.

Our mantra in health navigation is, "For them, with them and by them." The navigator first does things for the consumer while the consumer watches and listens. I typically help my consumers make a doctor's appointment by putting my telephone on speaker. In that way the consumer can listen to what I am saying and how the medical receptionist responds to me. The next time, the consumer makes the call and I provide coaching and support. This is called "with them." Finally, in the "by them" stage the consumer learns to make the calls on their own. The process takes up to 1 year of concentrated work with the navigator fading participation through time as the consumer becomes more and more capable. It is a joy to see consumers accomplishing things they never thought they could do. I am very fortunate to have such meaningful work. The consumers learn from me and I learn from them.

Evidence-Based Practice

Integrated Care for Individuals With Serious Mental Illness

Integrated care can improve health outcomes for people with SMI.

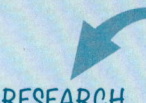

RESEARCH FINDINGS

Well-delivered, integrated care can enhance health outcomes for persons labeled with SMI. Adults with diabetes and comorbid SMI served in an integrated health-care delivery system had better cardiometabolic control than people with diabetes who did not have SMI (Mangurian et al., 2020). Despite improved outcomes, in an integrated health system SMI patients may need outreach strategies focused on disease prevention, screening and early diagnosis, and treatment to address medical comorbidities and associated poor health outcomes (Bahorik et al., 2017).

APPLICATIONS

➡ OTPs practicing in settings serving persons with SMI (e.g., community mental health, Clubhouses, Assertive Community Treatment [ACT] teams) should be aware that integrated care can improve health outcomes.

➡ Practitioners in these settings can ensure that their programs are integrated with primary care and work collaboratively with the PCPs as part of outreach strategies to ensure that the persons with whom they working are fully engaged with their PCP.

REFERENCES

Bahorik, A. L., Satre, D. D., Kline-Simon, A. H., Weisner, C. M., & Campbell, C. I. (2017). Serious mental illness and medical comorbidities: Findings from an integrated health care system. *Journal of Psychosomatic Research, 100*, 35–45. https://doi.org/10.1016/j.jpsychores.2017.07.004

Mangurian, C., Schillinger, D., Newcomer, J. W., Vittinghoff, E., Essock, S., Zhu, Z., Dyer, W., Young-Wolff, K. C., & Scmittdiel, J. (2020). Comorbid diabetes and severe mental illness: Outcomes in an integrated health care delivery system. *Journal of General Internal Medicine, 35*(1), 160–166. https://doi.org/10.1007/s11606-019-05489-3

Role of Occupational Therapy

Muir (2012) delineated some of the roles and functions of OTPs in primary care broadly as follows:

- Assist the physician to prevent disease or disability, reduce the negative impact of a disease process, and promote adherence with treatment regimens.
- Help to extend the holistic care of physicians and mid-level providers by identifying how symptoms are affecting function and participation.
- Improve patient satisfaction by focusing on the full range of issues facing the patient.
- Provide simple interventions that can be carried out at home.
- Improve occupational engagement through modification of activities and assistive and adaptive equipment.
- Provide group education.

More recently, efforts to frame the role of occupational therapy in primary care have been documented (Bolt et al., 2019; Donnelly et al., 2013; Halle et al., 2018). Most of these assert a role for occupational therapy in addressing behavioral health needs of primary care patients across the life span (AOTA, 2020b). Involvement of occupational therapy in an integrated behavioral health and primary care context in the United States may depend upon the creativity and initiative of OTPs to create their own connections and opportunities. Scharf and colleagues (2013) found that a small number of the SAMHSA's multiyear Primary Care and Behavioral Health Care (PCBH) Integration grants (i.e., 7%) included OTPs on their teams.

Over the last decade, more university-based occupational therapy researchers have partnered with other health professional educational programs to collaborate on PCBH projects. For example, in 2017, the University of New Hampshire's Departments of Occupational Therapy and Social Work were awarded a 4-year Health Resources and Services Administration, Behavioral Health Workforce, Education, and Training (HRSA BHWET) Grant to develop an interprofessional training program for graduate occupational therapy and social work students in integrated primary care. Alexis Trolley-Hansen, OTR/L, clinical assistant professor, served as the occupational therapy lead for this project.

This led to the development of the University of New Hampshire (UNH) Primary Care Behavioral Health Training program, which consisted of two graduate courses and a 6-month long clinical experience. Students applied for this 9-month training program and completed it in addition to their regular graduate program. Over the 4 years of the grant, occupational therapy students were placed at 14 different health-care organizations that had integrated care programs. These included federally qualified health-care centers, primary care organizations, substance use recovery organizations, community-based health-care programs, and community-based mental health-care centers. These organizations utilized a variety of integrated care models, including the collaborative care model, PCMH, integrated PCBH, and reverse integration. The type of program, organization, and integrated care model shaped occupational therapy student activities and programs. Some occupational therapy student activities included:

- Addressing functional participation needs of adults in an integrated PCBH setting, including interventions focused on health management, energy conservation, and occupational balance; and creating healthy activities of daily living (ADLs) and instrumental activities of daily living (IADLs) routines around eating, sleep, and exercise
- Developing and implementing an 8-week, holistic chronic pain management program for individuals as part of a collaborative care team
- Providing home-based occupational therapy services to seniors and adults with SMI as part of a PCMH. These interventions included developing IADL skills, building healthy habits and routines using the Action Over Inertia program (Krupa et al., 2021), and teaching about falls prevention.
- Completing developmental and sensory based screenings and using psychoeducation and coaching to help families build healthy family routines and address common pediatric challenges (eating, sleeping, attention, behaviors) in a PCBH pediatric primary care office
- Developing and implementing IADL, healthy living, prevocational program, healthy leisure, and creative self-expression group interventions as part of a substance use disorder recovery program using a reverse integration model

By the end of the grant, at least one organization had created a full-time occupational therapy position, and three others worked with the UNH Occupational Therapy Department to create programs that could be sustained through occupational therapy student fieldwork activities.

Challenges to occupational therapy in U.S.-based primary care include reimbursement, clarity around OTPs' role/value both within the profession as well as from other professionals, and the lack of specialized course work regarding primary care in entry-level educational programs (Halle et al., 2018). Internationally, Canada and Scandinavia offer examples of how OTPs have already established their presence in integrated care (Holmberg & Ringsberg, 2014; Smith-Carrier & Neysmith, 2014). In this section, the role of occupational therapy in integrated behavioral health and primary care is framed by distinguishing between health promotion and prevention and chronic disease management.

Health Promotion and Disease Prevention

Promotion and *prevention* are two broad perspectives in public health and medicine, with each emphasizing a particular directional impact for health and wellness interventions. Promotion efforts encourage individuals and communities to engage in healthy behaviors and to increase control over their own health, whereas prevention efforts focus on strategies to reduce impairments, disease, and disability. Each of these is focused on the overall health of populations and on mental health, in particular, by WHO (2004, 2007; WHO & UNICEF, 2018).

It is well understood that a variety of social factors that are multiple, complex, and interrelated, and can seem daunting impact health. These social determinants of health have been defined as "conditions in which people are born, grow, work, live, and age, and the wider set of forces and systems shaping the conditions of daily life. These forces and systems include economic policies and systems, development agendas, social norms, social policies and political systems" (WHO, 2016, para. 1). Fortunately, there is a depth and breadth of practice knowledge and interest in health promotion (Holmberg & Ringsberg, 2014; Letts et al., 1993) that OTPs in the IBHC context can use to understand and address these challenges. See Chapter 28: Social Determinants and Mental Health.

Efforts to address overall health and mental health promotion and prevention in the primary care context can be challenging given the nature of the primary care work environment (Calderon et al., 2011; McManus, 2013; Ramanuj et al., 2019). Primary care visits are short and expected to be infrequent, making it difficult for health-care practitioners to engage in health promotion education or to address lifestyle changes (Calderon et al., 2011; Grandes et al., 2008). On the other hand, there is evidence that outcomes of lifestyle interventions with a health promotion focus for persons with psychiatric disabilities are more durable when they continue 3 or more months (Bartels & Desilets, 2012).

A well-known example within the occupational therapy profession is Lifestyle Redesign™ (LRD; Clark et al., 1997). Jeanne Jackson, Ruth Zemke, and Florence Clark developed this approach at the Chan Division of the University of Southern California. Since its introduction into occupational therapy practice, this approach has been widely disseminated, including internationally, and the manual outlining the LRD approach with the well older adult was recently updated (Clark et al., 2015). In this approach, a direct link is made between occupational engagement and health, and participants engage in both a reflective and active process about their occupations to support their health.

Given that health is a key aspect of occupational therapy's scope of practice (AOTA, 2020a), particularly in primary care (AOTA, 2020b), OTPs practicing in the integrated behavioral health and primary care context need to understand these specific challenges (Halle et al., 2018).

Chronic Disease Management

Chronic disease management in the integrated behavioral health and primary care context refers to management of chronic medical conditions as well as chronic behavioral health conditions and substance abuse. Chronic illnesses can be defined as conditions that persist for 1 year or more and require ongoing medical attention and/or limit ADLs (National Center for Chronic Disease Prevention and Health Promotion, 2024). AOTA (2022) make clear that "occupational therapy practitioners are distinctly qualified to address the impact of chronic conditions on occupational performance and participation across the life span" (p. 1).

Self-management of such conditions to maintain health, manage symptoms, and delay or prevent complications is a particular focus of occupational therapy (AOTA, 2022). OTPs should use caution when using the language "chronic" in the specialty mental health service context, as its use has been criticized by persons labeled with mental illness as disempowering (Davidson et al., 2006, 2009). Persons identified as having a chronic illness may face a different level of stigmatization. "In the case of chronic illness stigma, the mark or attribute is the diagnosis of chronic disease. With this diagnosis, a person has transitioned from 'normal' to 'limited function'" (Salih & Landers, 2019, p. 132). Alternative terms have been proposed and are more commonly utilized in practice, including serious, severe, persistent, and enduring. In addition, the publicly funded specialty mental health service system has provided the equivalent of "chronic" disease management for persons with SMI for decades.

More than 25% of Americans are living with more than one chronic illness (Boersma et al., 2020). Over 60% of Medicare beneficiaries in the United States have more than one chronic medical condition, accounting for a high percentage of Medicare expenditures. The co-occurrence of major depressive disorder in older adults with medical conditions is associated with a higher risk of physical disability, increased health-care utilization, and higher medical costs (Huang et al., 2013).

Mercer and colleagues (2012) note that managing a cluster of conditions that can benefit from synergistic intervention is simpler than managing conditions separately in a nonsynergistic manner. However, they also note that, "When the mix of conditions experienced includes both physical and mental health problems, however, the poorly stitched seams of professional care are at their most threadbare. The stigma that surrounds mental ill health may prevent patients with physical conditions from disclosing mental health concerns, which compounds problems of management. For these patients' outcomes are usually worse" (p. 1).

Care Coordination

Care coordination is understood to be a key element of IBHC efforts, in particular for individuals with complex or high needs. Manning and Gagnon (2017) argue that "although patients deemed as complex exist, their emergence and prevalence in the biomedical literature may simply reflect a broadening of scope within health care rather than a new kind of patient" (p. 20). Complex patients have been identified as presenting with multiple chronic physical and mental health conditions and often struggle to manage them. They may have functional limitations, or a combination of vulnerabilities including social disadvantages such as homelessness, low income, behavioral health issues, or being a racial and ethnic minority. By coordinating care across the person's engagement in health and social care systems, health and social outcomes improve (Peterson et al., 2019).

Although care coordination has often been seen as a nursing or social work function, OTPs are well suited to this role, especially considering their Person-Environment-Occupation (PEO) frameworks. Occupational therapy brings a unique perspective to this role, given OTPs' knowledge and expertise in disability, function, and context (Dickson & Toto, 2018; Robinson et al., 2016). The narrative that appears in Box 34-3 describes Rosa's IBHC at a family health clinic and highlights both interdisciplinary teamwork and occupational therapy's distinct role in IBHC.

BOX 34-3 ■ Rosa's Story

Contributed by Alexis Trolley-Hanson, OTR/L, clinical assistant professor and codirector of UNH Primary Care Behavioral Health Training

Environment

The setting is a family health clinic designated as an FQHC. The clinic uses an integrated Primary Care Behavioral Health approach including regular team huddles and group problem-solving. Services are provided by an interdisciplinary team at one location, in overlapping visits if possible.

Person

In a routine morning huddle, the PCP shares her concerns about Rosa, who is coming in later that day for a follow-up health visit regarding her diagnosis of type 2 diabetes. Rosa is a 69-year-old small business owner, caregiver, and proud Latina woman. Three months ago, Rosa was diagnosed with type 2 diabetes by her PCP as part of a routine physical examination. She has struggled with weight management and had been prediabetic for 5 years before this diagnosis. After the diagnosis, the nurse provided her with a

glucose meter and showed her how to use it to monitor her blood sugar levels. Rosa was also prescribed insulin and shown how to self-administer it. Finally, she met with a nutritionist who provided information about type 2 diabetes and provided her with a meal plan and a few recipes.

Three-Month Follow-Up

This is a 3-month follow-up visit for Rosa, but previsit bloodwork shows her A1c levels remain unchanged. Rosa completed a previsit mental health screening (the Patient Health Questionnaire-9) and her answers suggest that she may be struggling with depressive symptoms. Rosa's PCP is concerned about how these symptoms impact her ability to manage her diabetes. The OTP and social worker on the team offer to participate in the visit. The team decides the social worker will begin the appointment and talk to Rosa about her mental health; the PCP will then follow up to complete a medical examination and go over Rosa's bloodwork and treatment plan. The OTP will go in at the end of the visit to better understand how Rosa's everyday activities are being impacted by and impacting her health.

Continued

BOX 34-3 ■ Rosa's Story—cont'd

Social Work

The social worker completes a more specific depression screening and confirms Rosa is struggling with depression. Rosa acknowledges she hasn't been testing her blood sugar, using insulin, or following the diet she was provided. She reports having trouble sleeping through the night, feeling sad and overwhelmed, and having trouble enjoying family activities. The social worker learns Rosa immigrated to the United States from Mexico when she was 20 years old and has been a U.S. citizen for 39 years. As a child in Mexico, she experienced trauma that has shaped who she is today. The social worker learns Rosa may have experienced previous periods of depression but never has received treatment.

Primary Care Provider

The PCP and nursing staff assess for any additional problems related to untreated diabetes. The PCP further explores Rosa's symptoms, rules out chronic pain, and orders some additional medical tests to rule out metabolic or endocrine concerns. The PCP discusses trialing an antidepressant medication with Rosa and provides her with a prescription. Nursing reviews blood sugar testing and insulin administration with Rosa. The PCP then invites the OTP into the treatment room as a "warm hand-off" and leaves to see other patients.

Occupational Therapy

The OTP completes an occupational profile and provides a brief intervention. Rosa is the owner of a Mexican bakery that specializes in wedding cakes and pastries and employs five people. She has owned this business for 20 years, and still works in the bakery 3 days a week. She has been married for 45 years. Her husband recently retired but struggles with chronic back pain that impacts his mobility and participation in daily activities. Rosa is the mother of two adult children, and has four grandchildren. She provides childcare for two of her grandchildren (ages 4 and 6) 2 days a week to support her daughter. Rosa reports she enjoys cooking and baking and that eating dinner together as a family is very important to her. She shares that she has tried to change the food that she prepares, but her family didn't like the dishes she prepared. She also states that the recipes that were provided were not foods that she or the family regularly eat or that she knows how to prepare.

When she is working or taking care of grandchildren, Rosa doesn't remember to test her blood sugar or eat on a regular schedule. In her free time, Rosa enjoys gardening and singing. She has a close group of women friends her age whom she has lunch with every Saturday. One of these friends also lives with type 2 diabetes and has been trying to help her with her sugar testing. Rosa says she frequently wakes at night or very early and can't fall back to sleep. She feels exhausted, sad, and doesn't enjoy her Saturday lunches as much as she used to. Rosa acknowledges the seriousness of her diagnosis but feels overwhelmed by the changes she is being asked to make.

The OTP recognizes the complex ways that food preparation and eating are embedded into Rosa's everyday roles and routines.

Food is involved in many aspects of Rosa's work, caregiving, and leisure occupations. The OTP notes the foods Rosa eats have cultural importance and this impacts her family's food preferences and her habits/routines around food preparation. The OTP weighs the potential impacts that daily stress and depression may be having on Rosa's ability to participate in behavioral change. In her brief intervention, the OTP recognizes and validates how hard it is to adjust to type 2 diabetes. She provides education about the process of behavioral change and the mind-body connection using a baking metaphor that Rosa connects to. They discuss taking small steps toward changing behavior. Rosa identifies creating a new habit around testing and treating her blood sugar levels as a short-term goal. The OTP brainstorms with Rosa regarding ways to set up environmental cues and reminders to support this goal of monitoring and treating her blood sugar. Rosa agrees to set up a follow-up appointment with the OTP to address occupational balance, symptom management, and health maintenance goals.

Plan of Care

The OTP, social worker, and PCP use the electronic health record to share data they learned in this visit. Based on this documentation, the team creates the following plan of care for Rosa.

- PCP/Nursing will follow-up with bloodwork and follow-up with a phone call in 3 weeks to check on antidepressant medication. They will schedule a follow-up appointment in 3 months to check on Rosa's diabetes management.
- Social work will set up individual social work visits to provide mental health interventions to address depression including cognitive behavioral therapy and trauma work.
- The OTP will follow up within a week to continue to promote engagement in activities that support health and wellness including health management related to diabetes management, new habits/routines around eating, and exploration of ways to embed healthier meals into existing meaningful routines.
- The health navigator will follow up with and connect Rosa to a certified diabetes educator and Latinx focused diabetes supports within the community.

12-Month Follow-Up

At this follow-up, Rosa is actively self-managing her type 2 diabetes and has established new eating habits. She has created new exercise routines with her group of friends and participates in a Latina diabetes support group. She continues to make foods that meet her family members' food preferences but has added in dishes that are healthier for her. Rosa reports a higher quality of sleep and more enjoyment in her everyday activities.

Reflective Questions

1. What strengths does Rosa have and how might the OTP have incorporated these into her interventions?
2. What unique knowledge and skills did the OTP bring to the integrated care team in this case study?

Homeless Health Care

It has been well-documented that people experiencing homelessness "face intersecting physical, mental and social burdens that greatly increase morbidity and mortality relative to the general population" (Liu & Hwang, 2021, p. 1). Specialized primary care settings have been developed to meet the needs of this population. In the United States, the Health Care for the Homeless (HCH) Program (authorized in Section 330(h) of the PHSA makes grants to community-based organizations in order to assist them in planning and delivering high-quality, accessible health care to people experiencing homelessness.

The HCH Program is a competitive grant program, funding primary health, mental health, addiction, and social services with intensive outreach and case management to link people with appropriate services. Examples of these programs include the Maryland Health Care for Homeless services in Baltimore; Central City Concern in Portland, Oregon; and the John Wesley Community Health Center in the Skid Row area of Los Angeles. All of these primary care settings are designated as HCH-FQHCs that have incorporated OTPs on their integrated health-care teams. Boxes 34-4 and 34-5 present two occupational therapy practice examples from the John Wesley Community Health (JWCH) Center. See Chapter 42: Homelessness and Housing Insecurity. 🤝

BOX 34-4 ■ The Home Visit

Contributed by Stephanie Moon, OTD, OTR/L

The JWCH Center licensed clinical social worker for pain management referred Jasmine to occupational therapy. Jasmine was experiencing severe pain in her lower back, knee, and shoulder. Medical interventions such as anti-inflammatory injections have helped previously, but Jasmine's follow-up appointment isn't for 3 months. She is currently unhoused and stays in a tent by a freeway overpass while her outreach team works on finding a permanent housing solution. Jasmine prefers the freedom of the streets over the rules and personalities at the shelters. Despite rowdy neighbors, Jasmine feels safe. She has a male friend who stays with her at times and beams when sharing about how she has become the point person on the block for aid volunteers. Jasmine cooks occasionally in her tent, toilets in her second tent or at the McDonald's next door, and reports no issues with navigating the community apart from her pain. Overall, Jasmine is satisfied with her interim living situation and is proud of her ability to keep her living area clean and her belongings safe.

Jasmine's pain impacts her ability to walk long distances, to sit for a meaningful duration of time, and to make transitions from lying down to sitting to standing. Grooming is also impacted as Jasmine is unable to lift her arms above shoulder level without pain and fatigue. Jasmine has a well-used endurance walker that she uses for walking, sitting, and carrying her belongings despite a broken brake, which concerns Stephanie, her OTP. Of the areas discussed to work on, Jasmine prioritizes transitioning out of bed in the morning, grooming, and walking longer distances.

Jasmine describes her bed as a collection of six pillows on the floor of her tent. In order to get out of bed, she often uses the sides of her tent and her endurance walker if it is within reach. Jasmine also describes a technique of launching herself out of bed while rocking her body and pumping her arms. Stephanie is concerned that Jasmine's sleeping arrangement, body mechanics, and use of the endurance walker while getting out of bed might contribute to and exacerbate her back pain. Additionally, using the walker and using body momentum to transition in and out of bed is a fall risk.

The OTP arranges with the outreach team to do a "home visit" to Jasmine's tent. Jasmine's bed is against the right side of the tent wall: six sofa cushions in a 2x3 arrangement with a bed sheet wrapped over the top of it. After asking Jasmine to demonstrate how she usually gets in and out of bed, the OTP provided patient education on proper body mechanics (i.e., log roll) and the dangers of using the walker as support to get out of bed.

Upon scanning the tent and its environment, the OTP begins identifying barriers and brainstorming modifications to support Jasmine's transition in and out of bed. First, considering Jasmine's sleeping surface: The gaps between the sofa cushions may cause further back pain and the unstable, dynamic, and uneven surface

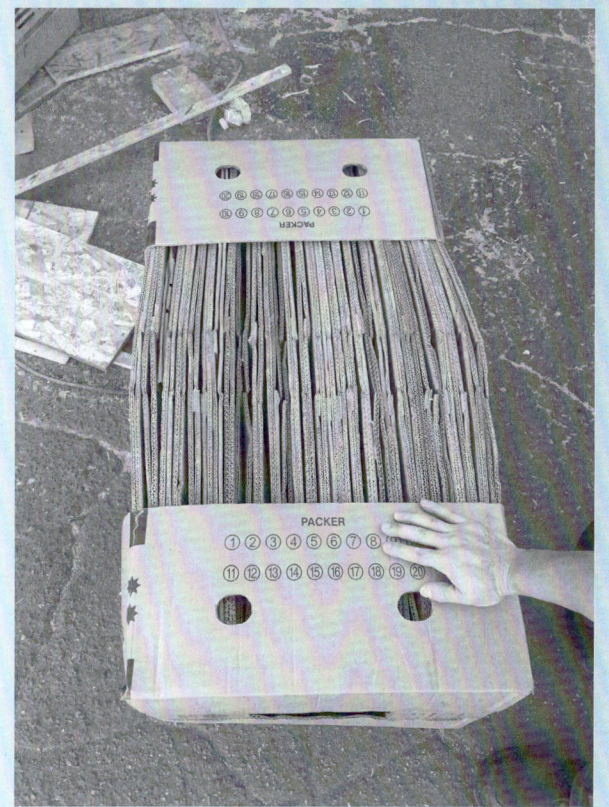

makes it difficult to transition in and out of bed. Additionally, the height of the sleeping surface is very low, which puts a lot of stress on many of Jasmine's joints while she tries to get out of bed. It is also a fall risk because her habit is to use either her walker or generate some body momentum to get out of bed.

The OTP looks for a stable surface that could be used to support Jasmine's transition but finds nothing, though she notices a nearby lamppost and an opening in the top of the tent. They consider fastening a strap to the post and hanging it above Jasmine's bedding so she could use it as leverage to get out of bed. However, Jasmine needs to move her tent to comply with law enforcement and street sweeping on occasion, and believes affixing personal items onto public ones is prohibited, though it is not. As they continue to explore options, the OTP and Jasmine decide that replacing her "mattress" to better support Jasmine's back with alternative materials is the best solution. The OTP can find cardboard slats (see photo) that were light enough for Jasmine to move.

BOX 34-5 ■ Transitioning From Street to Home

Contributed by Alicia McConnell Hatch, OTD, OTR/L

The PCP at the JWCH Center referred Barry, a male in his early 70s, to occupational therapy for support with mobility and resource seeking. Barry stated he was "ready for his retirement and his own little place" after experiencing chronic homelessness for 30 years. Barry has been living in his car and storing belongings in an abandoned shipping container. He was unwilling to enter a shelter or temporary housing because of restrictions of only being allowed to bring two bags. Barry presented with chronic left hip pain secondary to sciatica, as well as hypertension, and a diagnosis of schizophrenia. Barry expressed he had some distrust of medical providers and social workers and that he did not believe they could help him.

Barry's hip pain has worsened by sleeping in his car. He reported that he is not able to eat healthy foods to manage his hypertension because he can't store fresh groceries, and he finds it difficult to manage his medication because of his schedule being disrupted by the street environment. Barry's long-term goals are to get permanent housing, ride his bike again, and manage his health independently.

The OTP approached Barry's care by engaging with him over a long period of time to build rapport and establish trust. In this engagement phase, the OTP addressed functional mobility issues, connected Barry to a housing waitlist, introduced him to a mental health therapist on the JWCH team, and provided care coordination to address other medical issues that arose for Barry, such as an infected tooth. Through providing these interventions, the OTP kept Barry engaged with services while monitoring his housing status.

After 5 months of working with Barry on a weekly to biweekly basis, the OTP was contacted by a permanent housing site with an apartment for Barry. The OTP was given 48 hours to confirm that Barry would accept this housing; however, Barry did not come to his usual appointment that week. The OTP searched for Barry and found out he was very ill and had fallen inside his shipping container. Barry had to be persuaded to go to the hospital. He finally agreed, and at the hospital he was diagnosed with kidney stones. The OTP communicated with the hospital social worker that Barry had a match to permanent supportive housing but needed a safe place to discharge and recuperate such as a skilled nursing facility. The OTP also advocated to the housing site that Barry could live independently once discharged from skilled nursing.

After 6 weeks of hospitalization and skilled nursing care, Barry's apartment was ready for him to move in. The OTP picked Barry up and accompanied him to the bank to get checks to pay his rent using his Social Security Disability Income. After Barry moved in, the OTP began weekly home visits to check on Barry, often in collaboration with the mental health therapist. Interventions in these home sessions included IADL skills training with a focus on occupations such as laundry, grocery shopping, meal preparation, care coordination, and health management. Since his move, Barry's functional mobility improved and his pain has decreased because of his therapeutic exercise program and sleeping in a bed. He goes shopping each week for fresh food and can remember to take his medications and keep his medical appointments. He has even been able to ride his bike again!

Knowledge, Skills, and Competencies for Integrated Behavioral Health and Primary Care

In many ways, the knowledge, skills, and competencies that support an OTP's success in integrated behavioral health and primary care are not totally unique nor dissimilar to those used by practitioners in other areas. SAMHSA-HRSA has developed a set of core competencies to guide workforce development in all the health and behavioral health professions. Those competencies include:

- *Interpersonal communication:* the ability to establish rapport quickly and to communicate effectively with consumers of health care, their family members, and other providers
- *Collaboration and teamwork:* the ability to function effectively as a member of an interprofessional team that includes behavioral health and PCPs, individuals, and their family members
- *Screening and assessment:* the ability to conduct brief, evidence-based, and developmentally appropriate screening and to conduct or arrange for more detailed assessments when indicated
- *Care planning and care coordination:* the ability to create and implement integrated care plans, ensuring access to

an array of linked services and the exchange of information among individuals, family members, and providers
- *Intervention:* the ability to provide a range of brief, focused prevention, treatment, and recovery services, as well as longer-term treatment and support for individuals with persistent illnesses
- *Cultural competence and adaptation:* the ability to provide services that are relevant to the culture of the person and their family
- *Systems-oriented practice:* the ability to function effectively within the organizational and financial structures of the local system of health care
- *Practice-based learning and quality improvement:* the ability to assess and continually improve the services delivered as an individual provider and as an interprofessional team member
- *Informatics:* the ability to use information technology to support and improve integrated health care (Hoge et al., 2014, pp. 8–9)

AOTA "affirms that occupational therapy practitioners are well prepared to contribute to interprofessional collaborative care teams addressing the primary care needs of individuals across the life course." Furthermore, "occupational therapy practitioners' distinct knowledge of the significant impact that roles, habits, and routines have on health and wellness makes their contribution to primary care valuable" (AOTA, 2020b, p. 1). A summary of critical knowledge, skills, and areas of competence for practitioners in interprofessional

TABLE 34-4 | **Examples of Occupational Therapy Knowledge, Skills, and Competencies for Integrated Care**

Assessment and Intervention	Communication Skills	Teamwork and Collaboration	Systems Knowledge and Thinking	Cultural Competency and Professional Ethics
Assessing an individual's needs	Interviewing skills	Effective collaboration with interprofessional team and individual	Knowledge of available community resources	Cultural awareness and cultural competency
Assessing individual strengths and weaknesses	Ability to communicate empathy	Ability to guide individual in navigating systems	Understanding stages and systems of change	Understanding of ethical challenges unique to primary care
Collaborative and person-centered goal setting	Ability to quickly develop rapport with person and their family	Ability to teach and train others to work effectively across transprofessional boundaries	Quality and process improvement skills	Understands ethical care related to individuals, communities, and populations
Ability to determine plans of care appropriate in the primary care setting	Effectively communicate the distinct value of occupational therapy on the primary care team	Effective shared decision-making	Outcomes measurement and management	

From American Occupational Therapy Association. (2014). The role of occupational therapy in primary care. American Journal of Occupational Therapy, 68, 525–533. https://doi.org/10.5014/ajot.2014.686S06; Interorganizational Work Group on Competencies for Primary Care Psychology Practice. (2013). Competencies for psychology practice in primary care. http://www.apa.org/ed/resources/competencies-practice.pdf; Lawn, S., Battersy, M., Linder, H., Mathews, R., Morris, S., Wells, L., Litt, J., & Reed, R. (2009). What skills do primary health care professionals need to provide effect self-management support? Seeking consumer perspectives. Australian Journal of Primary Health, 15, 37–44. https://doi.org/10.1071/PY08053

primary care teams is provided in Table 34-4 (AOTA, 2020b; Interorganizational Work Group on Competencies for Primary Care Psychology Practice, 2013; Lawn et al., 2009).

Interprofessional Team-Based Collaboration

Interdisciplinary perspectives have been identified as critical when facing what are referred to as "wicked" problems. These problems are seen as being difficult to formulate and having more than one explanation; they are often seen as symptomatic of one or more other problems, are frequently unique, and do not resolve with a simple intervention (Drinka & Clark, 2000). Although the notion of wicked problems has focused mostly on societal issues, the nature of some IBHC practice contexts might be best understood as addressing wicked problems. Therefore, the need for interprofessional—interdisciplinary—teams becomes necessary.

The difference in training and perspective of members of *integrated care teams* can be challenging in practice. Being part of an integrated care team requires staying focused on the awareness that each team member cannot solve problem(s) alone and demands reflection and open dialogue among all team members. The focus of this communication and reflection is to help each team member understand the cognitive—what is the problem, how can it be solved—and the value—personal, professional, teamwork, organizational— maps of each of the other providers (Drinka & Clark, 2000; Rushmer & Pullis, 2003). Open dialogue and

clarity are important to minimize risk of "blurred boundaries" (Rushmer & Pallis, 2003), including:

- *Role uncertainty:* Who should be doing this "bit"?
- *Role ambiguity:* Is this really what I should be doing?
- *Feelings of inequity:* I feel they should have done this "bit."
- *Stress and anxiety:* Am I out of my depth here?
- *Feeling unprepared:* I didn't know I was going to be doing this now. (Rushmer & Pallis, 2003, p. 64)

The composition of the integrated behavioral health and primary care team can vary. Psychiatrists, medical physicians, nurses including advanced practice nurses (APNs), case managers or social workers, OTPs, and substance use counselors play primary roles. Other health professionals such as pharmacists and nutritionists may also serve on the team.

Screening and Assessment

Screening is an essential part of the routine intake process in health-care settings, including primary care, as it helps to identify care needs. In the United States, several national organizations have developed guidelines for what should be screened for and what screening tools are best for the primary care context. For example, the U.S. Preventive Services Task Force (USPSTF) recommends screening for behavioral health disorders in particular (Mulvaney-Day, et al., 2018). The Patient Health Questionnaire-9 (PHQ-9; Kroenke et al., 2001) is a commonly used self-report depression screening tool and is endorsed by the National Quality Forum (Mulvaney-Day et al., 2018).

Screening tools may also be used in the integrated behavioral health and primary care context to identify the need for more comprehensive occupational therapy assessment (Boone et al., 2022). For example, given occupational therapy's important role in functional cognition (Giles et al., 2020), the Menu Task (Edwards et al., 2019) was developed as "a brief, reliable, and valid screening measure of functional cognition that can be easily administered by a member of any health care discipline across both acute and post-acute treatment settings" (p. 3). It has been demonstrated to be a valid and reliable performance-based functional screen for community-dwelling older adults (Al-Heizan et al., 2022), a population often seen in the primary care practice context.

Although screening tools utilized in the primary care practice context have focused on condition management factors such as signs and symptoms, impact on daily life both from a functional and quality of life perspective may also be captured in such tools. The internationally recognized WHODAS 2.0 (WHO Disability Assessment Schedule, 2010; informed by the *International Classification of Functioning, Disability and Health [ICF]*) has also been identified as a screening tool to capture the functional impact of psychiatric disorders in the *Diagnostic and Statistical Manual of Mental Disorders* (5th ed., text revision; American Psychiatric Association, 2022).

Reimbursement and Documentation

Occupational therapy services are not often directly reimbursed in primary care (AOTA, 2020b) and the focus is often on physicians, physician assistants, and nurses. For example, within the FQHC, occupational therapy is incident to the service provided by designated billable providers (i.e., physicians, nurses, licensed clinical social workers [LCSWs]). As in most practice settings, maximizing available reimbursement requires clear and specific documentation. Implementation of the ACA has resulted in new payment structures, such as value-based purchasing including bundled payments for care and an increasing number of accountable care organizations. This makes demonstrating effectiveness in helping to lower costs, contributing to the improvement of outcomes,

and articulating occupational therapy's distinct value more important than ever.

As electronic health records (EHRs) are becoming commonplace, it is possible to document occupational therapy intervention in ways that are efficient and take advantage of the time-saving attributes of EHRs without losing focus on occupation-based practice. However, EHR workflows and policies are not always designed for primary care settings and can sometimes become cumbersome (Young et al., 2014).

OTPs need to learn about options that will allow for streamlining documentation while remaining occupation-based and able to capture and extract important information across individuals. For example, "smart phrases," which are phrases, sentences, or even paragraphs that are automatically entered as someone types the first few letters, are available in some documentation systems and can improve speed and standardization of documentation (Perez, 2014). Similar to other areas of knowledge, skills, and competency, effective and efficient documentation is not unique to primary care, but pressures may be particularly high because of the limited amount of time with each person.

Here's the Point

- Integrated care in mental health brings together behavioral health and primary care.
- Public policy initiatives have helped to create a political and social context where the operational challenges to delivering integrated behavioral health and primary care services can be overcome.
- The processes of providing integrated care and the roles of interprofessional team members are continually being delineated and refined.
- Approaches to the design and delivery of integrated behavioral health and primary care have been developed, yet challenges to their implementation still exist.
- OTPs have the necessary knowledge and skill sets to make valuable contributions to integrated behavioral health and primary care practices, but demonstrating their value will require effective documentation of the OTP's role.

Apply It Now

1. Reflections on John's Experiences With Integrated Behavioral Health Care

Reread Box 34-1: My Health: Making Sense of Integrated Care about John's experience receiving IBHC and serving as a peer provider at a local mental health center. Reflect and discuss John's experiences using the following guiding questions.

Reflective Questions
- How could an integrated primary care and behavioral health team—one that focuses on both John's physical health and behavioral health—support John's educational and health-care goals?

- What might an OTP working on an integrated primary care and behavioral health team do to support John's goals? Identify some specific areas of focus for the OTP.

2. Reflections on Street Medicine

Reread Box 34-2: Street Medicine for Grace, the story of Grace's interactions receiving integrated care from a homeless outreach service. This approach to health care is sometimes referred to as street medicine.

Explore resources that can help you better understand street medicine. Start at the Street Medicine Institute (https://www.streetmedicine.org). Pair up with a peer and discuss what you have learned. How might OTPs interface with street medicine?

Create two lists: one with all Grace's behavioral health risks and needs, and a second with all her physical health risks and needs. Review your lists and rank Grace's behavior and physical health risks and needs. Consider how an OTP could work to address Grace's most immediate risks and needs.

3. Reflections on Jasmine's Home Visit

Reread Box 34-4: The Home Visit, in which an OTP shares her experience organizing a home visit with an outreach team. The therapist meets Jasmine in the streets in a tent where she lives. Use the following prompts and guiding questions to reflect and discuss this story of a unique home visit.

Reflective Questions

■ Jasmine is in chronic pain. Knowing that chronic pain often interferes with problem-solving, mental agility, and mental endurance, how might impairments in these areas further put an individual living on the streets at increased risk? With peers, brainstorm various ways OTPs could help.

■ Jasmine "beams when sharing about how she has become the point person on the block for aid volunteers." How might her chronic pain interfere with this valued occupation?

■ How could an OTP address Jasmine's other concerns of grooming and walking longer distances?

4. Reflections on Transitioning From Street to Home

Reread Box 34-5: Transitioning From Street to Home, the story of an OTP working with Barry as he transitions from being chronically homeless for 30 years to moving into an apartment in a personal housing facility. Use the following prompts and guiding questions to reflect and discuss this story of transition.

Reflective Questions

■ The OTP describes her efforts at engaging Barry over a long period of time. Imagine you are the OTP in this story. What strategies would you use to engage a person who has physical and mental health challenges and has been homeless for 30 years?

■ Barry's long-term goals are to get permanent housing, ride his bike again, and independently manage his health. How might an OTP address Barry's self-defined goals?

■ Barry does get an apartment in a permanent housing facility. Make a list of ways that the OTP might work with Barry when he was unhoused and consider how the OTP's strategies and therapeutic interventions might shift (or stay the same) when Barry obtains housing. Review the story to find examples of how the OTP in this story engaged Barry in different spaces.

Resources

Books

• Hunter, C. L., Goodie, J. L., Oordt, M. S., & Dobmeyer, A. C. (2022). *Integrated behavioral health in primary care: Step-by-step guidance for assessment and intervention* (2nd ed.). American Psychological Association.

Organizations

• Agency for Healthcare Research and Quality (AHRQ) Academy—Integrating Behavioral Health & Primary Care: https://integrationacademy.ahrq.gov
This DHHS agency acts as a national resource and coordinating center for those interested in integrating behavioral health into primary care.

• Substance Abuse and Mental Health Services Administration (SAMHSA) National Center of Excellence for Integrated Health Solutions: https://www.samhsa.gov/national-coe-integrated -health-solutions
This DHHS agency leads public health efforts to advance the behavioral health of the nation.

• Rural Health Information Hub: Primary Care Behavioral Health Model: https://www.ruralhealthinfo.org/toolkits /services-integration/2/primary-care-behavioral-health
The Rural Health Information Hub, formerly the Rural Assistance Center, is funded by the Federal Office of Rural Health Policy to be a national clearinghouse on rural health issues.

• National Health Care for the Homeless Council: https://nhchc.org
The National Health Care for the Homeless Council is the premier national organization working at the nexus of homelessness and health care.

• AOTA's Homelessness Community of Practice: https://www .aota.org/community/communities-of-practice

This is one of several Communities of Practice hosted by AOTA to support networking and learning through a social environment.

References

Agency for Healthcare Research and Quality. (2015). *What is integrated behavioral health care?* https://integrationacademy.ahrq .gov/about/integrated-behavioral-health

Alegria, M., Frank, R. G., Hansen, H. B., Sharfstein, J. M., Shim, R. S., & Tierney, M. (2021). Commentary: Transforming mental health and addiction services. *Health Affairs, 40*(2), 226–234. https://doi.org/10.1377/hlthaff.2020.01472

Al-Heizan, M. O., Marks, T. S., Giles, G. M. & Edwards, D. F. (2022). Further validation of the menu task: Functional cognition screen for older adults. *OTJR: Occupational Therapy Journal of Research, 42*(4), 286–294. https://doi.org/10.1177/15394492221110546

American Occupational Therapy Association. (2012). *AOTA fact sheet on ACOs/medical homes.* http://www.aota.org/Advocacy -Policy/Health-Care-Reform.aspx

American Occupational Therapy Association. (2014). The role of occupational therapy in primary care. *American Journal of Occupational Therapy, 68,* 525–533. https://doi.org/10.5014 /ajot.2014.686S06

American Occupational Therapy Association. (2020a). Occupational therapy in the promotion of health and well-being. *American Journal of Occupational Therapy, 74,* 7403420010. https:// doi.org/10.5014/ajot.2020.743003

American Occupational Therapy Association. (2020b). Role of occupational therapy in primary care. *American Journal of Occupational Therapy, 74*(Suppl. 3), 7413410040. https://doi .org/10.5014/ajot.2020.74S3001

American Occupational Therapy Association. (2022). Occupational therapy's role in chronic conditions. *American Journal of Occupational Therapy, 74*(Suppl. 3), 7613410220. https://doi.org/10.5014/ajot.2022.76S3003

American Psychiatric Association. (2022). *Diagnostic and statistical manual of mental disorders* (5th ed., text rev.). American Psychiatric Publishing. https://doi.org/10.1176/appi.books.9780890425787

American Psychological Association. (2020). *Stress in America 2020: A national mental health crisis.* https://www.apa.org/news/press/releases/stress/2020/report-october

American Public Health Association. (2014). *Support for community health worker leadership in determining workforce standards for training and credentialing.* https://www.apha.org/policies-and-advocacy/public-health-policy-statements/policy-database/2015/01/28/14/15/support-for-community-health-worker-leadership

American Public Health Association. (2017). *Community health workers.* https://www.apha.org/apha-communities/member-sections/community-health-workers

Arias, D., Saxena, S., & Verguet, S. (2022). Quantifying the global burden of mental disorders and their economic value. *EClinicalMedicine, 54,* 101675. https://doi.org/10.1016/j.eclinm.2022.101675

Association of State and Territorial Health Officials. (2022, June). *State approaches to community health worker certification.* https://www.astho.org/topic/brief/state-approaches-to-community-health-worker-certification

Auxier, A., Runyan, C., Mullin, D., Mendenhall, T., Young, J., & Kesler, R. (2012). Behavioral health referrals and treatment initiation rates in integrated primary care: A Collaborative Care Research Network study. *Translational Behavioral Medicine, 2*(3), 337–344. https://doi.org/10.1007/s13142-012-0141-8

Bagalman, E., Dey, J., Jacobus-Kantor, L., Stoller, B., West, K. D., Radel, L., Schreier, A., Rousseau, M., Blanco, M., Creedon, T. B., Nye, E., Ali, M. M., Dubenitz, J. M., Schwartz, D., White, J. O., Swenson-O'Brien, A. J., Oberlander, S., Burnszynski, J., Lynch-Smith, M., . . . Haffajee, R. L. (2022, September 14). *HHS Roadmap for Behavioral Health Integration* (Issue Brief). Office of the Assistant Secretary for Planning and Evaluation, U.S. Department of Health and Human Services.

Bahorik, A. L., Satre, D. D., Kline-Simon, A. H., Weisner, C. M., & Campbell, C. I. (2017). Serious mental illness and medical comorbidities: Findings from an integrated health care system. *Journal of Psychosomatic Research, 100,* 35–45. https://doi.org/10.1016/j.jpsychores.2017.07.004

Bartels, S., & Desilets, R. (2012). *Health promotion programs for people with serious mental illness* (Prepared by the Dartmouth Health Promotion Research Team). SAMHSA-HRSA Center for Integrated Health Solutions.

Boersma, P., Black, L. I., & Ward, B. W. (2020). Prevalence of multiple chronic conditions among U.S. adults, 2018. *Preventing Chronic Disease, 17,* 200130. https://doi.org/10.5888/pcd17.200130

Bolt, M., Ikking, T., Baaijen, R., & Saenger, S. (2019). Occupational therapy and primary care. *Primary Health Care Research & Development, 20*(e27), 1–6. https://doi.org/10.1017/S1463423618000452

Boone, A. E., Henderson, W. L., & Dunn, W. (2022). Screening tools: They're so quick! What's the issue? *American Journal of Occupational Therapy, 76*(2), 7602347010. https://doi.org/10.5014/ajot.2022.049331

Brekke, J. S., Kelly, E., Duana, L., Cohen, H., Kiger, H., & Pancake, L. (2019). *Can people who have experience with serious mental illness help peers manage their health care?* Patient-Centered Outcomes Research Institute. https://doi.org/10.25302/4.2019.AD.13046650

Brekke, J. S., Siantz, E., Pahwa, R., Kelly, E., Tallne, L., & Fulginiti, A. (2013). Reducing health disparities for people with serious mental illness: Development and feasibility of a Peer Health Navigation intervention. *Best Practices in Mental Health, 9*(1), 62–82.

Brown, C., Cook, J. A., Jonikas, J. A., Steigman, P. J., Burke-Miller, J., Hamilton, M. M., Rosen, C., Tessman, D. C., & Santos, A. (2023). Nutrition and Exercise for Wellness and Recovery: A randomized controlled trial of a community-based health intervention. *Psychiatric Services, 74*(5), 463–471. https://doi.org/10.1176/appi.ps.202200038

Brown, C., Goetz, J., & Bledsoe, C. (2011a). *Nutrition and Exercise for Wellness and Recovery (NEW-R) leader manual.* https://www.cmhsrp.uic.edu/download/NEW-R%20Leader%20Manual%20for%20Web%20Posting_May%202017.pdf

Brown, C., Goetz, J., & Bledsoe, C. (2011b). *Nutrition and Exercise for Wellness and Recovery (NEW-R) participant manual.* https://www.cmhsrp.uic.edu/download/WeightWellnessParticipantManual.pdf

Brown, C., Goetz, J., Sciver, A. V., Sullivan, D., & Hamera, E. (2006). A psychiatric rehabilitation approach to weight loss. *Psychiatric Rehabilitation Journal, 29*(4), 267–273. https://doi.org/10.2975/29.2006.267.273

Brown, C., Read, H., Stanton, M., Zeeb, M., Jonikas, J. A., & Cook, J. A. (2015). A pilot study of the Nutrition and Exercise for Wellness and Recovery (NEW-R): A weight loss program for individuals with serious mental illnesses. *Psychiatric Rehabilitation Journal, 38*(4), 371–373. https://doi.org/10.1037/prj0000115

Brown, J., Breslau, J., Wishon, A., Miller, R., Kase, C., Dunbar, M., Stewart, K., Briscombe, B., Rose, T., Dehus, E., & DeWitt, K. (2021). *Implementation and impacts of the Certified Community Behavioral Health Clinic demonstration: Findings form the national evaluation* (Final report). Mathematica.

Butler, M., Kane, R. L., McAlpine, D., Kathol, R., Fu, S. S., Hagedorn, H., & Wilt, T. (2011). Does integrated care improve treatment for depression? A systematic review. *The Journal of Ambulatory Care Management, 34*(2), 113–125. https://doi.org/10.1097/JAC.0b013e31820ef605

Calderon, C., Balague, L., Cortada, J., & Sanchez, A. (2011). Health promotion in primary care: How should we intervene? A qualitative study involving both physicians and patients. *BMC Health Services Research, 11*(1), 62. https://doi.org/10.1186/1472-6963-11-62

Center for Mental Health Services. (2007). *The 10 by 10 Campaign: A national plan to improve life expectancy by 10 years in 10 years for people with mental illness: A report of the 2007 National Wellness Summit.* Center for Mental Health Services, Substance Abuse and Mental Health Services Administration.

Centers for Medicare & Medicaid Services. (2023). *The Mental Health Parity and Addiction Equity Act.* https://www.cms.gov/marketplace/private-health-insurance/mental-health-parity-addiction-equity

Cheung, S., Spaeth-Rublee, B., Shalev, D., Li, M., Docherty, M., Levenson, J., & Pincus, H. A. (2019). A model to improve Behavioral Health Integration into serious illness care. *Journal of Pain and Symptom Management, 58*(3), 503–514. https://doi.org/10.1016/j.jpainsymman.2019.05.017

Clark, F., Azen, S. P., Zemke, R., Jackson, J., Carlson, M., Mandel, D., Hay, J., Josephson, K., Cherry, B., Hessle, C., Palmer, J., & Lipson, L. (1997). Occupational therapy for independent-living older adults: A randomized controlled trial. *Journal of the American Medical Association, 278*(16), 1321–1326. https://doi.org/10.1001/jama.1997.03550160041036

Clark, F., Blanchard, J., Sleight, A., Cogan, A., Florindez, L., Gleason, S., Heymann, R., Hill, V., Holden, A., Murphy, M., Proffitt, R., Schepens-Niemiec, S., & Vigen, C. (2015). *Lifestyle Redesign: The intervention tested in the USC well elderly studies* (2nd ed.). AOTA Press.

Coffinbargar, M., Damian, A. J., & Westfall, J. M. (2022). *Risks and benefits to community health care worker certification.* Health Affairs. https://www.healthaffairs.org/do/10.1377/forefront.20220705.856203

Collins, C., Hewson, D. L., Munger, R., & Wade, T. (2010). *Evolving models of Behavioral Health Integration in primary care.* Milbank Memorial Fund.

Commonwealth Fund. (2022). *Integrating primary care and behavioral health to address the behavioral health crisis.* https://www.commonwealthfund.org/publications/explainer/2022/sep/integrating-primary-care-behavioral-health-address-crisis

Congressional Budget Office. (2013). *CBO's February 2013 estimate of the effects of the Affordable Care Act on health insurance coverage.* https://www.cbo.gov/sites/default/files/recurringdata/51298-2013-02-aca.pdf

Cutler, R. L., Fernandez-Llimos, F., Frommer, M., Benrimoj, C., & Garcia-Cardenas, V. (2018). Economic impact of medication non-adherence by disease groups: A systematic review. *BMJ Open, 8*(1), e016982. https://doi.org/10.1136/bmjopen-2017-016982

Davidson, L., O'Connell, M., Tondora, J., Styron, T., & Kangas, K. (2006). The top ten concerns about recovery encountered in mental health system transformation. *Psychiatry Services, 57*(5), 640–645. https://doi.org/10.1176/appi.ps.57.5.640

Davidson, L., Tondora, J., Lawless, M., O'Connell, M., & Rowe, M. (2009). *A practical guide to recovery-oriented practice: Tools for transforming mental health care.* Oxford University Press.

Dickson, K. L., & Toto, P. E. (2018). Feasibility of integrating occupational therapy into a care coordination program for aging in place. *American Journal of Occupational Therapy, 72,* 7204195020. https://doi.org/10.5014/ajot.2018.031419

Donnelly, C., Brenchley, C., Crawford, C., & Letts, L. (2013). The integration of occupational therapy into primary care: A multiple case study design. *BMC Family Practice, 14*(1), 60. https://doi.org/10.1186/1471-2296-14-60

Drake, R. E., Mueser, K. T., Brunette, M. F., & McHugo, G. J. (2004). A review of treatments for people with severe mental illnesses and co-occurring substance use disorders. *Psychiatric Rehabilitation Journal, 27*(4), 360–374. https://doi.org/10.2975/27.2004.360.374

Drinka, T. J., & Clark, P. G. (2000). *Health care teamwork: Interdisciplinary practice and teaching.* Praeger.

Edwards, D. F., Wolf, T. J., Marks, T., Alter, S., Larkin, V., Padesky, B. L., Spiers, M., Al-Heizan, M. O., & Giles, G. M. (2019). Reliability and validity of a functional cognition screening tool to identify the need for occupational therapy. *American Journal of Occupational Therapy, 73,* 7302205050. https://doi.org/10.5014/ajot.2019.028753

Firth, J., Siddiqi, N., Koyanagi, A., Siskind, D., Rosenbaum, S., Galletly, C., Allan, S., Caneo, C., Carney, R., Carvalho, A. F., Chatterton, M. L., Correll, C. U., Curtis, J., Garghran, F., Heald, A., Hoare, E., Jackson, S., Kisely, S., Lovell, K., . . . Stubbs, B. (2019). The Lancet Psychiatry Commission: A blueprint for protecting physical health in people with mental illness. *Lancet Psychiatry, 6*(8), 675–712. https://doi.org/10.1016/S2215-0366(19)30132-4

Gerrity, M., Zoller, E., Pinson, N., Pettinari, C., & King, V. (2014). *Integrating primary care into behavioral health settings: What works for individuals with serious mental illness.* Milbank Memorial Fund. https://www.milbank.org/wp-content/uploads/2016/04/Integrating-Primary-Care-Report.pdf

Gilbody, S., Bower, P., & Whitty, P. (2006). Costs and consequences of enhanced primary care for depression. Systematic review of randomised economic evaluations. *The British Journal of Psychiatry, 189*(4), 297–308. https://doi.org/10.1192/bjp.bp.105.016006

Giles, G. M., Edwards, D. F., Baum, C., Furniss, J., Skidmore, E., Wolf, T., & Leland, N. E. (2020). Making functional cognition a professional priority. *American Journal of Occupational Therapy, 74,* 7401090010. https://doi.org/10.5014/ajot.2020.741002

Goodell, S. (2014). *Mental health parity.* Health Affairs. http://www.healthaffairs.org/healthpolicybriefs/brief.php?brief_id=112

Grandes, G., Sanchez, A., Cortada, J., Balague, L., Calderon, C., Arrazola, A., Vergara, I., & Millan, E. (2008). Is integration of healthy lifestyle promotion into primary care feasible? Discussion and consensus sessions between clinicians and researchers. *BMC Health Services Research, 8,* 213. https://doi.org/10.1186/1472-6963-8-213

Grazier, K. L., Smiley, M. L., & Bondalapati, K. S. (2016). Overcoming barriers to integrating behavioral health and primary care services. *Journal of Primary Care & Community Health, 7*(4), 242–248. https://doi.org/10.1177/2150131916656455

Halle, A. D., Mroz, T. M., Fogelberg, D. J., & Leland, N. E. (2018). Health policy perspectives—Occupational therapy and primary care: Updates and trends. *American Journal of Occupational Therapy, 72,* 7203090010. https://doi.org/10.5014/ajot.2018.723001

Healthcare.gov. (2014). *Primary care.* https://www.healthcare.gov/glossary/primary-care

Health Resources and Services Administration. (2014). *The Affordable Care Act and health centers.* http://bphc.hrsa.gov/about/healthcenterfactsheet.pdf

Health Resources and Services Administration. (2016). *Health centers and the Affordable Care Act fact sheet.* http://bphc.hrsa.gov/about/healthcenterfactsheet.pdf

Heath, B., Wise Romero, P., & Reynolds, K. A. (2013). *Standard frameworks for levels of integrated healthcare.* SAMHSA-HRSA Center for Integrated Health Solutions.

Hoff, A., Hughes-Reid, C., Sood, E., & Lines, M. (2020). Utilization of integrated and colocated behavioral health models in pediatric primary care. *Clinical Pediatrics, 59*(14), 1225–1232. https://doi.org/10.1177/0009922820942157

Hoge, M. A., Morris, J. A., Laraia, M., Pomerantz, A., & Farley, T. (2014). *Core competencies for integrated behavioral health and primary care.* SAMHSA-HRSA Center for Integrated Health Solutions.

Holmberg, V., & Ringsberg, K. C. (2014). Occupational therapists as contributors to health promotion. *Scandinavian Journal of Occupational Therapy, 21*(2), 82–89. https://doi.org/10.3109/11038128.2013.877069

Huang, H., Russo, J., Bauer, A. M., Chan, Y. F., Katon, W., Hogan, D., & Unützer, J. (2013). Depression care and treatment in a chronically ill Medicare population. *General Hospital Psychiatry, 35*(4), 382–386. https://doi.org/10.1016/j.genhosppsych.2013.02.006

Insel, T. R., Collins, P. Y., & Hyman, S. E. (2015). Darkness invisible: The hidden global costs of mental illness. *Foreign Affairs, 94,* 127–135.

Interorganizational Work Group on Competencies for Primary Care Psychology Practice. (2013). *Competencies for psychology practice in primary care.* http://www.apa.org/ed/resources/competencies-practice.pdf

Kathol, R. G., deGruy, F., & Rollman, B. L. (2014). Value-based financially sustainable behavioral health components in Patient-Centered Medical Homes. *Annals of Family Medicine, 12*(2), 172–175. https://doi.org/10.1370/afm.1619

Kathol, R. G., Patel, K., Sacks, L., Sargent, S., & Melek, S. P. (2015). The role of behavioral health services in accountable care organizations. *The American Journal of Managed Care, 21*(2), e95–e98.

Kelly, E., Duan, L., Cohen, H., Kiger, H., Pancake, L., & Brekke, J. (2017). Integrating behavioral healthcare for individuals with serious mental illness: A randomized controlled trial of a Peer Health Navigator intervention. *Schizophrenia Research, 182,* 135–141. https://doi.org/10.1016/j.schres.2016.10.031

Kelly, E., Fulginiti, A., Pahwa, R., Tallen, L., Duan, L., & Brekke, J. (2014). A pilot test of a peer navigator intervention for improving the health of individuals with serious mental illness. *Community Mental Health Journal, 50*(4), 435–446. https://doi.org/10.1007/s10597-013-9616-4

Kessler, R. (2012). Mental health care treatment initiation when mental health services are incorporated into primary care practice. *Journal of the American Board of Family Medicine, 25*(2), 255–259. https://doi.org/10.3122/jabfm.2012.02.100125

Koyangi, C. (2004). *Get it together: How to integrate physical and mental health care for people with serious mental disorders.* Bazelon Center for Mental Health Law.

Kroenke, K., Spitzer, R. L., & Williams, J. B. (2001). The PHQ-9: Validity of a brief depression severity measure. *Journal of General Internal Medicine, 16* (9), 606–613. https://doi.org/10.1046/j.1525-1497.2001.016009606.x

Krupa, T., Edgelow, M., Chen, S., & Mieras, C. (2021). *Promoting activity and participation in individuals with serious mental illness: The Action Over Inertia approach.* Routledge Taylor & Francis Group.

Lawn, S., Battersy, M., Linder, H., Mathews, R., Morris, S, Wells, L., Litt, J., & Reed, R. (2009). What skills do primary health care professionals need to provide effective self-management support? Seeking consumer perspectives. *Australian Journal of Primary Health, 15,* 37–44. https://doi.org/10.1071/PY08053

Lemak, C. H., Johnson, C., & Goodrick, E. E. (2004). Collaboration to improve services for the uninsured: Exploring the concept of health navigators as interorganizational integrators. *Health Care Management Review, 29*(3), 196–206. https://doi.org/10.1097/00004010-200407000-00005

Letts, L., Fraser, B., Finlayson, M., & Walls, J. (1993). *For the health of it: Occupational therapy within a health promotion framework.* CAOT Publications ACE.

Levin, C., & Chisholm, D. (2016). Cost-effectiveness and affordability of interventions, policies, and platforms for the prevention and treatment of mental, neurological, and substance use disorders. In V. Patel, D. Chisholm, T. Dua, R. Laxminarayan, & M. Medina-Mora (Eds.), *Disease control priorities: Mental, neurological, and substance use disorders* (3rd ed., pp. 219–236). World Bank. https://doi.org/10.1596/978-1-4648-0426-7_ch12

Liu, M., & Hwang, S. W. (2021). Health care for homeless people. *Nature Reviews Disease Primers, 7*(1), 5. https://doi.org/10.1038/s41572-020-00241-2

Manderscheid, R., Druss, B., & Freeman, E. (2008). Data to manage the mortality crisis. *International Journal of Mental Health, 37*(2), 49–68. https://doi.org/10.2753/IMH0020-7411370202

Mangurian, C., Schillingger, D., Newcomer, J. W., Vittinghoff, E., Essock, S., Zhu, Z., Dyer, W., Young-Wolff, K. C., & Scmittdiel, J. (2020). Comorbid diabetes and severe mental illness: Outcomes in an integrated health care delivery system. *Journal of General Internal Medicine, 35*(1), 160–166. https://doi.org/10.1007/s11606-019-05489-3

Manning, E., & Gagnon, M. (2017). The complex patient: A concept clarification. *Nursing & Health Sciences, 19,* 13–21. https://doi.org/10.1111/nhs.12320

Mauer, B. J., & Jarvis, D. (2010). *The business case for bidirectional integrated care: Mental health and substance use services in primary care settings and primary care services in specialty mental health and substance use settings.* California Institute of Mental Health.

McManus, A. (2013). Health promotion innovation in primary health care. *The Australasian Medical Journal, 6*(1), 15–18. https://doi.org/10.4066/amj.2013.1578

Melek, S. P. (2012). *Bending the Medicaid healthcare cost curve through financially sustainable medical-behavioral integration.* Milliman Research Report. Milliman. https://www.milliman.com/en/insight/bending-the-medicaid-healthcare-cost-curve-through-financially-sustainable-medical-behavio

Mercer, S. W., Gunn, J., Bower, P., Wyke, S., & Guthrie, B. (2012). Managing patients with mental and physical multi-morbidity. *British Medical Journal, 345,* e5559. https://doi.org/10.1136/bmj.e5559

Mistry, S. K., Harris, E., & Harris, M. (2021). Community health workers as healthcare navigators in primary care chronic disease management: A systematic review. *Journal of General Internal Medicine, 36,* 2755–2771. https://doi.org/10.1007/s11606-021-06667-y

Muir, S. (2012). Occupational therapy in primary health care: We should be there. *American Journal of Occupational Therapy, 66*(5), 506–510. https://doi.org/10.5014/ajot.2012.665001

Mulvaney-Day, N., Marshall, T., Piscopo, K. D., Korsen, N., Lynch, S., Kamell, L. H., Moran, G. E. Daniels, A. S., & Ghose, S. S. (2018). Screening for behavioral health conditions in primary care settings: A systematic review of the literature. *Journal of General Internal Medicine, 33*(3), 335–346. https://doi.org/10.1007/s11606-017-4181-0

National Center for Chronic Disease Prevention and Health Promotion. (2024). *About chronic diseases.* Centers for Disease Control and Prevention. https://www.cdc.gov/chronic-disease/about/index.html

National Center for Health Statistics. (2021). *National hospital ambulatory medical care survey: 2020 emergency department summary tables.* https://www.cdc.gov/nchs/data/nhamcs/web_tables/2020-nhamcs-ed-web-tables-508.pdf

National Council for Mental Wellbeing. (2023). *Center of excellence for integrated health solutions.* https://www.thenationalcouncil.org/program/center-of-excellence

Office of the Assistant Secretary for Planning and Evaluation. (2011). *Essential health benefits: Individual market coverage.* U.S. Department of Health and Human Services. http://aspe.hhs.gov/health/reports/2011/individualmarket/ib.shtml

Padwa, H., Guerrero, E. G., Braslow, J. T., & Fenwick, K. M. (2014). Barriers to serving clients with co-occurring disorders in a transformed mental health system. *Psychiatric Services, 66*(5), 547–550. https://doi.org/10.1176/appi.ps.201400190

Perez, A. (2014). Abstract W P293: Using smart phrases in an electronic medical record to document the plan of care and decision-making process during time sensitive acute ischemic stroke patient interventions. *Stroke, 45*(Suppl. 1), AWP293. https://doi.org/10.1161/str.45.suppl_1.wp293

Pestaina, K. (2022). *Mental health parity at a crossroads.* KFF Issue Brief. https://www.kff.org/private-insurance/issue-brief/mental-health-parity-at-a-crossroads .

Peterson, K., Anderson, J., Bourne, D., Charns, M. P., Gorin, S. S., Hynes, D. M., McDonald, K. M., Singer, S. J., & Yano, E. M. (2019). Health care coordination theoretical frameworks: A systematic scoping review to increase their understanding and use in practice. *Journal of General Internal Medicine, 34,* 90–98. https://doi.org/10.1007/s11606-019-04966-z

Prince, M., Patel, V., Saxena, S., Maj, M., Maselko, J., Phillips, M. R., & Rahman, A. (2007). No health without mental health. *The Lancet, 370*(9590), 859–877. https://doi.org/10.1016/s0140-6736(07)61238-0

Ramanuj, P., Ferenchik, E., Docherty, M., Spaeth-Rublee, B., & Pincus, H. A. (2019). Evolving models of integrated behavioral health and primary care. *Current Psychiatry Reports, 21*(1), 1–12. https://doi.org/10.1007/s11920-019-0985-4

Reiss-Brennan, B., Briot, P. C., Savits, L. A., Cannon, W., & Staheli, R. (2010). Cost and quality impact of Intermountains' Mental Health Integration Program. *Journal of Healthcare Management, 55*(2), 97–113. https://doi.org/10.1097/00115514-201003000-00006

Robinson, M., Fisher, T. F., & Broussard, K. (2016). Health policy perspectives—Role of occupational therapy in case management and care coordination for clients with complex conditions. *American Journal of Occupational Therapy, 70,* 7002090010p1–7002090010p6. https://doi.org/10.5014/ajot.2016.702001

Rosenthal, E. L., Menking, P., St. John, J., Fox, D., Holderby-Fox, L. R., Redondo, F., Hirsch, G., Lee, L., Brownstein, J. N., Allen, C., Haywood, C., Ortiz Miller, J., Ibarra, J., Cole, M., Huxley, L., Palmer, C., Masoud, S., Uriarte, J., & Rush, C. H. (2022). *The Community Health Worker Core Consensus (C3) Project reports and website.* Texas Tech University Health Sciences Center El Paso. https://www.c3project.org

Ross, K. M., Klein, B., Ferro, K., McQueeney, D. A., Gernon, R., & Miller, B. F. (2019). The cost effectiveness of embedding a behavioral health clinician into an existing primary care practice to facilitate the integration of care: A prospective, case–control program evaluation. *Journal of Clinical Psychology in Medical Settings, 26*(1), 59–67. https://doi.org/10.1007/s10880-018-9564-9

Rushmer, R., & Pallis, G. (2003). Inter-professional working: The wisdom of integrated working and the disaster of blurred boundaries. *Public Money & Management, 23*(1), 59–66. https://doi.org/10.1111/1467-9302.00342

Salih, M. H., & Landers, T. (2019, July). The concept analysis of stigma towards chronic illness patient. *Hospice & Palliative Medicine International Journal, 3*(4), 132–136. https://doi.org/10.15406/hpmij.2019.03.00166

Scharf, D. M., Eberhart, N. K., Schmidt, N., Vaughan, C. A., Dutta, T., Pincus, H. A., & Burnam, M. A. (2013). Integrating primary care into community behavioral health settings: Programs and early implementation experiences. *Psychiatric Services, 64*(7), 660–665. https://doi.org/10.1176/appi.ps.201200269

Smith-Carrier, T., & Neysmith, S. (2014). Analyzing the interprofessional working of a home-based primary care team. *Canadian Journal on Aging/La Revue canadienne du vieillissement, 33*(3), 271–284. https://doi.org/10.1017/S071498081400021X

Sokol, M. C., McGuigan, K. A., Verbrugge, R. R., & Epstein, R. S. (2005). Impact of medication adherence on hospitalization risk and healthcare cost. *Medical Care, 43*(6), 521–530. https://doi.org/10.1097/01.mlr.0000163641.86870.af

Substance Abuse and Mental Health Services Administration. (2010). *Integrated treatment for co-occurring disorders evidence-based practices (EBP) kit.* http://store.samhsa.gov/product/Integrated-Treatment-for-Co-Occurring-Disorders-Evidence-Based-Practices-EBP-KIT/SMA08-4367

Substance Abuse and Mental Health Services Administration. (2012). *Understanding health reform: Integrated care and why you should care.* http://www.acgov.org/board/district3/documents/2012-07-23UnderstandingHealthReform.pdf

Substance Abuse and Mental Health Services Administration. (2016). *Wellness initiative.* http://www.samhsa.gov/wellness-initiative

Substance Abuse and Mental Health Services Administration. (2022). *Key substance use and mental health indicators in the United States: Results from the 2021 National Survey on Drug Use and Health* (HHS Publication No. PEP22-07-01-005, NSDUH Series H-57). Center for Behavioral Health Statistics and Quality, Substance Abuse and Mental Health Services Administration. https://www.samhsa.gov/data/report/2021-nsduh-annual-national-report

Unutzer, J., Schoenbaum, M., Druss, B. G., & Kanton, W. J. (2009). Transforming mental health care at the interface with general medicine: Report for the president's commission. *Psychiatric Services, 57*(1), 37–47. https://doi.org/10.1176/appi.ps.57.1.37

U.S. Department of Health and Human Services. (1999). *Mental health: A report of the surgeon general.* U.S. Public Health Services.

U.S. Department of Health and Human Services. (2003). *The President's New Freedom Commission on Mental Health. Achieving the promise: Transforming mental health care in America.* Author.

U.S. Department of Health and Human Services. (2005). *Transforming mental health care in America—The Federal Action Agenda: First steps.* Author.

Walker, E. R., McGee, R. E, & Druss, B. G. (2015). Mortality in mental disorders and global disease burden implications: A systematic review and meta-analysis. *JAMA Psychiatry, 72* (4), 334–341. https://doi.org/10.1001/jamapsychiatry.2014.2502

Wells, K. J., Valverde, P., Ustjanauskas, A. E., Calhoun, E. A., & Risdendal, B. C. (2018). What are patient navigators doing, for whom and where? A national survey evaluating the types of services provided by patient navigators. *Patient Education and Counseling, 101*(2), 285–294. https://doi.org/10.1016/j.pec.2017.08.017

Whiteford, H. A., Ferrari, A. J., Degenhardt, L., Feigin, V., & Vos, T. (2015). The global burden of mental, neurological and substance use disorders: An analysis from the Global Burden of Disease Study 2010. *PloS One, 10*(2), e0116820. https://doi.org/10.1371/journal.pone.0116820

Wittchen, H. U., Muhlig, S., & Beesdo, K. (2022). Mental disorders in primary care. *Dialogues in Clinical Neuroscience, 5*(2), 115–128. https://doi.org/10.31887/DCNS.2003.5.2/huwittchen

World Health Organization. (1948). *Preamble to the Constitution of the World Health Organization* as adopted by the International Health Conference, New York, 19-22 June 1946; signed on 22 July 1946 by the representatives of 61 states (Official Records of the World Health Organization, no. 2, p. 100) and entered into force on 7 April 1948.

World Health Organization. (2004). *Promoting mental health: Concepts, emerging evidence, practice.* Author.

World Health Organization. (2007). *Mental health.* https://www.who.int/en/news-room/fact-sheets/detail/mental-health-strengthening-our-response

World Health Organization. (2010). *Measuring health and disability: Manual for WHO Disability Assessment Schedule* (WHODAS 2.0). Author.

World Health Organization. (2016). *Social determinants of health.* http://www.who.int/social_determinants/en

World Health Organization. (2021). *Stories of change in four countries* https://www.who.int/publications/i/item/9789240037229

World Health Organization. (2022). *World mental health report: Transforming mental health for all.* Author. https://iris.who.int/bitstream/handle/10665/356119/9789240049338-eng.pdf?sequence=1

World Health Organization & United Nations Children's Fund (UNICEF). (2018). *A vision for primary health care in the 21st century: Towards universal health coverage and the Sustainable Development Goals.* World Health Organization. https://iris.who.int/handle/10665/328065

Young, R. A., Bayles, B., Hill, J. H., Kumar, K. A., & Burge, S. (2014). Family physicians' opinions on the primary care documentation, coding, and billing system. *Family Medicine, 46*(5), 378–384.

Zikos, D., & Afolayan-Oloye, O. (2021). Association between depressive disorder and hospital outcomes of care for elderly hospitalized patients. *Ageing International, 48*, 180–193. https://doi.org/10.1007/s12126-021-09455-5

Elizabeth Martin, Emily Petersen, Gina Baker, and Jaime Phillip Muñoz

The global prevalence of mental health issues such as depression, anxiety, posttraumatic stress disorder (PTSD), and stress and sleep disorders is significant (National Alliance on Mental Illness [NAMI], 2023b). These problems increased during the recent COVID-19 pandemic (GBD 2019 Mental Health Collaborators, 2022; Nochaiwong et al., 2021). Individuals seeking mental health services do so from different providers in a variety of service environments. Different settings are designed to meet specific needs, such as managing an immediate mental health crisis, connecting people to specific resources, or supporting daily roles such as home management and employment. A person's mental health and well-being can wax and wane over time, requiring different support services at different times. Access to these services varies across rural, city, and state contexts and in different countries.

This chapter describes occupational therapy's role in mental health settings across a continuum of care. It begins by presenting a continuum of mental wellness to mental illness that emphasizes the perspective that each person's mental health is unique and impacted greatly by their individual states of being and their social and physical contexts. This chapter explores the distinct role of occupational therapy in meeting mental health needs across this continuum. It discusses contextual features of various points of service, including hospital-based crisis management and behavioral health service and a range of community-based services and settings. Occupational therapy processes for evaluation and intervention are also described.

This chapter describes a continuum of mental health settings from a U.S. perspective. In other countries, settings where practitioners work will vary. However, both in the United States and internationally, there is strong evidence that most people who need mental health services lack access, face pervasive stigma, and live in places where the infrastructure for mental health service delivery is often limited or fragmented (Wainberg et al., 2017; World Health Organization [WHO], 2022). Occupational therapy practitioners (OTPs) have the knowledge and skill sets to step into existing positions in mental health settings and to create new opportunities.

Continuum of Mental Health and Wellness to Mental Illness

Chapter 1: Occupational Therapy Practice Across the Mental Health Continuum 🤝 presented a continuum of mental health using an image of a ruler. Figure 35-1 reflects this

same concept. On one end of this continuum, a person is in crisis experiencing symptoms of mental illness and difficulties functioning in daily life. On the other end, a person is excelling, participating, and flourishing. In between these two points, people demonstrate varying degrees of positive affect, social and occupational functioning, and capacity for adaptation and coping with the challenges of life. Because of the dynamic nature of mental health in a person's life, OTPs tune into and address the mental health needs of individuals in a variety of practice settings.

This mental health continuum is dynamic. Throughout life, every person may find themselves at different points on this continuum. The characteristics of mental health or mental illness one presents can be effectively addressed by setting and services that are designed to address specific levels of mental health needs. For example, a person who is suicidal is in crisis, struggling, and has likely really disengaged from life. Individuals on this end of the continuum may seek help through psychiatric inpatient hospitalization, where a key focus is providing a setting where they can be safe and receive needed supports. The focus shifts from managing the crisis to facilitating meaningful living with mental illness when a person is in a surviving mode and becoming unwell. At this point, intensive 24/7 intervention may not be needed, but effective supports can help move the person along the continuum from surviving to thriving, a stage of recovery that reflects more positive mental health.

These supports and interventions are typically provided in community mental health arenas. In these settings, the key focus is supporting the person's reintegration into everyday living, enhancing quality of life through meaningful occupations, and managing symptoms in a way that promotes mental health and supports personal recovery. Services are often less intense and support engagement in valued daily life roles and community participation. See Chapter 1: Occupational Therapy Practice Across the Mental Health Continuum. 🤝

The idea of a mental health continuum reminds practitioners that recovery is not a linear process. Each person's lived experience of mental health is unique and can fluctuate. The care settings highlighted in this chapter illustrate the different environments that exist to support individuals across the mental health continuum. Differences within and across settings can include how or where care is received, the specific services offered, the intensity of programming, and funding and payor sources. Ernie Mathis shares some of his lived experiences and demonstrates how a person can move through the continuum of care in mental health and access different support services depending on the need, and

Continuum of Care in Mental Health

Crisis	Struggling	Surviving	Thriving	Excelling
• Very anxious • Severely depressed • Detached from reality • Safety concerns • Poor sleep • Decreased ADLs • Getting through the day-to-day is taxing • Disengaged • Numb	• Anxious • Depressed • Tired • Safety risks still may be present • Poor sleep and low appetite • Decreased ADLs • Heavy • Slow • Engagement is a struggle	• Worried/nervous • Sad • Irritable • Distracted • Withdrawn • Difficulty with engagement with ADLs, IADLs, and meaningful occupations • Barriers with lifestyle balance	• Positive • Calm • Sleeping and eating well • Acceptance • Meaning in narrative, roles, and occupations • Purpose • Commitment to recovery • Social connections	• Cheerful • Connected to self, others, and environments of choice • Focused attention • Meaning in doing • Balance between enjoyment and mundane stressors • Enjoyment in everyday life

FIGURE 35-1. Continuum of care in mental health. *Adapted from Delphis. (2020, June 30). The mental health continuum is a better model for mental health. https://delphis.org.uk/mental-health/continuum-mental-health; Merryman, M. B., & Riegel, S. K. (2007). The recovery process and people with serious mental illness living in the community: An occupational therapy perspective.* Occupational Therapy in Mental Health, *23(2), 51–73. https://doi.org/10.1300/J004v23n02_03; Spaniol, L., & Wewiorski, N. J. (2012). Phases of the recovery process from psychiatric disabilities.* International Journal of Psychosocial Rehabilitation, *17(1); Sutton, D. J., Hocking, C. S., & Smythe, L. A. (2012). A phenomenological study of occupational engagement in recovery from mental illness.* Canadian Journal of Occupational Therapy, *79(3), 142–150. https://doi.org/10.2182/cjot.2012.79.3.3*

availability, of services. After reading Ernie's story on the next page, consider the following questions:

- What points on the continuum did Ernie move through (i.e., crisis, struggling, surviving, thriving, excelling)? Explain your answer to a peer.
- What specific mental health services did he access at different stages of recovery?
- How did these services support him to move through the recovery journey?

As readers learn about specific supports within the continuum of mental health care, come back to Ernie's story and ask, "How well did the settings Ernie lived in match the intensity of the mental health challenges he was experiencing at the time? Explain." Ernie will be referred to throughout the text to support readers' therapeutic reasoning about occupational therapy care within different mental health settings.

Hospital Settings

Individuals needing inpatient hospitalization are often experiencing a level of psychiatric symptomatology that can be overwhelming. In addition, safety concerns for the person or others can be substantial. On the continuum, these individuals are in crisis or struggling. Inpatient hospital settings are designed to meet the needs of individuals at risk of harming themselves or others. Many states use the words **gravely disabled** as a legal term to reflect functional status that can permit involuntary hospitalization (Mental Health America [MHA], 2023). Additionally, because of the state of mental health care in the United States, hospitalization often occurs because of the complex interaction between social determinants of health and mental illness (e.g., access to appropriate mental health care, basic needs). Crisis mental health interventions may be delivered by a variety of providers in different hospital settings such as an acute care unit on a medical floor, an inpatient psychiatric hospital, or a long-term residential care setting.

Acute Care and Medical Stabilization

The primary mission of the acute care setting is to save lives and medically stabilize the individual so they can begin their mental health recovery (Centers for Disease Control and Prevention [CDC], 2022). Acute care hospitals often have psychiatric departments located within the same building that are intended to treat individuals once medically stabilized. In the United States, the COVID-19 pandemic made glaringly apparent the challenge of providing care in acute settings given that the number of psychiatric hospital beds has steadily declined for more than 50 years (McBain et al., 2022). The combined death rates associated with alcohol, substance use disorders, and suicide increased by approximately 20% in 2020 during the COVID-19 pandemic, making it the highest year for substance use–related deaths (Trust for America's Health, 2020).

During the COVID-19 pandemic, visits to the emergency department (ED) increased by 31% for adolescents (NAMI, 2023a, 2023d), and hospitalizations for suicide attempt or self-injury rose by nearly 50% for adolescent girls (Zima et al., 2022). In the current U.S. health-care system, medical and mental health-care needs are frequently treated separately, often in different locations and with limited interdisciplinary engagement (Knickman & Elbel, 2019). Differences between medically focused and behavioral health-care–focused

The Lived Experience

Ernie Mathis

Growing up I had mood swings. It seemed as if I was angry most of the time. I had a quick temper and got into a lot of fights. My mood swings and temper caused a lot of difficulty in school. I ended up dropping out and going to work during my sophomore year. Eventually I got tired of working menial jobs so I went back and got my GED. I graduated in the top 2% in the state and was even asked to read my essay at the graduation ceremony. Still, during that time I had difficulty holding jobs. Sometimes it was my temper. Sometimes I wouldn't sleep for 4 days straight, and then I would crash for 2 days and miss work.

In 2007, my father passed away and I did not know how to cope. I got pretty depressed and angry at the world. I went to the hospital for help. The first time I was admitted I remember feeling trapped and alone. The staff took everything away from me, even my clothes, for several days until they felt I was safe to have them back. They took me into a padded room and made me take my clothes off to check my body for every tattoo, every little mark, scars, everything. I was so embarrassed. I was told I had to attend groups and they would lock my room door so I couldn't go in and lie down. I was told when to eat, when to sleep, and I had to ask for every little thing. I felt like a little kid again. I was in and out of hospitals for a while. Although it was embarrassing and I often felt like I was being treated like a child, I was able to talk to people and I was able to let stuff out that was bottled up inside me. It was in the hospital that I was diagnosed with bipolar disorder and the mood swings and anger started to make sense.

In 2008 my wife and I got a divorce. I had been in the hospital and no longer had a place to live. According to the hospital staff, my only real option was a nursing home. Living in a nursing home, you lose your freedom. Like the hospital, I was told when I could go out to smoke or when I could spend time with family. I was told what I could eat and what I was not allowed to eat. I shared a room with another guy and our rooms weren't locked. Some of the people that lived there would come into my space and take my things—my clothing, my DVDs, my toiletries, whatever they could find. The worst part of living in a nursing home was that they took my disability check and I lived off of $30.00 a month. I didn't think I would ever get out of there.

I was in the nursing home for about 5 years. In 2013 Thresholds (a community-based agency providing care and advocacy for people with psychiatric disabilities) came to the nursing home to tell us about a settlement in Illinois where we could get money to move out. I qualified for support through

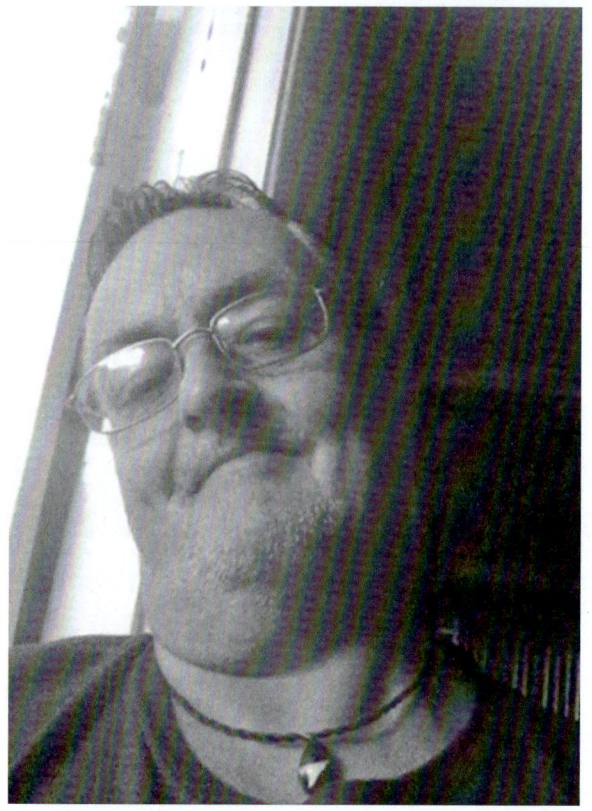

the ACT team so Thresholds offered me a chance to move out on my own. I got $2,000 to buy everything for my new apartment. The Thresholds ACT team helped me find and set up my apartment, shop for what I needed, and set up appointments with new doctors. They also helped me get on the right meds and helped me set up a system to make sure I have what I need to stay on them.

Now it's been almost 2 years on my own. I am grateful that I have staff I can talk to or call if I need something. Sometimes I get angry because I have to rely on them for transportation to doctor's appointments or support with a problem I can't do on my own and the staff doesn't always seem to find it as important as I do. I have become more independent in the last year. I now manage all my household needs. I recently remarried and my wife and I are working together to set up our home. I no longer need the ACT program and will be moving to the Thresholds' Community Support Team. The next step of being more independent is dealing with my own budget. I am working on that now and thank Thresholds for the opportunity!

service delivery models, highlighted in Table 35-1, further complicate health-care collaboration.

For OTPs, using a collaborative care model to support the physical and mental health needs of the individuals they serve is crucial. According to a Practice Analysis Executive Report in 2022 by the National Board for Certification in Occupational Therapy (NBCOT), only 3.1% of respondents

identified as working in mental health practice settings (NBCOT, 2022); however, few practitioners, regardless of practice setting, can say they have never provided occupational therapy services to individuals with psychiatric symptoms or a diagnosis. This indicates that every OTP has the potential to be considered a mental health clinician. In addition, occupational therapy services could bridge the gaps

TABLE 35-1	Medical Care Versus Behavioral Health-Care Settings
General/Medical Care Setting	**Psychiatric/Behavioral Care Setting**
• Hospitalization is disease focused.	• Providers apply a holistic approach in care.
• Care is provided in the individual's room.	• Environment encourages care in community spaces.
• Person is mostly encouraged to rest and remain in bed/room.	• Person is encouraged to limit time spent in room.
• Intervention is provided individually.	• Intervention is often provided in groups as well as individually.
• Medical equipment can pose safety risks.	• Safety risks are controlled and/or eliminated from environment.

between a medical and behavioral health model of care to support the needs of the whole individual. OTPs with behavioral health skills can support fellow clinicians working on medical floors through a care coordination model as described later in this chapter.

James Hill (he, him, his) works in an acute care hospital in the inpatient psychiatric unit in the suburbs of Chicago. His practice is described in his Practitioner Profile feature.

Inpatient Psychiatric Hospitalization

Inpatient mental health settings are structured, secure, and controlled environments that address the primary goals of crisis stabilization and safety and establishing aftercare services. The inpatient setting allows people to work through a crisis in a safe environment free from the everyday life stressors they were facing and provides opportunities for them to identify with others sharing similar problems, to understand their illness, and to begin treatment (MHA, 2023). In these settings, a person's fears and resistance are both acknowledged and challenged. Their mental health problems are framed as surmountable, and a vision of self-directed, mental health recovery is reinforced. Psychiatric treatment models and interventions commonly used during inpatient hospitalization may include medication management, psychotherapy, cognitive behavioral therapy (CBT), group therapy, and trauma therapy (McLean, 2023; NAMI, 2023a; Substance Abuse and Mental Health Services Administration [SAMHSA], 2021; Tyler et al., 2019).

Voluntary Versus Involuntary Admission

Criteria for admission to an inpatient setting can vary but typically the person is in crisis or at risk of self-harm or violence, has been stabilized in medical acute care, has a diagnosis of significant mental illness, or may not have other treatment options. Table 35-2 includes some of the terminology used when differentiating the criteria and processes for voluntary versus involuntary admission and for involuntary commitment.

Despite an individual's legal status, inpatient psychiatric hospitalization is often in a locked unit that is highly structured and contained to ensure the safety of the individual and staff. Inpatient hospitalization is a brief structured

intervention focused on transitioning the person into less restrictive care environments. From the moment a person comes into the hospital, the focus is on discharge and the follow-up care that will support the person as they continue their recovery. The average length of an inpatient psychiatric hospital stay is 3 to 10 days (Ruffalo, 2019). This evolution in the health-care system in combination with the emergent need for quality mental health services has resulted in a growing interest in evidence-based treatments. The recovery model, which emphasizes person-centered care and shared decision-making, has emerged as the gold standard for mental health care (Lyon, 2020).

Inpatient Hospital Environment

The inpatient environment includes spaces for individual and group treatment. Hospital rooms may be shared or private, and the unit is typically equipped with a large common room area often called the **dayroom**. Depending on the facility, other spaces on the unit may include group meeting rooms, a multipurpose room, a dining room and kitchen space, a sensory room, and/or an enclosed outdoor deck. Some hospitals have an area of containment for imminently dangerous behaviors, often called a seclusion or restraint room, although with the utilization of trauma-informed approaches, there is a strong movement in psychiatry to limit the use of these practices (Perers et al., 2022).

The behavioral health model of care is based on creating a **therapeutic milieu** that fosters participation and engagement as part of their recovery. The daily schedule can typically include individualized treatment, such as meetings with the treatment team or daily rounds, as well as interdisciplinary group therapy opportunities. Members of the treatment team may provide some foundational psychotherapy interventions, but it is very limited because of the time constraints and nature of the crisis episode during hospitalization. The interdisciplinary team provides awareness and education to identify stressors that lead to hospitalization and discharge planning for a safe transition back to the home/community.

Members of the Intervention Team

The composition of the intervention team in inpatient settings depends on the demographics of the population on the unit, regulatory or funding sources, and the intervention philosophy of the setting. The various members on the treatment team typically seen in an inpatient unit and some of the primary responsibilities of each team member are included in Table 35-3.

Specialized Treatment Hospitals or Units

Some inpatient hospitals or units are tailored to meet the specific needs of individuals based on the individual's age, diagnosis, or needs. Such settings may provide tailored interventions addressing substance use disorders, eating disorders, or dementia, or focused services for individuals with intellectual disabilities or older adults with neurocognitive disorders. For example, Sheppard Pratt Health System in Baltimore, Maryland (Sheppard Pratt, 2024), is a private hospital system

Practitioner Profile

Acute Inpatient Care

Contributed by James Hill, OTR/L (he, him, his), Linden Oaks Behavioral Health, Chicago, IL

Our team includes occupational, art, dance, music, and recreational therapists; psychiatrists; social workers; nurses; educators; and behavioral health technicians. Occupational therapy evaluates, then sets goals related to the person's occupational profile. We address psychological, cognitive, and sensory concerns impacting function in group and 1:1 sessions. Interventions are evidence-informed and guided by the Model of Human Occupation (MOHO), Person-Environment-Occupation (PEO) model, and ACT model. They include occupations such as arts, crafts, horticulture, and animal-assisted therapy (Figs. 35-2 and 35-3). We teach cognitive compensatory strategies and use verbal and experiential interventions to help people clarify values, or to promote greater awareness and acceptance of their circumstances.

Typically, I meet two to five new individuals daily to complete an initial interview, then gather information about their interests, routines, roles, and relationships. We explore their concerns, goals for hospitalization, and strategies they've found helpful in the past. I run two to three groups daily, often on different units, with different populations. I may have two to three individual

sessions to provide resources, such as reading materials or a weighted blanket, to assess functional cognition or sensory sensitivities, or to address concerns such as chronic pain, sleep hygiene, or routine planning. All interactions are documented.

My day often includes meetings, program development, or educating fieldwork students. I often present at conferences and universities and enjoy presenting to other professionals or to the public, usually related to my expertise with mindfulness-based cognitive behavioral approaches. A challenge of work in this setting is working in a culture where some don't understand or value occupational therapy. Despite this, I find it meaningful and fulfilling to witness transformative moments of hope or inspiration, and the process of facilitating such experiences never gets old.

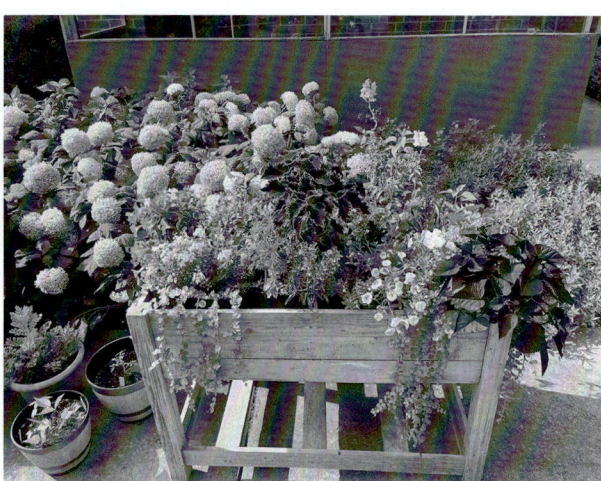

FIGURE 35-2. Horticulture is an occupation that can be used in many ways to regulate mood, promote social interaction, develop interests and routines, and cultivate a sense of purpose and meaning.

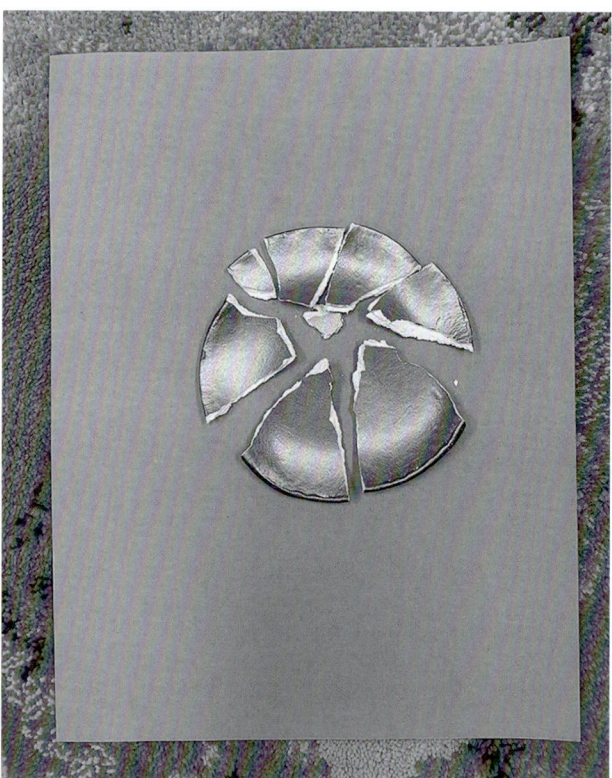

FIGURE 35-3. Creative arts occupations such as the kintsugi clay work pictured here can be used as a metaphor to help people explore themes such as brokenness, acceptance, and recovery.

that has specialized inpatient hospital programs subdivided by life stage (i.e., child, adolescent, young adult, adult, geriatric) or disability (crisis stabilization, eating disorder, psychotic disorder, co-occurring disorders, etc.). Although all programs share the basic inpatient hospitalization goals of safety, education, motivation, and transition, there are additional goals specific to the needs of these specific populations.

Specialty units often have additional staff for particular needs. For example, programs that serve people with

dementia employ team members who are specially trained in personal care techniques and provide activities of daily living (ADL) care, feeding, and other such needs. Dietitians are integral team members on units treating people with eating disorders. Many programs also include staff who care for spiritual needs, psychologists who provide psychiatric or neuropsychiatric testing, or volunteer opportunities for peer support personnel who may lead Alcoholics Anonymous (AA) or NAMI groups.

TABLE 35-2 | Admissions Terminology

Term	Definition
Voluntary Admission	Individual voluntarily signs legal paperwork for hospital admission.
Criteria for Involuntary Admission	*Danger to self (DTS):* The individual demonstrates intent and likelihood to harm themselves. *Danger to others (DTO):* The individual demonstrates intent and likelihood of inflicting harm to others. *Gravely disabled (GD):* The individual is unable to formulate a plan for their basic needs (food, clothing, and shelter) because of their mental illness.
Involuntary Admission Processes	Individual is in an emergency requiring hospitalization and is not willing or able to consent to treatment. *Emergency custody and evaluation:* Person is involuntarily held while a hospital team evaluates their need for treatment. Typically, this lasts 72 hours, but varies by state. *Right to appeal:* After the initial hold expires, a person can appeal any decision to continue involuntary hospitalization. This often involves going before a judge. *Outcome of appeal:* In some cases, there is a determination that the person does not meet criteria for admission and can be discharged if they do not want to sign in voluntarily. In other cases, the hold is justified, and the person is involuntarily committed to mental health treatment.
Involuntary Commitment	This involves court-ordered treatment in an inpatient or outpatient setting. A person's need for hospitalization is typically reevaluated at 14 days but may be up to 30 days. For individuals determined to be high risk for danger to others, there are lengthier legal psychiatric hold options available. *Right to refuse treatment:* Even when involuntarily admitted, the individual still has the right to refuse medications or certain treatment options, such as electroconvulsive therapy (ECT). *Reviews and patient advocates:* Some local departments of mental health may review legal holds to certify they are justified. Some also offer "patient advocates" to guarantee the person's rights are upheld during involuntary hospitalization.

TABLE 35-3 | Responsibilities of Interdisciplinary Team Members

Team Member/Discipline	Primary Role and Responsibilities
Doctor: Psychiatrists, medical doctors, psychologists (PhD or PsyD), physician assistants (PA), residents, and/or medical students	Diagnoses and manages psychiatric/medical conditions or symptoms, provides patient education and therapeutic interventions, manages medication, and guides the treatment team decisions.
Nurses: Registered nurse (RN), nurse practitioner (NP), licensed vocational nurse (LVN)	Administers medication, monitors positive or negative medication effects, and provides education. Expected to be routinely available to meet individual needs, provide therapeutic support, and address any medical needs. In some circumstances, an NP may direct and manage the individual's care.
Social worker or other licensed counselor: Social worker (MSW or LCSW), marriage and family therapist (LMFT), other licensed therapist/counselors	Provides family intervention, processes group therapy, and provides placement and referral support.
Therapy: Occupational therapy, recreation therapy (RT), music therapy, art therapy, pet therapy, and so on.	Each discipline has its own domain and therapeutic role. Practitioners provide various therapeutic activities that may focus on providing structure and routine, engagement in activities, socialization with others, opportunities for therapeutic self-expression, and movement.
Mental health workers: Mental health practitioners (MHPs), psychiatric technicians, and additional staff	Provides structure on the unit, helps with meals and daily scheduled activities, and leads educational groups.

Occupational Therapy in Inpatient Settings

Occupational therapy is a vital member of the inpatient interdisciplinary team. The history of occupational therapy has strong roots in the arts and crafts movement. These types of activities continue to be an effective way to observe an individual's functional cognition, including sequencing, planning, problem-solving, and the social-emotional components of engaging in a group with others. The OTP will work with the individual in a one-to-one or group setting to support them in their recovery process by collaborating with them

to identify their goals and empower them to participate in meaningful occupations (American Occupational Therapy Association [AOTA], 2016a).

Although the craft or task group may seem as if it is just an art group to the individual or other members on the treatment team, many intervention modalities can actually be targeted within this occupational therapy group. The treatment goals of occupational therapy directly align with the mental health recovery outcomes and WHO's promotion of mental health (AOTA, 2016b, 2017). The focus of treatment in inpatient care shifts as the individual moves along the recovery continuum. When admitted to an inpatient setting, individuals are often at the crisis or struggling end of the continuum,

TABLE 35-4 | Occupational Therapy Practitioner Focus Areas in an Inpatient Hospital Setting

Focus Area	Facilitating Occupations/Interventions
Evaluation to identify an individual's functional skills, cognition, strengths, and recovery goals	• Use strengths-based assessments. • Support autonomy and shared decision-making and identify goals that matter to the individual. • Explore character strengths and barriers (Niemiec & Pearce, 2021). • Build therapeutic rapport and use Motivational Interviewing to connect with the individual. • Employ Personal Recovery Outcome Measurement (PROM) to assist with measuring the individual's recovery needs (Barbic, 2015). • Survey interests, educate on meaningful occupations, and discuss and problem-solve barriers for engagement in interests. • Interview the individual and/or family and evaluate via observations during group or completion of occupation-based skills. • Monitor functional performance and changes in ability to complete occupation.
Independent living skills, ADLs, functional performance for day-to-day participation	• Promote ADL and IADL skills and participation in interventions. • Identify motivation and barriers for participation in everyday activities. • Utilize task analysis and break down or simplify the steps of the task.
Engagement in meaningful occupations	• Use data from occupational history to consider valued roles, habits, and routines. • Provide structure for engagement with the activity while on the unit. • Use simple tasks, such as crafts, to ground the individual with rhythmic occupations, increase attention to tasks, problem-solve, sequence, and so on (Leenerts et al., 2016; Merryman & Riegel, 2007). • Explore and educate on engagement in occupation and impact on recovery using occupational diary or activity reflection, such as the Occupational Experience Profile pre/post group (Atler & Berg, 2018; Bailliard et al., 2021). • Provide group skill building interventions on topics such as social behaviors, or problem-solving for community reintegration.
Exploration with personal narrative of mental illness	• Review the reasons for hospitalization and focus on occupations that were supporting/hindering their mental health symptoms. • Educate on diagnosis, symptoms, and understanding of illness; support autonomy in care; and engage person in discharge and referral decisions (Cheung et al., 2022). • Teach person to identify and use supports for managing symptoms to perform everyday occupations.
Coping skills for occupational performance	• Educate and practice coping skills to support function and occupational performance (AOTA, n.d.). • Support awareness of relationship between symptoms, triggers, feelings/interoception, and when to seek support. • Identify/provide referrals for available peer support networks including Wellness Recovery Action Plan (WRAP) groups (Advocates for Human Potential, 1995–2023). • Educate and practice CBT strategies to support occupational engagement (Tyler et al., 2019).
Environment and community considerations for discharge planning	• Frame expected discharge contexts using PEO or Person-Environment-Occupation Performance (PEOP) Models (Baum & Baptiste, 2002; Baum et al., 2015). • Utilize environmental assessments to explore triggers and barriers in the individual's environment and problem-solve before discharge (Lay et al., 2018; Schaub et al., 2018; Taylor et al., 2016). • Modify inpatient environment to support improved task completion. • Educate individual on recommended environmental modifications for their condition to support carryover into the community. • Educate/encourage person to assess social supports for community connectedness, access, resources, and safety. • Plan and practice problem-solving for community integration. • Engage in active discharge planning and exploration of appropriate community referrals (Duhig et al., 2017).

where day-to-day participation is difficult and the person may be only beginning to explore their own recovery narrative (Delphis, 2020; Spaniol & Wewiorski, 2012). OTPs meet the person where they are. Multiple ways that practitioners may intervene in inpatient hospital settings are included in Table 35-4.

Discharge From Inpatient Care

Discharge planning begins when an individual is admitted to the hospital and people can receive follow-up services in several ways. A variety of factors can influence the availability of and participation in follow-up services after discharge,

including the individual's motivation, their management of psychiatric symptoms, and their overall recovery. Personal and family resources, insurance coverage, and social determinants of health can also impact an individual's utilization of mental health services. The availability of services varies by location (i.e., urban vs. rural settings), and some settings may have specialized requirements based on the individual's diagnosis or their ability to participate in program activities.

A variety of discharge settings may be considered, such as the person's home or previous living situation, housing with family, a homeless shelter, a nursing home or residential care facility, a transitional housing program, an Assertive Community Treatment (ACT) program, or a home with

Evidence-Based Practice

Effective Occupational Therapy Approaches in Inpatient Settings

Occupational therapy services in inpatient settings should help people find ways to engage in occupations while an inpatient and after discharge.

RESEARCH FINDINGS

The length of stay in acute care and psychiatric inpatient settings is very short, so occupational therapy services in this setting include programs that focus on helping people find ways to engage and participate in occupations both within and when they leave the hospital setting. Research supports several approaches for OTPs in inpatient settings (Bailliard et al, 2021; Gallagher et al., 2023; Lipskaya-Velikovsky et al., 2016; Pereira et al., 2020; Synovec, 2015).

APPLICATIONS

➡ Implement a time-use diary tool and engage the person in occupational reflection on the structure of their day/habits by using the Occupational Experience Profile (OEP) during inpatient hospitalization.

➡ Use structured short-term interventions such as the Occupational Connections (OC) method to support community-based participation in daily living skills.

➡ Apply the Capabilities, Opportunities, Resources and Environments (CORE) approach, which defines strategies for promoting occupational engagement in acute behavioral health settings. This includes reviewing a person's barriers to participation through an inclusive lens, and practicing inclusive, occupation-based therapy.

➡ Apply practice-based inquiry with a Community of Practice Scholars (CoPS) to review the current occupation-based interventions in acute mental health settings to support individual and system-level change.

➡ Apply Recovery Model principles from the consumer perspective within short-term inpatient mental health hospitalization.

REFERENCES

Bailliard, A., Schafer, Z., & Hart, L. (2021). Occupational reflection as intervention in inpatient psychiatry. *The American Journal of Occupational Therapy, 75*(5), 7505205080. https://doi.org/10.5014/ajot.2021.043703

Gallagher, M., Bagatell, N., Godwin, K., & Peters, D. (2023). Using practice-based inquiry to enact occupation-centered, justice-oriented practice in an acute mental health setting. *The American Journal of Occupational Therapy, 77*(1), 7701205060. https://doi.org/10.5014/ajot.2023.050046

Lipskaya-Velikovsky, L., Kotler, M., & Krupa, T. (2016). Description of and preliminary findings for occupational connections, an intervention for inpatient psychiatry settings. *The American Journal of Occupational Therapy, 70*(6), 7006350010p1–7006350010p5. https://doi.org/10.5014/ajot.2016.014688

Pereira, R. B., Whiteford, G., Hyett, N., Weekes, G., Di Tommaso, A., & Naismith, J. (2020). Capabilities, Opportunities, Resources and Environments (CORE): Using the CORE approach for inclusive, occupation-centred practice. *Australian Occupational Therapy Journal, 67*, 162–171. https://doi.org/10.1111/1440-1630.12642

Synovec, C. E. (2015). Implementing recovery model principles as part of occupational therapy in inpatient psychiatric settings. *Occupational Therapy in Mental Health, 31*(1), 50–61. https://doi.org/10.1080/0164212X.2014.1001014

case management services. A critical determinant impacting discharge from the inpatient unit is the individual's capacity to safely return to their prehospitalization environment. The inpatient team will work with the individual to create a safety plan for discharge. This may include identifying triggers and social supports, defining activities or coping strategies to engage in when feeling overwhelmed, and education for the individual and their family on maintaining safety in the home by removing or locking up safety hazards. See Chapter 44: Addressing Suicide Across the Continuum. 🤝

Long-Term Care Facilities

Sometimes after a person is hospitalized in an inpatient unit, it is not safe for that person to return home. Long-term care facilities offer specialized, person-centered intervention within a 24/7 supervised setting for extended lengths of stay (NAMI, 2023c). For some, such as Ernie from this chapter's The Lived Experience feature, a long-term care facility may be needed to maintain safety or provide a stable living option. Long-term care facilities may have different names or specialized services, often based on the services offered or location, and include residential treatment centers (RTC), specialized skilled nursing facilities (SNF), or an institution for mental disease (California Department of Developmental Services, 2023). The purpose of these facilities is to provide a longer continuity of care and services for individuals while maintaining living in a restricted environment (NAMI, 2023c). Occupational therapy services in long-term care facilities may or may not be offered depending on the type of facility, state or local standards, and payor funding. See Chapter 41: State Hospitals.

Partial Hospitalization Programs and Intensive Outpatient Programs

Partial hospitalization programs (PHPs) and intensive outpatient programs (IOPs) are structured outpatient psychiatric services that are not physically located in a hospital setting, but they might be directly connected with psychiatric hospital. Similar to inpatient hospital settings, PHPs and IOPs provide structured mental health treatment, albeit with a reduction in the level of structure and care found in inpatient hospitals. These programs allow the individual to return to their living situation at the end of the program day. Typically, the person is cognitively and emotionally able to participate in therapy despite having a psychiatric condition that impacts their ability to participate fully in social, vocational, educational, and daily living occupations.

The focus of these programs is to provide the individual with a gradual stepdown of care to support recovery within the continuum from inpatient to community integration. These settings support transition with graded exposure to risks that exist within the home and community while still offering a supportive therapeutic environment. This is an appropriate intervention setting for individuals between struggling and thriving on the continuum, depending on their ability to maintain safety in a less restrictive environment.

Typically, PHPs function Monday through Friday for an average of 6 hours a day, whereas IOPs operate Monday through Friday for an average of 3 hours a day (Association for Ambulatory Behavioral Healthcare, n.d.). It is common for an individual to begin in the PHP and step down to the IOP as they progress through their recovery. In most cases, the only difference between a PHP and an IOP is the length of time a person spends at the facility; however, this difference can be important, especially for the person who needs the opportunity for longer, more frequent interventions to support their recovery. Whether a person participates in a PHP or IOP is often determined by their level of insurance coverage, availability of programs, space in a program in their geographic area, and life demands (e.g., work, parenting).

Similar to specialized care units, many PHPs and IOPs have different features to meet the needs of the individuals they serve. For example, at the Stewart and Lynda Resnick Neuropsychiatric Hospital at UCLA, there are PHPs and IOPs for individuals based on age, such as child, adolescent, and adult, as well as others focused on the needs of people with specific diagnoses, such as autism spectrum disorder (ASD), obsessive-compulsive disorder (OCD), perinatal care, and dual diagnosis for co-occurring mental health conditions and addiction (UCLA Health, 2023). Abigail Plotkin Kleiman describes her experience working in a PHP as the only OTP in her Practitioner Profile feature. Figures 35-4, 35-5, and 35-6 illustrate interventions from this setting. Depending on their recovery process, most people in PHPs and IOPs are encouraged to choose the days and hours of the program that most effectively address their needs.

The primary mission of PHPs and IOPs is both consistent with and extends inpatient care by addressing medication titration, education, and support for recovery. PHP/IOP settings typically offer far more therapeutic groups than an inpatient setting. The day is built on a schedule of back-to-back therapeutic groups, with less one-to-one contact with providers. Groups may provide psychotherapy, education, skill building, coping skills, symptom management, community transition, or recovery. This setting allows people to practice new skills and take supported risks in their natural living environment or home that are important in their continued recovery.

The treatment team consists of many of the same disciplines found in inpatient settings. Physicians often meet with participants weekly for medication management. Psychiatric nurses typically do not distribute medication, but do monitor vital responses to medication changes, provide education both individually and in groups, and assist with overall health needs. Social workers, counselors, and occupational, recreational, and expressive therapists lead group therapies. Depending on the location and insurance coverage, practitioners may be limited in the number of services they can bill in a PHP/IOP setting.

Community Mental Health

OTPs work in a variety of community mental health settings. Community mental health (a) encompasses a population approach; (b) views the individual in socioeconomic context; (c) practices individual as well as population-based prevention; (d) employs a systemic view of service provision; (e) advocates for open access to services; (f) provides team-based services; (g) takes a long-term, longitudinal, life-course perspective; and (h) is often a cost-effective, population-focused approach (Thornicroft et al., 2016).

An OTP can practice in various community settings and supports a person through each of the stages of the mental health continuum, depending on a person's needs and presentation at evaluation. An overarching goal of a community-based practitioner is to support a person's self-defined level of community integration and to promote recovery. Some common approaches used in the community include community case management, ACT, and psychosocial rehabilitation; these are used in a range of settings that can include psychosocial clubhouses, community mental health centers, group homes, and increasingly, social entrepreneurship or private mental health practice. Each approach and setting has unique benefits and challenges. The next section highlights some more universal approaches used in

Practitioner Profile

Adult Partial Hospitalization Program

Abigail N. Plotkin Kleiman, MS, OTR/L (she, her)

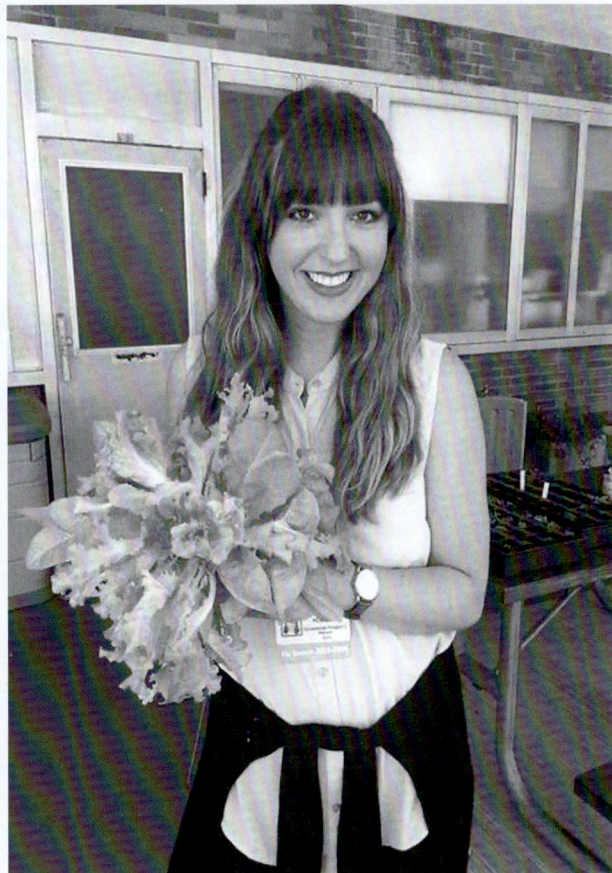

FIGURE 35-4. Abigail holding edible greens participants grew at the partial hospitalization program.

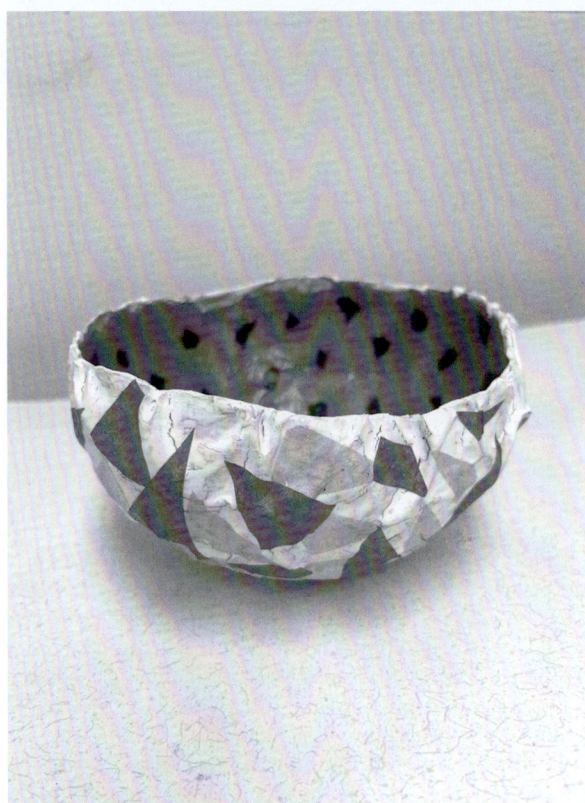

FIGURE 35-5. This paper maché bowl helped a person to improve their frustration tolerance and embrace imperfections.

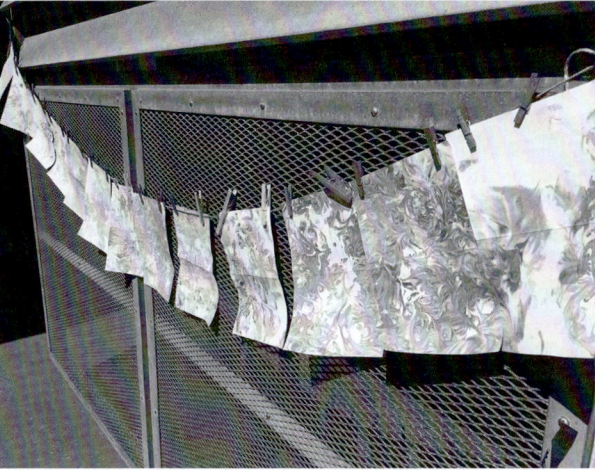

FIGURE 35-6. These marble papers were made with shaving cream and watercolors, encouraging a playful, open-ended sensory experience and promoting mental flexibility.

I work as an occupational therapist at an Adult Partial Hospital Program (PHP) in Los Angeles. Our program runs daily from 9:00 to 3:00. People who attend participate in different groups each hour of the day led by social workers and me. I see a variety of individuals with diagnoses that may include major depression, bipolar disorder, anxiety disorder, psychosis, or borderline personality disorder (and more). Our program also benefits individuals who have attempted suicide or struggle with suicidal ideation and/or self-harm. Most, but not all, were hospitalized in a psychiatric inpatient unit before coming to PHP. The PHP is part of their aftercare plan as they transition back into their lives outside of the hospital.

During my initial assessment, I complete an informal, narrative interview to learn what an individual is hoping to work on. I help them connect occupational therapy treatment to life outside of the program—their ADLs and IADLS, roles, and personal goals. If I think it will benefit, I sometimes conduct a sensory assessment. I provide education on sensory regulation, review their sensory profile, and provide opportunities for people to try out sensory strategies or to make sensory toys (stress balls, slime, fidgets, weighted blankets, etc.) that may support sensory regulation.

Continued

Practitioner Profile—cont'd

I run task and skills groups to build attention, planning, sequencing, and problem-solving; tolerate frustration; approach novel tasks; and tolerate imperfection. I maintain a craft room with every art or craft project imaginable (candle making, copper tooling, wood working, jewelry making, clay, painting, tile mosaics, weaving). I have participants help care for an outside garden with several garden beds and six aeroponic tower gardens, all with edible plants. I love working with adults in PHP because I can engage people in discussing how what we are working on connects to life outside of the program–how it reflects their routines and patterns and brings up similar challenges, and how these interventions can be used to take risks or shift responses and ways of relating.

Being a part of someone's journey as they move from crisis to surviving to thriving is gratifying, and occupational therapy has a unique role and potential for positive impact at this level of care. I love when individuals share stories about how their time in occupational therapy influenced them, or shifted their ways of thinking, or influenced their life outside the PHP by helping them get back to engaging in meaningful parts of their lives. I reinforce the power of focused doing, and often express that one may not initially understand how making a candle or learning how to sew during a session is helpful, but the positive domino effect speaks for itself. I feel I have the privilege of helping people reconnect with joy and reconnect with themselves—a special capability of occupational therapy that goes a long way.

community mental health, then describes the role of occupational therapy in some community mental health settings.

Occupational therapy has deep roots in community mental health and more and more practitioners are using their creativity and entrepreneurial spirit to create positions in community mental health (AOTA, 2016a). The distinct value practitioners contribute to community mental health is bolstered by their use of evidence-based and occupation-focused interventions. For example, in their systematic review of literature evaluating the effectiveness of interventions focused on improving occupational performance and participation for people with serious mental illness, D'Amico and colleagues (2018) reported moderate to strong evidence for occupation-based programs. Specifically, these authors concluded that practitioners should be aware that there is strong evidence supporting manualized programs using psychoeducation methods to improve and maintain ADL and instrumental ADL (IADL) performance, as well as moderate-to-strong evidence for the effectiveness of social, ADL, or IADL skills training (D'Amico et al., 2018).

In a systematic review and narrative synthesis of the literature, other researchers concluded that practitioners using supported employment approaches can feel confident in the strong evidence that exists for this approach and that employment and individual placement can result in competitive employment (Killaspy et al., 2022). There is also some evidence that supported education programs emphasizing goal setting, skill development, and cognitive training result in increased participation in educational pursuits. These same authors note outcomes are stronger when practitioners integrate cognition and social skills training in their interventions (Killaspy et al., 2022).

Brown and her colleagues completed a systematic review and meta-analysis of community-based weight loss interventions for people with serious mental illness and concluded various lifestyle-focused interventions had a significant effect on weight loss for this population (Brown et al., 2018). The take home point here is that OTPs, with their distinct focus on person-environment-occupation (PEO) interaction have the skills and training to contribute to community

mental health with a broad range of evidence-informed, occupation-focused interventions.

Community Case Management and Care Coordination

Case management is a person-centered, collaborative process of evaluation, planning, facilitation, and advocacy to meet an individual's health needs and promote population health management goals (Case Management Society of America, 2017). Case management is an individualized process. An effective case manager understands the strengths and needs of the person and their environments and is adept at developing trust in the relationship. **Care coordination** involves deliberately organizing care activities and sharing information among all the participants concerned with a person's care to achieve safe and effective care (Agency for Healthcare Research and Quality, 2018). Table 35-5 shares key components of case management and care coordination processes.

Occupational Therapy's Role in Care Coordination and Case Management

At its core, occupational therapy is an interprofessional practice with a focus on person-centered care and an individual's self-determination. Practitioners can and do play a unique role in case management and care coordination services. The OTP's focus on function and ability to assess occupational performance across multiple dimensions (e.g., cognitive, social, physical, sensory) ensures they can provide invaluable input when coordinating with other members of the care team. The OTP's ability to carefully consider the person-environment fit and to identify services that meet an individual's needs and match their functional capacities provides an invaluable functional perspective that supports the efforts of the entire team.

In community-based practice, practitioners motivate, guide, and promote a person's confidence through productive

TABLE 35-5 | Care Coordination Versus Case Management

Aspect of Practice	Case Management	Care Coordination
Focus	People receiving care	Providers
Goals	Connect the person with appropriate services	Increase collaboration between providers
Providers Involved	Primarily social workers, but it is an interdisciplinary effort	Interdisciplinary
Intended Outcomes	Person is connected to and engaged in the most appropriate service to support their recovery	Safer, more efficient, and effective care

TABLE 35-6 | Guiding Principles of Assertive Community Treatment

Principle	Description
1. Primary provider of services and fixed point of responsibility	This approach minimizes the need for coordination of numerous service providers within the mental health or social services organizations.
2. Services provided out of the office	Examples include working on cooking within the home, grocery shopping at the neighborhood grocery store, providing supports in the job place, or taking public transportation with an individual to support community mobility.
3. Highly individualized services	Team members place a great deal of importance on getting to know the values, wishes, goals, strengths, and problems of the person they are working with. Generally, the team provides services throughout the week according to the person's specific needs.
4. An assertive, "can do" approach	The team accepts responsibility to do whatever needs to happen to assist the person to meet their goals and desires. The team works to adapt the environment and their approaches to meet the needs of the person rather than expecting the person to adapt to the team or follow rules of a treatment program. Together with the person, the team establishes a treatment plan that addresses the person's goals and needs. This "transdisciplinary" approach depends on the members of the team being comfortable providing services outside their professional background (within legal limits) or comfort zone; for example, an OTP may help a person access social service resources for utility assistance, and a social worker might help an individual learn how to cook.
5. Continuous, long-term services	ACT services occur 24/7/365 and are not time limited. Frequency and duration of services are adaptable and fluid, allowing services to be tailored to a person's needs at particular points in time. The goal of providing continuous, long-term service is to have a positive impact on the course of the person's psychiatric disability so episodes of severe disability are less frequent or prolonged and functioning between episodes is improved.
6. Targeted population	ACT teams may have different focuses, but generally programs target individuals with one or more of the following characteristics: high-risk for hospitalization, frequently in crisis and requiring emergency intervention, severe and disabling symptoms and unresponsive to traditional outpatient programs, homeless, co-occurring substance use disorders, and at-risk of involvement with the criminal justice system (SAMHSA, 2024; Vanderlip et al., 2016). Individuals targeted by ACT are often those who have not been successful in case management with more traditional models such as the Broker Model or office-based models.

participation in roles, routines, and habits; education about goal setting and communication strategies; caregiver education to promote healthy and constructive relationships; resource utilization; and advocacy (AOTA, 2018). Many individuals are exposed to services that do not fit their needs adequately or that they are not ready to engage in at the time they are initially presented. Often case management involves discerning the person's readiness to engage and personally connecting the individual directly with a service provider instead of expecting them to independently connect.

Assertive Community Treatment and Program for Assertive Community Treatment

Since its inception in the 1980s, the effectiveness of ACT has been systematically evaluated. Multiple high-quality studies in the United States and internationally have established ACT as an evidence-based approach that can help many

individuals have more contact with their treatment team and improve mental health outcomes (Thoegersen et al., 2019), reduce the need for hospitalization (Clausen et al., 2016), stay housed (O'Campo et al., 2016), and improve their quality of life (Vanderlip et al., 2016).

Compared with traditional case management in which one individual works to support a large caseload of individuals, in the ACT approach, a multidisciplinary team provides community-based treatment, rehabilitation, and support services to a small caseload 24 hours a day, 365 days a year (Lama et al., 2021; Vanderlip et al., 2016). The small caseload is necessary because of the intense demand on individual team members' time serving individuals' various needs. The multidisciplinary team can include but is not limited to OTPs, social workers, nurses, psychiatrists, peer support workers, and vocational specialists. Each team member often holds the role of "case manager."

To understand the nature of ACT, practitioners must understand the underlying philosophy and principles that guide interactions between the person and the ACT team members. These principles are summarized in Table 35-6.

Occupational Therapy's Role on an ACT Team

An OTP may be included in an ACT team as a case manager, as an add-on service based on identified need and referral, or as a consultant. OTPs working on an ACT team can expect to experience some "role blurring." In fact, "role blurring" is part of the ACT model's philosophy. All ACT team members, including OTPs, often carry out duties that are traditionally identified with social work, particularly securing and referring the person to important resources. When working in an ACT model, the practitioner must be secure in their professional identity and frame their efforts as helping the person to live productively in the community, which is indeed "occupational therapy." The person may not know the specific professional backgrounds of each team member, but all individuals know that every team member is there to work with them to help develop skills and provide support each day.

Psychosocial Clubhouses

Clubhouses are local community centers that help adults living with mental illnesses pursue employment, education, housing, and community engagement. Recovery is not a linear process and each person's lived experience is different, even from day to day. Clubhouses are designed to meet the needs of individuals who are functioning at different points across the mental health continuum. Clubhouses are often a good setting for individuals who are struggling or surviving on the mental health continuum to find support and move toward thriving and excelling in a self-determined manner. However, if a person is in crisis, Clubhouses can support the person to access more intensive care, including hospitalization. Clubhouses frequently employ a psychosocial rehabilitation approach, meaning that the emphasis is on relationships and the belief that through relationships comes empowerment, engagement, productivity, and health and wellness.

Brief History of Clubhouses

The "Clubhouse Model" was purposely designed to differ from traditional medical model-based services. The Clubhouse Model began when six residents at Rockland State Hospital, a psychiatric hospital in New York City, formed a self-help group that met in the hospital "club room." Here, these individuals shared stories, read, and painted; socialized; and supported one another through their hospitalization and discharge planning. Once discharged, they recreated their "club room" on the steps of the New York Public Library and named their group "We Are Not Alone" (WANA), a message to a pervasive problem among those living with mental health conditions—social isolation. In 1948, WANA purchased a building to house their "Clubhouse" and named it Fountain House (Fountain House, n.d.). Fountain House still operates today, and learners can follow their great work by searching "Fountain House Bronx" on social media.

Initially ex-psychiatric patients, referred to as "members," staffed and operated all aspects of the Clubhouse. This peer support approach differed from hospital and other mental health services that were typically staffed by professionals who did not share these members' lived experiences. In 1955, Fountain House began hiring mental health professionals as

TABLE 35-7 | **Key Features of Clubhouses**

Feature	Description
Members	• Adults living with mental illness who attend the Clubhouse are not clients, consumers or patients; they're members. • Members must have a diagnosed mental illness, and this must be confirmed by a mental health professional upon application to be a Clubhouse member.
Work-ordered day	• The structure of the day-to-day activities in the Clubhouse mimic the workday. • The overall structure for the day depends on the culture in which the Clubhouse exists; however, in the United States, it usually parallels the structure of the Western workweek/workday, operating Monday through Friday 9:00 a.m. to 5:00 p.m. • Members engage in one or more "work units."
Work units	• Work units offer meaningful activities for Clubhouse members to work alongside each other, and paid staff, to contribute to the function of the Clubhouse. • The units structure the work-ordered day and may include a kitchen unit, a business unit, a wellness unit, an employment unit, and so on.
Staff	• Paid professionals within the Clubhouse are often referred to as "staff generalists." • Staff roles center around working alongside members and supporting them in whatever it is they need or want to do, such as working in the kitchen unit with members to prepare and serve lunch, driving the Clubhouse van to pick up or drop off members, assisting with transitional employment, or cofacilitating unit meetings.

staff. Their first director was John Beard, a social worker, whose methods perfectly fit the social approach of Fountain House. Through encouraging, equipping, and empowering members to work alongside one another in activities such as cleaning and painting the house, secretary tasks, preparing and serving lunch, and employment outside the Clubhouse, Beard transformed Fountain House from a social club to a comprehensive psychiatric rehabilitation program. John Beard's model is still used in Clubhouses to this day (Fountain House, 2023). Some key features of clubhouses are included in Table 35-7.

What started with six "psychiatric patients" in a hospital "club room" has now multiplied to over 300 Clubhouses worldwide. These Clubhouses are monitored and supported by Clubhouse International, a "non-profit organization that helps start and grow Clubhouses globally" (Clubhouse International, n.d.-b, para. 1). For Clubhouses to receive such support to start and grow, they must work toward and obtain accreditation, similar to how all occupational therapy programs work toward achieving and maintaining accreditation through the Accreditation Council for Occupational Therapy Education (ACOTE). Globally, accredited Clubhouses all work toward common goals, understandings, and standards of what it means to be a Clubhouse, ensuring quality for those who seek out the Clubhouse. To see what Clubhouses are in the readers' local area, go to the following link: https://club-house-intl.org/what-we-do/international-directory.

Outcomes and Impact of Clubhouses

In the past almost 75 years, Clubhouses have demonstrated that their psychosocial approach to rehabilitation promotes reduced hospitalizations and incarcerations, secured and maintained employment in the community, improved physical and mental health, and improved well-being, all at one-third of the cost of other models, such as community mental health centers, individual placement and support models of employment, and the ACT model (Clubhouse International, n.d.-a).

Additionally, literature examining Clubhouses has found that Clubhouse members and their families have experienced profound meaning from involvement with local Clubhouses. For example, Pernice-Duca and colleagues (2015) found that Clubhouse engagement afforded benefits to family members such as decreased family and caregiver burden, increased quality and effectiveness of family communication, and positive feelings associated with decreased depression or worry with an increased sense of hope. Brittany (she/her), a Clubhouse member, demonstrates some of these findings within

her own personal experience with both a Clubhouse and occupational therapy in Box 35-1. Figure 35-7 is an image of Brittany's art project while at the Clubhouse.

Clubhouses function on basic understandings such as "once a member, always a member" and that all engagement within the Clubhouse is entirely voluntary. There is no hierarchy among paid staff and members; in fact, per Clubhouse standards, staff and program directors are not allowed to have their own offices, as that would demonstrate that they are different from Clubhouse members. Clubhouse members, rather than mental health professionals, drive activities and decisions within Clubhouses. Nuances such as these can often cause ambiguity and role confusion among OTPs and students who get involved with a Clubhouse. However, these nuances are exactly what make Clubhouses the perfect fit for occupational therapy.

Occupational Therapy's Role Within Clubhouses

OTPs and students who are accustomed to traditional models of therapy and medicine, in which the health professional is in the "expert seat," does therapy *to* the person, or "leads"

BOX 35-1 ■ Brittany's Story: If I Can Do It, You Can Too!

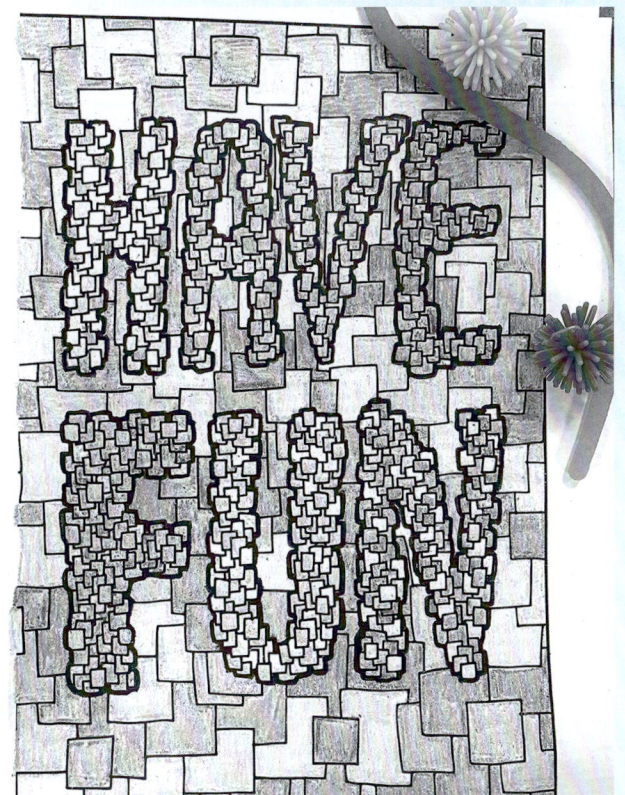

FIGURE 35-7. Brittany's "Have Fun" art project.

I started coming to Clubhouse in September 2020 while suffering from PTSD. Like going to any new place, especially being an introvert,

it was scary. Do they understand? I don't know anyone here. I don't want to talk about my struggles right away. That's intimidating.

Instead, I sat through a meeting and afterward I sat by myself coloring, and one of the staff members came over and just sat with me (Fig. 35-7). We didn't talk. She said she was here if I needed anything and that was it. She held space for me and that's all I needed. Clubhouse is very special. Everyone is very welcoming, but also very aware. This is the only place I have ever known where absolutely no one judges other people or cares what other people wear. It is the kindest group of people who could care less about materialistic things that "most other" people would care about way more.

It has helped coming to a place where I can be surrounded with people, especially since I live alone. It provides social activity, and supports me with different goals, such as getting a job, advocating for a schedule I'd normally not do, and just a place that can help me get out of those overwhelming feelings throughout the week until I could meet with my therapist.

Clubhouse also cooks meals together and that's another way to help my recovery by making sure I eat at least one nutritious meal a day. Occupational therapy students also come to help at Clubhouse. They help me by making plans for when I have down time and what I can do to stay off my depression instead of just sleeping and spiraling into a cycle that I can't get out of. Overall, Clubhouse has been a vital part of me continuing to get better. I would not be able to explain how much someone would need this program. I would just say you have to come, be consistent, and give it a chance. I was terrified. But if I can do it, you can too!

Reflective Questions

■ Examine Brittany's story of her experience within a Clubhouse and identify aspects of the Clubhouse that promote her health and well-being.

■ What occupations are used as means within the Clubhouse to support Brittany?

TABLE 35-8 | Examples of Clubhouse Activities

Occupation	Intervention Approach	Clubhouse Activities
IADL—communication management	Modify/adapt task by adding written and visual instructions.	With support of a step-by-step written guide made by an occupational therapy fieldwork student, a Clubhouse member creates a social media post reminding members of the upcoming holiday party next week.
IADL—financial management	Create/promote—everyone, no matter their health status, can benefit from financial wellness.	A Clubhouse member and occupational therapy fieldwork student cofacilitate a "Wellness Meeting" focused on financial wellness.
Health management—physical activity	Create/promote—everyone, no matter their health status, benefits from physical activity. Establish/restore—this involves establishing a physical activity routine, or restoring a valued routine.	Alongside, and at the suggestion of, Clubhouse members, the occupational therapy fieldwork student engages alongside Clubhouse members in taking a walk in the park during the scheduled "Wellness Unit." The occupational therapy fieldwork student offers social support and peer modeling within this activity.
Education—formal education participation	Modify/adapt the task; provide activity analysis.	A Clubhouse member wanting to pursue a college degree elicits support from the occupational therapy fieldwork student to initiate this task. The occupational therapy student "chunks" up this very large task and provides the just-right-challenge.
Work—employment interests and pursuits	Evaluating person, environment, and occupation fit; provides activity analysis.	A Clubhouse member identifies an interest in working part time. The occupational therapy fieldwork student assists in job exploration through supporting the member in considering their interests as well as supports and barriers within their contexts.
Leisure—leisure exploration	Evaluating person, environment, and occupation fit; provides activity analysis.	Members work together to choose leisure activities to include on the social calendar for the next month. The occupational therapy fieldwork student assists by considering group, context, and occupation factors.
Social participation—community participation IADL—meal preparation	Modify/adapt the task and environment; provides activity analysis.	The occupational therapy fieldwork student provides in-the-moment adaptations so that two individuals with differing needs can both work to prepare and serve the lunch meal, a necessary task within the Clubhouse community.

groups, might look at the Clubhouse Model and surmise that they have no place within a Clubhouse. However, occupational therapy and the Clubhouse Model share several values and approaches, including a value of occupation as means, person-centeredness, and promoting health and well-being. To further solidify this point, Table 35-8 provides examples of activities that have occurred among Clubhouse members and occupational therapy fieldwork students at a Clubhouse in Kansas. These activities tie directly to occupations and approaches used within occupational therapy practice, per the *Occupational Therapy Practice Framework* (*OTPF;* AOTA, 2020).

Most simply, an OTP's role within a Clubhouse is to use a lens of occupation to approach problems and situations and to do so alongside Clubhouse members and other professional staff.

Social Entrepreneurship

Occupational therapy addressing the needs of people along the mental health continuum has been a cornerstone of the occupational therapy profession since its inception (Meyer, 1922). Occupational therapy has deep roots in community mental health, and practitioners can be confident that since occupational therapy's inception their art and science has grown. OTPs have the knowledge, training, and skills to create and market evidence-informed, occupation-focused

services in community mental health (Armstrong, 2020; Kirsh et al., 2019; Smallfield & Molitor, 2018). Social entrepreneurship is the practice of using business principles and methods to create, fund, and implement innovative solutions to social, cultural, or environmental problems (Peek, 2020).

Social entrepreneurism is a practice area that is geared to offer occupational therapy services in a community mental health setting and specifically to historically underserved populations, including but not limited to black, Indigenous, People of Color (BIPOC), LGBTQIA2S+ (lesbian, gay, bisexual, transgender, queer and questioning, intersex, asexual and two-spirit), or adults living with HIV. Services can be structured in various ways. They could include a private practice, providing services within a community mental health clinic or nonprofit organization, or independent contracting, consulting, or coaching services.

One's private practice can also include helping other practitioners build their own practice in community mental health, or providing education, such as creating or offering a course or curriculum to an in-person or online audience. Entrepreneurial practitioners may offer mental health consultant services to facilities or other programs that do not yet offer occupational therapy services to support the development of an occupational therapy program. Consulting can also be done with other OTPs or clinicians to support their professional development. An entrepreneurial practitioner may offer education to the public that shares specific knowledge in their specialty area, which can support individuals or families to accomplish goals. For example, education programs can offer people with mental illness access to information on self-care, communication, leisure, or time management. Or a program can offer information to other providers on how to support a person with a specific diagnosis from an occupational perspective.

Although many opportunities exist for practitioners to develop a business related to the field of occupational therapy, there are also many occupational therapy skills that easily translate to roles outside of a clinic or agency.

OTPs who specialize in any area can develop a private clinical practice. Many create a private practice to fill the gaps that exist within traditional medical or mental health systems. A private clinical practice may accept insurance, or it may be a private pay clinic where the individual is responsible for all the fees associated with the service. Social entrepreneurism asserts that the service will help fill the gaps for historically underserved populations while providing a low-cost, sliding scale or free service to individuals. Often this means services are funded through a third party such as insurance, government programs, or subcontracting with other clinics or programs.

Dr. Elizabeth Martin—whose practice, Holistic Community Therapy (HCT), provides services and outreach to economically and culturally vulnerable populations (www.hctpdx.com)—is featured in her Practitioner Profile feature. Figures 35-8, 35-9, and 35-10 illustrate interventions from this setting. Other examples include

Practitioner Profile

Social Entrepreneurship

Dr. Elizabeth Martin, OTD, MHA, OTR/L, QMHP-C, CCTP-II, SEP™ (she, her)

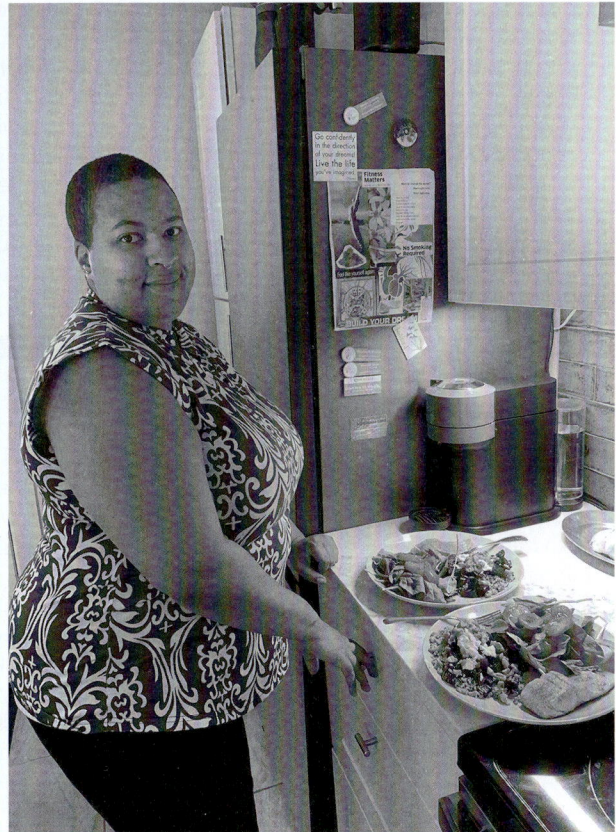

FIGURE 35-8. Spending time cooking and being in the kitchen with participants is a key and constant part of Dr. Martin's practice.

Holistic Community Therapy (HCT) is a virtual and community-based private practice specializing in helping adults aged 18 to 75 with cognitive changes and mental health concerns to address social determinants of health and regain their quality of life through virtual, in-home, and community-based

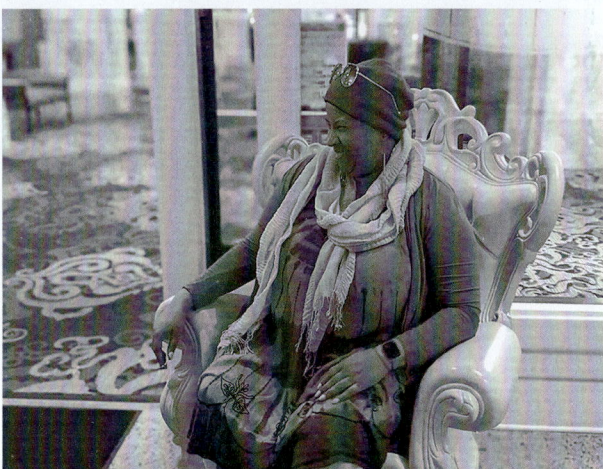

FIGURE 35-9. Fun, laughter, and participating in venues available in the community supports individuals to be aware of and engage in what their community has to offer.

cognitive rehabilitation and mental wellness services. HCT primarily works with BIPOC and LGBTQIA2S+ communities in Portland, Oregon. Individuals are typically in services 3 to 9 months and are referred to HCT from their primary care provider or other medical or mental health professionals or self-refer.

Most individuals at HCT experience mental health and/or medical challenges such as PTSD, attention deficit-hyperactivity disorder, autism, anxiety, depression, schizophrenia, or neurological conditions such as brain injury. Common challenges to occupational performance include executive dysfunction or disorganization, emotional dysregulation, and/or social isolation. Social determinants of health such as being from a racially marginalized community, limited social and economic supports, and barriers in receiving culturally responsive care negatively impact the access to adequate health care, basic resources, and self-care options for many at HCT. HCT is primarily funded through Medicare, Medicaid, and private insurance. In Oregon, occupational therapists are recognized as qualified mental health professionals (QMHPs) by Medicaid and must be competent in diagnosing mental illness to provide occupational therapy

Continued

Practitioner Profile—cont'd

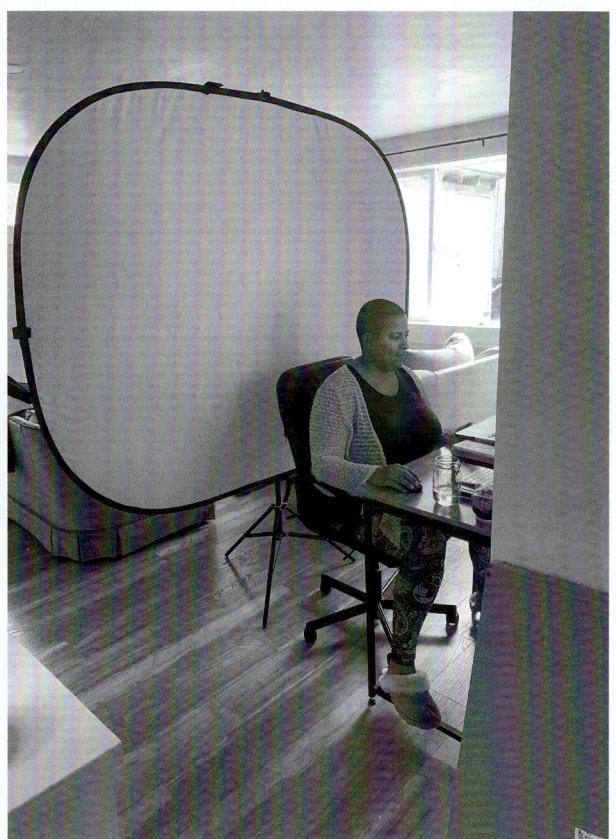

FIGURE 35-10. Dr. Martin provides virtual care services as well as community-based services in her private practice.

services to this population. It is inconclusive if occupational therapy assistants can be considered qualified mental health associates (QMHAs) by Medicaid at the time of this writing. These stakeholders influence and frame how services are delivered, monitored, and improved over time.

HCT routinely employs Maslow's Hierarchy of Needs and Person-Environment-Occupational Performance (PEOP) models to guide service provision for assisting individuals to meet their needs. Each person completes the World Health Organization Disability Assessment Schedule 2.0 (Ustün et al., 2010) and the *Diagnostic and Statistical Manual of Mental Disorders, Fifth Edition, Text Revision (DSM-5-TR)* Self-Rated Level 1 Cross-Cutting Symptom Measure—Adult (APA, 2022) for entry into practice. Services support individuals beyond traditional rehabilitation models and provide long-term, compensatory interventions. Program outcomes emphasize promoting individual self-advocacy and self-efficacy, mental wellness, chronic disease management, and effective health system navigation.

Many at HCT report experiencing disconnect from health providers, which often leads to difficulties with carryover to their home environments, particularly when receiving services in stressful medical clinics. Common HCT interventions include identifying needs around appointments, tracking appointments, identifying symptoms at home, identifying and documenting changes after starting a new medication, and problem-solving and role-playing self-advocacy and communication during a medical appointment. Assigned homework might be to attend an appointment, practice techniques, take notes, and write additional questions down. Follow-up sessions provide opportunities to review their appointment and to identify key information to implement into their current daily routine.

Dr. Tomeico Faison, who owns and operates Therapeutic Solutions of North Carolina (www.therapeuticsolutionsofnc. com), and Dr. Ariana Gonzalez, who founded and leads Life After Incarceration: Transition & Reentry (LAITR; www. lifeafterincarceration.com).

Occupational Therapy Across the Continuum of Need

There is a continuum of mental health services, from hospitalization to community access, available to individuals based on the person's needs. Access of services is variable based on location, and definitions and services differ across cities, states, and countries. Although this chapter attempts to present varied examples within the continuum, it is important to note that recovery is not linear, an individual's lived experience will change over time, changes may occur quick or proceed over a longer period, and individuals may be within any of the stages of the continuum in any of the therapeutic

settings mentioned throughout the chapter. An OTP uses clinical judgment, as well as their therapeutic rapport with individuals, to determine the best setting for the individual's mental health care.

OTPs have a deep understanding of how interactions between the individual, their desired occupational engagement, and their environments can influence mental health. Occupational therapy has a valuable role in the delivery of recovery-oriented care that supports the individual to establish meaningful roles and quality of life across the mental health continuum. Table 35-9 provides a summary of each area of practice highlighted in the chapter, and the role of occupational therapy within each setting. Table 35-10 offers common assessments used in these settings.

OTPs have access to a variety of assessment tools available to support practice in many settings across the continuum of care. The types of assessments and screenings span observational and performance-based screenings to subjective and self-reported questionnaires. Performance-based or observational assessments carry a unique application for OTPs that other mental health professionals do not regularly employ.

TABLE 35-9 | Continuum of Occupational Therapy Across Settings

Area of Practice	Mental Health Continuum	Key Areas of Focus
Acute care (general hospital)	Crisis	Meet the person's acute medical needs; consult and collaborate with mental health and medical setting practitioners.
Inpatient hospitalization (behavioral health)	Crisis to surviving	Evaluate function; identify goals, strengths, and barriers. Provide group interventions; manage/reduce acute symptoms within the inpatient setting. Apply psychoeducation approaches focused on knowing diagnoses, symptoms, and coping strategies and facilitate participation and routine engagement in everyday occupations. Ensure discharge planning includes environmental assessment, problem-solving of potential barriers, and appropriate referrals.
Partial hospitalization programs (PHPs) and intensive outpatient programs (IOPs)	Struggling to thriving	Evaluate function using tools focused on identifying individual's needs during transition from hospitalization; evaluate roles, habits, and routines; create occupational history and profile; evaluate environmental supports, barriers, and challenges. Intervene primarily in groups that are occupation focused such as building skills for reintegration posthospitalization, education, and identification of meaningful occupations, identifying supports, learning coping skills to maintain routines and responsibilities, and honing skills for mitigating risks within their posthospital environments. Support return to work/community settings, social connectedness, and peer supports.
Assertive Community Treatment (ACT)	Struggling to thriving	Contribute to interdisciplinary evaluation; contribute assessment data that is occupation-focused and that occurs within natural contexts (i.e., home and community). Ensure focus on social determinants impacting health and recognize roles can blur across disciplines (e.g., may need to assess medication adherence) Participate in interdisciplinary interventions; lead occupation-based treatments that occur in natural contexts. Address immediate needs (e.g., access to food) while also working toward short-term and long-term goals.
Clubhouses	Crisis to excelling	Evaluate with focus on optimizing occupational performance within the Clubhouse and immediate community contexts; most often occurs using informal interviewing and observation during activities in work-ordered day. Intervene in one-to-one and group contexts including modifying tasks and environments, supporting group exploration, and engaging person in the work-ordered day.
Social entrepreneurship	Crisis to excelling	Evaluation focuses on needs of the population served in the setting and often may include organizational and/or community needs assessment to identify a target market. Intervention focuses on providing specialized services that address the identified needs of the population the program or the organization served; can also include developing project proposals, negotiating contracts, developing program manuals, and determining budgets.

TABLE 35-10 | Therapeutic Reasoning Assessment Table: Practice Within the Continuum of Care

Which Tool?	Who Was This Tool Designed For?	Is This a Type of Tool the Person Can Do? What Is Required of the Person?	What Am I Measuring?	How Long Does It Take and Where Do I Administer This Assessment?	Is the Tool Associated With a Practice Model?
Occupational Circumstances Assessment–Interview and Rating Scale, Version 4.0 (OCAIRS; Forsyth et al., 2005)	Adults, older adults, and adolescents	This is a concrete occupation-based interview tool that can be used effectively for people with severe mental illness.	Occupation—interests, goals, values, role participation, and the impact of environment	Allow 45 minutes to an hour in any setting	Model of Human Occupation (MOHO)
Canadian Occupational Performance Measure (COPM; Law et al., 2019)	Children older than 8 years of age to adults with mental illness; persons with neurological or orthopedic conditions	Person can communicate their difficulty in performing tasks and prioritize concerns using rating scales.	A person's perceived problems in self-care, work, and leisure; person quantitatively rates perceived occupational performance and satisfaction with performance.	Allow 20–30 minutes for initial assessment, shorter for readministration; can administer in any space where the person and practitioner can discuss privately	Canadian Model of Occupational Performance

Continued

TABLE 35-10 | **Therapeutic Reasoning Assessment Table: Practice Within the Continuum of Care—cont'd**

Which Tool?	Who Was This Tool Designed For?	Is This a Type of Tool the Person Can Do? What Is Required of the Person?	What Am I Measuring?	How Long Does It Take and Where Do I Administer This Assessment?	Is the Tool Associated With a Practice Model?
Model of Human Occupation Screening Tool (MOHOST; Parkinson et al., 2006)	Adults, older adults, and adolescents	This is a tool used by therapists to report evaluation data collected through a variety of means.	In this screening tool ratings can be made after chart review, observation, and participation in a brief interview process.	Allow 10–15 minutes after data has been collected through other evaluations or observation	MOHO
World Health Organization Disability Assessment Schedule 2.0 (Üstün et al., 2010)	Adolescents and adults	Person answers questions about current ability to complete ADLs, IADLs, and other tasks; must be able to self-assess ability with moderate accuracy. Extended or brief options are available in multiple languages.	Person self-report of abilities to complete a daily task; assessment can be used as a subjective tool to assist with identifying an individual's quality of life and self-efficacy.	Can be self-administered or administered by clinician interview; requires 15–30 minutes	No specific occupational therapy model, but consistent with several models that include emphasis on quality of life
Adolescent/Adult Sensory Profile (Brown & Dunn, 2002)	Can be used with people 11 to 90 years old	Person must be able to report general responses to sensations.	Profile measures self-perceived sensory processing and associated behaviors related to taste or smell sensitivity; movement, visual, touch, and auditory processing as well as activity level.	Can be self-administered and takes typically 10–15 minutes	Dunn Sensory Processing Model

Table 35-10 provides a few examples of assessments OTPs can use to enhance understanding of an individual's performance patterns, engagement in various occupations, and quality of life.

Here's the Point

- Individuals seeking mental health support can access a variety of support services. Availability of services is dependent upon the locale, and the appropriateness of the support service is dependent upon the person's individual needs at their individual stage of well-being and recovery (i.e., in crisis, struggling, surviving, thriving, excelling).
- Mental health support services fall on a continuum from inpatient to community to settings such as social entrepreneurship through private practice, with the inpatient environment being the most highly controlled environment designed to maintain safety, help people manage their crisis, and engage them in the next level of service, depending on what they need. Community mental health is most appropriate when a person has progressed out of being in crisis into the community.
- OTPs work in settings across the continuum of care in mental health and have a distinct set of skills that can support a person's recovery and (re)engagement in occupation. These skills allow practitioners to function effectively in multiple

roles across the continuum of need, including roles such as service providers, case managers, and consultants.
- In acute care settings, the OTP can focus on identifying current skills and challenges related to role tasks, plan for meeting acute occupational needs after discharge, and identify and put resources in place to maintain a level of participation as individuals continue their recovery in the community.
- OTPs in community mental health work with people in their homes, community centers/agencies, and workplaces. This perspective allows practitioners to determine how the personal, occupational, and environmental factors merge to impact the person's participation. It also offers greater opportunities to address social determinants of health and gaps in mental health care, such as through serving BIPOC and LGBTQIA2S+ communities.

Acknowledgments

The authors want to acknowledge Dr. Lisa Mahaffey, PhD, OTR/L, FAOTA, and Jeanenne Dallas, MA, OTR/L, FAOTA, for their contributions to earlier versions of this chapter.

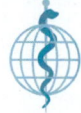 Visit the online resource center at FADavis.com to access the videos.

Apply It Now

1. Know Your State

Every state is different in terms of how much funding it allocates for care of people with psychiatric conditions and how those funds are distributed. Services for people can even vary widely from county to county within the state. For those with psychiatric conditions, this means trying to figure out where to go to get the support they need to continue their recovery. Individuals rely on practitioners to help them become aware of and access resources, and practitioners can only share knowledge about what they themselves have taken the time to learn. Take time to explore services that support recovery that are available in your area. Consider using "211" (call on your phone like you would with "911") to identify some of these resources, Additionally, considering the needs of Ernie, who was described earlier in this chapter, what supports will the person need to live, work, eat, go to school, attend church, and maintain his everyday life in the community? Begin with the premise that programs addressing these needs exist in your community. Identify the following information and put together a handout with a description of the available services and contact numbers. It may be useful to engage classmates in this project to collaborate on a recovery services directory for your community.

Reflective Questions

■ Identify the difference between Supplemental Security Income (SSI) and Social Security Disability Insurance (SSDI), as well as the difference between Medicaid and Medicare funding for services.
■ Develop an understanding of the state's system for calculating and distributing monies for food and other needs.
■ Identify special programs that qualify people for additional monies for specific services or populations such as education and training, medications, or to support employment for persons with a disability.

■ Understand the procedure that drug companies use in their indigent programs that distribute free or reduced-cost medications.
■ Learn about the community mental health programs in your local county and statewide. Include group homes, vocational rehabilitation, supported employment, supported work, supported living, and office of rehabilitation services. Get information on whom to contact, what they offer, how they are funded or what kind of funding they offer, and what criteria the person must meet to benefit from these services.
■ Develop a list of support groups in the area. Look for groups regarding chemical dependence, psychiatric conditions (e.g., bipolar disorder), attention deficit-hyperactivity disorder (ADHD), autism, self-injury, caregiver support groups, Alzheimer education programs, and so on.
■ Develop a list of supports for those in the process of career changes or needing additional role support, such as volunteer opportunities, leisure opportunities, church-related activities, sports, or other hobby groups, and so on.

2. Know the SAMHSA Evidence-Based Practices Resource Center

■ Explore the SAMHSA website (www.samhsa.gov).
■ Review the evidence-based programs that SAMHSA has deemed appropriate for using with people who have psychiatric conditions. These can be found under Publications/Professional & Research Topics at this link: https://www.samhsa.gov/resource-search/ebp.
■ Review the ACT Evidence-Based KIT information listed under the Treatment, Prevention & Recovery tab.
■ These are downloadable resources that are free of charge.
■ Develop a "job description" for an OTP as a case manager for a community mental health center to present to a team to make a case for hiring you as an OTP on the team.

Resources

- Assertive Community Treatment Association (ACTA) website: http://www.actassociation.org. This site provides information on the ACT model, the national ACT conference, model fidelity, ACT trainings, and other resources. ACTA organizes and supports a yearly conference on ACT services, which encourages service users and their families to join with practitioners and researchers to promote and improve ACT services. The resource link on this page is particularly helpful for finding ACT toolkits and summaries of evidence-based research on ACT.
- The Association of Therapeutic Communities (ATC): http://www.therapeuticcommunities.org. The mission of this professional organization in the United Kingdom is to support the work and continued development of therapeutic communities within the United Kingdom and internationally.

You can learn more about different types of therapeutic communities and find resources for education and training at their website.
- Clubhouse International: http://clubhouse-intl.org/what-we-do/overview. This nonprofit organization helps to start and grow Clubhouses around the world. Additionally, they grant and monitor accreditation of Clubhouses, provide training and mentoring to Clubhouses, educate communities, and conduct advocacy and research.
- Mental Health America (MHA): http://www.mentalhealthamerica.net. This nonprofit organization has lived its mission to "inform, advocate and enable access to quality behavioral health services for all Americans" for more than 100 years. The site provides many resources for advocacy, public education, and support services for people who have mental health conditions. It is a great site for mental health advocacy and for following U.S. legislation that impacts mental health care.

- National Alliance on Mental Illness (NAMI): http://www.nami.org. This site offers information about psychiatric disabilities and resources for education, family support, advocacy, and research. NAMI is a national organization with state affiliates. The site contains links to each state's NAMI office and other helpful websites. NAMI has been instrumental in advocating for Program of Assertive Community Treatment (PACT) teams in all states. This website also provides information on the PACT model and publications available through NAMI to learn how to start a PACT team.
- Psychiatric Rehabilitation Association (PRA): www.psychrehabassociation.org/determine-your-exam-eligibility-pathway. PRA offers OTPs certification as a certified psychiatric rehabilitation practitioner (CPRP).
- SAMHSA's Practitioner Training: https://www.samhsa.gov/practitioner-training. This component of the SAMHSA webpage directs practitioners to tools, trainings, and technical assistance to improve their skill in addressing mental health and substance use disorders.
- SAMHSA's Recovery to Practice: https://www.samhsa.gov/recovery-to-practice. This section of the SAMHSA website provides information for behavioral health and general healthcare practitioners to improve delivery of recovery-oriented services, supports, and treatment.

Videos

- "Child in Crisis" video. In this video, OTP Brittany shares her experience working in a psychiatric rehabilitation hospital's adolescent unit with Mikey, an 8-year-old boy presenting with a complex set of challenges. Diagnosed at birth with fetal alcohol syndrome, Mikey has a history of multiple adverse childhood experiences (ACEs), or potentially traumatic events that occurred in childhood (CDC, 2024). On admission, he presented with suicidal and homicidal ideation and symptoms consistent with PTSD. Brittany describes how she did her own research, learned more about Mikey, and developed an intervention that worked well for him and the other children in the group. Access the video at the online resource center at FADavis.com.
- "Student Panel Discusses Running Groups in Mental Health Settings" video. In this video, occupational therapy students discuss their first experience running groups for a 6-week period in a psychiatric day program. The students describe first being intimidated, but then feeling welcomed and surprised by how enjoyable and productive the groups were. They emphasize the team approach and the utility of the groups in developing their leadership skills. Access the video at the online resource center at FADavis.com.
- "Civic Engagement Group in an Inpatient Psychiatric Unit" video. In this video, OTP Jennifer speaks about her experience working as an occupational therapy assistant in an inpatient psychiatric unit for individuals with persistent mental illness. She describes a positive experience running civic engagement groups, which proved to do much more than give back to the community. In one project related to voting rights for individuals with felony histories, the group provided opportunities for the residents to practice life skills, feel empowered, and transcend the internalized stigma they faced as people living with mental illness. Access the video at the online resource center at FADavis.com.
- "First Fieldwork Experience in Inpatient Mental Health" video. In this video, Casey describes her first fieldwork experience in occupational therapy, which took place in an inpatient mental health setting. Casey shares what she was nervous about before her fieldwork coleading a group and then how things actually turned out. She emphasizes the benefit of creating detailed activity proposals before each group and learning to modify activities as needed on the spot. Access the video at the online resource center at FADavis.com.

References

Advocates for Human Potential. (1995–2023). *Wellness recovery action plan: Your wellness your way.* https://www.wellnessrecoveryactionplan.com/what-is-wrap

Agency for Healthcare Research and Quality. (2018, August). *Care coordination.* https://www.ahrq.gov/ncepcr/care/coordination.html

American Occupational Therapy Association. (n.d.). *Occupational therapy in mental and behavioral health.* https://www.aota.org/-/media/corporate/files/advocacy/federal/overview-of-ot-in-mental-health.pdf

American Occupational Therapy Association. (2016a). *Fact sheet: Occupational therapy's role with mental health recovery.* https://www.aota.org/-/media/Corporate/Files/AboutOT/Professionals/WhatIsOT/MH/Facts/Mental%20Health%20Recovery.pdf

American Occupational Therapy Association. (2016b). *Occupational therapy's distinct value: Mental health promotion, prevention, and intervention across the life span.* Author. https://www.aota.org/-/media/corporate/files/practice/mentalhealth/distinct-value-mental-health.pdf

American Occupational Therapy Association. (2017). Mental health promotion, prevention, and intervention in occupational therapy practice. *The American Journal of Occupational Therapy, 71*(2), 7112410035p1–7112410035p19. https://doi.org/10.5014/ajot.2017.716S03

American Occupational Therapy Association. (2018). Occupational therapy's role in case management. *American Journal of Occupational Therapy, 72*(Suppl. 2), 7212410050p1–7212410050p12. https://doi.org/10.5014/ajot.2018.72S206

American Occupational Therapy Association. (2020). Occupational Therapy Practice Framework: Domain and process—Fourth edition. *The American Journal of Occupational Therapy, 74*(Suppl. 2), 7412410010p1–7412410010p87. https://doi.org/10.5014/ajot.2020.74S2001

American Psychiatric Association. (2022). *Diagnostic and statistical manual of mental disorders* (5th ed., text rev.). American Psychiatric Publishing. https://doi.org/10.1176/appi.books.9780890425787

Armstrong, M. (2020). *Occupational therapy practice in community mental health: Four case examples.* American Occupational Therapy Association. https://www.aota.org/publications/student-articles/career-advice/community-mental-health

Association for Ambulatory Behavioral Healthcare. (n.d.). *An overview of the partial hospitalization modality.* https://www.aabh.org/partial-hospitalization-program

Atler, K., & Berg, B. (2018). *Occupational Experience Profile. Version 1.* Colorado State University.

Bailliard, A., Schafer, Z., & Hart, L. (2021). Occupational reflection as intervention in inpatient psychiatry. *American Journal of Occupational Therapy, 75*(5), 7505205080. https://doi.org/10.5014/ajot.2021.043703

Barbic, S. (2015). *Personal Recovery Outcome Measure (PROM).* https://emergencymedicinecases.com/wp-content/uploads/2022/07/PROM.pdf

Baum, C., & Baptiste, S. (2002). Reframing occupational therapy practice. In M. Law, C. Baum, & S. Baptiste (Eds.), *Occupation-based practice: Fostering performance and participation* (pp. 3–15). Slack.

Baum, C., Christiansen, C., & Bass, J. (2015). The Person-Environment-Occupation Performance (PEOP) model. In C. Christiansen, C. Baum, & J. Bass (Eds.), *Occupational* therapy: *Performance, participation, well-being* (4th ed., pp. 49–55). Slack.

Brown, C., & Dunn, W. (2002). *Adolescent/Adult Sensory Profile.* Psychological Corporation.

Brown, C., Geiszler, L. C., Lewis, K. J., & Arbesman, M. (2018). Effectiveness of interventions for weight loss for people with serious mental illness: A systematic review and meta-analysis. *American Journal of Occupational Therapy, 72,*

7205190030p1–7205190030p9. https://doi.org/10.5014/ajot .2018.033415

California Department of Developmental Services. (2023). *Institutions for mental disease.* https://www.dds.ca.gov/services /crisis-safety-net-services/institutions-for-mental-disease

Case Management Society of America. (2017). *Case Management Model Act: Supporting case management programs.* https://cmsali .org/pdf/public_policy/2014/Case%20Management%20Model %20Act.pdf

Centers for Disease Control and Prevention. (2022). *Suicide prevention resource for action.* https://www.cdc.gov/suicide/pdf /preventionresource.pdf

Centers for Disease Control and Prevention. (2024). *About adverse childhood experiences.* https://www.cdc.gov/aces/about/index .html

Cheung, E. H., Petersen, E., Zhang, L., Wilkerson, C., Barceló, N. E., Soderlund, P. D., Yerstein, M., & Wells, K. (2022). Drivers of shared decision making in inpatient psychiatry: An exploratory survey of patients' and multi-disciplinary team members' perspectives. *General Hospital Psychiatry, 79,* 7–14. https://doi .org/10.1016/j.genhosppsych.2022.08.004

Clausen, H., Landheim, A., Odden, S., Šaltytė Benth, J., Heiervang, K. S., Stuen, H. K., Killaspy, H., & Ruud, T. (2016). Hospitalization of high and low inpatient service users before and after enrollment into Assertive Community Treatment teams: A naturalistic observational study. *International Journal of Mental Health Systems, 10,* Article 14. https://doi.org/10.1186/s13033-016-0052-z

Clubhouse International. (n.d.-a). *Clubhouse outcomes.* https://club house-intl.org/our-impact/clubhouse-outcomes

Clubhouse International. (n.d.-b). *What we do—Clubhouse International.* https://clubhouse-intl.org/what-we-do/overview

D'Amico, M. L., Jaffe, L. E., & Gardner, J. A. (2018). Evidence for interventions to improve and maintain occupational performance and participation for people with serious mental illness: A systematic review. *American Journal of Occupational Therapy, 72*(5), 7205190020p1–7205190020p11. https://doi.org/10.5014/ajot .2018.033332

Delphis. (2020, June 30). *The mental health continuum is a better model for mental health.* https://delphis.org.uk/mental-health /continuum-mental-health

Duhig, M., Gunasekara, I., & Patterson, S. (2017). Understanding readmission to psychiatric hospital in Australia from the service users' perspective: A qualitative study. *Health Social Care Community, 25*(1), 75–82. https://doi.org/10.1111/hsc.12269

Forsyth, K., Deshpande, S., Kielhofner, G., Henriksson, C., Haglund, L., Olson, L., Skinner, S., & Kulkarni, S. (2005). *The Occupational Circumstances Assessment Interview and Rating Scale (OCAIRS). Version 4.0.* Model of Human Occupation Clearinghouse, University of Illinois at Chicago.

Fountain House. (n.d.). *Our history: Our founding story.* https:// fountainhouse.org/about/our-history

Fountain House. (2023, September 7). *How the visionary leadership of John Beard led to a groundbreaking new model for mental health.* https://www.fountainhouse.org/news/how-the-visionary -leadership-of-john-beard-led-to-a-groundbreaking-new-model -for-mental-health

Gallagher, M., Bagatell, N., Godwin, K., & Peters, D. (2023). Using practice-based inquiry to enact occupation-centered, justice-oriented practice in an acute mental health setting. *The American Journal of Occupational Therapy, 77*(1), 7701205060. https://doi.org/10.5014/ajot.2023.050046

GBD 2019 Mental Health Collaborators. (2022). Global, regional, and national burden of 12 mental disorders in 204 countries and territories, 1990–2019: A systematic analysis for the Global Burden of Disease Study 2019. *The Lancet Psychiatry, 9,* 137–150. https://doi.org/10.1016/S2215-0366(21)00395-3

Killaspy, H., Harvey, C., Brasier, C., Brophy, L., Ennals, P., Fletcher, J., & Hamilton, B. (2022). Community-based social interventions for people with severe mental illness: A systematic review and narrative synthesis of recent evidence. *World Psychiatry, 21,* 96–123. https://doi.org/10.1002/wps.20940

Kirsh, B., Martin, L., Hultqvist, J., & Eklund, M. (2019). Occupational therapy interventions in mental health: A literature review in search of evidence. *Occupational Therapy in Mental Health, 35*(2), 109–156. https://doi.org/10.1080/0164212X.2019.1588832

Knickman, J. R., & Elbel, B. (Eds.). (2019). *Jonas & Kovner's health care delivery in the United States* (12th ed.). Springer Publishing Company.

Lama, T. C., Fu, Y., & Davis, J. A. (2021). Exploring the ideal practice for occupational therapists on Assertive Community Treatment teams. *British Journal of Occupational Therapy, 84*(9), 582–590. https://doi.org/10.1177/03080226211026558

Law, M., Baptiste, S., Carswell, A., McColl, M. A., Polatajko, H., & Pollock, N. (2019). *Canadian Occupational Performance Measure* (5th ed., rev.). COPM Inc.

Lay, B., Kawohl, W., & Rossler, W. (2018). Outcomes of a psycho-education and monitoring programme to prevent compulsory admission to psychiatric inpatient care: A randomized controlled trial. *Psychological Medicine, 48,* 849–860. https://doi .org/10.1017/S0033291717002239

Leenerts, E., Evetts, C., & Miller, E. (2016). Reclaiming and proclaiming the use of crafts in occupational therapy. *The Open Journal of Occupational Therapy, 4*(4), Article 13. https://doi.org /10.15453/2168-6408.1194

Lipskaya-Velikovsky, L., Kotler, M., & Krupa, T. (2016). Description of and preliminary findings for occupational connections, an intervention for inpatient psychiatry settings. *The American Journal of Occupational Therapy, 70*(6), 7006350010p1–7006350010p5. https://doi.org/10.5014/ajot.2016.014688

Lyon, S. (2020, February 20). *The recovery model in mental health care.* Verywell Mind. https://www.verywellmind.com /what-is-the-recovery-model-2509979

McBain, R. K., Cantor, J. H., & Eberhart, N. K. (2022). Estimating psychiatric bed shortages in the US. *JAMA Psychiatry, 79*(4), 279–280. https://doi.org/10.1001/jamapsychiatry.2021.4462

McLean. (2023). *Depression.* https://www.mcleanhospital.org /treatment/depression

Mental Health America. (2023). *Hospitalization.* https://mhanational .org/hospitalization

Merryman, M. B., & Riegel, S. K. (2007). The recovery process and people with serious mental illness living in the community: An occupational therapy perspective. *Occupational Therapy in Mental Health, 23*(2), 51–73. https://doi.org/10.1300/J004v23n02_03

Meyer, A. (1922). The philosophy of occupational therapy. *Archives of Occupational Therapy, 1*(1), 1–10.

National Alliance on Mental Illness. (2023a). *Getting treatment during a crisis.* https://www.nami.org/Learn-More/Treatment /Getting-Treatment-During-a-Crisis

National Alliance on Mental Illness. (2023b). *Mental health by the numbers: The ripple effect on mental illness.* https://www.nami.org /mhstats

National Alliance on Mental Illness. (2023c). *Residential treatment.* https://www.nami.org/Your-Journey/Kids-Teens-and-Young -Adults/Kids/Residential-Treatment

National Alliance on Mental Illness. (2023d). *2020 Mental health by the numbers: Youth and Young Adults.* https://www.nami.org /mhstats

National Board for Certification in Occupational Therapy. (2022). *2022 practice analysis of the occupational therapist registered: The executive summary.* https://www.nbcot.org/-/media/PDFs/2022_ OTR_Practice_Analysis.pdf

Niemiec, R. M., & Pearce, R. (2021). The practice of character strengths: Unifying definitions, principles, and exploration of what's soaring, emerging, and ripe with potential in science and practice. *Frontiers in Psychology, 11,* 590220. https://doi .org/10.3389/fpsyg.2020.590220

Nochaiwong, S., Ruengorn, C., Thavorn, K., Hutton, B., Awiphan, R., Phosuya, C., Ruanta, Y., Wongpakaran, N., & Wongpakaran, T. (2021). Global prevalence of mental health issues among the general population during the coronavirus disease-2019 pandemic: A systematic review and meta-analysis. *Scientific Reports, 11,* 10173. https://doi.org/10.1038/s41598-021-89700-8

O'Campo, P., Stergiopoulos, V., Nir, P., Levy, M., Miser, V., Chum, A., Arbach, B., Nisenbaum, R., To, M. J., & Hang, S. W. (2016). How did a Housing First intervention improve health and social outcomes among homeless adults with mental illness in Toronto? Two-year outcomes from a randomised trial. *BMJ Open, 6,* e010581. https://doi.org/10.1136/bmjopen-2015-010581

Parkinson, S., Forsyth, K., & Kielhofner, G. (2006). *The Model of Human Occupation Screening Tool (MOHOST). Version 2.0.* Model of Human Occupation Clearinghouse, University of Illinois at Chicago.

Peek, S. (2020, July 30). *What is social entrepreneurship? 5 examples of businesses with a purpose.* U.S. Chamber of Commerce. https://www.uschamber.com/co/start/startup/what-is-social-entrepreneurship#:~:text=Social%20entrepreneurship%20is%20the%20process,in%20society%20or%20the%20world

Pereira, R. B., Whiteford, G., Hyett, N., Weekes, G., Di Tommaso, A., & Naismith, J. (2020). Capabilities, Opportunities, Resources and Environments (CORE): Using the CORE approach for inclusive, occupation-centred practice. *Australian Occupational Therapy Journal, 67,* 162–171. https://doi.org/10.1111/1440-1630.12642

Perers, C., Backstrom, B., Johansson, B. A., & Rask, O. (2022). Methods and strategies for reducing seclusion and restraint in child and adolescent psychiatric inpatient care. *Psychiatric Quarterly, 93,* 107–135. https://doi.org/10.1007/s11126-021-09887-x

Pernice-Duca, F., Biegel, D. E., Hess, H. R., Chung, C., & Chang, C. (2015). Family members' perceptions of how they benefit when relatives living with serious mental illness participate in Clubhouse community programs. *Family Relations, 64,* 446–459. https://doi.org/10.1111/fare.12127

Ruffalo, M. L. (2019, June 25). The dire state of inpatient mental health: The American mental health system is broken, and patients are paying the price. *Psychology Today.* https://www.psychologytoday.com/us/blog/freud-fluoxetine/201906/the-dire-state-inpatient-mental-health

Schaub, A., Goldmann, U., Mueser, T. K., Goerigk, G., Hautzinger, M., Roth, E., Charypar, M., Engel, R., & Möller, H. J. (2018). Efficacy of extended clinical management, group CBT, and group plus individual CBT for major depression: Results of a two-year follow-up study. *Journal of Affective Disorders, 238,* 570–578. https://doi.org/10.1016/j.jad.2018.05.081

Sheppard Pratt. (2024). *Inpatient programs and specialty services.* https://www.sheppardpratt.org/care-services/inpatient-specialty-services

Smallfield, S., & Molitor, W. L. (2018). Occupational therapy interventions supporting social participation and leisure engagement for community-dwelling older adults: A systematic review. *American Journal of Occupational Therapy, 72*(4), 7204190020p1–7204190020p8. https://doi.org/10.5014/ajot.2018.030627

Spaniol, L., & Wewiorski, N. J. (2012). Phases of the recovery process from psychiatric disabilities. *International Journal of Psychosocial Rehabilitation, 17*(1).

Substance Abuse and Mental Health Services Administration. (2021). *National Mental Health Services Survey (N-MHSS): 2020 data on mental health treatment facilities.* https://www.samhsa.gov/data/sites/default/files/reports/rpt35336/2020_NMHSS_final.pdf

Substance Abuse and Mental Health Services Administration. (2024). *Forensic Assertive Community Treatment (FACT): A service delivery model for individuals with serious mental illness involved with the criminal justice system* https://store.samhsa.gov/sites/default/files/pep19-fact-br.pdf

Sutton, D. J., Hocking, C. S., & Smythe, L. A. (2012). A phenomenological study of occupational engagement in recovery from mental illness. *Canadian Journal of Occupational Therapy, 79*(3), 142–150. https://doi.org/10.2182/cjot.2012.79.3.3

Synovec, C. E. (2015). Implementing recovery model principles as part of occupational therapy in inpatient psychiatric settings. *Occupational Therapy in Mental Health, 31*(1), 50–61. https://doi.org/10.1080/0164212X.2014.1001014

Taylor, C., Holsinger, B., Flanagan, J. V., Ayers, A. M., Hutchison, S. L., & Terhorst, L. (2016). Effectiveness of a brief care management intervention for reducing psychiatric hospitalization readmissions. *Journal of Behavioral Health Services & Research, 43*(2), 262–271. http://doi.org/10.1007/s11414-014-9400-4

Thoegersen, M. H., Morthorst, B. R., & Nordentoft, M. (2019). Assertive Community Treatment versus standard treatment for severely mentally ill patients in Denmark: A quasi-experimental trial. *Nordic Journal of Psychiatry, 73*(2), 149–158. https://doi.org/10.1080/08039488.2019.1576765

Thornicroft, G., Deb, T., & Henderson, C. (2016, October). Community mental health care worldwide: Current status and further developments. *World Psychiatry, 15*(3), 276–286. https://doi.org/10.1002/wps.20349

Trust for America's Health. (2020, May 21). *Annual deaths due to alcohol, drugs or suicide exceeded 150,000 according to the most recent data—And could get worse due to COVID-19.* https://www.tfah.org/article/annual-deaths-due-to-alcohol-drugs-or-suicide-exceeded-150000according-to-the-most-recent-data-and-could-get-worse-due-to-covid-19

Tyler, N., Wright, N., & Waring, J. (2019). Interventions to improve discharge from acute adult mental health inpatient care to the community: Systematic review and narrative synthesis. *BMC Health Services Research, 19*(1), 1–24. https://doi.org/10.1186/s12913-019-4658-0

UCLA Health. (2023). *Resnick neuropsychiatric hospital: Partial hospitalization (PHP) & intensive outpatient programs (IOP).* https://www.uclahealth.org/hospitals/resnick/patient-care/partial-hospitalization-and-intensive-outpatient-programs

Üstün, T. B., Chatterji, S., Kostanjsek, N., Rehm, J., Kennedy, C., Epping-Jordan, J., Saxena, S., von Korff, M., Pull, C., & WHO/NIH Joint Project. (2010, November). Developing the World Health Organization Disability Assessment Schedule 2.0. *Bulletin of the World Health Organization, 88*(11), 815–823. https://doi.org/10.2471/BLT.09.067231

Vanderlip, E. R., Henwood, B. F., Hrouda, D. R., Meyer, P. S., Monroe-DeVita, M., Studer, L. M., Schweikhard, A. J., & Moser, L., L. (2016). Systematic literature review of general health care interventions within programs of assertive community treatment. *Psychiatric Services, 68*(3), 218–224. https://doi.org/10.1176/appi.ps.201600100

Wainberg, M. L., Sforza, P., Shultz, J. M., Helpman, L., Mootz, J. J., Johnson, K. A., Neria, Y., Bradford, J. E., Oquendo, M. A., & Arbuckle, M. R. (2017). Challenges and opportunities in global mental health: A research-to-practice perspective. *Current Psychiatry Reports, 19*(5), Article 28. https://doi.org/10.1007/s11920-017-0780-z

World Health Organization. (2022, June). *Mental disorders.* https://www.who.int/news-room/fact-sheets/detail/mental-disorders

Zima, B. T., Edgcomb, J. B., Rodean, J., Cochran, S. D., Harle, C. A., Pathak, J., Tseng, C. H., & Bussing, R. (2022). Use of acute mental health care in U.S. children's hospitals before and after statewide COVID-19 school closure orders. *Psychiatric Services, 73*(11), 1202–1209. https://doi.org/10.1176/appi.ps.202100582

Early Intervention: A Practice Setting for Early Childhood Mental Health

Kate Barlow, Beth Mozolic-Staunton,
and Kris Pizur-Barnekow

Occupational therapy practitioners (OTPs) working in infant and toddler service settings routinely address the physical aspects of child development—such as strength, hand use, eye–hand coordination, and sensory-perceptual abilities—as they relate to engagement in occupations and co-occupations (American Occupational Therapy Association [AOTA], 2020). However, a concentrated focus on physical development in isolation, without recognition of social-emotional development and the impact of environmental, social, and cultural factors on child and family well-being, may result in oversight of important areas considered within the occupational therapy scope of practice in early intervention settings.

Healthy social-emotional development during early childhood is paramount for brain development and widely recognized as an antecedent for healthy developmental outcomes later in life (National Scientific Council on the Developing Child, 2020). Although healthy social-emotional development provides a foundation for later development, infants and young children who are experiencing adverse events, showing signs of developmental delays, or have diagnosed conditions may respond to nurturing caregiving differently than infants and toddlers who do not have these risks (Wolke et al., 2014).

These atypical responses may complicate relational interactions and lead to challenges with attachment and bonding. Problems related to attachment (e.g., clinging, calling), emotion regulation (e.g., fussiness, sleep problems), and cognitive development (e.g., responsiveness to stimuli) are all issues that can be considered in the realm of infant and early childhood mental health.

OTPs play a key role in promoting mental as well as physical health and well-being for all people across the life span (AOTA, 2020). This includes young children and their families and caregivers who may be experiencing risk factors for a broad range of mental health conditions. Children thrive in environments with supportive relationships and consistent routines. Young children who experience adverse events or do not feel physically and emotionally safe may have long-term impacts on physical and mental well-being, self-regulation, and learning abilities (National Scientific Council on the Developing Child, 2020).

Early intervention is a broad term to describe practice settings where services and support are provided to children and families during infancy and early childhood, when rapid development is occurring. OTPs who work with infants and young children partner with families and caregivers to support healthy development, well-being, and participation in childhood occupations and co-occupations including play, self-care, social interaction, learning, and self-regulation (Kingsley & Clark, 2020).

This chapter describes early intervention as a service delivery setting or context that incorporates principles of early childhood mental health into practice. It considers the mission of early intervention services, populations served, contemporary service-delivery models, evidence-based practices, and funding sources in the United States. Assessment and intervention related to mental health and well-being for infants and young children and their families is an emerging area of practice, globally, for pediatric OTPs. As such, best practices from global perspectives are included.

This chapter also presents methods and best-practice principles for monitoring the development of infants and young children as well as screening, assessment, and intervention methods that focus on the identification and support for young children and their caregivers. Finally, this chapter features several voices of early intervention practice around the world by sharing lived experiences from international pediatric OTPs and families who have received early intervention services.

Infant and Toddler Mental Health

Infant and early childhood mental health refers to healthy brain development for children from birth to age 5, including their ability to form healthy attachments with others and learn through sensory motor experiences. Infant and early childhood mental health utilizes a holistic view of the child's physical, mental, and emotional well-being. The phrase "infant and early childhood mental health" is used to depict a practice area concerned with the influence of social-emotional development on overall development. It is an evidence-based intervention approach for improving maternal responsiveness and the socioemotional outcomes of the child (Ribaudo et al., 2022).

Infant and early childhood mental health practice falls within occupational therapy's scope of practice and can be addressed when serving children from birth to age 5 and their families within early intervention settings. The families are not only included within the occupational therapy early intervention treatment session, but the concerns of the caregivers are also addressed (AOTA, 2020). Learners are encouraged to watch a 3-minute YouTube video entitled *What Is Infant Mental Health* (2020), where Dr. Sherri Alderman defines and emphasizes the critical importance of infant mental health: https://www.youtube.com/watch?v=PW3iLkGk4pU.

Influence of Chronic Stress on Brain Development

Through the study of epigenetics, researchers have found that high levels of maternal stress during pregnancy impact brain development in the unborn fetus, especially during the third trimester (DeSocio, 2018). Prenatal maternal stress has been associated with changes in the limbic and frontotemporal networks, including an enlarged amygdala (Lautarescu et al., 2020), which is associated with poor emotional regulation and increased fear responses (Lantz, 2020). Maternal postnatal mental health has an even greater impact on brain development (Burger et al., 2022; Uy et al., 2023), which is why the mother's mental health is vital during a child's first couple years of life. These early years are a critical period for brain development and too much negative stress, or toxic stress, can become "biological memories," which impact not only organ system function but also learning capabilities (de Magalhães-Barbosa et al., 2022).

A toxic stress response can occur when a child experiences "strong, frequent, and/or prolonged adversity, such as physical or emotional abuse, neglect, caregiver substance abuse or mental illness, exposure to violence and/or the accumulated burdens of family economic hardship" (Burke Harris, 2018, pp. 54–55). These traumatic events that children have been

The Lived Experience

The Impacts of the Sociopolitical Environment on Development

Contributed by Mary Musyoki, Occupational Therapist in Kenya

I am a pediatric occupational therapist practicing in Kenya. The growing global concern of childhood mental health is also seen in my country. In Kenya, there are rising concerns about children's behavior such as school dropouts, premarital sex, drug and substance abuse, and more, and this has brought heightened attention to the mental health of children and youth (Memiah et al., 2022). The general public in Kenya has little knowledge about child mental health. Providing proper mental health interventions is hampered by this lack of knowledge and by multiple other challenges that may include limited resources, infrastructure concerns, and lack of qualified providers. These challenges widen the gap between need and provision of care. In addition to economic constraints and limited knowledge about mental illness, systemic issues and the presence of stigma make it difficult to scale up mental health care (Getanda et al., 2017). In Kenya, mental health is looked at as a spiritual problem more than a medical one (Resilience Action, 2022). This in turn affects the acceptance of interventions as many consider religious approaches. There is a lack of awareness of mental health concerns in children among families and also in learning institutions.

There is a strong need to create awareness in the wider community about children's mental health and a need to lobby for facilities that may help children find intervention. Recently, there has been heightened successful suicide in children of "school-going" age in Kenya (Ongeri et al., 2022). If society can be made more aware of the signs of mental issues in children, early intervention will be an added advantage. This means key stakeholders in child mental health need to be involved in awareness campaigns. Stakeholders may include school administration, religious institutions, peers, and, most importantly, families.

One socioenvironmental factor that affects children's mental health is politics (Vertigans & Mueller-Hirth, 2022). Politics affects children's mental health both directly and indirectly.

Children are often caught in the middle of politics among family members and people around them. They may witness looting, fighting, tense political protests, and verbal abuse and their young minds are challenged to comprehend all the menace. These factors represent adverse childhood experiences that cause anxiety and stress to children. Their understanding of political affiliations and differences need to be explained to them to help them comprehend what is taking place around their environment. Children are never sure what the future holds during political upheaval, leading to uncertainty and imbalance. To help them with their mental stability, adults need to have a sit down to explain what it means and be intentional on their understanding of how, despite different political affiliations, there is a need to work together for the good of all.

References

Getanda, E. M., Vostanis, P., & O'Reilly, M. (2017). Exploring the challenges of meeting child mental health needs through community engagement in Kenya. *Child and Adolescent Mental Health, 22*(4), 201–208. https://doi.org/10.1111/camh.12233

Memiah, P., Wagner, F. A., Kimathi, R., Anyango, N. I., Kiogora, S., Waruinge, S., Kiruthi, F., Mwavua, S., Kithinji, C., Agache, J. O., Mangwana, W., Merci, N. M., Ayuma, L., Muhula, S., Opanga, Y., Nyambura, M., Ikahu, A., & Otiso, L. (2022). Voices from the youth in Kenya addressing mental health gaps and recommendations. *International Journal of Environmental Research and Public Health, 19*(9), 5366. https://doi.org/10.3390/ijerph19095366

Ongeri, L., Larsen, D., Jenkins, R., Shaw, A., Connolly, H., Lyon, J., Kariuki, S., Penninx, B., Newton, C., Sifuna, P., & Ogutu, B. (2022). Community suicide rates and related factors within a surveillance platform in Western Kenya. *BMC Psychiatry, 22*, 7. https://doi.org/10.1186/s12888-021-03649-6

Resilience Action. (2022). *Mental health in children and youths in Kenya.* https://www.resilienceaction.net/post/mental-health-in-children-and-youths-in-kenya

Vertigans, S., & Mueller-Hirth, N. (2022). *Children in peace-building and violence during political instability in a Kenyan informal settlement.* International Peace Support Training Centre (IPSTC). https://rgu-repository.worktribe.com/output/1920223/children-in-peace-building-and-violence-during-political-instability-in-a-kenyan-informal-settlement exposed to are referred to as **adverse childhood experiences** (ACEs; Felitti et al., 1998). This seminal research uncovered that the more ACEs a person experienced, the greater the risk to their health. In her TED talk *How Childhood Trauma Affects Health Across a Lifetime* (2015), Dr. Nadine Burke Harris emphasizes the connection between repeated ACEs and brain development in infants and children and the lifetime risk of chronic conditions such as heart disease and lung cancer. Learners are encouraged to take 15 minutes to review this important talk now: https://www.youtube.com/watch?v=95ovIJ3dsNk&t=2s.

The Centers for Disease Control and Prevention (CDC) reports that in addition to ACEs, **social determinants of health**, such as living in racially segregated neighborhoods and food insecurity, can also affect levels of toxic stress in children (2022). The World Health Organization (WHO) defines social determinants of health as "conditions in which people are born, grow, live, work and age, and people's access to power, money and resources" (WHO, 2024). OTPs must consider systemic racism as a possible source of trauma for the children and families they work with (Iruka et al., 2021) as well as the impact of poverty (Lee & Zhang, 2022).

Within the United States, low-income mothers have higher rates of postpartum depression and poorer maternal mental health outcomes (Klawetter et al., 2021). In addition to high stress levels and less access to resources, mothers with a migration background also experience social isolation (Samdan et al., 2021). During the coronavirus pandemic, pregnant and new mothers from marginalized communities experienced greater rates of isolation, depression, and stress (Choi et al., 2020). On a global scale, the ability for a mother to care for her child in a disadvantaged environment, such as without clean running water and continuous electricity in a low-income country, may also negatively impact an infant's development (Burger et al., 2022). In this chapter's The Lived Experience feature, an occupational therapist, Mary Musyoki, shares how social and political occupations in her home country of Kenya challenge the development of children and youth. See Chapter 5: Trauma-Informed Practice.

The Critical Role of Relationships

Living beyond the onset of the pandemic and with a focus on racial justice, there is a new paradigm shift to an emphasis on **early relational health** (Willis et al., 2022). Early relational health focuses on relationships in the early years as biologically fundamental to healthy growth and development. This framework views foundational relationships as being safe, stable, and nurturing for positive outcomes (American Academy of Pediatrics, 2022). Early relational health incorporates the knowledge from infant and early childhood mental health and related fields; its emphasis is on partnering with families to understand their lived experiences and social determinants of health that impact foundational relationships (Willis et al., 2022).

OTPs are responsible for focusing treatment on the "**safe, stable and nurturing relationships (SSNRs)** that buffer adversity and build resilience" (Garner et al., 2021, p. 1). Central to working on SSNRs, practitioners must consider that most, and possibly all, occupations during early childhood are co-occupations. *Co-occupations*, or shared engagement in activities and routines between

two or more people, are characterized by joint or mutual participation (Zemke & Clarke, 1996). Co-occupational routines are meaningful and, by their very nature, require active engagement between individuals. Pickens and Pizur-Barnekow (2009) described **co-occupation** as an activity in which individuals share a high level of physicality, emotionality and intentionality.

Communication is also a critical element of co-occupation (Beckinger et al., 2016). During early childhood, healthy co-occupational engagement enhances human connectedness. Daily shared routines (feeding, bathing, play, dressing) influence brain development, promote sensory health, and with proper scaffolding, increase the child's ability to self-regulate (Center on the Developing Child, 2021). It is critical that practitioners in pediatric settings attend to those elements that lead to healthy social and emotional development; this means addressing the quality of relationships that occur during co-occupational routines.

Maternal mental health is highly correlated with child mental health (Hagan et al., 2022) and the child's capacity for emotional regulation (Ribaudo et al., 2022). It is critical that OTPs in pediatric settings attend to caregivers' mental health and immediate concerns, which directly impact the quality of relationships that occur during co-occupational routines. OTPs can promote positive mental health for the mother–infant dyad, beginning with maternal mental health screening (Barlow & Sepulveda, 2020). "The power of relational health is that it not only buffers adversity when it occurs but also proactively promotes future resilience" (Garner et al., 2021, p. 2). Although practitioners take a family centered approach in early intervention, the shift to early relational health requires a widened lens from the individual child to the well-being of the family, which may involve developing new therapeutic approaches and screening practices.

Early Intervention Programs: Mission and Philosophy

Investment of resources by governments into early intervention and support programs that promote healthy early childhood development have been linked to substantial societal benefits including productivity, positive health outcomes across the life span, and social cohesion of populations and communities (Daelmans et al., 2017). WHO (2020) guidelines emphasize the promotion of mental health for young children and mothers through nurturing care as a central tenet. **Nurturing care** is defined as a stable environment that promotes health and optimal nutrition, protects children from threats, and provides opportunities for early learning through affectionate interactions and relationships. Although globally there is recognition that children, especially young children with disabilities, benefit from support for their development, gaps and inequalities in the provision of early developmental care persist in many parts of the world (Smythe et al., 2021).

The scope of occupational therapy practice in early intervention settings around the world has evolved in recent years to reflect occupational therapy's understanding of the impact of healthy early childhood development and supportive environments on long-term quality of life outcomes. Current practices vary among countries and jurisdictions in terms of service delivery models, professionals involved, and funding arrangements; however, best-practice principles based on international research inform practice and provide a framework for the development and delivery of universal and equitable, quality early intervention services.

Best Practices in Early Intervention

International research has identified several universal best-practice principles to be applied when working with young children and families in early childhood intervention settings (Early Childhood Intervention Australia, 2016). The following principles are considered best-practice for OTPs who provide early intervention services.

Family-centered care, a guiding philosophical and social model used in early intervention practice, promotes a partnership between providers and families (Kuo et al., 2012). This model recognizes that infants and young children depend upon family members for support, nurturance, and survival. Family-centered care is fully embraced when there is open communication; respect for diversity in knowledge, competence, and culture; negotiation and trust; and practice that is embedded in community settings (Kuo et al., 2012). Early intervention programs that use family-centered care models espouse the concept that families are experts on their child's habits and routines; therefore, family members need to be active team members.

Within a family-centered care model, therapy services are relevant to family priorities (Myers et al., 2015). Providers who use a family-centered approach include aspects of the caregiver–child relationship during problem identification and intervention planning. When considering the mental health and well-being of young children, the early intervention provider's work focuses on relationships through coaching in order to ensure the family's needs and concerns are addressed (Salisbury et al., 2018). See Chapter 29: Families. 🤝

Culturally responsive practice is a key component of family-centered care. Culturally responsive practitioners are respectful of diversity and provide services that are flexible and responsive to a family's cultural, racial, and socioeconomic backgrounds. The degree to which a family is involved in early intervention depends primarily on the family's structure, roles, beliefs, and family patterns. Practitioners are encouraged to reflect on their own value system to ensure that services are responsive to the family's characteristics.

Neurodiversity-affirming practice is a strengths-based approach to support young children with developmental delays and conditions. Neurodiversity is a term that is widely used to describe a broad range of characteristics that are associated with developmental conditions that impact the neurological system (Kapp, 2020). Neurodiversity-affirming practice is a social movement that has been likened to the civil rights movement and highlights the importance of addressing the role of social and environmental barriers to inclusion and participation of individuals rather than on interventions that focus on changing a child's behavior to meet social norms (Dawson et al., 2022).

A neurodiversity-affirming practitioner is a person who embraces the idea that people experience and interact with their environments in a myriad of different ways. They

---

BOX 36-1 ■ Five Top Tips for Supporting Neurodiversity in the Early Years

1. Use appropriate terminology and ask families what they prefer (e.g., autistic vs. child with autism spectrum disorder).
2. Assess individual differences in sensory processing and support families to create supportive environments to accommodate diverse sensory preferences.
3. Demonstrate and coach caregivers to support a variety of play activities.
4. Promote inclusive communities (e.g., advocate for a quiet hour at the local shop).
5. Avoid intervention focused on reducing deficits and aim to facilitate activities or skills that naturally lead to learning, social connection, and well-being.

---

understand that these are differences, not deficits to fix. Neurodiversity-affirming practitioners approach practice from the position that there is no one way or right way to interact and be in the world. They also actively facilitate and demonstrate their acceptance for diversity in ways of thinking, behaving, and learning.

Practitioners should apply neurodiversity-affirming practice when supporting individuals who are experiencing conditions that affect the development and function of the nervous system such as autism, fetal alcohol syndrome, adverse early childhood events, or intellectual impairment. Neurodiversity-affirming practice individuals are focused on identifying and building upon strengths and potential benefits of diversity in ways of thinking. Interventions that facilitate acceptance, inclusion, and participation in meaningful occupations are central to neurodiversity-affirming occupational therapy practice that supports mental health and well-being for young children and their families. Box 36-1 shares some key aspects of neurodiversity-affirming practice. See Chapter 27: Mental Health Stigma and Sanism and Chapter 28: Social Determinants and Mental Health. 🤝

Teletherapy in early intervention has grown since the onset of the COVID-19 pandemic in 2020. AOTA and leaders in the field identify teletherapy, telehealth, or telepractice as a means to prevent disabilities, evaluate for occupational and co-occupational performance challenges, intervene if challenges exist, and consult with family members and other professionals (Frolek Clark & Parks, 2021). Evidence shows that teletherapy practice can promote partnerships between OTPs and families of children diagnosed with autism as they collaborate to achieve child outcomes (Zylstra, 2013). In addition to providing occupational therapy assessments and interventions, through synchronous teletherapy, information can be transmitted via telehealth using asynchronous methods.

Telehealth can be provided asynchronously in the form of education and storing/forwarding information related to a child, family, or health-care professional (Maheu, 2022). Practitioners play an essential role in providing children and families with timely, comprehensive, and well-integrated **early intervention** support under a family-centered, best practice framework. Quality early childhood intervention with an early childhood mental health lens leads to better long-term outcomes for children and families, and promotes inclusion, a sense of belonging, and greater participation in their communities. See Chapter 33: Virtual Environments. 🤝

Populations Served in the United States

Early intervention programs, also known as Birth-to-Three programs in the United States, provide coordinated services to families with young children. Children referred to early intervention programs are at risk for or diagnosed with a condition that may impair their ability to fully participate in occupations or co-occupations experienced by typically developing peers. In the United States, **early intervention** refers to those services provided under Part C of the Individuals with Disabilities Education Act of 2004 (IDEA). According to Public Law 108-446 of IDEA, infants and toddlers at risk for or diagnosed with a disability can receive multiple services including, but not limited to, nutritional, educational, therapeutic, and psychological services. Early intervention programs serve families with infants or toddlers from the time they are born through their third birthday. Early intervention services may be provided in the home, an early child-care center, a Head Start Program, or in the community (AOTA, 2014).

Families become involved in early intervention services when their child has a developmental delay or has been diagnosed with a disability. In the United States, federal regulation through the IDEA indicates that the eligibility for early intervention services is decided by individual states, and therefore some states also include children who are deemed **at risk** (Early Childhood Technical Assistance [ECTA] Center, 2022). Children are considered at risk if they would experience a "substantial developmental delay if early intervention services were not provided" (U.S. Department of Education, 2019). Examples of factors that may consider a child at risk include low birth weight, respiratory distress as a newborn, history of abuse or neglect, or direct exposure to illegal substance abuse (National Center for Children in Poverty, 2020).

The U.S. government provides funding for early intervention programs under IDEA. Part C of IDEA regulates individual state policies and procedures for early intervention services. Early intervention is an entitlement program, which means that states are not obligated to provide the services. If a state chooses to provide early intervention services, it must follow the regulations established by the federal government. The U.S. Department of Education provides funding for early intervention services in tribal nations (ECTA Center, 2023).

Another requirement found within IDEA is development of an **Individualized Family Service Plan** (IFSP). The IFSP is developed *with* the family, and services should be family-centered, coordinated, and occur within the child's natural environments. The IFSP is a plan of care that identifies the family's resources, desired outcomes for their child, activities to achieve the noted outcomes, developmental strengths and needs of their child, and plans for transition if the child is approaching their third birthday.

Among children receiving early intervention services, inequities exist. Lack of access to educational support services and health care are social determinants that impede developmental screenings and early intervention services. For example, in the United States, "Black and Latino children with developmental delays are 78% less likely to have their need for early intervention services identified" and "Black children with developmental delays are 78% less likely to receive early intervention services" (Gillispie, 2021). Such disparities are a threat to child well-being (Garner et al., 2021).

Team Members and Approaches to Early Intervention Practice

Practitioners who work in early intervention programs collaborate with a variety of team members, including psychologists, social workers, physicians, special education teachers, physical therapists, nutritionists, and speech-language pathologists. Family members are a significant part of the team and play an important role in determining intervention priorities and outcomes (AOTA, 2014).

A variety of terms (e.g., Primary Service Provider [PSP] with Coaching Approach [Shelden & Rush, 2013], Routines-Based Early Intervention [McWilliam, 2010], and Everyday Children's Learning Opportunities [Dunst, 2000]) are used to describe models and approaches utilized in early intervention practice (ECTA Center, 2022). Each approach differs in philosophy, lines of communication, and service implementation. Although these approaches were developed over time, they are still currently used in early intervention today (ECTA Center, 2022).

Within the PSP with Coaching Approach, an early intervention specialist directs service provision and works with other team members to meet the family's goals and priorities. The PSP could be any team member (occupational therapy, physical therapy, speech-language pathology, etc.) who is identified as optimally suited to meet the family's desired outcomes (ECTA Center, 2022).

The Routines-Based Early Intervention approach (McWilliam, 2010) incorporates service provision in natural environments and inclusive settings. This approach emphasizes naturally occurring learning opportunities found in everyday routines that occur in home and preschool settings. McWilliam developed the Routines-Based interview, which guides the early intervention team in treatment planning and intervention (McWilliam et al., 2009). This approach aligns well with occupational therapy practice as routines are performance patterns that influence occupational engagement and well-being (AOTA, 2020).

The Everyday Children's Learning Opportunities approach (Dunst, 2000) utilizes the interests of children to identify activities that will be a source of learning. A goal of this approach is to engage children in opportunities that foster skill development through practice and exploration of naturally occurring activities within social and nonsocial environments (Dunst, 2000). This approach aligns well with occupational therapy practice as practitioners consider the person and their environments in therapeutic reasoning (AOTA, 2020).

Role of Occupational Therapy

When working in early intervention, occupational therapists follow the three-step occupational therapy process: (1) evaluation, (2) intervention, and (3) targeted outcomes (AOTA, 2020). During evaluation, interviewing occurs with the caregivers. When gathering information for the occupational profile, practitioners ask questions specific to key occupational routines of this population, such as their sleep, wake, feeding, and toileting schedules. Co-occupations of the child and caregiver's daily routines will require careful analysis to understand what the caregiver wants to be able to do and what the child can or cannot do.

It is important to ask the caregivers about their priorities, as they inform goal setting and guide intervention (AOTA, 2020). It is also important to ask open-ended questions to avoid bias in the question and sounding judgmental to the caregiver. For example, when asking caregivers about their child with feeding difficulties, parents are often already very stressed and anxious about this activity of daily living (ADL; Lamm et al., 2023). Practitioners must intentionally create a safe and supportive environment that invites the family to share their experiences.

The prevalence of pediatric feeding disorders (PFD) is now between 1 in 23 and 1 in 37 for children under 5 years of age, making PFD more common than autism or cerebral palsy (Kovacic et al., 2020). A key point to remember when utilizing an early childhood mental health approach in early intervention is that performance in child occupations and co-occupations, such as feeding, occur within the context of a relationship with a parent or caregiver. Therefore, models of co-occupation may provide a useful lens for a practitioner to consider key aspects such as the shared physicality, emotionality, and intentionality of co-occupation when engaged in important functional activities such as bedtime, feeding, or dressing routines (Pickens & Pizur-Barnekow, 2009). Practitioners in early intervention can maintain their focus on early childhood mental health, which is critical for promoting positive outcomes, by engaging in self-reflective practice (Caputo, 2016).

It is helpful for providers to understand the experiences and feelings of the parents, because they can influence the behavior they display and the quality of the interactions with their child. In addition, providers need to pay attention to their own feelings and their feelings in relation to the families they are serving. Self-reflection is at the core of all evaluation and intervention strategies in infant mental health practice. After each treatment session, the practitioner can reflect upon and may choose to journal about the session. Box 36-2 provides guiding reflective questions that practitioners may find helpful, and this chapter's The Lived Experience feature shares one family's experience navigating early intervention.

In addition to self-reflection and journaling, reflective supervision is recommended as best practice (ZERO TO THREE, 2016). Reflective supervision is provided to the early childhood mental health practitioner by an experienced supervisor who engages the practitioner in reflection and collaboration during regularly scheduled visits. The goal of reflective supervision is to promote awareness of feelings and perceptions during encounters with families and to better understand the experience in relation to providing optimal interventions. Research suggests that self-reflective practice

---

BOX 36-2 ■ Self-Reflective Practice in Early Childhood/Childhood Mental Health

Ten Questions to Foster Your Journey Toward Self-Reflection

1. What does it feel like to be in this situation?
2. With whom do I identify in this family?
3. Does this family's story press any "hot buttons" for me? Is there an emotional trigger for me? Consider similarities and differences.
4. What are my perspectives, assumptions, and personal beliefs and how might they be making an impact on my choices around my evaluation, treatment goals, and strategies?
5. Do I think I should play a particular role in this situation (i.e., educator, collaborator, advocator)?
6. What expectations do I have of myself? What other roles could I assume or are there other ways that I could be? How would it change my work with the family to shift my role or way of being? How might the experience shift for this family?
7. How do I explain the child's/family's/other professional's behavior? What are alternative explanations for their behaviors?
8. Given who I am, what do I bring to this family? How might I be influencing or having an impact upon this family in ways not at first apparent?
9. What am I taking for granted in this case?
10. How might I be getting in the way with this case?

Adapted from Nuzzo, 2006

---

enhances student and practitioner self-care, improves emotional health, and decreases workplace burnout (Curry & Epley, 2022).

Self-reflective practice and reflective supervision must be embedded in the pragmatics of assessment and intervention (ZERO TO THREE, 2016). Reflective supervision is an additional early childhood mental health service that can be provided using telepractice techniques. Practitioners should be intentional and proactive and seek mentoring relationships to support their professional development in situations where reflective supervision is not an accessible resource.

Conceptual Practice Models and Theoretical Frameworks

Various theoretical frameworks are available to guide a practitioner's evaluation and interventions and support their ability to effectively address early childhood mental health needs. This section presents four intervention models that provide frameworks for practice in settings that serve infants, toddlers, and their families. Psychobiological Attachment Theory (PAT; Kraemer, 1992) illustrates how the bond between caregiver and child regulates the child's physiology, behavior, emotion, and cognition. Sensory Health (The Star Institute, 2022) supports children's mental health, human connectivity, and resilience. In particular, the Sensory Processing

The Lived Experience

Steering the Way: A Mother's Story Coordinating Her Autistic Son's Health, Well-Being, and Family Life

My husband and I felt alone raising our little boy from the start, from my husband's panic attacks during my pregnancy to my anxiety that something will go wrong with the baby. We had difficulty with my son's sleep, only 45-minute naps when held in our arms; and difficulty breastfeeding and being unable to soothe him. I reached out to a local lactation parenting group and was told "breastfeeding takes some time" and "I was not alone," but it felt lonely and isolating. Nonetheless, our son continued to grow and thrive.

At 12 months old, I noticed language delays. He was not speaking enough. I brought my concerns to his pediatrician, who I assumed was up to date with evidence-based assessments and treatments, only to be dismissed and told to give our son more time because he is bilingual, and the only boy at home. By 18 months, the pediatrician was ready to refer him to early intervention. When I found out I could have self-referred him earlier, I felt devastated and angry because we lost a year of early intervention services. As an occupational therapist registered (OTR) now, I can say my son and family would have benefited from occupational therapy screenings in the primary care setting and being referred to the appropriate provider.

We were never asked about his sleep, eating, or socioemotional health. My son "fell through the cracks" a lot. My son's early intervention services were provided under the Primary Coaching Approach to Teaming (PCATT) model and a speech language provider (SLP), who lacked interdisciplinary training and up-to-date autism spectrum disorder (ASD) screening experience. They missed my son's signs of autism. I remember phrases such as "he connects with mom; he is a happy baby" to describe him during play, but the SLP was unable to assess his repetitive play and disruption to his sleep. We requested the provider collaborate with the team regarding his desire to play inside lying only, and we received a printout of heavy work; no further explanations and no rationale was given or occupational therapy follow-up. It felt like we were dismissed because that printout meant nothing to us—just two pages without education or an explanation of the continuum of care. It was a lot of things and we felt like we needed to be an expert just to put it together.

I don't think my husband and I ever were asked if we were doing OK. My husband and I struggle alongside our son. I have become the connector in the tripod between the spouse, the process, and the child. I felt I had been left to educating my husband while providing support. That was, I think, one of the hardest roles because then I was the one parent who became the expert on my son's care. I don't think professionals do a good job educating parents who are at their different levels of understanding neurodiverse development or at different stages of their journey. I think sometimes professionalism leads the providers to silence their concerns because they are afraid of stepping out of their lane. In our experience, those providers that were bold enough to care and expressed their concerns were the most helpful along the journey.

After countless efforts, including a developmental pediatric clinical evaluation, providers were hesitant and unwilling to sound the alarm for ASD. They did not "see it" as they did not use autism-specific screening or evaluation instruments. We eventually were scheduled for an ASD diagnostic evaluation which took place 2 months shy of our son's fifth birthday, even though we raised concerns about his development during his first year of life. My husband and I were consistently feeling a sense of loss for the child we did not have, processing and pushing because we must; we could not stagnate. We had to grieve and advocate for him all at once. We also learned to love his neurodivergent identity because this will lead him to self-acceptance and self-love; acceptance takes time. My son, now 8 years old, knows he is autistic and also knows he is loved for who he is no matter what.

Model (Dunn, 1997, 2004; Psimas, 2014) describes how the child's and caregiver's degree of processing sensory information during daily routines can influence the parent–child relationship.

The Intentional Relationship Model (IRM; Taylor, 2020) provides practitioners with a framework to reason about the therapeutic use of self. Taylor identifies six modes (advocating, collaborating, empathizing, encouraging, instructing, and problem-solving) that each depict a style of therapeutic interaction. Relationships should be deliberate and intentional, and the mode use should be flexible to meet the needs of the child and their respective caregivers (Taylor, 2020). Ecological Systems Theory (Bronfenbrenner, 1977; Vélez-Agosto et al., 2017) provides a blueprint of proximal and distal systems (microsystem, mesosystem, exosystem, and macrosystems) influencing child development. Vélez-Agosto and colleagues (2017) espouse that culture is inherent in everyday activities, settings, and routines. As such, culture becomes woven into all system levels from micro to macro.

From an early childhood mental health perspective, practitioners need to consider the influence of family, culture, early intervention, and preschool services embedded in a larger community and societal policies and practices. Dunn and colleagues (1994) applied Bronfenbrenner's theory to occupational therapy practice in the development of the Ecology of Human Performance (EHP) Model. The EHP Model transformed how practitioners approached early childhood intervention as there was recognition of the importance of context on task behaviors and performance outcomes. Using these models in early intervention practice can help the provider address mental health aspects of care.

Psychobiological Attachment Theory

PAT (Kraemer, 1992) and its associated frame of reference (Barnekow & Kraemer, 2005) contribute to the field of early intervention by identifying the influence of the sociocultural environment on early neurobiological development.

Caregiver–infant interactions regulate infant physiology through complex interactions between genomic expression, neurocircuitry, and demands or affordances of the contextual environment (Fleming & Kraemer, 2019). This theory extends John Bowlby's (1969) attachment theory for use in early intervention settings. Bowlby argued that the child's ability to form a strong relationship with at least one primary caregiver provided a secure foundation necessary for a child's development, and that parenting style predicts healthy or impaired attachment. Bowlby's theory informs practice when disruption in attachment is caused by inadequate caregiving, as it emphasizes the importance of warm responsive care.

The theory, however, does not fully account for disruptions in attachment when the caregiver is nurturing, yet the child responds differently. The variation in a child's response to nurturing care may be a direct result of impairment or disability (Wolke et al., 2014). Kraemer (1992) addressed attachment disruptions when the caregiver is nurturing and the child responds differently. Children with disabilities may not express behaviors and emotions in the same fashion as children without disabilities (Barnekow & Kraemer, 2005; Wolke et al., 2014; ZERO TO THREE, 2016). They may not respond to nurturing care with the same repertoire of behavior as children without disabilities.

Wolke and colleagues (2014) investigated differences in attachment security in very low birth weight and very preterm infants. They found that the infants' developmental delay predicted attachment security. Therefore, PAT and its associated frame of reference provide a way of considering infant and toddler mental health and relationships when a child has a disability or is at risk for developing a delay. Specifically, this theory includes four tenets that have implications for the child and caregivers' interactions (Barnekow & Kraemer, 2005).

First, Kraemer (1992) proposed that adaptive mechanisms present at birth foster attunement to a caregiver, and these mechanisms provide the foundation for development of prosocial behavior. Infants possess experience-expectant neural circuits that facilitate attention to highly relevant social stimuli found in the environment (Leppanan, 2011). When these circuits are disrupted, this affects the ability of the infant to tune into salient features of the caregiver that promote bonding. Consider Yengkong, a typically developing young child who became severely ill with an *Escherichia coli* infection at the age of 9 months, resulting in brain damage that caused cognitive impairment, cortical blindness, hearing loss, and fluctuating muscle tone. His parents told the therapist that they did not know if Yengkong knew who they were as Yengkong no longer demonstrated joint attention, visual tracking, or turning his head when they called his name.

Second, Kraemer (1992) stated that the child's nervous system is highly plastic. Nervous system development occurs within the context of the caregiver–child relationship (ZERO TO THREE, 2016), and social experiences facilitate neuronal connections (Greenough et al., 1987; Leppanan, 2011). Practitioners need to recognize that the social environment plays a significant role in neural maturation and facilitates parent–child social processes that occur during play and ADLs. In the case of Yengkong, as treatment progressed, the practitioner realized that Yengkong *did* know who his parents were, as he would become calm when he heard their voices. The practitioner helped the parents understand that his nervous system was recovering and was responsive to their loving care.

Third, Kraemer (1992) espoused that the caregiver serves as a psychobiological regulator of the child's physiology, neurobiology, and behaviors. In other words, a caregiver's capacity to provide structure and routine can influence the child's ability to regulate and self-organize. This point underscores the impact of caregiver responsiveness during daily routines. Initially, when Yengkong was discharged from the hospital, he was very agitated and cried much of the day. After 3 months, Yengkong began to sit when held by his father in a quiet alert state. His father provided for Yengkong's care and he regulated Yengkong's nervous system. He displayed separation anxiety when he was away from his father or primary caregiver, and when held by him, Yengkong gently nestled into his arms.

Fourth, Kraemer (1992) stated that caregiving styles are embedded within a sociocultural niche; therefore, sociocultural factors influence caregiver–child reciprocity. Ethnicity and culture play a significant role in parenting and caregiving characteristics, and the most adaptive parenting styles vary across cultures. For example, the Eastern medical traditions of the Hmong culture may be in direct conflict with practices of Western medicine (Carteret, 2012). Interpretation of caregiving patterns is best understood through the sociocultural influences on caregiving routines. In the story of Yengkong, because the family was Hmong and followed the practices of Eastern medicine, they had significant trust issues with professionals who practiced Western medicine. The parents believe that Yengkong's illness occurred at the hospital. They relied on shamanic spiritual practices of healing which included the belief that illness occurs because the soul is separated from the body.

The initial step in treating Yengkong within the context of the family was establishment of the professional–family relationship. The first home visit consisted of talking with the father for the entire visit. The practitioner did not physically handle the child until they were invited back for a second visit. Over time, the family and the practitioner established a relationship, and the parents became great teachers. They taught the practitioner about the Hmong culture, Eastern medicine, and the difficulties they encountered with Western health care.

Kraemer's theory aligns well with best practices in early intervention by encouraging cultural responsiveness and humility in practice; this involves learning about caregiving practices in other cultures. PAT addresses neurological differences in the child that may impact caregiver–child bonding and facilitate clinical reasoning about the role that attachment plays in the neurobiological development of the child.

Sensory Health and Sensory Processing Model

Sensory Health is demonstrated when a child can process the sensory information received from the environment in an adaptive manner that promotes emotional well-being and participation (The Star Institute, 2022). Many children have challenges processing the sensations they encounter in everyday life. Practitioners can use the Sensory Processing Model (Dunn, 1997, 2004; Psimas, 2014) to assist caregivers to understand their child's Sensory Health and processing. One good strategy is encouraging parents or caregivers to reflect on their own experiences with sensory stimuli as a way to understand their infant's sensory reactions during daily routines.

The *neurological threshold continuum* involves sensitization and habituation. If a child's neurological system primarily responds with sensitization, they may be readily distracted. Conversely, if a child's nervous system primarily responds to the environment by habituating, the child may not notice stimuli in the environment (Dunn, 2004). The *self-regulation strategy continuum* comprises passive and active categories. A child using a passive response strategy in respect to a sensory sensitivity may be distractible and highly responsive to stimulation in their environment (Psimas, 2014). Too much passivity may indicate that the stimuli are overwhelming.

A child using an active response strategy of sensory avoiding will engage in behaviors to manage the sensory stimuli inherent in their daily activities, such as forming rigid routines and rituals (Psimas, 2014).

When working with infants and toddlers in early intervention settings, practitioners consider the child's sensory processing profile while understanding the caregiver's sensory processing strategies. For example, a toddler utilizing a passive strategy to cope with stimuli in the environment may remain oblivious to events and stimuli. The toddler using this mode of regulation may present with a flat affect or seem self-absorbed. If the caregiver also presents with low registration, they may not readily notice the infant's signals, may be slower to respond to the infant, and may need cues to attend to the infant in a timely manner. In this chapter's Practitioner

Practitioner Profile

Contributed by Allison Bennet, OTR, Pediatric Care of Colorado

Pediatric Care of Colorado operates in the Greater Denver area with a mission to provide meaningful, individualized in-home pediatric services and assist children with disabilities and developmental delays in achieving inclusivity and an improved quality of life.

Children are referred here by pediatricians, care coordinators, related health professionals, and parents/caregivers. Occupational therapy focuses on supporting meaningful engagement in all occupations of childhood and family life. Practitioners work collaboratively with families and other professionals to address physical, sensory, and cognitive challenges and to overcome environmental barriers to participation.

Occupational therapy goals focus on optimizing occupational performance and well-being by providing individualized, holistic treatment tailored to each unique child and family. Practitioners here have expertise in:

- Family and caregiver education
- Coaching and parenting strategies
- Supporting healthy child development
- Motor skill development
- Self-care skill development
- Sensory and visual processing
- Cognitive delays and learning challenges
- Social interaction and play skills
- Movement, strength, or balance delays

Occupational therapy provides evaluation, prevention, diagnostic, and therapeutic services via interactive telecommunication technology or sessions in the child's home, preschool, or community settings (e.g., playgrounds, recreation centers, pools, local libraries). Providing telehealth services extends comprehensive, family-centered care to families living rurally.

The Sensory Processing and Intentional Relation Models are commonly used in our setting to understand a child's functioning, to build therapeutic rapport, and to support collaborative problem-solving with children and parents. For example, we encourage parents to be "sensory detectives" to gain a

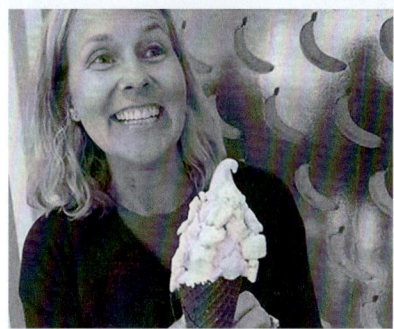

perspective of how their child perceives and filters sensory input in their daily activities. This awareness often helps the family to problem-solve new ways to support their child during challenging times of the day. Beginning sessions by asking parents what's been going well or has been challenging is a routine strategy for building an engaging relationship.

Evaluation often includes using the Routine-Based Inventory and the DAYC Supports IFSP reviews. Common approaches include play and routines-based interventions and co-occupation to foster relationship development, strong attachment, and bonding. Recognizing the links between positive social-emotional connections and the impact of relationships with mothers and caregivers on the well-being of children and families, we utilize coaching approaches. We coach families to engage in daily shared routines such as feeding, bathing, and play in ways that support healthy bonding and attachment. Mealtimes often provide opportunities to observe, problem-solve, and coach the family in real time.

Key professional practice skills in this setting include empathetic listening, communication, interviewing, playfulness, problem-solving, assessment, flexibility, advocacy, and coaching. Being able to problem-solve collaboratively and strong task analysis are also critical skills. Practitioners working closely with children and families must be mindful and look after their own well-being. Maintaining professional boundaries is essential for professional development as is setting aside time to have fun and develop health and sustainable self-care strategies.

Profile feature, Allison Bennet shares how Sensory Processing and Intentional Relation Models guide her interventions with children in her pediatric practice and support collaborative problem-solving with both children and parents.

The Intentional Relationship Model

The IRM (Taylor, 2020) assists practitioners as they serve children and families by providing a framework that creates a place for relationships. Within this model, therapeutic relationships and mindful empathy are central to enhancing occupational and co-occupational performance. They are the foundation of a healthy working alliance. Within IRM, the child and family identify if a relationship is successful.

Successful therapeutic use of self means that relationships are deliberate and intentional, and that the mode's use should be flexible to meet the needs of the child and their respective caregivers. Table 36-1 provides examples of each IRM mode's use in the context of early childhood mental health.

Central to IRM is mindful empathy, self-discipline, and flexible, intentional mode use. To assist practitioners with identification of their preferred mode use, Taylor developed a self-assessment tool. Understanding a practitioner's preferred mode is critical in clinical reasoning as this facilitates self-awareness and can facilitate adjustment if the practitioner's preferred mode is not a good fit for the needs of the child and family.

When using IRM to guide clinical reasoning, practitioners differentiate situational characteristics of the child and family within certain contexts and enduring characteristics of the child and family that may contribute to the relationship. Situational characteristics are characteristics unique to certain contexts. For example, a young child may be withdrawn at the onset of an initial visit with the practitioner and then actively engage with therapeutic activities at the end of the session. The context of the initial visit required rapport and relationship building. Enduring characteristics are seen consistently across contexts and tend to be personality traits. The child may become overwhelmed in multiple settings and demonstrate challenging behaviors across each setting.

Empathic breaks can occur when a practitioner isn't self-aware, or self-disciplined. An example of an empathic break may be when a parent frequently cancels therapy sessions, and the practitioner blames the parent versus taking a reflective stance and trying to understand why the parent is canceling therapy. When these challenges occur, they should be addressed, or the therapeutic relationship may be at risk. Early childhood mental health practice considers the role of multiple relationships (parent/child; parent/practitioner, and child/practitioner). Because relationships are central in early childhood mental health practice, the IRM is a critical model to use in early childhood mental health practice.

Bioecological Systems Theory and the Ecology of Human Performance Model

Urie Bronfenbrenner developed Ecological Systems Theory in 1977, and this theory transformed the view of child development and occupational therapy practice. Before 1977, scholars in the field of child development did not consider the impact of contextual factors that influence development. Figure 36-1 illustrates the use of concentric circles to represent proximal (those close to the child) and distal (those related to but surrounding the child) systems that impact development. In the 1990s, Bronfenbrenner (1995a, 1995b) made two important revisions to Ecological Systems Theory by adding the chronosystem (time elements) and additional postulates regarding the microsystem that included interactions between the child, other persons, objects, and symbols that are meaningful to the child (see Fig. 36-1). More recently, Vélez-Agosto and colleagues (2017) argued that the macrosystem is fluent throughout all of the systems and that cultural values and beliefs define the microsystem and are part of the proximal systems of development.

There is a direct relationship between Bronfenbrenner's Ecological Systems Theory and the EHP Model as espoused by Dunn and colleagues in 1994. In this seminal work, Dunn and colleagues provided practitioners with clinical reasoning when considering the interaction between context and the person engaging in occupations. The context includes temporal, physical, social, and

TABLE 36-1 | Using the Intentional Relationship Model in Early Childhood Mental Health

Mode	Definition	Example
Advocating	Facilitating access and opportunities for the child and family	The practitioner provides the family with a referral to obtain family therapy when they are struggling with discipline and challenging behaviors.
Collaborating	Allowing the family to lead the partnership by identifying goals	The parent identifies challenges with sleep and the practitioner provides resources on sleep routines.
Empathizing	Understanding and listening to the family and child in a nonjudgmental way	The parent describes their recovery process from opioid addiction and recognizes their role in their infant's neonatal abstinence syndrome. The practitioner listens carefully to the parents' story and understands that they are trying to do their best when caring for their child.
Encouraging	Utilizing positive reinforcement to increase performance	The practitioner praises a child or parent for completing a challenging task.
Instructing	Using educational strategies to enhance occupational or co-occupation engagement	The practitioner provides feeding techniques and strategies to a parent of a child with feeding challenges.
Problem-solving	Creating opportunities to reason or think about opportunities for success	The practitioner works with a mother who is experiencing anxiety about the pros and cons of going to a family celebration.

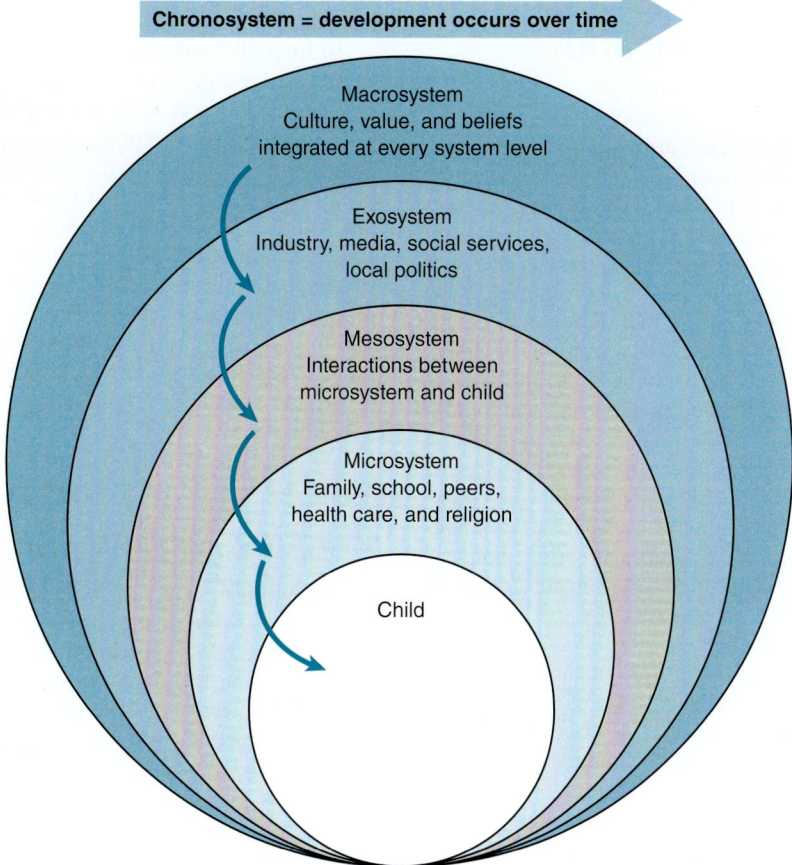

FIGURE 36-1. Bronfenbrenner's Ecological Systems Theory.

TABLE 36-2 | Applying the EHP Model in Childhood Mental Health

Strategy	Definition	Example
Establish and restore	This strategy focuses on changing "person" factors.	An infant is demonstrating difficulty with sucking, swallowing, and breathing during feeding, which is impacting the relationship between the caregiver and infant. The practitioner designs an intervention that improves coordinated feeding, which subsequently improves the maternal infant bond.
Alter	The practitioner looks at contextual opportunities to enhance development.	A foster care parent indicates that going out to eat is stressful and the child covers their ears and becomes dysregulated at dinner. The practitioner offers suggestions of restaurants that are sensory friendly.
Adapt	The practitioner identifies ways to change the environment or task to enhance co-occupational or occupational performance.	A mom of an infant recently discharged from the neonatal intensive care unit (NICU) is having difficulty holding the infant during bathing, which impacts her self-confidence. The practitioner recommends swaddle bathing, which is calming to the infant and facilitates maternal self-confidence.
Prevent	The practitioner employs strategies to prevent disease or disability.	The practitioner provides a local library with the CDC's "Learn the Signs. Act Early" 1-, 2-, and 3-year-old books to give to parents who attend a parenting class.
Create	The practitioner develops a strategy that enhances co-occupational and occupational performance for everyone involved.	The practitioner develops a classroom yoga routine with a preschool teacher to enhance self-regulation throughout the morning.

cultural aspects that interact with aspects of the person including values; beliefs; and sensorimotor, cognitive, and psychosocial aspects. The interaction between context and person results in completion of tasks; importantly, the three components (context, person, task) need to be understood together. In addition, Dunn and colleagues outlined novel intervention strategies of which many are included in the 4th edition of the *Occupational Therapy Practice Framework* (OTPF-4; AOTA, 2020). Table 36-2 provides the definitions and examples of each intervention strategy included in the EHP Model from an early childhood mental health approach.

Developmental Monitoring, Screening, Evaluation, and Intervention

The occupational therapy process utilizing an early childhood mental health approach in early intervention settings is similar to the process in other practice settings: Practitioners engage in developmental monitoring, screening, evaluation, intervention, and discharge (AOTA, 2020). However, when providing early childhood mental health services, the focus of these practices is guided by early childhood mental health principles (relationship and strengths-based, self-reflective practice). Various resources are available to practitioners, including the *Diagnostic Classification of Mental Health and Developmental Disorders of Infancy and Early Childhood* (*DC: 0–5*™; ZERO TO THREE, 2016, 2020), which assists the early childhood mental health practitioner with classifying mental health challenges during early childhood. Specifically, this categorization of conditions identifies Sensory Processing Disorder as a diagnosable condition and provides an understanding of the role of relationships and psychosocial stressors on early development.

Table 36-3 outlines key information about common evaluation tools to help guide the practitioner's therapeutic reasoning during the evaluation processes. Table 36-4 summarizes the core tenets of the four conceptual practice models described earlier, and describes scenario examples of application of the approach in evaluation and intervention.

Transition to Early Childhood and Inclusive Environments: Key Transitions and Mainstream Support

A critical role of the early intervention team is to coordinate a smooth transition from early intervention to early childhood education (Podvey & Myers, 2015). In early intervention in the United States, this transition occurs at the child's third birthday. Parents may feel insecure and even abandoned at this time, as their interactions with professionals in relation to their child significantly change. Families often become accustomed to professionals coming into their home and miss the close relationships that have been established with the early intervention team. The school setting differs from early intervention programming because the family loses the service coordination found in early intervention settings. Moreover, the emphasis in intervention shifts from play, ADLs, and school readiness to participation in activities and skills that are specific to the school environment.

Although play, ADLs, and school readiness may still pose challenges to a child's functional performance, the long-term goal is to help promote independence and functioning within the school environment. The concept of the natural environment also changes. In early intervention, natural environments include a child's home or early care and learning centers. As a child transitions out of early intervention into the school setting, professionals focus more on participation in various school environments such as the classroom, playground, or cafeteria (Podvey & Myers, 2015). See Chapter 37: School Mental Health.

To help alleviate this stress, the early intervention team can begin talking about transition services early. This planning should begin at 30 to 32 months (Wrightslaw, 2017). The OTP may be instrumental in setting up visits to the school and addressing the parents' concerns. Parents will need to be strong advocates for their children in school settings. The practitioner may assist through enabling the family to find its voice and advocate for their child (Podvey & Myers, 2015). It is important to remember that when taking a life-cycle approach to the family, transitions may be a challenging time. The practitioner's role may be to help the family develop a sense of balance and homeostasis by establishing new routines and habits.

Voices of Early Intervention Practice Around the World

In this section, OTPs from around the world share their experiences working with children and their families. The OTPs from Uganda, Rwanda, Guyana, and Kuwait are all members of an international mentorship program (https://libguides.aic.edu/OT_Resources) and attend regularly. The OTP from the Philippines, Lyle Duque, was a subject matter expert mentor on disaster management, who has presented for the mentorship program. These OTPs were interviewed and their stories were written from the perspective of a U.S.-based OTP. Some of them live and work in countries where health-care systems and resources are well developed and plentiful, whereas others work in resource-scarce environments. Despite the wide variety in health-care systems and funding sources for occupational therapy, OTPs from around the world share the goals of early intervention and family-centered care.

Low Resource Country: Uganda With George Bush

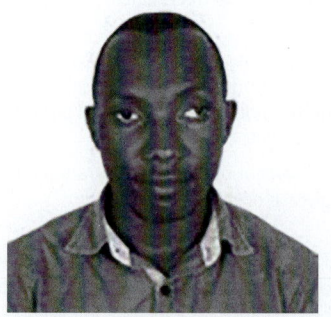

In Uganda, occupational therapy services are provided by the government and only in hospital settings. The government funds education for primary grades 1 to 7, for children ages 6 to 12, and for children with special needs who attend separate schools. Most schools sponsored or provided by the government focus primarily on visual and hearing impairment rather than physical or intellectual ones. Occupational therapy is currently not provided within the public school

TABLE 36-3 | Therapeutic Reasoning Assessment Table: Early Intervention

Which Tool?	Who Was This Tool Designed For?	What Is Required of the Person? Can They Use the Tool?	What Am I Measuring?	How Long Does It Take and Where Do I Administer This Assessment?	Is the Tool Associated With a Practice Model?
"Learn the Signs. Act Early" (CDC, 2023), https://www.cdc.gov/ncbddd/actearly	This free developmental monitoring program was designed for children 2 months to 5 years.	A parental checklist is used. Parent needs to be able to read or it can be read to parents. These tools can be used by health-care and child-care providers.	This tool tests for progress toward developmental milestones in language, cognition, social/emotion skills, and motor skills.	A checklist takes approximately 2–5 minutes to complete.	Psychobiological Attachment Theory: Children who are neurodiverse may respond differently, which could affect bonding and attachment. EHP: This considers aspects of the child that may influence social-emotional development.
Occupational Profile Template (AOTA, 2022)	This is available for individuals of all ages and abilities. It is a structured but informal method to better understand aspects of the family's internal experiences with the child.	The template is completed by trained OTPs. The parent or caregiver provides information to complete the profile.	It is used for parent or caregiver perception of the child, which is also informed by OTPs' observations of the child and parent/caregiver performing occupations.	It can be administered in the home in 10–20 minutes	No specific model but grounded in the *Occupational Therapy Practice Framework,* 4th ed. (*OTPF-4;* AOTA, 2020).
Ages and Stages Questionnaire, Third Edition (Squires & Bricker, 2009) Ages and Stages Questionnaire: Socialemotional, Second Edition (Squires et al., 2015)	It is used with infants and children 1 month to 6 years old. The parent or caregiver uses self-report screening instruments to determine if a child is at risk for developmental delay.	This questionnaire requires the parent or caregiver to read and understand written directions and instructions.	This identifies the parent or caregiver's perception of their child's development.	It can be administered in the home in 10–15 minutes or sent home with parent/caregiver to be scored and assessed upon next visit.	No specific model but consistent with family-centered care models
DC: 0–5™ Assessment of Dimensions of Caregiving, Infant Contributions to the Relationship and Dimensions of the Caregiving Environment (ZERO TO THREE, 2016)	It is used with infants and children from birth to 5 years old. It offers an interdisciplinary rating scale of relationship.	OTP observation during co-occupational engagement is essential.	Dimensions of the caregiving relationship are evaluated.	Observation can occur over 20–30 minutes.	No specific model but consistent with family-centered care models
DC: 0–5™ Psychosocial and Environmental Stressor Checklist (ZERO TO THREE, 2016)	It is used with infants and children from birth to 5 years old. It offers an interdisciplinary rating scale of psychosocial and environmental stressors.	The measure involves observation by treatment team members and history in multiple contexts–it is designed to capture exposure to cumulative stressors.	It evaluates for chronic or toxic stress.	Testing is continuous and ongoing.	No specific model but consistent with family-centered care models
ASDetect (2020), asdetect.org	This free app is designed to be completed by parents of children ages 11–30 months to identify early signs of autism.	ASDetect guides parents through assessment questions and simple activities using specially produced videos.	This highly accurate and evidence-based screening tool assesses key social, attentional, and communication milestones.	The assessment takes approximately 20–30 minutes and can be downloaded for free and administered at home by parents.	Consistent with best-practice principles of early intervention, this video-led self-assessment app is based on rigorous research conducted at the Olga Tennison Autism Research Centre and is 83% accurate in the early detection of autism (Barbaro et al., 2022).

Continued

TABLE 36-3 | Therapeutic Reasoning Assessment Table: Early Intervention—cont'd

Which Tool?	Who Was This Tool Designed For?	What Is Required of the Person? Can They Use the Tool?	What Am I Measuring?	How Long Does It Take and Where Do I Administer This Assessment?	Is the Tool Associated With a Practice Model?
Devereux Early Childhood Assessment: Infant version (DECA-I) Toddler version (DECA-T) Preschool version (DECA-P2)	It is used with: Infants 4 weeks to 18 months Toddlers 18–36 months Children 3–5 years	This parent/caregiver report measure can be read to the parent.	It measures emotional and behavioral adjustment and assesses positive and protective factors.	It takes approximately 5–10 minutes to administer.	It is a strengths-based approach grounded in resilience research.
Infant and Toddler Sensory Profile 2 (Dunn, 2014)	It is used with infants and children from birth to 14 years, 11 months old. Standardized assessment is designed to assess the person's sensory needs and preferences.	Questionnaire is completed by parents, caregivers, or teachers. Raters must be able to read and understand questions.	Sensory needs and preferences are recorded as observed by parents, caregivers, or teachers.	Observation of person completing occupation ranges from 15–45 minutes with approximately 20 minutes to score.	Dunn Model of Sensory Processing
Perinatal Posttraumatic Stress Disorder Questionnaire II (PPQ II; Callahan et al., 2006; DeMier et al., 2000)	The PPQ II is a self-report measure of symptoms of posttraumatic stress in mothers who have given birth to an infant requiring care in the NICU. Further evaluation by a trained psychologist is necessary to confirm a posttraumatic stress disorder (PTSD) diagnosis.	Questionnaire is completed by mothers more than 1 month after their infant is discharged from the NICU. Validity and reliability are established internationally.	The questionnaire measures symptoms of PTSD including intrusive thoughts, reliving, withdrawal and avoidance behaviors, numbness, hyperarousal, and feelings of guilt. When used clinically, early intervention providers should ensure that mental health services are available to the mothers.	It is a self-report measure; the person can complete the form in 20 minutes with approximately 10 minutes to score.	Psychobiological Attachment Theory: Maternal responsiveness may be impeded by PTSD symptoms, which may negatively impact attachment and bonding.
Edinburgh Postnatal Depression Scale (EPDS; Cox et al., 1987, 2014)	The EPDS is a screening instrument designed to identify if depressive symptoms are present 7 days before completing the screening. Further diagnostic evaluation is required to confirm a diagnosis of depression.	This self-report 10-item questionnaire has been translated in multiple languages.	The EPDS measures symptoms of depression, but does not measure somatic symptoms of depression. Early intervention providers should ensure that access to mental health services are available to mothers after screening is completed.	Questionnaire takes about 5 minutes to complete. It is frequently used during postnatal follow-up visits.	Psychobiological Attachment Theory: Symptoms of depression can impact maternal responsiveness and impede bonding.
Survey of Well-Being of Young Children (SWYC)	The SWYC is a free, developmental screen for children 2 months to 5 years of age.	The SWYC involves a parental checklist.	The SWYC measures developmental milestones, behavioral/emotional development, and family risk factors. Autism screening is also provided with 18-, 24-, and 30-month checklists.	A checklist takes approximately 10–15 minutes to complete.	https://www.tuftsmedicine.org/medical-professionals-trainees/academic-departments/department-pediatrics/survey-well-being-young-children

TABLE 36-4 | Theoretical Approaches in Early Intervention Table: Application to Assessment and Intervention

Approach	Core Tenets	Application Scenario
Psychobiological Attachment Theory (Kraemer, 1992)	The attachment bond between caregiver and child regulates the child's physiology, behavior, emotion, and cognition. Attachment bonds form within the context of co-occupational (shared physicality, emotionality, intentionality, and communicative) experiences.	***Scenario:*** A teenage mother lives with her mother and stepfather in a small rural home. She tends to play with her son very intrusively (e.g., tapping his face with toys, increasing the loudness of her voice). Her son eventually looks away from the mother and begins to cry. ***Assessment:*** • Use occupational profile to better understand daily routines and stress. • Observe using Dimension of Caregiving Relationship Scale and Psychosocial and Environment Stressors Checklist (DC: 0–5; ZERO TO THREE, 2016). • Observe co-occupational experiences and the interaction for shared physicality (motor responsiveness), emotionality (emotional responsiveness), and intentionality (purpose/goal of behavior). ***Intervention:*** • Video record the interaction and work with the mother to describe positive and challenging aspects during the co-occupation. • Develop a plan with the mother to achieve optimal developmental outcomes.
Sensory Processing Model (Dunn, 1997)	The ability to process sensory stimuli is related to self-regulation and functional engagement in young children. The sensory processing of caregivers and children falls on a continuum. Assessment is aimed at understanding sensory processing capacity of the child. The focus of intervention is promoting optimal self-regulation in the child and supporting the caregiver in functional engagement (Psimas, 2014).	***Scenario:*** A 2-year-old child is withdrawn and demonstrates significant sensory avoidance to tactile stimuli that is impairing engagement in early childhood/learning center activities. The child is quiet until overwhelmed and then will tantrum, disrupting classroom activities. ***Assessment:*** • Infant and Toddler Sensory Profile 2 • Observation of caregiver behaviors related to sensory processing ***Intervention:*** • Incorporate specific activities into the daily routine that are designed to address the sensory avoidance to tactile stimuli. • Intervention activities may include encouraging deep pressure/heavy work activities in the classroom (e.g., carrying objects, pushing a weighted cart) and holding the child firmly during dressing and cleaning up after eating (Psimas, 2014).
The Intentional Relationship Model (Taylor, 2020)	This person-centered tool utilizes mindful empathy as well as flexible and intentional modes.	***Scenario:*** A child diagnosed with Down syndrome (social and cognitive competence) requires assistance and longer time to get dressed in the morning (family interactions). Both parents are employed (family resources), and there is a 4-year-old sibling. Mother is being reprimanded by her employer because she is sometimes late to work because of slow dressing and stressful morning routine (family resources). Mother interacts with children abruptly, and their relationship is tense (parent-child interaction—social-emotional connectedness). ***Assessment:*** • Use the occupational profile to better understand daily routines and stress. • Observe using Dimensions of Caring Relationship Scale and Psychosocial and Environmental Stressors Checklist (DC: 0–5; ZERO TO THREE, 2016). ***Intervention:*** • Utilize the instructing mode to teach the mother strategies that positively impact morning routines (i.e., laying out clothing the night before).
Bioecological Systems Theory and EHP Model	Children develop within the context of the environment. Task performance is related to the interaction of the person, context, and the given task.	***Scenario:*** The OTP is providing consultation to the local Head Start Program. The early childhood education professional (ECEP) confides with the OTP that they are struggling with a 2-year-old child who is unable to self-regulate after their parent drops them off at the early care and learning setting. The OTP asks the ECEP what they perceive the child is feeling after being dropped off at the center and takes the child's psychosocial development into consideration (person). The OTP then asks what is happening at the center when the child is being dropped off (context) and helps the ECEP identify the importance of smooth transitions (task engagement) as this may be an important goal to address with the child to enhance the relationship between ECEP and the child. ***Assessment:*** • Ages and Stages Questionnaire: Social-Emotional, the Infant Toddler Sensory Profile, and observation during the time when children are dropped off. ***Intervention:*** • Prevent—The OTP and ECEP identify strategies that would prevent dysregulation when the child is dropped off. • Some ideas may be to see if the parent could stay a little longer or drop off the child earlier or allowing the child to bring a familiar toy or book to the center.

setting, primarily because of the limited number of OTPs in the country.

Children with special needs are often identified in the community from nongovernmental organization (NGO) outreach and education, as well as from a social worker going house to house (employed by the NGO). Once identified as having special needs, the child can receive NGO therapy services through home visiting, center-based services, and/or private preschool therapy services.

George works for an NGO called Soft Power Education, with children primarily 2 to 5 years of age. He works in a private preschool setting and in children's home. It is not common to see children under the age of 2, because they often have not yet been identified. Children are often identified around age 2, when they miss milestones and the parents become aware there is a problem. The NGOs are currently able to provide better therapy services and equipment than the public special education school, so many children receive services through the NGO. For example, the NGO can provide a child with a wheelchair, but the government school cannot.

Low Resource Country: Rwanda With Epiphanie Murebwayire

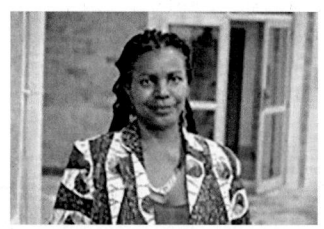

Epiphanie works at the Rwanda Military Hospital and provides outpatient pediatric services for children from birth to 4 years of age. Most children she treats are between the ages of 2 and 3; however, she does see children as young as a week old.

Epiphanie explains that a child with a diagnosis of Erb's palsy may come to the outpatient hospital as a newborn, compared with other children who are referred later. She is most likely to treat children with cerebral palsy, Down syndrome, attention deficit-hyperactivity disorder (ADHD), and ASD. Epiphanie stated that the OTPs take a family-centered approach with the families who come to outpatient therapy at the hospital. At this time, only physiotherapists work in the NICU.

Children in Rwanda start school at either age 2 or 5, depending on the child's ability to communicate (baby school or preschool). Public (government) school is partially paid for by the government; families have to pay a school fee and cover the cost of transportation. There are no occupational therapy services in the public schools currently. Epiphanie is hopeful that as the number of OTPs increases in the country, the services will expand into the school system. Children can receive occupational therapy in some of the private schools for children with disabilities. All schools for children with special needs are private;

therefore, the families have to pay for their children to receive therapy.

Occupational therapy services are covered by some, but not all, insurances. The Rwanda Occupational Therapy Association (RWOTA) is working closely with the Ministry of Health and company insurances advocating for occupational therapy services to be covered. The government does not provide free occupational therapy services. In 2015, there were only two practicing OTPs in Rwanda; today there are approximately 40. Epiphanie is one of only two OTPs in the hospital where she works. Epiphanie is hopeful though, because the number of occupational therapists is rising, and she is "happy to be an OT."

Middle Resource Country: Guyana With Errica Canterbury

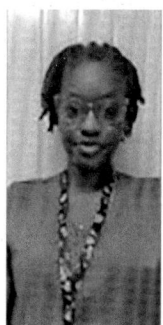

Occupational therapy in Guyana is provided within government centers free of charge to the public. The government center provides day care, outpatient therapy, and some home visiting when needed. Children at the center receive free occupational therapy from birth until they enter the school system at age 3. Children with special needs also receive the necessary equipment they need, such as a wheelchair, from the outpatient therapy centers run by the government.

Children with and without special needs receive a free education in Guyana; however, the children with special needs are in a separate school. OTPs do not currently work in the school systems because there are only six practicing OTPs in the country, and they all work in the government centers.

Errica works at the Ptolemy Reid Rehabilitation Center. The OTPs there educate the physicians in the NICUs in the local hospital about the services they can provide at the government center. Educating the doctors has been helpful in increasing the number of infants they see. Errica stated she has worked with an infant as young as 11 days old; however, most families recognize a delay around 1 year when the child has missed developmental milestones, such as walking. Children typically attend therapy two times per week, so the OTPs stress the importance of the parents continuing the therapy at home. Errica explains that they teach the parents a home program and then have them demonstrate competence as part of therapy. Home visits are also focused on parent education.

Middle Resource Country: Philippines With Lyle Duque

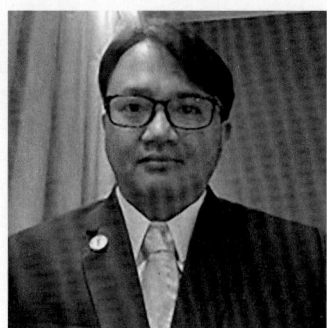

Lyle is a pediatric OTP in the Philippines where 95% of the approximately 5,000 OTPs work in pediatrics. Lyle explains that this is because of a combination of both culture and history. In Philippine culture, there is a large emphasis on child development and education, as well as an expectation that the family will care for older persons. The Philippine family has a large, extended setup. This facilitates care for older persons as well as extra hands for looking after children at home until they are school age.

Public education is free in the Philippines, and formal education begins at around 5 years with kindergarten.

Although OTPs work in private and international schools, they are not yet employed by the public schools. A few OTPs consult for the public schools, but it is not common practice. Lyle has been advocating for the implementation of the Inclusive Education Act (Republic Act 11650), which was signed into law in March 2022. The law mandates the establishment of inclusive learning resource centers across the country, and occupational therapy is one of the services to be offered in those centers. This is great advocacy work and will greatly expand occupational therapy into the public school system.

Although occupational therapy is growing in the country, less than half of the provinces in the Philippines have practicing OTPs. For example, Palawan province, the largest province in the Philippines, has only one. Most OTPs work in private pediatric centers in urban areas. Few OTPs work in the hospitals and even fewer work in home health.

Occupational therapy is largely not covered by most insurances, so therapy is paid mostly out of pocket. Lyle explained that the national insurance, The Philippine Health Insurance Corporation (PhilHealth), passed the Z Benefits package for children with disabilities in 2018 that covers occupational therapy services; however, it still covers a limited number of therapy sessions in a year. Even so, with the assistance of the extended family, most children from middle class backgrounds are able to afford the expense of therapy. Given the Filipino culture, Lyle explains that OTPs work with the immediate and extended family when providing pediatric occupational therapy services, which include providing mental health services for the child and family. Most children come in for services between 2 and 5 years of age, depending on the diagnosis and severity of symptoms.

High Resource Country: Kuwait With Nora Almadaj

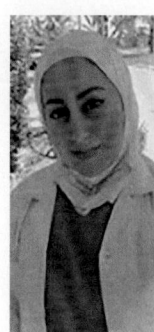

Nora is an OTP in Kuwait who has her "dream job." She works with infants in the NICU, the delivery room, on the maternity ward, and in the outpatient center at the Maternity Hospital. Nora has her breastfeeding certification from WHO and helps mothers with their first feed within the first hour after delivery. Occupational therapy in Kuwait takes a family-centered approach. Nora recites the mantra "Happy Family, Happy Baby." Nora explains how she not only helps new mothers with breastfeeding, but also helps new caregivers in the NICU with their fears and feelings of depression and anxiety. Nora feels that working with the families is a "gift." She helps the families learn how to hold their baby, position the baby, provide kangaroo care, provide massage therapy, and provide supporting and enhancing NICU sensory experiences (SENSE; Pineda et al., 2019).

Helping the families learn how to do the day-to-day care for their infant helps to reduce their fears and anxiety. When asked if the OTPs provide maternal mental health screenings, Nora reported that it is done informally, unless it is part of a research study. The OTPs do use the "Parenting Sense of Competence Scale" (Gibaud-Wallston & Wandersman, 1978) as an outcome measure, along with the Canadian Occupational Performance Measure (Law et al., 2017).

Occupational therapy is a free service for all Kuwaiti children and adults. In Kuwait, infants in the Maternity Hospital receive free care, as well as children on an outpatient basis at the Maternity Hospital. After the age of 2, children and adults can receive free therapy at the physical medicine rehabilitation hospitals. Non-Kuwaiti children and adults pay for therapy services.

Public school is also free for all Kuwaiti children, starting with preschool at age 4. Children enter primary school at age 6 and receive free schooling through their high school years. Education for college, master's, and doctorate degrees is also free for Kuwait people. The public schools have a special education program until children are 10 years of age, at which time they need to transfer to a private school. Children with special needs do not receive occupational therapy in the public schools. If children attend a private school, they can receive therapy services, but it is at a cost. Nora explains that there are only 150 OTPs currently in Kuwait, and they are trying to staff the hospitals. Nora is hopeful that in the future OTPs will also be in public schools.

High Resource Country: Australia With Analea Barnes

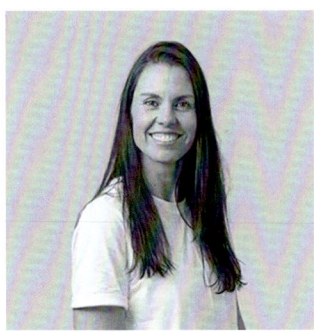

In the Australian health-care system, occupational therapy plays a significant role in early childhood intervention for children with developmental delay or disability. Early intervention supports for children with developmental delay or disability age 0 to 9 are funded by the Early Childhood Approach (ECA) as part of the National Disability Insurance Scheme (NDIS, n.d.).

The NDIS funding covers a range of supports, including assessments, therapy sessions, assistive technology, and other interventions identified in the child's support plan. Families have the flexibility to choose service providers that best meet their child's needs and goals.

Children under the age of 6 years do not need a diagnosis from a medical professional to access early intervention supports. Children may be referred for concerns about development by a child's doctor, early childhood educator, child health nurse, or parents/caregivers. Concerns about a child's development may include how they play and move, do things to take care of themselves, socialize with other children, and communicate what they want as compared with other children their age.

Analea Barnes is a graduate of the Master of Occupational Therapy program at Bond University, Gold Coast, Australia. Analea works as a pediatric OTP in private practice with children ages 3 to 7 years. Services are delivered in clinic, day-care, home, or school-based environments. Analea values working holistically with children and their families, focusing on the child's strengths, which allows the child to be authentically themselves while developing and learning new skills.

The NDIS aims to provide specialized support and services to children and their families to promote their capacity building and inclusion. The approach supports best practice in early childhood intervention (Early Childhood Intervention Australia, 2016) because it helps the child and family to build their capacity and supports greater inclusion in the community and everyday settings, meaning each child will be provided with opportunities to grow and learn.

This national scheme is focused on giving children and their families the right supports to enable them to have the best possible start in life. The Australian Early Childhood Approach focuses on being both family-centered and strengths-based. Families know their child best and are at the center of all services and supports.

As an OTP working with children and families in Australia, as part of the NDIS Early Childhood Approach, Analea's role includes:

- *Assessment:* OTPs assess the child's strengths, challenges, and developmental needs through both formal and informal assessment tools. They evaluate areas such as fine motor skills, sensory processing, self-care skills, play skills, and social interaction abilities.
- *Goal setting:* Through formal assessments, parent goal-setting meetings, discussions with educators, and informal assessments, OTPs work with the child and their family to set specific goals related to the child's development and functional abilities. These goals are individualized based on the child's environment, unique needs, and strengths; these areas allow the child to thrive and develop these skills, which are important for them and their families.
- *Intervention:* OTPs provide individualized interventions to help children achieve their goals. These may include education and coaching, motor skills, cognitive and learning skills, play-based interventions, strategies to enhance self-care skills, and social interaction, as well as participation in education and community activities.
- *Collaboration:* OTPs collaborate with other professionals involved in the child's care, such as speech therapists, physiotherapists, educators, and key workers/plan managers. These people work together to ensure a holistic and coordinated approach to the child's development and progress.
- *Family support:* OTPs also provide support and education to the child's family. They offer strategies and resources to promote the child's development and help the family navigate the NDIS system. At times, families require more support and coaching to assist with the child's goal achievement; therefore, more focus is around parent consultation rather than therapy intervention for the child.

Here's the Point

- Early childhood mental health includes physical, cognitive, and social development that occurs in a psychologically balanced family system and in the absence of disruption by harmful life events.
- Building SSNRs and healthy relationships, including but not limited to the practitioner–parent/caregiver relationships, parent–child relationships, and family–community relationships, is essential to early childhood mental health.
- Early intervention programs, which are also known as Birth-to-Three programs in the United States and include broader age ranges in some countries, provide coordinated services to families with young children. Children referred to early intervention programs are at risk for or diagnosed with a condition that may impact their ability to fully participate in occupations or

co-occupations that are meaningful for children and their families.
- Early intervention services in the United States are provided under Part C of the IDEA of 2004. Therapists working in other countries should review legislation relevant to the jurisdiction in which early intervention services are delivered.
- Being a self-reflective practitioner is essential to providing successful early intervention services, practicing self-care, and decreasing workplace burnout.

- Supporting families through transition from early intervention to early childhood programs is an important role for OTPs.

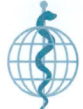

Visit the online resource center at FADavis.com to access the videos.

Apply It Now

1. Interview a Parent

Interview a parent regarding relationships with health professionals. Start by asking general questions, such as what qualities they look for in a health-care professional that foster trust. Ask them to reflect on positive and negative experiences that they have had with health-care professionals. What made those experiences good or bad, and how could the health professional have improved the interaction? Share/compare what you learned with peers who also completed this interview experience.

2. Know Your State's/Jurisdiction's Eligibility Determination

OTPs can inquire with their respective state's early intervention program to understand eligibility determination. Find your state's early intervention website and contact information through the CDC: https://www.cdc.gov/ncbddd/actearly/parents/state-text.html.

Reflective Questions
- What regulations impact early intervention practice in your area?
- Can an OTP evaluate and provide direct services?
- Can early intervention services be delivered in settings other than the home environment?
- Is a practitioner allowed to bring equipment to the home or must they use objects and materials within the home environment?

3. Infant Mental Health Endorsement

Many states offer Infant Mental Health Endorsement, which is a process of documenting competencies that are deemed important for infant mental health practice. OTPs can participate in endorsement programs to strengthen culturally responsive, relationship-based practice. Learn more about infant mental health endorsement at https://www.allianceaimh.org/endorsement-requirements-guidelines.

Reflective Questions
- What are some of the potential benefits of earning an endorsement credential?

- Different types of endorsement certifications can be earned. Which type do you think might best meet your career goals?

4. Video Exercise: Occupational Therapy Collaboration in Early Head Start

Pair up with another student in your class or form a small group of students. Access and watch the "Occupational Therapy Collaboration in Early Head Start" video at the online resource center at FADavis.com. Then, discuss and together answer the following questions.

Reflective Questions
- OTPs work with individuals across the life span and serve a variety of needs with a variety of skill sets/knowledge bases. The occupational therapist and occupational therapy assistant in this video described the importance of working on a team and knowing where one person's skill set ends and the other person's begins. This can necessitate reaching out to a practitioner who has more experience or calling in support from another profession. Why is a team-based approach so important, especially in educational settings and a program such as Head Start?
- Often individuals in mental health settings need support from a variety of provider types and in a variety of contexts to support them to successfully live, participate, and be. How are the occupational therapist and occupational therapy assistant in this video helping support the children they work with across the care continuum? What are the different strengths that the occupational therapist and occupational therapy assistant bring to the partnership?
- Early intervention and Head Start practice settings consider and address child development. When you think of these settings, you often think of development in the physical realm. What other forms of development need to be assessed and addressed, particularly when considering mental health and well-being?

Resources

- Annie E. Casey Foundation: http://www.aecf.org/kidscount. This foundation is dedicated to helping improve the lives of children, families, and communities across the United States.
- Mental Health America (MHA): https://mhanational.org. This community-based nonprofit, founded in 1909, addresses the needs of individuals living with mental illness and promoting the overall American mental health.
- World Association for Infant Mental Health: https://www .waimh.org. This organization "promotes education, research, and study of the effects of mental, emotional and social development during infancy on later normal and psychopathological development through international and interdisciplinary cooperation, publications, affiliate associations, and through regional and biennial congresses devoted to scientific, educational, and clinical work with infants and their caregivers" (para. 1).
- ZERO TO THREE Organization: https://www.zerotothree.org. This membership-based organization provides training and resources about social-emotional development for professionals who serve children ages birth to 3.
- Infant and Early Childhood Mental Health (IECMH) Resource Toolbox from the American Academy of Pediatrics Council on Early Childhood in partnership with ZERO TO THREE: https:// downloads.aap.org/AAP/PDF/Full%20toolbox.pdf. This toolkit provides free online resources for clinicians and families on building relationships and resiliency.
- Feeding Matters Infant and Child Feeding Questionnaire: https://questionnaire.feedingmatters.org. This online questionnaire offers a free tool parents can use to support early identification of children from birth to 3 years old with feeding disorders. It offers a way to connect children and at-risk infants to appropriate care.

Video

- "Child in Crisis" video. In this video, occupational therapist Brittany shares her experience working in a psychiatric rehab hospital's adolescent unit with Mikey, an 8-year-old boy presenting with a complex set of challenges. Diagnosed at birth with fetal alcohol syndrome, Mikey has a history of multiple ACEs. On admission, he presented with suicidal and homicidal ideation and symptoms consistent with PTSD. Brittany describes how she did her own research, learned more about Mikey, and developed an intervention that worked well for him and the other children in the group. Access the video at the online resource center at FADavis.com.
- "Occupational Therapy and Music Therapy in Early Head Start" video. In this video, an occupational therapist and music therapist discuss their unique and effective collaboration in a Head Start program. Running an 8-week group for infants and toddlers, the therapists assessed the children and established preventive goals linked to developmental milestones in areas such as self-regulation, awareness of self and others, attention, language, and motor movements. Access the video at the online resource center at FADavis.com.
- "Laura's Experience as a Mother of an Autistic Son" video. Laura is the mother of an adult son, Will, who was diagnosed with autism at age 3. In this video, she describes what Will was like as a baby and what signs she and day-care teachers first noticed. She explains what the evaluation process was like and how it felt when she learned that her loving, talkative, playful child had autism. Occupational therapy, social skills therapy, speech therapy, and other services—as well as intensely involved parents—laid the groundwork for Will to succeed in school and go on to fulfill his occupational dream as a young adult. Access the video at the online resource center at FADavis.com.

- "Tricks and Techniques From the Mother of an Autistic Son" video. In this video, Laura describes her and her family's creative and adaptive ways of helping their autistic son, Will, succeed. Giving several specific examples of solutions to common problem behaviors and challenges, Laura shares practical wisdom, "tricks and techniques" from 20 years of experience as the mother of a son with autism, with a focus on recognizing and focusing on Will's strengths. Access the video at the online resource center at FADavis.com.

References

American Academy of Pediatrics. (2022). *Early relational health.* https://www.aap.org/en/patient-care/early-childhood /early-relational-health

American Occupational Therapy Association. (2014). *What is the role of occupational therapy in early intervention?* https://www .aota.org/~/media/Corporate/Files/Practice/Children/Browse /EI/Role-of-OT_1/Early-Intervention-FAQ.pdf

American Occupational Therapy Association. (2020). Occupational therapy practice framework: Domain and process—Fourth edition. *American Journal of Occupational Therapy, 74*(Suppl. 2), 7412410010p1–7412410010p87. https://doi.org/10.5014/ajot .2020.74S2001

American Occupational Therapy Association. (2022). *AOTA Occupational profile template.* https://www.aota.org/~/media /Corporate/Files/Practice/Manage/Documentation/AOTA -Occupational-Profile-Template.pdf

ASDetect. (2020). *Home page.* https://asdetect.org

Barbaro, J., Sadka, N., Gilbert, M., Beattie, E., Li, X., Ridgway, L., Lawson, L. P., & Dissanayake, C. (2022). Diagnostic accuracy of the Social Attention and Communication Surveillance–Revised with preschool tool for early autism detection in very young children. *JAMA Network Open, 5*(3), e2146415. https://doi .org/10.1001/jamanetworkopen.2021.46415

Barlow, K., & Sepulveda, A. (2020). The promotion of positive mental health for new mothers during COVID-19. *World Federation of Occupational Therapy Bulletin, 76*(2), 86–89. https://doi.org/10 .1080/14473828.2020.1822577

Barnekow, K. A., & Kraemer, G. W. (2005). The psychobiological theory of attachment: A viable frame of reference for early intervention providers. *Physical and Occupational Therapy in Pediatrics, 25,* 3–15. PMID: 15760821

Beckinger, A., Overturf, A., & Pickens, N. (2016). Reliability and validity of the Complexity of Co-occupation Scale. *American Journal of Occupational Therapy, 70,* 7011500065. https://doi .org/10.5014/ajot.2016.70S1-PO6021

Bowlby, J. (1969). *Attachment and loss: Attachment* (Vol. 1). Basic Books.

Bronfenbrenner, U. (1977). Toward an experimental ecology of human development. *American Psychologist, 32,* 513–531. https:// doi.org/10.1037/0003-066X.32.7.513

Bronfenbrenner, U. (1995a). Developmental ecology through space and time: A future perspective. In P. Moen, G. H. Elder, Jr., & K. Lüscher (Eds.), *Examining lives in context: Perspectives on the ecology of human development* (pp. 617–649). American Psychological Association.

Bronfenbrenner, U. (1995b). The bioecological model from a life course perspective: Reflections of a participant observer. In P. Moen, G. H. Elder, Jr., & K. Lüscher (Eds.), *Examining lives in context: Perspectives on the ecology of human development* (pp. 599–616). American Psychological Association.

Burger, M., Einspieler, C., Niehaus, D. J. H., Unger, M., & Jordaan, E. R. (2022). Maternal mental health and infant neurodevelopment at 6-months in a low-income South African cohort. *Infant Mental Health Journal, 43,* 849–863. https://doi.org/10.1002 /imhj.22021

Burke Harris, N. (2018). *The deepest well: Healing the long-term effects of childhood adversity.* Houghton Mifflin Harcourt.

Callahan, J. L., Borja, S. E., & Hynan, M. T. (2006). Modification of the Perinatal PTSD Questionnaire to enhance clinical utility. *Journal of Perinatology, 26,* 533–539. https://doi.org/10.1038/sj.jp.7211562

Caputo, M. (2016). *Early childhood mental health consultation. Policies and practices to foster the social-emotional development of young children.* ZERO TO THREE. https://www.zerotothree.org/wp-content/uploads/2017/01/IECMH-Consultation-Brief.pdf

Carteret, M. (2012). *Dimensions of culture: Cross-cultural communications for healthcare professionals.* Author.

Center on the Developing Child. (2021, December 27). *Serve and return.* https//developing.child.harvard.edu/science/key-concepts/serve-and-return

Centers for Disease Control and Prevention. (2022). *Fast facts: Preventing adverse childhood experiences.* https://www.cdc.gov/violenceprevention/aces/fastfact.html

Centers for Disease Control and Prevention. (2023). *Learn the signs. Act early.* https://www.cdc.gov/ncbddd/actearly

Choi, K., Records, K., Low, L., Alhusen, J., Kenner, C., Bloch, J., Premji, S., Hannah, J., Anderson, C., Yeo, S., & Logsdon, C. (2020). Promotion of maternal-infant mental health and trauma-informed care during the COVID-19 pandemic. *Journal of Obstetric, Gynecologic & Neonatal Nursing, 49,* 409–415. https://doi.org/10.1016/j.jogn.2020.07.004

Cox, J., Holden, J., & Henshaw, C. (2014). *Perinatal mental health: The Edinburgh Postnatal Depression Scale (EPDS) Manual* (2nd ed.). Royal College of Psychiatrists. https://assets.cambridge.org/9781909726130_frontmatter.pdf

Cox, J., Holden, J., & Sagovsky, R. (1987). Detection of post-natal depression: Development of the ten item Edinburgh Postnatal Depression Scale. *British Journal of Psychiatry, 150,* 782–786. https://doi.org/10.1192/bjp.150.6.782

Curry, A., & Epley, P. (2022) "It makes you a healthier professional": The impact of reflective practice on emerging clinicians' self-care. *Journal of Social Work Education, 58*(2), 291–307. https://doi.org/10.1080/10437797.2020.1817825

Daelmans, B., Darmstadt, G. L., Lombardi, J., Black, M. M., Britto, P. R., Lye, S., Dua, T., Bhutta, Z. A., & Richter, L. M. (2017). Early childhood development: The foundation of sustainable development. *The Lancet, 389*(10064), 9–11. https://doi.org/10.1016/S0140-6736(16)31659-2

Dawson, G., Franz, L., & Brandsen, S. (2022). At a crossroads—Reconsidering the goals of autism early behavioral intervention from a neurodiversity perspective. *Archives of Pediatrics & Adolescent Medicine, 176*(9), 839–840. https://doi.org/10.1001/jamapediatrics.2022.2299

de Magalhães-Barbosa, M. C., Prata-Barbosa, A., & da Cunha, A. J. L. A. (2022). Toxic stress, epigenetics and child development. *Jornal de Pediatria, 98*(Suppl. 1), S13–S18. https://doi.org/10.1016/j.jped.2021.09.007

DeMier, R. L., Hynan, M. T., Hatfield, R. R., Varner, M. W., Harris, H. B., & Manniello, R. L. (2000). A measurement model of perinatal stressors: Identifying risk for postnatal emotional distress in mothers of high-risk infants. *Journal of Clinical Psychology, 56,* 89–100. https://doi.org/10.1002/(sici)1097-4679(200001)56:1<3.0.co;2-6

DeSocio, J. E. (2018). Epigenetics, maternal prenatal psychosocial stress, and infant mental health. *Archives of Psychiatric Nursing, 32,* 901–906. https://doi.org/10.1016/j.apnu.2018.09.001

Dunn, W. (1997). The impact of sensory processing abilities on the daily lives of young children and their families: A conceptual model. *Infants and Young Children, 9*(4), 23–25. https://doi.org/10.1097/00001163-199704000-00005

Dunn, W. (2004). A sensory processing approach to supporting infant–caregiver relationships. In A. J. Sameroff, S. C. McDonough, & K. L. Rosenblum (Eds.), *Treating parent–infant relationship problems* (pp. 152–187). Guilford.

Dunn, W. (2014). *The infant/toddler sensory profile 2.* Psimas Publishing.

Dunn, W., Brown, C., & McGuigan, A. (1994). The ecology of human performance: A framework for considering the effect of context. *American Journal of Occupational Therapy, 48,* 595–607. https://doi.org/10.5014/ajot.48.7.595

Dunst, C. (2000). *Everyday children's learning opportunities: Characteristics and consequences* (Vol. 2). Center for Dissemination and Utilization, Orelena Hawks Puckett Institute. http://www.puckett.org/everday_child_reports_lov2-1.php

Early Childhood Intervention Australia. (2016). *National guidelines for best practice in early childhood intervention.* https://www.eciavic.org.au/documents/item/1419

Early Childhood Technical Assistance Center. (2022). *Part C eligibility.* https://ectacenter.org/topics/earlyid/partcelig.asp

Early Childhood Technical Assistance Center. (2023). *Bureau of Indian Education (BIE).* https://ectacenter.org/topics/bie/bie.asp

Felitti, V. J., Anda, R. F., Nordenberg, D., Williamson, D. F., Spitz, A. M., Edwards, V., Koss, M. P., & Marks, J. S. (1998). Relationship of childhood abuse and household dysfunction to many of the leading causes of death in adults. The adverse childhood experiences (ACE) study. *American Journal of Preventive Medicine, 14*(4), 245–248. https://doi.org/10.1016/S0749-3797(98)00017-8

Fleming, A. S., & Kraemer, G. W. (2019). Molecular and genetic basis of mammalian maternal behavior. *Gender and the Genome, 3,* 114. https://doi.org/10.1177/2470289719827306

Frolek Clark, G., & Parks, S. (Eds.). (2021). *Best practices for occupational therapy in early childhood.* AOTA Press.

Garner, A., Yogman, M., & Committee on Psychosocial Aspects of Child and Family Health, Section on Developmental and Behavioral Pediatrics, Council on Early Childhood. (2021). Preventing childhood toxic stress: Partnering with families and communities to promote relational health. *Pediatrics, 148*(2), e2021052582. https://doi.org/10.1542/peds.2021-052582

Getanda, E. M., Vostanis, P., & O'Reilly, M. (2017). Exploring the challenges of meeting child mental health needs through community engagement in Kenya. *Child and Adolescent Mental Health, 22*(4), 201–208. https://doi.org/10.1111/camh.12233

Gibaud-Wallston, J., & Wandersman, L. P. (1978). *Parenting Sense of Competence Scale (PSOC).* [Paper presentation]. Meeting of the American Psychological Association, Toronto, Canada. https://www.bristol.ac.uk/media-library/sites/sps/documents/c-change/parenting-sense-of-competence-scale.pdf

Gillispie, G. (2021). *Our youngest learners: Increasing equity in early intervention.* The Education Trust. https://edtrust.org/increasing-equity-in-early-intervention

Greenough, W. T., Black, J. E., & Wallace, C. S. (1987). Experience and brain development. *Child Development, 15,* 539–559.

Hagan, M. J., Roubinov, D. R., Cordeiro, A., Lisha, N., & Bush, N. R. (2022). Young children's traumatic stress reactions to the COVID-19 pandemic: The long reach of mothers' adverse childhood experiences. *Journal of Affective Disorders, 318,* 130–138. https://doi.org/10.1016/j.jad.2022.08.061

Individuals with Disabilities Education Improvement Act, Pub. L. No. 108-446, 118 Stat. 2647 (2004). https://www.congress.gov/108/plaws/publ446/PLAW-108publ446.pdf

Iruka, I. U., Lewis, M. L., Lozada, F. T., Bocknek, E. L., & Brophy-Herb, H. E. (2021). Call to action: Centering blackness and disrupting systemic racism in infant mental health research and academic publishing. *Infant Mental Health Journal, 42,* 745–748. https://doi.org/10.1002/imhj.21950

Kapp, S. K. (2020). Introduction. In S. K. Kapp (Ed.), *Autistic community and the neurodiversity movement: Stories from the frontline* (pp. 1–19). Springer. https://doi.org/10.1007/978-981-13-8437-0

Kingsley, K. L., & Clark, G. F. (2020). Occupational therapy interventions for children ages birth–5 years. *American Journal of*

Occupational Therapy, 74(5), 7405390010p1–7405390010p4. https://doi.org/10.5014/ajot.2020.745001

Klawetter, S., Glaze, K., Sward, A., & Frankel, K. A. (2021). Warm connections: Integration of infant mental health services into WIC. *Community Mental Health Journal, 57,* 1130–1141. https://doi.org/10.1007/s10597-020-00744-y

Kovacic, K., Rein, L., Szabo, A., Kommareddy, S., Bhagavatula, P., & Goday, S. (2020). Pediatric feeding disorder: A nationwide prevalence study. *The Journal of Pediatrics, 228,* 126–131.e3. https://doi.org/10.1016/j.jpeds.2020.07.047

Kraemer, G. W. (1992). A psychobiological theory of attachment. *Behavioral and Brain Sciences, 15,* 493–541. https://doi.org/10.1017/S0140525X00069752

Kuo, D. Z., Houtrow, A. J., Arango, P., Kuhlthau, K. A., Simmons, J. M., & Neff, J. M. (2012). Family-centered care: Current applications and future directions in pediatric health care. *Maternal and Child Health Journal, 16*(2), 297–305. https://doi.org/10.1007/s10995-011-0751-7

Lamm, K., Kristensson Hallström, I., & Landgren, K. (2023). Parents' experiences of living with a child with paediatric feeding disorder: An interview study in Sweden. *Scandinavian Journal of Caring Science, 37*(4), 949–958. https://doi.org/10.1111/scs.13070

Lantz, A. J. (2020). Pediatric accidental trauma: Screening and reducing psychological impact. *Pediatric Nursing, 46*(3), 111–114, 118. https://cce.upmc.com/sites/default/files/Article%208%20-%20Pediatric%20Accidental%20trauma-%20Screening%20and%20Reducing%20Psychological%20Impact.pdf

Lautarescu, A., Craig, M. C., & Glover, V. (2020). Chapter two—Prenatal stress: Effects on fetal and child brain development. *International Review of Neurobiology, 150,* 17–40. https://doi.org/10.1016/bs.irn.2019.11.002

Law, M., Baptiste, S., Carswell, A., McColl, M., Polatajko, H., & Pollock, N. (2017). *Canadian occupational performance measure manual* (5th ed.). COPM Inc.

Lee, K., & Zhang, L. (2022). Cumulative effects of poverty on children's social-emotional development: Absolute poverty and relative poverty. *Community Mental Health Journal, 58,* 930–943. https://doi.org/10.1007/s10597-021-00901-x

Leppanan, J. M. (2011). Neuro and developmental basis of the ability to recognize social signals. *Emotion Review, 3,* 179–188. https://doi.org/10.1177/1754073910387942

Maheu, M. (2022, December 22). *What is asynchronous telehealth? Store-and-forward telehealth benefits.* Telehealth.org. https://blog.telehealth.org/asynchronous-telehealth

McWilliam, R. A. (2010). *Routines-based early intervention: Supporting young children and their families.* Brookes.

McWilliam, R. A., Casey, A. M., & Sims, J. (2009). The Routines-Based Interview: A method for gathering information and assessing needs. *Infants & Young Children, 22*(3), 224–233. https://doi.org/10.1097/IYC.0b013e3181abe1dd

Memiah, P., Wagner, F. A., Kimathi, R., Anyango, N. I., Kiogora, S., Waruinge, S., Kiruthi, F., Mwavua, S., Kithinji, C., Agache, J. O., Mangwana, W., Merci, N. M., Ayuma, L., Muhula, S., Opanga, Y., Nyambura, M., Ikahu, A., & Otiso, L. (2022). Voices from the youth in Kenya addressing mental health gaps and recommendations. *International Journal of Environmental Research and Public Health, 19*(9), 5366. https://doi.org/10.3390/ijerph19095366

Myers, C. T., Case-Smith, J., & Cason, J. (2015). Early intervention. In J. Case-Smith & J. C. O'Brien (Eds.), *Occupational therapy for children and adolescents* (7th ed., pp. 636–665). Elsevier Mosby.

National Center for Children in Poverty. (2020). *Infant and early childhood mental health in part C early intervention program.* https://www.nccp.org/mental-health-in-part-c

National Disability Insurance Scheme. (n.d.). *The early childhood approach for children younger than 9.* https://www.ndis.gov.au/understanding/families-and-carers/early-childhood-approach-children-younger-9

National Scientific Council on the Developing Child. (2020). *Connecting the brain to the rest of the body: Early childhood development*

and lifelong health are deeply intertwined. Working Paper No. 15. https://harvardcenter.wpenginepowered.com/wp-content/uploads/2020/06/wp15_health_FINALv2.pdf

Nuzzo, C. (2006). *Ten questions to foster your journey in self-reflection.* https://pacwrc.pitt.edu/curriculum/521%20SupervisorTrainingSeries-Module3-TheMiddleWorkPhase/HO33_QustnsFstrJrny.pdf

Ongeri, L., Larsen, D., Jenkins, R., Shaw, A., Connolly, H., Lyon, J., Kariuki, S., Penninx, B., Newton, C., Sifuna, P., & Ogutu, B. (2022). Community suicide rates and related factors within a surveillance platform in Western Kenya. *BMC Psychiatry, 22,* 7. https://doi.org/10.1186/s12888-021-03649-6

Pickens, N. D., & Pizur-Barnekow, K. (2009). Co-occupation: Extending the dialogue. *Journal of Occupational Science, 16,* 151–156. https://doi.org/10.1080/14427591.2009.9686656

Pineda, R., Raney, M., & Smith, J. (2019). Supporting and enhancing NICU sensory experiences (SENSE): Defining developmentally-appropriate sensory exposures for high-risk infants. *Early Human Development, 133,* 29–35. https://doi.org/10.1016/j.earlhumdev.2019.04.012

Podvey, M. C., & Myers, C. T. (2015). Early childhood transitions. In M. Orentlicher, S. Schefkind, & R. Gibson (Eds.), *Transitions across the lifespan: An occupational therapy approach* (pp. 51–74). AOTA Press.

Psimas, L. (2014). *Assessing sensory strengths and challenges.* Presentation at the Illinois Occupational Therapy Association Annual Conference. London, England.

Resilience Action. (2022). *Mental health in children and youths in Kenya.* https://www.resilienceaction.net/post/mental-health-in-children-and-youths-in-kenya

Ribaudo, J., Lawler, J. M., Jester, J. M., Riggs, J., Erickson, N. L., Stacks, A. M., Brophy-Herb, H., Muzik, M., & Rosenblum, K. L. (2022). Maternal history of adverse experiences and posttraumatic stress disorder symptoms impact toddlers' early socioemotional well-being: The benefits of infant mental health-home visiting. *Frontiers in Psychology, 12,* 792989. https://doi.org/10.3389/fpsyg.2021.792989

Salisbury, C., Woods, J., Snyder, P., Moddlemog, K., Mawdsley, H., Romano, M., & Windsor, K. (2018). Caregiver and provider experiences with coaching and embedded interventions. *Topics in Early Childhood Special Education, 38,* 17–29. https://doi.org/10.1177/0271121417708036

Samdan, G., Reinelt, T., Kiel, N., Mathes, B., & Pauen, S. (2021). Maternal self-efficacy development from pregnancy to 3 months after birth. *Infant Mental Health Journal, 43,* 864–877. https://doi.org/10.1002/imhj.22018

Shelden, M. L. L., & Rush, D. D. (2013). *The early intervention teaming handbook: The primary service provider approach.* Brookes Publishing Company.

Smythe, T., Zuurmond, M., Tann, C. J., Gladstone, M., & Kuper, H. (2021). Early intervention for children with developmental disabilities in low and middle-income countries: The case for action. *International Health, 13*(3), 222–231. https://doi.org/10.1093/inthealth/ihaa044

Squires, J., & Bricker, D. (2009). *Ages and Stages Questionnaires ASQ-3* (3rd ed.). Brookes Publishing Company.

Squires, J., Bricker, D., & Twombly, E. (2015). *Ages and Stages Questionnaires: Social-emotional ASQ:SE-2* (2nd ed.). Brookes Publishing Company.

Taylor, R. (2020). *The intentional relationship: Occupational therapy and use of self* (2nd ed.). F.A. Davis.

The Star Institute. (2022). *What is Sensory Health? Taking the stigma out of differences.* https://sensoryhealth.org/basic/about-spd

U.S. Department of Education. (2019). *Section 1432.* Individuals with Disabilities Education Act. https://sites.ed.gov/idea/statute-chapter-33/subchapter-iii/1432

Uy, J. P., Tan, A. P., Broeckman, B. B. F. P., Gluckman, P. D., Chong, Y. S., Chen, H., Fortier, M. V., Meaney, M. J., & Callaghan, B. L. (2023). Effects of maternal childhood trauma on child emotional health: Maternal mental health and frontoamygdala pathways. *Journal of Child Psychology and Psychiatry, 64,* 426–436. https://doi.org/10.1111/jcpp.13721

Vélez-Agosto, N. M., Soto-Crespo, J. G., Vizcarrondo-Oppenheimer, M., Vega-Molina, S., & Coll, C. G. (2017). Bronfenbrenner's Bioecological Theory revision: Moving culture from the macro into the micro. *Perspectives on Psychological Science, 12*(5), 900–910. https://doi.org/10.1177/1745691617704397

Vertigans, S., & Mueller-Hirth, N. (2022). *Children in peace-building and violence during political instability in a Kenyan informal settlement.* International Peace Support Training Centre (IPSTC). https://rgu-repository.worktribe.com/output/1920223/children -in-peace-building-and-violence-during-political-instability -in-a-kenyan-informal-settlement

Willis, D. W., Paradis, N., & Johnson, K. (2022). The paradigm shift to early relational health: A network movement. *ZERO TO THREE, 42*(4), 22–30.

Wolke, D., Eryigit-Madzwamuse, S., & Gutbrod, T. (2014). Very preterm/very low birthweight infants' attachment: Infant and maternal characteristics. *Archives of Disease in Childhood—Fetal and Neonatal Edition, 99*(1), F70–F75. https://doi.org/10.1136 /archdischild-2013-303788

World Health Organization. (2020). *Improving early childhood development: WHO guideline.* Author.

World Health Organization. (2024, February 19). *WHO releases new guidance on monitoring the social determinants of health equity.* https://www.who.int/news/item/19-02-2024-who-releases -new-guidance-on-monitoring-the-social-determinants -of-health-equity

Wrightslaw. (2017). *Early intervention: Part C of IDEA.* http://www .wrightslaw.com/info/ei.index.htm

Zemke, R., & Clarke, F. (1996). *Occupational science: The evolving discipline.* F. A. Davis.

ZERO TO THREE. (2016). *DC: 0–5*[TM]. *Diagnostic classification of mental health and developmental disorders of infancy and early childhood.* Author.

ZERO TO THREE. (2020). *DC: 0–5*[TM]. *Diagnostic classification of mental health and developmental disorders of infancy and early childhood* (Version 2.0). Author.

Zylstra, S. E. (2013). Evidence for the use of telehealth in pediatric occupational therapy. *Journal of Occupational Therapy, Schools and Early Intervention, 6,* 326–355. https://doi.org/10.1080/1941 1243.2013.860765

School Mental Health

Susan Bazyk and Lauren Thomas

Occupational therapy was founded on a commitment to mind–body unity contributing to a rich history of promoting mental health in all areas of practice using meaningful and enjoyable occupations (Bing, 1981; Ikiugu et al., 2022; Meyer, 1922). Despite this long-standing perspective, "mental health" practice is often implicitly interpreted to mean services provided to people with mental illness that focus on psychopathology in traditional behavioral health settings (Barry & Jenkins, 2007; Gutman & Raphael-Greenfield, 2014; von der Embse, 2018).

The way in which occupational therapy practitioners (OTPs) define mental health practice significantly impacts how services are perceived, articulated to others, and implemented. If addressing mental health refers only to intervention provided to individuals with identified mental disorders, services will be limited to this population and occur in only a small number of settings. In contrast, when addressing mental health involves helping all individuals develop and maintain positive mental health and prevent mental ill-health, occupational therapy services will extend to all people with and without identified mental illness in various school, health-care, and community settings (Bazyk, 2011b).

This chapter focuses on occupational therapy's role in addressing the mental health needs of children and youth in school settings from kindergarten through high school, typically ages 5 to 18. It provides a multitiered, public health framework for interpreting "mental health" services broadly, including mental health promotion, prevention, and provision of intensive interventions. Practical occupation-based strategies for implementing universal, targeted, and individualized interventions throughout the school day are provided, as well as ways to promote engagement in meaningful and enjoyable occupations in after-school programs.

Overview of School Mental Health

Although mental health services for children and youth were historically provided in hospitals and community mental health centers, during the past two decades there has been a movement nationally and internationally to develop and expand **school mental health (SMH)** supports and services (Atkins et al., 2010; Hoover & Bostic, 2021). The goal of education has moved beyond a focus solely on academic performance toward a broader focus on health, especially the social, emotional, and mental health of students (Marinucci et al., 2023).

School districts in the United States are mandated to provide **related services**, including occupational therapy, when students with disabilities and those with serious emotional disturbance require such services to benefit from special education.

Occupational therapy's scope of practice focuses on a broad range of occupational functioning (education, social participation, play, work, leisure, activities of daily living [ADLs], instrumental activities of daily living [IADLs], sleep hygiene, and health management), which results in a high demand for services; as such, schools are among the profession's primary work environments (American Occupational Therapy Association [AOTA], 2020; Cahill & Bazyk, 2019). In addition to serving students with disabilities, best practice in schools emphasizes the integration of occupational therapy services in the general education classroom and nonacademic settings (e.g., lunch, recess, after-school) when possible, offering opportunities to contribute to mental health promotion and prevention efforts in addition to addressing the needs of students with identified disabilities or mental health challenges (Cahill & Bazyk, 2019). Current legislation and factors shaping SMH services are described in the text that follows.

Legislation and Policies

The growth of SMH has been motivated by several factors, including the high prevalence of mental health conditions among youth, an awareness that more youths can be reached in schools, and the authorization of major federal initiatives (Adelman & Taylor, 2021; Kutash et al., 2006; Office of the Surgeon General, 2021). The Education of All Handicapped Children Act of 1975, later reauthorized as the Individuals with Disabilities Education Act (IDEA; 2004), was the first federal initiative to place significant responsibility on schools to meet the mental health needs of students with emotional challenges and provide prevention and early intervening services (EIS) for students at risk for academic or behavioral challenges (IDEA, 2004; Final Regulations, § 300.34, 2006). Therefore, it played a key role in expanding the responsibility for providing mental health services to children and youth in both health-care and education settings (Hoover & Bostic, 2021).

Additionally, Section 504 of the Rehabilitation Act of 1973 mandates that students with mental or physical impairments that substantially limit function must be provided with appropriate education and support in both general and special education (Cahill & Bazyk, 2019). Over two decades ago, the surgeon general's report (U.S. Department of Health and Human Services, 1999) on children's mental health concluded the nation lacked a coordinated infrastructure to help children with mental health concerns and labeled the situation a "health crisis" (U.S. Department of Health and Human Services, 1999). The most recent report from the Office of the Surgeon General (2021) continues to emphasize the mental health needs of children and youth, noting that the COVID-19 pandemic has further exacerbated the crisis. Several national health organizations followed suit, declaring children's mental health a national emergency (American Academy of Pediatrics [AAP], 2021).

Because of these and other national policies, most children who receive any mental health services obtain this care in school, making schools the de facto mental health system for children in the United States (Hoover & Bostic, 2021; Kutash et al., 2006).

In addition to focusing on the needs of special education students with identified mental health concerns, recent general education legislation has helped expand SMH to include mental health promotion and prevention. In 2015, the Every Student Succeeds Act (ESSA) was authorized to replace No Child Left Behind (NCLB). This legislation focuses on creating school environments that help all students succeed in school and advocates for embedding universal and targeted strategies that foster both mental and physical health (Cahill & Bazyk, 2019). Under ESSA, OTPs and other related service providers are named Specialized Instructional Support Personnel (SISP) and have the goal of working collaboratively with students and interdisciplinary school teams to ensure positive conditions for learning and to provide services that support mental and physical health and academic success (Laverdure et al., 2023; National Alliance of Specialized Instructional Support Personnel [NASISP], 2019).

ESSA legislation provides explicit support for OTPs, as SISPs, to contribute to health promotion and prevention efforts by helping all students participate successfully in health-promoting occupations in the classroom (e.g., sensory processing for self-regulation, stress-reduction activities), cafeteria (e.g., being a good friend and having meaningful conversations), recess (e.g., enjoying active play, teamwork), and after-school leisure (e.g., engaging in hobbies and interests).

In addition to legislation, international and national leaders and policymakers in education and mental health sectors increasingly recognize that health (mental and physical) and educational outcomes are closely connected and that schools are significant contributors to student, family, and community health. For example, the World Health Organization (WHO) and United Nations Educational, Scientific and Cultural Organization (UNESCO) have developed global standards for Health Promoting Schools (HPS) with evidence-based implementation strategies that can be applied worldwide (WHO & UNESCO, 2021). The HPS model supports a whole-school approach to promoting health and educational attainment by capitalizing on the organizational potential of schools to foster the physical, psychological, and social-emotional conditions for health and education success (Jané-Llopis & Barry, 2005).

Similarly, in the United States, the Whole School, Whole Community, Whole Child (WSCC) model is the Centers for Disease Control and Prevention's (CDC) framework, and advocates for collaboration between health and education to develop comprehensive school practices and environments that promote mental and physical health (CDC, 2021a, 2021b, 2023b). Specific to mental health, a recent U.S. Department of Education report highlighted challenges (e.g., negative stigma) and recommendations (e.g., enhance mental health literacy) for schools to support students' social, emotional, and mental health needs (U.S. Department of Education, Office of Special Education and Rehabilitative Services, 2021).

Based on current legislation and the emphasis on health, SMH has evolved to become a framework of multitiered systems of supports (MTSS) that expand on traditional services to emphasize mental health promotion, prevention, positive youth development, and schoolwide approaches (Atkins et al., 2010; Marsh & Mather, 2020). This framework promotes interdisciplinary collaboration among mental health providers, related service providers, school administrators, teachers, and families to meet the mental health needs of all students (Hoover & Bostic, 2021).

The fact that the absence of essential social-emotional skills is a major barrier to learning—and not necessarily a lack of sufficient cognitive skills (Koller & Bertel, 2006)—points to the critical need for schools to be active partners in the mental health of children and youth. "Education and mental health integration will be advanced when the goal of mental health includes effective schooling and the goal of effective schools includes the healthy functioning of students" (Atkins et al., 2010, p. 40).

Despite the growth of SMH, the field is still considered underdeveloped and emerging; far too many children remain underidentified and underserved in schools (Atkins et al., 2010). The failure to adequately provide mental health services for children is viewed as a major public health concern, causing leaders in the field to propose a multitiered public health framework to guide services in meeting the needs of all children (von der Embse, 2018).

Multitiered Approach to Mental Health

Although tiered systems of support have existed for several decades in school practice, school personnel are consistently challenged to make them work (Braun et al., 2020). Numerous terms have been used to describe tiered supports. For example, a public health approach to children's mental health emphasizing promotion, prevention, and intervention has been used internationally (WHO, 2022) and in the United States (Atkins & Frazier, 2011; Hoover & Bostic, 2021; Miles et al., 2010). The latest world mental health report advocates for public mental health—a global commitment to broadly address mental health promotion, prevention, and intervention across multiple sectors, including schools (WHO, 2022). Special education legislation (IDEA, 2004) uses Response to Intervention (RtI) as another way to describe tiered services to provide early intervening services for students demonstrating early signs of academic or behavioral delays (Cahill & Bazyk, 2019).

Over the last several years, many schools have been using MTSS to describe a three-tiered framework involving promotion, early identification and prevention, and intensive intervention (Hoover & Bostic, 2021). Occupational therapy publications (Bazyk, 2011b) and evidence-based reviews

(Arbesman et al., 2013; Bazyk & Arbesman, 2013) have applied a tiered public health approach regarding mental health to occupational therapy practice with children and youth. For this chapter, the phrase **multitiered approach to mental health** will be used.

A multitiered approach to mental health calls for a paradigm shift to better prepare *all* school personnel (e.g., teachers, administrators, psychologists, social workers, and related service providers) to proactively address the mental health needs of all students (Amudhan et al., 2021;

Koller & Bertel, 2006). This continuum of care can be envisioned within a three-tiered framework of mental health promotion, prevention, and intensive individualized interventions (see Fig. 37-1). The three major tiers of service are (1) Tier 1, universal, whole SMH promotion; (2) Tier 2, targeted, mental health prevention services for students identified as at risk of developing mental health challenges; and (3) Tier 3, individualized intensive services for students with identified mental disorders. A discussion of occupational therapy services at each tier is presented later in the chapter.

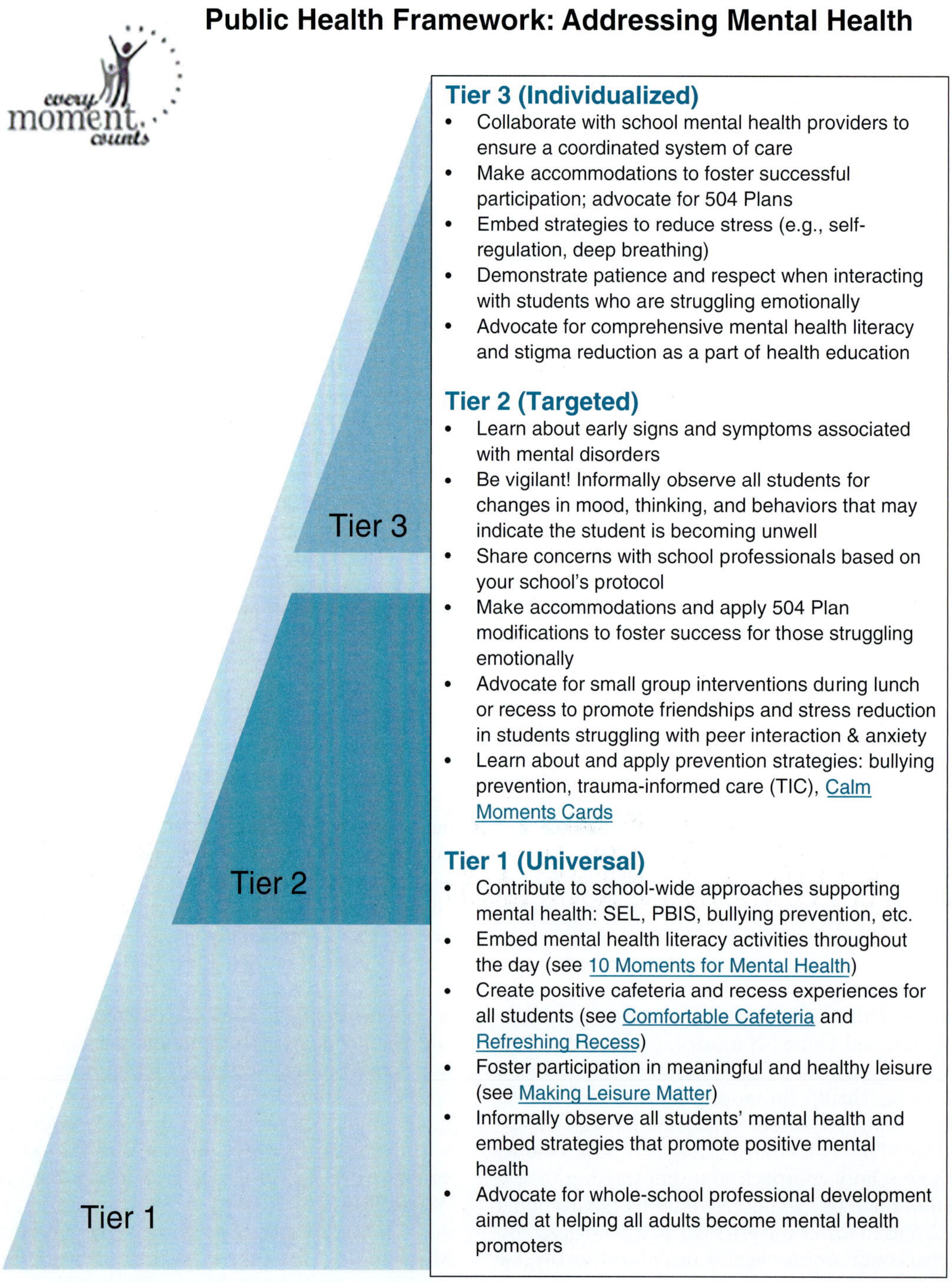

Public Health Framework: Addressing Mental Health

Tier 3 (Individualized)

- Collaborate with school mental health providers to ensure a coordinated system of care
- Make accommodations to foster successful participation; advocate for 504 Plans
- Embed strategies to reduce stress (e.g., self-regulation, deep breathing)
- Demonstrate patience and respect when interacting with students who are struggling emotionally
- Advocate for comprehensive mental health literacy and stigma reduction as a part of health education

Tier 2 (Targeted)

- Learn about early signs and symptoms associated with mental disorders
- Be vigilant! Informally observe all students for changes in mood, thinking, and behaviors that may indicate the student is becoming unwell
- Share concerns with school professionals based on your school's protocol
- Make accommodations and apply 504 Plan modifications to foster success for those struggling emotionally
- Advocate for small group interventions during lunch or recess to promote friendships and stress reduction in students struggling with peer interaction & anxiety
- Learn about and apply prevention strategies: bullying prevention, trauma-informed care (TIC), Calm Moments Cards

Tier 1 (Universal)

- Contribute to school-wide approaches supporting mental health: SEL, PBIS, bullying prevention, etc.
- Embed mental health literacy activities throughout the day (see 10 Moments for Mental Health)
- Create positive cafeteria and recess experiences for all students (see Comfortable Cafeteria and Refreshing Recess)
- Foster participation in meaningful and healthy leisure (see Making Leisure Matter)
- Informally observe all students' mental health and embed strategies that promote positive mental health
- Advocate for whole-school professional development aimed at helping all adults become mental health promoters

© Every Moment Counts (2020) www.everymomentcounts.org

FIGURE 37-1. Multitiered approach to mental health summary pyramid.

It is important to make distinctions between promotion, prevention, and intensive interventions within a multitiered approach to mental health. **Mental health promotion** efforts include creating supportive school, home, and community environments, as well as reducing stigma and discrimination, and educating children on how to develop and maintain positive mental health (Barry & Jenkins, 2007; Barry et al., 2019). Specifically, this means developing an interdisciplinary workforce that is knowledgeable about how to be mental health promoters throughout the school day by embedding evidence-based mental health promotion strategies in natural contexts.

Given the relationship between student academic achievement and mental health, school-based mental health promotion and prevention initiatives are expanding. A scoping review on interventions that promote mental health in schools found that most school-based programs aimed to prevent mental illness versus creating environments that support mental health (Enns et al., 2016). Quality implementation of Australia's KidsMatter schoolwide mental health promotion initiative during a 2-year span was found to improve students' social-emotional competencies and academic performance (Dix et al., 2012).

In a systematic review of universal approaches to mental health, positive evidence of effectiveness was achieved in programs that implemented whole school approaches for more than a year and emphasized mental health as opposed to prevention of mental illness (Wells et al., 2003). In a recent mixed methods study, school personnel, including teachers, indicated the need for interprofessional education and training in mental health literacy, identifying students at risk of mental illness, and strategies for promoting mental health during the school day (Marinucci et al., 2023).

Examples of schoolwide mental health promotion strategies include mental health literacy, social-emotional learning (SEL), positive behavioral interventions and supports (PBIS), and mindfulness strategies (Amudhan et al., 2021; Hoover & Bostic, 2021; Miller et al., 2008). Such schoolwide strategies are designed to meet the needs of all students with and without disabilities and/or mental health challenges. When all school personnel, including teachers, embed mental health promotion strategies, it helps to normalize conversations about mental health and fosters help-seeking behaviors (Marinucci et al., 2023).

Mental health prevention efforts focus on early identification and intervention to reduce the incidence and seriousness of problem behaviors and mental health disorders. This is accomplished by diminishing risk factors, such as bullying and stressful school environments, and enhancing protective factors, such as social and emotional competencies, coping strategies, and supportive environments (Moran, 2016). Embedding mental health promotion and prevention strategies at Tier 2 may be implemented by providing accommodations to modify the learning demands to decrease stress and small group interventions during lunch, recess, or after-school activities to promote social skills and friendships.

Intensive individualized interventions are services that reduce the effects of identified mental health challenges that limit participation and functioning at school. Intervention at this level often depends on the specific mental disorder and formal diagnosis. For example, for a student with an anxiety disorder, modifying the demands of the environment (e.g., breaking down assignments into manageable steps, giving more time on a test) and teaching coping strategies (e.g., deep breathing, thought stopping) can be effective in promoting successful participation throughout the school day (Downing, 2011).

For students with thought disorders or those at risk for developing psychosis, it is important to consult with school staff to make accommodations that reduce stress and enhance participation (e.g., reducing environmental stimulation, decreasing activity demands, and using a calm tone of voice to give simple and clear instructions). In addition to diminishing symptoms at this level, it is critical to also focus on promoting positive mental health. All school personnel, under the leadership of professionals with a background in mental health (e.g., school psychologists, social workers, OTPs, and school nurses), can embed Tier 3 strategies into everyday school experiences (Kutcher & Wei, 2017).

The Mental Health Continuum in Children and Youth

In order to address the mental health needs of all children and youth within a promotion, prevention, and intervention framework, it is important to understand the mental health continuum. Mental health represents a dynamic state of functioning separate from mental illness and can vary throughout life depending on situational stressors (e.g., bullying, academic challenges, and poverty; Cahill & Egan, 2017). Based on a large survey of U.S. adults between the ages of 25 and 74 (Keyes, 2007), the continuum of mental health can be viewed as ranging from mental illness or "languishing in life" at one end to "moderately mentally healthy" and "complete mental health and flourishing" at the other end. See Chapter 1: Occupational Therapy Practice Across the Mental Health Continuum.

Research findings suggest that mental health is not merely the absence of mental illness, but the presence of something positive (Keyes, 2007; Keyes et al., 2010; Wissing et al., 2021). In the same way that a diagnosis of major depressive disorder is based on symptoms of negative emotions and malfunctioning, a diagnosis of positive mental health consists of symptoms of positive emotions and positive psychological and social functioning. Higher degrees of impairment and disability have been noted in individuals without complete mental health and those who are languishing, even those without a diagnosed mental illness (Keyes, 2007). In contrast, people who are mentally healthy and feel happy demonstrate greater degrees of everyday functioning (Keyes, 2006; Wissing et al., 2021), healthy behaviors (Rasciute & Downward, 2010), and perceived good health (Sabatini, 2014).

Children and youth who experience positive mental health and well-being function better during academic and nonacademic times of the school day (Dix et al., 2012). As such, it is important for OTPs to be aware of this distinction and help school personnel, students, and families understand the emotional and behavioral indicators of mental health as well as the symptoms associated with mental illness (Bazyk, 2011b).

Positive Mental Health

Mental health is defined as a "state of successful performance of mental function, resulting in productive activities, fulfilling relationships with other people, and the ability to adapt to change and to cope with adversity" (U.S. Department of Health and Human Services, 1999, p. 4). Mental health in students encompasses more than demonstrating the presence of "good" behavior in school; it involves "feeling good emotionally" and "doing well" in everyday function (Bazyk, 2011b; Miles et al., 2010). Mental health, more than the absence of mental illness, is an integral part of overall health and a basic human right (WHO, 2022).

Research studying the dimensions of mental health and its measurement have identified the following cluster of characteristics associated with the presence of mental health: (a) positive affect (e.g., smiling, feeling happy or content); (b) positive psychological and social functioning (e.g., enjoying fulfilling relationships, having friends, and feeling positive about oneself); (c) engaging in productive activities (e.g., being able to complete everyday tasks at school and home such as attending in class); and (d) coping with life stressors and demonstrating resilience when challenged (e.g., bouncing back after a challenge, learning how to regulate emotions; Bazyk, 2011b; Fredrickson, 2009; Fredrickson & Joiner, 2018; Keyes, 2007). In addition, the development and growth of the field of positive psychology (Donaldson et al., 2011; Seligman & Csikszentmihalyi, 2000) has further enhanced OTPs' understanding of processes and conditions that promote optimal mental health.

Experiencing positive emotions (e.g., joy, gratitude, awe), for example, has been shown to broaden a person's habitual mode of thinking, reduce negative emotions, promote resilience, and fuel psychological and physical well-being (Fredrickson, 2001, 2004, 2009; Fredrickson & Joiner, 2018). Furthermore, Csikszentmihalyi's (1993) research confirms that people experience the most enjoyment in their lives when actively engaged in meaningful occupations. These findings reinforce occupational therapy's commitment to helping people engage in meaningful and enjoyable occupations to promote health and well-being. In schools, OTPs can strategically help create environments that promote enjoyable participation, such as the Comfortable Cafeteria program (see the Evidence-Based Practice feature).

Mental health is a dynamic state of functioning that can vary throughout a person's life based on several biological (e.g., genetics), environmental (e.g., abuse or neglect), and situational (e.g., death of a family member) factors (Barry et al., 2019; Barry & Jenkins, 2007; Bazyk, 2011a; WHO, 2022). For this reason, all school personnel must be vigilant for any marked changes in a student's affect, social functioning, and ability to adapt to daily challenges to promote early intervention.

Additionally, when working with children and youth, it is important to consider developmental factors such as age-related changes in several areas, including cognitive, emotional, and behavioral abilities. Competencies gained at one stage of development provide a foundation for future competencies as young people face new challenges and opportunities. Understanding the age-related patterns of competence and disorder is important for developing promotion

and prevention interventions (National Research Council [NRC] & Institute of Medicine [IOM], 2009).

Mental Ill-Health

Mental ill-health is a broad term that includes a continuum from mild symptomatology to severe disorders of differing duration and intensity (Barry et al., 2019). The terms "mental illness" and "mental health disorders" are commonly used to refer to diagnosable psychiatric conditions that significantly interfere with a person's functioning, such as schizophrenia, bipolar disorder, and dementia. "Mental health challenges" often refer to milder issues such as situational anxiety and depression, which may be of shorter duration but, if left unattended, may develop into a diagnosable mental illness (Barry et al., 2019). The demographics of mental health challenges in children and youth, with and without disabilities, follow.

General Population

Several research studies and national surveys reported a steady increase in mental health disorders since the 2000s (Bitsko et al., 2022). Approximately one in every six children and adolescents experiences a mental health disorder each year (Bitsko et al., 2022; CDC, 2023a). This number is greater for children living in poverty, with nearly 22% of children experiencing mental health, behavioral, or developmental disorders (CDC, 2023a). According to the CDC (2023a), the most diagnosed disorders among children ages 3 to 17 are attention deficit-hyperactivity disorder (ADHD; 9.8%), anxiety problems (9.4%), behavior problems (8.9%), and depression (4.4%). Notably, from 2016 to 2020, the percentage of children diagnosed with an emotional disorder increased from 8.0% to 10.2%, with the most significant increase noted for children 12 to 17 years old (HRSA Maternal & Child Health, 2021).

Nearly 50% of mental health disorders have onset by 14 years of age (Bitsko et al., 2022). Moreover, approximately two in five youths will meet the criteria for a mental disorder by 18 years old. The likelihood that mental health disorders in adults first develop in childhood and adolescence signifies the need for prevention as well as early identification and intervention services in schools.

There is increased awareness of the impact of technology on children and youth, particularly on social media platforms such as Facebook, Snapchat, Instagram, and Twitter. Although these tools can enhance friendships and decrease loneliness, institutions in the United Kingdom and United States have raised concerns that children and youth who overuse these tools can experience mental health challenges such as lowered self-esteem, less life satisfaction, and increased depression, anxiety, and suicidality (Child Mind Institute, 2017; Frith, 2017). Less than 1 hour of gaming a day has been associated with positive mental health effects (Przybylski, 2014), whereas 10 or more hours per week on social media are associated with negative mental health effects and a negative impact on sleep, which can also contribute to poor mental health (Kann et al., 2016; Twenge, 2017). See Chapter 33: Virtual Environments.

Children and Youth With Disabilities

Students with disabilities are at greater risk of experiencing mental health challenges when compared with their nondisabled peers. Results from a U.S. national survey indicated children with special needs are 9 times more likely to have anxiety and 16 times more likely to have depression compared with their nondisabled peers (HRSA Maternal & Child Health, 2020). The reasons for a higher prevalence of mental health conditions in children and youth with developmental disabilities may be related to genetic predisposition combined with additional situational and daily living stressors associated with disability (Lebrun-Harris et al., 2022; Yang et al., 2022). Children with disabilities are more likely than their nondisabled peers to encounter negative social environments and experiences well into their adulthood (Fang et al., 2022; Petrenchik et al., 2011).

The co-occurrence of mental health disorders with specific developmental disabilities has also been reported. Lai and colleagues (2019) noted greater prevalence of mental health disorders in the autism population compared with the general population. Increased rates of ADHD, anxiety disorders, sleep–wake disorders, conduct disorders, depressive disorders, obsessive-compulsive disorder, bipolar disorders, and schizophrenia have been identified in children with autism spectrum disorder (ASD). Children with co-occurring autism and ADHD diagnosis are more likely to experience other mental health conditions (Casseus et al., 2023; Hong et al., 2021).

Co-occurrence often exists between ADHD, learning disabilities (LD), and developmental coordination disorders (DCD), which may also coexist with other conditions, such as Tourette syndrome; sleep, depression, and anxiety disorders; and overweight and obesity (Hansen et al., 2018; Poulsen, 2011). Children with physical disabilities are more vulnerable to mental health problems than their peers (Hwang et al., 2020).

Two studies reported the high frequency of anxiety and depression among children, adolescents, and young adults with cerebral palsy because of risk factors such as limited physical participation, pain, and sleep (Hanes et al., 2019; Whitney et al., 2019). Lastly, in an extensive literature review of psychopathology and intellectual impairment (ID), 38% to 49% of children with ID had a co-occurring mental health disorder (Buckley et al., 2020). The most prevalent diagnoses included ADHD, conduct disorder, and anxiety disorders. "Understanding the co-occurrence of mental health challenges is important for designing effective prevention, early intervening, and individualized intensive intervention programs" (Crabtree & Delany, 2011, p. 167).

Challenge of Early Identification and Intervention

Because many disorders share common symptoms, early identification and diagnosis of mental illness is challenging and presents a major obstacle to providing responsive services for children and youth (Koppelman, 2004; von der Embse, 2018). For example, difficulty concentrating, changes in sleep, and social withdrawal may occur in children experiencing depression or anxiety. Accurate identification relies on information obtained from multiple sources, including the child, family, teachers, and physicians. Unfortunately, most children who need mental health care do not receive services (over 50%), and for those receiving care, less than one-half receive adequate care (Hoover & Bostic, 2021; Masia-Warner et al., 2006). Without intervention, mental health issues tend to become more severe over time, causing further emotional pain, functional challenges, and increased risk of alcohol and drug use.

Occupational Therapy in School Mental Health

"An important component of integrating mental health efforts into the ongoing routines of schools is the identification and support of indigenous persons and resources within schools as agents of change" (Atkins et al., 2010, p. 42). OTPs are among the few team members in schools who have specialized knowledge and skills in addressing individuals' psychosocial and mental health needs; as such, they are indigenous resources for integrating mental health efforts in schools (Atkins et al., 2010; Cahill & Bazyk, 2019).

With occupational therapy's rich history of addressing mental health in all areas of practice, along with the call for all school personnel to proactively address children's mental health, the role of occupational therapy in SMH seems clear (Bazyk, 2011b). "The psychosocial perspective in occupational therapy is not an add-on or special technique but is rather an integrated, everyday way of thinking about what the client needs and wants to do" (Jackson & Arbesman, 2005, p. 5). It is essential that OTPs expand services in schools to include mental health promotion, prevention, and intervention and advocate for such shifts in service provision.

Occupation-Based Services

Although many specific approaches to mental health promotion, prevention, and intervention are important to know about and apply, all occupational therapy services emphasize using meaningful occupation to promote participation in needed and desired occupations within their full scope of practice (e.g., education, play, leisure, work, social participation, ADLs, IADLs, sleep/rest, health management, see Fig. 37-2) within a variety of contexts (AOTA, 2020; Bazyk, 2023).

Participation in School Occupations

OTPs are distinctly qualified to provide occupation-based services because of their expertise in activity design, task analysis, human development, and group processes (Bazyk, 2011b). "As such, OTPs use activities as the means to 'occupation' and for participation within a variety of contexts" (Jackson & Arbesman, 2005, p. 31).

When interacting with other mental health providers in schools (e.g., psychologists, social workers, and school counselors), it is vital that OTPs articulate the distinct value of evidence-based meaningful activities in promoting participation in occupations reflecting their full scope of practice (Bazyk, 2022b). The findings of an evidence-based review, for example, indicate that activity-based interventions such as arts and crafts, play, and games help improve students'

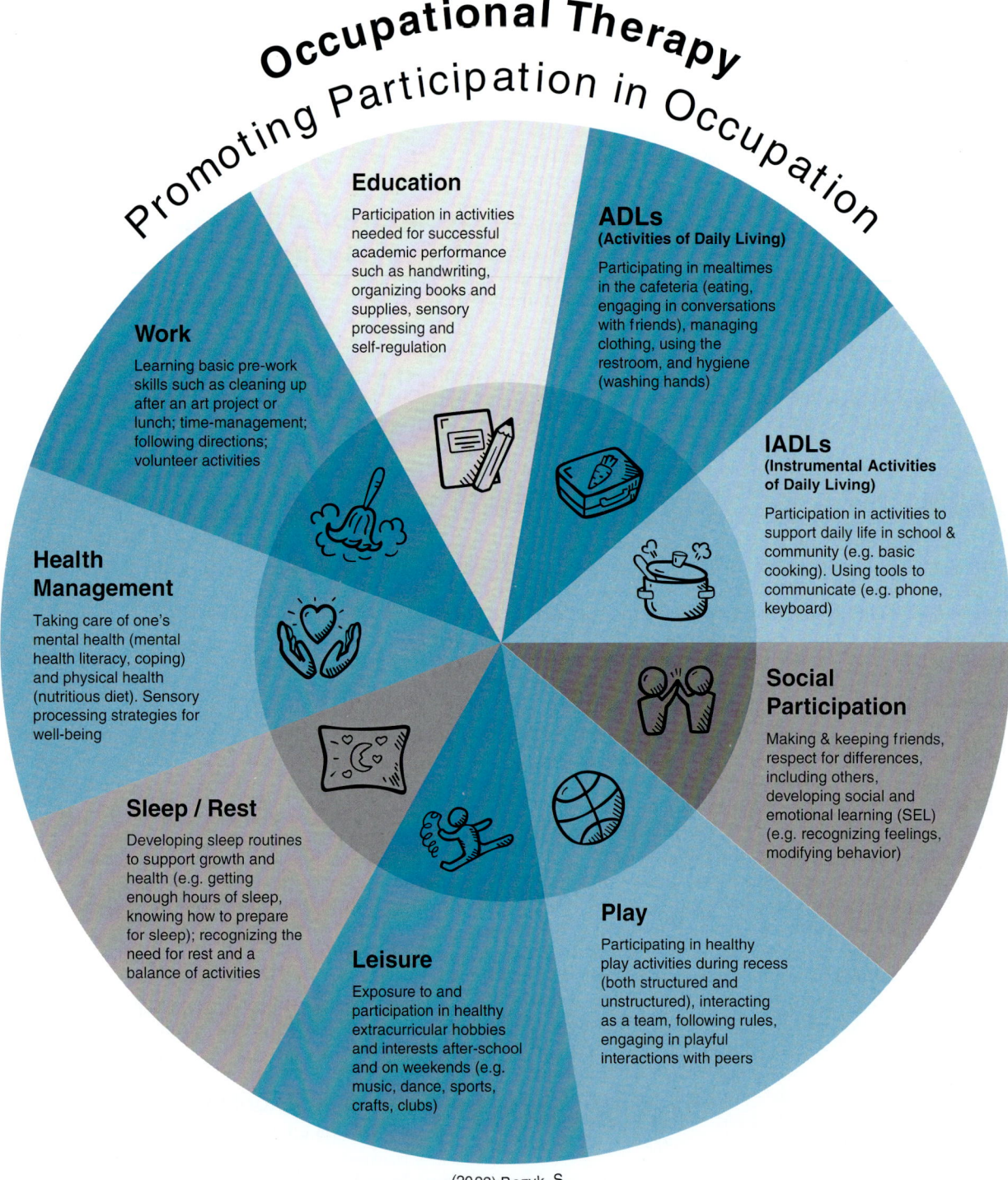

FIGURE 37-2. Occupational therapy: Promoting participation in occupation. *From Bazyk, S. (2022). Occupational therapy: Promoting participation in occupation. www.everymomentcounts.org*

peer interactions, task-focused behaviors, and conformity to social norms (Bazyk & Arbesman, 2013).

The suggested intervention strategies cited in the research include using a variety of activities to teach and encourage skill development. Also recommended are the use of peer models to foster new skills, supportive adults to provide coaching, and a long enough intervention program to allow ample opportunity for practicing emergent skills (Bazyk & Arbesman, 2013).

Activities intended to promote participation should fit the student's interests and developmental level as well as encourage the desired social and emotional skills. The use of small groups tends to be the most powerful form of intervention for promoting social competence and mental well-being (Bazyk & Bazyk, 2009). An effective OTP assumes the role of activity designer and facilitator as well as positive model, coach, and source of emotional support (Bazyk & Arbesman, 2013).

Positive Emotions and Mental Health

Experiencing positive emotions is thought to contribute to mental health (Fredrickson, 2009; Fredrickson & Joiner, 2018; Seligman, 2002). Individuals can experience positive emotions about the past, such as contentment, and about the future, such as happy anticipation. Such experiences can be enhanced and prolonged through reflection, discussion, and daydreaming.

Positive emotions in the present can be elicited in several ways. Sensory pleasures, such as eating a favorite meal, can bring about positive emotions in a momentary fashion. However, Seligman (2011) recommends other routes to happiness that are more enduring—all of which involve engagement in meaningful and enjoyable activities. Participation in occupations that enlist character strengths (e.g., love of learning, curiosity, humor) and talents (e.g., painting, puzzle-making) is associated with positive emotions and feelings of joy (Bazyk, 2010).

Researchers have examined *how* positive emotions influence mental health. Major theorists' models of emotion focus on the idea that emotions are associated with specific action tendencies (Levenson, 1994). Anger, for example, is associated with the urge to attack, disgust with the urge to repel, and fear with the urge to escape. However, traditional approaches to the study of emotion have tended to ignore positive emotions. Fredrickson (2004) proposed a new model of positive emotions—the *broaden-and-build theory*—"because positive emotions appear to *broaden* peoples' momentary thought-action repertoires and *build* their enduring personal resources" (p. 1369).

For example, joy creates an urge to play and be creative, contentment creates the urge to relax and savor life circumstances, interest creates an urge to explore and take in new information, and love creates recurring urges to play with, explore, or savor one's loved ones. These thought-action tendencies can potentially broaden habitual modes of thinking or acting. For example, play can lead to shared moments of social interaction, enjoyment, and attachment. Based on a phenomenological study by Bazyk and Bazyk (2009), occupation-based groups involving creativity and choice were described by children as "fun," resulting in positive emotions and a desire to engage in more of the same activities. Fredrickson (2004) presented foundational evidence supporting many mental health benefits of positive emotions.

Research suggests that positive emotions broaden attention and thinking, reduce negative emotions, promote emotional resilience, fuel mental and physical well-being, and foster human flourishing. In sum, when positive emotions are prominent in daily life, people become "generative, creative, resilient, ripe with possibility and beautifully complex" (Fredrickson, 2004, p. 1375).

Csikszentmihalyi's (1990) years of research studying thousands of people around the world to identify when people experience the most enjoyment in their lives concluded that optimal experience occurs when people are actively versus passively engaged in meaningful activity. Specifically, enjoyment or fun occurs with engagement in occupations that involve several major characteristics:

- Have clear goals (e.g., making greeting cards)
- Involve concentration (e.g., thinking about how to design the card)
- Are doable (e.g., students have a clear chance of completing the cards)
- Allow for choice (e.g., choosing colors)
- Provide immediate feedback (e.g., seeing the end product and giving the card to family or friends)

Challenge is another important element of enjoyment—where "the opportunities or action perceived by the individual are equal to his or her capabilities" (Csikszentmihalyi, 1990, p. 53). OTPs have traditionally valued the use of occupations that provide the "just-right" challenge—a concept inspired by A. Jean Ayres (1998).

Occupational Enrichment

The concept of **occupational enrichment** can be used to promote participation among school-age children in occupations that foster positive emotions and build strengths. Occupational enrichment involves the deliberate modification of the environment to support engagement in a meaningful array of occupations; this concept is especially critical in situations involving occupational deprivation (Molineux & Whiteford, 1999). For youth experiencing significant mental health issues or developmental disabilities, ensuring access to a range of community-based leisure occupations and supporting successful participation are recommended (arts, theatre, dance, sports, etc.; Bazyk & Arbesman, 2013).

Individuals with a variety of developmental disabilities can recognize and develop artistic talents. Art developed by young adults with autism (https://sethchwast.storenvy.com/) and those with various developmental disabilities (Pure Vision Arts at www.purevisionarts.org) is shown at the noted websites. See Chapter 30: Natural Environments.

OTPs can apply occupational enrichment concepts in everyday practice in schools by (a) recognizing features of activities associated with positive emotions (i.e., those that utilize personal strengths, offer a just right challenge, and allow choice); (b) consciously designing occupations for children and youth that lead to enjoyment and positive emotions; and (c) observing and articulating the mental health outcomes of such participation to students, families, and other health-care providers.

For individuals with severe and persistent mental illness or developmental disabilities, it is important to guard against focusing solely on reducing problem behaviors. Attention to participation in meaningful occupations that foster positive emotions and signature strengths will enhance a sense of emotional well-being, happiness, and quality of life (Bazyk, 2010). For an example of an occupational therapy–led initiative emphasizing participation in meaningful and enjoyable occupations within a multitiered mental health framework, read about Every Moment Counts in Box 37-1.

Integrating Occupational Therapy Services in Schools

The role of occupational therapy in schools is to help students benefit from their education, participate successfully in academic and nonacademic activities, and promote health. The nature of occupational therapy practice in schools is complex because of the considerable variability in service provision, including the target of services (who), place of delivery (where), types of services (what), ways in which services are

---

BOX 37-1 ■ Every Moment Counts: Promoting Mental Health Throughout the Day

Every Moment Counts: Promoting Mental Health Throughout the Day is an occupational therapy–led mental health promotion initiative funded by the Ohio Department of Education, Office of Exceptional Children (2012–15). Guided by a multitiered public health approach to mental health, the focus of this initiative is to help all children and youth become mentally healthy to succeed in school, at home, and in the community. A major goal of Every Moment Counts has been the development and implementation of model programs (Comfortable Cafeteria, Refreshing Recess, Making Leisure Matters, Calm Moment Cards) and embedded strategies designed to promote successful and enjoyable participation throughout the day. The use of enjoyable occupations to promote positive emotions and mental health provides the foundation for all the model programs and embedded strategies. A second major goal has been to build the capacity of OTPs and occupational therapy students to address the mental health needs of children and youth (Bazyk et al., 2015, 2020). The project director is Susan Bazyk, PhD, OTR/L, FAOTA.

Model Programs:

- *Comfortable Cafeteria:* This 6-week, 1-day/week program is embedded during lunchtime with the purpose of creating a positive cafeteria environment so that all students can enjoy their meal and socialize with friends. The goal of the 6-week program is to provide the cafeteria staff and students with the necessary knowledge, skills, and resources to sustain a Comfortable Cafeteria environment.
- *Refreshing Recess:* This 6-week program was developed by OTPs to be embedded during recess with the purpose of creating a positive recess experience so that all students can enjoy playing

and socializing with friends. The goal of the 6-week program is to provide the recess supervisors and students with the necessary knowledge, skills, and resources to sustain a positive recess environment. Specifically, Refreshing Recess was designed to support school personnel during recess and to give them strategies for fostering friendships, engaging children in a variety of play activities, resolving conflicts, promoting positive behavior, and creating opportunities for inclusion of all students. Any structured activities that are provided are strictly optional, so students may choose whether they want to participate.

- *Calm Moments Cards:* The Calm Moments Cards provide user-friendly information for frontline school personnel on how to recognize stress reactions in children and youth and embed simple evidence-based strategies to promote emotional well-being throughout the school day (thinking, focusing and calming, and sensory strategies).
- *Making Leisure Matters:* The focus of Making Leisure Matters is to help *all* children and youth explore, select, and participate in extracurricular leisure activities to develop enjoyable hobbies and interests. Occupational Therapy Leisure Coaching is the process used either *individually* with a child/youth and family, or within a *small group* context to educate youth and families about the health benefits of participation in enjoyable hobbies and interests, facilitate the change process used to explore and participate in leisure activities, and advocate for inclusive leisure participation in integrated school and community-sponsored extracurricular activities.

For more details, refer to the Every Moment Counts website at www.everymomentcounts.org.

---

delivered (how), and scheduling of services (when; Cahill & Bazyk, 2019).

Another factor influencing occupational therapy service provision is a consideration of the different *approaches to intervention*—to promote health; prevent disability; restore function; adapt, or modify the task; or maintain function. Traditionally, occupational therapy's role in schools focused on restoring function and adapting the task or environment to promote participation for students with disabilities. However, the reauthorization of IDEA (2004) and authorization of ESSA (2015) have created new opportunities for occupational therapy to contribute to health promotion and prevention in *all* students. The shift to include promotion and preventive models of service delivery has broadened the definition of "client" for OTPs to include *all* children and youth in general and special education (Cahill & Bazyk, 2019).

Traditionally, services in schools were provided directly to the student in an isolated therapy setting such as clinical practice. This type of service delivery involved primarily one person—the student. However, IDEA (2004) does not mandate any one service delivery model. It allows for a range of services, including those provided directly with the student (direct), on behalf of the student (indirect), and as program supports or modifications for teachers and other staff working with the student (indirect; Cahill & Bazyk, 2019).

Integrated services involve providing occupational therapy in the student's natural environment to emphasize nonintrusive methods and common goals (Conway et al., 2015).

Such services give OTPs access to all students, not just those on their caseload, maximizing the ability to reach students who are at risk of developing mental health challenges. Integrated services also benefit therapists. By working in natural settings, OTPs learn about the curriculum, academic and behavioral expectations, teacher preferences, and the unique culture of each classroom.

Observing and interacting with students in the classroom and other school settings enables practitioners to fully analyze the relationships among the student's abilities, the activity expectations, and the physical and social environment, and gives practitioners access to all students with and without mental health challenges. A combination of informal and formal strategies can be used in integrated services. Informal strategies include modifying the environment (physical, social, sensory) and/or the task to foster successful participation and mental health. Formal strategies include coteaching, coaching, small group interventions, and universal programs (Cahill & Bazyk, 2019).

Integrated services can be embedded in several natural contexts throughout the day, including the classroom, cafeteria (e.g., lunch groups, Comfortable Cafeteria program), recess (e.g., game clubs, Refreshing Recess program), art, music, and physical education, as well as after-school programs. Table 37-1 provides information on six occupational therapy–developed programs designed to be integrated into the classroom to help students self-regulate emotional and sensory needs, cope with stress, and learn relaxation

TABLE 37-1 | Classroom-Based Occupational Therapy Embedded Programs

Program	Description	Additional Information and Resources
Calm Moment Cards	**What:** Teachers, paraeducators, and students learn to recognize and respond to common situational stressors at school to reduce stress and enhance emotional well-being. **Type of Collaboration:** OTPs can implement *Calm Moment Cards* activities with the whole class, small groups, or individuals. They can also educate and coach any school personnel to implement thinking, calming and focusing, and sensory strategies through-out the day. **Program Contents:** Informational sheets focus on 17 situational stressors prevalent at school (e.g., test taking, starting the school day) and provide user-friendly strategies and activities in thinking (cognitive behavioral), focusing and calming (mindfulness and yoga), and sensory strategies to reduce stress and triggers that may cause stress. Teaching moments (explanations) support the use of strategies. Appendices include activity templates, yoga poses, and links to useful videos for teaching deep breathing and mindfulness.	**Materials:** Kolic, S., Deininger, A., Young, D., & Bazyk, S. (2016). *Calm Moments Cards booklet. An Every Moment Counts initiative.* http://s3.us-east-2.amazonaws.com/s3.everymomentcounts.com/wp-content/uploads/2021/01/24211256/CMC_Booklet_Final_1-24-21.pdf **Website:** https://everymomentcounts.org/calm-moments-cards **Research:** Visit website to learn more about study outcomes by Kolic and colleagues.
The Interoception Curriculum & Interoception Activity Cards	**What:** Interoception-based resources that help children and adults identify and understand emotions, recognize signs of distress, develop healthy habits and coping mechanisms, and recognize and respond to body signals (e.g., toilet training, recognizing hunger, fullness, or thirst, and pain). **Program Contents:** *The Interoception Curriculum:* A book and digital resource with 25 lessons to empower people to understand and respond to their personal body sensations and emotions. *The Interoception Activity Cards:* This evidence-based card deck includes 100 activities to supplement lessons or practice interoception awareness. Yoga cards and exercise cards are also available. *The Body Check Ring:* A card ring with visual and verbal language support to assist people in expressing or communicating their sensations.	**Website:** https://www.kelly-mahler.com **Book:** Mahler, K. (2019). *The Interoception Curriculum: A step-by-step guide to developing mindful self-regulation.* Mahler. **Selected Research:** Koch, A., & Pollatos, O. (2014). Interoceptive sensitivity, body weight and eating behavior in children: A prospective study. *Frontiers in Psychology, 5,* 1003. https://doi.org/10.3389/fpsyg.2014.01003 Palser, E. R., Fotopoulou, A., Pellicano, E., & Kilner, J. M. (2018). The link between interoceptive processing and anxiety in children diagnosed with ASD: Extending adult findings into a developmental sample. *Biological Psychology, 136,* 13–21. https://doi.org/10.1016/j.biopsycho.2018.05.003
Zones of Regulation	**What:** Curriculum providing a systematic, cognitive behavioral approach to teach children about their emotional and sensory needs to self-regulate and control emotions and impulses, manage sensory needs, and improve the ability to problem-solve conflicts. The Zones of Regulation combines Social Thinking concepts and visual supports to help students identify feelings, understand how behaviors impact others, and learn tools that can be used to move to a more acceptable state. **Type of Collaboration:** Any school personnel can lead whole class, small group, or individual lessons. OTPs can train or lead with any school personnel including teachers, para-educators, counselors, and so on. **Program Contents:** Strategies for regulating emotional and sensory needs to meet the demands of the context and succeed academically and socially. The Four Zones: • *Red Zone:* Heightened state of alertness and intense emotions resulting in being "out of control." • *Yellow Zone:* A less heightened state of alertness and elevated emotions allowing for some control, but that results in stress, anxiety, silliness, or nervousness. • *Green Zone:* A calm state of alertness associated with being happy, content, focused, and ready to learn. • *Blue Zone:* A low state of alertness that may occur when one feels sad, sick, bored, or tired.	**Website:** http://www.zonesofregulation.com **Book:** Kuypers, L. (2011). *The Zones of Regulation: A curriculum designed to foster self-regulation and emotional control.* Social Thinking Publishing.

Continued

TABLE 37 1 | Classroom-Based Occupational Therapy Embedded Programs—cont'd

Program	Description	Additional Information and Resources
Drive Thru Menus • Relaxation & Stress Busters • Attention & Strength	**What:** Similar to how drive thru restaurants quickly provide food, these drive thru menus were developed to help students engage in meaningful activities that take only a short amount of class time. **Type of Collaboration:** Consultation to educate the teacher about the program and how and when to embed it in the classroom. **Length of Time:** Each activity takes approximately 3–5 minutes of class time to help the students manage stress and relax or engage in active movement to attend. **Program Contents:** Each program consists of a large, laminated colorful poster with 10 activities, a DVD of the author's overview of the program, and a leader's manual that explains the purpose, how to prepare for the activity, how to do the activity, and suggested adaptations. • *Relaxation Menu* activities use visualization and meditation to bring about a sense of peacefulness and tranquility. • *Stress Buster Menu* activities involve active movements to relieve stress. • *Strength Menu* activities help students who have difficulty completing fine motor tasks because of muscle weakness. • *Attention Menu* activities help students who struggle with attention and keeping their bodies quiet enough to learn.	**Products:** Bowen-Irish, T. (n.d.-a). *Drive thru menus: Exercises for attention and strength.* Therapro. Bowen-Irish, T. (n.d.-b). *Drive thru menus: Relaxation and stress busters.* Therapro.
Alert Program for Self-Regulation of Arousal	**What:** The Alert Program was initially developed for children with attention and learning difficulties, ages 8–12, but has been adapted for preschool through adult-age individuals with and without a variety of disabilities. The purpose of the program is to teach individuals (children and youth, school personnel, and parents) how to understand their unique sensory processing style to help them use sensory strategies to maintain optimal states of alertness for successful functioning throughout the day. **Program Contents:** An engine analogy is used to teach children and adults how to self-regulate levels of alertness throughout the day to participate in activities they need or want to do. • Three car engine levels are taught: High: feeling "hyper," Low: feeling lethargic, Just right: able to attend and focus on the task at hand. • Five strategies for changing "engine speeds" and alertness are (a) put something in the mouth, (b) move, (c) touch, (d) look, and (e) listen. Children analyze how their engine speeds vary throughout the day and learn how to use sensory strategies to regulate their alertness to feel good and function well for the task at hand.	**Website:** http://www.alertprogram.com **Book:** Williams, M. S., & Shellenberger, S. (1996). *How does your engine run?® A leader's guide to the Alert Program® for self-regulation.* Therapy Works, Inc. **Products:** leaders guide, introductory booklet, games (Alert Bingo), songs (Alert Program CD) **Selected Research:** Barnes, K. J., Vogel, K. A., Beck, A. J., Schoenfeld, H. B., & Owen, S. V. (2008). Self-regulation strategies of children with emotional disturbance. *Physical & Occupational Therapy in Pediatrics, 28*(4), 369–387. https://doi.org/10.1080/01942630802307127 Bertrand, J. (2009). Interventions for children with fetal alcohol spectrum disorders (FASDs): Overview of findings for five innovative research projects. *Research in Developmental Disabilities, 30*(5), 986–1006. https://doi.org/10.1016/j.ridd.2009.02.003
Get Ready to Learn	**What:** Research-based yoga curriculum combines yoga, movement, and mindfulness to address students' behavioral and learning needs from preschool to high school. **Length of Time:** The program is embedded into a teaching period as the warmup for learning, such as a morning routine. Students participate in the session for 20 minutes. The length of **intervention** ranges from 4–26 weeks, with the best results occurring with at least 16 weeks of implementation. **Program Contents:** The program offers a 2-day training (in-person or virtual), streaming services, online coaching support, and program resources such as online tools or data collection services. • *Foundation Series:* A "warm-up" video series designed for young learners to prepare their body and brain for optimal learning states. • *Floor Series:* A video series designed for students of all levels and abilities to reinforce early development patterns to build body awareness and self-regulation. • *Seated Series:* A chair practice series inclusive to address the needs of nonambulatory students. The seated series can complement the floor series or provide therapeutic movement in classrooms with limited space. • *Ready Break Series:* A free short series of yoga movements ranging from 5–13 minutes that can be used to prepare students to engage in learning at home, in the community, or at school.	**Website:** https://www.thegetreadyproject.com/school-program **Selected Research:** Garg, S., Buckley-Reen, A., Alexander, L., Chintakrindi, R., Ocampo Tan, L.V., & Patten Koenig, K. (2013). The effectiveness of a manualized yoga intervention on classroom behaviors in elementary school children with disabilities: A pilot study. *Journal of Occupational Therapy, Schools, & Early Intervention, 6*(2), 158–164. https://doi.org/10.1080/19411243.2013.810942 Milton, L. E., Bantel, S., Calmer, K., Friedman, M., Haley, E., & Rubarts, L. (2019). Yoga and autism: Students' perspectives on the Get Ready to Learn yoga program. *The Open Journal of Occupational Therapy, 7*(4), 1–10. https://doi.org/10.15453/2168-6408.1560

strategies. In addition to the traditional school day, increased emphasis is placed on participation in extracurricular leisure activities, opening the doors wider for OTPs to help children and youth develop and participate in structured leisure interests during recess and after-school hours (Bazyk, 2022a).

The Occupational Therapy Process

An understanding of occupation-based practice, positive psychology, positive youth development, and mental health promotion contributes to the development of occupational therapy services in addressing the mental health needs of students in schools (Bazyk, 2011d). The first step involves gaining *awareness, knowledge, and skills* necessary for addressing the mental health needs of children and youth at each tier. For example, at Tier 1 in a school setting, it is important to obtain information about schoolwide programs relevant to mental health and behavior and support implementation in everyday practice. This may include applying PBIS, for example. At Tiers 2 and 3, the OTP needs to become *aware* of the mental health continuum, including the signs and symptoms associated with various mental illnesses and their impact on school functioning.

The second step involves *appraisal* specific to each tier. This may include a range of evaluation strategies, including structured observation or gathering information using assessment tools specific to each tier. Table 37-2 outlines key information about common assessment tools to help guide the practitioner's therapeutic reasoning when choosing to add these tools to the evaluation processes.

At Tier 1, appraisal might involve using various strategies to evaluate students' mental health and the qualities of the physical and social environments. At the most basic level, OTPs should pay attention to every student's mental health by specifically observing emotions: Does the student demonstrate periods of happiness, joy, or satisfaction throughout the day? Patterns of occupational participation should also be noted: Does the student engage in a range of healthy and enjoyable occupations throughout the day? Does the student have special interests or hobbies that foster a sense of joy and personal well-being? The quality of the settings should also be noted: Do the settings involve caring adults who promote character strengths and positive emotions (Bazyk, 2011d)? By incorporating these questions into the evaluation process, the practitioner can capture the student's experiences, values, perspectives, and strengths, creating an occupational profile that describes a holistic view of the child.

Practitioners may consider additional evidence from the student's record, such as attendance, academics, and behavior data. Many schools administer universal social, emotional, and behavioral (SEB) screening tools as a systematic and multitiered approach to improving student well-being (Romer et al., 2020). OTPs are encouraged to review existing data to complete a comprehensive assessment of the child. Overall, the evaluation process is driven by a strengths-based, person-centered approach, which leads to collaborative goal setting to support the well-being of students at school. See Chapter 4: Person-Centered Evaluation.

The third step involves *action*, that is, indirect and direct intervention strategies that are specific to each tier. *Actions* are based on the appraisal process and refer to interventions and conditions that promote optimal mental health. An example of an action used to promote mental health at Tier 1 is occupational therapy consultation with teachers to understand behaviors associated with sensory defensiveness, followed by the modification of interactions and the environment to enhance social interaction and feelings of emotional well-being (Bazyk, 2011d; Lynch et al., 2023).

Diversity, Equity, and Inclusion in School Mental Health

Given the prevalence of mental health concerns in schools coupled with disproportionality in special education, it is vital that OTPs use their advocacy skills and knowledge in mental health promotion and prevention to uphold diversity, equity, and inclusion (DEI). Advocacy efforts can include contributing to policy-level changes, professional development, curriculum design, and school climate initiatives, as well as providing consultation, education, or training to school teams, parents, and community members. Collaboration is the common thread in the literature discussing DEI and SMH. Research shows that the student is best supported when the family, school teams, and community work together (Tucker & Matson, 2022). This collaboration includes sharing perspectives, giving the family and student a voice, and partnering with community providers. Using the multitiered approach to mental health assessment, planning, and intervention demands a collaborative approach.

Diversity

OTPs must demonstrate a commitment to educating themselves about the diverse backgrounds of students and families to meet their needs. OTPs must also embrace cultural humility, use culturally responsive practices, avoid assumptions and norms, and understand culturally based beliefs and language barriers to successfully collaborate for students' mental health needs (Agner, 2020; Lynch et al., 2023). Finally, OTPs must be conscious that the assessments and interventions reflect the daily life activities, skills, and values of marginalized groups (Silverman et al., 2023). This includes awareness of cultural beliefs, languages, and other factors that may impact student participation and success. See Chapter 27: Mental Health Stigma and Sanism and Chapter 28: Social Determinants and Mental Health.

Under the MTSS model, team members, including OTPs, collaborate to select and implement culturally and linguistically relevant interventions for diverse learners (Tucker & Matson, 2022). Tucker and Matson (2022) reported that mental health is perceived differently in different cultural groups; creating a shared understanding between the school and family is essential to the collaborative relationship. When school teams work together to discuss the mental health needs of all students, conversations can shift to a proactive, strengths-based, and integrative approach that supports students'

TABLE 37-2 | **Therapeutic Reasoning Assessment Table: Social Participation and Social and Emotional Functioning in School**

Name of Tool	Population/ Age	Description and Administration	Target Area	Time and Location for Administration	Associated Practice Model
Evaluation of School Environment					
Comfortable Cafeteria Environmental Analysis (Demirjian et al., 2021)	School environments for students grades K–12	Nonstandardized structured observations by OTPs in collaboration with relevant school personnel of the cafeteria context as a part of the Comfortable Cafeteria program in the areas of routines, supervisor interactions, behavioral interactions, the social environment including mealtime conversations and friendships, inclusion, and sensory factors including auditory input (noise), visual input (lighting), quality of food, and tactile input.	Useful in identifying positive and negative aspects of the lunch experience in order to tailor program implementation to the specific school context.	Naturalistic observations of student participation and enjoyment during lunch; ½ hour to complete written analysis	Physical and mental health promotion, MTSS
Refreshing Recess Environmental Analysis (Bazyk et al., 2021)	School environments for students grades K–12	Nonstandardized structured observation by OTPs in collaboration with relevant school personnel of the recess context as a part of the Refreshing Recess program in the areas of play materials and equipment, supervisor interactions, behavior expectations, students' social interaction and friendships, physical activity, play activities and games, opportunities for structured and unstructured play, inclusion of students with disabilities or emotional challenges, and transition to and from recess.	Useful in identifying positive and negative aspects of recess to tailor program implementation to the specific recess context.	Naturalistic observation of student participation, healthy occupations, and enjoyment during indoor or outdoor recess; ½ hour to complete written analysis	Physical and mental health promotion, MTSS
Child or Youth Social Participation or Social and Emotional Functioning					
Devereux Student Strengths Assessment (DESSA; LeBuffe et al., 2009)	Students grades K–8	• Standardized norm-referenced, strengths-based rating scale of social-emotional competencies as displayed by students in classrooms or the community. • Completed by parents or guardians, teachers, or out of school staff. • Assesses competencies in eight dimensions: self-awareness, social awareness, self-management, goal-directed behavior, relationship skills, personal responsibility, decision-making, and optimistic thinking.	Can be used individually or with a whole class to identify social-emotional skills to build on strengths to enhance competencies in weaker areas needing instruction and support.	Mini-DESSA takes 1 minute per student and has eight items. Full DESSA assessment has 72 items and provides deeper data on strengths across the eight dimensions.	Social-emotional learning (SEL); strengths-based approaches
School Function Assessment (SFA; Coster et al., 1998)	Students grades K–6	• This is a standardized criterion-referenced assessment. • Judgment-based questionnaire is completed by one or more school personnel. • Assesses social and physical function in nonacademic tasks in classroom, recess, bathroom activities, mealtimes, or snacks; transitioning to and from class; and transportation to and from school and home. • Evaluates students' participation, task supports, and activity performance.	Identifies the strengths and needs in important nonacademic functional tasks in elementary school students with disabilities to enhance academic and social aspects of school function.	Takes 1.5–2 hours in a school setting; individual scales can be done in 5–10 minutes.	Developmental; functional

TABLE 37-2 | **Therapeutic Reasoning Assessment Table: Social Participation and Social and Emotional Functioning in School—cont'd**

Name of Tool	Population/ Age	Description and Administration	Target Area	Time and Location for Administration	Associated Practice Model
Children's Assessment of Participation and Enjoyment (CAPE) and Preferences for Activities of Children (PAC; King et al., 2004)	6–21 years	Requires individual to read and write or be able to understand verbal directions and communicate for interview-assisted version.	Measures the child's or youth's exposure to and preferences in out-of-school recreational, social, active, physical, skill-based, and self-improvement activities to plan leisure participation.	Can be administered in school or home settings in 30–45 minutes	Person-Environment-Occupation (PEO) model
School Setting Interview (SSI; Hemmingsson et al., 2005)	Elementary (7 years) to high school students	• This is a nonstandardized structured interview. • A person-centered semistructured interview is used to assess student-environment fit and identify the need for accommodations in physical or social contexts such as classroom, playground, gym, and field trips.	This can be used to identify the student's perceptions of their social participation and enjoyment of school throughout the day with accommodations that can facilitate greater participation.	Time not specified; interview at school	Model of Human Occupation (MOHO); person-centered model
School Companion Sensory Profile 2 (Dunn, 2014)	3–14 years	Teacher completes the form based on observation and teaching experiences.	Sensory processing preferences are observed through participation in daily life.	Allow 30 minutes at school	Dunn Model of Sensory Processing
Social Profile–Child Version (Donohue, 2013)	Students grades K–12 and adulthood	• This is completed by a skilled OTP who observes social participation in a group. • A 40-item scale is divided into three areas: activity participation, social interaction, and group membership/roles; child version is 27 items. • The focus is on interaction within a group.	The profile can help evaluate a student's cooperation and participation in group activities throughout the day (classroom, lunch, recess).	Can be done in home, school, community, and clinical settings, wherever groups occur; time to complete not specified	Psychosocial or developmental
Pediatric Interest Profile: Surveys of Play for Children and Adolescents • Kid Play Profile • Preteen Play Profile • Adolescent Leisure Interest Profile (Henry, 2000)	Kid: 6–9 years Preteen: 9–12 years Adolescent: 12–21 years	• The profile utilizes nonstandardized interview checklists. • Three age-appropriate profiles—play, leisure interests, and participation—can be used with children and adolescents with and without disabilities. • Child self-reports interest and participation in activities. • Examples of activity categories: sports, outdoor, creative, social, lessons, winter, intellectual, and so on.	The profile can assist in identifying a student's play and leisure participation and help identify potential areas of interest.	Can be done in home, school, community, and clinical settings; time to complete not specified	Can be applied to MOHO, developmental
Occupational Therapy Psychosocial Assessment of Learning (OT PAL; Townsend, 1999)	6–12 years	This assessment uses a nonstandardized observational rating scale and interview of the child, teacher, and parents around the student's ability to make choices, their roles and routines, and the environmental fit within the classroom setting.	To measure the psychosocial aspects of a student's performance within the classroom as a part of the occupational therapy evaluation and to determine student-environment "fit."	40-minute classroom observation	MOHO
Canadian Occupational Performance Measure (COPM; Law et al., 2014)	All ages with and without disabilities	This performance-based measure identifies and prioritizes the person's occupational performance limitations related to daily activities, leisure, or productivity using standardized rating scales. The information guides collaborative goal setting.	Three categories of occupational performance: (1) self-care: personal care, functional mobility, and community management;	15–30 minutes; semistructured interview	The Canadian Model of Occupational Performance and Engagement (CMOP-E)

Continued

TABLE 37 2 | **Therapeutic Reasoning Assessment Table: Social Participation and Social and Emotional Functioning in School—cont'd**

Name of Tool	Population/ Age	Description and Administration	Target Area	Time and Location for Administration	Associated Practice Model
			(2) productivity: paid/unpaid work, household management, and play/school; (3) leisure: quiet recreation, active recreation, and socialization.		
Child Occupational Self-Assessment (COSA; Kramer et al., 2014)	Research based on children 7–17 years but may be suitable for children 6–21 years, with the ability to self-reflect	A self-rating scale assists the therapist in understanding the child's sense of competence and facilitates collaborative goal setting with the child. Three administration formats: • A youth rating form with symbols • A youth rating form without symbols • A card sort option	Captures the child's perception of occupational competence and value of everyday activities related to school, home, and in the community.	25 minutes; self-report, structured interview	MOHO
Visual Activity Sort (VAS; Gutman et al., 2022; O'Day, 2020)	Adolescents, young adults 13–25 years	This qualitative and quantitative visual interpretation tool facilitates discussion about the person's strengths and barriers to participation in desired daily life activities. The people sort cards with visual images and narrow the selection to 7–10 occupations. Next, they rate the occupations based on participation, satisfaction, motivation, and perceived competence level using a 0–2 point scale. Results are used to discuss strengths and barriers that create an occupational profile that leads to collaborative goals.	The cards are divided into seven categories of occupations based on the *Occupational Therapy Practice Framework*, 4th Edition (OTPF-4): (1) ADLs, (2) IADLs, (3) health management, (4) social participation, (5) work, (6) school, and (7) leisure.	Not specified	Occupation-based
The Comprehensive Assessment of Interoceptive Awareness, 3rd Edition (Mahler, 2021)	All ages, preschool through adulthood	• This self-report tool explores each learner's unique interoceptive awareness. • There are three sub-assessments. • *The Interoceptive Awareness Interview (self-report):* A series of open-ended and Likert-scale questions about the student's experience noticing and understanding body signals. • *The Assessment of Self-Regulation + Picture Cards (self-report):* A series of picture cards with questions about a student's perspective and experience regulating to body signals, emotions, and regulation actions. • *The Caregiver Questionnaire for Interoceptive Awareness (observation/ caregiver report):* Administered when the student cannot self-report; therefore, a caregiver or someone that knows the student well answers questions that explore various interoception experiences and observations related to emotions such as hunger, thirst, toileting, anxiety, and so on. • The assessment can be adapted for use with various communication styles, allowing students to speak, write, draw, color, or act out their responses.	It is designed to gather the student's perspective and a baseline for the student's interoceptive relationship.	Not specified; can be administered in schools, therapy clinics, mental health facilities, and home	Interoception, participation, and health

TABLE 37-2 | Therapeutic Reasoning Assessment Table: Social Participation and Social and Emotional Functioning in School—cont'd

Name of Tool	Population/ Age	Description and Administration	Target Area	Time and Location for Administration	Associated Practice Model
Universal Screeners for Student's Social-Emotional Well-Being					
Strengths and Difficulties Questionnaire (SDQ; Goodman, 1999, 2005)	3–18 years and adults	• Brief behavioral screening questionnaire that has several versions for researchers, clinicians, and educators; ages 11+ also have self-report. • All versions focus on 25 attributes in five areas: emotional symptoms, conduct problems, hyperactivity and inattention, peer social relationships, and prosocial behavior.	This is an easy-to-use measure that addresses both problem behaviors as well as strengths.	Primarily used as a research tool; can be used clinically and in schools; time to complete not specified.	Mental health and well-being
Behavioral and Emotional Rating Scale–Second Edition (BERS-2; Epstein, 2004)	5–18 years	• Standardized multimodal assessment with a youth rating scale, parent rating scale, and teacher/professionals rating scale. • This strengths-based assessment identifies interpersonal strengths, family involvement, intrapersonal strengths, school functioning, affective strength, and career strength.	This can help identify behavioral and emotional strengths and areas needing development.	10 minutes to complete the scale; used in school, home, and juvenile justice settings	Behavioral; developmental
Social Skills Improvement System: Rating Scales (SSRS), Student Form (SSRS; Elliott & Gresham, 2008)	3–18 years	• This is a standardized norm-referenced assessment and intervention system to help students develop, improve, and maintain important social skills. • It offers teacher, parent, and student forms. • It provides a universal screening tool as well as targeted and comprehensive assessments. • Areas assessed include social skills (cooperation, empathy, self-control); competing problem behaviors (bullying, hyperactivity, externalizing or internalizing); academic competence (reading and math achievement, motivation to learn).	This enables targeted assessment of individual students and small groups to evaluate social skills, problem behaviors, and academic competence. It provides intervention guides.	Allow 10–25 minutes in school and home setting	Social-emotional learning (SEL); developmental

overall well-being, reducing retroactive approaches rooted in stigma, shame, and isolation.

Furthermore, the literature suggested that collaborative multitiered interventions yield the greatest outcomes when the home, school, and community all work together to meet the needs of diverse learners (Enns et al., 2016; Tucker & Matson, 2022). This includes ensuring families and community partners are represented and heard at individualized education plan (IEP) meetings or other school events.

Equity

Historically, students of diverse racial and ethnic backgrounds, students from low-income households, and students with disabilities experience inequities in school systems (National Center for Learning Disabilities [NCLD], 2020). These groups are referred to special education, placed in more restrictive environments, and disciplined (e.g., restraint or suspension) at a higher rate than their peers, resulting in overrepresentation in special education (NCLD, 2020; Tucker & Matson, 2022).

In 2017, the Obama administration authorized the Equity in IDEA (2004) regulations that set standard practices for how all states address racial and ethnic disparities in identification, placement, and use of discipline for students of color with disabilities. States were mandated to abide by the new regulation by March 2019. OTPs need to remain informed of factors that may impact the special education eligibility process, such as linguistic, cultural, or economic disadvantages (NCLD, 2020). Teams that regularly communicate with the family and use universal and evidence-based assessments to measure learning and track progress can reduce bias when identifying students with disabilities.

Second, OTPs can play a key role in Tier I initiatives, such as collaborating with school teams to perform universal screenings (Cahill & Egan, 2017). Research has shown that districts providing universal screeners and approaches promote equity for diverse learners (Romer et al., 2020). Screening for both characteristics of positive mental health and mental illness symptoms can lead to early detection, proactive intervention, and improved educational outcomes (Cahill & Egan, 2017). Effective screening and progress monitoring can help practitioners determine the need to intensify or reduce tiered services for diverse students.

Similarly, Lynch and colleagues (2020) reported that OTPs using a trauma-informed care perspective could work with school staff to promote a positive school climate and create equitable discipline practices, thereby decreasing disparities. OTPs can play a vital role in educating school-based staff on evidence-based interventions for each tier to promote positive mental health. Practitioners can help school teams create learning environments that foster student engagement and teach prosocial behaviors and restorative practices (e.g., building healthy relationships; NCLD, 2020).

At the Tier 2 and Tier 3 level, schoolwide mental health prevention and intervention is critical for students from underserved communities with low income and minority backgrounds who may not receive or have access to services (Raval et al., 2019). These youth are at greater risk for developing mental health concerns, especially the Latinx population, which is one of the fastest growing ethnic groups in the United States (Montañez et al., 2015; Raval et al., 2019).

In an effort to mitigate the unmet mental health needs of Latinx students living in an underserved area of Northern Manhattan, the Turn 2 Us (T2U) program developed as a partnership between families, elementary schools, and community stakeholders. The program aimed to improve student social, behavioral, and academic functioning while also building the knowledge and support of teachers and families (Montañez et al., 2015). T2U recognized the benefits of a multisystem approach that met cultural needs by providing a continuum of services and intervention tracks tailored to the social and emotional needs of the Latinx students and families. Student services included sports, dance, arts, and drama before or after school, lunch time mentorship groups with interactive skill building during recess, and ongoing feedback and monitoring for behavioral and academic performance.

Students experiencing internalizing behaviors participated in a creative arts track, whereas students experiencing externalizing behaviors participated in a sports or dance track. Through the school year, teachers and families received training that focused on mental health literacy. Consultation between community partners, schools, and families also served as a key component of the program.

Research has shown that the T2U program led to significant improvements in students' social skills and classroom performance, especially for those at highest risk for both internalizing and externalizing behaviors. This research highlights the importance of building comprehensive school-based mental health promotion and intervention services that include collaboration among families, teachers, and community; culturally relevant intervention; and attention to a positive school climate.

Inclusion

OTPs can help schools promote policies, procedures, and programming that ensure all students feel safe and connected to the community (Lynch et al., 2020). As previously noted, dynamic school team collaboration supports inclusive practices. Tier 1 initiatives strongly support inclusion efforts, emphasizing the importance of OTP involvement in school teams that promote mental health and well-being.

Practitioners can work with school teams to ensure students feel safe and share a sense of belonging with the school community and can identify, advocate for, and promote inclusive programs, such as antibullying (Conway et al., 2015; Njelesani et al., 2022). In addition to programming, OTPs have a unique lens in environmental and activity analysis to promote inclusion. OTPs can work with school staff to adapt or create positive learning environments that foster social participation, self-regulation, and social-emotional functioning for all students (e.g., apply universal design for learning principles, create sensory-friendly classrooms and cafeterias, or develop buddy systems for walking to school or accessing playgrounds; Conway et al., 2015). When analyzing school occupations or environments, OTPs must consider if the occupations pose barriers, further trauma, or exclude marginalized groups (Gutman et al., 2022).

Practitioners can ensure that all students receive consistent opportunities to participate in the general education setting. For students with disabilities, IDEA (2004) mandates that services are delivered in the general education setting to the greatest extent possible. Practitioners can facilitate inclusion through an integrated service delivery model by providing student services in the natural environment (Conway et al., 2015). By advocating for placement in the least restrictive environment (LRE), OTPs can ensure inclusion opportunities for students to participate in a rigorous curriculum with their general education peers.

Key Takeaway

Practitioners can practice self-reflection that includes accepting cultural humility and avoiding assumptions, norms, stigma, shame, or isolation. OTPs can focus on developing relationships with families that include creating open communication to better understand the student's familial, social, and cultural background to elevate the family and student voice in the evaluation, intervention, and decision-making processes (NCLD, 2020). Research shows that a collaborative team approach using multitiered systems for mental health is essential to meet the needs of diverse learners, reduce inequities, and promote inclusion in school systems. Several studies articulated the importance of sharing information with stakeholders (Helseth & Frazier, 2018; Montañez et al., 2015; Raval et al., 2019).

Major Approaches Used in School Mental Health

In addition to traditional occupational therapy intervention approaches (e.g., sensory processing, occupation-based practice), other whole school approaches developed in the fields of public health, psychology, and education can be used to address the mental health needs of students. These include sensory processing; mental health literacy; positive youth development and structured leisure participation; SEL; mindfulness, yoga, and relaxation; PBIS; and cognitive behavioral thinking strategies (Bazyk, 2011c). Table 37-3 describes these approaches and provides examples of application to practice, as well as supporting literature. These approaches can be applied individually or in combination to guide occupational therapy individual, small group, and whole school interventions (Fig. 37-3). Interdisciplinary collaboration and implementation of whole school strategies is key to obtaining successful outcomes (Marinucci et al., 2023).

TABLE 37-3 | Major Whole School Approaches Used in Mental Health Promotion, Prevention, and Intervention

Approach	Description	Implications for Occupational Therapy	Supporting Evidence and Resources
Sensory Processing	Sensory processing is a person's way of noticing and responding to sensory messages from their body and the environment (Dunn, 2007). Persons with disabilities or mental health difficulties may experience everyday sensations with more or less intensity than those without such challenges. Such sensory differences may influence a person's behavior, social interaction, and regulation of emotions. It is important to teach all students and adults to respect one another's sensory needs (e.g., less noise, more movement, less eye contact). Self-regulation is the ability to manage and control our emotions and behavior. Self-regulation helps us do what we need to do throughout the day. OTPs are distinctly qualified to apply this knowledge and skill at the universal, targeted, and intensive levels to promote successful participation in school and community settings. They play an important role in helping children, families, and professionals develop a working knowledge of sensory processing. This will help others to understand children's behaviors and modify everyday interactions and environments to foster success and well-being (Dunn, 2007).	• Educate school personnel, students, and parents about sensory processing, impact on mental health, and accommodations. • Educate relevant stakeholders to enhance their understanding of self-regulation and participation from a sensory perspective. • Evaluate and modify environments (e.g., classroom, cafeteria, playground) to meet a range of sensory needs. • Collaborate with educators and students to identify patterns of sensory processing (overresponsive, underresponsive) and offer embedded sensory strategies to promote participation and enjoyment. • Use available occupational therapy programs to create sensory-friendly environments and promote self-regulation.	Dunn, W. (2007). Supporting children to participate successfully in everyday life by using sensory processing knowledge. *Infants & Young Children, 20*(2), 84–101. https://doi.org/10.1097/01.IYC.0000264477.05076.5d Kuypers, L. (2011). *The Zones of Regulation.* Social Thinking Publishing. This curriculum can be used by an interdisciplinary team. See http://www .zonesofregulation .com/index.html. Mahler, K. (2015). *Interoception: The eighth sensory system.* AAPC Publishing. Mahler, K. (2019). *The Interoception Curriculum: A step-by-step framework for developing mindful self-regulation.* Mahler. Williams, M. S., & Shellenberger, S. (1996). *"How does your engine run?®"* A leader's guide to the Alert Program® for self-regulation. Therapy Works, Inc.
Mental Health Literacy	Mental health literacy refers to providing all people with a working knowledge of mental health as an essential part of overall health (Barry & Jenkins, 2007). It includes many components, such as learning about mental health and strategies for improving and maintaining mental health; recognizing when a disorder is developing and where to seek help; effective self-help strategies for mild problems; and how to support others facing a mental health crisis (Jorm, 2019). Youth Mental Health First Aid (YMHFA) training courses for youth educate adults on how to provide support for adolescents showing symptoms of a mental health disorder until professional help is obtained (Kelly et al., 2011). Randomized controlled trials comparing Mental Health First Aid course attendees with wait-list controls found improvements in knowledge, helping behaviors, and stigmatizing attitudes (Jorm, 2012).	• Talk about mental health to help all students and adults develop a working knowledge of positive mental health as well as the signs of mental illness. • Reinforce the attitudes and actions associated with mental health such as participating in enjoyable occupations, exercising, thinking positively, and keeping stress in check. • Host Children's Mental Health Awareness Day events every May (http://www.samhsa.gov/children). • Collaborate with health educators, teachers, and school nurses to embed educational activities related to mental health literacy into the school ecology. • Bring a training course such as YMHFA to your school.	Jorm, A. (2012). Mental health literacy: Empowering the community to take action for better mental health. *American Psychologist, 67*(3), 231–243. https://doi.org/10.1037/a0025957 Jorm, A. F. (2019). The concept of mental health literacy. In O. Okan, U. Bauer, D. Levin-Zamir, P. Pinheiro, & K. Sørensen (Eds.), *International handbook of health literacy: Research, practice and policy across the life-span* (pp. 53–66). Policy Press. https://doi.org/10.51952/9781447344520.ch004 Jorm, A. F., Korten, A. E., Jacomb, P. A., Christensen, H., Rodgers, B., & Pollitt, P. (1997). "Mental health literacy": A survey of the public's ability to recognize mental disorders and their beliefs about the effectiveness of treatment. *Medical Journal of Australia, 166*(4), 182–186. https://doi.org/10.5694/j.1326-5377.1997.tb140071.x Kelly, C. M., Mithen, J. M., Fischer, J. A., Kitchener, B. A., Jorm, A. J., Lowe, A., & Scanlan, C. (2011). YMHFA: A description of the program and an initial evaluation. *International Journal of Mental Health Systems, 5*(4), 1–9. https://doi.org/10.1186/1752-4458-5-4

Continued

TABLE 37-3 | **Major Whole School Approaches Used in Mental Health Promotion, Prevention, and Intervention—cont'd**

Approach	Description	Implications for Occupational Therapy	Supporting Evidence and Resources
Positive Youth Development and Structured Leisure Participation	Positive youth development emphasizes building and improving assets that enable youth to grow and flourish throughout life (Moore, 2017). Larson (2000) emphasizes the development of initiative as a core quality of positive youth development and makes a case for participation in structured leisure activities (e.g., sports, arts, organized clubs) as an important context for such development. An important aspect of occupation-based practice when promoting mental health in children is attention to the development of structured leisure participation during out-of-school time. Extracurricular participation may be included as a standard item on IEPs. Highly structured leisure activities are associated with regular participation schedules, rule-guided interaction, direction by one or more adult leaders, an emphasis on skill development that increases in complexity and challenge, and performance that requires sustained active attention and the provision of feedback (Bazyk, 2022a). Correlational research has demonstrated a positive relationship between participation in structured leisure and positive outcomes such as diminished delinquency, greater achievement, and increased self-efficacy and self-control (Larson, 2000).	• Encourage students to explore and participate in out-of-school interests (arts, music, sports, clubs, etc.). Commit to helping all students engage in at least one meaningful hobby and interest. • Conduct environmental scans to identify a range of extracurricular participation options for students—both school and community-sponsored options. • Provide coaching to help students with disabilities and mental health challenges successfully participate in structured leisure interests. Coaching may involve adapting entry into the activity and educating the coach or adult leader about strategies for promoting successful participation based on the individual needs of the child or youth.	Larson, R. W. (2000). Toward a psychology of positive youth development. *American Psychologist, 55*(1), 170–183. https://doi.org/10.1037/0003-066X.55.1.170 McNeil, D. A., Wilson, B. N., Siever, J. E., Ronca, M., & Mah, J. K. (2009). Connecting children to recreational activities: Results of a cluster randomized trial. *American Journal of Health Promotion, 23*(6), 376–387. https://doi.org/10.4278/ajhp.071010107 Moore K. A. (2017). Commentary: Positive youth development goes mainstream. *Child Development, 88*(4), 1175–1177. https://doi.org/10.1111/cdev.12874
Social-Emotional Learning (SEL)	SEL is a framework used to guide the process of helping children and youth develop critical skills for life: how to get along with others, handle challenges, and behave ethically. Programs that foster SEL help children recognize feelings and think about how feelings influence behavior. Specifically, these programs help children to recognize and manage emotions, think about their feelings and how one should act, regulate behavior based on thoughtful decision-making, and acquire important social skills for developing healthy relationships in life. Five core SEL skills are developed: self-awareness, self-management, social awareness, relationship skills, and responsible decision-making. For more information, refer to the Collaborative for Academic, Social, and Emotional Learning (CASEL) at www.casel.org. Currently, all 50 states have preschool SEL standards, and many states have SEL integrated in their academic standards. Evidence-based reviews provide strong support for the use of SEL programming at the universal level to improve social-emotional functioning, increase academic success, and reduce emotional distress and problem behaviors.	• Investigate whether the school has adopted an SEL curriculum. If so, become involved in schoolwide implementation. • Tune into students' feelings daily. Simply asking "How is your day going?" or "How are you feeling?" can communicate an interest in the child's emotional life. • Help students develop a feeling vocabulary and use words to express feelings. Foster the ability to recognize and respond to others' emotions. • Refer to Illinois SEL academic standards in order to determine age-appropriate SEL expectations and intervention supports. • Embed SEL goals and activities into all interventions.	Carter, E. W., & Hughes, C. (2005). Increasing social interaction among adolescents with intellectual disabilities and their general education peers: Effective interventions. *Research and Practice for Persons With Severe Disabilities, 30*(4), 179–193. https://doi.org/10.2511/rpsd.30.4.179 Durlak, J. A., Mahoney, J. L., & Boyle, A. E. (2022). What we know, and what we need to find out about universal, school-based social and emotional learning programs for children and adolescents: A review of meta-analyses and directions for future research. *Psychological Bulletin, 148*(11-12), 765–782. https://doi.org/10.1037/bul0000383
Mindfulness, Yoga, and Relaxation Approaches	Mindfulness, yoga, and relaxation approaches are found to be promising practices in school settings for improving coping abilities and reducing anxiety. Such practices help students "step back" from stressful situations by teaching them how to purposefully and nonjudgmentally "be in the moment." Kabat-Zinn (2003) suggests that mindfulness helps calm and clear the mind and help focus attention. There is promising evidence that school-based mindfulness can positively impact students' mindfulness and self-regulation skills, reduce students' internalizing distress, and improve students' physical health and healthy relationships (Roeser et al., 2023).	• Consider embedding whole class or whole school mindfulness strategies during transitions or before tests. These activities can be as short as 1–2 minutes or as long as 5–10 minutes. Important calming strategies include deep breathing, yoga, short meditations, sensory strategies, creative arts activities, and time spent in green spaces.	Kabat-Zinn, J. (2003). Mindfulness-based interventions in context: Past, present, future. *Clinical Psychology: Science and Practice, 10*(2), 144–156. https://doi.org/10.1093/clipsy.bpg016

TABLE 37-3 | **Major Whole School Approaches Used in Mental Health Promotion, Prevention, and Intervention—cont'd**

Approach	Description	Implications for Occupational Therapy	Supporting Evidence and Resources
	Learning how to cope with stressful situations and everyday challenges is an important life skill for all children and youth. All children and youth experience stress to varying degrees because of situational challenges (taking a test, entering a noisy environment, being teased, completing a difficult assignment, etc.). Feeling stressed and anxious can negatively impact student learning (e.g., difficulty concentrating) and everyday functioning (sleeping, eating, and socializing).	• *Deep breathing:* Have students take three to five deep belly breaths. Teach a variety of deep breathing strategies. • *Yoga:* Have students stop and do a yoga pose. Suggested program: Yoga4classrooms Card Deck and training programs (www.yoga4classrooms.org)	Roeser, R.W., Greenberg, M. T., Frazier, T., Galla, B. M., Semenov, A. D., & Warren, M. T. (2023). Beyond all splits: Envisioning the next generation of science on mindfulness and compassion in schools for students. *Mindfulness, 14,* 239–254. https://doi.org/10.1007/s12671-022-02017-z Weare, K. (2023). Where have we been and where are we going with mindfulness in schools? *Mindfulness, 14,* 293–299. https://doi.org/10.1007/s12671-023-02086-8
Positive Behavioral Interventions and Supports (PBIS) Website: www.pbis.org	PBIS is a framework for promoting positive behavior by creating school environments that proactively encourage appropriate behavior and prevent problem behaviors. PBIS approaches are based on evidence-based behavioral interventions and are applied at a whole school level, providing a continuum of strategies and supports at the universal (all students), targeted (for those at-risk), and intensive (for those with identified behavioral challenges) levels. This approach recognizes that several relevant factors can influence a student's behavior, including those existing within the child and those reflected in the interaction between the child and the environment. Schoolwide PBIS systems support all students along a continuum of need based on the three-tiered prevention model.	• Determine whether your school has adopted PBIS as the behavioral framework. If so, explore opportunities to participate in and contribute to schoolwide PBIS committees. • Help create environments that focus on proactively promoting positive behavior. • Collaborate with all school personnel to foster consistency in communicating behavioral expectations and reinforcing positive behaviors in classroom and nonclassroom settings.	Bradshaw, C. P., Mitchell, M. M., & Leaf, P. J. (2010). Examining the effects of schoolwide PBIS on student outcomes: Results from a randomized controlled effectiveness trial in elementary schools. *Journal of Positive Behavioral Interventions, 12*(3), 133–148. https://doi.org/10.1177/1098300709334798 Horner, R. H., & Sugai, G. (2015). School-wide PBIS: An example of applied behavior analysis implemented at a scale of social importance. *Behavior Analysis in Practice, 8,* 80–85. https://doi.org/10.1007/s40617-015-0045-4
Cognitive Behavioral Thinking Strategies	For children and youth with mental health challenges, Cognitive Behavioral Therapy (CBT) is provided because it is one of the most extensively researched and applied forms of therapy. CBT is a relatively short-term, focused approach that teaches people how to modify thought patterns to change troublesome feelings and behavior. The emphasis is on helping the person identify cognitive distortions (i.e., inaccurate beliefs), learn effective self-help skills, and practice them in daily life. Although OTPs need additional training to be called a cognitive behavioral therapist, OTPs can provide simple cognitive behavioral strategies embedded in services. Sometimes changing how students think helps to change how they feel and behave. People who think positive tend to be happier, healthier, and cope better during challenging times, but it's important to be a "realistic optimist." It's not realistic to pretend that everything is fine during difficult times. Being a realistic optimist requires being able to put situations in perspective by using thinking skills to help develop a positive outlook.	• Help students pay attention to "self-talk" and recognize negative thinking "traps." Thinking traps represent faulty thinking that can lead to feeling sad, anxious, or angry. • Help the young person develop "realistic thinking" and "reframe the situation in a balanced way, identifying both the negative and positive aspects of the situation." • Encourage gratitude and optimism. Help the young person think about one or two good things happening at that moment, being mindful of what can be seen, heard, or felt that is positive. • Look for opportunities to learn from the situation. Help young people view difficult situations as a challenge to overcome and opportunities to learn and become more resilient.	Ginsburg, G. S., & Kingery, J. N. (2007). Evidence-based practice for childhood anxiety disorders. *Journal of Contemporary Psychotherapy, 37*(3), 123–132. https://doi.org/10.1007/s10879-007-9047-z Kuypers, L. (2011). *The Zones of Regulation.* Social Thinking Publishing. See http://www.zonesofregulation.com/the-book.html Lyubomirsky, S. (2007). *The HOW of happiness: A new approach to getting the life you want.* Penguin Books. Madrigal, S., & Winner, M. G. (2008). *Superflex: A superhero social thinking curriculum.* Social Thinking Publishing.

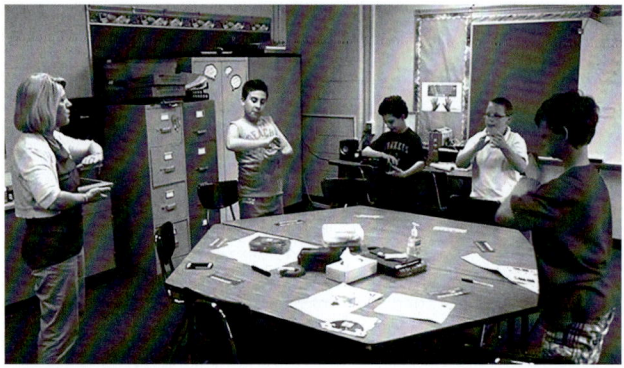

FIGURE 37-3. Embedding mental health literacy into an occupation-based self-regulation group for students with developmental disabilities.

Intervention Strategies for Mental Health Promotion, Prevention, and Intervention

Within a multitiered approach to mental health, OTPs provide a continuum of services geared toward mental health promotion, prevention, early identification, and intervention (Bazyk, 2011c). Intervention strategies are integrated into the student's classroom schedule, school routines, and curriculum. The application of the occupational therapy process within this multitiered public health framework is summarized in the following sections (Bazyk, 2011c, 2019).

Tier 1: Universal, Whole School Services for Mental Health Promotion and Prevention

Universal Tier 1 services, implemented collaboratively by interdisciplinary teams, are geared toward the entire student body, including many students who do not demonstrate mental health or behavioral challenges. Universal services reflect a dual commitment to the promotion of mental health and the prevention of mental illness (Atkins & Frazier, 2011).

OTPs have ample opportunities to promote positive mental health given that engagement in meaningful occupations fosters the development of needed and desired occupations. Overall strategies for promoting positive mental health include individual or small group and whole classroom or school interventions.

Individual or small group interventions embed strategies and activities into existing individualized or group interventions that specifically promote positive mental health, such as talking about mental health and teaching coping skills. *Whole classroom or school interventions* embed services that focus on creating social, emotional, and physical environments and activities that are enjoyable for all students and enhance mental well-being (e.g., creating sensory and emotionally friendly contexts using programs described in Table 37-1, such as Drive Thru Menus or Zones of Regulation, and implementing the Comfortable Cafeteria or Refreshing Recess programs; Bazyk, 2019).

The contexts in which students participate in activities throughout the day are evaluated: Does the social and physical context support successful participation and enjoyment? If not, what adaptations or accommodations might the OTP offer? For example, how might the cafeteria be modified to support positive social interaction and successful participation in the mealtime occupation? How is positive behavior fostered in school hallways, recess, restrooms, and on the bus?

Tier 1 interventions also emphasize obtaining information about and supporting existing whole school approaches, such as SEL, PBIS, and mental health literacy, which foster positive mental health in all students (refer to Table 37-3). It is critical for OTPs to work collaboratively with a wide variety of individuals, including administrators, teachers, health educators, school nurses, and families, to provide Tier 1 services. In addition to the schoolwide approaches described in Table 37-3, other evidence-based mental health promotion strategies that can be embedded throughout the day include:

- Foster the identification and use of character strengths such as persistence, curiosity, and creativity (Park & Peterson, 2008).
- Encourage caring connections and foster friendships throughout the day. People with strong social relationships are healthier and happier (Denworth, 2020).
- Promote participation in enjoyable occupations. Aim for a 3 to 1 ratio of positive to negative emotions throughout the day (Fredrickson, 2009).
- Embed enjoyable movement breaks throughout the day. Foster active play during recess. Even short doses of movement help to reduce anxiety and depression, elevate mood, and improve concentration (Otto & Smits, 2011; Peluso & Andrade, 2005).
- Promote acts of kindness in big and small ways. Being kind to others increases levels of happiness in the giver and receiver. Acts of kindness build a sense of cooperation, trust, and safety (Layous et al., 2012).

Additional specific examples of Tier 1 strategies include:

- *Informally observe all students.* Make a point to observe signs of positive mental health (e.g., positive affect, successful participation throughout the day, ability to cope with challenges). Look for behaviors that might suggest mental health concerns or limitations in social or emotional development (e.g., changes in affect, academic and social functioning, behavioral changes, Fig. 37-4).
- *Promote mental health literacy.* Support and promote health education initiatives offered in the school to increase mental health literacy. Embed information and activities focusing on mental health literacy into everyday occupational therapy practice. Make mental health part of everyday conversation with students and teachers. Collaborate with health educators, school counselors, and teachers to educate children and youth about how to develop and maintain mental health and what to do if one begins to feel mentally unstable.
- *Clearly articulate the scope of occupational therapy practice to all school personnel, students, and families.* Articulate the scope of occupational therapy as including social

BOX 37-2 ■ Application in Practice: Participating in School Leadership

The American Federation of Teachers (AFT) recognized that school staff members need a voice in education policy. To empower teachers and school personnel to assume active leadership positions in schools, the AFT created a program called the Teacher Leadership Program. In this program, a group of union members dedicated one Saturday per month to discuss education policy, network and advocate with local leaders and stakeholders, and develop strategic action plans that address school needs and build community support.

Lauren Thomas, an occupational therapist in Boston, dedicated the year to informing various stakeholders about OTPs' role in mental health and inclusive practices, specifically citing the ESSA as a key policy. By participating in the program, Lauren developed the skills to connect policy with practice and advocate for OTPs in public schools. Therefore, school leaders, faculty, and community members gained awareness and knowledge about occupational therapy's role under ESSA. Additionally, this program provided a platform for Lauren to highlight OTPs' role in district initiatives, such as inclusion and MTTS, to better serve students of diverse backgrounds.

OTPs can have a role in advocacy at the district level to educate stakeholders and promote mental health initiatives.

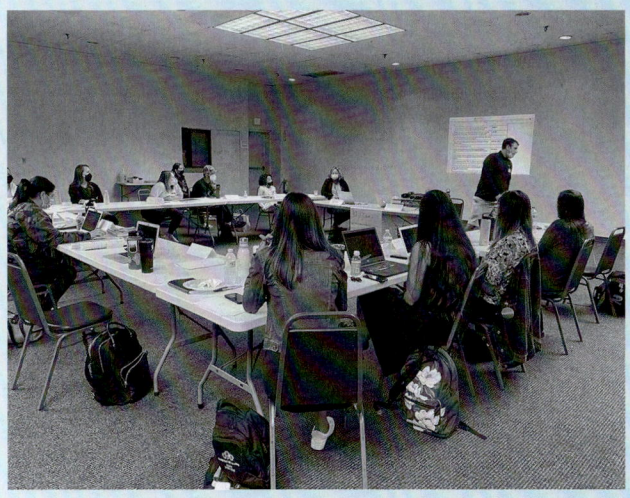

For more information, visit https://www.aft.org/position/teacher-leadership.

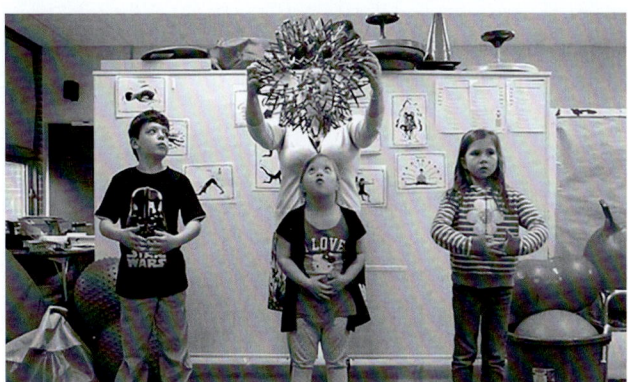

FIGURE 37-4. Tier 1: Embedding mental health promotion strategies in the classroom.

participation, social-emotional function, and mental health. Discuss the OTP's role in promoting participation in a range of occupations and interactions to promote health (e.g., play, leisure, sleep/rest; refer to Fig. 37-2)

- *Collaborate with teachers, administrators, and other school personnel.* Talk with teachers and other school personnel about mental health promotion and how to embed simple strategies into the classroom (e.g., calming and focusing activities). Ask them if they have concerns about the mental health and social participation of any students and offer suggestions and supports.
- *Evaluate lunch and recess.* Identify factors that may support or impede social participation or promote dysfunction for a student. Implement universal programs such as Every Moment Counts, Comfortable Cafeteria, and Refreshing Recess (see this chapter's Evidence-Based Practice feature).
- *Provide in-service education.* Educate teachers, staff, administrators, parent councils, or community partners on topics such as positive mental health, mental health promotion, sensory processing, and self-regulation, including strategies to help reduce stress and cope with sensory challenges and emotional regulation.
- *Participate on school, district, or statewide educational teams.* OTPs can partner with school teams to support student well-being at a systems level. By participating on school teams, OTPs can contribute to school policies, procedures, and initiatives that support health promotion. Work at this level may include developing partnerships with community organizations or universities to develop and implement mental health promotion or prevention programming. Practitioners may also participate on school teams, such as MTSS or student support teams (SST), to review school data and become involved in interdisciplinary tiered intervention planning. At the systems level, OTPs contribute to mental health advocacy for the well-being of all students (Box 37-2).

Tier 2: Targeted Prevention Services for At-Risk Students

Targeted services (Tier 2) are designed to support students who are at risk for developing mental health challenges or who are showing early signs of not doing well emotionally. Early identification and intervention are critical at this point to prevent emotional challenges from becoming more severe. Intervention at this level focuses on modifying the environment to foster success, employing embedded strategies to reduce symptoms and promote feelings of emotional well-being, and developing small activity groups to promote participation. Practitioners may collaborate with teachers, school counselors, and other mental health providers to develop and cofacilitate targeted interventions (Bazyk, 2011b).

Evidence-Based Practice

Tier 1: The Comfortable Cafeteria

The program significantly improved participation in and enjoyment for students, and cafeteria supervisors expressed feeling able to promote social participation and healthy eating.

RESEARCH FINDINGS

The Comfortable Cafeteria program is a universal, schoolwide program developed by OTPs to build the capacity of cafeteria supervisors in developing the knowledge and skills needed to create positive lunch experiences, help all students participate successfully in and enjoy lunch, and foster inclusion of students with disabilities or mental health challenges (Bazyk et al., 2018).

Results of a mixed methods design exploring the outcomes of this 6-week, occupational therapy–led program found statistically significant improvements in pretest–posttest ratings of participation in and enjoyment for students with low and mid-range scores at the outset. Cafeteria supervisor pretest–posttest ratings demonstrated statistically significant improvements in perceptions of having the knowledge and skills to supervise and to encourage healthy eating (Fig. 37-5).

Qualitative findings suggest that students learned prosocial values (e.g., being kind, helping others), supervisors actively encouraged positive social interaction, and OTPs enjoyed implementing the Comfortable Cafeteria program and recognized positive supervisor and student changes because of integrating services in the cafeteria.

APPLICATIONS

➡ OTPs can enhance students' social participation, enjoyment, and emotional well-being by integrating services in the cafeteria.

➡ OTPs should work collaboratively with cafeteria supervisors to build their capacity to be effective supervisors and actively create positive environments for participation and enjoyment.

REFERENCES

Bazyk, S., Demirjian, L., Horvath, F., & Doxsey, L. (2018). The Comfortable Cafeteria program for promoting student participation and enjoyment: An outcome study. *American Journal of Occupational Therapy, 72*(3), 7203205050p1–7203205050p9. https://doi.org/10.5014/ajot.2018.025379

It is important for OTPs to be aware of the variety of conditions and situational stressors that increase a student's risk of struggling emotionally or developing a mental health disorder. Some of these include:

- Situational stressors (friendship challenges, taking a test, academic struggles, natural disasters)
- Physical and/or developmental disabilities, such as ADHD, autism, or cerebral palsy (Children with disabilities may struggle because of chronic stress or low self-esteem. They are at higher risk of being bullied than nondisabled peers. Some have a higher incidence of mental health challenges associated with the diagnosis [e.g., higher incidence of anxiety in those with ADHD and autism].)

- Living in poverty (because of chronic stress)
- Trauma (violence in the home, parent with a mental illness or substance use disorder)
- Experiencing loss and grieving (e.g., loss of a family member, friend, or pet; parental divorce)
- Bullying (e.g., physical or verbal aggression)
- Overweight or obese (higher incidence of self-esteem issues and depression; Bazyk & Winne, 2013)
- Genetic predisposition to mental illness (e.g., family history of depression or anxiety)

Students at the Tier 2 level may show beginning signs of not doing well emotionally but are generally not identified as needing mental health services. For this reason, it is critical for all school personnel, including OTPs, to be able to identify

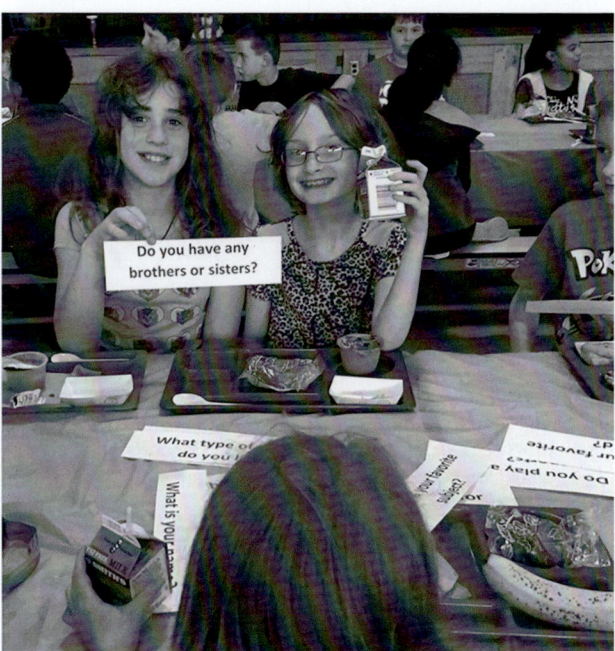

FIGURE 37-5. Comfortable Cafeteria program: Promoting participation and health during lunch.

and know how to respond to a young person's early signs and symptoms of mental health challenges, such as changes in:

- *Affect or mood* (e.g., from generally happy to looking sullen or sad, feeling lethargic, moody, anxious)
- *Thinking* (e.g., difficulty concentrating, inability to complete work, drop in grades)
- *ADLs* (e.g., difficulty sleeping or sleeping too much, loss of appetite, changes in grooming)
- *Social and leisure participation* (e.g., withdrawn from friends, limited engagement in occupations that are typically enjoyed)

Tier 2 Intervention and Supports

Students at risk of or demonstrating early signs of mental health challenges are generally not eligible for special education under IDEA (2004) unless the student has a comorbid disability that qualifies them for services. However, general education students at risk of or demonstrating behavioral or learning difficulties because of mental health challenges may be provided *coordinated early intervening services,* according to IDEA (2004). Another way to offer services is through Section 504 of the Rehabilitation Act of 1973. For many students with mild mental disorders, 504 accommodations are sufficient for enhancing school functioning. At this level, close collaboration among all school personnel and mental health providers to develop and cofacilitate targeted interventions is essential. When integrating services in natural school contexts, related service providers (OTPs, speech-language pathologists [SLPs], physical therapists, and school counselors) can embed strategies to promote mental health within a whole class or in small groups to benefit students at risk for mental health challenges.

Educating school and community providers on how to recognize and respond to early signs of mental health challenges

is an important Tier 2 strategy. Youth Mental Health First Aid (YMHFA) is a manualized 8-hour training course designed to educate the public about mental health disorders among youth and provide tools to help a young person in emotional distress. The five strategies, referred to by the acronym ALGEE, are (A) assess risk of suicide or self-harm, (L) listen nonjudgmentally, (G) give reassurance and support, (E) encourage appropriate professional help, and (E) encourage self-help or other support strategies.

In a pretest–posttest study of 384 social service employees who completed the YMHFA training, results indicated significant improvements in the application of four out of five of the ALGEE strategies and increased confidence in, likelihood of, and comfort with helping a young person in emotional distress or crisis (Aakre et al., 2016). A controlled trial of 149 parents and 118 adolescents 3 years after the training indicated significant improvements in parental knowledge of youth mental health problems and adolescent perceptions of parental support (Morgan et al., 2020). Embedding mental health promotion and prevention strategies at Tier 2 may also involve the provision of the following:

- **Accommodations** can reduce or simplify academic routines to foster successful participation and promote positive psychological functioning. Two examples of accommodations for a student with ADHD are providing color-coded notebooks and encouraging movement breaks throughout the day. For students with anxiety, reasonable accommodations may include breaking down school assignments and giving one part at a time, teaching relaxation strategies, and giving extra time to complete tests and assignments (Moran, 2016).
- **Small group interventions** during lunch, recess, or after school can be used to promote social skills, friendships, hobbies and interests, and mental health promotion. Related service providers (e.g., occupational therapist, physical therapist, SLP, school counselors) may colead small integrated groups, including special education students and those who are at risk for developing mental health challenges. Lunch bunch groups might focus on social interaction, respecting differences, and inclusion. For low-income urban youth, small activity-based groups focusing on SEL and mental health promotion have been shown to enhance positive emotions, group cohesion, and healthy leisure (Bazyk & Bazyk, 2009). Embedded in the activity is the OTP's facilitation of group process, targeting psychosocial abilities such as the development of social skills, identification and expression of feelings, and development of a positive group identity (Box 37-3). Research suggests that children who demonstrate personal or social difficulties benefit more from small groups that provide a supportive environment and an opportunity to develop positive relationships with caring adults than those who receive individual interventions (Bazyk & Arbesman, 2013; Shechtman, 2001).
- **Co-teaching** involves two or more school professionals providing instruction. OTPs, for example, might co-teach the Zones of Regulation with the school counselor or the special education teacher. In this way, all students in the classroom learn self-regulation strategies, not just those who may be struggling emotionally (Fig. 37-6). A recess group focusing on yoga and mindfulness might be cotaught by occupational and physical therapists.

BOX 37-3 ■ Tier 2 Application in Practice: Occupational Therapy Friendship and Leisure Promotion Group During Recess

OTPs need to be vigilant in identifying the need for occupation-based services to address the mental health needs of students in schools and offer services to meet those needs. Teri LaGuardia, MOT, OTR/L, did just that in the Westlake City Schools. Teri states, "OTs need to look for the open doors." While participating in an IEP meeting for a second-grade girl on her caseload (Heather), the mother shared concern regarding her daughter's experience of being bullied by a peer, resulting in anxiety about attending school. The mother also indicated that her daughter struggled with making friends and felt alone during recess. The IEP team explored possible options to help her daughter. Although the school counselor offers small group interventions to address social and emotional challenges, she indicated that her schedule was full.

Teri saw this as an opportunity to expand her services in mental health promotion and prevention. She offered to develop and facilitate a small recess group focusing on friendship promotion, SEL, and healthy hobbies. The team agreed and the principal gave permission. Teri developed the 8-week "Friendship Ambassadors" group including Heather and eight other students at risk of social and emotional challenges (e.g., students identified as "bullies," those who struggle with social interaction, and those with identified anxiety). The occupation-based groups focused on playing table-top and outdoor games and embedding child-friendly information on how to be a good friend, healthy hobbies and interests, and SEL.

Students enjoyed the groups and Heather became more confident in socializing with peers. Her mother noticed a positive change in Heather, stating "She's happier overall and wants to go to school." The principal was so pleased with the outcome that he asked Teri to expand to other grades and continue implementation throughout the school year.

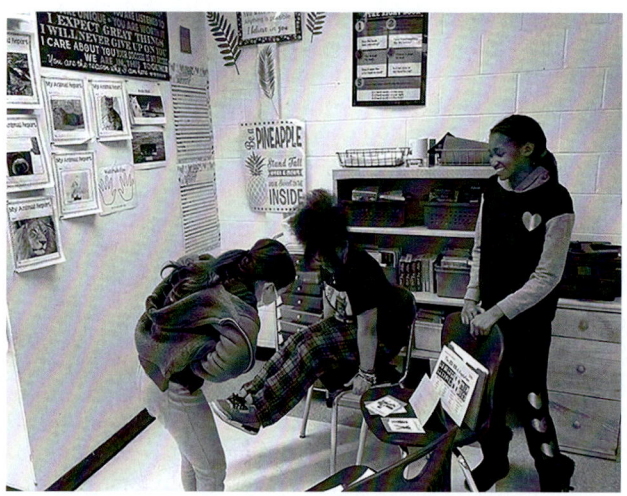

FIGURE 37-6. Zones of Regulation station in the classroom: Student practicing movement tools including chair push-ups, wall push-ups, and jumping jacks.

Additional specific targeted strategies appropriate for Tier 2 include (Table 37-4):

- *Learn about the early signs of common mental illnesses and mental health problems* (e.g., depression, anxiety, obsessive compulsive disorder, schizophrenia) and how such symptoms might influence occupational performance in school and home settings. Refer to the Minnesota Children's Mental Health Fact Sheets and other reliable resources listed in the Resources section.
- *Use both informal and formal evaluation strategies* to identify risk, changes in behavior or functional skills, or the early presence of mental health problems.
- *Provide Early Intervention Services* for students who demonstrate behavioral or learning difficulties because of mild mental health disorders or psychosocial issues.
- *Consult with teachers* to modify learning demands and academic routines to foster successful participation and promote positive psychological functioning

(e.g., breaking down school assignments and giving one part at a time to minimize anxiety; teaching relaxation strategies; Downing, 2011).
- *Provide parent education* on how to adapt family routines or activities to support students' mental health, especially with high-risk children and youth, including their use of gaming and social media.

Tier 3: Individualized Intensive Mental Health Interventions

When targeted interventions do not meet the needs of students, *individualized intensive interventions* are provided for students with identified mental, emotional, or behavioral disorders that limit their participation in needed and desired areas of occupational performance throughout the school day. At this level, in addition to diminishing symptoms, it is critical to also focus on promoting positive mental health. All school personnel under the leadership of professionals with a background in mental health intervention (e.g., OTPs, school psychologists, school nurses, and guidance counselors) can embed Tier 3 interventions into everyday school experiences (Atkins et al., 2010; Bazyk, 2011d). It is critical that a collaborative perspective be adopted because children and youth with mental disorders often receive services from both school and community providers.

OTPs need to maintain an in-depth knowledge of a range of mental health and behavioral disorders, how the disorders influence a young person's functioning in a variety of occupational areas, current medical and psychosocial interventions, and school and community services. Moreover, it is also important to become aware of the mental health disorders commonly present in children and youth with various developmental disorders. For example, as noted earlier, many autistic children have one or more comorbid psychiatric disorders (Lai et al., 2019; Salazar et al., 2015).

A variety of evaluation strategies, such as observation, interviews, and formal assessment, can be used to analyze the factors that limit occupational performance (see Table 37-2).

TABLE 37-4 | Tier 2: Targeted Prevention Efforts for Students At Risk for Mental Health Challenges

At-Risk Condition	Associated Mental Health Risks	Occupational Performance Risks	Suggested Occupational Therapy Intervention Strategies and Supports
Physical disabilities (Anaby et al., 2016; Adair et al., 2015; Imms et al., 2017; Petrenchik et al., 2011)	• Overemphasis on rehabilitation of physical impairments overshadows attention to social and emotional needs. • More likely than typical peers to encounter negative social environments (stigmatized, marginalized, socially excluded, and bullied). • Approximately one in three children with developmental disabilities are identified as having a co-occurring mental health condition such as anxiety and depression.	• May have fewer opportunities to participate in extracurricular activities, resulting in boredom and delayed skill development. • Social isolation may result in delayed social skills, lack of friends, and limited opportunities to develop extracurricular interests. • Poor self-confidence, depression, or anxiety may contribute further to social isolation.	• Promote a balanced view of health including attention to both physical and emotional needs of the child. • Foster sustained participation in enjoyable neighborhood- and community-based out-of-school activities to promote the development of interests, friends, and to build on strengths and talents. Encourage the child to express and process feelings related to reduced physical functioning. Focus on consistent attendance and engagement with an emphasis on social participation rather than physical capacity building to increase feelings of success and belonging. • Help create school and community environments that are inclusive, stimulating, satisfying, and enjoyable. Work with the student, family, and school teams to increase inclusion opportunities by reducing environmental barriers or activity demands. • Contribute to whole school approaches emphasizing disability awareness and acceptance of differences. • Facilitate occupation-based small groups using coaching and mentoring to foster self-determination, inclusive friendships, and engagement in school or community activities (e.g., meaningful leisure and work).
Autism Spectrum Disorders (Bernier et al., 2022; Crabtree & DeLany, 2011; Dean, & Chang, 2021; Tanner et al., 2015; Vermeulen, 2014)	• Social-cognitive challenges may lead to difficulties in making and keeping friends. • Higher rates of anxiety, depression, obsessive-compulsive, and ADHD disorder than the typical population. • Over 90% experience sensory processing challenges, which are associated with increased stress and social and communication challenges.	• Challenges occur with social participation, making and keeping friends, and social isolation because of sensory modulation and communication difficulties. • *ADL:* People may see restricted diets and clothing choices because of sensory modulation issues. • Delays may develop in academic, independent living, and work skills because of social, cognitive, and sensory challenges.	• Promote social and leisure participation in natural contexts with peers to foster generalization of skills. • Foster participation in extracurricular activities to promote the development of interests and meaningful friendships. • Create sensory-friendly environments to reduce stress and enhance emotional well-being. • Apply cognitive behavioral strategies to foster social awareness and manage emotions. Use Social Stories to teach the child how to respond in a specific situation. • Develop peer support programs such as Circle of Friends (https://www.circleofriends.org), lunchtime clubs, and Best Buddies (Best Buddies International, https://www.bestbuddies.org) to prevent isolation and bullying while fostering friendships. Provide group-based social-emotional learning in natural school contexts (e.g., recess, lunch) including peer-mediated participation. Offer staff coaching and consultation to enhance their ability to implement groups focusing on social skills and inclusion. • Promote participation in creative leisure activities (e.g., drawing, painting, music, and theater) and meaningful work in inclusive community settings to foster skill development and strengths.
Attention Deficit-Hyperactivity Disorder, Learning Disorders, and Developmental Coordination Disorder (Fox et al., 2020; Kim et al., 2020; Levanon-Erez et al., 2019; Poulsen, 2011)	• Low self-esteem because of difficulties in school and home performance • Social exclusion • Anxiety • Depression	• *School:* Failure to attend to details, careless errors, avoids challenging academic tasks that require sustained mental effort, frequent shifts in attention, difficulty organizing school materials in locker or desk, forgets homework • *ADLs:* Messy eating or drinking; irregular sleeping	• Encourage the identification and expression of feelings by applying SEL strategies. • Help children explore and successfully participate in extracurricular leisure interests based on areas of strength to enhance feelings of competence and autonomy. Provide leisure coaching if necessary. • Analyze the student's sensory needs and develop a sensory diet to successfully function in home, community, and school context. • Consult with teachers to modify classroom expectations and assignments based on the specific sensory and behavioral needs of the child (breaking down assignments into manageable pieces, taking tests in a distraction-free area, etc.). These accommodations may take the form of a 504 Plan.

Continued

TABLE 37-4 | Tier 2: Targeted Prevention Efforts for Students At Risk for Mental Health Challenges—cont'd

At-Risk Condition	Associated Mental Health Risks	Occupational Performance Risks	Suggested Occupational Therapy Intervention Strategies and Supports
		• *IADLs:* Disorganized bedroom and study space, homework incomplete, poor follow through with chores • *Leisure:* Inattention to instructions, performance erratic, difficulty waiting turn, may have coordination problems (DCD) • *Social participation:* May be teased or bullied for poor performance	• Help parents and teachers understand the reasons for the child's behaviors and offer support and solutions for changing and adapting the unwanted behaviors. • Promote social-emotional learning using peer intervention groups to improve play, communication, and prosocial behaviors for social participation. • For ADHD, support positive behaviors through small group coaching that includes executive functioning (organization), self-awareness, and prosocial behaviors. Examples include the CLAS program (culturally and linguistically appropriate services) or Cog-Fun (cognitive functional intervention).
Obesity (~19.7% of children ages 2–19 in the United States; CDC, 2024b) Overweight (~25%) Children at greatest risk of obesity are those living in poverty or who have a disability (Bazyk, 2011d; Bazyk & Winne, 2013; Pizzi et al., 2014)	• Poor self-esteem and body image • Anxiety • Depression • May experience the negative effects associated with weight bias • Eating disorders (binge dieting and eating)	• Social participation challenges; difficulty making and keeping friends because of weight bias • Higher risk of being bullied • Sleep or rest challenges because of risk of sleep apnea • Limited play and leisure; may find physical activities too challenging	• Emphasize "health at any size" versus weight loss, and support a school climate that accepts diverse abilities and encourages positive body image. • Teach children about healthy food choices. • Work with school officials to decrease the availability of foods high in fat and sugar in the cafeteria and in vending machines. Community partnerships for fruit and vegetable programs can support availability of healthy food options. • Develop after-school programs that foster participation in enjoyable physical activities, healthy cooking, or gardening. • Consult with school personnel to develop enjoyable physical activities during recess. • Work with school officials to prevent weight-biased bullying. • Embed SEL strategies to help children identify feelings and develop positive coping strategies. • Analyze the school environment to ensure access to safe spaces and equipment for physical activity and availability of nonfood rewards (e.g., extra recess time or class game time).
Grieving loss The conflicted feelings caused by change because of loss. Examples: death of parent, friend, or pet; parental divorce; moving to a new home; and so on (Bazyk, 2011d; Eftoda, 2021; Fluegeman et al., 2013; Scaletti & Hocking, 2010)	• Stress associated with loss may result in a range of behavioral changes (emotional withdrawal, regressive behaviors) • Anxiety • Depression • Difficulty concentrating at school • Psychosomatic complaints (headaches, stomachaches)	• ADL changes (altered eating patterns, bedwetting) • Altered sleep and rest including excessive or limited sleep • Difficulty concentrating in school; drop in grades • Social withdrawal and friendship issues • Loss of interest in play and leisure activities	• Teach children how to provide support to friends who are grieving. • Help teachers recognize emotional and behavioral changes associated with grieving and suggest strategies for modifying expectations and providing support. • Work with teams to create a transition plan that helps to ease student's return to school • Encourage participation in enjoyable but low-stress activities with close friends to minimize feelings of isolation. • Use creative arts occupations to help children express feelings of loss either in small group or individual sessions (e.g., journaling, memory boards, storytelling, sand trays, music). Therapeutic listening programs can also promote self-regulation after loss. • Mention the person who died in everyday conversation to encourage the student to talk about what they valued in the relationship. • Be aware of "grief triggers" such as birthdays and holidays. Reassure children that heightened emotions during these times are a natural part of grieving. • Connect students and families with community programs, such as Camp Erin, that focus on fostering relationships and healthy occupations. • Work with school teams to provide grief and bereavement training that includes education about how different age groups respond to death and misconceptions about death. A proactive approach can help normalize conversations about death.

TABLE 37-4 | Tier 2: Targeted Prevention Efforts for Students At Risk for Mental Health Challenges—cont'd

At-Risk Condition	Associated Mental Health Risks	Occupational Performance Risks	Suggested Occupational Therapy Intervention Strategies and Supports
Poverty: ~16.9% of families with children under 18 (Benson, 2022) Low income: ~37% of U.S. population (Bazyk, 2011d; Ma et al., 2023)	• Depression • Anxiety • Substance abuse • Aggressive behavior	• Sleep problems caused by stressful environment • Obesity caused by limited access to fresh fruits, vegetables, and safe playgrounds • Limited opportunities to engage in extracurricular leisure activities, resulting in boredom and participation in risky behavior	• Help parents consciously steer children away from street influences by monitoring free time and friendships. • Promote engagement in structured leisure activities outside of school such as sports, church groups, and creative arts in positive environments. • Foster SEL-identifying feelings and reflect on how feelings influence behavior. • Incorporate mental health literacy interventions into practice, including knowledge and availability of mental health resources.
Children who have experienced trauma or adverse childhood experiences (ACEs) Domestic violence; homelessness; physical abuse, sexual abuse; neglect; natural disasters; medical trauma; parental instability (Bloom, 1995; CDC, 2024a; Lynch et al., 2020; Whiting, 2018)	• Posttraumatic stress disorder (PTSD) • ADHD • Anxiety • Depression • Communication disorder • Conduct disorder • Eating disorders • Oppositional defiant disorder • May engage in self-destructive and risky behaviors	• Sleep disorders • *ADL:* may demonstrate poor hygiene and self-care • Social participation, social withdrawal, and isolation; may have difficulty trusting people • *School:* poor attendance, low grades, difficulty concentrating, and behavioral challenges • *Play or leisure:* loss of interest in leisure activities and play • Increased high-risk behaviors as coping mechanism (e.g., substance or alcohol abuse)	• Modify home and school environments to create trauma-sensitive spaces that are safe, secure, predictable, and sensory friendly (e.g., weighted lap pads, fidget toys, rocking chairs, bean bag chairs, calming music or noise reduction tools, and soothing lights). • Apply the Sanctuary Model to help create collaborative and healing environments that promote recovery from trauma (www.sanctuaryweb.com). • Structure predictable routines in home and school. • Tune into the child's affect and emotional responses, triggers to problem behaviors, sensory regulation, interoceptive skills, signs of dysregulation, and strengths. Lead or colead small groups to build their awareness and develop strategies to modify them. • Offer small occupation-based groups to provide opportunities to share feelings, learn new coping strategies, and engage in enjoyable creative occupations. • Provide leisure coaching to help children identify and participate in enjoyable extracurricular activities. • Teach relaxation skills including yoga, deep breathing, and progressive relaxation. • Foster opportunities for connection through after-school or mentoring programs

The goal is not to diagnose, but to be aware of the symptoms and their impact on participation. An important part of the evaluation includes observations in natural contexts. All school personnel need to tune into signs and symptoms that may be present in students who are experiencing mental health challenges. Significant and sudden changes need to be noted. A "sign" is something observable (e.g., crying, withdrawal), and a "symptom" is something that is felt that may not be observable (e.g., anxiety, sadness, delusions, hallucinations; Kutcher & Wei, 2017). Signs and symptoms may include:

- *Emotions:* depressed mood, excessive irritability, anxiety, feeling hopeless
- *Thinking:* pessimism, difficulty making decisions, rigid thinking, poor concentration
- *Functional behavior:* social withdrawal, appetite changes, sleep changes, academic difficulties
- *Physical:* headaches, nausea, excessive movement

General education students demonstrating diagnosed mental health challenges may be provided with accommodations under Section 504 to enhance school functioning (Bazyk, 2019).

Students with disabilities who have comorbid mental health disorders will receive services to address their mental health and behavioral needs as determined by the IEP (Cahill & Bazyk, 2019).

Although services at Tier 3 are individualized to meet the specific needs of children and youth based on their mental health conditions and symptoms, a systems perspective is critical because children and youth often benefit from supports and services provided by multiple systems within the school and community. *Systems of care* approaches provide a framework for youth, families, schools, and community partners to provide individualized services and supports that help children and youth with serious emotional disturbances and their families achieve their desired goals (Stroul et al., 2021). Such approaches are necessary because children and youth with serious mental health disorders typically receive services from two or more public agencies, such as juvenile justice, child welfare, special education, and state and local mental health departments.

The overall focus of occupational therapy services, as compared with counseling, is to provide services that help students with mental disorders participate successfully in academic and nonacademic aspects of the school day

BOX 37-4 ■ Tier 3 Application in Practice: Occupational Therapy Leisure Coaching

Kelson is a 14-year-old boy who lives with multiple diagnoses including anxiety, ASD, optic nerve hypoplasia, and a rare chromosomal disorder. He lives with his mother, Sonia, on the second floor of a two-family home. Although he is close to his biological father, he has inconsistent contact with him, which causes anxiety. Kelson attends a special school, the Positive Education Program's (PEP) Prentiss Autism Center, for children and youth who demonstrate severe and challenging behaviors and have other complex developmental disabilities and significant communication impairments. The school provides integrated special education and mental health services that emphasize strengths and the generalization of socially appropriate self-management skills in community-based settings.

Kelson is a very social person who enjoys being helpful, playing, and being praised by his mother and teachers. He loves art and sports—especially watching football and basketball. Despite these strengths, he has had a history of aggressive and violent behavior at home, resulting in frequent 911 calls to the police and hospitalizations because of the violent outbursts.

David Weiss, OTR/L, is Kelson's occupational therapist at PEP. He also provides occupational therapy leisure coaching as a part of the Every Moment Counts: Promoting Mental Health Throughout the Day initiative. David identified Kelson as a candidate for leisure coaching because Kelson has significantly limited access to extracurricular community-based leisure. Although he has a variety of toys and art supplies at home, Kelson has limited opportunities to play outside because his family lives on a busy urban street. When discussing Kelson's leisure needs with David, Sonia expressed a concern about his social isolation and her desire for him to have positive adult male role models and to be on a sports team.

To begin the leisure coaching process, David shared information with Sonia and Kelson about the mental and physical health benefits of participation in structured extracurricular activities outside of school to develop and engage in healthy hobbies and interests. Using an informal leisure interest inventory, David talked with Kelson about potential extracurricular activities. Kelson indicated a desire to play football. The next step of the process involved David and Sonia exploring community-based options based on Kelson's abilities and needs. They agreed that an adaptive football league would be a good match. David helped Sonia access and complete the necessary registration materials and then attended the first few sessions to share strategies with the coach for helping Kelson regulate behavior and participate successfully. Kelson participated in the entire 3-month weekly adaptive football sessions.

Sonia has been happy to see Kelson's successful participation and enjoyment in being a part of a football team. In a short, videotaped interview, she stated that playing football "has made a tremendous difference in my son." Participation has helped him be more focused and patient in working toward a goal and learning that "if he can control himself, he is able to participate. . . . That he looks forward to football and that it makes him happy." David adds that Kelson's participation in adaptive football gives him an opportunity to practice the skills learned in school (e.g., self-regulation and calming strategies, motor skills). He adds that when Kelson participates in football, he's joyful, laughing, and smiling, which contributes to his positive mental health. Because Kelson's experience with adapted football was so successful, Sonia enrolled him in an adapted soccer program in the Spring. To view a video of Kelson playing soccer, go to https://youtu.be/zzJwNEc6ryQ.

(Box 37-4). Occupational therapy suggestions for modifying activities and the environment to reduce stress and foster successful participation provide distinct contributions to services at Tier 3 (Mental Health America, 2017). Additional specific Tier 3 services for students with identified mental health challenges include:

■ *Evaluate school function* (e.g., classroom participation, ADLs, play and leisure, social participation, beginning work skills) in a variety of natural contexts (e.g., classroom, lunchroom, recess).
■ *Promote the development of individual interests* by exploring extracurricular activities and providing the necessary supports to enhance successful participation.
■ *Assist in the functional behavior assessment* process and contribute to developing and implementing the behavioral intervention plan.
■ *Collaborate with the other SMH providers, teachers, and administrators* to ensure a coordinated *system of care* for children needing intensive interventions.
■ *Provide tips to promote successful functioning throughout the school day,* including transitioning to classes, organizing workspaces such as a desk or locker, handling stress, and developing strategies for time management.
■ *Collaborate with teachers* in modifying classroom expectations based on the student's specific mental health needs.
■ *Offer individual or group interventions* for students with serious emotional disturbance through special education

or Section 504 to enhance participation in education, social participation, play and leisure, and ADLs.
■ *Analyze the student's unique sensory needs* and develop intervention strategies to promote sensory processing and successful function in multiple school contexts (e.g., classroom, cafeteria).

Services should focus on helping students engage in activities that promote feelings of emotional well-being and modifying environments to reduce stress. It is also important to help students develop reasonable goals for maintaining participation and daily routines that include good nutrition and some physical exercise (Downing, 2011). Table 37-5 outlines mental health diagnoses, associated symptoms, occupational performance risks, and intervention strategies that focus on minimizing the symptoms of the disorders and promoting mental health and well-being.

Building Capacity of Occupational Therapy Practitioners and Students to Address Mental Health in Schools

"The interplay between knowledge and its implementation is complex." (Cramm et al., 2013, p. 119)

TABLE 37-5 | Tier 3: Intensive, Individualized Interventions for Students With Identified Mental Health Challenges

Mental Health Diagnosis	Associated Symptoms	Occupational Performance Risks	Suggested Occupational Therapy Interventions
Generalized Anxiety Disorder (Chan et al., 2017; Enns et al., 2016; Kugel et al., 2016; Moran, 2016; Vassilopoulos et al., 2013)	• Excessive anxiety and worry that is difficult to control, causing disability in social, work, school, or other important areas of functioning • Feeling "keyed up" or "on edge" • Difficulty concentrating, or mind "going blank" • Irritability • Muscle tension • Easily fatigued • Difficulty falling or staying asleep, or restless unsatisfying sleep	• Tendency to isolate from others and withdraw from activities to reduce anxiety—may refuse school or work or drop out of extracurricular activities • Difficulty completing tasks because of fatigue, distractibility, poor concentration, low frustration tolerance • May forget thoughts when talking • May appear restless or have difficulty engaging in tasks • Peers may avoid because of irritability • May complain of soreness in different body areas, or may appear stiff during physical activities (even when walking or sitting)	• Practice Mindfulness. Explore enjoyable, calming activities, especially deep breathing, meditation, and physical exercise. • Identify tasks the person needs to complete, then break them into easy, manageable steps with a realistic time frame (i.e., extra time allowed, but within a finite period). Posting a daily schedule can help reduce anxiety because expectations and tasks are clear. • Discuss ways to decrease muscle tension (e.g., warm baths, yoga, stretching, heating pads on muscles). • Encourage writing thoughts on paper before speaking so there is a "reference" and to increase confidence. • Help establish a bedtime routine that prepares for restful sleep (e.g., no caffeine 5–6 hours before sleep—includes soda and chocolate), no TV 1 hour before bed, consistent bedtime, and so on. • Interventions that include creativity, play, or physical activity can reduce anxiety and promote self-esteem. • School-based psychoeducational and CBT small groups can reduce social anxiety.
Depression (Chan et al., 2017; Sung-Min & Byoung-Jin, 2022)	• Sadness that lingers • Irritability • Low energy • Loss of interest in activities • Difficulty initiating tasks • Withdrawal from friends and social activities • Sleep and appetite disturbances • Children and adolescents may refuse school attendance • Decreased mental functioning • Thoughts of death and suicide	• Affect appears sad • Can appear argumentative or short-tempered, which impacts social relationships • Falls asleep easily, in class, at work, in social situations • May not be able to get out of bed all day • Overeats or refuses to eat • Difficulty initiating and sustaining attention to tasks or processing information; may fall behind at school or work • Difficulty making decisions • Decrease in quality of friendships, limiting social interactions • May experience overdependence on smartphone	• Eliminate decision-making to increase activity-engagement and reduce stress. • Offer simple, structured, familiar tasks to promote self-efficacy and productivity—one at a time. • Encourage the development of daily routines that include good nutrition and some physical activity. • Advocate for shorter school and work days, with reduced tasks and expectations, even if only temporarily. • Offer to consult with employers, school personnel, and service providers to help with accommodations. • Keep conversations short and simple. • Set reasonable goals within the person's reach (e.g., "try doing this in the next 10 minutes"). • Be alert to signs and talk of suicide. Get help quickly. • School-based psychoeducational and CBT small groups that focus on thoughts, feelings, and beliefs can reduce depression symptoms
Children at-risk of psychosis and demonstrating signs of prodromal phase Subtle, experiential symptoms may ebb and flow in frequency and intensity up to 4 years before the onset of an illness (Cendrero-Luengo et al., 2021; Read et al., 2018)	• Cognitive changes in functioning such as difficulty concentrating or remembering information; may experience jumbled thoughts or confusion • May experience perceptual distortions such as hearing one's name called or increased sensitivity to sounds	• *Social participation:* deteriorating social function altering relationships with family and friends; may become socially isolated • *School:* problems staying focused in class or during studies; may demonstrate a drop in grades	• Offer in-services to school personnel and families about sensory preferences and how to modify the environment to decrease stress and promote positive functioning. Research supports leading or coleading family psychoeducational groups to enhance participation in meaningful occupations.

Continued

TABLE 37-5 | **Tier 3: Intensive, Individualized Interventions for Students With Identified Mental Health Challenges—cont'd**

Mental Health Diagnosis	Associated Symptoms	Occupational Performance Risks	Suggested Occupational Therapy Interventions
	• May demonstrate behavioral changes such as withdrawal or increased irritability • May become suspicious of others or fearful for no good reason • May demonstrate jumbled speech or writing	• *Work:* may demonstrate declining performance such as tardiness and a failure to complete work assignments • *Leisure:* may drop out of extracurricular activities • *ADLs:* may demonstrate dramatic changes in appetite and difficulty in dressing or hygiene • *Sleep or rest:* may demonstrate dramatic changes in sleep—either difficulty sleeping or excessive sleep	• Offer small group sessions to foster participation in enjoyable activities to reduce stress and promote socialization. • Consult with teachers and parents to make accommodations to reduce stress and enhance participation such as decreasing activity demands, assisting with organization of a task, and reducing environmental stimulation. • Assist school personnel and families in developing routines that include exercise, healthy nutrition, and good sleep hygiene. Consult with outside stakeholders if necessary. • Adolescents benefit from vocational education and training to promote prosocial skills. • Cognitive remediation for early psychosis improves cognition, self-esteem, and social and occupational functioning at school. • Promote occupational balance and foster good habits by helping adolescents establish habits, routines, and roles that are driven by their own volition.
Thought Disorders (Peak age of onset is between 16 and 25 years) • Schizophrenia • Schizoaffective Disorder *Note:* Medication and other therapies may be prescribed to treat these disorders—suggestions made here are to help guide occupational therapy interventions (Downing, 2011; Kirby et al., 2020; Read et al., 2018)	• *Hallucinations:* visual, auditory, olfactory, or tactile sensory distortions • *Delusions:* beliefs that are fixed and false • Paranoia or suspiciousness • Low registration • Reduced sense of smell • Poor insight about symptoms • Reduced ability to process information • Slowed visual scanning abilities • Mood fluctuations • Reduced facial expressions ("blunting")	• Distracted by internal stimulation, making it difficult to orient to tasks and stay focused, and adding to the appearance of being "odd" • Difficulty organizing thoughts and articulating well, which affects school and work performance and social relationships • Isolation and difficulties making and keeping friends because of moodiness, sensory sensitivities, suspiciousness, delayed responses, and odd behaviors • Tendency to miss key information because of poor awareness of visual cues and surroundings, as well as slowed information processing • Difficulty reading facial expressions, which can lead to inappropriate emotional responses and poor understanding of social situations • Difficulty multitasking and understanding complex directions	• Use activities to help organize thoughts and behaviors, such as deep proprioceptive tasks (calisthenics, yoga, physical work, weightlifting; kneading dough; etc.). • Use environments with few distractions in which to perform school or work tasks (e.g., quiet spaces, few interruptions, predictable changes, and not crowded). • Use simple and clear instructions that are repeated or written down to ensure success—use a calm tone, but not patronizing. • Demonstrate new tasks and allow the individual to practice several times, offering extra demonstrations and practice sessions as needed. • Create and support opportunities for socialization with peers and coworkers, especially when social situations are not overwhelming (e.g., small gatherings). Introduce student to one person who shares a common interest and assist with "small talk." • Respond to signs of depression and talk of suicide. Help the person seek professional assistance when necessary. • Adolescents benefit from vocational education and training to promote prosocial skills.

Focus is on minimizing symptoms associated with the mental health disorder and promoting mental health and well-being.

Despite the availability of evidence-based publications devoted to learning about and applying a multitiered approach to mental health in occupational therapy with children and youth, there is a concern about the efficient transfer of this knowledge to practice (Cramm et al., 2013). It is estimated that it takes an average of 17 years for only about 14% of new evidence to be applied to clinical practice (Westfall et al., 2007). Because the value of new knowledge is only attained when it is applied in practice and leads to change, it is important to consider how to best bring about knowledge translation (KT; Lencucha et al., 2007).

The need for OTPs to have a framework and language for describing the profession's role related to mental health is essential for ensuring that such efforts are recognized (Nielsen & Hektner, 2014). Practitioners are encouraged to strategically engage in activities designed to build their capacity to address the mental health needs of children and youth (Jané-Llopis & Mittlemark, 2005).

In order to reduce the gap between new knowledge and action, a 6-month *building capacity process* was developed and implemented throughout Ohio to foster KT and implementation of a public health approach to mental health among OTPs participating in a Community of Practice (CoP). A one-group ($n = 117$) mixed methods design using quantitative (pretest–posttest survey) and qualitative methods (phenomenological analysis of written reflections) was used to explore the meaning and outcomes of participation in the *building capacity process* involving reading, discussion (in-person and online), practice reflection, and community building. Statistically significant improvements ($p <0.02$) in pretest–posttest scores of knowledge, beliefs, and actions related to a public health approach to mental health were found.

Four major themes reflecting the meaning and impact of the *building capacity process* emerged from the qualitative data: (1) The *building capacity process* was both meaningful and enjoyable. (2) New knowledge regarding mental health resulted in a change in thinking about the term "mental health" to include promotion and prevention. (3) The experience evoked strong emotions regarding participants' occupational therapy identity, reconnecting them to the "OT roots." (4) Changes in practice occurred: Greater confidence empowered practitioners to actively advocate for and address mental health in big and small ways (Bazyk et al., 2015).

In a similar study of 19 occupational therapy Level II fieldwork students, a virtual building capacity process aimed at promoting KT of a tiered approach to mental health in schools was found to be effective. Statistically significant improvements in knowledge, beliefs, and actions were found. The building capacity process expanded student knowledge of a public health approach to mental health, resulting in increased awareness and application of embedded strategies to address the emotional needs of students during a Level II fieldwork experience in school settings (Bazyk et al., 2020).

Here's the Point

- Children and youth who experience positive mental health and well-being function better during academic and non-academic times of the school day.
- Approximately one in five children (22%) between the ages of 9 and 17 have a diagnosable behavioral or emotional disorder. A higher prevalence (33%) of mental health conditions occurs in children and youth with developmental disabilities.
- SMH services have grown during the past two decades with approximately three-fourths of youth who receive mental health services obtaining this care in schools.
- Addressing the mental health needs of all students can be envisioned within a multitiered public health framework of mental health promotion, prevention, and intensive individualized interventions.
- OTPs are among the few team members in schools who have specialized knowledge and skills in addressing mental health and serve as indigenous resources for integrating mental health strategies in schools.
- Best practice in schools emphasizes the integration of occupational therapy services in the general education classroom and nonacademic settings (e.g., lunch and recess) when possible, as well as offering opportunities to contribute to mental health promotion and prevention efforts in addition to addressing the needs of students with identified disabilities or mental health challenges.
- Although the focus of occupational therapy services varies based on the tier, all efforts share a common belief in the positive relationship between participation in a balance of meaningful and enjoyable occupations and positive mental health.
- OTPs need to create opportunities for expanding new knowledge and strategically reflect on and apply new knowledge to practice to articulate, advocate for, and implement practice changes reflecting occupational therapy's role in addressing the student's mental health in everyday practice.

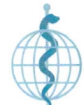

Visit the online resource center at **FADavis.com** to access the videos.

Apply It Now

1. Mental Health Promotion and Literacy

Refer to the Embedded Strategies section of the Every Moment Counts website (https://everymomentcounts.org /embedded-strategies). Read through the 10 Moments for Mental Health, refer to the downloadable materials (books, coloring sheets, information sheets), and watch the short video vignettes. Write down and plan to implement five strategies that you will embed in your everyday practice with children and youth. Identify ways that you can use these in your school setting to help students learn about positive mental health and coping strategies.

2. Helping At-Risk Students

This activity involves recognizing students at risk for mental health challenges and situational stressors and planning how to embed strategies to reduce stress and enhance feelings of emotional well-being. Refer to Table 37-4 on targeted prevention efforts for students at risk for mental health challenges. Select two student groups who are at risk and plan to embed appropriate intervention strategies as described in the table. Go to the Calm Moments Cards program on the Every Moment Counts website (https://everymomentcounts.org/calm-moments-cards). Read about the program and 17 cards based on situational stressors. Select three or four of the listed cards and identify the thinking, focusing and calming, and sensory strategies that you can embed in practice to reduce stress and enhance feelings of well-being in the students you serve.

3. Comfortable Cafeteria

Read through the program information, 10 Steps to Success, and the six weekly lesson plans for the Comfortable Cafeteria program (https://everymomentcounts.org/comfortable-cafeteria). Think about the need for and feasibility of implementing this program with one grade level of students and complete the Comfortable Cafeteria Environmental Analysis (http://s3.us-east-2.amazonaws.com/s3.everymomentcounts.com/wp-content/uploads/2021/03/01192619/CC_Environment_FINAL_fillable_3-1-21.pdf).

4. Refreshing Recess

Read through the program information, 10 Steps to Success, and the six weekly lesson plans for the Refreshing Recess program (https://everymomentcounts.org/refreshing-recess). Think about the need for and feasibility of implementing this program with one grade level of students. Complete the Refreshing Recess Environmental Analysis (https://everymomentcounts.org/refreshing-recess).

5. Building Capacity of Occupational Therapists and School Personnel to Address the Mental Health Needs of Students

Consider how you might build capacity of OTPs and school personnel to learn about and apply a public health approach to mental health using this chapter's content and the Creating Change Leaders section of the Every Moment Counts website (https://everymomentcounts.org/creating-change-leaders). Refer to the *Building Capacity of School Personnel to Promote Positive Mental Health in Children and Youth* online course developed by Sarah Nielsen, PhD, OTR/L, and Susan Bazyk, PhD, OTR/L, FAOTA. Developed for the Mountain Plains Mental Health Technology Transfer Center (MHTTC) and funded by the Substance Abuse and Mental Health Services Administration (SAMHSA) in 2019, this five-part webinar series is free (https://mhttcnetwork.org/centers/mountain-plains-mhttc/product/building-capacity-school-personnel-promote-positive-mental). Identify four or five colleagues that you know have a vested interest in student mental health to complete the building capacity course together.

Resources

Online Resources

- Every Moment Counts: Promoting Mental Health Throughout the Day: http://www.everymomentcounts.org. Free, downloadable information and material on how to apply a public health approach to mental health and implement occupation-based embedded strategies and model programs.
- Building Capacity of School Personnel to Promote Positive Mental Health in Children and Youth: https://mhttcnetwork.org/centers/mountain-plains-mhttc/product/building-capacity-school-personnel-promote-positive-mental. This online course was developed by Sarah Nielsen, PhD, OTR/L, and Susan Bazyk, PhD, OTR/L, FAOTA. Developed for the Mountain Plains Mental Health Technology Transfer Center (MHTTC) and funded by the Substance Abuse and Mental Health Services Administration (SAMHSA) in 2019, this five-part webinar series is free.
- AOTA's School Mental Health Toolkit: https://www.aota.org/practice/clinical-topics/school-mental-health-toolkit. This toolkit is a resource for OTPs working with children and youth in school and community settings to obtain specific knowledge about mental health promotion, prevention, and intervention and to guide service provision. Each topic in the toolkit provides an overview of the topic, implications for occupational therapy, and strategies for mental health promotion, prevention, and intervention in a variety of settings.
- Action for Happiness: http://www.actionforhappiness.org. This site provides practical strategies, research, and resources committed to helping people build a happier and more caring society in their homes and communities. Ten keys for happier living backed by research are provided.
- Bully Prevention: http://www.pbis.org. The OSEP Technical Assistance Center on PBIS offers free downloadable manuals: *Bully Prevention Manual: Elementary School Level; Bully Prevention Manual: Middle School Level*—Authors: B. Stiller, S. Ross, and R. Horner.
- Children's Mental Health Fact Sheets (Minnesota Children's Mental Health Association): https://macmh.org/publications/mental-health-fact-sheets. This site offers free, downloadable fact sheets on mental health conditions, the impact on function, and strategies to foster successful participation in schools.
- Mental Health Literacy: http://www.mentalhealthliteracy.org. This Canadian resource provides high-quality mental health literacy information, research, education, and resources. Materials are provided in a variety of mediums that include videos, animations, brochures, e-books, face-to-face training programs, and online training programs. Resources are specifically designed to meet the needs of children, youth, young adults, families, educators, community agencies, and health-care providers. Refer to the *Mental Health and High School Curriculum Guide* (Version 3); a free download is available at https://mentalhealthliteracy.org/product/mental-health-high-school-curriculum.
- Mindful Schools: www.mindfulschool.org. This site provides education and resources for schools to cultivate mindful and heart-centered learning communities so that all members are supported and thrive.
- Random Acts of Kindness: https://www.randomactsofkindness.org. This nonprofit provides free resources to foster kindness in schools, at home, and at work. An evidence-based Kindness in the Classroom® curriculum gives students the social and emotional skills needed to live more successful lives. Kindness lesson plans, posters, and projects are provided to foster kindness throughout the school.

National Organizations and Technical Assistance Centers

- Centers for School Mental Health—Technical Assistance Centers: www.smhp.psych.ucla.edu (UCLA) and www.csmh.umaryland.edu (University of Maryland at Baltimore). In 1995, two national training and technical assistance centers focused on mental health in schools were established with partial support from the U.S. Department of Health and Human Services and the Center for Mental Health Services. One center is at UCLA and the other is at the University of Maryland at Baltimore. The websites for each of these centers include information and resources on school-based mental health programs.

- Collaborative for Academic, Social, and Emotional Learning (CASEL): http://www.casel.org. CASEL is the nation's leading organization devoted to expanding the development and implementation of evidence-based SEL as an integral part of education from preschool through high school. Readers can use this site to learn about and access research and resources on SEL.
- The Center for Health and Health Care in Schools (CHHCS): https://healthinschools.org. This nonpartisan policy, resource, and technical assistance center is housed within the Milken Institute School of Public Health at The George Washington University. The purpose is to advance policies, systems, and environments to build and sustain strategies that bridge health and learning for all students.
- National Council for Mental Wellbeing: https://www.thenationalcouncil.org. This association advocates for policy and social change on behalf of mental health and substance use treatment organizations in the United States. This organization oversees Mental Health First Aid (MHFA) programs that help people in the United States to identify, understand, and respond to signs and symptoms of mental health and substance use challenges in youth and adults.
- Caring for Every Child's Mental Health Substance Abuse and Mental Health Services Agency (SAMHSA): http://www.samhsa.gov/children. This organization supports a comprehensive system of care approach to children's mental health. It sponsors an annual Children's Mental Health Awareness Day every May.
- Positive Behavioral Interventions and Supports (PBIS): https://www.pbis.org. The technical assistance center on PBIS is established by the U.S. Department of Education's Office of Special Education (OSEP) to develop, implement, and evaluate a multitiered approach to promoting positive behavior and academic outcomes for all students.

Videos

- Every Moment Counts (EMC) video vignettes: https://www.youtube.com/channel/UCYfut1MBrm47DHjOADkOCPQ. These 2- to 5-minute videos depict OTPs working in collaboration with school personnel to implement occupation-based mental health promotion strategies and programs throughout the school day—classroom, lunch, recess, and extracurricular leisure.
- "Child in Crisis" video. In this video, occupational therapist Brittany shares her experience working in a psychiatric rehab hospital's adolescent unit with Mikey, an 8-year-old boy presenting with a complex set of challenges. Diagnosed at birth with fetal alcohol syndrome, Mikey has a history of multiple ACEs. On admission, he presented with suicidal and homicidal ideation and symptoms consistent with PTSD. Brittany describes how she did her own research, learned more about Mikey, and developed an intervention that worked well for him and the other children in the group. Access the video at the online resource center at FADavis.com.
- "Occupational Therapy Collaboration in Early Head Start" video. In this video, an occupational therapist and occupational therapy assistant (OTA) describe their partnership while working collaboratively at an Early Head Start program. They explain the importance of a team approach to tiered intervention services and how they work together to support children, parents, and staff. This includes strategizing on how to implement creative intervention ideas and address challenges with individual children, some of whom have experienced

trauma. Access the video at the online resource center at FADavis.com.
- "Managing Challenging Behaviors in Young Children" video. In this video, an occupational therapist and OTA discuss the OTA's work in an Operation Breakthrough program within Head Start. The OTA works with young children from at-risk families; together with teachers and other therapists, she helps to catch any developmental delays and intervene as necessary. She describes a particularly challenging behavior in one child and the strategies she uses to help him feel comfortable, safe, and loved, allowing him to better participate in the classroom and individual sessions. Access the video at the online resource center at FADavis.com.
- "Jenny's Lived Experience of Sensory Processing Differences" video. Jenny is an occupational therapy degree (OTD) student with the lived experience of sensory differences, anxiety, and depression. In this video, she describes how she discovered her diagnosis, how it affects her in the classroom, and what interventions she uses to manage her reactions to stimuli. Importantly, she discusses the need to advocate for herself and for practitioners to help people across the life span to understand their sensory processing needs in order to improve their mental health and overall quality of life. Access the video at the online resource center at FADavis.com.
- "Laura's Experience as a Mother of an Autistic Son" video. Laura is the mother of an adult son, Will, who was diagnosed with autism at age 3. In this video, she describes what Will was like as a baby and what signs she and day-care teachers first noticed. She explains what the evaluation process was like and how it felt when she learned that her loving, talkative, playful child had autism. Occupational therapy, social skills therapy, speech therapy, and other services—as well as intensely involved parents—laid the groundwork for Will to succeed in school and go on to fulfill his occupational dream as a young adult. Access the video at the online resource center at FADavis.com.

References

Aakre, J. M., Lucksted, A., & Browning-McNee, L. (2016). Evaluation of Youth Mental Health First Aid USA: A program to assist young people in psychological distress. *Psychological Services, 13*(2), 121–126. https://doi.org/10.1037/ser0000063

Adair, B., Ullenhag, A., Keen, D., Granlund, M., & Imms, C. (2015). The effect of interventions aimed at improving participation outcomes for children with disabilities: A systematic review. *Developmental Medicine and Child Neurology, 57*(12), 1093–1104. https://doi.org/10.1111/dmcn.12809

Adelman, H., & Taylor, L. (2021). *Embedding mental health as schools change.* University of California at Los Angeles: The Center for Mental Health in Schools & Student/Learning Supports. http://smhp.psych.ucla.edu/pdfdocs/mh20a.pdf

Agner, J. (2020). The issue is—Moving from cultural competence to cultural humility in occupational therapy: A paradigm shift. *American Journal of Occupational Therapy, 74*(4), 1–7. https://doi.org/10.5014/ajot.2020.038067

American Academy of Pediatrics. (2021). *AAP, AACAP, CHA declare national emergency in children's mental health.* AAP News. https://publications.aap.org/aapnews/news/17718?autologincheck=redirected

American Occupational Therapy Association. (2020). Occupational therapy practice framework: Domain and process—Fourth edition. *American Journal of Occupational Therapy, 74*(Suppl. 2), 7412410010p1–7412410010p87. https://doi.org/10.5014/ajot.2020.74S2001

Amudhan, S., Jangam, K., Mani, K., Murugappan, N. P., Sharma, E., Mahapatra, P., Burma, A. D., Tiwari, H. K., Ashok, A., Vaggar, S., & Rao, G. N. (2021). Project SUM (scaling up of mental health in schools): Design and methods for a pragmatic, cluster randomized waitlist-controlled trial on integrated school mental health intervention for adolescents. *BMC Public Health, 21*(2034), 1–11. https://doi.org/10.1186/s12889-021-12086-9

Anaby, D. R., Law, M. C., Majnemer, A., & Feldman, D. (2016). Opening doors to participation of youth with physical disabilities: An intervention study. *Canadian Journal of Occupational Therapy, 83*(2), 83–90. https://doi.org/10.1177/0008417415608653

Arbesman, M., Bazyk, S., & Nochajski, S. (2013). Systematic reviews of occupational therapy and mental health promotion, prevention, and intervention for children and youth. *American Journal of Occupational Therapy, 67*(6), e120–e130. https://doi.org/10.5014/ajot.2013.008359

Atkins, M. S., & Frazier, S. L. (2011). Expanding the toolkit or changing the paradigm: Are we ready for a public health approach to mental health? *Perspectives on Psychological Science, 6*(5), 483–487. https://doi.org/10.1177/1745691611416996

Atkins, M. S., Hoagwood, K. E., Kutach, K., & Seidman, E. (2010). Toward the integration of education and mental health in schools. *Administration and Policy in Mental Health, 37*, 40–47. https://doi.org/10.1007/s10488-010-0299-7

Ayres, A. J. (1998). The art of therapy. *Sensory Integration Special Interest Section Quarterly, 21*(4), 1–6. https://sensoryproject.org/wp-content/uploads/2021/06/SISIS1298.pdf

Barnes, K. J., Vogel, K. A., Beck, A. J., Schoenfeld, H. B., & Owen, S. V. (2008). Self-regulation strategies of children with emotional disturbance. *Physical & Occupational Therapy in Pediatrics, 28*(4), 369–387. https://doi.org/10.1080/01942630802307127

Barry, M. M., Clarke, A. M., Petersen, I., & Jenkins, R. (2019). *Implementing mental health promotion* (2nd ed.). Springer International Publishing. https://doi.org/10.1007/978-3-030-23455-3

Barry, M. M., & Jenkins, R. (2007). *Implementing mental health promotion*. Elsevier.

Bazyk, S. (2010, September). Promotion of positive mental health in children and youth with developmental disabilities. *OT Practice, 15*(7), CE-1–CE-8.

Bazyk, S. (2011a). Enduring challenges and situational stressors during the school years: Risk reduction and competence enhancement. In S. Bazyk (Ed.), *Mental health promotion, prevention, and intervention with children and youth: A guiding framework for occupational therapy* (pp. 119–139). AOTA Press.

Bazyk, S. (2011b). *Mental health promotion, prevention, and intervention with children and youth: A guiding framework for occupational therapy*. AOTA Press.

Bazyk, S. (2011c). The occupational therapy process: A public health approach to promoting mental health in children and youth. In S. Bazyk (Ed.), *Mental health promotion, prevention, and intervention with children and youth: A guiding framework for occupational therapy* (pp. 21–44). AOTA Press.

Bazyk, S. (2011d). The promotion of positive mental health in children and youth: A guiding framework for occupational therapy. In S. Bazyk (Ed.), *Mental health promotion, prevention, and intervention with children and youth: A guiding framework for occupational therapy* (pp. 3–20). AOTA Press.

Bazyk, S. (2019). Best practices in school mental health. In G. F. Clark, J. E. Rioux, & B. Chandler (Eds.), *Best practices for occupational therapy in schools* (2nd ed., pp. 153–160). AOTA Press.

Bazyk, S. (2022a). Leisure and play in adolescence. In H. Kuhaneck & S. Spitzer (Eds.), *Making play just right: Activity analysis, creativity, and playfulness in pediatric occupational therapy* (pp. 347–373). Jones & Bartlett Publishers.

Bazyk, S. (2022b). *Occupational therapy: Promoting participation in occupation*. Every Moment Counts. https://everymomentcounts.org/about/about-occupational-therapy

Bazyk, S. (2023, March 29). *About occupational therapy*. Every Moment Counts. https://everymomentcounts.org/about/about-occupational-therapy

Bazyk, S., & Arbesman, M. (2013). *Occupational therapy practice guidelines for mental health promotion, prevention, and intervention for children and youth*. AOTA Press. https://doi.org/10.7139/2017.978-1-56900-446-3

Bazyk, S., & Bazyk, J. (2009). The meaning of occupational therapy groups for low-income youth: A phenomenological study. *American Journal of Occupational Therapy, 6*(1), 69–80. https://doi.org/10.5014/ajot.63.1.69

Bazyk, S., Demirjian, L., Horvath, F., & Doxsey, L. (2018). The Comfortable Cafeteria program for promoting student participation and enjoyment: An outcome study. *American Journal of Occupational Therapy, 72*(3), 7203205050p1–7203205050p9. https://doi.org/10.5014/ajot.2018.025379

Bazyk, S., Demirjian, L., LaGuardia, T., Thompson-Repas, K., Conway, C., & Michaud, P. (2015). Building capacity of occupational therapy practitioners to address the mental health needs of children and youth: Mixed methods study of knowledge translation. *American Journal of Occupational Therapy, 69*(6), 6906180060p1–6906180060p10. https://doi.org/10.5014/ajot.2015.019182

Bazyk, S., Kerns, S., & Mohler, R. (2021). *Refreshing Recess environmental analysis*. Every Moment Counts. http://s3.us-east-2.amazonaws.com/s3.everymomentcounts.com/wp-content/uploads/2021/03/01192600/RR_EnvironmentalAnalysis_FINAL_fillable_3-1-21.pdf

Bazyk, S., Pataki, K., & DeBoth, K. (2020). Building capacity of occupational therapy students to address the mental health needs of children and youth during a level II fieldwork in a school setting. *Journal of Occupational Therapy, Schools, & Early Intervention, 13*(4), 443–461. https://doi.org/10.1080/19411243.2020.1776186

Bazyk, S., & Winne, R. (2013). A multi-tiered approach to addressing the mental health issues surrounding obesity in children and youth. *Occupational Therapy in Health Care, 27*(2), 84–98. https://doi.org/10.3109/07380577.2013.785643

Benson, C. (2022, October 4). *Poverty rate of children higher than national rate, lower for older populations*. Census.gov. https://www.census.gov/library/stories/2022/10/poverty-rate-varies-by-age-groups.html

Bernier, A., Ratcliff, K., Hilton, C., Fingerhut, P., & Li, C.-Y. (2022). Art interventions for children with autism spectrum disorder: A scoping review. *American Journal of Occupational Therapy, 76*, 1–9. https://doi.org/10.5014/ajot.2022.049320

Bertrand, J. (2009). Interventions for children with fetal alcohol spectrum disorders (FASDs): Overview of findings for five innovative research projects. *Research in Developmental Disabilities, 30*(5), 986–1006. https://doi.org/10.1016/j.ridd.2009.02.003

Bing, R. (1981). 1981 Eleanor Clarke Slagle lecture: Occupational therapy revisited: A paraphrastic journey. *American Journal of Occupational Therapy, 35*(8), 499–518. https://doi.org/10.5014/ajot.35.8.499

Bitsko, R. H., Claussen, A. H., Lichstein, J., Black, L. I., Jones, S. E., Danielson, M. L., Hoenig, J. M., Davis Jack, S. P., Brody, D. J., Gyawali, S., Maenner, M. J., Warner, M., Holland, K. M., Perou, R., Crosby, A. E., Blumberg, S. J., Avenevoli, S., Kaminski, J. W., & Ghandour, R. M. (2022). Mental health surveillance among children—United States, 2013–2019. *MMWR Morbidity and Mortality Weekly Report, 71*(Suppl. 2), 1–42. https://doi.org/10.15585/mmwr.su7102a1

Bloom, S. L. (1995, October). Creating sanctuary in the school. *Journal for a Just and Caring Education, 1*(4), 403–433. https://sandrabloom.com/wp-content/uploads/1995-Bloom-Creating-Sanctuary-in-the-School.pdf

Bowen-Irish, T. (n.d.-a). *Drive thru menus: Exercises for attention and strength*. Therapro.

Bowen-Irish, T. (n.d.-b). *Drive thru menus: Relaxation and stress busters*. Therapro.

Bradshaw, C. P., Mitchell, M. M., & Leaf, P. J. (2010). Examining the effects of schoolwide PBIS on student outcomes: Results from a randomized controlled effectiveness trial in elementary schools. *Journal of Positive Behavioral Interventions, 12*(3), 133–148. https://doi.org/10.1177/1098300709334798

Braun, G., Kumm, S., Brown, C., Walte, S., Tejero Hughes, M., & Maggin, D. M. (2020). Living in Tier 2: Educators' perceptions of MTSS in urban schools. *International Journal of Inclusive Education, 24*(10), 1114–1128. https://doi.org/10.1080/13603116.2018.1511758

Buckley, N., Glasson, E. J., Chen, W., Epstein, A., Leonard, H., Skoss, R., Jacoby, P., Blackmore, A. M., Srinivasjois, R., Bourke, J., Sanders, R. J., & Downs, J. (2020). Prevalence estimates of mental health problems in children and adolescents with intellectual disability: A systematic review and meta-analysis. *Australian & New Zealand Journal of Psychiatry, 54*(10), 970–984. https://doi.org/10.1177/0004867420924101

Cahill, S., & Bazyk, S. (2019). School-based occupational therapy. In J. C. O'Brien & H. Kuhaneck (Eds.), *Case-Smith's occupational therapy for children and adolescents* (8th ed., pp. 627–658). Mosby.

Cahill, S. M., & Egan, B. E. (2017). Identifying youth with mental health conditions at school. *OT Practice, 22*(5), CE 1–7.

Carter, E. W., & Hughes, C. (2005). Increasing social interaction among adolescents with intellectual disabilities and their general education peers: Effective interventions. *Research and Practice for Persons With Severe Disabilities, 30*(4), 179–193. https://doi.org/10.2511/rpsd.30.4.179

Casseus, M., Kim, W. J., & Horton, D. B. (2023). Prevalence and treatment of mental, behavioral, and developmental disorders in children with co-occurring autism spectrum disorder and attention-deficit/hyperactivity disorder: A population-based study. *Autism Research, 16*(4), 855–867. https://doi.org/10.1002/aur.2894

Cendrero-Luengo, C., Jiménez-Palomares, M., Rodríguez-Mansilla, J., & Garrido-Ardila, E. M. (2021). Cross-sectional descriptive pilot study on the risk of psychotic disorders among adolescents. *Children, 8*(10), 1–13. https://doi.org/10.3390/children8100916

Centers for Disease Control and Prevention. (2021a, June 28). *About mental health.* https://www.cdc.gov/mentalhealth/learn/index.htm

Centers for Disease Control and Prevention. (2021b, February 15). *School health guidelines.* https://www.cdc.gov/healthyschools/npao/strategies.htm

Centers for Disease Control and Prevention. (2023a, March 8). *Data and statistics on children's mental health.* https://www.cdc.gov/childrensmentalhealth/data.html

Centers for Disease Control and Prevention. (2023b, February 9). *Whole School, Whole Community, Whole Child (WSCC).* https://www.cdc.gov/healthyschools/wscc/index.htm

Centers for Disease Control and Prevention. (2024a, May 16). *About adverse childhood experiences.* https://www.cdc.gov/aces/about/?CDC_AAref_Val=https://www.cdc.gov/violenceprevention/aces/fastfact.html

Centers for Disease Control and Prevention. (2024b, April 2). *Childhood obesity facts.* https://www.cdc.gov/obesity/php/data-research/childhood-obesity-facts.html?CDC_AAref_Val=https://www.cdc.gov/obesity/data/childhood.html

Chan, C., Dennis, D., Kim, S. J., & Jankowski, J. (2017). An integrative review of school-based mental health interventions for elementary students: Implications for occupational therapy. *Occupational Therapy in Mental Health, 33*(1), 81–101. https://doi.org/10.1080/0164212X.2016.1202804

Child Mind Institute. (2017). *2017 Children's mental health report.* https://childmind.org/awareness-campaigns/childrens-mental-health-report/2017-childrens-mental-health-report

Conway, C. S., Kanics, I. M., Mohler, R., Giudici, M., & Wagenfeld, A. (2015). *Inclusion of children with disabilities: Occupational therapy's role in mental health promotion, prevention, & intervention with children and youth.* American Occupational Therapy Association. https://www.aota.org/~/media/Corporate/Files/Practice/Children/Inclusion-of-Children-With-Disabilities-20150128.PDF

Coster, W., Deeney, T., Haltiwanger, J., & Haley, S. (1998). *School Function Assessment (SFA).* Psychological Corporation.

Crabtree, L., & Delany, J. (2011). Autism: Promoting social participation and mental health. In S. Bazyk (Ed.), *Mental health promotion, prevention, and intervention with children and youth: A guiding framework for occupational therapy* (pp. 163–187). AOTA Press.

Cramm, H., White, C., & Krupa, T. (2013). From periphery to player: Strategically positioning occupational therapy within the knowledge translation landscape. *American Journal of Occupational Therapy, 67*(1), 119–125. https://doi.org/10.5014/ajot.2013.005678

Csikszentmihalyi, M. (1990). *Flow: The psychology of optimal experience.* Harper & Row.

Csikszentmihalyi, M. (1993). Activity and happiness: Towards a science of occupation. *Journal of Occupational Science, 1,* 38–42. https://doi.org/10.1080/14427591.1993.9686377

Dean, M., & Chang, Y. C. (2021). A systematic review of school-based social skills interventions and observed social outcomes for students with autism spectrum disorder in inclusive settings. *Autism, 25*(7), 1828–1843. https://doi.org/10.1177/13623613211012886

Demirjian, L., Baird, L., & Bazyk, S. (2021). *Comfortable Cafeteria Environmental Analysis.* Every Moment Counts. http://s3.us-east-2.amazonaws.com/s3.everymomentcounts.com/wp-content/uploads/2021/03/01192619/CC_Environment_FINAL_fillable_3-1-21.pdf

Denworth, L. (2020). *Friendship: The evolution, biology, and extraordinary power of life's fundamental bond.* W. W. Norton & Company.

Dix, K. L., Slee, P. T., Lawson, M. J., & Keeves, J. P. (2012). Implementation quality of whole-school mental health promotion and student's academic performance. *Child and Adolescent Mental Health, 17*(1), 45–51. https://doi.org/10.1111/j.1475-3588.2011.00608.x

Donaldson, S. I., Csikszentmihalyi, M., & Nakamura, J. (2011). *Applied positive psychology: Improving everyday life, health, schools, work, and society.* Routledge Academic.

Donohue, M. V. (2013). *Social profile: Assessment of social participation in children, adolescents, and adults.* AOTA Press.

Downing, D. (2011). Occupational therapy for youth at risk of psychosis and those with identified mental illness. In S. Bazyk (Ed.), *Mental health promotion, prevention, and intervention with children and youth: A guiding framework for occupational therapy* (pp. 141–161). AOTA Press.

Dunn, W. (2007). Supporting children to participate successfully in everyday life by using sensory processing knowledge. *Infants & Young Children, 20*(2), 84–101. https://doi.org/10.1097/01.IYC.0000264477.05076.5d

Dunn, W. (2014). *School Companion Sensory Profile 2.* Psychological Corporation.

Durlak, J. A., Mahoney, J. L., & Boyle, A. E. (2022). What we know, and what we need to find out about universal, school-based social and emotional learning programs for children and adolescents: A review of meta-analyses and directions for future research. *Psychological Bulletin, 148*(11–12), 765–782. https://doi.org/10.1037/bul0000383

Eftoda, K. (2021). Addressing grief in the classroom: A complicated equalizer. *BU Journal of Graduate Studies in Education, 13*(4), 3–10. https://www.brandonu.ca/master-education/files/2021/10/BU-Journal-of-Graduate-Studies-in-Education-2021-vol-13-issue-4.pdf

Elliott, S. N., & Gresham, F. M. (2008). *Social Skills Improvement System (SSIS) performance screening guide.* Pearson.

Enns, J., Holmqvist, M., Wener, P., Halas, G., Rothney, J., Schultz, A., Goertzen, L., & Katz, A. (2016). Mapping interventions that promote mental health in the general population: A scoping review of reviews. *Preventive Medicine, 87,* 70–80. https://doi.org/10.1016/j.ypmed.2016.02.022

Epstein, M. H. (2004). *Behavioral and Emotional Rating Scale—Second Edition (BERS-2).* PRO-ED, Inc.

Every Student Succeeds Act, 20 U.S.C. § 6301 (2015). https://www.congress.gov/114/plaws/publ95/PLAW-114publ95.pdf

Fang, Z., Cerna-Turoff, I., Zhang, C., Lu, M., Lachman, J. M., & Barlow, J. (2022). Global estimates of violence against children with disabilities: An updated systematic review and meta-analysis. *The Lancet. Child & Adolescent Health, 6*(5), 313–323. https://doi .org/10.1016/S2352-4642(22)00033-5

Fluegeman, J., Schrauben, A., & Cleghorn, S. (2013). Bereavement support for children: Effectiveness of Camp Erin from an occupational therapy perspective. *Bereavement Care. 32*(2), 78–81. https://.doi.org/10.1080/02682621.2013.812820

Fox, A., Dishman, S., Valicek, M., Ratcliff, K., & Hilton, C. (2020). Effectiveness of social skills interventions incorporating peer interactions for children with attention deficit hyperactivity disorder: A systematic review. *American Journal of Occupational Therapy, 74*(2), 1–19. https://doi.org/10.5014/ajot.2020 .040212

Fredrickson, B. L. (2001). The role of positive emotions in positive psychology: The broaden-and-build theory of positive emotions. *American Psychologist, 56*(3), 218–226. https://doi .org/10.1037/0003-066X.56.3.218

Fredrickson, B. L. (2004). The broaden-and-build theory of positive emotions. *Philosophical Transactions of the Royal Society B: Biological Sciences, 359*(1449), 1367–1377. https://doi .org/10.1098/rstb.2004.1512

Fredrickson, B. L. (2009). *Positivity: Groundbreaking research reveals how to embrace the hidden strength of positive emotions, overcome negativity, and thrive.* Crown Publishing Group.

Fredrickson, B. L., & Joiner, T. (2018). Reflections on positive emotions and upward spirals. *Perspectives in Psychological Science, 13*(2), 194–199. https://doi.org/10.1177/1745691617692106

Frith, E. (2017). *Social media and children's mental health: A review of the evidence.* Education Policy Institute. https://epi.org .uk/wp-content/uploads/2018/01/Social-Media_Mental-Health_ EPI-Report.pdf

Garg, S., Buckley-Reen, A., Alexander, L., Chintakrindi, R., Ocampo Tan, L. V., & Patten Koenig, K. (2013). The effectiveness of a manualized yoga intervention on classroom behaviors in elementary school children with disabilities: A pilot study. *Journal of Occupational Therapy, Schools, & Early Intervention, 6*(2), 158–164. https://doi.org/10.1080/19411243.2013.810942

Ginsburg, G. S., & Kingery, J. N. (2007). Evidence-based practice for childhood anxiety disorders. *Journal of Contemporary Psychotherapy, 37*(3), 123–132. https://doi.org/10.1007/s10879-007-9047-z

Goodman, R. (1999). The extended version of the Strengths and Difficulties Questionnaire as a guide to child psychiatric caseness and consequent burden. *Journal of Child Psychology and Psychiatry, 40*(5), 791–801. https://doi.org/10.1111/1469-7610.00494

Goodman, R. (2005). *Strengths and Difficulties Questionnaire.* https://www.sdqinfo.org/a0.html

Gutman, S. A., O'Day, K., & Rogers, S. (2022, December 2–3). Examining and selecting assessments that are inclusive of diverse service recipients. [Conference Session]. AOTA Specialty Conference: Mental Health, Columbus, Ohio. https://www.aota.org/-/media /corporate/files/conferencedocs/2022/mental-health/2022-mental -health-specialty-conference-program-guide.pdf

Gutman, S. A., & Raphael-Greenfield, E. I. (2014). Five years of mental health research in the *American Journal of Occupational Therapy,* 2009–2013. *American Journal of Occupational Therapy, 68*(1), e21–e36. https://doi.org/10.5014/ajot.2014.010249

Hanes, J. E., Hlyva, O., Rosenbaum, P., Freeman, M., Nguyen, T., Palisano, R. J., & Gorter, J. W. (2019). Beyond stereotypes of cerebral palsy: Exploring the lived experiences of young Canadians. *Child Care Health Development, 45*(5), 613–622. https://doi .org/10.1111%2Fcch.12705

Hansen, B. H., Oerbeck, B., Skirbekk, B., Petrovski, B. E., & Kristensen, H. (2018). Neurodevelopmental disorders: Prevalence and comorbidity in children referred to mental health services. *Nordic Journal of Psychiatry, 72*(4), 285–291. https://doi.org /10.1080/08039488.2018.1444087

Helseth, S. A., & Frazier, S. L. (2018). Peer-assisted social learning for diverse and low-income youth: Infusing mental health promotion into urban after-school programs. *Administration and Policy in Mental Health, 45*(2), 286–301. https://doi.org/10.1007 /s10488-017-0823-0

Hemmingsson, H., Egilson, S., Hoffman, O., & Kielhofner, G. (2005). *School Setting Interview (SSI).* Model of Human Occupation Clearinghouse, University of Illinois at Chicago.

Henry, A. (2000). *Pediatric Interest Profiles.* Model of Human Occupation Clearinghouse, University of Illinois at Chicago. https:// moho-irm.uic.edu/productDetails.aspx?aid=43

Hong, J. S., Singh, V., & Kalb, L. (2021). Attention deficit hyperactivity disorder symptoms in young children with autism spectrum disorder. *Autism Research, 14*(1), 182–192. https://doi .org/10.1002/aur.2414

Hoover, S. H., & Bostic, J. (2021). Schools as a vital component of the child and adolescent mental health system. *Psychiatric Services, 72*(1), 37–48. https://doi.org/10.1176/appi.ps.201900575

Horner, R. H., & Sugai, G. (2015). School-wide PBIS: An example of applied behavior analysis implemented at a scale of social importance. *Behavior Analysis in Practice, 8,* 80–85. https://doi .org/10.1007/s40617-015-0045-4

HRSA Maternal & Child Health. (2020, July). *Children with special health care needs.* https://mchb.hrsa.gov/sites/default/files/mchb /programs-impact/nsch-cshcn-data-brief.pdf

HRSA Maternal & Child Health. (2021, October). *National survey of children's health.* https://mchb.hrsa.gov/sites/default/files/mchb/ data-research/national-survey-childrens-health-2021-overview -fact-sheet.pdf

Hwang, A. W., Chang, C. H., Granlund, M., Imms, C., Chen, C. L., & Kang, L. J. (2020). Longitudinal trends of participation in relation to mental health in children with and without physical difficulties. *International Journal of Environmental Research and Public Health, 17*(22), 8551. https://doi.org/10.3390/ijerph 17228551

Ikiugu, M. N., Molitor, L., & Feldhacker, D. F. (2022). The feasibility of interventions based on meaningful and psychologically rewarding occupations in improving health and well-being. *Occupational Therapy in Mental Health, 38*(3), 258–272. https://doi .org/10.1080/0164212X.2022.2042454

Imms, C., Granlund, M., Wilson, P. H., Steenbergen, B., Rosenbaum, P. L., & Gordon, A. M. (2017). Participation, both a means and an end: A conceptual analysis of processes and outcomes in childhood disability. *Developmental Medicine and Child Neurology, 59*(1), 16–25. https://doi.org/10.1111/dmcn.13237

Individuals with Disabilities Education Act, 20 U.S.C. §1400 *et seq.* (2004). https://www.govinfo.gov/content/pkg/PLAW -108publ446/pdf

Jackson, L. L., & Arbesman, M. (2005). *Occupational therapy practice guidelines for children with behavioral and psychosocial needs.* AOTA Press.

Jané-Llopis, E., & Barry, M. M. (2005). What makes mental health promotion effective? *Promotion & Education, 12*(Suppl. 2), 47–55. https://doi.org/10.1177/10253823050120020108

Jané-Llopis, E., & Mittlemark, M. B. (2005). No health without mental health. *Promotion & Education, 12*(Suppl. 2), 4–5. https://doi .org/10.1177/10253823050120020101x

Jorm, A. F. (2012). Mental health literacy: Empowering the community to take action for better mental health. *American Psychologist, 67*(3), 231–243. https://doi.org/10.1037/a0025957

Jorm, A. F. (2019). The concept of mental health literacy. In O. Okan, U. Bauer, D. Levin-Zamir, P. Pinheiro, & K. Sørensen (Eds.), *International handbook of health literacy: Research, practice and policy across the life-span* (pp. 53–66). Policy Press. https://doi .org/10.51952/9781447344520.ch004

Kabat-Zinn, J. (2003). Mindfulness-based interventions in context: Past, present, future. *Clinical Psychology: Science and Practice, 10*(2), 144–156. https://doi.org/10.1093/clipsy.bpg016

Kann, L., McManus, T., Harris, W. A., Shanklin, S. L., Flint, K. H., Hawkins, J., Queen, B., Lowry, R., Olsen, E. O., Chyen, D., Whittle, L., Thornton, J., Lim, C., Yamakawa, Y., Brener, N., & Zaza, S. (2016). Youth risk behavior surveillance—United States, 2015. *MMWR Morbidity and Mortality Weekly Report Surveillance Summary, 65*(6), 1–174. https://doi.org/10.15585/mmwr.ss6506a1

Kelly, C. M., Mithen, J. M., Fischer, J. A., Kitchener, B. A., Jorm, A. J., Lowe, A., & Scanlan, C. (2011). YMHFA: A description of the program and an initial evaluation. *International Journal of Mental Health Systems, 5*(4), 1–9. https://doi.org/10.1186/1752-4458-5-4

Keyes, C. L. (2006). Mental health in adolescence: Is America's youth flourishing? *American Journal of Orthopsychiatry, 76*(3), 395–402. https://doi.org/10.1037/0002-9432.76.3.395

Keyes, C. L. (2007). Promoting and protecting mental health as flourishing: A complementary strategy for improving national mental health. *American Psychologist, 62*(2), 95–108. https://doi.org/10.1037/0003-066X.62.2.95

Keyes, C. L., Dhingra, S. S., & Simoes, E. J. (2010). Change in level of positive mental health as a predictor of future risk of mental illness. *American Journal of Public Health, 100*(12), 2366–2371. https://doi.org/10.2105/AJPH.2010.192245

Kim, M. J., Park, H. Y., Yoo, E. Y., & Kim, J. R. (2020). Effects of a cognitive-functional intervention method on improving executive function and self-directed learning in school-aged children with attention deficit hyperactivity disorder: A single-subject design study. *Occupational Therapy International, 2020,* 1–9. https://doi.org/10.1155/2020/1250801

King, G., Law, M., King, S., Hurley, P., Rosenbaum, P., Hanna, S., Kertoy, M., & Young, N. (2004). *Children's Assessment of Participation and Enjoyment (CAPE) and Preferences for Activities of Children (PAC)*. PsychCorp.

Kirby, A. V., Henderson, J., Schwartz, A., Kramer, J., Whitaker, B. N., & Terrill, A. L. (2020). Youth suicide prevention and occupational therapy: What can we do? *SIS Quarterly Practice Connections, 5*(3), 6–8.

Koch, A., & Pollatos, O. (2014). Interoceptive sensitivity, body weight and eating behavior in children: A prospective study. *Frontiers in Psychology, 5,* 1003. https://doi.org/10.3389/fpsyg.2014.01003

Kolic, S., Deininger, A., Young, D., & Bazyk, S. (2016). *Calm Moments Cards booklet*. Every Moment Counts. http://s3.us-east-2.amazonaws.com/s3.everymomentcounts.com/wp-content/uploads/2021/01/24211256/CMC_Booklet_Final_1-24-21.pdf

Koller, J. R., & Bertel, J. M. (2006). Responding to today's mental health needs of children, families and schools: Revisiting the preservice training and preparation of school-based personnel. *Education and Treatment of Children, 29*(2), 197–217.

Koppelman, J. (2004). *Children with mental disorders: Making sense of their needs and systems that help them*. Issue Brief, No. 799. National Health Policy Forum. https://www.ncbi.nlm.nih.gov/books/NBK559784

Kramer, J., Ten Velden, M., Kafkes, A., Basu, S., Federico, J., & Kielhofner, G. (2014). *Child Occupational Self-Assessment (COSA)*. Version 2.2. Model of Human Occupation Clearinghouse, University of Illinois at Chicago.

Kugel, J., Hemberger, C., Krpalek, D., & Javaherian-Dysinger, H. (2016). Occupational therapy wellness program: Youth and parent perspectives. *The American Journal of Occupational Therapy, 70*(5), 1–8. https://doi.org/10.5014/ajot.2016.021642

Kutash, K., Duchnowski, A. J., & Lynn, N. (2006). *School-based mental health: An empirical guide for decision-makers*. University of South Florida; The Louis de la Parte Florida Mental Health Institute; Department of Child & Family Studies; Research and Training Center for Children's Mental Health. http://rtckids.fmhi.usf.edu/rtcpubs/study04/SBMHfull.pdf

Kutcher, S., & Wei, Y. (2017). *Mental Health & High School Curriculum Guide* (Version 3). https://mhlcurriculum.org/wp-content/uploads/2020/11/fixed-guide-dec-2017-online-cover-and-interior-1.pdf

Kuypers, L. (2011). *The Zones of Regulation: A curriculum designed to foster self-regulation and emotional control*. Social Thinking Publishing.

Lai, M. C., Kassee, C., Besney, R., Bonato, S., Hull, L., Mandy, W., Szatmari, P., & Ameis, S. H. (2019). Prevalence of co-occurring mental health diagnoses in the autism population: A systematic review and meta-analysis. *The Lancet. Psychiatry, 6*(10), 819–829. https://doi.org/10.1016/S2215-0366(19)30289-5

Larson, R. W. (2000). Toward a psychology of positive youth development. *American Psychologist, 55*(1), 170–183. https://doi.org/10.1037/0003-066X.55.1.170

Laverdure, P., VanCamp, A. B., & LeCompte, B. (2023, April). Empowering ESSA's value in schools: Leveraging competencies of Fieldwork and Capstone students. *OT Practice, 28*(4), 15–19.

Law, M., Baptiste, S., Carswell, A., McColl, M., Polatajko, H., & Pollock, N. (2014). *Canadian Occupational Performance Measure* (5th ed.). CAOT Publication.

Layous, K., Nelson, S. K., Oberle, E., Schonert-Reichl, K. A., & Lyubomirsky, S. (2012). Kindness counts: Prompting prosocial behavior in preadolescents boosts peer acceptance and well-being. *PLoS One, 7*(12), 1–3. https://doi.org/10.1371/journal.pone.0051380

Lebrun-Harris, L. A., Ghandour, R. M., Kogan, M. D., & Warren, M. D. (2022). Five-year trends in US children's health and well-being, 2016–2020. *JAMA Pediatrics, 176*(7), 1–11. https://doi.org/10.1001/jamapediatrics.2022.0056

LeBuffe, P. A., Shapiro, V. B., & Naglieri, J. A. (2009). *The Devereux Student Strengths Assessment (DESSA)*. Kaplan Press.

Lencucha, R., Kothari, A., & Rouse, M. (2007). The issue is– Knowledge translation: A concept for occupational therapy? *American Journal of Occupational Therapy, 61*(5), 593–596. https://doi.org/10.5014/ajot.61.5.593

Levanon-Erez, N., Kampf-Sherf, O., & Maeir, A. (2019). Occupational therapy metacognitive intervention for adolescents with ADHD: Teen Cognitive-Functional (Cog-Fun) feasibility study. *British Journal of Occupational Therapy, 82*(10), 618–629. https://doi.org/10.1177/0308022619860978

Levenson, R. W. (1994). Human emotions: A functional view. In P. Ekman & R. Davidson (Eds.), *The nature of emotion: Fundamental questions* (pp. 123–126). Oxford University Press.

Lynch, A. K., Ashcraft, R., Mahler, K., Whiting, C. C., Schroeder, K., & Weber, M. (2020). Using a public health model as a foundation for trauma-informed care for occupational therapists in school settings. *Journal of Occupational Therapy, Schools, & Early Intervention, 13*(3), 219–235. https://doi.org/10.1080/19411243.2020.1732263

Lynch, H., Moore, A., O'Connor, D., & Boyle, B. (2023). Evidence for implementing tiered approaches in school-based occupational therapy in elementary schools: A scoping review. *American Journal of Occupational Therapy, 77*(1), 1–11. https://doi.org/10.5014/ajot.2023.050027

Lyubomirsky, S. (2007). *The HOW of happiness: A new approach to getting the life you want*. Penguin Books.

Ma, K. K. Y., Burn, A.-M., & Anderson, J. K. (2023). Review: School-based mental health literacy interventions to promote help-seeking—A systematic review. *Child and Adolescent Mental Health, 28*(3), 408–424. https://doi.org/10.1111/camh.12609

Madrigal, S., & Winner, M. G. (2008). *Superflex: A superhero social thinking curriculum*. Social Thinking Publishing.

Mahler, K. (2015). *Interoception: The eighth sensory system*. AAPC Publishing.

Mahler, K. (2019). *The Interoception Curriculum: A step-by-step guide to developing mindful self-regulation*. Author.

Mahler, K. (2021). *The Comprehensive Assessment of Interoceptive Awareness* (3rd ed.). Mahler Autism Services.

Marinucci, A., Grove, C., & Allen, K. (2023). Australian school staff and allied health professional perspectives of mental health literacy in schools: Mixed methods study. *Educational Psychology Review, 35*(3), 1–30. https://doi.org/10.1007/s10648-023-09725-5

Marsh, R. J., & Mathur, S. R. (2020). Mental health in schools: An overview of multi-tiered systems of supports. *Intervention in School and Clinic, 56*(2), 67–73. https://doi.org/10.1177/1053451220914896

Masia-Warner, C., Nangle, D. W., & Hansen, D. J. (2006). Bringing evidence-based child mental health services to the schools: General issues and specific populations. *Education and Treatment of Children, 29*(2), 165–172.

McNeil, D. A., Wilson, B. N., Siever, J. E., Ronca, M., & Mah, J. K. (2009). Connecting children to recreational activities: Results of a cluster randomized trial. *American Journal of Health Promotion, 23*(6), 376–387. https://doi.org/10.4278/ajhp.071010107

Mental Health America. (2017). *Tips for teachers: Ways to help students who struggle with emotions or behavior.* http://www.mentalhealthamerica.net

Meyer, A. (1922). The philosophy of occupational therapy. *Archives of Occupational Therapy, 1*(1), 1–10.

Miles, J., Espiritu, R. C., Horen, N., Sebian, J., & Waetzig, E. (2010). *A public health approach to children's mental health: A conceptual framework.* Georgetown University Center for Child and Human Development, National Technical Assistance Center for Children's Mental Health. https://gucchd.georgetown.edu/products/PublicHealthApproach.pdf

Miller, D. N., Gilman, R., & Martens, M. P. (2008). Wellness promotion in the schools: Enhancing students' mental and physical health. *Psychology in the Schools, 45*(1), 5–15. https://doi.org/10.1002/pits.20274

Milton, L. E., Bantel, S., Calmer, K., Friedman, M., Haley, E., & Rubarts, L. (2019). Yoga and autism: Students' perspectives on the Get Ready to Learn yoga program. *The Open Journal of Occupational Therapy, 7*(4), 1–10. https://doi.org/10.15453/2168-6408.1560

Molineux, M. L., & Whiteford, G. (1999). Prisons: From occupational deprivation to occupational enrichment. *Journal of Occupational Science, 6*(3), 124–130. https://doi.org/10.1080/14427591.1999.9686457

Montañez, E., Berger-Jenkins, E., Rodriguez, J., McCord, M., & Meyer, D. (2015). Turn 2 Us: Outcomes of an urban elementary school-based mental health promotion and prevention program serving ethnic minority youths. *Children & Schools, 37*(2), 100–107. https://doi.org/10.1093/cs/cdv004

Moore, K. A. (2017). Commentary: Positive youth development goes mainstream. *Child Development, 88*(4), 1175–1177. https://doi.org/10.1111/cdev.12874

Moran, K. (2016). Anxiety in the classroom: Implications for middle school teachers. *Middle School Journal, 47*(1), 27–32. https://doi.org/10.1080/00940771.2016.1059727

Morgan, A. J., Fischer, J. A. A., Hart, L. M., Kelly, C. M., Kitchener, B. A., Reavely, N. J., Yap, M., & Jorm, A. F. (2020). Long-term effects of Youth Mental Health First Aid training: Randomized controlled trial with 3-year follow-up. *BMC Psychiatry, 20,* 487. https://doi.org/10.1186/s12888-020-02860-1

National Alliance of Specialized Instructional Support Personnel. (2019). *Home page.* http://nasisp.org

National Center for Learning Disabilities. (2020). *Significant disproportionality in special education: Current trends and actions for impact.* https://ncld.org/wp-content/uploads/2023/07/2020-NCLD-Disproportionality_Trends-and-Actions-for-Impact_FINAL-1.pdf

National Research Council & Institute of Medicine. (2009). *Preventing mental, emotional, and behavioral disorders among young people: Progress and possibilities.* National Academies Press. https://nap.nationalacademies.org/catalog/12480/preventing-mental-emotional-and-behavioral-disorders-among-young-people-progress

Nielsen, S. K., & Hektner, J. M. (2014). Understanding the psychosocial knowledge and attitudes of school-based occupational therapists. *Journal of Occupational Therapy, Schools, & Early Intervention, 7*(2), 136–150. https://doi.org/10.1080/19411243.2014.930615

Njelesani, J., Faulkner, A., Schweitzer, B., & Jeon H. (2022). A call to the front: Occupational therapy practice in addressing school bullying. *OTJR: Occupational Therapy Journal of Research, 42*(2), 99–104. https://doi.org/10.1177/15394492211058723

O'Day, K. (2020). *Visual Activity Sort (VAS).* https://www.visualactivitysort.com/product-page/visual-activity-sort

Office of the Surgeon General. (2021). *Protecting youth mental health: The U.S. surgeon general's advisory.* U.S. Department of Health and Human Services. https://www.ncbi.nlm.nih.gov/books/NBK575984

Otto, M. W., & Smits, J. A. (2011). *Exercise for mood and anxiety: Proven strategies for overcoming depression and enhancing well-being.* Oxford University Press.

Palser, E. R., Fotopoulou, A., Pellicano, E., & Kilner, J. M. (2018). The link between interoceptive processing and anxiety in children diagnosed with autism spectrum disorder: Extending adult findings into a developmental sample. *Biological Psychology, 136,* 13–21. https://doi.org/10.1016/j.biopsycho.2018.05.003

Park, N., & Peterson, C. (2008). Positive psychology and character strengths: Application to strength-based school counseling. *Professional School Counseling, 12*(2), 85–92. https://doi.org/10.5330/PSC.n.2010-12.85

Peluso, M. A., & Andrade, L. H. (2005). Physical activity and mental health: The association between exercise and mood. *Clinics, 60,* 61–70. https://doi.org/10.1590/s1807-59322005000100012

Petrenchik, T. M., King, G. A., & Batorowicz, B. (2011). Children and youth with disabilities: Enhancing mental health through positive experiences of doing and belonging. In S. Bazyk (Ed.), *Mental health promotion, prevention, and intervention with children and youth: A guiding framework for occupational therapy* (pp. 189–205). AOTA Press.

Pizzi, M., Vroman, K. G., Lau, C., Gill, S. V., Bazyk, S., Suarez-Balcazar, Y., & Orloff, S. (2014). Occupational therapy and the childhood obesity epidemic: Research, theory and practice. *Journal of Occupational Therapy, Schools, & Early Intervention, 7*(2), 87–105. https://doi.org/10.1080/19411243.2014.930605

Poulsen, A. (2011). Children with attention deficit hyperactivity disorder, developmental coordination disorder and learning disabilities. In S. Bazyk (Ed.), *Mental health promotion, prevention, and intervention with children and youth: A guiding framework for occupational therapy* (pp. 231–265). AOTA Press.

Przybylski, A. K. (2014). Electronic gaming and psychosocial adjustment. *Pediatrics, 134*(3), e716–e722. https://doi.org/10.1542/peds.2013-4021

Rasciute, S., & Downward, P. (2010). Health or happiness? What is the impact of physical activity on the individual? *Kyklos, 63*(2), 256–270. https://doi.org/10.1111/j.1467-6435.2010.00472.x

Raval, G., Montañez, E., Meyer, D., & Berger-Jenkins, E. (2019). School-based mental health promotion and prevention program "Turn 2 Us" reduces mental health risk behaviors in urban, minority youth. *The Journal of School Health, 89*(8), 662–668. https://doi.org/10.1111/josh.12805

Read, H., Roush, S., & Downing, D. (2018). Early intervention in mental health for adolescents and young adults: A systematic review. *American Journal of Occupational Therapy, 72*(5), 1–8. https://doi.org/10.5014/ajot.2018.033118

Rehabilitation Act, Pub. L. No. 93-112, 87 Stat. 355 (1973). https://www.govtrack.us/congress/bills/93/hr8070

Roeser, R. W., Greenberg, M. T., Frazier, T., Galla, B. M., Semenov, A. D., & Warren, M. T. (2023). Beyond all splits: Envisioning the next generation of science on mindfulness and compassion in schools for students. *Mindfulness, 14,* 239–254. https://doi.org/10.1007/s12671-022-02017-z

Romer, N., von der Embse, N., Eklund, K., Kilgus, S., Perales, K., Splett, J. W., Suldo, S., & Wheeler, D. (2020). *Best practices in universal social, emotional, and behavioral screening: An implementation guide*. Version 2.0. School Mental Health Collaborative. https://smhcollaborative.org/universalscreening

Sabatini, F. (2014). The relationship between happiness and health: Evidence from Italy. *Social Science & Medicine, 114,* 178–187. https://doi.org/10.1016/j.socscimed.2014.05.024

Salazar, F., Baird, G., Chandler, S., Tseng, E., O'Sullivan, T., Howlin, P., Pickles, A., & Simonoff, E. (2015). Co-occurring psychiatric disorders in preschool and elementary school-aged children with ASD. *Journal of Autism & Developmental Disorders, 45,* 2283–2294. https://doi.org/10.1007/s10803-015-2361-5

Scaletti, R., & Hocking, C. (2010). Healing through story telling: An integrated approach for children experiencing grief and loss. *New Zealand Journal of Occupational Therapy, 57*(2), 66–71.

Seligman, M. E. P. (2002). *Authentic happiness*. Free Press.

Seligman, M. E. P. (2011). *Flourish: A visionary new understanding of happiness and well-being*. Free Press.

Seligman, M. E. P., & Csikszentmihalyi, M. (2000). Positive psychology: An introduction. *American Psychologist, 55*(1), 5–14. https://doi.org/10.1037/0003-066X.55.1.5

Shechtman, Z. (2001). Prevention groups for angry and aggressive children. *Journal of Specialists in Group Work, 26,* 228–236. https://doi.org/10.1080/01933920108414214

Silverman, D. M., Rosario, R. J., Hernandez, I. A., & Destin, M. (2023). The ongoing development of strength-based approaches to people who hold systemically marginalized identities. *Personality and Social Psychology Review, 27*(3), 255–271. https://doi.org/10.1177/10888683221145243

Stroul, B. A., Blau, G. M., & Larsen, J. (2021). *The evolution of the system of care approach*. The Institute for Innovation and Implementation, School of Social Work, University of Maryland. https://nyssoc.com/wp-content/uploads/2021/10/SOC-Website-Resources-The-Evolution-of-the-SOC-Approach-.pdf

Sung-Min, S., & Byoung-Jin, J. (2022). Effects of smartphone overdependence and the quality of friendship on depression among high school students. *Occupational Therapy International, 2022,* 1–7. https://doi.org/10.1155/2022/3932326

Tanner, K., Hand, B. N., O'Toole, G., & Lane, A. E. (2015). Effectiveness of interventions to improve social participation, play, leisure, and restricted and repetitive behaviors in people with autism spectrum disorder: A systematic review. *American Journal of Occupational Therapy, 69*(5), 1–12. https://doi.org/10.5014/ajot.2015.017806

Townsend, S. (1999). *Occupational Therapy Psychosocial Assessment of Learning (OT PAL)*. Model of Human Occupation Clearinghouse, University of Illinois at Chicago.

Tucker, V. E., & Matson, L. J. (2022). Collaboration for school mental health needs: A case for high-leverage practices in a culturally responsive framework. *TEACHING Exceptional Children, 56*(3), 148–158. https://doi.org/10.1177/00400599221115623

Twenge, J. M. (2017). *iGen: Why today's super-connected kids are growing up less rebellious, more tolerant, less happy—and completely unprepared for adulthood (and what this means for the rest of us)*. Simon & Schuster, Inc.

U.S. Department of Education & Office of Special Education and Rehabilitative Services. (2021). *Supporting child and student social, emotional, behavioral, and mental health needs*. https:// www2.ed.gov/documents/students/supporting-child-student-social-emotional-behavioral-mental-health.pdf

U.S. Department of Health and Human Services. (1999). *Mental health: A report of the surgeon general*. National Institute of Mental Health. https://profiles.nlm.nih.gov/101584932X120

Vassilopoulos, S. P., Brouzosb, A., Damerc, D. E., Melloub, A., & Mitropouloub, A. (2013). A psychoeducational school-based group intervention for socially anxious children. *The Journal for Specialists in Group Work, 38*(4), 307–329. https://doi.org/10.1080/01933922.2013.819953

Vermeulen, P. (2014). The practice of promoting happiness in autism. In G. Jones & E. Hurley (Eds.), *Good autism practice: Autism, happiness and wellbeing* (pp. 7–16). BILD.

von der Embse, N. (2018). The promise of school-based mental health within multi-tiered systems of support: A response to Humphrey. *The Psychology of Education Review, 42,* 39–44.

Weare, K. (2023). Where have we been and where are we going with mindfulness in schools? *Mindfulness, 14,* 293–299. https://doi.org/10.1007/s12671-023-02086-8

Wells, J., Barlow, J., & Stewart-Brown, S. (2003). A systematic review of universal approaches to mental health in schools. *Health Education, 103*(4), 197–220. https://doi.org/10.1108/09654280310485546

Westfall, J. M., Mold, J., & Fagnan, L. (2007). "Blue Highways" on the NIH roadmap. *Journal of the American Medical Association, 297*(4), 403–406. https://doi.org/10.1001/jama.297.4.403

Whiting, C. C. (2018). Trauma and the role of the school-based occupational therapist. *Journal of Occupational Therapy, Schools, & Early Intervention, 11*(3), 291–301. https://doi.org/10.1080/19411243.2018.1438327

Whitney, D. G., Warschausky, S. A., & Peterson, M. D. (2019). Mental health disorders and physical risk factors in children with cerebral palsy: A cross-sectional study. *Developmental Medicine & Child Neurology, 61*(5), 579–585. https://doi.org/10.1111/dmcn.14083

Williams, M. S., & Shellenberger, S. (1996). *"How does your engine run?"" A leader's guide to the Alert Program*® *for self-regulation*. Therapy Works, Inc.

Wissing, M. P., Schutte, L., Liversage, C., Entwisle, B., Gericke, M., & Keyes, C. (2021). Important goals, meanings, and relationships in flourishing and languishing states: Towards patterns of well-being. *Applied Research in Quality of Life, 16,* 573–609. https://doi.org/10.1007/s11482-019-09771-8

World Health Organization. (2022, June 16). *World mental health report: Transforming mental health for all*. https://www.who.int/publications/i/item/9789240049338

World Health Organization & the United Nations Educational, Scientific and Cultural Organization. (2021, June 22). *Making every school a health-promoting school: Global standards and indicators for health-promoting schools and systems*. https://www.who.int/publications/i/item/9789240025073

Yang, Y., Zhao, S., Zhang, M., Xiang, M., Zhao, J., Chen, S., Wang, H., Han, L., & Ran, J. (2022). Prevalence of neurodevelopmental disorders among US children and adolescents in 2019 and 2020. *Frontiers in Psychology, 13,* 1–12. https://doi.org/10.3389/fpsyg.2022.997648

Early Psychosis Programs for Adolescents and Young Adults

Sean Roush and Michelle De Oliveira

Psychosis affects an estimated 1.5% to 3.5% of the population and is characterized by symptoms that cause a misunderstanding about the nature of reality (Calabrese & Al Khalili, 2022). An individual's brain may experience a change in its ability to process information, including changes in sensory perception, organizing information, and expressing information (Sage, 2019). Individuals may experience hallucinations (seeing, hearing, tasting, or feeling things that others around them don't perceive), delusions (believing in things that those around them do not believe in), disorganized behavior (including emotional responses that are incongruent with the situation), disorganized thought (observed through disorganized speech patterns), or negative symptoms (loss of energy, interest, concentration, and/or enjoyment of activities; Calabrese & Al Khalili, 2022; McClellan, 2018).

Psychosis is ubiquitous and "can affect individuals of any race, gender, sex, nationality, religion, educational background, cultural identity, age, socioeconomic status, and ability" (Sage, 2019, p. 55). Most psychotic disorders have their onset during late adolescence or early adulthood, with a profound impact on nearly all aspects of functioning (Early Psychosis Guidelines Writing Group and EPPIC National Support Program, 2016; McClellan, 2018). Young people with psychosis and their families have historically suffered in isolation and faced a poor prognosis because of the marginalization caused by the negative stigma surrounding psychosis. Current research is showing that early detection and intervention with a focus on recovery can greatly improve outcomes for individuals who experience, or are at high risk for developing, psychosis. Early psychosis programs offer a primary prevention approach, hope, and opportunities for autonomy.

This chapter introduces early psychosis. It details an overview of early psychosis, describes programs designed for this population, and highlights the role of occupational therapy. Because addressing early psychosis has been a global effort, international programs are also profiled. Lastly, the chapter notes an international focus beyond psychosis to youth mental health in general.

Overview of Early Psychosis

Although psychotic disorders were first defined approximately a century ago, until recently there was very little focus on the early stages of disorders. Examples of psychotic disorders include schizophrenia, schizophreniform disorder, schizoaffective disorder, delusional disorder, brief psychotic disorder, and mood disorders with psychotic features such as bipolar disorder and depression with psychotic features. **Early psychosis programs** focus on two consecutive periods of time, the prodrome and the first-episode psychosis (FEP), which together compose the critical period.

Research has shown that most of the functional decline occurs during the critical period, and that functional status achieved during the first 2 to 5 years after the onset of symptoms tends to persist long term and may predict life long functioning (Birchwood et al., 1998; Crumlish et al., 2009; Jackson & McGorry, 2009; Keshavan et al., 2003). However, more recent studies add to the complexity of this picture and indicate that early intervention programs that help individuals to stay engaged in education and maintain or develop strong peer relationships can improve long-term functioning (Hansen et al., 2023; Xu et al., 2020).

Prodrome Period

The **prodrome period**, in which early signs of dysfunction begin to appear but diagnostic criteria for a psychotic disorder are not yet met, has long been recognized but has not been historically well studied. This is in part because there is not yet a reliable method for determining which individuals showing potential signs of an impending psychotic episode will progress to a diagnosable condition. Because of the lack of a diagnostic tool, the prodrome can only be dependably authenticated after the individual has progressed to full-blown psychosis. This challenge is analogous to, for instance, symptoms such as widespread body pain and fatigue, which could eventually lead to a diagnosis of fibromyalgia but may also be precursors to other conditions, such as multiple sclerosis. For some, early signs of dysfunction may be time limited and resolve completely on their own. For others, these prodrome symptoms eventually lead to a diagnosis of a psychotic condition (American Psychiatric Association [APA], 2022; Hansen et al., 2023).

In the early 1990s, researchers began to address limitations of the prodrome concept by focusing on a **clinical high risk (CHR)** state for psychosis (also known as "ultra-high risk" [UHR] or "at-risk mental state" [ARMS]). Approximately 25% of individuals identified as CHR develop a psychotic disorder within 2 to 3 years of being identified as CHR, and approximately 35% do so within 10 years (de Pablo et al., 2021).

BOX 38-1 ■ Hal's Story

Hal was a typical teenager who was actively involved in high school sports (wrestling in the fall and track and field in the spring) and activities (president of the student council and a member of the debate team), and he earned excellent grades until his junior year. During his junior year, Hal began to withdraw from his sports and activities, and his grades declined from A's and B's to C's and D's. He spent less time with his friends and more time isolating himself in his room. Hal's mood became unpredictable, and he seemed to have little desire to participate in his favorite activities. His behavior became erratic, and he was suspicious of others while sometimes referring to the "mystical power" of numbers. Hal's parents suspected he had begun smoking marijuana on a regular basis but didn't know how to handle the situation. By the end of his junior year, Hal had stopped going to school and rarely left the house. Hal's grandfather had been diagnosed with schizophrenia and other close family members had experienced other symptoms of other mental illnesses. Taken together, this information indicates that Hal was at CHR of developing psychosis.

In order to be identified as CHR, an individual must display at least one of the following (Fusar-Poli, 2017; Fusar-Poli et al., 2013):

- Psychotic symptoms that are below the threshold required for diagnosis (**attenuated psychotic symptoms [APSs]**)
- A brief limited intermittent psychotic episode (BLIP)
- A genetic risk (close relative with a psychotic disorder) with a significant decline in functioning

In Box 38-1. Hal's story reflects the changes in perception, functioning, and thinking that often precede a first episode of psychosis.

Two primary assessment tools have been developed for identifying the CHR state: the Comprehensive Assessment of At-Risk Mental State (CAARMS) and the Structured Interview for Prodromal Symptoms (SIPS). The CAARMS is most widely used in Australia and Asia, whereas the SIPS and its companion scale, the Scale of Prodromal Symptoms (SOPS), are more commonly used in the United States. Both the CAARMS and SIPS/SOPS are commonly used in Europe (de Pablo et al., 2021; Fusar-Poli et al., 2013, 2020).

Ideally, biological markers, such as measuring differences in specific sensory event-related potentials (i.e., electrical brain activity in response to sensory stimuli that is measured by electroencephalography; Bodatsch et al., 2015), **sensory gating deficiencies** (i.e., the inability to effectively screen out redundant and irrelevant sensory input; Shaikh et al., 2015), specific sensory processing patterns (Pfeiffer et al., 2014; Roush et al., 2014), and changes in brain structures that can be detected by neuroimaging studies (Sun et al., 2009), eventually may be defined that allow clinicians to more accurately identify the prodrome. However, until such markers are discovered, the construct of the CHR state enables the possibility of early detection of individuals who are most likely to develop psychosis using the SIPS or the CAARMS (Fusar-Poli et al., 2020; Worthington & Cannon, 2021).

The goal of early detection is to provide minimal-risk interventions that can potentially prevent or delay conversion to full-blown psychosis without exposing the 53% to 70% of individuals identified as CHR who would not naturally progress to a psychotic disorder to treatments that they don't need (Fusar-Poli et al., 2020; Worthington & Cannon, 2021). The APA considered adding a diagnosis of attenuated psychosis syndrome to the *Diagnostic and Statistical Manual of Mental Disorders,* Fifth Edition *(DSM-5);* however, because of the limited amount of research available, the syndrome was instead placed in Section III: Emerging Measures and Models (APA, 2022).

First-Episode Psychosis

First-episode psychosis (FEP) refers to the first time that an individual reaches diagnostic criterion for psychosis and includes the first 2 to 5 years after the diagnosis. Research into early psychosis began emerging in the early 1990s in Australia, with clinical programs beginning to see and assist people in the mid-1990s. Research and therapeutic interest have increased and spread to numerous other countries worldwide (Early Psychosis Guidelines Writing Group and EPPIC National Support Program, 2016; Fusar-Poli et al., 2020; International Early Psychosis Association [IEPA], 2008; McGorry, 2015; Worthington & Cannon, 2021).

Most psychotic disorders begin to manifest in the teens and early 20s, a time when other health issues are at a minimum and young people are generally considered relatively healthy compared with their other periods in life (Sage, 2019). Common signs and symptoms of psychosis include decreases in school performance, withdrawal from previously enjoyed activities, anxiety, restlessness, changes in sleep patterns, mood swings, trouble with concentration and attention, forgetfulness, delusions, hallucinations, and impulsivity (Early Psychosis Guidelines Writing Group and EPPIC National Support Program, 2016). Left untreated, these early signs of psychosis may develop into much more serious *DSM-5* diagnoses such as schizophrenia, schizoaffective disorder, delusional disorder, or a mood disorder such as bipolar disorder or major depression with psychotic features. See Chapter 23: Schizophrenia Spectrum and Psychotic Disorders.

Early Psychosis Programs

To address the needs of individuals who are at CHR or experiencing a first episode of psychosis, specialized programs have emerged that focus on keeping individuals in meaningful, age-appropriate roles and routines. Early psychosis programs are primarily outpatient in nature, but clinicians work closely with inpatient facilities to provide youth-targeted services that are focused on returning the youth to their natural environment as quickly as possible. Hospitalization is avoided whenever possible and is reserved for the most severely affected individuals.

Programs are designed to provide culturally relevant services to late adolescents and young adults to help them maintain participation in activities that are typical for their age cohort. Recovery and maintaining a typical psychosocial developmental path are the driving forces behind early psychosis programs. Meetings may occur in the clinic or the community, but engaging in the youth's natural environments is preferred whenever possible.

PhotoVoice

A Standstill

"The meaning behind it is the feeling I get when I see something and can't get away from it."

As an OTP, what could you learn about a person's experience of mental illness using artistic expression occupations such as the one featured in the PhotoVoice box?

Describe how you might use other occupations involving artistic expression to help an individual work through the impact that the onset of symptoms might have on everyday occupations and relationships.

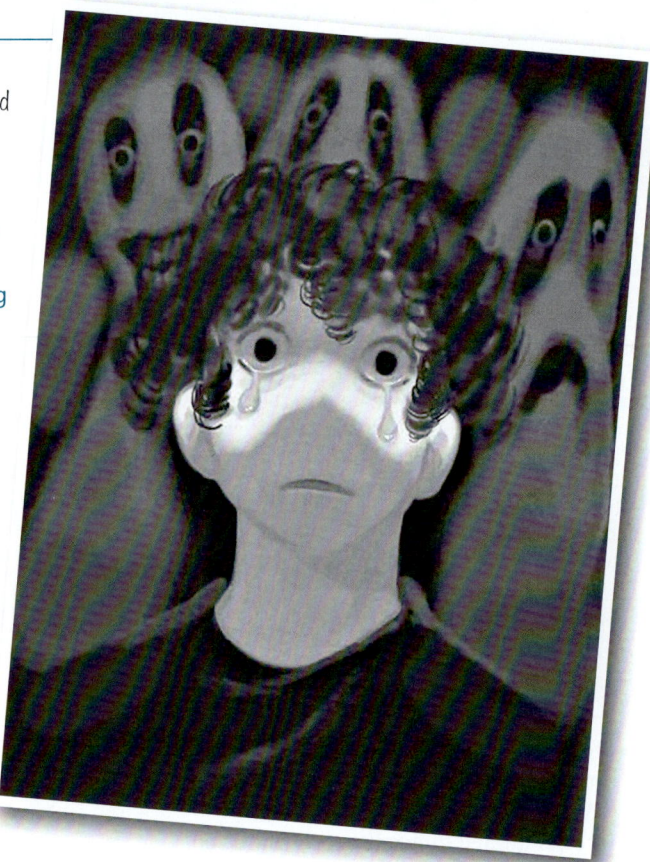

Mission and Philosophy

Early psychosis programs use a transdisciplinary team approach and embrace the Recovery Model to focus on returning young people to a typical developmental trajectory (Addington, 2021; Early Psychosis Guidelines Writing Group and EPPIC National Support Program, 2016; Sage, 2019). Early psychosis programs are based on a growing body of evidence that indicates that services aimed at treating the first episode of psychosis are cost effective (McGorry, 2014) and improve both symptomatic and functional recovery (Fusar-Poli et al., 2017; Kane et al., 2016; Sage, 2019). Evidence that services for people at CHR for psychosis lead to improvements is emerging, but further study needs to be undertaken before solid conclusions regarding efficacy at the CHR stage can be made (Correll et al., 2018; Puntis et al., 2020).

In addition to an emphasis on recovery, early psychosis services focus on the **duration of untreated psychosis (DUP),** the period between the onset of early symptoms and the initiation of treatment. Several studies have found that shorter DUP correlates with decreased severity of positive and negative symptoms, better social and vocational functioning, and increased quality of life (Fusar-Poli et al., 2017; Gonzalez-Valderrama et al., 2017; Johannessen et al., 2011; Kane et al., 2016; McGorry, 2014). Also see Chapter 2: Recovery and Wraparound Models.

Program Components

Early psychosis programs worldwide share a set of fundamental principles and components to promote recovery (Table 38-1).

Program staff typically includes:

- A psychiatrist or nurse practitioner to evaluate the need for, prescribe, and oversee medication
- Nurses to monitor the metabolic effects of medications and provide nutritional counseling
- Social workers or psychologists to provide coordination of resources and counseling
- Supported employment and education specialists to assist with obtaining or maintaining work and school participation
- An occupational therapy practitioner (OTP) to focus on functional performance
- Peer support to provide feedback and ideas through shared experience with mental health challenges

The number of staff members within each discipline depends on the size of the program and number of individuals served. Small person-to-staff ratios are prioritized to maintain high-quality service. In addition, any staff member may be trained as a "screener" or "intake coordinator." This person administers assessments, such as the CAARMS and SIPS/SOPS, and conducts interviews with individuals and families

Evidence-Based Practice

First-Episode Programs

> *Growing evidence supports the effectiveness of early intervention services (EIS) and the valuable role that OTPs play within EIS through providing evidence-based services.*

RESEARCH FINDINGS

Early intervention services (EIS) for psychosis have spread rapidly around the world in recent years and evidence is mounting regarding their effectiveness. Correll and colleagues (2018) completed a systematic review of randomized trials that compared EIS for early psychosis with treatment as usual (TAU). Ten studies met their inclusion criteria and the results indicated that individuals in EIS were much more likely to remain in services, were less likely to be hospitalized, spent less time in the hospital if they were hospitalized, had better symptom improvements, and displayed higher improvements in global functioning than those in TAU. Puntis and colleagues (2020) had similar results in their review of four studies focused on early intervention for recent-onset psychosis in the Cochrane Schizophrenia study-based register of trials. They also found that individuals engaged in early intervention programs were more likely to stay engaged in services, likely had fewer hospitalizations, and had a greater increase in global functioning than those in TAU.

Two systematic reviews, Read et al. (2018) and Frawley and colleagues (2023), focused on the effectiveness of psychosocial interventions on occupational functioning in early psychosis. Both reviews found that cognitive remediation, supported employment/supported education, and family-based therapy/family psychoeducation led to statistically significant improvements in occupational functioning. Both reviews also found mixed evidence for the effectiveness of Cognitive Behavioral Therapy (CBT) for psychosis. Frawley and colleagues (2023), however, identified that CBT for psychosis originally focused on clinical symptoms and relapse rates, but that specialized CBT focused on social recovery demonstrated better improvements in functioning than traditional CBT.

APPLICATIONS

➡ When compared with TAU, participating in a recovery-oriented, specialized comprehensive FEP program leads to:
- Increased functioning
- Greater improvement in quality of life
- Increased work and school participation
- Improved family relationships that may have a preventive effect on psychosis
- Reduced psychopathology

➡ OTPs contribute to early psychosis teams by using their specialized skills in activity analysis to create "just right challenges" for people in early FEP programs.

➡ OTPs should use evidence-based interventions such as cognitive remediation, supported employment/supported education, and family-based therapy/family psychoeducation in their work with individuals experiencing early psychosis.

➡ OTPs should use their knowledge of the PEO interaction to conduct research on the efficacy of early psychosis programs.

Continued

Evidence-Based Practice—cont'd

First-Episode Programs

REFERENCES

Correll, C. U., Galling, B., Pawar, A., Krivko, A., Bonetto, C., Ruggeri, M., Craig, T. J., Nordentoft, M., Srihari, V. H., Guloksuz, S., Hui, C. L. M., Chen, E. Y. H., Valencia, M., Juarez, F., Robinson, D. G., Schooler, N. R., Brunette, M. F., Mueser, J. T., Rosenheck, R. A., . . . Kane, J.M. (2018). Comparison of early intervention services vs treatment as usual for early-phase psychosis. *JAMA Psychiatry, 75*(6), 555–565. https://doi.org/10.1001/jamapsychiatry.2018.0623

Frawley, E., Cowman, M., Lepage, M., & Donohoe, G. (2023). Social and occupational recovery in early psychosis: A systematic review and meta-analysis of psychosocial interventions. *Psychological Medicine, 53,* 1787–1798. https://doi.org/10.1017/S003329172100341X

Puntis, S., Minichino, A., De Crescenzo, F., Harrison, R., Cipriani, A., & Lennox, B. (2020). Specialised early intervention teams for recent-onset psychosis (review). *Cochrane Database of Systematic Reviews, 11*(11), CD013288. https://doi.org/10.1002/14651858.CD013288.pub2

Read, H., Roush, S., & Downing, D. (2018). Early intervention in mental health for adolescents and young adults: A systematic review. *American Journal of Occupational Therapy, 72*(5), 7205190040p1–7205190040p8. https://doi.org/10.5014/ajot.2018.033118

TABLE 38-1 | Core Principles and Components of Early Psychosis Programs

Core Principle	Components
Promoting recovery	• All activities are focused on recovery from illness and minimizing disruptions to normal, age-appropriate occupations. • Focus is on functional recovery, emphasizing return to full social, educational, and vocational functioning. • Interventions should take place in the community whenever possible. • Home-based assessment and care are available. • Natural supports should be maximized. • Youth should identify their own goals and determine their own life trajectory.
Increasing public awareness and decreasing stigma	• Active public education campaigns • Specific education targeting high-risk groups • Awareness of appropriate and relevant cultural contexts
Easy access to care	• Networking with public and private providers; partnerships in the community to enhance support for youth • Outreach to schools and other contexts where youth gather • Rapid access to services • Anyone can refer to services
Family engagement and support	• Strong collaboration with person's identified family • Family peer supports • Training for family members around mental health and advocacy
Practitioner training	• Recovery-oriented focus • Focus on specific early intervention principles and interventions • Focus on youth culture and age-appropriate techniques
Early assessment and intervention	• Biopsychosocial approach • Comprehensive strategies • Best-practices driven • Normalization of mental illness and recovery • Stage-specific interventions in least restrictive environment • Minimal use of medications • Multidisciplinary team approach

Addington, D. (2021). The first episode psychosis services fidelity scale 1.0: Review and update. Schizophrenia Bulletin Open, 2(1), sgab007. *https://doi.org/10.1093 /schizbullopen/sgab007; Early Psychosis Guidelines Writing Group and EPPIC National Support Program. (2016).* Australian clinical guidelines for early psychosis *(2nd ed. updated). Orygen, The National Centre of Excellence in Youth Mental Health. Australian-Clinical-Guidelines-for-Early-Psychosis.aspx (orygen.org.au); McGorry, P. D. (2015). Early intervention in psychosis: Obvious, effective, overdue.* The Journal of Nervous and Mental Disease, 203(5), 310–318. *https://doi .org/10.1097/NMD.0000000000000284; Orygen Youth Health. (n.d.). Principles. http://oyh.org.au/about-us/principles; Sage, M. G. (Ed). (2019). EASA team manual. EASA Center for Excellence. https://easacommunity.org/wp-content/uploads/2024/05/EASA-Team-Manual.pdf*

to determine the appropriateness of early psychosis services and gather detailed medical and social histories.

Access to early psychosis programs is purposefully designed to remove as many barriers as possible. Anyone can refer an individual for screening, and participants may self-refer after learning about programs through public education campaigns. Despite efforts to remove barriers to services, recent research shows that there are inequities in access related to race and socioeconomic status. Oluwoye et al. (2021) found that black individuals in the United States had more police involvement and exposure to traumatic experiences that led to longer DUP than their white counterparts. Lilford et al. (2020) identify that individuals in low- and middle-income countries also have longer delays in accessing early interventions that lead to longer DUP. Both studies identify that there is a paucity of research in this area and that further study is required to better understand and combat these inequities.

Criteria for admission to early psychosis programs vary slightly by program but typically include age 15 to 25 years old, recent onset of symptoms (i.e., within 1 year and ideally within the last 30 days), and no medical condition or substance use that could account for the current symptoms. Upon admittance to a program, participants are assessed to identify their skills and needs. Assessment is then continuous throughout the program, during which participants typically receive specialized services for 2 to 5 years. Services are time-limited and focused from the start on building natural supports for the individual's transition out of the program. Multiple specialized services are offered to the person and their family, such as counseling (with a cognitive behavioral focus), psychoeducation about mental illness and recovery, occupational therapy, supported employment and education, psychiatry and nursing, and multifamily group (MFG) therapy aimed at teaching problem-solving skills and providing peer support.

Although hospitalization may be necessary for some participants if the person displays symptoms severe enough to cause concern of harm to self or others, most services are provided in the community and focus on maintaining as much normalcy as possible in routines and habits that are typical for adolescents and young adults.

The Clinical Staging Approach

Psychosis often develops gradually, and it may be weeks, months, or even years before an individual has symptoms of psychosis that meet *DSM-5* diagnostic criteria. Initial changes may be more subtle and are often difficult to tie together diagnostically. For example, the person may experience cognitive issues, such as slowed processing or short-term memory lapses, changes in affect, or slight sensory perception alterations. These changes are often subclinical initially, may be transient, and not all will reach a clinical threshold (Cross et al., 2014; Hickie et al., 2013; Jackson & McGorry, 2009). Traditional diagnostic systems do not adequately address the incipient nature of developing psychosis, as they were initially defined using well-established symptomology. A clinical staging approach was developed by researchers in Australia to better define the onset and early stages of psychosis to determine and apply the most effective treatments (Cross et al., 2014; Hickie et al., 2013; McGorry et al., 2006, 2010).

In the **clinical staging model**, early psychosis is broken down into stages, beginning with high risk but no symptoms or help-seeking (stage 0) to severe persistent mental illness (stage 4; Fusar-Poli, 2017; Hickie et al., 2013; McGorry et al., 2006, 2010). Initial research into this approach supports validity (Berendsen et al., 2021). Treatment strategies begin at the lowest level with a benign, educational approach for the person and family or caregiver. Interventions progress along with the person's symptoms to include more and more assertive strategies that are focused on long-term stabilization, including medication management. Occupational therapy interventions should be introduced at the earliest possible stage to assist in preventing or delaying transition to higher levels of symptomatology. Table 38-2 outlines the levels and potential interventions of the Clinical Stages Model.

Psychopharmacology

Early psychosis programs espouse a conservative approach to the use of antipsychotic medications. Because of the lack of a reliable tool with which to predict who in the CHR population will progress to a psychotic episode, recommended interventions at stages 0 to 1a are typically psychologically or psychosocially based. In this stage, the use of antipsychotic medications is generally not recommended to avoid increasing the risk of exposure to unnecessary treatment and making differential diagnosis more challenging (McClellan, 2018). Practice guidelines recommend that medications be reserved for the most severe cases in level 1b and typically not introduced until at least level 2 (Early Psychosis Guidelines Writing Group and EPPIC National Support Program, 2016; Fusar-Poli et al., 2013; McGorry, 2014).

When antipsychotic medications are appropriate, a conservative approach is implemented, and polypharmacy (i.e., the use of multiple medications) is avoided whenever possible. Individuals at CHR and those experiencing a first episode of psychosis tend to be more sensitive to the side effects of medications than older individuals, so a low dose of a second-generation antipsychotic may be prescribed by the team psychiatrist with careful monitoring of metabolic functioning because of the increased risk of metabolic issues from this class of medication (Early Psychosis Guidelines Writing Group and EPPIC National Support Program, 2016; Jackson & McGorry, 2009; McClellan, 2018; Melton et al., 2013).

Role of Occupational Therapy

Within early psychosis programs, the overall role of the OTP is to help the person maintain a sense of self through engagement in meaningful activities that are designed for success in areas of education, vocation, and socialization (Lloyd et al., 2000, 2008). Adolescents and young adults experience high levels of biological change during this developmental period. In addition to these bodily changes associated with the transition from child to adult, existential questions such as "Who am I?" "What do I want to be?" or "Where am I going from here?" are common.

Because of the nature of psychosis and its effects on social, cognitive, and sensory processing skills, OTPs provide opportunities for people to utilize feedback from

TABLE 38-2 | Clinical Stages Model: Levels and Potential Interventions

Stage	Level of Symptoms/Risk Factors	Focus of Intervention	Focus for Occupational Therapy
0—Increased risk of psychosis	• No symptoms • First-degree relative with psychosis • Teenager • No help-seeking	• Increase mental health literacy • Family education • Brief cognitive skills training • Substance use education • Antipsychotic medications not recommended because of potential side effects and lack of diagnostic certainty	• Maintain a sense of self • Facilitate engagement in education, vocation, and socialization • Maintain engagement in established roles, and facilitate development of new roles, habits, and routines associated with transition to adulthood • Develop or improve sleep routine and hygiene
1a—Possible prodrome	• Help-seeking • Mild symptoms of psychosis, including neurocognitive deficits • Mild functional impact	• Formal mental health literacy • Family psychoeducation • CBT • Substance use reduction • Antipsychotic medications not recommended because of potential side effects and lack of diagnostic certainty	All the previously noted items, plus: • Education on how prodrome can affect roles, habits, and routines • Build coping skills based on sensory needs • Cognitive adaptations and skill building to support engagement in occupations
1b—Possible prodrome	• UHR • Moderate, subthreshold symptoms • Moderate neurocognitive deficits • Chronic poor functioning	All the 1a interventions, plus: • Omega-3 fatty acids • Potential medications (reserved for most severe cases) Atypical antipsychotics Antidepressants Mood stabilizers	All the previously noted items, plus: • Education on symptoms and managing symptoms to support engagement in occupations • Maintenance and development of living skills, school and work skills, and interventions • Engagement in and exploration of lost and new occupations
2—First-episode psychosis or mood disorder	• Clear episode of psychotic, manic, or severe depression • Diagnosable *DSM-5* disorder • Moderate-severe symptoms • Moderate-severe neurocognitive deficits • Clear decline in functioning (social, educational, occupational)	All the 1b interventions, plus: • Greater consideration of use of medications • Vocational rehabilitation	All the previously noted items, plus: • Strengths identification • Groups skills training on social, educational, and vocational related skills • Engagement in age-appropriate and preferred occupations • Medication management • Lifestyle and wellness interventions • Facilitate development of identity with integration of mental illness experience • Career exploration and planning of future occupations Facilitate creation of new roles, habits, and routines to promote engagement in occupations within new identity
3—Recurrent or persistent disorder	• Incomplete remission from first episode 12 months from admission • Recurrence of severe episode after recovery • Deteriorating neurocognitive function • Continued clear decline in functioning	Same as the stage 2 interventions but with increased emphasis on: • Medical and psychosocial strategies to encourage full remission • Relapse prevention and focus on early warning signs of relapse • Long-term stabilization	All the previously noted items, plus: • Define recovery and create a wellness action plan. • Identify early warning signs and practice using those coping skills. Maintenance planning and how to care for basic activities of daily living (ADLs) and instrumental activities of daily living (IADLs) when in episode of illness
4—Severe, persistent, and unremitting illness	• Severe, persistent, unremitting illness • Severe decline in neurocognitive functioning • Marked decline in functioning	Same as the stage 3 interventions but with emphasis on: • Clozapine as drug of choice • Other treatments and social participation despite ongoing disability	All the previously noted items, plus: • Maintain gained illness management skills. • Define and utilize individual recovery plan. • Encourage exploration of other leisure or recreational activities. • Perform wellness interventions to ensure balance of health and well-being.

Cross, S. P. M., Hermens, D. F., Scott, E. M., Ottavio, A., McGorry, P. D., & Hickie, I. B. (2014). A clinical staging model for early intervention youth mental health services. Psychiatric Services, 65(7), 939–943. https://doi.org/10.1176/appi.ps.201300221; Hickie, I. B., Scott, E. M., Hermens, D. F., Naismith, S. L., Guastella, A. J., Kaur, M., Sidis, A., Whitwell, B., Glozier, N., Davenport, T., Pantelis, C., Wood, S. J., & McGorry, P. D. (2013). Applying clinical staging to young people who present for mental health care. Early Intervention in Psychiatry, 7, 31–43. https://doi.org/10.1111/j.1751-7893.2012.00366.x; McGorry, P. D., Dodd, S., Purcell, R., Yung, A., Thompson, A., Goldstone, S., & Killackey, E. (2010). Australian clinical guidelines for early psychosis (2nd ed.). Orygen, The National Centre of Excellence in Youth Mental Health; McGorry, P. D., Hickie, I. B., Yung, A. R., Pantelis, C., & Jackson, H. J. (2006). Clinical staging of psychiatric disorders: A heuristic framework for choosing earlier, safer, and more effective interventions. Australian and New Zealand Journal of Psychiatry, 40(8), 616–622. https://doi.org/10.1080/j.1440-1614.2006.01860.x

The Lived Experience

Nicholas Buekea

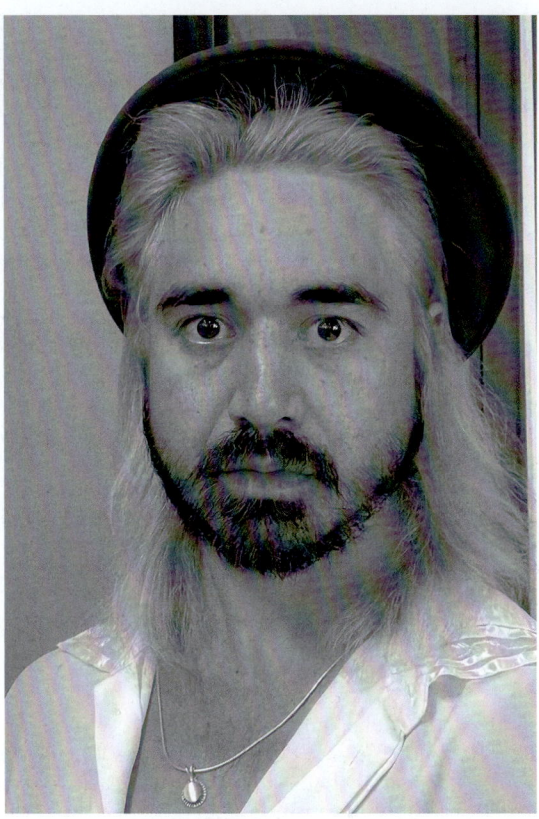

My father was born in the Federated States of Micronesia. He passed away in 2018. The biggest thing we shared was the love for our family, but we also shared the pain of being misunderstood, he far more so than I. Unlike me, my father's schizophrenia was untreated. The generational gap between us was apparent when looking at the self-perceptive attitudes of his diagnosis. The deal was, he never talked about it. Not once. Around the age of 12, I discovered he had schizophrenia, but I had no idea what it even meant. I still don't know what parts of his personality were attributed to having schizophrenia and which parts were cultural or unique to just him. I know he lacked any support other than my mom. When it came to his mental illness, he didn't have anyone to relate to, no community, no way to bounce thoughts back and forth, and no medium to express his innermost mind.

He was isolated throughout his adulthood, turning to booze and a bad temper, turning to a frustrated state of loneliness and separation from the mainstream. He would often yell outside on our apartment balcony; my mother informed us that he was hearing things that weren't there.

My father would talk to himself (his voices) more than he would talk to his children. I don't want to make my father out as a bad guy, because he wasn't, but he was distant for most of my life, almost unreachable. I didn't know how to talk to him for the longest time and there were times I lived in fear of his emotive states. Growing up, I would rather just ignore him all together, rather than engage in conversation that could potentially turn for the worst.

Around the age of 21 my own life turned for the worst. I was sent to the hospital and diagnosed with the dreaded schizophrenia myself. After swearing that I would never turn out like him, I could not believe how this was possible. How was it that I would share the same fate as him? I grew up witnessing the pain he endured, and now doctors were telling me I was about to carry the same weight. If I was going to tread along the same journey that my father trekked, then I needed answers if I was going to survive.

I began to insist upon deeper conversations with my father to understand the mind. I remember asking him in the car during a road trip to my grandparents, what the meaning of life was. I insisted upon gathering the depths of knowledge from my own creator, from my own god. He responded with something along the lines of, "to find your own purpose." In a sense, this set me up for my own self-discovery, one that was just beginning. It was one of the few lessons my father ever instilled.

I started to bond with my father over more philosophical questions. I asked him what it was like on the islands where he grew up. He told a few stories and painted a better picture of his boyhood. Why did I wait so long to ask these questions? Because I was waiting for him to come to me. I was waiting for him to start the conversations, without knowing that he had probably been yearning himself for someone to ask him about his own life experiences.

I think my father feared talking about his deepest thoughts because he lived in an era where mental illness was to be hushed. He lived in an era where having schizophrenia was a death curse, the fatal black spot, the end of progress, where dreams would stop, and the nightmares were the only thing to look forward to. The amount of anxiety and frustration he expressed existed in darkness, but where my own quest through the shadowy mind differed from his was the community that stood right beside me. I had support where he had none. As I stood next to my father, I think he was finally relieved from the idea that he was simply crazy. He had finally come across a person who was equally lost in the world, and he had seen a reflection in himself through me. Moreso, he saw the people that were seeing me through the darkness and into the light. He saw that there were people who truly cared about me, despite my shortcomings, and he witnessed the comradery for battling stigma that he unfortunately had missed during all those years in isolation.

There was no EASA in his day. He had no occupational therapists by his side. There was no path to recovery. It wasn't until toward the end of his life that he saw it was possible to make it out of the diagnosis, to become reintegrated into society and to be treated as equal. Although it pains me that he had to withstand the harsh reality of his time, I am comforted that he was able to see the beginning of systemic change.

EASA strives to make change. It is an FEP recovery organization built with an interdisciplinary approach. Being an outpatient mental health program that stresses person-centeredness, peer support, and strengths of its people, it calls upon multiple professions such as nursing, psychiatry, art therapy, employment specialists, drug counselors, case management, and occupational therapy to work together toward healthier individual lives. EASA works with families

Continued

The Lived Experience—cont'd

and their communities to build a sense of trust and groundedness, maintaining warmth and therapeutic comfort away from stigma and blame. EASA and other organizations such as Cascadia Behavioral Health are well situated in the mental health culture to provide people with dignity and respect as they recover from a world of misunderstanding, delusions, hallucinations, traumas, and pain caused by unwelcomed psychoses brought about by historic and societal illness, stress, and pressure that the world puts on youth and young adults that are still forming their realities and identities.

EASA and Cascadia are foundations of healing, using shared decision-making, as people relearn reality and formulate ways to express themselves positively, and in some cases find remedies to the shame of battling addictions and for some even legal consequences for actions made during loss of reality. These organizations utilize occupations to bring meaning and healing to their patrons.

My father witnessed my own healing from psychosis with the help of occupational therapy. He witnessed that it is possible to have people stand by your side, even through your darkest of times, to be there with compassion, deep listening, and understanding without judgment. I am happy to know that he saw me come full circle in my own understanding of why I was hospitalized, as I pursued a career in occupational therapy myself, graduating from Pacific University and now licensed to practice occupational therapy in Oregon after passing my NBCOT (National Board for Certification in Occupational Therapy) examination. The examination took me four attempts to pass, but like life itself and its many challenges, it isn't the number of failures that count, it's the number of times you are willing to get back up and try again. Even after the mind is broken, you can regain a sense of being and healing, perhaps becoming even more resilient and belonging to an even deeper sense of community and tribe.

My father was a beautiful soul. I may have children of my own someday. Perhaps they too will be struck with schizophrenia. Perhaps the genetics are inescapable. But where schizophrenia was a death curse in his day, perhaps in my child's future it will be similar to getting the flu: Something to worry about, sure, but nothing to lose hope over.

---

their physical, social, and cultural environments to improve functioning. In a systematic review by D'Amico et al. (2018), it was found that OTPs are well suited to provide evidence-based interventions that are person-centered, occupation-based, cognition-based, skills-based, and psychoeducation-focused, which lead to better occupational performance and better health outcomes.

OTPs use many forms of assessment and treatment to aid young people experiencing early psychosis in maintaining engagement in the occupations they cherish, along with promoting self-exploration at a time when socially and developmentally appropriate (Lloyd et al., 2008; Wen, n.d.). The role of OTPs in early psychosis programs around the world varies somewhat depending on the country, but all maintain a focus on engagement in meaningful occupations as the core of practice. In this chapter's Practitioner Profile feature, one practitioner working in an early psychosis program shares some of her experiences. Box 38-2 describes the role of occupational therapy in Australian early psychosis programs.

Importance of Rapport

An OTP's first step in intervention is to build rapport with the person and their family. Using therapeutic use of self, the individual and practitioner build trust so that the young person feels safe and comfortable discussing their fears and dreams (American Occupational Therapy Association [AOTA], 2020). OTPs are recommended to engage the person in an activity of the individual's choosing as part of building rapport. Adolescents and young adults will share more when treated as equals and engaged in meaningful occupations. One other crucial aspect to building rapport is ensuring the person feels comfortable and safe during therapy.

Once rapport has been established with the person, the OTP can pursue rapport building with the family. Engaging family members in discussions of their experiences since illness or symptom onset and providing opportunities for the individual to have the family hear their experiences or concerns are recommended rapport building strategies. The practitioner's goal is to nurture a collaborative relationship dynamic in which the young person is the expert on their recovery and the family continues to be a critical natural support.

Models of Practice

Adolescence and young adulthood are times of role change and identity formation. When a person experiences symptoms of psychosis, the impact on role development can be manifested in multiple areas of occupational performance, including motivation, habit formation, sensory processing, and social development. Models of practice most frequently used in early psychosis programs include the Person-Environment-Occupation (PEO) model, the Model of Human Occupation (MOHO), Dunn's Model of Sensory Processing, and the Kawa model.

Young adults engaged in occupations can develop a sense of mastery. Mastery is most effectively achieved when environmental demands match the person's individual factors and occupational demands. The PEO model guides intervention for this population by providing a framework for teaching adaptation to changing environmental input to enhance occupational performance. See Chapter 3: Person-Environment-Occupation Model. 🤝

As a member of early psychosis teams, the OTP is the only professional who specifically evaluates the PEO interaction. The PEO model drives many of the therapeutic decisions

Practitioner Profile

Occupational Therapy's Role in an Early Psychosis Program

Contributed by Michelle De Oliveira, OTD, OTR/L, QMHP

I'm an occupational therapist in a community-based, grant-funded, early psychosis intervention program in Oregon, USA. An individual can be in our program for up to 2 years. We can use grant funds to cover services, which helps to reduce barriers for those with low or no insurance. Occupational therapy can also bill insurance as Qualified Mental Health Providers (QMHPs) using behavioral health procedure codes.

Our program serves 15- to 25-year-olds who are at risk for developing psychosis, or who have had a first full episode of psychosis within the last 12 months. Individuals are commonly diagnosed with unspecified psychosis, bipolar with psychotic features, major depression with psychotic features, or a schizophrenia spectrum disorder. People experiencing psychosis can present positive and negative symptoms. Negative symptoms impact social engagement, hygiene, sleep, academic participation, and vocational participation, and impede progress toward life goals.

Our treatment team includes people from a broad range of professions including a screener, mental health therapist, licensed medical provider for medication management, nurse, occupational therapist, skills trainer, peer support, supported employment specialist, and supported education specialist. We support recovery from multiple disciplinary perspectives.

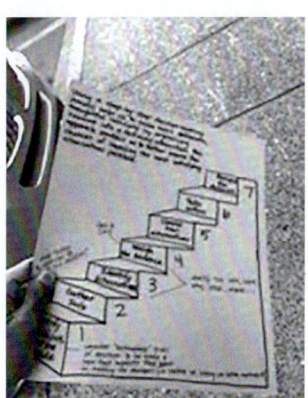

Goal setting ladder

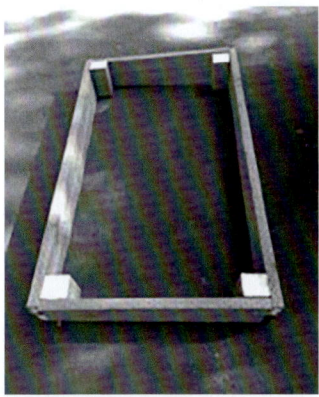

Building a planter box

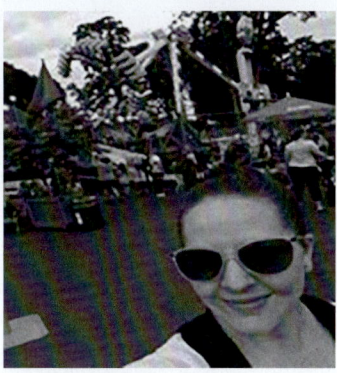

Community engagement

Occupational therapy models of practice used in our setting include PEO, MOHO, and Kawa, and common assessments are the Adolescent/Adult Sensory Profile, OCAIRS, MOHOST (Model of Human Occupation Screening Tool), PASS (Performance Assessment of Self-care Skills), and SLUMS (Saint Louis University Mental Status Exam). A person's sensory preferences are routinely assessed to identify strategies matching sensory needs. Occupational therapy helps people structure their daily activities and manage routines including finding enjoyable activities or developing healthy sleep habits. We encourage participation in daily activities, work, school, and healthy social relationships. Functional cognition, memory and attention, and low motivation challenges are addressed by offering skill building in self-awareness, problem-solving, time management, and mental flexibility.

Practitioners work independently with individuals, lead groups, and collaborate with the team to help support a person's goals. For example, we may encourage use of a goal setting ladder to practice a step-by-step process for setting and achieving goals. It is essential to provide a range of opportunities for participation, from quiet productive activities such as constructing a planter box for gardening to more active engagement at a community amusement park.

We do all of this by collaborating with each person and prioritizing engagement in meaningful and important occupations that they choose. Outcomes are measured through engagement: Are they spending more time with friends after isolating? Are they attending classes more regularly? Are they improving their sleep habits? Are they preparing and eating meals/snacks daily? Are they managing their routine and making it to appointments on time? Have they returned to a favorite occupation that they set aside because of low motivation?

Skills that are key for working in this setting include the ability to connect and build rapport, adjust communication, grade activities to meet people where they're at, and adapt intervention strategies on the go, as young people's goals can change daily. This can be challenging, in that it limits the time a practitioner spends on developing specific interventions, but can be an opportunity to think creatively about ways to support young people in participating in what is important to them day to day. When approaching this work from a mind that keeps occupation front and center through incorporating practice guidelines and models of practice and emphasizing the young person's choice, OTPs really have an opportunity to help young people to be successful in multiple different ways, which is especially rewarding.

BOX 38-2 ■ Description of Occupational Therapy Services in Australian Early Psychosis Programs

The *Australian Clinical Guidelines for Early Psychosis* (Early Psychosis Guidelines Writing Group and EPPIC National Support Program, 2016) direct early psychosis services in Australia. Occupational therapists are employed as case managers or clinicians in early psychosis community mental health teams, assertive outreach teams, or in crisis assessment and treatment teams. Some are also employed in discipline-specific roles (either part time or full time) in teams or services, although this is less common. More commonly, occupational therapists employed in discipline-specific roles work in hospital inpatient settings. They are employed to work with young people who have experienced a first episode of psychosis, as well as young people who are at UHR of developing psychosis.

Occupational therapists as case managers administer a standard suite of psychological assessments and interventions including mental state assessment and monitoring, functional assessment and intervention, psychosocial interventions, and care coordination. Because of the varied roles that occupational therapists can be employed in within early psychosis services, the duties they perform are dictated by the role in which they are employed.

In some services, occupational therapists may provide specific occupational therapy assessment and intervention as well as secondary consultation. Occupational therapists employed in community or outpatient settings use a variety of therapeutic approaches, including psychological interventions such as CBT and Motivational Interviewing (MI), guided by early intervention principles and the phase-based approach to early psychosis management.

More specifically, occupational therapists may provide specialized assessment and interventions for sensory processing (Adolescent/Adult Sensory Profile Assessment), functional assessment and interventions (Assessment of Motor and Process Skills [AMPS]), or driving assessment in the case of occupational therapists who have undertaken driver assessor training. Occupational therapists are also generally involved in the development and implementation of group programs in both inpatient and outpatient or community settings. These groups aim to provide young people with developmentally appropriate settings to develop skills and engage in meaningful activities across a variety of domains. In some services, occupational therapists may also be involved in vocational supports and services.

made in the occupational therapy process to create the best fit between the person, environment, and occupation, aiding the person in successfully reaching their goals (Sage, 2019).

The MOHO model assumes the person is part of an open system and is receiving feedback from the environment, which in turn serves to help motivate the person to engage in behaviors that build a sense of self through establishing meaningful roles and generating productive habits and routines (Taylor, 2017). When a psychotic disorder manifests, the young person struggles with making life choices, defining desires, and maintaining a sense of control and self-efficacy—all of which lead to difficulty planning and working toward goals. This negative effect on motivation can impact the development of roles and satisfying routines; healthy habits can take longer to develop, and the individual can respond in potentially unhealthy ways to the environment (e.g., maladaptive coping skills, loss of student role; Lloyd et al., 2000, 2008). Working under this model, OTPs in early psychosis programs facilitate healthy role and routine development to promote people's functioning and perceived performance.

Dunn's Model of Sensory Processing is used by OTPs working in early psychosis programs to understand the sensory preferences and needs of the person, family members, and other important people in the person's life. Understanding the sensory preferences and needs of those engaged in early psychosis programs enables the OTP to facilitate the best match for those involved.

Recent research also supports the findings of Brown and coworkers (2002), who identified very specific sensory patterns in individuals diagnosed with schizophrenia. Parham and colleagues (2019) found that individuals at CHR for psychosis displayed the same pattern of higher scores on low registration, sensation sensitivity, and sensation avoiding, with lower scores on sensation seeking for individuals with schizophrenia. Individuals with this sensory processing pattern require a higher volume or intensity of sensory input (e.g., louder music, brighter lights) to engage their nervous system (low registration) but then can become quickly overwhelmed if the intensity continues at that level or continues to increase. These individuals may fall asleep or have difficulty focusing on low stimulation environments (e.g., lecture classes, movie theaters), but also can become irritable or distracted in environments with too much stimulation, such as a busy laboratory section of a class and a shopping mall during the holidays.

The optimal range of sensory input is much narrower for a person with early psychosis or schizophrenia than is typical (Brown et al., 2002; Parham et al., 2019), making this an important area for OTPs, who can help modify environments to provide the "just right" sensory input. Further research is needed, but these findings suggest that disruptions in a person's sensory pattern may precede the psychotic diagnosis and therefore may serve as a biomarker that, when combined with other biomarkers, can help predict which individuals at CHR for psychosis are more likely to convert to a *DSM-5* diagnosable psychotic disorder (Parham et al., 2019). A study by Harrison et al. (2019) suggests that challenges in modulating sensory sensitivity may be a key etiological factor in many mental health conditions, including schizophrenia. See Chapter 9: Sensory Processing and the Lived Sensory Experience.

Dr. Michael Iwama and colleagues developed the Kawa model to support a culturally responsive approach to providing occupational therapy services (Ober et al., 2022). The model uses the metaphor of a river to learn about a person's contexts, strengths, challenges/barriers, and occupational goals.

Evaluation

The goal of occupational therapy during the initial evaluation in early psychosis is to determine the person's baseline functioning, what they want to do, where they see themselves going, current strengths and abilities, and goals for the future

(Sage, 2019). This is accomplished through a collaborative process involving interviewing the young person, as well as their family or immediate supporters, and completing standardized and nonstandardized assessments. After baseline functioning is established, ongoing assessment monitors for change and effectiveness regarding the interventions.

Gathering information through open-ended questions that facilitate discussion with the person surrounding values, interests, patterns of daily life, and occupational history is the recommended starting point. Several semistructured occupational therapy interviews are suitable assessment choices, such as the Occupational Circumstances Assessment Interview and Rating Scale—OCAIRS (Forsyth et al., 2006), the Occupational Performance History Interview II—OPHI-II (Kielhofner et al., 2004), the Canadian Occupational Performance Measure—COPM (Law et al., 2005), and the Kawa model approach (Iwama, 2006). Establishing the occupational profile may also begin with an informal interview process that engages the young person in dialogue that encourages them to tell their own story, thus building rapport. The Kawa model may be particularly helpful in developing rapport and can be used as a guide for an informal interview to learn about a person's contexts, strengths, challenges/barriers, and occupational goals.

A person-centered, collaborative evaluation approach allows for better matching of the person's needs to facilitate occupational participation. For example, paying close attention to the person's experiences of stress in the context of daily living skills can clarify the role stress plays in their experience of the illness and, in turn, how that relationship affects their performance (Krupa et al., 2010). Once this foundation is established, it can then inform the clinician's decision-making process regarding which assessments to use. Specific assessments have been found particularly useful in eliciting information about the young person, their environment, and how the onset of psychotic symptoms has affected occupational performance. Table 38-3 outlines key information about common evaluation tools to help guide the practitioner's therapeutic reasoning during the evaluation processes.

Many times, the symptoms of psychosis, particularly negative symptoms such as apathy and anhedonia, can affect a person's ability to self-reflect and express aspects of themself. More importantly, living with symptoms of psychosis at a time when independent self-identity is only beginning to emerge can negatively impact the ability to identify goals and make decisions about the future. The Occupational Self-Assessment (OSA; Baron et al., 2006) is a person-centered tool that encourages collaborative goal setting and enables the OTP to elicit how the individual perceives their own competence in daily occupations and how important each of those occupations are (value).

Assessment of cognitive performance is a major focus of early psychosis intervention teams (Early Psychosis Guidelines Writing Group and EPPIC National Support Program, 2016; McFarlane, 2011; Melton et al., 2013) and falls within the domain of occupational therapy. From problem-solving and planning to organization and memory, occupational therapy assesses cognition to reveal how a person's symptoms may impact their ability to use feedback from the environment to complete tasks and initiate and maintain engagement in occupations. Cognitive assessments such as the Contextual Memory Test and Allen's Cognitive Level Screen are appropriate choices for determining cognitive functioning and needs. Cognition and cognitive assessments used by OTPs are covered in previous chapters in this text. See Chapter 7: Cognition and Chapter 8: Cognitive Beliefs. 🤝

OTPs working in early psychosis also assess for sensory needs and preferences using tools such as the Adolescent/Adult Sensory Profile (Early Assessment and Support Alliance [EASA], 2013). Assessment of sensory preferences and needs can be helpful in setting up accommodations in the school or work setting, preparing for social experiences, and improving family relationships. Practitioners have found that there are often competing sensory needs within families and that unmet sensory preferences and needs often create barriers to success in school, work, and social situations.

Intervention

OTPs play a unique role on early psychosis intervention teams, providing multiple forms of intervention and executing occupational therapy from a true transdisciplinary approach. For example, suppose a person is struggling to maintain employment because environmental and sensory processing factors are not addressed at work. This person is then evaluated by the OTP. Using the results of the Adolescent/Adult Sensory Profile and observation of the individual's work environment, the OTP generates a list of recommendations. The OTP shares assessment results and recommendations with the person, along with education and training on self-advocacy. In addition to education on self-advocacy, the OTP provides recommendations to the supported employment specialist or works directly with the individual's work supervisor to make the needed changes in the work environment. This example highlights the many ways in which OTPs intervene in this practice setting. From one-on-one intervention to community-based intervention with employers, OTPs engage people in regaining a sense of self and learning healthy life skills.

When targeting a person's integration into the community, the OTP works with the individual to gather resources that identify local groups of interest for the person. To encourage and support participation, the therapist and individual initially attend the group together and slowly transition to meet a goal of independent participation. Another example of direct, community-based, one-on-one intervention is collaborative problem-solving concerning how to maintain attention and motivation to complete weekly grocery shopping. The OTP can support the person's goals by grading essential elements of the activity, including travel to the store, writing a shopping list, and gathering and purchasing items in the store.

Facilitating MFGs (McFarlane, 2002; Sage, 2019) is another area of intervention in which OTPs engage with individuals with early psychosis and their families and/or supporters. In MFG, multiple individuals and their family members work on learning problem-solving skills. The long-term goal of MFG is to teach problem-solving skills, and the immediate goal of each group is to solve specific problems brought to the group that day. The MFG has a clear structure and process, typically beginning with each person sharing what is going well and what could be better in the next 2 weeks. An OTP and a social worker, counselor, or supported employment specialist often cofacilitate such group sessions. They engage the group in a transparent discussion to select an issue to problem-solve.

TABLE 38-3 | Therapeutic Reasoning Assessment Table: Early Psychosis Programs

Which Tool?	Who Was This Tool Designed For?	Is This a Type of Tool the Person Can Do? What Is Required of the Person?	What Am I Measuring?	How Long Does It Take and Where Do I Administer This Assessment?	Is the Tool Associated With a Practice Model?
Structured Interview for Prodromal Syndromes (SIPS; McGlashan et al., 2014)	Teens and adults experiencing positive psychotic symptoms or having first episode of psychosis	Administered by trained occupational therapists. Uses narrative interviewing to assess level of severity of symptoms, if being experienced.	Existing positive psychosis symptoms, negative symptoms, anxiety and depression symptoms, and level of impairment caused by symptoms	Allow 1–2 hours for administration, conducted one-on-one with the person and family/caregiver; can be done in home, clinic, or community.	Psychodynamic Model
Occupational Self-Assessment (OSA; Baron et al., 2006)	Teens and adults who are receiving occupational therapy services. The OSA is not designated for a specific diagnostic group but rather a wide range of individuals.	Self-questionnaire requires the person to rate their competence in each occupation and the value each occupation holds. The person then prioritizes goals based on these ratings.	Self-concept, insight, values, volition, and goal-setting skills	Can be administered in 15–30 minutes; results should be used collaboratively to set goals, build rapport, and plan out person's care.	Model of Human Occupation
Allen Cognitive Level Screen (ACLS) and Large Cognitive Level Screen (LCLS; Allen et al., 2007)	Adults with psychiatric disorders, adults with dementia, people with disruption in cognitive processing skills; use LCLS for visually impaired	Leather Lacing Task requires person to follow verbal or visual directions.	Global cognition as it affects occupational performance; it corresponds to the Allen Scale of Cognitive Performance Levels 3.0–5.8.	Can be administered in the clinic in 10–20 minutes to screen possible limitations in information processing impacting function; results of screening should be verified with other tools.	Cognitive Disabilities Model
Adolescent/Adult Sensory Profile (Brown & Dunn, 2002)	Age 11 to older adult	Self-report completed by the participant independently or therapist can read items and circle responses	Sensory processing preferences as observed through participation in daily life	30 minutes at home or clinic	Dunn's Model of Sensory Processing
Contextual Memory Test (Toglia, 1993)	Adults with brain injury of psychiatric conditions	Questionnaire of individual's awareness of memory	Assesses awareness of memory problems and recall memory. Includes a dynamic component to determine if individual can learn strategies to improve performance.	Takes 10–20 minutes to measure, administered in a clinical setting	Toglia's Dynamic Interactional Approach

For example, a father may report wanting to worry less about the amount of sleep his daughter is getting each night. His worrying is a constant stressor that is inhibiting his ability to support his daughter. The cofacilitators lead the group in a process that rewords the father's concern into a "what" or "how" statement, such as "What can the father do to reduce his worry about his daughter's sleeping habits in the next 2 weeks?" Using this question, the group then brainstorms up to 10 potential solutions, all of which are written for all to see and received without judgment or discussion. The group then examines each solution, listing the disadvantages and advantages of each option. In the final step, the person who raised the selected issue chooses one or two solutions they will implement in the next 2 weeks. In this example, the group's collective problem-solving informs the specific plan this father creates.

PhotoVoice

Kane's Story

Kane: When I'm stressed I work on my cars. It is time consuming and therapeutic, and it keeps me moving.

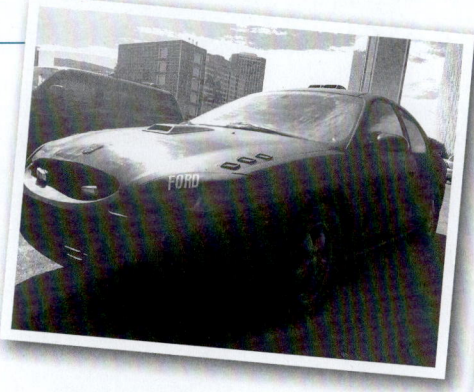
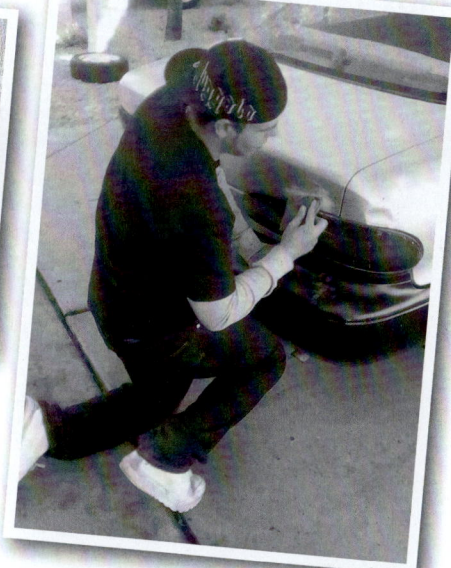

Building rapport has been identified within this chapter as the first step in intervention. Describe multiple ways of how you might use Kane's interest in working on cars to build rapport with him.

Occupational therapy assessment and intervention in early psychosis is based on specific models of practice that are described in this chapter. Use those models to describe Kane's occupation of working on cars and how working on cars helps him to adapt to stress in his life.

How could you use Kane's interest in working on cars to inform interventions in other areas of occupation that he wants to do, needs to do, or is expected to do?

The outcomes are also monitored by the group when the father reports outcomes at the next meeting. This process is repeated every 2 weeks and provides an effective means for the OTP to assist the individual and their family to build problem-solving skills, reduce family stress, and increase successful outcomes in areas of the person's life (McFarlane, 2002; Melton et al., 2013; O'Brien Cannon et al., 2023).

Group intervention is an effective tool for OTPs in early psychosis programs, and they can design and implement many types of group interventions, ranging from processing groups to skills training groups. The design of group interventions must account for the teenage through early adulthood age range and consider unique developmental needs, strengths, challenges, and opportunities to use altruism to build trust and rapport among members. Box 38-3 shows an example of a group activity.

Groups can be used to build stress management skills, independent living skills, work readiness skills, and academic functional skills. For example, an OTP working with young adults who are not sure what job they want or career path they are interested in could create a career exploration group. In this group, the people would volunteer each week at a different community site to learn about the job requirements and what, if any, education is required. By using the natural environments of young people, teaching group dynamics and processes, and using activity-based interventions, OTPs provide individualized interventions within the group setting and ultimately promote improved social functioning of their people.

Case Management, Community Education, and Advocacy

In addition to typical occupational therapy intervention, the OTP on early psychosis teams may provide case management, many times in the form of supported education. In supported education, the OTP provides case management by identifying resources for the person that are available at the school or in the community to increase academic achievement. As case managers, OTPs may collaborate with the person and college admission offices, a specific school or department in the college, or even individual professors to educate and to establish supports that can facilitate the person's success. OTPs may also join middle school or high school Section 504 or individualized education program (IEP) meetings to help advocate for the person's needs and accommodations. They also help people learn skills to advocate for their own needs within academic settings.

The early warning signs or symptoms of psychosis can sometimes go unseen or be disregarded as representing another issue, such as typical teenage behavior. As a member of the early psychosis team, OTPs have the knowledge and skill sets to provide prevention-focused education to community members regarding the specific perceptual, behavioral, and functional changes indicative of a young person at CHR or who may be experiencing FEP. Educational and advocacy efforts may be directed at schoolteachers, counselors, administrators, primary care doctors, members of the local faith-based community, and anyone interested in the mental health of adolescents and young adults.

Advocacy may require the OTP to develop effective, culturally responsive, health literacy materials and engage in assertive networking, in which the OTP goes to community groups to provide information on what psychosis is, how to identify the warning signs, and how to refer to an early psychosis program. This form of outreach not only increases community awareness of mental illness, which reduces stigma, but it also can support early identification efforts, which have the potential to prevent the long-term, disabling effects of serious mental illness on young people in the community. See Chapter 37: School Mental Health.

BOX 38-3 ■ Example of Group Activity: Sculpting

This group at EASA is conducting a "sculpting exercise." The participants choose a topic or theme (e.g., pride, anxiety, good vs. evil). One person acts as the sculptor and, without speaking, uses touch to mold the other members of the group into a sculpture that they feel represents that topic or idea. Participants take turns acting as sculptor and clay.

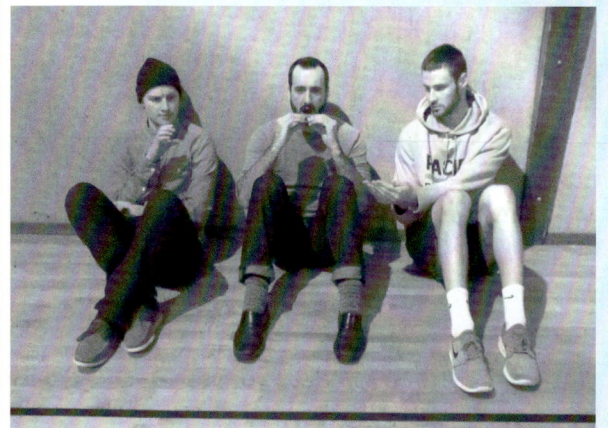
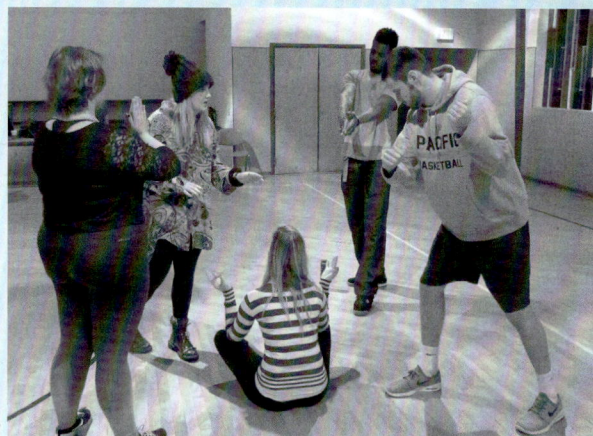
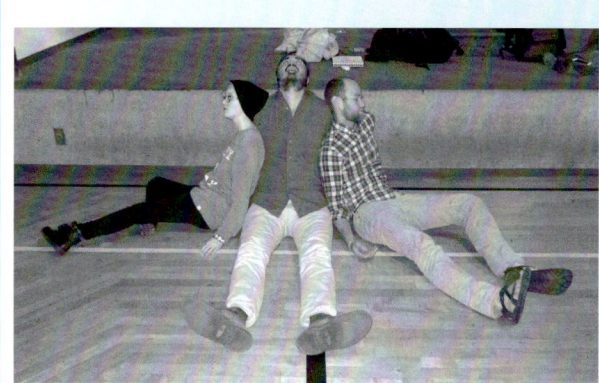
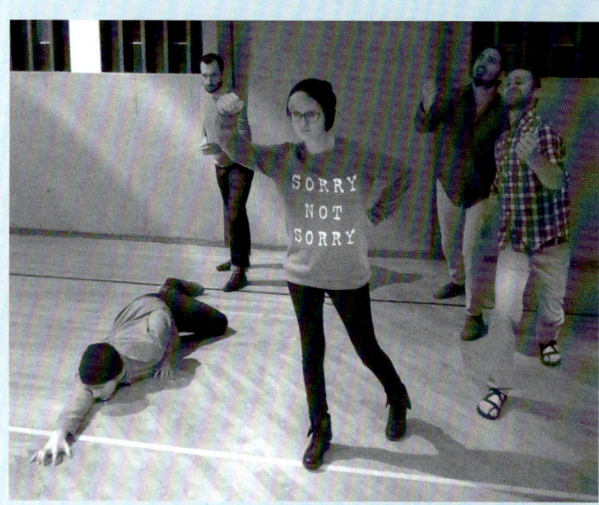

Emerging Broader Focus on Youth Mental Health

Although this chapter focuses on psychosis, there are growing national and international efforts to address youth mental health in general. The growing attention paid to youth mental health stems from recognition that this issue has been largely ignored historically, and more recently impacted by global events such as an ongoing pandemic, population migration, fragile economies, and climate change (Fusar-Poli et al., 2021).

Mental disorders affect about 1 billion people of the total population, and young people account for 41% of the total population. Thus, mental disorders largely impact young people, with 75% having onset before age 24, and may have a profound impact on their future functioning (Fusar-Poli et al., 2021). Failing to address this health crisis results in a major decrease in productive years for those impacted (McGorry, 2014). Countries such as Australia, New Zealand, and the United Kingdom have adopted national guidelines to address this issue, but the United States has not adopted national policy at the time of this publication. However, some individual states have programs; currently, Oregon is the only state attempting a statewide early psychosis program.

The International Association for Youth Mental Health held its first conference in 2011 and now hosts an international conference every other year. In Australia, the first national youth mental health initiative, *headspace,* was launched in 2006 to help youth ages 12 to 25 who are having mental health difficulties of any type. Physical *headspace* centers are spread throughout Australia, with 90 operating in 2015. For youth who can't access a center or who don't feel comfortable showing up in person, *eheadspace* provides support via online chat, e-mail, or telephone. The idea of *headspace* has spread internationally, with programs operating in New Zealand, Denmark, and Ireland.

Here's the Point

- Early psychosis services began in Australia in the 1990s and have been adopted in other countries around the world. Emerging research shows that early intervention can reduce disability in those impacted by psychosis.
- Early psychosis services are designed to be culturally responsive and focus on keeping the individual engaged in age-appropriate activities.
- Early psychosis services are for individuals approximately 15 to 25 years old who are within 1 year of first experiencing signs and symptoms.
- Early psychosis services provide supportive counseling, resource coordination, supported employment and education, family support, medications when appropriate, and advocacy to help individuals maintain or regain a typical developmental path in life.
- OTPs within early psychosis programs help individuals maintain a sense of self through engagement in meaningful activities that are designed for success in areas of education, vocation, and socialization.
- Practitioners provide both specialized assessment and intervention, such as focusing on sensory needs, and generalized services, such as cofacilitating multifamily groups.
- Although health-care professionals are not yet able to reliably predict which individuals who are at CHR for psychosis will go on to develop *DSM-5* psychotic disorders, programs focusing on the prodrome period show that they are effective at delaying, and sometimes preventing, the onset of a diagnosable psychotic disorder, such as schizophrenia, bipolar disorder, or major depression with psychotic features.
- Programs focusing on identifying and treating FEP can reduce the DUP and improve functioning during the "critical period."
- Improving functioning during the critical period often results in improved postpsychosis functioning for those affected.
- Longer-term studies are needed to determine whether the positive outcomes achieved in early psychosis programs are long-lasting or if service duration and intensity need to be modified to maximize outcomes.
- OTPs can play a unique and valuable role in early psychosis programs but there is very little occupational therapy–specific research to date. Early studies looking at sensory processing and early psychosis are promising but more work remains to be done in this practice area.
- Internationally, the focus is turning from just psychosis to the broader range of mental health challenges that adolescents and young adults are susceptible to by addressing youth mental health overall.

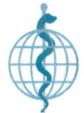 Visit the online resource center at **FADavis.com** to access the videos.

Apply It Now

1. Person-Environment-Occupation (PEO) Analysis

After reading this chapter's The Lived Experience about Nicholas and his father, complete a PEO analysis using the template in Appendix A. Consider the following guiding questions.

Reflective Questions
- What occupations are most important to Nicholas?
- What changes are observed in the personal factors?
- How did environmental factors contribute to their experiences before and after receiving care?

2. International Early Psychosis Virtual Conference

Go to the IEPA Early Intervention in Mental Health YouTube site at https://www.youtube.com/@iepaearlyinterventionin men8232/videos and choose at least one video that interests you. View the presentations and reflect on what you learn in your journal.

3. Watch and Reflect

Go to the IEPA Early Intervention in Mental Health You-Tube site at https://www.youtube.com/@iepaearlyinterven tioninmen8232/videos and search for "Mental Health in an Uncertain World." Watch the first video in the symposium titled "How Racism Shapes Risk Factors and Outcomes for Black Americans Diagnosed With Psychosis" and reflect in your journal about the intersection of racism and mental health diagnosis, treatment, and outcomes in early psychosis.

4. Develop an Occupational Therapy in Early Psychosis Brochure

Explore the websites for current early psychosis programs in the United States and then design a fact sheet or brochure identifying what occupational therapy has to offer to an early psychosis program. When creating the fact sheet or brochure, consider including the role of occupational therapy in mental health, areas where occupational therapy can support goals, common functional barriers someone with psychosis might experience, and types of interventions that can be used. Also, consider the audience you are creating the fact sheet or brochure for, and adjust the information provided accordingly.

5. Develop a Group Protocol for Using Artistic Expression of Mental Health Experiences

Design a group that allows members to use a specified form of artistic medium to express their explanatory model and/or experiences with mental health symptoms. Consider including group leader/coleader, group title, intervention setting, intervention population, purpose of the group, occupational therapy models/frames of reference used, group goals/rationale, outcome/evaluation method, group outline (e.g., warmup, introduction of activity, activity, sharing, processing, applying, closing), and any supplies and costs.

6. Become a Member of the IEPA Early Intervention in Mental Health

Go to the IEPA webpage at http://iepa.org.au/about-us/membership and join the association. Membership is free to anyone with an interest in early psychosis and includes a free subscription to the journal *Early Intervention in Psychiatry*. Once you subscribe, explore the Early Intervention Resources, and review a resource for either families/carers/friends, professionals, or individuals. While reviewing, consider factors such as the readability of the resource, the functional cognition that may be required of the reader, and the accessibility of the materials and what might support or limit the accessibility. Discuss your thinking with a peer who has evaluated the same resource.

Resources

- IEPA Early Intervention in Mental Health: http://iepa.org.au
  This network of clinicians, policymakers, and other individuals with an interest in the field of early psychosis aims to increase awareness of early psychosis recovery through communication and collaboration on the development of best practices for early psychosis. The association hosts an international conference every other year (even years).
- National Council for Mental Wellbeing – Early Onset Schizophrenia Community of Practice https://www.thenationalcouncil.org/program/early-intervention-treatments-for-psychosis/
  Nearly a decade ago this organization developed and continues to support an Early Onset Community of Practice to focus efforts and information about early intervention models of care for the treatment of psychosis. This site includes useful links and slideshows for workforce trainings focused on early intervention, referral and outreach, models of practice and model early psychosis programs.
- Orygen: The National Centre of Excellence in Youth Mental Health: https://orygen.org.au
  This Australian youth mental health and research program provides direct treatment, research, and training of professionals working in youth mental health.
- Psychosis Risk and Early Psychosis Program Network (PEPPNET): https://med.stanford.edu/peppnet/whoweare.html
  This organization supports the development and dissemination of evidence-based practices and evaluation standards.

U.S. Early Psychosis Programs

- Early Assessment and Support Alliance (EASA): http://www.easacommunity.org
  This Oregon-based program is aimed at providing information and support to young people experiencing symptoms of psychosis for the first time. EASA uses a fidelity, evidence-based tool to support community-based mental health programs in running these transdisciplinary teams.
- Early Psychosis Intervention Network (EPINET): https://nationalepinet.org/about-epinet
  This National Institute of Mental Health (NIMH) initiative includes multiple regional hubs and early psychosis clinics across multiple states in the United States.
- National Early Psychosis Program Directory: https://med.stanford.edu/peppnet/interactivedirectory.html
  This is a directory of early psychosis programs across the United States.

Adolescent/Young Adult Mental Health

- headspace Australia: http://www.headspace.org.au
  This website is designed and developed for young people in Australia who may be experiencing symptoms themselves or who may have friends or family who are experiencing symptoms.

Ancillary Teaching Materials

- International Association for Youth Mental Health (IAYMH): http://www.iaymh.org
  The IAYMH was established in 2012 to assist in advocating and collaborating for the mental health needs of young people across the world.

Additional Adolescent/Young Adult Mental Health

- Jigsaw, Young People's Health in Mind: https://www.jigsaw.ie
  Jigsaw provides supports to youth around mental health issues in Ireland.

U.S.-Based Early Psychosis Research and Intervention Programs

- Lieber Schizophrenia Research Clinic: http://columbiapsychiatry.org/researchclinics/lieber-schizophrenia-research-clinic
  The Lieber Center website is a repository of contemporary, multidisciplinary research focused on understanding the etiology of schizophrenia and treatment effectiveness.
- NAVIGATE: https://navigateconsultants.org
  NAVIGATE programs, implemented across the United States and in many countries around the world, are designed to support individuals with a first episode of psychosis and help their families navigate a path to well-being and needed mental health services.
- Program for Early Psychosis (PATH): https://www.ucsfhealth.org/en/clinics/path-program-for-early-psychosis
  This clinic focuses on identifying and treating psychosis early, to connect people and their families with resources, and to prevent symptoms from escalating.

Videos

- "Student Panel Discusses Running Groups in Mental Health Settings" video. In this video, occupational therapy students discuss their first experience running groups for a 6-week period in a psychiatric day program. The students describe first being intimidated, but then feeling welcomed and surprised by how enjoyable and productive the groups were. They emphasize the team approach and the utility of the groups in developing their leadership skills. Access the video at the online resource center at FADavis.com.
- "Nicholas' Lived Experience of Schizophrenia" video. Nicholas is an occupational therapist living with the lived experience of schizophrenia. In this video, he describes his first episode of psychosis and the crucial role that occupational therapy played in his recovery. Nicholas emphasizes the importance of engaging with other people during rehabilitation and how, through occupational engagement, he discovered reconnection, felt loved, and found a sense of meaning and purpose. Access the video at the online resource center at FADavis.com.

References

Addington, D. (2021). The first episode psychosis services fidelity scale 1.0: Review and update. *Schizophrenia Bulletin Open, 2*(1), sgab007. https://doi.org/10.1093/schizbullopen/sgab007

Allen, C. K., Austin, S. L., David, S. K., Earhart, C. A., McCraith, D. B., & Riska-Williams, L. (2007). *Allen Cognitive Level Screen-5 (ACLS-5) and Large Allen Cognitive Level Screen-5 (LACLS-5).* ACLS and LACLS Committee. https://www.allencognitive.com/wp-content/uploads/web-13-ACLS-5-Handout-Eng1.pdf

American Occupational Therapy Association. (2020). Occupational therapy practice framework: Domain and process—Fourth edition. *American Journal of Occupational Therapy, 74*(Suppl. 2), 7412410010p1–7412410010p87 https://doi.org/10.5014/ajot.2020.74S2001

American Psychiatric Association. (2022). *Diagnostic and statistical manual of mental disorders* (5th ed., text rev.). https://doi.org/10.1176/appi.books.9780890425787

Baron, K., Kielhofner, G., Iyenger, A., Goldhammer, V., & Wolenski, J. (2006). *The Occupational Self-Assessment.* Version 2.2. Model of Human Occupation Clearinghouse, Department of Occupational Therapy, College of Applied Health Sciences, University of Illinois at Chicago.

Berendsen, S., Van, H. L, van der Paardt, J. W., de Peuter, O. R., van Bruggen, M., Nusselder, H., Jalink, M., Peen, J., Dekker, J. J. M., & de Haan, L. (2021). Exploration of symptom dimensions and duration of untreated psychosis within a staging model of schizophrenia spectrum disorders. *Early Intervention in Psychiatry, 15,* 669–675. https://doi.org/10.1111/eip.13006

Birchwood, M., Todd, P., & Jackson, C. (1998). Early intervention in psychosis: The critical period hypothesis. *International Clinical Psychopharmacology, 13*(Suppl. 1), S31–S40. https://doi.org/10.1192/S0007125000297663

Bodatsch, M., Brockhaus-Dumke, A., Klosterkotter, J., & Ruhrmann, S. (2015). Forecasting psychosis by event-related potentials—Systematic review and specific meta-analysis. *Biological Psychiatry, 77,* 951–958. https://doi.org/10.1016/j.biopsych.2014.09.025

Brown, C., Cromwell, R. L., Filion, D., Dunn, W., & Tollefson, N. (2002). Sensory processing in schizophrenia: Missing and avoiding information. *Schizophrenia Research, 55,* 187–195. https://doi.org/10.1016/s0920-9964(01)00255-9

Brown, C. E., & Dunn, W. (2002). *Adolescent/Adult Sensory Profile.* Pearson.

Calabrese, J., & Al Khalili, Y. (2022). Psychosis. In: *StatPearls.* StatPearls Publishing. https://www.ncbi.nlm.nih.gov/books/NBK546579

Correll, C. U., Galling, B., Pawar, A., Krivko, A., Bonetto, C., Ruggeri, M., Craig, T. J., Nordentoft, M., Srihari, V. H., Guloksuz, S., Hui, C. L. M., Chen, E. Y. H., Valencia, M., Juarez, F., Robinson, D. G., Schooler, N. R., Brunette, M. F., Mueser, J. T., Rosenheck, R. A., . . . Kane, J. M. (2018). Comparison of early intervention services vs treatment as usual for early-phase psychosis. *JAMA Psychiatry, 75*(6), 555–565. https://doi.org/10.1001/jamapsychiatry.2018.0623

Cross, S. P. M., Hermens, D. F., Scott, E. M., Ottavio, A., McGorry, P. D., & Hickie, I. B. (2014). A clinical staging model for early intervention youth mental health services. *Psychiatric Services, 65*(7), 939–943. https://doi.org/10.1176/appi.ps.201300221

Crumlish, N., Whitty, P., Clarke, M., Browne, S., Kamali, M., Gervin, M., McTigue, O., Kinsella, A., Waddington, J. L., Larkin, C., & O'Callaghan, E. (2009). Beyond the critical period: Longitudinal study of 8-year outcomes in first-episode non-affective psychosis. *British Journal of Psychiatry, 194*(1), 18–24. https://doi.org/10.1192/bjp.bp.107.048942

D'Amico, M. L., Jaffe, L. E., & Gardner, J. A. (2018). Evidence for interventions to improve and maintain occupational performance and participation for people with serious mental illness: A systematic review. *American Journal of Occupational Therapy,* 72(5), 7205190020p1–7205190020p11. https://doi.org/10.5014/ajot.2018.033332

de Pablo, G. S., Radua, J., Pereira, J., Bonoldi, I., Arienti, V., Besana, F., Soardo, L., Cabras, A., Fortea, L., Catalan, A., Vaquerizo-Serrano, J., Coronelli, F., Kaur, S., Da Silva, J., Shin, J. I., Solmi, M., Brondino, N., Politi, P., McGuire, P., & Fusar-Poli, P. (2021). Probability of transition to psychosis in individuals at clinical high risk: An updated meta-analysis. *JAMA Psychiatry, 78*(9), 970–978. https://doi.org/10.1001/jamapsychiatry.2021.0830

Early Assessment and Support Alliance. (2013). *EASA practice guidelines.* Portland State University.

Early Psychosis Guidelines Writing Group and EPPIC National Support Program. (2016). *Australian clinical guidelines for early psychosis* (2nd ed. updated). Orygen, The National Centre of Excellence in Youth Mental Health. https://www.orygen.org.au/Campus/Expert-Network/Resources/Free/Clinical-Practice/Australian-Clinical-Guidelines-for-Early-Psychosis.aspx

Forsyth, K., Deshpande, S., Kielhofner, G., Henriksson, C., Haglund, L., Olson, L., Skinner, S., & Kulkarni, S. (2006). *A user's manual for the Occupational Circumstances Assessment Interview and Rating Scale (OCAIRS).* Version 4.0. University of Illinois.

Frawley, E., Cowman, M., Lepage, M., & Donohoe, G. (2023). Social and occupational recovery in early psychosis: A systematic review and meta-analysis of psychosocial interventions. *Psychological Medicine, 53,* 1787–1798. https://doi.org/10.1017/S003329172100341X

Fusar-Poli, P. (2017). The clinical high-risk state for psychosis (CHR-P), version II. *Schizophrenia Bulletin, 43*(1), 44–47. https://doi.org/10.1093/schbul/sbw158

Fusar-Poli, P., Borgwardt, S., Bechdolf, A., Addington, J., Riecher-Rossler, A., Schultze-Lutter, F., Keshavan, M., Wood, S., Ruhrmann, S., Seidman, L. J., Valmaggia, L., Cannon, T., Velthorst, E., De Haan, L., Cornblatt, B., Bonoldi, I., Birchwood, M., McGlashan, T., Carpenter, W., . . .Yung, A. (2013). The psychosis high-risk state: A comprehensive state-of-the-art review. *JAMA Psychiatry, 70*(1), 107–120. https://doi.org/10.1001/jamapsychiatry.2013.269

Fusar-Poli, P., Correll, C. U., Arango, C., Berk, M., Patel, V., & Ioannidis, J. P. A. (2021). Preventive psychiatry: A blueprint for improving the mental health of young people. *World Psychiatry, 20*(2), 200–221. https://doi.org/10.1002/wps.20869

Fusar-Poli, P., de Pablo, G. S., Correll, C. U., Meyer-Lindenberg, A., Millan, M. J., Bogwardt, S., Galderisi, S., Bechdolf, A., Pfennig, A., Kessing, L. V., van Amelsvoort, T., Nieman, D. H., Dornschke, K., Krebs, M. O., Koutsouleris, N., McGuire, P., Do, K. Q., & Arango, C. (2020). Prevention of psychosis: Advances in detection, prognosis, and intervention. *JAMA Psychiatry, 77*(7), 755–765. https://doi.org/10.1001/jamapsychiatry.2019.4779

Fusar-Poli, P., McGorry, P. D., & Kane, J. M. (2017). Improving outcomes of first-episode psychosis: An overview. *World Psychiatry, 16*(3), 251–265. https://doi.org/10.1002/wps.20446

Gonzalez-Valderrama, A., Castaneda, C. P., Mena, C., Undurraga, J., Mondaca, P., Yanez, M., Bedregal, P., & Nachar, R. (2017). Duration of untreated psychosis and acute remission of negative symptoms in a South American first-episode psychosis cohort. *Early Intervention in Psychiatry, 11,* 77–82. https://doi.org/10.1111/eip.12266

Hansen, H. G., Andersen, N. K., Nordentoft, M., & Albert, N. (2023). Long-term development and outcome of early-onset psychosis. In I. Agartz & R. E. Smelror (Eds.), *Adolescent psychosis: Clinical and scientific perspectives* (pp. 299–318). Elsevier.

Harrison, L.A., Kats, A., Williams, M. E., & Aziz-Zadeh, L. (2019). The importance of sensory processing in mental health: A proposed addition to the research domain criteria (RDoC) and suggestions for RDOC 2.0. *Frontiers in Psychology, 10,* Article 103. https://doi.org/10.3389/fpsyg.2019.00103

Hickie, I. B., Scott, E. M., Hermens, D. F., Naismith, S. L., Guastella, A. J., Kaur, M., Sidis, A., Whitwell, B., Glozier, N., Davenport, T.,

Pantelis, C., Wood, S. J., & McGorry, P. D. (2013). Applying clinical staging to young people who present for mental health care. *Early Intervention in Psychiatry, 7,* 31–43. https://doi.org/10.1111/j.1751-7893.2012.00366.x

International Early Psychosis Association. (2008). *EP services: Country list.* https://iepa.org.au/services

Iwama, M. (2006). *The Kawa model: Culturally relevant occupational therapy.* Churchill Livingstone Elsevier.

Jackson, H., & McGorry, P. D. (2009). *The recognition and management of early psychosis: A preventive approach* (2nd ed.). Cambridge University Press.

Johannessen, J. O., Joa, I., Auestad, B., Haahr, U., Larsen, T. K., Melle, I., Opjordsmoen, S., Simonsen, P., Rund, B. R., Simonsen, E., Vaglum, P., Friis, S., & McGlashan, T. (2011). First-episode patients recruited into treatment via early detection teams versus ordinary pathways: Course and health service use during 5 years. *Early Intervention in Psychiatry, 5,* 70–75. https://doi.org/10.1111/j.1751-7893.2010.00201.x

Kane, J. M., Robinson, D. G., Schooler, N. R., Mueser, K. T., Penn, D. L., Rosenheck, R. A., Addington, J., Brunette, M. F., Correll, C. U., Estroff, S. E., Marcy, P., Robinson, J., Meyer-Kalos, P. S., Gottlieb, J. D., Glynn, S. M., Lynde, D. W., Pipes, R., Kurian, B. T., Miller, A. L., . . . Heinssen, R. K. (2016). Comprehensive versus usual community care for first-episode psychosis: 2-year outcomes from the NIMH RAISE early treatment program. *American Journal of Psychiatry, 173*(4), 362–372. https://doi.org/10.1176/appi.ajp.2015.15050632

Keshavan, M. S., Haas, G., Miewald, J., Montrose, D. M., Reddy, R., Schooler, N. R., & Sweeney, J. A. (2003). Prolonged untreated illness duration from prodromal onset predicts outcome in first episode psychosis. *Schizophrenia Bulletin, 29,* 757–769. https://doi.org/10.1093/oxfordjournals.schbul.a007045

Kielhofner, G., Mallinson, T., Crawford, C., Nowak, M., Rigby, M., Henry, A., & Walens, D. (2004). *The Occupational Performance History Interview-II (OPHI-II).* Version 2.1. University of Illinois.

Krupa, T., Woodside, H., & Pocock, K. (2010). Activity and social participation in the period following a first episode of psychosis and implications for occupational therapy. *British Journal of Occupational Therapy, 73*(1), 13–20. https://doi.org/10.4276/030802210X12629548272

Law, M., Baptiste, S., Carswell, A., Mccoll, M. A., Polatajko, H., & Pollock, N. (2005). *Canadian Occupational Performance Measure.* (4th ed.). Canadian Association of Occupational Therapists.

Lilford, P., Bimalka, O., Rajapakshe, W., & Singh, S. P. (2020). A systematic review of care pathways for psychosis in low-and middle-income countries. *Asian Journal of Psychiatry, 54,* 102237. https://doi.org/10.1016/j.ajp.2020.102237

Lloyd, C., Bassett, J., & Samra, P. (2000). Rehabilitation programmes for early psychosis. *The British Journal of Occupational Therapy, 63*(2), 76–82. https://doi.org/10.1177/030802260006300205

Lloyd, C., Waghorn, G., Williams, P. L., Harris, M. G., & Capra, C. (2008). Early psychosis: Treatment issues and the role of occupational therapy. *The British Journal of Occupational Therapy, 71*(7), 297–304. https://doi.org/10.1177/030802260807100708

McClellan, J. (2018). Psychosis in children and adolescents. *Journal of the American Academy of Child & Adolescent Psychiatry, 57*(5), 308–312. https://doi.org/10.1016/j.jaac.2018.01.021

McFarlane, W. R. (2002). *Multi-family groups in the treatment of severe psychiatric disorders.* Guilford Press.

McFarlane, W. R. (2011). Prevention of the first episode of psychosis. *Psychiatric Clinics of North America, 34*(1), 95–107. https://doi.org/10.1016/j.psc.2010.11.012

McGlashan, T. H., Walsh, B. C., & Woods, S. W. (2014). *The psychosis risk syndrome: Handbook for diagnosis and follow-up.* Oxford University Press.

McGorry, P. D. (2014, November 19). *Preventive strategies in emerging mental disorders in young people: Clinical staging and translational research.* Presented at the 9th International Conference on Early Psychosis—(2014). *The International Journal of Neuropsychopharmacology, 17,* 2.

McGorry, P. D. (2015). Early intervention in psychosis: Obvious, effective, overdue. *The Journal of Nervous and Mental Disease, 203*(5), 310–318. https://doi.org/10.1097/NMD.0000000000000284

McGorry, P. D., Dodd, S., Purcell, R., Yung, A., Thompson, A., Goldstone, S., & Killackey, E. (2010). *Australian clinical guidelines for early psychosis* (2nd ed.). Orygen, The National Centre of Excellence in Youth Mental Health.

McGorry, P. D., Hickie, I. B., Yung, A. R., Pantelis, C., & Jackson, H. J. (2006). Clinical staging of psychiatric disorders: A heuristic framework for choosing earlier, safer, and more effective interventions. *Australian and New Zealand Journal of Psychiatry, 40*(8), 616–622. https://doi.org/10.1080/j.1440-1614.2006.01860.x

Melton, R. P., Roush, S. N., Sale, T. G., Wolf, R. M., Usher, C. T., Rodriguez, C. L., & McGorry, P. D. (2013). Early intervention and prevention of long-term disability in youth and adults: The EASA model. In K. Yeager, D. Cutler, D. Svendsen, & G. M. Sills (Eds.), *Modern community mental health: An interdisciplinary approach* (pp. 256–275). Oxford University Press.

Ober, J. L., Newbury, R. S., & Lape, J. E. (2022). The dynamic use of the Kawa model: A scoping review. *The Open Journal of Occupational Therapy, 10*(2), 1–12. https://doi.org/10.15453/2168-6408.1952

O'Brien Cannon, A. C., Caporino, N. E., O'Brien, M. P., Miklowitz, D. J., Addington, J. M., & Cannon, T. D. (2023). Family communication and the efficacy of family focused therapy in individuals at clinical high risk for psychosis with comorbid anxiety. *Early Intervention in Psychiatry, 17*(3), 281–289. https://doi.org/10.1111/eip.13326

Oluwoye, O., Davis, B., Kuhney, F. S., & Anglin, D. M. (2021). Systematic review of pathways to care in the U.S. for Black individuals with early psychosis. *NPJ Schizophrenia, 7,* Article 58. https://doi.org/10.1038/s41537-021-00185-w

Orygen Youth Health. (n.d.). *Principles.* http://oyh.org.au/about-us/principles

Parham, L. D., Roush, S., Downing, D. T., Michael, P. G., & McFarlane, W. R. (2019). Sensory characteristics of youth at clinical high risk for psychosis. *Early Intervention in Psychiatry, 13*(2), 264–271. https://doi.org/10.1111/eip.12475

Pfeiffer, B., Brusilovskiy, E., Bauer, J., & Salzer, M. S. (2014). Sensory processing, participation, and recovery in adults with serious mental illnesses. *Psychiatric Rehabilitation Journal, 37,* 289–296. https://doi.org/10.1037/prj0000099

Puntis, S., Minichino, A., De Crescenzo, F., Harrison, R., Cipriani, A., & Lennox, B. (2020). Specialised early intervention teams for recent-onset psychosis (review). *Cochrane Database of Systematic Reviews, 11*(11), CD013288. https://doi.org/10.1002/14651858.CD013288.pub2

Read, H., Roush, S., & Downing, D. (2018). Early intervention in mental health for adolescents and young adults: A systematic review. *American Journal of Occupational Therapy, 72,* 7205190040p1–7205190040p8. https://doi.org/10.5014/ajot.2018.033118

Roush, S., Parham, D., Downing, D., & Michael, P. (2014, November). *Sensory characteristics of youth at clinical high risk for psychosis.* Poster presented at the 9th International Conference on Early Psychosis—To the New Horizon, Tokyo, Japan.

Sage, M. G. (Ed.). (2019). *EASA team manual.* EASA Center for Excellence. https://easacommunity.org/wp-content/uploads/2024/05/EASA-Team-Manual.pdf

Shaikh, M., Dutta, A., Broome, M. R., Vozmediano, A. G., Ranlund, S., Diez, A., Caseiro, O., Lappin, J., Amankwa, S., Carletti, F., Fusar-Poli, P., Walshe, M., Hall, M.-H., Howes, O., Ellett, L., Murray, R. M., McGuire, P., Valmaggia, L., & Bramon, E. (2015). Sensory gating deficits in the attenuated psychosis syndrome. *Schizophrenia Research, 161,* 277–282. https://doi.org/10.1016/j.schres.2014.12.021

Sun, D., Phillips, L., Velakoulis, D., Yung, A., McGorry, P. D., Wood, S. J., van Erp, T. G., Thompson, P. M., Toga, A. W.,

Cannon, T. D., & Pantelis, C. (2009). Progressive brain structural changes mapped as psychosis develops in "at risk" individuals. *Schizophrenia Research, 108,* 85–92. https://doi.org/10.1016/j.schres.2008.11.026

Taylor, R. R. (2017). *Kielhofner's Model of Human Occupation* (5th ed.). Lippincott Williams, & Wilkins.

Toglia, J. P. (1993). *Contextual Memory Test.* Therapy Skill Builders.

Wen, V. (n.d.). *Occupational therapy manual.* https://easacommunity.org/pro-resource/ot-mental-health-assessment

Worthington, M. A., & Cannon, T. D. (2021). Prediction and prevention in the clinical high-risk for psychosis paradigm: A review of the current status and recommendations for future directions of inquiry. *Frontiers in Psychiatry, 12,* 770774. https://doi.org/10.3389/fpsyt.2021.770774

Xu, L., Guao, Y., Cao, Q., Li, X., Mei, T., Ma, Z., Tang, X, Ji, Z., Yang, L., & Liu, J. (2020). Predictors of outcome in early onset schizophrenia: A 10-year follow-up study. *BMC Psychiatry, 20,* Article 67. https://doi.org/10.1186/s12888-020-2484-x

Karen Rebeiro Gruhl

Adults and youth who experience a mental health or substance use disorder need not be destined to dismal prognoses and futures. Many go on to live full lives, often with limited or no professional intervention. Diagnoses are not a reason for hopelessness—people can and do recover! Individuals who have recovered from a mental illness or addiction have unique insights into what was most helpful to them on their journey, and in the mental health system of care. In her seminal paper, Patricia Deegan (1988) candidly wrote about her experiences within the mental health system and described recovery as a process of moving beyond a state of dependency upon the system and toward a state of being empowered, hopeful, and self-determined regarding one's prognosis and future.

Deegan (2001) also articulated aspects of professional care that got in the way of her recovery. Specifically, she wrote about a lack of hopefulness on the part of the health provider, an almost exclusive focus on illness and diagnostic labels to inform care, and the continued (over)reliance on experts, rather than people determining the care that was best for them and their future recovery pathway. Unfortunately, occupational therapy practitioners (OTPs) have been complicit in illness-centered models of care in the past (Rebeiro Gruhl, 2005). Also see Chapter 2: Recovery and Wraparound Models. 🤝

Contributing to the **recovery** process are **peer support workers** and peer-led programs and services. It is important to note at the onset of this chapter that peers contribute a different knowledge and perspective than OTPs—equally valid and important, but different. This chapter describes types of peer-led models of service, their benefits, evidence supporting their work, and some of the current challenges faced by peer support workers in a stand-alone peer service or as an integrated service within mainstream mental health programs. The chapter also provides an historical context for the development and growth of peer-led services.

Most of the examples of programs and organizations described in this chapter have been developed and led by people who have a mental health or substance use disorder and their families who support them. Some have been collaboratively developed with an OTP. One such program is highlighted because of the involvement of an occupational therapist in its program development; this individual currently remains involved in collaborative research with this peer-led program (Rebeiro et al., 2001; Rebeiro Gruhl et al., 2021).

Why should OTPs be interested in **peer support** and **peer-led services**? For starters, peer support is an evolving occupation facing exponential growth. Peer support workers will undoubtedly become an OTP colleague at some point in

their careers. Second, peer support faces some growing pains as they assert their place within the continuum of mental health services. Third, peer support workers, as an evolving occupation, continue to experience some degree of stigma and discrimination within the health-care arena from other providers—and they need strong allies!

OTPs, because of their focus on occupation and interest in egalitarian, collaborative relationships with people who experience mental health and substance use disorders, are natural allies for peer support workers and their peer-led services. OTPs may collaborate with peer support workers in the design, delivery, and evaluation of peer-led service models to support their value to mental health systems. Roles and opportunities for OTPs to support peer support workers and peer-led services have been described elsewhere (Bibyk et al., 1999; Rebeiro et al., 2001; Rebeiro Gruhl et al., 2021; Swarbrick & Pratt, 2006; Wright & Rebeiro, 2003) and are further detailed later in this chapter, including roles in consultation, instrumental support, research, advocacy, and program development.

Historical Context

Peer-led services have their own history, tracing the evolution of mutual support and service user empowerment over at least two centuries (Ansell & Insley, 2013; Ostrow & Adams, 2012). According to Martin and Associates (2016), significant changes have occurred within the peer support movement in Canada and globally, wherein peer support has shifted from "an alternative to mental health services to a recognized best practice and recommended element of mainstream mental health services" (p. 1). The expansion of peer-led services began when peer leaders formed networks and groups to advocate for changes in the mental health system, paralleling other civil rights advocacy efforts in the 1970s (Chamberlain, 1978; Clay, 2005).

The mental health consumer-survivor (peer) movement was organized by people with lived experience who were largely dissatisfied with the existing mental health service system, which they viewed as paternalistic and lacking in a range of options and opportunities (Deegan, 1988; Rebeiro, 1999). The collective efforts of mental health service users, their families, and their allies continue to transform federal and state mental health systems both at home and globally. An overview of the key historical points that have defined occupational therapy's role across the mental health continuum is provided in Chapter 1: Occupational Therapy Practice Across the Mental Health Continuum. 🤝

Overview of Peer-Led Services

Peer-led services were developed based on the key recommendations of the Mental Health Commission of Canada's Workforce Advisory Committee (Cyr et al., 2016) and were highlighted as a way to transform the mental health system in Canada. The concept of "peer" typically refers to someone belonging to the same or similar social group especially based on age, grade, or status (Merriam-Webster Dictionary, n.d.). For example, a student might refer to their classmates as their peers. Among this group, some of their peers might offer reliable, tangible support that the student draws strength from, whereas others might not be as supportive. Although the student's professor also provides reliable, tangible supports, that individual is not the student's peer.

In mental health settings, people who identify with the title of peer do so precisely because they have their own lived experiences in recovery from a mental illness. Lived experience provides peers with an empathy for others as a basis of the relationship, an inclination to listen versus providing advice or judgment, a personal interest to support others in managing the struggles of living with a mental illness and their recovery, and experience in navigating the mental health system.

A key foundational concept in peer-led service models is that support for recovery is provided by peers who have experienced recovery themselves. In peer-led models, support for recovery is offered by someone who has personal lived experiences with a mental health or a substance use disorder; who has experience using community, social, and clinical resources; and who has the capacity to connect with others in an egalitarian relationship that has the potential to foster growth and learning (Bibyk et al., 1999; Repper & Carter, 2011).

Underlying Concepts

Peer-led services are based on the premise of *people in recovery helping others* pursue their recovery. A basic underlying belief of peer support is that peers foster hope in the potential for recovery. This is because people who have similar experiences can relate to one another, and peers who are doing well provide a living role model of the potential of recovery to others (Rebeiro Gruhl et al., 2016).

Peer-led services may be offered before, during, or after treatment provided by mental health professionals, or collaboratively with nonpeers to facilitate long-term recovery in the community. The following list paraphrases work by Cronise and coworkers (2016, p. 215), who reported that peer-led services in the United States are offered in a variety of settings, are extensive, and may include the following:

- Community and/or peer-run programs (e.g., community support programs, recovery centers, peer-run organizations, or drop-in centers)
- Outpatient mental health and substance abuse treatment settings (e.g., day treatment, outpatient clinics, or assertive community treatment)
- Inpatient mental health and substance abuse treatment settings (e.g., acute inpatient units, detox facilities, emergency departments (EDs), and residential rehabilitation programs)
- Less restrictive residential settings (e.g., assisted living programs, supported housing, and programs for populations that are homeless)
- More restrictive residential settings (e.g., skilled nursing facilities, residential programs, and group homes)
- Precrisis and crisis settings (e.g., mobile crisis units, peer crisis centers or crisis respite centers, EDs, and warm lines)
- Employment or educational settings (e.g., supported employment and supported educational programs in schools, universities, or the workplace)
- Criminal justice settings from more restrictive settings (e.g., forensic mental health units and jails to less restrictive settings including mental health or substance abuse courts)
- Varied other locations (e.g., primary care settings, independent practice, government/state offices or agencies, or health insurance companies)

The term "peer-led services" also indicates that people in recovery provide a leadership role in the development, control, and provision of services. Peers may aid in developing coping and problem-solving strategies for illness self-management—drawing on their lived experiences and empathy to promote hope, insights, and the development of skills. Peers may also help to link individuals with supports in the community to help them develop support networks beyond the mental health system. However, increasingly, the peer community has raised concerns that peer services within mainstream mental health systems are drifting from their foundational roots and are being required to provide more generic tasks that detract from authentic peer support (Mulvale et al., 2019; Rebeiro Gruhl et al., 2023; Watson, 2017).

Rebeiro Gruhl and colleagues (2023) found that the social location of peer-led services was related to whether or not peers practiced authentically—that is, in harmony with their core values. Peer-led services are based on the core concepts summarized in Table 39-1, many of which parallel principles and values of the profession of occupational therapy.

Stakeholders

People who are directly, and sometimes indirectly, impacted by peer-led services are considered stakeholders. In the context of this chapter, stakeholders are individuals with a vested interest in developing, implementing, and evaluating peer-led services. There are many stakeholders including the people using the services, the people who care about them, service providers and administrators ensuring service delivery, the funders of those services (often government and, by extension, taxpayers), policymakers, and researchers who evaluate service quality and outcomes.

However, two of the most directly affected stakeholder groups are people in recovery and their family supporters. Historically, these two stakeholder groups have been largely excluded from the process of service design, delivery, and evaluation. The inclusion of these voices adds an important perspective—ensuring that services are relevant, meaningful, and effective. A growing cohort of stakeholders, including individuals with mental health and substance use disorders, caregivers, and family members, have become influential leaders in designing and delivering peer-led models

TABLE 39-1 | Key Concepts in Peer-Led Services

Concept	Description
Peer support is voluntary.	• People using peer support services participate according to their own volition, rather than being required or coerced to attend. • Service users are not required to take medications or attend traditional service programs to participate.
Peer support is person driven.	• The person using the services sets the goals and has some choice over what issues to address, if any, and how best to address them. • This concept reflects a philosophy of empowerment and the ethical principle of **autonomy**, indicating that people have the right to make decisions about the things that affect them directly. • Peers understand from their **lived experience** that truly effective helpers explore a person's internal motivation, and support the person's desires, rather than trying to persuade or coerce someone to do what others think needs to be done.
Peer supporters are hopeful and open-minded.	• Peer-led services are optimistic and based on a heartfelt and deep-seated belief that "recovery is real." • Recognizing that each recovery journey is unique, peer-led services often consider whatever approaches might benefit the people using services, rather than prescribing standard interventions based on diagnosis.
Peer support is strengths focused.	• The emphasis of peer-led services is on the individual's strengths and competencies. • The focus is not on symptoms or remediating impairments, but on quality of life. • The peer neither diagnoses nor provides therapy.
Peer supporters facilitate change.	• Peer service providers and peer-led organizations are invested in transforming mental health service systems in ways that promote recovery and empowerment. • The role of change agent is an important aspect of peer services.

International Association of Peer Supporters. (2013). National practice guidelines for peer supporters. *https://inaops.org/national-standards*

of service (e.g., Cyr et al., 2016—see Chamberlain, 1978 and Deegan, 2001). These individual stakeholders have transformed their own lives and the mental health service delivery system to address the social, emotional, occupational, and other practical needs of individuals with mental health and substance use disorders. The voices of these pioneer stakeholders continue to be a force in the evolution of peer-led services.

Peer Support

Peer support is a way of giving and receiving help, based on the "key principles of respect, shared responsibility, and mutual agreement of what is helpful" (Mead et al., 2001, p. 6). More recently, Rebeiro Gruhl and colleagues (2016) defined peer support as "work that draws upon one's lived experience and the therapeutic use of self, is reciprocal and mutually beneficial, and is led by the recipient of peer services" (p. 5). People using mental health or substance use services (and their family supporters) often provide each other with support and fellowship and have long shared coping strategies and resources. Increasingly, the impact that peer relationships can have on sustaining recovery is being recognized and, in many countries, formalized and integrated into mental health services (Cyr et al., 2016; Davidson et al., 2012).

Some peer support programs are grassroots groups that operate without public funding. Descriptions of peer support practices can be found in Australia (Franke et al., 2010), Canada (Cyr et al., 2016), the United Kingdom (Repper, 2013), New Zealand (Scott et al., 2011), and Scandinavian countries (Castelein et al., 2008). Practice guidelines and

training procedures for peer supporters are available in the United States (Daniels et al., 2010), Canada (Peer Support Accreditation and Certification Canada, 2016), and internationally (Creamer et al., 2012). Efforts to clarify the role of peer support workers include a list of competencies (Substance Abuse and Mental Health Services Administration [SAMHSA], n.d.) and the development of formal peer specialist certification programs (Kaufman et al., 2014).

Peer support specialists have received training on how to inspire and support others in one-to-one connections using shared experiences. In order to access training and become certified, a person must have been in recovery for some time and must have learned enough from that experience to be able to use it in a way that will support others. Serving as a role model for others, and often collaborating with nonpeer colleagues, peer specialists can support recovery-oriented programs. Many countries have defined the core competencies expected of peer support staff, such as those listed in Table 39-2. Across nations, these competencies consistently reflect core values of being recovery-oriented, person-centered, and trauma-informed.

Peer support services can enhance or complement professional services, including occupational therapy. Peers can help to support by being a mentor, coach, or peer resource specialist—not serve as a counselor, case manager, sponsor, or therapist. Terms of reference are also important and align with the consumer-survivor movement mentioned earlier. Hence, supports are provided to a peer, mentee, or member—not to a client, consumer or patient. The language used in peer support reflects the nature of the helping relationship. A focus on terminology is important, as language both reflects and influences attitudes.

TABLE 39-2 | Core Competencies for Peer Support Workers

Competency	Critical Behaviors
Interpersonal Relations and Communication	Interacts respectfully, honors the dignity of others, and demonstrates acceptance and respect by listening without judgment, adjusts to meet the situation, and uses recovery and strengths-based language.
Shares Lived Experiences of Recovery	Demonstrates nonjudgmental empathy and selectively self-discloses own lived experiences, knowing when to share and when to listen.
Links to Resources and Supports	Supports others to connect with behavioral health and community supports, resources, and services that support their recovery.
Critical Thinking	Looks at issues from multiple perspectives and helps peers consider implications of decisions and possible consequences of taking various options.
Hope	Expresses confidence in peer's success in recovery and models realistic optimism.
Self-Management and Resiliency	Recognizes signs of distress, stays calm, and diffuses stressful situations; encourages and models self-care and stress management practices.
Flexibility and Adaptability	Maintains an open attitude that accepts ambiguity and adjusts behavior to situation.
Self-Awareness and Confidence	Is reflective and considers how their thoughts and actions can influence behaviors and interacts in a self-confident manner.
Initiative and Commitment	Demonstrates dependability, carries through on commitments to complete tasks, and recognizes when to seek insight or assistance from others.
Teamwork	Cooperates and collaborates; shares their knowledge, ideas, and experiences while also respecting the roles and experiences of other team members.
Continuous Learning and Development	Remains curious, defines areas for personal growth and development, and engages in opportunities for skill development.

Adapted from Peer Support Canada. (n.d.). Peer supporter competencies. *https://peersupportcanada.ca/wp-content/uploads/2019/06/Peer_Supporter_Competencies-ENG.pdf; Substance Abuse and Mental Health Services Administration. (2015).* Core competencies for peer workers in behavioral health services. *https://www.samhsa.gov/sites/default/files/programs_campaigns/brss_tacs/core-competencies_508_12_13_18.pdf*

PhotoVoice

Mary from S.I.D.E.

I am vice president of the board of S.I.D.E. which stands for socialization, interdependence, development, empowerment. Being part of the organization has been a successful feeling. S.I.D.E. is a consumer-led organization for members diagnosed with a mental illness. S.I.D.E. to me is a place where I feel I totally belong. S.I.D.E. provides leadership skills, educational skills, and fun activities such as Halloween, Christmas, and the Super Bowl gatherings. A lot of members have no family for celebrations during the year. So S.I.D.E. compensates for the lack of family gatherings. I feel fortunate to be a member of a wonderful consumer-led organization that deeply cares about its members.

—Mary

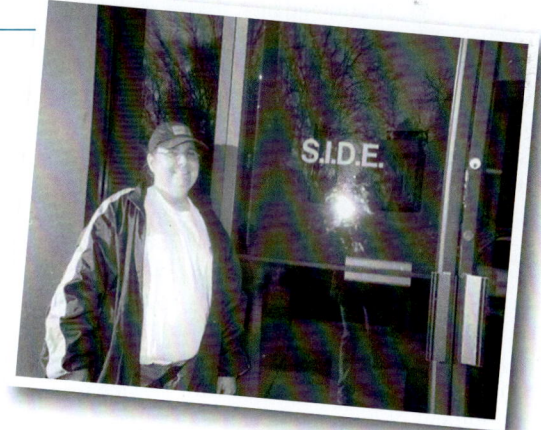

Consider Mary's words from a Person-Environment-Organization (PEO) perspective. How might her involvement with this consumer-led organization impact her as a person? What opportunities might this environment provide?

Are there specific occupations that become available for Mary because of her participation in this setting?

Underlying Evidence

There is a growing body of literature describing the benefits of peer-led services in the behavioral health and the addictions field, as well as for people living with various other medical conditions (Bellamy et al., 2017). The Northern Initiative for Social Action (NISA) is a peer-led program that has been extensively studied. Research has demonstrated positive impacts of peer-led services on the lives of persons with lived experience seeking services, those peer support workers providing services, and the mental health system in general (Rebeiro Gruhl et al., 2021).

Much of the contemporary research on peer support has highlighted the importance of peer-led services to the empowerment, self-efficacy, and recovery of persons with a lived experience of mental illness (Mahlke et al., 2017; Rebeiro Gruhl et al., 2016; Rooney et al., 2016; Taylor et al., 2018). The literature has also shown that peer support provides a complementary service to mainstream mental health providers (Bellamy et al., 2017; Chien et al., 2019; Pitt et al., 2013;

Walker & Bryant, 2013; Watson, 2017; White et al., 2020; Wrobleski et al., 2015), fulfills an important gap in the provision of emotional support or affective labor (Voronka, 2017), and in rural contexts, facilitates rural mental health help-seeking behavior (Cheesmond et al., 2020).

The evidence about peer support is not limited to qualitative studies. Although Lloyd-Evans and colleagues (2014) found peer services to be less effective on hospitalization rates, overall symptoms, and satisfaction with services, many peer support workers suggest these to be more system-driven than peer-driven outcomes of interest (Watson, 2017). In contrast, Cyr and colleagues (2016) reported on a robust and growing research base that shows peer support to be associated with reductions in hospitalizations for mental health problems, reductions in symptom distress, improvements in social support, and improvements in quality of life. Mahlke and colleagues (2017) conducted a randomized clinical trial using trained peer support workers to evaluate 1:1 peer support as compared with usual treatment, and reported several positive outcomes. They identified that one-to-one peer support delivered by trained peer supporters can improve self-efficacy of people with severe mental illnesses over a 1-year period.

Otte and colleagues (2020a) reported beneficial effects of peer support to include less professional distance, more time for one-on-one attendance, and a role model for recovery. Mental health professionals participating in the study reported that peer support added a new perspective to the team, improved continuity in treatment offers, and was helpful in preserving a respectful tone in team meetings within mental health services (Otte et al., 2020a). And a systematic review conducted by Cabassa et al. (2017) identified that the more promising peer-led interventions for persons with serious mental illness were self-management of health conditions and peer-navigator interventions. Yet, despite the documented benefits of peer support to mental health systems, studies reveal that peer support workers remain underutilized in formal mental health systems because of a variety of barriers and influences on the implementation of their role (Otte et al., 2020b)—potentially limiting the full participation of peer-led services in the mental health workforce (Gillard et al., 2017; Mirbahaeddin & Chreim, 2022; Watson, 2017).

Occupational therapy research on peer support and led services includes collaboration with service users in the redevelopment of a peer drop-in/self-help group into a peer-led community wellness center (Swarbrick & Duffy, 2000), and in the development of a peer-run, occupation-based mental health program (Rebeiro et al., 2001; Rebeiro Gruhl et al., 2021). Occupational therapy researchers have worked collaboratively with peer members of a community wellness center to identify sensory preferences of members (Gardner, Swarbrick, Kearns et al., 2017); understand how one's physical limitations affect occupational functioning (Gardner, Swarbrick, Ackerman et al., 2017), sleep habits, and routines (Gardner et al., 2021); and evaluate a financial management program (Gardner et al., 2019).

Occupational therapist Rebeiro Gruhl remains involved in participatory action research with a peer-led organization in program evaluation (Rebeiro Gruhl et al., 2018; Rebeiro Gruhl et al., 2020) and in investigating the benefits and challenges of peer support work within mainstream mental health systems (Rebeiro Gruhl et al., 2016; Rebeiro Gruhl et al., 2023).

Types of Peer-Led Services

Peer-led services encompass a wide variety of service types. Some are offered within a traditionally funded and structured mental health service agency that was founded and run by nonpeer-credentialed professionals. Other peer-led services are part of a peer-led organization, defined as "an incorporated, independent nonprofit organization or a nonincorporated organization that operates independently from a parent organization; at least 51% of the board of directors or advisory board are peers; the director is a peer; and most staff members or volunteers are peers" (Ostrow & Leaf, 2014, p. 240).

Although advocacy groups and organizations have been an important part of the history of the peer movement and could be considered a type of peer-led service, this section focuses on direct peer-led service models. Similarly, policy, research, and evaluation efforts—such as participatory action research (PAR)—led or co-led by peers (Rebeiro Gruhl et al., 2021; Rogers & Delman, 2014; Roush et al., 2015) are not examples of direct services. They are, however, an important component of a recovery-oriented service system that ensures active stakeholder involvement and that the perspectives of service users are heard.

Four types of peer-led services are described here, although others may cluster peer-led services differently. Examples of each type of peer-led service are provided as well as a few suggestions for how OTPs might engage with them. Peer-led services may be categorized as follows:

- Self-help: individual and groups
- Peer community-based services
- Peer-professional partnerships
- Peer-led organizations

Self-Help: Individual and Groups

Self-help support groups are also known as **mutual-aid** or **mutual-help support groups** because the primary dynamic is peers helping one another. Self-help is based on the idea that people facing the same problem learn from and support one another when they share their experiences and strengths within an understanding and nonjudgmental community of peers.

The term "self-help support group" has been used to distinguish member-run support groups from professionally run support groups. Self-help groups are a valuable source of ongoing support, education, and connection to a community for people in recovery. Group meetings are typically held outside the publicly funded mental health system and located in informal local community settings. In addition to being centrally located, these groups are also financially accessible because they typically have no fees and minimal, if any, dues. Groups can serve as bridges to professional treatment through provision of referral information from peers; alternately, OTPs may want to link people they are working with to self-help for ongoing support beyond occupational therapy.

Evidence-Based Practice

Benefits of Mental Health Peer Support

Research highlights OTPs as important allies to peer support workers.

RESEARCH FINDINGS

The wide array of peer-led supports and services described in this chapter are supported by evidence-based research and promising practices. Peer support, as an occupation, continues to evolve as this chapter is written—as does the research in its support.

The demonstrated benefits of receiving mental health peer support include increased engagement in services and reductions in hospital admissions and ED use (Bellamy et al., 2017). Much of the contemporary research on peer support has highlighted the importance of peer-led services to addressing gaps within the mental health system and to the empowerment, self-efficacy, hope, and recovery of persons with lived experience of mental illness (Mahlke et al., 2017; Rebeiro Gruhl et al., 2016; Rooney et al., 2016; Taylor et al., 2018).

A systematic review conducted by Cabassa and colleagues (2017) identified that the more promising peer-led interventions for persons with serious mental illness were self-management of health conditions and peer-navigator interventions. Longitudinal research on peer-led warm line services shows positive impacts on primary physician contact, accessing social and leisure occupations, and socialization (Dalgin et al., 2018). This research also underscores the complexity of psychiatric recovery and the critical role that peer support may play.

APPLICATIONS

➡ Research highlights OTPs as important allies to peer support workers.
➡ The occupational therapy profession is well suited to collaborating with peer support workers and within peer-led services.
➡ OTPs need to be mindful of the role and scope of peer support, the importance of creating egalitarian relationships with peer support workers/specialists, and the need for mutual respect for the knowledge each brings to the table.

REFERENCES

Bellamy, C., Schmutte, T., & Davidson, L. (2017). An update on the growing evidence base for peer support. *Mental Health and Social Inclusion, 21*(3), 161–167. https://doi.org/10.1108/MHSI-03-2017-0014

Cabassa, L. J., Camacho, D., Vélez-Grau, C. M., & Stefancic, A. (2017). Peer-based health interventions for people with serious mental illness: A systematic literature review. *Journal of Psychiatric Research, 84*, 80–89. https://doi.org/10.1016/j.jpsychires.2016.09.021

Dalgin, R. S., Dalgin, M. H., & Metzger, S. J. (2018). A longitudinal analysis of the influence of a peer-run Warm Line phone service on psychiatric recovery. *Community Mental Health Journal, 54*(4), 376–382. https://doi.org/10.1007/s10597-017-0161-4

Mahlke, C. I., Priebe, S., Heumann, K., Daubmann, A., Wegscheider, K., & Bock, T. (2017). Effectiveness of one-to-one peer support for patients with severe mental illness—A randomized controlled trial. *European Psychiatry: The Journal of the Association of European Psychiatrists, 42*, 103–110. https://doi.org/10.1016/j.eurpsy.2016.12.007

Rebeiro Gruhl, K. L., Lacarte, S., & Calixte, S. (2016). Authentic peer support: Challenges to an evolving occupation. *Journal of Mental Health, 25*(1), 78–86. https://doi.org/10.3109/09638237.2015.1057322

Rooney, J., Miles, N., & Barker, T. (2016). Patients' views: Peer support worker on inpatient wards. *Mental Health and Social Inclusion, 20*(3), 160–166. https://doi.org/10.1108/MHSI-02-2016-0007

Taylor, A., Dorer, G., & Gleeson, K. (2018). Evaluation of a peer support specialist led group. *Mental Health and Social Inclusion, 22*(3), 141–148. https://doi.org/10.1108/MHSI-03-2018-0012

A significant number and variety of member-run self-help groups have evolved since the formation of Alcoholics Anonymous (AA) in 1935 (AA, 2024) and Recovery Inc., in 1937 (Recovery International, 2017). Self-help groups have become an important means of providing a cost-effective adjunct to the traditional mental health service system. They are widely available for a variety of challenging life experiences, including many serious illnesses, addictions, disabilities, bereavement situations, abuse experiences, parenting problems, and other stressful life problems.

Peer-led, mutual-aid, self-help initiatives have continued to evolve in mental health and include, but are not limited

PhotoVoice

NISA Staff Having Fun

What I get out of NISA is equally essential, is to feel that I belong, that I have a social existence. The belongingness here has been very much at the heart of things for me. If I don't feel like I belong, then I can't begin anywhere. If I don't belong, I don't exist.

—NISA Member

Based on the image, the quote, and the content in this chapter, what kinds of things help facilitate a sense of belonging in peer-led services?

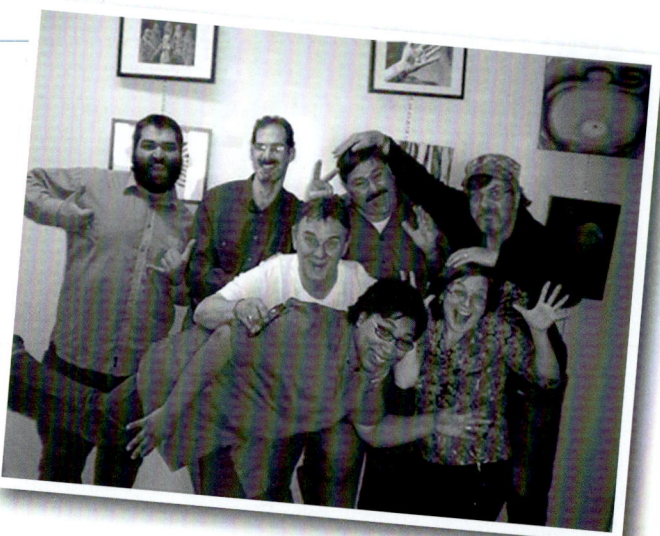

to, the following: *Wellness Recovery Action Plans* (WRAP; Advocates for Human Potential, Inc., 2016), Schizophrenics Anonymous (National Schizophrenia Foundation, n.d.), the Depression and Bipolar Support Alliance (DBSA; 2016), GROW (GROW in America, n.d.), Double Trouble in Recovery (Vogel, 2010), Dual Diagnosis Anonymous (DDA; n.d.); Hearing Voices Network (Hearing Voices Network–USA, n.d.), and many local, independent grassroots groups.

Some peer-led self-help services are provided on an as-needed basis for individuals at drop-in centers, or more formally through ongoing or structured groups. In these settings, people can "drop-in" at times of their choosing. Collaborative Support Programs of New Jersey Inc. (CSPNJ, 2024) is a peer-led not-for-profit organization that provides flexible, community-based services that promote responsibility, recovery, and wellness through the provision of community wellness centers, supportive and respite housing, human rights advocacy, and educational and innovative programs for people with the lived experience of behavioral health conditions. The text that follows provides a few examples of the many existing peer self-help groups available.

Boothroyd and Fisher (2010) have promoted peer support globally as a key part of health, health care, and prevention. Initially focused on diabetes, **Peers for Progress** (Peersforprogress.org) has expanded to include mental health and a variety of complex health conditions. The mission of Peers for Progress is to accelerate the availability of best practices in peer support, which is done by conducting and disseminating research, creating networks to share knowledge and experience, and advocating for more peer support services.

Online self-help support groups have also proliferated. Many of these online mutual support networks were developed independently over the years by persons with lived experience. The website www.self.com provides some examples; readers may search for those close to where they live and work. Support groups are gatherings of people (virtually or in real life [IRL]) who share common ground in some way, and can offer emotional support to one another. Participants may share a similar experience or they may share a common identity.

OTPs can search for support groups at https://heypeers.com, which curates support groups from the National Alliance on Mental Illness (NAMI) and oneMind.org. Online self-help networks eliminate many of the barriers that limit people from participating in community-based groups (e.g., lack of any local support group, a lack of transportation, or a need for day care).

Some peer-led self-help groups are time-limited and educational in nature. Using a peer-led group format, peers meet to acquire new information or gain new skills related to recovery and advocacy. Educational programs may provide a more informal sharing of information or courses that follow an established curriculum, such as the WRAP.

The **Wellness Recovery Action Plan (WRAP)** is a simple and powerful tool designed for creating the life and wellness an individual desires for themselves. WRAP was founded in Vermont in 1997, developed by peers for peers, and is now recognized as an evidence-based practice (Cook et al., 2010). WRAP is globally regarded as an important tool for addressing many of life's issues, not just those pertaining to mental health. Learn more about WRAP at www.wellnessrecoveryactionplan.com.

Another example is the *National Alliance on Mental Illness (NAMI) Family-to-Family* program. The *NAMI Family-to-Family* program is a free, 12-session, evidence-based educational program for families, partners, and friends of individuals diagnosed with a mental illness (Mercado et al., 2016; NAMI, 2017). The course is designed to facilitate a better understanding of mental health conditions, increase coping skills, and empower participants to become advocates for their family members. *NAMI Family-to-Family* is taught by NAMI-trained family members who have firsthand experience with a family member with a mental illness and includes presentations, discussion, and interactive exercises. To learn more, check out https://www.nami.org/Support-Education/Mental-Health-Education/NAMI-Family-to-Family.

In summary, self-help groups are widely available and can help to address some of the gaps within mainstream mental health systems and services—especially those that limit access because of availability, transportation, and affordability. An OTP's knowledge of local and national self-help groups can be a helpful resource to share with persons seeking ongoing support and education beyond their involvement with the mental health system. OTPs can advocate for peer-led self-help groups in hospital settings where they do not already exist, and work collaboratively with peer support providers, peer support group leaders, and peer specialists in service delivery. OTPs can also help to bridge recovery-based services and supports by providing instrumental support to peer-led groups, access to goods and services that they may be denied (e.g., securing free meeting spaces), and, where needed, supporting the peer support worker's participation in this valued occupation.

Peer Community-Based Services

With the advent of the deinstitutionalization movement of the 1960s and 1970s, people with mental illnesses—who had lived many years in institutions—were deinstitutionalized into a community that lacked the services and supports that people needed for successful living in the community. The history of the consumer-survivor movement also paralleled that of the disability, feminist, and queer advocacy movements, and, importantly, their civil and rights-based lenses. Also see Chapter 26: The Public Policy Environment and Chapter 27: Mental Health Stigma and Sanism. 🤝

Judy Chamberlain, a consumer-survivor pioneer and early organizer, stated that the goal of the consumer-survivor movement was self-definition (reflected in the many terms used at that time to refer to an individual with lived experience of mental illness) and **self-determination** (reflected in the focus of advocacy on ownership and direction of future lives). Consequently, a variety of services have evolved at this time to help individuals with mental illnesses to live in the community, to address these service gaps, and to ensure that people with lived experience had a say in their futures.

Peers initially met informally in churches and community centers to support one another. Programs, such as the "peer-bridger" program, evolved to help people transition out of a long-term inpatient facility and integrate into the community. It was first introduced in 1994 by the New York Association for Psychiatric Rehabilitation Services (NYAPRS) to provide support for individuals with long or repeated psychiatric hospitalizations as they made the transition back to their home communities. It is a manualized model that focuses on four topics:

1. Outreach and engagement
2. Crisis stabilization
3. Wellness and self-management skills
4. Community support

To learn more about the peer-bridger program, and whether there is a program near you, check out https://rightsandrecovery.org/nyaprs-peer-bridger-program.

Peer-Run Precrisis and Respite

Peer-run precrisis programs are another community-based service to meet the needs of adults experiencing distress or crisis in the community. A variety of programs are now implemented across the United States and globally. For some individuals, these programs provide an alternative to an inpatient psychiatric hospital.

Crisis often leads to disruptions in balance of self-care occupations. To restore this balance in one's self-care occupations, the respite services offer intensive peer support and involvement in wellness activities. Staff help guests to plan for adjustments to their home, their associated valued roles, and their community activities. If there is a waiting list, or if a guest chooses to remain at home in the community to adjust to the crisis, the respite services can provide continued face-to-face or phone contact and outreach for up to 1 month.

A peer-run **warm line** is a telephone precrisis support service available in some locations, whereby callers can connect with a person with lived experience of a mental health condition (Dalgin et al., 2011). Local and national warm lines are available, and are typically staffed by paid peer support workers. Some warm lines also provide virtual support groups through Skype, Zoom, blogs, or chat rooms. In Canada, warm lines—designed by peers, for peers—provide an essential outreach mental health support, especially to rural and remote places where peer support programs might not be available (NISA, n.d.).

In summary, individuals with mental health issues and addictions will experience challenges of daily living in the community beyond the mental health clinic and occupational therapy services. Hence, knowledge of local, regional, and national warm lines and the availability of peer-led community supports and services will assist the OTP to ensure that the people they work with have the tools they require to live well and to be supported in their community. For more information, see Chapter 35: Practice Across the Continuum of Service Needs. 🤝

Peer-Professional Partnerships

Peer-led services are, by definition, peer-managed, although some peer-based services, referred to as "peer-professional partnerships," incorporate the use of nonpeer professionals in certain areas of planning, implementation, and evaluation (Solomon, 2004). This may take the form of groups that are led by both peer and nonpeer professionals or may use a dedicated peer support provider as a member of a service team that also includes nonpeer workers (e.g., Assertive Community Treatment Teams [ACTT]) or Flexible Assertive Community Treatment Teams (FACTT). Peer-professional partnerships have the benefit of drawing upon both clinical knowledge and lived experience.

To illustrate, NISA was initially a peer-professional partnership involving an occupational therapist and four people who identified as consumer-survivors of the mental health system. This partnership created the program, developed a theoretical model in its support, and collaboratively carried out research and program evaluation. Today, the program is 100% peer-led, and the occupational therapist only remains involved peripherally, in research and evaluation (Rebeiro Gruhl et al., 2021).

The **Vet-to-Vet program** is another example of a peer-professional partnership model in which peer services are embedded in a mental health setting (Resnick et al., 2004). *Vet-to-Vet* is a partnership program that utilizes veterans in recovery in a peer-counseling capacity to help other veterans. Vet-to-Vet is administered by veterans who themselves have been consumers of Veterans Administration mental health services. Vet-to-Vet provides a 6-week, peer-facilitator training program that teaches veterans how to facilitate peer group sessions and deliver program learning topics. In Canada, Stephane Grenier, a retired veteran who had experienced posttraumatic stress disorder (PTSD) after his tour in Rwanda, strongly advocated for peer support in the military and other workplaces (https://stephanegrenier .com).

A **wellness coach** (Brice et al., 2014; Swarbrick, 2013; Swarbrick et al., 2011) is a specialized type of peer-professional partnership in which peer support workers help an individual to link to a primary health-care professional and provide support and encouragement to help that individual set and achieve a desired short-term wellness or health-related goal (Perez & Kidd, 2015). Peer support workers are increasingly represented as members of mental health community support teams, where they deliver services that are coordinated with services offered by other nonpeer team members. Although peer roles on service teams differ, some commonalities exist (U.S. Department of Health and Human Services, 2015). In some states, Medicaid reimbursement is available for peer support services; however, some funders, such as state and insurance companies, require peer specialist certification in order to be funded (Kaufman et al., 2014).

Some examples of occupational therapists collaborating in peer-professional relationships include the development of a manual on diet and exercise (Brown et al., 2017)—producing a program manual and series of videos (Brown et al., 2015). A second example is a manual on wellness activities, developed collaboratively by occupational therapy students and members of a peer-run wellness center (Swarbrick, 2016).

Peer support workers are likely to be occupational therapy colleagues on the job. Accordingly, OTPs can draw upon peer support worker knowledge for feedback and guidance to ensure that their services are recovery-oriented and person-centered. OTPs who work in behavioral health treatment programs, as well as in the community, may collaborate with peer support workers to provide recovery-oriented services and supports. Integrating the unique perspectives of clinical and lived experience has become increasingly important to addressing the complex issues of daily living and recovery for those experiencing mental illnesses and addictions within the community.

Peer-Led Organizations

Peer-led organizations, or peer-led programs within larger organizations, are often independent of the larger mental health system, are fully peer-led, and offer a variety of services and opportunities. These organizations are often known as consumer-operated services (U.S. Department of Health and Human Services, 2011) or peer-run organizations. For example, CSPNJ is a peer-led, not-for-profit, statewide mental health agency in New Jersey that was incorporated in 1984 (Swarbrick, 2009a). CSPNJ offers services that are community-based and flexible. It places a strong emphasis on recovery, relationship building, self-sufficiency, and overall health and wellness for people with the lived experience of behavioral health conditions. Programs are inclusive and emphasize human rights advocacy and the dignity of every person. Services are offered in community wellness centers as well as supportive and respite care housing settings, where they address a myriad of challenging needs for individuals who are unhoused and people living with substance use and/or behavioral health conditions (CSPNJ, 2024).

CSPNJ is nationally recognized for its innovative design and delivery of housing, employment, and economic development services that address poverty. Innovative antipoverty services at CSPNJ include programs designed to help people pursue goals of budgeting, investing, controlling their debt,

---

PhotoVoice

Izzy

Making the invisible seen and the silent heard
Robbed of identity and spoken voice
Living in obscurity as if by choice
None would listen none could see
Invisible to self as well as thee
Recovery Innovations was then found
Hope and love and more abound
Never alone surrounded by peers
Strength of resolve not ruled by fears
Life now has meaning I'm undeterred
Making the invisible seen and the silent heard

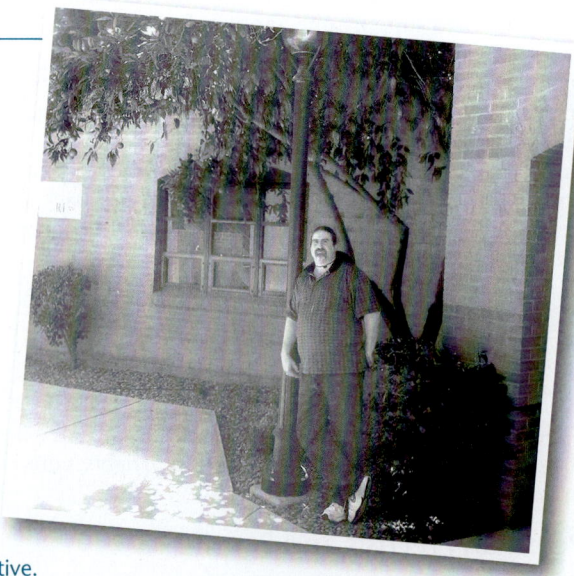

What does this image of Izzy and his poem evoke for you?

What is your interpretation of his poem?

The poem mentions Recovery Innovations, which offers peer support and recovery education programs. Apply a PEO perspective.
How would attending a peer support program influence the person? As an environment, what might the peer support program provide? What occupations might be available, and how do these support recovery?

PhotoVoice

S.I.D.E. Recovery Quilt

Members of the peer-led organization S.I.D.E. in Kansas City, Kansas, standing in front of a quilt they created that depicts recovery.

The quilt patches depicted in this photo facilitate self-expression and reflect multiple and diverse perspectives on recovery. What other types of activities might an OTP use to facilitate creative self-expression?

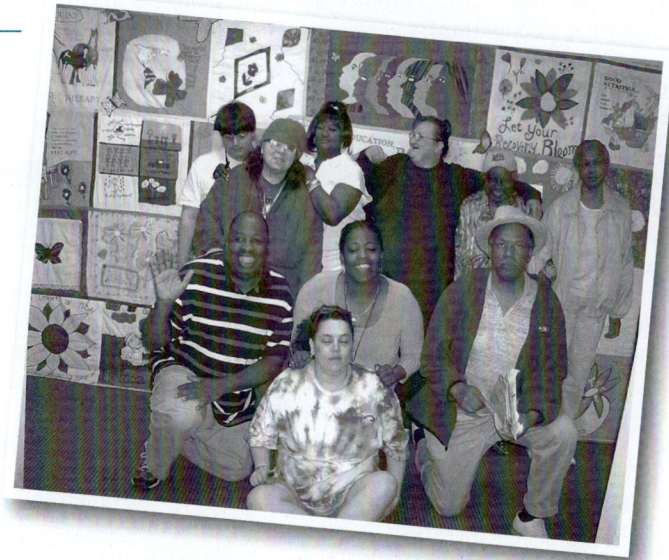

building wealth, and accumulating assets. They offer financial literacy education, match savings programs, financial management accounts, credit counseling, and emergency microloans. Honoring the lived experiences of individuals working through their own recovery is a consistent and core component of CSPNJ's mission, vision, and values. Wellness and recovery-oriented services offer people opportunities to live, learn, and work in their own communities. The agency is directed, managed, and staffed by people with the lived experience of mental health conditions. CSPNJ's vision is one of healing and hope, which is promoted by choice, freedom, inclusion, and destigmatization.

Family-Run Organizations

Family-run organizations across the country are lead providers of family and youth peer support services. Most are grassroots organizations developed and run by the parents and caregivers of youth and young adults affected by serious emotional and behavioral challenges. The mission of most family-run organizations is family support, education, public awareness, and local and state policy advocacy to ensure that an effective and evidence-based service delivery infrastructure is in place.

Family support providers offer peer support to parents and caregivers. They often help with system navigation by phone and in person, such as helping families to secure basic needs and access to health insurance or social service benefits. Family-run organizations also ensure the family and youth voice is prominent in shaping the state's health-care system infrastructure. As an example, the New Jersey Alliance of Family Support Organizations seeks to strengthen and promote the wellness of families with children and youth who have emotional, behavioral, or mental health challenges. This umbrella organization supports family-led organizations offering education, support, and advocacy.

Peer support for youth recognizes that the concept of "peer" may be more than a shared experience of a mental

health condition. For many young people, connecting with others of the same age is important. Youth Motivating Others through Voices of Experience National (Youth M.O.V.E.) is a youth and young adult–led national advocacy organization. Youth M.O.V.E. is focused on preparing young people to speak up for system change to benefit themselves and others and to provide peer support. The organization is working to develop national peer support standards and provide technical assistance to states to expand the quality and accessibility of peer support services.

Some of these organizations provide local networking opportunities for peers and nonpeer allies and may offer educational materials that OTPs could use. In the peer-led service model, the inclusion of nonpeer professionals (including OTPs) is a choice that is made by the individual peer organizations and programs. The next section provides an exploration of how occupational therapy might be involved with peer-led services.

Role of Occupational Therapy

Many opportunities exist for OTPs to collaborate with and support peer-led services and peer support workers. Research on peer-run, occupation-based services indicated that the occupational therapist's initial role involved supporting the group to obtain goods and services and spaces that they did not have access to. The occupational therapist was also involved in helping the group to establish an environment conducive to addressing their being, belonging, and becoming needs (Bibyk et al., 1999; Rebeiro et al., 2001; Rebeiro Gruhl et al., 2021). The provision of occupational opportunity was a foundational consideration at NISA—building upon previous research and an evolving understanding of the paucity of opportunities available in the community to become involved in meaningful occupation (Rebeiro, 1999).

Many of these occupational opportunities evolved organically and were required for the daily operation of NISA (e.g., office/receptionist, computer technician, OMQ Editor, etc.). Other occupations were purposefully created based upon members' interests or unmet social needs in the community (Warm Hearts, Warm Bodies Program; Artists Loft). Over time, and based upon the needs of new members, other occupational opportunities were developed—most notably, an extensive peer support network.

Sometimes, the occupational therapist took the lead when it involved occupational opportunities or advocacy to funders or the media; but mostly, the occupational therapist took direction from the membership. This was achieved through one-on-one discussions, membership surveys, and a robust research program known as ParNorth (Rebeiro Gruhl et al., 2018).

In the United States, OTPs working in behavioral health care, including inpatient state and county hospital settings, Veterans Administration services, and community-based settings, might use their knowledge and skills to collaborate with peer support workers to develop, implement, and evaluate peer-led services. OTPs would not be providing direct services to peer support workers in this context, but rather might provide a consultative or a train-the-trainer approach. For example, OTPs may consult on designing a drop-in center space or support a peer support training program.

As an initial step to becoming involved with peer-led services, the OTP needs to determine what peer-led services are already available in the community. This can be accomplished in a couple of ways—the easiest, perhaps, is to do an initial internet search using the key words of "peer support"; "peer services"; and "consumer mental health groups." One can also contact the state consumer or peer liaison at the local, county, or state mental health authority and inquire which peer-led programs are listed in the directory.

Becoming familiar with existing peer-led services in the OTP's local community is an important first step to understanding any gaps and services—from the perspective of the service user—as well as any potential roles for occupational therapy. There is great benefit in relationship-building with local peer groups/leaders through phone contact and by visiting these programs to learn more about them. OTPs might compile an inventory of the program information and peer-contacts to share with individuals they are working with who might benefit from participating in peer-led programs. This is also a great student project. OTPs can provide student intern support to peer-led programs to codevelop marketing materials, such as brochures and websites that can assist people with mental or substance use disorders to find their way to a local peer-led group or program.

OTPs can also support peer-led program leadership in their work in collaborating with traditional mental health programs, as well as in advocating for peer-led programs and services to be included as a part of the more formal mental health referral networks. If the search leads the OTP to conclude that there are no peer-led programs available locally, they should consider advocating for the funding of peer support workers and the development of peer-led programs. They can connect with other OTPs who have been involved with peer-led services for ideas, search the literature and understand the evidence in its support, and inquire broadly. However, most importantly, they should meet with, listen to, and take the lead from people with lived experience about what their needs are as a basis for getting started.

Finally, OTPs might assist with knowledge translation about the benefits of peer support and peer-led services among the people they work with, their professional colleagues, and their professional and personal community. To do so, they might invite peer-led program participants or peer leaders to visit settings where OTPs are employed to inform people and staff about the availability of peer-led services in the community. Alternately, OTPs can visit peer-led settings to learn more about what is involved in establishing a successful program. For example, in New Jersey, the peers from local community wellness centers collaborate with OTPs to educate current inpatients about the variety of free resources that are available to them in the community when they are discharged.

OTPs may find themselves as coworkers of a peer or family support specialist if they are working on an ACTT or in a case management or early intervention program. Some peer and family specialists report feelings of isolation and discrimination from treatment team members and other nonpeer colleagues (Gates & Akabas, 2007; Rebeiro Gruhl et al., 2023). OTPs can become important allies for peer colleagues and help to shift the attitudes of unsupportive nonpeer workers and the sometimes-disempowering culture of mental health service programs through their support of and advocacy for peer-led services.

This instrumental support can happen in a few ways. OTPs might help peer-led programs link with nonpeer mental health provider agencies, family groups, and other community resources to expand their reach and influence. OTPs can support peer leaders in developing presentations and outreach activities to educate health-care professionals at mental health service agencies about the role of peer-led programs in providing social support for people with mental health and substance use disorders living in the community.

Advocating for peer-led services can take many forms; however, one of the more powerful ways to advocate for new programs is to provide evidence of their effectiveness. Occupational therapists working at research centers or universities can contribute to research on peer-led endeavors (Rebeiro Gruhl et al., 2023; Swarbrick et al., 2016). PAR is an empowering form of applied research whereby the people being studied are fully engaged in the process of investigation. PAR is a method of inquiry consistent with the peer–self-help ethos that explores practical problems of importance to service users and is the foundational methodology used by ParNorth at NISA (Rebeiro et al., 2001).

The PAR approach involves maximum participation of stakeholders in the systematic collection and analysis of information for the purposes of taking action and making change. Using a participatory research approach, such as PAR, occupational therapy researchers can play an important role in assisting peer-led groups to evaluate the benefits (and challenges requiring attention) of peer-led services.

OTPs can take a leadership role in establishing peer support on university and college campuses by supporting peer-led recovery colleges, such as the Collaborative Learning Centre at the Centre for Addiction and Mental Health (CAMH; https://clc.camh.ca) and educational programs that provide training, education, or certification of the peer support occupation. To learn more, check out https://campusmentalhealth.ca/wp-content/uploads/2020/02/CICMH-Peer-Support-Toolkit-EN.pdf.

The Lived Experience

Marty

In December 2013, Marty Hadge spoke to hundreds of delegates from across the world at the Alternatives 2013 peer conference in Austin, Texas. Her story is an example of how effective peer support can be in instilling hope and rescuing the potential lying dormant in someone struggling with the effects of illness, poverty, trauma, and medication. Excerpts from her speech are captured in the text that follows. Readers are encouraged to listen to her full speech at https://youtu.be/eX15aHflgrU.

I came into this world under adverse conditions. I had early experiences of visions and voices and as a child they served me well, in a way that the people around me did not. I came to the realization that no one was going to rescue or fix me, that I had to rescue myself, that I had to figure out my own way of being able to walk through this world. That the experts—despite their claims and certainty—did not know me or have all the answers. I was told that I had a serious mental illness and that the most I could hope for was to have some periods of time not in the hospital, that I needed to take medication for the rest of my life and would not be able to work. This was not the life I wanted to live!

When I first met folks at the Western Mass Recovery Learning Community (WMRLC), I found that there were people who had gone through similar things as me, who were told by providers the same things as me and yet were changing their lives in positive

ways and living lives they were told were not possible. I began to believe it might be a possibility for me to create a life worth living beyond the trauma, beyond the addiction, beyond the labels and beyond the medical model.

I did not have much going on when I started visiting RLC spaces, but people still said hello. I did not feel judged, and my participation was not based on any diagnosis. Instead, the focus was on, What's your story? What do you want to do? and How can we support that? I was included and offered opportunities. People had a vision of wellness and ability for me that I did not have for myself. I finally found a safe place to share my experiences. It was safe in that it was nonjudgmental. People were coming from a place of curiosity, and no one was trying to fix or correct me or reacting to me in a fear-based way. My own opinion of what I was going through was valued and I was met wherever I was at.

At the WMRLC, we work to build an inclusive community. People are allowed their own beliefs and agreement is not required, but respect and self-determination are honored. A person's right to determine what is helpful to oneself is respected. Now, [as a peer support worker] in the same institutions I was previously confined to, I am happy to share the possibility of recovery and perspectives beyond the medical model.

To learn more about the WMRLC, now known as the Wildflower Alliance, check out their website at https://wildflower alliance.org.

Here's the Point

- Peer- and family-led services are important components of a recovery-oriented service system. Peers provide elements of care that have been either abandoned by the traditional mental health system or significantly reduced because of clinical protocols and funding (e.g., listening time). Peers also embody a missing component in mainstream services—that is, that recovery is possible (e.g., the embodiment that recovery is visible to service users).
- Peer-led services often address social and emotional needs that are left unmet by more traditional service delivery models.
- OTPs' interest in meaningful occupation (which peer support is for many) and person-driven services complement OTPs working with peer support workers and within peer-led services.

- Knowledge of the variety of peer-led services at the local, state, and national level will provide OTPs, especially those working in community-based mental health practices, with the ability to provide meaningful links to a host of supportive networks for the people they treat.
- OTPs, while respecting the autonomy and self-determination of peer-led groups, are encouraged to seek out and foster collaborative partnerships with peer-led services in their area to provide support in the development, implementation, and evaluation of peer-led models.

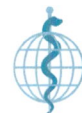

Visit the online resource center at **FADavis.com** to access the videos.

Apply It Now

1. Experience a Peer-Led Program

Research a peer-led program in your area. You can check your state or county website or visit the National Empowerment Center website (www.power2u) to determine peer-led programs in your area. Take the following steps:

- Review the website for the program you want to visit to see what type of services they offer, which populations

they serve, and whether a visit might be appropriate. You might want to see if they provide occupational opportunities at their services.
- Contact the peer-led service by e-mail or by phone to discuss your interest in their program as an OTP and the possibility of a site visit. It is likely a good idea to have some ideas of other programs and what you might have to offer the program.

■ You might want to gain an overall impression of the service before you dive into questions; however, here are a few to get you started:
  ● What type of peer support services do you offer?
  ● How long have you offered each of these peer support services?
  ● How does someone access your service? Does it cost anything?
  ● What are the benefits of these services for the people who use them?
  ● Do you work directly with formal mental health services in the area? How does this work (e.g., do you take referrals, can someone drop in, do other mental health providers provide support to your service)?
  ● Do you collaborate with other mental health providers and services? How does this work? What is helpful and not-so-helpful?
■ Write a summary about the program and what you learned about the service. Reflect upon your experience and your understanding of how peer-led services fit within the recovery continuum.

2. Watch Videos on Peer Support

In groups of three or four, go to http://www.intentionalpeer support.org/videos and select a few videos to watch.
■ Discuss among your peers your overall reaction to the videos after watching them.
■ Discuss how occupational therapy might support peer-led services.
■ Identify what makes peer support different from other mental health services and other helping relationships.

3. Contact a Peer-Led or Family-Led Advocacy Organization in Your Area

Research local peer- or family-led advocacy organizations. This may require both web searching and phone calls to locate a local group.
■ Identify what their key advocacy issues are.
■ Reflect on whether these issues might also be important to occupational therapy.
■ Prepare a brief presentation for your classmates, providing an overview of the organization, their key issues, and those occupations that they engage in to support their advocacy. Identify a role for occupational therapy (if any) and the steps you would take to become involved.

4. Reflect on Lived Experience Stories

After reading the feature about Marty, brainstorm ways that an OTP might support the individual in this story, or perhaps the peer-led organization that they belong to.

Reflective Questions
■ Think about how you, as a licensed health-care professional, might be intimidating. How might you reduce this power differential?
■ Think about experiences that individuals might have had within the health-care system before you arrived in their lives. What have you personally witnessed?
■ How would you feel about your potential for having a good life based upon what Marty was repeatedly told?
■ What are some of the strategies you could employ to reduce the power differential and to make yourself and your vision of occupation more accessible and, possibly, more palatable to peer-led groups?

Resources

General Peer Technical Assistance and Training Resources
• National Empowerment Center: http://www.power2u.org. This site provides many resources for peer supporters and professionals who support peer-led services.
• Warm Lines: National Empowerment Center: Peer-Run Warm Lines & Resources: https://power2u.org/resources. This site provides information as well as a directory.

Support for Veterans
• The Vet-to-Vet program: http://www.vet2vetusa.org. This site describes the Vet-to-Vet program, provides resources, and has contact information.

Funding for Family- and Peer-Led Services
• Center for Health Care Strategies' resource: Medicaid Financing for Family and Youth Peer Support: A Scan of State Programs at https://www.chcs.org/resource/medicaid -financing-for-family-and-youth-peer-support-a-scan-of -state-programs-3.

Family Support Organizations
• Parent Support Provider Certification: https://www.ffcmh.org (click on "certification"). This is a certification for parent support providers administered by the National Federation of Families for Children's Mental Health.

• New Jersey Alliance of Family Support Organizations: http:// NJFamilyAlliance.org. Through this site, individuals can sign up for trainings in New Jersey that support peer-led services.
• National Alliance on Mental Illness: NAMI Family-to-Family: https://www.nami.org/Find-Support/NAMI-Programs /NAMI-Family-to-Family. This website provides information about the NAMI Family-to-Family program.

Youth
• Youth Motivating Others Through Voices of Experience (Youth M.O.V.E.) National: https://youthmovenational.org. This youth and young adult–led national advocacy organization is devoted to improving services and systems that support young people. They focus on empowering young people to partner with adults to create meaningful change in mental health, juvenile justice, education, and child welfare systems. The organization represents over 75 chapters across 39 states. This group has supported several initiatives.
  • *What Helps What Harms* is an initiative for young adults in each of Youth M.O.V.E. National's chapters to spend time in facilitated discussions, analyzing their community network, resources, services, and environment. Discussions are framed with two simple questions: *What is helping us? What is harmful to us?* These questions are applied to systems, service providers, education settings, homes, and so on. All answers received from youth are right—from the simple (how appointments are scheduled) to the complex (how school environments can foster bully-free environments). Responses

are categorized into themes, as identified by the young adult participants.

- The *National Young Leaders Network* (NYLN) consists of youth leaders and advocates who have passion and experience to provoke positive change within youth serving social systems through utilizing authentic youth voice. The young people nominated and accepted into the NYLN will be offered opportunities to share their voices of experience at the national level. Opportunities may include participation in national speaking engagements and work groups, research studies, educational opportunities, and the chance to join the Youth M.O.V.E. National delegate and consultant communities.

Older Adults
- Older Adult Peer Support: https://nisa.on.ca/programs /older-adult-peer-support. This is a peer-led initiative that focuses on senior's mental health and well-being.

LGBTQIA2S+
- LGBTQIA2S+ Youth Community Resources: https://www. nami.org/Find-Support/LGBTQ. This NAMI site provides information for the LGBTQIA2S+ community on mental health issues, addictions, stigma, suicide, youth issues, and choosing service providers. The site includes links to:
  - The *Association for Lesbian, Gay, and Bisexual & Transgender Issues in Counseling* offers a list of resources for LGBTQIA2S+ individuals: https://www.pridecounseling.com.
  - The *Association of Gay and Lesbian Psychiatrists* offers numerous resources for LGBTQIA2S+ people who are experiencing mental health conditions, including a directory of LGBTQIA2S+-friendly therapists: http://www.aglp.org.
  - The *GLBT National Help Center* provides multiple resources and access to a hotline and a youth chat line.
  - The *Gay, Lesbian and Straight Education Network* provides an annual report called the *National School Climate Survey,* which reports on the experiences of lesbian, gay, bisexual, and transgender youth in U.S. schools.
  - The *Pride Institute* is an unlocked, LGBTQIA2S+-exclusive facility that offers a residential treatment program, including psychiatric care for depression, anxiety, and other needs.
  - The *Rainbow Access Initiative* works to inform and educate health-care providers on LGBTQIA2S+-specific issues.
  - The *Trevor Project* is a multimedia support network for LGBTQIA2S+ youth providing crisis intervention and suicide prevention.
- Youth*in*Mind: https://youthinmind.com. Youth*in*Mind is a collection of psychologists, educators, and experts in integrated testing (IT). Their aim is to promote the psychological well-being of people everywhere through the provision of information, assessment, treatment, and research.

Peer-Led Respite Resources
- Collaborative Support Programs of New Jersey (CSPNJ) Respite Services: https://cspnj.org/about
- People Inc.: http://www.people- inc.org/disabilities_services_home /respite_services/respite_programs/index.html
  - This organization features respite houses and in-home respite services in western New York for individuals with developmental disabilities in need of planned or emergency care.
  - The target audience is children and adults with developmental disabilities.
- Peer-Run Crisis Respites: https://power2u.org/peer-respite -resources
  - Peer-run crisis respites (PRCR) are emerging forms of acute residential crisis services for people with psychiatric disorders. PRCRs are an alternative to psychiatric inpatient hospitalization, and are completely peer-run; that is, they are staffed and operated by other people with lived experience of mental illness.

- This manual contains information, resources, and strategies that can help mental health agencies to successfully introduce the peer wellness coach role into the array of services offered.
- Hospital Diversion Services: Developing a Peer-Respite Diversion Service in Your Area: https://youtu.be/FnPEdy30uro
  - This webinar serves as a guide to opening and operating a peer-operated hospital diversion service in an OTP's area. It is intended only as a guide; OTP's may choose to make modifications that better serve their purpose and the needs of their community. They may also choose to modify or enhance the design so that it is culturally appropriate for the environment and philosophy of their community.
- Peer Support in the Emergency Department: https://www .sinaihealth.ca/news/innovative-peer-support-program-helps -young-adults-visiting-the-emergency-department. Accessing services for mental health and addiction services in a hospital ED can be overwhelming and challenging. Having the opportunity to talk and connect with someone who has been in similar circumstances can create a sense of belonging and understanding for those who may feel they are alone in their journey.
- Peer Respite Services: https://power2u.org/directory-of-peer -respites
  - This site features a directory of peer respites in the United States. This site also contains information and links related to evaluation tools, technical assistance, research, resources, and training directly related to peer respites.
  - The target audience is consumers, program staff and administrators, students, researchers, and other stakeholders.
- Peer Respite Toolkit: https://www.hsri.org/publication/peer -respite-toolkit
  - The Toolkit for Evaluating Peer Respites is written for evaluators, government officials, and peer-to-peer program staff and managers. It can be used to document program operations and outcomes and to build evidence for the efficacy of peer respites. This resource includes recommendations on best practices in evaluation and data monitoring based on techniques used by other peer respites. It encompasses a range of strategies for collecting and reporting data. In this context, data is any information collected from guests who use the peer respite or people working there, regardless of whether programs use the information for research or for reporting to constituents or funders.
- Campus Peer Support Development: https://campusmental health.ca/wp-content/uploads/2020/02/CICMH-Peer-Support -Toolkit-EN.pdf. This site provides information on how to develop a peer support program on university and college campuses.

International Peer-Led Organizations
- Intentional Peer Support UK: https://www.intentionalpeer support.org/?v=b8a74b2fbcbb
- Peer Support Australia: https://peersupport.edu.au. Peer Support Australia is a national nonprofit organization that has been working with schools across Australia for almost 50 years to support student well-being.
- Peer Support Canada: https://peersupportcanada.ca. This site provides a variety of resources, certifications, and standards of practice for peer support work in Canada.
- Ontario Peer Development Initiative (Peer Works): https://www .peerworks.ca
- Peer Support New Zealand: http://www.peersupport.org.nz
- Peer Support Wales: https://mhmwales.org.uk/peer-support-1
- Peer Support Germany: https://www.mhinnovation.net /resources/peer-begleitung-d-ch-peer-support-germany

• Peer Support International: https://www.coe.int/en/web/bioethics/other-initiatives-toward-reduction-of-coercion/-/highest_rated_assets/ZaFHEPWjPcNI/content/peer-support-and-the-peer-workforce. This site contains linkages to several other peer support organizations in Europe.

Videos

• "Life Skills Groups in an Unhoused Population" video. Kailin is an occupational therapist who works in community mental health and homeless services. In this video, she describes the impactful life skills groups she runs in a women's shelter and how the use of a group facilitates peer-to-peer support. Kailin offers several creative examples of life skill group activities. She emphasizes the need to employ trauma-informed practices and harm-reduction strategies in this population, meeting clients where they truly are. Access the video at the online resource center at FADavis.com.

• "Jordan's Lived Experience of Anxiety and Depression" video. In this video, occupational therapist Jordan describes her lived experience of anxiety and depression. She touches on many issues critical to recovery and occupational therapy practice, including social determinants of health, peer support, and how mental health labels can adversely affect an individual's medical treatment. Importantly, she explains how she has learned to blend her lived experience with her work as an occupational therapist while ensuring she takes care of herself and manages her symptoms. Jordan also offers priceless words of wisdom to OTPs regarding establishing a therapeutic connection with individuals with whom they practice. Access the video at the online resource center at FADavis.com.

• "Mary's Lived Experience as an Unhoused Individual and Her Occupational Therapist's Perspective" video. In this video, Mary provides a first-person account of being unhoused and the tremendous impact occupational therapy services have had on her life. In addition, occupational therapist Quinn Tyminski describes working with Mary and shares her perspective on Mary's journey and transformation, including her improved conflict resolution and emotion regulation skills. Access the video at the online resource center at FADavis.com.

Acknowledgment

The first author would like to acknowledge Peggy Swarbrick for her work on previous editions of this chapter, some of which have been retained.

References

Advocates for Human Potential, Inc. (2016). *WRAP is . . ..* https://www.wellnessrecoveryactionplan.com/what-is-wrap

Alcoholics Anonymous. (2024). *Origins.* https://www.aa.org/aa-timeline

Ansell, D. I., & Insley, S. E. (2013). *Youth peer-to-peer support: A review of the literature.* Ansell & Associates. https://youthmovenational.org/wp-content/uploads/2019/05/Youth-Peer-to-Peer-Literature-Review.pdf

Bellamy, C., Schmutte, T., & Davidson, L. (2017). An update on the growing evidence base for peer support. *Mental Health and Social Inclusion, 21*(3), 161–167. https://doi.org/10.1108/MHSI-03-2017-0014

Bibyk, B., Day, D. G., Morris, L., O'Brien, M. C., Rebeiro, K. L., Seguin, P., Semeniuk, B., Wilson, B., & Wilson, J. (1999, Sept/Oct). Who's in charge here? The client's perspective on client-centered care. *Occupational Therapy Now,* 11–12.

Boothroyd, R. I., & Fisher, E. B. (2010, June). Peers for Progress: Promoting peer support for health around the world. *Family Practice, 27*(Suppl. 1), i62–i68. https://doi.org/10.1093/fampra/cmq017

Brice, G. H., Swarbrick, M. A., & Gill, K. J. (2014). Promoting wellness of peer providers through coaching. *Journal of Psychosocial Nursing and Mental Health Services, 52*(1), 41–45. https://doi.org/10.3928/02793695-20130930-03

Brown, C., Goetz, J., & Bledsoe, C. (2017). *Nutrition and exercise for wellness and recovery NEW-R. Leader manual.* University of Illinois at Chicago, National Research and Training Center on Psychiatric Disability and Co-Occurring Medical Conditions.

Brown, C., Read, H., Stanton, M., Zeeb, M., Jonikas, J., & Cook, J. (2015). A pilot study of the Nutrition and Exercise for Weight Loss and Recovery (NEW-R): A weight loss program for individuals with serious mental illness. *Psychiatric Rehabilitation Journal, 38,* 371–373. https://doi.org/10.1037/prj0000115

Cabassa, L. J., Camacho, D., Vélez-Grau, C. M., & Stefancic, A. (2017). Peer-based health interventions for people with serious mental illness: A systematic literature review. *Journal of Psychiatric Research, 84,* 80–89. https://doi.org/10.1016/j.jpsychires.2016.09.021

Castelein, S., Bruggeman, R., van Busschbach, J. T., van der Gaag, M., Stant, A. D., Knegtering, H., & Wiersma, D. (2008). The effectiveness of peer support groups in psychosis: A randomized controlled trial. *Acta Psychiatrica Scandinavica, 118*(1), 64–72. https://doi.org/10.1111/j.1600-0447.2008.01216.x

Chamberlain, J. (1978). *On our own: Patient-controlled alternatives to the mental health system.* Hawthorn Books.

Cheesmond, N., Davies, K., & Inder, K. (2020). The role of the peer support worker in increasing rural mental health help-seeking. *Australian Journal of Rural Health, 28*(2), 203–208. https://doi.org/10.1111/ajr.12603

Chien, W. T., Clifton, A. V., Zhao, S., & Lui, S. (2019). Peer support for people with schizophrenia or other serious mental illness. *Cochrane Database of Systematic Reviews, 4*(4), CD010880. https://doi.org/10.1002/14651858.CD010880.pub2

Clay, S. (2005). *On our own together: Peer programs for people with mental illness.* Vanderbilt Press.

Collaborative Support Programs of New Jersey. (2024). *Peer led. Recovery focused. Wellness driven.* https://cspnj.org

Cook, J. A., Copeland, M. E., Corey, L., Buffington, E., Jonikas, J. A., Curtis, L. C., Grey, D. D., & Nichols, W. H. (2010). Developing the evidence base for peer-led services: Changes among participants following Wellness Recovery Action Planning (WRAP) education in two statewide initiatives. *Psychiatric Rehabilitation Journal, 34*(2), 113–120. https://doi.org/10.2975/34.2.2010.113.120

Creamer, M. C., Varker, T., Bisson, J., Darte, K., Greenberg, N., Lau, W., Moreton, G., O'Donnell, M., Richardson, D., Ruzek, J., Watson, P., & Forbes, D. (2012). Guidelines for peer support in high-risk organizations: An international consensus study using the Delphi method. *Journal of Traumatic Stress, 25,* 134–141. https://doi.org/10.1002/jts.21685

Cronise, R., Teixeira, C., Rogers, E. S., & Harrington, S. (2016). The peer support workforce: Results of a national survey. *Psychiatric Rehabilitation Journal, 39*(3), 211–221. https://doi.org/10.1037/prj0000222

Cyr, C., Mckee, H., O'Hagan, M., & Priest, R. (2016). *Making the case for peer support: Report to the Peer Support Project Committee of the Mental Health Commission of Canada* (2nd ed.). Mental Health Commission of Canada.

Dalgin, R. S., Dalgin, M. H., & Metzger, S. J. (2018). A longitudinal analysis of the influence of a peer-run Warm Line phone service on psychiatric recovery. *Community Mental Health Journal, 54*(4), 376–382. https://doi.org/10.1007/s10597-017-0161-4

Dalgin, R. S., Maline, S., & Driscoll, P. (2011). Sustaining recovery through the night: Impact of a peer-run Warm Line. *Psychiatric Rehabilitation Journal, 35*(1), 65–68. https://doi.org/10.2975/35.1.2011.65.68

Daniels, A., Grant, E., Filson, N., Powell, I., Fricks, L., & Goodale, L. (2010). *Pillars of peer support: Transforming mental health systems*

of care through peer support services. www.pillarsofpeersupport
.org

Davidson, L., Bellamy, C., Guy, K., & Miller, R. (2012). Peer support among persons with mental illness: A review of evidence and experience. *World Psychiatry, 11,* 123–128. https://doi.org/10.1016/j.wpsyc.2012.05.009

Deegan, P. (1988). Recovery: The lived experience of rehabilitation. *Psychosocial Rehabilitation Journal, 11*(4), 11–19. https://doi.org/10.1037/h0099565

Deegan, P. (2001). Recovery as a self-directed process of healing and transformation. *Occupational Therapy in Mental Health, 17*(3-4), 5–21. https://doi.org/10.1300/j004v17n03 02

Depression and Bipolar Support Alliance. (2016). *About the Depression and Bipolar Support Alliance.* http://www.dbsalliance.org

Dual Diagnosis Anonymous. (n.d.). *Home page.* https://ddainc.org

Franke, C. C. D., Paton, B. C., & Gassner, L. J. (2010). Implementing mental health peer support: A South Australian experience. *Australian Journal of Primary Health, 16*(2), 179– 186. https://doi.org/10.1071/py09067

Gardner, J., Swarbrick, M., Ackerman, A., Church, T., Rios, V., Valente, L., & Rutledge, J. (2017). Effects of physical limitations on daily activities among adults with mental health disorders. *Journal of Psychosocial Nursing and Mental Health Services, 55*(10), 45–51. https://doi.org/10.3928/02793695-20170818-05

Gardner, J., Swarbrick, M., Dennis, S., Franklin, M., Pricken, M., & Palmer, K. (2021). Sleep habits and routines of individuals diagnosed with mental and/or substance-use disorders. *Occupational Therapy in Mental Health, 37*(2), 158–177. https://doi.org/10.1080/0164212X.2021.1877592.

Gardner, J., Swarbrick, M., Kearns, D., Suero, L., Moscoe, E., Harder, P., … Rutledge, J. (2017, March). *Sensory preferences of community wellness center members.* Poster presentation at American Occupational Therapy Association Annual Conference, Philadelphia, Pennsylvania.

Gardner, J., Swarbrick, M., Olker, S., Ben-Baruch, M., Beronio, A., Malinak, J., Pignataro, L., & Rodar, S. J. (2019). *Impacts of financial management programs for adults with substance use and mental disorders. American Journal of Occupational Therapy, 73*(4_Suppl._1), 7311520388p1. https://doi.org/10.5014/ajot.2019.73S1-PO2028

Gates, L. B., & Akabas, S. H. (2007). Developing strategies to integrate peer providers into the staff of mental health agencies. *Administration Policy in Mental Health and Mental Health Services Research, 34,* 293–306. https://doi.org/10.1007/s10488-006-0109-4

Gillard, S., Foster, R., Gibson, S., Goldsmith, L., Marks, J., & White, S. (2017). Describing a principles-based approach to developing and evaluating peer worker roles as peer support moves into mainstream mental health services. *Mental Health and Social Inclusion, 21*(3), 133–143. https://doi.org/10.1186/1471-244X-14-39

GROW in America. (n.d.). *About us.* https://www.growinamerica.org/home/about-us

Hearing Voices Network–USA. (n.d.). *Home page.* http://www.hearingvoicesusa.org/links

International Association of Peer Supporters. (2013). *National practice guidelines for peer supporters.* https://inaops.org/national-standards

Kaufman, L., Brooks, W., Bellinger, J., Steinley-Bumgarner, M., & Stevens-Manser, S. (2014). *Peer specialist training and certification programs: A national overview.* Texas Institute for Excellence in Mental Health, School of Social Work, University of Texas at Austin. https://doi.org/10.5014/ajot.55.1.90

Lloyd-Evans, B., Mayo-Wilson, E., Harrison, B., Istead, H., Brown, E., Pilling, S., Johnson, S., & Kendall, T. (2014). A systematic review and meta-analysis of randomised controlled trials of peer support for people with severe mental illness. *BMC Psychiatry, 14*(1), Article 39. https://doi.org/10.1186/1471-244X-14-39

Mahlke, C. I., Priebe, S., Heumann, K., Daubmann, A., Wegscheider, K., & Bock, T. (2017). Effectiveness of one-to-one peer support for patients with severe mental illness—A randomized controlled trial. *European Psychiatry: The Journal of the Association of European Psychiatrists, 42,* 103–110. https://doi.org/10.1016/j.eurpsy.2016.12.007

Martin, N., & Associates. (2016, March). *Closing the gap: Strengthening the state of peer support in Ontario. Recommendations in response to the findings from "Investigating the State of Peer Support in Ontario."* OPDI.

Mead, S., Hilton, D., & Curtis, L. (2001). Peer support: A theoretical perspective. *Psychiatric Rehabilitation Journal, 25*(2), 134–141. https://doi.org/10.1037/h0095032

Mercado, M., Fuss, A. A., Sawano, N., Gensemer, A., Brennan, W., McManus, K., Dixon, L. B., Haselden, M., & Cleek, A. F. (2016). Generalizability of the NAMI Family-to-Family Education Program: Evidence from an efficacy study. *Psychiatric Services, 67,* 591–593. https://doi.org/10.1176/appi.ps.201500519

Merriam-Webster Dictionary. (n.d.). *Peer.* https://www.merriam-webster.com/dictionary/peer

Mirbahaeddin, E., & Chreim, S. (2022). A narrative review of factors influencing peer support role implementation in mental health systems: Implications for research, policy and practice. *Administration and Policy in Mental Health 49*(4), 596–612. https://doi.org/10.1007/s10488-021-01186-8

Mulvale, G., Wilson, F., Jones, S., Green, J., Johansen, K.-J., Arnold, I., & Kates, N. (2019). Integrating mental health peer support in clinical settings: Lessons from Canada and Norway. *Healthcare Management Forum, 32*(2), 68–72. https://doi.org/10.1177/0840470418812495

National Alliance on Mental Illness. (2017). *NAMI Family-to-Family.* https://www.nami.org/Find-Support/NAMI-Programs/NAMI-Family-to-Family

National Schizophrenia Foundation. (n.d.). *Home page.* https://www.nsfoundation.org

Northern Initiative for Social Action. (n.d.). *Regional Warm Line.* Retrieved June 22, 2023 from https://nisa.on.ca/programs/regional-warm-line

Ostrow, L., & Adams, N. (2012). Recovery in the USA: From politics to peer support. *International Review of Psychiatry, 24*(1), 70–78. https://doi.org/10.3109/09540261.2012.659659

Ostrow, L., & Leaf, P. J. (2014). Improving capacity to monitor and support sustainability of mental health peer-run organizations. *Psychiatric Services, 65*(2), 239–241. https://doi.org/10.1176/appi.ps.201300187

Otte, I., Werning, A., Nossek, A., Vollman J., Juckel, G., & Gather, J. (2020a). Beneficial effects of peer support in psychiatric hospitals. A critical reflection on the results of a qualitative interview and focus group study. *Journal of Mental Health, 29*(3), 289–295. https://doi.org/10.1080/09638237.2019.1581349

Otte, I., Werning, A., Nossek, A., Vollman J., Juckel, G., & Gather, J. (2020b). Challenges faced by peer support workers during the integration into hospital-based mental health-care teams: Results from a qualitative interview study. *International Journal of Social Psychiatry, 66*(3), 263–269. https://doi.org/10.1177/0020764020904764

Peer Support Accreditation and Certification Canada. (2016). *National certification handbook.* Author. https://peersupportcanada.ca/wp-content/uploads/2019/06/Certification_Handbook_v3-ENG.pdf

Peer Support Canada. (n.d.). *Peer supporter competencies.* https://peersupportcanada.ca/wp-content/uploads/2019/06/Peer_Supporter_Competencies-ENG.pdf

Perez, J., & Kidd, J. (2015). Peer support workers: An untapped resource in primary mental health care. *Journal of Primary Health Care, 7*(1), 84–87. https://doi.org/10.1071/HC15084

Pitt, V., Lowe, D., Hill, S., Prictor, M., Hetrick, S. E., Ryan, R., & Berends, L. (2013). Consumer providers of care for adult clients of statutory mental health services. *Cochrane Database of Systematic Reviews, 2013*(3), CD004807. https://doi.org/10.1002/14651858.CD004807.pub2

Rebeiro, K. L. (1999). The labyrinth of community mental health: In search for meaningful occupation. *Psychiatric Rehabilitation Services, 23*(2), 143–152. https://doi.org/10.1037/h0095177

Rebeiro, K. L., Day, D. G., Semeniuk, B., O'Brien, M. C., & Wilson, B. (2001). Northern Initiative for Social Action: An occupation-based, mental health program. *American Journal of Occupational Therapy, 55*, 493–500. https://doi.org/10.5014/ajot.55.5.493

Rebeiro Gruhl, K. L. (2005). Reflections on…The recovery paradigm: Should occupational therapists be interested? *Canadian Journal of Occupational Therapy, 72*(2), 96–102. https://doi.org/10.1177/000841740507200204

Rebeiro Gruhl, K. L., Boucher, M., & Lacarte, S. (2021). Evaluation of an occupation-based, mental-health program: Meeting being, belonging and becoming needs. *Australian Occupational Therapy Journal, 68*(1), 78–89. https://doi.org/10.1111/1440-1630.12707

Rebeiro Gruhl, K. L., Lacarte, S., & Boucher, M. (2023). Mainstream integration of mental health peer support in Canada: A mixed method study. *Canadian Journal of Community Mental Health, 42*(1), 75–95. https://doi.org/10.7870/cjcmh-2023-007

Rebeiro Gruhl, K. L., Lacarte, S., Boucher, M., & Ledrew, L. (2018). Being, belonging and becoming: Development of the 3B Scale. *Australian Occupational Therapy Journal, 65*(5), 354–362. https://doi.org/10.1111/1440-1630.12468

Rebeiro Gruhl, K. L., Lacarte, S., & Calixte, S. (2016). Authentic peer support: Challenges to an evolving occupation. *Journal of Mental Health, 25*(1), 78–86. https://doi.org/10.3109/09638237.2015.1057322

Recovery International. (2017). *Recovery International celebrates 80th year.* https://www.recoveryinternational.org/inthenews/recovery-international-celebrates-80th-year

Repper, J. (2013). *Peer support workers: A practical guide to implementation.* Mental Health Network, NHS Confederation. https://imroc.org/resources/7-peer-support-workers-practical-guide-implementation

Repper, J., & Carter, T. (2011). A review of the literature on peer support in mental health services. *Journal of Mental Health, 20*(4), 392–411. https://doi.org/10.3109/09638237.2011.583947

Resnick, S., Armstrong, M., Sperrazza, M., Harkness, L., & Rosenheck, R. (2004). A model of peer-provider partnership: Vet-to-Vet. *Psychiatric Rehabilitation Journal, 28*(2), 185–187. https://doi.org/10.2975/28.2004.185.187

Rogers, E. S., & Delman, J. (2014). Research, evaluation, and evidence-based practices. In P. B. Nemec & K. Furlong-Norman (Eds.), *Best practices in psychiatric rehabilitation* (pp. 47–63). Psychiatric Rehabilitation Association.

Rooney, J., Miles, N., & Barker, T. (2016). Patients' views: Peer support worker on inpatient wards. *Mental Health and Social Inclusion, 20*(3), 160–166. https://doi.org/10.1108/MHSI-02-2016-0007

Roush, S., Monica, C., Pavlovich, D., & Drake, R. E. (2015). Community engagement research and Dual Diagnosis Anonymous. *Journal of Dual Diagnosis, 11*(2), 142–144. https://doi.org/10.1080/15504263.2015.1025214

Scott, A., Doughty, C., & Kahi, H. (2011, March). *Peer support practice in Aotearoa New Zealand.* https://ir.canterbury.ac.nz/items/d58b2329-6adc-48a0-b301-00c696eefd6c

Solomon, P. (2004). Peer support/peer provided services: Underlying processes, benefits, and critical ingredients. *Psychiatric Rehabilitation Journal, 27*(4), 392–402. https://doi.org/10.2975/27.2004.392.401

Substance Abuse and Mental Health Services Administration. (n.d.). *Core competencies for peer workers.* https://www.samhsa.gov/brss-tacs/recovery-support-tools/peers/core-competencies-peer-workers

Swarbrick, M. (2009). Collaborative support programs of New Jersey. *Occupational Therapy in Mental Health, 25*(3-4), 224–238. https://doi.org/10.1080/01642120903083952

Swarbrick, M. (2013). Wellness-oriented peer approaches: A key ingredient for integrated care. *Psychiatric Services, 64*(8), 732–726. https://doi.org/10.1176/appi.ps.201300144

Swarbrick, M. (2016). *Wellness activity lessons: A guide for group facilitators.* Collaborative Support Programs of New Jersey, Wellness Institute.

Swarbrick, M., & Duffy, M. (2000). Consumer-operated organizations and programs: A role for occupational therapists. *Mental Health Special Interest Quarterly, 23*, 1–4.

Swarbrick, M., Gill, K. J., & Pratt, C. W. (2016). Impact of peer delivered wellness coaching. *Psychiatric Rehabilitation Journal, 39*(3), 234–238. https://doi.org/10.1037/prj0000187

Swarbrick, M., Murphy, A. A., Zechner, M., Spagnolo, A. B., & Gill, K. J. (2011). Wellness coaching: A new role for peers. *Psychiatric Rehabilitation Journal, 34*(4), 328–331. https://doi.org/10.2975/34.4.2011.328.331

Swarbrick, M., & Pratt, C. (2006, March 20). *Consumer-operated self-help services: Roles and opportunities for occupational therapy practitioners.* OT Practice, 11(5), CE1–CE7.

Taylor, A., Dorer, G., & Gleeson, K. (2018). Evaluation of a peer support specialist led group. *Mental Health and Social Inclusion, 22*(3), 141–148. https://doi.org/10.1108/MHSI-03-2018-0012

U.S. Department of Health and Human Services. (2011). *Consumer-operated services evidence-based practice toolkit.* Substance Abuse and Mental Health Services Administration, Center for Mental Health Services. https://store.samhsa.gov/product/Consumer-Operated-Services-Evidence-Based-Practices-EBP-KIT/SMA11-4633CD-DVD

U.S. Department of Health and Human Services. (2015, December 7). *Core competencies for peer workers in behavioral health services.* Substance Abuse and Mental Health Services Administration, Center for Mental Health Services. https://www.samhsa.gov/brss-tacs/recovery-support-tools/peers/core-competencies-peer-workers

Vogel, H. (2010). *Double trouble in recovery: Basic Guide.* Hazelden Publishing.

Voronka, J. (2017). Turning mad knowledge into affective labor: The case of the peer support worker. *American Quarterly, 69*(2), 333–338. https://doi.org/10.1353/aq.2017.0029

Walker, G., & Bryant, W. (2013). Peer support in adult mental health services: A meta-synthesis of qualitative findings. *Psychiatric Rehabilitation Journal, 36*, 28–34. https://doi.org/10.1037/h0094744

Watson, E. (2017). The growing pains of peer support. *Mental Health and Social Inclusion, 21*(3), 129–132. https://doi.org/10.1108/MHSI-03-2017-0017

White, S., Foster, R., Marks, J., Morshead, R., Goldsmith, L., Barlow, S., Sin, J., & Gillard, S. (2020). The effectiveness of one-to-one peer support in mental health services: A systematic review and meta-analysis. *BMC Psychiatry, 20*, 1–20. https://doi.org/10.1186/s12888-020-02923-3

Wright, C., & Rebeiro, K. L. (2003). Exploration of a single case in a consumer-governed mental health organization. *OT in Mental Health, 19*(2), 19–32. https://doi.org/10.1300/J004v19n02_02

Wrobleski, T., Walker, G., Jarus-Hakak, A., & Suto, M. (2015). Peer support as a catalyst for recovery: A mixed methods study. *Canadian Journal of Occupational Therapy, 82*(1), 64–73. https://doi.org/10.1177/0008417414551784

CHAPTER 40

Criminal Justice Systems

Jaime Phillip Muñoz and Lisa A. Jaegers

A country's **criminal justice system** typically includes law enforcement agencies, courts and lawyers, and institutions to supervise and detain individuals. These institutions are responsible for interpreting and applying laws; apprehending, prosecuting, and/or defending those accused of crimes; detaining individuals who are convicted; and providing rehabilitation that may prevent future crimes. Occupational therapy practitioners (OTPs) working within judicial system settings require specialized knowledge of the criminal justice system in their country and unique skill sets, attitudes, and perspectives to inform their practice.

Occupational therapy has an important role in criminal justice and may provide services throughout the criminal justice system. This role includes tasks such as applying occupational therapy processes of functional assessment, skill building, and facilitating transitions that lead to meaningful community participation. Practitioners apply an occupational perspective in the courts systems, juvenile detention centers, jails, prisons, secured units of state hospitals, forensic hospital settings, and various community-based settings that focuses on prevention, deflection and diversion, and/or community reentry (Ferrazzi, 2019; Gonzalez et al., 2023; Muñoz et al., 2020; Schindler, 2019).

This chapter employs a Person-Environment-Occupation (PEO) lens to describe occupational therapy practice in criminal justice settings. It examines the person component by exploring populations in or at-risk of entering criminal justice settings and surveys the specific needs of persons with mental illness. This chapter explores the environment by surveying the range of judicial system settings where practitioners may intervene and the occupational risk factors that can impact recovery. Occupation is investigated by describing occupational therapy roles and processes in the judicial system, including recovery pre- and postrelease. The chapter presents models of practice and evaluation and intervention processes often employed by practitioners in judicial settings. Table 40-1 reviews terminology used throughout this chapter. Readers are encouraged to familiarize themselves with these terms now, as becoming familiar with these terms can help make this chapter's content and this unique practice context more accessible.

The Person: Criminal Justice System Demographics

Incarcerating people suspected of criminal behaviors who are awaiting trial or have been convicted of crimes is a worldwide practice. The objectives for incarceration vary by country; however, the common goals are typically related to public safety and rehabilitation. Incarceration maintains secure control of a person and deprives the person of certain liberties and occupations. While incarcerated, the rehabilitative process is intended to address issues that led to criminal behavior and to reduce recidivism, or the repetition of criminal behavior, that results in reincarceration. In practice, rehabilitation is often limited; however, national initiatives are supporting the practices of restorative justice, rehabilitation, and reentry in criminal justice settings (Council of State Governments [CSG], 2023; Domestic Policy Council, 2023). This section focuses on the person in the PEO framework by examining who is incarcerated or at-risk of incarceration in judicial system settings.

The rate of incarceration or imprisonment in the United States exceeds that of every other nation in the world. The United States has a higher rate of incarceration than Germany, Canada, France, Italy, Norway, and Mexico combined (Fair & Walmsey, 2021). In 2021, more than 1.2 million people were in U.S. state and federal prisons (Carson, 2022), more than 650,000 were in jail (Sawyer & Wagner, 2022), and nearly 4.2 million others were on probation or parole (Kaeble, 2021). In 2021, nearly 25,000 youth were detained in various U.S. juvenile facilities (Office of Juvenile Justice and Delinquency Prevention [OJJDP], 2023).

For individuals living in a jail, prison, or forensic hospital, roles, habits, and routines differ significantly from those they may have had when living in the community. Occupations during incarceration are limited by the policies and procedures enforced within each facility that are intended to restrict occupational participation; remove and detain one from their community environment; limit their access to communicating with those outside the facilities; and adjust to the schedules, rules, and routines of the system, ultimately significantly curtailing occupations.

In addition to individuals incarcerated, the criminal justice system includes a workforce of individuals addressing security, health care, education, and behavioral and mental health services, to name a few. Facilities are staffed by correctional officers, case managers, social workers, teachers, and health professionals including physicians, nurses, and a growing number of OTPs. Workers in corrections or the criminal justice system also experience limitations in occupational performance based on facility policies and procedures. Employees also have limited access to the outside world when inside the institution. Examples of workplace policies include no use of a personal smartphone (e.g., texting, use of social media, access to phone calls), internet access, or bringing in

TABLE 40-1 | Criminal Justice Terminology

Term	Definition
Acquitted	A judgment, by a judge or a jury, that the person being charged has been found not guilty of the offense(s)
Adjudication	The formal delivery of judgment about whether a law was broken and, if so, the sentence for the person convicted of the crime
Appeal	A challenge to a previous legal determination in which a person found guilty of a crime petitions for a rehearing in an appeals court, which has the jurisdiction to review the conviction decision
Arraignment	The first step in a criminal proceeding in which a person is officially called to court, informed of their charge(s), and given the opportunity to enter a plea or response to the charges
Bail bond	Financial obligation signed by the accused to ensure they appear at trial; the accused will lose this money if they do not appear for the trial
Bench warrant	A judge's order for the arrest of a person
Churning	The constant movement of people in and out of the criminal justice system, especially jails
Community reintegration planning	Planning a person's return to the community; ideally, the process begins when the person is incarcerated, follows the person through release, and includes aftercare and interagency coordination
Correctional officer (CO)	A person who maintains custody and security of justice-involved individuals, usually within the confines of a correctional institution
Defendant	In court, the person accused of a crime
Deflection	Typically occurs before a person is arrested or has contact with the justice system; intended to provide a path for treatment that averts the need for action by law enforcement agencies
Deposition	Testimony of a witness or a party taken under oath outside the courtroom
Disposition	The action taken as a result of the defendant's court appearance (e.g., dismissed, acquitted, convicted, or sentenced, placed on probation)
Diversion	Typically occurs after a person is arrested and can take place before charges are filed, before a person appears in court, and before adjudication; individuals may complete a work, rehabilitation, or educational diversion program instead of being incarcerated
Felony	A serious crime, often involving violence, punishable by imprisonment of at least 1 year; can also result in a death sentence
Forensic psychiatry	The branch of psychiatry that focuses on the study of crime and criminality
Halfway or transitional house	A transitional facility where the returning citizen lives and is involved in school, work, training, and so on, while stabilizing for reentry to the community
Incarceration	Being held in a jail, prison, or other judicial system setting to serve a sentence or await disposition
Misdemeanor	An offense that is less serious than a felony but punishable by a fine or incarceration, usually in a local jail and typically for 1 year or less
Parole	A period of control and monitoring that occurs after a person's release from incarceration
Probation	A judicial sentence of community-based supervision or a requirement that a person fulfill certain conditions of behavior in lieu of incarceration; probation can include a fine, a jail sentence, or both
Problem-solving court	Courts designed to address a defendant's underlying problems and assign remediation, restitution, or rehabilitation as alternatives to incarceration (e.g., drug courts, mental health courts, and veterans courts)
Recidivism	Repetition of criminal behavior resulting in a return to incarceration
Relapse prevention	Strategies to help people learn coping and other skills for diminishing stress and resisting environmental triggers that can lead them back into drug use, as well as illegal or nonsanctioned activities
Risk management	A process of identifying, controlling, and minimizing the impact of negative events, such as systematically applying policies, procedures and practices, and vigilance when identifying, evaluating, addressing, and monitoring risk
Work release	An alternative to continuous incarceration whereby an individual works for pay in the community but returns to the correctional institution during nonworking hours

items from outside a facility. All these policies are intended to prevent misuse in the corrections environment.

Mental Illness and the Criminal Justice System

Juveniles and adults with mental illness represent a vulnerable and overrepresented population in criminal justice system settings (Beaudry et al., 2021; Puzzanchera et al., 2022).

For example, in their analysis of 2016 survey data, Maruschak et al. (2021b) found 41% of those in prison self-reported a history of mental health problems. Commonly reported disorders included depression, bipolar disorder, anxiety disorders, posttraumatic stress disorder (PTSD), personality disorder, and schizophrenia. Co-occurring mental illness with substance use disorder are also prevalent (Fazel et al., 2017). Among youth in juvenile detention, the most common disorders noted include conduct disorder, depression, and PTSD in females and conduct disorder, attention deficit-hyperactivity disorder (ADHD), and depression in males (Beaudry et al., 2021). Prevalence rates for psychiatric disorders in older adult populations that are incarcerated, when compared with older people in the community, reflect higher rates for depression; PTSD; psychoses; and bipolar, anxiety, and personality disorders (di Lorito et al., 2018).

Notably, correctional staff working in judicial system settings also report mental health challenges. For example, in an online survey, Canadian judicial system employees, such as correctional officers, probation officers, nurses, or program officers screened positive for disorders such as PTSD, depression, and generalized anxiety disorder (Carleton et al., 2020). Correctional workplace health is a major issue with disproportionately high rates of mental health challenges including suicide, PTSD, depression, and burnout (Ellison & Jaegers, 2022; Jaegers et al., 2022). Recent initiatives from the National Institute of Corrections (NIC) are seeking resources to address staff trauma and organizational stress among employees working directly with people held in prisons and jails (Stewart et al., 2022).

Prevalence rates for mental illnesses among people in criminal justice systems are significantly higher than rates in the general population (Gómez-Figueroa & Camino-Proaño, 2022). These individuals experiencing mental health disorders while incarcerated are often untreated, and substance misuse and trauma are frequent co-occurring lived experiences. There is clear evidence that the number of people with mental illness in U.S. jails and prisons is substantial and the provision of sufficient mental health services is inadequate (Hockenberry et al., 2016; Hopkin et al., 2018). For many individuals, entering the criminal justice system represents the first opportunity to access substance abuse treatment and mental health counseling as well as other aspects of health care (Bonfine et al., 2020).

Disparities in Criminal Justice Systems: Race, Gender, Economics, and Education

The demographics of individuals who are incarcerated are similar worldwide: People who are economically and socially disadvantaged (Rucker & Richeson, 2021; Wang et al., 2022) are overrepresented in jails and prisons. These individuals are most often poor, live in substandard housing, or are unhoused. Many have disorganized family structures and histories that can include mental illness, substance misuse, and domestic violence (Beech et al., 2021; Sutton & Routon, 2023).

Systemic injustices exist in the lives of so many who have been affected by pathways to the criminal justice system, and this recognition has led to conceptualizing the relationships between school, foster care or trauma, juvenile detention, and incarceration in jails and prisons (Grooms, 2020; Jaegers et al., 2019; Muñiz, 2021; Sinko et al., 2021). These relationships have been described using terms such as the "school to prison pipeline" (Bacher-Hicks et al., 2021; Morgan, 2021), the "trauma to prison pipeline" (Sinko et al., 2021), or the "foster care to prison pipeline" (Yi & Wildeman, 2018).

There is a clear overrepresentation of racial and ethnic minorities in the U.S. criminal justice system (Beech et al., 2021; Sutton & Routon, 2023). The arrest rate of blacks and Latinx individuals is three to five times higher than that for whites (Carson, 2022). From an economic perspective, if the individuals who are arrested and detained were contributing to the household economics and food security of their families, after release these racial and ethnic minorities are likely to return to their community unhoused, unemployed, and in debt, which in turn can lead to recommitting a crime (Mears & Cochran, 2015; Sundaresh et al., 2021).

One of the fastest growing incarcerated populations in the United States has been women. For example, in the past three decades the number of females incarcerated increased by more than 585% (Monazzam & Budd, 2023) and over half of these women (58%) had a child under 18 years of age (Maruschak et al., 2021b). Women in jail are disproportionately poor or low income, survivors of domestic violence and trauma (Rodda & Beichner, 2017), and have high rates of physical and mental illnesses and substance use (Nowotny et al., 2014). Many parents who are in jail have not been charged with a crime but cannot afford bail; therefore, they remain detained while they are awaiting trial (Sawyer, 2018).

The existence of educational disparities of people who are incarcerated is an established fact (Sheehan, 2019; Wildeman & Wang, 2017). In analyses of available data, Couloute (2018) reported that 55% of the public in the United States had completed some college education or achieved a bachelor's degree or higher, whereas only 23% of the incarcerated population had done so. Further, only 13% of the public had not attained a high school diploma or equivalency, whereas nearly twice as many of those who were incarcerated (25%) had not attained this level of education (Couloute, 2018).

Boen and colleagues (2022) found that poor parental education increased the risk of arrest, probation, and incarceration among black and Latinx youth, Education attainment levels for women were about the same as those for men, except that females were more likely to have some college or have graduated with a degree; however, regardless of race, ethnicity, or gender, people incarcerated in U.S. jails and prisons are drawn primarily from the least educated segments of society (Nowotny et al., 2016).

Many U.S. state prisons, and to a lesser degree federal prisons, offer some form of educational program, and many take advantage of such programs during their incarceration (Davis, 2019; Gould & Brent, 2020). Education is a route of social mobility. Limited access to occupations of schooling and the roles of students and education that may occur in less enriched educational environments has consequences before and after incarceration (Cai et al., 2019). On the other hand, education both reduces the probability of arrest and incarceration (Bozick et al., 2018; Schuster & Stickle, 2023) and is a consistent factor in reducing recidivism (Cai et al., 2019; Magee, 2021).

Persons with disabilities are also overrepresented in criminal justice systems (Bixby et al., 2022). Maruschak and colleagues (2021a) determined that 38% of the individuals in U.S. state and federal prisons had at least one disability. Most often, these included cognitive (23%), ambulatory (12%), or vision (11%) disabilities. About one quarter (24%) of those surveyed reported that at some point in their life a teacher, doctor, or psychologist told them they had an attention deficit disorder, and the same percentage indicated that they had attended special education classes (Maruschak et al., 2021a). Reingle Gonzalez and her colleagues (2016) similarly reported that 40% of individuals in prison self-identified a non-psychiatric disability; that these were often learning, sensory, and speech-related disabilities; and that those reporting at least one type of disability were more likely to be from minoritized populations. See Chapter 27: Mental Health Stigma and Sanism and Chapter 28: Social Determinants and Mental Health.

The Environment: Key Elements in Criminal Justice Systems

The role of a criminal justice system in any country is to ensure an ordered society and standards of behavior that safeguard individuals, property, and the public. The justice system delineates what constitutes criminal behavior, legislates laws and policies that prevent or limit crime, ensures laws are enforced, tries those accused, and sanctions those convicted of committing crimes. Justice systems reflect the culture, history, traditions, and needs of the country that created them. No two systems are exactly alike; however, broadly speaking, they share consistent elements.

In order to understand the criminal justice system in their countries, practitioners can examine three components inherent in all criminal justice systems: the legislative system that creates laws, the courts responsible for judging and sentencing law breakers, and the correctional institutions that enforce sentencing. Figure 40-1 provides a basic overview of the processes that may occur when a person enters the justice system, and Box 40-1 shares Esteban's story as he enters and progresses through the justice system. It is challenging to visually represent all possible permutations of these processes, but Figure 40-1 lays out the basic structures of the process.

Legislators

In democratic countries, legislatures or parliaments hold authority to make new laws or refine old ones. Legislators crafting these laws are often cognizant of societal concerns and political pressures for addressing criminal behavior. For example, at the end of the 20th century, U.S. legislators passed laws that took clear and significant steps toward more punitive policies. Sentences got longer and, in many cases, were made mandatory, and legislation was adopted that made it more likely for juveniles to be prosecuted as adults. OTPs need to appreciate how laws and policies reflect the country's values and beliefs, as well as their approaches toward crime prevention; punishment and rehabilitation; and the social, political, and economic realities of their country.

Courts

A country's court system is responsible for **adjudication**, or making judgments about whether a law was broken and, if so, defining the sentence for the person convicted of a crime. How a court system works depends on which part of the system has **jurisdiction**, or the authority to make a judgment. In the United States, for example, jurisdiction can occur at the local, city, state, or federal levels and can also be determined by a tribal government or the military. Systems differ across countries. For example, in the United Kingdom, England and Wales have one system, whereas Scotland has its own, and

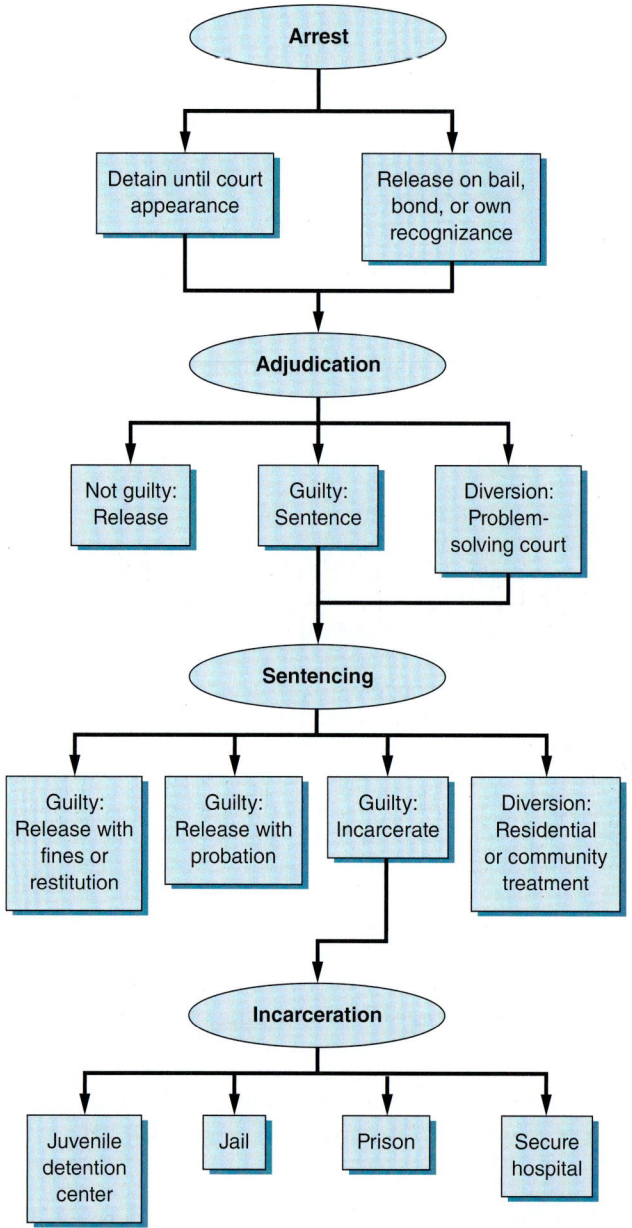

FIGURE 40-1. Entering and moving through the justice system.

all differ from the system in Northern Ireland. Most people have a general understanding that their country has a hierarchical system of courts; Supreme or High Courts are the highest courts in the country, and they render rulings that cannot be appealed in lower courts. As an OTP working in a justice-based setting, it is useful to have a general understanding of the hierarchy of courts and a specific understanding of adjudication in problem-solving courts.

Problem-Solving Courts

Problem-solving courts are designed to address a defendant's underlying problems and assign remediation, restitution, or rehabilitation as alternatives to incarceration. Examples include drug courts, mental health courts, and veterans' courts, which have existed in the United States for nearly

BOX 40-1 ■ Esteban's Story of Moving Through the System

Esteban is a 37-year-old male. He is pacing in front of an Army recruitment office, which is closed, and is observed repeatedly shaking and kicking the doors. Police arrive and order Esteban to "get down and show your hands." Esteban cowers, begins to wail, and repeatedly slaps his hands over his ears. The officers approach, barking orders for Esteban to "be still" but he flails his arms wildly, striking an officer.

Esteban is arrested and charged with vagrancy, unlawful trespass, resisting arrest, and assaulting an officer. Mental health professionals reviewing Esteban's arrest paperwork arrange for him to appear in mental health court. There the mental health court team ensures Esteban, a veteran, is diverted from incarceration and sentenced to treatment.

Esteban will likely have to agree to voluntary inpatient or outpatient treatment, case management, and continued supervision for at least as long as he would have been sentenced to incarceration. If he accepts these conditions, charges may be dismissed, or his sentence can be reduced. His other choice is to be incarcerated and await trial. If he chooses jail, he will receive whatever level of mental health care is available at the jail.

---

40 years and have proliferated in the past decade (Council of State Governments Justice Center, 2009). The common denominator in problem-solving courts is that they all seek to divert individuals from traditional criminal justice processes of court proceedings and incarceration. Collectively, they are judge-centered and nonadversarial, meaning that the individual can expect more direct conversation with a judge to problem-solve the approach to the offense (National Institute of Justice, 2020).

Problem-solving courts exist in many countries, and even though some differences related to jurisdictional processes exist, all are characterized by sentencing processes that include discussions on treatment options and monitoring processes. These facilitate collaboration between the person and their mental health team and assume community engagement (Miller et al., 2020).

Mental Health Courts

Mental health courts are designed to address the mental health needs of the individual. They combine judicial supervision, community mental health, and support services to both reduce crime and address the mental health needs of the perpetrator (American Psychiatric Association [APA], 2021; Bullard & Thrasher, 2016). There are over 300 mental health courts operating in the United States and others that specifically address the mental health needs of juveniles (Substance Abuse and Mental Health Services Administration [SAMHSA], 2018). Mental health courts connect people with mental illness who are suspected of or detained for committing a crime to the resources they need for medication, employment, social functioning, housing, and other support services in lieu of incarceration.

Veterans courts are a specific type of mental health court that is designed to keep veterans with mental illnesses from being incarcerated by diverting them to mental health services. It is important for OTPs to understand how problem-solving courts operate and to understand that even though these courts may divert people from incarceration, the larger systemic problems that lead to the arrest and detention of people with mental illnesses persist and advocacy for timely access to services that may avoid a court appearance altogether remains a continuing need.

People who are addicted may be sentenced in a **drug court**. As in other problem-solving courts, the individual voluntarily agrees to be diverted from confinement, is expected to receive treatment, must meet obligations of their sentence, often must submit to random drug testing, and always risks being returned to the traditional justice system if they fail to meet their obligations (Dollar et al., 2018).

Practitioners should develop a good understanding of the adjudication processes in problem-solving courts. These courts offer opportunities to demonstrate how the inclusion of OTPs can improve the mental health care of individuals adjudicated in these courts and may support improved outcomes.

Deflection and Diversion

Deflection changes the course. Deflection programs in the criminal justice system can change a person's course before the individual is arrested, a law is enforced, or contact with the criminal justice system is initiated (Widgery, 2023). The goal behind these programs is to create a path that replaces arrest with outreach to community-based service providers, especially for persons with mental health or substance use conditions. Deflection programs avert a response from law enforcement. Programs typically involve law enforcement, peer support specialists, recovery coaches, clinical staff, case managers, or social workers.

Diversion is a defining characteristic of sentencing in problem-solving court proceedings (Widgery, 2023). Diversion from prosecution and incarceration requires the person to agree to meet sentencing guidelines for completing restitution, education, work, drug, or mental health treatment programs. Diversion can sometimes occur before the person is charged. In these situations, the police officer or teams of mental health professionals respond to potential arrest situations that involve mental health crises and divert the person from arrest procedures to treatment (Freudenberg & Heller, 2016). Diversion may also occur after charges are recorded. Postcharge diversion processes require that specialized personnel, including OTPs (Ferrazzi, 2019), work in concert with prosecutors, judges, and defense attorneys to divert people with mental illness or addiction to community-based mental health providers (Landess & Holoyda, 2017).

Diversion takes many forms. Some jurisdictions only consider individuals with misdemeanor charges as candidates for diversion, whereas others may accept someone with a more serious felony charge (Freudenberg & Heller, 2016). The type and level of supervision can vary. For example, a person can be sentenced to community service or a work release program, expected to report on weekends, monitored electronically, or referred to residential treatment (Landess & Holoyda, 2017).

Upon successful completion of the conditions of their diversion, some individuals may have their charges dropped, and some may have their records expunged or the charges erased from their record. Others will have records that reflect a guilty plea but recognize that the sentence was deferred. Some will be required to complete a period of probation. Failure to complete the program or meet obligations can result in incarceration, additional court hearings, or stricter conditions (Widgery, 2023).

The team approach in diversion that pairs law enforcement and mental health personnel provides OTPs with opportunities to advocate roles as members of these community evaluation and treatment teams. Rebecca Lord presents a firsthand account of occupational therapy practice in a diversion program in this chapter's first Practitioner Profile feature.

Practitioner Profile

The DOVE Program (Diversion, Occupation, Vocation, and Education)

Trails Ministries, https://trailsministries.org

Rebecca S. Lord, OTD, OTR/L

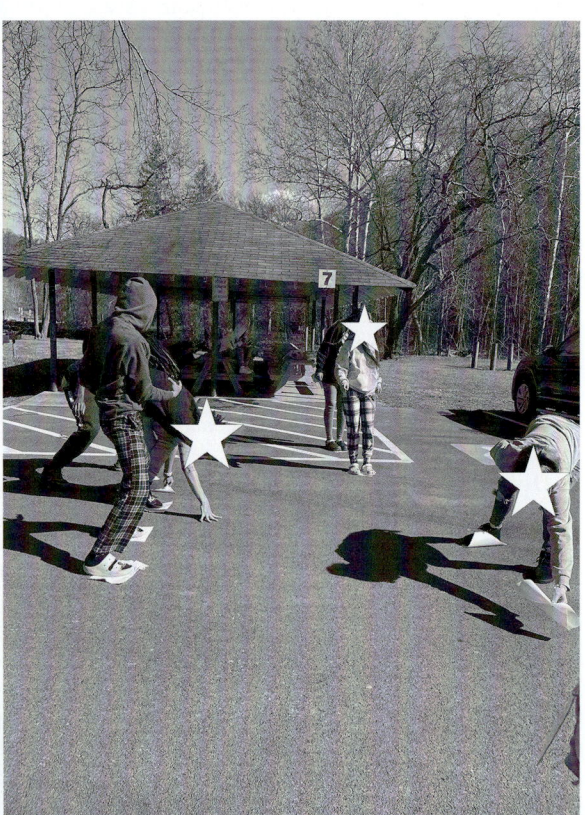

This DOVE session emphasized team building, communication, and critical thinking skills. The task is to flip the sheet onto the other side without stepping on the pavement or using their hands.

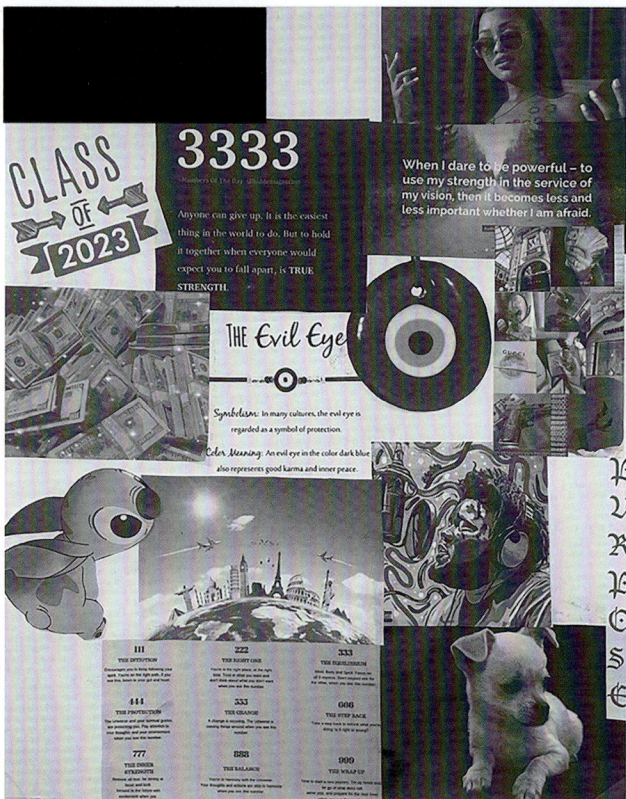

A DOVE participant made this occupational identity poster utilizing newspaper cutouts and printing out images she felt reflected who she is and/or who she wants to be.

DOVE (Diversion, Occupation, Vocation, and Education) is a diversion-based program featuring education n-based and job-readiness tracks. Ultimate program outcomes are reentry into school or obtaining a job. Grants offered by CYS (Child Youth Services) and the PACCT Program (Pennsylvania Academic, Career, and Technical Training) support my occupational therapy position.

Youth are ages 12+ and all have a history of trauma. Most live in stressful environments where they often experience ongoing trauma and all live below the poverty line. Referrals to DOVE come from the juvenile justice system, from CYS, or through schools. Primary reasons for referral include truancy and externalizing behaviors preventing participation in routines

Practitioner Profile—cont'd

and age-appropriate roles. Typical occupational challenges include difficulties engaging socially with peers/family, following routines, engagement in "dark" occupations, occupational imbalances, and difficulty managing psychosocial health. Oppositional defiant disorder, ADHD, PTSD, anxiety, depression, and autism are common diagnoses in this population. I am the only occupational therapist on a team with a program director, behavioral specialist, two facilitators (teachers), and two drivers. We all collaborate with probation officers/CYS case managers.

The MOHO and principles of trauma-informed care guide our programming. The evaluation process includes assessments such as the Role Checklist, a time log screening, Beck's Depression Inventory, GAD-7 screening, the Kawa Model, the MOHOST, and the Sensory Profile. The Double OT is utilized for youth on the vocation track or with those interested in obtaining a job. Motivational Interviewing and reflective listening are key interpersonal approaches. Occupational therapy interventions target sensory regulation, attention, psychosocial health, positive social interactions, occupational balance, occupational identity, self-efficacy, participation, goal setting, and increasing a participant's ability to meet school-based or employment-based expectations. These intervention areas are integrated into sessions that include movement or creative activities to increase motivation and task engagement.

Solid therapeutic use of self is critical for establishing rapport with the youth. Skills in Motivational Interviewing, trauma-informed care, and culturally responsive care are also essential for understanding the complexities of occupational deprivation the participants face in their lives. Some are restricted by parole/probation requirements, which limit engagement in meaningful occupations, but poverty, discrimination, and limitations in the neighborhood environment also present challenges to overcome.

Most participants have difficulty identifying strengths and thinking about the future. However, as a strengths-based occupational therapist, I help them focus on all the incredible facets of their personality, skills, and dreams. Channeling this energy into achievable short-term and long-term goals increases their self-efficacy and ability to think about the future. We celebrate success daily and the best part of this job is seeing the visible shifts in motivation and inspiring hope in participants. This transformation is incredible to witness and support.

Probation and Parole

Probation and **parole** are alternatives to incarceration, but also place limits on participation. Probation is a judicial sentence of community-based supervision or a requirement that a person fulfill certain conditions of behavior in lieu of incarceration; probation can include a fine, a jail sentence, or both. Parole is a period of control and monitoring that occurs after a person's release from incarceration. Both probation and parole represent a contract between the justice system and the person, as they require varying levels of supervision and rules the person must follow to meet the terms of the contract. These conditions can negatively impact participation in multiple ways such as making it more difficult to secure employment, find housing, access health care, or qualify for educational supports (Harding et al., 2022).

The Environment: Criminal Justice System Settings

An OTP may engage individuals involved in the criminal justice system in a variety of settings, including courts, juvenile detention or correctional facilities, jails, prisons or penitentiaries, forensic mental health hospitals, drug and alcohol treatment facilities, military detention centers, immigration detention centers, halfway houses, and community corrections facilities. OTPs are most likely to work in juvenile justice facilities, jails, prisons, secure psychiatric hospitals, and community-based correctional settings (Kapoor et al., 2018; Muñoz et al., 2020). Terms to describe individuals held in these facilities vary widely, such as "offender," "prisoner," "inmate," or "criminal." More person-centered humanizing terms include a person who is justice-involved, incarcerated, resident of a facility, or returning citizen.

Jails

In the United States, jails are facilities operated at the city or county level rather than by the state or federal government. There are far more jails than prisons in the United States, and they hold individuals immediately after their arrest, typically for a short-term period. Jails tend to be smaller than prisons, although large U.S. cities such as Los Angeles and Chicago have huge jail complexes that house thousands of individuals. Jails confine people who are awaiting trial or a hearing for parole, probation, or bail revocation. Some people can be confined in jails temporarily while they await transfer to a juvenile facility, a prison, or an immigration facility. Most people in U.S. jails are charged but not convicted (incarcerated). They are legally innocent and awaiting trial, but most cannot afford bail, which on average is $10,000 for a felony charge (Sawyer & Wagner, 2022). Jails are also a place where people serve their sentence. Jail sentences are often 1 year or less.

Jails confine people shortly after arrest, a time when both stress levels and health and mental health-care needs are high. If a person with a mental illness is arrested, it is very possible that acute symptoms that may have contributed to poor behavior and led to their arrest are still present (Lamb & Weinberger, 2014). Many U.S. jails are ill equipped to respond with mental health treatment or to manage issues that can include the need for seclusion or restraint, medication, and keeping the person, jail personnel, and other detainees safe (Bronson & Berzofsky, 2017).

Practitioner Profile

Hancock County Justice Center and Community Forensic Mental Health Team

Miranda Tippie, EdD, OTR/L

At the Hancock County Justice Center (HCJC, jail based), OTPs and students work with individuals involved in the justice system. Individuals are self-referred or referred by jail staff with identified needs focused on life skills, self-regulation, or executive functioning. Individuals with or without a psychiatric diagnosis are eligible for services. In the jail, occupational therapy students completing level 2 fieldwork provided unreimbursed interventions under the supervision of faculty from The University of Findlay.

Occupational therapy is also part of a forensic mental health team that includes case managers; counselors; and forensic, assertive community treatment, and prevention team members. Team members operate at a local community mental health facility. Here, individuals diagnosed with mental illnesses such as bipolar disorder, schizophrenia, anxiety, depression, or substance use disorders receive services within the facility, in their homes, or anywhere in the community that meets the person's needs. Referrals for occupational therapy are to address areas such as life skills and self-regulation, or to improve functional independence and participation. Occupational therapy services are billed as case management and reimbursed though insurance. The team also seeks grants to purchase supplies and additional services.

Assessments, such as the Allen Cognitive Level Screen, Sensory Profile, ACEs, PTSD Checklist, and the Rhode Island Change Assessment Scale are used to generate an occupational profile and an individualized intervention plan. Typical challenges to occupational functioning in both settings include the inability to complete activities of daily living (ADLs)/IADLs (e.g., financial and home management, self-care), limited/lack of roles and routines, coping skills, and limited exploration of/participation in leisure, education, and work/volunteer occupations.

Occupational therapy may address sensory modulation, self-awareness, emotional regulation, role development, executive functioning, coping skills, mindfulness, ADLs/IADLs, or participation (leisure, work, education). Broad intervention outcomes include improving independence and function in daily living, improved coping, symptom management, better self-awareness and emotional regulation, and meaningful engagement in valued routines of occupation. Therapeutic conversations routinely stress problem-solving and

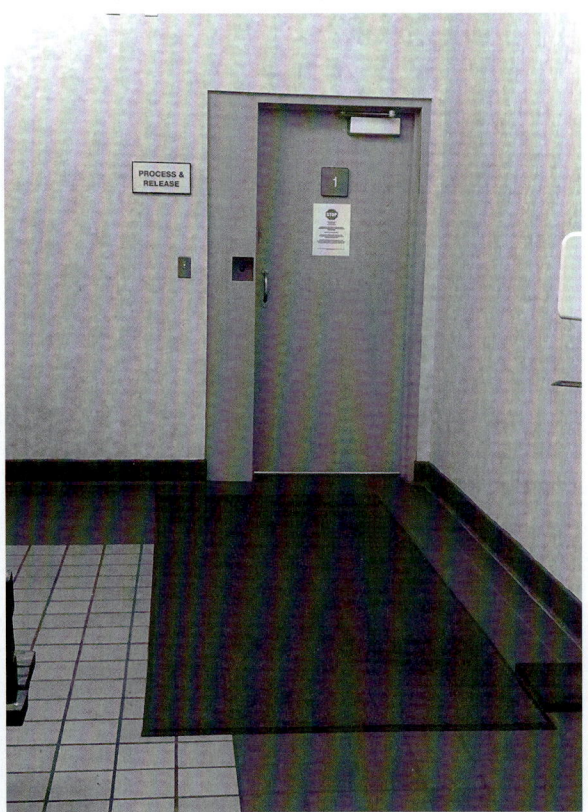

Jails are secure facilities. Each day, OTPs are escorted to the occupational therapy office by correctional officers to begin programming.

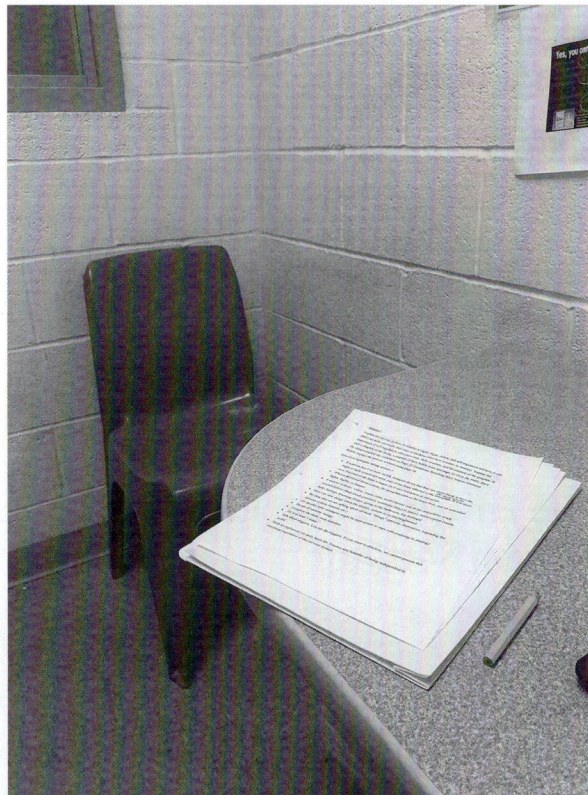

Residents attend 1:1 sessions in our county jail with occupational therapy level 2 fieldwork students.

Practitioner Profile—cont'd

decision-making. Engagement in simple occupations is key. That is, playing a game with the person or having them take a walk, clean their kitchen, or practice a mindfulness or sensory strategy can be effective intervention,

Flexibility and problem-solving are two main skills practitioners working in this setting need. Flexibility requires creativity to meet a person where they are despite sometimes considerable barriers to participation. Modeling

problem-solving that maintains a person's dignity and agency helps facilitate function and independence is key.

Individuals in these settings can experience intense emotions and engage in or consider self-harm or suicide. These are difficult conversations to have with a person, but it is rewarding to help individuals develop their own safety plan and use coping or sensory strategies they have learned to find purpose in life.

Jails are high-volume facilities that serve as correctional distribution hubs filtering people to and from courts, community programs, and other correctional institutions while simultaneously confining many who have already been sentenced. In the United States, jail admissions routinely exceed 10 million people per year (APA, 2016; Sawyer & Wagner, 2022). Jail environments feature a steady stream of family members; visitors; and legal, social, and faith-based human service personnel moving in and out daily, all of whom must adhere to visitation protocols and are subjected to security scrutiny and searches. Compared with prisons, jails offer more opportunity for social participation with a wider range of individuals.

The physical environment in jails varies, but most are structured by classification of individuals to minimum, medium, and maximum security levels with housing separated by floors or units. Depending on the facility, there will be more or fewer designated areas for medical, mental health, educational, leisure, or drug and alcohol programs. Each floor may include space for staff offices, and some have an open multipurpose or gym area. Eggers and colleagues (2006) described the physical structure of a county jail in which occupational therapy was included in a community reintegration program. In that setting, each floor of the jail was subdivided into cellblocks or "pods," a common area allowed for some interaction among residents. In general, activities were limited to watching television, playing cards or table games, reading, writing letters, talking on the payphone, and playing basketball or walking in the small gym area on the pod.

Jails are mandated to provide basic mental health screening, and some jails have beds designated for people with mental illness; however, the availability of comprehensive mental health services in jails (e.g., crisis intervention, referral services, ability to segregate consumers) varies considerably (Bronson & Berzofsky, 2017). OTPs have developed effective programing in jail settings (Dillon et al., 2020; Eggers et al., 2006; Jaegers, Ahmad et al., 2020). An occupational therapist, Miranda Tippie, shares one example of an occupational therapy program in a county jail setting in the chapter's second Practitioner Profile feature.

Prisons

Prisons are secure institutions that confine individuals who, in general, have been convicted of a felony and have been sentenced to at least 1 year of incarceration. In the United States,

a person can be sentenced to a state or federal prison depending on the type of offense committed and the jurisdiction of the sentencing court.

Compared with jails, prisons are generally larger and more stable environments with much less movement in and out of the facility. A primary objective of any prison facility is to confine the person and protect the safety of the public, the residents, and the correctional staff. In contrast to most people in jails, people in prison have often been in the criminal justice system longer, are more likely to experience geographic separation from their home communities, experience social and psychological adjustment related to longer incarceration, and can experience different postrelease challenges (Prins, 2014).

Prisons are classified by their level of security. The Federal Bureau of Prisons (BOP; 2018b) designates levels of security as high, medium, low, and minimum security, according to the presence of various security features in the institution. Security features often include armed external patrols, security towers, fences and other security barriers, electronic detection devices, and staff-to-resident ratios. Most people in U.S. prisons are housed in low- or minimum-security (55%) and medium-security prisons (30%). Relatively few are housed in high-security prisons (12%), and a very small minority (3%) are housed in unclassified settings (BOP, 2018b).

High-security prisons often house the individuals who are classified as the most dangerous and have the most significant security features. In these settings, individuals can be confined for long periods of the day. Each cell typically has a toilet bolted to the floor, and residents may take brief showers up to three times a week. Movement out of the cellblock area often does not occur without further restrictions such as handcuffs, leg irons, and correctional officer escorts. These facilities have the highest staff-to-resident ratio of all prisons (BOP, 2018a).

Medium-security prisons provide more opportunity for movement, activity, and interaction among individuals. A prison yard or recreational areas, libraries, showers, health-care services, and other facilities are typically available. Medium-security prisons can offer a variety of work-oriented and treatment programs. In some medium-security prisons, individuals sleep in dormitories and have access to communal showers, toilets, and sinks.

Low- and minimum-security prisons have consistent security routines, but residents generally have opportunities for

Practitioner Profile

Occupational Therapy in the Federal Prison System

Catherine Kaminski, MS, OTR/L, BCMH

Editor's Note: The opinions expressed in this article are those of the author and do not necessarily represent the opinions of the Federal Bureau of Prisons or the U.S. Department of Justice.

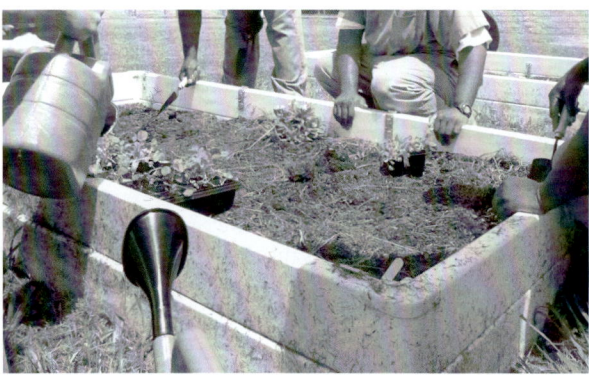

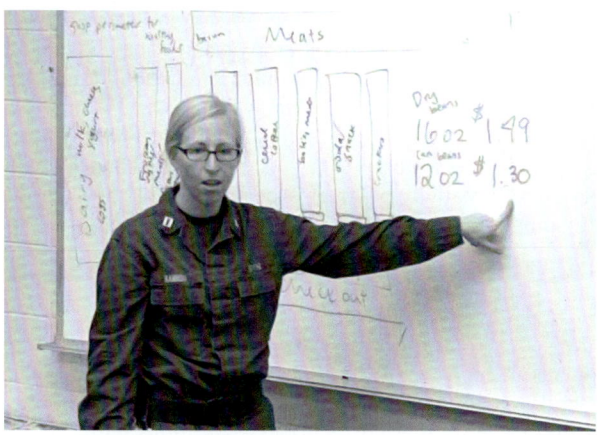

The BOP is the federal government agency responsible for the confinement and rehabilitation of approximately 155,000 individuals throughout the United States. Within the BOP, OTPs work in multiple settings to include acute care, inpatient rehab, orthopedics, and mental health. Although OTPs may have a primary practice area at their institution, the holistic nature of our profession enables us to support a variety of health-care issues this population faces.

OTPs work primarily within mental health at three BOP facilities in the United States. Here they address a range of needs with people having a variety of serious mental illnesses including schizophrenia, anxiety, depression, substance abuse, schizoaffective disorder, bipolar disorder, and antisocial or borderline personality disorder. Individuals receiving occupational therapy may be housed on a locked inpatient psych unit, or, as support needs decrease, progress through a series of residential programs such as the Step Down Program and ultimately into a more traditional outpatient approach.

Occupational therapy within BOP mental health is grounded in the recovery model and interventions use a holistic approach to improve an incarcerated individual's ability to live with mental illness both in the prison and once transitioned to the community. During the initial evaluation, OTPs generate an occupational profile and administer assessments such as the OCAIRS, AMPS, Routine Task Inventory, or the COPM to identify an individual's strengths, weaknesses, and other occupational concerns. OTPs may use resources such as SAMHSA's 8 Dimensions of Wellness model to aid in the discussion of different domains that may be incorporated into the treatment plan.

Common individual factors impacting capacity for occupational engagement include poor emotional regulation, maladapted communication and social skills, limitations in cognition, avolition, and low sense of self-efficacy. In addition, the correctional environment limits occupational choice, which affects an individual's habits, daily routine, and overall well-being. Together, the OTP and the individual set goals for their recovery. Depending on what level of support the individual needs, treatment plans may include facilitating opportunities to return to work through supported employment; establishing a routine to manage symptoms and/or addiction cravings; or, for someone who is struggling with severe avolition, focusing on activity exploration through the MOHO-driven Remotivation Process to reignite a desire for engagement in life tasks.

Practice within the prison setting is challenging because it requires navigating strict safety requirements daily to provide comprehensive care. However, 95% of incarcerated individuals will return to the community. Being a part of the change process that allows these individuals to adapt to new health-promoting, law-abiding lifestyles needed for successful community reintegration is rewarding.

movement, interaction, work, and treatment. There is often more open space, and perimeter security tends to be less extensive. Individuals in these settings may work on agricultural, transportation, and conservation projects.

Prisons are mandated to provide a basic level of psychiatric service, including screening, assessment, referral, evaluation, intervention, and community reentry planning, but the frequency, quality, and availability of these services vary among institutions (APA, 2016; SAMHSA, 2022). Many individuals enter U.S. jails and prisons with histories of trauma, mental illness, difficulties controlling impulses and managing emotions, and poor problem-solving (Butler et al., 2022; SAMHSA, 2022). Carceral environments can exacerbate symptoms, especially when a majority of those with mental illness do not receive mental health treatment or continue psychiatric medications they may have been taking before incarceration (National Alliance on Mental Illness [NAMI], 2023; Ring & Gill, 2017). OTPs can and do provide services in prisons, as described in the chapter's third Practitioner Profile feature, which is contributed by Catherine Kaminski.

Secure Psychiatric Hospitals

Secure psychiatric hospitals are facilities that evaluate, treat, and rehabilitate individuals with mental illnesses who have entered the criminal justice system or those who, because of their conditions, are considered unfit for trial or are deemed not criminally responsible (Galappathie et al., 2017; Ozkan et al., 2018; Pinals & Callahan, 2020). In the United Kingdom, secure hospitals may house individuals with co-morbid disorders associated with their criminal behaviors, such as personality disorders and substance use, but can also include people with significant neurodevelopmental disorders and learning disabilities (Royal College of Occupational Therapists, 2017). Secure hospitals in the United Kingdom are clearly differentiated, and can include low secure units, medium secure regional hospitals, high secure special hospitals, and dangerous and severe personality disorder units (McNeil & Bannigan, 2014).

Some individuals who have not committed crimes but who present with a complex set of disorders and behavior that may be too challenging to address in a general psychiatry ward may also be confined in a forensic hospital (Kapoor et al., 2018). A primary difference between secure psychiatric hospitals and mental health care for individuals who have not committed a crime is that these settings have the dual responsibility to treat the mental illness and address the individual's offense. Secure settings use the physical environment, person-staff relationships, and procedural measures within the setting to deliver interventions in a safe and protected environment (Galappathie et al., 2017; Royal College of Occupational Therapists, 2017).

Some correctional settings house individuals with mental illness separately only when the person is in crisis or acutely symptomatic; when the person exhibits severe decompensation in the general population; or when the person is considered dangerous, suicidal, or at significant risk of self-harm (Adams & Ferrandino, 2008). In some states, individuals with mental illness are not housed in a mental health unit but in segregated disciplinary sections of the prison or they are assigned to a high-security prison setting (Fellner, 2008; Haney, 2008).

Both prisons and jails do transfer the most severely mentally ill to secure units in state mental hospitals or public forensic psychiatric hospitals (Fitch, 2014). Within these secure forensic hospitals there is great diversity in the available treatment; some facilities have considerable resources and space directed toward mental health services and programming, whereas others have much less. In the United States, the number of people admitted to forensic units in state hospitals because they are found incompetent to stand trial, require competency evaluations, and/or are in need of restoration services has continued to increase (Wik et al., 2017). In a review from 2020 to 2021, over half the residents in state hospitals (56%) had a forensic status (National Association of State Mental Health Program Directors Research Institute [NRI], 2021). It is important for learners reading these data to bear in mind that, worldwide, there is a high prevalence of people with mental illness who are incarcerated and that in the United States a person with severe mental illness is more

likely to be in jail or prison than in a facility providing rehabilitative services (Timme & Nowotny, 2021).

In addition to treatment of their mental illness, forensic psychiatric hospitals address the person's offense-related treatment needs. For example, individuals who are convicted sex offenders require specialized intervention to address these types of offenses (Galappathie et al., 2017). When forensic units are housed in state hospitals, OTPs can encounter many of the same resources found in large mental health institutions. Security concerns will always add a layer of watchfulness, protection, and safety, but practitioners may offer comprehensive programming such as life skill, prevocational, or social skills training (Kapoor et al., 2018; White et al., 2013). See Chapter 41: State Hospitals.

Community-Based Justice Settings

Community-based justice settings may be federally contracted **residential reentry centers** where individuals are sent as an alternative to incarceration or placed just before or upon their release. They can also be residential or nonresidential community-based programs funded by a combination of state and local government and community nonprofit organizations that are funded by private and public foundations. Community-based correction settings can be a heterogeneous mix of programs developed to serve the needs of varied populations including but not limited to juveniles, adults, people with addictions, women, children of offenders, elders, sex offenders, and people who are at risk for entering or returning to the criminal justice system or who are transitioning to the community after incarceration.

In the United States, the BOP contracts with community-based residential reentry centers to provide structured, supervised community reentry services (BOP, 2018a). These centers are not specifically designed to address the unique needs of a person with mental illness; however, it is a well-established finding that people formerly incarcerated have a high rate of mental illness (Hoke, 2015; Hopkin et al., 2018), that those attempting to reintegrate into the community face a multitude of challenges that can negatively impact their mental health (Kelly et al., 2017; Western et al., 2015), and that women (Pedlar et al., 2018), veterans (Finlay et al., 2019), people with addictions (Gunnison & Helfgott, 2017), and sex offenders (Yoder & Farkas, 2017) all experience significant mental health challenges.

Community reentry centers assist residents with reintegration planning, job placement, and financial management; help them to locate permanent housing; and connect residents with an array of community services that can support their recovery and return to the community (BOP, 2018a). These centers expect rigid adherence to a strict schedule, and periodic, random head counts are common. Residents are not restricted to the center, but they must sign in and out of the facility, and random calls or visits to employment sites can be used to monitor their location. Random drug and alcohol tests can also be administered to people sentenced to a community reentry center.

The level of security at community reentry is similar to a minimum-security setting, and multiple strategies are used to monitor the movements of the residents. Those with noncompliant behavior can be restricted to the center, whereas at the other end of the continuum, those who are meeting

BOX 40-2 ■ **Reentry and Recovery—Joel**

Joel is a 43-year-old white male who has been convicted and sentenced for various crimes since he was a teenager. He has been diagnosed with bipolar disorder and has battled substance abuse for 27 years. He is the single father of a 14-year-old son. His wife died of an overdose when his son was 7. Joel is on a path of recovery and has not used alcohol or drugs for 4 years. Joel completed an occupational therapy community reintegration program while in the county jail and he lived in supervised housing postrelease. He and his son now live with Joel's aunt. Joel's reflections on what helps and what gets in the way of his recovery and reintegration appear in the text that follows.

Strategies for Reintegration

- "I avoid my relatives. Anybody, any of my friends in the past that used drugs. I am finding new people and places to be without drinking and drugs."
- "You have to work hard. Everybody is proud of a paycheck. I know mine's not gonna equal theirs [from selling on the street],

but who has to walk around and worry? Not me, 'cause all mine is legal. All his is illegal."
- "The first thing that has to happen is that you have to *want to* inside. That'll get you clean, but it won't keep you clean. Now, to stay clean, you gotta discipline yourself."

Family and Social Environments

- "My dad was into numbers and used to collect money for people. . . . He used to hurt people and he always had card games at the house. My uncles were cocaine dealers and drug dealers. I basically come from a family of criminals."
- "I decided I couldn't keep running in and out of my son's life. 'Cause how you think a kid feels when his dad is not around? It's not good for the kid, I can speak from experience on that one."
- "People, places, and things. You can't go back into the same environment. I cannot go to, like, my relatives still sell drugs, use drugs. I haven't visited them since I got out. No. People, places, and things will get you in trouble or keep you out of trouble."

---

obligations and who have a release plan may be able to spend extended time at their own or a family member's home to support their transition. "Community-based program" is a term used to describe a wide variety of different services designed and developed to address the needs of youth and adults in justice-based systems. This includes programs addressing the needs of those who are at risk of entering or reentering criminal justice settings. These programs are funded by a variety of public and private sources. Some are faith-based programs.

Community-based programs may target a specific population such as women, mothers, youth, individuals with intellectual disabilities, those with addiction problems, sex offenders, or elders released after serving long prison sentences. Some programs are specifically designed for people with serious mental illness and the majority target mental health. In Box 40-2, Joel shares some strategies that supported his recovery and reintegration that he learned in a community-based program.

The services provided at community-based programs vary. They may emphasize employment by providing job-seeking classes, organizing job fairs, and developing connections with local employers and industries willing to hire people with criminal histories. Many programs support returning citizens as they look for housing. A critical component of many of these programs is offering substance abuse and mental health treatment and counseling. Such services can be offered on-site, or these programs may contract with local providers to deliver these services. Family support services and financial and legal planning may also be provided at such settings.

Community-based settings may provide one of the best contexts for authentic occupational therapy intervention. The focus on reintegrating into the daily routines of community life and the development of the skill sets necessary to support reintegration resonate with the basic mission and philosophy on which the profession was founded. An evaluation of occupational performance and a thorough occupational profile reflecting the person's potential for functional and prosocial occupational performance can support the person's recovery

and reentry and provide their defense attorney with a vision of participation that lets the attorney advocate for sentencing that considers the person's rehabilitation potential.

Practitioners who can create evidence-based, person-centered programs can find a place in community-based settings, but they will need to prove their program's effectiveness and earn their place. Programs that help demonstrate a clear link between incarceration alternatives, functional occupational performance, and reduced recidivism can elicit the attention of the many communities searching for and experimenting with alternatives to incarceration. Practitioners need to market their skill sets within justice-based systems, with judges, lawyers, reentry program directors, and community programs that are already addressing the needs of this population and advocate for occupational therapy's place in the development and delivery of these programs. The chapter's fourth Practitioner Profile feature presents an OTP who has created her own business and is successfully proving the distinct value of occupational therapy in a community-based setting.

Foster Care Settings

Over 600,000 children and youth were living in foster care in the United States in 2021 (Anne E. Casey Foundation [AECF], 2022). Foster care is meant to provide safe, temporary living arrangements and support services for children who have been removed from their families because of maltreatment, lack of safety, or inadequate care. Children and youth in foster care are most likely to live in a nonrelative foster family's home or at the home of a relative, but many live in institutions or a group home and some may live in a supervised independent living situation (U.S. Department of Health and Human Services [USDHHS], 2022). The foster care-to-prison pipeline refers to the channeling of youth from foster care to juvenile detention or adult incarceration (Williams et al., 2021; Yang et al., 2021).

Youth in the foster care system have a higher risk for pathways to incarceration as compared with their peers because of

Practitioner Profile

Life After Incarceration: Transition and Reentry (LAITR)

https://www.lifeafterincarceration.com/

Ariana Gonzalez, OTD, OTR/L, CTP

LAITR is an entrepreneurial private practice providing 1:1 and group occupational therapy services to individuals who are incarcerated or were previously incarcerated. Occupational therapists work in a county jail and with a community reentry team that includes case managers, housing specialists, and peer supports. Some referrals come from state and nonprofit organizations for individuals on parole or living in the community postincarceration.

The population served at LAITR is, on average, 33.5 years old, 88% male, and 90% report substance use difficulty with an average ACE score of 4.17. Almost half (49%) our population reports at least one mental health diagnosis; 28.57% report ADHD, and 35% have had one or more traumatic brain injuries (TBIs). Other commonly reported diagnoses include anxiety, PTSD, and depression. Data from varied PROMIS (Patient-Reported Outcomes Measurement Information System) person-centered measures reflect a population with high stress and anxiety, low general self-efficacy, difficulties managing emotions, minimal social supports, trouble setting achievable goals, and poor time management skills.

LAITR Life Skills groups occur inside the jail on consumer-identified topics such as emotional management, time management, budgeting, sleep, leisure, health management, pain management, communication, and goal setting. The core focus of individual sessions is on building life skills and healthy habits and routines. Most of what we do is related to behavior change. Our practice uses problem-solving and guided discovery approaches and models (e.g., Motivational Interviewing, Cognitive Orientation to Occupational Performance, MOHO, and the Stages of Change model) in every session, so people learn to independently problem-solve barriers to their goals.

For example, a person may continually forget to use their habit tracker during the week and only complete it right before arriving for their session, despite their desire to use it daily. Instead of outright instructing the person to put the tracker somewhere visible, such as the fridge, we use guided questioning to facilitate problem-solving, so the person independently identifies this or a similar solution. This increases buy-in and, most importantly, increases opportunities to build executive functioning skills and ultimately progress to a point where occupational therapy is unneeded. Our main goal is to improve justice-involved individuals' quality of life (QOL) and overall health in multiple dimensions to increase the probability that people will live the lives they want to live in the community and stay out of the judicial system.

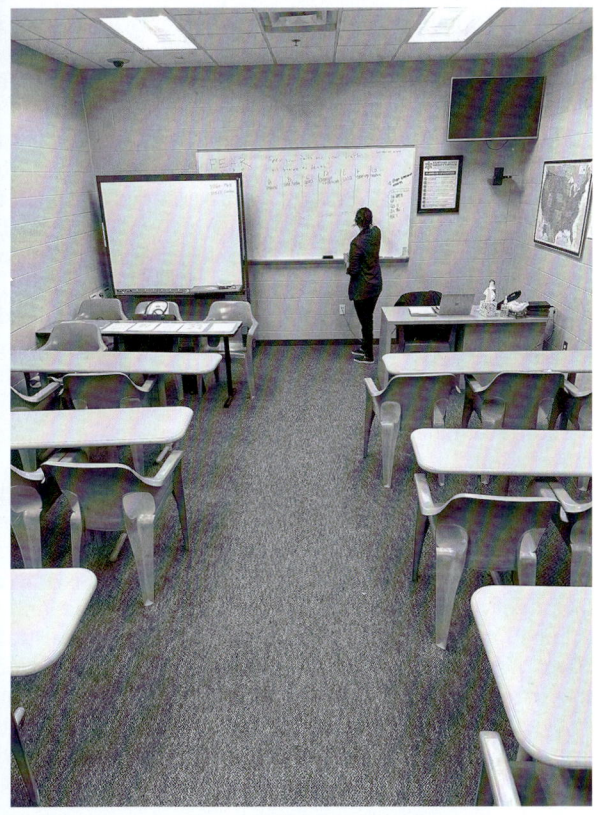

Dr. Gonzalez preps for a LAITR Life Skills group.

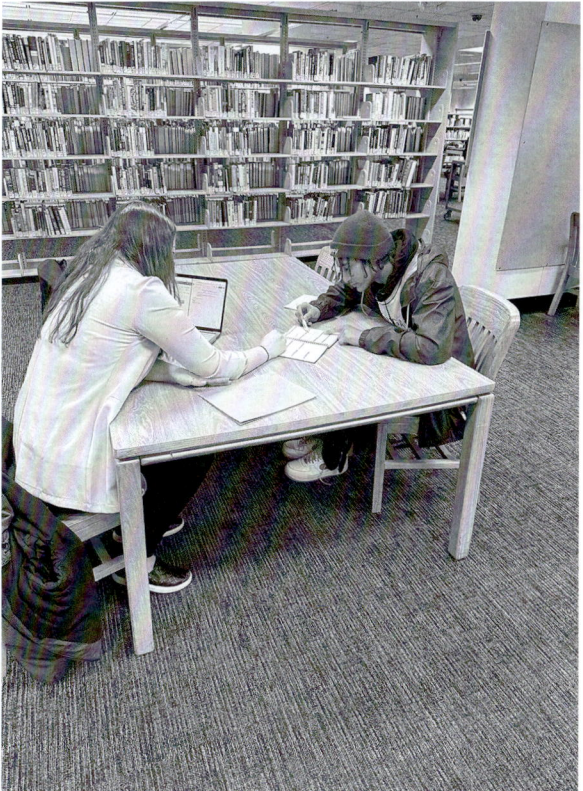

A practitioner meets 1:1 with a participant to focus on time management.

Continued

Practitioner Profile—cont'd

This work is difficult, but extremely rewarding. I enjoy being an entrepreneur in a niche area of practice, working toward advocacy for a stigmatized and underserved population, and educating future practitioners on their role with this population. Advocacy is a skill that I use every day, advocating against injustices faced by the people we serve, for new programming, for funding, and for occupational therapy's seat at the table.

vulnerable situations when lacking caregiver support, a stable home, and treatment to address adverse childhood trauma (Muñiz, 2021; Sinko et al., 2021). In fact, half of the youth living in foster care (50%) will be arrested, convicted, or detained by the time they reach the age of 17, and 25% will encounter the criminal legal system within 2 years of leaving foster care (Juvenile Law Center, 2018; Perez, 2023). When transitioning out of foster care, those young adults experience higher rates of incarceration (AECF, 2022).

Systemic inequities are reflected in the demographics of the foster system and juvenile justice system (Children's Bureau, 2021). Minoritized youth, particularly black, American Indian, and Alaskan Native youth, are overrepresented among those entering foster care and the juvenile justice system (Cénat et al., 2020; Puzzanchera & Taylor, 2020). LGBTQ+ youth more frequently experience physical, sexual, and emotional abuse both in foster and in secure settings than their cisgendered peers (Baams et al., 2019; Matarese et al., 2021). Youth in foster care who have a neurodisability tend to enter foster care earlier, experience more caregiver relinquishment, and experience cumulative maltreatment and trauma; these factors contribute to criminal activity and charges (Baidawi & Piquero, 2021). Foster care youth are also at higher risk for suicide, chronic health issues, homelessness, and unemployment than their same-aged peers (AECF, 2022). The trauma experiences of youth in foster care can affect their long-term development, mental health, education, and everyday occupational performance (AECF, 2022).

OTPs will encounter juveniles who are at risk of or who are already involved in the foster care system or juvenile justice system in schools, in community programs, in juvenile detention centers, or in juvenile correction facilities. A juvenile detention center is designed for secure, short-term confinement where youth are held after being arrested, but before adjudication, disposition, or transfer. Juvenile correctional facilities are secure institutions designed for longer-term placements. Youth in correctional facilities are charged, found delinquent, and a judge has ordered their confinement (AECF, 2021).

It is essential that practitioners approach their practice in a trauma-informed manner and understand that youth in these systems are very likely to have histories that include adverse childhood experiences (ACEs) and trauma. Having OTPs to address the occupational needs and development of youth in the foster care system and to support caregiver roles may prevent or reduce entry to the criminal justice system. Useful descriptions of occupational therapy programs and practices in foster care and juvenile justice can be found in the professional literature (Armstrong-Heimsoth et al., 2020; Dowdy et al., 2023; George-Paschal & Bowen, 2019; Jaegers et al., 2019; Shea et al., 2019; Smith, 2022). This chapter's final Practitioner Profile feature shares one example of occupational therapy practice with criminal justice–involved juveniles in a community-based setting.

Environment: Occupational Risk Factors

Justice-based settings are contexts that create unique problems and obstacles to implementing occupation-based practice. These settings are established to confine; therefore, the primary goal is to maintain order and security, not to provide rehabilitation. Practices for maintaining security often significantly restrict opportunities for engagement in occupations (Whiteford et al., 2020). A person with mental illness experiencing prolonged confinement may feel isolated, bored, and frustrated at the lack of opportunities for participation in activity (Ring & Gill, 2017).

At its worst, the environment can be one where a person is routinely victimized by others or overloaded with sensory stimulation (NAMI, 2023). A small, cramped cell is an ineffective refuge from an overstimulating environment. The images in Figure 40-2 provide two visual examples of confinement spaces. Readers should compare and contrast the physical structure and the objects pictured in these environments to those that they have in their own living spaces. Note that a single-occupancy cell has a floor space of 70 square feet (7 feet by 10 feet). Half of this space is taken up by a bed, a desk or writing space, and a toilet (American Correctional Association, 2016).

Occupational science literature contains useful concepts for deepening practitioners' understanding of how justice environments limit engagement in occupation and for designing interventions to address these limitations. These concepts include occupational imbalance, occupational alienation, and occupational deprivation (Occupational Therapy Australia, 2016; Whiteford et al., 2022; Wilcock, 1998); occupational restriction and reconciliation (Galvaan, 2005); occupational apartheid (Kronenberg & Pollard, 2005; Simaan, 2021); and occupational enrichment (Molineux & Whiteford, 1999).

Practitioner Profile

Occupational Therapy in a Juvenile Detention Center Occupational Therapy Training Program (OTTP-SF): http://ottp-sf.org

Colleen McNeil, OTR/L; Emily Tunnat, OTR/L; and Janelle Buccat, OTR/L

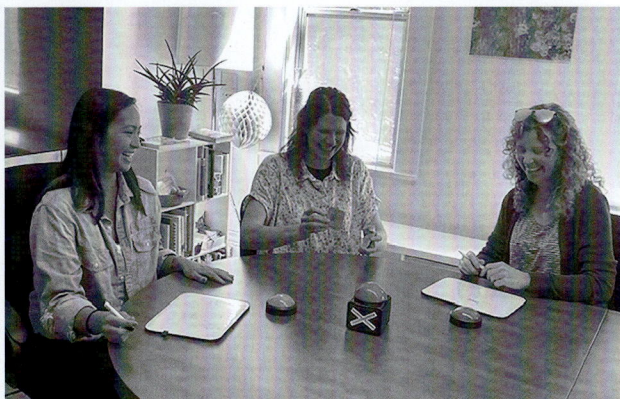

Colleen, Emily, and Janelle, OTTP-SF practitioners, trying out a modified Family Feud Harm Reduction Edition game.

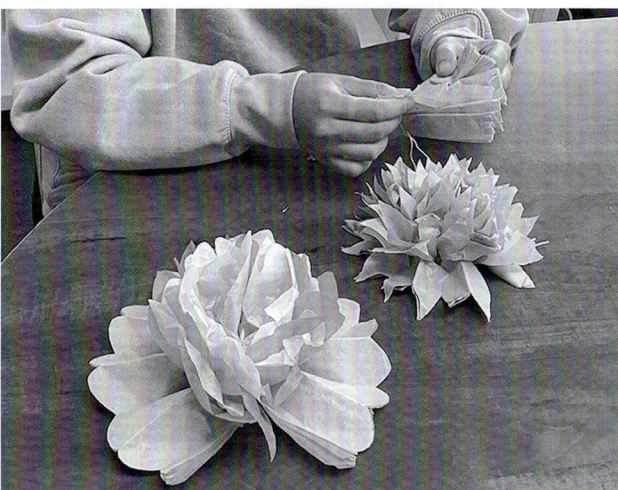

Using an art activity for focused skill building and for use in a celebration of youths' accomplishments.

OTTP-SF has served youth ages 13 to 25 at the Juvenile Justice Center (JJC) in San Francisco for several years. Services are grant funded through San Francisco's Department of Children, Youth and Families (DCYF). OTTP-SF routinely responds to DCYF requests for proposals that identify a population, define a specific purpose, and offer funding for a 3- to 5-year cycle.

At the JJC, youth charged with a criminal offense are detained for lengths of stay that range from 24 hours to several years. All youth have Individual Rehabilitation Plans (IRPs). Occupational therapy provides group and individual skill-building interventions that address these IRPs. Occupational therapy services target skills for self-regulation, self-awareness, positive self-concept, activity tolerance, anger management, empathy, perspective taking, communication, conflict resolution, and life skills.

Occupational therapists use nonstandardized assessments that build on each youth's strengths-based personal narrative. Occupational therapists assess needs and interests to plan effective and relevant interventions. Trauma-informed care, the MOHO, harm reduction, and strengths-based models guide practice. Typical occupational challenges include exposure to compound traumatic experiences, impulse control, isolation from familiar relationships, lack of roles and routines, challenged coping, unpredictable and chaotic environments, and hopelessness. Occupational therapists work collaboratively on a team to provide services at the JJC, operating under the supervision of correctional officers and JJC program directors/managers. OTTP-SF Occupational therapists meet weekly to share treatment ideas, offer support, and problem-solve challenges.

Occupational therapists harness youth's interests and practice decision-making to promote their skill-building and engagement in self-directed therapeutic activities as a form of healing through activity. Some barriers to skill-building are the passivity of some youth and occupational deprivation of detention settings such as restrictions on the unit. This year, occupational therapy recognized accomplishments by planning an appreciation event on each long-term commitment unit. Youth made many tissue paper flowers to decorate for the event. This activity presented an opportunity to experience mastery in an artistic hands-on task that challenged their frustration tolerance but led to the creation of something meaningful. Each youth was provided a just-right challenge and activity demands were graded to promote problem-solving, healthy risk taking, and accomplishment.

In a system that defines youth as criminals to be punished, OTPs can model empowerment for each youth and affirm them as individuals with strengths and potential for skill-building. Key practitioner skills required in settings such as this include a strong capacity for activity analysis and the ability to harness each person's motivations and interests to build transferable skills by offering choices and building trust. Being able to recognize youth as experts of their own experience, and being present to witness agency and strengths in the face of incredibly vulnerable and adversarial situations, is powerful and rewarding.

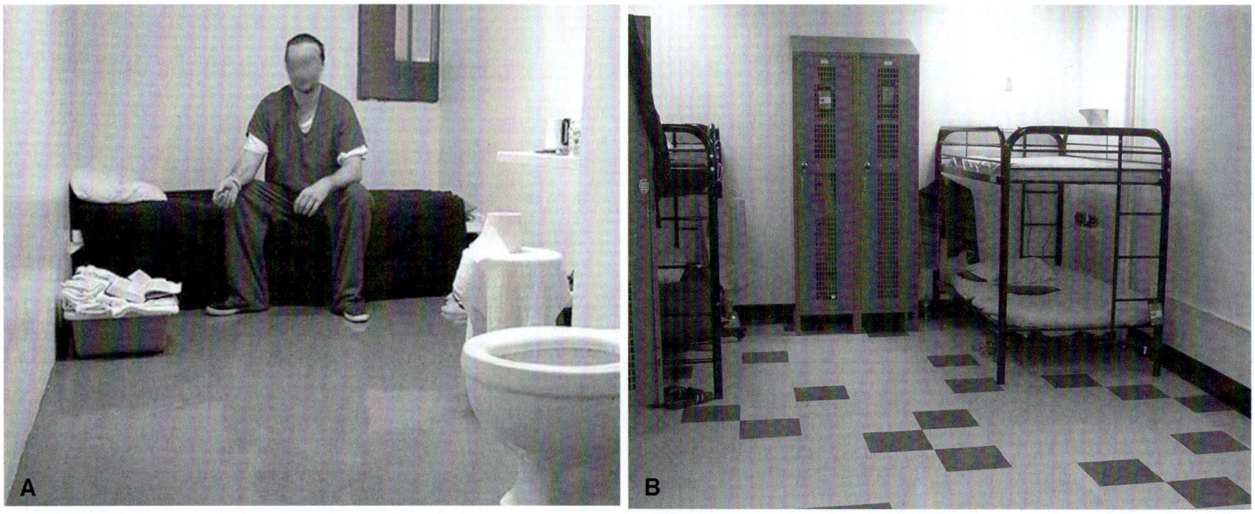

FIGURE 40-2. Two examples of confinement spaces. A. Individual cell at a county jail. B. Dormitory room in a community corrections site.

Brief definitions of several of these concepts and examples of how they may be applied are listed in Table 40-2.

Each of these occupational science concepts has relevance for understanding and intervening with people in correctional settings (Jaegers et al., 2019). Occupational deprivation in particular provides a useful conceptual framework for understanding the environmental contexts of justice-based settings (Phelps & Aldrich, 2022). Occupational engagement provides a conceptual lens for designing skill-building and role-development interventions that can provide opportunities for participation despite contextual limitations and may help practitioners create successful skill building approaches within justice-based settings and in the community postrelease (Gunarathne et al., 2022).

Occupational Deprivation

Occupational deprivation is a tacit dimension of the environment in correctional institutions (Whiteford et al., 2020). Occupational deprivation not only limits opportunities for participation while the person is incarcerated but can also pose significant barriers to successful community reintegration postrelease. While incarcerated, individuals can become so estranged from productive, social, leisure, and relationship roles that they may lose their capacity to structure their own time to meet the challenges of daily life and community participation, skills that are necessary for adaptive community reintegration. Occupational deprivation can lead to diminished capacities, reduced self-efficacy, and significant loss of identity as a citizen of the community (Farnworth & Muñoz, 2009; Whiteford, 1997, 2000).

Occupational Enrichment

About 25 years ago, Molineux and Whiteford (1999) offered the concept of occupational enrichment as a guiding principle to enhance settings where occupational deprivation is a consistent characteristic of an environment. **Occupational enrichment** in justice-based settings creatively generates opportunities for the person (P) to engage in occupations (O) despite limitations that often exist in justice-based environments (E). Justice-based settings place significant restrictions on a person's opportunities for engagement in meaningful activities. The typical daily routine, especially in the most secure settings, is structured by a strict schedule for meals, showering, security checks, staff shift changes, and lights out.

In some settings, in-house jobs such as cooking or washing dishes in the staff cafeteria, janitorial tasks, laundry, and assisting in a library may be available to well-disciplined individuals on the recommendation of correctional officers. Different settings may provide varied offerings of literacy, educational and computer instruction, religious services, recovery support groups, and reintegration planning services, which can offer welcome diversion from the structured security routine.

Unique challenges to occupational enrichment exist in justice settings requiring practitioners to creatively generate possibilities for participation. For example, it is difficult to find ways to individualize interventions in a context where conformity is a valued method for confinement and control. Modification of the physical and social environment can be challenging when the environment and rhythm of routine are designed to severely restrict one's capacity to gain any measure of control over their environment. Finally, it is challenging to provide people with choices regarding how they orchestrate their daily routines in an environmental context where nearly every activity is completed in a manner dictated by the correctional institution.

Occupation: The Occupational Therapy Process in Criminal Justice Systems

OTPs around the world have recognized for nearly 75 years that the profession has an important role to play in the rehabilitation of people within justice-based systems

TABLE 40-2 | Occupational Science Concepts Applied to Justice-Based Settings

Concept	Definition	Example of Application to Incarcerated Populations
Occupational alienation	"Sense of isolation, powerlessness, frustration, loss of control, estrangement from society or self because of engagement in occupation which does not satisfy inner needs" (Wilcock, 1998, p. 257).	Mr. Hardy was challenged to feel connected or to have a sense of purpose when his rhythm of life in a justice-based setting was monotonous and repetitive. Once released, he continued his pattern of isolation he demonstrated in prison. Despite having a vibrant community center operating literally next door to his home, his sense of immobilization and inertia made it very difficult for him to utilize this resource.
Occupational apartheid	"Refers to the segregation of groups of people through the restriction or denial of access to dignified and meaningful participation in occupations of daily life on the basis of race, color, disability, national origin, age, gender, sexual preference, religion, political beliefs, status in society, or other characteristics" (Kronenberg & Pollard, 2005, p. 67).	A practitioner working with Mr. Hardy would need to examine the social, economic, and political conditions that deny or restrict opportunities for participation. For example, in the state he lives, because of his felony conviction he is disqualified from registering to vote, may not vote, and cannot run for office. He is also restricted or not eligible for federal loans or grants for education and is ineligible for government assistance such as welfare or supplemental nutrition assistance programs.
Occupational deprivation	"Deprivation of occupational choice and diversity because of circumstances beyond the control of individuals or communities" (Wilcock, 1998, p. 257). "Deprivation is distinguished from a disruption in occupational choice because it is a process that occurs over a long period of time" (Whiteford, 1997).	Occupational deprivation is an implicit characteristic of correctional settings. For years Mr. Hardy has been systematically denied the ability to make choices for participation in meaningful and health-promoting occupations and this impacts his reintegration. Postrelease, Mr. Hardy is easily overwhelmed as he adjusts to unstructured time, open spaces, and crowded environments, which trigger his anxiety and feelings of incompetence.
Occupational enrichment	"The deliberate manipulation of environments to facilitate and support engagement in a range of occupations congruent with those that the individual might normally perform" (Molineux & Whiteford, 1999, p. 127).	The practitioner learns Mr. Hardy once loved to garden and looks to directly address occupational deprivation by modifying Mr. Hardy's immediate environment. Together they construct a raised garden box and add plants to rekindle his interest in gardening. Some neighbors also garden, and eventually Mr. Hardy may engage neighbors when he shares or trades his produce.
Occupational imbalance	"A lack of balance or disproportion of occupation resulting in decreased well-being" (Wilcock, 1998, p. 257).	During years of incarceration Mr. Hardy rarely experienced a balance of physical, mental, social, and restful occupations. Now trying to reintegrate, for Mr. Hardy, a "busy" day is when he cleans his small apartment and takes a walk to a local park where he sits for hours watching squirrels play.
Occupational reconciliation	This concept describes a person's submissive response to stifling environmental conditions. Loneliness, lack of stimulation, and limited resources can lead a person to "give way to their circumstances and engage in limited occupations because of their restricted opportunities" (Galvaan, 2005, p. 436).	Mr. Hardy experienced the prison environment as overcrowded, boring, and dangerous. His reaction to this environment was to "just do the time." Now released, Mr. Hardy has resigned himself to a routine where he spends a lot of his time alone. He chooses not to engage in opportunities to develop his potential. He is alone when he eats. He does not walk or exercise, read, or participate in any community activities.

Galvaan, R. (2005). Domestic workers' narratives: Transforming occupational therapy practice. In F. Kronenberg, S. S. Algado, & N. Pollard (Eds.), Occupational therapy without borders: Learning from the spirit of survivors (pp. 429–439). Elsevier Churchill Livingstone; Kronenberg, F., & Pollard, N. (2005). Overcoming occupational apartheid: A preliminary exploration of the political nature of occupational therapy. In F. Kronenberg, S. S. Algado, & N. Pollard (Eds.), Occupational therapy without borders: Learning from the spirit of survivors (pp. 58–86). Elsevier Churchill Livingstone; Molineux, M. L., & Whiteford, G. (1999). Prisons: From occupational deprivation to occupational enrichment. Journal of Occupational Science, 6(3), 124–130. https://doi.org/10.1080/14427591.1999.9686457; Whiteford, G. (1997). Occupational deprivation and incarceration. Journal of Occupational Science, 4(3), 126–130. https://doi.org/10.1080/14427591.1997.96 86429; Wilcock, A. (1998). An occupational perspective of health. Slack.

(British Columbia Society of Occupational Therapy, 1949). Descriptions of occupational therapy's unique role in U.S. (Bartholomew, 1976; Penner, 1978), Australian (Farnworth et al., 1987; Lloyd, 1987a), and New Zealand prisons and forensic mental health settings (Seek, 1989; Tse, 1990) began appearing in occupational therapy professional journals in the mid-1970s. National (Schindler, 2019) and international (Muñoz, 2019b; Muñoz, Farnworth, & Dielman, 2016) journals have devoted full issues to this practice setting, sharing examples of occupational therapy in justice settings with contributions from practitioners from Australia, Brazil, Canada, and the United States.

Despite recognition of occupational therapy's potential role in justice systems, the profession has moved slowly to articulate clear roles and establish guidelines for the scope of occupational therapy services within criminal justice systems. One exception is the practice guidelines developed in the United Kingdom (Royal College of Occupational Therapists, 2012, 2017), which offer recommendations for occupation-focused practice in secure hospital settings.

Models of Practice

There are several models of practice for occupational therapy that could effectively be used to address the needs of people incarcerated. The Model of Human Occupation (MOHO; Taylor, 2017), PEO models (Christiansen et al., 2015; Law et al., 1996), and the Canadian Model of Occupational Performance (Townsend & Polatajko, 2013) are three practice models in particular that are identified most often in the occupational therapy literature and in recent surveys of justice-based practice in the United Kingdom (McQueen, 2011; Royal College of Occupational Therapists, 2012, 2017), the United States (Muñoz, Moreton, & Sitterly, 2016), and Canada (Chui et al., 2016). Other models include the Occupational Adaptation Model (Schkade & Schultz, 1992; Stelter & Whisner, 2007) and the Kawa Model (Iwama, 2006).

Each of these models can be described as comprehensive models of occupational functioning. Each, to a greater or lesser degree, offers specific concepts for considering the physical and social environment and provides one or more assessment tools for evaluation. See Chapter 3: Person-Environment-Occupation Model, Chapter 4: Person-Centered Evaluation, Chapter 7: Cognition, and Chapter 11: Motivation for detailed information about these models of practice. 🤝

Evaluation and Assessment

Practitioners in criminal justice settings use a wide variety of assessment tools to determine individual needs in areas of juvenile detention, specialty court conditions (i.e., family, substance abuse, or mental health courts), forensic mental health, jail, or prison reentry; probation or parole; community corrections; and related areas of practice. In addition to community and mental health–informed practice areas, OTPs also provide typical rehabilitation services in prisons and jails similar to acute, inpatient, outpatient, skilled nursing, and long-term care therapy. OTPs working in criminal justice settings can work with people across the life span, from juveniles to older people. Given the wide range of populations and practice settings within criminal justice, it is critical for OTPs to choose assessment tools that allow them to tailor their evaluation processes to ensure person-centered, contextually informed intervention plans.

Evaluation may be considered at the individual, group, organization, and population levels, depending upon the area of focus. For instance, when working with a person who is returning to the community after a long-term stay in prison, the OTP would choose assessment tools to develop a reentry plan (Gonzalez et al., 2023). For group level interventions, the OTP would use assessments informed by the group and a related interprofessional team. At the organizational level, an OTP performs a participatory workplace needs assessment with multiple key informants and a variety of stakeholders to gain an understanding of workplace mental health risk factors to reduce work stress and trauma (Jaegers, Ahmad et al., 2020).

Practitioners working in UK forensic settings overwhelmingly utilize assessments grounded in the MOHO (Cassidy & Garrick, 2012; Duncan et al., 2003; Royal College of

Occupational Therapists, 2012, 2017). Muñoz, Moreton and Sitterly (2016) reported similar preferences for MOHO in their survey of U.S. practitioners. Chui and colleagues (2016) sampled Canadian practitioners who also frequently reported using MOHO assessments but were most likely to use the Canadian Occupational Performance Measure (Law et al., 2014). This preference was also reported by U.S. practitioners in recent studies (Jaegers, Neff et al., 2020; Patel et al., in press).

As with any person receiving occupational therapy, practitioners must consider the activities that individuals need, want, and have to do in order to support everyday living. Criminal justice occupational therapy is no exception. Practitioners use their lens for exploring occupations with individuals in order to determine their goals. In one study reviewing the goals explored with people who were incarcerated ($n = 21$), 84 subcategories of goals were identified (Fig. 40-2; Jaegers, Neff et al., 2020).

Most identified goals could be categorized as instrumental activities of daily living (IADLs; $n = 195$) goals and included ambitions such as driving, using technology, learning how to budget, and establishing a home routine. Health management ($n = 120$) goals included finding a primary care physician, mental health services, health insurance, addiction treatment, and relationship counseling. Other leading categories of goals were work ($n = 53$), social participation ($n = 34$), education ($n = 22$), and leisure ($n = 9$). The study results not only show the need for skilled occupational therapy intervention but also the complexity in individual needs when in the criminal justice system (Fig. 40-3).

The evaluation process with people may be ongoing and initially may take multiple sessions. As the practitioner learns more from the person, additional assessments may be indicated by actions, interests, and problems expressed by the person. For instance, when working with a person on jail-to-community reentry planning, the practitioner would begin with a "chart review" if available by the jail case manager to reduce extra questions to ask the person and consider the jail and community contexts. A trauma-informed approach seeks to reduce repeated questions by multiple professionals in an effort to reduce trauma.

Next, an interview and, if possible, observation during an occupational profile would be informative to a Canadian Occupational Performance Measure to gain baseline satisfaction and performance of tasks before the person's short-term stay in jail. Then the practitioner can determine if additional cognitive, mental health, sensory, physical, or other assessments are indicated to further inform the evaluation and guide goal setting and intervention planning. Readers should review Chapter 4: Person-Centered Evaluation 🤝 to further inform their consideration of the variety of assessment tools that can be used with individuals in the criminal justice system. This evaluation process, depending on the format—in person (at a facility or in the community) or telehealth (phone or video)—may take multiple sessions to complete.

Researchers studying occupational therapy practice in criminal justice settings have urged practitioners to utilize reliable and valid outcomes measures (McQueen, 2011; Muñoz et al., 2020; O'Connell & Farnworth, 2007; Royal College of Occupational Therapists, 2017; Schindler, 2019). Evidence

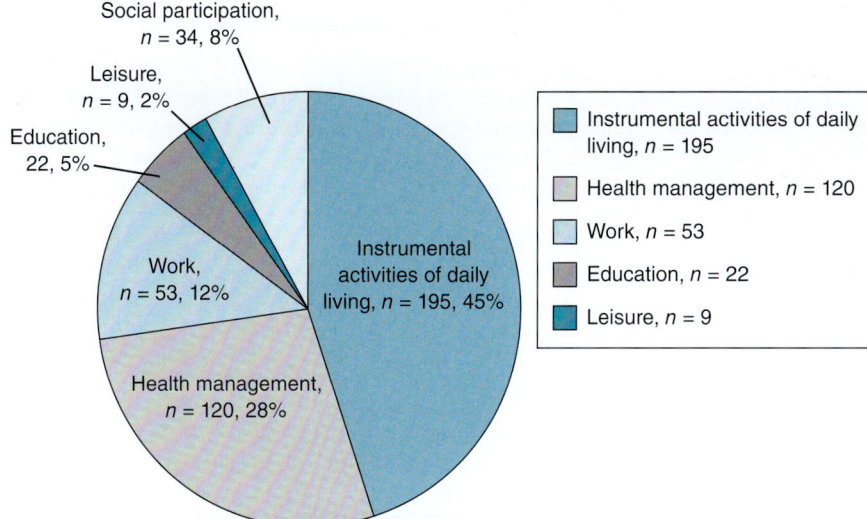

Occupation-Based Client Reentry Goals, *n* = 21 Clients
Number of Goals in Each Category

FIGURE 40-3. Distribution of occupation-based reentry goals.

from recent surveys of practice in the United States (Muñoz, Moreton, & Sitterly, 2016) and reviews of evidence in secure hospital settings in the United Kingdom (Royal College of Occupational Therapists, 2017) suggest that some practitioners are using tested assessment tools, whereas others do so less routinely. It is important to consider both validated assessment tools in combination with strong interview and observation skills when performing an evaluation. Overall, practitioners need to use their best therapeutic reasoning skills and choose assessment tools that fit the person, level of intervention, and the context.

Specific Assessment Tools

This section will focus on individual level assessment tools that have been used by practitioners in criminal justice settings including but not limited to the MOHO Screening Tool (MOHOST; Fitzgerald, 2011), the Occupational Self-Assessment (OSA; Baron et al., 2006), the Assessment of Motor and Process Skills (Fisher, 2014), the Assessment of Communication and Interaction Skills (Fitzgerald et al., 2012), the Occupational Questionnaire (Stewart & Craik, 2007), the Occupational Therapy Task Observation Scale (Smith et al., 2010), the Occupational Circumstances Assessment Interview and Rating Scale (OCAIRS; Ozkan et al., 2018), and the Allen Cognitive Level Screen (Lindstedt et al., 2011).

Overall, occupational therapy has not designed and tested assessment tools specifically tailored to people involved in criminal justice. Nonetheless, there are a variety of valid and reliable tools appropriate for use in these settings, a selected number of which are outlined in Table 40-3. Because descriptions and considerations for using most of these tools appear in other chapters, only a selected number of assessments are listed here and included in Table 40-4.

An interview guided by an American Occupational Therapy Association (AOTA) occupational profile can help a

practitioner develop a comprehensive understanding for the person's perceptions, need for services, surrounding contexts, performance patterns, related factors, and goals. One interview tool designed to assess the explicit needs of justice-based populations is the OCAIRS (Forsyth et al., 2005). The OCAIRS includes interview questions modified for use with forensic populations. Questions are designed to elicit data on roles, habits, personal causation, values, readiness for change, interests, skills, goals, interpretation of past experiences, and the physical and social environment (Parkinson et al., 2006). To date, no published studies have examined the specific usefulness of this tool in forensic practice.

For individuals who understand the metaphors used when considering one's life as a flowing river, the Kawa Model interview process (Iwama, 2006) can be a useful interview approach. This method asks the person to portray their life as a river that has problems (rocks) to contend with and elicits useful data for understanding how the person's social and physical contexts (riverbanks) impact their life and problem-solving. In this process, the person identifies assets and attributes (driftwood) that they bring to managing their life situation. The overall image that is created can help better understand the person in context, and a skilled practitioner can use the image as the basis for focused interviewing and collaborative intervention planning.

As an interview method, the Kawa Model interview process is flexible. Most often, it is used in a way to help the person portray their current life situation, but it can also be used to encourage the individual to represent their life history. Examples of this approach with one justice-involved individual are shown in Figure 40-4. See Chapter 4: Person-Centered Evaluation. 🤝

The *Barriers to Reentry Success Inventory,* 3rd ed. (BRSI; Liptak, 2022) is an example of a self-report tool specifically designed for justice populations. The Outcome Rating Scale (ORS) measures the apprehensions and barriers that people facing reentry are concerned about. It is structured to be

TABLE 40-3 | Selected Assessment Tools Used in Criminal Justice Settings

Type of Assessment	Examples
Interview	• AOTA Occupational Profile (AOTA, 2021) • Canadian Occupational Performance Measure (Law et al., 2014) • Kawa Model Interview Process (Iwama, 2006) • Occupational Therapy Circumstances Assessment Interview and Rating Scale (Forsyth et al., 2005) • Occupational Performance History Interview II (Kielhofner et al., 2004)
Self-Report	• Assessment of Occupational Functioning Modified Interest Checklist (Role Checklist Version 3; Scott et al., 2019) • Occupational Self-Assessment (Baron et al., 2006) • Barriers to Reentry Success Inventory, 3rd ed. (Liptak, 2022) • Sensory Profile (Brown & Dunn, 2002)
Performance	• Double OT (Haworth & Cyrs, 2017) • Executive Function Performance Test (Baum et al., 2008) • Kohlman Evaluation of Living Skills (Thomson & Robnett, 2016) • Montreal Cognitive Assessment (Nasreddine et al., 2005) • Texas Functional Living Scale (Cullum et al., 2009)
Observational	• Assessment of Motor and Process Skills (Fisher, 2014) • Model of Human Occupation Screening Tool (Parkinson et al., 2006) • Occupational Therapy Task Observation Scale (Margolis et al., 1996)

Synthesized from multiple sources including: Chui, A., Wong, C. I., Maraj, S. A., Fry, D., Jecker, J., & Jung, B. (2016). Forensic occupational therapy in Canada: The current state of practice. Occupational Therapy International, 23(3), 229–240. https://doi.org/10.1002/oti.1426; Couldrick, L., & Aldred, D. (2003). Forensic occupational therapy. Whurr; Haworth, C., & Cyrs, G. (2017, August 21). Supporting transitions to the workforce for at-risk youth: Developing and using an occupation–based work assessment. OT Practice, 22, 21–24; McNeil, S., & Bannigan, K. (2014). Forensic and prison services. In W. Bryant, J. Fieldhouse, & K. Bannigan, Creek's occupational therapy and mental health (5th ed., pp. 424–438). Churchill Livingstone Elsevier; Moore, M. (2014). Forensic psychiatry and occupational therapy. In R. Crouch & V. Alers (Eds.), Occupational therapy in psychiatry and mental health (pp. 106–114). Wiley Blackwell; Muñoz, J. P., Catalano, A., Wang, Y., & Phillips, G. A. (2020). Justice-based occupational therapy: A scoping review. Annals of International Occupational Therapy, 3(4), 162–174. https://doi.org/10.3928/24761222-20200924-02; Muñoz, J. P., Moreton, E. M., & Sitterly, A. M. (2016). The scope of practice of occupational therapy in U.S. criminal justice settings. Occupational Therapy International Journal, 23(3), 241–254. https://doi.org/10.1002/oti.1427

self-scored and self-interpreted; however, similar to most self-report tools, an effective approach is for the practitioner to complete this tool collaboratively with the person. Reviewing the results of this measure with the person can help ensure meaningful transition planning. The BRSI surveys the respondents' concerns for basic needs, job searching, family relationships, life skills, and career development.

The MOHOST provides an expansive overview of a person's occupational participation (Parkinson et al., 2006). The MOHOST is a good choice when the practitioner has regular opportunities to interact with the person and the person can participate in meaningful occupations that allow the practitioner to effectively evaluate performances. When the practitioner has sufficient evaluation information, the MOHOST helps identify challenges a person may have in their occupational performances. It helps a practitioner focus on areas where follow-up with specific assessments can support the development of a comprehensive occupational profile. As new assessment information is generated, the MOHOST becomes a useful repository of the knowledge the practitioner develops about the person through time.

Risk/Needs Assessment

One area of assessment specific to the criminal justice setting is risk/needs assessment. At a practical, everyday level, practitioners working in justice settings need to recognize that assessment of risk is a dynamic process, and vigilance to ensure safety and security is a consistent component of the environmental context in these settings (Cordingley & Ryan, 2009; McNeil & Bannigan, 2014). Risk assessment involves therapeutic reasoning about whether the person may carry out high-risk behaviors that can include harm to self or others (Castaneda, 2010). The risk-need-responsivity model for offender assessment and rehabilitation (Andrews & Dowden, 2007) has guided the development of risk assessment instruments and attempts to explain why some interventions work and others do not.

Although occupational therapy does not have a specific practice model addressing risk and needs of people incarcerated, Cordingley and Ryan (2009) proposed that PEO models (Christiansen et al., 2015; Townsend & Polatajko, 2013) could frame risk assessment in secure settings for occupational therapy practice. When assessing person factors, the practitioner would consider aspects such as the person's history, especially if it includes violent behavior; the person's current state of mind (e.g., one of motivation and purpose or frustration and resentment); and the person's self-regulation behaviors.

Practitioners need to proactively consider criminogenic risk by maintaining a secure environment, considering how the therapy environment is structured and maintained, and limiting access to equipment and supplies to ensure accountability for these materials. Managing risk can also be accomplished through effective activity analysis and thoughtful consideration of the occupations presented in therapy. A practitioner who considers the person and the environment and remains vigilant about risk management

TABLE 40-4 | Therapeutic Reasoning Assessment Table: Justice-Based Systems

Which Tool?	Who Was This Tool Designed For?	Is This a Type of Tool the Person Can Do? What Is Required of the Person?	What Am I Measuring?	How Long Does It Take and Where Do I Administer This Assessment?	Is the Tool Associated With a Practice Model?
AOTA Occupational Profile (AOTA, 2021)	Person, group, or population being treated	Functional cognition to respond to a range of interview questions	Perceptions of need for services, contexts, performance patterns, individual factors, and goals	Varies, can be performed in 45 minutes to 1 hour in any setting, and can be performed in multiple sessions	*Occupational Therapy Practice Framework: Domain and Process* (4th ed.)
Kawa Model (Iwama, 2006)	Use with youth to adult populations; can be tailored to assess a person's perceptions specifically related to release and reintegration	Functional cognition to communicate and reason at a basic level with metaphors used in this approach	A person's perceptions of problem situations, personal strengths, and environmental factors that aid or undermine performance	Varies, but a drawing can be made in fewer than 20 minutes with 15–20 minutes of discussion to understand the person's perspectives	Kawa Model
Occupational Circumstances Assessment–Interview and Rating Scale Version 4.0 (OCAIRS; Forsyth et al., 2005)	Adults/Older adults and adolescents	Functional cognition to respond to a range of interview questions	Assesses occupation, interests, goals, values, role participation, and the impact of the environment	Allow 45 minutes to 1 hour in any setting	MOHO
Model of Human Occupation Screening Tool (MOHOST; Parkinson et al., 2006)	Adults/Older adults and adolescents	A screening tool on which ratings can be made after chart review, observation, and participation in a brief interview process	Practitioner synthesizes data to rate multiple performance, habituation, volition, and environmental factors impacting function	Allow 10–15 minutes after data have been collected through other evaluations or observation	MOHO
Barriers to Reentry Success Inventory, 3rd ed. (Liptak, 2022)	Adults/Older adults and adolescents	A self-report tool that can be self-scored or used as a practitioner checklist; person must be able to read and participate in an interview	Identifies challenges people may experience postrelease and includes items assessing basic needs: job, family, wellness, and career	Administer in quiet, private space; time varies depending on the administration format used, but generally 15–30 minutes	No specific model; consistent with Canadian Occupational Performance Model (COPM), MOHO, and PEO models in occupational therapy

uses therapeutic reasoning to know when it may be appropriate to present activities that may be higher risk (Cordingley & Ryan, 2009). Box 40-3 provides a variety of approaches for practitioners to consider to ensure proactive risk management.

Risk assessment is also a crucial management function in justice settings because it is a means to gauge a person's potential to commit another offense and evaluate the risk of violence (Ho et al., 2009; James, 2015). Risk assessment is typically performed by psychologists and psychiatrists. Practitioners should have a working understanding of the purpose and intent of risk assessments and know primary tools used to measure risk. Practitioners can proactively contribute

their observations to improve the interdisciplinary team's risk management decisions. Common risk assessment measures include the Ohio Risk Assessment System (ORAS; Latessa, 2010) and the Level of Service Inventory-Revised (LSI-R; Andrews & Bonta, 1995).

Occupation: Occupational Therapy Interventions

Occupational therapy has a very long history of recognizing and responding to the needs of individuals in the criminal justice system (Penner, 1978), a history that dates

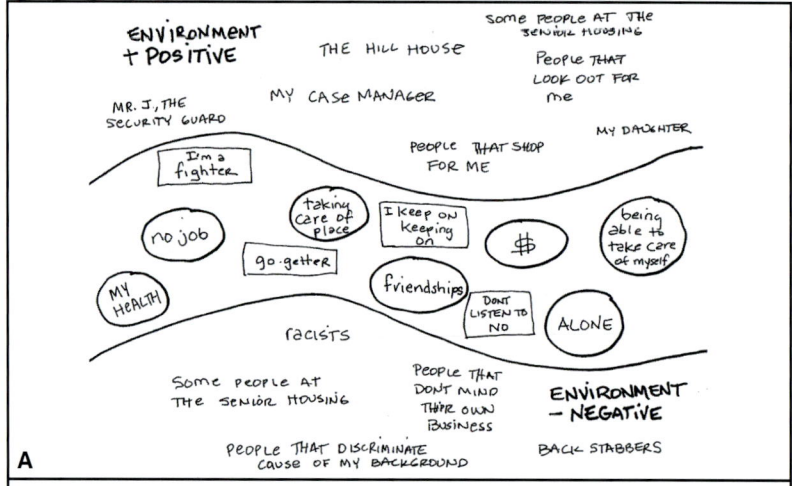

Mr. Clarke is a 65-year-old male released from prison almost 2 years ago. With the help of a local nonprofit agency, he has secured housing in a low-income neighborhood. Circles represent his primary problem situations; he is most concerned about his health, as he needs a hip replacement. Rectangles are personal strengths; these collectively reflect his drive to engage in life regardless of the obstacles. He notes the people and places in his environment that both provide supports (+) and create challenges (-).

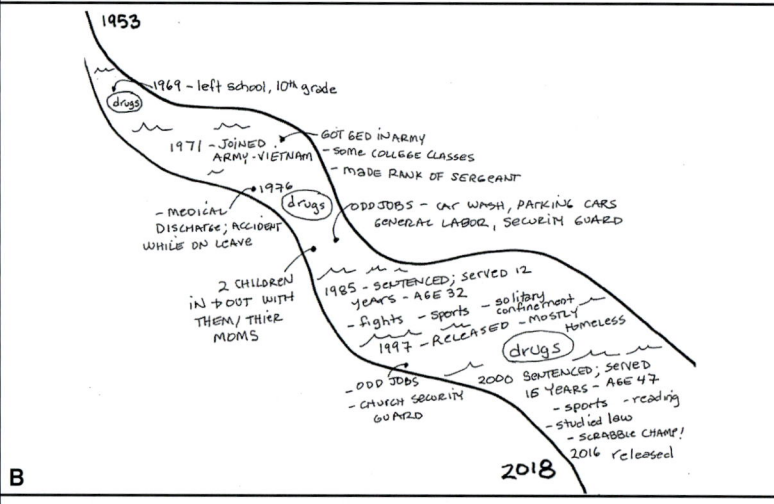

The KAWA was used to reflect Mr. Clarke's occupational, educational, vocational, and criminological histories. He left school early but is not uneducated. His performances and leadership helped him get promoted to sergeant while in the military. His employment record is limited, and he has mostly held nonskilled positions. He has been incarcerated for nearly 60% of his adult life. His drug use has waxed and waned over the years, but it has been a consistent pattern in his life for nearly 50 years. His drawing identifies "key turns" in his river of life and patterns in occupational role performances. It helped open the conversation for where his river of life may flow next.

FIGURE 40-4. Using the Kawa Model interview process to understand the person in context.

back more than 75 years (Muñoz et al., 2020). Early publications were descriptive, portraying interventions focused on skill building, employment, and education issues in justice settings (Chackersfield & Forshaw, 1997; Farnworth et al., 1987; Garner, 1995; Lloyd, 1985, 1987a, 1987b, 1988, 1989).

Many of these programs used group interventions to address problem-solving and social skills (Garner, 1995) and sought to develop work-related skills individuals could use to reenter the community and the job market (Lloyd, 1988). Practitioners can now access book resources describing occupational therapy services in criminal justice settings that focus on skill development, relapse prevention, community reintegration, and employment, all of which are appropriate interventions for occupational therapy programming in criminal justice settings (McNeil & Bannigan, 2014; Moore, 2014; Muñoz, 2019a; Ozkan et al., 2018; White et al., 2013).

BOX 40-3 ■ Reflection on Safety and Security

OTPs who work with persons in, or recently released from, a correctional setting should be aware that there are some risks, and this is particularly true of postrelease work. The chances of a significant problem arising and the risk of being put in a seriously dangerous situation are small, and one can reduce risk by knowing and following security and safety procedures. This reflective exercise is designed to help practitioners consider knowledge, attitudes, and skill sets that support success in justice-based settings. Review the two lists of strategies with another peer or in a small group. Discuss how each strategy represents a specific method for maintaining personal safety and security.

General Strategies for Working With Individuals in Criminal Justice Systems

- Wear appropriate, modest clothing.
- Do not make promises that you may not or will not keep.
- Know the person; seek out information about any risk that any person may represent.
- Do not give or accept gifts.
- Guard personal information (e.g., personal circumstances, family details, home address, telephone number).
- If the person is distressed or escalating at the end of your therapy session, make sure to communicate this to corrections staff.
- Always share information when a person discloses any intention of self-harm, suicide, physical violence, uprising, or escape.
- Always disclose to staff if a person at your setting is a friend or relative.
- Do not do favors (e.g., run errands, mail letters, make phone calls) or ask for favors.
- In community settings, do not agree to transport a resident anywhere if you have not read a detailed risk assessment; even then,

make sure you carry a mobile phone and that other staff know your travel plan, including expected departure and arrival times.
- Avoid meetings in your own community, and do not give details that disclose where you live.

Strategies for Reducing Risk and Maintaining Security

- Any keys should be concealed and secured. Never put keys down anywhere.
- Educate yourself to know how people in justice settings can use keys, tools, food, chemicals, and cleaning or medical supplies to escape or cause injury to self or others.
- Know how to call for emergency assistance if needed and be clear on how you should respond should an alarm sound.
- Understand procedures for maintaining and controlling materials and tools within the occupational therapy environment.
- Organize workspace to always maintain clear access to an exit and to emergency alarm systems.
- Always double-check gates, doors, cabinets, windows, and so on, to confirm that the lock is functioning.
- It is your responsibility to fully understand security procedures and requirements, to find out when you are not sure, to ask when you visit a new facility, and to make sure you always follow procedures (e.g., policies for escape prevention, emergency response, custody escorts, lockup units, tool control, syringe counts, key control).
- Strictly observe rules for what can and cannot be taken into a correctional setting and limit the personal possessions you carry as much as possible.

Throughout the world, an ever-increasing number of articles in professional journals address evaluation processes and interventions regarding the needs of populations at risk of entering, or in, criminal justice settings. Muñoz and colleagues (2020) used key terms and controlled vocabulary related to occupational therapy and criminal justice settings/populations to broadly search the role of occupational therapy as portrayed in the literature from 1940 to 2019. These researchers identified 139 sources—74 studies and 65 nonstudy sources. Half of these sources (50%) originated in the United Kingdom, United States, or Canada, and another 11% described forensic occupational therapy practice in Australasia.

Studies focused on the characteristics of the populations being served, explored occupational therapy processes or the impact of interventions, audited occupational therapy processes, or reported service users' perspectives of occupational therapy (Muñoz et al., 2020). The nonstudy sources portrayed assessment or intervention processes, provided group or program descriptions, described the role of occupational therapy in criminal justice, or offered critiques of justice system practices through an occupational lens (Muñoz et al., 2020).

In this scoping review, Muñoz and colleagues (2020) found that, even though most nonstudy sources (78%)

were published more than two decades ago, nearly all of the studies (87%) were published in the last two decades. This finding reflects that the effectiveness of occupational therapy in criminal justice settings is a growing topic in the profession's literature internationally (Collingwood et al., 2021; Garzón-Sarmiento et al., 2017; Pereira et al., 2020; Soeker et al., 2021; Whiteford et al., 2020).

In the past decade, researchers have surveyed practitioners working in criminal justice settings in Canada (Chui et al., 2016), the United States (Muñoz, Moreton, & Sitterly, 2016), and the United Kingdom (Connel, 2016). The results of these studies allow practitioners to understand the scope of occupational therapy practices and common intervention approaches as well as to envision potential ways to demonstrate occupational therapy's distinct role in criminal justice. Collectively, practitioners responding to these surveys report developing intervention programs that focus on skill development, primarily vocational skills, as well as time management, self-awareness, leisure, and life skills. To a lesser extent, they also focus on education, family, social skills, and role functioning (Muñoz et al., 2020). The focus of occupational therapy interventions in criminal justice settings is visually represented in Figure 40-5, and key areas of knowledge and skill sets that practitioners need to develop to function effectively in criminal justice settings are outlined in Table 40-5.

Occupational therapy practice has become increasingly evidence-based, and practitioners are more routinely using valid and reliable tools to measure outcomes of their programs and providing descriptions that model the way for other OTPs to contribute to this growing area of practice

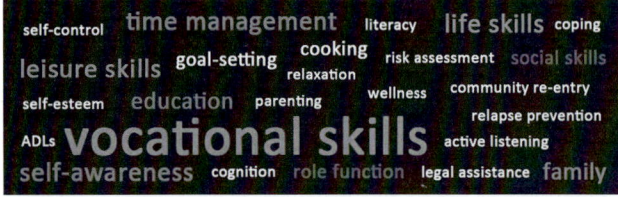

FIGURE 40-5. This image reflects the results of a scoping review of literature focused on occupational therapy practice in criminal justice settings/populations as depicted in 139 sources appearing in publications between 1940 and 2019. Terms that appear in larger font are areas of intervention that were most prominently discussed in the literature. *Muñoz, J. P., Catalano, A., Wang, Y., & Phillips, G. (2020). Justice-based occupational therapy: A scoping review.* Annals of International Occupational Therapy, 4, *162–174. https://doi.org /10.3928/24761222-20200924-02*

(Crabtree et al., 2016; Dillon et al., 2020; Ferrazzi, 2019; Garzón-Sarmiento et al., 2017; George-Paschal & Bowen, 2019; Jaegers, Skinner et al., 2020; Shea & Siu, 2016). Increasingly, practitioners and students are developing programs addressing the needs of people in or at risk of entering the criminal justice system and are presenting these at professional conferences. In addition, students are including programs they develop in repositories of capstone projects at various universities. Brief descriptions of some programs described in the occupational therapy literature from around the world appear in Table 40-6.

In the United States, several universities with community-university partnerships are focused on meeting the needs of people in criminal justice systems. Duquesne University in Pittsburgh, Pennsylvania; Indiana University in Indianapolis, Indiana; Pacific University in Forest Grove, Oregon; Saint Louis University in St. Louis, Missouri; and The University of Findlay in Findlay, Ohio, are all programs with significant records of focusing on building evidence for occupational therapy practice in criminal justice settings. These programs meet this critical need while simultaneously educating new generations of occupational therapists.

TABLE 40-5 | Key Knowledge and Skill Sets for Practitioners in Criminal Justice Settings

Knowledge Area or Type of Skill	Specific Skills
Evaluation	• Choose measures that reliably assess performance and measure change. • Generate an occupational history and profile inclusive of social, educational, vocational, and criminal histories. • Elicit the person's perspectives on performance, employment, and social participation. • Assess and address culture and gender-specific needs.
Interpersonal	• Collaborate effectively with justice-based personnel. • Practice effective listening skills. • Develop strong de-escalation strategies. • Cultivate and use strong culturally responsive communications skills.
Intervention	• Collaboratively develop occupation-based, recovery-focused plans and interventions. • Facilitate the person's ability to constructively use their time and self-structure daily routines. • Deliver interventions that emphasize skill and that build habits for productive role functioning, self-care, and employment. • Utilize interventions emphasizing health, wellness, and mindfulness.
Judicial Systems	• Learn about justice systems, including structure, processes, and terminology. • Become familiar with justice subculture and criminogenic lifestyles. • Understand processes and methods for risk assessment and management and recognize the range of prerelease and postrelease options. • Understand social, occupational, and restorative justice perspectives.
Practical Skills	• Document clearly and concisely, and always maintain confidentiality. • Practice self-care coping skills to manage institutional and environmental stressors. • Be vigilant and proactively recognize, assess, and manage risk and learn basic self-defense to ensure personal safety. • Scan community environments to be able to access programs having expertise serving returning citizens with mental illness.
Professional Development	• Practice consistent professionalism and show confidence in your professional identity. • Demonstrate a strong commitment to ongoing professional development. • Promote the creation of occupationally enriched environments within the structures of secure environments. • Advocate by defining occupational therapy's distinct role and delineating how occupational therapy contributes to the intervention team and the person's success at recovery.

TABLE 40-6 | **Examples of Occupational Therapy Programming in Criminal Justice Settings**

Setting and Population	Focus of Occupational Therapy Interventions
Men and women incarcerated in a county jail in Findlay, Ohio, United States, many with histories of trauma, mental health challenges, and substance use (Dillon et al., 2020)	• Evaluation includes creating an occupational profile, administering the Allen Cognitive Level Screen and the Adolescent/Adult Sensory Profile, and determining an ACE score. • Participants frequently defined goals including improved skills in concentration, time management, goal setting, and coping, as well as the ability to develop healthy lifestyles and supports. • The OT Life Skills Program included modules on interpersonal communication, employment, finance, leisure, and community resources.
Adolescent males in maximum-security juvenile corrections facility demonstrating sensory processing issues and histories of trauma and violence (Dowdy et al., 2023)	• Examined outcomes for youth with self-regulation difficulties and propensity to commit acts of violence who received at least 5 hours of sensory based occupational therapy interventions. • The majority of youth receiving sensory based occupational therapy interventions (e.g., making rain sticks, meditation, creating rhythmic music) had fewer violent behaviors. • The youth self-reported they enjoyed occupational therapy, found it helpful, and that occupational therapy helped them learn to manage feelings and act differently.
Adolescents involved in a juvenile drug court (George-Paschal & Bowen, 2019)	• Provided an 11-week mentoring program based on Occupational Adaptation for juveniles under the jurisdiction of a local drug court. • Included 1:1 sessions that encouraged participants to self-assess and engage in their own intervention planning and group enrichment activities such as touring a college campus, learning study habits, exploring leisure, preparing a meal, or preparing to get a driver's license. • Most participants demonstrated increased mastery in regard to self-identified goals.
Community-based forensic service center in the United Kingdom serving men with learning disabilities who had committed serious sexual offenses (Graham et al., 2016)	• Partnered with multiple disciplines in care planning and risk assessment. Provided a MOHO-based program offering graded levels of support and care to encourage independence and skill development. • Ensured a calm, consistent, supportive environment where workers could experience a sense of belonging and inclusion. • Focused on skills development and building self-confidence.
Men and women incarcerated in a city jail in St. Louis, Missouri, United States; OTPs provided both prerelease and postrelease programming (Jaegers, Skinner, et al., 2020)	• The occupational therapy program provided 8 weeks of modules on topics such as job seeking, literacy, communication skills, healthy relationships, and community transition planning. • Prerelease, participants created individualized plans with goals addressing employment, education, leisure, and social participation, and a detailed postrelease plan that included contact with the postrelease, community-based occupational therapist. • Study reinforced the feasibility of delivering an occupational therapy program in a county jail and identified key barriers (e.g., public policies, availability of community level supports) as well as critical facilitators (e.g., city support for funding, community partnerships) for program success.
Men with psychiatric disorders, forensic histories, chronic unemployment, and low levels of education in a low secure mental health setting in the United Kingdom (Roberts et al., 2015)	• Addressed atrophy of skills through community-based, skill-focused, and physical activity programs and supported individual risk assessment and risk management planning. • Implemented the "Down to Earth" vocational program through completing woodcraft, outdoor activities, dry stone walling, construction training, and community projects. • Implemented "Kick Start" physical activity and exercise program for individuals with varied fitness levels. Program included sessions of Nordic walking, cycling, and, occasionally, kayaking.
Adult women diagnosed with an intellectual and developmental disability who were incarcerated in a state prison in the southwest region of the United States (Stelter & Evetts, 2020)	• Evaluated occupational performance and participation using the Volitional Questionnaire, Goal Attainment Scaling, the Social Profile, and a relative mastery scale. • Implemented a 12-week occupational therapy workshop program designed to encourage prosocial occupational roles and structured, graded activities in a supported work environment. • Participants chose and joined a therapeutic work crew focused on horticulture, cooking, crafts, or technology. Participation in the occupational therapy workshop significantly curtailed adverse behavioral incidents of all program participants.
Men incarcerated in a forensic mental health hospital in a prison setting in Singapore (Tan et al., 2015)	• Occupational therapy developed opportunities for work role exploration in food service, supervised cleaning tasks, and varied worker roles within the prison. • Practitioners contributed to risk assessment by providing detailed reports of task behaviors such as engagement, following instructions, initiative, concentration, cooperation, interpersonal skills, and communication. • Group interventions addressed life management and social skills; provided individualized supports; and encouraged self-assessment of performance, self-esteem, and pride in performance.

Dillon, M. B., Dillon, T. H., Griffiths, T., Prusnek, L., & Tippie, M. (2020). The distinct value of occupational therapy in corrections: Implementation of a life skills program in a county jail. Annals of International Occupational Therapy, 4, 185–193. https://doi.org/10.3928/24761222-20200309-01; Dowdy, R., Estes, J., McCarthy, C., Onders, J., Onders, M., & Suttner, A. (2023). The influence of occupational therapy on self-regulation in juvenile offenders. Journal of Child and Adolescent Trauma, 16, 221–232. https://doi.org/10.1007/s40653-022-00493-y; George-Paschal, L., & Bowen, M. R. (2019). Outcomes of a mentoring program based on occupational adaptation for participants in a juvenile drug court program. Occupational Therapy in Mental Health, 35(3), 262–286. https://doi.org /10.1080/0164212X.2019.1601605; Graham, A., Harbottle, C., & King, D. (2016). Resolve: A community-based forensic learning disability service specialising in supporting male sex offenders—Our model, approach and evidence base for effective intervention. Journal of Intellectual Disabilities and Offending Behaviour, 7(4), 186–194. https://doi.org/10.1108/JIDOB-10-2014-0014; Jaegers, L. A., Skinner, E., Conners, B., Hayes, C., West-Bruce, S., Vaughn, M. G., Smith, D. L., & Barney, K. F. (2020). Evaluation of the jail-based Occupational Therapy Transition and Integration Services program for community reentry. American Journal of Occupational Therapy, 74(3), 7403205030p1–7403205030p11. https://doi.org/10.5014/ajot.2020.035287; Roberts, C., Davies, J., & Maggs, R. G. (2015). Structured community activity for forensic mental health: A feasibility study. Journal of Forensic Practice, 17(3), 180–191. https://doi.org/10.1108/JFP-12-2014-0049; Stelter, L., & Evetts, C. (2020). Effect of an occupation-based program for women with intellectual and developmental disabilities who are incarcerated. The Annals of International Occupational Therapy, 3(4), 175–184. https://doi.org/10.3928/24761222-20190910-01; Tan, B. L., Kumar, V. R., & Devaraj, P. (2015). Development of a new occupational therapy service in a Singapore prison. British Journal of Occupational Therapy, 78(8), 525–529. https://doi.org/10.1177/0308022615571083

Evidence-Based Practice

Occupational Therapy Reentry Services

> *Occupational therapy is a viable and effective service in criminal justice settings.*

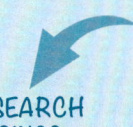

RESEARCH FINDINGS

When considering occupational therapy reentry services as an emerging and growing area of practice, it is important to consider the extent to which occupational therapy can be implemented in a criminal justice setting, and the impact of providing these services. Program evaluation studies are important for establishing the feasibility of providing occupational therapy reentry services, considering the design of programming, offering details on barriers and facilitators to implementation, and evaluating efficacy. A variety of occupational therapy studies have shown the viability of services for reentry in jail, prison, and community supervision settings (Gonzalez et al., 2023; Jaegers et al., 2020).

APPLICATIONS

➡ Evaluation of prerelease reentry services in an urban jail setting ($N = 63$) indicated facilitators through jail workplace and community partners and the need to overcome institutional policy and environmental barriers (Jaegers et al., 2020).

➡ Of the people participating in a jail-based occupational therapy reentry program who completed prerelease interventions while incarcerated ($N =24$, 38%), all initiated postrelease occupational therapy upon their release to the community (Jaegers et al., 2020).

➡ In a pre-/posttest study, men ($N = 5$) involved in a community supervision center experienced significant improvements in self-efficacy, management of emotions, and reduction in anxiety and sleep disturbances (Gonzalez et al., 2023).

REFERENCES

Gonzalez, A. V., Eikenberry, J., Griess, C., Jaegers, L., & Baum, C. M. (2023). Evaluation of an occupational therapy reentry program: Achieving goals to support employment and community living after incarceration. *Work* (Reading, Mass.), *75*(2), 639–656. https://doi.org/10.3233/WOR-220035

Jaegers, L. A., Skinner, E., Conners, B., Hayes, C., West-Bruce, S., Vaughn, M. G., Smith, D. L., & Barney, K. F. (2020). Evaluation of the jail-based Occupational Therapy Transition and Integration Services program for community reentry. *American Journal of Occupational Therapy, 74*, 7403205030p1–7403205030p11. https://doi.org/10.5014/ajot.2020.035287

Here's the Point

- The criminal justice system includes institutions that make laws and pass judgments to sentence people when laws are broken, as well as settings where people are detained when these sentences include incarceration.
- In the United States in particular, and worldwide, there are millions of individuals who are incarcerated and/or under some form of supervision that limits their ability to engage in meaningful and productive occupations.
- Services for people with mental illnesses who are incarcerated or supervised in criminal justice settings are often inadequate.
- OTPs can provide individual and group interventions that facilitate the development of skill sets that support full community reintegration, social participation, and attainment of the individual's highest level of recovery.

- Opportunities for addressing occupational performance challenges in criminal justice populations can occur in a variety of settings, including jails, prisons, secure psychiatric hospitals, and community-based justice settings such as residential reentry centers and community-based programs.
- In order to strengthen occupational therapy's access to and position in criminal justice settings, practitioners must design evidence-based, occupation-focused programs and use valid reliable assessments to measure intervention outcomes.

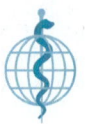

Visit the online resource center at **FADavis.com** to access the videos.

Apply It Now

1. Build an Occupationally Focused Jail Diversion Program

Jail diversion programs divert people with serious mental illness away from incarceration and toward community-based treatment and support services. Form a small group of peers, discuss what you have learned about the needs of people incarcerated with mental illness, and then complete the following exercises. Begin with a perspective that you are addressing the needs of an adult male population. Consider searching the internet for a recent arrest story that involves a person experiencing a mental health crisis.

Keep in mind the principles of community needs assessment are the first steps in program development. In a full needs assessment, you would explore city, county, or state level data to inform your team of the main populations arrested recently to understand the needs of the local community.

The process would also involve identifying city or county departments and community agencies that may inform a needs assessment and consider key stakeholders and people with lived experience for informing the specific needs for a jail diversion program in your community.

For the purposes of this activity, collectively create an outline that includes content your team believes could be part of a successful occupationally focused diversion program. For example, your team's program may include reentry goal setting, housing, employment, or drug and alcohol counseling. When you have collectively created a list that has at least 10 areas of possible occupational therapy interventions, have each member independently rank order the list from most to least essential.

Have each member share the five areas they prioritized, then discuss and debate the rationales for your choices. Now discuss whether your choices will change if the population is female. How will it change if the population is juvenile?

2. Debating an Occupational Therapy Role Within Juvenile Justice

Juveniles convicted of crimes can be confined in juvenile correction centers, residential group homes, and in a variety of "camps" run similar to military boot camps or wilderness training programs. YouthBuild is a U.S. federally funded program focused on building the potential of low-income youth in underserved communities. Read about their program at https://youthbuild.org/our-programs.

Examine the approaches employed by YouthBuild (e.g., alternative school, job-training, community service). Create two groups of two to three peers. One group wants to propose to YouthBuild that there is a role for occupational therapy in their organization. Your task is to develop your best arguments that your skill sets are needed.

The second group must remain skeptical that there is any need for occupational therapy. Your task is to generate arguments against occupational therapy involvement. Each group should take a few minutes to define their talking points, then verbally share these points with the other group without debate. Once the positions have been outlined, meet again in small groups to strengthen your arguments, and consider counterarguments to the other group's main points. Debate a role for occupational therapy.

3. Perspectives on Crime, Punishment, and Rehabilitation

This chapter recommends considering how the criminal justice policies in your nation reveal some of your nation's perspectives on criminal justice. In a small group of your peers, do a quick search to find the answers to the following questions, and then compare how the answers you find may reflect differing perspectives about criminal justice worldwide.

Reflective Questions
■ How many countries have criminal laws against the sexual activity of gay, lesbian, or transgendered people? Can you think of any other examples of human behavior that may be considered legal in one context but deemed illegal in another?
  ● #OUTLAWED–"The Love That Dare Not Speak Its Name": https://features.hrw.org/features/features/lgbt_laws
■ Define the practice of using *sentencing circles,* as is done by Canadian First Nation aboriginal people. What values and beliefs about the person incarcerated and options for rehabilitation are reflected in the practice of sentencing circles? Would it be possible for *sentencing circles* to operate effectively in your community? Explain.
  ● Sentencing Circle: https://www.edmontonpolice.ca/News/SuccessStories/SentencingCircle
■ The United States is the only country in the world where a person can spend their entire life behind bars for a crime committed before reaching the age of 18. In a small group, discuss how this fact may reflect perceptions about accountability, rehabilitation potential, and punishment in the United States and elsewhere. The point of this discussion is not to debate whether a juvenile life sentence without parole policy is right or wrong, but to reflect on sentencing practices that may reflect societal views on incarceration and rehabilitation.
  ● Juvenile Life Without Parole: An Overview: https://www.sentencingproject.org/policy-brief/juvenile-life-without-parole-an-overview
  ● What Are Different Countries in the World Doing in the Field of Juvenile Justice System and Care? https://judicateme.com/what-are-different-countries-in-the-world-doing-in-the-field-of-juvenile-justice-system-and-care

4. Occupational Enrichment

Occupational enrichment is defined as a "deliberate manipulation" of an environment such that individuals could engage in a range of occupations (Molineux & Whiteford, 1999, p. 127). Envision the confining environment of a criminal justice setting. Now identify some adjustments that could make this context a more ideal therapeutic environment for justice-involved individuals with mental illness. Consider the social environment and the opportunities that should exist to support social participation. Visualize the physical environment and how the built environment could be organized to support occupation and participation.

Reflective Question

■ What could realistically be included in the physical space, taking into consideration the use of color, sound, natural lighting, and plants? Your task is to imagine therapeutic activities and spaces that can have personal and cultural meaning for an individual while also considering the realities of the need for security and safety in carceral environments.

5. Video Exercise: Fieldwork Experience in a Juvenile Correction Setting

Pair up with another student in your class or form a small group of students. Access and watch the "Fieldwork Experience in a Juvenile Correction Setting" video at the online resource center at FADavis.com. Then, discuss and together answer the following questions.

Reflective Questions

■ Why was it important for Maggie to reflect on the concept of the therapeutic use of self, and how could it be used with the juveniles in the program?
■ How do you feel about your strengths and styles of relating as explained in the Intentional Relationship Model and Therapeutic Use of Self?
■ What are some boundaries that Maggie could have set to ensure her well-being as a practitioner?
■ How might you set boundaries with your fieldwork and work as you transition into the field; that is, what steps or measures will you have in place to make sure you can separate the two?
■ Maggie felt least prepared for what the therapeutic purpose of her work would be. How could she have been better prepared in that way?

Resources

Organizations

- The Federal Bureau of Prisons: https://www.bop.gov. This website provides an excellent overview of various types of prison facilities, updated statistics on the U.S. prison population, and research reports on a variety of topics such as prison populations, mental health and drug treatment, and postrelease employment.
- The GAINS Center for Behavioral Health and Justice Transformation (SAMHSA): https://www.samhsa.gov/gains-center. This is a source for the collection and dissemination of resources about evidence-based mental health and substance abuse interventions for people with co-occurring disorders in the criminal justice system.
- Justice-Based Occupational Therapy (JBOT): https://linktr.ee/ot4justice. The JBOT network is a grassroots, informal effort by OTPs to expand education, research, resources, and advocacy and policy in criminal justice occupational therapy. The network seeks to promote occupational engagement and participation among people incarcerated and those working in corrections to promote community health and well-being. Other related social media sites include Instagram: https://www.instagram.com/justice_ot and FaceBook: https://www.facebook.com/JusticeOT1.
- The Prison Policy Initiative: https://www.prisonpolicy.org. This nonprofit organization is dedicated to criminal justice reform. It analyzes and disseminates data using accessible reports and strong graphics that document the harm related to mass incarceration.
- Restorative Justice International: https://www.restorativejusticeinternational.com. This international organization is focused on systematic justice reform grounded in restorative justice practices designed to restore individuals and communities injured by crime as much as possible while also addressing accountability.
- The Sentencing Project: https://www.sentencingproject.org. This national organization has advocated for a fair and effective criminal justice system for over 20 years. This website provides a wealth of research, publications, and policy reviews on a variety of topics, including inequities in the U.S. criminal justice system, sentencing laws and practices, and alternatives to incarceration.

Video

- "Civic Engagement Group in an Inpatient Psychiatric Unit" video. In this video, occupational therapist Jennifer speaks about her experience working as an occupational therapy assistant in an inpatient psychiatric unit for individuals with persistent mental illness. She describes a positive experience running civic engagement groups, which proved to do much more than give back to the community. In one project related to voting rights for individuals with felony histories, the group provided opportunities for the residents to practice life skills, feel empowered, and transcend the internalized stigma they faced as people living with mental illness. Access the video at the online resource center at FADavis.com.

References

Adams, K., & Ferrandino, J. (2008). Managing mentally ill inmates in prisons. *Criminal Justice and Behavior, 35*(8), 913–927. https://doi.org/10.1177/0093854808318624

American Correctional Association. (2016, November). *2016 standards supplement.* Commission on Accreditation for Corrections. https://www.aca.org/common/Uploaded%20files/2016%20Standards%20Supplement.pdf

American Occupational Therapy Association. (2021). Improve your documentation and quality of care with AOTA's updated occupational profile template. *American Journal of Occupational Therapy, 75*(Suppl. 2), 7502420010p1–7502420010p3. https://doi.org/10.5014/ajot.2021.752001

American Psychiatric Association. (2016). *Psychiatric services in correctional facilities* (3rd ed.). American Psychiatric Publishing.

American Psychiatric Association. (2021, February). *Examining mental health courts.* Author. https://www.psychiatry.org/news-room/apa-blogs/examining-mental-health-courts

Andrews, D. A., & Bonta, J. (1995). *LSI-R: The Level of Service Inventory–Revised.* Multi-Health Systems.

Andrews, D. A., & Dowden, C. (2007). The risk-need-responsivity model of assessment and human service in prevention and corrections: Crime-prevention jurisprudence. *Canadian Journal of Criminology and Criminal Justice, 49*(4), 439–464. https://doi.org/10.3138/cjccj.49.4.439

Anne E. Casey Foundation. (2021, March). *Juvenile detention explained.* Author. https://www.aecf.org/blog/what-is-juvenile-detention

Anne E. Casey Foundation. (2022, May 16). *Child welfare and foster care statistics.* Author. https://www.aecf.org/blog/child-welfare-and-foster-care-statistics.

Armstrong-Heimsoth, A., Hahn-Floyd, M., Williamson, H. J., & Lockmiller, C. (2020). Toward a defined role for occupational therapy in foster care transition programming. *Open Journal of Occupational Therapy, 8*(4), 13. https://doi.org/10.15453/2168-6408.1726

Baams, L., Wilson, B. D. M., & Russell, S. T. (2019). LGBTQ youth in unstable housing and foster care. *Pediatrics, 143*(3), e20174211. https://doi.org/10.1542/peds.2017-4211

Bacher-Hicks, A., Billings, S., & Deming, D. (2021). Proving the school-to-prison pipeline: Stricter middle schools raise the risk of adult arrest. *Education Next, 21*(4), 52–57. https://www.educationnext.org/proving-school-to-prison-pipeline-stricter-middle-schools-raise-risk-of-adult-arrests

Baidawi, S., & Piquero, A. R. (2021). Neurodisability among children at the nexus of the child welfare and youth justice system. *Journal of Youth and Adolescence, 50,* 803–819. https://doi.org/10.1007/s10964-020-01234-w

Baron, K., Kielhofner, G., Iyenger, A., Goldhammer, V., & Wolenski, J. (2006). *A user's manual for the Occupational Self-Assessment (OSA)* (Version 2.2). Model of Human Occupation Clearinghouse, Department of Occupational Therapy, College of Applied Health Sciences, University of Illinois at Chicago.

Bartholomew, A. (1976). The need for recreational activity in forced confinement. *Australian Occupational Therapy Journal, 23,* 62–69. https://doi.org/10.1111/j.1440-1630.1976.tb01045.x

Baum, C. M., Connor, L. T., Morrison, T., Hahn, M., Dromerick, A. W., & Edwards, D. F. (2008). Reliability, validity, and clinical utility of the Executive Function Performance Test: A measure of executive function in a sample of people with stroke. *American Journal of Occupational Therapy, 62,* 446–455. https://doi.org/10.5014/ajot.62.4.446

Beaudry, G., Yu, R., Långström, N., & Fazel, S. (2021). An updated systematic review and meta-regression analysis: Mental disorders among adolescents in juvenile detention and correctional facilities. *Journal of the American Academy of Child & Adolescent Psychiatry, 60*(1), 46–60. https://doi.org/10.1016/j.jaac.2020.01.015

Beech, B. M., Ford, C., Thorpe, R. J., Jr., Bruce, M. A. & Norris, K. C. (2021). Poverty, racism, and the public health crisis in America. *Frontiers in Public Health, 9,* 9:699049. https://doi.org/10.3389/fpubh.2021.699049

Bixby, L., Bevan, S., & Boen, C. (2022). The links between disability, incarceration, and social exclusion. *Health Affairs, 41*(10), 1460–1469. https://doi.org/10.1377/hlthaff.2022.00495

Boen, C. E., Graetz, N., Olson, H., Ansari-Thomas, Z., Bixby, L., Schut, R. A., & Lee, H. (2022). Early life patterns of criminal legal system involvement: Inequalities by race/ethnicity, gender, and parental education. *Demographic Research, 46,* 131–146. https://doi.org/10.4054/demres.2022.46.5

Bonfine, N., Wilson, A. B., & Munetz, M. R. (2020). Meeting the needs of justice-involved people with serious mental illness within community behavioral health systems. *Psychiatric Services, 71*(4), 355–363. https://doi.org/10.1176/appi.ps.201900453

Bozick, R., Steele, J., Davis, L., & Turner, S. (2018). Does providing inmates with education improve postrelease outcomes? A meta-analysis of correctional education programs in the United States. *Journal of Experimental Criminology, 14,* 389–428. https://doi.org/10.1007/s11292-018-9334-6

British Columbia Society of Occupational Therapy. (1949). From coast to coast: Report of the British Columbia Society of Occupational Therapy. *Canadian Journal of Occupational Therapy, 16*(4), 144–149. https://doi.org/10.1177/000841744901600408

Bronson, J., & Berzofsky, M. (2017, June). *Indicators of mental health problems reported by prisoners and jail inmates 2011–2012.* U.S. Department of Justice, Office of Justice Programs, Bureau of Justice Statistics. https://www.bjs.gov/content/pub/pdf/imhprpji1112.pdf

Brown, C., & Dunn, W. (2002). *Adolescent/Adult Sensory Profile.* Psychological Corporation.

Bullard, C. E., & Thrasher, R. (2016). Evaluating mental health court by impact on jurisdictional crime rates. *Criminal Justice Policy Review, 27*(3), 227–246. https://doi.org/10.1177/0887403414562420

Butler, A., Nicholls, T., Samji, H., Fabian, S., & Lavergne, M. R. (2022). Prevalence of mental health needs, substance use, and co-occurring disorders among people admitted to prison. *Psychiatric Services, 73*(7), 737–744. https://doi.org/10.1176/appi.ps.202000927

Cai, J., Ruhil, A. V. S., & Gut, D. M. (2019). *Prison-based education: Programs, participation and proficiency in literacy/numeracy.* PIAAC Gateway. https://static1.squarespace.com/static/51bb74b8e4b0139570ddf020/t/5e4192c89a480e7dee6da3d9/1581355720733/2019_Cai_Ruhil_Gut_Prison-Based_Education.pdf

Carleton, R. N., Ricciardelli, R., Taillieu. T., Mitchell, M. M., Andres, A., & Afifi, T. O. (2020). Provincial correctional service workers: The prevalence of mental disorders. *International Journal of Environmental Research and Public Health, 17*(7), 2203. https://doi.org/10.3390/ijerph17072203

Carson, E. A. (2022, December). *Prisoners in 2021—Statistical tables.* Bureau of Justice Statistics, U.S. Department of Justice. https://bjs.ojp.gov/sites/g/files/xyckuh236/files/media/document/p21st.pdf

Cassidy, K., & Garrick, I. (2012). *An exploration of standardised assessments including risk assessments used by occupational therapists in forensic mental health.* [Unpublished honors dissertation.] York St. John University, York, UK.

Castaneda, R. (2010). Therapeutic relationships in difficult contexts: Involuntary commitment, forensic settings and violence. In M. Scheinholz (Ed.), *Occupational therapy in mental health: Considerations for advanced practice* (pp. 199–213). AOTA Press.

Cénat, J. M., McIntee, S., Mukunzi, J. N., & Noorishad, P. (2020). Overrepresentation of Black children in the child welfare system: A systematic review to understand and better act. *Children and Youth Services Review, 120,* 105714. https://doi.org/10.1016/j.childyouth.2020.105714

Chackersfield, J., & Forshaw, D. (1997). Occupational therapy and forensic addictive behaviors. *British Journal of Therapy and Rehabilitation, 4*(7), 381–386. https://doi.org/10.12968/bjtr.1997.4.7.14417

Children's Bureau. (2021, April). *Child welfare practice to address racial disproportionality and disparity.* https://www.childwelfare.gov/pubPDFs/racial_disproportionality.pdf

Christiansen, C. H., Baum, C. M., & Bass, J. D. (2015). *Occupational therapy: Performance, participation and well-being.* Slack.

Chui, A., Wong, C. I., Maraj, S. A., Fry, D., Jecker, J., & Jung, B. (2016). Forensic occupational therapy in Canada: The current state of practice. *Occupational Therapy International, 23*(3), 229–240. https://doi.org/10.1002/oti.1426

Collingwood, E., Messina, A., Dam, A., Bernard, T., Cockburn, L., & Penney, S. (2021). Experiences of recovery for Canadian forensic mental health patients and staff participating in a horse stables program. *The Journal of Forensic Psychiatry & Psychology, 32*(5), 641–657. https://doi.org/10.1080/14789949.2021.1881582

Connell, C. (2016). Forensic occupational therapy to reduce risk of reoffending: A survey of practice in the United Kingdom. *Journal of Forensic Psychiatry & Psychology, 27*(6), 907–928. https://doi.org/10.1080/14789949.2016.1237535

Cordingley, K., & Ryan, S. (2009). Occupational therapy risk assessment in forensic mental health practice: An exploration. *British Journal of Occupational Therapy, 72*(12), 531–538. https://doi.org/10.4276/030802209X12601857794736

Couldrick, L., & Aldred, D. (2003). *Forensic occupational therapy.* Whurr.

Couloute, L. (2018, October). *Getting back on course: Educational exclusion and attainment among formerly incarcerated people.* Prison Policy Initiative. https://www.prisonpolicy.org/reports /education.html

Council of State Governments. (2023, November). *Advancing safety and second chances.* Author. https://csgjusticecenter.org

Council of State Governments Justice Center. (2009). *Mental health courts: A guide to research-informed policy and practice.* Author. https://csgjusticecenter.org/wp-content/uploads/2009/09 /Mental_Health_Court_Research_Guide.pdf

Crabtree, J. L., Wall, J. M., & Ohm, D. (2016). Critical reflections on participatory action research in a prison setting: Toward occupational justice. *OTJR: Occupational Therapy Journal of Research, 36*(4), 244–252. https://doi.org/10.1177/1539449216669132

Cullum, M., Saine, K., & Weiner, M. (2009). *Texas functional living scale.* APA PsycTests. https://doi.org/10.1037/t15157-000

Davis, L. M. (2019). *Higher education programs in prison: What we know now and what we should focus on going forward.* RAND Corporation. http://www.jstor.com/stable/resrep19903

Dillon, M. B., Dillon, T. H., Griffiths, T., Prusnek, L., & Tippie, M. (2020). The distinct value of occupational therapy in corrections: Implementation of a life skills program in a county jail. *Annals of International Occupational Therapy, 4,* 185–193. https://doi .org/10.3928/24761222-20200309-01

di Lorito, C., Völlm, B., & Dening, T. (2018). Psychiatric disorders among older prisoners: A systematic review and comparison study against older people in the community. *Aging and Mental Health, 22*(1), 1–10. https://doi.org/10.1080/13607863.2017 .1286453

Dollar, C. B., Ray, B., Hudson, M. K., & Hood, B. J. (2018). Examining changes in procedural justice and their influences on problem solving court outcomes. *Behavioral Sciences and the Law, 36*(1), 32–45. https://doi.org/10.1002/bsl.2329

Domestic Policy Council. (2023, April). *The White House alternatives, rehabilitation, and reentry strategic plan.* https://www .whitehouse.gov/wp-content/uploads/2023/04/The-White-House-Alternatives-Rehabilitation-and-Reentry-Strategic-Plan.pdf

Dowdy, R., Estes, J., McCarthy, C., Onders, J., Onders, M., & Suttner, A. (2023). The influence of occupational therapy on self-regulation in juvenile offenders. *Journal of Child and Adolescent Trauma, 16,* 221–232. https://doi.org/10.1007/s40653-022-00493-y

Duncan, E. A., Munro, K., & Nicol, M. M. (2003). Research priorities in forensic occupational therapy. *British Journal of Occupational Therapy, 66*(2), 55–64. https://doi.org/10.1177/03080 2260306600203

Eggers, M., Muñoz, J. P., Sciulli, J., & Crist, P. A. H. (2006). The community reintegration project: Occupational therapy at work in a county jail. *Occupational Therapy in Health Care, 20*(1), 17–37. https://doi.org/10.1080/J003v20n01_02

Ellison, J. M., & Jaegers, L. A. (2022). Suffering in silence: Violence exposure and post-traumatic stress disorder among jail correctional officers. *Journal of Occupational and Environmental Medicine, 64*(1), e28–e35. https://doi.org/10.1097 /JOM.0000000000002432

Fair, H., & Walmsley, R. (2021). *World prison population list* (13th ed.). Institute for Crime and Justice Policy Research. https://www.prisonstudies.org/sites/default/files/resources /downloads/world_prison_population_list_13th_edition.pdf

Farnworth, L., Morgan, S., & Fernando, B. (1987). Prison-based occupational therapy. *Australian Occupational Therapy Journal, 34*(2), 40–46. https://doi.org/10.1111/j.1440-1630.1987.tb01567.x

Farnworth, L., & Muñoz, J. P. (2009). An occupational and rehabilitation perspective for institutional practice. *Psychiatric Rehabilitation Journal, 32*(3), 192–198. https://doi.org/10.2975 /32.3.2009.192.198

Fazel, S., Yoon, I. A., & Hayes, A. J. (2017). Substance use disorders in prisoners: An updated systematic review and meta-regression analysis in recently incarcerated men and women. *Addiction, 112,* 1725–1739. https://doi.org/10.1111/add.13877

Federal Bureau of Prisons. (2018a). *About our facilities.* https://www. bop.gov/about/facilities/federal_prisons.jsp

Federal Bureau of Prisons. (2018b). *Prison security levels.* https://www. bop.gov/about/statistics/statistics_inmate_sec_levels.jsp

Fellner, J. (2008). Afterwords: A few reflections. *Criminal Justice and Behavior, 35,* 1079–1087. https://doi.org/10.1177/00938548 08318907

Ferrazzi, P. (2019). Occupational therapy and criminal court mental health initiatives: An important emerging practice setting. *Occupational Therapy in Mental Health, 35*(3), 238–261. https://doi.or g/10.1080/0164212X.2019.1571467

Finlay, A. K., Owens, M. D., Taylor, E., Nash, A., Capdarest-Arest, N., Rosenthal, J., Blue-Howells, J., Clark, S., & Timko, C. (2019). A scoping review of military veterans involved in the criminal justice system and their health and healthcare. *Health & Justice, 7,* Article 6. https://doi.org/10.1186/s40352-019-0086-9

Fisher, A. G. (2014). *Assessment of Motor and Process Skills: Vol. 2. User manual* (6th ed.). Three Star Press.

Fitch, W. L. (2014). *Forensic mental health services in the United States, 2014.* National Association of State Mental Health Program Directors. https://www.nasmhpd.org/sites/default/files /Assessment%203%20-%20Updated%20Forensic%20Mental%20 Health%20Services.pdf

Fitzgerald, M. (2011). An evaluation of the impact of a social inclusion programme on occupational functioning for forensic service users. *British Journal of Occupational Therapy, 74*(10), 465–472. https://doi.org/10.4276/030802211X13182481841903

Fitzgerald, M., Ratcliffe, G., & Blythe, C. (2012). Family work in occupational therapy: A case study from a forensic service. *British Journal of Occupational Therapy, 75*(3), 152–155. https://doi.org /10.4276/030802212X13311219571864

Forsyth, K., Deshpande, S., Kielhofner, G., Henriksson, C., Haglund, L., Olson, L., Skinner, S., & Kulkarni, S. (2005). *A user's manual for the Occupational Circumstances Assessment Interview and Rating Scale.* Version 4.0. Model of Human Occupation Clearinghouse, Department of Occupational Therapy, College of Applied Health Sciences, University of Illinois at Chicago.

Freudenberg, N., & Heller, D. (2016). A review of opportunities to improve the health of people involved in the criminal justice system in the United States. *Annual Review of Public Health, 37,* 311–333. https://doi.org/10.1146/annurev-publhealth-032315-021420

Galappathie, N., Khan, S. T., & Hussain, A. (2017). Civil and forensic patients in secure psychiatric settings: A comparison. *BJ Psychiatric Bulletin, 41*(3), 156–159. https://doi.org/10.1192 /pb.bp.115.052910

Galvaan, R. (2005). Domestic workers' narratives: Transforming occupational therapy practice. In F. Kronenberg, S. S. Algado, & N. Pollard (Eds.), *Occupational therapy without borders: Learning from the spirit of survivors* (pp. 429–439). Elsevier Churchill Livingstone.

Garner, R. (1995). Prevocational training within a secure environment: A programme designed to enable the forensic patient to prepare for mainstream opportunities. *British Journal of Occupational Therapy, 58*(1), 2–6. https://doi.org/10.1177/030802269505800102

Garzón-Sarmiento, A. M., Pérez-Miranda, C. C., Torres-Zaque, Y. A., Tunaroza-Chilito, Y. P., & Peñas-Felizzola, O. L. (2017). El terapeuta ocupacional en el ámbito penitenciario Colombiano [Occupational therapists in the Colombian penitentiary system]. *Revista de la Facultad de Medicina, 65*(1), 81–88. https://doi .org/10.15446/revfacmed.v65n1.54153

George-Paschal, L., & Bowen, M. R. (2019). Outcomes of a mentoring program based on occupational adaptation for participants in a juvenile drug court program. *Occupational Therapy in Mental Health, 35*(3), 262–286. https://doi.org/10.1080/0164212X.2019.1601605

Gómez-Figueroa, H., & Camino-Proaño, A. (2022). Mental and behavioral disorders in the prison context. *Revista Española de Sanidad Penitenciaria, 24*(2), 66–74. https://doi.org/10.18176/resp.00052

Gonzalez, A. V., Eikenberry, J., Griess, C., Jaegers, L., & Baum, C. M. (2023). Evaluation of an occupational therapy reentry program: Achieving goals to support employment and community living after incarceration. *Work, 75*(2), 639–656. https://doi.org/10.3233/WOR-220035

Gould, L. A., & Brent, J. J. (2020). *Handbook on American prisons.* Routledge.

Graham, A., Harbottle, C., & King, D. (2016). Resolve: A community-based forensic learning disability service specialising in supporting male sex offenders—Our model, approach and evidence base for effective intervention. *Journal of Intellectual Disabilities and Offending Behaviour, 7*(4), 186–194. https://doi.org/10.1108/JIDOB-10-2014-0014

Grooms, J. (2020). No home and no acceptance: Exploring the intersectionality of sexual/gender identities (LGBTQ) and race in the foster care system. *The Review of Black Political Economy, 47*(2), 177–193. https://doi.org/10.1177/0034644620911381

Gunarathne, G. P. C., Rodrigo, M. D. A., & Mendis, T. S. S (2022). *Occupational engagement in prisons: An evaluation of time-use in Sri Lankan correctional settings.* General Sir John Kotelawala Defence University. http://192.248.104.6/handle/345/2881

Gunnison, E., & Helfgott, J. B. (2017). Critical keys to successful offender reentry: Getting a handle on substance abuse and mental health problems. *Qualitative Report, 22*(8), 2152–2172. https://doi.org/10.46743/2160-3715/2017.3260

Haney, C. A. (2008). Culture of harm: Taming the dynamics of cruelty in supermax prisons. *Criminal Justice and Behavior, 35,* 956–984. https://doi.org/10.1177/0093854808318585

Harding, D. J., Western, B., & Sandelson, J. A. (2022). From supervision to opportunity: Reimagining probation and parole. *The Annals of the American Academy of Political and Social Science, 701,* 8–25. https://doi.org/10.1177/00027162221115486

Haworth, C., & Cyrs, G. (2017, August 21). Supporting transitions to the workforce for at-risk youth: Developing and using an occupation-based work assessment. *OT Practice, 22*(15), 21–24.

Ho, H., Thomson, L., & Darjee, R. (2009). Violence risk assessment: The use of the PCL-SV, HCR-20 and VRAG to predict violence in mentally disordered offenders discharged from a medium secure unit in Scotland. *Journal of Forensic Psychiatric Psychology, 20*(4), 523–541. https://doi.org/10.1080/14789940802638358

Hockenberry, S., Wachter, A., & Sladky, A. (2016). *Juvenile residential facility census, 2014: Selected findings.* U.S. Department of Justice, Office of Justice Programs, Office of Juvenile Justice and Delinquency Prevention. https://www.ojjdp.gov/pubs/250123.pdf

Hoke, S. (2015). Mental illness and prisoners: Concerns for communities and healthcare providers. *The Online Journal of Issues in Nursing, 20*(1), Manuscript 3. https://doi.org/10.3912/OJIN.Vol20No01Man03

Hopkin, G., Evans-Lacko, S., Forrester, A., Shaw, J., & Thornicroft, G. (2018). Interventions at the transition from prison to the community for prisoners with mental illness: A systematic review. *Administration and Policy in Mental Health and Mental Health Services Research, 44*(2), 177–187. https://doi.org/10.1007/s10488-018-0848-z

Iwama, M. (2006). *The Kawa Model: Culturally relevant occupational therapy.* Churchill Livingstone Elsevier.

Jaegers, L. A., Ahmad, S. O., Scheetz, G., Bixler, E., Nadimpalli, S., Barnidge, E., Katz, I. M., Vaughn, M. G., & Matthieu, M. M. (2020). Total Worker Health® needs assessment to identify workplace mental health interventions in rural and urban jails. *American Journal of Occupational Therapy, 74,* 7403205020p1–7403205020p12. https://doi.org/10.5014/ajot.2019.036400

Jaegers, L. A., Barney, K. F., & Aldrich, R. M. (2019). The role of occupational science and occupational therapy in the juvenile justice system. In M. G. Vaughn, C. P. Salas-Wright, & D. B. Jackson (Eds.), *Routledge international handbook of delinquency and health* (pp. 291–304). Taylor & Francis. https://doi.org/10.4324/9780429289194-21

Jaegers, L. A., El Ghaziri, M., Katz, I. M., Vaughn, M. G., Ellison, J. M., & Cherniack, M. G. (2022). Critical incident exposure among custody and non-custody correctional workers: Prevalence and impact of violent exposure to work-related trauma. *American Journal of Industrial Medicine, 65*(6), 500–511. https://doi.org/10.1002/ajim.23353

Jaegers, L. A., Neff, J., Hayes-Picker, C., Blank, S., Murphy, M., Schur, N., & Barney, K. F. (2020). Community transition goal setting for adults in long-term prison: Reentry needs of people sentenced as juveniles to life without the option of parole. *American Journal of Occupational Therapy, 76*(Suppl. 1), 7610500003p1. https://doi.org/10.5014/ajot.2022.76S1-RP3

Jaegers, L. A., Skinner, E., Conners, B., Hayes, C., West-Bruce, S., Vaughn, M. G., Smith, D. L., & Barney, K. F. (2020). Evaluation of the jail-based Occupational Therapy Transition and Integration Services program for community reentry. *American Journal of Occupational Therapy, 74*(3), 7403205030p1–7403205030p11. https://doi.org/10.5014/ajot.2020.035287

James, N. (2015). *Risk and needs assessment in the criminal justice system.* Congressional Research Service. https://www.everycrsreport.com/files/20150724_R44087_0c47cc191ecc982888fa182c82ef0099a86eca8d.pdf

Juvenile Law Center. (2018, May). *What is the foster care to prison pipeline?* https://jlc.org/news/what-foster-care-prison-pipeline

Kaeble, D. (2021, December). *Probation and parole in the United States, 2020.* Bureau of Justice Statistics. https://bjs.ojp.gov/content/pub/pdf/ppus20.pdf

Kapoor, R., Dike, C. C., & Norko, M. A. (2018). Psychiatric treatment in forensic hospital and correctional settings. *Psychiatric Annals, 48*(2), 102–108. https://doi.org/10.3928/00485713-20180110-01

Kelly, B. L., Barrenger, S. L., Watson, A. C., & Angell, B. (2017). Forensic assertive community treatment: Recidivism, hospitalization, and the role of housing and support. *Social Work in Mental Health, 15*(5), 567–597. https://doi.org/10.1080/15332985.2016.1261754

Kielhofner, G., Mallison, T., Crawford, C., Nowak, M., Rigby, M., Henry, A., & Walens, D. (2004). *Occupational Performance History Interview-II (OPHI-II).* Version 2.1. Model of Human Occupation Clearinghouse, Department of Occupational Therapy, College of Applied Health Sciences, University of Illinois at Chicago.

Kronenberg, F., & Pollard, N. (2005). Overcoming occupational apartheid: A preliminary exploration of the political nature of occupational therapy. In F. Kronenberg, S. S. Algado, & N. Pollard (Eds.), *Occupational therapy without borders: Learning from the spirit of survivors* (pp. 58–86). Elsevier Churchill Livingstone.

Lamb, H. R., & Weinberger, L. E. (2014). Decarceration of U.S. jails and prisons: Where will persons with serious mental illness go? *Journal of the Academy of Psychiatric Law, 42*(4), 489–494.

Landess, J., & Holoyda, B. (2017). Mental health courts and forensic assertive community treatment teams as correctional diversion programs. *Behavioral Sciences and the Law, 35*(5–6), 501–511. https://doi.org/10.1002/bsl.2307

Latessa, E., Lemke, R., Makarios, M., & Smith, P. (2010). The creation and validation of the Ohio Risk Assessment System (ORAS). *Federal Probation, 74*(1), 16–22. https://www.ojp.gov/ncjrs/virtual-library/abstracts/creation-and-validation-ohio-risk-assessment-system-oras

Law, M., Baptiste, S., Carswell, A., McColl, M. A., Polatajko, H., & Pollock, N. (2014). *Canadian Occupational Performance Measure* (5th ed.). CAOT Publications.

Law, M., Cooper, B., Strong, S., Stewart, D., Rigby, P., & Letts, L. (1996). The Person–Environment–Occupation model: A transactive approach to occupational performance. *Canadian Journal of Occupational Therapy, 66,* 9–23. https://doi.org/10.1177/000841749606300103

Lindstedt, H., Grann, M., & Soderlund, A. (2011). Mentally disordered offenders' daily occupations after one year of forensic care. *Scandinavian Journal of Occupational Therapy, 18*(4), 302–311. https://doi.org/10.3109/11038128.2010.525720

Liptak, J. J. (2022). *Barriers to Reentry Success Inventory* (3rd ed.). Impact Publications. https://www.impactpublications.com/product/barriers-to-reentry-success-inventory-third-edition

Lloyd, C. (1985). Evaluation and forensic psychiatric occupational therapy. *British Journal of Occupational Therapy, 48*(5), 137–140. https://doi.org/10.1177/030802268504800509

Lloyd, C. (1987a). The role of occupational therapy in the treatment of the forensic psychiatric patient. *Australian Occupational Therapy Journal, 34*(1), 20–25. https://doi.org/10.1111/j.1440-1630.1987.tb01561.x

Lloyd, C. (1987b). Working with a female offender: A case study. *British Journal of Occupational Therapy, 50*(2), 44–46. https://doi.org/10.1177/030802268705000203

Lloyd, C. (1988). A vocational rehabilitation programme in forensic psychiatry. *British Journal of Occupational Therapy, 51*(4), 123–126. https://doi.org/10.1177/030802268805100407

Lloyd, C. (1989). Parenting: A group programme for abusive parents. *Australian Occupational Therapy Journal, 36*(1), 24–33. https://doi.org/10.1111/j.1440-1630.1989.tb01636.x

Magee, G. (2021). Education reduces recidivism. *Technium Social Sciences Journal, 16,* 175–182. https://doi.org/10.47577/tssj.v16i1.2668

Margolis, R. L., Harrison, S. A., Robinson, H. J., & Jayaram, G. (1996). Occupational Therapy Task Observation Scale (OTTOS): A rapid method for rating task group function of psychiatric patients. *American Journal of Occupational Therapy, 50*(5), 380–385. https://doi.org/10.5014/ajot.50.5.380

Maruschak, L. M., Bronson, J., & Alper, M. (2021a). *Disabilities reported by prisoners.* Bureau of Justice Statistics. https://bjs.ojp.gov/content/pub/pdf/drpspi16st.pdf

Maruschak, L. M., Bronson, J., & Alper, M. (2021b). *Parents in prison and their minor children: Survey of prison inmates, 2016.* Bureau of Justice Statistics. https://bjs.ojp.gov/library/publications/parents-prison-and-their-minor-children-survey-prison-inmates-2016

Matarese, M., Greeno, E., Weeks, A., & Hammond, P. (2021). *The Cuyahoga youth count: A report on LGBTQ+ youth experience in foster care.* The Institute for Innovation & Implementation, University of Maryland School of Social Work. https://theinstitute.umaryland.edu/our-work/national/lgbtq/cuyahoga-youth-count

McNeil, S., & Bannigan, K. (2014). Forensic and prison services. In W. Bryant, J. Fieldhouse, & K. Bannigan (Eds.), *Creek's occupational therapy and mental health* (5th ed., pp. 424–438). Churchill Livingstone Elsevier.

McQueen, J. (2011). *Towards work in forensic mental health: National guidance for allied health professionals. A review to government.* Carstairs: The Forensic Network. http://www.forensicnetwork.scot.nhs.uk/wp-content/uploads/2012/08/Towards-Work-in-Forensic-Mental-Health-Publication.pdf

Mears, D. P., & Cochran, J. C. (2015). *Prisoner reentry in the era of mass incarceration.* Sage Publications.

Miller, M. K., Block, L. M., & DeVault, A. (2020). Problem-solving courts in the United States and around the world: History, evaluation, and recommendations. In M. K. Miller & B. H. Bornstein (Eds.), *Advances in psychology and law* (Vol. 5, pp. 301–371). Springer. https://doi.org/10.1007/978-3-030-54678-6_9

Molineux, M. L., & Whiteford, G. (1999). Prisons: From occupational deprivation to occupational enrichment. *Journal of Occupational Science, 6*(3), 124–130. https://doi.org/10.1080/14427591.1999.9686457

Monazzam, N., & Budd, K. M. (2023). *Incarcerated women and girls.* The Sentencing Project. https://www.sentencingproject.org/fact-sheet/incarcerated-women-and-girls

Moore, M. (2014). Forensic psychiatry and occupational therapy. In R. Crouch & V. Alers (Eds.), *Occupational therapy in psychiatry and mental health* (pp. 106–114). Wiley Blackwell.

Morgan, H. (2021). Restorative justice and the school-to-prison pipeline: A review of existing literature. *Education Sciences, 11*(4), 159. https://doi.org/10.3390/educsci11040159

Muñiz, J. O. (2021). Exclusionary discipline policies, school-police partnerships, surveillance technologies and disproportionality. A review of the school to prison pipeline literature. *The Urban Review, 53,* 735–760. https://doi.org/10.1007/s11256-021-00595-1

Muñoz, J. P. (2019a). Mental health practice in criminal justice systems. In C. Brown, V. Stoffel, & J. P. Muñoz (Eds.), *Occupational therapy in mental health: A vision for participation* (2nd ed., pp. 615–641). F.A. Davis.

Muñoz, J. P. (2019b). Toward a critical mass: Justice-based occupational therapy. *Annals of International Occupational Therapy, 3*(4), 160–161. https://doi.org/10.3928/24761222-20200924-01

Muñoz, J. P., Catalano, A., Wang, Y., & Phillips, G. A. (2020). Justice-based occupational therapy: A scoping review. *Annals of International Occupational Therapy, 3*(4), 162–174. https://doi.org/10.3928/24761222-20200924-02

Muñoz, J. P., Farnworth, L., & Dieleman, C. (2016). Harnessing the power of occupation to meet the needs of people in criminal justice settings. *Occupational Therapy International, 23,* 221–228. https://doi.org/10.1002/oti.1439

Muñoz, J. P., Moreton, E. M., & Sitterly, A. M. (2016). The scope of practice of occupational therapy in U.S. criminal justice settings. *Occupational Therapy International, 23*(3), 241–254. https://doi.org/10.1002/oti.1427

Nasreddine, Z. S., Phillips, N. A., Bedirian, V., Charbonneau, S., Whitehead, V., Collin, I., Cummings, J. L., & Chertkow, H. (2005). The Montreal Cognitive Assessment, MoCA: A brief screening tool for mild cognitive impairment. *Journal of the American Geriatrics Society, 53,* 695–699. https://doi.org/10.1111/j.1532-5415.2005.53221.x

National Alliance on Mental Illness. (2023). *Mental health treatment while incarcerated.* Author. https://www.nami.org/Advocacy/Policy-Priorities/Improving-Health/Mental-Health-Treatment-While-Incarcerated

National Association of State Mental Health Program Directors Research Institute (NRI). (2021, September). *Use of state psychiatric hospitals.* NRI Analytics Improving Behavioral Health. https://www.nri-inc.org/media/ju5ld0hx/nri_2020_profiles_-_use_of_state_psychiatric_hospitals-_september_2021.pdf

National Institute of Justice. (2020, February). *Problem solving courts.* Author. https://nij.ojp.gov/topics/articles/problem-solving-courts

Nowotny, K. M., Belknap, J., Lynch, S., & DeHart, D. (2014). Risk profile and treatment needs of women in jail with co-occurring serious mental illness and substance use disorders. *Women and Health, 54*(8), 781–795. https://doi.org/10.1080/03630242.2014.932892

Nowotny, K. M., Masters, R. K. & Boardman, J. D. (2016). The relationship between education and health among incarcerated men and women in the United States. *BMC Public Health, 16*(1), 916. https://doi.org/10.1186/s12889-016-3555-2

Occupational Therapy Australia. (2016). *Position paper: Occupational deprivation.* https://otaus.com.au/publicassets/5e5829df-2503-e911-a2c2-b75c2fd918c5/Occupational%20Deprivation%20(April%202016).pdf

O'Connell, M., & Farnworth, L. (2007). Occupational therapy in forensic psychiatry: A review of the literature and a call for a united and international response. *British Journal of Occupational Therapy, 70*(5), 184–191. https://doi.org/10.1177/030802260707000502

Office of Juvenile Justice and Delinquency Prevention. (2023, November). *Trends and characteristics of youth in residential placement, 2021.* Author. https://www.ojjdp.gov/ojstatbb/snapshots/DataSnapshot_CJRP2021.pdf

Ozkan, E., Belhan, S., Yaran, M., & Zarif, M. (2018). Occupational therapy in forensic settings. IntechOpen. https://doi.org/10.5772/intechopen.79366

Parkinson, S., Forsyth, K., & Kielhofner, G. (2006). *A user's manual for the MOHOST; The Model of Human Occupation Screening Tool* (Version 2.0). Model of Human Occupation Clearinghouse, Department of Occupational Therapy, University of Illinois at Chicago.

Patel, S., Barnes, M. A. & Jaegers, L. A. (2024). Occupational therapy in carceral settings: Qualitative study of practitioner experiences and perspectives. *OTJR: Occupational Therapy Journal of Research.* https://doi.org/10.1177/15394492241268850

Pedlar, A., Arat, S., Yuen, F., & Fortune, D. (2018). *Community re-entry: Uncertain futures for women leaving prison.* Routledge.

Penner, D. A. (1978). Correctional institutions: An overview. *American Journal of Occupational Therapy, 32*(8), 517–524.

Pereira, R. B., Whiteford, G., Hyett, N., Weekes, G., Di Tommaso, A., & Naismith, J. (2020). Capabilities, Opportunities, Resources and Environments (CORE): Using the CORE approach for inclusive, occupation-centred practice. *Australian Occupational Therapy Journal, 67,* 162–171. https://doi.org/10.1111/1440-1630.12642

Perez, J. (2023). The foster care-to-prison pipeline: A road to incarceration. *The Criminal Law Practitioner.* https://www.crimlawpractitioner.org/post/the-foster-care-to-prison-pipeline-a-road-to-incarceration

Phelps, E. M., & Aldrich, R. M. (2022). Incarceration during a pandemic: A catalyst for extending the conceptual terrain of occupational deprivation. *Journal of Occupational Science, 29*(3), 430–440. https://doi.org/10.1080/14427591.2022.2060286

Pinals, D., & Callahan, L. (2020). Evaluation and restoration of competence to stand trial: Intercepting the forensic system using the sequential intercept model. *Psychiatric Services, 71*(7), 698–705. https://doi.org/10.1176/appi.ps.201900484

Prins, S. J. (2014). Prevalence of mental illness in U.S. state prisons: A systematic review. *Psychiatric Services, 65*(7), 862–872. https://doi.org/10.1176/appi.ps.201300166

Puzzanchera, C., Hockenberry, S., & Sickmund, M. (2022, December). *Youth and the juvenile justice system: 2022 national report.* National Center for Juvenile Justice. https://ojjdp.ojp.gov/publications/2022-national-report.pdf

Puzzanchera, C., & Taylor, M. (2020). *Disproportionality rates for children of color in foster care dashboard.* National Center for Juvenile Justice. http://ncjj.org/AFCARS/Disproportionality_Dashboard.aspx

Reingle Gonzalez, J. M., Cannell, M. B., Jetelina, K. K., & Froehlich-Grobe, K. (2016). Disproportionate prevalence rate of prisoners with disabilities: Evidence from a nationally representative sample. *Journal of Disability Policy Studies, 27*(2), 106–115. https://doi.org/10.1177/1044207315616809

Ring, K., & Gill, M. (2017, June). *Using time to reduce crime: Federal prisoner survey results show ways to reduce recidivism.* Families Against Mandatory Minimums. https://www.prisonpolicy.org/scans/famm/Prison-Report_May-31_Final.pdf

Roberts, C., Davies, J., & Maggs, R. G. (2015). Structured community activity for forensic mental health: A feasibility study. *Journal of Forensic Practice, 17*(3), 180–191. https://doi.org/10.1108/JFP-12-2014-0049

Rodda, J., & Beichner, D. (2017). Identifying programming needs of women detainees in a jail environment. *Journal of Offender Rehabilitation, 56*(6), 373–393. https://doi.org/10.1080/10509674.2017.1339161

Royal College of Occupational Therapists. (2012). *Occupational therapists' use of occupation-focused practice in secure hospitals: Practice guideline.* Author.

Royal College of Occupational Therapists. (2017). *Occupational therapists' use of occupation-focused practice in secure hospitals: Practice guideline* (2nd ed.). Author.

Rucker, J. M., & Richeson, J. A. (2021). Toward an understanding of structural racism: Implications for criminal justice. *Science, 374,* 286–290. https://doi.org/10.1126/science.abj7779

Sawyer, W. (2018). *How does unaffordable money bail affect families?* Prison Policy Initiative. https://www.prisonpolicy.org/blog/2018/08/15/pretrial

Sawyer, W., & Wagner, P. (2022, March). *Mass incarceration: The whole pie.* Prison Policy Institute. https://www.prisonpolicy.org/reports/pie2022.html

Schindler, V. P. (2019). Introduction to the issue on OT and the criminal justice system. *Occupational Therapy in Mental Health, 35*(3), 217–218. https://doi.org/10.1080/0164212X.2019.1644719

Schkade, J. K., & Schultz, S. (1992). Occupational adaptation: Toward a holistic approach for contemporary practice, part 1. *American Journal of Occupational Therapy, 46,* 829–837. https://doi.org/10.5014/ajot.46.9.829

Schuster, S. S., & Stickle, B. (2023). *Are education programs in prison worth it? A meta-analysis of the highest quality academic research.* Policy Brief Mackinac Center. https://www.mackinac.org/archives/2023/s2023-01.pdf

Scott, P. J., McKinney, K. G., Perron, J. M., Ruff, E. G., & Smiley, J. L. (2019). The Revised Role Checklist: Improved utility, feasibility, and reliability. *OTJR: Occupational Therapy Journal of Research, 39*(1), 56–63. https://doi.org/10.1177/1539449218780618

Seek, N. (1989). The New Zealand prison system: The potential role of occupational therapy. *Journal of the New Zealand Association of Occupational Therapists, 40,* 16–19.

Shea, C., Jackson, N., & Haworth, C. (2019). Serving high-risk youth in context: Perspectives from Hong Kong. *The Open Journal of Occupational Therapy, 7*(3), 1–16. https://doi.org/10.15453/2168-6408.1566

Shea, C.-K., & Siu, A. M. (2016). Engagement in play activities as a means for youth in detention to acquire life skills. *Occupational Therapy International, 23*(3), 276–286. https://doi.org/10.1002/oti.1432

Sheehan, C. M. (2019). Education and health conditions among the currently incarcerated and the non-incarcerated populations. *Population Research and Policy Review, 38*(1), 73–93. https://doi.org/10.1007/s11113-018-9496-y

Simaan, J. (2021) Occupational apartheid in Palestine, global racism, and transnational solidarity: Update on Simaan (2017). *Journal of Occupational Science, 28*(3), 435–440. https://doi.org/10.1080/14427591.2021.1880265

Sinko, L., He, Y., & Tolliver, D. (2021). Recognizing the role of healthcare providers in dismantling the trauma-to-prison pipeline. *Pediatrics, 147*(5), e2020035915. https://doi.org/10.1542/peds.2020-035915

Smith, A., Petty, M., Oughton, I., & Alexander, R. T. (2010). Establishing a work-based learning programme: Vocational rehabilitation in a forensic learning disability setting. *British Journal of Occupational Therapy, 73*(9), 431–436. https://doi.org/10.4276/030802210X12839367526174

Smith, M. N. (2022). Occupational therapy's role in the foster care system. *The Open Journal of Occupational Therapy, 10*(1), 1–6. https://doi.org/10.15453/2168-6408.1850

Soeker, M. S., Hare, S., Mall, S., & van der Berg, J. (2021). The value of occupational therapy intervention for the worker roles of forensic mental healthcare users in Cape Town, South Africa. *Work, 68*(2), 399–414. https://doi.org/10.3233/WOR-203381

Stelter, L., & Evetts, C. (2020). Effect of an occupation-based program for women with intellectual and developmental disabilities who are incarcerated. *The Annals of International Occupational Therapy, 3*(4), 175–184. https://doi.org/10.3928/24761222-20190910-01

Stelter, L., & Whisner, S. M. (2007). Building responsibility for self through meaningful roles: Occupational adaptation theory applied in forensic psychiatry. *Occupational Therapy in Mental Health, 23*(1), 69–84. https://doi.org/10.1300/J004v23n01_05

Stewart, B., Owens, D. M., El Ghaziri, M., Jaegers, L., Cherniack, M. G., & Fallon, P. (2022). *Current and innovative practices in reducing staff trauma and organizational stress in corrections for correctional officers.* National Institute of Corrections. https://nicic.gov/resources/nic-library/webinars-broadcasts/current-and-innovative-practices-reducing-staff-trauma

Stewart, P., & Craik, C. (2007). Occupation, mental illness and medium security: Exploring time-use in forensic regional secure units. *British Journal of Occupational Therapy, 70*(10), 416–425. https://doi.org/10.1177/030802260707001002

Substance Abuse and Mental Health Services Administration. (2018). *GAINS Center for behavioral health and justice transformation: Treatment court locators.* https://www.samhsa.gov/gains-center/mental-health-treatment-court-locator/adults

Substance Abuse and Mental Health Services Administration. (2022, March). *About criminal and juvenile justice.* https://www.samhsa.gov/criminal-juvenile-justice/about

Sundaresh, R., Yi, Y., Harvey, T. D., Roy, B., Riley, C., Lee, H., Wildeman, C., & Wang, E. A. (2021). Exposure to family member incarceration and adult well-being in the United States. *JAMA Network Open, 4*(5), e2111821. https://doi.org/10.1001/jamanetworkopen.2021.11821

Sutton, M. B., & Routon, P. W. (2023). Poverty, inequality, and incarceration: Estimates from state and prison level data. *Journal of Poverty, 28*(5), 436–453. https://doi.org/10.1080/10875549.2023.2235336

Tan, B. L., Kumar, V. R., & Devaraj, P. (2015). Development of a new occupational therapy service in a Singapore prison. *British Journal of Occupational Therapy, 78*(8), 525–529. https://doi.org/10.1177/0308022615571083

Taylor, R. (2017). *Kielhofner's Model of Human Occupation: Theory and application* (5th ed.). Lippincott Williams & Wilkins.

Thomson, L. K., & Robnett, R. (2016). *Kohlman Evaluation of Living Skills (KELS).* American Occupational Therapy Association.

Timme, A., & Nowotny, K. M. (2021). Mental illness and mental health care treatment among people with criminal justice involvement in the United States. *Journal of Health Care for the Poor and Underserved, 32*(1), 397–422. https://doi.org/10.1353/hpu.2021.0031

Townsend, E., & Polatajko, H. J. (2013). *Enabling occupation II: Advancing an occupational therapy vision for health, wellbeing and justice through occupation* (2nd ed.). CAOT Publications ACE.

Tse, S. S. (1990). Occupational therapy in forensic psychiatric units. *New Zealand Journal of Occupational Therapy, 41*(2), 18–22.

U.S. Department of Health and Human Services. (2022, June). *The adoption and foster care analysis and reporting system report–2021.* Administration for Children and Families, Administration on Children, Youth and Families, Children's Bureau. https://www.acf.hhs.gov/sites/default/files/documents/cb/afcars-report-29.pdf

Wang, L., Sawyer, W., Herring, T., & Widra, E. (2022). *Beyond the count: A deep dive into state prison populations.* Prison Policy Initiative. https://www.prisonpolicy.org/reports/beyondthecount.html

Western, B., Braga, A. A., Davis, J., & Sirois, C. (2015). Stress and hardship after prison. *American Journal of Sociology, 120*(5), 1512–1547. https://doi.org/10.1086/681301

White, J., Grass, C. D., Hamilton, T. B., & Rogers, S. (2013). Occupational therapy in criminal justice. In E. Cara & A. MacRae (Eds.), *Psychosocial occupational therapy: An evolving practice* (3rd ed., pp. 715–773). Delmar Cengage Learning.

Whiteford, G. (1997). Occupational deprivation and incarceration. *Journal of Occupational Science, 4*(3), 126–130. https://doi.org/10.1080/14427591.1997.9686429

Whiteford, G. (2000). Occupational deprivation: Global challenge in the new millennium. *British Journal of Occupational Therapy, 63*(5), 200–204. https://doi.org/10.1177/030802260006300503

Whiteford, G. E., Jones, K., Weekes, G., Ndlovu, N., Long, C., Perkes, D., & Brindle, S. (2020). Combatting occupational deprivation and advancing occupational justice in institutional settings: Using a practice-based enquiry approach for service transformation. *British Journal of Occupational Therapy, 83*, 52–61. https://doi.org/10.1177/0308022619865223

Whiteford, G. E., Parnell, T., Ramsden, L., Nott, M., & Vine-Daher, S. (2022). Understanding and advancing occupational justice and social inclusion. In P. Liamputtong (Ed.), *Handbook of social inclusion* (pp. 181–210). Springer. https://doi.org/10.1007/978-3-030-89594-5_10

Widgery, A. (2023). *The legislative primer series for front-end justice: Deflection and diversion.* National Conference of State Legislators. https://documents.ncsl.org/wwwncsl/Criminal-Justice/Deflection-Diversion-f02.pdf_

Wik, A., Hollen, V., & Fisher, W. H. (2017). *Forensic patients in state psychiatric hospitals: 1999-2016.* National Association of State Mental Health Program Directors. https://www.nasmhpd.org/sites/default/files/TACPaper.10.Forensic-Patients-in-State-Hospitals_508C_v2.pdf

Wilcock, A. (1998). *An occupational perspective of health.* Slack.

Wildeman, C., & Wang, E. A. (2017). Mass incarceration, public health, and widening inequality in the USA. *The Lancet, 389*, 1464–1474. https://doi.org/10.1016/S0140-6736(17)30259-3

Williams, F. S., Martinovich, Z., Kisiel, C., Griffin, G., Goldenthal, H., & Jordan, N. (2021). Can the development of protective factors help disrupt the foster care-to-prison pipeline? An examination of the association between justice system involvement and the development of youth protective factors. *Journal of Public Child Welfare, 15*(2), 223–250. https://doi.org/10.1080/15548732.2019.1696912

Yang, J., McCuish, E., & Corrado, R. (2021). Is the foster care-crime relationship a consequence of exposure? Examining potential moderating factors. *Youth Violence and Juvenile Justice, 19*(1), 94–112. https://doi.org/10.1177/1541204020939643

Yi, Y., & Wildeman, C. (2018). Can foster care interventions diminish justice system inequality? *The Future of Children, 28*(1), 37–58. https://doi.org/10.1353/FOC.2018.0002

Yoder, J., & Farkas, M. A. (2017). Unique challenges of reentry for convicted sex offenders. In S. Stojkovic (Ed.), *Prisoner reentry: Critical issues and policy decisions* (pp. 13–84). Palgrave Macmillan. https://doi.org/10.1057/978-1-137-57929-4_2

State Hospitals

Janice Hinds, Valerie Wen, and Nikki Hancock

State psychiatric hospitals play an essential role in the continuum of mental health services. Modern state hospitals strive to be recovery-oriented facilities offering trauma-informed, culturally responsive caring in the least restrictive environment possible. State hospitals are often staffed with a diverse set of health professionals, including occupational therapy practitioners (OTPs), who address a person's health and wellness and work diligently to integrate with community-based mental health services. State hospital facilities are not intended to be a person's home or a terminal placement. They are a vital, safe space designed to support each person's recovery; they are a space where people can stabilize and receive services that promote successful transitions to community life. Many individuals return to the community when they do not need the 24/7 structure, support, and safety provided by a state hospital.

This chapter begins with a demographic description of the people served in state hospitals in the United States and describes the range of interdisciplinary treatment team members providing care in these settings. It reviews frameworks, such as the Recovery Model and trauma-informed care, which can guide intervention and illustrates the expanding role of occupational therapy in state hospitals. Evaluation and intervention planning considerations, including models of practice that can work well for OTPs in this setting, are defined. This chapter shares common individual and group interventions and supporting evidence for occupational therapy practice and outlines opportunities for applying occupational therapy knowledge and skill sets to improve care in state hospital systems.

Overview of State Hospitals in the United States

State hospitals are public establishments, providing inpatient psychiatric services to individuals diagnosed with mental illness. Each state has inpatient commitment laws determining standards for admission. Methods of admission include involuntary **civil commitment**, involuntary **forensic commitment**, and voluntary admission. Criteria for involuntary civil commitment include symptoms of a serious mental illness indicating the likelihood the person is a danger to self or others, or an inability to provide for basic personal needs (Substance Abuse and Mental Health Services Administration [SAMHSA], 2019a).

Involuntary forensic commitment involves individuals being accused of committing a crime and then having a judge determine they are not competent to stand trial, or being judged as either **not guilty by reason of insanity** or **guilty except for insanity** (Lutterman, 2022). Most state laws also require individuals to receive services in the least restrictive setting (SAMHSA, 2019a). Briefly reflecting on the history of how state hospitals evolved in the continuum of care in the United States is helpful for understanding current circumstances and potential opportunities in state hospitals.

A Brief History

In the United States, state-run mental health facilities were established in the late 1700s to treat individuals with mental illness who could not afford to pay for care at private hospitals. At this time, inhumane conditions existed in many state hospitals and asylums globally. People were often chained, beaten, or starved (Peloquin, 1989). Conditions and treatment began to change in the 1800s as Philippe Pinel introduced and championed **moral treatment** in France. This approach, which influenced care in U.S. state hospitals, advocated for structured, individualized, and humane interventions with the goal of returning individuals to the community (Benjamin & Baker, 2004).

In the United States in the 1840s, Dorothea Dix documented inhumane conditions in Massachusetts and demanded reform. In doing so, she started a movement to improve conditions for individuals both in state hospitals and in prisons and to increase the number of state hospitals across the country (Avila, 2017). Although this movement led to an overall improvement in conditions, racially segregated treatment and discriminatory practices continued to result in substandard care for black individuals in these settings (Geller, 2020).

The total number of individuals in U.S. state hospitals reached a peak in 1955, numbering approximately 559,000 (Manderscheid et al., 2009). Overcrowding was a major issue. In the 1960s, public policies were initiated that impacted state hospital care. In 1961, The Joint Commission on Mental Illness and Mental Health (1961) emphasized deinstitutionalization and promoted community-based treatment. Two years later, the federal government passed the Community Mental Health Centers Act (Benjamin & Baker, 2004). Around the same time, Title VI of the Civil Rights Act of 1964, which prohibited discrimination based on race, put states at risk for losing funding for publicly funded institutions. After reports of violations and several lawsuits, the last remaining state institutions were desegregated by 1969 (Geller, 2020).

These events initiated a shift in funding away from state hospitals and toward community-based programs, resulting in a dramatic decrease in individuals in state facilities to fewer than 200,000 by 1980 (Manderscheid et al., 2009). The 1990 U.S. Supreme Court *Olmstead* decision contributed to continued decline in state hospital populations. This ruling determined the Americans with Disabilities Act (ADA) applied to individuals in state psychiatric hospitals. States were required to make reasonable accommodations to support the community integration of individuals clinically appropriate for community-based settings (Lutterman, 2022). By 2020, state hospital populations in the United States had been reduced by over half a million people, and there were now only approximately 39,900 individuals receiving services at 177 state hospitals (Lutterman, 2022). See Chapter 26: The Public Policy Environment. 🤝

State Hospital Demographics

State facilities serve children, adolescents, adults, and older adults. Some hospitals serve all age groups, whereas others have separate facilities for children and adolescents. According to SAMHSA's National Mental Health Services Survey (SAMHSA, 2019b), the people served in the public psychiatric hospitals were primarily adults 18 to 64 years (85%), but the overall demographics also included adults 65 years and older (12%) and children and adolescents (3%). In 2020, 51% of admissions were involuntarily forensically committed, 38% were involuntarily civilly committed, and only 11% were voluntary admissions to state and county hospitals (Lutterman, 2022). Recent aggregated demographics on psychiatric diagnoses for people requiring hospitalization across public state hospitals, as well as private and general hospitals, could not be found (SAMHSA, 2021).

SAMHSA now collects data about substance use and mental health facilities using the National Substance Use and Mental Health Service Survey (N-SUMHSS); individual facilities tend to track their data in the same reporting manner. The most recent survey to track the demographics of psychiatric disorders reported most individuals hospitalized in psychiatric facilities were diagnosed with schizophrenia (46%) or an affective disorder (39%; National Association of State Mental Health Program Directors [NASMHPD] Research Institute, 2013).

As state hospital populations are decreasing in size, there continues to be an increase in involuntary treatment for sex offenders and forensic involvement, resulting in a 36% increase in funding to address these people (NASMHPD, 2014). Funding sources for state mental health hospitals usually include state general funds, state special appropriations, and Medicaid and Medicare revenues, plus other federal funds such as Medicaid Disproportionate Share Hospital (DSH) provisions (Lutterman, 2022; NASMHPD, 2014). Learners are encouraged to refer to the plethora of reports and data found on SAMHSA's N-MHSS website, which also contains a link to the SAMHSA data website (https://www.datafiles.samhsa.gov/dataset/national-mental-health-services-survey-2020-n-mhss-2020-ds0001).

Models Guiding Practice in State Hospitals

The Recovery Model is the standard in mental health care. It is a person-centered approach that supports people to make decisions about their own lives that promote their recovery and well-being. This model focuses on providing choice, achieving self-identified goals, and supporting individuals in feeling empowered to make their own choices (SAMHSA, 2023). The use of trauma-informed care in state hospitals recognizes that trauma is prevalent, often in multiple ways, in the lives of those needing mental health care and has a widespread and lasting impact. Interventions using a trauma-informed approach seek to create an environment of safety, are person-centered and strengths-based, prioritize building trust, and promote collaboration in the treatment process. OTPs in state hospitals seamlessly link the Recovery Model and trauma-informed approaches with occupational therapy models of practice. See Chapter 5: Trauma-Informed Practice and Chapter 25: Trauma- and Stressor-Related Disorders. 🤝

Useful occupational therapy models of practice in state hospitals include the Person-Environment-Occupation (PEO) model (Law et al., 1996), the Person-Environment-Occupation-Performance (PEO-P) model (Baum et al., 2015), and the Occupational Therapy Intervention Process Model (OTIPM; Fisher & Marterella, 2019). Other occupational therapy models that may guide practice include the Ecology of Human Performance (EHP; Dunn et al., 1994), Model of Human Occupation (MOHO; Taylor et al., 2023), Canadian Model of Occupational Performance and Engagement (CMOP-E; Polatajko et al., 2007), and Allen Cognitive Disabilities Model (ACDM; Allen et al., 1992).

Each of these models considers the transaction between the individual and their environments while engaging in occupations and how these interactions impact performance. In state hospitals, these models support person-centered evaluation and the inclusion of individuals in their own treatment planning process so that goals and interventions are valuable and meaningful.

State hospital environments emphasize safety and security, which can present limitations and restrictions to participation in some daily occupations. OTPs must creatively find ways to maximize an individual's independence and self-efficacy in the state hospital setting. Examples include encouraging individuals to plan meals in cooking groups, which may reflect their own family or cultural history; supporting individuals who want to share about their lived experiences on panels or in peer-led groups; and guiding individuals in identifying strategies and tools that promote self-regulation in stressful situations, thereby decreasing the potential for repeated traumatic seclusion and restraint.

The Interdisciplinary Treatment Team

The interdisciplinary treatment team is key to the care and services provided in state hospitals. Each member of the team brings a specific perspective and skill set to an individual's care. The team composition and size may vary based on the

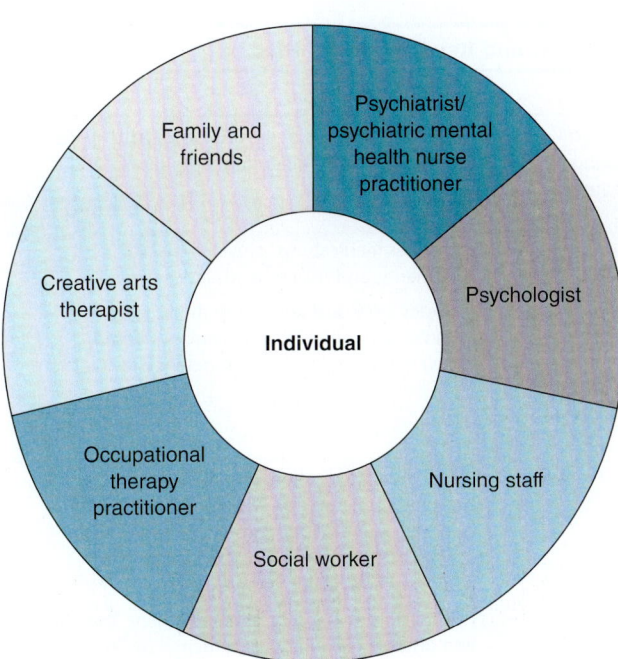

FIGURE 41-1. Members of the interdisciplinary team.

state and funding; however, there are minimum members needed to make up the team. The interdisciplinary treatment team starts with the individual receiving services. Figure 41-1 illustrates the various members that may make up the team.

Required members of the team include a psychiatrist or psychiatric mental health nurse practitioner, a nurse, and a social worker. OTPs provide input and are frequently part of the team. Occupational therapy addresses daily activities, functional cognition, sensory processing concerns, the person-environment fit, and other impacts on occupational performance, with a focus on transition back to the community. Table 41-1 describes the roles and interventions used by professionals working in state hospitals.

In addition to these personnel, medical and other health-care providers may be available on site to create ease of access to care. This can include primary care providers (e.g., medical doctor, physician assistant, nurse practitioner), dentists, dietitians, physical therapists, or speech therapists. Peer support specialists, chaplains, and community liaisons can also be found in many state hospital settings to promote recovery and successful transition. Addiction services are frequently offered at state hospitals to meet individual needs. Certified addiction specialists evaluate and provide recommendations and treatment for people who benefit from recovery-oriented groups or individual counseling.

Forensic services have become a consistent component of mental health treatment in many state hospitals because of shifts in populations. Between 1999 and 2014, there was a 76% national increase in the number of individuals admitted through involuntary forensic commitment, with the largest increase for people accused of committing a crime and determined by a court not to be competent to stand trial (Wik et al., 2020). Forensic staff include psychiatrists and psychologists, who evaluate individuals for competency to stand trial and provide results and recommendations to the legal system. Additional forensic staff may overlap with members found in

the interdisciplinary treatment team, including OTPs, who tailor interventions based on treatment requirements as dictated by legal status.

Vocational services in state hospitals provide environments for learning and reinforcing work habits and behaviors. OTPs may provide some of these services, or there may be other specialized staff. Staff teach and provide constructive feedback on job skills such as time management, work quality, dependability, and flexibility. They provide individuals with the opportunity to practice interpersonal and communication skills such as listening, talking, collaborating, and handling conflict. Vocational services staff work with individuals and their teams to support successful transition of the worker role into community settings.

Role of Occupational Therapy

OTPs working in state psychiatric facilities provide services to individuals with severe and persistent mental illnesses designed to improve their occupational performance and the quality of their lives. Mental health practitioners provide direct care with individuals and groups, and indirect care that consists of advocacy and/or consultative services that could also include large group training with unit staff, hospital personnel, and/or community agencies. The occupational therapy process is reflected in occupational therapy services, which may include:

- Screening for medical necessity and readiness for occupational therapy intervention.
- Person-centered evaluation that may include gathering occupational profile data, reviewing the medical records, observing the person in the treatment milieu, discussing treatment status and needs with the interdisciplinary team, and/or administering assessments and interpreting their outcomes, all relative to the individual consumer's needs and the reasons for referral.
- Establishing an intervention plan and selecting relevant preparatory and/or occupation-based interventions, ideally in collaboration with the individual.
- Implementing the interventions, modifying the treatment plan and/or modalities with the individual and at times in consultation with the treatment team, and/or (re)administering assessments as indicated, all to best reflect and support the individual's strengths, abilities, and needs to reach and sustain their goals. At times, therapeutic interventions might also address the goals of the treatment team and/or collaborating agencies, such as conducting a home assessment, contributing data to a guardianship hearing or need for potential community services, and/or recommending staff education via an outside agency consultation.
- Discontinuing the treatment plan when the reason for referral has been met, the individual's goals have been met, person and caregiver education has been completed, and/or the person is discharged from the treatment unit or hospital.
- Using outcome measures to assist in treatment aspects such as discharge planning and making referrals, providing caregiver education on the influence of the environment on occupational performance or instructing

TABLE 41-1 | State Hospital Interdisciplinary Treatment Team Roles and Key Responsibilities

Team Member	Role	Key Responsibilities
Individual	Person receiving services; seen as the expert of their own life; contributes to establishing treatment goals and engages in the treatment process	Recommends focus of interventions; participates in treatment and monitoring of outcomes and progress
Psychiatrist/Psychiatric mental health nurse practitioner	Primary diagnostician, team leader, and medication manager	Prescribes medications, provides specific treatments, and recommends levels of care
Psychologist	Performs psychological evaluations and assessments to help individuals identify their concerns or needs; identifies risk factors, including suicidal ideation, self-injurious behavior, anger or low frustration tolerance, violence or homicidal ideation, and history of impulsivity	Provides individual and group therapy; consults with the team on a behavioral plan, trauma recovery services, and/or competency restoration
Nursing staff: Registered nurse (RN), licensed practical nurse (LPN), direct care staff	Responsible for maintaining a safe and therapeutic environment; manages daily operations of the state hospital units	Administers medication, monitors changes in response to medication, tracks ADL completion or needs, and facilitates groups on topics such as medication management, understanding diagnosis, and health and wellness
Social worker	Facilitates connection to and use of supports available to the individual, including family, financial, spiritual, cultural, and community resources	Key role in providing case management, transition and discharge planning, and mental health counseling
Occupational therapist, and/or occupational therapy assistant	Administers assessments and facilitates successful engagement with activities of daily living and instrumental activities of daily living in the hospital environment and in preparation for community transition	Uses interventions within the context of functional performance to address a variety of areas including functional cognition, social interactions, self-care, sensory processing, home management, and vocational and community living skills
Recreation therapist, music therapist, art therapist, dance/movement therapist	Uses specific therapeutic modalities (e.g., leisure, music, art, movement) to facilitate and address emotional, cognitive, and social needs	*Recreation therapist:* Uses recreation and activity-based interventions to provide leisure education, exercise programs, and recreation skills development *Music therapist:* Provides interventions that may include improvisation, drumming, lyric analysis, music listening, and singing *Art therapist:* Guides art processes using a variety of art forms to address consumers' needs *Dance/Movement therapist:* Focuses activities that emphasize movement, posture, breathing, and interaction with the environment
Family and friends	Maintain connection with the individual through in-person and/or virtual visits, phone calls, and mail to promote recovery	May provide essential background/historical information; can provide suggestions and ideas for improving their loved one's care

on a safety measure (e.g., use of gait belt with transfers, durable medical equipment [DME] for showering), and/or serving on the interdisciplinary treatment team to provide information on the scope of occupational therapy.

Each component of the occupational therapy process requires communication with the individual, their self-identified family members or significant others, and the treatment team. Skilled service documentation is a necessary and vital part of the OTP's responsibilities, with requirements that vary from individual session notes to weekly or monthly documentation. Documentation standards are established by accreditation organizations, facility procedures, or specific treatment programs. It may also be necessary for OTPs to document specific incidents or events such as self-injury; aggression; physical, verbal, or sexual assaults; accidents; or

medical emergencies, doing so according to facility procedures. Additionally, per state law, OTPs may be mandatory reporters, and in these cases will work in consultation with their supervisor for reporting and documentation processes and support.

The opportunities for practitioners in state mental health facilities are broad, challenging, and professionally stimulating. Most discipline-specific practitioners are clinical evaluators, providers of direct services, and advocates for the person within the treatment team. Unique to an OTP voice is the focus on occupation, and specifically how the individual's functional cognition, the task demands, the environment, and the person's sensory processing preferences and modulation strategies impact occupational performance. OTPs also have an opportunity to impact the treatment context by contributing to the facility's implementation of the Recovery Model and trauma-informed care approaches. As a direct service provider, the OTP can help to alter an individual's role expectations from that of a passive recipient to one who is able to influence events and have some agency regarding their daily living experiences.

State hospital settings offer additional opportunities that match the knowledge and skill sets of OTPs.

- One example is collaborating with the architect responsible for ensuring the remodel of a unit meets facility and state codes as well as access requirements for persons with disabilities. An OTP who understands the ADA as well as how people typically use a space can make recommendations for adequate room in a shower to allow for a bariatric-sized chair. They can also advocate that universal design principles be employed, such as recommending that hallway and community room flooring glare be minimized, and act as a resource for decisions on room signage coloring, size, and location for people who ambulate as well as those who use wheeled mobility devices.

- Health-care facilities, including state hospitals, typically include fall rates as a quality indicator for quality service. Practitioners can design fall prevention programs and aid with identification of people at risk for falls in addition to making recommendations regarding education, training, adaptation, and environmental modification needs. This may include providing in-services to staff on the use of gait belts or transfers to/from elevated bed platforms or other DME, observing for and removing potential trip and fall hazards in the milieu such as tree skirts around a Christmas tree, showing consumers how to roll up their long pant legs, or being a member of a multidisciplinary falls prevention committee.

- Practitioners may serve on discharge planning committees alongside other members such as the in-hospital social workers and community-based case managers. The committees' purposes can range from discussions about global and specific needs of individuals discharging to the community, a referral system for hospital- and community-based services (e.g., medication management, home- and community-based services [HCBS]), and/or caregiver education consultation. These needs might include specific community reintegration concerns, types of settings ranging from skilled nursing facilities (SNFs) and assisted living facilities (ALFs) to subsidized apartments, and the type of environmental supports, transportation, and staff assistance that supports an individual to function at their best.

A variety of other administrative responsibilities may be integrated into an OTP's role. All hospitals have a variety of committees that exist to better the physical working environment, provide staff resources and support systems, and support the recovery work provided. Using a PEO/PEO-P framework may assist the OTP to conceptualize contributions to these administrative roles and lend a distinct occupational therapy perspective when sharing recommendations with other committee members. PEO/PEO-P is a unique organizing construct that provides a well-rounded and balanced viewpoint, and one that non-occupational therapy colleagues readily understand.

- Medical records committees are responsible for the content, format, and review of medical records;

subcommittees are charged with updating the electronic health records' documents and processes to reflect current practice. The Compliance Committee acquires and disseminates education and processes that align with The Joint Commission, Culturally and Linguistically Appropriate Services (CLAS), and/or management of protected health information (PHI) violations. Committees such as these determine if the facility's records are complete, accurate, and in compliance with legal and accreditation requirements.

- Justice, Equity, Diversity, and Inclusion (JEDI) committees address both consumer and staff concerns. They might write staff guidelines for responding to racist and bigoted language and/or behaviors and provide in-services for implementation; provide awareness about microaggressions and education to eliminate—or minimize—their use and impact; and consult with other departments to celebrate secular, nonsecular, and state or federal holidays. For example, the nutrition services department can serve a special meal, or treatment team nursing staff can lead a current events group with education provided by the committee.

- Committees that boost staff morale might host Spirit Week, organize a chili tasting, or create a fundraising event such as a bake sale or distribute carnations and chocolates to team members, with the proceeds supporting another event such as an annual barbecue for staff and other people. Other staff-focused committees might exist as conduits of information between staff and management or to collect recruitment or retention suggestions for the human resources department.

Additional roles for OTPs can include:

- Testifying in court, such as guardianship hearings, administrative reviews, and certification disputes. Practitioners working in forensic settings receive additional education about neutral and objective documentation to not unduly influence a court evaluator.

- Specific to state hospital settings is the use of low- and high-level interventions to assist a person in maintaining or regaining control over their safe behaviors. All clinical staff are required to participate in annual training in a variety of team-based techniques. After a crisis episode, which may be an attempt to self-harm or act of aggression, staff debrief the de-escalation techniques used. Debriefing may include an assessment of potential triggers so the person can be supported earlier in any subsequent situation (e.g., change to an individualized behavior plan), safety reassurance needs for the rest of the unit's community, and/or offering staff members trauma support. Debriefing with individuals on the unit is vital; answering their questions while maintaining privacy and confidentiality and reassuring their safety is imperative to creating and maintaining a therapeutic treatment milieu.

- With the COVID-19 pandemic, the use of telehealth-type service delivery methods became prevalent in state hospital settings. This included conducting in-hospital interventions via the telephone or video (e.g., Health Insurance Portability and Accountability Act [HIPAA] compliant electronic rooms for treatment planning, individual treatment sessions, virtual court) and supporting a person's use of technology to meet with their family, providers, and community-based care managers. Many of these role adaptations remained in place as the hospital's state government agencies conservatively lifted pandemic guidelines.

■ Practitioners may also serve as fieldwork educators for OTP students, and/or as capstone mentors for occupational therapy doctoral students. Interns typically undergo a more rigorous application and acceptance process because of government agency requirements to protect the vulnerable populations treated at state-run facilities.

Evaluation

State psychiatric hospitals across the United States share many similarities, and yet they differ in size, treatment focus, funding, and community resources that can impact some of the day-to-day aspects of occupational therapy practice (e.g., bed capacity ranging from less than 100 to more than 450, separate units or integrated forensic individual treatment, transition services via grant funding). Therefore, evaluation focus is influenced by a combination of these various overarching factors. Ideally, settings are staffed with enough OTPs to support routine initial screenings or evaluations upon admission, robust treatment, and regular reassessments during an annual review period.

Some settings have a lower OTP-to-consumer ratio, and therefore a single OTP may be responsible for providing consultative services to multiple treatment units. In such a setting, an OTP must prioritize and may only offer evaluations and treatment sessions for individuals with highly specific treatment needs. OTPs working in state hospital settings need to be familiar with the occupational therapy process for persons, groups, and populations provided in the *Occupational Therapy Practice Framework: Domain and Practice,* Fourth Edition (*OTPF-4;* American Occupational Therapy Association [AOTA], 2020), as well as the hospital's policies on the role of occupational therapy, funding, and documentation.

In other state hospital settings, there is an OTP assigned to each treatment unit who conducts evaluations with each person in that unit. In either situation, thoughtful consideration needs to be given to the value of using standardized assessments and when nonstandardized assessments are beneficial. The OTP who uses sound therapeutic reasoning administers assessments that support the reason for referral and contribute to the person's treatment and/or discharge planning in a meaningful way. For some individuals, this may be a battery of assessments that identify their global functioning ability for living in a community setting, and for others it may be an assessment that focuses on a single aspect important to the individual, such as a healing hand injury, potential need for specific DME for self-care activities of daily living (ADLs), or an individualized sensory modulation program.

Additionally, the evaluation process has become more person-centered and holistic, focusing on global functioning of the individual, performance patterns, environment in the hospital, and the discharge environment, as well as the occupations that are of value and interest to the consumer

(AOTA, 2020). The evaluation results guide interventions to improve quality of life while in the hospital, promote health and wellness, prepare for discharge into the community, and minimize the need for further hospitalizations. See Chapter 4: Person-Centered Evaluation. 🤝

Initial Evaluation

When an individual is referred for "occupational therapy eval and treat," the OTP typically begins the evaluation process through observation and interaction with the person. Additional data for the evaluation may be gathered through input from other members of the treatment team, including a discussion with the provider as to the reason for the referral as well as a brief chart review.

Given these varied data sources, the evaluating OTP is often able to familiarize themself with the person's prior living conditions, education, social and legal history, and social support systems. Past traumatic experiences are typically documented, and in these cases the OTP can maintain a trauma-informed approach by not posing trauma history questions. When more guidance is needed, whether in the initial evaluation phases or subsequent sessions, the OTP might use the current edition of the *OTPF* and other professional documents to guide the evaluation process (e.g., state practice act, code of conduct, level of competency, facility standards and practices).

The OTIPM (Fisher & Marterella, 2019) can guide an occupation-centered evaluation approach that is top-down and considers specific person factors when indicated. The astute OTP will tease out aspects of a person's functional abilities in reading, writing, and comprehension; visual acuity; visual perception; executive function and cognition; and expressive and receptive language during evaluation. The OTP is responsible for communicating an individual's functional abilities and needs to the treatment team, and, when indicated, for assessing further and making referrals to other multidisciplinary team members.

This holistic process supports building a therapeutic rapport; maximizes the person's attending and concentration; and assists the treatment team, and the person, in better understanding the type and content of written educational materials and verbal directions that best convey information to individual consumers. This may minimize frustration and confusion for the treatment team and for the person throughout the individual's hospitalization.

Interpretations of initial assessment data are documented and filed in the medical record to ensure accurate information is communicated with the treatment team. When the evaluation process is completed, the practitioner can collaborate with the individual, the occupational therapy assistant, and the entire treatment team to design the individual's plan of care that addresses intervention recommendations and discharge plans. The occupational therapy evaluation may be used to guide the treatment team's decisions for discharge planning. Standardized assessment tools can help develop an in-depth occupational profile with analysis of specific areas of occupational performance while remaining focused on the person's overall needs and goals (AOTA, 2020). Table 41-2 includes a partial summary of standardized assessments, organized into a referral-based listing of assessments, that may be utilized by OTPs in state psychiatric facilities.

TABLE 41-2 | **Therapeutic Reasoning Assessment Table: State Hospitals**

Reason for Administering; What Am I Measuring?	Tool	Logistical Considerations (Always Consider Safety With Regard to PEO-P) Perspective)	Contribution to Treatment Perspective	Associated Practice Model	Additional Assessment Tools to Consider
Functional cognition	Allen Cognitive Level Screen (ACLS); Allen Diagnostic Modules (ADM; e.g., Bead Kits I & II, Bargello Bookmark, Fabric-Covered Notebook; Earhart, 2006; Earhart et al., 2022)	Portable tool(s); 10–20 minutes to administer ACLS; screening results to be verified by other means (e.g., ADM, ACLS readministration); store completed ADM projects versus allowing them in consumer's room (e.g., elastic lacing used in Bead Kits)	Eliminates OTP's trial and error to understand a person's information processing ability, and therefore provide interventions at person's "best ability to function"; readministration measures stability or change in functional cognition (e.g., because of medication regimen)	Allen Cognitive Disabilities Model (ACDM)	Executive Function Performance Test (original and alternate versions; Baum et al., 2003) Cognitive Performance Test (CPT; Burns, 2018)
Occupational performance, life skills	Assessment of Motor and Process Skills (AMPS) and Assessment of Compared Qualities–Occupational Performance (ACQ-OP; Fisher & Jones, 2014)	Access to ADL/IADL equipment and supplies (e.g., linens, washer/dryer, kitchen); rater certification and scoring/documentation software; for use across the life span	Occupation-based; measures the quality of ADL/IADL task performance (e.g., independence, efficiency, effectiveness, safety of their occupational performance embedded in familiar, everyday occupations; use of ACQ-OP addressed discrepancies between person and OTP that can impact treatment focus [e.g., remediation, education, environment modification])	Occupational Therapy Intervention Process Model (OTIPM)	Independent Living Scales (ILS; Loeb, 1996) Kohlman Evaluation of Living Skills (KELS), 4th edition (Thomson & Robnett, 2016) Performance Assessment of Self-Care Skills (PASS; Rogers & Holm, 1989)
Sensory processing, sensory modulation	Adult/Adolescent Sensory Profile, Self-Questionnaire (Brown & Dunn, 2002)	Self-report; reading comprehension to independently complete pen-and-paper assessment (or complete with OTP)	Self-identified sensory processing preferences with OTP observing for potential impact on daily functioning	Dunn's Model of Sensory Processing Ayres Sensory Integration Theory (SPM)	Sensory Processing Measures (Parham et al., 2021) Sensory Defensiveness Screening for Adults; Sensory Defensiveness Evaluation (Moore, 2005)
Social interactions	Evaluation of Social Interactions (ESI); Assessment of Compared Qualities–Social Interaction (ACQ-SI; Fisher & Griswold, 2008)	Person's choice of social interactions; rater certification and scoring/documentation software; for use across the life span	Measurement of quality of person's social interactions in natural and self-chosen situations with social partners; use of ACQ-SI to address discrepancies between person and OTP that can impact treatment focus	OTIPM	Social Profile: Assessment of Social Participation in Children, Adolescents, and Adults (Donohue, 2013)

Informal and Formal Reevaluation

Evaluation is an ongoing aspect of the occupational therapy process; an effective OTP is always trying to develop the most complete, accurate, and current occupational profile for every individual they work with. The use of formal and informal observation to assess an individual's behaviors in the milieu, in one-to-one interactions, and in therapy groups is just one example of ongoing efforts to refine the profile. These observations and treatment interactions are documented in the medical record.

This ongoing assessment process guides changes in treatment focus and interventions. The practitioner might choose a specific assessment tool to fill a gap in the occupational profile, to compare progress against the assessments administered upon admission or at the beginning of individual treatment sessions, and/or to address a specific treatment or discharge planning need. These assessments might focus on functional cognition embedded in occupational performance, social interactions with various social partners (e.g., staff vs. family members), or a home and community assessment.

Because of the severity of illness seen in individuals admitted to state psychiatric hospitals, it is common to work with people who have had multiple long-term hospitalizations throughout their life. People may also have been incarcerated in between hospitalizations and community living. These types of institutional living can affect the person's self-care skills and ability to perform instrumental activities of daily living (IADLs); they also may hinder the person's ability to perform time management tasks and make choices and decisions.

A person's social interaction skills, self-efficacy, and how they imagine their future are also often impacted. Therefore, periodically, readministration of assessments with process and outcome comparisons may assist in gauging progression and regression in occupational performance. The OTP can document changes in function and modify the treatment plan, as well as recommend adaptations in occupations or the environment to guide interventions to assist the individual in relearning or adapting for these skills. Different state hospitals may require formal evaluations at different intervals or at the request of the court for persons with forensic involvement.

Intervention

Initial and ongoing evaluation processes guide intervention and discharge planning. Accurate, person-centered, holistic evaluation provides the data needed to build meaningful and successful interventions for individuals receiving state psychiatric services. Intervention is a rewarding process by which the OTP utilizes their creativity, capitalizes on their therapeutic use of self, and builds rapport with individuals. Although there are broad trends in occupational therapy intervention within the state psychiatric hospital system, interventions need to continue to be occupation-based, person-centered, and focused on the identified strengths, needs, goals, and context (AOTA, 2020). Overall, the purpose of intervention is to promote well-being, health, and participation (AOTA, 2020).

Interventions in this section are examined through the service delivery approaches of direct and indirect services. Note that direct services can occur at the person level, group level, or population level and include direct contact with the individual through interventions provided. Indirect services can include consultation or advocacy work that occurs on behalf of the individual by the OTP to address a specific need (AOTA, 2020). This section addresses the general goals of intervention within the context of occupations, considerations for intervention planning and implementation, use of group intervention, types of rehabilitation programming, and emerging areas of focus in state hospitals.

General Goals

The goals of occupational therapy intervention tend to focus on increasing an individual's independence with identified occupations and are tailored to the individual's identified strengths, needs, and context, but general goals remain the same in most inpatient psychiatric settings. Although admissions criteria are unique to each state system, the acute inpatient state psychiatric setting is designed for individuals who are a serious harm to self or others and/or unable to care for self at the time of admission. Because of the acute stage of illness experienced by individuals receiving services in this setting, they often present with paranoid or delusional thinking and/or aggressive behaviors (Fisher et al., 2009).

Other individuals may present with catatonia or selective mutism, stable and healing medical conditions such as hand injuries or status post hip fractures, withdrawal from recent substance use, or severe depressive symptoms. Practitioners in acute care units must therefore work on interdisciplinary teams with the common goal of providing a safe, stable daily routine for individuals experiencing an exacerbation of their psychiatric symptoms to facilitate progress toward recovery. Acute care intervention strategies are influenced by the individual's occupational performance and center on improving orientation functions, impulse control, and emotional functions. They seek to establish medication routines and diagnosis education, all while preparing the person for discharge back to the community (AOTA, 2020).

In addition to acute mental illness, many individuals admitted to state hospitals have forensic involvement. These individuals with mental illness are sometimes first diagnosed following an arrest triggered by bizarre or violent behavior stemming from symptoms of their illness (Fisher et al., 2009). In a few states, individuals at high risk for hurting themselves or others and who are unable to provide for their basic needs such as food, shelter, or clothing are identified as having a **grave disability**, a legal status reflecting the previously listed criteria. In this context, intervention may also focus on helping people cope and manage themselves within the legal system.

There continues to be a shift in funding and focus away from inpatient state hospitals and into community rehabilitation settings to assist individuals in receiving treatment services in less restrictive and more natural environments (Lutterman, 2022; SAMHSA, 2022). However, there also continues to be a need for the state hospital system, with its more restrictive environment, to treat individuals with severe mental illness safely and effectively. With the availability of community rehabilitation settings, individuals who become stable can reenter the community with more frequency and efficiency. Therefore, some individuals are discharged within weeks after being admitted to state hospitals.

However, there are individuals who have utilized and exhausted many of the local community resources and are unable to return to prior living environments. It may take a longer duration of time to locate appropriate placement for these individuals. Therefore, they may spend additional time being hospitalized even though they are clinically and psychiatrically stable and ready for discharge from the more restrictive setting of a state hospital. The remaining individuals in the state hospital system are those whose mental illness is so chronic and severe that they often require inpatient care for many months or years or require conditional release within the court system. These individuals are transferred to long-term stay programs, which may be unique to state psychiatric hospitals.

Long-term hospitalization creates additional challenges for reentry into the community. During hospitalization, hospital personnel may provide for many of the individuals' needs, such as meal preparation and medication management, and may even assist with basic ADLs. Although staff members encourage individuals to be as independent as possible in the setting, the opportunities for independence are limited, which can result in loss of skills and learned helplessness. However, to successfully reenter the community, individuals are expected to be able to care for themselves at a level consistent with the expected discharge placement context. Therefore, intervention in long-term programs is focused on building the functional living skills people will need upon discharge to community settings, such as home with family or nursing homes.

Goal areas in long-term programs at state hospitals are similar to those in any psychiatric setting, such as improving ADLs (e.g., grooming and hygiene) and IADLs (e.g., financial management, home establishment and management, meal preparation and clean-up, safety procedures, and emergency responses). Other goal areas include developing employment interests or acquiring skills, improving job performance, participating in volunteer activities, pursuing play and leisure activities, and improving social participation (AOTA, 2020). Refer to Table 41-3 for examples of interventions based on different service delivery approaches. Even though the general goal areas in state hospitals are similar to those in other psychiatric settings, the course of intervention to achieve them typically occurs at a much slower pace and training begins and proceeds using more basic, structured approaches, with outcomes likely dependent upon the person's level of psychiatric stability and symptomatology.

Considerations for Intervention Planning

The unique setting of a state hospital requires special considerations for intervention planning. The diverse population includes individuals in both acute and chronic phases of mental illness, forensic or legal involvement, and comorbid diagnoses; the level of impairment of hospitalized individuals varies widely. In addition, state hospitals typically have limited resources because of the financial structure of the setting and the safety considerations. These limitations must be considered when designing interventions.

Strategies for Successful Intervention

Always focus on function. Some individuals in state hospitals will continue to present active symptoms, such as delusions, hallucinations, and disorganized thinking, even while on medications. Others may present severe negative symptoms (e.g., catatonic behavior, impoverished speech, and slowed cognitive and motor responses). Psychiatric medications can contribute to, cause, or exacerbate negative symptoms.

When planning interventions, recognize that these symptoms may impact memory, problem-solving, and abstract thinking, and can make it difficult for a person to attend to activities or organize their behavior and speech. Sometimes administering a specific functional cognition assessment such as the Allen Cognitive Level Screen (ACLS) or Allen Diagnostic Modules (ADM) can help a practitioner more accurately gauge the impact of symptomatology. Applying skills in activity, task, or performance analysis can help a OTP match their interventions with the individual's performance and to grade the task and the environment. See Chapter 7: Cognition, Chapter 12: Emotion Regulation, and Chapter 23: Schizophrenia Spectrum and Psychotic Disorders.

In state hospital settings, an OTP who presents information in a concrete manner is more likely to create successful interventions. It can take practice for an OTP to learn to choose their words deliberately, to communicate in clear and short sentences, and to provide an individual time to process the message. During communication, it is often helpful to focus the person's attention on tangible, real-world characteristics and to information that connects to one of their senses.

Individuals with severe mental illness often have difficulty processing auditory information by simply hearing it alone. For example, a verbal discussion about stress management techniques may result in the person speaking off-topic, misunderstanding information, or falling asleep. However, when information is delivered in a more multimodal way (e.g., through visual examples on a video, pictures and words on a worksheet, or hands-on activities), individuals are often more engaged and integrate the information more effectively. Generally, individuals with disorganized thought are more likely to process information successfully if several of their senses are stimulated. Therefore, it is important for OTPs to provide information in ways that allow people to hear, see, do, and say as much as possible.

Successful interventions apply activity analysis principles, breaking down tasks into one- or two-step subtasks and chaining steps for individual success. During forward chaining, the next step of a task is not attempted until the first step is successfully accomplished, and when the next step is presented, supports are in place to promote success. For example, during an intervention related to meal preparation, the OTP may need to provide visual demonstration of a subtask, such as breaking an egg into a bowl, before expecting the person to do so correctly. Only after this step is accomplished is the individual encouraged to move on to the next step, using a fork to scramble the egg, for example.

Also, the OTP may need to perform large segments of the activity (e.g., cooking the egg) for the individual to engage in the subtasks appropriate for their current level of ability. During backward chaining, the individual will be provided prompts from the beginning through the last step and is then expected to complete the final step independently. Using the egg example, the OTP would prompt the individual to get the eggs out of the fridge, break an egg into a bowl, scramble the egg with a fork, and cook the egg in a pan, but would not prompt the individual to use the spatula to move the scrambled egg onto a plate (to serve and/or eat), as that would be the final step.

Errorless learning is another successful intervention strategy. Through errorless learning, individuals are provided the "just right" level of prompts (e.g., number of prompts, quality, type, steps in a prompt, augmented with gesture or not) to successfully complete a specific task correctly every time. For example, to continue with the cooking task of scrambled eggs, the OTP would tell the individual that they will be scrambling an egg today and allow the individual to complete the tasks independently until they demonstrate a need for assistance, at which point the OTP would then provide prompts and cuing (e.g., verbal, visual, and/or tactile) so that

TABLE 41-3 | **Common Intervention Approaches and Therapeutic Reasoning Prompts for Individuals in State Hospitals**

Occupation	Service Delivery	Example Intervention	Therapeutic Reasoning Prompts
ADLs (e.g., bath/shower, toilet, dress, eat/feed, functional mobility, personal hygiene/grooming)	Direct care	Toilet training to address incontinence	*AE/DME:* Are you able to provide, can the individual keep it in their room, will the individual discharge with it? *Environmental adaptations:* Can any be made, is there anything in the environment impacting independence with ADLs?
	Indirect care (consultation or advocacy)	Provide consultation on environmental modifications to bathrooms	
	Group	*Hygiene group:* Psychoeducational approach for situational dressing/attire (e.g., court appearances, interview for housing or employment)	
IADLs (e.g., manage communication, community mobility, financial responsibilities, home management, meal prep; engage in spiritual activities; understand/recognize safety risks; and shop)	Direct care	Utilizing AE to increase participation in meal prep activities; graded or simplified task steps; box mix with figure directions	What opportunities exist within the state hospital to practice IADL skills? Can the individual leave the facility to engage in IADL training within a community setting?
	Indirect care (consultation or advocacy)	Collaboration with chaplain to provide spiritual services to meet individual needs	
	Group	Social skills Cooking Community outing	
Health management (e.g., self-regulate, manage symptoms [both psychiatric and medical], manage medication[s], engage in physical activity, manage nutrition, and manage any personal care items/devices)	Direct care	Practice medication management with use of pill box	Does the individual have capacity to complete these health management activities independently or will they require some level of assistance in the community (e.g., appropriately grading the task)? Are there any safety concerns related to use of sensory diet/modulation items?
	Indirect care (consultation or advocacy)	Design and implement sensory, comfort, or relaxation room in facility or on treatment unit	
	Group	Physical fitness Yoga Tai chi Movement Symptom management Medication management Sensory regulation Nutrition WRAP (Wellness and Recovery Action Plan) Stress management	
Rest and sleep	Direct care	Provide education on sleep hygiene techniques and practice skills	How might a sleep diet appear different in an inpatient psychiatric setting versus in the community/home setting? Are there any safety concerns related to the use of a sleep diet routine in the inpatient setting? How might an OTP partner with the night staff who needs to check on individuals every 30 minutes?
	Indirect care (consultation or advocacy)	Member of environment of care team to address lighting and noise impacting sleep	
	Group	Sleep hygiene Relaxation techniques	
Education	Direct care	Assist individual in identifying learning style and utilize compensatory strategies to increase learning	Are General Educational Development (GED) classes available at the facility or does a referral need to be made? Does the individual need to further their academic education to reach a vocational goal, or could they do so through online courses or on-the-job-training? What learning styles best match an individual's functional cognition so they are successful?
	Indirect care (consultation or advocacy)	Make referral to appropriate GED courses/instruction Invite a community-based organization to provide in-hospital education sessions (e.g., math for budgeting)	
	Group	GED preparation Basic computer skills	
Work	Direct care	Provide skills training and education on building a resume and interviewing for a job	Is there a work program already offered at the facility? If not, is this something that can be started by an OTP? Are there community mental health center supported work programs the individuals can tour and/or apply to as part of discharge planning?
	Indirect care (consultation or advocacy)	Assist in the development of a vocational/work program Consult with a vocational rehabilitation agency for job-specific training.	
	Group	Job skills Volunteer opportunities to learn work skills Gardening group Library group	

TABLE 41-3 | **Common Intervention Approaches and Therapeutic Reasoning Prompts for Individuals in State Hospitals—cont'd**

Occupation	Service Delivery	Example Intervention	Therapeutic Reasoning Prompts
Play/Leisure	Direct care	Assist individual in modifying environment to increase participation in leisure activity	What leisure opportunities are available to the individual in the facility? What leisure opportunities are available in the community? What does the individual want to do?
	Indirect care (consultation or advocacy)	Provide recommendations to safety team about appropriate/safe leisure opportunities that are accessible to all	
	Group	Leisure education Indoor/outdoor recreation Gardening Knitting Craft	
Social participation	Direct care	Provide education to increase social skills related to social etiquette	What cultural barriers are not being addressed or limiting participation? Are certified interpreters available for small talk social interactions, leisure pursuits, and therapy groups?
	Indirect care (consultation or advocacy)	Provide educational training to staff on how to assist individuals with developmental disorders to appropriately engage in social activities	
	Group	Social skills	

the individual could continue to make the scrambled eggs safely and correctly. The individual might demonstrate the ability to start and end the task independently but require additional prompts in the middle of the task. Over time with continued repetitions of the same task, the prompts and cues should decrease as the individual demonstrates increased independence with completing this task correctly every time.

Many individuals who continue to present with negative symptoms, such as catatonic behavior, experience decreased verbalization. For these individuals, it is important to incorporate motor activities as a precursor to verbal activities. For example, during group introductions, the OTP might throw a ball to members of the group when it is their turn to introduce themselves. For those who are nonverbal, motor stimulation often provides an alerting response that can trigger the person to verbalize when they otherwise might not.

Sensory Approaches

"The experience of being human is imbedded in sensory events of everyday life" according to Dunn (2001, p. 608); as such, it is essential for OTPs to utilize their unique skill set to address not only the sensory needs of the individual, but the sensory environment that exists within the inpatient psychiatric setting. The Massachusetts Department of Mental Health, the NASMHPD, and The Joint Commission have all recognized the need for responsible and skilled use of sensory approaches, identifying OTPs as the professionals most qualified to provide consultation to create and carry out these services (AOTA, 2020).

The sensory environment in a clinic or treatment setting, such as that of the state inpatient psychiatric facility, can impact the mental health of the individuals being served in this setting (Bailliard, 2015). Therefore, as the OTP in this setting, there is an opportunity to create a positive sensory experience. Following the evaluation and assessment process, the OTP may start to work with an individual to develop an individualized sensory diet; make environmental modifications and recommendations; utilize a sensory room or develop one if there is not one currently; and

incorporate sensory modalities, such as weighted blankets, into treatment.

Additionally, OTPs may assist in creating positive sensory experiences in this setting through consultation with facility directors and managers, quality or risk management specialists, environmental services, security, and other important interested parties. For example, observing that the lights in the facility are bright and reflect off the even brighter white walls, an OTP could explain that this might be visually overstimulating or alerting to some individuals and that it can ultimately impact that individual's mood. They might also make recommendations for ways to modify the visual sensory environment by adding cloud covers over the ceiling lights or adding cool or warm color tones to the walls. Other options might include painting a mural of a mountain scape on a wall in the day room, securing a painting of a forest scene to a conference or waiting room wall, and using velcro or magnets to hang an image of flowers or a sunset on a bathroom door.

Another way the OTP can create positive sensory experiences is through individualized sensory interventions. Given the same scenario as previously noted, this may involve providing an individual with sunglasses or a ball cap to shade their eyes and/or spending time with this individual in a comfort room or sensory room with decreased visual stimuli.

Sensory approaches can also be utilized in a group setting as well. Knight and colleagues (2010) reported sensory intervention via a group setting can effectively assist in introducing the concept of sensory processing and help to explain tools and strategies that are useful for self-regulation for individuals with mental illness. An OTP may lead a sensory group where each group session addresses a different sensory system (e.g., auditory, visual, tactile) and allows exploration of sensory strategies or tools related to that sensory system. For example, one group session may focus on the olfactory system, or sense of smell, and OTPs might utilize various essential oils to educate on alerting versus calming scents (e.g., lemon vs. lavender). The end goal of a sensory

Evidence-Based Practice

Holistic, Person-Centered Interventions in State Hospitals

> *OTPs can facilitate interventions that improve and maintain occupational performance and participation in people with serious mental illness in the hospital setting.*

RESEARCH FINDINGS

Research suggests that providing holistic and person-centered programming can improve performance in social participation, ADLs, IADLs, rest and sleep, and leisure, whether provided individually or in the group setting (D'Amico et al., 2018). Occupational therapy interventions in mental health aim to enhance quality of life and resilience, reduce health disparities, teach risk reduction strategies, assist in the development of healthy habits and routines, teach coping strategies and relaxation techniques, engage in skill development, and provide adaptations to tasks and contexts (Reitz & Scaffa, 2020). Interventions commonly focus on health promotion through primary, secondary, and tertiary prevention means, which might include education on stress management strategies within the everyday routines for adults with mood disorders or training people with mental illness on independent living skills for community reintegration (Reitz & Scaffa, 2020). Evidence exists to support the use of cooking interventions in this setting to improve psychosocial outcomes and increase positive socialization when used in a group setting (Farmer et al., 2018).

APPLICATIONS

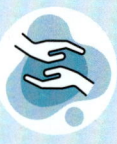

➡ OTPs can use their expertise to develop skills training groups, such as cooking groups or independent living skills groups, to help with community reintegration.

➡ OTPs can use their expertise of group facilitation to create and develop group protocols, lead groups within the treatment mall, and serve as role models and trainers for other staff in the program.

➡ Occupational therapists can use their expertise of functional assessment to accurately refer people to relevant groups and provide outcomes data regarding the effectiveness of interventions to meet treatment goals.

REFERENCES

D'Amico, M. L., Jaffe, L. E., & Gardner, J. A. (2018). Evidence for interventions to improve and maintain occupational performance and participation for people with serious mental illness: A systematic review. *American Journal of Occupational Therapy, 72*(5), 1–11. https://doi.org/10.5014/ajot.2018.033332

Farmer, N., Touchton-Leonard, K., & Ross, A. (2018). Psychosocial benefits of cooking interventions: A systematic review. *Health Education & Behavior, 45*(2), 167–180. https://doi.org/10.1177/1090198117736352

Reitz, S. M., & Scaffa, M. E. (2020). Occupational therapy in the promotion of health and well-being. *American Journal of Occupational Therapy, 74*(3), 7403420010p1–7403420010p14. https://doi.org/10.5014/ajot.2020.743003

group series might be for individuals to create sensory diets that work for them based on their unique sensory preferences that can be utilized as an effective strategy in the community setting as well.

Overall, sensory tools and interventions are used to assist individuals with the following: (a) understanding sensory processing, (b) identifying appropriate sensory tools and/or strategies, (c) utilizing sensory tools and/or strategies effectively, (d) identifying the regulation level of the body, (e) understanding and utilizing the sensory strategies to regulate the body appropriately, and (f) improving the ability to self-regulate overall (Champagne, 2011; Moore, 2016). Additionally, Scanlan and Novak (2015) reported that sensory approaches can be empowering, self-directed, and a less invasive way for OTPs to support an individual in their recovery. In the following Practitioner Profile, Sara Pickett, OTR/L, shares some of her insights about practice in a state hospital setting. See also Chapter 9: Sensory Processing and the Lived Sensory Experience, Chapter 12: Emotion Regulation, and Chapter 30: Natural Environments.

Practitioner Profile

Sara Pickett, OTR/L

Oregon State Hospital (OSH) is a state-run psychiatric hospital with locations in Salem and Junction City. The two campuses have a total of 728 beds across 30 units. The primary sources of funding come through the state budget and the Centers for Medicare & Medicaid Services. OSH serves adults ages 18 and older who are commonly diagnosed with schizophrenia, schizoaffective disorder, bipolar disorder, depression, anxiety disorders, neurocognitive disorder, or a personality disorder. Many individuals enter OSH with substance use issues and histories of unstable housing, which often further exacerbate symptoms and prolong acuity.

Individuals present with challenges in self-care, managing symptoms, social interactions, and life skills. Individuals are admitted through involuntary civil commitment, voluntary commitment by guardian, or involuntary forensic commitment, which is broken up into guilty except for insanity and "aid and assist," meaning an individual accused of a crime is ordered by a judge to receive treatment. An individual's length of stay can be anywhere from 30 days to many years.

Approximately 20 OTPs work across the OSH campuses. All are part of the treatment services department, and all collaborate in treatment teams with psychiatrists, psychologists, nurses, creative arts therapists, social workers, and other staff. Primary practice models used at OSH include PEO, MOHO, ACDM, and Dunn's Model of Sensory Processing. Most individuals receive occupational therapy in a group setting and are encouraged to attend groups daily in a treatment mall format based on their needs and interests.

Groups focus on emotional regulation, communication and social skills, legal understanding, mental wellness, life skills, addiction recovery, and health and wellness. Offered groups include tai chi, yoga, sensory connections, crafts, cooking, fitness, computer skills, gardening, healthy leisure, or newsletter groups. Some individuals gain privileges to go outside OSH and build community transition skills, first on the broader grounds of the hospital and

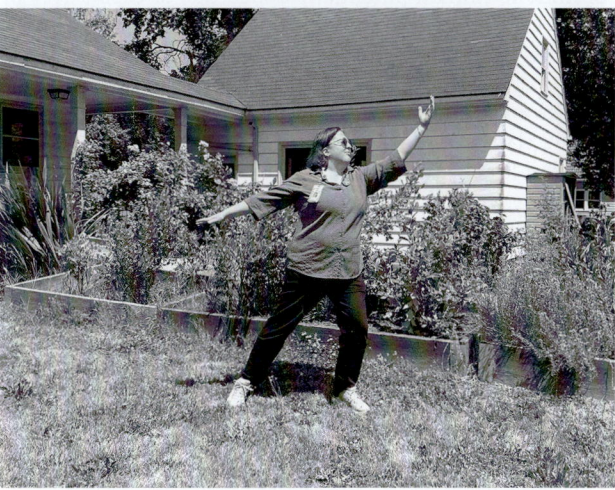

then further into the community to go shopping, get coffee, and visit museums, parks, or community placement sites.

Tai chi is a particularly effective intervention that not only improves balance and decreases fall risk, but also improves emotional regulation and symptom management. Individuals say they feel calmer and more centered after the groups. Some report decreased auditory hallucinations and improved focus for daily tasks.

I like working at OSH because occupational therapy is valued in this setting. We are known for our holistic approaches that address all aspects of an individual's life, including sexuality. Individual occupational therapy primarily focuses on sensory regulation and functioning, functional cognition, functional living skills, and addressing fall risk/physical rehabilitation needs. Common assessments include the Adolescent/Adult Sensory Profile, Allen Cognitive Level Screen, and Kohlman Evaluation of Living Skills. This setting is challenging but as a practitioner here I like it because it challenges me to be flexible, adapt quickly, and hone my skills at grading activities as acuity changes.

Additional Service Delivery Methods

Several types of modalities or interventions might lend themselves to an OTP developing or incorporating a theme for a variety of service delivery options, and collaborating with various members of the interdisciplinary treatment team, involving hospital management, and involving community-based partners as indicated. These could include:

- Highlighting the impact of occupational performance on transition to the community, including administering standardized assessments of occupational performance; assisting with the Supports Intensity Scale (SIS; Thompson et al., 2015); interviewing persons with mental illnesses and an intellectual/developmental disability (IDD) diagnosis; training with SNF staff on interacting with people with serious mental illness (SMI)

to promote person-centered care while maintaining a safe environment; and/or partnering with hospital social workers and community-based case managers for community reintegration sessions.

- Organizing an in-house prevocational program that includes hospital personnel serving as job coaches in areas of housekeeping, gardening, and landscaping; dining services; or making sellable items and working alongside volunteer auxiliary staff in the gift shop.

- Advocating for trauma-informed care through staff education, environmental modifications, or adaptations; actively involving the individual in their treatment process; and making appropriate referrals to additional services and resources as needed (Menschner & Maul, 2016).

Unique Considerations of Context

Because individuals in state psychiatric hospital settings can continue to remain potentially dangerous to themselves or others, OTPs must address certain contextual considerations when planning an intervention. Although this can be challenging at times, it also allows the OTP to be creative in their practice and provide interventions with limited resources at times. Let's look at safety concerns as they relate to the PEO Model of Practice.

P—Person

When providing any intervention, it is always essential to understand and know enough about the individual who will be receiving the intervention to remain safe. For example, an individual admitted to the state facility because of self-harming in the community by cutting their wrists is likely not going to be safe initially with use of sharp objects, such as scissors or forks. Upon admission, this individual may be directly supervised by a staff person but require finger foods and additional safety measures to ensure that they do not continue to engage in cutting or other self-harm behaviors. Another example might be an individual who is experiencing tremors or drooling as a side effect of their psychiatric medications. The OTP may need to provide compensatory interventions and/or adaptive equipment (AE) to assist with this new challenge the individual is experiencing.

E—Environment

Numerous environmental challenges or considerations exist in the state inpatient psychiatric setting. For example, some individuals are unable to leave their locked units without close supervision, if at all. Also, in areas such as the occupational therapy clinic, potentially dangerous materials such as scissors and kitchen knives must be carefully managed and accounted for before, during, and after an activity, and safely secured in a locked area. Finally, many items people take for granted, such as balloons, pipe cleaners, and aluminum foil, are identified as contraband in the hospital setting. Therefore, OTPs must carefully consider the materials and modalities used for intervention during the planning process. For example, an OTP leading a task group must ensure that all project ideas are free of contraband materials so that individuals will be allowed to keep their project once finished.

Additional environmental considerations include the need for ligature-resistant items, such as ligature-resistant doors and doorknobs, picture frames, handrails, and shower curtains, as these are important considerations for an individual who has been deemed to be at risk or is currently suicidal. Other items that may be considered a ligature risk include belts, shoelaces, straps, necklaces, ropes, string, and corded earbuds. From a fire safety standpoint, papers or drawings are not to be taped to walls or doors and items cannot be hanging from the ceilings. This can have a visual impact on the individuals in this setting as it creates an institutional appearance that is not warm or welcoming.

As the OTP in this setting, there may be an opportunity to advocate and provide consultation for environmental changes that are needed to help individuals with regulation, coping, rest and sleep, and so on. This may include something as simple as a painted area on the wall of their bedroom on which they can tape their drawings. It is common for state hospitals to have various "privilege" levels based on clinical status that allow individuals to access less supervised spaces and additional resources within or outside the facility based on their clinical status. The OTP must also check individuals' clinical statuses, indicating their level of safe behavior, before taking them off the unit for a group or individual intervention sessions held in the clinic or elsewhere on the hospital grounds such as the rec room or treatment mall.

O—Occupation

When an individual is admitted into the state hospital system, many of their occupations are left behind in the community setting and they may be unable to engage in them while hospitalized. For example, individuals are typically not able to keep shoelaces in their shoes and may walk around in shoes that are not secured properly, increasing their risk of falling. There is often a set list of preapproved hygiene items, and an individual's preferred hygiene products might not be on the list, ultimately impacting their desire or motivation to complete their personal hygiene. Additionally, while hospitalized, an individual who engages in paid employment, is a parent, or has a pet to care for is unable to engage in those roles while in the state facility, which could impact their overall recovery.

However, there are occupations that an individual can continue to engage in or can do in a modified or slightly different way. For example, an individual may choose to attend advocacy council meetings and represent their unit of individuals to request positive changes for the hospital. In this role, an individual may develop leadership skills, public speaking skills, and communication skills. An individual may invite their family members to visit while they are hospitalized, either virtually or in person. For someone in school at the time of hospitalization, classes may continue to be taken virtually through a media center or computer laboratory area. Additionally, an individual with community level privileges may be working or volunteering in the community but continue to live at the hospital until they are able to transition fully back into the community.

Because context is an important aspect of meaningful occupation, OTPs try to provide intervention in the most natural context possible. However, OTPs are often limited in where interventions can take place because of safety restrictions or limited ability to go into the community. For example, the most effective context in which to teach money-handling skills would be in a setting such as a grocery store. However, for an individual who is unable to leave the hospital building, the OTP might start by challenging the individual to figure out the correct change needed to purchase a snack from the lobby vending machine instead.

The OTP may work with individuals on various IADL skills to include laundry, meal preparation, and budgeting, and they may be able to utilize the laundry machines on the unit or a kitchen that is available to individuals in a supervised space. The OTP and individuals might also work on budgeting money to spend in the canteen for the week or month ahead. This setting challenges the OTP to be creative at times to assist individuals in further developing their meaningful occupations.

Technology

Technology is constantly advancing and is potentially a resource for OTPs to utilize in an environment with increased restrictions and limitations. However, access to technology for individuals may be minimal because of limited resources or safety and security concerns. It is important to recognize the individual's experiences with technology may vary. For individuals with limited experience, graded intervention on the use of items such as computers, cell phones, tablets, or microwaves is generally required before the occupation can be independently performed.

Computers can be utilized to provide individuals with a way to plan their transition to the community around work and leisure, as well as education on how to research community resources, create resumes, search for jobs, and even apply for jobs online. They can also be used as a teaching tool for individuals with limited computer skills or poor access to technology in the community setting. The OTP may also utilize handheld devices, such as a basic MP3 player or Bluetooth headphones that do not have batteries or cords, as a coping mechanism for individuals to listen to music or relaxing sounds. During the COVID-19 pandemic, facilities were required to discontinue live or in-person visits, which further isolated individuals from their family, friends, and community resources. Technology was heavily utilized during this time to bridge the gap by providing virtual visits through Zoom, Google Meets, and other virtual platforms that were approved for use at the facility. See Chapter 33: Virtual Environments. 🤝

Group Intervention

Group intervention continues to be the most common intervention technique used in state hospital systems. Logistically, group intervention offers efficient services in a setting where staffing is quite often limited. Groups are less expensive to provide, allow OTPs to see more people at one time, and deliver services to a larger population than individual interventions. Group treatment sessions also provide opportunities for peer collaboration, teaching-learning, and support.

With group intervention, the focus is often around screening, health promotion, and prevention. Group interventions may include various topics; for example, educational services such as training people to use the internet in a computer skills group, self-management training to learn new coping skills in a group setting or anger management techniques, and providing education about environmental modifications to make in the day room and people's bedrooms to prevent trips, slips, and falls (AOTA, 2020). It is important to structure groups based on the interests, abilities, strengths, and challenges of the individuals in the group.

Group sessions can provide social benefits to individuals who often have very limited social networks. Those with disorganized thoughts may be so focused internally that they are unaware of the people around them, making it difficult to form social relationships. Group intervention encourages individuals to talk with each other, cooperate, and help one another, thus offering opportunities for social participation and feedback. In addition, offering a variety of intervention groups throughout the day provides a structured routine for individuals, and these balanced routines can be a healthy and organizing part of daily life.

Group intervention is a hallmark of service delivery in state hospitals. It continues to be an effective and efficient way to meet the needs of many individuals receiving services. Practitioners in this setting must have a strong skill set for planning and leading occupation-centered group interventions and be able to readily adapt groups to a diverse population of individuals who may attend the group (Fisher & Marterella, 2019).

Treatment Mall Approach

A *treatment mall approach* is a decentralized programming area, meaning that individuals come from different areas (e.g., units, wards) of a hospital to attend the psychosocial programming offered. It is typically structured around an educational or classroom model with a large selection of courses available to individuals. The treatment mall supports many recovery practices, such as occupational engagement, socialization, skill learning, sense of choice, sense of wellness, and change in environment (Estrella et al., 2019). The physical layout of a treatment mall may vary from one hospital to the next; however, the concept of utilizing treatment malls to provide therapeutic, evidence-based, and person-centered group programming remains the same.

The treatment mall approach was designed as an alternative to unit-based or ward-based programming. Previous research showed that a highly structured, locked unit or ward tended to increase individuals' dependence on staff, isolation from the community, and general boredom (Bartholomew & Cook, 2013; McLoughlin et al., 2010). Treatment malls offer an alternative environment for individuals in much the same way that work, school, or volunteering does for members of the general community. The mall is typically held in an easily accessible, locked building or location separate from the unit on which individuals live.

Programs offered by treatment malls vary by hospital, but they are typically based on an academic or psychoeducational model in which individuals participate in groups or courses designed to assist them in improving life skills (Ballard, 2008). A wide variety of multidisciplinary groups are offered, and individuals are encouraged to take an active role in creating their own treatment schedule to address their personal goals (Matthews et al., 2015). In addition to activity rooms and classrooms, treatment malls may offer resources such as a fitness center, gymnasium, boutique or gift shop, hair salon, library, media center, and kitchen. Such resources not only allow for a change of context from the unit but also for broader social opportunities, as individuals from several different units may attend the same treatment mall program. Box 41-1 provides a snapshot of a day in the life of one OTP working in a state psychiatric hospital, and this chapter's The Lived Experience feature shares the perspectives of Sean, who shares his state hospital experiences in occupational therapy.

BOX 41-1 ■ A Day in the Life—State Hospital

Contributed by Jonathan Isco, OTR/L

I am an occupational therapist working at a state psychiatric hospital. In my setting, most individuals discharge within a year, although a small percentage may stay for many years. I provide occupational therapy as part of the treatment services department and collaborate as a member of an interdisciplinary treatment team that includes psychiatry, nursing, social work, clinical psychology, and other professionals. We all engage in weekly leadership meetings where we discuss and problem-solve some of the most complex challenges that affect individuals. The hospital I work at uses a treatment mall approach that is sometimes described as a "college for mental health." A variety of different treatment groups are provided in this format and individuals choose the groups they prefer to participate in. There are many choices including addiction recovery, community transition, emotional wellness, health and wellness, communication and social skills, mental wellness, and legal understanding groups. Here is a snapshot of one day in my practice.

7:30 a.m.—*Sensory Garden.* I come in early to water the garden for an early individual session. Gardening is an effective intervention used to increase access to nature and to support an individual's sensory diet, habit/routine building, and healthy leisure exploration. It is a peaceful start to the day.

8:00—*Orienting to the Day.* This is the time to check in with fellow clinicians and read the unit nursing reports. Team members are scurrying, making coffee/tea, yawning, and scrambling.

8:15—*Treatment Mall Huddles.* I gather with other staff who provide services on the treatment mall. We review unit nursing reports, group schedules, staffing, and any issues needing problem-solving.

8:45—*Group Set-Up or Leadership Meetings.* Leadership meetings review all individuals on a unit and their treatment progress, and problem-solve unit concerns.

9:00—*Sensory Connections Group.* I lead a sensory-focused group to support individuals' emotional regulation. The group focuses on grounding strategies and provides individuals an opportunity to explore their sensory preferences.

10:00—*Cooking Group.* This is one type of life skills group in our mall. It is often a favorite among the participants because it supports their ability to perform ADLs and IADLs. Other life skills groups focus on gardening, money management, grooming/hygiene, and community integration skills.

11:00—*Documentation Attempt #1.* This is the time to process and document the events that happened during groups earlier in the morning. Usually a time to collect myself, then . . .

CODE GREEN! CODE GREEN!

Oh darn, a code green!! A code green is a common emergency code that is called out throughout the campus during a behavioral incident. Staff may hear this throughout the day at the state hospital. We all start running toward the unit and notice other staff scurrying from other directions. A common sight once staff enter the unit is to see an individual being manually restrained or on a stretcher with restraints and being wheeled into the seclusion room.

During a code it is every staff's job to "stay cool" and to help manage the milieu. There are frequently many individuals present during the incident. Some look at the code incident like a spectacle, whereas others are visibly upset because they were either directly involved in the incident or witnessed what happened. Every staff's responsibility is to provide support, redirection, and consolation when appropriate. Afterward, we all debrief in the nursing hub, discuss what happened, and engage in problem-solving.

12:30—*Lunch.*

12:45—*CODE GREEN! CODE GREEN!* It's the same drill: Staff will leave their lunch and start running over to the unit. Right before staff enter the unit, they observe other staff leaving and saying, "false alarm."

1:00—*Individual Sessions.* For the next 2 to 3 hours, I have individual sessions. I might be responding to an evaluation referral I received or provide individual interventions. I could be addressing sensory regulation, functional cognition, or fall risk/physical rehabilitation needs; exploring meaningful engagement within the hospital; or evaluating the level of assistance an individual requires for participating in ADLs/IADLs to support safe discharge planning. I like the variety.

3:00—*Meetings and Documentation Attempt #2.* Afternoon meetings are usually scheduled during this time, whether they are treatment mall huddles or department meetings. This is also a time to debrief and process with colleagues to solve challenges with certain individuals or address any issues that came up during the day. This is also the second attempt to document and cross fingers that there will not be another code green.

Although the concept of a treatment mall and the evidence behind the use of it is promising, there are many factors that impact a facility's ability to truly implement treatment mall programming the way that it was originally intended. Because of this, many facilities utilize a modified approach to offering treatment programming based on the physical infrastructure of the facility and staffing limitations. For example, many state hospital buildings were built before the research of treatment mall approaches and do not have this designated, separate treatment space built in. Over time, some facilities have adjusted or made small changes to the building, when possible, to create "off-unit" or "off-ward" treatment areas.

In addition to infrastructure limitations, staffing limitations impact the ability for a facility to fully operate their treatment areas. Staffing limitations have resulted, in part, because consequences of the COVID-19 pandemic have impacted coverage across all disciplines within this setting. These personnel limitations might impact the number of groups or treatment offered, the type of treatment offered, and the ability to escort and supervise individuals in these off-unit treatment areas.

The OTPs providing interventions in off-unit settings, such as the treatment mall approach or a modified version, frequently cofacilitate groups with other disciplines such as nursing, social work, psychology, music therapy, art therapy, and therapeutic recreation. This cooperation strengthens the occupational therapy intervention by providing a wider scope of expertise and resources to support individuals' engagement more fully in occupation. OTPs working within this approach may also be called upon to help manage and assess treatment mall programming and develop new groups or courses to meet the needs of the individuals receiving services more fully.

The Lived Experience

Sean

Sean is a 38-year-old single African American male who currently resides in a state psychiatric hospital in the recovery program. Sean attends the treatment mall program 4 days per week and is involved in a variety of multidisciplinary groups at the treatment mall. His occupational therapy groups have included independent living skills, consumer skills, Spanish, creative stress relief, explore your world, and cooking group. One day per week Sean works with occupational therapy and vocational adjustment services in the Spring Rock Café as the grill cook. The following interview with Sean took place in a quiet conference room and gym area at the treatment mall. The purpose of the interview was explained to Sean before the meeting took place, and he agreed to participate. Some dialogue has been left out for brevity.

Occupational therapist: Sean, I thought first we could talk about your hospitalizations. I was wondering if you could tell me how many times you have been hospitalized?

Sean: I've been in and out probably five or six times. As I get older, each time it seems like I'm in shorter before I leave again.

Occupational therapist: How old were you when you were first hospitalized?

Sean: Twenty-three.

Occupational therapist: Is Springfield the only state hospital you've ever been in?

Sean: Yep. I've been to hospitals in Baltimore before coming here but only for a day or two. I like coming here to the same place when I need to, to people I know and who know me.

Occupational therapist: Do you think you have benefited from your time in the hospital?

Sean: Each time I come in I learn new skills, so yeah. It gives me time to think and to reflect too.

Occupational therapist: Can you tell me a little about your hobbies and interests?

Sean: I like to be independent. To just do my own thing—listen to music, smoke a cigarette, go for a walk, or work.

Occupational therapist: Sean, can you tell me about your experiences with the rehabilitation department and occupational therapy? Any favorite things that stick out in your mind that you've learned?

Sean: I loved when I was in Gateway [Assisted Living Program held at Springfield Hospital Center] before it was closed. I went out in the community every week with the occupational therapist, and she really taught us how to get around, budget our money, get the best deal—she kept it real. I also love cooking group. It's not just about learning the skills to shop or cook—it's about the being together and doing it as group too . . . the togetherness and conversation.

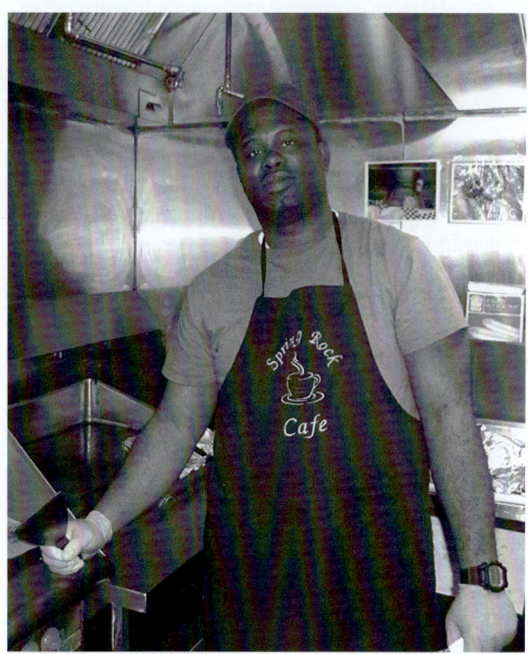

Occupational therapist: Do you think your groups and experiences with rehabilitation improve your quality of life while you are at the hospital?

Sean: Oh yeah. That's why when I know I need to come back to the hospital I know you have my back.

Occupational therapist: What kind of work have you done in the past?

Sean: McDonald's, Popeyes, grocery store.

Occupational therapist: You work at Spring Rock Café as the grill cook. Do you like your job now?

Sean: I love it! Sometimes I sit back and look at all the people when it's a slow time on the grill and for just a short period of time a good feeling comes over me just watching everyone enjoying themselves.

Occupational therapist: How did you get the job?

Sean: It was the occupational therapist. She recommended me, told me that they needed me to be there working and knew I could do it. She had faith in me and had worked with me in cooking group . . . this time and before [previous admissions].

Occupational therapist: Do you plan to work when you are discharged to the community?

Sean: Of course! It keeps me busy and helps me save money. I'm from Jamaica and sometime in the next 20 years I want to be able to go back there to visit. I want to have learned a skill by then and have enough money so I can stay for a nice visit.

Occupational therapist: What about housing, Sean? Where would you like to live?

Continued

The Lived Experience—cont'd

Sean: I have a conditional release that says I must live in a RRP [Residential Rehabilitation Program]. I've done that before and I'm just waiting on a bed to open, but it's so far away from my family I don't know if I want to go.

Occupational therapist: I have one last question for you. If you could give advice to anyone who is studying and learning to become an occupational therapist, what would you tell them to help work with you better?

Sean: When I first come in the hospital, I know everyone needs to meet with me and do their assessments and ask their questions but treat me like I'm a person and not a number. I know I'm a patient and that I'm sick—I have paranoid schizophrenia. Take the time to look at your papers and know what you want to know from me and talk to me like I matter, like I'm more than just the questions on your paper.

Here's the Point

- State hospitals have continuously changed over the last 70 years, which is reflected in staffing, access, and funding directed to mental health care for persons who rely on public assistance for their health-care and community living needs. These factors have impacted the current number of state-run hospitals, bed capacity, and duration of hospitalization, as well as led to an increase in consumers who enter mental health treatment through the legal system.
- People hospitalized in state facilities are often more psychiatrically ill, have co-occurring conditions that add to the complexity of their treatment and disposition planning needs, and tend to face inequities in access to resources because of a variety of social determinants of health.
- The Recovery Model, strengths-based occupational therapy models of practice, and trauma-informed care approaches are foundational guides for providing occupational therapy care in these settings. These frameworks all emphasize providing individuals with voice and choice in achieving self-identified goals, as well as person-centered supports that empower individuals to make their own decisions.
- As a member of the interdisciplinary treatment team, OTPs promote holistic care, skill building, environmental adaptation, and a focus on quality of life.

- Occupational therapy's focus on occupation, functional cognition, sensory processing preferences and teaching of sensory regulation strategies, and emphasis on personal agency adds a distinct and valuable perspective in state hospital teams.
- Successful interventions rely on creativity and positivity, collaborative interactions with the person and their support system, and therapeutic use of self to adhere to inherent challenges based on context and safety.
- OTPs working in state psychiatric hospital settings often find job satisfaction when they balance delivery of quality care with engagement in opportunities such as effectively using crisis prevention techniques, developing decentralized and transitional programs (e.g., modified treatment mall approaches, community reintegration sessions), being a fieldwork educator or capstone mentor, and serving in leadership or member roles in hospitalwide committees.

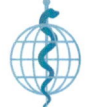 Visit the online resource center at **FADavis.com** to access the videos.

Apply It Now

1. Limited Freedoms and Choices

Try to imagine being admitted to a state psychiatric hospital. Similar to Sean in this chapter's The Lived Experience feature, you just "want to do your own thing." You would prefer to eat now but are told that meals are served only at certain times, and there is no food available right now. You decide you would enjoy some time to lie down alone, so you go into your bedroom. However, you now share a room with two other people, and they are talking, so you cannot lie down and rest as you would prefer to do. You really need a cigarette because you are a smoker, but there is no smoking allowed. A shower might feel good, but you realize the showers are being cleaned, and you will not be able to take one any time soon. You want to watch television, but the group decides together what to watch and you are not very

interested in the show they have chosen. How do you feel right now? Reflect on how living with these limited freedoms and choices would make you feel, using the following guiding questions.

Reflective Questions
- If you were working on such a unit, what could you do to give Sean greater freedom and more choices?
- As an OTP, how could you assist Sean in a situation such as this? How could you collaborate with the other staff working on the unit?
- How can the treatment team ensure safety and set appropriate limits yet still allow individuals as many choices and freedoms as possible?
- What do you think may happen to Sean's ability to problem-solve and make choices if he lives with limited

opportunities to do so for a long period of time? How do you think this would affect Sean's self-esteem?

■ What activities might an OTP do with Sean to give him opportunities to problem-solve and make choices so he may improve upon these skills?

2. Evaluation/Assessment

Consider the value that the administration processes and outcomes of standardized assessments offer to occupational therapy intervention planning and implementation, and for holistic multidisciplinary treatment and discharge planning. At the time of the interview, Sean indicated that his group treatment involvement and one-day-a-week work schedule supported his values of working, learning skills, experiencing togetherness, engaging in conversation (with peers, work colleagues), saving money, and envisioning a nice visit in Jamaica. The intention is to discharge Sean to community living in a residential rehabilitation program (RRP) and he is "waiting for a bed to open up."

As a new OTP assigned to Sean's treatment team, you receive an "occupational therapy eval and treat" order to focus on readiness for discharge. What factors might you consider, and which assessment tools might provide information that will assist with the transition from being an inpatient in a state hospital to living in the community? Consider using a PEO-P model and clinical reasoning to guide your thinking to determine which assessments might combine to give you data on which to base your recommendations.

Reflective Questions
■ What do you want to know about Sean that will help determine his abilities and needs to continue engaging in life aspects he values (e.g., semistructured interview with MOHO tool, ACDM for functional cognition)?

■ The interview was conducted in a quiet conference room. What might that tell you? What do you want to know about his grill cook job and work environment? How will you find out about the work environments, and task expectations, of jobs available to people in the RRP? Anticipate realistic suggestions you could make for environmental modifications (e.g., SPM, task, and occupation analyses; home assessment; AMPS; ILS, PASS, and ACQ-OP).

■ Sean is likely independent with his self-care ADLs within the structure of the state hospital setting. What IADLs will he be responsible for when he lives in the RRP community setting? Based on what you know about Sean (e.g., functional cognition, values, occupational performance quality), what assessment tools might guide occupational therapy treatment for transitioning current skills, modifying the environment, providing caregiver education, and/or teaching him new skills (e.g., ACDM, ACQ-SI, ESI, ILS, PASS)?

■ Sean will be living with different people than he has been accustomed to, in a setting with different house rules, and in a different neighborhood. How might you best support this change in Sean's social environment and opportunities (e.g., ESI and ACQ-SI, Social Profile, "community assessment")?

3. Shopping on a Budget

Sean went out in the community every week when he was in the assisted living program. Budgeting was an important skill to learn. Your assignment is to go shopping for items needed to make chili for a group of five people. Consider all expenses from the time you leave your home to meal completion. You have $35.00 to spend.

Reflective Questions
■ What skills were required to plan the shopping trip? To use transportation? To find the ingredients? To pay for the ingredients? Did you feel competent in these skills?

■ Did you ask others for any kind of assistance? If so, were the individuals helpful?

■ What challenges did you experience during this shopping trip?

■ What feelings did you experience during the shopping trip?

■ What other challenges would an individual with severe mental illness who has not lived in the community for 10 years have faced?

4. Motivation

Sean described his hesitancy to relocate far from his family following discharge.

Many states have few state hospitals, making it difficult for family and friend visitation during long hospitalizations because of location. Also, limited community resources can provide a challenge in availability for discharge options.

Reflective Questions
■ What are the benefits of maintaining a support system? Who is your support system?

■ As an OTP, what resources can you help Sean explore as he transitions to a new community so that he maintains motivation to continue in his recovery process?

■ How can you help prepare Sean to maintain contact with his family that is too far away to visit?

5. Video Exercise: Cooking Group in a State Mental Hospital

Pair up with another student in your class or form a small group of students. Access and watch the "Cooking Group in a State Mental Hospital" video at the online resource center at FADavis.com. Then, discuss and together answer the following questions.

Reflective Questions
■ How does Samuel use the cooking group intervention to assess the group members' occupational performance? How does he assess their physical health in the group? Why would an OTP in a state mental hospital be concerned about the physical health of the residents?

■ Why do you think the cooking group is particularly meaningful to the residents in this state hospital? In what other settings might a group such as this be possible and effective?

■ How is the cooking group effective in building community as well as developing functional skills? Why do you think Samuel asks each person to identify something for which they are grateful?

■ Samuel mentions the "countless gaps in the systems in which these incredible souls fell through." What specific gaps do you think he is referring to? Why is it so important for OTPs to be aware of such gaps?

Resources

Movies/Books

- *A Beautiful Mind* by Sylvia Nasar (book and movie): https://en.wikipedia.org/wiki/A_Beautiful_Mind_(book)
- *An American's Resurrection, My Pilgrimage From Child Abuse and Mental Illness to Salvation* by Eric C. Arauz (book): https://www.amazon.com/Americans-Resurrection-Pilgrimage-Illness-Salvation-ebook/dp/B00AUA9R9K?ref_=ast_author_mpb
- *Brain on Fire, My Month of Madness* by Susannah Cahalan (book): https://www.amazon.com/Brain-Fire-My-Month-Madness/dp/1451621388
- *An Unquiet Mind, A Memoir of Moods and Madness* by Kay Redfield Jamison (book): https://www.amazon.com/Unquiet-Mind-Memoir-Moods-Madness/dp/0679763309
- *Awakenings* by Oliver Sacks (book and movie): https://en.wikipedia.org/wiki/Awakenings
- *Girl, Interrupted* by Susanna Kaysen (book and movie): https://en.wikipedia.org/wiki/Girl,_Interrupted_(film)
- Minds on the Edge: http://mindsontheedge.fredfriendly.org [Fred Friendly Seminar for PBS, 2009]
- *Ordinary People* by Judith Guest (book and movie): https://en.wikipedia.org/wiki/Ordinary_People
- *Sometimes Amazing Things Happen* by Elizabeth Ford (book): https://www.amazon.com/Sometimes-Amazing-Things-Happen-Psychiatric/dp/1941393438
- *The Center Cannot Hold, My Journey Through Madness* by Elyn R. Saks (book): https://www.amazon.com/Center-Cannot-Hold-Journey-Through/dp/1401309445

Videos

- "Student Panel Discusses Running Groups in Mental Health Settings" video. In this video, occupational therapy students discuss their first experience running groups for a 6-week period in a psychiatric day program. The students describe first being intimidated, but then feeling welcomed and surprised by how enjoyable and productive the groups were. They emphasize the team approach and the utility of the groups in developing their leadership skills. Access the video at the online resource center at FADavis.com.
- "Sensory Garden in Geriatric Psychiatric Unit" video. In this video, occupational therapist Callie Ward showcases the sensory garden at an inpatient psychiatric facility. The multisensory garden was designed for occupational therapy groups with a goal of helping participants identify the effects the garden and its related tasks have on their level of arousal. Callie offers specific examples of the many positive effects of the garden on residents, such as collaborating on tasks, problem-solving, encouraging routines, working on cognition, and assisting with self-regulation, among others. She explains how she uses it for active and passive group interventions and in one-to-one sessions. Access the video at the online resource center at FADavis.com.

Websites

- Every Moment Counts: https://everymomentcounts.org
- It's Never 2 Late: Dignity Through Technology system: https://in2l.com
- Man Therapy: https://mantherapy.org
- Minds on the Edge: http://mindsontheedge.fredfriendly.org
- National Association of State Mental Health Program Directors Publications: https://www.nasmhpd.org/content/publications
- Occupational Therapy Toolkit: https://www.ottoolkit.com/links
- OT-Innovations: https://www.ot-innovations.com
- The Community Guide: https://www.thecommunityguide.org Search for the Community Tool Box: https://ctb.ku.edu/en (The Community Tool Box is a service of the Center for Community Health and Development at the University of Kansas.)
- The Struggle of Mental Health, TED Playlist: https://www.ted.com/playlists/175/the_struggle_of_mental_health

Podcasts

- Blog Talk Radio: https://www.blogtalkradio.com/aotainc/2021/05/10/everyday-evidence-serious-mental-illness-with-dr-liz-griffin-lannigan
- Hidden Brain: https://hiddenbrain.org
- Occupied: https://occupiedpodcast.com
- OT & Chill: https://radiopublic.com/ot-chill-6BJxoR/episodes (or any platform where people get their podcasts, such as Apple or Spotify)

Resource List for National Association of State Mental Health Program Directors (NASMHPD: see https://nasmhpd.org/content/publications)

- Lutterman, T. (2022). *Trends in psychiatric inpatient capacity, United States and each state, 1970 to 2018.* Technical Assistance Collaborative Paper No. 2. National Association of State Mental Health Program Directors. https://www.nasmhpd.org/sites/default/files/2023-01/Trends-in-Psychiatric-Inpatient-Capacity_United-States%20_1970-2018_NASMHPD-2.pdf
- Menschner, C., & Maul, A. (2016). *Key ingredients for successful trauma-informed care implementation.* Substance Abuse and Mental Health Services Administration. https://www.samhsa.gov/sites/default/files/programs_campaigns/childrens_mental_health/atc-whitepaper-040616.pdf
- National Alliance on Mental Illness. (2023). *Mental health by the numbers.* https://www.nami.org/about-mental-illness/mental-health-by-the-numbers
- National Association of State Mental Health Program Directors. (2022). *From crisis to care: Building from 988 and beyond for better mental health outcomes.* https://www.nasmhpd.org/sites/default/files/2023-01/NASMHPD-2022-Compendium-508-V2.pdf

References

Allen, C. K., Earhart, C., & Blue, T. (1992). *Occupational therapy treatment goals for the physically and cognitively disabled.* American Occupational Therapy Association.

American Occupational Therapy Association. (2020). Occupational therapy practice framework: Domain and process—Fourth edition. *American Journal of Occupational Therapy, 74*(Suppl. 2), 7412410010p1–7412410010p87. https://doi.org/10.5014/ajot.2020.74S2001

Avila, R. (2017). Dix, Dorothea (1802–1887). In P. A. Lamphier & R. Welch (Eds.), *Women in American history: A social, political, and cultural encyclopedia and document collection* (Vol. 2, pp. 43–44). ABC-CLIO.

Bailliard, A. L. (2015). Habits of the sensory system and mental health: Understanding sensory dissonance. *The American Journal of Occupational Therapy, 69*(4), 1–8. https://doi.org/10.5014/ajot.2015.014977

Ballard, F. A. (2008). Benefits of psychosocial rehabilitation programming in a treatment mall. *Journal of Psychosocial Nursing, 46*(2), 26–32. https://doi.org/10.3928/02793695-20080201-01

Bartholomew, T., & Cook, R. (2013). Toward a fidelity scale of inpatient treatment malls. *American Journal of Psychiatric Rehabilitation, 16*(3), 179–198. https://doi.org/10.1080/15487768.2013.813872

Baum, C. M., Christiansen, C. H., & Bass, J. D. (2015). The Person-Environment-Occupation-Performance (PEOP) model. In C. H. Christiansen, C. M. Baum, & J. D. Bass (Eds.),

Occupational therapy: Performance, participation, and well-being (4th ed., pp. 49–56). Slack.

Baum, C. M., Morrison, T., Hahn, M., & Edwards, D. F. (2003). *Executive Function Performance Test (EPFT)*. Washington University Medical School.

Benjamin, L. T., Jr., & Baker, D. B. (2004). *From seance to science: A history of the profession of psychology in America*. Wadsworth /Thomson.

Brown, C., & Dunn, W. (2002). *Adolescent–Adult Sensory Profile: User's manual*. Therapy Skill Builders: Psychological Corp.

Burns, T. (2018). *Cognitive Performance Test (CPT), revised manual*. Maddak SP Ableware.

Champagne, T. (2011). The influence of posttraumatic stress disorder, depression, and sensory processing patterns on occupational engagement: A case study. *Work, 38,* 67–75. https://doi .org/10.3233/WOR-2011-1105

D'Amico, M. L., Jaffe, L. E., & Gardner, J. A. (2018). Evidence for interventions to improve and maintain occupational performance and participation for people with serious mental illness: A systematic review. *American Journal of Occupational Therapy, 72*(5), 1–11. https://doi.org/10.5014/ajot.2018.033332

Donohue, M. (2013). *Social profile: Assessment of social participation in children, adolescents, and adults*. AOTA Press.

Dunn, W. (2001). The sensations of everyday life: Empirical, theoretical, and pragmatic considerations. *American Journal of Occupational Therapy, 55*(6), 608–620. https://doi.org/10.5014 /ajot.55.6.608

Dunn, W., Brown, C., & McGuigan, A. (1994). The ecology of human performance: A framework for considering the effect of context. *American Journal of Occupational Therapy, 48*(7), 595–607. https://doi.org/10.5014/ajot.48.7.595

Earhart, C. A. (2006). *Allen Diagnostic Module: Manual* (2nd ed.). S&S Worldwide. https://www.allen-cognitive-network.org/index .php/allen-model/assessments/76-allen-diagnostic-modeul -second-edition-adm-2

Earhart, C. A., McCraith, D. B., & Riska-Williams, L. (2022). *Manual for Version 5 of the Allen Cognitive Level Screen* (2nd ed.). ACLS and LACLS Committee.

Estrella, M. J. E., Vatsya, M., Tsuda, M., & Roby, R. C. L. (2019). Exploring the experiences of individuals with serious mental illness in a modified treatment mall: Centralized off-unit programing with extended hours, a mixed methods study. *Occupational Therapy in Mental Health, 35*(4), 361–385. https://doi.org/10.1080/01 64212X.2019.1648226

Farmer, N., Touchton-Leonard, K., & Ross, A. (2018). Psychosocial benefits of cooking interventions: A systematic review. *Health Education & Behavior, 45*(2), 167–180. https://doi .org/10.1177/1090198117736352

Fisher, A. G., & Jones, K. B. (2014). *Assessment of motor and process skills. User manual* (Vol. 2, 8th ed.). Three Star Press.

Fisher, A. G., & Griswold, L. A. (2018). *Evaluation of social interaction* (4th ed.). Three Star Press.

Fisher, A. G., & Marterella, A. (2019). *Powerful practice: A model for authentic occupational therapy*. Center for Innovative OT Solutions.

Fisher, W. H., Geller, J., & Pandianini, J. A. (2009). The changing role of the state psychiatric hospital. *Health Affairs, 28,* 676–685. https://doi.org/10.1377/hlthaff.28.3.676

Geller, J. (2020, September 9). Structural racism in American psychiatry and APA: Part 6. *Psychiatric News, 55*(18), 2. https://doi .org/10.1176/appi.pn.2020.9b17

Knight, M., Adkison, L., & Kovach, J. S. (2010). A comparison of multisensory and traditional interventions on inpatient psychiatry and geriatric neuropsychiatry units. *Journal of Psychosocial Nursing, 48*(1), 24–31. https://doi.org/10.3928/02793695-20091204-03

Law, M., Cooper, B., Strong, S., Stewart, D., Rigby, P., & Letts, L. (1996). Person–Environment–Occupation Model: A transactive

approach to occupational performance. *Canadian Journal of Occupational Therapy, 63,* 9–23. https://doi.org/10.1177 /000841749606300103

Loeb, P. A. (1996). *Independent Living Scales (ILS) manual*. Psychological Corp.

Lutterman, T. (2022). *Trends in psychiatric inpatient capacity, United States and each state, 1970 to 2018*. National Association of State Mental Health Program Directors. https://www.nasmhpd.org /sites/default/files/2023-01/Trends-in-Psychiatric-Inpatient -Capacity_United-States%20_1970-2018_NASMHPD-2.pdf

Manderscheid, R., Atay, J., & Crider, R. (2009). Changing trends in state psychiatric hospital use from 2002 to 2005. *Psychiatric Services, 60*(1), 29–34. https://doi.org/10.1176/ps.2009.60.1.29

Matthews, A., Beecher, B., Hofer, P. J., & Short, R. (2015). An exploratory evaluation of a treatment mall at a state psychiatric hospital. *American Journal of Health Sciences, 6*(1), 83–90. https://doi .org/10.19030/ajhs.v6i1.9272

McLoughlin, K. A., Webb, T., Myers, M., Skinner, K., & Adams, C. H. (2010). Developing a psychosocial rehabilitation treatment mall: An implementation model for mental health nurses. *Archives of Psychiatric Nursing, 24*(5), 330–338. https://doi.org/10.1016 /j.apnu.2009.12.001

Moore, K. (2005). *Sensory defensiveness screening for adults*. https://www.sensoryconnectionprogram.com/pdf/sensory _defensiveness_assessment_tools_moore.pdf

Moore, K. (2016). *Following the evidence: Sensory approaches in mental health*. http://www.sensoryconnectionprogram.com /sensory_treatment.php

National Association of State Mental Health Program Directors Research Institute. (2013). *Characteristics of state operated or supported psychiatric hospital inpatient care: A topical public report*. Author. https://nri-inc.org/our-work/nri-reports/characteristics -of-state-operated-or-supported-psychiatric-hospital-inpatient -care

National Association of State Mental Health Program Directors. (2014). *The vital role of state psychiatric hospitals*. Author. https:// www.nasmhpd.org/sites/default/files/The%20Vital%20Role%20 of%20State%20Psychiatric%20HospitalsTechnical%20Report _July_2014.pdf

Parham, L. D., Ecker, C. L., Kuhaneck, H., Henry, D. A., & Glennon, T. J. (2021). *Sensory processing measure (SPM-2)*. Western Psychological Services.

Peloquin, S. M. (1989). Moral treatment: Contexts considered. *American Journal of Occupational Therapy, 43,* 537–544. https:// doi.org/10.5014/ajot.43.8.537

Polatajko, H. J., Townsend, E. A., & Craik, J. (2007). Canadian Model of Occupational Performance and Engagement (CMOP-E). In E. A. Townsend & H. J. Polatajko (Eds.), *Enabling occupation II: Advancing an occupational therapy vision of health, well-being, & justice through occupation* (pp. 22–36). CAOT Publications ACE.

Reitz, S. M., & Scaffa, M. E. (2020). Occupational therapy in the promotion of health and well-being. *American Journal of Occupational Therapy, 74*(3), 7403420010p1–7403420010p14. https://doi.org/10.5014/ajot.2020.743003

Rogers, J. C., & Holm, M. B. (1989). *Performance assessment of self-care skills (PASS)*. University of Pittsburgh.

Scanlan, J. N., & Novak, T. (2015). Sensory approaches in mental health: A scoping review. *Australian Occupational Therapy Journal, 62*(5), 277–285. https://doi.org/10.1111/1440-1630.12224

Menschner, C., & Maul, A. (2016). *Key ingredients for successful trauma-informed care implementation*. Substance Abuse and Mental Health Services Administration. https://www.samhsa .gov/sites/default/files/programs_campaigns/childrens_mental _health/atc-whitepaper-040616.pdf

Substance Abuse and Mental Health Services Administration. (2019a). *Civil commitment and the mental health care continuum:*

Historical trends and principles for law and practice. Office of the Chief Medical Officer. https://www.samhsa.gov/sites/default/files/civil-commitment-continuum-of-care.pdf

Substance Abuse and Mental Health Services Administration. (2019b). *National Mental Health Services Survey (N-MHSS): 2018. Data on mental health treatment facilities.* https://www.samhsa.gov/data/sites/default/files/cbhsq-reports/NMHSS-2018.pdf

Substance Abuse and Mental Health Services Administration. (2021). *National Mental Health Services Survey (N-MHSS): 2020 data on mental health treatment facilities.* Department of Health and Human Services. https://www.samhsa.gov/data/sites/default/files/reports/rpt35336/2020_NMHSS_final.pdf

Substance Abuse and Mental Health Services Administration. (2022). *Biden-Harris administration announces millions of dollars in new funds for states to tackle mental health crisis* [Press release]. https://www.samhsa.gov/newsroom/press-announcements/20221018/biden-harris-administration-announces-funding-states-tackle-mental-health-crisis

Substance Abuse and Mental Health Services Administration. (2023, February 16). *Recovery and recovery support.* U.S. Department of Health and Human Services. https://www.samhsa.gov/find-help/recovery

Taylor, R., Bowyer, P., & Fisher, G. (2023). *Kielhofner's Model of Human Occupation* (6th ed.). Wolters Kluwer.

The Joint Commission on Mental Illness and Mental Health. (1961). *Action for mental health: Final report, 1961.* Basic Books.

Thompson, J. R., Bryant, B. R., Schalock, R. L., Shogren, K. A., Tassé, M. J., Wehmeyer, M., Campbell, E. M., Craig, E. M., Hughes, C., & Rotholz, D. A. (2015). *Supports Intensity Scale—Adult Version: User's manual.* American Association on Intellectual and Developmental Disabilities.

Thomson, L. K., & Robnett, R. H. (2016). *KELS: Kohlman Evaluation of Living Skills* (4th ed.). American Occupational Therapy Association.

Wik, A., Hollen, V., & Fisher, W. H. (2020). Forensic patients in state psychiatric hospitals: 1999–2016. *CNS Spectrums, 25*(2), 196–206. https://doi.org/10.1017/S1092852919001044

Homelessness and Housing Insecurity

Christine A. Helfrich and Caitlin E. Synovec

Occupational therapy practitioners (OTPs) work with individuals with mental health diagnoses in a wide range of settings, including homeless shelters, transitional living, and medical respite programs. Individuals in these settings may experience acute or persistent psychological symptoms. They have often transitioned through a series of housing arrangements and, by the time they encounter an OTP, have experienced severe disruptions to their habits and daily routines. A person experiencing acute symptoms of mental illness can have challenges engaging in social interactions, performing activities of daily living (ADLs), and managing more complex instrumental activities of daily living (IADLs). However, symptoms of a mental health diagnosis alone do not cause a person to become homeless; stories of becoming unhoused are typically complex and person, health, and environmental factors all play a role in the story.

This chapter explores the lives of individuals with the lived experience of mental illness who enter homeless shelters or transitional living programs. It examines reasons people become and remain homeless in the context of person, environment, and occupational factors. It presents occupational therapy practice theories and describes application of the occupational therapy process to those who are living unhoused. See Chapter 7: Cognition, Chapter 13: Communication and Social Skills, and Chapter 46: Activities of Daily Living, Instrumental Activities of Daily Living, and Health Management Occupations. 🤝

What Does It Mean to Be Homeless?

Often individuals who are labeled homeless or unhoused are viewed as if that is their only identity. However, being unhoused, or homeless, suggests that an individual does not have a home to *live in* or that they currently do not have "housing," but it does not *define* their identity. Almost anyone can find themselves in a circumstance where they temporarily or permanently do not have housing. A discussion of what it means to be homeless and some of the causes follows; later in the chapter, examples are used to reinforce the argument that homelessness is not an identity.

The United Nations (UN) Secretary General defines **homelessness** as "a condition where a person or household lacks habitable space with security of tenure, rights and ability to enjoy social relations, including safety" (UN, 2020, p. 2). In the United States, the Department of Housing and

Urban Development (HUD) offers a specific definition of *homeless* as describing "An individual or family who lacks a fixed, regular, and adequate nighttime residence, meaning the individual or family:

1. Has a primary nighttime residence that is a public or private place not meant for human habitation;
2. Is living in a publicly or privately operated shelter designated to provide temporary living arrangements (including congregate shelters, transitional housing, and hotels and motels paid for by charitable organizations or by federal, state, and local government programs); or
3. Is exiting an institution where they have resided for 90 days or less and resided in an emergency shelter or place not meant for human habitation immediately before entering that institution." (HUD, 2023)

These definitions do not comprehensively describe the specific population OTPs may see in homeless shelters. People who are unhoused are not a homogeneous group and may differ in demographics, subgroups, and their patterns of homelessness.

In the United States, the onset of the COVID-19 pandemic shifted the demographics of this population; more individuals are living unsheltered, and the number of older adults experiencing homelessness has increased whereas homelessness among veterans has decreased (Henry et al., 2022; Kushel, 2020). These statistics are estimates and the numbers are likely to be much higher. Point-in-time (PIT) estimates only count individuals seen on one night per year and include only those staying in shelters or who are outside and visible to PIT volunteers. Research on homelessness can also be difficult to interpret because researchers use different definitions and methods for counting. Many statistics do not include individuals who are "doubling up" with relatives or acquaintances, or who are in unstable housing situations and cannot count on having a consistent place to stay.

Person and Population Factors

This section examines five subgroups of individuals who are at higher risk of experiencing homelessness and who are more likely to be encountered by OTPs: adults with behavioral health conditions, people with disabilities, people who identify as LGBTQIA+, people who are survivors of family violence, and youth. Practitioners work with these populations in many types of settings including inpatient, outpatient, rehabilitation, skilled nursing facilities, and schools.

Yet, they are often identified by their housing situations as simply "homeless" or "staying in a shelter." It is important to note that for each of these subgroups, the risk of experiencing homelessness is significantly influenced by person and environmental factors. Although presented separately in this text, OTPs should understand the intersection of policy, societal priorities, and person factors that culminate in a person becoming homeless.

Adults With Behavioral Health Conditions

Adults with mental health diagnoses are at risk for becoming homeless. In addition, being unhoused exacerbates mental health symptoms, which makes managing them significantly more challenging. In higher income countries, 75% of those experiencing homelessness have a mental health disorder; comparatively, in the United States 20% of the general population has a mental health disorder (Gutwinski et al., 2021). Substance use disorders occur at three times the rate in adults experiencing homelessness than in the general U.S. population; however, substance use may be either an effect or cause of being unhoused (Gutwinski et al., 2021). Similarly, rates of posttraumatic stress disorder (PTSD) are significantly higher in adults experiencing homelessness than in the general population; and similar to substance use, being unhoused increases the likelihood of experiencing trauma/traumatic events (Ayano et al., 2020).

Individuals who are homeless with psychiatric symptoms often present with other comorbidities, including traumatic or acquired brain injury, and chronic health conditions. The existence of comorbidities can complicate and worsen symptoms, affect cognition, and are more complicated to manage when unhoused (Fazel et al., 2014; Stone et al., 2019; Stubbs et al., 2020). Adults experiencing homelessness who have health comorbidities experience early mortality; the presence of substance use and mental health diagnoses increases this risk (Fazel et al., 2014; National Health Care for the Homeless Council [NHCHC], 2021). Veterans experiencing chronic homelessness also have high rates of mental health and substance use disorders and are likely to have a history of brain injury (Greer et al., 2020).

Although veterans are eligible for specific services, some may be encountered in settings such as the general unhoused population because of their service discharge status or lack of connection to services (Holliday & Pederson, 2017). See Chapter 24: Substance-Related and Addictive Disorders and Chapter 43: Serving Veterans and Service Members.

People With Disabilities

People who experience **chronic homelessness** are those that "are single *disabled* individuals who have been continuously homeless for more than 1 year or have experienced at least four episodes of homelessness in the past 3 years" (HUD, 2015). One-third of those experiencing homelessness in the United States meet the definition of chronically homeless, and this population is more likely to be unsheltered than others experiencing homelessness, in part because of a lack of accessibility in shelter settings (Henry et al., 2022). Disability experienced by unhoused individuals can be a result of physical, cognitive, and

behavioral health conditions, and can impact daily functioning (Rider et al., 2022). In high-income countries, adults experiencing homelessness have higher rates of chronic conditions, such as cardiovascular disease or diabetes, and these conditions worsen much more quickly when a person is unhoused; this can then result in significant health events (such as a stroke) that impact overall function (Fazel et al., 2014).

Unhoused adults with physical conditions experience health and functional decline 15 to 20 years earlier than the general housed population, have high rates of falls, vision and hearing loss, and incontinence. They also have less access to treatment; one-third of older adults experiencing homelessness report at least some difficulty completing ADLs (Brown et al., 2017). At least 25% of adults experiencing homelessness have an identified cognitive impairment (Stone et al., 2019). Causes of cognitive impairment may include a history of brain injury, intellectual and developmental disability, age-related conditions, and behavioral health conditions (Brown & McCann, 2020; Brown et al., 2017; Stone et al., 2019). See Chapter 7: Cognition.

Experiencing a disability increases the risk for becoming homeless for many reasons, including not being able to earn a living wage, the loss of social support systems, increased risk for engagement in the criminal justice system, and decreased access to health-care and rehabilitation services to address conditions and functional skills (Brown & McCann, 2020; Stone et al., 2019). For example, an adult with an intellectual disability who has lived with a parent for their entire life may lose their home if this parent passes away. Further, once someone with a cognitive disability becomes homeless, they are more likely to remain homeless for longer periods of time than those without a cognitive impairment, in part because of the complexity of service systems that can be difficult to navigate (Synovec et al., 2022). See Chapter 26: The Public Policy Environment.

Gender and Sexual Identity

Those who are part of the lesbian, gay, bisexual, transgender, queer, intersex, asexual, and other sexual and gender minorities (LGBTQIA+) are at increased risk of experiencing homelessness. This is a result of discrimination that often causes job and housing loss, as well as loss of family and social networks, because of nonacceptance of the person's gender identity or sexual orientation, along with other population-risk factors such as physical or mental health (Fraser et al., 2019). Once unhoused, they are also more likely to experience additional discrimination and violence, primarily because of their gender identity and/or sexual orientation (HUD, 2021). Thirty percent of LGBTQIA+ individuals who seek shelter report having been turned away from shelters, and 20% of those who stay in shelters are victims of harassment and sexual assault (HUD, 2021).

Those who can access shelters may feel unsafe, especially if they are required to stay in areas designated for their sex assigned at birth instead of their identity, and because shelters lack privacy, especially for self-care activities (Fraser et al., 2019; HUD, 2021). Although all people experiencing homelessness experience bias and stigma in health-care settings, this is especially prevalent for LGBTQIA+ individuals (Fenway Institute et al., 2021). This results in limited access to primary and basic medical and behavioral health care and means that many individuals also do not receive gender-affirming care. Bias and discrimination in housing programs may also result in those with LGBTQIA+ identities remaining unhoused longer and having reduced access to permanent housing (Fenway Institute et al., 2021). See Chapter 27: Mental Health Stigma and Sanism. 🤝

Families and Youth

Families with children make up 70% of the homeless population internationally (UN, 2020). Internationally, countries with the best social protections have the lowest rates of unhoused families. In the United States, they are one of the largest subgroups at 30% (de Sousa et al., 2022; National Alliance to End Homelessness [NAEH], 2021). The phrase "families with children" refers to households composed of at least one adult and one child under age 18. Overall, the number of U.S. families that are unhoused decreased between 2012 and 2022 by 27%; however, 50% of unaccompanied youth remain unsheltered (de Sousa et al., 2022; NAEH, 2021). Youth ages 15 to 24 are the population at highest risk for becoming homeless because of economic factors, migration, and those issues discussed previously (UN, 2020). Youth homelessness in the United States has reached epidemic proportions, with estimates reaching 2.5 million (Bassuk et al., 2014) and nearly 100,000 for PIT estimates (Henry et al., 2022).

The challenges of single parenting and traumatic experiences, particularly domestic violence (28%), precede and prolong homelessness for women and children (Bassuk et al., 2014). Single women who are homeless as an immediate result of domestic violence account for approximately 12% of the homeless population (NAEH, 2015) and nearly 80% of homeless families (SAMHSA, 2016). Women who experience domestic abuse report substantial difficulty with daily activities often because they have not acquired life skills or because their abusers controlled the household, allowing them little opportunity for responsibility and decision-making (SAMHSA, 2016).

Domestic violence has both health and functional consequences. Physical injuries are most common to the head, neck, and face, followed by musculoskeletal and genital injuries; these often increase in severity through time (Nemeth et al., 2019; World Health Organization [WHO], 2013). The psychological consequences of abuse are broad, with PTSD and depression occurring most frequently (WHO, 2013). More than 44% of domestic violence survivors living in a shelter (compared with only 2.6% of U.S. women) reported their mental conditions resulted in difficulties functioning in work, school, and social environments (Helfrich et al., 2008). Women's abilities to interact effectively with others may also be limited by psychological symptoms. Their behavior may be misunderstood by employers, coworkers, and service providers as "attitudinal" rather than resulting from trauma and treatable symptoms. This misunderstanding contributes to stigma and feelings of powerlessness (Helfrich et al., 2008).

Although 93% of homeless mothers have a lifetime history of interpersonal trauma (Hayes et al., 2013), at least 25% of homeless children have witnessed violence (McCoy-Roth et al., 2012). The experience of trauma in addition to being transient or unhoused places children at risk for a myriad of health and development problems. They are four times more likely to experience significant developmental delays in language, gross and fine motor skills, and psychosocial milestones and have a higher incidence of medical, social, psychological, and behavioral issues compared with children with stable housing (Bassuk et al., 2014; Clark et al., 2019).

Transition-Age and Unaccompanied Youth

Transition-age youth are young adults between the ages of 16 and 24. "Unaccompanied youth" refer to those experiencing homelessness who are not connected to a family/

PhotoVoice

You Hit, I Hurt

10/31/2008 was the last time my ex-husband beat me. While I lost my unborn child, I know that I will see her again. I spent 4 months in a coma. He spent 22 days in jail. Eight years later, I still have nightmares. I have PTSD. While domestic violence is in my past, that is where it is going to stay. I attend the CHEERS program to help with preventing isolation. I go to cooking class and art class to help with my recovery. I hope that this PhotoVoice will help others get out of similar situations, and to know that there is life worth living after you get out of the situation.

The author in this PhotoVoice shares some of the ways that domestic violence impacted and continues to affect her life. What can we learn from this woman who has moved from being a victim to being a survivor?

Do you believe that the occupations of cooking and art classes have helped this person find healing? Explain.

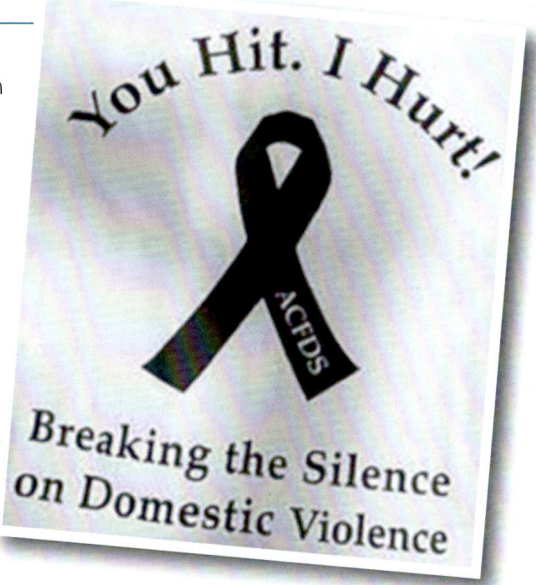

You Hit. I Hurt!

ACFDS

Breaking the Silence on Domestic Violence

support system (Henry et al., 2022). About half these youth stay in shelter services, whereas the other half are unhoused (Henry et al., 2022). The approximate number of youths experiencing homelessness is likely undercounted, as they may be staying in unstable housing situations (e.g., staying with friends or acquaintances). Unaccompanied youth may overlap with other populations at risk of homelessness; 20% to 45% of youth identify as LGBTQIA+ and 44% report experiencing sexual violence before becoming homeless (Fenway Institute, 2020; Fraser et al., 2019).

Youth transitioning out of foster care systems and/or who have disabilities are also more likely to be homeless (Baams et al., 2019; Baker Collins et al., 2018). Older youth and young adults may be required to separate from their families at shelter settings because of age or gender limitations, especially young adults who identify as male. Youth living on the streets are at risk for unsafe situations, including physical and sexual assault and sex trafficking. They may acquire hazardous survival skills, such as sex work, theft, drug use, and gang membership, while living on the street. These skills are gained at the expense of life skills needed for independent living or employment, which would support a transition from homelessness. In addition, these situations limit opportunities to develop life skills that promote mainstream roles such as student, family member, and worker, despite this population's identification of these skills and roles as a priority (Aviles de Bradley, 2011; Simpson et al., 2020).

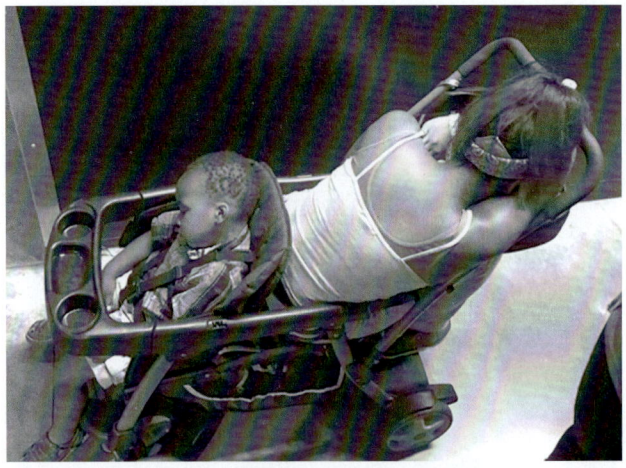

A pregnant teen with a 2-year-old child uses a stroller for rest while waiting for shelter. *Photo courtesy of Gineen Hecht-Sander, Chicago, IL.*

Environmental Factors Affecting Homelessness

There are multiple environmental factors that strongly contribute to a person or family becoming unhoused. Policies and societal events play a significant role in homelessness rates and can make it more difficult for someone to exit homelessness. Across the globe, low living wages and social support benefits, housing costs, and access to health care all contribute to homelessness (UN, 2020). Although the impact of these variables depends on local and national policies, the UN (2020) has identified that a lack of affordable housing is a significant contributor to homelessness across the world.

Income and Living Wages

In the United States, a "living wage" is the hourly wage needed to spend no more than 30% of one's income on housing costs. In almost all communities in the United States, the minimum wage is significantly lower than the living wage, and in all communities the Social Security benefit amount for people with disabilities falls far below this amount (National Low Income Housing Coalition [NLIHC], 2022). In fact, the annual income of those who rely solely on Social Security benefits falls within extreme poverty, and people with disabilities live in poverty at more than twice the rate of those without disabilities (National Council on Disability, 2017; NLIHC, 2022). In economically developing countries, almost 60% of those experiencing homelessness are employed working full-time jobs, but their wages are not sufficient to pay for adequate housing (UN, 2020). In other areas of the world, most people who work earn a sufficient income to pay for housing (UN, 2020).

Lack of Affordable Housing

There is a significant lack of affordable housing in most countries (UN, 2020). In the United States, housing prices for rentals and homeownership have expanded far beyond the living wage (NLIHC, 2024). In major urban areas, the stock of designated affordable housing does not meet the demand and waitlists are often several years long. Therefore, families and individuals may "double up," sharing space within dwellings with few bedrooms and bathrooms for many people.

Eligibility criteria for affordable housing or housing assistance programs is based on strict definitions of homelessness, which reduces individuals' eligibility. Additionally, only 3.5% of low-income rental homes are accessible, which is far lower than the number of people with disabilities who need affordable housing (NLIHC, 2021). This results in individuals making difficult decisions to take housing that is available but may not be safe or fully meet their accessibility needs or remain homeless because housing is not accessible. Those who are living in poverty are at great risk of becoming homeless when they experience job loss and/or significant health events or illness, as social and family networks may not have economic resources to support the person. Occupancy criteria for affordable housing may also be restrictive, limiting someone's ability to utilize natural supports or other economic benefits, such as roommates.

Access to Health Care

Those who are low-income and living in poverty face significant barriers to accessing sufficient health, including lack of insurance, lack of medical providers, inability to afford medical treatment or medications, limited ability to attend appointments, and stigma when receiving services (Allen et al., 2017; Ford et al., 2018; Gilmer & Buccieri, 2020). This can often result in the development of chronic health conditions or significant health events, which can then lead to job loss or inability to continue to work. A person may become homeless while admitted to the hospital following a significant health event if they lose their job because of an inability to return to work.

Access to mental health services is even more limited than primary physical care, especially for those who are homeless, low income, minoritized, or part of the LGBTQIA+ community; and available services may not be culturally appropriate or include those from the community (Coombs et al., 2021; Skosireva et al., 2014). A lack of access to mental health services limits early intervention that may prevent worsening of symptoms and loss of self-care skills and can make it difficult to get medications as needed (National Alliance on Mental Illness [NAMI], 2023).

Punitive approaches to substance use disorders and limited availability of harm reduction and recovery-oriented interventions also make it more challenging to address substance use and its effects. Once unhoused, there is a continued lack of access to care as well as increased experiences of bias and stigma, which perpetuates health disparities. Managing health conditions while unhoused is difficult as one does not have a place to store medications, engage in self-care, manage routines, or eat recommended and nutritious meals. This results in deterioration of health, disability, and early mortality (NHCHC, 2021). See Chapter 23: Schizophrenia Spectrum and Psychotic Disorders and Chapter 25: Trauma- and Stressor-Related Disorders. 🤝

Natural Disasters and Extreme Weather Events

Natural disasters and extreme weather events are global issues that result in temporary and chronic homelessness. Floods, fires, hurricanes, and earthquakes cause an immediate loss of housing, belongings, and income. Although everyone in a community may experience displacement because of a disaster or weather event, those with a disability, those who live in poverty, persons with limited social and economic resources, and those who are renters are more likely to become homeless long term (Internal Displacement Monitoring Centre, 2021). Government and local responses to disasters influence the supports available after a disaster and who is eligible for these resources.

Political and Societal Responses

Political and societal perceptions and attitudes toward those who are unhoused determine how a community responds to and addresses the needs of people experiencing homelessness. In some cases, policies may be broad and not specific to the person (such as not enforcing laws that require housing developers to develop affordable housing or not increasing the minimum wage to ensure all citizens are able to make a living wage). Some countries and local governments have policies that directly affect those experiencing homelessness by criminalizing activities a person may do while homeless, such as eating, camping, sitting, or asking for money in public spaces, resulting in fines, arrests, and incarceration (Aykanian & Fogel, 2019; Diamond et al., 2022).

These policies and regulations further prevent individuals from finding employment or qualifying for housing programs; this often perpetuates, instead of resolves, homelessness. One example of this is the disruption of "encampments," which exist when unhoused individuals congregate in one area of a community. The reasons why encampments

occur are complex; there are many individuals who do not feel safe or whose needs cannot be met in congregate or emergency shelter settings, including those with more acute mental health needs. However, frequently the community and governmental response is to "sweep" and clear out encampment areas, disrupting those who are unsheltered and often resulting in trauma and loss of belongings without being paired with appropriate housing and resources (NHCHC, 2022).

Governments will also develop different support systems and resources for people experiencing homelessness; for example, some countries provide housing for people with disabilities. In Taiwan, individuals with mental illness are not discharged to the street; if they do not have other supports, there is sufficient institutional support for them (A.W. Pan, 2023, personal communication). This chapter is limited to a brief overview of the many physical and societal environmental factors that contribute to homelessness. Readers are encouraged to review the 2020 UN report (UN, 2020), which provides a thorough discussion and analysis of the social, cultural, and intrapersonal factors that contribute to homelessness and the theories that help explain these factors.

Homeless Shelters and Transitional Housing Environments

In general, the primary mission of **homeless shelters** is to provide temporary, safe housing, and shelters are typically the first place people access social and mental health services. An emergency shelter is defined as "any facility, the primary purpose of which is to provide a temporary shelter for the homeless in general or for specific populations of the homeless and which does not require occupants to sign leases or occupancy agreements" (Definitions, 2023). The length of stay, physical, and service arrangements at each shelter vary. For example, a person may need to wait in line to secure a bed for the night, then exit the shelter by a specified time and then return to wait in line the next night for another bed. Other shelters admit a person for up to 30 days and provide a locker for personal belongings.

Most shelters are "congregate," which means the beds are in a large, open space with minimal privacy and many individuals staying in close quarters. Some settings may serve meals, offer showers, or provide other services such as health care or clothing. Many shelters are in older or repurposed buildings and may be focused on ensuring overall safety of shelter residents and meeting basic functions (bathing facilities, meals). They may not be fully accessible to those with different disabilities or gender identities or located in neighborhoods close to other resources.

Some emergency shelters have a specific approach or are designed to respond to specific needs, which may determine requirements to stay at the shelter, such as paying a fee or participating in programs or groups. These are dependent on the organization operating the shelter and how the shelter itself is funded. For example, the focus may be on a specific population, such as veterans, older adults, youth, or survivors of domestic and interpersonal violence. Eligibility for these programs requires the person to meet the program's definition of their target population. In contrast, **low barrier shelters** do not require a person to pass a background check, have identification, refrain from substance use, or participate in programs to access the shelter or services. Low barrier shelters may be the only place some people can access shelter services. These settings require staff to have expertise in trauma-informed approaches and deescalation skills. See Chapter 5: Trauma-Informed Practice. 🤝

Medical Respite Care Programs

Medical respite care programs offer acute and postacute medical care for people experiencing homelessness who are too ill or frail to recover from a physical illness or injury on the streets, but who are not ill enough to be in a hospital. These programs provide short-term residential services coupled with support services and access to medical care (National Institute for Medical Respite Care [NIMRC], 2021). Medical respite programs may be in a standalone space, a specific part of the shelter, or a transitional housing program. Individuals transition or discharge from the medical respite program once their medical conditions are stable, and the person can safely return to the shelter. Ideally, program participants would transition into stable housing, but this is variable and dependent on housing availability in the community. Figure 42-1 shows various types of shelter sites.

Transitional Housing

Transitional housing programs are designed to promote housing stability and provide temporary housing for up to 2 years (HUD, 2024.). In addition to offering housing, they

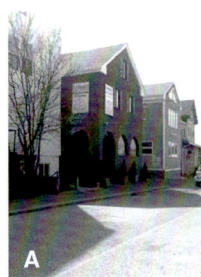
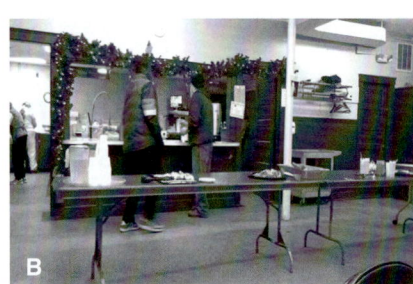
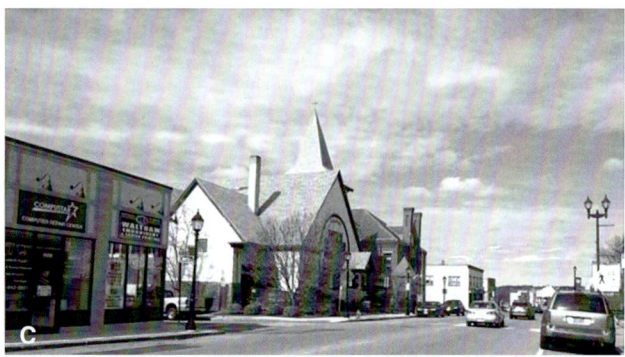
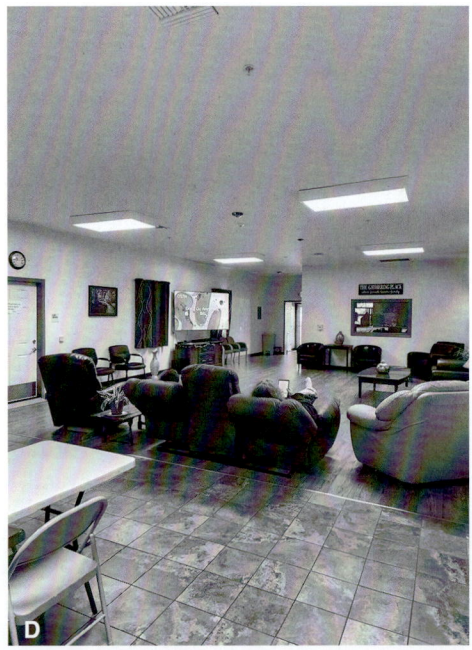
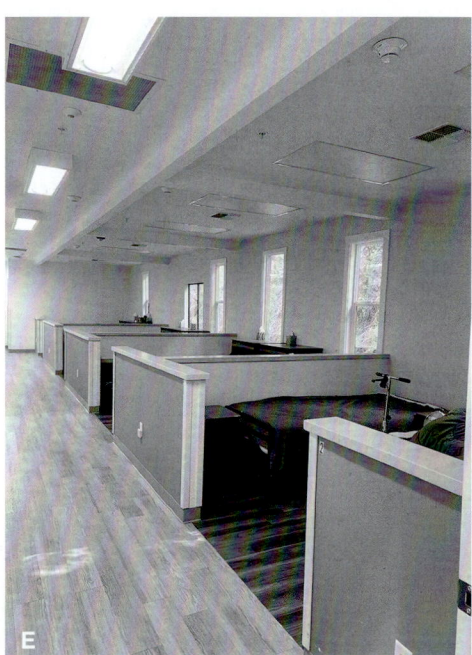

FIGURE 42-1. Types of shelter sites. A. Shelter site (row of buildings): The second floor of this building is used as a day center where people can receive mail, lunch, and connections to services for 3 hours daily. In extreme weather, it doubles as an emergency shelter. B. People who are living on the street or in shelters come to a soup kitchen daily for warmth, socialization, and sustenance. C. Soup kitchen: The basement of this church discreetly serves as a year-round soup kitchen and warming center. A medical respite program provides a place for people to stay and recover, focusing on their health after a hospitalization. Medical respite programs often include common living areas (D) and a sleeping/dorm space (E). *A, B, C: Photos courtesy of Christine Helfrich, Waltham, MA. C, D: Photos courtesy of Caitlin Synovec.*

BOX 42-1 ■ **Additional Sites Where Occupational Therapy Practitioners Can Work With Populations That Are Unhoused**

There are many places where individuals and families experiencing homelessness engage with services. Although this chapter is focused on the shelter setting, OTPs may also work directly with this population in:

- **Federally Qualified Health Centers or Health Care for the Homeless Programs** provide integrated primary and behavioral health care. These are federally funded entities that provide health-care services regardless of a person's insurance status or ability to pay for care (https://nhchc.org).
- **Street Medicine Teams** focus on providing care to those who are living unsheltered and may have difficulty engaging with traditional health-care entities. Street medicine teams may operate out of health care for the homeless (HCH) programs,

universities/medical student programs, and local hospitals or health-care organizations (https://www.streetmedicine.org).

- **Drop-In Centers** focus on providing day services, which often include meals, telephone access, bathrooms and/or places to shower/bathe, and may include additional services such as laundry facilities, mail services, and case management (e.g., https://www.communitydaycenter.org).

Occupational therapy practice within these settings is emerging but growing, as the value and distinct role of occupational therapy has become more widely recognized, and OTPs are able to advocate and integrate their practice.

---

typically offer varied services, and some programs address the specific needs of persons with mental illness, individuals in substance abuse recovery, or women and children who are survivors of domestic violence. Participants in transitional housing programs are often required to participate in job training or educational programs, be employed, or participate in treatment services for substance use, mental health diagnoses, or recovery. These settings often include their own programs and services, which may focus on skill building and rehabilitation, behavioral changes, education, or addressing barriers to occupational performance.

Ideally, someone who has accessed shelter services will move into permanent housing, or permanent supportive housing. Often, however, individuals and families may remain homeless for many years before they are able to access and move into housing. Finally, it is important to note that although this chapter focuses on shelters, many individuals experiencing homelessness do not stay within shelter settings. The reasons are complex and varied, but may be because of histories of trauma, lack of low barrier services causing ineligibility to stay in shelters, a desire to stay with social supports and not be separated in the shelter, having a vehicle to live in, or having pets who cannot join the shelter. Providers, including OTPs, can work to engage those who are unsheltered in services through other entities, such as those presented in Box 42-1. See Chapter 31: The Home Environment: Permanent Supportive Housing.

Team Members

Shelter and transitional living program staff members include individuals with varying levels of education and experience. Staff receive specialized training related to the population the shelter serves (e.g., survivors of domestic violence or substance abuse). The number, credentials, titles, and roles of staff vary greatly according to funding and availability, but the need nearly always exceeds the available staffing. Case managers primarily focus on supporting individuals in accessing services, such as housing and income, but may have

large caseloads that make it difficult to meet the individual needs of each person. Staff turnover tends to be high because of the high stress level placed on frequently overworked, undertrained, and underpaid staff.

Most shelters and transitional programs depend on volunteers and administrative or office staff for completion of the daily tasks that maintain shelter functioning. Transitional programs may additionally employ housing supervisors or managers to ensure residents are able to pay rent and follow housing rules and obligations. Individuals staying at shelters often engage with a variety of staff and providers addressing different needs within the shelter, in health care, and in social services. It is important for staff and providers to coordinate care and work collaboratively, when possible, to minimize the complications of navigating multiple providers and systems.

Funding Sources

Most shelters and housing programs are operated by not-for-profit agencies, requiring them to seek funding from multiple sources, including government, foundations, and private fundraising. This is a constant challenge and is usually supported by at least one full-time development staff member. HUD is the primary U.S. federal agency providing funding to shelters. The U.S. Department of Health and Human Services (DHHS), which includes several specific branches (e.g., Health Resources and Services Administration, Bureau of Primary Health Care, SAMHSA, Center for Mental Health Services, Centers for Disease Control and Prevention, Administration for Children and Families, the U.S. Department of Labor, and the U.S. Department of Education), also provides funding for various programs.

In addition, state, regional, county, and city governments may provide government funding. Most shelters and transitional living programs also seek funding from foundations and private contributors, including businesses and individuals. Some shelters are funded by a particular religious organization or by other social welfare groups. Stories regarding the unhoused experience can be found in Box 42-2.

PhotoVoice

Mental Health and Homelessness in Phoenix

When I became homeless, I went to Central Arizona Shelter Services (C.A.S.S.). I told them I have issues with behavioral and medical health. They suggested I go to a different shelter. I was sad, mad, and confused. So I called four different shelters and they all turned me away. I believe that this is the norm here in Phoenix. There needs to be more outreach to our community so that this doesn't happen to one more person.

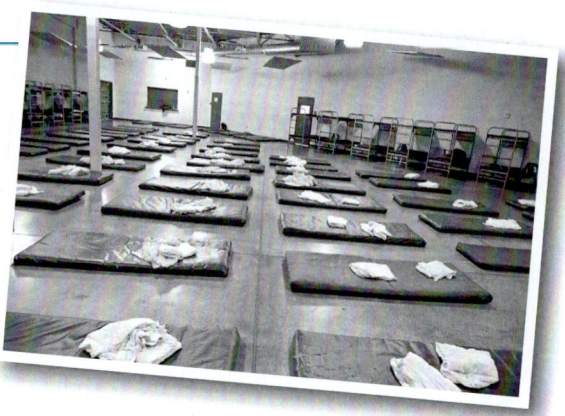

John suggests advocacy and outreach to the community. Does occupational therapy have a role in such activities? Explain.

Examine the image that John provides. Using a person-environment interaction perspective, imagine how ADLs such as eating, dressing, medication management, or sleeping might be impacted within this environment.

BOX 42-2 ■ In Their Voice: Individuals Who Are Unhoused Share Experiences

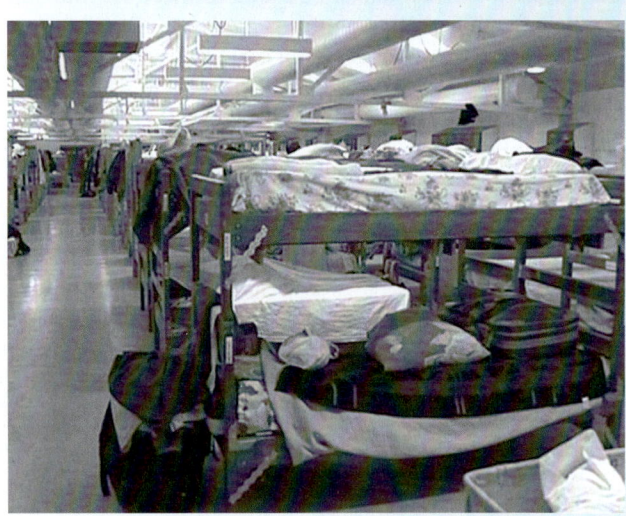

If you have never been unhoused yourself, you might wonder what it is like to spend a night in a shelter. An honest answer is, "It depends." Shelters for the unhoused can offer a variety of services and enforce different house rules, such as curfews, drug testing, or mandatory chores. The quotes here are from people with lived experiences in shelters:

Pete—"They would wake you up at 5 in the morning, and there was one floor where they had all these bunkbeds, um, you would wake up at 5 in the morning, and the first thing you would do when you woke up in the morning was you would run downstairs and sign up, to get a room, to stay again for the next night. You had to sign up then, they only took so many signatures. So you had to sign up as early as you could, to stay the next night."

Fancy—"Oh God, you know you have no privacy, . . . for one thing I wasn't used to sleeping with so many people. That was my main thing you know, trying to sleep with all these other people around. That was my biggest problem, because I wasn't used to it. You know and then, well you gotta shower around a whole bunch of strange people, and I found that kind of hard."

Mike—"And so I had to sleep with my girlfriend, and when she kicked me out, I was on the streets, slept under bridges. Piers. Parks. Backyards, dumpsters. Sold myself. Till you can get a, just a place to sleep. Went in the um laundry, laundromats. Stayed up all day, slept and you stayed up all night, slept all day. You do what you have to."

Understanding Occupational Participation of People Experiencing Homelessness

It is important for OTPs to understand that there are a variety of factors that contribute to homelessness and to honestly reflect on one's own biases and beliefs about the prevailing stereotypes regarding people who are unhoused and their occupations. These include ideas that they are lazy, dangerous, and that they choose to be homeless. First impressions can be distorted. For example, when an individual describes their homelessness as a "choice," it may be difficult for an OTP to comprehend this choice. Considering issues associated with living in a shelter, such as a loss of freedom, experiencing triggers to trauma, and requirements to follow strict rules, may help the OTP understand the perspective.

Individuals who are homeless often have a history of unstable housing dating back to childhood; many have experienced trauma in some form before becoming homeless and continue to experience trauma because of being homeless (Ayano et al., 2020). Most OTPs have never personally experienced homelessness, which highlights the importance of using a trauma-informed approach and using tools to build relationships to understand each person's individual experience. See Chapter 25: Trauma- and Stressor-Related Disorders.

Practitioners must consider the intersectionality of issues that contribute to a person's risk for homelessness in order to be sensitive to cultural differences and practice using cultural

The Lived Experience

A City Shelter Resident

Editor's Note: At the time of the interview, the person was staying on the convalescent care floor of a city shelter.

Around 11½ years ago I became homeless. I got divorced. The people I lived with lost their homes because of drugs; they weren't working and didn't pay bills. I'm not going to lie, I did drugs too, but they were worse off than me, and I was the only one working. My youngest boy lived there, he wore diapers and had to catheterize himself. I stopped working 6 to 9 hours a day because I couldn't leave my disabled child out in a wheelchair all day long on the street by himself. I had no place for him. His SSI [Supplemental Security Income] pays for him to be in a nursing home. Then things fell downhill.

I couldn't find work. I couldn't apply for a job in old, dirty, nasty clothes, I smelled to heck. When you're out on the street there aren't bathrooms you can go into: people know you're homeless, and they're not going to let you into their facilities. You have to learn to go in different places, and you have accidents. I started taking clothes from other people, realizing I need to clean up a bit. That's the way I lived out there. People don't understand how I done it, but I did it. You have to learn how to respect people and get respected. People fed me, gave me water if I needed water. You learn how to live.

I gave up drugs after I was homeless because of the way I was living. I looked at myself, and talked to myself, and said it was time, "I don't want to be around that." I had enough problems in my life now, being on the streets, sleeping here and there, what do I need them for? I still drink 2 days a week, Wednesdays and Saturdays, I need to get enjoyment out of my life.

I slept outside under an overhang to keep out of the weather and protected from the snow and rain. During the hurricane I went to a park with a giant canopy and slept there. The winds blew my blankets off, I got wet. Then I caught hypothermia, went to the hospital, stayed there 7 hours the last time. I caught hypothermia three times when I was on the street. But after that I just kept living.

A few years ago I got frostbite and lost half my foot. It got amputated. I went to a rehab program for about 2 months, learned how to walk again, go down steps. I still hate steps. They didn't help find housing there, they were just a rehab place, gave medicine for pain, and took care of an infection that set in. I went right back out there walking around with half a foot. I got frostbite again, my left foot got worse, and both my knees. They started really hurting. They sent me to the hospital and cut a whole big silver dollar scab off my knee, took care of my feet, and I went back out on the street again.

I went to go home, and I fell face first in the street—three stitches above my left eye, scraped my head up pretty good. They took me to the hospital again. I told them to let me die. I was tired of living. I tried to commit suicide three times, I can't take this no more. I had everything in life, and now I'm just alone, living on the street. They sent me to the f'ing psych ward for about a month and a half.

They sent me here, the convalescent program at the shelter, 3 months ago. I want to live, get back out on my feet again. I'm

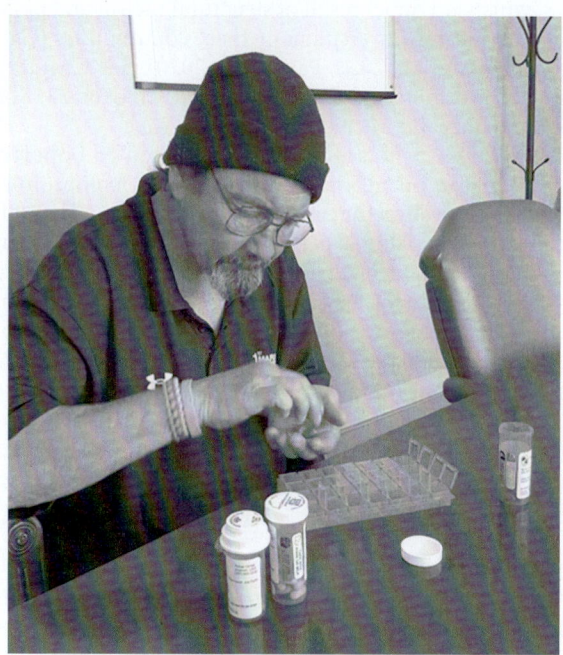

very excited about my apartment (I'm getting). It's a nice place, not right in the city. Out my living room window I can see trees and grass. It's got a washer, refrigerator, and a stove. I haven't cooked a meal in almost 12 years. I'm one heck of a cook. I'm just happy gas and electric is included. I can walk out of my apartment door, and right there's the laundry room. Take my dirty clothes and put them in the washer, go to my apartment, watch a little boob tube, go back and put them in the dryer, watch some more boob tube, get them, fold, and put them away. I had help from an outreach worker. She helped me get vouchers and Section 8 and all, and come up here and took me to a couple of apartments. She had a car to take me places. It would have been hard to walk. I'm only allowed out 1 day besides Wednesday from 11–4 in the afternoon. I couldn't have done it by myself. I wouldn't have been able to keep track of the paperwork. She helped me a lot. I only get $185 a month, and my food stamps. I lived on just my food stamps when I was out there.

When I get my place, I'll probably slow down the drinking. I am going to put a bird feeder outside my window and watch the birdies. And I'm going to get a TV, so I can watch what I want to watch, not what everyone else wants to watch. I will walk around my neighborhood, there's big rich homes there. I've come a long way; other people, they don't understand how I made it out there, with bitter cold down into the zeroes, blizzards, hurricanes, and whatever nature felt like throwing down on me. I prayed to that Man every day, and I still pray to that Man every day.

I'll miss this place. It's my second time here, but I'll like my apartment too. I'll be able to go see my son, I can't go now because he'd want me to stay all day and I have to be back here so early. We used to go crabbing and fishing when we were on the street. His place has a van, they could take him to me and we could spend the day together. We could go fishing again.

humility. In the United States, BIPOC (black, Indigenous, and people of color) and Indigenous communities are overrepresented in the population of people experiencing homelessness, which is a direct result of structural racism and policies that have created poverty among these communities (Carter, 2011; Henry et al., 2022; Paul et al., 2020). See Chapter 27: Mental Health Stigma and Sanism and Chapter 28: Social Determinants and Mental Health. 🤝

Individuals who are homeless have limited opportunities to engage in meaningful occupations, compromising their health, well-being, and social integration. They often experience occupational performance problems and occupational deprivation related to finances, housing, personal care, difficulties satisfying basic needs, health concerns, coping skills, education and employment, and leisure engagement (Helfrich & Chan, 2013). While unhoused, many individuals will focus on "occupations of survival" and "occupations of self-management," which focus on acquiring basic needs (such as shelter or food), determining where to do self-care (such as take medications), and attending appointments (Illman et al., 2013).

In between meeting these basic needs, people experiencing homelessness have limited ways to structure and spend their time (Marshall et al., 2019). However, those experiencing homelessness who have engaged in occupational therapy services have identified a range of occupational priorities, including ADLs, IADLs, leisure participation, and health management (Synovec et al., 2020). This diversity in priorities supports the need for an individualized, person-centered occupational therapy process.

Many individuals are perceived as not "housing ready" because their providers or shelter staff have difficulty determining if the person is able to effectively manage their own home. Assessment of readiness may be made based on the person's acuity of symptoms, cognition, and engagement with providers. However, Adair and colleagues (2017) found there is not a predictor of who will be successful in housing, regardless of mental health or substance use diagnosis, cognitive skills, or time spent homeless before housing. Instead of focusing on potential deficits and diagnoses, shelters and homeless services should utilize a strengths-based approach to identify skills and potential needed supports to prepare individuals to move into housing.

This approach aligns with the occupational therapy process. When a person is transitioning into housing, occupational priorities may shift to focus on adjusting time use and routines, managing health conditions, learning and utilizing independent living skills, connecting to a new community, and focusing on longer-term life goals (Helfrich & Chan, 2013; Marshall et al., 2020; Marshall & Rosenberg, 2014). Although positive, the preparation and transition into housing can be difficult after someone has experienced occupational deprivation and trauma related to homelessness. Continued support once the person is housed can improve outcomes and support the person in staying housed long term (Aubry et al., 2016). See Chapter 31: The Home Environment: Permanent Supportive Housing. 🤝

The nature of transitional housing and homelessness causes families to renegotiate routines, living environments, and family roles, especially for men and adolescent boys who may not be allowed to stay in the same shelter. Practitioners should always ask about family members who are not

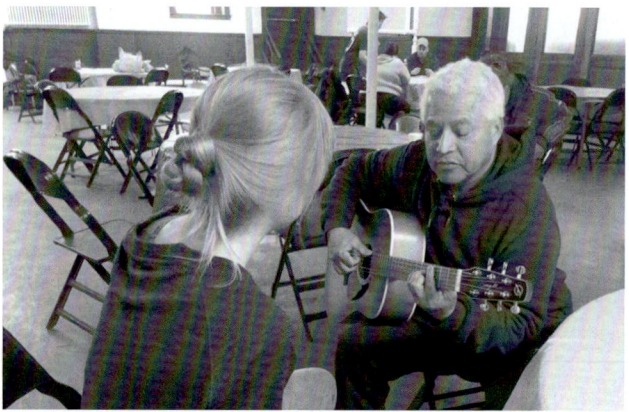

A precariously housed man comes to the soup kitchen daily for 3 hours to socialize, eat, and get warm. An occupational therapy student engages him in a former leisure occupation of guitar playing. *Photo courtesy of Christine Helfrich, Waltham, MA.*

currently with the sheltered family to understand the whole family network. The physical setting and materials present in the environment are instrumental in shaping interactions that support children's play activities, which are known to foster life skills development (The Homeless Children's Playtime Project, n.d.). Children who are homeless frequently have difficulty routinely attending school, causing delays in basic skills learned in elementary education and impacting the development of skills necessary for adult roles (McCoy-Roth et al., 2012). See Chapter 29: Families.

Role of Occupational Therapy

The role of occupational therapy in shelters is diverse and determined by the setting, funding sources, existing staffing, and the specific population at each shelter. As is true for the types and roles of staff members who work in shelters, the role of OTPs in these settings also varies. The most involved role is that of **direct service provider**. As a direct service provider, the OTP is integrated into the shelter staffing model and spends most of their time engaging the residents. They may also have additional roles and responsibilities that include supporting shelter staff, maintaining operations of the shelter, and participating in team meetings and care planning. Practitioners need a broad range of knowledge and competencies to work in these settings and support individuals experiencing homelessness or transitioning to housing (Marshall et al., 2021).

The role of **consultant** is a common and complex role for OTPs in shelters. This often occurs because shelters in general have limited funding to employ staff and are likely unable to bill for services as would happen in medical settings. The consultant role may be time limited (e.g., for a specific project or time duration) or have limited hours (e.g., 1–2 days at the shelter setting). In this model, the OTP may be employed by an outside agency that serves the shelter or work as an independent contractor who is paid by the shelter for limited services.

As a consultant, the OTP may only interact with the shelter staff that support the individuals they are working with (e.g., a specific case manager) to share recommendations or contribute to the shelter's case management plan.

Practitioners working in a consulting role and conducting specific groups may not have a complete understanding of the individuals they work with; therefore, it is important for OTPs to communicate effectively with other staff to share and acquire additional information,

As a consultant, an OTP may take a role in program development. They might be tasked to identify gaps in services with staff and shelter residents. Often this includes identifying occupational therapy services that can address these gaps. A key task for the consultant may be to establish the role of occupational therapy in the shelter setting from the ground up. This would include establishing an evaluation and referral process, completing a thorough needs assessment to identify needs, and defining and implementing occupational therapy interventions to meet critical needs. For example, a consultant may collaborate with program administrators to set realistic parameters on a caseload size and routinely complete evaluations and ongoing interventions.

An OTP working as a consultant has the knowledge and skill set to participate in resource development and staff training that can extend the services or capabilities of the shelter's program and staff. Staff training would move beyond the expected provision of education about occupational therapy services. It might include training on co-occurring conditions affecting the populations served by the shelter or focus on a range of other topics such as education on accommodations and Americans with Disabilities Act (ADA) compliance, functional cognition, health management, suicide prevention, mental health first aid, or trauma-informed care.

Another key aspect of the consultant's role may be to evaluate outcomes not only for the occupational therapy programming but also for existing programs in the shelter. An OTP's capacity to design outcomes and evaluations can help ensure program funding. Finally, an OTP's consultant role may be to use their person-environment-occupation (PEO) focus to address overall environmental design at the shelter. A consultant could collaborate with staff to help structure the routines or environment to enhance the resident's functioning and promote normative routines and habits. Responsibilities might also include completing an environmental evaluation on accessibility of the shelter, considering the physical, cognitive, and emotional needs of residents. They might make recommendations on ways to create a trauma-informed environment that includes quiet zones, places for use of coping skills, and calming or comfortable designs in the shelter environment (e.g., plants, paint colors).

Table 42-1 provides some examples of how one occupational therapy consultant addressed program development, staff training, and environmental design to help transform a shelter.

Shelter case managers and direct staff often support shelter residents with life skills. It is essential for the OTP to explain and differentiate their distinct role and how occupational therapy can complement other services. For example,

---

TABLE 42-1 | Occupational Therapy Practitioner in the Consultant Role

As a PhD student, Christine Helfrich, MS, OTR/L, was hired as the onsite evaluator for the Chicago Homeless Children's Project Head Start Ethnographic Evaluation. She spent 20 hours each week conducting Participatory Action Research (PAR) activities in the Head Start Program. She quickly identified occupational needs of the children and their families and was able to introduce occupational therapy students into the setting to help integrate occupational therapy services into the shelter setting in multiple ways, as noted in the text that follows.

Program Development

- Oversaw changes in the gross motor room to ensure a safe, structured, indoor activity space to ensure physical activity.
- Implemented standardized developmental testing for all children and trained staff to better understand normal developmental milestones.
- After conducting a full needs assessment of the shelter's *Before & After* school program, implemented environmental adaptations to enhance the use of the space and introduced social/emotional learning activities and healthy physical activities.
- Developed a life skills program for the mothers who had all experienced domestic violence.
- Developed Level I and II Field Work (FW) programs for occupational therapy students.
- Introduced interprofessional education (IPE) with physical therapy (PT) and nutrition students to develop programing for families.
- Created a binder of activities for staff to do with children with directions, supplies needed, and suggestions of different ways to engage the children.

Staff Training

- Provided a weekly in-service to shelter staff to provide education on cognition, cognitive impairment, and its prevalence in people experiencing homelessness.
- Organized in-service meetings to teach strategies that shelter staff could use to support individuals with cognitive impairment, facilitate effective communication, introduce environmental strategies for memory (such as posted schedules), and educate on health and trauma-informed care.
- Encouraged staff to bring situations from their day-to-day work to be discussed and processed as a group to help everyone learn and apply the strategies.

Environmental Design

- Recommended ways to organize the shelter space to be more accommodating (e.g., large, clear signs about where to find essential items or staff).
- Worked with staff to identify areas where conflicts among residents were most likely to occur and used environmental and activity analysis to identify issues and provide recommendations.
- Shared analyses that revealed a primary source of conflict at the shelter was that those with mobility needs were frustrated when other residents used the accessible shower stalls, creating conflict in the chaotic morning time when residents were all getting ready for the day.
- Recommended a universal design approach to address this conflict. Oversaw the installation of grab bars within all showers and the purchase of additional, removable shower chairs to increase accessibility in all showers.
- Recommended that residents sign up for the most accessible shower stall and advocated with shelter staff to allow residents to use the stall throughout the day to ensure all residents that needed full accessibility had adequate time to use it.

a peer support specialist might pair with the OTP to lead a group on basic home management skills in preparation for transitioning into housing. The peer specialist would have critical knowledge and awareness of strategies to manage transitions, community resources, and group members' concerns. The OTP could help create or modify activities that meet different cognitive needs and learning styles, explain home or activity modifications that address physical needs or disabilities, ensure materials meet health and functional literacy guidelines, and identify group members who might benefit from individual evaluation and intervention.

The OTP would bring their expertise in these areas while recognizing the expertise of the peer specialist, whose lived experiences may include having previously navigated the transition from housing instability into housing stability themselves. Together, they would make important contributions to make the housing transition group comprehensive and accessible for all shelter residents.

As an OTP, both the direct service and consultative model would use the occupational therapy process to inform delivery of services (American Occupational Therapy Association [AOTA], 2020). Table 42-2 illustrates how the OTP may implement both consultative and direct service roles in the shelter setting by introducing Belinda, a shelter resident. Belinda's story continues in subsequent sections on evaluation and intervention to reinforce chapter content.

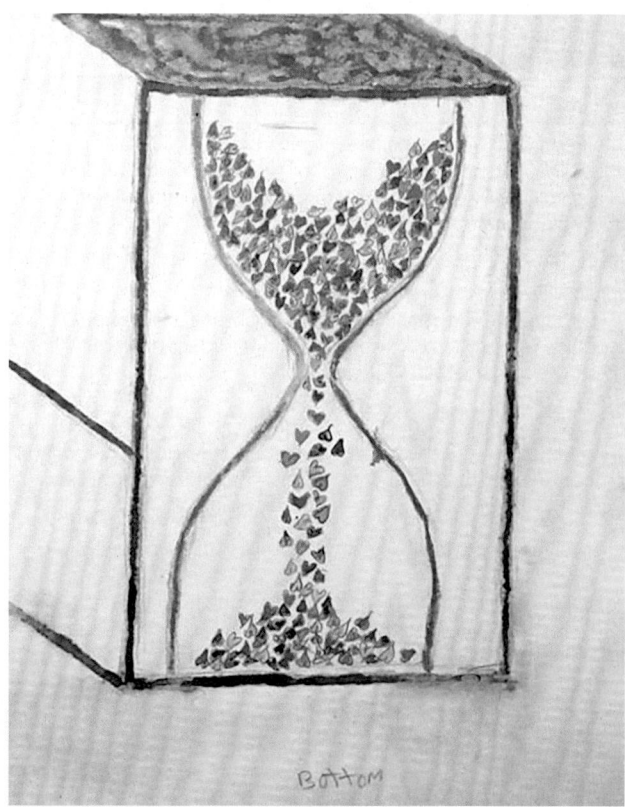

When two occupational therapy students interned at a soup kitchen, they brought adult coloring books. A gentleman who had been isolative retrieved a drawing pencil from his pocket and proceeded to teach the students about drawing with perspective and how to use water colors to make a drawing more attractive. Creating the opportunity to reengage in a former interest opened the door to understanding this individual. Over the day, the man shared his past history of supporting himself as an artist. *Photo courtesy of Christine Helfrich, Waltham, MA.*

Evaluation

The goal of evaluation in shelters is to identify an individual's strengths and limitations related to independent functioning and determine what skills and supports the person needs to manage and transition to different environments they choose. The hallmark of occupational therapy evaluation in shelters is holism, focusing on both the person's strengths and needs. The OTP may be the only professional in the shelter or transitional housing program with the training to assess medical, functional, and social aspects of performance and the ability to analyze person–environment interaction. It is important to screen for the broad range of physical, mental, cognitive, social, and functional challenges a person might encounter in their current and future environments.

It is particularly vital to assess strengths in these areas for both personal and staff awareness. Occupational therapy may be the only area where an individual has an opportunity to show their skills and view current barriers as an opportunity for skill building instead of deficits. Practitioners need to be trauma informed and consider the information they are asking. Building rapport and using positive feedback throughout the evaluation can be critical, as individuals may perceive themselves to have poor performance on assessments or identify assessments as barriers to housing. One good approach is framing evaluation in a person-centered manner that helps an individual see the process to understand their concerns and perceptions of their situation. Key questions an OTP can ask themselves are presented in Table 42-3.

Evaluation in the shelter setting should include completing an occupational profile and ensuring the person identifies current occupations and their priorities. Evaluation could begin with a general conversation, a practitioner rating (e.g., Model of Human Occupation Screening Tool [MOHOST]), a semistructured interview tool (e.g., Canadian Occupational Performance Measure [COPM], Occupational Circumstances Assessment Interview and Rating Scale [OCAIRS]), or an interactive self-report tool (e.g., Activity Card Sort-Advancing Inclusive Participation; Law et al., 1994; Parkinson & Forsyth, 2002; Tyminski et al., 2020). Following the occupational profile, the practitioner may select specialized assessment tools to assess specific functional and independent living skills such as medication management or ADLs, executive functioning, cognition, and physical skills.

Assessments that focus on skills for completing functional tasks as well as underlying performance strengths or barriers are beneficial for developing ongoing interventions or providing recommendations to other providers, as screening tools may not capture an individual's full capabilities (Synovec, 2020). A few assessments appropriate to use with populations in shelters and therapeutic reasoning questions that support assessment selection are included in Table 42-4.

Although several areas of function could be assessed, prioritizing assessments is critical, as residents in shelters often have multiple appointments or have a lower tolerance for engaging in lengthy assessments. The need to build rapport and gain the trust of a person living in a shelter can also impact an OTP's therapeutic reasoning about how to proceed with the evaluation process. Because the shelter environment is often restrictive and limits engagement in occupations, occupational therapy assessments allow for both the individual and staff to understand what the person

TABLE 42-2 | Occupational Therapy Roles in a Shelter Setting

Shelter Resident Presentation	Example of Consultation/Direct Service Roles
Belinda (she/her/hers) was staying in an emergency shelter that allowed residents to store their belongings and stay in the same bed for 30 days at a time. Each day, residents left the floor where they slept by 7:30 a.m. and could return at 4:00 p.m. During the day, residents stayed in the day area of the shelter or spent time in the community. Belinda's case manager received several complaints from floor staff about Belinda's bed and storage area. Other residents also complained about Belinda's belongings encroaching on their space. Belinda often had food wrappers or empty bottles in her belongings, which were not allowed on the floor. Belinda frequently approached shelter staff is a distressed state, worried that she left important items by her bed, such as medications, ID, phone, and so on, that she needed during the day. These recurring issues frustrated shelter staff, and Belinda too often became upset. She filed a complaint stating that "staff are keeping me from my medications that I need every day and it's affecting my health." Belinda's case manager referred her to the shelter's occupational therapist to assess Belinda and recommend how to address these issues with Belinda.	Diana is an adjunct professor in an occupational therapy program. As part of her academic role, she spends 2 days per week at a men's shelter. Her position is thus funded by the academic programs who hired her. In her role, Diana advocates for how occupational therapy can engage in a service role at the shelter. She primarily supervises Level I fieldwork rotations throughout the year on the 2 days she is in the shelter. She oversees both occupational therapists and occupational therapy assistant (OTA) students who work collaboratively to provide the groups. Diana's students spend the initial part of the semester determining the topic and structures of the groups to be delivered. Diana wants to make sure that the groups are relevant and address the needs of the shelter residents while still providing a learning experience for her students. As a consultant, she provides a report of the students' performances and the effectiveness of their interventions to shelter administration to advocate for more consistent occupational therapy services at the shelter. As a consultant, Diana is occasionally asked to complete evaluations for individuals specifically referred to her. Often these people are having difficulty managing within the shelter or following their case management plan. Other times the referral is to help the shelter better understand a resident's capacities to ensure a person's success when transitioning into housing.

TABLE 42-3 | Therapeutic Reasoning Questions About the Evaluation Processes

- What other services is the person receiving and what evaluation data already exists?
- What person factors may impact evaluation (e.g., will performance capacities or symptoms of mental illness impact the person's participation in the evaluation process)?
- Where will the evaluation take place and what resources are available in the spaces?
- What assessment tools are readily available, and which of these gather the data needed, include tasks that are familiar to the person, and are appropriate for their age/diagnoses, education, and literacy levels?
- What goal could be met by having the person engaging in occupational therapy services?
- What are the shelter's/program's/other providers' goals for the person being evaluated?

may be capable of within a less restricted environment. Limited private space and access to assessment tools that require functional performance may hinder the evaluation process. In these cases, OTPs must be cognizant to not make significant inferences or generalizations if performance of skills cannot be analyzed.

For an example of how an OTP might proceed in the evaluation process, see Table 42-5 where Belinda's story continues. See also Chapter 4: Person-Centered Evaluation and Appendix B: Index of Assessments. 🤝

Synthesizing the Evaluation and Setting Goals

Synthesizing involves consolidating evaluation data collected through the various assessment tools a practitioner employs. The endpoint of this analysis is the creation of evaluation

reports that share findings in a way that multiple audiences will find accessible. An OTP can use strategies such as those in Table 42-6 to produce a synthesis of evaluation data that is accessible to other shelter staff and demonstrate the distinct value of occupational therapy.

The OTP can use the person's performance on assessments to help identify appropriate settings in which to transition and the supports, services, and consultations necessary to move successfully into independent living. Although people experiencing homelessness may present with many needs and goals, it is important to help the individual prioritize two to three goal areas at a time. The OTP must be aware of what the person will be working on with other providers to encourage synergy and avoid redundancy. For example, a peer support specialist might be working with the person on using public transportation to go to appointments. Instead of prioritizing this as a goal, the OTP might collaborate with the staff if the person has difficulty learning the skill or if there is a strategy identified that supports the person while using public transit (such as a sensory-based coping skill to manage anxiety in crowded spaces). An example of how an OTP synthesized data from an evaluation of Belinda is included in Table 42-7.

Intervention

When selecting interventions in the shelter setting, OTPs must consider the specifics of the shelter setting they are in, the person's goals, and all relevant person or population factors. For example, in a shelter setting serving transition-age youth, occupational therapy may focus on developing work/employment skills, budgeting skills, and independent living skills. Conversely, a shelter that primarily serves middle-aged and older adults experiencing homelessness might focus on managing health and adapting to functional changes related to aging in addition to transitions into housing.

TABLE 42-4 | Therapeutic Reasoning Assessment Table: Functional Assessments Within a Shelter Setting

Which Tool?	Who Was This Tool Designed For?	What Is Required of the Person?	What Am I Measuring?	How Long Does It Take and Where Do I Administer This Tool?	Is the Tool Associated With a Practice Model?
Kohlman Evaluation of Living Skills (KELS; Kohlman Thomson & Robnett, 2016)	Initially designed for adults within inpatient psychiatric facilities. Newest version was tested in a variety of environments and adult populations.	Requires skills of reading and writing, self-care, safety and health, money management, community mobility, telephone use, and employment and leisure.	Standardized tool to evaluate both basic ADLs and IADLs by assessing living skills grouped into categories of self-care, safety and health, money management, community mobility, telephone, and work and leisure.	Typically, 30 minutes is needed. Easy to administer in tabletop setting or limited space setting. Requires computer to assess online banking skills.	No specific model but consistent with several models that include an emphasis on functional performance.
ManageMed Screening (Robnett et al., 2007)	Community dwelling adults are responsible for self-managing medications. Typically used in adults age 65 and older but appropriate for anyone who may have cognitive impairment and is responsible for medication management.	Ability to answer verbal questions regarding medications based on labels and handouts provided. Ability to manipulate medications, medication bottles, and a pill box.	A quick screen to determine if someone can manage a moderately difficult medication routine (Robnett et. al. 2007).	Typically, 20 minutes is needed. Easy to administer in tabletop setting or limited space setting. Requires basic reading abilities.	The development of this tool came from the lens of functional cognition. It models the cognitive processes assessed on the Mini-Mental Status Exam or Cognistat but includes assessment of functional skills and metacognition.
Performance Assessment of Self-Care Skills (PASS; Rogers & Holm, 2014)	Can be used with adolescents and adults with cognitive, physical, or behavioral impairments.	Person completes PASS tasks that are relevant to their life situation.	Person's ability to live independently and safely in the community is evaluated by assessing performance on various ADLs and IADLs.	Practitioner must have several types of items on hand but can also develop tasks that fit within setting. May not be private space to assess ADLs.	No specific model but consistent with several models that include an emphasis on functional performance.

TABLE 42-5 | Initiating the Evaluation Processes With Belinda

- The OTP chooses to begin evaluation with an informal conversation and a visit to Belinda's sleeping space in the shelter. Belinda reports feeling "groggy" in the morning because of her medications and that she has "difficulty waking up" even when the lights are on and staff are waking residents.
- Belinda says she often "feels rushed" in the morning and feels this is why she does not have enough time to shower, dress, and complete basic hygiene before it is time to leave the floor.
- Belinda describes "scrambling" to gather her things to leave the floor on time and to avoid being "written up" by staff. She often doesn't realize she is missing important personal items until she needs them later in the day. She is motivated to "figure this problem out" as she had missed appointments, left the floor without her bus pass, and has been inconsistent with her medications.
- Belinda identified three priorities: (1) avoid confrontations with staff about violating shelter rules, (2) take medications consistently to manage health, and (3) have what she needs throughout the day when she leaves the floor.
- The OTP and Belinda assess her bed area together and examine how Belinda organizes her belongings. The OTP observes that Belinda's bed area is disorganized (e.g., personal items and paperwork are mixed with clothes and plastic bags with her personal effects). Belinda's belongings spread to the adjacent bed area and impede the walkway space to her neighbor's bed. Belinda's medication is stored in pharmacy bottles and stuffed in a plastic bag in a locked storage area.
- When the OTP asks Belinda to demonstrate her morning routine, Belinda demonstrates decreased attention and executive functioning skills. She becomes distracted when coming across certain items and overall has difficulty finding her supplies. The OTP does not observe any motor limitations, though they note Belinda moves at a slow pace and her hands become shaky when she moves quickly or seems more distressed. She also fatigues easily as evidenced by her need to sit down after 5 to 6 minutes of standing.
- The OTP makes a mental note to use the Allen Cognitive Level Screen (ACLS-5) to assess Belinda's functional cognition, or the Assessment of Motor and Process Skills for a performance-based assessment to further evaluate motor and processing skills.

TABLE 42-6 | Strategies for Reporting Synthesized Data

- Report assessment results and document goals in terms that non–occupational therapists will understand. Convert occupational therapy language to terms commonly used in the setting, especially if the evaluation may be used by other providers to support the person in accessing resources, such as SSI or housing.
- Provide recommendations that are clear, and which can be understood and used by the individual and/or their providers to identify areas for skill development and support functional performance in the shelter. Recommendations may include strategies to support performance, adaptive equipment, and suggestions for community resources as appropriate.
- Occupational therapy goals should reflect the person's priorities and the needs of the program/shelter, as well as address occupational performance concerns identified during evaluation. Goals should be feasible to address and meet within the shelter setting.

TABLE 42-7 | Synthesizing Data to Generate Intervention Goals

- The OTP concludes that Belinda faces functional cognition challenges. She interprets her score of 4.8 on the ACLS-5 as a reflection of Belinda's need for support to establish routines and respond to new situations, particularly in the shelter environment where schedules are often inconsistent. On the Assessment of Motor and Process Skills (AMPS) ADL motor ability measure, the OTP observed mild to moderate clumsiness and increased physical effort and fatigue during ADL task performances. Belinda's ADL process ability measure was consistent with the ACLS-5 findings and reflected moderate to marked inefficiency and time–space disorganization.
- The OTP documents Belinda's decreased planning, organization, and sequencing. She notes a relative strength is that Belinda has a fair ability to problem-solve when given time to process information, but also notes that these skills decrease when Belinda is feeling anxious, stressed, or rushed. The AMPS confirmed that Belinda's fine motor skills and endurance were also decreased and exacerbated under stress and impacted her ability to continue her participation in ADLs.
- Based on the findings and incorporating Belinda's concerns, the OTP identified intervention goals which included:
  - Maintain her bed space to meet the criteria of the shelter.
  - Complete ADLs to Belinda's preference and with minimal anxiety.
  - Increase consistency in taking medications so that medications are taken on time at least 6 out of 7 days per week.
  - Leave her shelter bed each day with her essential belongings and medications at least 5 out of 7 days per week.

Although occupational therapy may be an ideal service to learn and expand skills (Synovec et al., 2020), not all interventions or occupations are feasible in this setting. For example, a person may have a goal to learn how to cook meals but does not have access to a space to do so. Instead of cooking, the OTP could focus on preparatory skills such as learning about meal planning or kitchen safety. Ideally, the person would have access to occupational therapy services when they transition into housing where they would have the opportunity to then learn cooking skills in their own kitchen. In Table 42-8, several questions are provided that can support an OTP's therapeutic reasoning when implementing interventions.

Interventions may be delivered through individual and group sessions, which may be "open" or "closed." In an "open"

TABLE 42-8 | Therapeutic Reasoning Questions for Implementing Interventions

- What evidence-based interventions can be applied or adapted for this person in this setting?
- Is this skill or occupation relevant to the person and consistent with their goals?
- Is this a skill or occupation that can be addressed within the shelter setting?
  - Is there space or supplies to work on the identified skills during occupational therapy sessions?
  - Is the person able to practice and apply skills learned in occupational therapy within the shelter setting?
  - What strategies can effectively and realistically be used within the shelter space?
  - How can the OTP support the person to use and apply skills outside of occupational therapy sessions?
- What resources or supplies does the person have access to that can be used?
  - If supplies are a limitation, are there resources that can help the person acquire the supplies?
- What resources are available within the shelter setting that can be used for the intervention?
- Is another provider or staff person already addressing these skills with the person?
  - If yes, what are they working on? Has it been effective?
  - How might the OTP collaborate with this provider?

group, anyone can attend any week; a "closed" group, in contrast, is one in which a set number of participants will join each week. In open groups, the topic and intervention should be such that the knowledge and skills can be gained within one group session, whereas closed groups are better for more topic continuity. A closed group might focus on life skill development such as the Life Skills Modules discussed further in this section. Individual sessions will be based on the goals determined by the evaluation process and may occur within the shelter or relevant community settings. In Table 42-9, Belinda's story is continued; reflect on the identified goals that Belinda and her OTP agreed on.

Discharge Planning

Discharge may be complicated as shelter residents may stay for long durations while waiting for housing. A resident may need to pause or discontinue occupational therapy services until they are closer to transitioning into housing, where the transition and change would require a need to reengage in services. Considerations for discharge planning are reviewed in Table 42-10. The conclusion of Belinda's case in Table 42-11 demonstrates discharge and transition planning within a shelter setting.

Theoretical Approaches for Interventions

Occupational therapy in shelter settings is often guided by public health approaches and adult learning strategies. Common and successful approaches discussed here include trauma-informed care, situated learning theory, and harm reduction. Within this broader framework, OTPs use specific approaches such as the Model of Human Occupation

TABLE 42-9	Implementing Interventions With Belinda

- To address self-organization of belongings
  - The OTP and Belinda first received permission from staff to access Belinda's bed area to organize and clean out the bed space and items.
  - Essential items were situated in one space in a locked drawer near the bed.
  - Colored tape was used to mark where items should go in the drawer at the end of the day.
  - The OTP helped Belinda decide what items were unneeded and these were discarded.
  - Plastic bags were reused to sort/organize/separate additional belongings within her drawer.
- To address medication management
  - The OTP worked with Belinda to learn how to utilize a pillbox for medications that she needed to have with her throughout the day.
  - The OTP coordinated with Belinda's psychiatrist who recommended to take nighttime meds 1 hour earlier to decrease morning drowsiness.
- To minimize rushing with ADLs and ensure Belinda had essential items for the day
  - The OTP helped Belinda hang a checklist by her bed with essential items (identified by Belinda) that needed to be double checked before leaving the bed area each morning.
  - Belinda agreed to the OTP's suggestion to shift her routines to shower at night and pick out/lay out her clothes for the next day.
  - The OTP provided education on energy conservation and how to use deep breathing to manage distress and fatigue.
  - The OTP communicated strategies to floor staff and case managers to help with follow-through and show that their concerns were addressed.

TABLE 42-10	Therapeutic Reasoning Questions for Discharge Planning

- Have the identified occupational therapy goals been met?
- Are there additional areas of need that could be addressed? Would the person benefit from a new testing measure or reevaluation?
- What does the person need in preparation for discharge from occupational therapy services to be able to continue the strategies and skills developed?
- What needs to be communicated to the shelter staff as part of the discharge process?

Important note: Ensure the person is aware of the discharge plan and has adequate time to prepare for discontinuing with occupational therapy to ensure the discharge or transition is trauma informed. Considerations for transitioning the person:
- Is the person transitioning from the shelter or to other services (such as permanent supportive housing)?
- What do other staff need to support the person to implement skills?
- Is the person transitioning to a new occupational therapy in a different setting, and have the goals and plan been communicated?

If the goals have not been met while the person is in the shelter:
- Are the originally established goals feasible to be met within the shelter space?
- Is it more appropriate to address these when the person transitions from the shelter?
- If the goals are not feasible to be met, is it because of the person's capacity to complete the skill independently?
  - If so, the OTP needs to work with the person's team to identify and establish ongoing supports as appropriate, especially for a transition into a shelter space.
  - Have the person's skills appeared to decrease since the initial evaluation, and is a new evaluation warranted to assess for the change?
  - Would the person benefit from a medical evaluation for potential health changes impacting functional skills?

TABLE 42-11	Implementing Interventions With Belinda

Once the OTP had supported the organization process over 1 week, they met with Belinda twice a week for 3 weeks to assess her follow-through on changed routines, review strategies, and to support problem-solving for new encounters.

Belinda was on a housing waiting list and was approved to stay in the shelter for another 60 days while waiting for housing. The OTP followed up with Belinda one additional session to confirm no new needs had come up, and then Belinda was discharged from occupational therapy services. Belinda's case manager was reminded she could refer Belinda again as needed or when she was transitioning into housing to address self-organization in preparation for housing.

(MOHO; Taylor, 2017) or the Allen Cognitive Disabilities Model (Allen, 2016). An example of how these approaches can be integrated to complement an occupational therapy life skills curriculum is included here while the occupational therapy models are explained in multiple other chapters in this text.

Trauma-Informed Approaches

Trauma-informed approaches (trauma-informed care) are strengths-based service delivery approaches emphasizing physical, psychological, and emotional safety for survivors of trauma and their providers. It considers the impact of trauma and creates opportunities for survivors to rebuild a sense of control and empowerment (Hopper et al., 2010). This approach focuses on anticipating and avoiding institutional processes and individual practices that are likely to retraumatize individuals with histories of trauma, and it upholds the importance of consumer participation in the development, delivery, and evaluation of services (SAMHSA, 2015). Trauma-informed care includes six basic principles:

1. Safety
2. Trustworthiness and transparency
3. Peer support
4. Collaboration and mutuality
5. Empowerment, voice, and choice
6. Cultural, historical, and gender issues

Trauma-informed care serves as an organizing framework for creating an environment in which people who have not experienced others as welcoming or safe can engage in treatment designed to meet their needs. People experiencing trauma often develop characteristic behaviors and survival coping strategies such as learning to push others away to avoid being a victim or sleeping on top of one's belongings to keep them from being stolen during the night. These behaviors, which help the person survive being homeless, may appear odd and are often ineffective in other contexts; however, understanding how and why they exist enhances the OTP's ability to help the individual develop healthier alternatives.

Helfrich, Peters, and Chan (2011) found that while trauma symptoms decreased during participation in a life skills intervention, they spiked during times of transition, such as moving out of a shelter or into a new home. The *Trauma-Informed Organizational Toolkit* (Guarino et al., 2009) is a resource for organizations and service delivery settings to become trauma-informed. The toolkit includes the Self-Assessment and User's Guide as well as a consumer evaluation. The reader is referred to an Apply It Now activity at the end of this chapter to learn more about this approach. See also Chapter 5: Trauma-Informed Practice and Chapter 25: Trauma- and Stressor-Related Disorders. 🤝

Evidence-Based Practice

Functional Cognition in Unhoused Individuals

OTPs can play an important role in evaluating and addressing functional cognition within the unhoused population.

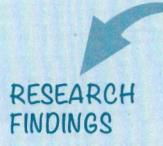

RESEARCH FINDINGS

Functional cognition is "the cognitive ability to perform daily life tasks; incorporating metacognition, executive function, other domains of cognitive functioning, performance skills (e.g., motor skills that support action), and performance patterns" (e.g., habits, routines; Giles et al., 2020, p. 2). Functional cognition encompasses the range of cognitive impairments identified in adults experiencing homelessness (Depp et al., 2015; Stone et al., 2019). Within the shelter setting, a person may not be identified as having cognitive impairment yet may struggle to meet shelter rules or guidelines because of their cognition. When someone is identified as having a cognitive impairment, their ability to live independently may be questioned and may impact their ability to access housing or other services. Occupational therapy has a distinct role in evaluating and addressing functional cognition within this population.

APPLICATIONS

➡ Although most occupational therapy referrals identified cognitive impairments, individuals' functional skills varied (Synovec, 2020).

➡ Performance-based assessments identified that cognition was related to performance of ADLs/IADLs, but not other occupational domains (Synovec et al., 2022).

➡ Functional cognition assessments should be used to identify existing skills and supports needed for housing transition, shifting away from a deficits-based approach that may keep individuals from moving into housing.

➡ OTPs should utilize their skills to evaluate for functional cognition in people experiencing homelessness, with the goal of identifying skills and supports needed to access and transition into housing.

REFERENCES

Depp, C. A., Vella, L., Orff, H. J., & Twamley, E. W. (2015). A quantitative review of cognitive functioning in homeless adults. *The Journal of Nervous and Mental Disease, 203*(2), 126–131. https://doi.org/10.1097/NMD.0000000000000248

Giles, G. M., Edwards, D. F., Baum, C., Furniss, J., Skidmore, E., Wolf, T., & Leland, N. E. (2020). Making functional cognition a professional priority. *The American Journal of Occupational Therapy, 74*(1), 7401090010p1–7401090010p6. https://doi.org/10.5014/ajot.2020.741002

Stone, B., Dowling, S., & Cameron, A. (2019). Cognitive impairment and homelessness: A scoping review. *Health & Social Care in the Community, 27*(4), e125–e142. https://doi.org/10.1111/hsc.12682

Synovec, C. (2020). Evaluating cognitive impairment and its relation to function in a population of individuals who are homeless. *Occupational Therapy in Mental Health, 36*(4), 330–352. https://doi.org/10.1080/0164212X.2020.1838400

Synovec, C. E., Westover, L., & Boland, L. (2022). Evaluation of functional cognition in people experiencing homelessness: A scoping review. *American Journal of Occupational Therapy, 76*(Suppl. 1), 7610505122p1. https://doi.org/10.5014/ajot.2022.76S1-PO122

Situated Learning Theory

Social cognitive learning theory using a situated learning approach provides an intervention model wherein adult learners gain knowledge and skills by immersing themselves in a social learning community (Lave, 1988; Ormrod, 2020). Situated learning places the learner in contexts that reflect the real world with application to everyday situations (Helfrich, 2023). The occupational therapy student will find this reflected in fieldwork: The supervisor explains the intervention to be performed, demonstrates, and then the student tries it. It is a familiar process for learning many life skills. The process follows a logical sequence of providing information, observing the skill performed, and practicing the skill in a desired context (Helfrich, 2023). Situated learning allows for:

- An individual's choice and involvement to address those skills the person wants and needs to learn
- Didactic learning with modeling and practice in a context preferred by the individual
- Evaluation of the skill in a specific context to identify barriers and supports needed to be successful in the skill
- An individualized process that considers the person's level of functioning

Harm Reduction

The literature describes the benefits of harm reduction principles and strategies for people who are homeless and for people with mental illness and substance addictions in a variety of settings (Logan & Marlatt, 2010); however, harm reduction is also being applied to health care (Hawk et al., 2017) and occupational therapy practice (Helfrich & Halverson, 2011). Harm reduction emphasizes the importance of accepting a behavior or value without judgment to reduce the harm associated with a risky behavior. Rather than attempting to reduce or eliminate the behavior itself, the individual's choice to engage in certain behaviors is honored. The focus of the intervention is on setting realistic goals in treatment. The International Harm Reduction Association (IHRA) defines **harm reduction** as: "policies, programmes and practices that aim primarily to reduce the adverse health, social and economic consequences of the use of legal and illegal psychoactive drugs without necessarily reducing drug consumption" (IHRA, 2010, p. 1).

The five key principles and ideas of harm reduction are:

1. Accepting that drugs and risky behaviors are a part of society that will never be eliminated
2. Placing the focus on reducing the harm associated with risky behaviors rather than reducing or eliminating the behavior itself
3. Meeting the individual where they are at and working with the individual to minimize the effects of a harmful behavior
4. Honoring individual choices, resisting condemnation, and refraining from judgment
5. Setting practical goals by focusing on immediate, achievable objectives rather than abstinence or other unrealistic expectations

Three areas of harm reduction were identified by Helfrich and Hellman (2013) in their qualitative study of individuals

---

BOX 42-3 ■ Applying Harm Reduction Principles With Blanche

Blanche, a client in a life skills program at a single room occupancy (SRO) residence, was very distrustful of authority figures and institutions. When she entered therapy, she was having her Social Security check mailed to her sister's house, which was a 90-minute bus ride away. She would cash her monthly check, buy alcohol and food, pay bills, and then hide the rest in her room. She attended life skills groups on money management and community safety. She learned about banking and direct deposit. After making significant changes in therapy she reported, "It was a positive experience. . . . I used to have my Social Security check mailed to my sister's house, but since then I've gotten direct deposit. I write a check for the rent first and then get enough to do a little extra shopping, and then I don't have a lot of money in my room."

Using direct deposit reduced Blanche's financial, physical, and psychological harm. She experienced *financial harm reduction* by writing her rent check first, rather than having cash that she might otherwise spend on other things. Limiting her access to cash helped her limit the money she spent on alcohol, which provided *physical harm reduction* as she drank less. Finally, she experienced *psychological harm reduction* because she no longer had to worry about her room being robbed.

---

who were or had been homeless: financial harm reduction, physical harm reduction, and psychosocial harm reduction. Financial harm reduction includes strategies aimed at reducing the financial harm associated with attaining and maintaining necessary goods and services. Physical harm reduction consists of strategies intended to reduce the physical harm associated with behaviors, choices, and living situations. Psychosocial harm reduction includes strategies that are meant to reduce symptoms such as anxiety, stress, guilt, or self-blame. Examples of how to apply harm reduction principles are included in a case story in Box 42-3.

Life Skills: An Evidence-Based Intervention

Occupational therapy treatment for individuals who are homeless or unstably housed is targeted at regaining or developing independent living skills. In response to a lack of resources available for adults who desire to learn the practical life skills necessary to live independently in the community, Helfrich (2006a, 2006b, 2006c, 2006d) developed an evidence-based, manualized, life skills intervention curriculum that includes four critical areas:

1. The *Food and Nutrition Management* module features activities to learn strategies for preparing healthy meals and snacks, eating healthily on a budget, and identifying food resources in the community.
2. The *Money Management* module features strategies for budgeting, saving money, and protecting one's credit and identity.
3. The *Home and Self-Care* module features activities to increase knowledge and skills on topics such as personal hygiene, management of health conditions,

maintaining one's living space, and obtaining and caring for one's clothing.

4. The *Safe Community Participation* module features topics such as personal, home, and community safety, as well as how to handle emergencies.

The curriculum content was created in partnership with individuals who were homeless, individuals who were transitioning to housing, service delivery workers from a range of disciplines who work with individuals for whom life skills are challenging, peer leaders, peer recovery specialists, and various consultants to create an effective, feasible, and age-appropriate curriculum. The curriculum is designed to be implemented in six group sessions with an individual workbook to help participants individualize the group content at their own pace. Each module includes a participant workbook and facilitator manuals for both group and individual sessions. The life skills intervention has demonstrated effectiveness with individuals experiencing homelessness at various cognitive levels (Helfrich, Chan, & Sabol, 2011) and stages of change (Helfrich, Chan, Simpson, & Sabol, 2011).

The intervention models and techniques described earlier can be used to complement and inform an occupational therapy life skills curriculum. For example, an OTP employing a trauma-informed care approach would remain open and nonjudgmental, recognizing how trauma may have impacted a person's occupations and habits related to food, finances, self-care, and safety in the community.

Using situated learning approaches, OTPs would help guide group interventions by ensuring everyone can participate meaningfully in the group activity. Practitioners would create opportunities for consumers to assume different roles within a group session depending on their life experiences. Approaching life skill development from a harm reduction stance conveys an accepting attitude and realistic expectations. This is especially critical if the OTP is to develop rapport with an individual who is homeless, has experienced trauma, and may have little reason to trust anyone in authority. This approach requires the OTP to accept the person's choices when they reduce harm, even when these choices may not reduce or eliminate behaviors that are maladaptive.

Each approach allows the OTP to view the individual holistically and collaboratively to determine their treatment needs and priorities. These are consumer-driven approaches that recognize an individual as the central force in determining the direction for treatment. None of these models specifically dictates treatment priorities; rather, they encourage the OTP to provide opportunities for the person to direct their own care.

For example, an OTP was working on money management with three men living in shelters. She taught the men to use coupons and scan ads for cigarettes to teach them how to save money and avoid scams while not giving up their smoking habits. When her supervisor questioned the ethics of using cigarette coupons in a life skills intervention, she explained her narrative clinical reasoning: All three men said they would NOT join the group if she was going to tell them they had to stop buying cigarettes. She engaged them by using harm reduction principles of decreasing the *financial harm* of their habit. An unexpected secondary *physical harm* reduction occurred when the men learned that rolling their own cigarettes was least expensive and ultimately used less tobacco, thus decreasing their nicotine intake.

Transition into Housing

Preparation and the transition into housing is a critical time for support and intervention. Although the move from homelessness into housing is a positive change to improve quality of life and health, it can also be challenging as the person moves into a new environment, may lose or change professional supports, and be located away from previous social support networks.

In response to this need and recognizing the role of occupational therapy in supporting people in navigating life transitions, Marshall and colleagues (2020) established *Bridging the Transition From Homelessness to Housed: A Social Justice Framework to Guide the Practice of Occupational Therapists*. This framework was established through evidence-based practice and by engaging with people with lived experience of homelessness and OTPs working with this population (Marshall et al., 2020). The framework identifies Four Processes of Leaving Homelessness. They are specifically identified as processes, not steps or phases, as the transition is often not linear, and transition may happen in phases. The Four Processes are:

- *Survival:* This process describes a period when a person is homeless. This phase covers the time when the person is most likely focused on occupations of survival.
- *Adaptation:* In this process, one has recently left homelessness and has been living in transitional or permanent housing. The person is adapting to living in a new environment outside the shelter or the street.
- *Integration:* During this process, individuals who have left homelessness have been living in transitional or permanent housing and have overcome the initial period of transition to being housed.
- *Precarity:* This is the process during which one's tenancy is at risk, which can be experienced by a person who has been homeless before, but also by a person who has never lost their housing. This framework recognizes that loss of one's tenancy can be prevented; however, if appropriate supports are not available, the person may become homeless or return to homelessness, and will proceed through the processes of *Survival, Adaptation,* and *Integration.*

Within each of these processes, there are four occupational priorities:

- Time use and participation in meaningful activity
- Managing mental health and substance use
- Emotional growth and change
- Creating connection and community

The framework does not prescribe specific interventions although it offers examples of how OTPs may address each of the priorities within each phase, based on the person's needs, experiences, and available resources. OTPs within the shelter and transitional shelter setting primarily focus on the processes of Survival and Adaptation, providing opportunity and skill-building to facilitate and promote engagement in each of the occupational priorities. Development of skills and continued support once housed can contribute to prevention of precarity and housing loss. See Chapter 31: The Home Environment: Permanent Supported Housing.

Here's the Point

- Occupational therapy has a valuable role within the homeless shelter setting. In order to provide effective and supportive services, OTPs should understand the multiple complex factors that contribute to someone becoming homeless and how these factors continue to impact engagement in daily life roles.

- OTPs can be a vital resource supporting those who are unhoused in identifying and engaging in meaningful occupations and ideally supporting the transition into permanent housing.

- People who are homeless are a heterogeneous population and may have a variety of physical and mental health–care issues.

- Individuals who are homeless may be seen in a variety of shelter settings, and the services they receive are dependent on the shelter structure and staffing. Individuals living in temporary settings frequently have significant needs related to independent living, child-care skills, and work skills.

- Emergency shelters, transitional housing, and medical respite programs are practice areas OTPs can expand into; the Affordable Care Act creates opportunities to support this expansion.

- Trauma-informed care, situated learning theory, and harm reduction are all intervention approaches that complement occupational therapy models and emphasize the provision of a respectful, empowering environment for intervention.

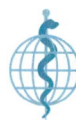 Visit the online resource center at FADavis.com to access the videos.

Apply It Now

1. Life Skills Acquisition Exercise

Listed in the table that follows are five common IADLs that most people are expected to complete. Please consider each one and complete the worksheet based on your own experience. *After* you have filled in the table, answer the reflective questions that follow.

Life Skill	Where Did You Learn This?	Who Taught You?	When Did You Learn This?	Do You Currently Receive Any Assistance With This Activity?
How to open a bank account				
How to grocery shop on a budget				
How to repair your clothing				
How to manage your health-care needs				
How to do your laundry				

Reflective Questions

- How would having a serious mental illness impact learning these skills?
- How would living in an institution impact learning these skills?
- How would living with an abusive partner who controlled all your actions impact learning these skills?
- How would growing up living on the street or in a shelter impact your ability to learn these skills?

Learning strategy developed by Christine Helfrich.

2. Count Your Losses

The experience of individuals who are in a domestic violence situation can be very challenging. This exercise will help you get a glimpse of how one might feel if they were homeless because of domestic violence.

- Take out a piece of paper and number it 1 to 5.
- Write down the name of your best friend after number 1.
- Write down your most supportive coworker after number 2.
- Write down your closest family member after number 3.
- Write down your favorite possession after number 4.
- Write down your dream for the future after number 5.

You are in an abusive relationship that you have tried to keep hidden from your friends, family, and coworkers. Last night, your partner came home in a rage and punched your face until you were bleeding because you did not have the house clean. Your 2-year-old child's toys were not all put away. After beating you, your partner threatened to beat your child for being so messy with their toys. You keep your child safe from your partner (at the expense of a few more bruises) and vow to yourself that you will leave the relationship as soon as it is safe to go.

- You call your best friend that night and ask if you and your child can come and stay because your partner has beaten you and threatened to hurt your child. They ask you why you were beaten, and after you explain, they tell you that your partner is a really good person and that you must have deserved to be hit. They advise you to stay in the relationship and keep your house cleaner. You end the phone call feeling ashamed and hurt and wonder why your friend cannot understand what you are going through.

You have just lost your best friend. Tear your best friend's name off your paper and crumple it up.

■ You decide to stay at home that night even though you feel very afraid for the safety of both you and your child. In the morning, you try to cover your bruises and cuts with makeup. You take your child to day care and go to work. When you get there, your coworkers ask you what happened. You decide to tell them, and they respond similarly to your friend the night before. During lunch with coworkers, they give you the cold shoulder and tell you that you should not be making such accusations about your partner. When you try to explain, they tell you that it is probably your fault for not being a better partner.

You have just lost your support system at work. Tear off your most supportive coworker's name and crumple up the paper.

■ You go home very upset; fortunately, your partner is not there, so you call your closest family member (say, your sibling) and explain why you are upset. When they finish listening to you, they tell you that you're crazy and ask what you expected by trying to work full time, go to school, and maintain a household for your partner. They tell you they are sorry and wish they could help, but just can't. You need to learn to be a better partner and parent yourself. You're going to have to figure out what to do with this one: maybe reparative therapy is an option.

You've just lost your closest family member and what you thought would be an option for shelter. Tear off your family member's name and crumple up the paper.

■ You see your partner walking up to the front door with flowers, and you realize you must leave now or never. As you start to gather your things frantically in a bag, you wonder where you will spend the night. As your partner walks in the front door, you walk out the back. You realize that you have left behind your favorite possession, but you are too afraid to turn back.

You've just lost your favorite possession. Tear off your favorite possession and crumple up the paper.

■ You now realize that your dreams are being destroyed: Your most basic needs are not even being met, you have no money, no financial support, only the clothes on your back and a few personal belongings in a grocery bag. You wonder if you should just go back and try to make it work.

You have just lost all your hopes and dreams for the future. Tear off your dreams and crumple up the last piece of paper.

Reflective Questions

■ How did it feel to do this exercise?
■ How did it feel to lose the things you lost?
■ Were some things more difficult to lose than others?
■ How will you help a person dealing with these issues?
Learning strategies adapted by Christine Helfrich.

3. Trauma-Informed Organizational Self-Assessment and Consumer Self-Assessment

Download the *Trauma-Informed Organizational Toolkit* (Guarino et al., 2009) from http://www.air.org/sites/default /files/downloads/report/Trauma-Informed_Organizational _Toolkit_0.pdf and familiarize yourself with the organizational and consumer self-assessment forms. Select either an organization that provides services to individuals who may have experienced trauma or a consumer who participates in a program that identifies itself as providing trauma-informed services and complete the following:

■ Visit a setting serving individuals experiencing homelessness in your community and arrange a meeting with the director to complete the trauma-informed self-assessment.
■ If you are doing fieldwork or observation in a setting that identifies itself as providing trauma-informed care, ask permission to have a consumer complete the self-assessment from the *Trauma-Informed Organizational Toolkit*.
■ Identify situations in which people's trauma symptoms may be exacerbated by everyday life activities when they participate in treatment.

Reflective Questions

■ What was the individual's response to the completed self-assessment?
■ What surprised you?
■ What did you learn?
■ How can you apply trauma-informed care in your current practice setting?
■ Identify strategies to improve at least three items on the self-assessment.

4. The Role of Occupational Therapy in Shelters for the Unhoused

■ Identify three service agencies within your community that serve individuals who are homeless or at risk of becoming homeless.
■ Select one of these agencies, and identify the specific services they offer, including if they offer occupational therapy services.
■ Identify what current roles or positions an OTP could fill and explain how an OTP could enhance this identified role.
■ Identify how an OTP could supplement existing services and the types of interventions that would be beneficial to the people.
■ Develop a "pitch" to the board of the organization as to how an OTP could benefit their people and program, and how this role could be integrated and funded.

5. Video Exercise: Mary's Lived Experience as an Unhoused Individual and Her Occupational Therapist's Perspective

Pair up with another student in your class or form a small group of students. Access and watch the "Mary's Lived Experience as an Unhoused Individual and Her Occupational Therapist's Perspective" video at the online resource center at FADavis.com. Then, discuss and together answer the following questions.

Reflective Questions

■ Why do you think occupational therapy services were so transformative for Mary? What is it about the structure and dynamics of occupational therapy–facilitated groups that can sometimes make the experience more powerful than one-to-one services?
■ One of the main skills that Mary worked on both in the occupational therapy group and during her one-to-one occupational therapy sessions was emotional regulation. How do you think improving her emotion regulation helped Mary gain an overall sense of stability?
■ How did Mary use the skills she gained from occupational therapy services to help her peers with a lived experience? How can OTPs facilitate peer-to-peer interactions and colearning?

Resources

Books

- Helfrich, C. A. (2001). *Domestic abuse across the lifespan.* Haworth Press.
- Kidder, T. (2023). *Rough sleepers.* Random House.
- Lopez, S. (2010). *The soloist: A lost dream, an unlikely friendship, and the redemptive power of music.* The Berkley Publishing Group.
- Swenson Miller, K., Herzberg, G. L., & Ray, S. A. (2007). *Homelessness in America: Perspectives, characterizations and considerations for occupational therapy.* Taylor & Francis.

Movies

- Bailey, M. (Producer), Gere, R. (Producer), Inglee, L. (Producer), Kaplan, C. (Producer), Pohlad, B. (Producer), Walson, E. (Producer), & Moverman, O. (Director). (2014). *Time out of mind* [Motion Picture]. Gere Productions.
- Fellner, E. (Producer), Heffron, E. (Producer), Foster, G. (Producer), Skoll, J. (Producer), Davies, J. (Producer), & Wright, J. (Director). (2009). *The soloist* [Motion Picture]. Dreamworks Video. (Special features on the DVD include the documentary featurette: *One Size Does Not Fit All: Addressing Homelessness in Los Angeles.*)

Organizations

- ARC4Justice: https://arc4justice.org. This organization's goal is to advance a vision of society where the systemic roots of inequities in housing and community systems have been addressed; where power and resources are held and allocated by those who have been most marginalized; where all cultures are appreciated; and where wholeness, rather than scarcity, is the guiding principle.
- The National Alliance to End Homelessness: http://www.endhomelessness.org. This organization works to prevent and end homelessness by advocating for improved federal homelessness policy; building capacity to assist communities to develop best practices; and educating policymakers, practitioners, and the public about homelessness and its solutions.
- The National Child Traumatic Stress Network: http://www.nctsn.org. This organization provides information on evidence-based mental health interventions.
- National Coalition for the Homeless (NCH): http://www.nationalhomeless.org. This is a national network of people who are currently experiencing or who have experienced homelessness, activists and advocates, community-based and faith-based service providers, and others committed to a single mission. The NCH engages in public education, policy advocacy, and grassroots organizing with work in the following four areas: housing justice, economic justice, health-care justice, and civil rights.
- National Harm Reduction Coalition: https://harmreduction.org. This organization works to uplift the voices and experiences of people who use drugs and bring harm reduction strategies to scale.

Videos

- "Occupational Therapy Approaches in a Shelter for Unaccompanied Refugee Youth" video. In this video, occupational therapist Claudette Fette shares the impactful work she, volunteer students, and staff performed in a massive unaccompanied minor shelter in Texas in 2021. Many of the minors, mostly from Central America, had histories of trauma, and the conditions in the shelter were dismal—lack of meaningful occupations, bullying, untrained staff, and so on. Claudette describes her approach to assessing the environment, training staff, recruiting volunteers, responding to the minors' trauma responses, and creating and supporting occupations and leisure activities. Access the video at the online resource center at FADavis.com.
- "Student Perceptions of Bias and Stigma" video. In this video, four occupational therapy students reflect on how they came to recognize and work through their own biases against people who are unhoused. Each describes meeting and working in a student-run occupational therapy clinic with individuals who were unhoused and/or experiencing mental illness. They explain how engaging with these individuals and learning their stories became the impetus for transformative learning. Access the video at the online resource center at FADavis.com.
- "Leisure Occupations for Unhoused Individuals" video. In this video, Kailin, an occupational therapist who works in community mental health and homeless services, describes the power of leisure activities to the individuals whom she serves. Kailin talks about the barriers to engaging in leisure that often exist for people who are unhoused. She explains how she integrates the evaluation of leisure in her occupational profile and provides several examples of realistic leisure activities that OTPs can use to support individuals' mental health. Access the video at the online resource center at FADavis.com.

References

Adair, C. E., Streiner, D. L., Barnhart, R., Kopp, B., Veldhuizen, S., Patterson, M., Aubry, T., Lavoie, J., Sareen, J., LeBlanc, S. R., & Goering, P. (2017). Outcome trajectories among homeless individuals with mental disorders in a multisite randomized controlled trial of housing first. *The Canadian Journal of Psychiatry, 62*(1), 30–39. https://doi.org/10.1177/0706743716645302

Allen, C. K. (2016). *Allen App.* Version 0.8. [Mobile application software]. Retrieved from https://acdmweb.com

Allen, M. E., Call, K. T., Beebe, T. J., McAlpine, D. D., & Johnson, P. J. (2017). Barriers to care and healthcare utilization among the publicly insured. *Medical Care, 55,* 207–214. https://doi.org/10.1097/MLR.0000000000000644

American Occupational Therapy Association. (2020). Occupational therapy practice framework: Domain and process—Fourth edition. *American Journal of Occupational Therapy, 74*(Suppl. 2), 7412410010p1–7412410010p87. https://doi.org/10.5014/ajot.2020.74S2001

Aubry, T., Goering, P., Veldhuizen, S., Adair, C. E., Bourque, J., Distasio, J., Latimer, E., Stergiopoulos, V., Somers, J., Streiner, D. L., & Tsemberis, S. (2016). A multiple-city RCT of Housing First with Assertive Community Treatment for homeless Canadians with serious mental illness. *Psychiatric Services (Washington, D.C.), 67*(3), 275–281. https://doi.org/10.1176/appi.ps.201400587

Aviles de Bradley, A. M. (2011). Unaccompanied homeless youth: Intersections of homelessness, school experiences and educational policy. *Child & Youth Services, 32*(2), 155–172. https://doi.org/10.1080/0145935X.2011.583176

Ayano, G., Solomon, M., Tsegay, L., Yohannes, K., & Abraha, M. (2020). A systematic review and meta-analysis of the prevalence of post-traumatic stress disorder among homeless people. *Psychiatric Quarterly, 91,* 949–963. https://doi.org/10.1007/s11126-020-09746-1

Aykanian, A., & Fogel, S. J. (2019). The criminalization of homelessness. In H. Larkin, A. Aykanian, & C. L. Streeter (Eds.), *Homelessness prevention and intervention in social work* (pp. 185–205). Springer. https://doi.org/10.1007/978-3-030-03727-7_9

Baams, L., Wilson, B. D. M., & Russell, S.T. (2019). LGBTQ youth in unstable housing and foster care. *Pediatrics, 143,* e20174211. https://doi.org/10.1542/peds.2017-4211

Baker Collins, S., Fudge Schormans, A., Watt, L., Idems, B. & Wilson, T. (2018) The invisibility of disability for homeless youth. *Journal of Social Distress and Homelessness, 27*(2), 99–109. https://doi.org/10.1080/10530789.2018.1480892

Bassuk, E. L., DeCandia, C. J., Beach, C. A., & Berman, F. (2014). *America's youngest outcasts: A report card on child homelessness.* National Center on Family Homelessness. http://www.air.org/sites/default/files/downloads/report/Americas-Youngest-Outcasts-Child-Homelessness-Nov2014.pdf

Brown., M., & McCann, E. (2020). Homelessness and people with intellectual disabilities: A systematic review of the international research evidence. *Journal of Applied Research in Intellectual Disabilities, 34*(2), 390–401. https://doi.org/10.1111/jar.12815

Brown, R. T., Hemati, K., Riley, E. D., Lee, C. T., Ponath, C., Tieu, L., Guzman, D., & Kushel, M. B. (2017). Geriatric conditions in a population-based sample of older homeless adults. *The Gerontologist, 57*(4), 757–766. https://doi.org/10.1093/geront/gnw011

Carter, G. R. (2011). From exclusion to destitution: Race, affordable housing, and homelessness. *Cityscape, 13*(1), 33–70. https://doi.org/10.2139/ssrn.1808950

Clark, R. E., Weinreb, L., Flahive, J. M., & Seifert, R. W. (2019). Infants exposed to homelessness: Health, health care use, and health spending from birth to age 6. *Health Affairs, 38,* 721–728. https://doi.org/10.1377/hlthaff.2019.00090

Coombs, N. C., Meriwether, W. E., Caringi, J., & Newcomer, S. R. (2021). Barriers to healthcare access among U.S. adults with mental health challenges: A population-based study. *SSM - Population Health, 15,* 100847. https://doi.org/10.1016/j.ssmph.2021.100847

Definitions: Emergency shelter. 24 C.F.R. § 91.5. (2023). https://www.ecfr.gov/current/title-24/subtitle-A/part-91/subpart-A/section-91.5

Department of Housing and Urban Development. (2015). Homeless emergency assistance and rapid transition to housing: Defining "chronically homeless." 80 *Federal Register,* 75791–75806 (24 C.F.R. Pts. 91 and 578). https://www.federalregister.gov/documents/2015/12/04/2015-30473/homeless-emergency-assistance-and-rapid-transition-to-housing-defining-chronically-homeless

Department of Housing and Urban Development. (2021). *Equal access for transgender people: Supporting inclusive housing and shelters.* https://files.hudexchange.info/resources/documents/Equal-Access-for-Transgender-People-Supporting-Inclusive-Housing-and-Shelters.pdf

Department of Housing and Urban Development. (2023). *Homeless definition.* https://files.hudexchange.info/resources/documents/HomelessDefinition_RecordkeepingRequirementsandCriteria.pdf

Department of Housing and Urban Development. (2024). *Continuum of Care (CoC) program eligibility requirements.* https://www.hudexchange.info/programs/coc/coc-program-eligibility-requirements

Depp, C. A., Vella, L., Orff, H. J., & Twamley, E. W. (2015). A quantitative review of cognitive functioning in homeless adults. *The Journal of Nervous and Mental Disease, 203*(2), 126–131. https://doi.org/10.1097/NMD.0000000000000248

de Sousa, T., Andrichik, A., Cuellar, M., Marson, J., Prestera, E., & Rush, K. (2022). *The 2022 Annual Homeless Assessment Report (AHAR) to Congress: PART 1—Point-in-time estimates of homelessness.* The U.S. Department of Housing and Urban Development, Office of Community Planning and Development. https://www.huduser.gov/portal/sites/default/files/pdf/2022-AHAR-Part-1.pdf

Diamond, B., Burns, R., & Bowen, K. (2022). Criminalizing homelessness: Circumstances surrounding criminal trespassing and people experiencing homelessness. *Criminal Justice Policy Review, 33*(6), 563–583. https://doi.org/10.1177/08874034211067130

Fazel, S., Geddes, J. R., & Kushel, M. (2014). The health of homeless people in high-income countries: Descriptive epidemiology, health consequences, and clinical and policy recommendations. *Lancet (London, England), 384*(9953), 1529–1540. https://doi.org/10.1016/S0140-6736(14)61132-6

Fenway Institute. (2020). *Supportive housing and health services for LGBTQIA+ youth experiencing homelessness: Promising*

practices. https://www.lgbtqiahealtheducation.org/wp-content/uploads/2020/07/Supportive-Housing-and-Health-Services-for-LGBTQIA-Youth-Experiencing-Homelessness.pdf

Fenway Institute, Corporation for Supportive Housing, National Center for Equitable Care for Elders, & National Health Care for the Homeless Council. (2021). *Housing, health, and LGBTQIA+ older adults 2021.* https://nhchc.org/wp-content/uploads/2021/09/Housing-Health-and-LGBTQIA-Older-Adults-2021-_9.20_21.pdf

Ford, J. A., Turley, R., Porter, T., Shakespeare, T., Wong, G., Jones, A. P., & Steel, N. (2018). Access to primary care for socio-economically disadvantaged older people in rural areas: A qualitative study. *PLoS One, 13,* e0193952. https://doi.org/10.1371/journal.pone.0193952

Fraser, B., Pierse, N., Chisholm, E., & Cook, H. (2019). LGBTIQ+ homelessness: A review of the literature. *International Journal of Environmental Research and Public Health, 16*(15), 2677. https://doi.org/10.3390/ijerph16152677

Giles, G. M., Edwards, D. F., Baum, C., Furniss, J., Skidmore, E., Wolf, T., & Leland, N. E. (2020). Making functional cognition a professional priority. *The American Journal of Occupational Therapy, 74*(1), 7401090010p1–7401090010p6. https://doi.org/10.5014/ajot.2020.741002

Gilmer, C., & Buccieri, K. (2020). Homeless patients associate clinician bias with suboptimal care for mental illness, addictions, and chronic pain. *Journal of Primary Care & Community Health, 11,* 1–7. https://doi.org/10.1177/2150132720910289

Greer, N., Sayer, N., Spoont, M., Taylor, B. C., Ackland, P. E., MacDonald, R., McKenzie, L, Rosebush, C., & Wilt, T. (2020). Prevalence and severity of psychiatric disorders and suicidal behavior in service members and veterans with and without traumatic brain injury: Systematic review. *Journal of Head Trauma Rehabilitation, 35*(1), 1–13. https://doi.org/10.1097/HTR.0000000000000478

Guarino, K., Soares, P., Konnath, K., Clervil, R., & Bassuk, E. (2009). *Trauma-Informed Organizational Toolkit.* Center for Mental Health Services, Substance Abuse and Mental Health Services Administration, Daniels Fund, National Child Traumatic Stress Network, W.K. Kellogg Foundation. https://www.air.org/sites/default/files/downloads/report/Trauma-Informed_Organizational_Toolkit_0.pdf

Gutwinski, S., Schreiter, S., Deutscher, K., & Fazel, S. (2021). The prevalence of mental disorders among homeless people in high-income countries: An updated systematic review and meta-regression analysis. *PLoS Medicine, 18*(8), e1003750. https://doi.org/10.1371/journal.pmed.1003750

Hawk, M., Coulter, R. W. S., Egan, J. E., Fisk, S., Reuel Friedman, M., Tula, M., & Kinsky, S. (2017). Harm reduction principles for healthcare settings. *Harm Reduction Journal, 14,* 70. https://doi.org/10.1186/s12954-017-0196-4

Hayes, M., Zonneville, M., & Bassuk, E. (2013). *The SHIFT study: Final report.* The National Center on Family Homelessness. https://www.air.org/sites/default/files/SHIFT_Service_and_Housing_Interventions_for_Families_in_Transition_final_report.pdf

Helfrich, C. A. (2006a). *Food management: A life skills intervention.* University of Illinois at Chicago. http://naric.com/?q=en/content/order-life-skills-manual

Helfrich, C. A. (2006b). *Home and self-care: A life skills intervention.* University of Illinois at Chicago. http://naric.com/?q=en/content/order-life-skills-manual

Helfrich, C. A. (2006c). *Money management: A life skills intervention.* University of Illinois at Chicago. http://naric.com/?q=en/content/order-life-skills-manual

Helfrich, C. A. (2006d). *Safe community participation: A life skills intervention.* University of Illinois at Chicago. http://naric.com/?q=en/content/order-life-skills-manual

Helfrich, C. A. (2023). Principles of learning and behavior change. In G. Gillen, & C. Brown (Eds.), *Willard and Spackman's occupational therapy* (14th ed., pp. 667–682). Lippincott, Williams & Wilkins.

Helfrich, C. A., & Chan, D. V. (2013). Changes in self-identified priorities, competencies, and values of adults with psychiatric disabilities who were recently homeless. *American Journal of Psychiatric Rehabilitation, 16,* 22–49. https://doi.org/10.1080/15487768.2013.762298

Helfrich, C. A., Chan, D. V., & Sabol, P. (2011). Cognitive predictors of life skill interventions: Outcomes for adults with mental illness at risk for homelessness. *American Journal of Occupational Therapy, 65*(3), 277–286. https://doi.org/10.5014/ajot.2011.001321

Helfrich, C. A., Chan, D. V., Simpson, E. K., & Sabol, P. (2011). Readiness-to-change cluster profiles among adults with mental illness who were homeless participating in a life skills intervention. *Community Mental Health Journal, 48*(6), 673–681. https://doi.org/10.1007/s10597-011-9383-z

Helfrich, C. A., Fujiura, G., & Rutkowski, V. (2008). Mental health characteristics of women in domestic violence shelters. *Journal of Interpersonal Violence, 23,* 437–453. https://doi.org/10.1177/0886260507312942

Helfrich, C. A., & Halverson, A. (2011, April). *Occupational therapy's role in using a harm reduction approach with a homeless population.* Workshop presented at the American Occupational Therapy Association Annual Conference, Philadelphia, PA.

Helfrich, C. A., & Hellman, M. (2013). *Use of harm reduction strategies in an occupational therapy life skills intervention: A qualitative study* [Unpublished thesis]. Department of Occupational Therapy, Boston University.

Helfrich, C. A., Peters, C. Y., & Chan, D. V. (2011). Trauma symptoms of individuals with mental illness at risk for homelessness participating in a life skills intervention. *Occupational Therapy International, 18*(3), 115–123. https://doi.org/10.1002/oti.308

Henry, M., de Sousa, T., Tano, C., Dick, N., Hull, R., Shea, M., Morris, T., & Morris, S. (2022). *The 2021 Annual Homeless Assessment Report (AHAR) to Congress.* Department of Housing and Urban Development. https://www.huduser.gov/portal/sites/default/files/pdf/2021-AHAR-Part-1.pdf

Holliday, S. B., & Pederson, E. R. (2017). The association between discharge status, mental health, and substance misuse among young adult veterans. *Psychiatry Research, 256,* 428–434. https://doi.org/10.1016/j.psychres.2017.07.011

Hopper, E. K., Bassuk, E. L., & Olivet, J. (2010). Shelter from the storm: Trauma-informed care in homelessness services settings. *The Open Health Services and Policy Journal, 3,* 80–100. https://doi.org/10.2174/1874924001003020080

Illman, S. C., Spence, S., O'Campo, P., & Kirsh, B. (2013). Exploring the occupations of homeless adults living with mental illnesses in Toronto. *Canadian Journal of Occupational Therapy, 80*(4), 215–223. https://doi.org/10.1177/0008417413506555

Internal Displacement Monitoring Centre. (2021). *2021 Global report on internal displacement.* https://www.internal-displacement.org/sites/default/files/publications/documents/grid2021_idmc.pdf

International Harm Reduction Association. (2010). *What is harm reduction?* A position statement from the International Harm Reduction Association. https://www.hri.global/files/2010/08/10/Briefing_What_is_HR_English.pdf

Kohlman Thomson, L., & Robnett, R. (2016). *Kohlman Evaluation of Living Skills (KELS)* (4th ed.). AOTA Press.

Kushel, M. (2020). Homelessness among older adults: An emerging crisis. *Generations: Journal of the American Society on Aging, 44*(2). https://escholarship.org/uc/item/5601g730

Lave, J. (1988). *Cognition in practice.* Cambridge University Press.

Law, M. B., Baptiste, S., Carswell, A., McColl, M., Polatajko, H., & Pollock, N. (1994). *Canadian Occupational Performance Measure* (2nd ed.). CAOT Publications ACE.

Logan, D., & Marlatt, G. (2010). Harm reduction therapy: A practice-friendly review of research. *Journal of Clinical Psychology, 66*(2), 201–214. https://doi.org/10.1002/jclp.20669

Marshall, C. A., Cooke, A., Gewurtz, R., Barbic, S., Roy, L., Ross, C., Becker, A., Lysaght, R., & Kirsh, B. (2021). Bridging the transition from homelessness: Developing an occupational therapy framework. *Scandinavian Journal of Occupational Therapy, 30*(7), 953–969. https://doi.org/10.1080/11038128.2021.1962970

Marshall, C. A., Davidson, L., Li, A., Gewurtz, R., Roy, L., Barbic, S., Kirsh, B., & Lysaght, R. (2019). Boredom and meaningful activity in adults experiencing homelessness. *Canadian Journal of Occupational Therapy, 86*(5), 357–370. https://doi.org/10.1177/0008417419833402

Marshall, C. A., Gewurtz, R., Barbic, S., Roy, L., Lysaght, R., Ross, C., Becker, A., Cooke, A., & Kirsh, B. (2020). *Bridging the transition from homeless to housed: A social justice framework to guide the practice of occupational therapists.* Social Justice in Mental Health Research. https://www.sjmhlab.com/publications

Marshall, C. A. & Rosenberg, M. W. (2014). Occupation and the process of transition from homelessness. *Canadian Journal of Occupational Therapy, 81*(5), 330–338. https://doi.org/10.1177/0008417414548573

McCoy-Roth, M., Mackintosh, B., & Murphey, D. (2012). *When the bough breaks: The effects of homelessness on young children.* http://www.childtrends.org/?publications-when-the-bough-breaks-the-effects-of-homelessness-on-young-children

National Alliance on Mental Illness. (2023). *Facts & statistics.* https://namica.org/what-is-mental-illness/facts-statistics

National Alliance to End Homelessness. (2015). *Domestic violence.* http://www.endhomelessness.org/pages/domestic_violence

National Alliance to End Homelessness. (2021). *Children and families.* https://endhomelessness.org/homelessness-in-america/who-experiences-homelessness/children-and-families

National Council on Disability. (2017). *Highlighting disability: Poverty connection, NCD urges Congress to alter federal policies that disadvantage people with disabilities.* https://www.ncd.gov/2017/10/26/highlighting-disability-poverty-connection-ncd-urges-congress-to-alter-federal-policies-that-disadvantage-people-with-disabilities

National Health Care for the Homeless Council. (2021). *Homeless Mortality Data Toolkit: Understanding and tracking deaths of people experiencing homelessness.* https://nhchc.org/wp-content/uploads/2020/12/Homeless-Mortality-Toolkit-FULL-FINAL.pdf

National Health Care for the Homeless Council. (2022). *Impact of encampment sweeps on people experiencing homelessness.* https://nhchc.org/wp-content/uploads/2022/12/NHCHC-encampment-sweeps-issue-brief-12-22.pdf

National Institute for Medical Respite Care. (2021). *Medical respite care: Defining characteristics.* National Health Care for the Homeless Council. https://nimrc.org/wp-content/uploads/2021/09/Defining-Characteristics-of-MRC2.pdf

National Low Income Housing Coalition. (2021). *The shortage of affordable, available, and accessible rental homes.* https://nlihc.org/resource/shortage-affordable-available-and-accessible-rental-homes

National Low Income Housing Coalition. (2022). *Out of reach: The high cost of housing.* https://nlihc.org/oor

National Low Income Housing Coalition. (2024). *The gap: A shortage of American homes.* https://nlihc.org/gap

Nemeth, J. M., Mengo, C., Ramirez, R., Kulow, E., & Brown, A. (2019). Provider perceptions and domestic violence (DV) survivor experiences of traumatic and anoxic-hypoxic brain injury: Implications for DV advocacy service provision. *Journal of Aggression, Maltreatment & Trauma, 28*(6), 744–763. https://doi.org/10.1080/10926771.2019.1591562

Ormrod, J. E. (2020). *Human learning: Principles, theories and educational applications* (8th ed.). Pearson.

Parkinson, S., & Forsyth, K. (2002). *Model of Human Occupation Screening Tool.* Version 1.0. Model of Human Occupation Clearinghouse.

Paul, D. W., Knight, K. R., Olsen, P., Weeks, J., Yen, I. H., & Kushel, M. B. (2020). Racial discrimination in the life course of older adults experiencing homelessness: Results from the HOPE HOME Study. *Journal of Social Distress and the Homeless, 29*(2), 184–193. https://doi.org/10.1080/10530789.2019.1702248

Rider, J. V., Selim, J., & Garcia, A. (2022). Health and disability among persons experiencing homelessness. *Occupational Therapy in Mental Health, 38*(1), 49–66. https://doi.org/10.1080/0164212X .2021.1975010

Robnett, R. H., Dionne, C., Jacques, R., Lachance, A., & Mailhot, M. (2007). The ManageMed Screening. *Clinical Gerontologist, 30*(4), 1–23. https://doi.org/10.1300/J018v30n04_01

Rogers, J. C., & Holm, M. B. (2014). *The Performance Assessment of Self-Care Skills (PASS).* Version 4.0. https://www.ono.ac.il /wp-content/uploads/PASS-Home-Test-Manual.pdf

Simpson, E. K., McDermott, C. P., & Hild, L. E. (2020). Needs of transitionally housed young people to promote occupational participation. *Occupational Therapy in Health Care, 34*(1), 62–80. https://doi.org/10.1080/07380577.2020.1737895

Skosireva, A., O'Campo, P., Zerger, S., Chambers, C., Gapka, S., & Stergiopoulos, V. (2014). Different faces of discrimination: Perceived discrimination among homeless adults with mental illness in healthcare settings. *BMC Health Services Research, 14,* 376. https://doi.org/10.1186/1472-6963-14-376

Stone, B., Dowling, S., & Cameron, A. (2019). Cognitive impairment and homelessness: A scoping review. *Health & Social Care in the Community, 27*(4), e125–e142. https://doi.org/10.1111/hsc .12682

Stubbs, J. L., Thornton, A. E., Sevick, J. M., Silverberg, N. D., Barr, A. M., Honer, W. G., & Panenka, W. J. (2020). Traumatic brain injury in homeless and marginally housed individuals: A systematic review and meta-analysis. *The Lancet. Public Health, 5*(1), e19–e32. https://doi.org/10.1016/S2468-2667(19)30188-4

Substance Abuse and Mental Health Services Administration. (2015). *Trauma-informed approach and trauma-specific interventions.* http://www.samhsa.gov/nctic/trauma-interventions

Substance Abuse and Mental Health Services Administration. (2016). *Trauma and trauma-informed care: Domestic violence.* http://www.samhsa.gov/homelessness-housing/trauma -informed-care

Synovec, C. (2020). Evaluating cognitive impairment and its relation to function in a population of individuals who are homeless. *Occupational Therapy in Mental Health, 36*(4), 330–352. https:// doi.org/10.1080/0164212X.2020.1838400

Synovec, C. E., Merryman, M., & Brusca, J. (2020). Occupational therapy in integrated primary care: Addressing the needs of individuals experiencing homelessness. *The Open Journal of Occupational Therapy, 8*(4), 1–14. https://doi.org/10.15453/2168-6408.1699

Synovec, C. E., Westover, L., & Boland, L. (2022). Evaluation of functional cognition in people experiencing homelessness: A scoping review. *American Journal of Occupational Therapy, 76*(Suppl. 1), 7610505122p1. https://doi.org/10.5014/ajot.2022.76S1-PO122

Taylor, R. R. (2017). *Kielhofner's Model of Human Occupation* (5th ed.). Lippincott Williams & Wilkins.

The Homeless Children's Playtime Project. (n.d.). *Family homelessness.* http://www.playtimeproject.org

Tyminski, Q. P., Drummond, R. R., Heisey, C. F., Evans, S. K., Hendrix, A., Jaegers, L. A., & Baum, C. M. (2020). Initial development of the activity card sort-advancing inclusive participation from a homeless population perspective. *Occupational Therapy International, 2020,* Article 9083082. https://doi.org/10.1155/2020 /9083082

United Nations. (2020). *Affordable housing and social protection systems for all to address homelessness.* Report of the Secretary General, Economic and Social Council. E/CN.5/2020/3. https:// digitallibrary.un.org/record/3840349?ln=en

World Health Organization. (2013). *Global and regional estimates of violence against women: Prevalence and health effects of intimate partner violence and non-partner sexual violence.* Author. https:// www.who.int/publications/i/item/9789241564625

Monica Ayala, Jillian Taxman, and Amy M. Mattila

The role of occupational therapy as part of the mental health team in the United States military dates to World War I, when occupational therapists were introduced as reconstruction aides. Today, occupational therapy practitioners (OTPs) treat both active service members and veterans in a variety of settings—from austere environments, to large military medical centers, to community clinics and home settings. Regardless of the setting, the principles and primary treatment goals remain constant: utilize evidence-based practice and occupation-based interventions to increase the individual's independence, restore function, and uphold the identity of the service member or veteran.

This chapter provides an overview of occupational therapy services provided to service members and veterans in a variety of settings and describes how to establish a plan of care efficacious to a military member's needs and occupations. The chapter begins by examining occupational therapy's historical role in the military and defining the skill sets that OTPs bring to providing care within the unique culture of military settings. It reviews the current needs of the active-duty service members and veterans, as well as a range of best practice interventions that support this population. Additionally, in the context of the military culture, this chapter describes the skills, occupations, and artful structuring of the rhythms and routines common to military environments used by OTPs to refine skills, build confidence, and sharpen resilience to enable success.

The thoughts, content, and opinions expressed in this chapter belong solely to the authors and not to the authors' employers. Monica Ayala and Jillian Taxman are employed by the **Veterans Health Administration (VHA)**. This work is independent of their roles and not affiliated with the VHA.

History of Occupational Therapy in the Military

The integration of occupational therapy into the United States military can be traced to the Civil War (Dunton, 1919). In these early days, purposeful activities provided occupation for the mind and body to manage what the U.S. military now calls posttraumatic stress disorder (PTSD) or **combat operational stress reaction (COSR)**. These phenomena refer to symptoms that emerge in response to combat that can manifest in physiological (e.g., somatic signs), mental (e.g., difficulty concentrating, loss of concentration), emotional

(e.g., anxiety, anger), or behavioral (e.g., recklessness, hypervigilance) symptoms (Friedman, 2015). Although both COSR and PTSD are expected and predictable reactions to combat experiences, they differ in how long their symptoms persist. COSRs are adaptive and more temporary in nature, whereas PTSD symptoms last longer than 1 month and interfere with daily functioning. See Chapter 25: Trauma- and Stressor-Related Disorders.

The first civilian occupational therapists were called reconstruction aides and they brought military application of occupational therapy interventions to the U.S. Army in June 1918 (Dunton, 1919). Reconstruction aides were civilian women who worked stateside in military hospitals to treat the wounded and were deployed near the front lines to treat service members with neuropsychiatric conditions (Ellsworth et al., 1993). Their mission was to rehabilitate physically and mentally war-injured service members using curative crafts, such as basketry and beadwork, and workshop activities, such as carpentry, painting, and modeling (Crane, 1927). Their interventions went far beyond wound care to assist service members to recapture purpose in their lives. Their efforts on and off the battlefield influenced the growth of the occupational therapy profession and helped establish the role of occupational therapy in the military.

Today, in many nations, OTPs continue to engage service members in purposeful activity and occupations on and off the battlefield to facilitate recovery and return them to duty or to a productive civilian life (Kerr et al., 2020). See Chapter 1: Occupational Therapy Practice Across the Mental Health Continuum.

Military Culture

Effectively treating a service member or veteran requires an understanding of **military culture**, including a unique set of values, beliefs, symbols, language, dress, behaviors, relationships, and work. OTPs working with these individuals must be knowledgeable of the different branches of service, rank structure, and military occupations or specialties. Understanding the basic tenets of the military, including their work environments, the importance of unit cohesiveness, and the resolute temperament of the service member seeking mental health services, greatly assists the OTP in establishing rapport, fostering therapeutic relationships, and developing and implementing individual treatment plans (Gregg et al., 2015).

Aspects of military culture vary between each branch of service; nonetheless, there are core values common to all uniformed services and these values are grounded in the enlistment oath all service members take "to support and defend the United States Constitution against all enemies, foreign and domestic" (U.S. Army Center of Military History, n.d.). Fundamental values for all military services include honor, selfless service, and integrity. Another common element is the hierarchical organization of military leadership. Finally, the performance requirements of all service members, regardless of their branch of service, are dictated by comprehensive and detailed regulations, instructions, and field manuals that delineate expectations for behaviors ranging from an individual's personal grooming standards to conducting military operations on a global scale.

Maintaining a national defense force requires a workforce that is broad and diverse. Some military specialties are similar to trades and professions in the civilian workforce, such as mechanics, construction personnel, engineers, lawyers, or health professionals. Other military occupations are quite different, such as those related to combat; for example, specialists in infantry, artillery, or Special Forces. Regardless of their job specialty, all service members are required to maintain a certain level of physical fitness and operational readiness, and those standards may be higher or lower depending on the military specialty, geographic location, and assigned unit.

A general understanding of a service member's specific occupation and assigned unit can assist the OTP in developing and implementing an effective treatment plan. For example, a service member involved in a combat unit likely adheres to a vastly different work schedule than the traditional 40-hour/5-day work week and requires intense physical fitness and operational training to maintain overall combat readiness.

In civilian life, every job and lifestyle has its own set of unique stressors; this is no different in the military, but service members are exposed to a variety of additional stressors specific to the military culture. Throughout their careers, service members may experience multiple relocations, which may include overseas and stateside. Career advancement and promotion may require competition for needed training and educational programs to support advancement. Depending on the political climate, service members may be required to participate in numerous training exercises, predeployment trainings, and deployments to hostile or nonhostile environments. The constant need to adapt to new environments, occupational stressors, and family separation can impact even the most resilient service member's mental health and well-being, potentially leading to a variety of psychosocial issues.

Critical Issues Impacting Service Members and Veterans Across the Mental Health Continuum

Because of the lifestyle demands and experiences based around the military culture, nearly one in four active-duty service members exhibits signs of a mental health condition (Kessler et al., 2014). Service members often do not seek out appropriate mental health care for fear of being perceived as "weak" or incompetent (Hamilton et al., 2017). In addition, the stigma associated with mental health disorders further discourages service members from seeking care (Hoge et al., 2004). Common diagnoses that disproportionately affect veterans include PTSD, substance use disorders (SUDs), depression, and traumatic brain injury (TBI). Similarly, veterans are at greater risk for suicidality and insomnia. It is also important to consider the experiences that may lead to PTSD, including **military sexual trauma (MST)**. Lastly, this section examines the intersection between physical disabilities and mental health in the military personnel population. It is imperative for the OTP to understand how these diagnoses specifically affect participation in meaningful occupations in the service member and veteran populations.

Posttraumatic Stress Disorder

PTSD can result from a variety of traumatic experiences, including but not limited to war zone deployment, training accidents, and MST. Statistics show that veterans experience PTSD at slightly higher rates compared with the civilian population. Additionally, PTSD is more common among female veterans versus male veterans (U.S. Department of Veterans Affairs, 2018). In general, service members reported symptoms such as sleep issues, anger, nightmares, hypervigilance, and substance use, which are symptoms similar to those experienced by their civilian counterparts. A growing body of research suggests that **survivor's guilt** is associated with more severe PTSD symptoms. Those who experience survivor's guilt tend to take on a sense of responsibility related to the death or injury of their fellow comrade, even when they had no actual control over the outcome of the situation (Murray et al., 2021; Wang et al., 2018). Additionally, research indicates that those with PTSD are at increased risk for depression and substance use disorders (Smith et al., 2016).

Further research indicates that black and Latinx individuals develop PTSD at higher rates compared with white individuals. Additionally, nonwhite individuals experience greater severity and chronicity of symptoms, yet are less likely to seek treatment (Roberts et al., 2011). Given the well-documented nature of these health disparities (Beydoun et al., 2016), a growing number of VHA hospitals have begun to implement Race-Based Stress and Trauma Empowerment groups to address these gaps in care and to promote a more culturally responsive approach (Wang et al., 2023). By better understanding the compounding ways that stress impacts minoritized communities, the OTP can be more prepared to deliver both individualized and group services that promote inclusive and equitable care. See Chapter 20: Mood Disorders and Chapter 28: Social Determinants and Mental Health. 🤝

Military Sexual Trauma

MST is defined as sexual assault or sexual harassment that occurs during one's military service. Those with MST may experience nightmares, self-blame, reduced self-esteem, difficulty feeling safe, and difficulty expressing strong emotions, such as anger. Research reveals that one in three women and

The Lived Experience

Breaking Free From PTSD

Contributed by Nikki S., U.S. Army Veteran

I admitted I was powerless over my PTSD . . . my life had become unmanageable.

Imagine a picture of a jail cell. I envision this picture as a strong metaphor for the way my PTSD holds me back. Being confined behind bars is like how my PTSD confines me in my body and mind. I've been trapped in this cell for far too long. It wasn't until I admitted my life had become unmanageable that the cell door slightly opened, just as I imagine in my mind.

In this situation, "powerless" to me means the lack of control. Being powerless makes me feel insignificant, hopeless, and frustrated. I was incapable of making a meaningful decision or any decision, for that matter. I was unable to take action in all aspects of my life. I was powerless.

My feeling of being powerless over my PTSD impacted my everyday life. It was so significant that I knew the only way to get that steel bar door open was to seek professional help. My counselor and I are actively working on gaining control over my life again. He's giving me the guidance to develop a mindset where I will feel empowered.

I'm trying to focus on what I can control and accept the things that I can't. . . . Easier said than done, of course. I'm putting my energy into things like my physical health. I can control my workouts and what I put into my body. I'm concentrating on my mental health. I can control whether I take my medication or go to counseling. I'm setting small goals that are achievable to build up my self-esteem. These simple things can add up to more profound situations. However, these simple things can also be the most challenging when my PTSD holds me back.

Gaining control back over my life, I really have had to be willing—willing to be open and honest. I've had to be willing to trust the process that my counselor is taking me through. I have had to have the willingness to delve deep into all my comprehensive memories. This is a marathon, not a sprint. I'll celebrate small victories along the way to keep myself motivated on this journey.

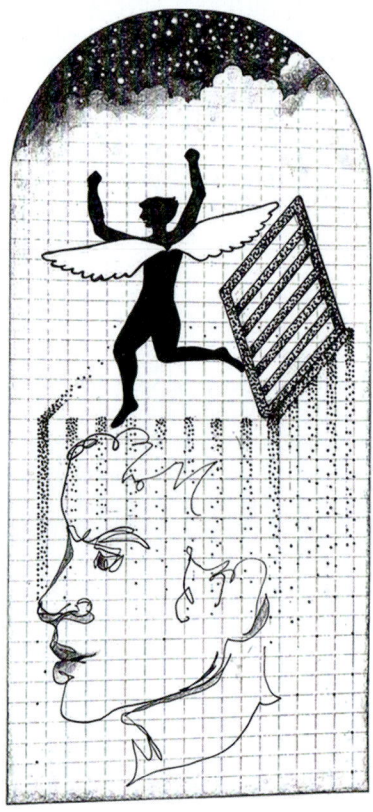

Image contributed by Stephanie Muñoz-O'Neil

It's important while on my journey to keep a routine of some sort. The lack of structure will only hinder my recovery process. I also know that I need to be kind to myself when I'm faced with obstacles and presented with triggers. I know these are inevitable. If I'm too hard on myself, I know it'll discourage me and that could be detrimental to my success. I can see the light through the window—the door is ajar and I'm moving forward.

---

1 in 50 men report experiences of MST at some point during their military service (Street et al., 2018). Rates of MST are even higher in certain minoritized groups, including transgender service members and lesbian, bisexual, and gay service members (Lucas et al., 2018; Shipherd et al., 2021). Those who experienced MST are likely to also meet the diagnostic criteria for PTSD and are at increased risk for suicidal ideation (Tannahill et al., 2020).

MST can lead to difficulty with community reintegration, challenges with building or maintaining close relationships, and reduced participation in meaningful activities (Katz et al., 2012; Pavao et al., 2013). The OTP must consider how MST may impact the person's comfort to engage in interventions that target activities of daily living (ADLs), specifically bathing and dressing.

Often an OTP will only know of an MST diagnosis if it is specifically documented in the veteran's medical chart, or if the veteran feels comfortable enough to disclose that information. Practitioners should adjust their approach based upon knowledge of this information and should employ therapeutic use of self and trauma-informed care to build rapport and guide the plan of care. Additionally, it is imperative to practice within the scope of the profession and to know when to offer referrals to other disciplines. For example, every VHA medical facility has a dedicated MST coordinator, who assists veterans in accessing care, such as outpatient MST-related counseling, residential treatment for MST, and other mental health services to support veterans with MST. See Chapter 25: Trauma- and Stressor-Related Disorders. 🤝

Suicidality

In the United States in 2020, the average number of veteran suicides per day was 16.8, which is 1.5 times greater than the nonveteran population (U.S. Department of Veterans Affairs, 2023). Furthermore, the rate of suicide is two times greater in women veterans than in nonveteran women (Kimerling et al., 2016). The VHA offers a variety of resources to support suicide prevention, including the Veterans Crisis Line, which is a 24-hour hotline for crisis support. Additional efforts include comprehensive mental health-care services and dedicated staff who serve as suicide prevention coordinators. Within the VHA's medical records, providers will see a "suicide flag" for those veterans who have been identified as being at high risk. The risk assessment and flag are based upon prior behaviors and serve as a visual cue for the provider who anticipates caring for the veteran (Krishnamurti et al., 2023). See Chapter 44: Addressing Suicide Across the Continuum.

Substance Use Disorders

SUDs are of growing concern in the veteran population. When looking at data from the wars in Iraq and Afghanistan, nearly 1 in 10 returning veterans in VHA care were found to struggle with alcohol or other drugs. In fact, deployment is negatively associated with smoking initiation, unhealthy alcohol consumption, drug use, and high-risk behaviors. Societal stigma, along with a variety of military-related rules and regulations, is known to discourage those who need treatment (Mattila et al., 2022).

Because SUD is so frequently found to be comorbid with PTSD, much of the developing research on SUD in the veteran population examines SUD in conjunction with PTSD (U.S. Department of Veterans Affairs, 2017). A growing body of research suggests that veterans with comorbid SUD and PTSD are at heightened risk for lifetime homelessness, violent behaviors, and suicide. Furthermore, post 9/11 veterans with co-occurring SUD and PTSD face worse vocational, financial, and social well-being when compared with post 9/11 veterans with only one or neither diagnosis (Blakey et al., 2022).

Although many veterans report using substances to help with sleep, stress management, pain management, relaxation, or facing difficult situations, it is historically known that substance use leads to worsened outcomes in all of those domains. For example, a veteran who suffers from sleep disturbances related to PTSD may choose to "self-medicate" with substances, without realizing that substance use will likely contribute to worsened sleep hygiene. As OTPs, it is important to not only consider the primary diagnosis, but also the co-occurring conditions that may impact the overall picture of health. See Chapter 24: Substance-Related and Addictive Disorders.

Insomnia

Sleep disturbances are commonly associated with the stressors of military training, deployment, combat, and community reintegration. Data from a variety of sources reveal that 27% to 54% of service members and veterans struggle with insomnia (Hoge et al., 2008; Mysliwiec et al., 2013), which is more than two times the prevalence seen in the general U.S. adult population (Ford et al., 2015; Roth, 2007). Sleep disturbances in service members may be attributed to a variety of causes including irregular schedules; ongoing physical, social, and emotional demands; combat exposure; and frequent traveling, which disrupts the circadian rhythm. Insomnia is further compounded by stress related to military separation and community reintegration in the veteran population (Hughes et al., 2018). Poor sleep significantly impacts the person's ability to function and to engage in meaningful occupations, making this an emerging area of focus for occupational therapy intervention. See Chapter 52: Sleep.

Traumatic Brain Injury

According to the U.S. Department of Defense, over 450,000 service members were diagnosed with TBI between the years 2000 to 2021. Most of these diagnoses are categorized as mild TBIs (U.S. Department of Defense Office of Inspector General, 2023). Although most acute symptoms of TBI usually resolve within 3 months from the injury, 15% to 20% of these individuals continue to suffer from cognitive, physical, and emotional impairments (Carroll et al., 2014; Williams et al., 2010). In contrast with the civilian population, TBI among service members often co-occurs with psychological trauma associated with their environmental context. If the TBI is acquired on the battlefield, the service member may not be afforded the privilege of attending to their symptoms in the moment. Likely, they will need to remain focused on avoiding further danger, responding to commands, or providing instruction to others.

The high-stress nature of their environment may be associated with late-onset symptoms and delayed seeking of medical services (Cogan et al., 2019). Recent research found that service members diagnosed with TBI are at increased risk for development of PTSD, depressive disorders, SUD, and anxiety disorders. Furthermore, the research points to increased rates of suicide attempts for those service members with TBI compared with those without TBI (Greer et al., 2020). For these reasons, it is important for the OTP to consider how the veteran acquired the TBI and how the environmental or situational context may impact overall mental health and occupational functioning. See Chapter 7: Cognition.

Spinal Cord Injury

The VHA provides robust care for veterans who have experienced SCI. OTPs working with this population are generally physical rehabilitation specialists; however, addressing mental health falls well within the occupational therapy scope, and should not be overlooked when evaluating and designing interventions for veterans and service members with SCI. Rates of mental health diagnoses, including depression, anxiety, and substance abuse, tend to be higher in the population of individuals with SCI compared with the general population (Cadel et al., 2020; Sandalic et al., 2022). This trend is consistent in the veteran population with SCI (McDonald et al., 2017) and further research indicates that the most common diagnoses are depressive disorders (19.3%), PTSD (11.7%), SUDs (8%), adjustment disorders (6.8%), pain disorders

(4.5%), anxiety disorders (3%), and personality disorders (3%), with comorbidities common (Bombardier et al., 2020).

Veterans and people with SCI and a comorbid mental health diagnosis more commonly report worse health functioning (e.g., higher risk of pressure ulcer, urinary tract infection) and lower life satisfaction (Bombardier et al., 2020; McDonald et al., 2017). In addition to these clinically diagnosed mental health conditions, people with SCI also experience mental health challenges with coping and adjustment, grief, and cognitive impairment (Bombardier et al., 2020; Sandalic et al., 2022).

In the population of veterans with SCI, an interdisciplinary approach to mental health is most effective in treating the behavioral and functional manifestations of these diagnoses (Bombardier et al., 2020; Sandalic et al., 2022). Referral to a mental health provider is essential for determination of pharmacological and intensive therapy interventions. OTPs can utilize nonspecific therapeutic strategies, including facilitating hope through goal setting, promoting self-efficacy,

assisting engagement in meaningful activities, and promoting the development of supportive relationships (Sandalic et al., 2022). Practitioners can also promote physical activity, including resistance exercises, aerobic training, adaptive sports, and yoga, all of which have been shown to improve life satisfaction (Bombardier et al., 2020; Boyce & Fleming-Castaldy, 2012). Cognitive behavioral strategies, such as coping effectiveness training, has also been shown to be effective in managing depressive symptoms in people with SCI (Pisegna et al., 2022).

To facilitate adjustment and coping, OTPs should help individuals understand that their SCI specific deficits are manageable (Sandalic et al., 2022), which can be achieved through person-centered goal setting and interventions that are constructed to be the just-right challenge. Grief is considered an acceptable response to SCI, and when present in the first 6 months, OTPs should employ skills with therapeutic use of self to empathize with the person's frustrations. If it sustains

---

Being a Psychosocial OT Practitioner

Contributed by Monica Ayala, MS, OTR/L

Engineering Hope With Empathy and Validation

Identifying Psychosocial Strengths and Needs

OTPs working with individuals experiencing spinal cord injury (SCI) may prioritize goals related to physical rehabilitation; however, it is equally important to address psychosocial needs. These individuals often face significant changes in their IADL and ADL independence, social roles, and how they engage in meaningful activities. Consider the story of Theo, a middle-aged Marine Corps veteran who was recently diagnosed with C4 complete tetraplegia. While helping his battle buddy restore his garage roof, Theo fell from a 20-foot ladder, resulting in his SCI. Because of the extent of his injury, he will require long-term, around-the-clock care.

Theo lost sensory and motor function below the level of his injury. He requires total assistance for nearly all ADLs. He demonstrates trace bilateral upper extremity (BUE) motor function in specific muscle groups, suggesting the potential for functional gains in self-feeding and grooming. While undergoing inpatient rehabilitation at the Veterans Health Administration SCI center, Theo participated in occupational therapy interventions one to two times a day, 5 days per week. After 2 months of occupational therapy intervention, including BUE strengthening and several trials of low-tech adaptive equipment training, Theo has progressed from total assistance to maximum assistance with self-feeding. His long-term goal is to self-feed at the level of setup assistance with adaptive equipment.

Despite notable functional gains, Theo regularly shares frustrations related to his perceptions of the slow nature of his progress and his reliance on others to meet his personal needs. He expresses feelings of worthlessness and regularly presents as irritable when he makes errors during self-feeding interventions. At times, he impulsively terminates occupational therapy sessions out of anger and disappointment.

Using a Holistic Occupational Therapy Approach

Using a Motivational Interviewing approach, the OTP initiates a semistructured interview related to Theo's frustrations with self-feeding. This conversation explores how these feelings and emotions contribute to his occupational performance and self-esteem. Furthermore, the OTP aims to facilitate hope through goal setting and navigating the just-right challenge.

Theo shares that he was a highly respected captain during his military service. He has always viewed himself as a strong, self-sufficient leader who can inspire others. He reflects on his retirement plans, including a bucket list of rock-and-roll concerts to attend and a cross-country motorcycle trip. He grows tearful as he shares, "Now I won't be able to do any of that . . . I'll be confined to this bed, relying on others for my every want and need. . . . This is so embarrassing."

The OTP uses empathetic listening, assesses Theo for suicidal ideation, and offers validation, specifically surrounding his altered sense of independence. With Theo's permission, the OTP offers feedback rooted in Cognitive Behavioral Therapy (CBT) and invites Theo to consider how his thoughts influence his occupational performance. Together, they complete the following TIC TOC Activity.

TIC TOC Activity

Activity: Home management tasks

Task-Interfering Cognitions (TICs)	Thought Distortions	Task-Oriented Cognitions (TOCs)
• "I can't do anything for myself anymore." • "Everyone is looking at me with pity." • "This is as good as it's ever going to get." • "I should be able to feed myself without any help."	• All-or-nothing thinking (if it's not perfect, it is a failure) • Catastrophizing (overestimating negative outcomes and ruminating) • Fortune telling (thinking negative outcomes are inevitable) • "Should" statements (fixed statements about how self, others, or the world should operate)	• "How I feed myself is different now, but it is still possible with adaptive equipment." • "I don't know what others think about me, and I can't control their thoughts." • "Slow progress is still progress." • "I want to be more independent in feeding myself, and I'm working on it."

Being a Psychosocial OT Practitioner—cont'd

Along with challenging these cognitive distortions, the OTP validates the grief associated with Theo's new diagnosis (reduced independence with self-care, altered sense of self, and changed plans for his future). Theo seems to appreciate this acknowledgment and asks for clarification on realistic expectations for goal attainment. The OTP takes a strengths-based approach, reviewing his progress from total assistance to maximum assistance with self-feeding and highlighting additional functional gains, such as improved assertive communication. The OTP explains that, although Theo may not be able to physically move through his self-care independently, he continues to improve his skills for directing his care in ways that promote safety and personal satisfaction.

The OTP and Theo completed a task analysis of his feeding routine to promote greater self-efficacy. They outline areas for improvement, and they work with the team's assistive technology professional to create a high-tech plate rotator system designed to reduce the margin for error and maximize functional independence. After developing this customized equipment,

Theo continues to make progress over the next 2 months. Theo can complete a meal at the level of setup assist using the plate rotator system, a plate guard, custom orthosis, and custom silverware. Additionally, he demonstrates improved insight into maladaptive thinking patterns and can independently challenge these thoughts, resulting in improved self-esteem and stress management.

Reflective Questions

1. During an interdisciplinary meeting, the nursing staff shared that Theo barely sleeps at night. He is frequently observed crying inconsolably, leaving him fatigued and irritable in the morning. How might the OTP collaborate with the nursing staff and Theo to address his sleep hygiene?
2. How might the OTP address Theo's disappointment with his retirement bucket list? Aside from Motivational Interviewing and cognitive behavioral strategies, what other interventions might be beneficial to address Theo's feelings of frustration and hopelessness?

TABLE 43-1 | Military Settings and Occupational Therapy Roles On and Off the Battlefield

Setting	Service Member Profile	Occupational Therapy Roles and Responsibilities	Primary Interventions
On the Battlefield			
Combat Operational Stress Control (COSC) unit	Deployed service members who are experiencing acute or posttraumatic stress	Develop occupation-based interventions that align with the "military setting" and roles of the service member to address functional performance and support RTD.	Work hardening and life skills (e.g., coping skills, leisure management, communication skills)
Off the Battlefield			
Veterans Health Administration (VHA)	Veterans who require access to health-care services for physical, psychiatric, vocational, educational, or social problems in hospital or outpatient settings	Identify the current challenges or dysfunction and create a plan to improve coping skills and transitional care to the community.	ADLs, leisure exploration, professional development, goal setting, medication management, financial management, falls prevention, adaptive equipment needs, social skills, coping skills, and home exercise programs
Community-based services	Veterans living in the community who are working through mental health challenges associated with dysfunction, disorganization, or a transition into civilian life	Address prevention and promotion of healthy occupations in the community, which may include transition to civilian life. Aim to utilize the community not only as the practice setting, but also as part of the intervention.	ADLs, leisure exploration, professional development, goal setting, medication management, financial management, falls prevention, adaptive equipment needs, social skills, coping skills, and home exercise programs

for greater than 6 months, referral to a psychologist for intensive therapy is recommended (Sandalic et al., 2022).

It is important to screen for mild cognitive impairment in the SCI population initially and annually, as research continues to develop and demonstrates that people with SCI are experiencing premature cognitive aging (Alcántar-Garibay et al., 2022; Chiaravalloti et al., 2020). Practitioners should take this into consideration when setting goals, as individuals with mild cognitive impairment show greater difficulty with adjustment to SCI and are likely to have decreased independence with ADLs and instrumental activities of daily living (IADLs). In this chapter's Being a Psychosocial OT Practitioner feature, an OTP shares some of her experiences addressing the psychosocial needs of service veterans. See Chapter 16: Acquired Physical Disability and Mental Health. 🤝

Continuum of Care for Service Members and Veterans

Some service members may receive mental health-care services on the battlefield in **Combat and Operational Stress Control (COSC) units**. In a COSC unit, the OTP's goal is to support the service member with return to duty (RTD). Off the battlefield, OTPs work with those who have transitioned to civilian life and may be eligible for care at the VHA or have access to community-based care. In the next part of this chapter, several settings along this continuum of care are discussed in more detail. Table 43-1 provides brief outlines of some key settings where a service member or veteran may receive care, provides profiles of service members and veterans commonly encountered, and identifies typical roles, responsibilities, and primary interventions employed by OTPs in these settings. Regardless of the setting, the primary mission of mental health occupational therapy in the military is to keep service members and veterans operational and functional within their occupations or communities.

Combat and Operational Stress Control Units

Combat operations can require service members to react to life and death challenges daily. Combat units can have exhausting deployment schedules and continuous operations that may physically and emotionally deplete even the most resilient service member. The toll of war is frequently characterized by physical injuries such as gunshot wounds, loss of limbs, and TBI; however, the psychological and emotional effects can be even more devastating, debilitating, and longer lasting than many physical injuries (Tanielian & Jaycox, 2008). The multiple complexities of the combat environment and its subsequent impact on functional performance were the impetus for providing mental health services on the battlefield.

In the early 1990s, the Army Medical Department recognized that education and awareness of COSR were instrumental in preventing more severe mental health pathology (U.S. Army, 2016). The need for unit commanders to offer an expedient intervention to service members who present with COSR, which focuses on normalizing reactions and reinforcing coping mechanisms, led to the formation of COSC units. A couple examples of COSC units are presented in Figure 43-1.

COSC units provide restoration, reconditioning, reconstitution, and stabilization focusing on returning service members to duty. The units are multidisciplinary and include psychiatrists, psychiatric nurses, psychologists, social workers, OTPs, chaplains, chaplain assistants, and mental health specialists from all branches of service. Service members who are unable to RTD may be evacuated to a combat support hospital located near the battlefield or to a larger military treatment facility overseas or in the United States.

Role of Occupational Therapy

The role of occupational therapy in COSC units is largely guided by the Person-Environment-Occupation (PEO) model. Practitioners provide creative and innovative environments of care, ensuring that mental health interventions are focused on the service member (person), the deployed setting (environment), the service member's military tasks/responsibilities (occupation), and the interactions among each. Occupational therapy provides a unique perspective that emphasizes the use of occupation to keep service members functional and engaged in their military routines. Practitioners employ treatment strategies that address occupational performance and therapeutic interventions focused on improving coping skills, enhancing self-care, facilitating recognition of significant problems, and managing combat and operational stressors to optimize a service member's ability to return to and function on the battlefield.

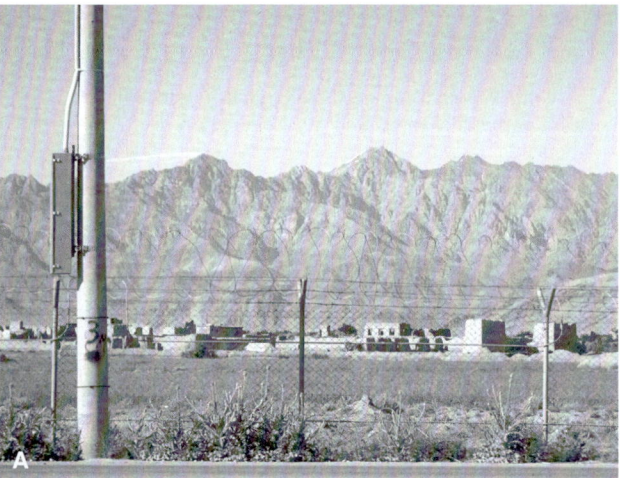

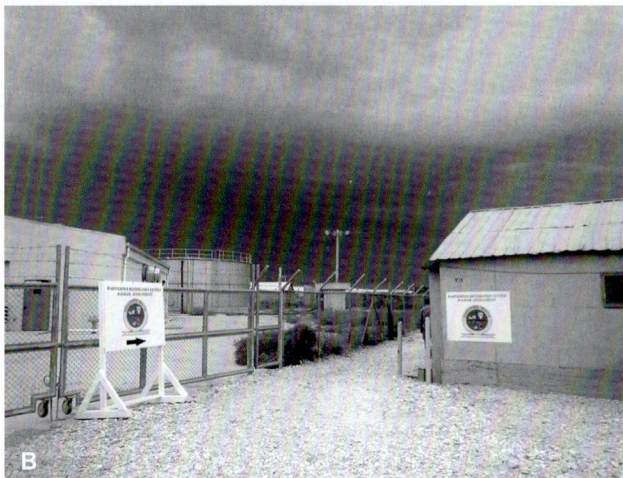

FIGURE 43-1. COSC units. A. View from the forward operating base. B. A COSC unit in Afghanistan.

During interventions, it is critical that the OTP "set the environment" to prevent service members from adopting a "patient" or "sick" role. Figure 43-2 provides examples of how OTPs use the expectations of the environment to support the service member's recovery. Participating in these roles helps the individual maintain their identity as a service member. The individual is also encouraged to balance work and rest activities, allowing them to acquire a sense of emotional grounding and enhancing the opportunity to reduce stress.

Practitioners in COSC units consistently employ purposeful activities, such as team building exercises and life skills, to meet the service member's goals. Service members typically enjoy participation in purposeful activities that foster competition, which is a routine element of military culture. These activities serve as an emotional outlet to reduce stress (Fig. 43-3). To keep the interventions occupation-based, this could involve participation in a physical fitness program or military training exercises. Planning and participation in such events give service members a sense of accomplishment while helping to restore their minds and bodies.

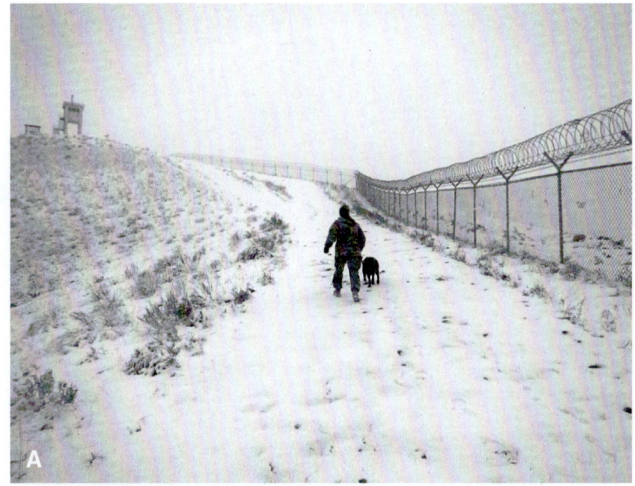

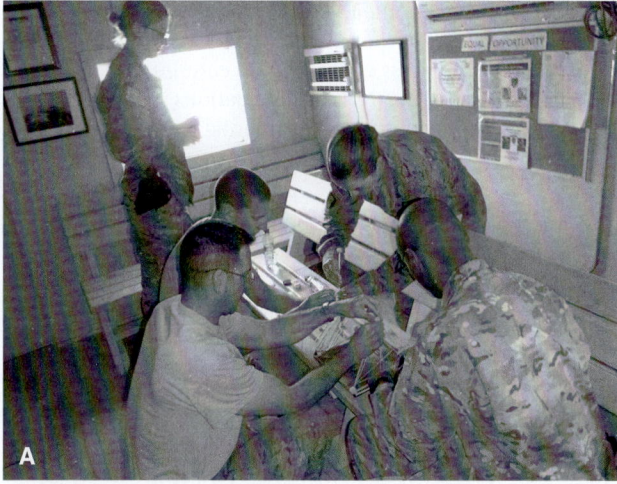

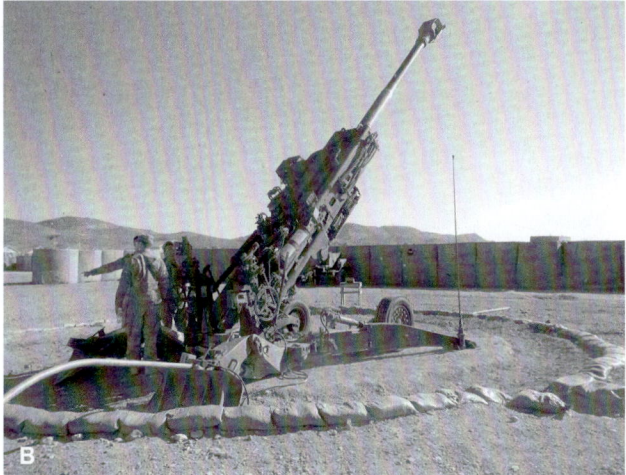

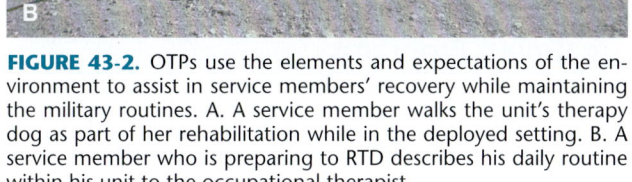

FIGURE 43-2. OTPs use the elements and expectations of the environment to assist in service members' recovery while maintaining the military routines. A. A service member walks the unit's therapy dog as part of her rehabilitation while in the deployed setting. B. A service member who is preparing to RTD describes his daily routine within his unit to the occupational therapist.

Empirically understood as a powerful therapeutic tool, therapeutic use of self is a necessity in occupation-based processes (Taylor et al., 2009). In a group setting, therapeutic use of self empowers service members by integrating new thought considerations, alternate insight, and a sense of belonging under the guidance of a facilitator (Holmqvist et al., 2013). Combined with purposeful activity, this method becomes a powerful tool that solidifies abstract concepts into tangible applications. At an individual level, ADLs, such as sleep, eating, personal hygiene, and basic work tasks, continue to be important occupations that support the service member's resumption of normal routines and overall recovery. Practitioners conducting restoration and reconditioning programs increasingly emphasize the use of higher level, social-oriented, team-building activities as practice tools to enhance functional performance and integrate behavioral change via application (Gindi et al., 2016).

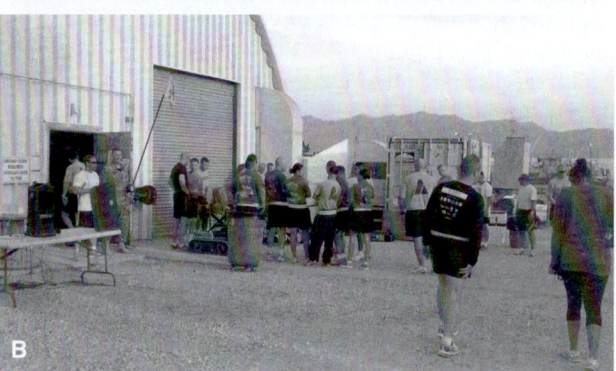

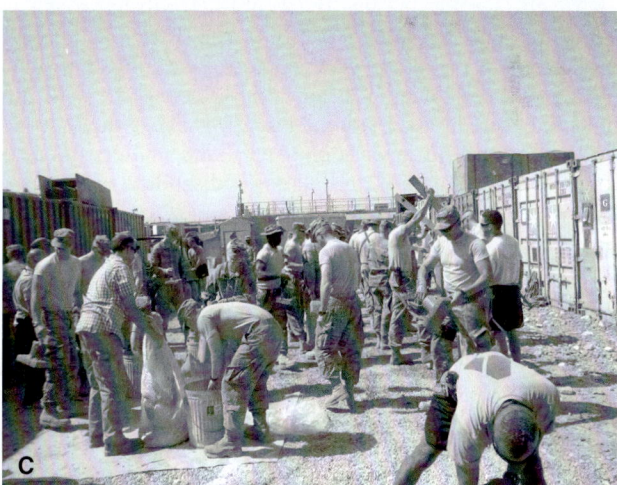

FIGURE 43-3. Purposeful activities in military context. A. Occupational therapy activity emphasizing teamwork and communication. B. Service members participating in a 5K run to improve morale and encourage continued physical fitness. C. Service members volunteering to make fire starters for the local nationals.

Although the value of occupational therapy on the battlefield is well documented, there is limited evidence to describe services designed to minimize mental health concerns before they arise. This paucity of research indicates a service gap, suggesting opportunities for occupational therapy in preventive care for service members with mental health concerns.

In this role, occupational therapy could promote early intervention strategies tailored to the unique needs of military personnel, including stress management, communication skills, and engagement in meaningful occupations. See Chapter 46: Activities of Daily Living, Instrumental Activities of Daily Living, and Health Management Occupations. 🤝

Veterans Health Administration

Once the service member has separated from the service, an option for continuum of care is the VHA. The VHA serves over 9 million veterans each year at 1,321 facilities across the country (VHA, 2023a). The VHA mission is to "honor America's veterans by providing exceptional health care that improves their health and well-being" (VHA, 2023a).

The VHA offers comprehensive mental health services, including, but not limited to, residential rehabilitation, outpatient care, housing programs, physical fitness programs, and vocational rehabilitation. The VHA system provides mental health services and programs that include inpatient and outpatient mental health care, homeless programs, substance use programs, and specialized PTSD services, all of which are programs OTPs can either consult with or provide as direct services. Regarding the role of mental health consultation, many OTPs in the VHA serve on the National VHA Occupational Therapy Field Advisory Council, which partners with the American Occupational Therapy Association (AOTA) to advocate for positive changes in veterans' health care at the national level.

The VHA provides health care using a Whole Health approach (see Fig. 43-4). The Whole Health approach is a person-centered and evidence-based, interdisciplinary model of care that empowers people to take control of their health and well-being. This approach is consistent with the holistic nature of occupational therapy because the focus is on the person and what is important and matters most to them. The focus is not on diagnosis, disability, or disease. As can be seen in Figure 43-4, the person is in the center of this approach. This approach to care encourages the person to engage in self-reflections of their core values and to strive toward their personal well-being goals (Reddy et al., 2021). Under this umbrella of care, OTPs may employ interventions such as biofeedback, meditation, mindfulness, tai chi, and yoga.

Role of Occupational Therapy

The VHA is the single largest employer of OTPs in the United States, accounting for over 1,700 OTPs. In collaboration with AOTA, the VHA offers over 15 occupational therapy fellowship programs across a variety of practice settings. These programs are designed to provide OTPs with specialized training through clinical experience and intensive mentorship. OTPs work in a variety of VHA settings, including acute care, driver rehabilitation, geriatrics and psychogeriatrics, mental health, neurology, pain management, substance use, TBI, and inpatient rehabilitation. The following sections outline the role of occupational therapy in several practice settings that are unique to the VHA.

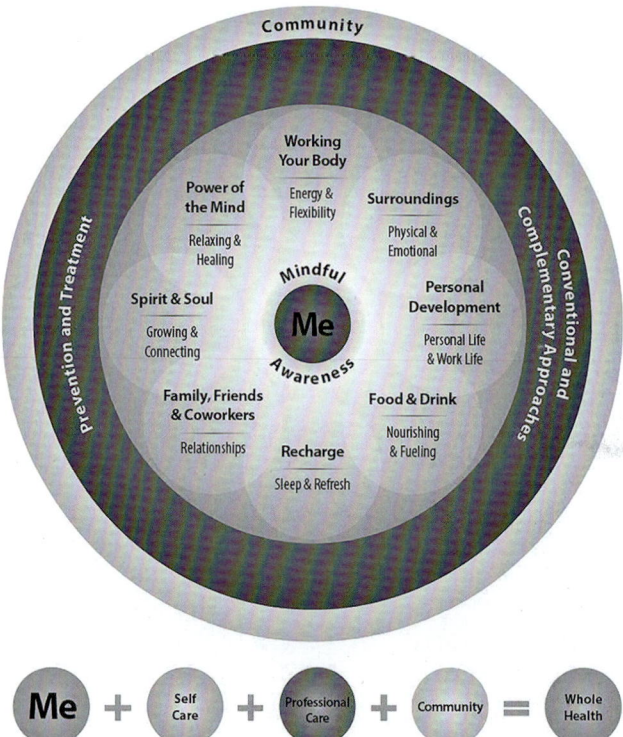

FIGURE 43-4. The VHA's Whole Health Circle of Health is a visual tool used to guide a person's self-reflection on their health and well-being. OTPs can utilize this tool to guide collaborative discussions between people and other members of the interdisciplinary team. *From U.S. Department of Veterans Affairs. (2024). Whole health library.* https://www.va.gov/wholehealthlibrary

Mental Health Residential Rehabilitation Treatment Programs

According to the Substance Abuse and Mental Health Services Administration (SAMHSA), over 5 million veterans experienced a mental health condition in 2020 and more than half of veterans with a mental illness did not receive care, including 90% of those with an SUD (Owens, 2022).

One unique area of practice within the VHA is Mental Health Residential Rehabilitation Treatment Programs (MHRRTP). These facilities provide a multidisciplinary, structured housing environment to address issues such as homelessness, SUDs, vocational training, and other mental health-care needs. Typically, residential treatment is group-based, with group facilitators including psychologists, social workers, chaplains, recreational therapists, art therapists, nursing, and OTPs. The OTP will lead groups that target coping strategies, stress and anger management, social skills, leisure exploration, community reintegration, executive functioning, and general life skills. As veterans transition from residential treatment to the community, they are encouraged to engage in a variety of options for outpatient programming. In this chapter's first Practitioner Profile feature, Monica Ayala, an occupational therapist, shares some of her experiences working with service veterans in an MHRRTP.

Practitioner Profile

Occupational Therapy in the Mental Health Residential Rehabilitation Treatment Program

Monica Ayala, MSOT, OTR/L

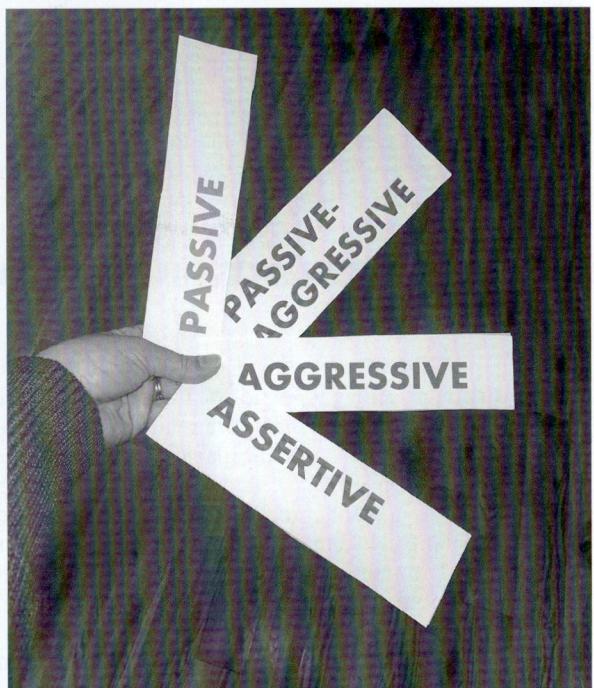

This Living Skills for Recovery Group activity invites veterans to examine communication styles through role-play. Two veterans act out a scenario, and peers identify and discuss the impact of each communication style.

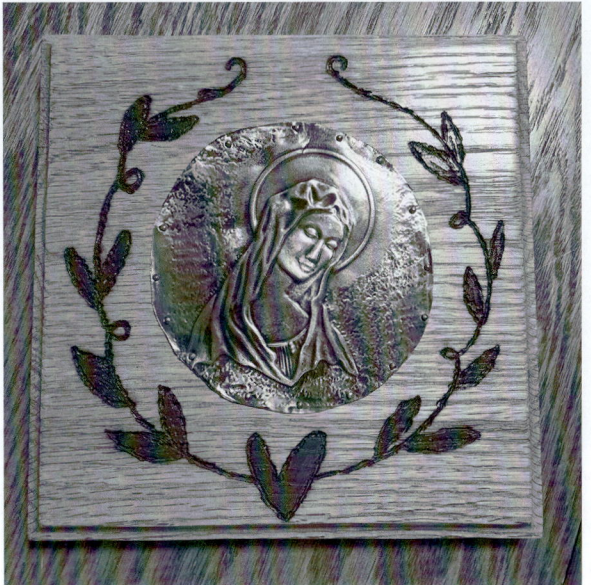

This Work Skills Group project challenged a veteran to plan, problem-solve, and ask for help as he combined wood burning, copper tooling, and painting, which were all new experiences for him.

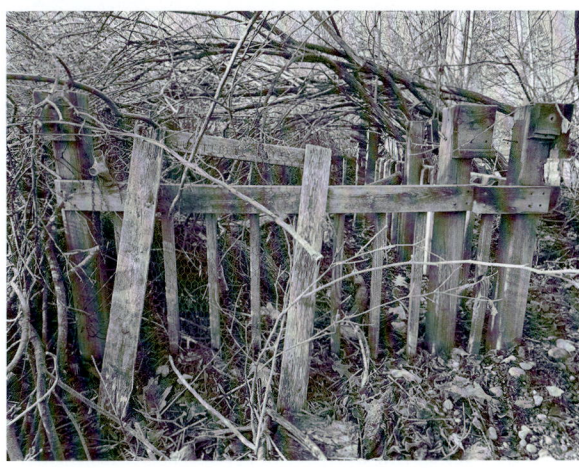

For PhotoVoice Group, a veteran submitted this image of a broken fence to symbolize the need for stronger personal boundaries. The branches represent outside forces that have encroached on the veteran's boundaries.

I work at a Mental Health Residential Rehabilitation Treatment Program (MHRRTP) at a Veterans Affairs Medical Center in Wisconsin. The MHRRTP is a 125-bed facility servicing veterans with substance use disorders (SUDs) and other mental health diagnoses, including but not limited to PTSD, depression, and anxiety.

OTPs at this facility work primarily with the SUD team. Most of the veterans admitted to the MHRRTP are dual diagnosed. Veterans often admit to our program following a period of detoxification in the hospital's acute mental health medical floor. The MHRRTP is a 6-week-long residential treatment program with mandatory group programming 6 days per week. Most days, veterans are required to attend 4 hours of group therapy, with each group lasting 45 minutes. All groups are delivered by interdisciplinary team members. The group may be led by OTPs, social workers, psychologists, recreation therapists, art therapists, kinesiotherapists, chaplains, peer support specialists, or nurses.

Before seeing veterans in the group setting, the OTP completes a semistructured, informal interview to gain a clear understanding of their reason for admission and personal goals. The OTP then uses this information to create an occupational profile and tailor treatment that supports individual needs. OTPs offer three different groups in this setting.

The Living Skills for Recovery Group (1x/week) is a discussion-based group using self-assessment tools, educational worksheets, and interactive activities to help veterans understand the relationship between codependency and self-esteem and to build skills for communication, stress management, and goal setting. The purpose of this group is to promote healthy relationships and performance patterns that support one's recovery.

Continued

Practitioner Profile—cont'd

The Work Skills Group (3x/week) is a hands-on, art-based group that encourages veterans to put their newly acquired skills to practice. In collaboration with the OTP, the veteran plans and creates a complex therapeutic media project plan (ceramics, wood-burning, leather work, mosaics, or copper tooling) which is completed over the course of their 6-week program. Participation in art-based activities is a new experience for many veterans. The group structure and long-term nature of the projects provides multiple opportunities to practice healthy help-seeking behaviors for completing novel task-work, challenges patience and stress management, promotes socialization, and improves self-esteem.

The PhotoVoice Group (1x/week) offers a creative way to express thoughts, feelings, and emotions using photos.

Each week there is a different topic, which aligns with the Living Skills for Recovery curriculum (Precin, 2015). Veterans are asked to find a photo that represents how the topic (e.g., self-esteem, boundary setting, coping skills) relates to themselves and their recovery. During group, each person shares their photo and their reflections and offers feedback to peers.

Though each group is unique in structure and format, the overarching therapeutic goals remain the same—to support the veteran to improve their health and wellness, to live an independent and meaningful life, and to strive to reach their full potential. These principles are deeply rooted in the Mental Health Recovery Model and are thoughtfully examined through the PEO model of occupational performance.

Psychosocial Rehabilitation and Recovery Center

Compared with the rest of the population, individuals with serious mental illnesses (SMI) are hospitalized and use emergency services more frequently; often use primary care and preventive services less often, including for nonpsychiatric medical illnesses; and have poorer health outcomes (Ronaldson et al., 2020: Young et al., 2022). The VHA has a long history of advocating for and establishing recovery-oriented approaches in mental health care (Goldberg & Resnick, 2010). The VHA has established Psychosocial Rehabilitation and Recovery Centers (PRRCs) as recovery-oriented outpatient programs designed specifically for veterans living with SMI, such as schizophrenia, schizoaffective disorder, bipolar disorder, severe depression, or PTSD.

By providing interventions rooted in skills development and goal setting, PRRC programming strives to inspire hope for recovery from SMI, which can have debilitating impacts on functional performance and overall engagement in meaningful activities. PRRC services include peer-led groups, health and wellness classes, family education, recreation therapy, vocational services, community reintegration activities, and both group-based and individual psychotherapy (VHA, 2023b).

Housing and Urban Development–VA Supportive Housing Program

According to the U.S. Department of Housing and Urban Development, there are 33,129 unhoused veterans living in the United States (2022). Although this number represents a 55% reduction since 2009, veterans continue to be at increased risk of homelessness compared with the general U.S. population. The lowered prevalence of homeless veterans is because of a combination of a lower number of U.S. veterans in general and the U.S. government's development of supportive housing organizations for veterans.

Housing and Urban Development–VA Supportive Housing Program (HUD-VASH) is a partnership between the U.S. Department of Veterans Affairs and the Department of

Housing and Urban Development that coordinates services for veterans who utilize a Section 8 Voucher. The goal of HUD-VASH is to help support veterans and their families to obtain and maintain safe and affordable housing. Additionally, the program helps with accessing health care and specific mental health services that promote long-term housing security. The program takes a multidisciplinary approach, including social work, nursing, peer support specialists, recreation therapy, and occupational therapy.

In this setting, OTPs may provide group therapy at community-based facilities or individually through home-based care. Interventions vary greatly depending on individual needs, but may include medication management, financial management, falls prevention, adaptive equipment needs, social skills, coping skills, ADLs, and home exercise programs. Utilizing the PEO model of care, OTPs are well placed to examine and address the environmental barriers to participation in meaningful occupations that are needed to support the homeless veteran's well-being.

Evaluation of Service Members and Veterans

Assessment of military personnel for inpatient, outpatient, or group therapy mental health intervention is similar to that of the civilian population. The evaluation process is typically initiated by thoroughly screening the service member's or veteran's medical chart to gain an understanding of their medical, military, and occupational histories. During the initial sessions, the OTP may use standardized or nonstandardized screening measures, similar to any mental health setting, to determine the most appropriate assessment tools to use. See Chapter 4: Person-Centered Evaluation. 🤝

An initial intake interview is typically utilized to generate the occupational profile of the service member or veteran. Commonly, tools discussed in prior chapters such as the Canadian Occupational Performance Measure (COPM) or the Occupational Circumstances Interview and Rating Scale (OCAIRS) may be used to develop an in-depth occupational

BOX 43-1 ■ Personal Health Inventory

The PHI is a self-reported examination of one's mission, aspirations, and purpose. It can be completed in collaboration with the OTP, which would include goal setting and provision of resources that support the individual toward their unique health plan. The PHI uses the Whole Health Circle (see Fig. 43-4) to encourage the individual to take a comprehensive look at their health. By doing so, the OTP may generate questions such as:

■ Are you able to rest sufficiently to feel energized each day?

■ Do you move your body with physical activity in ways that allow you to continue to engage in daily life?

■ Does your environment leave you feeling supported so you may participate in meaningful activities?

■ Are you spending time with people who support you mentally and physically?

■ Are you continuing to learn and grow on your own and with others?

Based on the veteran or service member's answers to these questions, the OTP collaborates with them to develop a plan of care, including identification of areas of growth, personal goals, and interventions to address these goals. The PHI can be repeated at a predetermined date to measure progress and to revise goals as needed.

From U.S. Department of Veterans Affairs. (2022). Personal health inventory. https://www.va.gov/WHOLEHEALTH/docs/PHI_Jan2022_Final_508.pdf

---

profile (Forsyth et al., 2005; Law et al., 2014). None of these assessments were designed specifically for service members or veterans, but practitioners with an understanding of military culture can deepen their understanding of the individual by intentionally considering their occupational history and performances through the lens of the military culture and mindset. For example, the service member's or veteran's rank provides a cue for their current or previous roles and responsibilities. A deeper understanding of the service member or veteran can be gained by considering potential work stressors or role identity challenges.

The OTP's evaluation process would also collect data on the individual's living arrangements, which may further inform the amount of social support available. Knowing their assigned unit will provide additional insight into their operational tempo (e.g., schedule of deployments and training cycles) and potential work or family separation stressors. Box 43-1 presents the Personal Health Inventory (PHI). This is a VHA Whole Health assessment tool that is commonly used by the interdisciplinary team and is reflective of the holistic approach of occupational therapy.

Informally, the OTP will need to be familiar with screening for suicide risk, anxiety, depression, and PTSD. Additionally, the OTP will need to learn to interpret assessment tools that may be part of the service member's medical record. These assessments are often completed by other members of the mental health team, such as psychologists, neuropsychologists, or psychiatrists, and may include the PTSD Checklist (PCL-5), the PTSD Checklist–Military Version (PCL-M), and the Mississippi Scale for Combat-Related PTSD (M-PTSD; Weathers et al., 2013).

Interventions for Service Members and Veterans

With consideration for critical issues impacting the military personnel population, such as PTSD, MST, SUDs, TBI, depression, and anxiety, OTPs treating the service member and veteran will often target specific performance areas, such as stress and pain management, sleep hygiene, and living skills for recovery. An overview of the common functional performance areas that are affected by these diagnoses and how they are commonly addressed through occupational therapy intervention are discussed in the following sections. Table 43-2 provides detailed examples of occupational therapy interventions addressing some of these common performance challenges. See Chapter 10: Coping and Resilience and Chapter 52: Sleep. 🤝

With the population of service members and veterans growing, an increasing number of evidence-based, emerging practice interventions are being implemented to meet their unique needs. Generally speaking, OTPs working with this population utilize the PEO, Model of Human Occupation (MOHO), or Kawa models to develop occupation-based interventions in conjunction with psychological therapies. Although research focused on occupational therapy mental health intervention in the service member and veteran populations remains limited, the consensus is to focus on addressing quality of life, self-confidence, self-identity, and social interaction, particularly for those with PTSD. One systematic review (Kerr et al., 2020) also highlighted the recommendation for OTPs working with people with PTSD to pursue further training in trauma-informed care.

Many of the interventions discussed in the text that follows can be delivered on either an individual or group basis, with service delivery being dictated by practice setting and population needs. The benefits of mental health group therapy for the military personnel population are well documented (Sunderlin et al., 2022). According to a growing body of research, veterans and service members benefit from having a shared experience with others as they can offer support to one another. Particularly for veterans, some of whom may struggle with socialization after transitioning to civilian life, group intervention can offer a newfound sense of belonging, identity, routine-building, overall well-being, and quality of life (Derefinko et al., 2019; Drebing et al., 2018; Gorman et al., 2018), all of which positively reflect values of military culture.

Mindfulness

Service members and veterans can benefit from occupational therapy–led relaxation interventions, such as **mindfulness-based cognitive therapy (MBCT)** and

TABLE 43-2 | Interventions in Common Performance Areas

Performance Area	Functional Impact	Example	Intervention
Pain	Pain is common after a traumatic event and may indicate stress and anxiety. Practitioners can gain insight on a person's tolerance for specific activities or times of the day by evaluating pain levels before, during, and after treatment sessions. This can assist the OTP and service member in planning daily activities.	A service member suffers from frequent migraines. After tracking her daily activities and pain levels for 1 week she realizes that if she does not eat anything for more than 5 hours, then becomes increasingly physically active, she will experience a migraine.	By assisting the service member to identify a correlation between daily activities and migraines, the service member was able to make a change. The OTP encouraged setting cues, such as an alarm, to remind her to eat regularly and encouraged her to participate in local relaxation classes to manage her stress levels.
Sleep	Many service members and veterans find it difficult to maintain a healthy sleep routine. This can be associated with any one or combination of the following factors: pain, nightmares, restlessness, or insomnia.	A service member experiences night terrors because of his combat experience during deployment. This leads him to avoid sleeping in the same bed as his partner, for fear that he may involuntarily cause them harm. After waking from a night terror, his mind is racing, so he decides to get out of bed to go watch television.	Within a group setting, the OTP takes a Cognitive Behavioral Therapy for Insomnia (CBT-I) approach. The OTP educates the service member on proper sleep hygiene and relaxation techniques, such as guided meditation, grounding, or diaphragmatic breathing.
Global functioning	Because of their military experience, military personnel members may experience deficits in psychological, social, and occupational functioning.	A service member sustained a femur fracture during a vehicle accident. She describes difficulty walking more than a block without experiencing leg pain. She reports increased isolation because of the pain and is concerned she could be discharged from the military because of reduced engagement. These fears lead to feelings of depression, fatigue, and lowered self-worth.	After assessing the service member's insight into her injury, the OTP structures therapy to focus on performance. For example, they grade interventions to encourage energy conservation, maximize productivity, and support safety, pain management, and sense of independence.
Stress	Service members or veterans may experience stress for a variety of reasons, including stress associated with the environment, job duties, family separation, community reintegration, and so on.	A service member has been in the military for 13 years and recently returned from his third deployment. His partner is expecting their first child, and he is struggling with adjustment to civilian life, as well as questioning his capacity to raise a child. The service member's perceived stress scale score is high.	The OTP and service member discuss his concerns about his ability to raise a child. Using principles of CBT, these beliefs are challenged through group therapy and purposeful activity. Guiding this conversation in a low-stress setting, where the service member feels relaxed, will facilitate better outcomes.

mindfulness-based stress reduction (MBSR). Mindfulness training generally involves purposeful attention, regulation, and awareness of the present moment along with a non-judgmental acceptance of one's present stream of thoughts, sensations, or emotions. These approaches encourage the individual to focus on the present moment, proving particularly beneficial in addressing symptoms of TBI and PTSD in service members and veterans (Cole et al., 2015).

For individuals with TBI, mindfulness-based interventions support cognitive processing such as working memory and concentration, while also promoting quality of life, perceived self-efficacy, and reduced symptoms of depression (Azulay et al., 2013; Lovette et al., 2022). In a recent study, Stephenson and colleagues (2017) reported that increases in mindfulness were significantly associated with reduced PTSD symptoms. This is consistent with a growing set of literature that finds mindfulness training enhances coping mechanisms, relaxation, and overall reduction of symptoms. See Chapter 45: Self-Care and Well-Being Occupations and Chapter 53: Spiritual Occupations.

Cognitive-Based Therapy

Support groups and group therapy are often primary interventions used in settings that serve veterans with mental health issues (Hundt et al., 2015). The most common frame of reference when conducting PTSD-based groups is a **Cognitive Behavioral Therapy (CBT)** approach. Using this approach, OTPs can reinforce concepts learned and skills introduced in individual sessions while fostering social bonds with other group members. Figure 43-5 provides a brief overview of the key structures in CBT.

One method used in group interventions is addressing the irrational thoughts that individuals with PTSD often have about their abilities or beliefs about their environment. These thoughts and beliefs often lead to behaviors that ultimately interfere with their performance in meaningful occupations. By utilizing a cognitive-based approach in occupational therapy group sessions, OTPs can help people control their thoughts and behaviors to promote improved emotional regulation and participation in meaningful occupations.

Cognitive Behavioral Therapy Model
Implemented at the 254th COSC, Kandahar, Afghanistan 2012–2013

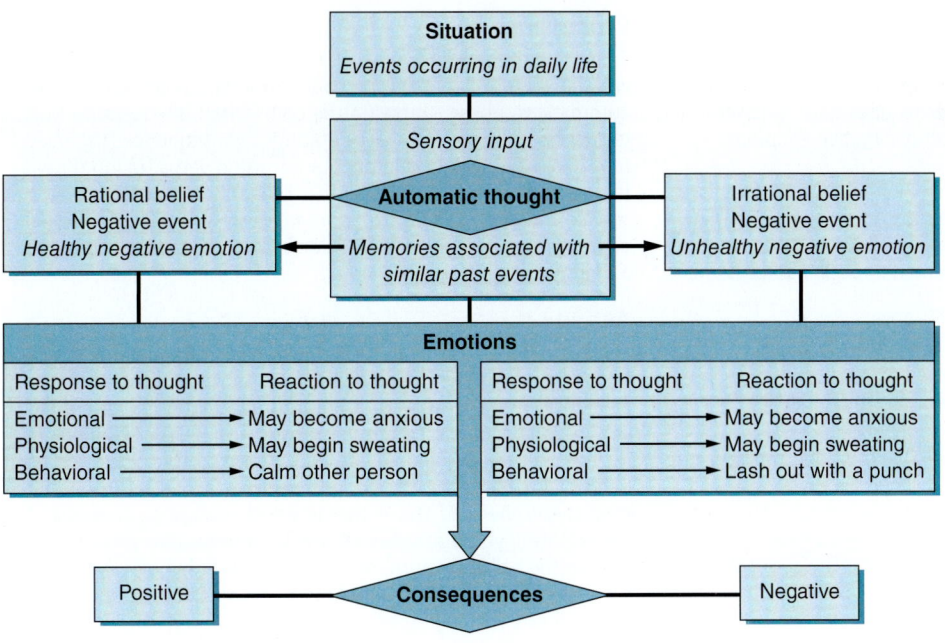

FIGURE 43-5. Cognitive Behavioral Therapy Model. CBT Training is an evidence-based approach used to intervene when service members present with thoughts and behaviors that interfere with their ability to effectively discharge their duties. Using CBT, service members learn to recognize and interrupt automatic, negative, and irrational thoughts and to use interpersonal skills to help counteract negative beliefs and behaviors.

An example of such an intervention, Think Before You Act, is presented in Box 43-2. See also Chapter 8: Cognitive Beliefs.

Living Skills

Through group therapy, occupational therapy can focus on "Living Skills for Recovery" (Precin, 2015), which involves provision of education and skill development in building self-esteem, promoting improved emotional regulation through stress and anger management, and addressing communication skills to enhance interpersonal relationships. Occupational therapy interventions in these areas are specifically designed to support the person with the dual diagnosis of substance abuse and mental illness (Doğu & Özkan, 2023).

For so many service members, the transition to civilian life is accompanied by a significant adjustment period. The transition from a highly structured daily routine with established expectations to civilian life can be challenging as the veteran learns to independently occupy their time in productive and meaningful ways. These difficulties can lead to trouble with finding or maintaining employment and lowered participation in preferred activities. Similarly, service members grow accustomed to social norms and styles of communication that are consistent with military culture, differing from those of the general public. For this reason, it is helpful to target assertive communication and social skills training in the group setting. Lastly, it is critical to consider the ways that the service member's sense of identity changes as they transition out of their military service. Utilizing the Living Skills framework, occupational therapy can address altered self-esteem, which impacts all areas of daily functioning.

Developing research indicates that occupational therapy–led group intervention for living skills is significantly correlated with improved time and stress management, social skills, and ADLs. Furthermore, the study points to increased sober time in those who received the Living Skills for Recovery Curriculum versus the control group (Precin, 2018). In this chapter's second Practitioner Profile, Erik S. Johnson, an occupational therapist, shares examples of holistically addressing service members' life skills and leisure participation.

The Managing Overweight Veterans Everywhere (MOVE!) Program

The Managing Overweight Veterans Everywhere (MOVE!) Program is a multidisciplinary effort to assist veterans in achievement of weight management goals. Within the veteran population, 78% are classified as overweight or obese based on the body mass index (BMI) chart. Obesity is linked to various chronic diseases such as type 2 diabetes mellitus, heart disease, and certain cancers. Rates of any mental health diagnosis are higher among women than men (52% vs. 36%) and people with obesity versus those without obesity (women 54% vs. 50%; men 38% vs. 35%). For example, there is a 25% higher PTSD diagnosis rate among men with obesity versus those without. Obesity and related comorbidities can interfere with veteran participation in leisure, vocational, and social occupations (Breland et al., 2020).

OTPs possess a unique skill set appropriate for treating veterans with a primary diagnosis of obesity. Within the MOVE! Program, OTPs are part of a team of health-care providers working with veterans to focus on forming personally meaningful health habits and routines to support weight reduction and chronic disease management. OTPs provide care through individual and group settings within this program. Sessions may include one-on-one counseling and supportive care for health behavior goal setting or group opportunities

BOX 43-2 ■ Think Before You Act

Therapeutic Goal

This activity creates an opportunity for the service member to experientially understand CBT and the impact of thinking distortions. The goal is for the service member to distinguish between the consequences of healthy and unhealthy negative emotions.

Environment

The activity is performed outdoors under a tent canopy, independent of weather conditions. Safety is paramount. Water rations and protective gear are used as indicated through risk assessment.

Materials: Six 12-inch cinder blocks
Three 16-foot long 12" × 2" wooden planks
Handheld stress ball

Applications: Planks are set up on the cinder blocks, forming a triangle
One stress ball per service member, representing a situation

Instruction

The OTP begins by reviewing CBT specifically; the connection between situations, emotions, and thoughts or beliefs; and how these influence behavior. The impact of exaggerated or irrational thought (distorted thinking) on one's psychological state is discussed, and expectations for group processing are reiterated. Service members are given a stress ball and asked to let it represent their current stressful situation. Service members are reminded, "Each situation leads to a thought. Sometimes thoughts occur that cannot be stopped; these are automatic thoughts. Depending on the significance you place on that situation, the thoughts can be followed by reactions that are multifactorial, incorporating behavior, emotion, and physiology, and which result in a response. This activity is designed to reinforce CBT principles you have been learning through activity."

Activity I

The activity occurs in silence. All service members stand on a plank of their choice. Service members are instructed, "You must throw the ball [situation] as soon as you get it [response]. Throwing the ball represents your response. There is no verbal communication. If you throw the ball and it is missed, the thrower must get off the plank, pick up the ball, and return to the board. Stepping off the plank represents your consequence. Count the number of times you get off the board to retrieve your ball." The activity continues for 2 minutes; upon completion, each service member reports the number of times they stepped off the plank.

Processing

Processing the activity focuses on reinforcing CBT principles. Faced with unwanted situations (the ball), the service members used an automatic response (throwing the ball). Often, the response was unsuccessful (not caught), generating a consequence (the need to retrieve the ball). The impact of not using verbalization during the activity and the frustration this generated is considered. The service member's ability to spontaneously integrate nonverbal communication into the activity as a strategy to reduce frustration and improve success is also noted.

Activity II

Service members are instructed, "Each of you has a stress ball. It represents a current stressful situation. Each situation leads to a thought. This time instead of an automatic thought, give yourself an opportunity to communicate and engage the situation. To do this, say the person's name you intend to throw the ball to before throwing the ball; this represents a 'processed thought,' then throw the ball. This is the only rule change for this part of the activity. If you throw the ball and it is not caught, you must go pick up the ball and return to the plank. The action of stepping off the plank still represents your consequence. Count the number of times you are required to get off the board." The activity continues for 2 minutes; upon completion, each service member reports the number of dropped balls.

Processing

The group observes that there are fewer dropped balls in Activity II. Service members are asked to process the activity focusing on how communication impacted the situation, processed thought, reaction, consequence cycle they learned in CBT training. Service members are encouraged to compare and contrast the first and second activity with specific focus on communication. Practitioners using this activity note this simplified way of experiencing CBT principles can become a very cathartic experience for some service members, and many gain a deeper understanding of the importance of becoming engaged with the situation and implementing healthy communication. Application is emphasized by supporting the service members as they summarize their own learning during the activity. Inevitably, service members articulate the need to take time in each situation to think about what is occurring, that "thinking before you act" saves time, that they are in control of how they choose to communicate, and that application of their CBT training can help reduce frustration and negative consequences in normal circumstances.

---

such as didactic lecture-style with discussion groups, physical activity, and cooking groups. Much of the curriculum is tailored by a national program, though it leaves an opportunity for individualization. Care is provided in person and over telehealth platforms, allowing this care to be provided to veterans in rural settings further from VHA clinics.

Leisure Exploration

Conditions such as anxiety, depression, or PTSD may lead to isolation and loss of interest in activities. This often results in increased stress, anger, and fear, while decreasing self-esteem

and quality of interpersonal relationships through maladaptive behaviors. Leisure and social participation intervention have been identified to have a positive effect on veterans with PTSD, such as a decrease in symptoms of PTSD and depression, increase in positive mood and affect, a heightened awareness of their emotions, and overall reports of increased quality of life (Dustin et al., 2011; Vella et al., 2013). Moreover, mounting evidence suggests a significant connection between engagement in meaningful activities, social and community-based participation, and both psychological and subjective well-being in the veteran population. This study indicates that when veterans participate in activities of greater personal interest, as well as

Evidence-Based Practice

Cognitive Behavioral Therapy for Insomnia (CBT-I)

Occupational therapy–delivered CBT-I can promote improved sleep, reduced symptoms of depression, and greater participation in meaningful occupations for service members and veterans.

RESEARCH FINDINGS

Occupational therapy (AOTA, 2020) and occupational science (Leive & Morrison, 2020) have recognized sleep and rest as foundational to health and well-being. OTPs can play a vital role in addressing sleep problems with individuals across the life span (Leland et al., 2014) and across the mental health continuum (Yoo, 2023). Ho and Siu (2018) proposed a model using PEO to frame sleep interventions. Reviews of occupational therapy interventions addressing sleep conclude that using cognitive approaches, physical activity, and modification of the sleep environment, as well as restructuring daily routines, can be effective (Ho & Siu, 2018; Leland et al., 2014; Nasiri et al., 2023). For example, Eakman and colleagues (2022) reported significant positive outcomes of their REST (Restoring Effective Sleep Tranquility) program, which used 1:1 and group formats to address sleep disturbances, psychological symptoms (e.g., depression), and participation in meaningful activities with veterans. The positive effects of their cognitive-based program were maintained at a 3-month retesting.

APPLICATIONS

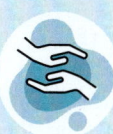

➡ Sleep is a restorative occupation, and OTPs must ensure that they train to address sleep problems and use evidence-based interventions when appropriate.

➡ OTPs can pursue advanced training in CBT-I, which typically implements sleep restriction therapy, stimulus control therapy, cognitive therapy, psychoeducation, and sleep hygiene for individuals, including veterans and service members.

➡ CBT-I in group and individual formats can be used to promote improved sleep, reduced symptoms of depression, and greater participation in meaningful occupations of veterans and service members.

REFERENCES

American Occupational Therapy Association. (2020). Occupational therapy practice framework: Domain and process (4th ed.). *American Journal of Occupational Therapy, 74*(Suppl. 2), 7412410010. https:// doi.org/10.5014 /ajot.2020.74S2001

Eakman, A. M., Schmid, A. A., Rolle, N. R., Kinney, A. R., & Henry, K. L. (2022). Follow-up analyses from a wait-list controlled trial of occupational therapist–delivered cognitive–behavioral therapy for insomnia among veterans with chronic insomnia. *American Journal of Occupational Therapy, 76*, 7602205110. https://doi.org/10.5014/ajot .2022.045682

Ho, E. C. M., & Siu, A. M. H. (2018). Occupational therapy practice in sleep management: A review of conceptual models and research evidence. *Occupational Therapy International, 8637498*. https://doi.org/10.1155 /2018/8637498

Leive, L., & Morrison, R. (2020). Essential characteristics of sleep from the occupational science perspective. *Cadernos Brasileiros de Terapia Ocupacional, 28*(3), 1072–1092. https://doi.org/10.4322/2526-8910 .ctoARF1954

Leland, N. E., Marcione, N., Schepens Niemiec, S. L., Kelkar, K., & Fogelberg, D. (2014). What is occupational therapy's role in addressing sleep problems among older adults? *Occupational Therapy Journal of Research, 34*(3), 141–149. https://doi.org/10.3928/15394492-20140513-01

Nasiri, E., Karbalaei-Nouri, A., & Hosseini, S. A. (2023). Occupation-based sleep interventions for improving sleep quality in individuals with severe mental disorders: A scoping review. *The Scientific Journal of Rehabilitation Medicine, 12*(5), 832–843. https://doi.org/10.32598/SJRM.12.5.10

Yoo, I. (2023). A scoping review of sleep management as an occupational therapy intervention: Expanding a niche area of practice in mental health. *Irish Journal of Occupational Therapy, 51*(2), 22–34. https://doi.org/10.1108 /IJOT-01-2023-0001

Practitioner Profile

Occupational Therapy for Service Members with Polytraumatic Injuries

Erik S. Johnson, OTD, OTR/L

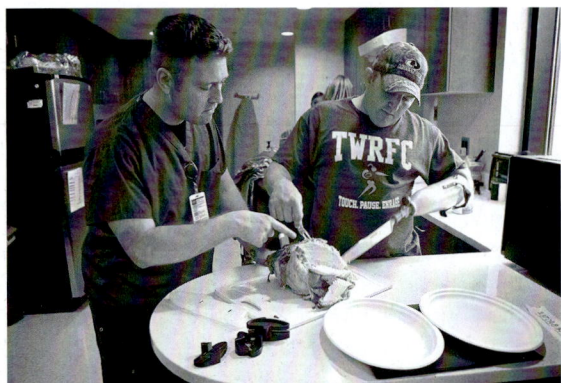

Dr. Johnson works with a service member on advanced prosthetic training focused on food preparation.

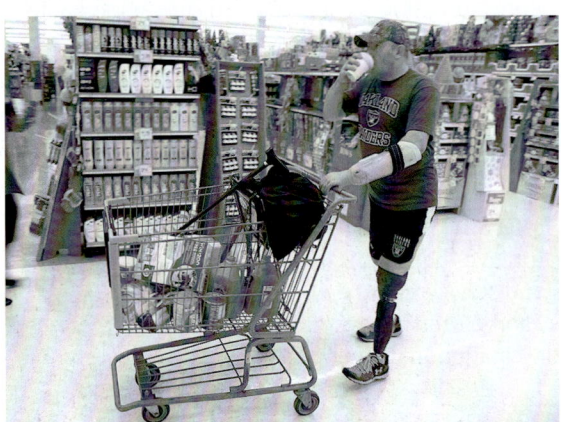

A veteran navigates a grocery store during a community reentry treatment session.

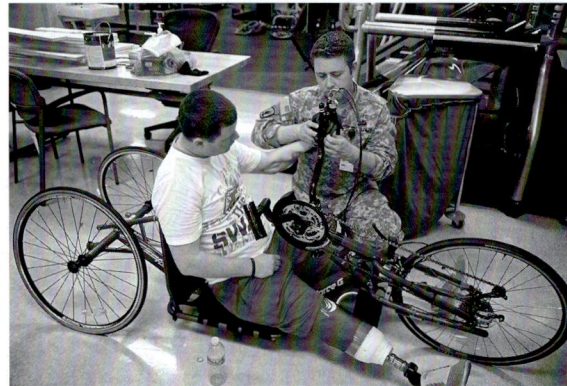

Dr. Johnson works with a service member to gain independence on a hand cycle for leisure participation.

Occupational therapy plays a vital role in the rehabilitation of service members and military veterans who are amputees. Walter Reed National Military Medical Center, renowned for its comprehensive care, hosts the Military Advanced Training Center (MATC). Here, military and civilian-trained OTPs embark on a transformative journey with service members who have suffered amputations as well as complex polytraumatic injuries. The Department of Defense funds the program, ensuring the best resources and care are available for service members.

At Walter Reed, the occupational therapy process of building a new occupational identity after such injuries is multifaceted, addressing physical, emotional, and social challenges. If a service member was injured in a blast, there are often multiple layers of injury the OTP will need to consider. The therapeutic process begins by evaluating the unique needs of each person and creating a thorough occupational profile. This assessment process considers physical implications of amputation, but also focuses on the psychological impact, a common aspect in war-related injuries. The OTP collaborates with each service member to develop a personalized rehabilitation plan, aiming to restore independence and building confidence.

The MATC is equipped with state-of-the-art facilities, enabling OTPs to employ a variety of therapeutic techniques. One critical aspect of rehabilitation is prosthetic training. Practitioners guide service members as they adapt to prosthetic limbs, which is vital for their independence. Training includes activities to enhance motor skills, balance, and coordination, ensuring that patients can navigate everyday tasks confidently.

Using a holistic, whole-body approach, OTPs also focus on helping service members and veterans develop coping strategies to manage pain and emotional distress, a frequent byproduct of traumatic injuries. Group therapy sessions provide a platform for social interaction and peer support, which are essential for psychological healing. An innovative aspect of occupational therapy services at Walter Reed is the incorporation of technology in rehabilitation. Practitioners have access to video games, virtual reality systems, and advanced simulation tools that are utilized to create realistic scenarios, aiding in a person's adaptation to their prosthetics and enhancing problem-solving and other cognitive skills. This technology-driven approach accelerates physical recovery and often provides a boost to confidence and motivation.

Education for the service member and caregivers is paramount as the person looks to return home. This includes identifying and practicing strategies for all aspects of life and ensuring the home environment is safe and can support the service member to take on new life challenges with confidence.

The MATC includes a comprehensive community reintegration component. This part of the program takes service members outside the walls of the hospital and engages them in scenarios and contexts designed to instill confidence in themselves and their abilities. Practitioners accompany service members into the community to engage in IADLs like shopping and using transportation and to explore new leisure interests. By offering comprehensive and individualized care, OTPs play an instrumental role in helping service members with amputations to adapt to and overcome physical injuries and psychological challenges and pave the way for participation in a fulfilling and independent postinjury life.

The Lived Experience

I'm Going to Be OK

In January of 2005, my patrol was ambushed by an IED (improvised explosive device) strike in Iraq. The blast detonated directly on the right side of my vehicle at point blank range. When the smoke cleared from the blast, I knew I'd been hammered; I just had no idea how severely I was wounded. I could tell my arm was broken, but I couldn't see through my right eye, so I couldn't see that most of the flesh under my right forearm had been blown off. I remember being unable to move my right hand. I thought it was because my arm was guarding my fractures. I didn't learn until later that my median and ulnar nerves were severed, which paralyzed my hand.

The docs put me into a drug-induced coma and I woke up 6 days later at a Military Medical Center in Germany. That's when I knew it was bad. I'd been around long enough to know that if you were sent to Germany from the battlefield, you were done. You weren't going back to your platoon. I had failed my soldiers. I had left them in the sand without me. That was the beginning of years of heart break.

I was a Ranger-qualified, prior-enlisted Army Infantry Officer. I was no stranger to discomfort, misery, and pain. I could handle the physical pain while harboring the hope that I would recover, regain function, and return to the fight. About a month later, the docs came to my room and leveled with me. "Listen up, Lieutenant. You've lost the nerves that control dexterity and grip to your hand. The damage to your elbow is extensive. We'll continue to do our best to heal you, but you're never going to regain full function of your arm. Realistically, you won't be back in the fight anytime soon." At that moment, my soul was taken hostage by three unforgiving grips—Anger, Anxiety, and Depression. The emotional pain was overwhelming. At times, I expressed that it was all too much to bear—that I should have bled out on the battlefield. I was in hell. The misery consumed me. I could only focus on the negative aspects of my wounds. I had left the war in Iraq only to return home to a war with myself.

Eventually, the skin grafts would take, the incisions would close, and the bones would mend. I still couldn't use my hand, and my elbow was locked up. My new disability was permanent. I spent a considerable amount of time in the occupational therapy clinic. One day, I strolled into the occupational therapy clinic and was approached by the chief of occupational therapy. He knew I was a fly fisherman from Montana; he was a fly fisherman himself. He insisted on shaking my wounded hand; the Colonel required a semblance of normalcy with all his Wounded Warriors. Years later, I'm grateful. "Lieutenant, I want to introduce you to Captain Ed, U.S. Navy Retired. I told him you're a fly fisherman, and he would like to take you fishing."

On a clear May morning in 2005, 5 months after I was wounded, volunteers wrangled three of us Wounded Warriors into vehicles and we convoyed to Maryland to fish a stretch of Beaver Creek, a small limestone stream near the border of West Virginia. As we drew near, my anxiety was at an all-time high. I'd never experienced this level of apprehension—not even while rolling through Baghdad. As we approached the

creek, I heard the familiar sound of the water trickling by. I dropped two feet into the chilly water. Instantaneously, the sensation caused flashbacks of being submerged in ice-cold water with my dad in Montana. OK. Here I go. I did not realize until later that I was ignoring my anxiety and focusing on the task at hand. There was no time for anger or depression. I was wading in a beautiful stretch of water, and I was there to catch a fish. One of the volunteers helped me land a 10-inch rainbow trout. We released the trout back into the creek to live another day. And that was it. I was back. I'm gonna be OK. That was the beginning of my recovery—my return to the Eivind Forseth that my family and friends knew and loved. That experience saved my life.

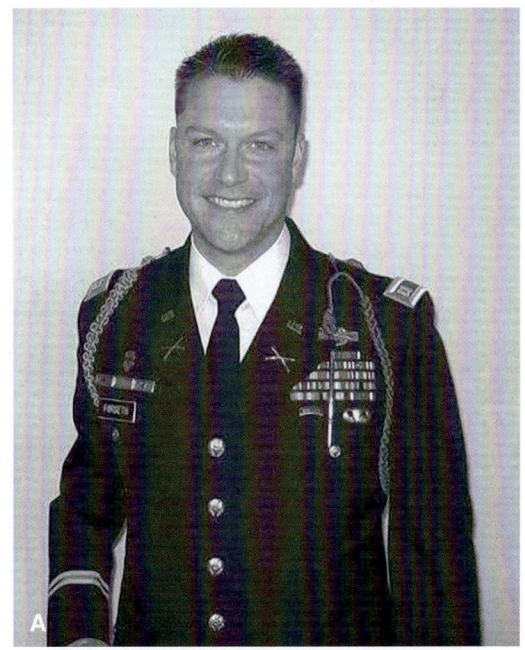

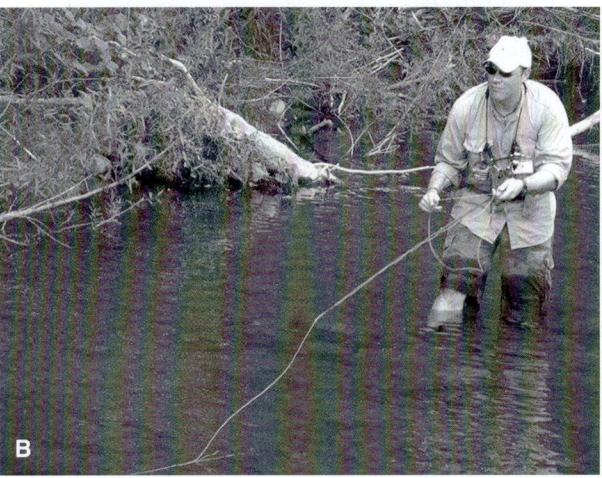

A. Eivind gets promoted to captain following his injury. B. Eivind fly-fishing as part of his recovery process.

ones that foster social connection, they are more likely to experience a meaningful and satisfying life (Kinney et al., 2020).

Vella and associates (2013) examined the effectiveness of a recreational fly-fishing program in reducing psychological symptoms such as anxiety, depression, and somatic stress in postwar veterans with a diagnosis of PTSD. They found these group-based outdoor recreation interventions provided psychosocial benefits. Specifically, their measures found significant improvements in attentiveness and positive mood states, as well as a significant reduction in PTSD symptoms and associated qualities such as depression, anxiety, and negative mood states. For OTPs, these results have potential implications for PTSD treatment as well as further examination of outdoor and nature-based recreation as a therapeutic tool. In this chapter's The Lived Experience feature, "I'm Going to Be OK," the veteran in this story shares his personal experience and the impact of nature-based therapy on his own recovery. See also Chapter 30: Natural Environments and Chapter 51: Leisure and Creative Occupations.

Community-Based Programming

A truly person-centered approach is realized when the OTP can use the individual's environment as part of the focus of the intervention to address their unique needs. For this reason, occupational therapy in nontraditional, community-based settings is an emerging practice area. The same is true for occupational therapy to address mental health needs in the service member and veteran populations.

Community-based programming in these settings is diverse. For example, occupational therapy services for homeless veterans could include support to find and maintain permanent housing, build ADL and IADL skills, and/or address vocational rehabilitation. When comparing different homeless veteran programs, participants rated their experiences higher with the programs that were tailored to their specific needs (Kertesz et al., 2013). Similarly, recent studies

examined occupational therapy driving interventions for combat veterans who returned to civilian life with maladaptive driving practices because of evasive driving behaviors learned during combat. In these studies, OTPs successfully used a driving simulation tool to reduce aggressive driving strategies, ultimately leading to safer participation in meaningful occupations (Classen, Cormack et al., 2014; Classen, Monahan et al., 2014).

Practitioners working with veteran populations in community-based settings can address several of the performance patterns found in the *Occupational Therapy Practice Framework* (AOTA, 2020), such as habits, routines, rituals, and role identity. Specific areas of occupational performance to address through intervention can include financial management, meal preparation, safe community participation, grocery shopping, household chores, or self-care. Addressing these key areas of functioning can help develop and expand the role of occupational therapy with this population. See Chapter 32: The Neighborhood and Community and Chapter 42: Homelessness and Housing Insecurity.

Biofeedback

Biofeedback teaches self-regulation that highlights the mind–body connection. By using sensors to provide information (feedback) about the body (bio), this intervention helps the individual to use their mind to regulate their body to prevent, reduce, or eliminate symptoms of stress-related conditions. Above all, biofeedback helps people to feel more in control of their body and to make healthy changes. OTPs use a variety of interventions to implement biofeedback principles, including, but not limited to, diaphragmatic breathing, progressive muscle relaxation, and visualization.

A growing body of research indicates that biofeedback results in reduced perceived pain, stress, negative emotions, and physical activity limitations in veterans who suffer from chronic pain (Berry et al., 2014). A more recent study (Schuman et al., 2023) demonstrated the use of heart rate

---

PhotoVoice

Guitar

The guitar is a great representation of what University of Wisconsin-Milwaukee is doing for vets. Also with the creative writing class, these classes allowed a smoother transition into civilian life. Similar to the guitar, I feel sometimes that I stand alone in a civilian world, the isolation, and not quite getting what is going on in civilian life. By offering these classes (Guitar for Vets and creative writing class) it brought me away from a feeling of isolation and into a smoother transition. More schools and communities need to understand the needs of veterans. We have a high unemployment and drop-out rate. It is not because we cannot do it. We need the community and people to understand that we volunteered to serve our country, but do not feel as if we belong at times.

The veteran in this story indicates that they use playing the guitar and creative writing as ways to deal with feeling isolated and to support transition. What other creative and self-expression activities might be used to address isolation and support transition to civilian life?

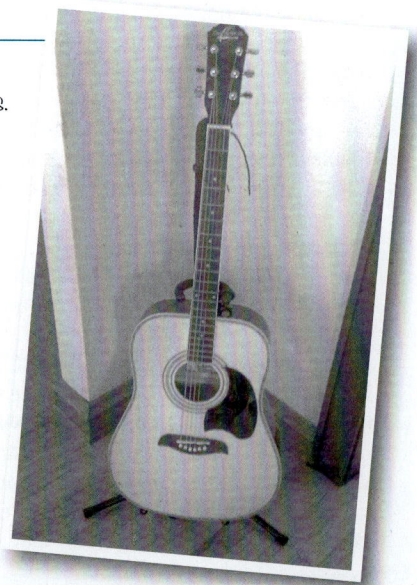

variability biofeedback, a breathing-based cardiorespiratory training technique, in addressing a variety of mental health and general health concerns facing the veteran population. In combination with clinical training, heart rate variability biofeedback was found to reduce depression and improve overall autonomic functioning in veterans with PTSD.

OTPs who are interested in providing biofeedback intervention must complete specialized training. Although OTPs are not the only health-care providers who may pursue biofeedback certification, their educational background and holistic lens make them well-suited candidates to address the gap in nonpharmacological interventions for pain, stress, anxiety, PTSD, insomnia, and anger management in the veteran and service member populations.

Here's the Point

- Throughout history, the utility of occupational therapy theory and practice has been appreciated by the military, on and off the battlefield, advancing practice and developing interventions.
- Understanding the unique military culture is essential for effectively treating the service members and veterans who OTPs will encounter in military and nonmilitary health-care settings.
- A unique continuum of care exists within the military health-care system, starting on the battlefield and continuing through transition out of service, the VHA, and into communities in all aspects of care.
- A high rate of service members, especially compared with civilian counterparts, exhibit signs of mental health issues. Prevalent conditions to consider include PTSD, depression, anxiety, MST, SUDs, and TBI.

- As related to these diagnoses, service members and veterans often report symptoms such as sleep issues, anger, nightmares, hypervigilance, and substance use.
- Successful, evidence-based interventions to address these issues in service members and veterans include, but are not limited to, work hardening, life skills, goal setting, mindfulness, and social and leisure participation.
- Although the military environment is constantly changing and an increasing number of veterans enter people's communities each day, the occupational therapy philosophies that guide the assessment and intervention for service members and veterans remain perpetually effective.
- Occupational therapy continues to play a significant role in treating service members on and off the battlefield and is instrumental in providing them with the skills they need to RTD or lead productive civilian lives.

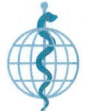

Visit the online resource center at **FADavis.com** to access the videos.

Acknowledgment

The authors acknowledge Teresa L. Brininger, Charles D. Quick, Amy M. Mattila, Michelle J. Nordstrom, Robert D. Montz, and Arthur F. Yeager who all contributed to this chapter in an earlier edition of this text. Some of their contributions were retained. The authors also want to recognize Julia Eckhoff and Erik Johnson for early contributions in framing the content of this chapter.

Apply It Now

1. Reflecting on Military Culture

Imagine applying for a 2- to 6-year contract job at a large corporation that won't hire you unless you meet published physical standards in height and weight ratios, physical appearance (i.e., appropriate tattoos/piercings), fitness, and overall health. Meeting those requirements gets you into an 8- to 13-week common skills course where you will live 24 hours a day and train hard with at least 40 people you've never met before.

Your classmates are between 18 and 35 years old; may be single, married, divorced, with or without children; and represent a diverse variety of socioeconomic, educational, and cultural backgrounds that may be unfamiliar to you. All of you will become a team required to adhere to exacting fashion and grooming standards that limit self-expression and promote unity. You will relinquish some of your constitutional freedoms and swear to abide by and uphold a code of justice more stringent than civilian laws.

During this initial training, you will have very little free time and limited access to your phone or e-mail. You will need to function without your traditional support networks, and leisure pursuits you previously used to cope

will likely be unavailable to you. Each day will begin early with a challenging group workout to prepare you for an age- and gender-based physical fitness test you must pass every 6 months while employed by this organization. For many, completing the initial training is a challenging rite-of-passage and a source of lifelong camaraderie regardless of branch or specialty.

Following common skills training, you will attend advanced individual training (AIT), which may require you to temporarily move and change stations for 2 to 12 months depending on your occupational specialty. During this time, you might resume a typical work week with reduced physical training and be granted visits to family and friends. Once this training is complete, however, you must be ready for your first assignment, which hopefully will be one of your top three choices for locations around the world. During peacetime, currently unknown to almost an entire generation, your employment affords you a variety of unique benefits as well as a typical American lifestyle. However, contingent on the needs of the nation, your job assignments may take you to harsh hazardous environments where you will apply your new skills to a humanitarian or combative mission.

■ Reflect on how you would respond to this type of culture and context.
■ Generate a list of pros and cons for committing to this kind of professional and personal experience.
■ Create a list of the unique stressors that would be the most challenging for you.
■ List the coping strategies you would use to mitigate these stressors and be successful in this unique corporation.

2. Exploring Services for Veterans in My Community

Contact a local veterans hospital, clinic, or community organization. Learn as much as you can about the mental health services they offer. Ask specifically about whether the VA offers housing and what emergency resources are available.

Ask questions to help you learn how a veteran qualifies for the available programs (e.g., does the veteran need to have a specific prior level of service to qualify? Do they need to have an honorable discharge? What do you need to do as a health-care professional to be able to connect people who are veterans to available services?).

Create a resource brochure for veterans and providers in your area with the information you gain.

Once you have gathered information on these resources, think about what aspects of these programs would be beneficial from an occupational therapy perspective. Do any of these programs employ OTPs? If they do not, how would you advocate for a role for occupational therapy?

3. Design a Group Protocol Using Mindfulness Best Practices

Think about the unique aspects of military culture that can impact practice with service members and veterans that have been discussed in this chapter. You are an OTP assigned to run an anger management group for an outpatient PTSD program in your community. Given what you have learned about military culture and PTSD, work with a partner to create a list of:
■ Interpersonal approaches you might use with this veteran population, while keeping in mind the military identity of the people in your group
■ Mindfulness approaches you want to integrate into the session
■ Potential community resources that could be accessed as naturally occurring environments for the service members to participate in

4. Eivind's Story Through a PEO Lens

Consider Eivind's story from this chapter's The Lived Experience feature, "I'm Going to Be OK." Leisure therapy is supported by the PEO model and combines the person's occupations with the outdoors to create a safe environment to support well-being. Complete a PEO analysis using the template in Appendix A. You may refer to Chapter 3: Person-Environment-Occupation Model 🗨 and consider the following guided questions.
■ *Person:* Describe Eivind with consideration of his roles and identity. Does he have any performance deficits? If so, describe the motor, process, or communication or interaction issues he faces.
■ *Environment:* How is the environmental context affecting Eivind? Describe the physical, social, cultural, and organizational contexts that influence this case.
■ *Occupation:* What are the activities, tasks, and occupations that make up Eivind's everyday life?
■ Finally, how do all the previously noted areas influence Eivind's occupational performance? Think about his performance immediately following the IED versus 5 months later. What was the impact of the leisure activity on that performance?

5. Video Exercise: Veteran's Caregiver on Advocacy and VA Support

Pair up with another student in your class or form a small group of students. Access and watch the "Veteran's Caregiver on Advocacy and VA Support" video at the online resource center at FADavis.com. Then, discuss and together answer the following questions.

Reflective Questions
■ Do you think Nancy's story about her husband's surprising diagnosis of early-onset Alzheimer disease is unique or common? Why? What clues to his cognitive disorder might she have noticed over the years?
■ What did receiving a service-related connection ruling from the VA mean to Nancy and her husband? What will it mean in the future?
■ How can OTPs advocate for their veteran clients to ensure they receive support and resources from the VA?
■ Nancy has supports and advocates to help her navigate the health-care system and take care of her husband. She advocates for OTPs to work with social workers to access health-care benefits. How would you delineate the role of the OTP versus the role of a social worker when providing supports for someone like Nancy?

Resources

Web-Based Resources
• Guide to VA Mental Health Services for Veterans and Families: https://www.mentalhealth.va.gov/docs/MHG_English.pdf. This handbook provides an overview of the guiding principles of mental health care in the VHA system, the context of MH services available, and the types of treatment most used for veterans. It also provides links to resources and VHA hospitals and clinics that provide mental health services to veterans.

• Military OneSource: http://www.militaryonesource.mil. Military OneSource provides medical and nonmedical confidential information across all aspects of military life. Their services include counseling for the service members and their family, financial and legal assistance, health and wellness, education and employment, and deployment and separation transitions.
• The National Center for PTSD: www.ptsd.va.gov. The National Center for PTSD has vast resources on research and education on trauma and PTSD. The center works to ensure that they share

the latest research findings for consumers and professionals to assist those exposed to trauma. The site also provides resources on benefits and veterans' service organizations.

- Tricare Online: https://www.tricare.mil. Tricare Online provides information on a variety of benefits and services to military service members, veterans, and their families. Services include assistance with health and wellness, finding a physician, and life events.
- Veterans Benefits Administration: www.benefits.va.gov. The VBA provides a variety of benefits and services to military service members, veterans, and their families. Programs include insurance services, education, vocational rehabilitation, housing, and many others.
- VHA Whole Health Home: www.va.gov/wholehealth. The VHA Whole Health Home page introduces this person-centered approach to care. The site provides access to patient and provider educational handouts and resources that encourage the veteran to take charge of their health and well-being.

Videos

- "Student Panel Discusses Running Groups in Mental Health Settings" video. In this video, occupational therapy students discuss their first experience running groups for a 6-week period in a psychiatric day program. The students describe first being intimidated, but then feeling welcomed and surprised by how enjoyable and productive the groups were. They emphasize the team approach and the utility of the groups in developing their leadership skills. Access the video at the online resource center at FADavis.com.
- "Two Practitioners Discuss Their Work in Suicide Prevention" video. In this video, two occupational therapists, Nadine and Kim, discuss their work in suicide prevention. They share reflections and pearls of wisdom gained in years of practice in this area—both observations about people in crisis and how they have responded as OTPs. They express the role that the occupational lives of these individuals have in their recovery and crisis plans, as well as serving as a springboard for interventions. Nadine and Kim also describe what is rewarding about this work and the crucial need to meet their self-care and well-being needs in order to stay connected to this work. Access the video at the online resource center at FADavis.com.

Books

- Blaisure, K. R., Saathoff-Wells, T., Pereira, A., Wadsworth, S. M., & Dombro, A. L. (2012). *Serving military families in the 21st century*. Routledge. This text provides an overview of the unique culture of military families, their resilience, and the challenges of military life. The authors include personal stories from nearly 70 active duties, reservists, veterans, and their families from all branches and ranks of the military. A review of the latest research, theories, policies, and programs better prepares readers for understanding and working with the military.
- Stahl, B., & Goldstein, E. (2010). *A Mindfulness-Based Stress Reduction workbook*. New Harbinger Publications. This workbook is based around the Mindfulness-Based Stress Reduction (MBSR) program created by Jon Kabat-Zinn, author of *Full Catastrophe Living*. The workbook provides a variety of resources to teach individuals how to replace stress-promoting habits with mindful ones in a systematic and practical way.
- Williams, M. B., & Poijula, S. (2016). *The PTSD workbook: Simple, effective techniques for overcoming traumatic stress symptoms* (3rd ed.). New Harbinger Publications. Written by psychologists and trauma experts, this workbook outlines techniques and interventions to address the most common symptoms of PTSD. This new edition features chapters focused on veterans with PTSD.

References

Alcántar-Garibay, O. V., Incontri-Abraham, D., & Ibarra, A. (2022). Spinal cord injury-induced cognitive impairment: A narrative review. *Neural Regeneration Research, 17*(12), 2649–2654. https://doi.org/10.4103/1673-5374.339475

American Occupational Therapy Association. (2020). Occupational therapy practice framework: Domain and process—Fourth edition. *American Journal of Occupational Therapy, 74*(Suppl. 2), 7412410010p1–7412410010p87. https://doi.org/10.5014/ajot.2020.74S2001

Azulay, J., Smart, C. M., Mott, T., & Cicerone, K. D. (2013). A pilot study examining the effect of mindfulness-based stress reduction on symptoms of chronic mild traumatic brain injury/postconcussive syndrome. *Journal of Head Trauma Rehabilitation, 28*(4), 323–331. https://doi.org/10.1097/htr.0b013e318250ebda

Berry, M. E., Chapple, I. T., Ginsberg, J. P., Gleichauf, K. J., Meyer, J. A., & Nagpal, M. L. (2014). Non-pharmacological intervention for chronic pain in veterans: A pilot study of heart rate variability biofeedback. *Global Advances in Health and Medicine, 3*(2), 28–33. https://doi.org/10.7453/gahmj.2013.075

Beydoun, M. A., Beydoun, H. A., Mode, N., Dore, G. A., Canas, J. A., Eid, S. M., & Zonderman, A. B. (2016). Racial disparities in adult all-cause and cause-specific mortality among US adults: Mediating and moderating factors. *BMC Public Health, 16,* Article 1113. https://doi.org/10.1186/s12889-016-3744-z

Blakey, S. M., Dillon, K. H., Wagner, H. R., Simpson, T. L., Beckham, J. C., Calhoun, P. S., & Elbogen, E. B. (2022). Psychosocial well-being among veterans with posttraumatic stress disorder and substance use disorder. *Psychological Trauma: Theory, Research, Practice, and Policy, 14*(3), 421–430. https://doi.org/10.1037/tra0001018

Bombardier, C. H., Hurt, S. M., & Peters, N. (2020). A primary care provider's guide to depression after spinal cord injury: Is it normal? Do we treat it? *Topics in Spinal Cord Injury Rehabilitation, 26*(3), 152–156. https://doi.org/10.46292/sci2603-152

Boyce, K. O., & Fleming-Castaldy, R. P. (2012). Active recreation and well-being: The reconstruction of the self-identity of women with spinal cord injury. *Occupational Therapy in Mental Health, 28*(4), 356–378. https://doi.org/10.1080/0164212x.2012.708603

Breland, J. Y., Frayne, S. M., Timko, C., Washington, D. L., & Maguen, S. (2020). Mental health and obesity among veterans: A possible need for integrated care. *Psychiatric Services (Washington, D.C.), 71*(5), 506–509. https://doi.org/10.1176/appi.ps.201900078

Cadel, L., DeLuca, C., Hitzig, S. L., Packer, T., Lofters, A., Patel, T., & Guilcher, S. J. T. (2020). Self-management of pain and depression in adults with spinal cord injury: A scoping review. *Journal of Spinal Cord Medicine, 43*(3), 280–297. https://doi.org/10.1080/10790268.2018.1523776

Carroll, L. J., Cassidy, J. D., Cancelliere, C., Côté, P., Hincapié, C. A., Kristman, V. L., Holm, L. W., Borg, J., Nygren-de Boussard, C., & Hartvigsen, J. (2014). Systematic review of the prognosis after mild traumatic brain injury in adults: Cognitive, psychiatric, and mortality outcomes: Results of the International Collaboration on Mild Traumatic Brain Injury Prognosis. *Archives of Physical Medicine and Rehabilitation, 95*(Suppl.), S152–S173. https://doi.org/10.1016/j.apmr.2013.08.300

Chiaravalloti, N. D., Weber, E., Wylie, G., Dyson-Hudson, T., & Wecht, J. M. (2020). Patterns of cognitive deficits in persons with spinal cord injury as compared with both age-matched and older individuals without spinal cord injury. *Journal of Spinal Cord Medicine, 43*(1), 88–97. https://doi.org/10.1080/10790268.2018.1543103

Classen, S., Cormack, N. L., Winter, S. M., Monahan, M., Yarney, A., Lutz, A. L., & Platek, K. (2014). Efficacy of an occupational therapy driving intervention for returning combat veterans. *OTJR: Occupation Therapy Journal of Research, 34*(4), 176–182. https://doi.org/10.3928/15394492-20141006-01

Classen, S., Monahan, M., Canonizado, M., & Winter, S. (2014). Utility of an occupational therapy driving intervention for a combat veteran. *American Journal of Occupational Therapy, 68*(4), 405–411. https://doi.org/10.5014/ajot.2014.010041

Cogan, A. M., Haines, C. E., Devore, M. D., Lepore, K. M., & Ryan, M. (2019). Occupational challenges in military service members with chronic mild traumatic brain injury. *The American Journal of Occupational Therapy, 73*(3), 7303205040p1–7303205040p9. https://doi.org/10.5014/ajot.2019.027599

Cole, M. A., Muir, J. J., Gans, J. J., Shin, L. M., D'Esposito, M., Harel, B. T., & Schembri, A. (2015). Simultaneous treatment of neurocognitive and psychiatric symptoms in veterans with post-traumatic stress disorder and history of mild traumatic brain injury: A pilot study of mindfulness-based stress reduction. *Military Medicine, 180*(9), 956–963. https://doi.org/10.7205/MILMED-D-14-00581

Crane, A. G. (1927). Physical reconstruction and vocational education. In F. W. Weed & A. M. McAfee (Eds.), *Medical Department of the United States Army in the World War* (Vol. XIII). U.S. Government Printing Office.

Derefinko, K. J., Hallsell, T. A., Isaacs, M. B., Colvin, L. W., Salgado Garcia, F. I., & Bursac, Z. (2019). Perceived needs of veterans transitioning from the military to civilian life. *The Journal of Behavioral Health Services & Research, 46*(3), 384–398. https://doi.org/10.1007/s11414-018-9633-8

Doğu, S. E., & Özkan, E. (2023). The role of occupational therapy in substance use. *Nordic Studies on Alcohol and Drugs, 40*(4), 406–413. https://doi.org/10.1177/14550725221149472

Drebing, C. E., Reilly, E., Henze, K. T., Kelly, M., Russo, A., Smolinsky, J., Gorman, J., & Penk, W. E. (2018). Using peer support groups to enhance community integration of veterans in transition. *Psychological Services, 15*(2), 135–145. https://doi.org/10.1037/ser0000178

Dunton, W. (1919). *Reconstruction therapy.* Saunders.

Dustin, D., Bricker, N., Arave, J., Wall, W., & Wendt, G. (2011). The promise of river running as a therapeutic medium for veterans coping with post-traumatic stress disorder. *Therapeutic Recreation Journal, 45*(4), 326–340. https://www.bctra.org/wp-content/uploads/tr_journals/2439-9558-1-PB.pdf

Eakman, A. M., Schmid, A. A., Rolle, N. R., Kinney, A. R., & Henry, K. L. (2022). Follow-up analyses from a wait-list controlled trial of occupational therapist–delivered cognitive–behavioral therapy for insomnia among veterans with chronic insomnia. *American Journal of Occupational Therapy, 76*, 7602205110. https://doi.org/10.5014/ajot.2022.045682

Ellsworth, P., Sinnott, M., Laedtke, M., & McPhee, S. (1993). Utilization of occupational therapy in combat stress control during the Persian Gulf War. *Military Medicine, 158*(6), 381–385. https://doi.org/10.1093/milmed/158.6.381

Ford, E., Cunningham, T., Giles, W., & Croft, J. (2015). Trends in insomnia and excessive daytime sleepiness among US adults from 2002 to 2012. *Sleep Medicine, 16*(3), 372–378. https://doi.org/10.1016/j.sleep.2014.12.008

Forsyth, K., Deshpande, S., Kielhofner, G., Henriksson, C., Haglund, L., Olson, L., Skinner, S. C., & Supriya, K. (2005). *The Occupational Circumstance Assessment Interview and Rating Scale* (Version 4.0). Model of Human Occupation Clearinghouse, Department of Occupational Therapy, College of Applied Health Sciences, University of Illinois at Chicago.

Friedman, M. J. (2015). *Posttraumatic and acute stress disorders* (6th ed.). Springer International Publishing.

Gindi, S., Galili, G., Volovic-Shushan, S., & Adir-Pavis, S. (2016). Integrating occupational therapy in treating combat stress reaction within a military unit: An intervention model. *Work, 55*(4), 737–745. https://doi.org/10.3233/WOR-162453

Goldberg, R. W., & Resnick, S. G. (2010). US Department of Veterans Affairs (VA) efforts to promote psychosocial rehabilitation and recovery. *Psychiatric Rehabilitation Journal, 33*(4), 255–258. https://doi.org/10.2975/33.4.2010.255.258

Gorman, J., Scoglio, A., Smolinsky, J., Russo, A., & Drebing, C. (2018). Veteran coffee socials: A community-building strategy for enhancing community reintegration of veterans. *Community Mental Health Journal, 54*(8), 1189–1197. https://doi.org/10.1007/s10597-018-0288-y

Greer, N., Sayer, N. A., Spoont, M., Taylor, B. C., Ackland, P. E., MacDonald, R., McKenzie, L., Rosebush, C., & Wilt, T. J. (2020). Prevalence and severity of psychiatric disorders and suicidal behavior in service members and veterans with and without traumatic brain injury: Systematic review. *The Journal of Head Trauma Rehabilitation, 35*(1), 1–13. https://doi.org/10.1097/HTR.0000000000000478

Gregg, B., Howell, D., Quick, C., & Iwama, M. (2015). The Kawa River model: Applying theory to develop interventions for combat and operational stress control. *Occupational Therapy in Mental Health, 31*, 366–384. https://doi.org/10.1080/0164212X.2015.1075453

Hamilton, J. A., Coleman, J. A., & Davis, W. J. (2017). Leadership perspectives of stigma-related barriers to mental health care in the military. *Military Behavioral Health, 5*(1), 81–90. https://doi.org/10.1080/21635781.2016.1257964

Ho, E. C. M., & Siu, A. M. H. (2018). Occupational therapy practice in sleep management: A review of conceptual models and research evidence. *Occupational Therapy International, 8637498*. https://doi.org/10.1155/2018/8637498

Hoge, C. W., Castro, C. A., Messer, S. C., McGurk, D., Cotting, D. I., & Koffman, R. L. (2004). Combat duty in Iraq and Afghanistan, mental health problems and barriers to care. *New England Journal of Medicine, 351*, 13–22. https://doi.org/10.1056/NEJMoa040603

Hoge, C. W., McGurk, D., Thomas, J. L., Cox, A. L., Engel, C. C., & Castro, C. A.. (2008). Mild traumatic brain injury in US soldiers returning from Iraq. *New England Journal of Medicine, 358*, 453–463. https://doi.org/10.1056/NEJMoa072972

Holmqvist, K., Holmefur, M., & Ivarsson, A. B. (2013). Therapeutic use of self as defined by Swedish occupational therapists working with clients with cognitive impairments following acquired brain injury: A Delphi study. *Australian Occupational Therapy Journal, 60*(1), 48–55. https://doi.org/10.1111/1440-1630.12001

Hughes, J. M., Ulmer, C. S., Gierisch, J. M., Hastings, S. N., & Howard, M. O. (2018). Insomnia in United States military veterans: An integrated theoretical model. *Clinical Psychology Review, 59*, 118–125. https://doi.org/10.1016/j.cpr.2017.11.005

Hundt, N. E., Robinson, A., Arney, J., Stanley, M. A., & Cully, J. A. (2015). Veterans' perspectives on benefits and drawbacks of peer support for posttraumatic stress disorder. *Military Medicine, 180*(8), 851–856. https://doi.org/10.7205/MILMED-D-14-00536

Katz, L. S., Cojucar, G., Davenport, C. T., Clarke, S., & Williams, J. C. (2012). War experiences inventory: Initial psychometric and structural properties. *Military Psychology, 24*, 48–70. https://doi.org/10.1080/08995605.2012.642291

Kerr, N. C., Ashby, S., Gerardi, S. M., & Lane, S. J. (2020). Occupational therapy for military personnel and military veterans experiencing post-traumatic stress disorder: A scoping review. *Australian Occupational Therapy Journal, 67*, 479–497. https://doi.org/10.1111/1440-1630.12684

Kertesz, S. G., Holt, C. L., Steward, J. L., Jones, R. N., Roth, D. L., Stringfellow, E., Gordon, A. J., Kim, T. W., Austin, E. L., Henry, S. R., Johnson, N. K., Granstaff, U. S., O'Connell, J. J., Golden, J. F., Young, A. S., Davis, L. L., & Pollio, D. E. (2013). Comparing homeless persons' care experiences in tailored versus non-tailored primary care programs. *American Journal of Public Health, 103* (Suppl. 2), S331–S339. https://doi.org/10.2105/AJPH.2013.301481

Kessler, R. C., Heeringa, S. G., Stein, M. B., Colpe, L. J., Fullerton, C. S., Hwang, I., Naifeh, J. A., Nock, M. K., Petukhova, M., Sampson, N. A., Schoenbaum, M., Zaslavsky, A. M., Ursano, R. J.; for the Army

STARRS Collaborators. (2014). Thirty-day prevalence of *DSM-IV* mental disorders among nondeployed soldiers in the US Army: Results from the Army Study to Assess Risk and Resilience in Servicemembers (Army STARRS). *JAMA Psychiatry, 71*(5), 504–513. https://doi.org/10.1001/jamapsychiatry.2014.28

Kimerling, R., Makin-Byrd, K., Louzon, S., Ignacio, R. V., & McCarthy, J. F. (2016). Military sexual trauma and suicide mortality. *American Journal of Preventive Medicine, 50*(6), 684–691. https://doi.org/10.1016/j.amepre.2015.10.019

Kinney, A. R., Graham, J. E., & Eakman, A. M. (2020). Participation is associated with well-being among community-based veterans: An investigation of coping ability, meaningful activity, and social support as mediating mechanisms. *American Journal of Occupational Therapy, 74*(5), 7405205010p1–7405205010p11. https://doi.org/10.5014/ajot.2020.037119

Krishnamurti, L. S., Denneson, L. M., Agha, A., Beyer, N., Mitchell, S., & Dichter, M. E. (2023). Improving suicide prevention for women veterans: Recommendations from VHA Suicide Prevention Coordinators. *General Hospital Psychiatry, 84,* 67–72. https://doi.org/10.1016/j.genhosppsych.2023.05.014

Law, M., Baptiste, S., Carswell, A., McColl, M. A., Polatajko, H., & Pollock, N. (2014). *Canadian Occupational Performance Measure* (5th ed.). Canadian Association of Occupational Therapists.

Leive, L., & Morrison, R. (2020). Essential characteristics of sleep from the occupational science perspective. *Cadernos Brasileiros de Terapia Ocupacional, 28*(3), 1072–1092. https://doi.org/10.4322/2526-8910.ctoARF1954

Leland, N. E., Marcione, N., Schepens Niemiec, S. L., Kelkar, K., & Fogelberg, D. (2014). What is occupational therapy's role in addressing sleep problems among older adults? *Occupational Therapy Journal of Research, 34*(3), 141–149. https://doi.org/10.3928/15394492-20140513-01

Lovette, B. C., Kanaya, M. R., Bannon, S. M., Vranceanu, A. M., & Greenberg, J. (2022) "Hidden gains"? Measuring the impact of mindfulness-based interventions for people with mild traumatic brain injury: A scoping review. *Brain Injury, 36*(9), 1059–1070. doi:10.1080/02699052.2022.2109745

Lucas, C. L., Goldbach, J. T., Mamey, M. R., Kintzle, S., & Castro, C. A. (2018). Military sexual assault as a mediator of the association between posttraumatic stress disorder and depression among lesbian, gay, and bisexual veterans. *Journal of Traumatic Stress, 31*(4), 613–619. https://doi.org/10.1002/jts.22308

Mattila, A., Santacecilia, G., & Lacroix, R. (2022). Perceptions and knowledge of substance use disorders and the role of OT: A national survey. *The American Journal of Occupational Therapy, 76*(Suppl. 1), 7610510156p1. https://doi.org/10.5014/ajot.2022.76s1-po156

McDonald, S. D., Mickens, M., Goldberg-Looney, L. D., Mutchler, B., Ellwood, M. S., & Castillo, T. (2017). Mental disorder prevalence among U.S. Department of Veterans Affairs outpatients with spinal cord injuries. *Journal of Spinal Cord Medicine, 41*(6), 691–702. https://doi.org/10.1080/10790268.2017.1293868

Murray, H., Pethania, Y., & Medin, E. (2021). Survivor guilt: A cognitive approach. *Cognitive Behaviour Therapist, 14,* e28. https://doi.org/10.1017/S1754470X21000246

Mysliwiec, V., McGraw, L., Pierce, R., Smith, P., Trapp, B., & Roth, B. J. (2013). Sleep disorders and associated medical comorbidities in active-duty military personnel. *Sleep, 36*(2), 167–174. https://doi.org/10.5665/sleep.2364

Nasiri, E., Karbalaei-Nouri, A., & Hosseini, S. A. (2023). Occupation-based sleep interventions for improving sleep quality in individuals with severe mental disorders: A scoping review. *The Scientific Journal of Rehabilitation Medicine, 12*(5), 832–843. https://doi.org/10.32598/SJRM.12.5.10

Owens, S. (2022, November 8). *Supporting the behavioral health needs of our nation's veterans.* Substance Abuse and Mental Health Services Administration, SAMHSA Blog. https://www.samhsa.gov/blog/supporting-behavioral-health-needs-our-nations-veterans

Pavao, J., Turchik, J. A., Hyun, J. K., Karpenko, J., Saweikis, M., McCutcheon, S., Kane, V., & Kimerling, R. (2013). Military sexual trauma among homeless veterans. *Journal of General Internal Medicine, 28,* S536–S541. https://doi.org/10.1007/s11606-013-2341-4

Pisegna, J., Anderson, S., & Krok-Schoen, J. L. (2022). Occupational therapy interventions to address depressive and anxiety symptoms in the physical disability inpatient rehabilitation setting: A systematic review. *American Journal of Occupational Therapy, 76*(1), 7601180110. https://doi.org/10.5014/ajot.2022.049068

Precin, P. (2015). *Living skills recovery workbook.* Echo Point Books and Media.

Precin, P. (2018). Effectiveness of the living skills recovery curriculum for dual diagnosis clients. *The American Journal of Occupational Therapy, 72*(4 Suppl. 1), 7211520332p1. https://doi.org/10.5014/ajot.2018.72s1-po8002

Reddy, K. P., Schult, T. M., Whitehead, A. M., & Bokhour, B. G. (2021). Veterans Health Administration's Whole Health System of care: Supporting the health, well-being, and resiliency of employees. *Global Advances in Health and Medicine, 10,* 1–6. https://doi.org/10.1177/21649561211022698

Roberts, A. L., Gilman, S. E., Breslau, J., Breslau, N., & Koenen, K. C. (2011). Race/ethnic differences in exposure to traumatic events, development of post-traumatic stress disorder, and treatment-seeking for post-traumatic stress disorder in the United States. *Psychological Medicine, 41*(1), 71–83. https://doi.org/10.1017/S003329 1710000401

Ronaldson, A., Elton, L., Jayakumar, S., Jieman, A., Halvorsrud, K., & Bhui, K. (2020). Severe mental illness and health service utilisation for nonpsychiatric medical disorders: A systematic review and meta-analysis. *PLoS Medicine, 17*(9), e1003284. https://doi.org/10.1371/journal.pmed.1003284

Roth, T. (2007). Insomnia: Definition, prevalence, etiology, and consequences. *Journal of Clinical Sleep Medicine, 3*(5), S7–S10.

Sandalic, D., Arora, M., Pozzato, I., Simpson, G., Middleton, J., & Craig, A. (2022). A narrative review of research on adjustment to spinal cord injury and mental health: Gaps, future directions, and practice recommendations. *Psychology Research and Behavior Management, 15,* 1997–2010. https://doi.org/10.2147/prbm.s259712

Schuman, D. L., Lawrence, K. A., Boggero, I., Naegele, P., Ginsberg, J. P., Casto, A., & Moser, D. K. (2023). A pilot study of a three-session heart rate variability biofeedback intervention for veterans with posttraumatic stress disorder. *Applied Psychophysiology and Biofeedback, 48*(1), 51–65. https://doi.org/10.1007/s10484-022-09565-z

Shipherd, J. C., Lynch, K., Gatsby, E., Hinds, Z., DuVall, S. L., & Livingston, N. A. (2021). Estimating prevalence of PTSD among veterans with minoritized sexual orientations using electronic health record data. *Journal of Consulting and Clinical Psychology, 89*(10), 856–868. https://doi.org/10.1037/ccp0000691

Smith, S. M., Goldstein, R. B., & Grant, B. F. (2016). The association between post-traumatic stress disorder and lifetime *DSM-5* psychiatric disorders among veterans: Data from the National Epidemiologic Survey on Alcohol and Related Conditions-III (NESARC-III). *Journal of Psychiatric Research, 82,* 16–22. https://doi.org/10.1016/j.jpsychires.2016.06.022

Stephenson, K. R., Simpson, T. L., Martinez, M. E., & Kearney, D. J. (2017). Changes in mindfulness and posttraumatic stress disorder symptoms among veterans enrolled in mindfulness-based stress reduction. *Journal of Clinical Psychology, 73*(3), 201–217. https://doi.org/10.1002/jclp.22323

Street, A., Skidmore, C., Gyuro, L., & Bell, M. (2018, August 20). *Military sexual trauma.* U.S. Department of Veterans Affairs. https://www.ptsd.va.gov/professional/treat/type/sexual_trauma_military.asp#one

Sunderlin, C., Kennedy, K., Sehring, K., Blair, T., Atkinson-Smith, C., Plumley, P., & Foley, M. (2022). Supporting our troops—The use of peer support with veterans with mental health conditions: A systematic review. *The American Journal of Occupational Therapy, 76*(Suppl. 1), 7610510200p1. https://doi.org/10.5014/ajot.2022.76s1-po200

Tanielian, T., & Jaycox, L. (2008). *Invisible wounds of war: Psychological and cognitive injuries, their consequences, and services to assist recovery.* RAND Corporation.

Tannahill, H. S., Livingston, W. S., Fargo, J. D., Brignone, E., Gundlapalli, A. V., & Blais, R. K. (2020). Gender moderates the association of military sexual trauma and risk for psychological distress among VA-enrolled veterans. *Journal of Affective Disorders, 268,* 215–220. https://doi.org/10.1016/j.jad.2020.03.017

Taylor, R., Lee, S., & Kielhofner, G. (2009). Therapeutic use of self: A nationwide survey of practitioners' attitudes and experiences. *American Journal of Occupational Therapy, 63,* 198–207. https://doi.org/10.5014/ajot.63.2.198

U.S. Army. (2016). *Force health protection.* Department of the Army. http://www.apd.army.mil/ProductMaps/PubForm/ATP.aspx

U.S. Army Center of Military History. (n.d.). *Oaths of enlistment and oaths of office.* https://history.army.mil/html/faq/oaths.html

U.S. Department of Defense Office of Inspector General. (2023). *Evaluation of the DoD's management of traumatic brain injury* (DODIG-2023-059). https://media.defense.gov/2023/Mar/30/2003190188/-1/-1/1/DODIG-2023-059V2.PDF

U.S. Department of Housing and Urban Development. (2022). *The 2022 Annual Homelessness Assessment Report (AHAR) to Congress.* U.S. Government Printing Office. https://www.huduser.gov/portal/datasets/ahar/2022-ahar-part-1-pit-estimates-of-homelessness-in-the-us.html

U.S. Department of Veterans Affairs. (2017, May 15). *Treatment of co-occurring PTSD and substance use disorder in VA.* PTSD: National Center for PTSD. https://www.ptsd.va.gov/professional/treat/cooccurring/tx_sud_va.asp

U.S. Department of Veterans Affairs. (2018, July 24). *How common is PTSD in veterans?* PTSD: National Center for PTSD. https://www.ptsd.va.gov/understand/common/common_veterans.asp

U.S. Department of Veterans Affairs. (2019). *MyStory: Personal Health Inventory.* https://www.va.gov/wholehealth/docs/PHI_Jan2022_Final_508.pdf

U.S. Department of Veterans Affairs. (2023). *National veteran suicide prevention annual report.* Office of Mental Health and Suicide Prevention. https://www.mentalhealth.va.gov/docs/data-sheets/2023/2023-National-Veteran-Suicide-Prevention-Annual-Report-FINAL-508.pdf

Vella, E. J., Milligan, B., & Bennett, J. L. (2013). Participation in outdoor recreation program predicts improved psychosocial well-being among veterans with post-traumatic stress disorder: A pilot study. *Military Medicine, 178*(3), 254–260. https://doi.org/10.7205/MILMED-D-12-00308

Veterans Health Administration. (2023a). *About VHA.* U.S. Department of Veterans Affairs. https://www.va.gov/health/aboutVHA.asp

Veterans Health Administration. (2023b). *Psychosocial Rehabilitation and Recovery Center.* U.S. Department of Veterans Affairs. https://www.va.gov/san-francisco-health-care/programs/psychosocial-rehabilitation-and-recovery-center-prrc-0

Wang, C., Malaktaris, A., McLean, C. L., Kelsven, S., Chu, G. M., Ross, K. S., Endsley, M., Minassian, A., Liu, L., Hong, S., & Lang, A. J. (2023). Mitigating the health effects of systemic racism: Evaluation of the Race-Based Stress and Trauma Empowerment intervention. *Contemporary Clinical Trials, 127,* 107118. https://doi.org/10.1016/j.cct.2023.107118

Wang, W., Wu, X., & Tian, Y. (2018). Mediating roles of gratitude and social support in the relation between survivor guilt and posttraumatic stress disorder, posttraumatic growth among adolescents after the Ya'an earthquake. *Frontiers in Psychology, 9,* Article 2131. https://doi.org/10.3389/fpsyg.2018.02131

Weathers, F. W., Litz, B. T., Keane, T. M., Palmieri, P. A., Marx, B. P., & Schnurr, P. P. (2013). *The PTSD Checklist for DSM-5 (PCL-5).* National Center for PTSD. https://www.ptsd.va.gov/professional/assessment/adult-sr/ptsd-checklist.asp

Williams, W. H., Potter, S., & Ryland, H. (2010). Mild traumatic brain injury and postconcussion syndrome: A neuropsychological perspective. *Journal of Neurology, Neurosurgery, and Psychiatry, 81,* 1116–1122. https://doi.org/10.1136/jnnp.2008.171298

Yoo, I. (2023). A scoping review of sleep management as an occupational therapy intervention: Expanding a niche area of practice in mental health. *Irish Journal of Occupational Therapy, 51*(2), 22–34. https://doi.org/10.1108/IJOT-01-2023-0001

Young, A. S., Chang, E. T., Cohen, A. N., Oberman, R., Chang, D. T., Hamilton, A. B., Lindamer, L. A., Sanford, J., & Whelan, F. (2022). The effectiveness of a specialized primary care medical home for patients with serious mental illness. *Journal of General Internal Medicine, 37*(13), 3258–3265. https://doi.org/10.1007/s11606-021-07270-x

Addressing Suicide Across the Continuum

Nadine Larivière, Kim Hewitt-McVicker,
Theresa Straathof, Linda Bowden, Ellen Nicholson,
Mansi Patel, Lindsay Sinclair, Heather Vrbanac-Cress,
and Catherine M. White

This chapter is written by a collective of occupational therapy practitioners (OTPs) spanning different areas of practice, different years of practice, and different countries of practice. The common thread is that all authors are practitioners deeply invested in life and meaningful living, as defined by those they serve. This chapter identifies factors that protect one from suicide (prevention), strategies to accompany a person going through suicidal ideation and suicide attempts (crisis intervention), and ways of healing after a suicide attempt (postvention).

Throughout the chapter, a practice scenario is integrated to illustrate compassionate approaches in suicide care across the suicide continuum. The practitioner in the scenario, Cara, shares her experiences of working through the **suicide prevention continuum** (prevention, intervention, postvention) with Evan. Both names are pseudonyms. The scenario shares Evan's story and Cara's inner dialogue of therapeutic reasoning. This chapter focuses solely on suicide and is delineated from other related complex, difficult issues in practice such as medical assistance in dying and self-harm. The critical importance of someone understanding their own biases, comfort, and competence for addressing suicide across the continuum is emphasized.

Safety for Readers

Each person has the potential to be pushed beyond their threshold of managing; this is not the intent of this chapter. However, some content in this chapter can be challenging and even triggering for some and it is important to be aware and keep safe. One strategy for maintaining personal safety is to identify informal and formal supports. Informal supports could include a trusted friend, family member, coach, or colleague, whereas formal supports might be a primary care provider, OTP, or student services on campus. Practitioners often encourage individuals they work with to put these resources into their phone or wallet; consider doing the same. All practitioners, from the most recent graduate to the seasoned clinician, in all practice settings should be educated in suicide prevention. The reflection in Box 44-1 from a recent occupational therapy graduate emphasizes this point.

Worldwide Overview of Suicide

Suicide, according to the National Center for Injury Prevention and Control (NCIPC) within the Centers for Disease Control and Prevention in the United States (NCIPC, 2022), refers to death caused by self-directed injurious behavior with any intent to die because of the behavior. It can be situated as an extreme of self-directed violence, which includes nonfatal acts of suicidal behaviors (suicide attempts), **suicidal ideation** (which can be active [including thoughts about suicide, which may include determining the method and having a plan and/or an intent to act] or can be passive thoughts about death [without intent or plan]), and/or nonsuicidal intentional **self-harm** (e.g., deliberate self-injurious actions without an intent to die; NCIPC, 2022).

Worldwide, every 40 seconds, someone dies by suicide (World Health Organization [WHO], 2019). Suicide is a delicate, sensitive part of the human experience that remains taboo, although many countries around the world have made great efforts to understand it better. In some cultures, suicide is seen as a sin, a crime, or a symptom of a psychiatric problem (Pompili, 2010). In other cultures, it carries the negative connotation that it is a dangerous or weak behavior (Tzeng & Lipson, 2004).

At the heart of this deep, complex, and intimate human experience is an existential questioning about life and death triggered by unbearable suffering. Suicide can be imagined as painful fractures with oneself, other people, and nature (Pompili, 2010). In the Indigenous (tangata whenua) perspective of suicide in Aotearoa New Zealand, mauri (life force), mauri ora (flourishing), and mauri noho (languishing) are key concepts. Notably, these te reo Māori (Māori language) terms mirror those used in the very first chapter of this text, where the continuum of mental health to mental illness was presented. Within Mātauranga Māori[1] one's life force is believed to constantly change and can influence a person's being, as well as how they relate to themselves, their world, and the wider environment (Durie, 2017).

---

[1] Mātauranga Māori is a term used to refer to the traditional knowledge of the Māori people including their culture, values, identity, and world view (Hikuroa, 2017).

BOX 44-1 ■ Reflections of a New Grad: A Call to Action

Contributed by *Meghan Lees, OT Reg. (Ont.), MScOT, HBSc (she/her/hers)*
Occupational Therapist
Community Rehabilitation Services

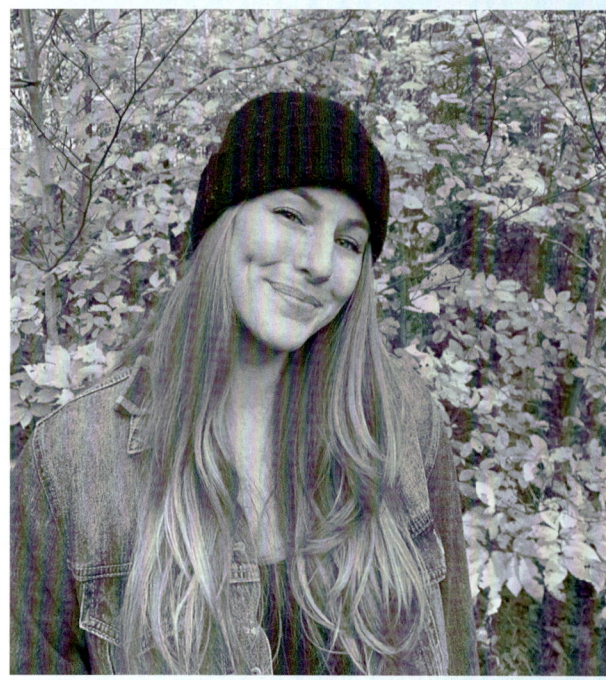

When starting my professional degree, I did not anticipate that occupational therapy would be deemed a key player in addressing suicide. I had chalked this role up to psychiatrists, psychologists, psychotherapists, or social workers. However, I came to appreciate that as holistic providers, OTPs are in fact mental health providers, too. Further, I have recalled the quote, "Medicine adds days to life, occupational therapy adds life to days." A key tenet in addressing and intervening in suicide is to find a turning point that connects to life and to assist with life. As such, I believe practitioners are primed to play a pivotal role in addressing suicide and promoting hope for living. We understand the importance of meaning in our day-to-day lives and of doing, being, becoming, and belonging.

As a new grad clinician, I urge students to seek opportunities to acquire knowledge and skills to equip you with the competence to address suicide, both in your clinical practicums and future practice. I currently work in community mental health and the topic of suicide has come up on various occasions within my first 6 months of practice. In considering these instances, I would also like to gently remind both new and seasoned practitioners that we can be competent yet sometimes lack the confidence. I recall many of these conversations being difficult and doubting myself, though through experiential learning and practice, I have carried with me the comfort of knowing I did my part in initiating a difficult conversation and assisting with life.

Mauri ora (flourishing, well-being), the ultimate state of mauri, is a state of positive vitality, with connections to people, place, and society that bring a sense of purpose and meaning (Durie, 2017). In the state of mauri noho, one's mauri (life force) has been weakened. Mauri noho encompasses the painful feelings and emotions of languishing, where low physical and mental energy is observed and there is a lack of participation in society, weakening the life force and will to live. See Chapter 1: Occupational Therapy Practice Across the Mental Health Continuum.

In North America, Marsha Linehan is a well-known psychologist who developed Dialectical Behavior Therapy (DBT). This evidence-based therapy for persons with borderline personality disorder is designed to help them manage their self-harm and suicidal thoughts and behaviors. Linehan personally lived with suicidal thoughts and behaviors and in her 2020 biography she shared her lived experience of suicidality:

> Like someone trapped in a small room with high walls that are stark white. The room has no lights or windows. The room is hot and humid, and the boiling heat of the floor of hell is excruciatingly painful. The person searches for a door out to a life worth living but cannot find it. Scratching and clawing on the walls do no good. Screaming and banging bring no help. Falling to the floor and trying to shut down and feel nothing gives no relief. Praying to God and all the saints one knows brings no salvation. The room is so painful that enduring it for even a moment longer appears impossible; any exit will do. The only door out the individual can find is the door of suicide. The urge to open it is great indeed. (Linehan, 2020, p. 24)

Epidemiology Worldwide

The latest data provided by WHO for the year 2019 indicates that 703,000 persons died by suicide (WHO, 2021b). Rates varied between countries from fewer than two deaths by suicide per 100,000 to over 80 per 100,000. Globally, the age-standardized suicide rate was 2.3 times higher in men than in women. Most deaths by suicide occurred in low- and middle-income countries (77%), where most of the world's population live. More than half of global suicides (58%) occurred before the age of 50 years (Fig. 44-1).

The iceberg in Figure 44-2 is a way to conceptualize the impact of suicide. This image alerts readers to intervention potential across the suicide continuum. This includes considerations of **suicide prevention** (for people affected by a suicide), **intervention** (for people with thoughts of suicide), and **postvention** (for people with nonfatal suicidal behaviors and loved ones of those who die by suicide). It is important to realize that these are not stages that occur in a hierarchy. A brief description of intervention at each point of the continuum follows in Table 44-1 and is expanded on throughout this chapter.

Continuum: Prevention

WHO is working to mobilize countries to engage in suicide prevention interventions. The LIVE LIFE program, endorsed by WHO, aims to encourage countries to develop national

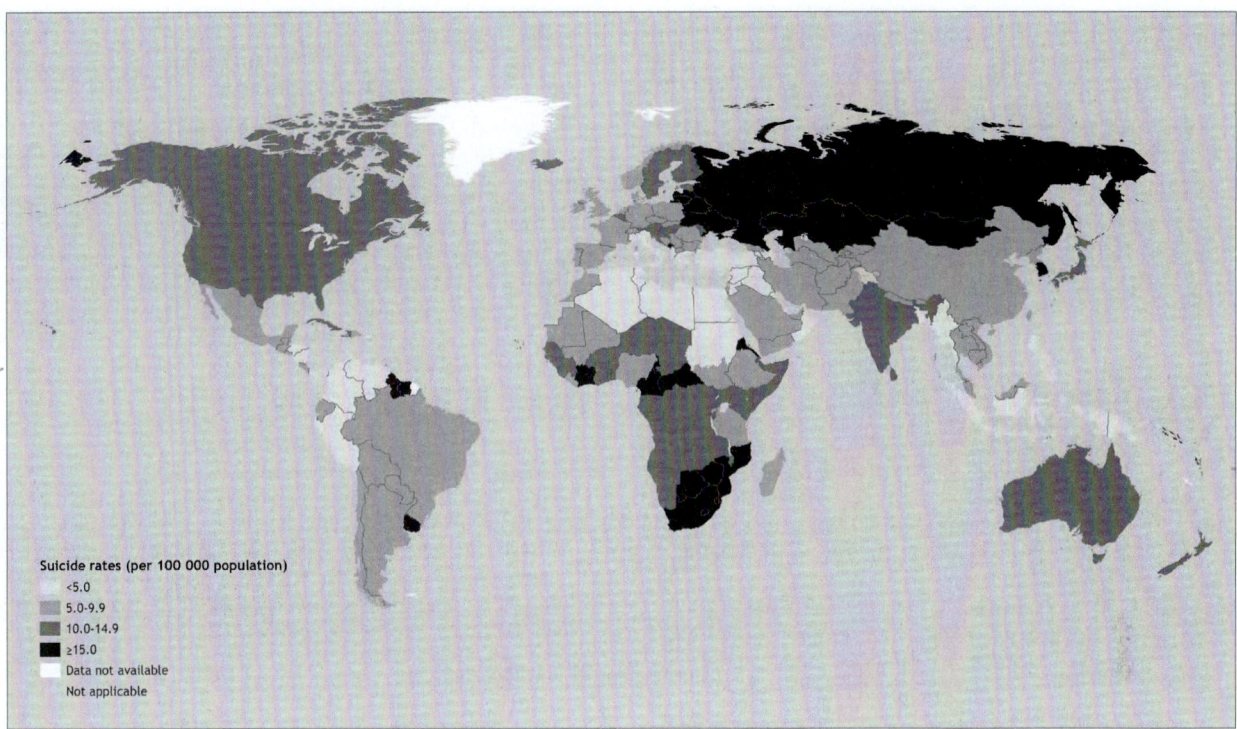

Source: WHO Global Health Estimates 2000-2019

FIGURE 44-1. Global epidemiology of suicide. *Courtesy of World Health Organization. (2021).* LIVE LIFE: An implementation guide for suicide prevention in countries. *Author. https://www.who.int/publications/i /item/9789240026629.*

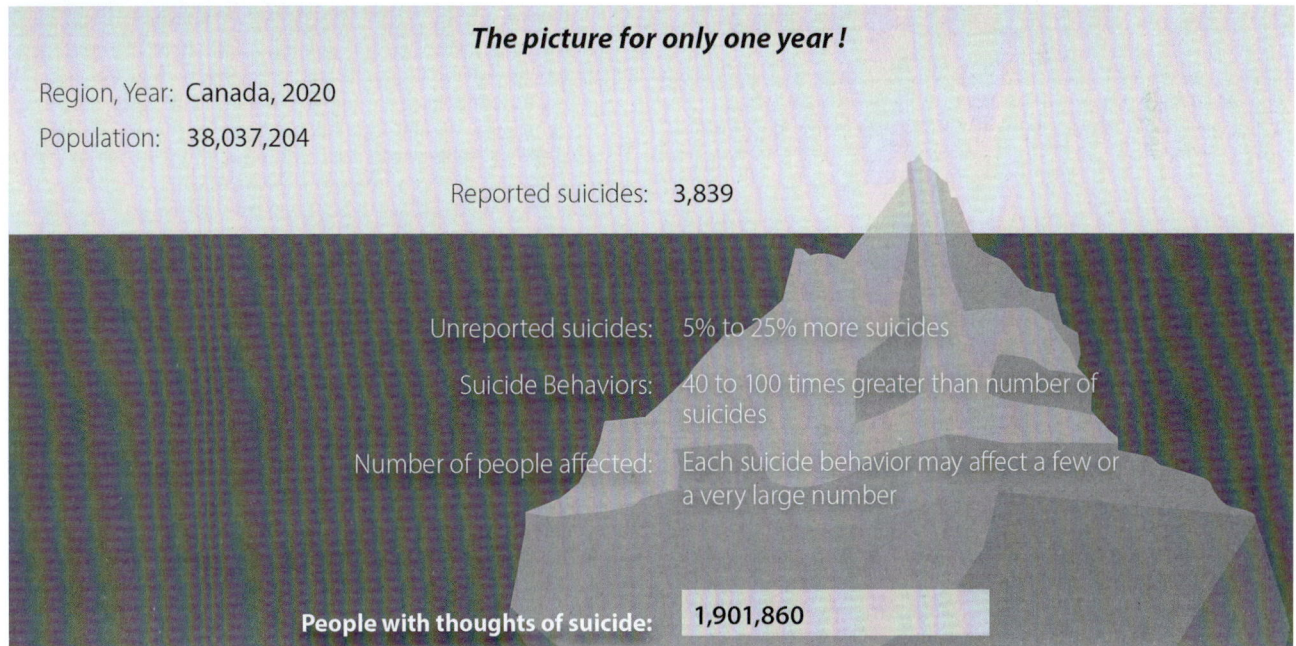

FIGURE 44-2. The impact of suicide. LivingWorks Education. (2018). *ASIST Applied Suicide Intervention Skills Training: Trainer manual with update insert.* https://livingworks.net/training/livingworks-asist

suicide prevention strategies using the core pillars of situation analysis; multisectoral collaboration; awareness-raising and advocacy; capacity-building; financing; and surveillance, monitoring, and evaluation (WHO, 2021a). LIVE LIFE endorses the following key effective interventions for suicide prevention: "limit access to means of suicide, interaction with the media for responsible reporting of suicide,

foster socio-emotional life skills in adolescents, early identify, assess, manage and follow up anyone who is affected by suicidal behaviours" (WHO, 2021a, p. 4).

An inspirational example of a community-built prevention approach comes from Aotearoa New Zealand. Te Tiriti o Waitangi, and recognition of the special relationship between Māori and the Crown, is key to achieving pae ora (healthy

TABLE 44-1 | Stage of Continuum and Focus of Interventions

Stage	Intervention Focus
Suicide prevention	• Provide identification; early detection, and action on personal, social, and collective risk factors. • Offer support programs for persons who are more at risk (e.g., marginalized groups, persons with mental health and addiction issues). • Provide socioeconomic and cultural conditions for life promotion and mental wellness in a population.
Suicide intervention	• Address the risk of suicide, focusing on how best to respond early when someone has thoughts of suicide or suicide-related behaviors. • Provide intervention if suicide screening/assessment indicates that there is a risk of suicide. • Consider the nature of intervention based on the current level of risk, the practitioner's personal comfort and skill level, and monitor/modify with changing levels of risk.
Suicide postvention	• Support those affected after the loss or experience of suicide and provide follow-up education/prevention to reduce the risk of future crises. • Provide support for family and friends after a death by suicide, involve staff when there is death by suicide, and reevaluate risk management procedures.

Canadian Association for Suicide Prevention. (2023). Home page. *https://suicideprevention.ca/resource/suicide-is-everyones-business-steps-in-prevention*

futures) and equity for Māori. Tūramarama ki te Ora (Durie et al., 2017) provides the foundation for dialogue and partnership between government agencies and Māori to address the unacceptably high Māori suicide rate. The wider aim of Tūramarama ki te Ora is to contribute to Māori well-being, Māori resilience and flourishing whānau, through a commitment to promote Māori ownership of Māori well-being and suicide prevention (Durie et al., 2017).

The main concepts include the following: to build on the strengths of Māori whānau, hapū, iwi, and communities; deliver culturally safe supports and services; prioritize whānau-centered treatment and management models; acknowledge intergenerational trauma, grief, and loss of mana; provide suicide bereavement responses that protect the continuation of whakapapa, hapū, and iwi structures; and build the evidence base and Mātauranga Māori of what works for Māori (Durie et al., 2017).

Whether at the systems level as in the previous examples or working at the individual person level as in the story with Cara and Evan introduced in the text that follows (Boxes 44-2 and 44-3), a common challenge exists within the prevention point on the continuum regarding identifying who is at risk for suicide, protective factors, and what screens may help define level of risk. Engage the application story and person-environment-occupation (PEO) oriented

---

BOX 44-2 ■ Application Story—Cara and Evan Part A

My name is Cara, and I am an OTP. When I met Evan, I was working for a large mental health hospital in an outpatient setting, specifically around gambling addiction. Evan was in his early 30s and was wanting to reduce his gambling because of significant financial, legal, and emotional challenges he was experiencing. When I began as an OTP on the problem gambling team, I oriented myself to the specific needs of the practice environment, including the increased risk of suicide for the people I would be serving. In addition to having gambling as a risk factor, Evan's additional risk factors included being diagnosed with bipolar disorder and having a history of past suicide attempts. He also had limited protective factors, as he was not employed and had no purposeful activity in his day.

Cara's Therapeutic Reasoning: When I met Evan, I knew I would have to keep a close eye on him. He had several risk factors and limited protective factors. I made the clinical decision to see him more often than other people on my caseload and refer him to groups I was facilitating to keep an even closer watch. I had to also set boundaries and remind myself that there was a limit to what I could do.

BOX 44-3 ■ Application Story—Cara and Evan Part B

I collaborated with Evan to establish a treatment plan that he felt would provide him with enhanced meaning and purpose in his life. Two of his main triggers to gambling were boredom and loneliness. We set occupational goals for him to volunteer at an animal shelter, reach out to his friend once a week, and engage in his previous interests in creative writing and hiking. Secondly, I referred Evan to our team psychiatrist and the emotion regulation program facilitated by our team. Ensuring that Evan had the appropriate medical intervention and coping skills to manage his emotional challenges was going to be fundamental to his safety. I also worked with Evan to develop a crisis plan. Although we had not yet experienced a crisis together, I wanted to ensure there was a safety plan in place should a crisis occur. He provided me with the phone numbers of two emergency contacts and we spoke about which hospital he would prefer to go to if he ever needed to go.

Some days Evan came to our meetings, and he had clearly put effort into his appearance, he used humor, and he was eager to set goals. Each visit I assessed for suicide, considering various factors including Evan's mood. When Evan reported feeling "great" and was "future oriented," I had increased confidence his current safety plan was sufficient. During other meetings he appeared downcast, tired, and slightly disheveled. On those days, I always asked explicitly about his suicidal ideation and revisited his safety plan to determine if adjustments were needed.

Cara's Therapeutic Reasoning: I was proud of the work I was doing with Evan, and I was deeply hoping it would be enough to prevent his passive suicidal ideation from escalating. The part of me that wants to rescue people was coming on strong in my work with Evan, and I desperately wanted to help him change his life and keep him safe. Every time I saw him, I braced myself for a bad day, and relished the good days when he had them.

TABLE 44-2 | Risk Factors Through a PEO Lens

Person (Characteristics)	• Gender: Men (suicide)
	• Age: Adolescents
	• Current or history of adverse childhood experiences
	• History of suicidal behavior
	• Mental health disorders, including substance-related and addictive disorders (e.g., gambling)
	• Brain-related disorders (e.g., cognitive decline in seniors, traumatic brain injury)
	• Certain personality traits: hopelessness, impulsivity, neuroticism, anxiety
	• Groups vulnerable to stigmatization and marginalization (e.g., LGBTQ+; Indigenous)
	• Loneliness
	• Grief from loss of relatives and friends who passed away from COVID-19
Environment (Social, Physical, Political)	• Exposure to violence (bullying, child abuse)
	• Groups vulnerable to stigmatization and marginalization (e.g., LGBTQ+; Indigenous)
	• Social isolation (loneliness)
	• Season (spring, summer)
	• Carceral institutions (e.g., juvenile detention, jails, prisons)
	• Internet and media information which reports on suicides
	• Marital status (single, divorced, and widowed) and marital conflicts
	• Economic insecurity and hardship
	• Family dynamics
	• Access to lethal means (e.g., handguns, medications)
	• Lack of access to health care and stigma associated with help-seeking and mental illness
Occupation (Features of Occupations)	• Unemployment
	• Certain types of jobs: first responders, police, military, frontline health professionals (e.g., during the COVID-19 pandemic)
	• Certain working conditions (e.g., shifts, temporary position, lack of task variety)
	• Boredom
	• Loss of independence to accomplish ADLs in older adults
	• Insomnia

Harris, L. M., Huang, X., Linthicum, K. P., Bryen, C. P., & Ribeiro, J. D. (2020). Sleep disturbances as risk factors for suicidal thoughts and behaviours: A meta-analysis of longitudinal studies. Scientific Reports, 10*(1), 13888. https://doi.org/10.1038/s41598-020-70866-6; Mental Health Commission of Canada (2018).* Research on suicide and its prevention: What the current evidence reveals and topics for future research. *Public Health Agency Canada; Mohanty, S., Sahu, G., Mohanty, M. K., & Patnaik, M. (2007). Suicide in India: A four year retrospective study.* Journal of Forensic and Legal Medicine, 14*(4), 185–189. https://doi.org/10.1016/j.jcfm .2006.05.007; National Center for Injury Prevention and Control. (2022).* Suicide Prevention Resource for Action: A compilation of the best available evidence. *Centers for Disease Control and Prevention. https://www.cdc.gov/suicide/pdf/preventionresource.pdf; Rurup, M. L., Pasman, H. R. W., Goedhart, J., Deeg, D. J. H., Kerkhof, A. J. F. M., & Onwuteaka-Philipsen, B. D. (2011). Understanding why older people develop a wish to die.* Crisis, 32*(4), 204–216. https://doi.org/10.1027 /0227-5910/a000078; Zalsman, G., Stanley, B., Szanto, K., Clarke, D. E., Carli, V., & Mehlum, L. (2020). Suicide in the time of COVID-19: Review and recommendations.* Archives of Suicide Research, 24*(4), 477–482. https://doi.org/10.1080/13811118.2020.1830242*

Tables 44-2 and 44-3 to begin to identify some high risk and protective factors.

This part of Cara and Evan's story emphasizes the practitioner's need to have a clear and holistic picture of a person's situation. For Cara to operate as an evidence-informed practitioner, she needed to assess and discuss what could increase Evan's risk of suicide and be aware of the research on factors that could buffer and protect Evan. For example, knowing how Evan cultivated resilience was essential to assess.

Risk Factors for Suicide

It is very often a combination of **risk factors** that will strain a person to a point of contemplating suicide (Gunnell & Chang, 2016). A qualitative study involving 31 older adults illustrates this finding (Rurup et al., 2011). The participants shared that going through many losses and other adverse events over time accumulated reasons to develop a wish to die. These individuals expressed a sense of resignation for not being able to find a new purpose in life and not feeling useful because of health challenges and related impairments and disabilities affecting their capacity to accomplish many activities of daily living (ADLs; Rurup et al., 2011). Table 44-2 builds on these findings and shows that risk factors for suicide can be viewed through a PEO lens and are often related to personal characteristics, environmental influences, and features of occupations.

At a collective level, examples of risk factors for suicide in Indigenous communities include loss of culture (e.g., language), insecure cultural identity, spiritual disconnection, and colonization (e.g., oppression, alienation from ancestral lands, and loss of self-determination; Durie, 2001, 2017). At the prevention point on the continuum, a focus on large groups at greater risk of suicide is an important health

TABLE 44-3 | Protective Factors Through a PEO Lens

Person (Characteristics)	• Positive attributional style
	• Personal sense of agency
	• Having coping strategies
	• Strong sense of cultural identity
Environment (Social, Physical, Political)	• Stable and favorable socioeconomic situation
	• Loving parent–child relationship
	• Social connectedness
	• Sense of belonging
	• Services that treat symptoms and/or offer support
	• Residential stability
Occupation (Features of Occupation)	• Leisure activities (hobbies)
	• Having a pet
	• Having a job; employment stability
	• Sports
	• Feeling connected to school, community, social institutions

Beaudoin, V., Séguin, M., Chawky, N., Affleck, W., Chachamovich, E., & Turecki, G. (2018). Protective factors in the Inuit population of Nunavut: A comparative study of people who died by suicide, people who attempted suicide, and people who never attempted suicide. International Journal of Environmental Research and Public Health, 15(1), 144. https://doi.org/10.3390/ijerph15010144; Deuter, K., Procter, N., & Evans, D. (2020). Protective factors for older suicide attempters: Finding reasons and experiences to live. Death Studies, 44(7), 430–439. https://doi.org/10.1080/07481187.2019.1578303; Johnson, J., Wood, A. M., Gooding, P., Taylor, P. J., & Tarrier, N. (2011). Resilience to suicidality: The buffering hypothesis. Clinical Psychology Review, 31(4), 563–591. https://doi.org/10.1016/j.cpr.2010.12.007; Mental Health Commission of Canada (2018). Research on suicide and its prevention: What the current evidence reveals and topics for future research. Public Health Agency Canada; National Center for Injury Prevention and Control. (2022). Suicide Prevention Resource for Action: A compilation of the best available evidence. Centers for Disease Control and Prevention. https://www.cdc.gov/suicide/pdf/preventionresource.pdf; Odom, K. (2016). Combating the suicide epidemic: The effects of leisure engagement on the incidence of depression and poor life satisfaction in soldiers. Occupational Therapy in Mental Health, 32(1), 70–85. https://doi.org/10.1080/0164212X.2015.1082172

promotion perspective that could make a significant impact on coping and trajectory (LivingWorks, 2014).

Occupations and Suicide—Work

Certain types of jobs are related to increased risks of suicide because of the nature of the work responsibilities, the environment, and the conditions of the job. People working in emergency services, law enforcement, or the military can experience repeated stressful and potentially traumatic situations that increase their risk of having mental health issues (e.g., depression, posttraumatic stress disorder [PTSD], anxiety; Reger et al., 2020).

Exposure to death or pain may have the effect of decreasing inner fear and make the person more at risk of contemplating suicide as an option to cope (Chu et al., 2017). Available access to lethal means can also be a factor, such as medications/drugs for health-care workers, carbon monoxide for bus or truck drivers, or firearms for law enforcement officers (Milner et al., 2017). Finally, the case of family physicians indicates that a job with moral loneliness, conflicts with

family life, constant interruptions both at home and at work, constraints (e.g., administrative), and high expectations from management and people are conditions that can affect job satisfaction and mental health (Dutheil et al., 2019).

Unemployment, having a fragile work status, and engaging in shift work have also been associated with increased suicidal ideation and risk (Dalglish et al., 2015; Faria et al., 2020; Park, 2019). This instability may bring financial stress and insecurity for the future (Dalglish et al., 2015; Park, 2019). Shift work often interferes with socialization aligned with traditional working hours, leads to feelings of disconnection and isolation (Park, 2019; Vogel et al., 2012), and disrupts the quality of sleep (Vogel et al., 2012). Unemployment can affect self-esteem, reduce social contacts, and take away structure in routines and daily schedules (Gunnell & Chang, 2016). Within the work environment, lack of job autonomy and task variety as well as ongoing struggles to balance work and family life obligations can influence suicidal ideation and depression and, thus, suicide attempts (Howard & Krannitz, 2017).

Regardless of the context surrounding work, social support within the job and outside the work environment appear to be important protective factors (Faria et al., 2020).

Occupations and Suicide—Sleep

In an analysis of a cohort of 394,000 Taiwanese adults, Gunnell and colleagues (2013) found that fewer than 6 hours of sleep, difficulty falling asleep, being easily awoken, active dreaming, and reported use of sleep medications were markers for suicide risk. Similarly, a recent meta-analysis showed that insomnia significantly predicted suicide ideation and nightmares, which significantly predicted suicide attempts (Harris et al., 2020).

Protective Factors for Suicide

Resilience and meaning in life, assessed through perceptions of aspects of life which are fulfilling and satisfactory, as well as life goals and purposes have been shown to buffer the association between suicide risk factors and hopelessness in persons living with mental health conditions (Marco et al., 2016). Belonging, safety, dignity, and hope also support resilience (NCIPC, 2022). **Protective factors** for suicide also include personal characteristics, occupational features, and environmental influences, as shown in Table 44-3.

At the personal level, having an overall positive attributional style (i.e., explaining negative events by causes that are external, likely to change, and specific) and a high level of agency (controlling and governing one's actions and decisions) have been associated with resilience (Johnson et al., 2011). A qualitative study involving persons with a lived suicidal experience informs OTPs that having close relationships is important in that they provide someone to share one's life with and express one's abilities in relationships, such as taking care or helping. Different types of pleasures, such as intellectual ones to contact harmony, beauty, and creativity, as well as nonintellectual pleasures, including sports, recreational activities, convivial occasions, and travel, contribute to give life meaning (Constanza et al., 2020). Being employed or engaged as a student is an occupation that supports self-realization and a positive self-image (Constanza et al., 2020).

An increasing amount of evidence indicates that aspects of culture and cultural identity are important protective factors for Indigenous persons in North America (Beaudoin et al., 2018) and Aotearoa New Zealand (Ihimaera & MacDonald, 2009). Strong cultural identity has been associated with better overall well-being and fewer depressive symptoms in young Māori (Williams et al., 2018).

When examining the two tables listing risk and protective factors, it is interesting to note that some factors, such as work, can protect or enhance risk. Religion is also that type of factor. Regardless of one's religion, a common value message, to varying degrees, is condemnation of taking one's life (Nelson et al., 2012). Still, religions also offer explanations about the complexities and mysteries of life, death, and the universe, which serves as a source of comfort and meaning and can appease existential anxiety for some (Eskin et al., 2019). Religious practices, such as prayer, meditation, or listening to music/chanting associated with the religion, can alleviate anxiety or depressive symptoms (Nelson et al., 2012).

Religion also allows social affiliation by practicing in a community with shared beliefs or a network of support in challenging life situations (Eskin et al., 2019). However, in some groups, such as the LGBTQ+ (lesbian, gay, bisexual, transgender, queer [and in some cases, "questioning"], plus others yet to be defined), religiosity can trigger additional conflicting feelings because of negative attitudes and beliefs toward homosexuality and exclusion from religious groups (Gibbs, 2015). Understanding the personal meaning of protective and risk factors is critical.

Ethical Considerations for Addressing Suicide in Practice

As Cara's self-dialogue shows, when a practitioner is addressing the suicide continuum it can trigger different types of fears and questions. A specific fear is doubting whether one is doing the right thing and the potential repercussions of one's actions. Severe distress, including high levels of depression, guilt, grief, inadequacy, and anxiety, was found among a group of psychologists, psychiatrists, and social workers when surveyed about their reactions when a person they work with dies by suicide (Hendin et al., 2004). In her story, Cara models the importance of person-centered care emphasizing Evan's strengths and preferences and actively engaging him in creating his own safety plan.

A critical action step for all practitioners working with people with thoughts of suicide is to ensure a comprehensive suicide safety plan is created and reviewed periodically. Examples of components for a practitioner to consider are demonstrated in Cara's reflection. Table 44-7 includes more specific resources to understand how to develop a suicide safety plan.

Impact of Media

Many people get their informal training about suicide from social media or television/film, which often contributes to unhelpful views of suicide and the stigma that is too often associated with suicide. WHO (2021a) identifies media reporting as critical in reducing suicide as suicide imitation becomes a risk if not reported responsibly. This chapter's Mental

Health in Culture and Society feature reviews the television program *13 Reasons Why* to illustrate the very dangerous consequences that can occur when suicide is discussed and represented poorly in the media. The Recommendations for Reporting on Suicide list indicates what to do and what not to do when sharing information about suicide in the media (Reporting on Suicide, 2020).

Mental Health in Culture and Society

Contributed by Aster Harrison

Impact of Media and Ethical Reporting—*13 Reasons Why*

In 2017, the first season of the TV show *13 Reasons Why* (McCarthy, 2017) caused a controversy for its representation of suicide. The show's main character, a teenager named Hannah, dies by suicide. Before her death, Hannah records 13 cassette tapes for people who she deems responsible (at least in part) for her suicide. The first season begins after Hannah's death and follows the suspenseful reveal of the content of the tapes. This dramatic unfolding of events after her death is intercut with flashbacks to the memories Hannah describes on the tapes.

Although suicide is certainly an important issue to discuss in media for teenagers, scientific research shows that the way *13 Reasons Why* depicts suicide is dangerous. Public suicides have a documented *contagion effect,* meaning that when people learn of a suicide, this often spurs an increase in suicides in the group of people who learn this death (Reporting on Suicide, 2020). This is particularly true when a great deal of information is shared about the suicide, including the method of death and the content of the suicide note (or video or tape). Contagion effects have also been shown to be more powerful when the person who dies by suicide is a well-liked, well-known person, such as a celebrity or a close friend that people admired. If the method of death is reported, there is a 30% increase in risk of death by that same method (Niederkrotenthaler et al., 2020). Suicide contagion can happen because of both fictional depictions of suicide (Niederkrotenthaler et al., 2021) and reporting on the suicides of real people (Niederkrotenthaler et al., 2020).

Because of the risks of suicide contagion, a team of scientists, suicide prevention organizations, public health organizations, and journalism organizations teamed up to publish the Recommendations for Reporting on Suicide (Reporting on Suicide, 2020). These recommendations are a list of what to do and what not to do when sharing information about suicide in the media. For example, responsible media reporting about suicide should not share the methods or location of the suicide, glamorize the suicide, present suicide as an appropriate response to hardship, or provide specific details about the person who died. They encourage media to share resources for support and treatment and to emphasize that help is effective and available (Reporting on Suicide, 2020).

Experts on suicide prevention were extremely concerned about *13 Reasons Why,* because the show does nearly everything that experts suggest that people avoid. The show depicts suicide as Hannah's way of exacting revenge on the people who mistreated her in high school.

It positions Hannah as the likeable main character and romanticizes the way her classmates and school are affected by her death. And in the final episode of Season 1, the original version of the series showed the character's suicide on screen in graphic detail.

Unfortunately, research suggests that the way the creators of *13 Reasons Why* chose to depict suicide contributed to a notable increase in teen suicides. Soon after the season was released, research indicated that Google searches for methods of dying by suicide (e.g., "how to commit suicide," "how to kill yourself") were significantly higher in the 19 days following the release of *13 Reasons Why* (Ayers et al., 2017). And in 2019, a study found that there was a 28.9% increase in completed suicides among 10- to 17-year-olds in the month following the release of *13 Reasons Why* (Bridge et al., 2019). The researchers controlled for seasonal effects and general trends of increasing suicides among youth and concluded that this uptick in suicides was linked to the show.

Two months after the study by Bridge and colleagues was published, Netflix removed the graphic 3-minute suicide scene from the final episode of *13 Reasons Why*. At the time of this writing, the series begins with a recorded message from the actors warning viewers about the content and encouraging them to watch with a trusted adult or seek help if they are struggling with the issues depicted in the show. At several points in the first series, a link to a website with resources about sexual assault and suicide (13ReasonsWhy.info) is shared. Although the deletion of the suicide scene and the addition of content warnings and resources are steps in the right direction, *13 Reasons Why* still represents suicide in a glamorized fashion that does not conform with reporting guidelines and could increase risk of suicide among viewers.

Media guidelines play a critical role in preventing future suicides, and many countries have defined reporting guidelines (Reporting on Suicide, 2020). For example, within Aotearoa New Zealand, there are some restrictions on what can be made public about a suicide or suspected suicide (Mental Health Foundation of New Zealand, 2023). Unless an exemption is issued by the chief coroner, no one is able to make public the method or suspected method of the death, any detail (such as the place of death) that might suggest the method or suspected method of the death, or a description of the death as a suicide before the coroner has released their findings and stated the death was a suicide (although the death can be described as a suspected suicide before then). "Making public" does not just mean news reports and other media—it also includes things such as public posts on Facebook, too. Whether or not someone has died from suicide is a legal decision made by coroners, not a medical decision made by doctors.

Within Canada, there are guidelines for reporting on mental health called Mindset (Canadian Journalism Forum on Violence and Trauma, 2020). The purpose of this document is to reduce stigma around suicide by equipping journalists with the background and language needed for safe reporting. OTPs can advocate for sounder representation of suicide in the media by being mindful of these reporting guidelines in their own communications with others in their communities.

It is important to break the silence around suicide, but it is equally important to do so in a responsible manner. See Chapter 33: Virtual Environments.

Occupational Therapy Within Suicide Prevention Care

Although OTPs are rarely cited in the literature as a discipline equipped to prevent and support people with suicidal thinking and/or recovery from suicidal actions, there is a clear role for OTPs at the individual and population levels. The Canadian Association of Occupational Therapists published a role paper outlining the important role occupational therapy has across the suicide prevention continuum, which is discussed alongside common occupational therapy process frameworks. The paper identifies a vision for the profession and for the individual practitioner (Hewitt et al., 2019). For the profession, the vision outlines that OTPs are well positioned to address suicide in their practice, consider mental health wellness as a foundational aspect of care, and that all practitioners be minimally equipped with gatekeeper training (GKT) to address suicide across all practice settings (Hewitt et al., 2019). GKT is discussed in more detail later in this chapter.

For the individual practitioner, the role paper outlines a vision in which all OTPs are oriented to key suicide prevention resources, ask directly about suicide, acknowledge suffering as a barrier to living, apply current occupational therapy models, and engage in self-care (Hewitt et al., 2019).

When examining the strategies and approaches to achieve and sustain substantial reductions in suicide recommended by the NCIPC (2022), many target intervention on occupational aspects of life and align with the occupational therapy contributions described in the role paper. These may include creating protective environments, stabilizing housing, engaging community members in shared activities and healthy connections, teaching coping and problem-solving skills, and supporting resilience through education programs.

Continuum: Crisis Intervention

In 2014, a survey of 585 Canadian OTPs practicing in various settings demonstrated that 88% of the respondents identified that they had to provide suicide intervention in their occupational therapy careers (Collins et al., 2014). Despite this, a substantial number of health-care professionals feel that their training is inadequate to appropriately address the topic of suicide in their practice (Canady, 2018; Cross et al., 2019). Although suicide ideation and behaviors have primarily been associated with mental health practice, individuals at risk are identified across a range of occupational therapy practice settings and include veterans, individuals with chronic illnesses, marginalized populations, and those who have suffered physical or emotional trauma or stressors (Aquila et al., 2020; Collins et al., 2014; Kashiwa et al., 2017).

A survey of 12 Canadian occupational therapy programs (out of 14) revealed that a broad range of pedagogical methods were being used by programs to educate their students on suicide prevention; however, there was a lack consistency on how and what education was provided (Larivière et al., 2021). Only one school out of the 12 required their students to participate in a formal training program (Larivière et al., 2021). However, 10 other programs did suggest training for their students, which was not mandatory, and students were expected to organize and pay for the training out of pocket (Larivière et al., 2021). As such, many novice practitioners might lack the skills, knowledge, and self-efficacy to effectively address suicide in their practice.

One approach to filling this knowledge gap across the various areas of practice in occupational therapy is **gatekeeper training** (GKT; Isaac et al., 2009). Gatekeepers are individuals who have primary contact with individuals at risk for suicide. Gatekeepers can be health professionals, school personnel, family members, religious leaders, coaches, law

enforcement personnel, and other community members (Burnette et al., 2015; Isaac et al., 2009). GKT is an approach to suicide prevention that teaches gatekeepers how to identify people at risk for suicide by recognizing suicidal risk factors (Isaac et al., 2009). The training also teaches gatekeepers how to manage the risk of suicide by referring the individuals to appropriate support services (Burnette et al., 2015; Isaac et al., 2009). These training programs are modeled on the fact that individuals who are at the highest risk of suicide often do not seek help and that gatekeepers can help identify and manage the risk (Isaac et al., 2009). This chapter's Evidence-Based Practice feature summarizes current research on the efficacy of gatekeeping programs.

Evidence-Based Practice

Gatekeeper Training

GKT programs are evidence-based and widely accessible for individuals seeking to gain competency in suicide risk assessment and management.

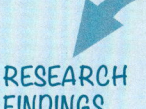

RESEARCH FINDINGS

GKT is an effective approach to helping individuals learn to identify, assess, and connect people at risk of suicide with appropriate care (Holmes et al., 2019; Yonemoto et al., 2019). Patel and Degagne's (2017) review of the literature identified seven GKT programs with evidence for increasing a clinician's self-efficacy, knowledge, skills, and attitudes toward suicide risk assessment and management: Question, Persuade, Respond (QPR); Applied Suicide Intervention Skills Training (ASIST); Skills Training On Risk Management (STORM); Counseling Access to Lethal Means (CALM); Recognizing and Responding to Suicide Risk (RRSR); Suicide Awareness and Intervention Program (SAIP); and the Collaborative Assessment and Management of Suicidality (CAMS). Content and training processes in these programs differ, and Patel and Degagne (2017) did not identify a gold standard program. However, a minimum set of GKT competencies that are organized around knowledge, skills and abilities, attitudes, and self-efficacy has been proposed by other researchers (Hawgood et al., 2021).

Some of the strongest outcomes of GKT programs involve a practitioner's knowledge, attitudes, and self-efficacy around suicide prevention (Hawgood et al., 2021; Zinzow et al., 2018). Systematic reviews of GKT programs often recommend periodic retraining (Holmes et al., 2019; Yonemoto et al., 2019). GKT approaches that provide opportunities for role-play and behavioral practice can be among the most effective approaches (Morton et al., 2021). GKT programs, using methods such as lectures, discussions, and role-play to target family and friends caring for individuals at risk for suicide, and for college students, for whom suicide is one of the leading causes of death, have been shown to be effective interventions to prevent suicide (Khadijah et al., 2023; Morton et al., 2021; Zinzow et al., 2018).

APPLICATIONS

➡ OTPs who participate in GKT can expect their knowledge and skills for recognizing and discussing suicide and for referring individuals at risk for suicide to improve.

➡ Practitioners are encouraged to seek out training that includes ample opportunities for role-play and for practicing the implementation of suicide prevention knowledge and skills.

➡ OTPs are encouraged to periodically refresh their GKT to keep their knowledge, skills, and self-efficacy for suicide prevention sharp.

Continued

Evidence-Based Practice—cont'd

REFERENCES

Hawgood, J., Woodward, A., Quinnett, P., & De Leo, D. (2021). Gatekeeper training and minimum standards of competency. *Crisis, 43*(6), 516–522. https://doi.org/10.1027/0227-5910/a000794

Holmes, G., Clancy, A., Hermens, D. F., & Lagopoulos, J. (2019). The long-term efficacy of suicide prevention gatekeeper training: A systematic review. *Archives of Suicide Research, 25*(2), 177–207. https://doi.org/10.1080/13811118.2019.1690608

Khadijah, S., Martono, M., & Tarnoto, K. W. (2023). Results of professional interventions of gatekeeper training programs for college student suicide prevention: A systematic review. *GSC Advanced Research and Reviews, 17*(3), 23–39. https://doi.org/10.30574/gscarr.2023.17.3.0443

Morton, M., Wang, S., Tse, K., Chung, C., Bergmans, Y., Ceniti, A., Flam, S., Johannes, R., Schade, K., Terah, F., & Rizvi, S. (2021). Gatekeeper training for friends and family of individuals at risk of suicide: A systematic review. *Journal of Community Psychology, 49*(6), 1838–1871. https://doi.org/10.1002/jcop.22624

Patel, M., & Degagne, C. (2017). *Supporting occupational therapists in practice: A review of suicide intervention training.* Canadian Association of Occupational Therapists. https://caot.ca/site/rc/caot-bc/practiceresources/suicideinterventiontraining?language=fr_FR&nav=sidebar

Yonemoto, N., Kawashima, Y., Endo, K., & Yamada, M. (2019). Implementation of gatekeeper training programs for suicide prevention in Japan: A systematic review. *International Journal of Mental Health Systems, 13*(1), Article 2. https://doi.org/10.1186/s13033-018-0258-3

Zinzow, H. M., Thompson, M. P., Fulmer, C. B., Goree, J., & Evinger, L. (2018). Evaluation of a brief suicide prevention training program for college campuses. *Archives of Suicide Research, 24*(1), 82–95. https://doi.org/10.1080/13811118.2018.1509749

There is great variability among GKT programs in terms of content, pedagogical approach, training length, cost, and availability. All suicide training programs provide basic rudimentary knowledge about facts and myths about suicide and risk and protective factors for suicide. Often, organizations or institutions may develop their own training programs, in collaboration with appropriate stakeholders, to support the gatekeepers in their communities. For example, because of the increasing concern of high rates of suicide among Aboriginal people in Australia, a culturally appropriate and sensitive GKT program, Shoalhaven Aboriginal Suicide Prevention Program (SASPP), was developed and implemented. This culturally responsive training program provided education about facts and myths about suicide, warning signs and risk factors, and referral strategies (Capp et al., 2001; National Academies of Science, Engineering and Medicine, 2022).

Finally, specific intervention approaches (e.g., DBT, Acceptance and Commitment Therapy [ACT], and Mentalization) include components related to managing suicide and offer knowledge and skills that can be generalized and applied by OTPs when working with individuals across the suicide continuum. When exploring additional training, practitioners should consider jurisdiction-related factors (provision of psychotherapy, training requirements for more intensive vs. less intensive intervention approaches, licensure laws, etc.). Examples of GKT programs are provided in the Resources at the end of the chapter.

Asking About Suicide: Introducing the Conversation

Asking directly about suicide is best practice and there is no evidence that asking directly about suicide will make people suicidal or make them engage in self-harm. Broaching the subject allows the person to talk about their feelings. Direct questioning can also assist the practitioner to assess how high the risk is for suicide (Table 44-4). For example, if a person

TABLE 44-4	Examples of Screening Questions for Suicide
Seniors	• "Are you thinking about suicide?" • "If you did not wake up the next morning, would that be a good thing? If yes, would you do anything to help that along?"
General Adult Population (From the PHQ-9; Kroenke et al., 2001)	• "Are you thinking about hurting yourself or killing yourself?" • "Have you ever thought you would be better off dead?"
Children 12+ Years Old (From the ASQ; Horowitz et al., 2012)	• "In the past few weeks, have you wished you were dead?" • "In the past few weeks, have you felt that you or your family would be better off if you were dead?" • "Have you been having thoughts about hurting yourself or killing yourself?"
Children (Under the Age of 12 Years)	• "Are you thinking about hurting yourself or killing yourself?" • "Are you depressed or very sad lately?" • "Did you ever feel so upset or sad that you wanted to die?"

has had previous suicide attempts and/or thoughts of suicide, has developed a series of actions toward committing suicide, and organized the means, then the individual may be much more prepared to follow through on suicide action.

Addressing the Risk of Suicide: Safety Plan

If suicide screening/assessment indicates that there is a risk of suicide, intervention is needed. The nature of the intervention depends on the current level of risk, the practitioner's personal

TABLE 44-5 | Coping Strategy Foundations

Coping Category	Purpose	Coping Strategy Examples
Maintain health and wellness routines.	Reduce stress by reducing change. Ensure basic physical needs are met.	Schedule healthy, balanced routines; address sleep hygiene and medication management.
Change the situation.	Choose action initiatives to gain control.	Set goals, communicate needs, set limits, and practice time management.
Change the body's response to stress.	Reduce fight/flight/freeze symptoms to assist with reasoning and problem-solving ability.	Identify stress symptoms, build distress tolerance, and practice relaxation and mindfulness.
Change attitude.	Manage thoughts to reduce emotion intensity; positive thoughts decrease emotional distress.	Recognize the thought-feeling-behavior connection, practice gratitude, reframe negative thinking, and use positive affirmations.

McNamara, M., & Straathof, T. (2017). Coping strategies to promote occupational engagement and recovery: A program manual for occupational therapists and other care providers. CAOT Publications ACE; Tubesing, N., & Tubesing, D. (1983). Structured exercises in stress management (Vol. 1). Whole Person Associates.

comfort and skill level of intervention, and the person's needs/abilities. Interventions are monitored and modified based on changing levels of risk. All people with suicidal thoughts or actions need a **safety plan,** because it will decrease the risk of a suicide attempt (Marshall et al., 2023; Moscardini et al., 2020). When a person seems to have lost purpose for life, practitioners use suicide safety plans to reengage individuals in meaningful occupations. Strategies that focus on reducing factors that increase risk of suicide and multiplying factors that promote coping and meaningful (protective) occupations are recommended (Marshall et al., 2023).

When a person has functional cognition and insight, they are likely to benefit from collaborating to complete a comprehensive suicide safety plan. If cognition is impaired, the practitioner must consider the environment that the person is living in and increase the support available to decrease suicide risk (e.g., limit access to lethal means). Many factors impact a person's ability to participate in suicide safety planning. For example, if an individual is not eating meals or not sleeping, they may have difficulty with the cognitive effort and problem-solving for creating a suicide safety plan. Completion of a safety plan may need to be deferred until functioning improves. Readiness for completion of a suicide safety plan begins with assessment of the person related to the following (Straathof et al., 2019):

- *Behavior activation:* The person follows basic routines for sleep and nutrition, tolerates some social interactions, and is somewhat activated during the day.
- *Cognitive function:* The person demonstrates insight, working memory, and ability to engage in problem-solving.
- *Coping strategies:* The person has knowledge/skill of some basic coping strategies from each of the four coping categories (Table 44-5).
- *Community integration:* The person has an interest in suicide safety planning and sharing the safety plan with community supports.

Components of a Comprehensive Suicide Safety Plan

A high-quality suicide safety plan (Box 44-4) has recommended components to include, is completed in advance of an event to manage a crisis, and is reviewed/updated

TABLE 44-6 | Examples of Ways to Reduce Lethal Means

Risk	Strategy to Reduce Access
Overdose	Work with supports to lock medications and remove excess medications; use a weekly medication blister pack.
Motor vehicle accident	Provide car keys to partner when symptoms are present.
Hanging	Work with supports to remove ropes/cords from home.
Power tools	Store at a support person's home.
Jumping from bridge	Choose a safe destination and constructive purpose when walking.
Knives	Remove excess sharps; lock drawers.
Handguns	Store unloaded in a locked gun safe, store handgun and ammunition separately, secure with locking device, and make a list of trusted family members to help reduce access during high-risk periods (e.g., transfer to them temporarily).

Note: Further training on this topic is recommended—see Counseling of Access to Lethal Means (CALM) at https://sprc.org/online-library/calm-counseling-on-access-to-lethal-means

periodically (Moscardini et al., 2020). See Table 44-6 for strategies for reducing access to lethal means and Table 44-7 for a summary of best practices for content and process for creating safety plans.

Documenting Interventions

Documentation is important for the security of the person receiving service and for the practitioner. Regulations for documentation from the professional association/regulatory body that a practitioner answers to must be respected. Such regulations may vary by jurisdiction, so the practitioner should verify guiding documents in their geographic area. Using a suicide prevention planning tool that is already in existence eases documentation time and effort. A practitioner using such a tool can refer to this in their documentation without needing to restate the full content and process. Sample documentation language might read: "The person completed a

TABLE 44-7 | Content and Process for a Suicide Safety Plan

- Recognize warning signs of an impending suicide crisis.
- Remind self of reasons to live.
- Employ internal coping strategies.
- Use social activity for distraction.
- Work with family or friends to manage the crisis.
- Include emergency contacts: names and contact information.
- Restrict/remove access to lethal means.

(Stanley & Brown, 2012)

- Words of others as to why the person is valued and appreciated
- Acts of kindness or gratitude

(Crowley et al., 2019)

- Personal and delegated responsibilities
- Coping strategy foundations (Table 44-5)
- Storage information of the plan with various stakeholders including informing personal and professional supports that a safety plan exists
- Clear timeline for review by self, and/or with personal and professional supports

(Straathof, 2022b)

- Monitoring and follow-up with named personal and professional supports, and modification of safety plan as needed (when there is a change in level of risk)

(Brodsky et al., 2018)

- Use a collaborative approach rather than self-administration.
- Include the person's own wording.
- Use a manual to guide the practitioner in completion of a safety plan.
- Consider following a teaching process such as Kolb's Adult Learning Model that supports partnership in training.
- Identify protocols for completion of suicide safety plans.

(Kolb, 2015; Moscardini et al., 2020)

BOX 44-4 ■ Mohammed: Implementing a Suicide Safety Plan

Mohammed is a 21-year-old university student admitted to inpatient psychiatry with suicide thoughts. The OTP assists him to develop coping foundations such as health and wellness routines, relaxation techniques, and reframing negative thinking to reduce anxiety. He is then ready to complete a suicide safety plan using the teaching module, sample plan, and template for the Suicide Safety Plan for Occupational Engagement and Recovery (SSP-OEAR; Straathof, 2022a).

Suicide Safety Plan for Occupational Engagement and Recovery (SSP-OEAR)

Name: Mohammed   *Date: March 28, 2023*

MISSION STATEMENT: What is my reason to live? What brings me meaning and purpose? *To explore my potential and see where I can go in life, to travel, my family*

WORDS OF OTHERS: Why do others appreciate me, and say I am important and valuable?
I am kind and generous—my friend Sam
I have a sense of humor—my roommates

WARNING SIGNS OF SUICIDE RISK

Triggers: *Failure, conflict with others*
Negative thoughts: *Life is too hard, my family is disappointed in me*
Emotions: *Overwhelmed, sad, anxious*
Physical symptoms: *Crying spells, loss of sleep, no appetite, pacing*
Actions: *Isolate from others, ruminate on negatives, research suicide methods*

BOX 44-4 ■ Mohammed: Implementing a Suicide Safety Plan—cont'd

COPING STRATEGIES—I can take these steps when warning signs are present to stay safe:

A balanced thought: *My family and friends care for me and love me, I can find solutions*

To manage emotions: *Deep breathing, go for a walk*

To manage physical symptoms: *Listen to calming music, follow consistent sleep/wake times*

Constructive actions: *Ask for help, talk to my friend about how I am feeling*

A social interaction for distraction: *Play basketball with my friend Mitch*

An act of kindness or gratitude: *Thank my mom for support*

How can I make my environment safe? Remove lethal means. Add healthy means.
Return extra medications to pharmacy with my friend's help, use weekly blister packs

Name my responsibility in using this safety plan:
Let friend or counselor know if suicide thoughts are present, take medication correctly

Name two people I will share the plan with and state what support they could provide:

1. *Friend Sam—do something fun for distraction such as watch a comedy show together*

2. *Counselor—help me break down the problem and find solutions*

Supports (Name) and Health-Care Services	Phone Number/Location
Emergency contact: **Father**	**777-777-7777**
Emergency response services:	911
Crisis line:	**1-866-996-0991**
Emergency department: **General hospital**	**Main Street**
Family physician: **Dr. Family MD**	**City Centre**
Psychiatrist: **Dr. Mi Psychiatrist**	**First Street**
Counselor/sponsor/other: **University counselor**	**University Campus**
Pharmacy: **Pharmacy**	**Second Street**

Healthy Lifestyle Checklist for Review (McNamara & Straathof, 2017)

(Check off two to three activities to prioritize for maintaining health, wellness, and resilience)

☐ Eating regular nutritious meals

☒ Maintaining a healthy sleep routine

☐ Exercising regularly

☐ Taking medications as prescribed

☐ Limiting substance use (alcohol, street drugs, caffeine, other)

☐ Keeping in touch with the people who support me

☐ Participating in meaningful social and leisure activity

☐ Keeping appointments with my doctors and counselors

☒ Using assertive communication

☐ Doing deep breathing

☒ Encouraging myself with positive or balanced self-talk

Name places where I could keep copies of this plan:
My phone, with my roommate and counselor, on my desk, on my electronic health record

I commit to reviewing my plan (circle 1) (Straathof, 2022a): daily  weekly monthly other:

Straathof, T. (2022b). *Suicide safety plans: Content and process for implementation.* Occupational Therapy Now, 24, 8–10. *https://www.proquest.com/docview/2825889091?sourcetype=Trade%20Journals*

For more information about the development of the SSP-OEAR, see Straathof, T. (2022b).

Reprinted with permission from CAOT Publications.

Adapted from: Crowley, P., Carmichael. D., Marshall, C.. & Murphy, S. 2019; Stanley & Brown, 2012. Crowley, P., Carmichael, D., Marshall, C., & Murphy, S. (2019, May 31). Safety planning for suicide prevention: A scoping review. Canadian Association of Occupational Therapists Annual Conference, *Niagara Falls, Ontario;* McNamara, M., & Straathof, T. (2017). Coping strategies to promote occupational engagement and recovery: A program manual for occupational therapists and other care providers. Ontario; Stanley, B., & Brown, G. (2012). Safety planning intervention: A brief intervention to mitigate suicide risk. *Cognitive and Behavioral Practice, 19*(2), 252–264. *https://doi.org/10.1016/j.cbpra.2011.01.001;* Straathof, T. (2022a). Coping strategies to promote mental health: Training modules for occupational therapists and other care providers. *Oxfordshire, UK:Routledge:Taylor & Francis.;* Straathof, T. (2022b). *Suicide safety plans: Content and process for implementation.* Occupational Therapy Now, 24, 8–10. *https://www.proquest.com/*

suicide safety plan using the prescribed module and template for the SSP-OEAR." Further suggestions of documentation considerations follow:

- Document level of risk based on assessment that may include a standardized risk assessment tool and score. Include specific words used by the person related to thoughts, plans, actions, and access to lethal means and intervention provided. Include a time stamp of when assessment was completed.
- Document that informed consent was obtained to complete a suicide safety plan. Using a prescribed script for gaining informed consent is recommended.
- Describe the person's level of engagement while completing the plan, reaction to the completion of the plan, and likelihood of using the plan based on what the individual says and what is observed.
- Include revisions to the suicide safety plan when there is a change in level of risk.
- If there is an option to scan the safety plan to the electronic health record, ensure informed consent is obtained and documented, and indicate where the plan can be found in the record.
- Document all places where a copy of the safety plan will be kept.
- Include clear information on how the person will reduce or eliminate lethal means, plans for the storage and review of the safety plan, and plans to inform named supports that a safety plan exists.
- Include communication that occurs with other health professionals for safety considerations.
- Complete a follow-up session to ensure the person confirms lethal means restriction has occurred and that supports have been notified of information in the suicide safety plan.
- Document any information related to what the person refuses such as refusing to have a copy scanned onto the electronic health record.

Resources in the Community

In addition to utilizing their knowledge and skills in occupation, practitioners must develop a foundational understanding of community resources and know how to navigate them. This knowledge can increase a practitioner's confidence and competence when addressing suicide across the continuum. When connecting individuals with helping resources in the community, effective communication about the resources is important. This can help individuals understand what to expect from accessing the resource, and address questions or concerns they have. In doing so, practitioners are using their relationship to help promote safety and reduce risk. Consider the following when looking at helping resources in the community.

- Regional distress or crisis phone numbers, many of which also have chat-based options
- Mental health outreach teams or support services affiliated with local hospitals, mental health service agencies, or police services
- Organizations providing population-targeted services (youth, Indigenous, older adults, etc.)

- Government organizations or those referenced by government sources
- Organizations affiliated with local hospitals or health units (e.g., crisis centers)
- Regional chapters of national organizations for specific services in a community
- Call resources to ensure that the information available about the service is accurate and up to date

It is essential that practitioners familiarize themselves with the helping resources and services that exist in their own community. OTPs should consider the following steps to be well prepared when sharing resources with the individual they are supporting and when communicating and collaborating with community resources and partners.

- Call resources such as distress centers or crisis lines to better understand what individuals can expect when placing a call; consider calling with the person for the first time.
- If accessing emergency services, obtain first responders' information and communicate key information about safety concerns.
- If accessing hospital services, call ahead to communicate key information about safety concerns.
- Obtain consent for communication with community partners.

In addition to the previously mentioned formal resources, it is important to also consider informal resources available to help practitioners be well positioned to help others. Informal supports can include interdisciplinary teams and colleagues, supports within a practitioner's personal network, and self-care. Self-care for practitioners, taking care of themselves by participating in activities that promote individual health and well-being, is an essential tool to remain ready, willing, and able to support individuals along the suicide continuum (Box 44-5).

Continuum: Postvention

Because so many are lost to suicide each year, millions are left behind to grieve the loss (Spillane et al., 2017). These individuals are known as *survivors of suicide* (Honeycutt & Praetorius, 2016). A survivor is "a person who has lost a significant other (or a loved one) by suicide, and whose life is changed because of the loss" (Andriessen, 2009, p. 43). Some people are *exposed* to suicide (such as learning of the suicide of a classmate or acquaintance), whereas others are *affected* by suicide (such as the suicide of a family member or close friend; Cerel et al., 2014). Typically, those who are affected by the suicide will experience emotional distress and are bereaved, but those who are exposed may also be affected. Historically, the seminal work of Edwin Shneidman, who coined the term "postvention" in the 1960s, and Albert Cain, who published the book *Survivors of Suicide* in 1972, has evolved considerably to modern-day postvention and bereavement support.

The challenges faced by survivors can be felt in the days and weeks leading up to the suicide, from the trauma of learning of the suicide itself, including in some cases being the person who is present or discovers the remains of the deceased individual, and during the period following the

BOX 44-5 ■ Application Story—Cara and Evan Part C

During one of our interactions, I developed an agenda for the session before our meeting. We were going to use our time to call the volunteer organization Evan had been interested in and to book his first meeting with them to get the ball rolling. However, when I saw him, I quickly recognized that the plan for our meeting would have to change. He appeared tearful and tired. I asked how he was doing, and he expressed "not good, I am feeling hopeless." In that moment my mind shifted into crisis intervention mode. I next asked him, "Can you tell me more about the hopeless feeling?" He replied, "Nothing works for me, there is no point in trying anymore." I asked him outright, "Are things so bad that you are thinking of ending your life?" I wanted to leave no room for misinterpretation or confusion. He responded, "Yes I am."

I then asked, "On a scale from 1 to 10, how intense are the thoughts, with 10 meaning you are feeling a strong urge to act on the thoughts and 1 meaning you have the thought, but it passes, and you don't have any intention to act?" He responded that her thoughts were at a 7 on the scale. I asked if he had thought about a plan about how he might end his life and he mentioned he would take multiple weeks of medication because he had a monthly blister pack with 3 weeks left. I then asked when he thought he might act on this plan. He said, "I am pretty sure I will be safe tonight, I don't think I will actually do it, I hope I won't." At this point I wanted to highlight the hope that was starting to shine in for him. I asked, "What makes you hope you won't? What makes you confident you won't take your own life?" He responded, "I have people who care about me who would be upset, and my mother lives with me so I am pretty confident she would notice if I took all my pills." I asked him how confident he was in being safe tonight out of 10. He said, "7/10, because I am pretty sure my mom will help, but also she might fall asleep at some point so I will be alone at times."

At this point I shared with Evan my thoughts on the situation: "Evan, based on what we have been talking about, I would like you to go to our hospital emergency department tonight to check in and have an assessment with a psychiatrist. I know this is probably not what you want to hear, but we must do everything we can to keep you safe, and right now I am not confident that you are safe on your own." Evan said, "I really don't want to go to the

hospital, I am probably safe, I don't think I need it." I could hear the worry in his voice. At this point I tried to provide comfort and reassurance. I said, "Evan, the hospital will only keep you there if you need to stay. Sometimes just going and talking to someone can be the most helpful thing you can do. At this point you do need to go to the hospital, so let's plan some things you can bring to help you be comfortable while you are there."

I put a detailed note in his chart for the hospital emergency staff to read to have the full context of the situation when he arrived. He was able to be assessed and was discharged the same night because of their assessment that his suicidal ideation had lessened in intensity over time. They recommended he switch his medication to one blister pack per week rather than monthly blister packs to reduce the risk of harm. They ensured his mother had possession of his medication until this change was made at the pharmacy. He returned home with the support and supervision of his mother.

Cara's Therapeutic Reasoning: *When I hung up the phone with Evan and his mother, my heart was beating out of my chest. I could feel the adrenaline pumping through my body. I tried to frantically write down everything we both said so I wouldn't forget as the adrenaline threatened my recollection of events. I questioned everything; "Was it fair that I sent him to the hospital? Was it smart to have his mother bring him instead of police? Could I have done more for him? Did I make the right decisions? Will he be mad at me? Will he be safe?"*

Looking back on the situation now I know that this debrief in my own brain is a normal response to a highly charged situation. At all steps in the process there were clinical decisions that weighed on me, and it's impossible to go back and think about every possible outcome. The truth is that we make the best decisions in the moment with the information we have available. I chose to err on the side of caution when deciding he needed to go to the hospital, and gave Evan some trust in letting him go with his mother, which was a calculated risk I took. At the end of the day, I led with compassion and wanting the best for Evan, so knowing that is what guided my decision-making gave me peace. I knew that it would be helpful to seek out support from colleagues and planned to contact my supervisor to review my decision-making and actions.

---

death (Harrington-LaMorie et al., 2018). As one person stated, "Emotions surge, bodies shake, legs buckle. Call it a grenade, an earthquake, or an avalanche. Plans evaporate" (Walker, 2017, p. 635). Unlike other deaths, in suicide bereavement guilt and blame may be accompanied by feeling rejected, abandoned, and angry, and constant questioning "Why?" (Honeycutt & Praetorius, 2016). Family members play over their last encounters with the loved one, and question if something they said or did may have pushed the person to act. In addition to emotional upheaval, the routines of daily life are disrupted and must be gradually reconstructed, incorporating the loss (Dransart, 2017).

Depending on the relationship, those bereaved by suicide can be at increased risk for suicide themselves, with parents who have lost a child being at greatest risk because of the intensity and duration of symptoms, such as depression and prolonged grief (Hamdan et al., 2020). Bereaved mothers who lost a child to suicide spoke of internalizing blame while idealizing the deceased offspring, a never-ending search for answers, navigating the pain while trying to be there for other family members, and finally finding hope

(Shields et al., 2019). In a study of children who lost a parent to suicide, mental health, functional problems, and physical health required increased attention, and drug and alcohol misuse, suicidal ideation, self-injury, and emotional distress were observed in adolescents who experienced a parental suicide at higher rates than those who had not lived this experience (Cerel et al., 2008).

The suicide loss of military members creates additional challenges related to primary and secondary losses (Harrington-LaMorie et al., 2018). Spouses and children must cope with the tragedy of the immediate loss and often have to navigate a future where a breadwinner is removed from the family. Their way of life is challenged as they envision a future often separate from a well-structured military lifestyle. Military suicides are often seen as dishonorable, "a disgrace to the victim and the profession," adding an additional challenge (Harrington-LaMorie et al., 2018, p. 145). See Chapter 43: Serving Veterans and Service Members.

Coping with the resulting emotional pain and eventually trying to incorporate the loss into a new identity, revising life goals, finding meaning and purpose relative to the loss, and navigating the ongoing bond with the deceased person also characterize the experience of suicide bereavement (Shields et al., 2017). These experiences hold similarities to other forms of grieving and friends and family struggle to know what to do or say. Jordan (2017) discusses the *social ambiguity* they may feel—not knowing what is considered appropriate behavior in this circumstance. A form of *social helplessness* may arise, as even well-established social supports pull back or stay away because of lack of capacity for sharing in another's grief and pain (Grad et al., 2004).

As suicide survivors navigate the bereavement process, they sometimes experience complicated grief; this intense grief lasts longer than expected and causes impacts on daily functioning, such as sleep disruption (Levi-Belz & Lev-Ari, 2023). Along with shame and guilt, some may develop PTSD, placing them at increased risk for depression, substance abuse, suicidal ideation, and suicide themselves (Honeycutt & Praetorius, 2016; Spillane et al., 2017).

Helping Those Who Have Experienced Loss to Suicide

People bereaved by a suicide loss experience intense emotional responses that can be prolonged. As they struggle to make sense of what happened, they often feel the need to formulate a new identity, examine and revise life goals, be there for others, and search for meaning and purpose in the face of unfathomable loss. Needs of survivors will vary and encompass practical, psychological, social, and spiritual domains (Andriessen, 2009). Postvention is intended to "buffer the burden of distress" by assisting survivors to manage the immediate crisis and navigate the longer-term consequences (Harrington-LaMorie et al., 2018, p. 144). It includes "those activities developed by, with, or for suicide survivors, in order to facilitate recovery after suicide, and to prevent adverse outcomes including suicidal behavior" (Andriessen, 2009, p. 43).

The current approaches most accessed as postvention include individual therapy and support groups (both suicide-specific and non–suicide-specific; Honeycutt & Praetorius, 2016). Although some people prefer the individualized approach, participants in a study by Shields and colleagues (2019) found the group setting helped them to make meaning out of their experiences by providing an environment where they could share their story with others similarly bereaved in a nonjudgmental supportive environment. Peer support can help people to normalize their grief experiences and share ways of coping with the death (Ali & Lucock, 2020) as well as contribute to posttraumatic growth (Smith et al., 2011). However, some survivors may become overly entrenched in the "activist" role and may need support to reorient their lives toward other activities (Dransart, 2017).

Some have found informal internet-based support groups helpful because of their 24-hour-a-day availability (especially when support is needed to get through anniversaries of key events) and the opportunity to remain anonymous and support others. Unhelpful or inappropriate input may happen in virtual environments, and people who experience this may become more distressed (Bailey et al., 2017). Active

outreach programs offering connections to practical supports such as funeral planning, financial services, and legal advice are proving to be beneficial (Hill et al., 2022). Survivors also rely on informal help from friends and family, individual psychotherapy, information and referral services, talking one-on-one with another suicide survivor, and medication (Ligier et al., 2020).

Ensuring cultural relevance of postvention interventions is critical (Goebert et al., 2018). This was exemplified in a study of Native Hawaiian youth, in which appropriate postvention was found to increase hope for suicide survivors. "A rainbow is waiting: In moments when darkness is all around, and it's hard to see beyond it, a rainbow or preserver of life for youth is waiting" (Goebert et al., 2018, p. 337) is a quote taken from a song that was used to convey "cultural pride as source of nourishment, healing and strength" (Goebert et al., 2018, p. 337).

Although people bereaved by suicide may be up to nine times more in need of professional help than those mourning other causes of death, many neither seek nor receive the help needed (Froese et al., 2020). Services may be nonexistent, inconsistently available (timewise and geographically), or they may not be perceived as suitable or helpful, leaving many to cope on their own. Still, formalized postvention programs exist such as Yvonne Bergmans' Skills for Safer Living program (2016). Skills for Safer Living (Bergmans, 2016) incorporates strategies used in cognitive behavioral therapy and DBT. The goal of this program is to decrease the intensity, duration, and frequency of suicide-related behaviors by enhancing coping strategies, emotional literacy, and language to describe feelings rather than focus on deterring suicidal thinking.

Occupations to Support a Way Forward After a Suicide Loss

Many people who have experienced a suicide loss are likely to experience occupational disruptions. After a loss, roles and routines can change and occupations and co-occupations can be significantly transformed. Whalley Hammell (2020) points out an unexpected biographical disruption such as bereavement may "puncture the mundane and taken-for-granted routines of daily living and the performance of valued roles and activities" (p. 134). This in turn could impact self-identity and self-worth, and lead to feeling useless and disconnected from others (Whalley Hammell, 2020).

Practitioners can collaborate to mitigate the impacts of suicide loss and support survivors in this challenging circumstance. Froese and colleagues (2020) have proposed that leisure may have a potential role in the bereavement recovery by using leisure to contribute to meaning-making and by providing opportunities to break the grief cycle by (re-)engagement with life. Meaning can be derived from engaging in personally, spiritually, socially, and/or culturally valued activities. Leisure participation is commonly linked to well-being, suggesting a tremendous potential role in postvention. Machado and Swank (2019) discussed how engaging with nature can contribute to healing in suicide bereavement. Specifically, they discussed therapeutic gardening, incorporating the interaction with gardening materials, and later

TABLE 44-8 | Dimensions of Occupational Experience in Bereavement

Dimension	Definition	Examples
Restoration	"Occupational experiences that contribute to well-being, especially for those confronting difficult life challenges" (Whalley Hammell, 2009, p. 110).	• Use of poems, letters, and journals can contribute to the desensitization of traumatic memories and help the bereaved move beyond anguish (Stepakoff, 2009). • "Recuperative conditioning" or engaging in a restorative activity such as a hobby or exercising and repeating those that impact emotions in a positive way (Kasahara-Kiritani et al., 2017, p. 447).
Contribute and connect	"The ability to contribute to others in reciprocal relationships . . . and a sense of connection and belonging are important to one's sense of well-being" (Whalley Hammell, 2009, p. 110). Connect and contribute may include "belonging, connecting, contributing, caring, and feeling cared for and needed" (Whalley Hammell, 2009, p. 111).	• By participating in a support group, survivors were able to "remove the mask that they had to wear in front of others who had not been bereaved by suicide and share their stories in a nonjudgmental supportive environment" (Shields et al., 2017, p. 196). • Activities such as social projects and volunteering to help others served as a resource in the grieving process (Parente & Ramos, 2020). • Survivors are committed to suicide prevention and survivor support groups and other social causes, eventually taking a leadership role (Dransart, 2017).
Engaging in doing	"Occupations that contribute to a sense of purpose and meaning in everyday life" (Whalley Hammell, 2009, p. 111).	• Engaging with nature can contribute to healing in suicide bereavement (e.g., therapeutic gardening, incorporating the interaction with gardening materials, and later reflecting on the experience). Some might plant a commemorative tree to memorialize the person lost (Machado & Swank, 2019). • Use of art, scrapbooking, writing songs, and journaling as a means of processing painful suicide loss (bear similarities with restorative activities; Wilks, 2014). • Activities such as walking, socializing, or going to the park can provide a sense of hope and optimism that helps to maintain coping efforts even after the activity has ended (Froese et al., 2020).
Connect the past and present to a hopeful future	Connecting the past and the present to a hopeful future involves envisioning a future when the person will be "engaged in meaningful occupations and working towards goals that generated a feeling of hope" (Whalley Hammell, 2009, p. 111).	• Belief that death was not an eternal split may lead to reconstruction of a bond with the deceased (Kawashima & Kawano, 2017). • The person living a redefined life feels as if something is missing: "There is a hole in me" (Kasahara-Kiritani et al., 2017, p. 452). • "Leisure may be one such needle through which to re-thread together the two worlds and create a meaningful, re-discovered life" (Froese et al., 2020, p. 329).

reflecting on the experience. The participants in the study by Honeycutt and Praetorius (2016) engaged in reading, writing, and outdoor activities—chosen because they contribute to occupying time and allow the opportunity to process thoughts. See Chapter 30: Natural Environments. 🤝

Engaging in occupations is a key factor that can aid in navigating the disruptions and charting a path toward recovery, which some may envision as regaining a past reality and others may envision as something new as they revise priorities (Whalley Hammell, 2020). A framework of categories or "dimensions of occupational experience" proposed by Whalley Hammell (2009, p. 107) draws on the subjective qualities of occupational engagement in hopes of creating a more visible link between occupations and well-being (Box 44-6). This framework serves as a valuable tool to identify occupations that may support well-being and be beneficial in suicide bereavement (Table 44-8).

Advocacy Efforts

OTPs are working together at the systems level to integrate the occupational lens. Examples of such collaboration include encouraging discussions at the World Federation of Occupational Therapists Congress in 2022, creation of national networks of practitioners working to address suicide in occupational therapy practice, and creation of national position statements advocating for occupational therapy in suicide prevention. For example, in Canada, the *CAOT Position Statement: Occupational Therapy to Prevent and Support Recovery From Suicide* (Hewitt-McVicker et al., 2023) calls for the following actions:

1. Advocate for life promotion through occupational therapy among persons and communities at high risk for suicide.
2. Promote equitable access to occupations to increase living opportunities and decrease death by suicide.
3. Embed suicide prevention, intervention, and postvention within occupational therapy curriculum and professional development across all practice settings.
4. Lobby for systematic access to occupational therapy to promote life through occupational engagement in a cost-effective manner.
5. Fund occupational therapy to be integrated in social and health-care initiatives to promote occupation beyond surviving.

BOX 44-6 ■ Application Story—Cara and Evan Part D

The next day I checked the hospital notes to find out what happened from a clinical perspective while Evan was there. I then called Evan to check in. Evan explained that his suicidal ideation had significantly reduced compared with his heightened distress the day before. He still was feeling down and hopeless, but no longer had any intention or plan to end his life. I asked how Evan felt from his perspective during the crisis intervention the previous day. Evan responded, "I know you did what you had to do. I really did not want to go to the hospital, but at least I didn't have to get taken by police, which happened to me before and it was difficult. So, I liked that I had the option to go with my mom. I just wish I had more time at home before I had to go because I already felt better by the time I got to the hospital, so it was kind of a waste of time."

I validated his feelings and thanked him for his honesty. At our next meeting, we created together a plan with explicit instructions of what should happen next time he is having strong suicidal ideation. For example, we added that if he expresses suicidal ideation, he would like to stay on the phone with me, a crisis line, or his family/friends for at least an hour before he is forced to go to the hospital (because he reported usually feeling better within the

hour). We added that his preference is to go to the hospital with a family or friend rather than police. I added that if he consistently refused to go that police would have to be called at that point and he was aware of that. We wrote out a list of what he might bring to the hospital next time in his comfort bag.

Involving Evan in this plan helped him to be part of his own plan and maintain his power in the situation. At our meetings following this crisis intervention, Evan's mood continued to improve slightly. We continued to work on developing a meaningful routine for him moving forward. He continued to come to therapy groups to work on coping skills and I ensured that every time we met, I was looking out for red flags.

Cara's Therapeutic Reasoning: *When I spoke with Evan the next day and he sounded in a better headspace, there was a feeling of relief that washed over me. I felt in that moment I was justified in the decisions I had made the day before. Most importantly, he was safe. I was also relieved to find out he was not mad at me. This might seem inconsequential to some, but for me I was deeply worried about hurting our therapeutic relationship. Evan was understanding of the situation, because he knew that I was acting from a place of care, so we were able to continue to work together with trust and respect.*

Here's the Point

- The value of occupation has been demonstrated across the continuum of suicide prevention, intervention, and postvention.
- OTPs are skilled at supporting people to navigate life transitions.
- Occupation to recovery and occupation as an outcome (e.g., returning to work or other daily routines) can be critical tethers to a meaningful life.
- Focusing on restoration, connections, and contributions; rediscovering purpose; engaging in doing; and connecting to a hopeful future hold great promise in this regard.
- Within prevention at an individual or community level, it is essential to apply a PEO lens to foster an understanding of what puts people at risk for suicide and simultaneously what fosters safety and meaning to protect life.
- As gatekeepers, practitioners benefit from engaging in GKT to gain skills and knowledge about suicide prevention and intervention to support individuals across various practice areas. There are several training programs that practitioners can choose from; however, several factors need to be considered to identify one that supports their knowledge needs.

- Safety plans are needed for those presenting with suicide risk and are most effective if coping foundations are addressed, appropriate content is included, and when made collaboratively in line with a person's coping style, strengths, and meaningful occupations. It is also important to consider how the physical and social environment shapes safety. When having this crucial conversation, it is important to address suicide directly, in a compassionate way.
- The needs of survivors of suicide loss will vary, and encompass practical, psychological, social, and spiritual domains. Practitioners can play a valuable role in helping survivors to rebuild a meaningful life.

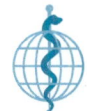 Visit the online resource center at **FADavis.com** to access the videos.

Acknowledgments

The authors want to acknowledge Marc Rouleau (editing and review), Meghan Lees (new grad reflection), and Aster Harrison (media reflection) for their contributons.

Apply It Now

1. Reflecting on Risk

Reread the section of this chapter that discusses risk and protective factors. Answer the following reflective questions for yourself and ask a friend to do the same, then share and discuss your perspectives.

Reflective Questions
- What information on suicide risk and protective factors was new to you?
- Could some protective factors mask risk factors? Explain.
- How could using a PEO lens help a practitioner to understand risk and protective factors?

■ The authors suggested that some factors may operate to increase risk in one person while being a protective factor in another person or can be both a risk and protective factor in the same individual. How can that be? Try to create scenarios where a single factor operates in this way. Discuss your thinking with a colleague.

2. Self-Assessment: Am I Ready to Intervene?

Take a pause with yourself at this point if you need to. Breathe. Most things about suicide intervention do not need to be done in fast forward. Slow things down. Breathe. Then consider skills you have and skills you may need to develop to prepare yourself to address suicide across the continuum. Answer the following reflective questions for yourself and ask a friend to do the same, then share and discuss your perspectives.

Reflective Questions
■ Why is it important to ask people directly about suicide?
■ Am I ready to be direct in such conversations? What are one to two steps I can take to bolster my readiness?
■ When could using language of "harming oneself" be unhelpful?
■ Think about your "script"—how you would introduce the conversation and ask about suicide. How does that script sound? Identify one question you would use when opening a conversation about suicide.

3. Video Exercise: Aster's Lived Experience of Suicidality

Pair up with another student in your class or form a small group of students. Access and watch the "Aster's Lived Experience of Suicidality" video at the online resource center at FADavis.com. Then, discuss and together answer the following questions.

Reflective Questions
■ There were several factors that Aster described as leading to the episode of major depression and suicidality, including starting a new medication with a black box warning. As an OTP, what did you learn from that part of Aster's story?
■ What were some of the resources and tools that helped Aster get through the crisis? Can you identify any others that you would have recommended to them?
■ Aster had previous experience in a hospital setting that they describe as being inaccessible, uncomfortable, and actually worsening their mental health symptoms. How would you address the decision-making process related to treatment in an individual who was suicidal? What options are available?
■ What plans did Aster work to put into place to keep them safe and inform their brother in the event they could not care for themselves?
■ One thing Aster learned that particularly resonated with them was that, when people are suicidal, they need to hear basic messages such as, "You matter to me," and "I'm glad I know you." Why do you think those simple words are so powerful to individuals experiencing mental health crises?

4. Video Exercise: Two Practitioners Discuss Their Work in Suicide Prevention

Pair up with another student in your class or form a small group of students. Access and watch the "Two Practitioners Discuss Their Work in Suicide Prevention" video at the online resource center at FADavis.com. Then, discuss and together answer the following questions.

Reflective Questions
■ How do these two OTPs connect with individuals who are in crisis and/or contemplating suicide? What is unique about the way an OTP might connect with people who are questioning "the meaning of life"?
■ How did occupational deprivation affect many of the people with whom these OTPs worked? How might the OTPs help individuals increase their awareness of the power of occupation?
■ One therapist describes the realization that she could not take a "one size fits all" approach. How did that affect her approach to working with individuals in distress? What role does compassion on the part of the occupational therapists play in their work?
■ These practitioners described suicide prevention work as "heavy," "intense," and "emotionally draining," and they advocate for practitioners to be intentional about their own self-care. Why is self-care so crucial for these occupational therapists in their suicide prevention practice? What strategies might you use to replenish and take care of yourself?
■ The practitioners in the video emphasized the importance of zeroing in on "occupational issues" in crisis plans. What language might you include in a crisis intervention plan that prioritizes occupation as a strategy?
■ Flexibility, compassion, and the ability to connect were key tools these practitioners said they used in suicide prevention work, and they noted that, "Conversations about suffering are intimate conversations." Create a list of key interpersonal skills a practitioner needs to effectively engage in these intimate conversations. Critically self-assess your own skills to identify strengths and areas to build up.

5. Self-Assessment: Reflecting on My Own Safety and Self-Care

This chapter begins with a prompt to think about your wellness and well-being. It ends with these same two considerations. Consider these self-care reflections:

Reflective Questions
■ What goals have you made regarding your self-care?
■ What does spiritual self-care mean to you?
Remember this is a team effort:
■ Get support from colleagues.
■ Two-person interventions can work.
■ It doesn't always have to be you to intervene, but you need to know enough to get the person at risk for suicide to someone who can help.
I am only one; but still I am one. I cannot do everything; but still I can do something; and because I cannot do everything, I will not refuse to do the something that I can do (Hale, 1902, p. 172).

Resources

International Resources
- American Foundation for Suicide Prevention: https://afsp.org
- Canadian Association for Suicide Prevention: www.suicideprevention.ca
- Mental Health Foundation of New Zealand: https://mentalhealth.org.nz/suicide-prevention

Gatekeeper Programs
- Applied Suicide Intervention Skills Training (ASIST): https://livingworks.net/training/livingworks-asist
- Question, Persuade, Refer (QPR): https://qprinstitute.com
- Shoalhaven Aboriginal Suicide Prevention Program (SASPPP): https://www.sspan.org.au

Canadian Organizations
- Canadian Association of Occupational Therapists Addressing Suicide in OT Practice Network: https://caot.ca/site/prac-res/otn/sot?nav=sidebar&banner=4. This is a national network of OTPs collaborating and advocating to increase the connection between occupational therapy and suicide prevention.

Opportunities to Participate in World Suicide Prevention Day (September 10)
- Visit www.who.int to read about world suicide prevention initiatives.
- Search your local resources for who is carrying out an event endorsing September 10. Look for the butterfly, which is a common symbol in suicide prevention healing work.
- Gather with others or take a quiet moment for yourself on September 10 to honor the work and healing that can be connected to suicide postvention.

Videos
- "Life Skills Groups in an Unhoused Population" video. Kailin is an OTP who works in community mental health and homeless services, a population that often experiences trauma and stressors that can lead to suicidal ideation. In this video, she describes the impactful life skills groups she runs in a women's shelter and how the use of a group facilitates peer-to-peer support. Kailin offers several creative examples of life skills group activities. She emphasizes the need to employ trauma-informed practices and harm-reduction strategies in this population, meeting clients where they truly are. Access the video at the online resource center at FADavis.com.
- "Jordan's Lived Experience of Anxiety and Depression" video. In this video, OTP Jordan describes her lived experience of anxiety and depression. She touches on many issues critical to recovery and occupational therapy practice, including social determinants of health, peer support, and how mental health labels can adversely affect an individual's medical treatment. Importantly, she explains how she has learned to blend her lived experience with her work as an occupational therapist, while ensuring she takes care of herself and manages her symptoms. Jordan also offers priceless words of wisdom to practitioners regarding establishing a therapeutic connection with individuals with whom they practice. Access the video at the online resource center at FADavis.com.

References

Ali, F., & Lucock, M. (2020). 'It's like getting a group hug and you can cry there and be yourself and they understand'. Family members' experiences of using a suicide bereavement peer support group. *Bereavement Care, 39*(2), 51–58. https://doi.org/10.1080/02682621.2020.1771951

Andriessen, K. (2009). Can postvention be prevention? *Crisis: The Journal of Crisis Intervention and Suicide Prevention, 30*(1), 43–47. https://doi.org/10.1027/0227-5910.30.1.43

Aquila, I., Sacco, M. A., Ricci, C., Gratteri, S., Montebianco Abenavoli, L., Oliva, A., & Ricci, P. (2020). The role of the COVID-19 pandemic as a risk factor for suicide: What is its impact on the public mental health state today? *Psychological Trauma: Theory, Research, Practice, and Policy, 12*(Suppl. 1), S120–S122. https://doi.org/10.1037/tra0000616

Ayers, J. W., Althouse, B. M., Leas, E. C., Dredze, M., & Allem, J.-P. (2017). Internet searches for suicide following the release of *13 Reasons Why. JAMA Internal Medicine, 177*(10), 1527–1529. https://doi.org/10.1001/jamainternmed.2017.3333

Bailey, E., Krysinska, K., O'Dea, B., & Robinson, J. (2017). Internet forums for suicide bereavement: A cross-sectional survey of users. *Crisis: The Journal of Crisis Intervention and Suicide Prevention, 38*(6), 393–402. https://doi.org/10.1027/0227-5910/a000471

Beaudoin, V., Séguin, M., Chawky, N., Affleck, W., Chachamovich, E., & Turecki, G. (2018). Protective factors in the Inuit population of Nunavut: A comparative study of people who died by suicide, people who attempted suicide, and people who never attempted suicide. *International Journal of Environmental Research and Public Health, 15*(1), 144. https://doi.org/10.3390/ijerph15010144

Bergmans, Y. (2016). *Understanding and responding to recurrent suicide attempts* [Doctoral thesis]. School of Nursing and Human Sciences, Dublin City University. http://doras.dcu.ie/21547/1/YB_thesissubmitted._dec.12.16.pdf

Bridge, J. A., Greenhouse, J. B., Ruch, D., Stevens, J., Ackerman, J., Sheftall, A. H., Horowitz, L. M., Kelleher, K. J., & Campo, J. V. (2019). Association between the release of Netflix's *13 Reasons Why* and suicide rates in the United States: An interrupted time series analysis. *Journal of the American Academy of Child & Adolescent Psychiatry, 59*(2), 236–243. https://doi.org/10.1016/j.jaac.2019.04.020

Brodsky, B. S., Spruch-Feiner, A., & Stanley, B. (2018). The Zero Suicide Model: Applying evidence-based suicide prevention practices to clinical care. *Frontiers in Psychiatry, 9*(33), 1–7. https://doi.org/10.3389/fpsyt.2018.00033

Burnette, C., Ramchand, R., & Ayer, L. (2015). Gatekeeper training for suicide prevention: A theoretical model and review of the empirical literature. *Rand Health Quarterly, 5*(1), 16.

Cain, A. (1972). *Survivors of suicide.* Charles C Thomas.

Canadian Association for Suicide Prevention. (2023). *Home page.* https://suicideprevention.ca/resource/suicide-is-everyones-business-steps-in-prevention

Canadian Journalism Forum on Violence and Trauma. (2020). *Mindset: Reporting on mental health.* Mindset+third+edition_2020.pdf

Canady, V. (2018). Suicide prevention training needed for MH professionals, journal reports. *Mental Health Weekly, 28*(14), 1–8. https://doi.org/10.1002/mhw.31405

Capp, K., Deane, F. P., & Lambert, G. (2001). Suicide prevention in Aboriginal communities: Application of community gatekeeper training. *Australian and New Zealand Journal of Public Health, 25*(4), 315–321. https://doi.org/10.1111/j.1467-842x.2001.tb00586.x

Cerel, J., Jordan, J. R., & Duberstein, P. R. (2008). The impact of suicide on the family. *Crisis: The Journal of Crisis Intervention and Suicide Prevention, 29*(1), 38–44. https://doi.org/10.1027/0227-5910.29.1.38

Cerel, J., McIntoshosh, J., Neimeyer, R. A., Maple, M., & Marshall, D. S. (2014). The continuum of "survivorship": Definitional issues in the aftermath of suicide. *Suicide & Life-Threatening Behavior, 44*(6), 591–600. https://doi.org/10.1111/sltb.12093

Chu, C., Buchman-Schmitt, J. M., Stanley, I. H., Hom, M. A., Tucker, R. P., Hagan, C. R., Rogers, M. L., Podlogar, M. C., Chiurliza, B., Ringer, F. B., Michaels, M. S., Patros, C. H. G., & Joiner, T. E. (2017). The interpersonal theory of suicide: A systematic review and meta-analysis of a decade of cross-national research. *Psychological Bulletin, 143*(12), 1313–1345. https://doi.org/10.1037/bul0000123

Collins, R., Vrbanac, H., & Hewitt, K. (2014). *Addressing the gap of suicide in occupational therapy practice.* Paper presented at Canadian Association of Occupational Therapists Annual Conference 2014: Reflection on occupation: Enabling healthy communities, Fredericton, New Brunswick, Canada.

Costanza, A., Amerio, A., Odone, A., Baertschi, M., Richard-Lepouriel, H., Weber, K., Di Marco, S., Prelati, M., Aguglia, A., Escelsior, A., Serafini, G., Amore, M., Pompili, M., & Canuto, A. (2020). Suicide prevention from a public health perspective. What makes life meaningful? The opinion of some suicidal patients. *Acta Biomedica, 10;91*(3 Suppl.), 128–134. https://doi.org/10.23750/abm.v91i3-S.9417

Cross, W. F., West, J. C., Pisani, A. R., Crean, H. F., Nielsen, J. L., Kay, A. H., & Caine, E. D. (2019). A randomized controlled trial of suicide prevention training for primary care providers: A study protocol. *BMC Medical Education, 19*(1), 1–9. https://doi.org/10.1186/s12909-019-1482-5

Crowley, P., Carmichael, D., Marshall, C., & Murphy, S. (2019, May 31). *Safety planning for suicide prevention: A scoping review.* Canadian Association of Occupational Therapists Annual Conference, Niagara Falls, Ontario, Canada.

Dalglish, S. L., Melchior, M., Younes, N., & Surkan, P. J. (2015). Work characteristics and suicidal ideation in young adults in France. *Social Psychiatry Psychiatric Epidemiology, 50*(4), 613–620. https://doi.org/10.1007/s00127-014-0969-y

Deuter, K., Procter, N., & Evans, D. (2020). Protective factors for older suicide attempters: Finding reasons and experiences to live. *Death Studies, 44*(7), 430–439. https://doi.org/10.1080/07481187.2019.1578303

Dransart, D. A. C. (2017). Reclaiming and reshaping life: Patterns of reconstruction after the suicide of a loved one. *Qualitative Health Research, 27*(7), 994–1005. https://doi.org/10.1177/1049732316637590

Durie, M. (2001). *Mauri ora: The dynamics of Māori health.* Oxford University Press.

Durie, M. (2017). Indigenous suicide: The Tūramarama declaration. *Journal of Indigenous Wellbeing: TeMauri–Pimatisiwin, 2*(2), 59–67.

Durie, M. H., Lawson-Te Ahn, K. R., Naera, M. H., & Waiti, J. (2017). *Tūramarama ki te ora: National Māori strategy for addressing suicide 2017–2022.* Te Rūnanga o Ngāti Pikiao Trust.

Dutheil F., Aubert C., Pereira B., Dambrun M., Moustafa F., Mermillod M., Baker, J. S., Trousselard, M., Lesage, F. X., & Navel, V. (2019) Suicide among physicians and health-care workers: A systematic review and meta-analysis. *PLoS One, 14*(12), e0226361. https://doi.org/10.1371/journal.pone.0226361

Eskin, M., Poyrazli, S., Janghorbani, M., Bakhshi, S., Carta, M. G., Moro, M. F., Tran, U. S., Voracek, M., Mechri, A., Aidoudi, K., Hamdan, M., Nawafleh, H., Sun, J. M, Flood, C., & Phillips, L. (2019). The role of religion in suicidal behavior, attitudes and psychological distress among university students: A multinational study. *Transcultural Psychiatry, 56*(5), 853–877. https://doi.org/10.1177/1363461518823933

Faria, M., Remédios Santos, M., Sargento, P., & Branco, M. (2020). The role of social support in suicidal ideation: A comparison of employed vs. unemployed people. *Journal of Mental Health, 29*(1), 52–59. https://doi.org/10.1080/09638237.2018.1487538

Froese, J. E., McDermott, L., & Iwasaki, Y. (2020). The other side of suicide loss: The potential role of leisure and meaning-making for suicide survivors. *Annals of Leisure Research, 23*(3), 322–338. https://doi.org/10.1080/11745398.2019.1616572

Gibbs, J. (2015). Religious conflict, sexual identity, and suicidal behaviors among LGBT young adults. *Archives of Suicide Research, 19*(4), 472–488. https://doi.org/10.1080/13811118.2015.1004476

Goebert, D., Alvarez, A., Andrade, N. N., Balberde-Kamalii, J., Carlton, B. S., Chock, S., Chung-Do, J. J., Eckert, M. D., Hooper, K., Kaninau-Santos, K., Kaulukukui, G., Kelly, C., Pike, M. J.,

Rehuher, D., & Sugimoto-Matsuda, J. (2018). Hope, help, and healing: Culturally embedded approaches to suicide prevention, intervention and postvention services with native Hawaiian youth. *Psychological Services, 15*(3), 332–339. https://doi.org/10.1037/ser0000227

Grad, O. T., Clark, S., Dyregrov, K., & Andriessen, K. (2004). What helps and what hinders the process of surviving the suicide of somebody close? *Crisis, 25*(3), 134–139. https://doi.org/10.1027/0227-5910.25.3.134

Gunnell, D., & Chang, S. S. (2016). Economic recession, unemployment, and suicide. In R. C. O'Connor & J. Pirkis (Eds.), *The international handbook of suicide prevention* (2nd ed., pp. 284–300). Wiley Blackwell.

Gunnell, D., Chang, S. S., Tsai, M. K., Tsao, C. K., & Wen, C. P. (2013). Sleep and suicide: An analysis of a cohort of 394,000 Taiwanese adults. *Social Psychiatry Psychiatric Epidemiology, 48,* 1457–1465. https://doi.org/10.1007/s00127-013-0675-1

Hale, E. (1902). I am only one; but still I am one. In J. A. B. Greenough, *A year of beautiful thoughts* (p. 172). Thomas Y. Crowell.

Hamdan, S., Berkman, N., Lavi, N., Levy, S., & Brent, D. (2020). The effect of sudden death bereavement on the risk for suicide: The role of suicide bereavement. *Crisis: The Journal of Crisis Intervention and Suicide Prevention, 41*(3), 214–224. https://doi.org/10.1027/0227-5910/a000635

Harrington-LaMorie, J., Jordan, J. R., Ruocco, K., & Cerel, J. (2018). Surviving families of military suicide loss: Exploring postvention peer support. *Death Studies, 42*(3), 143–154. https://doi.org/10.1080/07481187.2017.1370789

Harris, L. M., Huang, X., Linthicum, K. P., Bryen, C. P., & Ribeiro, J. D. (2020). Sleep disturbances as risk factors for suicidal thoughts and behaviours: A meta-analysis of longitudinal studies. *Scientific Reports, 10*(1), 13888. https://doi.org/10.1038/s41598-020-70866-6

Hawgood, J., Woodward, A., Quinnett, P., & De Leo, D. (2021). Gatekeeper training and minimum standards of competency. *Crisis, 43*(6), 516–522. https://doi.org/10.1027/0227-5910/a000794

Hendin, H., Haas, A. P., Maltsberger, J. T., Szanto, K., & Rabinowicz, H. (2004). Factors contributing to therapists' distress after the suicide of a patient. *The American Journal of Psychiatry, 161*(8), 1442–1446. https://doi.org/10.1176/appi.ajp.161.8.1442

Hewitt, K., Hébert, M., Vrbanac, H., & Canadian Association of Occupational Therapists. (2019). *CAOT role paper: Suicide prevention in occupational therapy.* CAOT. https://caot.ca/document/7445/Role%20Paper-Suicide%20Prevention_ENG_Sept5_2019.pdf

Hewitt-McVicker, K., Rouleau, M., Straathof, T., Larivière, N., Vrbanac-Cress, H., Froese, D., White, C., Hébert, M. L., Patel, M., Shimmell, L., Schooley, R., & Canadian Association of Occupational Therapists. (2023). *CAOT Position Statement: Occupational therapy to prevent and support recovery from suicide.* CAOT.

Hikuroa, D. (2017). Mātauranga Māori—The ūkaipō of knowledge in New Zealand. *Journal of the Royal Society of New Zealand, 47*(1), 5–10. https://doi.org/10.1080/03036758.2016.1252407

Hill, N. T. M., Walker, R., Andriessen, K., Bouras, H., Tan, S. R., Amaratia, P., Woolard, A., Strauss, P., Perry, Y., & Lin, A. (2022). Reach and perceived effectiveness of a community-led active outreach postvention intervention for people bereaved by suicide. *Frontiers in Public Health, 10,* 1040323. https://doi.org/10.3389/fpubh.2022.1040323

Holmes, G., Clancy, A., Hermens, D. F., & Lagopoulos, J. (2019). The long-term efficacy of suicide prevention gatekeeper training: A systemic review. *Archives of Suicide Research, 25*(2), 177–207. https://doi.org/10.1080/13811118.2019.1690608

Honeycutt, A., & Praetorius, R. T. (2016). Survivors of suicide: Who they are and how do they heal? *Illness, Crisis & Loss, 24*(2), 103–118. https://doi.org/10.1177/1054137315587646

Horowitz, L. M., Bridge, J. A., Teach, S. J., Ballard, E., Klima, J., Rosenstein, D. L., Wharff, E. A., Ginnis, K., Cannon, E., Joshi, P., &

Pao, M. (2012). Ask Suicide-Screening Questions (ASQ): A brief instrument for the pediatric emergency department. *Archives of Pediatrics & Adolescent Medicine, 166*(12), 1170–1176. https://doi.org/10.1001/archpediatrics.2012.1276

Howard, M., & Krannitz, M. (2017). A reanalysis of occupation and suicide: Negative perceptions of the workplace linked to suicide attempts. *The Journal of Psychology, 151*(8), 767–788. https://doi.org/10.1080/00223980.2017.1393378

Ihimaera, L., & MacDonald, P. (2009). *Te Whakauruora. Restoration of health: Māori suicide prevention resource.* Ministry of Health.

Isaac, M., Elias, B., Katz, L. Y., Belik, S. L., Deane, F. P., Enns, M. W., & Sareen, J. (2009). Gatekeeper training as a preventative intervention for suicide: A systematic review. *The Canadian Journal of Psychiatry, 54*(4), 260–268. https://doi.org/10.1177/070674370905400407

Johnson, J., Wood, A. M., Gooding, P., Taylor, P. J., & Tarrier, N. (2011). Resilience to suicidality: The buffering hypothesis. *Clinical Psychology Review, 31*(4), 563–591. https://doi.org/10.1016/j.cpr.2010.12.007

Jordan, J. R. (2017). Postvention is prevention—The case for suicide postvention. *Death Studies, 41*(10), 614–621. https://doi.org/10.1080/07481187.2017.1335544

Kasahara-Kiritani, M., Ikeda, M., Yamamoto-Mitani, N., & Kamibeppu, K. (2017). Regaining my new life: Daily lives of suicide-bereaved individuals. *Death Studies, 41*(7), 447–454. https://doi.org/10.1080/07481187.2017.1297873

Kashiwa, A., Sweetman, M. M., & Helgeson, L. (2017). Occupational therapy and veteran suicide: A call to action. *American Journal of Occupational Therapy, 71*(5), 1–6. https://doi.org/10.5014/ajot.2017.023358

Kawashima, D., & Kawano, K. (2017). Meaning reconstruction process after suicide: Life-story of a Japanese woman who lost her son to suicide. *Omega: Journal of Death and Dying, 75*(4), 360–375. https://doi.org/10.1177/0030222816652805.

Khadijah, S., Martono, M., & Tarnoto, K. W. (2023). Results of professional interventions of gatekeeper training programs for college student suicide prevention: A systematic review. *GSC Advanced Research and Reviews, 17*(3), 23–39. https://doi.org/10.30574/gscarr.2023.17.3.0443

Kolb, D. A. (2015). *Experiential learning: Experience as the source of learning and* development (2nd ed.). Pearson.

Kroenke, K., Spitzer, R. L., & Williams, J. B. (2001). The PHQ-9: Validity of a brief depression severity measure. *Journal of General Internal Medicine, 16*(9), 606–613. https://doi.org/10.1046/j.1525-1497.2001.016009606.x

Larivière, N., Rouleau, M., Hewitt-McVicker, K., Shimmell, L., & White, C. (2021). Addressing suicide in entry-to-practice occupational therapy programs: A Canadian picture. *Journal of Occupational Therapy Education, 5*(3), 1–12. https://doi.org/10.26681/jote.2021.050310

Levi-Belz, Y., & Lev-Ari, L. (2023). Thinking for healing: The role of Mentalization deficits as moderator in the link between complicated grief and suicide ideation among suicide-loss survivors. *Death Studies, 47*(3), 360–369. https://doi.org/10.1080/07481187.2022.2065707

Ligier, F., Rassy, J., Fortin, G., van Haaster, I., Doyon, C., Brouillard, C., Séguin, M., & Lesage, A. (2020). Being pro-active in meeting the needs of suicide-bereaved survivors: Results from a systematic audit in Montréal. *BMC Public Health, 20*(1), 1–13. https://doi.org/10.1186/s12889-020-09636-y

Linehan, M. (2020). *Building a life worth living: A memoir.* Random House.

LivingWorks. (2014). *ASIST (Applied Suicide Intervention Skills Training) 11.1: Trainer manual, 1EN1011.1.* LivingWorks Education. https://livingworks.net/training/livingworks-asist

Machado, M. M., & Swank, J. M. (2019). Therapeutic gardening: A counseling approach for bereavement from suicide. *Death Studies, 43*(10), 629–633. https://doi.org/10.1080/07481187.2018.1509908

Marco, J. H., Pérez, S., & García-Alandete, J. (2016). Meaning in life buffers the association between risk factors for suicide and hopelessness in participants with mental disorders. *Journal of Clinical Psychology, 72*(7), 689–700. https://doi.org/10.1002/jclp.22285

Marshall, C. A., Crowley, P., Carmichael, D., Goldszmidt, R., Aryobi, S., Holmes, J., Easton, C., Isard, R., & Murphy, S. (2023). Effectiveness of suicide safety planning interventions: A systematic review informing occupational therapy. *Canadian Journal of Occupational Therapy, 90*(2), 208–236. https://doi.org/10.1177/00084174221132097

McCarthy, T. (Director, Writer). (2017). *13 Reasons Why* [Television series]. Netflix.

McNamara, M., & Straathof, T. (2017). *Coping strategies to promote occupational engagement and recovery: A program manual for occupational therapists and other care providers.* CAOT Publications ACE.

Mental Health Commission of Canada (2018). *Research on suicide and its prevention: What the current evidence reveals and topics for future research.* Public Health Agency Canada.

Mental Health Foundation of New Zealand. (2023). *Reporting and portrayal of suicide.* https://mentalhealth.org.nz/media/reporting-and-portrayal-of-suicide

Milner, A., Witt, K., Maheen, H., & LaMontagne, A. D. (2017). Access to means of suicide, occupation and the risk of suicide: A national study over 12 years of coronial data. *BMC Psychiatry, 17*(1), Article 125. https://doi.org/10.1186/s12888-017-1288-0

Mohanty, S., Sahu, G., Mohanty, M. K., & Patnaik, M. (2007). Suicide in India: A four year retrospective study. *Journal of Forensic and Legal Medicine, 14*(4), 185–189. https://doi.org/10.1016/j.jcfm.2006.05.007

Morton, M., Wang, S., Tse, K., Chung, C., Bergmans, Y., Ceniti, A., Flam, S., Johannes, R., Schade, K., Terah, F., & Rizvi, S. (2021). Gatekeeper training for friends and family of individuals at risk of suicide: A systematic review. *Journal of Community Psychology, 49*(6), 1838–1871. https://doi.org/10.1002/jcop.22624

Moscardini, E. H., Hill, R. M., Dodd, C. G., Do, C., Kaplow, J. B., & Tucker, R. P. (2020). Suicide safety planning: Clinician training, comfort and safety plan utilization. *International Journal of Environment Research & Public Health, 17*(18), 6444. https://doi.org/10.3390%2Fijerph17186444

National Academies of Sciences, Engineering, and Medicine. (2022). *Suicide prevention in Indigenous communities: Proceedings of a workshop.* National Academies Press. https://doi.org/10.17226/26745

National Center for Injury Prevention and Control. (2022). *Suicide Prevention Resource for Action: A compilation of the best available evidence.* Centers for Disease Control and Prevention. https://www.cdc.gov/suicide/pdf/preventionresource.pdf

Nelson, G., Hanna, R., Houri, A., & Klimes-Dougan, B. (2012). Protective functions of religious traditions for suicide risk. *Suicidology Online, 3*(1), 59–71.

Niederkrotenthaler, T., Braun, M., Pirkis, J., Till, B., Stack, S., Sinyor, M., Tran, U. S., Voracek, M., Cheng, Q., Arendt, F., Scherr, S., Yip, P. S. F., & Spittal, M. J. (2020). Association between suicide reporting in the media and suicide: Systematic review and meta-analysis. *BMJ, 368*, m575. https://doi.org/10.1136/bmj.m575

Niederkrotenthaler, T., Kirchner, S., Till, B., Sinyor, M., Tran, U. S., Pirkis, J., & Spittal, M. J. (2021). Systematic review and meta-analyses of suicidal outcomes following fictional portrayals of suicide and suicide attempt in entertainment media. *EClinicalMedicine, 36*, 100922. https://doi.org/10.1016/j.eclinm.2021.100922

Odom, K. (2016). Combating the suicide epidemic: The effects of leisure engagement on the incidence of depression and poor life satisfaction in soldiers. *Occupational Therapy in Mental Health, 32*(1), 70–85. https://doi.org/10.1080/0164212X.2015.1082172

Parente, N. T., & Ramos, D. G. (2020). The influence of spiritual-religious coping on the quality of life of Brazilian parents who have lost a child by homicide, suicide, or accident. *Journal of Spirituality in Mental Health, 22*(3), 216–239. https://doi.org /10.1080/19349637.2018.1549525

Park, S. M. (2019). Effects of work conditions on suicidal ideation among middle-aged adults in South Korea. *International Journal of Social Psychiatry, 65*(2), 44–150. https://doi .org/10.1177/0020764019831327

Patel, M., & Degagne, C. (2017). *Supporting occupational therapists in practice: A review of suicide intervention training.* Canadian Association of Occupational Therapists. https://caot.ca/site/rc/caot-bc/practiceresources /suicideinterventiontraining?language=fr_FR&nav=sidebar

Pompili, M. (2010). Exploring the phenomenology of suicide. *Suicide and Life-Threatening Behavior, 40*(3), 234–244. https://doi.org /10.1521/suli.2010.40.3.234

Reger, M. A., Piccirillo, M. L., & Buchman-Schmitt, J. M. (2020). COVID-19, mental health, and suicide risk among health care workers: Looking beyond the crisis. *The Journal of Clinical Psychiatry, 81*(5), 3915. https://doi.org/10.4088/JCP.20com13381

Reporting on Suicide. (2020). *Best practices and recommendations for reporting on suicide.* https://reportingonsuicide.org /recommendations

Rurup, M. L., Pasman, H. R. W., Goedhart, J., Deeg, D. J. H., Kerkhof, A. J. F. M., & Onwuteaka-Philipsen, B. D. (2011). Understanding why older people develop a wish to die. *Crisis, 32*(4), 204–216. https://doi.org/10.1027/0227-5910/a000078

Shields, C., Kavanagh, M., & Russo, K. (2017). A qualitative systematic review of the bereavement process following suicide. *Omega: Journal of Death & Dying, 74*(4), 426–454. https://doi .org/10.1177/0030222815612281

Shneidman, E. (1973). *On the nature of suicide.* San Francisco, CA: Jossey-Bass.

Shields, C., Russo, K., & Kavanagh, M. (2019). Angels of courage: The experiences of mothers who have been bereaved by suicide. *Omega: Journal of Death & Dying, 80*(2), 175–201. https://doi.org /10.1177/0030222817725180

Smith, A., Joseph, S., & Das Nair, R. (2011). An interpretative phenomenological analysis of posttraumatic growth in adults bereaved by suicide. *Journal of Loss & Trauma, 16*(5), 413–430. https://doi.org/10.1080/15325024.2011.572047

Spillane, A., Larkin, C., Corcoran, P., Matvienko-Sikar, K., Riordan, F., & Arensman, E. (2017). Physical and psychosomatic health outcomes in people bereaved by suicide compared to people bereaved by other modes of death: A systematic review. BMC *Public Health, 17*(1), 939. https://doi.org/10.1186/s12889-017-4930-3

Stanley, B., & Brown, G. (2012). Safety planning intervention: A brief intervention to mitigate suicide risk. *Cognitive and Behavioral Practice, 19*(2), 256–264. https://doi.org/10.1016 /j.cbpra.2011.01.001

Stepakoff, S. (2009). From destruction to creation, from silence to speech: Poetry therapy principles and practices for working with suicide grief. *The Arts in Psychotherapy, 36*, 105–113. https://doi .org/10.1016/j.aip.2009.01.007

Straathof, T. (2022a). *Coping strategies to promote mental health: Training modules for occupational therapists and other care providers.* Routledge.

Straathof, T. (2022b). Suicide safety plans: Content and process for implementation. *Occupational Therapy Now, 24,* 8–10. https://www.proquest.com/trade-journals/suicide-safety-plans -content-process/docview/2825889091/se-2

Straathof, T., Simoneau, E., & McNamara, M. (2019). Occupational therapy in acute mental health: Proposal for practice. *Occupational Therapy Now, 21,* 14–16. https://www.proquest.com/trade-journals /occupational-therapy-acute-mental-health-proposal/docview /2317914102/se-2

Tubesing, N., & Tubesing, D. (1983). *Structured exercises in stress management* (Vol. 1). Whole Person Associates.

Tzeng, W. C., & Lipson, J. G. (2004). The cultural context of suicide stigma in Taiwan. *Qualitative Health Research, 14*(3), 345–358. https://doi.org/10.1177/1049732303262057

Vogel, M., Braungardt, T., Meyer, W., & Schneider, W. (2012). The effects of shift work on physical and mental health. *Journal of Neural Transmission, 119*(10), 1121–1132. https://doi.org/10.1007 /s00702-012-0800-4

Walker, R. S. (2017). After suicide: Coming together in kindness and support. *Death Studies, 41*(10), 635–638. https://doi.org /10.1080/07481187.2017.1335549

Whalley Hammell, K. (2009). Self-care, productivity, and leisure, or dimensions of occupational experience? Rethinking occupational "categories". *The Canadian Journal of Occupational Therapy, 76*(2), 107–114. https://doi.org/10.1177/000841740907 600208

Whalley Hammell, K. R. (2020). *Engagement in living: Critical perspectives on occupation, rights, and wellbeing.* CAOT.

Wilks, D. (2014). Autobiographical case study: Using art and poetry therapy to process family member suicide. *Journal of Poetry Therapy, 27*(4), 213–216. https://doi.org/10.1080/08893675.2014. 949524

Williams, A. D., Clark, T. C., & Lewycka, S. (2018). The associations between cultural identity and mental health outcomes for Indigenous Māori youth in New Zealand. *Frontiers in Public Health, 6,* 319. https://doi.org/10.3389/fpubh.2018.00319

World Health Organization. (2019). *Suicide: One person dies every 40 seconds.* https://www.who.int/news/item /09-09-2019-suicide-one-person-dies-every-40-seconds

World Health Organization. (2021a). *LIVE LIFE: An implementation guide for suicide prevention in countries.* Author. https://www.who .int/publications/i/item/9789240026629

World Health Organization. (2021b). *Suicide worldwide in 2019: Global health estimates.* Author. https://www.who.int /publications/i/item/9789240026643

Yonemoto, N., Kawashima, Y., Endo, K., & Yamada, M. (2019). Implementation of gatekeeper training programs for suicide prevention in Japan: A systematic review. *International Journal of Mental Health Systems, 13*(1), Article 2. https://doi.org/10.1186 /s13033-018-0258-3

Zalsman, G., Stanley, B., Szanto, K., Clarke, D. E., Carli, V., & Mehlum, L. (2020). Suicide in the time of COVID-19: Review and recommendations. *Archives of Suicide Research, 24*(4), 477–482. https://doi.org/10.1080/13811118.2020.1830242

Zinzow, H. M., Thompson, M. P., Fulmer, C. B., Goree, J., & Evinger, L. (2018). Evaluation of a brief suicide prevention training program for college campuses. *Archives of Suicide Research, 24*(1), 82–95. https://doi.org/10.1080/13811118.2018.1509749

Occupation

This part of the text comprehensively addresses areas of occupational performance by covering the more familiar occupations of work, play, self-care, and leisure, as well as some areas of occupation that may be neglected, such as sleep, volunteering, creative occupations, health management occupations, and spirituality. Attention is paid to the character or purpose of different occupations across the life span. Most of these chapters include descriptions of specific assessments and intervention approaches used by occupational therapy practitioners (OTPs). Therapeutic reasoning assessment tables are often included for easy reference to assessment tools specific to different areas of occupation.

Self-Care and Well-Being Occupations

Evguenia S. Popova, Bridget J. Hahn,
and Margaret (Peggy) Swarbrick

This chapter describes how occupational therapy practitioners (OTPs) can promote well-being at the person, group, and population levels. The chapter also explores opportunities to promote well-being across occupational therapy settings based on the **eight dimensions of wellness** (Swarbrick & Yudof, 2015): (1) emotional/mental, (2) environmental, (3) financial, (4) intellectual, (5) occupational, (6) physical, (7) social, and (8) spiritual. The influence of individual and environmental contributors to well-being occupations, including social determinants of health, are explored. These concepts are applied to clinical reasoning while working with persons in each stage of the occupational therapy process, including evaluation, intervention, and outcome tracking. Lastly, the chapter explores the literature on professional well-being among OTPs and students.

Overview of Well-Being Concepts

Occupational therapy is a client-centered health profession concerned with promoting health and wellbeing through occupation (World Federation of Occupational Therapists [WFOT], 2018). Although **well-being** is a common term in occupational therapy and health care, it can be challenging to operationalize and define in practice (Aldrich, 2011). People often use terms such as "happy," "content," and "healthy" to describe well-being.

The World Health Organization (WHO) describes well-being as "a positive state experienced by individuals and societies" and "similar to health, it is a resource for daily life and is determined by social, economic and environmental conditions" (WHO, n.d.-b, para. 1). The WHO definition of well-being has been recognized as the guiding definition for OTPs and is incorporated into the *Occupational Therapy Practice Framework* (American Occupational Therapy Association [AOTA], 2020). These definitions reinforce the importance of person-centered care and remind OTPs that well-being (a) is best defined by the person and (b) should be considered in light of contextual influences. Consistent with person-centered practice, OTPs must refrain from assigning their values to occupations to promote a person's well-being (Stewart et al., 2016).

In health care, well-being has been operationalized using five measurable elements: positive emotion, engagement, relationships, meaning, and achievement (Seligman, 2011). Each element is a critical outcome of occupational therapy

practice and can be independently defined and measured during evaluation. OTPs work to address these elements by engaging persons in meaningful occupations that foster a sense of mastery and achievement. Occupational therapy practice acknowledges the influence of the person's context on the state of well-being and recognizes the dynamic relationship between the person's physical, social, and occupational environments.

In occupational therapy literature, well-being is often linked to **health and wellness, quality of life,** and **flourishing**, all of which can describe the continuum of positive and negative experiences in everyday life. WHO (n.d.-a, para. 1) defines health as "a state of complete physical, mental, and social well-being and not merely the absence of disease or infirmity." Similarly, wellness focuses on the importance of mind, body, and spirit connection; the need for satisfaction, value, and purpose; and a view of health that extends beyond nonillness. Rather than looking to attain wellness, this definition recognizes that wellness is a direction in progress toward one's greatest potential. Wellness is not the absence of disease, illness, and stress. Instead, wellness encompasses life purpose, satisfaction, and perception of happiness.

Health and wellness concepts are frequently incorporated into the definition of quality of life, which aims to capture a self-reported sense of well-being on individual and community levels (Teoli & Bhardwaj, 2022). Common descriptions of "quality of life" include having a sense of general well-being, enjoying life, and being healthy and able to participate in activities of daily living. Additionally, the concept of flourishing has been gaining attention in health-care literature. In research, flourishing has been operationalized according to five core features: positive emotions, engagement, interest, meaning, and purpose (Huppert & So, 2013; Seligman, 2011). Additional features encompassed in flourishing include self-esteem, optimism, resilience, vitality, self-determination, and positive relationships (Huppert & So, 2013; Seligman, 2011).

The growing emphasis on quality of life and flourishing in occupational therapy calls for practitioners to embrace strengths-based and solution-focused approaches in practice that prioritize empowering mental well-being over attempting to eliminate mental illness. These approaches expand beyond reductionistic disease management and into the expansive opportunities to collaborate with individuals and populations to maximize their unique perspectives on what makes their life good. Focusing on well-being allows OTPs to expand their impact by partnering to identify what a "good life" means for the person and ways to achieve such a state.

Eight Dimensions of Wellness

This chapter explores well-being through the lens of wellness. **Wellness** is defined as a conscious and deliberate process that requires a person to become aware of and make choices for a more satisfying lifestyle. A wellness lifestyle includes a self-defined balance of wellness routines and habits, including participation in meaningful occupations such as health management, work, leisure, rest and sleep, and social participation. Similar to well-being, wellness is often self-defined, and OTPs recognize the uniqueness of each individual's needs and preferences. Swarbrick and Yudof (2015) proposed eight dimensions of wellness: (1) emotional/mental, (2) environmental, (3) financial, (4) intellectual, (5) occupational, (6) physical, (7) social, and (8) spiritual (Fig. 45-1).

OTPs can use the eight dimensions of wellness to guide occupational therapy evaluation, intervention, and outcome tracking. These dimensions are dynamic and intertwined, reminding OTPs of the interconnectedness between contributors to wellness. For example, while working toward an occupational therapy degree, a graduate student may experience increased anxiety and stress (*emotional/mental*) from the increased cognitive demands of studying (*intellectual*) and the financial burdens of student loans (*financial*).

To support their well-being, the student may seek out more opportunities for self-care, such as exercising (*physical*), spending time outside (*environmental*), and staying connected with their friends, family, and peers (*social*). They may also take time to reflect on the values that empowered them to seek out the occupational therapy degree (*spiritual*)

to bolster their identity as an occupational therapy student and future OTP (*occupational*). Table 45-1 provides definitions and examples of each of the eight dimensions as they may be applied by OTPs in practice.

This chapter's The Lived Experience feature shows well-being as an occupation in relation to the eight dimensions of wellness. The sections that follow take a closer look at the individual and environmental contributors to well-being occupations.

Individual Contributors to Well-Being

Well-being is influenced by a multitude of factors, including the impact of a person's motivation, occupational balance, occupational participation and performance, and co-occurring health conditions. The following sections explore how these individual contributors can affect well-being as an occupation.

Motivation

People are driven to pursue well-being occupations that align with their values, interests, and motivations. Playfulness, for example, is a strong predictor of well-being (Farley et al., 2020; Parker et al., 2022), and playful adults and children are much more likely to participate in fun, engaging activities that foster their sense of well-being. Research suggests that motivation, occupational participation, and a sense of well-being are strongly intertwined.

A study by Burton and colleagues (2006) explored the association between intrinsic and identified motivation,

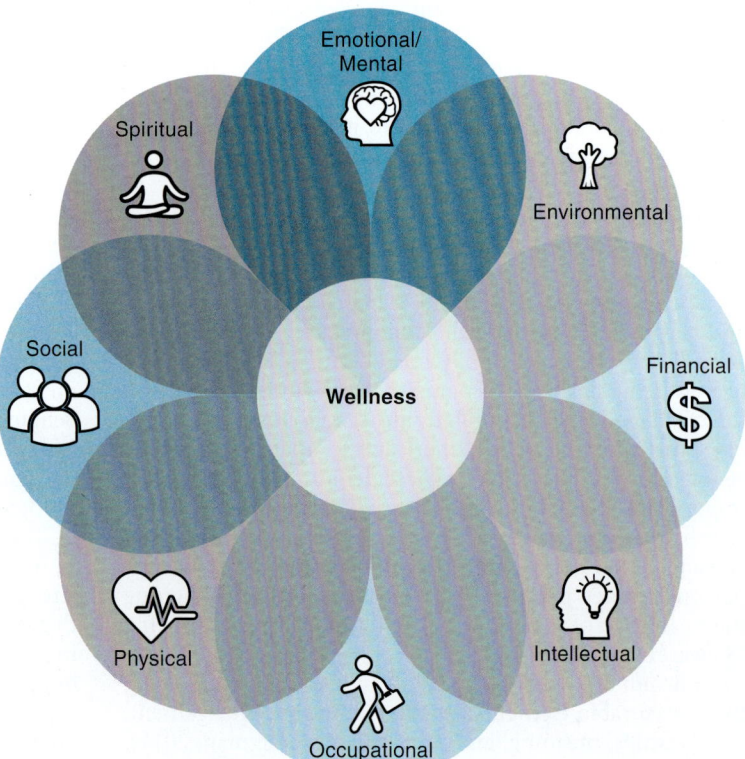

FIGURE 45-1. The Wellness Model in Community Mental Health Practice includes eight dimensions of wellness. This framework can be used to address the health disparities facing people with or at risk of developing mental and substance use disorders.

TABLE 45-1 | Eight Dimensions of Wellness

Dimension	Description
Physical	• Recognizing the need for physical activity, a healthy diet, and good nutrition • Discouraging the use of tobacco, drugs, and excessive alcohol consumption • Attention to physical and physiological signs of stress • Creating a self-defined daily routine • Learning to assume personal responsibility and care for minor illnesses and knowing when professional medical attention is needed
Spiritual	• Personal beliefs and values, having meaning and purpose, developing a sense of balance and peace • An appreciation for the depth and expanse of life and natural forces that exist in the universe • Often closely related to cultural, religious, and/or spiritual traditions
Social	• Contributing to the environment and community • Emphasizing the interdependence between ourselves, others, and nature • Communicating our needs and ideas with people who support and care about us • Personal relationships, important friendships, and connection with people, pets, and the community • Often involves a sense of reciprocity *and* equality
Intellectual	• Recognizing our creative abilities and finding ways to expand our knowledge and skills while discovering the potential for sharing those gifts with others • Lifelong learning, application of knowledge learned, and sharing knowledge
Emotional	• Capacity to recognize our feelings • Ability to express feelings, adjust to emotional challenges, and cope with life's stressors • Ability to assess our strengths, limitations, and areas we want to develop further • Tolerance of, awareness of, and acceptance of a wide range of feelings in ourselves and in other people, including recognizing conflict as being potentially healthy
Occupational	• Not just work, but participating in activities that are meaningful and rewarding, as well as provide meaning and purpose • Experiencing personal satisfaction and enrichment in one's life from participation in work and volunteer activity, as well as other activities and tasks from which we derive pleasure and satisfaction
Environmental	• Our living, learning, and working spaces and the larger communities where we participate as citizens • Ability to be and feel physically safe in safe and clean surroundings • Access to clean air, food, and water • Good health fostered by occupying pleasant, stimulating environments that support our well-being; enhanced by places and spaces that promote learning and contemplation and that elicit the relaxation response
Financial	• Both the *objective* perceptions and *subjective* indicators of individuals' personal financial status • *Objective indicators:* income, debt, savings, and aspects of financial capability, such as knowledge of financial products and services, planning ahead, and staying on budget • *Subjective indicators:* an individual's perception of satisfaction with their current and potential future financial situation

From Swarbrick, M., & Yudof, J. (2009). Words of wellness. Occupational Therapy in Mental Health, 25(3–4), 367–412. https://doi.org/10.1080/01642120903084158

The Lived Experience

Mike

When it comes to wellness, I think of being in a situation where you do not feel anxiety, stress, or stuff like that. Where your situation is calm, not bothered by a lot of stuff. You have everything in order. Where my current illnesses do not hinder me, and I can do what I want, when I want. I think I'm on the road to that.

Recently I have not been good at a lot of things. I've been behind on getting paperwork done. I hadn't gotten my health card for like 2 years, and the health card is the thing you need to go to doctor's appointments in Ontario, Canada. And to start, you know, going to see the doctor. I want to get back on my medication for ADHD (attention deficit hyperactivity disorder) because it helps me focus more. Having more focus will get me to exercise more. And you know it's the domino effect.

I'm 42 now. So probably about 10 years ago, I was relatively normal. Had a job, living on my own, self-sufficient, you know, doing well, getting paid a decent salary. I mean, I wasn't the

healthiest person, but I wasn't the worst off either. And then, one day, we were coming back from a trip, and I was feeling super sick. I couldn't explain why because I hadn't drunk or done any drugs. I was perfectly fine and then it progressively got worse to throwing up all the time. Feeling incredibly uncomfortable. High anxiety. Just super stressed, and everything just from that point started falling apart. My health went downhill. I couldn't go to work because I'd get up in the morning, and there would be probably 3 hours that I had to sit at the corner of my bed with a bucket beside me, just waiting to throw up.

Then it progressively got worse, and the only thing that was really helping was marijuana. But at that point, you're super high, and you can't do anything anyway, right? So you're locked in this endless cycle of being unable to do anything. And then I started getting way worse, ending up at the hospital every other day and staying there. The only thing working on me was hydromorphone, or Dilaudid, and I became very

Continued

The Lived Experience—cont'd

addicted to that. Not really much you can do about that. That's the reality of things. And then, at a certain point, I went to see my doctor, who recommended taking small doses of morphine. It made things a lot better to the point where I wasn't in the hospital all the time. I was still throwing up daily, and not being able to keep food down. I was only able to eat certain types of food and had to switch to a diet of pretty much all carbs. So at this point, I'm also struggling with weight gain. Plus, now my back is really messed up, which is super uncomfortable. So you know it's lots of stretching and yoga and stuff like that. I need to talk to somebody, especially nutrition. Not merely for the weight loss, but also for what can I actually eat. Right now I'm on a high-carb diet and proteins. I can't really eat any vegetables. I can't eat anything too fibrous. So many fruits and vegetables are out of the question. It's such a weirdly limiting diet. It's also super expensive. At this point, I'm living way beyond my means. If I didn't have the people who help me on a month-to-month basis I would probably be homeless.

Besides feeling physically ill, I have ADHD, and I used to depend heavily on ADHD medication. When I couldn't work anymore, I didn't see any point in keeping that medication going. It felt like because I was not working, I didn't need to focus on anything. Why would I need this medication? I'm now discovering that that was probably a bad idea. I have zero motivation and zero attention span. So that makes it very hard for me to get stuff done. Things that are super easy feel insurmountable. Like the idea of keeping my apartment tidy. It's so hard. I have to clean in spurts. I did have a mental health specialist for a while, but I wasn't getting the results I wanted from the relationship with that doctor. She helped with a lot of things, but at the time I had way too much going on in my life. I wasn't ready to deal with that stuff. If my doctor gave me another opportunity to speak to someone like that. I would totally take advantage of that. I think I'm in a better head space to work with someone on my mental health.

Right now is sort of the comeback phase. I've got a few things on the horizon. My doctor has recommended bariatric surgery because of the condition I have, which is gastroparesis. This condition might be related to diabetes, which I also have. The doctor said it might be neuropathy in my stomach. I haven't been to the hospital in probably a year. And that's a good thing, as long as I'm not in the hospital. There are certain things that I still have hang-ups on, like leaving my apartment. I have a lot of social anxiety. I would say agoraphobia. I never used to be like that. I'm a very extroverted person but have become an incredibly closed-off person when it comes to getting out of my safe zone.

I'm doing everything in my power to distract myself from my current situation. I play games a lot on my computer and try to hang out with people as much as possible online. I have a great group of friends I connect with online at night and, you know, I socialize with them. I tend to read a lot, around four to five books a month. Just to stay engaged in something. I feel like if you don't exercise your brain by doing some things, things tend to get a little dark, and you get into a dark emotional state. I also watch TV and a lot of Netflix. Sometimes I go outside and walk for a bit. I also spend time with my bird, Coby. He has his routine. I usually wake up around 6 a.m., and I get him out of his cage. He likes to come and cuddle in bed

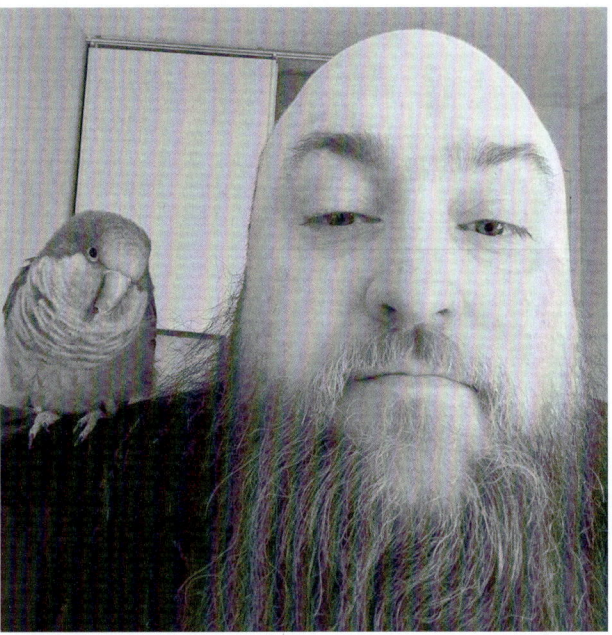

Mike and his bird Coby.

and sleep with me for a little bit. Then he goes on his routine and likes to play with his toys. He also likes to join me for all meals. He is very much entwined in my life.

Thankfully I have a very good support network. I have a lot of really good friends whom I can count on. When the chips are down and I need help, they are there. One of my good friends is a social worker, so I tend to talk to them about like my day-to-day stuff. They're the one that has been giving me motivational stuff to get out and do stuff. He's the reason why I got out and did all this stuff with the health card and the ID, so he's been invaluable. I don't like to bother him about things like that, but he tends to be the one who's always checking up on me. I am trying to get out more socially. I have friends that play "Magic the Gathering," the card game. They get together every couple of weeks. I medicate myself, and then someone comes to pick me up. But that is the one time out of the house, where there are no unknowns and I'm comfortable. Everything is great, and I'm having a good time.

I would love to work if I could. If I could pick any job, I would probably work in a shelter for parrots. There are a couple of shelters around my city, but they're not convenient places to get to. Transportation is a barrier and some of them are 30 minutes outside of town. I actually just gave up my ability to legally drive the other day. My passport, my driver's license, and all of my government IDs have expired. And because of my financial situation, and everything going on, it made more sense for me to get the government ID instead of spending $120 on a driver's license. I haven't driven in 10 years. Part of it is my fault. There's no reason why I should have let my government cards expire. And it was just another thing. Things tend to compound on one another. That is essentially what was happening, and it just keeps getting bigger and bigger and bigger. And everything starts to feel insurmountable. That's where I am, and I'm clawing my way back from that.

PhotoVoice

Mike

Coby [is] obviously my little rock. He keeps me going. It's helpful to have something to care for.

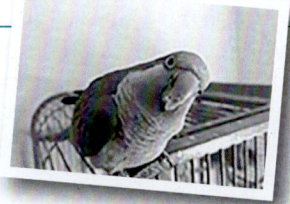

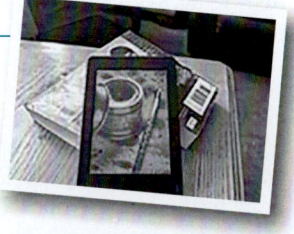

Reading is the other side of staying fit. Working out the mind really helps to keep intrusive thoughts out and keep me happy.

Exercise, trying to stay fit, is just as important as keeping your mind fit. Although it can be hard at times I always come out the other side feeling happy that I exercised.

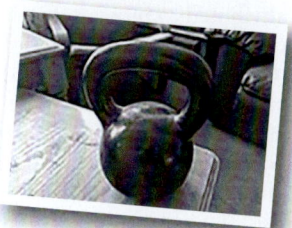

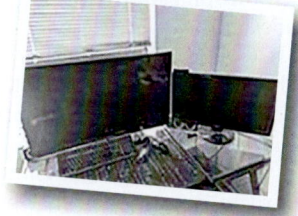

Lastly, my PC is one thing that is really important to me. It's basically my window to the outside world. It gives me lots of comfort being able to socialize with people all over the world. It allows me to escape into these grand stories from the video games I play. And it allows me to watch all sorts of shows and movies. A one stop shop of all my entertainment and social needs.

Which dimensions of wellness do you notice in Mike's lived experience narrative and PhotoVoice? How might an OTP further evaluate Mike's self-care and wellness occupations in his home health setting? Which dimensions of wellness might the OTP prioritize in their intervention and outcome tracking for Mike?

well-being, and academic performance of elementary school children. The researchers found that intrinsic motivation (e.g., "I enjoy doing my homework") predicted well-being independent of academic performance (Burton et al., 2006). Identified motivation (e.g., "It's important to me to do my homework"), on the other hand, predicted academic performance, and the student's self-reported well-being was contingent on performance (Burton et al., 2006). In practice, OTPs can support well-being by exploring motivations and interests that drive participation and ensuring an adaptive response to successes and challenges in everyday life. Chapter 11: Motivation takes a closer look at this factor. Chapter 51: Leisure and Creative Occupations also explores this link.

Occupational Balance

Everyday routines and habits bring structure to one's days and are at the core of occupational participation, including participation in well-being occupations. Health behaviors and lifestyle patterns significantly affect an individual's wellness. Positive health habits, such as getting restful sleep, brushing and flossing teeth, walking regularly at a brisk pace, making nutritious food choices, and avoiding alcohol, are common ways to promote a sense of mental and physical well-being. See Chapter 14: Time Use and Habits.

In examining well-being, OTPs should be cognizant of the person's **occupational balance**, a perception of having the "right" amount and variability between daily occupations (Wagman et al., 2011), and consider individuals' performance patterns as they relate to the time being spent in productive, restorative, and leisure occupations (AOTA, 2020). Perception of occupational balance is associated with lower stress and higher mental and physical health (Yu et al., 2018).

In discussing occupational balance, individuals may reflect on their well-being regarding the occupations in which they participate, the characteristics of the occupations, and the time dedicated to each occupation (Wagman et al., 2011). For example, a person may reflect on being satisfied with the variety of occupations they do throughout their week. At the same time, the same person may also experience decreased well-being because of the high productivity demands of each occupation and insufficient time dedicated to rest and leisure.

In mental health settings, occupational balance has been strongly associated with self-reported quality of life (Doğu & Örsel, 2022). People with psychiatric disabilities living independently in the community with housing support have been reported to perceive themselves as underoccupied in home management and self-care occupations (Eklund et al., 2019). In these situations, self-mastery has been recognized as an important contributor to occupational balance in relation to work, home management, and self-care (Eklund et al., 2019).

Occupational Participation and Performance

In supporting self-care as an occupation, OTPs should be mindful of the impact occupational participation and performance in self-care occupations may have on well-being. For example, in women, perception of sleep quality and fatigue is significantly associated with perceived occupational balance (specifically among physical, social, intellectual, and restful occupations) and satisfaction with the number of occupations in a typical week (Magnusson et al., 2020). Additionally, occupational participation in prosocial occupations (such as volunteerism and helping) is associated with psychological well-being, with informal helping being linked with more well-being benefits (Hui et al., 2020).

Beyond looking at the positive impact of occupational participation and performance, OTPs can also examine the impact of self-reported "yellow flags" on well-being. People with depression and anxiety are more likely to report low levels of occupational performance and satisfaction, especially in the areas of household management, self-care, and social participation (Gunnarsson et al., 2021). In research, yellow flags (such as worry, fear, avoidance, vigilance, and catastrophization) to health in community settings are associated with interference with daily life and time off work (Buck et al., 2010). OTPs working across different settings should be mindful of yellow flags as reported by individuals and provide concrete support to empower their participation in valued occupations.

When dealing with emotional distress, people may also turn to occupations that may have a negative impact on well-being such as heavy use of alcohol, tobacco, and drugs; excessive or unusual eating; and self-injury. A national survey conducted in 2021 found that approximately 45% of adults with serious mental disorders and 34% of adults with mental disorders also experienced substance dependence or abuse in a single year (Center for Behavioral Health Statistics and Quality [CBHSQ], 2022). Additionally, according to the 2021 National Survey on Drug Use and Health (NSDUH), youth (12–17 years old) and adults (18+ years old) with a reported mental health disorder were much more likely to report illicit drug use compared with the general population.

For example, 27.7% of youth with a major depressive episode were reported to use illicit drugs in the past year compared with 10.7% of youth without a major depressive disorder (Substance Abuse and Mental Health Services Administration [SAMHSA], 2021). In adults, it was estimated that 50.2% of adults with serious mental illness and 38.7% of adults with any mental illness used illicit drugs, compared with 17.7% of adults without any reported mental illness (SAMHSA, 2021). Also see Chapter 24: Substance-Related and Addictive Disorders.

Additionally, people with serious mental illness are reported to have lower physical activity and are less likely to meet the established criteria for physical activity levels compared with the general population (Vancampfort et al., 2017). Sedentary lifestyles may also be related to medication side effects, and medications used to treat the symptoms of mental disorders are reported to have multiple negative side effects, including short- and long-term weight gain (Dayabandara et al., 2017). Children are especially vulnerable to these negative side effects and, although switching medications and turning to nonpharmacological treatment is an option, it presents the risk of relapse (Dayabandara et al., 2017). Chapter 20: Mood Disorders and Chapter 23: Schizophrenia Spectrum and Psychotic Disorders offer deeper insights.

Co-Occurring Health Conditions

Research repeatedly points to a 10- to 25-year "mortality gap," with reduced life expectancy for people with serious mental illness compared with the general population (Plana-Ripoll et al., 2020). Specifically, people with co-occurring mental and medical health conditions are reported to have shorter life expectancy than (a) the general population or (b) people with only mental health or medical health conditions (Momen et al., 2022). Among co-occurring health conditions, of particular concern is the high rate of metabolic syndrome, a cluster of symptoms that increases the risk for diabetes and heart disease, including increased obesity, triglycerides and cholesterol, hypertension, and glucose (Beyazyüz et al., 2013; Riordan et al., 2011).

Research examining nutritional well-being in people with serious mental illness suggests significantly higher caloric and sodium intake (Teasdale et al., 2019), which has been attributed to increased weight gain and obesity rates for this population. Children, adolescents, and adults with serious mental illness are reported to have a greater prevalence of obesity compared with the general population (Afzal et al., 2021; Kokka et al., 2023). Metabolic syndrome has been reported in 68% of individuals with schizophrenia, 42% of people with schizoaffective disorder, and 22% to 30% of people with bipolar disorder (De Hert et al., 2011; Kelly et al., 2007). These conditions are often further impacted by high smoking rates and, in turn, can contribute to a sedentary lifestyle, symptom burden, poor self-care skills, higher disability status, and lower (poorer) quality of life. OTPs should be mindful of these risk factors in their work with individuals and ensure appropriate support, resources, and referrals as risk factors are identified.

In examining well-being, it is important to consider the impact of comorbid health conditions that influence well-being across the life span. In children and youth with intellectual and developmental disabilities, for example, mental health and social-emotional well-being are major considerations for pediatric OTPs. Adolescents with intellectual and developmental disabilities report more mental health challenges and fewer positive social experiences with family and peers, with girls reporting greater mental health challenges and fewer positive social experiences than boys (Boström et al., 2018).

Research examining the lived experiences of autistic children and youth suggests similar findings. Compared with neurotypical peers, autistic adolescents report lower quality of friendships, less school participation, and greater experience of anxiety and loneliness (Chang et al., 2018). Additionally, compared with non-autistic adults, autistic adults report significantly lower self-compassion (including self-kindness, common humanity, and mindfulness), and lower self-compassion has been associated with lower psychological well-being and greater levels of depression (Cai et al., 2023).

In older adulthood, many people experience social isolation (Cudjoe et al., 2020), and research suggests a reciprocal relationship between physical and mental health in older adulthood (Luo et al., 2019) and benefits of intergenerational communities on social, health, and cognitive outcomes (Peters et al., 2021). In response to these findings, OTPs have been called to reevaluate opportunities to support the work-to-retirement transition, including support for meaningful occupational engagement and lifestyle modification (Eagers et al., 2022). Additionally, occupational therapy researchers have been exploring opportunities to support meaningful occupational engagement and social participation through day centers (Österholm et al., 2022). Chapter 17: Chronic Health Conditions and Mental Health and Chapter 49: Connectedness and Belonging take a closer look at these factors.

Environmental Contributors to Well-Being

Quality of life, health, and wellness are affected by the economic and social conditions under which people live. The impact of the environment on well-being can be explored through the lens of trauma, as well as the **social determinants of health**, including health-care access and quality, neighborhood and built environment, social and community context, economic stability, and education access and quality (U.S. Department of Health & Human Services, n.d.).

Research examining social determinants of mental illness highlights a high prevalence of violence and maltreatment, adverse life events and experiences, racism and discrimination, inequality in structural policies, and a financial burden (Huggard et al., 2023). Additionally people experience lower rates of social support and employment and suboptimal housing and living conditions (Huggard et al., 2023). Older adults (50+ years) living in the community are significantly more likely to report not having enough money at the end of the month, not liking where they live, and being unhappy with community-based support (Kellett et al., 2020).

Trauma Exposure

When considering environmental and contextual contributors to well-being, a major emphasis is placed on the negative impact of adverse childhood experiences (ACEs), which are traumatic experiences such as violence, abuse, and neglect in childhood (Felitti et al., 1998). Contextual risk factors are major contributors to ACEs, including an association with childhood socioeconomic status (Walsh et al., 2019). Research repeatedly highlights the negative effect of ACEs on health and well-being, including increased posttraumatic stress symptoms, depressive symptoms, anxiety symptoms, and lower quality of life (Nelson et al., 2021). ACEs are associated with a multitude of conditions that impact physical well-being, including developmental delay (Cprek et al., 2020), decreased cognitive functioning (Hawkins et al., 2021), increased risk for obesity (Tabone et al., 2022), and headaches (Mansuri et al., 2020).

Beyond immediate and long-term effects, research suggests the possibility of intergenerational effects, with parental ACEs positively associated with lower parental mental health, greater parental body mass index (BMI), and greater child BMI (Berge et al., 2023). The effects of trauma are further amplified in children and youth with disabilities and those who experience barriers to occupational participation. Specifically, research suggests that children and youth who experience trauma and lower occupational participation are more likely to report clinical depression (Berg et al., 2018). Chapter 5: Trauma-Informed Practice looks more closely at this topic, including the principles of trauma-informed care.

People with mental health diagnoses often report trauma histories; therefore, many avoid health-care settings where they fear they may be retraumatized. People who have received treatment against their will or have been physically restrained in a health-care setting (both common among people with mental disorders) are more likely to fear (and avoid) medical retraumatization (Cusack et al., 2018). A history of trauma may include the use of physical restraints for routine medical and dental procedures. People with such experiences are naturally less comfortable placing themselves in settings where they may be fully undressed or physically restrained. Adopting trauma-informed care practices in health-care settings can increase access to needed medical services for individuals with a trauma history (SAMHSA, 2014).

Health-Care Access and Quality

People with mental health diagnoses are at risk for developing chronic medical conditions and often are not receiving the quality medical care they need. Research suggests that mental health providers may not be adequately equipped to support people with mental health diagnoses, including insufficient support within the health-care system, limited competency in evaluation and diagnostics, and limited understanding of the lived experience of people with mental illness (Molloy et al., 2023). Additionally, from the consumer perspective, people with mental illness might have limited awareness of whether their symptoms are physical or mental, and they experience challenges navigating the health-care system (Molloy et al., 2023).

Practitioners may also become overly focused on the mental disorder, overlooking symptoms or concerns related to other medical conditions, a phenomenon known as **diagnostic overshadowing** (Lester et al, 2005; Viron & Stern, 2010). Reported barriers to preventive medical services (including screening tests) include a lack of physician recommendations and poor communication with providers (Rockson et al., 2016; Swarbrick et al., 2015).

In light of these findings, health-care providers are called to advocate for health-care systems that offer coordinated physical and mental health services and access to case managers that can help guide the system navigation process (Lawrence & Kisely, 2010). Additionally, people may not seek health-care services because of mental health stigma, which could be addressed through education and peer-mediated interventions (Lawrence & Kisely, 2010). OTPs can address this

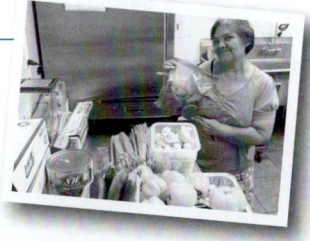

PhotoVoice

Margarita
Here I am getting ready to prepare for our delicious dinner and serving the community. Serving food to the community makes me happy and puts smiles on people's faces.

I enjoy being around food and preparing it. I like to work with all the colors of food because it makes the food healthy. Working in the kitchen showed me many different spices and how to use them. As I prepare food, it reminds me of when I was small, helping my mother prepare dinner for my family. Also, it taught me to help others. This is why I love to cook!

Eating healthy can be challenging for everyone. What additional barriers to healthy eating might people with mental health concerns face?

gap in service by supporting the person through transition points in care and serving in the role of case managers and service navigation support.

Neighborhood and Built Environment

Geographic location and living conditions within a person's home substantially affect health and well-being across physical, mental, and social domains. The neighborhood's socioeconomic status and personal/crime-related safety can substantially affect its role in mental health, including an increased likelihood of depressive symptoms (Barnett et al., 2018).

This relationship between the built environment and health might be due in part to access to spaces that promote a sense of well-being. For example, green spaces (including spaces such as parks, nature, sports, and recreation) are associated with greater mental well-being (Wood et al., 2017), and research suggests that approximately one-third of adults with cardiometabolic disease reside in neighborhoods that are not activity friendly (Gupta et al., 2023). Persistent housing problems are associated with decreased mental health outcomes (Pevalin et al., 2017), and supported housing has been shown to be an important contributor to a sense of well-being, social identity, and privacy, all of which are essential for mental health recovery (Friesinger et al., 2019). Several chapters offer deeper insights, such as Chapter 31: The Home Environment: Permanent Supportive Housing and Chapter 32: The Neighborhood and Community. 🤝

Social and Community Context

Social support is critical for health and well-being and often plays a critical role in recovery and capacity to cope with acute and chronic stressors. An association exists between a sense of trust and satisfaction with relationships in the family and depression (Han & Lee, 2015), and people value not only the relationships themselves but also the places and the activities within which the social participation takes place (Sweet et al., 2018). Although at an increased risk for social isolation, people with mental health diagnoses consistently report "yearning for connection," "connecting intensely," "encountering rejection and exclusion," "choosing isolation," and "finding peers/helping others" (Hine et al., 2018). Despite this drive for social connectedness and belonging, past experiences of trauma and rejection may create a significant barrier to social connectedness, especially in women (Hine et al., 2018). Chapter 49: Connectedness and Belonging takes a closer look at these factors. 🤝

Economic Stability

Economic stability is a major contributor to health and well-being and often serves as the primary support or a barrier to access and quality of health-care services. Beyond impacting one's ability to pay for quality health care, a lack of financial resources can create difficulties with transportation and the inability to pay for medication. People with very limited incomes often do not have disposable income to purchase recommended over-the-counter medications, vitamin supplements, and nonprescription appliances.

Limited discretionary spending also often restricts options for food choices or health-promoting activities, including a lack of access to healthy foods or safe spaces for engaging in regular exercise. People with mental illness may also experience difficulty with maintaining paid employment, resulting in increased economic hardship. A study by Hennekam and colleagues (2021) concluded that even though employees with mental illness excelled in many areas of their employment, they were also at a greater risk for overworking, resulting in increased stress and reduced capacity to cope.

Education Access and Quality

Education and academic achievement contribute to economic stability and health-care access. In addition, education quality impacts individuals' health literacy and, therefore, capacity to effectively navigate the health-care system and play an active role in personal health management. For example, attitudes toward mental health care and mental health literacy are associated with psychotherapy use and psychiatric medication adherence (Bonabi et al., 2016).

Internationally, evidence suggests that the general public may lack access to knowledge about the prevention of mental illness and mental health promotion, including knowledge of self-help strategies, help-seeking behaviors, mental health first aid, and treatment options (Jorm, 2012). However, mental health campaigns in community and education settings are showing promise in improving mental health literacy (Jorm, 2012). For example, research examining the benefits of mental health education for college students suggests that formal education on mental health effectively changes beliefs and awareness toward mental health and decreases mental health stigma (Shim et al., 2022).

Well-Being and the Occupational Therapy Process

Promotion of health and well-being are foundational to occupational therapy practice, and practitioners strive to support a person's well-being across physical, mental, and social domains. Additionally, occupational therapy practice emphasizes occupational balance, and practitioners have an opportunity to support individuals' well-being across multiple settings, including well-being in the workplace and the community.

Throughout the occupational therapy evaluation, intervention, and outcome tracking, OTPs emphasize well-being as a process and outcome of everyday life. In doing so, OTPs consider the intricacies of what it means to be well. In addition to examining the role and impact of everyday occupational participation in activities of daily living (ADLs), instrumental activities of daily living (IADL), health management, rest and sleep, education, work, play, and leisure on well-being, OTPs can explore and consider well-being as an occupation in itself. Exploration of well-being as an occupation opens up opportunities for practitioners to expand beyond the traditional view of health and wellness promotion (such as a focus on physical activity, nutrition, and sleep) and expand into exploring:

- Contexts and environments that embody and promote well-being on person, group, and population levels
- Routines and habits that sustain well-being, as well as roles and rituals that are integral to well-being occupations

Being a Psychosocial OT Practitioner

Supporting Well-Being in Primary Care Settings

Identifying Psychosocial Strengths and Needs

OTPs in primary care settings have a unique opportunity to support individual well-being through addressing health-promoting habits, routines, and lifestyle management of chronic conditions, enabling maximal participation and satisfaction with occupations. OTPs are called to provide holistic and preventive services in primary care, which must address psychosocial concerns as well as physical health (Sit et al., 2023), and preliminary efficacy is providing evidence of well-being interventions in primary care, including stress management (Connolly et al., 2018).

Consider the story of Claudia, a 68-year-old woman who was receiving a routine primary care visit with her primary care provider for her annual visit. Claudia has a past medical history of diabetes, disc disorder, hepatitis A, hyperlipidemia, hypertension, and sleep apnea. Her primary care provider referred her for a clinic visit with the OTP for chronic disease self-management because of Claudia's uncontrolled diabetes. She reports left hip and knee pain, for which she received physical therapy but stopped attending because of the $45 copay.

During the occupational profile, Claudia describes herself as lazy, stating, "I do everything for others. I don't have the energy to do for myself." Claudia is retired and lives with her husband, son, daughter-in-law, and two grandchildren. She reports her health management as "terrible" and that she loves sweets too much. The OTP collaborates with Claudia to assess her current health holistically and determine in what areas of her health she may be ready to make a change.

Using a Holistic Occupational Therapy Approach

Claudia and the OTP further discuss her daily life and routine. She reported wanting to start to make changes to start caring for herself more as she saw the impact her current health was having on her role as a grandmother and wife. She reported beginning to lose interest in playing with her grandson because of the pain in her leg, and her vision was starting to become impacted. She loves her time playing Bunco and getting together with friends but was beginning to worry about her ability to continue participating in these activities with the ongoing decline of her health.

The OTP had Claudia consider the following holistic health considerations in managing her diabetes:

- Food and drink choices
- Social supports
- Managing emotions (depression, worry, anxiety, stress)
- Physical activity
- Caring for your body (eyes, tooth/gum care, foot care)

Claudia reports feeling that changing her physical activity may be the easiest change for her to make at this time. Both Claudia and the OTP felt a small increase in her physical activity could have a wide range of effects on her health, including supporting her ability to manage emotions and increasing her ability to care for her body. Claudia had previously been enjoying her physical therapy sessions and was interested in joining a gym, but she did not continue with either because of the financial cost.

The OTP presents Claudia with some low/no-cost options for her to consider, including walking with a friend or family member, low-cost classes at the local community center, or online classes. Claudia reports an interest in yoga, and the two identify a short free 15-minute seated yoga and mindfulness class online. The OTP guided Claudia to complete an action plan, which she had at least a 7/10 confidence in completing, to support her in establishing the yoga practice as part of her routine. As part of her action plan, Claudia identifies a device and confirms internet access to view the video as part of her action plan. She identifies a space within her home to complete the yoga practice. She anticipates the best time of day to complete the practice to be right before lunch on Mondays and Fridays when she has the least amount of responsibilities. Claudia rates herself as 8/10 in confidence in her plan to complete the yoga session twice weekly.

Three weeks later, the OTP followed up with Claudia by phone to check on how her action plan was working. Claudia reports completing the yoga and mindfulness online session as planned for 2 out of the past 3 weeks. One day she reported she was busy with her grandson's school concert, but she even could sneak in an extra session 1 week. With more physical energy and increased motivation, Claudia's leg pain decreased. She began using the breathing and self-compassion techniques she had been practicing to help her manage stress and remind herself that, like her family, she too was worthy of care.

Reflective Questions

1. What other strategies to support well-being might be useful to explore with Claudia?
2. How might the OTP address the eight dimensions of wellness during the evaluation and intervention process in a primary care setting?
3. What other outcomes may be useful for the OTP to track to demonstrate treatment efficacy?

- Education, coaching, and supports that facilitate skills associated with well-being occupations, including self-management and goal setting
- Values and beliefs that guide well-being occupations, including spiritual beliefs and practices

This shift in perspective can also support practitioners in examining their own implicit and explicit biases toward health and wellness and empower a more person-centered, inclusive, and equitable health-care approach. Box 45-1 offers a perspective on how Certified Community Behavioral Health Clinics (CCBHCs) offer opportunities for expanding the role of occupational therapy in promoting well-being as a part of a CCBHC interprofessional team.

OTPs can apply occupation-focused models, such as the Canadian Model of Occupational Performance and Engagement (CMOP-E; Townsend & Polatajko, 2007) or the Model of Human Occupation (MOHO; Taylor et al., 2017) to guide their understanding of well-being as an occupation throughout the occupational therapy process.

Practitioners can also use frameworks such as the Occupational Perspective of Health (OPH; Wilcock, 2006) and the Pan Occupational Paradigm (POP; Hitch & Pepin, 2021) to explore concepts that are integral to occupational therapy practice and extend beyond conceptual practice models by emphasizing the intersectional nature of *doing, being, becoming,* and *belonging* in their exploration of well-being (Gruhl, 2020). In fact, these concepts appear to be so relevant to

> ## BOX 45-1 ■ Opportunities for Occupational Therapy in Certified Community Behavioral Health Clinics
>
> OTPs are critical members of community mental health clinics, and opportunities exist to expand occupational therapy roles on integrated primary care teams and in CCBHCs. The CCBHCs are designed to provide coordinated, person-centered, and recovery-oriented care that integrates physical and behavioral health-care approaches (SAMHSA, 2023). The services have been designed with social determinants of health in mind, and CCBHCs are required to offer services to anyone in need of mental health, whether mental health or substance use services, regardless of their ability to pay. Additionally, CCBHCs offer services to people regardless of age, including developmental approach health-care services for children and youth.
>
> OTPs working in CCBHCs can use a wellness-oriented approach that engages people in their health management and promotes a balanced and satisfying life. OTPs have the expertise to ensure that interprofessional teams identify and address commonly overlooked barriers to wellness, including social, cognitive, and physical barriers to occupational participation in ADLs, IADLs, work, and leisure.
>
> Each of these performance areas impacts goals related to housing, education, employment, and other valued occupational roles. As part of a CCBHC team, OTPs can contribute to individuals' evaluation and treatment by:
>
> - Identifying individual strengths, goals, skills, and other factors important for wellness and recovery planning
> - Performing psychosocial evaluations, including housing, vocational, and educational status, as well as social support networks and community participation
> - Promoting health and wellness through the use of everyday activities
> - Offering adapted and compensatory strategies that mitigate the impact of the illness and methods for reducing symptoms through engagement in wellness roles and routines
> - Developing person, group, and population health promotion interventions to support mental health and chronic disease management

well-being that even young children endorse them. For example, in a study by Vidal-Sanchez and colleagues (2021), most children described well-being as related to their participation in play and a sense of belonging within their community.

In exploring the **doing** dimension of well-being, practitioners can focus on the person's perceived participation and competence in well-being occupations, including associated routines and habits. Within the **being** dimension, practitioners can consider the person's performance of well-being occupations, including values, motivations, and roles associated with the occupation. Within the **becoming** dimension, practitioners can explore the process of occupational adaptation and the influence of the person's context on their capacity to engage in valued well-being occupations.

Lastly, in examining the **belonging** dimension, practitioners can explore the person's connectedness to others in their family, friends, and people in the wider community associated with the well-being occupations. For example, an individual may identify listening to music as essential to their well-being. They may talk about listening to music at home and going out to see live shows and concerts (*doing*) and how this process has evolved in making them music lovers and situating music as an integral part of their daily self-care (*becoming*). They may also reflect on their value of music and art as the core driver behind participation (*being*) and how these values were instilled in them through their family and later reinforced through their friend groups (*belonging*).

The concept of wellness as an occupation has been something that has been applied within and outside of occupational therapy practice, including its application to providing wellness in occupational therapy students (Larson, 2020).

Evaluation

Throughout the evaluation process, OTPs are asked to critically reflect on the person's occupational participation and well-being across physical, mental, and social domains. Incorporating the eight dimensions of wellness into occupational therapy evaluation ensures that practitioners gain a holistic understanding of the person's strengths, challenges, and self-determined goals.

When the assessment process involves collaboration between the provider and the person in recovery, it promotes a focus on health and personal responsibility that can strengthen optimism and a belief in the capacity for self-management. This approach can lead individuals to feel more empowered to manage life crises, stress, and disappointments and to direct attention to personal strengths, resources, and goals. A positive and strengths-based approach can result in people assuming an active role in self-monitoring health and increasing activity in the dimensions where they perceive there may be an imbalance.

Several tools have been developed that practitioners can use to support person-centered evaluation and goal setting in relation to well-being occupations. OTPs can begin the evaluation process by gathering a comprehensive occupational profile and learning more about the individual's strengths, opportunities, and goals related to their self-care and well-being. Additionally, a variety of assessment instruments have been developed that can be used to guide evaluation data gathering using interviews, observation, and self-report, and OTPs can choose from occupation-based and performance-based measures.

The evaluation process should take a top-down approach focused on occupation. While working with adults, OTPs can choose an interview-based assessment such as the Canadian Occupational Performance Measure (COPM; Law et al., 1990), a self-report assessment such as the Occupational Self-Assessment (OSA, Baron et al., 2006), or an observational assessment such as the Model of Human Occupation Screening Tool (MOHOST; Parkinson et al., 2006). A similar set of tools can be used in pediatric settings, including the COPM, Child Occupational Self-Assessment (COSA; Kramer et al., 2014), and Short Child Occupational Profile (SCOPE; Bowyer et al., 2005). If performance level challenges are suspected, the OTP can also administer additional assessments such as the Evaluation of Social Interaction Skills (ESI; Fisher & Griswold, 2018). Additionally, if challenges appear to be related to routines, habits, and roles, OTPs may administer self-reported tools such as the Role Checklist Version 3 (Scott, 2019) or the Occupational Questionnaire (Smith et al., 1986).

Beyond occupations, assessments can be administered to evaluate general well-being, such as the World Health Organization Five Well-Being Index (WHO-5; WHO Collaborating Centre in Mental Health, 1998), and quality of life, such as Health-Related Quality of Life-14 (HRQOL-14) (Centers for Disease Control and Prevention [CDC], 2018). The practitioner may also be interested in gaining additional insight into how the individual participates in health and wellness routines. Assessments such as the Mindful Self-Care Scale (Cook-Cottone & Guyker, 2017) can help practitioners better understand their individuals' self-care practices. Additionally, administering the Health Promoting Lifestyle Profile II (HPLP-II; Walker et al., 1995) can offer insights into unique life habits.

Table 45-2 summarizes occupation-based assessment tools that OTPs can use to evaluate participation in well-being occupations across pediatric and adult practice settings.

Intervention

OTPs use various methods to promote well-being, including occupations and activities, preparatory activities, education and training, and advocacy. Occupational therapy interventions span a variety of formats, including person, group, and population-based interventions. Furthermore, OTPs have been successful at advocating for increased health-care access and equity by expanding telehealth in response to decreased access to in-person services resulting from the COVID-19 pandemic. When it comes to empowering change in health behaviors, it has been recognized that simply changing the knowledge of health behaviors does not necessarily translate into observable behavioral change (Happell et al., 2014). These findings present a perfect opportunity for OTPs, whose interventions specialize in going beyond knowing and into knowledge generalization and translation through doing.

One example of an occupation-based intervention that has been gaining attention in occupational therapy literature is Lifestyle Redesign®. Lifestyle Redesign® interventions are aimed at promoting health and wellness habits and routines. These interventions have been shown to improve mental health, leisure, and social participation in older

---

TABLE 45-2 | Therapeutic Reasoning Assessment Table: Well-Being Occupations

Which Tool?	Whom Was This Tool Designed For?	What Is Required of the Person? Can They Use the Tool?	What Am I Measuring?	How Long Does It Take to Administer This Assessment?	Is the Tool Associated With a Practice Model?
Canadian Occupational Performance Measure (COPM; Law et al., 1990)	• Adults (18+ years) • Children and youth 8+ years • Parents of young children (0–8 years)	The assessment is completed in a format of a semistructured interview with support from an OTP.	A measure of occupational satisfaction and performance in self-care, leisure, and productivity	30–60 minutes	Canadian Model of Occupational Performance (CMOP-E; Townsend & Polatajko, 2007)
Occupational Self-Assessment (OSA; Baron et al., 2006) or Child Occupational Self-Assessment (COSA; Kramer et al., 2014)	• Adults (18+ years) • Children and youth 5+ years	The assessment can be completed as a self-report assessment or in a format of a semistructured interview with support from an OTP.	Self-reported competency and value across various occupations	30–60 minutes	Model of Human Occupation (Taylor, 2017)
Evaluation of Social Interaction Skills (ESI; Fisher & Griswold, 2018)	• Adults (18+ years) • Children and youth 3+ years	The assessment is completed by the OTP following a structured observation of an occupation.	A measure of occupational performance specific to social interaction skills	30–60 minutes	Transactional Model and Occupational Therapy Intervention Process Model (OTIPM; Fisher & Marterella, 2019)
Model of Human Occupation Screening Tool (MOHOST; Parkinson et al., 2006) or Short Child Occupational Profile (SCOPE; Bowyer et al., 2005)	• Adults (18+ years) • Children and youth (0–18 years)	The assessment is completed by the OTP following a semistructured interview and a structured observation of an occupation.	A measure of supports and barriers to occupational participation across volition, habituation, communication, and interaction skills, process skills, motor skills, and environment	30–60 minutes	Model of Human Occupation (Taylor, 2017)

adults (65+ years) with and without disabilities (Levasscur et al., 2019). Additionally, in adults with fibromyalgia, participation in a Lifestyle Redesign® program resulted in significant improvements in activity participation, life balance, mental domains of quality of life, depression, and pain self-efficacy (Lagueux et al., 2021). Additionally, Lifestyle Redesign® is effective across different formats of program delivery. For example, Lifestyle Redesign® programs delivered via telehealth demonstrated significant improvements in occupational performance, satisfaction, and health management (Mitchell et al., 2023).

Significant benefits have also been associated with interventions that incorporate leisure participation, including crafts, nature, and sports. Research exploring the benefits of participation in crafts demonstrated positive health and well-being benefits from participation in knitting (Brooks et al., 2019) and embroidering (von Kürthy et al., 2022). Similarly, participation in gardening and horticulture has been shown to promote a positive sense of being, including a greater sense of belonging (Suto et al., 2021) and decreased loneliness (Mourão et al., 2021).

Despite these positive findings, research also suggests that participation in leisure can be inhibited by marginalization and stigma within the community. For example, in football (or soccer), players who experienced mental distress perceived community-based football leagues as promoting a sense of belonging and reducing stigma and exclusion within the community (Pettican et al., 2021, 2022). See Chapter 51: Leisure and Creative Occupations for a deeper look at leisure and creative occupations and their link to well-being. 🤝

Throughout the evaluation and intervention process, OTPs can guide their individuals to reflect on what the person already does to promote their well-being (daily routines, habits, and valued life roles and activities) and opportunities to continue expanding their wellness routines and occupations. At the core of well-being occupations is self-care. Although often challenging to define, according to research, many OTPs align self-care with participation in ADLs. Occupation-based interventions incorporating self-care through peer-mediated learning have improved well-being and general self-efficacy.

The following section outlines examples of occupational therapy intervention opportunities to promote well-being across the eight domains of wellness. Table 45-3 offers examples of interventions across the eight dimensions in occupational therapy practice. Box 45-2 provides a description of how health fairs can be used to engage persons, communities, and populations in primary and public health-care settings to promote well-being.

Review of the Eight Dimensions of Wellness

Emotional/Mental Dimension

OTPs can support emotional well-being by designing interventions that promote awareness of emotional-well-being and the capacity to cope with life's stressors. Specifically, mindfulness-based interventions can promote the individual's self-reflection on strengths, challenges, and support

systems through individual education and coaching. Practitioners can also support individuals in reflecting on the emotional impact of daily routines and habits and consider ways to adjust their experience to create more optimal fit and balance in everyday life.

Mindfulness-based programs have been shown to improve anxiety, depression, distress, and well-being, with the greatest impact of mindfulness-based programs being targeted to the individual needs of a high-risk population (Galante et al., 2021). In occupational therapy, mindfulness-based approaches such as the Zentangle® intervention have been shown to significantly reduce anxiety and improve self-compassion in the general population of adults (Chung et al., 2022). Additionally, occupation-based interventions that incorporate mindfulness components (including creative arts and yoga) have been shown to be increasingly effective in pediatric settings in supporting mental health, positive behavior, and social participation (Cahill et al., 2020).

Environmental Dimension

In addition to providing individualized support, OTPs can consider ways to design interventions that promote well-being through the therapeutic use of everyday spaces at home, school, work, and community. Practitioners can help individuals structure and adapt their environment to promote well-being and safety and help individuals explore new environments for occupational engagement. For example, occupational participation in arts- and nature-based spaces has been shown to significantly improve the emotional well-being of children (Chiumento et al., 2018) and adults (Thomson et al., 2020).

Beyond physical environments, practitioners can also consider the therapeutic use of virtual environments. Specifically, practitioners can consider ways to support individuals through structured support using virtual technology, such as cell phones. For example, research suggests that interventions that utilize text messaging can be effective in promoting medication adherence and clinical outcomes in individuals with mental illness (Simon et al., 2022). Practitioners can consider ways to incorporate virtual environments, including text messaging, to support individuals' participation in wellness routines and health management.

Financial Dimension

OTPs can support individuals' capacity and skills associated with financial management. Education and coaching interventions can include budgeting or pursuing employment to promote financial independence. Additionally, OTPs can support the person's long-term planning and support their knowledge and awareness of life planning or the implications of high-risk behaviors on financial health.

Practitioners can also use advocacy and apply their knowledge of community resources to support individuals' access to support and services available in their community. For example, people might not be aware of all the financial supports available and may need assistance navigating health care and social systems in their community. An example of such intervention is highlighted by Schmelzer and Leto (2018), who found that interventions that supported individuals' capacity to maximize food resources during meal

TABLE 45-3 | Examples of Wellness Interventions in Occupational Therapy Practice by Dimension

Dimension of Wellness	Example of Intervention
Emotional/Mental Dimension	Amari (they/them; 48 years old) was recently diagnosed with thyroid cancer, resulting in a decreased capacity to effectively respond to and cope with stress and anxiety. The OTP works with Amari to explore ways to integrate yoga practice into the health management routine. They work together to reflect on the psychosocial impact of cancer treatment and consider ways to promote effective coping and recovery. The practitioner also uses coaching and education to empower the individual's self-advocacy for mental health support during their rehabilitation stay and upon return to work.
Environmental Dimension	Rowan (he/him; 57 years old) reports increased PTSD symptoms and decreased capacity to participate in rest and sleep occupations. The OTP supports Rowan's knowledge and use of sleep hygiene strategies, including progressive relaxation techniques and environmental redesign of the bedroom to promote increased relaxation in preparation for bed. Rowan and the practitioner explore how the sleep environment can be adjusted to facilitate increased participation in sleep hygiene routines and reflect on the positive and negative impact of technology (including screen time) as part of the nighttime routine. They also consider ways that Rowan can advocate for increased opportunities for mindfulness breaks during the day.
Financial Dimension	Asher (he/him; 19 years old) has an autism diagnosis and has been experiencing increased social isolation and decreased community participation after graduating from high school. As the OTP and Asher work on exploring new employment opportunities, the therapist uses coaching to support Asher's capacity to explore budget-friendly options for community transportation. The therapist supports Asher by sharing resources on accessible and public transportation services for people with disabilities.
Intellectual Dimension	Deven (he/him; 24 years old) reports increased symptoms of anxiety and depression because of the growing demands of graduate school. Deven and the OTP explore ways to adjust Deven's study routine to best capitalize on the use of memory aids and environmental supports to organize studying. The practitioner also recommends that Deven explore workshops on school-work-life balance that are offered through the counseling center and resources on wellness supports and services for students, including services for students in crisis.
Occupational Dimension	Nico (they/them; 37 years old) reports that following experiencing a first-time psychosis episode, they have been struggling to stay focused at work. They also report that they have been increasingly afraid that others might find out about their mental health condition, and in order to "stay off the radar," they have been saying yes to more work projects. The OTP works with Nico to explore ways to create boundaries and structure in the workday that incorporate intentional moments of mindfulness breaks, including opportunities for walking meetings. Nico and the therapist discuss ways mindfulness would support Nico and their coworkers, including the benefits of wellness routines and advocacy for flexible work schedules.
Physical Dimension	Ira (she/her; 9 years old) has been experiencing increased social anxiety and decreased participation in social and play opportunities with peers at school and in the community. The OTP works with Ira's parents and teachers to offer education on the benefits of occupational participation in activities that incorporate physical activities (such as yoga and sports) for mental health and social well-being in children and youth. Together, they explore ways to support Ira's participation in structured and unstructured play and physical activities at school and as part of extracurricular activities.
Spiritual Dimension	Charlie (she/her; 66 years old) reports increased depressive symptoms and decreased community participation since her retirement. The OTP uses coaching to help Charlie explore opportunities for Charlie to reengage in valued occupations. Charlie identifies an interest in getting more involved in community service and her church. Together, the practitioner and Charlie explore opportunities for service at Charlie's church, including incorporating her past experience as an early childhood teacher and volunteering to support evening and weekend programming for young children.
Social Dimension	Rita (she/her; 73 years old) recently transitioned from independent community living to a supported living community. The OTP works with Rita to explore ways for her to engage in activities and groups available to residents and recommends that Rita enjoys several groups led by other residents. Together, they explore Rita's interests and opportunities for leisure pursuits.

preparation effectively increased both satisfaction and performance associated with food resource management.

Intellectual Dimension

Education and coaching are critical components of occupational therapy intervention, and practitioners support individuals' capacity for lifelong learning, problem-solving, and self-direction. In addition to designing interventions that empower people to explore formal and informal education, practitioners can use coaching to guide individuals' self-reflection on strengths and opportunities to expand their learning. Self-reflection on personal health narratives has been recognized as a valuable tool in working with people with intellectual and developmental disabilities (Caudill et al., 2022), and practitioners can support individuals' use of health narratives to empower increased knowledge and health-care access. Additionally, practitioners can be mindful of differences in self-directed learning patterns as they work with individuals (Therrien et al., 2020) and consider how to support self-directed learning throughout the occupational therapy process.

BOX 45-2 ■ Health Fairs to Promote Wellness

An increasing number of community-based programs are partnering with primary care and federally qualified health centers for communitywide education campaigns. In addition to education initiatives, community-based programs are increasingly integrating health screening into their facilities by sponsoring health and wellness fairs, empowering participation in health management, and normalizing the idea of health maintenance for both service providers and service users.

Health fairs help people in recovery learn how to better manage medical conditions that can be improved with screening, education, and support. They also provide personalized health information that participants can share with their physicians, family members, and other supporters. Through education and awareness building, health fairs can encourage people to make healthier choices that lead to a satisfying lifestyle centered on wellness. OTPs can play an important role in coordinating health fairs, and this tool can be a useful roadmap for planning a successful event, regardless of size and complexity.

For example, OTPs, faculty, and students can take the opportunity to participate in back-to-school fairs to support family and child education on best health management practices, including backpack fitting and sharing of best practices of building confidence, self-efficacy, and self-determination in children and youth.

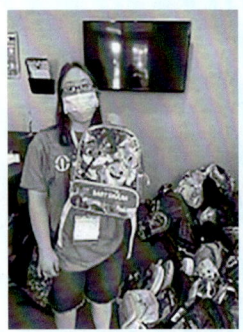 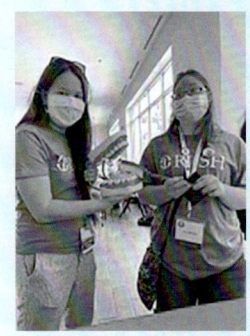 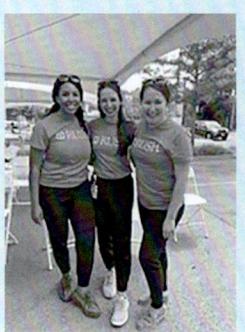

Occupational therapy faculty, students, and interns volunteer at a back-to-school health-care fair providing wellness education and backpack fittings in preparation for going back to school.

Occupational Dimension

Occupational therapy interventions are uniquely designed to create opportunities to participate in a wide array of occupations that are fulfilling and rewarding to individuals. Occupational therapy interventions are designed to support people in identifying and engaging in occupations that bring meaning and purpose to life. Beyond supporting interest exploration, participation, and engagement in occupations, practitioners can also consider using advocacy and empowering occupational environments that support well-being.

For example, research suggests that employment and well-being are influenced by both experience of stigma at work (van Beukering et al., 2021) and a person's perspective on their decision to disclose (or not to disclose) a mental health diagnosis (Bogaers et al., 2023). Practitioners can consider how they can design individual interventions that promote self-advocacy and work on community and organizational levels to address mental health stigma and advocate for increased equity and inclusion of people with mental illness in the community.

Physical Dimension

OTPs can design interventions that help people to establish or reestablish health habits and routines. For example, practitioners can consider opportunities to address well-being across physical, mental, and social domains and promote health management of chronic and comorbid conditions through routine health screenings and routine preventive health services. Practitioners can also prioritize evidence-based strategies that decrease common risk factors, including interventions that promote healthy nutrition and weight management (Conn et al., 2019; Doğu et al., 2023; Ellison et al., 2020; Jessen-Winge et al., 2021; Lunt et al., 2022).

Additionally, research suggests that peer-mediated interventions delivered in individual and group formats may be especially effective. For example, in people with schizophrenia, peer-mediated interventions (with peers involved as primary or coleaders) are effective in increasing physical activity and capacity, with intervention effects ranging from self-reported physical health, nutrition, and BMI (Coles et al., 2022). Research findings on the benefits of nutrition-based interventions for addressing metabolic syndrome risk factors in people with serious mental illness remain inconclusive, with limited evidence highlighting the benefits of individual interventions and those delivered by dietitians (Rocks et al., 2022). Chapter 46: Activities of Daily Living, Instrumental Activities of Daily Living, and Health Management Occupations takes a closer look at this dimension. 🤝

Social Dimension

Social connectedness and a sense of belonging are key components of well-being, and practitioners can consider ways to empower social participation. Research suggests that an increased focus on health management following a first-episode psychosis can negatively impact social participation by shifting a person's focus away from larger life goals (Fox & Bailliard, 2021). Practitioners can assist individuals in social participation, helping them to maintain and improve personal relationships and important friendships and to maintain connections with others and the community.

Practitioners can also consider ways to promote positive social interactions and support within the individual's home, work (or school), and community environments. For example, occupational therapy interventions that facilitate participation in positive social environments have been found to increase occupational well-being, including a sense of content, competence, belonging, identity, and autonomy in adults with intellectual disability (Milbourn et al., 2020). For example, OTPs can consult with community-based organizations on opportunities to increase social connectedness and support through integration of peer mentor groups. Chapter 49: Connectedness and Belonging offers insights regarding this dimension. 🤝

Spiritual Dimension

Within the spiritual dimension, OTPs can support individuals' reflection and goal-directed behaviors that align with their personal beliefs and values. Practitioners can also consider ways to support individuals' engagement, or reengage, in activities, habits, and rituals closely related to cultural, religious, or spiritual traditions. Practitioners can help people prioritize actions that empower a sense of meaning and purpose, as well as consider strategies to create a sense of peace and balance. For example, research examining resilience in student veterans found that students who reported a greater perception of life meaning reported greater engagement in meaningful activities, social support, and coping abilities (Kinney et al., 2020). The students also reported fewer somatic symptoms and fewer depressive and posttraumatic stress disorder (PTSD) symptoms (Kinney et al., 2020). Chapter 53: Spiritual Occupations takes a closer look at this dimension. 🤝

Evidence-Based Practice

Applying Mindfulness for Health and Wellness Promotion in OTPs

Daily mindfulness practice can reduce anxiety, depression, and stress in health-care practitioners.

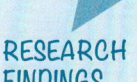

RESEARCH FINDINGS

With the rise of burnout and stress in health-care practitioners, mindfulness-based stress reduction strategies, including mindfulness meditation and yoga, have been gaining increased attention as an intervention strategy to promote psychological functioning in health-care professionals. A systematic review conducted by Kriakous and colleagues (2020) examined the benefits of mindfulness-based stress reduction interventions for health-care providers, including daily formal mindfulness practice.

The study findings suggested that mindfulness-based stress reduction can be effective in reducing anxiety, depression, and stress in health-care practitioners (Kriakous et al., 2020). However, there was insufficient evidence to support the effectiveness of this approach in reducing burnout or increasing resilience (Kriakous et al., 2020). The researchers noted that the majority of programs spanned 8 weeks; however, positive outcomes were also noted for shortened 2- and 4-week programs (Kriakous et al., 2020).

APPLICATIONS

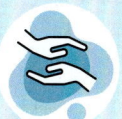

➡ Daily formal mindfulness practice is an effective strategy for reducing anxiety, depression, and stress in health-care practitioners.

➡ Mindfulness-based stress reduction interventions are most effective when they integrate multiple opportunities for experiential learning and practice through 2 to 8 weeks of intervention.

➡ Opportunities exist to expand evidence on strategies that can be effectively used to reduce burnout and resilience.

REFERENCES

Kriakous, S. A., Elliott, K., Lamers, C., & Owen, R. L. (2020). The effectiveness of mindfulness-based stress reduction on the psychological functioning of healthcare professionals: A systematic review. *Mindfulness, 12*(1), 1–28. https://doi.org/10.1007/s12671-020-01500-9

Well-Being and Occupational Therapy Outcomes

OTPs support well-being outcomes through an emphasis on occupational performance and participation as well as role competency in valued occupations. Occupational therapy interventions to support well-being vary widely and range from disease prevention to health and wellness promotion initiatives delivered at person, group, and population levels. Through empowering participation in health and wellness routines, practitioners can empower well-being and quality of life. Most importantly, practitioners can work with organizations and communities to empower occupational justice and equitable access to supports and services necessary for well-being.

Research examining individuals' desired outcomes within occupation-based preventive programs highlights the importance of weight management, disease management, mental health and well-being, stress management, financial management, and social connectedness with family, friends, and the wider community (Schepens-Niemiec et al., 2015). In fact, opportunities for OTPs to promote well-being through social participation have been highlighted across occupational therapy settings, including settings that support women with chronic fatigue syndrome (Rosenberg et al., 2023), women with cancer diagnoses (Maher & Mendonca, 2018), and people with nontraumatic spinal cord injury (Barclay et al., 2018).

In addition to working with individuals, practitioners can reflect upon and consider their role in supporting caregivers. Research examining the perspectives of caregivers for people with mental illness suggests that caregivers experience an impact of caregiving on their own occupational participation and identity, requiring support for coping and achieving occupational balance (Howes & Ellison, 2021). Findings such as these are especially prominent in pediatrics, with parents of children with developmental disabilities repeatedly reporting negative mental health and well-being outcomes because of the difficulty in maintaining a sense of occupational balance and self-care (Günal et al., 2021; McAuliffe et al., 2018; Smith et al., 2023).

To support positive family and caregiver outcomes, practitioners can consider advocating for increased health promotion and coaching programs for caregivers of children and adults with disabilities. One example of such a program includes Health Promoting Activity Coaching, an intervention within the Healthy Mothers Healthy Families (HMHF-HPAC) program (Harris et al., 2022). At the end of the study, mothers reported decreased stress and anxiety, as well as increased participation in health-promotion activities, mood, activity levels, self-awareness, and participation in leisure activities with their children (Harris et al., 2022).

PhotoVoice

Reflections From Occupational Therapy Students

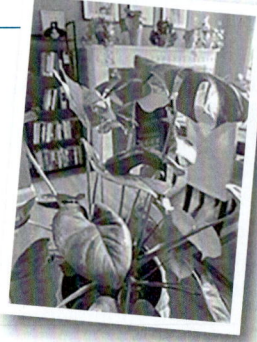

As health-care providers, so much of our value is placed on how productive we are and how much we can provide to others, which is wonderful! But . . . reading and indoor gardening are just for me. I'm "producing" and cultivating my own joy at my own pace.

— Ashley B., OTD, OTR/L

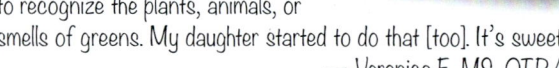

Well-being to me is slowing down enough to get outdoors and enjoy nature with my family or alone. The elements stimulate all my senses. It's a time of prayer and gratitude. When I go for walks with the kids, I stoop to recognize the plants, animals, or smells of greens. My daughter started to do that [too]. It's sweet.

— Veronica F., MS, OTR/L

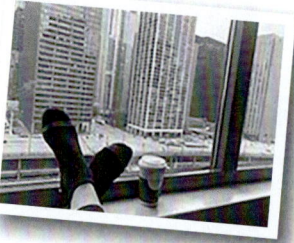

This is me relaxing on Mother's Day morning at a downtown hotel with my family in near proximity. My daughter and her friends had a fun and safe after-prom gathering in the rooms next door, and my son, just back from college before heading to D.C., is sleeping in our room. A late checkout means no rushing. I know where the kids are, that they are safe and well, and that we will have some quality time together today. That's well-being for me!

— Veronica L., OTD, OTR/L

Which self-care and well-being occupations are prioritized in the practitioners' PhotoVoice contributions? Which dimensions of wellness do you notice in the practitioners' PhotoVoices? How could these self-care and well-being occupations be integrated into the practitioners' work days to support their professional quality of life?

Practicing What Is Taught: Reflections on Health and Well-Being After the COVID-19 Pandemic

The COVID-19 pandemic brought the importance of health and well-being to the forefront of health care, impacting communities worldwide. The pandemic had a negative impact regardless of whether or not a particular person got sick with COVID-19, including negative health impacts across mental, physical, and social health domains. Survivors of COVID-19 reported decreased social participation and increased feelings of isolation and fear (Cavaliere et al., 2023). People of all ages found themselves in situations where they had to adapt to challenges associated with lockdown measures and newfound participation restrictions, as well as increased reliance on technology to stay connected with their families, friends, and other members of the community (Lee et al., 2022).

Families and caregivers of children with disabilities experienced an increased negative impact on mental health and well-being (Lee et al., 2021), and adults with developmental disabilities experienced increased mental health problems and decreased access to developmental disability services (Rosencrans et al., 2021).

Occupational therapy service recipients and OTPs alike experienced the negative impact of the pandemic on mental health and well-being. In North America, South America, and Europe, OTPs and students experienced decreased occupational participation, which was associated with perceptions of cultural, environmental, and lifestyle conditions as well as financial concerns (Alvarez et al., 2021). In the United States, although OTPs and students reported "normal" resilience, they perceived a sense of well-being "less than half of the time" while managing "moderate" levels of stress (Popova et al., 2022). Although practitioners experienced decreased well-being and quality of life because of moral distress (Howard et al., 2023), students had to adapt to the changing demands of online and blended learning (Brown et al., 2022; Guszkowska & Dąbrowska-Zimakowska, 2022).

Here's the Point

- OTPs apply multiple lenses to understanding self-care and well-being occupations, including theoretical foundations informing their understanding of health and wellness, quality of life, and flourishing.
- OTPs have an opportunity to support self-care and well-being occupations across the eight dimensions of wellness: emotional/mental, environmental, financial, intellectual, occupational, physical, social, and spiritual.
- Self-care and well-being occupations are influenced by multiple individual factors, including motivation for occupation, perception of occupational balance, subjective and objective experience, occupational performance, and the impact of co-occurring health conditions.
- Social determinants of health should be assessed as supports and barriers to participation and performance of self-care and well-being occupations, including considerations of health-care access and quality, neighborhood and built environment, social and community context, economic stability, and education access and quality.
- Occupational therapy evaluation of self-care and well-being occupations should incorporate gathering of the occupational profile and evaluation using performance and occupation-based assessment tools that incorporate a person's self-report and lived experience.
- Mindfulness and occupation-based approaches have been increasingly gaining attention as evidence-based practices for supporting self-care and well-being occupations.
- OTPs should consider different ways of tracking the efficacy of interventions, including evaluation of the impact of self-care and well-being interventions on health, wellness, and quality of life on the person, group, and population levels.
- OTPs and students report increasing rates of stress and burnout, highlighting the importance of increased emphasis on individual and environmental supports to promote professional quality of life.

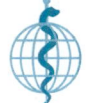

Visit the online resource center at **FADavis.com** to access the videos.

Apply It Now

1. Eight Dimensions of Wellness Workbook

Reflect on the eight dimensions of wellness in your life by completing a *Wellness Wheel Worksheet:* https://jflowershealth.com/8-dimensions-of-wellness

2. Reflection on Implicit and Explicit Bias

Reflect on the impact of implicit and explicit bias on OTPs' capacity to support the health and wellness of people across health-care settings. How have implicit and explicit biases impacted your participation and performance in health and wellness occupations? To guide your reflection, consider taking the Implicit Association Test (IAT) developed by the University of Virginia: https://implicit.harvard.edu/implicit/takeatest.html. The website offers a multitude of implicit bias sets, such as the Weight IAT, that explores the influence of "Fat–Thin" implicit biases.

3. Reflective Journaling Exercise

Apply your knowledge of the eight dimensions of wellness by journaling using the following prompts: "Describe a time when you experienced a state of flourishing in your life. How was that experience influenced by your emotional/mental, environmental, financial, intellectual, occupational, physical, social, and spiritual wellness?

4. PhotoVoice Partner Activity

With a partner, reflect on individual and environmental contributors to your individual health and wellness. Individually reflect upon your experience and take photos that represent self-care and well-being occupations in your life. Share your photos and lived experience with your partner.

5. Applying the Occupational Therapy Process to a Case Study

Review Mike's The Lived Experience narrative in the chapter. Apply the information presented by developing an evaluation, intervention, and outcome tracking plan to support Mike's occupational performance and participation in self-care and well-being occupations. Consider how your therapeutic reasoning might change based on if you were working with Mike in an acute, outpatient, or home health setting.

6. Exploring Evidence-Based Practices in Occupational Therapy

Expand your knowledge of doing, being, becoming, and belonging by conducting your own literature review on health and wellness occupations in occupational therapy science literature. Consider how these research findings can be applied in your everyday life and integrated into your clinical practice.

7. Knowledge Translation in Occupational Therapy Practice

Apply the research findings from Popova and colleagues (2022) and Kriakous and colleagues (2020) to develop a proposal for empowering participation and performance of self-care and well-being occupations in OTPs and students. Consider what evaluations, interventions, and outcome measures you might recommend on individual, group, and organizational levels.

Resources

- American Occupational Therapy Association—Maintain Your Optimal Health: https://www.aota.org/career/career-center /wellness-for-life-and-career/maintain-your-optimal-health
- *Healthy People 2030*—Social Determinants of Health: https:// health.gov/healthypeople/priority-areas/social-determinants -health
- National Institutes of Health (NIH) Mindfulness for Your Health: https://newsinhealth.nih.gov/2021/06/mindfulness-your -health
- Northwestern University—Eight Dimensions of Wellness Overview: https://www.northwestern.edu/wellness/8-dimensions
- Self-Compassion by Dr. Kristin Neff: https://self-compassion.org including a Self-Compassion Test: https://self-compassion.org /self-compassion-test

Videos

- "Fieldwork Experience in Juvenile Correction Setting" video. In this video, occupational therapist Maggie reflects on how she felt prepared and unprepared for her fieldwork experience. She touches on topics such as trauma, emotional regulation, and sensory processing, and emphasizes the need to be aware of her own self-care by setting boundaries. Access the video at the online resource center at FADavis.com.
- "Will Horowitz: Lived Experience of Autism" video. In this video, a young adult with autism describes his childhood interest in trains and how it has translated into an adult volunteer opportunity. He explains that, although an autistic individual can seem to have a "one-track mind" about a subject, it can also become an advantage in that they can become very specialized, as has been true for him with the Steam Into History project at a local railroad. Access the video at the online resource center at FADavis.com.
- "Life Skills Groups in an Unhoused Population" video. Kailin is an occupational therapist who works in community mental health and homeless services. In this video, she describes the impactful life skills groups she runs in a women's shelter and how the use of a group facilitates peer-to-peer support. Kailin offers several creative examples of life skill group activities. She emphasizes the need to employ trauma-informed practices and harm-reduction strategies in this population, meeting clients where they truly are. Access the video at the online resource center at FADavis.com.
- "Two Practitioners Discuss Their Work in Suicide Prevention" video. In this video, two occupational therapists, Nadine and Kim, discuss their work in suicide prevention. They share reflections and pearls of wisdom gained from years of practice in this area—both observations about people in crisis and how they have responded as practitioners. They express the role that the occupational lives of these individuals have in their recovery and crisis plans, as well as serving as a springboard for interventions. Nadine and Kim also describe what is rewarding about this work and the crucial need to meet their self-care and well-being needs

in order to stay connected to this work. Access the video at the online resource center at FADavis.com.
- "Jordan's Lived Experience of Anxiety and Depression" video. In this video, occupational therapist Jordan describes her lived experience of anxiety and depression. She touches on many issues critical to recovery and occupational therapy practice, including social determinants of health, peer support, and how mental health labels can adversely affect an individual's medical treatment. Importantly, she explains how she has learned to blend her lived experience with her work as an occupational therapist, while ensuring she takes care of herself and manages her symptoms. Jordan also offers priceless words of wisdom to practitioners regarding establishing a therapeutic connection with individuals with whom they practice. Access the video at the online resource center at FADavis.com.
- "Leisure Occupations for Unhoused Individuals" video. In this video, Kailin, an occupational therapist who works in community mental health and homeless services, describes the power of leisure activities to the individuals whom she serves. Kailin talks about the barriers to engaging in leisure that often exist for people who are unhoused. She explains how she integrates the evaluation of leisure in her occupational profile and provides several examples of realistic leisure activities that OTPs can use to support individuals' mental health. Access the video at the online resource center at FADavis.com.

References

Afzal, M., Siddiqi, N., Ahmad, B., Afsheen, N., Aslam, F., Ali, A., Ayesha, R., Bryant, M., Holt, R. I. G., Khalid, H., Ishaq, K., Koly, K. N., Rajan, S., Saba, J., Tirbhowan, N., & Gomez, G. A. Z. (2021). Prevalence of overweight and obesity in people with severe mental illness: Systematic review and meta-analysis. *Frontiers in Endocrinology, 12*. https://doi.org/10.3389/fendo.2021.769309

Aldrich, R. M. (2011). A review and critique of well-being in occupational therapy and occupational science. *Scandinavian Journal of Occupational Therapy, 18*(2), 93–100. https://doi.org/10 .3109/11038121003615327

Álvarez, N. M., Villoria, E. D., Arberas, E. J., Pérez, A. M., & Izquierdo, A. L. (2021). Limitations on participation and their relation to social determinants of health among occupational therapists and occupational therapy students during coronavirus lockdown. *The American Journal of Occupational Therapy, 75*(6). https://doi.org/10.5014/ajot.2021.049050

American Occupational Therapy Association. (2020). Occupational therapy practice framework: Domain and process —Fourth edition. *American Journal of Occupational Therapy, 74*(Suppl. 2), 7412410010p1–7412410010p87. https://doi.org/10 .5014/ajot.2020.74S2001

Barclay, L., Lentin, P., Bourke-Taylor, H., & McDonald, R. (2018). The experiences of social and community participation of people with non-traumatic spinal cord injury. *Australian Occupational Therapy Journal, 66*(1), 61–67. https://doi.org/10.1111/1440-1630.12522

Barnett, A. H., Zhang, C. J. P., Johnston, J. M., & Cerin, E. (2018). Relationships between the neighborhood environment and depression in older adults: A systematic review and meta-analysis. *International Psychogeriatrics, 30*(8), 1153–1176. https://doi .org/10.1017/s104161021700271x

Baron, K., Kielhofner, G., Iyenger, A., Goldhammer, V., & Wolenski, J. (2006). *The Occupational Self-Assessment (OSA).* Version 2.2. Model of Human Occupation Clearinghouse, Department of Occupational Therapy, College of Applied Health Sciences, University of Illinois at Chicago. https://moho-irm.uic .edu/products.aspx?type=allA

Berg, K. L., Medrano, J., Acharya, K., Lynch, A., & Msall, M. E. (2018). Health impact of participation for vulnerable youth with disabilities. *The American Journal of Occupational Therapy, 72*(5), 7205195040p1–7205195040p9. https://doi.org/10.5014/ajot.2018 .023622

Berge, J. M., Tate, A., Trofholz, A., & Kunin-Batson, A. (2023). Intergenerational pathways between parental experiences of adverse childhood experiences (ACEs) and child weight: Implications for intervention. *Journal of the American Board of Family Medicine, 36*(1), 39–50. https://doi.org/10.3122/jabfm.2022 .220134r1

Beyazyüz, M., Albayrak, Y., Eğilmez, O. B., Albayrak, N., & Beyazyüz, E. (2013). Relationship between SSRIs and metabolic syndrome abnormalities in patients with generalized anxiety disorder: A prospective study. *Psychiatry Investigation, 10*(2), 148–154. https://doi.org/10.4306/pi.2013.10.2.148

Bogaers, R., Geuze, E., van Weeghel, J., Leijten, F., van De Mheen, D., Rüsch, N., Rozema, A., & Brouwers, E. P. M. (2023). Workplace mental health disclosure, sustainable employability and well-being at work: A cross-sectional study among military personnel with mental illness. *Journal of Occupational Rehabilitation, 33*(2), 399–413. https://doi.org/10.1007/s10926-022-10083-2

Bonabi, H., Müller, M., Ajdacic-Gross, V., Eisele, J. F., Rodgers, S., Seifritz, E., Rössler, W., & Rüsch, N. (2016). Mental health literacy, attitudes to help seeking, and perceived need as predictors of mental health service use. *Journal of Nervous and Mental Disease, 204*(4), 321–324. https://doi.org/10.1097/nmd.0000000000000488

Boström, P. J., Johnels, J. Å., & Broberg, M. (2018). Self-reported psychological well-being in adolescents: The role of intellectual/developmental disability and gender. *Journal of Intellectual Disability Research, 62*(2), 83–93. https://doi.org/10.1111/jir.12432

Bowyer, P., Ross, M., Schwartz, O., Kielhofner, G., & Kramer, J. (2005). *The Short Child Occupational Profile (SCOPE).* Version 2.1. Model of Human Occupation Clearinghouse, Department of Occupational Therapy, College of Applied Health Sciences, University of Illinois. https://moho-irm.uic.edu/products.aspx ?type=allA

Brooks, L. A., Ta, K. N., Townsend, A., & Backman, C. L. (2019). "I just love it": Avid knitters describe health and well-being through occupation. *Canadian Journal of Occupational Therapy, 86*(2), 114–124. https://doi.org/10.1177/0008417419831401

Brown, T., Robinson, L., Gledhill, K., Yu, M., Isbel, S., Greber, C., Parsons, D., & Etherington, J. (2022). 'Learning in and out of lockdown': A comparison of two groups of undergraduate occupational therapy students' engagement in online-only and blended education approaches during the COVID-19 pandemic. *Australian Occupational Therapy Journal, 69*(3), 301–315. https:// doi.org/10.1111/1440-1630.12793

Buck, R., Barnes, M., Cohen, D. A., & Aylward, M. (2010). Common health problems, yellow flags and functioning in a community setting. *Journal of Occupational Rehabilitation, 20,* 235–246. https://doi.org/10.1007/s10926-009-9228-6

Burton, K. A., Lydon, J. P., D'Alessandro, D. A., & Koestner, R. (2006). The differential effects of intrinsic and identified motivation on well-being and performance: Prospective, experimental, and implicit approaches to self-determination theory. *Journal of Personality and Social Psychology, 91*(4), 750–762. https://doi .org/10.1037/0022-3514.91.4.750

Cahill, S. M., Egan, B. E., & Seber, J. (2020). Activity- and occupation-based interventions to support mental health, positive behavior, and social participation for children and youth: A systematic review. *American Journal of Occupational Therapy, 74*(2), 7402180020p1–7402180020p28. https://doi.org/10.5014 /ajot.2020.038687

Cai, R. Y., Gibbs, V., Love, A. M. A., Robinson, A., Fung, L. K., & Brown, L. D. (2023). "Self-compassion changed my life": The self-compassion experiences of autistic and non-autistic adults and its relationship with mental health and psychological well-being. *Journal of Autism and Developmental Disorders, 53*(3), 1066–1081. https://doi.org/10.1007/s10803-022-05668-y

Caudill, A. A., Hladik, L., Gray, M. M., Dulaney, N., Barton, K., Rogers, J. A., Noblet, N., & Ausderau, K. (2022). Health narratives as a therapeutic tool for health care access for people with intellectual and developmental disabilities. *Occupational Therapy in Health Care, 38*(3), 750–767. https://doi.org/10.1080/07380577 .2022.2099603

Cavaliere, C., Damiao, J., Pizzi, M. A., & Fau, L. (2023). Health, well-being, and health-related quality of life following COVID-19. *Occupational Therapy Journal of Research, 43*(2), 188–193. https:// doi.org/10.1177/15394492221111733

Center for Behavioral Health Statistics and Quality. (2022). *Key substance use and mental health indicators in the United States: Results from the 2021 National Survey on Drug Use and Health* (HHS Publication No. PEP 22-07-01-005. NSDUH Series H-57). Substance Abuse and Mental Health Services Administration. https://www .samhsa.gov/data/sites/default/files/reports/rpt39443/2021NS DUHFFRRev010323.pdf

Centers for Disease Control and Prevention. (2018). *Healthy Days Core Module: HRQOL-14 Measure.* https://www.cdc.gov/hrqol /hrqol14_measure.htm

Chang, Y., Chen, C., Huang, P. J., & Lin, L. Y. (2018). Understanding the characteristics of friendship quality, activity participation, and emotional well-being in Taiwanese adolescents with autism spectrum disorder. *Scandinavian Journal of Occupational Therapy, 26*(6), 452–462. https://doi.org/10.1080/11038128.2018.1449887

Chiumento, A., Mukherjee, I., Chandna, J., Dutton, C., Rahman, A., & Bristow, K. (2018). A haven of green space: Learning from a pilot pre-post evaluation of a school-based social and therapeutic horticulture intervention with children. *BMC Public Health, 18*(1), 836. https://doi.org/10.1186/s12889-018-5661-9

Chung, S., Ho, F. Y. Y., & Chan, H. C. (2022). The effects of Zentangle® on affective well-being among adults: A pilot randomized controlled trial. *American Journal of Occupational Therapy, 76*(5), 7605205060. https://doi.org/10.5014/ajot.2022.049113

Coles, A., Maksyutynska, K., Knezevic, D., Agarwal, S. M., Strudwick, G., Dunbar, J. A., Druss, B., Selby, P., Banfield, M., Hahn, M. K., & Castle, D. J. (2022). Peer-facilitated interventions for improving the physical health of people with schizophrenia spectrum disorders: Systematic review and meta-analysis. *The Medical Journal of Australia, 217*(Suppl. 7), S22–S28. https://doi.org /10.5694/mja2.51693

Conn, A., Bourke, N., James, C., & Haracz, K. (2019). Occupational therapy intervention addressing weight gain and obesity in people with severe mental illness: A scoping review. *Australian Occupational Therapy Journal, 66*(4), 446–457. https://doi.org /10.1111/1440-1630.12575

Connolly, D., Anderson, M., Colgan, M., Montgomery, J., Clarke, J., & Kinsella, M. (2018). The impact of a primary care stress management and wellbeing programme (RENEW) on occupational participation: A pilot study. *British Journal of Occupational Therapy, 82*(2), 112–121. https://doi.org/10.1177/0308022618793323

Cook-Cottone, C. P., & Guyker, W. M. (2017). The development and validation of the Mindful Self-Care Scale (MSCS): An assessment of practices that support positive embodiment. *Mindfulness, 9,* 169–175. https://doi.org/10.1007/s12671-017-0759-1

Cprek, S. E., Williamson, L. H., McDaniel, H., Brase, R. M., & Williams, C. M. (2020). Adverse childhood experiences (ACEs)

and risk of childhood delays in children ages 1–5. *Child & Adolescent Social Work Journal, 37*(1), 15–24. https://doi.org/10.1007/s10560-019-00622-x

Cudjoe, T. K., Roth, D., Szanton, S. L., Wolff, J. L., Boyd, C. M., & Thorpe, R. J. (2020). The epidemiology of social isolation: National health and aging trends study. *The Journals of Gerontology: Series B, Psychological Sciences and Social Sciences, 75*(1), 107–113. https://doi.org/10.1093/geronb/gby037

Cusack, P., Cusack, F., McAndrew, S., McKeown, M., & Duxbury, J. (2018). An integrative review exploring the physical and psychological harm inherent in using restraint in mental health inpatient settings. *International Journal of Mental Health Nursing, 27*(3), 1162–1176. https://doi.org/10.1111/inm.12432

Dayabandara, M., Hanwella, R., Ratnatunga, S., Seneviratne, S., Suraweera, C., & de Silva, V. A. (2017). Antipsychotic-associated weight gain: Management strategies and impact on treatment adherence. *Neuropsychiatric Disease and Treatment, 13,* 2231–2241. https://doi.org/10.2147/NDT.S113099

De Hert, M., Correll, C. U., Bobes, J., Cetkovich-Bakmas, M., Cohen, D., Asai, I., Detraux, J., Gautam, S., Möller, H. J., Ndetei, D. M., Newcomer, J. W., Uwakwe, R., & Leucht, S. (2011). Physical illness in patients with severe mental disorders. I. Prevalence, impact of medications and disparities in health care. *World Psychiatry, 10,* 52–77. https://doi.org/10.1002/j.2051-5545.2011.tb00014.x

Doğu, S. E., Kokurcan, A., & Örsel, S. (2023). An occupation-based healthy nutrition and wellness program for individuals with schizophrenia. *PubMed,* 15394492231153112. https://doi.org/10.1177/15394492231153113

Doğu, S. E., & Örsel, S. (2022). The relationship between psychopathology, occupational balance, and quality of life among people with schizophrenia. *OTJR: Occupational Therapy Journal of Research, 43*(4), 626–636. https://doi.org/10.1111/1440-1630.12855

Eagers, J., Franklin, R. C., Broome, K., Yau, M. K., & Barnett, F. (2022). Potential occupational therapy scope of practice in the work-to-retirement transition in Australia. *Australian Occupational Therapy Journal, 69*(3), 265–278. https://doi.org/10.1111/1440-1630.12788

Eklund, M., Brunt, D., & Argentzell, E. (2019). Perceived occupational balance and well-being among people with mental illness living in two types of supported housing. *Scandinavian Journal of Occupational Therapy, 27*(6), 450–461. https://doi.org/10.1080/11038128.2019.1622771

Ellison, N., Keesing, S., & Harris, C. (2020). Understanding occupational engagement for individuals with bariatric needs: The perspectives of Australian occupational therapists. *Australian Occupational Therapy Journal, 67*(5), 417–426. https://doi.org/10.1111/1440-1630.12657

Farley, A., Kennedy-Behr, A., & Brown, T. (2020). An investigation into the relationship between playfulness and well-being in Australian adults: An exploratory study. *OTJR: Occupational Therapy Journal of Research, 41*(1), 56–64. https://doi.org/10.1177/1539449220945311

Felitti, V. J., Anda, R. F., Nordenberg, D., Williamson, D. P., Spitz, A. M., Edwards, V. J., Koss, M. P., & Marks, J. G. (1998). Relationship of childhood abuse and household dysfunction to many of the leading causes of death in adults. *American Journal of Preventive Medicine, 14*(4), 245–258. https://doi.org/10.1016/s0749-3797(98)00017-8

Fisher, A. G., & Griswold, L. A. (2018). *Evaluation of Social Interaction* (4th ed.). Three Star Press Inc.

Fisher, A. G., & Marterella, A. (2019). *Powerful practice: A model for authentic occupational therapy.* Center for Innovative OT Solutions.

Fox, V., & Bailliard, A. (2021). Liminal space of first-episode psychosis: Health management and its effect on social participation. *American Journal of Occupational Therapy, 75*(6), 7506205090. https://doi.org/10.5014/ajot.2021.046953

Friesinger, J. G., Topor, A., Bøe, T. D., & Larsen, I. B. (2019). Studies regarding supported housing and the built environment for people with mental health problems: A mixed-methods literature review. *Health & Place, 57,* 44–53. https://doi.org/10.1016/j.healthplace.2019.03.006

Galante, J., Friedrich, C., Dawson, A., Montero-Marin, J., Gebbing, P., Delgado-Suárez, I., Gupta, R., Dean, L. D., Dalgleish, T., White, I. R., & Jones, P. B. (2021). Mindfulness-based programmes for mental health promotion in adults in nonclinical settings: A systematic review and meta-analysis of randomised controlled trials. *PLoS Medicine, 18*(1), e1003481. https://doi.org/10.1371/journal.pmed.1003481

Gruhl, K. R., Boucher, M., & Lacarte, S. (2020). Evaluation of an occupation-based, mental-health program: Meeting being, belonging and becoming needs. *Australian Occupational Therapy Journal, 68*(1), 78–89. https://doi.org/10.1111/1440-1630.12707

Günal, A., Pekçetin, S., Wagman, P., Håkansson, C., & Kayihan, H. (2021). Occupational balance and quality of life in mothers of children with cerebral palsy. *British Journal of Occupational Therapy, 85*(1), 37–43. https://doi.org/10.1177/0308022621995112

Gunnarsson, A. B., Hedberg, A., Håkansson, C., Hedin, K., & Wagman, P. (2021). Occupational performance problems in people with depression and anxiety. *Scandinavian Journal of Occupational Therapy, 30*(2), 148–158. https://doi.org/10.1080/11038128.2021.1882562

Gupta, N., Crouse, D. L., Miah, P., & Takaro, T. (2023). Individual physical activity, neighbourhood active living environment and mental illness hospitalisation among adults with cardiometabolic disease: A Canadian population-based cohort analysis. *BMJ Open, 13*(2), e067736. https://doi.org/10.1136/bmjopen-2022-067736

Guszkowska, M., & Dąbrowska-Zimakowska, A. (2022). Occupational balance, changes in occupations and psychological well-being of university students during the COVID-19 pandemic. *Scandinavian Journal of Occupational Therapy, 30*(4), 463–474. https://doi.org/10.1080/11038128.2022.2143892

Han, S., & Lee, H. (2015). Social capital and depression. *Asia-Pacific Journal of Public Health, 27*(2), NP2008–NP2018. https://doi.org/10.1177/1010539513496140

Happell, B., Stanton, R., Hoey, W., & Scott, D. (2014). Knowing is not doing: The relationship between health behaviour knowledge and actual health behaviours in people with serious mental illness. *Mental Health and Physical Activity, 7*(3), 198–204. https://doi.org/10.1016/j.mhpa.2014.03.001

Harris, V. C., Bourke-Taylor, H., & Leo, M. (2022). Healthy Mothers Healthy Families, Health Promoting Activity coaching for mothers of children with a disability: Exploring mothers' perspectives of programme feasibility. *Australian Occupational Therapy Journal, 69*(6), 662–675. https://doi.org/10.1111/1440-1630.12814

Hawkins, M. A., Layman, H. M., Ganson, K. T., Tabler, J., Ciciolla, L., Tsotsoros, C. E., & Nagata, J. M. (2021). Adverse childhood events and cognitive function among young adults: Prospective results from the national longitudinal study of adolescent to adult health. *Child Abuse & Neglect, 115,* 105008. https://doi.org/10.1016/j.chiabu.2021.105008

Hennekam, S., Follmer, K. B., & Beatty, J. E. (2021). The paradox of mental illness and employment: A person-job fit lens. *The International Journal of Human Resource Management, 32*(15), 3244–3271. https://doi.org/10.1080/09585192.2020.1867618

Hine, R., Maybery, D., & Goodyear, M. (2018). Challenges of connectedness in personal recovery for rural mothers with mental illness. *International Journal of Mental Health Nursing, 27*(2), 672–682. https://doi.org/10.1111/inm.12353

Hitch, D., & Pepin, G. (2021). Doing, being, becoming and belonging at the heart of occupational therapy: An analysis of theoretical ways of knowing. *Scandinavian Journal of Occupational Therapy, 28*(1), 13–25. https://doi.org/10.1080/11038128.2020.1726454

Howard, B. S., Beckmann, B., Flynn, D., Haller, J., Pohl, M., Smith, K., & Webb, S. (2023). Moral distress in the time of

COVID-19: Occupational therapists' perspectives. *Occupational Therapy in Health Care, 38*(3), 513–529. https://doi.org/10.1080/07380577.2023.2181625

Howes, M., & Ellison, D. M. (2021). Understanding the occupational identity of care-givers for people with mental health problems. *British Journal of Occupational Therapy, 85*(4), 274–282. https://doi.org/10.1177/03080226211018153

Huggard, L., Murphy, R., O'Connor, C., & Nearchou, F. (2023). The social determinants of mental illness: A rapid review of systematic reviews. *Issues in Mental Health Nursing, 44*(4), 302–312. https://doi.org/10.1080/01612840.2023.2186124

Hui, B. P. H., Ng, J. C. K., Berzaghi, E., Cunningham-Amos, L. A., & Kogan, A. (2020). Rewards of kindness? A meta-analysis of the link between prosociality and well-being. *Psychological Bulletin, 146*(12), 1084–1116. https://doi.org/10.1037/bul0000298

Huppert, F. A., & So, T. T. (2013). Flourishing across Europe: Application of a new conceptual framework for defining well-being. *Social Indicators Research, 110*(3), 837–861. https://doi.org/10.1007/s11205-011-9966-7

Jessen-Winge, C., Ilvig, P. M., Jonsson, H., Fritz, H., Lee, K., & Christensen, J. R. (2021). Obesity treatment: A role for occupational therapists? *Scandinavian Journal of Occupational Therapy, 28*(6), 471–478. https://doi.org/10.1080/11038128.2020.1712472

Jorm, A. F. (2012). Mental health literacy: Empowering the community to take action for better mental health. *American Psychologist, 63*, 231–243 https://doi.org/10.1037/a0025957

Jorm, A. F., Kitchener, B. A., Fischer, J., & Cvetkovski, S. (2010). Mental Health First Aid Training by e-Learning: A randomized controlled trial. *Australian and New Zealand Journal of Psychiatry, 44*(12), 1072–1081. https://doi.org/10.3109/00048674.2010.516426

Kellett, K., Ligus, K., Baker, K., & Robison, J. (2020). Social determinants of health for people with serious mental illness after transitioning to the community. *Innovation in Aging, 4*(Suppl._1), 32–33. https://doi.org/10.1093/geroni/igaa057.105

Kelly, D. L., Boggs, D. L., & Conley, R. R. (2007). Reaching for wellness in schizophrenia. *Psychiatric Clinics of North America, 30*, 453–479. https://doi.org/10.1016/j.psc.2007.04.003

Kinney, A. R., Schmid, A. A., Henry, K. L., Coatsworth, J. D., & Eakman, A. M. (2020). Protective and health-related factors contributing to resilience among student veterans: A classification approach. *The American Journal of Occupational Therapy, 74*(4), 7404205040p1–7404205040p11. https://doi.org/10.5014/ajot.2020.038331

Kokka, I., Mourikis, I., & Bacopoulou, F. (2023). Psychiatric disorders and obesity in childhood and adolescence—A systematic review of cross-sectional studies. *Children (Basel), 10*(2), 285. https://doi.org/10.3390/children10020285

Kramer, J., ten Velden, M., Kafkes, A., Basu, S., Federico, J., & Kielhofner, G. (2014). *The Child Occupational Self Assessment (COSA). Version 2.2.* Model of Human Occupation Clearinghouse, Department of Occupational Therapy, College of Applied Health Sciences, University of Illinois at Chicago. https://moho-irm.uic.edu/products.aspx?type=allA

Kriakous, S. A., Elliott, K., Lamers, C., & Owen, R. L. (2020). The effectiveness of mindfulness-based stress reduction on the psychological functioning of healthcare professionals: A systematic review. *Mindfulness, 12*(1), 1–28. https://doi.org/10.1007/s12671-020-01500-9

Lagueux, É., Levasseur, M., Tousignant-Laflamme, Y., Dépelteau, A., Pagé, R., Pinard, A.-M., Lévesque, M.-H., & Masse, J. (2021). French-Canadian adaptation of Lifestyle Redesign® for chronic pain management: A pre-experimental pilot study. *The American Journal of Occupational Therapy, 74*(4_Suppl._1), 7411515366p1. https://doi.org/10.5014/ajot.2020.74s1-po2715

Larson, E. (2020). Threshold occupational science concepts for lifestyle change: "Doing" wellness in a course for US college students. *Journal of Occupational Science, 27*(2), 274–287. https://doi.org/10.1080/14427591.2019.1689529

Law, M., Baptiste, S., McColl, M., Opzoomer, A., Polatajko, H., & Pollock, N. (1990). The Canadian Occupational Performance Measure: An outcome measure for occupational therapy. *Canadian Journal of Occupational Therapy, 57*(2), 82–87. https://doi.org/10.1177/000841749005700207

Lawrence, D., & Kisely, S. (2010). Review: Inequalities in healthcare provision for people with severe mental illness. *Journal of Psychopharmacology, 24*(4_Suppl.), 61–68. https://doi.org/10.1177/1359786810382058

Lee, P. N., How, J. A., & Xu, T. (2022). Exploring the impacts of COVID-19 on the lifestyles of community-living adults in Singapore: A qualitative study. *Australian Occupational Therapy Journal, 69*(5), 546–558. https://doi.org/10.1111/1440-1630.12812

Lee, V., Albaum, C., Tablon Modica, P., Ahmad, F., Gorter, J. W., Khanlou, N., McMorris, C., Lai, J., Harrison, C., Hedley, T., Johnston, P., Putterman, C., Spoelstra, M., & Weiss, J. A. (2021). The impact of COVID-19 on the mental health and wellbeing of caregivers of autistic children and youth: A scoping review. *Autism Research: Official Journal of the International Society for Autism Research, 14*(12), 2477–2494. https://doi.org/10.1002/aur.2616

Lester, H., Tritter, J. Q., & Sorohan, H. (2005). Patients' and health professionals' views on primary care for people with serious mental illness: Focus group study. *BMJ, 330*, 1122. https://doi.org/10.1136/bmj.38440.418426.8F

Levasseur, M., Filiatrault, J., Larivière, N., Trépanier, J., Lévesque, M.-H., Beaudry, M., Parisien, M., Provencher, V., Couturier, Y., Champoux, N., Corriveau, H., Carbonneau, H., & Sirois, F. (2019). Influence of Lifestyle Redesign® on health, social participation, leisure, and mobility of older French-Canadians. *The American Journal of Occupational Therapy, 73*(5), 7305205030p1–7305205030p18. https://doi.org/10.5014/ajot.2019.031732

Lunt, A., Foy, M., & White, C. (2022). Working with clients of higher weight in Australia: Findings from a national survey exploring occupational therapy practice. *Australian Occupational Therapy Journal, 69*(4), 403–413. https://doi.org/10.1111/1440-1630.12799

Luo, M. S., Chui, E. W. T., & Li, L. W. (2019). The longitudinal associations between physical health and mental health among older adults. *Aging and Mental Health/Aging & Mental Health, 24*(12), 1990–1998. https://doi.org/10.1080/13607863.2019.1655706

Magnusson, L., Håkansson, C., Brandt, S., Öberg, M., & Orban, K. (2020). Occupational balance and sleep among women. *Scandinavian Journal of Occupational Therapy, 28*(8), 643–651. https://doi.org/10.1080/11038128.2020.1721558

Maher, C., & Mendonca, R. J. (2018). Impact of an activity-based program on health, quality of life, and occupational performance of women diagnosed with cancer. *The American Journal of Occupational Therapy, 72*(2), 7202205040p1–7202205040p8. https://doi.org/10.5014/ajot.2018.023663

Mansuri, F., Nash, M. C., Bakour, C., & Kip, K. E. (2020). Adverse childhood experiences (ACEs) and headaches among children: A cross-sectional analysis. *Headache: The Journal of Head and Face Pain, 60*(4), 735–744. https://doi.org/10.1111/head.13773

McAuliffe, T., Thomas, Y., Vaz, S., Falkmer, T., & Cordier, R. (2018). The experiences of mothers of children with autism spectrum disorder: Managing family routines and mothers' health and wellbeing. *Australian Occupational Therapy Journal, 66*, 68–76. https://doi.org/10.1111/1440-1630.12524

Milbourn, B., Mahoney, N., Trimboli, C., Hoey, C., Cordier, R., & Wilson, N. J. (2020). "Just one of the guys." An application of the Occupational Wellbeing framework to graduates of a Men's Shed Program for young unemployed adult males with intellectual disability. *Australian Occupational Therapy Journal, 67*(2), 121–130. https://doi.org/10.1111/1440-1630.12630

Mitchell, S., Sideris, J., Blanchard, J., Granados, G., Díaz, J., & Pyatak, E. (2023). Telehealth Lifestyle Redesign occupational therapy for diabetes: Preliminary effectiveness, satisfaction, and engagement. *OTJR: Occupational Therapy Journal of Research, 43*(3), 426–434. https://doi.org/10.1177/15394492231172933

Molloy, R., Brand, G., Munro, I., & Pope, N. (2023). Seeing the complete picture: A systematic review of mental health consumer and health professional experiences of diagnostic overshadowing. *Journal of Clinical Nursing, 32*(9–10), 1662–1673. https://doi.org/10.1111/jocn.16151

Momen, N. C., Plana-Ripoll, O., Agerbo, E., Christensen, M. K., Iburg, K. M., Laursen, T. M., Mortensen, P. B., Pedersen, C. B., Prior, A., Weye, N., & McGrath, J. J. (2022). Mortality associated with mental disorders and comorbid general medical conditions. *JAMA Psychiatry, 79*(5), 444. https://doi.org/10.1001/jamapsychiatry.2022.0347

Mourão, I., Mouro, C. V., Brito, L. M., Costa, S. R., & Almeida, T. C. (2021). Impacts of therapeutic horticulture on happiness and loneliness in institutionalized clients with mental health conditions. *British Journal of Occupational Therapy, 85*(2), 111–119. https://doi.org/10.1177/03080226211008719

Nelson, S. M., Beveridge, J. K., Mychasiuk, R., & Noel, M. (2021). Adverse childhood experiences (ACEs) and internalizing mental health, pain, and quality of life in youth with chronic pain: A longitudinal examination. *The Journal of Pain, 22*(10), 1210–1220. https://doi.org/10.1016/j.jpain.2021.03.143

Österholm, J., Andreassen, M., Gustavsson, M. K., & Ranada, Å. L. (2022). Older people's experiences of visiting social day centres: The importance of doing and being for health and well-being. *Scandinavian Journal of Occupational Therapy, 30*(1), 76–85. https://doi.org/10.1080/11038128.2022.2130423

Parker, C., Kennedy-Behr, A., Wright, S., & Brown, T. (2022). Does the self-reported playfulness of older adults influence their well-being? An exploratory study. *Scandinavian Journal of Occupational Therapy, 30*(1), 86–97. https://doi.org/10.1080/11038128.2022.2145993

Parkinson, S., Forsyth, K., & Kielhofner, G. (2006). *The Model of Human Occupation Screening Tool (MOHOST).* Version 2.0. Model of Human Occupation Clearinghouse, Department of Occupational Therapy, College of Applied Health Sciences, University of Illinois. https://moho-irm.uic.edu/products.aspx?type=allA

Peters, R., Ee, N., Ward, S., Kenning, G., Radford, K., Goldwater, M. B., Dodge, H. H., Lewis, E., Xu, Y., Kudrna, G., Hamilton, M., Peters, J., Anstey, K. J., Lautenschlager, N. T., Fitzgerald, A., & Rockwood, K. (2021). Intergenerational programmes bringing together community dwelling non-familial older adults and children: A systematic review. *Archives of Gerontology and Geriatrics, 94*, 104356. https://doi.org/10.1016/j.archger.2021.104356

Pettican, A., Speed, E., Bryant, W., Kilbride, C., & Beresford, P. (2022). Levelling the playing field: Exploring inequalities and exclusions with a community-based football league for people with experience of mental distress. *Australian Occupational Therapy Journal, 69*(3), 290–300. https://doi.org/10.1111/1440-1630.12791

Pettican, A., Speed, E., Kilbride, C., Bryant, W., & Beresford, P. (2021). An occupational justice perspective on playing football and living with mental distress. *Journal of Occupational Science, 28*(1), 159–172. https://doi.org/10.1080/14427591.2020.1816208

Pevalin, D. J., Reeves, A., Baker, E., & Bentley, R. (2017). The impact of persistent poor housing conditions on mental health: A longitudinal population-based study. *Preventive Medicine, 105*, 304–310. https://doi.org/10.1016/j.ypmed.2017.09.020

Plana-Ripoll, O., Musliner, K. L., Dalsgaard, S., Momen, N. C., Weye, N., Christensen, M. K., Agerbo, E., Iburg, K. M., Laursen, T. M., Mortensen, P. B., Pedersen, C. B., Petersen, L., Santomauro, D., Vilhjálmsson, B. J., Whiteford, H., & McGrath, J. J. (2020). Nature and prevalence of combinations of mental disorders and their association with excess mortality in a population-based cohort study. *World Psychiatry, 19*(3), 339–349. https://doi.org/10.1002/wps.20802

Popova, E. S., Hahn, B., Morris, H. R., Loomis, K., Shy, E., Andrews, J., Iacullo, M., & Peters, A. (2022). Exploring well-being: Resilience, stress, and self-care in occupational therapy practitioners and students. *OTJR: Occupational Therapy Journal of Research, 43*(2), 159–169. https://doi.org/10.1177/15394492221091271

Riordan, H. J., Antonini, P., & Murphy, M. F. (2011). Atypical antipsychotics and metabolic syndrome in patients with schizophrenia: Risk factors, monitoring, and healthcare implications. *American Health & Drug Benefits, 4*(5), 292–302.

Rocks, T., Teasdale, S. B., Fehily, C., Young, C., Howland, G., Kelly, B., Dawson, S., Jacka, F., Dunbar, J. A., & O'Neil, A. (2022). Effectiveness of nutrition and dietary interventions for people with serious mental illness: Systematic review and meta-analysis. *The Medical Journal of Australia, 217*(Suppl. 7), S7–S21. https://doi.org/10.5694/mja2.51680

Rockson, L. E., Swarbrick, M. A., & Pratt, C. (2016). Cancer screening among peer-led community wellness center enrollees. *Journal of Psychosocial Nursing and Mental Health Services, 54*(3), 36–40. https://doi.org/10.1177/1078390319877227

Rosenberg, M., Bar-Shalita, T., Weiss, M., Rahav, G., & Bar, M. A. (2023). Associations between daily routines and social support among women with chronic fatigue syndrome. *Scandinavian Journal of Occupational Therapy, 30*(7), 1037–1046, https://doi.org/10.1080/11038128.2023.2200580

Rosencrans, M., Arango, P., Sabat, C., Buck, A., Brown, C., Tenorio, M., & Witwer, A. (2021). The impact of the COVID-19 pandemic on the health, wellbeing, and access to services of people with intellectual and developmental disabilities. *Research in Developmental Disabilities, 114*, 103985. https://doi.org/10.1016/j.ridd.2021.103985

Schepens-Niemiec, S. L., Carlson, M., Martínez, J., Guzmán, L., Mahajan, A., & Clark, F. (2015). Developing occupation-based preventive programs for late-middle-aged Latino patients in safety-net health systems. *The American Journal of Occupational Therapy, 69*(6), 6906240010p1–6906240010p11. https://doi.org/10.5014/ajot.2015.015958

Schmelzer. L., & Leto, T. (2018, July/August). Promoting health through engagement in occupations that maximize food resources. *American Journal of Occupational Therapy, 72*(4), 7204205020p1–7204205020p9. https://doi.org/10.5014/ajot.2018.025866

Scott, P. J. (2019). *Role Checklist Version 3: Participation and Satisfaction (RCv3).* Model of Human Occupation Clearinghouse, Department of Occupational Therapy, College of Applied Health Sciences, University of Illinois at Chicago. https://moho-irm.uic.edu/products.aspx?type=allA

Seligman, M. (2011). *Flourish: A visionary new understanding of happiness and well-being.* Free Press.

Shim, Y. R., Eaker, R., & Park, J. (2022). Mental health education, awareness and stigma regarding mental illness among college students. *Journal of Mental Health & Clinical Psychology, 6*(2), 6–15. https://doi.org/10.29245/2578-2959/2022/2.1258

Simon, E., Edwards, A. M., Sajatovic, M., Jain, N., Montoya, J. L., & Levin, J. B. (2022). Systematic literature review of text messaging interventions to promote medication adherence among people with serious mental illness. *Psychiatric Services (Washington, D.C.), 73*(10), 1153–1164. https://doi.org/10.1176/appi.ps.202100634

Sit, W., Wheeler, C., & Pickens, N. (2023, October). Occupational therapy in primary health care for underserved populations: A scoping review. *Occupational Therapy in Health Care, 37*(4), 552–575. https://doi.org/10.1080/07380577.2022.2081752

Smith, J., Halliwell, N., Laurent, A., Tsotsoros, J., Harris, K., & DeGrace, B. (2023). Social participation experiences of families raising a young child with autism spectrum disorder: Implications for mental health and well-being. *The American Journal of Occupational Therapy, 77*(2), 770218509. https://doi.org/10.5014/ajot.2023.050156

Smith, N. R., Kielhofner, G., & Watts, J. H. (1986). The relationships between volition, activity pattern, and life satisfaction in the elderly. *American Journal of Occupational Therapy, 40*(4), 278–283. https://doi.org/10.5014/ajot.40.4.278

Stewart, K. E., Fischer, T. M., Hirji, R., & Davis, J. A. (2016). Toward the reconceptualization of the relationship between occupation and health and well-being. *Canadian Journal of Occupational Therapy, 83*(4), 249–259. https://doi.org/10.1177/0008417415625425

Substance Abuse and Mental Health Services Administration. (2014). *SAMHSA's concept of trauma and guidance for a trauma-informed approach.* Author. https://ncsacw.acf.hhs.gov/userfiles/files/SAMHSA_Trauma.pdf

Substance Abuse and Mental Health Services Administration. (2021). *2021 National Survey of Drug Use and Health (NSDUH) releases.* https://www.samhsa.gov/data/release/2021-national-survey-drug-use-and-health-nsduh-releases

Substance Abuse and Mental Health Services Administration. (2023, April 24). *Certified Community Behavioral Health Clinics (CCBHCs).* https://www.samhsa.gov/certified-community-behavioral-health-clinics

Suto, M. J., Smith, S., Damiano, N., & Channe, S. (2021). Participation in community gardening: Sowing the seeds of well-being: Participation au jardinage communautaire: Pour semer les graines du bien-être. *Canadian Journal of Occupational Therapy, 88*(2), 142–152. https://doi.org/10.1177/0008417421994385

Swarbrick, M., Rockson, L., Pratt, C., Yudof, J., & Nemec, P. (2015). Perceptions of overall health and recency of screenings. *American Journal of Psychiatric Rehabilitation, 18*(1), 5–18. https://doi.org/10.1080/15487768.2015.1001703

Swarbrick, M., & Yudof, J. (2009). Words of wellness. *Occupational Therapy in Mental Health, 25*(3–4), 367–412. https://doi.org/10.1080/01642120903084158

Swarbrick, P., & Yudof, J. (2015). *Wellness in eight dimensions. Collaborative Support Programs of New Jersey.* https://www.center4healthandsdc.org/uploads/7/1/1/4/71142589/wellness_in_8_dimensions_booklet_with_daily_plan.pdf

Sweet, D., Byng, R., Webber, M., Enki, D. G., Porter, I., Larsen, J., Huxley, P., & Pinfold, V. (2018). Personal well-being networks, social capital and severe mental illness: Exploratory study. *The British Journal of Psychiatry, 212*(5), 308–317. https://doi.org/10.1192/bjp.bp.117.203950

Tabone, J. K., Cox, S., Aylward, L., Abunnaja, S., Szoka, N., & Tabone, L. E. (2022). The roles of depression and binge eating in the relationship between adverse childhood experiences (ACEs) and obesity. *Obesity Surgery, 32*(9), 3034–3040. https://doi.org/10.1007/s11695-022-06192-9

Taylor, R. (2017). *Kielhofner's Model of Human Occupation: Theory and application* (5th ed.). Wolters Kluwer.

Teasdale, S., Ward, P. B., Samaras, K., Firth, J., Stubbs, B., Tripodi, E., & Burrows, T. (2019). Dietary intake of people with severe mental illness: Systematic review and meta-analysis. *British Journal of Psychiatry, 214*(5), 251–259. https://doi.org/10.1192/bjp.2019.20

Teoli, D., & Bhardwaj, A. (2022). Quality of life. In *StatPearls.* StatPearls Publishing. https://www.ncbi.nlm.nih.gov/books/NBK536962

Therrien, D., Corbière, M., & Collette, K. (2020). Workers with severe mental illness coping with clinical symptoms: Self-directed learning of work-health balance strategies. *Australian Occupational Therapy Journal, 67,* 341–349. https://doi.org/10.1111/1440-1630.12662

Thomson, L. J., Morse, N., Elsden, E., & Chatterjee, H. J. (2020). Art, nature and mental health: Assessing the biopsychosocial effects of a 'creative green prescription' museum programme involving horticulture, artmaking and collections. *Perspectives in Public Health, 140*(5), 277–285. https://doi.org/10.1177/1757913920910443

Townsend, E. A., & Polatajko, H. J. (2007). *Enabling occupation II: Advancing an occupational therapy vision for health, well-being and justice through occupation.* CAOT Publications ACE.

van Beukering, I. E., Smits, S. J., Janssens, K. M., Bogaers, R. I., Joosen, M. C., Bakker, M., van Weeghel, J., & Brouwers, E. P. (2021). In what ways does health related stigma affect sustainable employment and well-being at work? A systematic review. *Journal of Occupational Rehabilitation, 32*(3), 365–379. https://doi.org/10.1007/s10926-021-09998-z

Vancampfort, D., Firth, J., Schuch, F. B., Rosenbaum, S., Mugisha, J., Hallgren, M., Probst, M., Ward, P. B., Gaughran, F., De Hert, M., Carvalho, A. F., & Stubbs, B. (2017). Sedentary behavior and physical activity levels in people with schizophrenia, bipolar disorder and major depressive disorder: A global systematic review and meta-analysis. *World Psychiatry, 16*(3), 308–315. https://doi.org/10.1002/wps.20458

Vidal-Sánchez, M., Laborda-Soriano, A., Cambra-Aliaga, A., Sanz-Valer, P., & Gasch Gallén, Á. (2021). Childhood health assets in a Spanish neighborhood: Children and families' perception. *OTJR: Occupational Therapy Journal of Research, 41*(3), 185–195. https://doi.org/10.1177/15394492211011188

Viron, M. J., & Stern, T. A. (2010). The impact of serious mental illness on health and healthcare. *Psychosomatics, 51,* 458–465. https://doi.org/10.1176/appi.psy.51.6.458

von Kürthy, H., Aranda, K., Sadlo, G., & Stew, G. (2022). Embroidering as a transformative occupation. *Journal of Occupational Science, 30*(4), 647–660. https://doi.org/10.1080/14427591.2022.2104349

Wagman, P., Håkansson, C., & Björklund, A. (2011). Occupational balance as used in occupational therapy: A concept analysis. *Scandinavian Journal of Occupational Therapy, 19*(4), 322–327. https://doi.org/10.3109/11038128.2011.596219

Walker, S., Sechrist, K., & Pender, N. (1995). Health promotion model—Instruments to measure health promoting lifestyle: Health-Promoting Lifestyle Profile [HPLP II] (Adult Version). *PsycTESTS Dataset.* https://doi.org/10.1037/t44576-000

Walsh, D., McCartney, G., Smith, M. J., & Armour, G. (2019). Relationship between childhood socioeconomic position and adverse childhood experiences (ACEs): A systematic review. *Journal of Epidemiology and Community Health, 73*(12), 1087–1093. https://doi.org/10.1136/jech-2019-212738

WHO Collaborating Centre in Mental Health. (1998). *WHO-5 questionnaires.* https://www.psykiatri-regionh.dk/who-5/who-5-questionnaires/Pages/default.aspx

Wilcock, A. A. (2006). *An Occupational Perspective of Health* (2nd ed.). Slack.

Wood, L., Hooper, P., Foster, S., & Bull, F. (2017). Public green spaces and positive mental health—Investigating the relationship between access, quantity and types of parks and mental wellbeing. *Health & Place, 48,* 63–71. https://doi.org/10.1016/j.healthplace.2017.09.002

World Federation of Occupational Therapists. (2012). About occupational therapy. https://wfot.org/about/about-occupational-therapy

World Health Organization. (n.d.-a). *Constitution of the World Health Organization.* Author. https://www.who.int/about/governance/constitution

World Health Organization. (n.d.-b). *Promoting well-being.* Author. https://www.who.int/activities/promoting-well-being

Yu, Y., Manku, M., & Backman, C. L. (2018). Measuring occupational balance and its relationship to perceived stress and health. *Canadian Journal of Occupational Therapy, 85*(2), 117–127. https://doi.org/10.1177/0008417417734355

CHAPTER 46

Activities of Daily Living, Instrumental Activities of Daily Living, and Health Management Occupations

Lauren A. Selingo and Jaclyn K. Schwartz

Consider if, in addition to the sensory overload of the grocery store, someone also hears voices. What if they experience social anxiety? What if problem-solving and decision-making are an everyday challenge? What if they don't have transportation to the store? What if they face the stigma of using food stamps to purchase their groceries? An everyday task such as grocery shopping can be a real hardship for someone dealing with these factors.

Activities of daily living (ADLs), instrumental activities of daily living (IADLs), and **health management** can be holistically affected for people dealing not only with mental health conditions, but also with complex health conditions such as stroke, diabetes, cancer, and compromised lungs, as these also impact overall mental health and well-being. Occupational therapy practitioners (OTPs) can help individuals with mental health challenges perform basic ADLs and more complex IADLs by addressing both personal and environmental factors that interfere with a successful and satisfying daily life and manage their health so as to be able to participate in everyday life based on their wants and needs.

Across this chapter, readers will engage with the text, which provides detailed descriptions of ADLs, IADLs, and health management within the contexts of individuals with mental health conditions. Readers will also become familiarized with the effect of various mental health and physical conditions on occupational engagement across these areas, as well as current assessment tools that OTPs can implement to assess individuals' strengths and barriers to occupational performance.

The chapter also explores current evidence-based interventions targeting ADL, IADL, and health management performance, as well as preparatory skills needed to engage in desired daily care occupations and critical skill sets such as financial management skills. After learning more about assessment and interventions and the evidence surrounding their implementation, readers will have the opportunity to apply the content they have been engaging with to a case study. The chapter concludes with resources for addressing areas for potential additional learning and some questions to encourage further reflection on the chapter material.

As readers engage with the text, they should consider the following:

- What are some of the ways in which a person's mental health affects their engagement in ADLs, IADLs, and health management occupations?

- What are some social and environmental barriers and supports to individuals' occupational engagement in ADLs, IADLs, and health management tasks?
- Consider settings and populations people work with or plan on working with. What assessment tools might be beneficial to integrate into their practice?
- Have readers had experiences using any of the interventions noted? Were they beneficial for the individual with whom they were collaborating? What interventions are they interested in learning more about and what resources might be helpful for this continued learning?
- How do readers plan on applying the chapter content to their own practice as an OTP?

Overview of Activities of Daily Living, Instrumental Activities of Daily Living, and Health Management

ADLs include basic activities of daily life. Also referred to as self-care skills, ADLs are tasks that are typically performed in a habitual manner across age groups and genders; they may differ by culture. The *Occupational Therapy Practice Framework (OTPF)* identifies eight ADLs: bathing or showering, toileting and toilet hygiene, dressing, eating and swallowing, feeding, functional mobility, personal hygiene and grooming, and sexual activity (American Occupational Therapy Association [AOTA], 2020). In mental health practice, ADL concerns are likely to be related to cognitive, psychological, or sensory issues and less frequently due to motor impairments. Issues can range from minor challenges such as poor nail care to total dependence across all ADLs during the later stages of dementia.

IADLs are activities that support daily life that are more complex than ADLs (AOTA, 2020). The *OTPF* defines 11 IADLs: care of others, care of pets and animals, child rearing, communication management, driving and community mobility, financial management, home establishment and management, meal preparation and cleanup, religious and spiritual expression, safety and emergency maintenance, and shopping.

The *OTPF* has now designated health management, or "activities related to developing, managing, and maintaining health and wellness routines," as its own category of activity as of the updated 2020 framework (AOTA, 2020, p. 32). This includes seven activities: social and emotional health promotion and maintenance, symptom and condition management, communication with the health-care system, medication management, physical activity, nutrition management, and personal care device management.

OTPs have a duty to ensure consistent access and the ability to engage in an individual's preferred and needed ADLs, IADLs, and health management practices. The therapeutic process requires collaboration to ensure person-centered care. To be able to effectively serve people with mental health challenges, OTPs must first understand the influence of mental health on participation in these occupations.

Influence of Mental Health on Activities of Daily Living, Instrumental Activities of Daily Living, and Health Management Performance

Successful performance of ADLs, IADLs, and health management is based on the complex interaction of the skills and knowledge of the person, the demands of the task, and the barriers and supports present in the environment. For example, memory or attentional impairments can cause safety challenges when cooking. A socially demanding task, such as riding a crowded city bus, can be difficult for persons with anxiety. Environmental and societal factors, such as systemic racism, biases, and poverty, may mean that individuals lack resources for accomplishing IADLs (e.g., a vacuum cleaner to keep their home clean).

Mental health challenges are often associated with impaired performance of ADLs, IADLs, and health management. Individuals with varying mental health diagnoses can experience different impairments and subsequently have a variety of impairment profiles (Aniserowicz et al., 2022; Moore et al., 2010). The next section demonstrates

the relationship between mental health challenges and impairments in ADL, IADL, and health management performance by exploring the research on persons with dementia, depression, anxiety, substance use disorders, schizophrenia, obsessive-compulsive disorder (OCD), and eating disorders. For a full discussion across diagnoses, see Part II: The Person of this textbook.

Mental Health Diagnoses That Can Affect Activities of Daily Living, Instrumental Activities of Daily Living, and Health Management Abilities

Dementia

Individuals with dementia typically lose ADL, IADL, and health management skills because of declining cognitive abilities. Poor performance of ADLs and IADLs is a core problem associated with late-stage dementia (Delva et al., 2016). Although memory loss is a key feature of dementia, executive dysfunction (i.e., problems with high-level cognitive processes such as planning, problem-solving, and initiating activity) is most predictive of functional impairment in dementia. Difficulties in completing more "advanced" ADLs, such as reading the newspaper or writing a letter, can begin and denote the potential for a dementia diagnosis years before a formal diagnosis is made (Fieo et al., 2018).

In a study of 1,026 older adults with dementia and their caregivers, researchers found declines in bathing, dressing, toileting, transfers, continence, and feeding (Giebel et al., 2014). Specifically, they discovered that functional impairments worsen with the course of the disease and that impairments are more pronounced in tasks with higher cognitive load (i.e., bathing and dressing). In another study of 3,547 individuals, researchers found that ADL performance is associated with dementia and is also predictive of a later dementia diagnosis (Fauth et al., 2013).

PhotoVoice

Alexander

This is a market store near Buckeye and 5th Ave. At times it's beautiful there, but it's quiet now. In this picture it glows. It was well organized and easy to find what I wanted. The market helped my community grow in a good way. It helped to build trust because all different types of people shopped there.

IADL performance often occurs in business and social places. Are there businesses or social spaces that you frequent that act as sources of support for you?

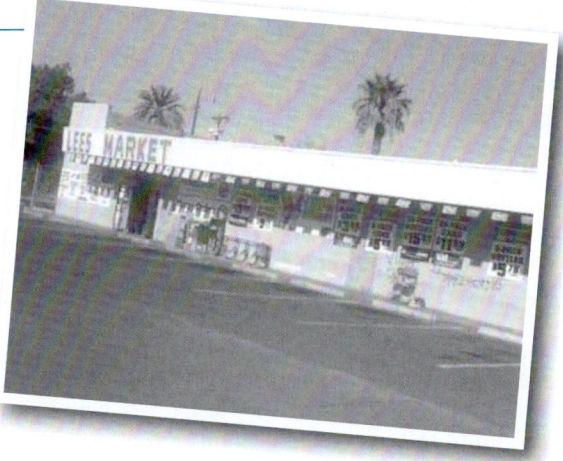

Health management occupations are also impacted. Despite evidence that up to 50% of individuals with dementia experience some form of pain (Corbett et al., 2012), assessing pain for persons with dementia can be difficult, leading to pain management challenges for health-care team members and caregivers (Achterberg et al., 2013). Changes in motor skills, cognition, and executive functioning can challenge other aspects of health management, such as seeking out resources when needed, accessing personal health information, making decisions about one's health, and acting on those decisions (Ibrahim et al., 2017).

Depression

Depression can also have an impact on the performance of daily occupations. Baune and colleagues (2010) compared the health and function among persons with active depression, a history of depression, and no depression. Adults with active depression demonstrated cognitive impairments in memory, visuospatial, language, and attention skills. Although symptoms are worse during active depression, cognitive impairments in memory and attention persist even after the end of a depressive episode.

Although more research is needed, Evans and colleagues (2014) found that cognitive impairment was associated with impaired performance in ADLs and IADLs. They suggest that in mild depression, ADL and IADL impairments may be associated with cognitive deficits, whereas in major depression, impairments may be associated with symptoms of depression (e.g., lack of motivation, hopelessness). Depression is also associated with other physical conditions such as stroke. For all individuals with impaired mood, promoting personal well-being, satisfaction with care, and successful engagement in ADLs, IADLs, and health management are important outcomes (Simpson et al., 2018).

Brijnath and Antoniades (2016) found that health management occupations for persons with depression, such as seeking medical assistance for the management of one's symptoms, can be impacted because of severe depressive episodes as well as challenges operating in health-care systems that emphasize that it is the responsibility of the individual to seek out resources. Efforts to engage in health management can be further hampered by health-care systems that are costly and looking to balance health management with the responsibilities of everyday life. Also see Chapter 20: Mood Disorders.

Anxiety

Anxiety has been tied to challenges in ADL and IADL functioning. Brenes and colleagues (2005) found that older women who reported anxiety symptoms are 28% to 67% more likely to have difficulty with ADLs and IADLs compared with those who did not have anxiety. Anxiety can also co-occur with changes in physical status, such as a stroke (Juniper et al., 2022). Anxiety, when coupled with depression and neurological impairments that result from a major health event such as a stroke, can lead to perceptions of worse ADL and IADL functioning (Juniper et al., 2022). Anxiety can limit the ability to take part in rehabilitation services, an

aspect of one's health management (Pisegna et al., 2022). Also see Chapter 18: Anxiety Disorders.

Substance Use Disorders

Performance of ADLs, IADLs, and health management occupations can be neglected by individuals who are experiencing harmful substance use and substance use disorders (Rawat et al., 2021). Substance use becomes so paramount that it replaces other occupations (Cloete & Ramugondo, 2015). Substance use can also be a health management strategy by using illicit substances to treat issues such as depression, pain, anxiety, or inattention (Cloete & Ramugondo, 2015; Fishman, 2002).

Extended substance use can directly impact individuals' ability to perform ADLs, IADLs, and health management occupations because of physical impairments such as tremors, blurred vision, and a lack of balance. Cognitive impairments such as memory difficulties and a lack of focus can also affect performance across these occupational areas. Also see Chapter 24: Substance Related and Addictive Disorders.

Schizophrenia

Persons with schizophrenia can demonstrate challenges in ADLs, IADLs, and health management because of their symptoms, cognitive deficits, and environmental and social considerations. Schizophrenia is associated with positive symptoms (e.g., hallucinations and delusions) and negative symptoms (e.g., apathy and social withdrawal). In their study of 81 adults with schizophrenia, Lipskaya and colleagues (2011) found that ADL and IADL performance was associated with negative symptoms of schizophrenia and cognitive impairment. Specifically in their model of IADL performance, negative symptoms explained 13%, memory and abstract thinking explained 13.5%, and executive functioning explained 21% of the variance.

Individuals with schizophrenia may also experience poor performance in ADLs, IADLs, and health management because of a lack of opportunity to learn these life skills. Schizophrenia often begins in the late teens or early 20s and can result in numerous health-care admissions (Walker et al., 2004). Therefore, individuals may not have had the naturally occurring opportunities to, for example, learn how to manage their finances, use a microwave, or take the bus. Roach and colleagues (2021) conducted interviews and surveys with decision-makers across the spectrum of health-care and payer professions about barriers to health management for individuals with schizophrenia. Participants reported that barriers to health management include inconsistently taking one's medication and coping with health-care costs. Also see Chapter 23: Schizophrenia Spectrum and Psychotic Disorders.

Obsessive-Compulsive Disorder

The time involved in attending to obsessive thoughts and compulsive behaviors can interfere with participation in ADLs, IADLs, and health management occupations. Obsessive and compulsive behaviors can make it so persons overly engage in activities, such as washing hands. It can negatively impact other ADLs and IADLs because obsessive and compulsive behaviors can make it too difficult to leave the home either given the time-consuming nature of the behaviors or because of the social stigma of completing obsessive and compulsive behaviors in the public environment.

A qualitative study examining women with OCD's lived experiences surrounding sex and sexuality, and ADLs, found that women may abstain from engaging in sexual and intimate activities as a way of managing symptoms of OCD, including compulsions and negativistic, intruding cognitions (Boulton, 2020). Qualitative research on young peoples' (ages 14–17) experiences surrounding OCD found that given the stigma surrounding mental health and unique experiences with one's symptoms, younger individuals with OCD may hide their obsession(s) from others (Keyes et al., 2018). Also see Chapter 21: Obsessive Disorders.

Eating Disorders

Persons with eating disorders experience dysfunction in ADLs, IADLs, and health management that are associated with food and eating (Bradford et al., 2015). Persons with eating disorders may engage in inappropriate eating behaviors and avoid social eating settings. Further, they may have limited cooking skills and difficulty in purchasing food. Also see Chapter 19: Eating Disorders.

Evaluation

Although specific diagnoses tend to be associated with different impairments in ADLs, IADLs, and health management, performance is ultimately a function of the person's skills, environment, and desired occupations. Therefore, it is important to understand the individualized needs of each person. A variety of assessment tools are available to help occupational therapists, often in collaboration with occupational therapy assistants, identify individuals in need of occupational therapy services and to plan intervention.

Upon referral, the evaluation should initiate and place emphasis on determining the individual's needed and desired occupations, evaluating their current and past occupational performance, and exploring the individual's barriers and supports surrounding their health, occupational engagement, and overall well-being (AOTA, 2020). The evaluation should include an occupational profile and assessment of the individual's occupational profile (AOTA, 2020; Brown, 2012; Hinojosa et al., 2014). Then the therapist should evaluate the individual's occupational performance, performance skills, personal factors, performance patterns, contexts and environments, and activity demands. The evaluation should consist of tools that are standardized and have demonstrated reliability and validity. Further, when possible, the evaluation process should occur in an environment in which the person will actually perform the skill (Zayat et al., 2011).

A variety of assessment tools are available to help OTPs evaluate the ADL, IADL, and health management skills of persons with mental health challenges. Table 46-1 outlines key information about common evaluation tools to help guide the practitioner's therapeutic reasoning during the evaluation process.

Katz Index of Independence in Activities of Daily Living Scale

The Katz Index of Independence in Activities of Daily Living Scale (Katz, 1983) is a very brief assessment of self-care. The therapist scores an individual's ability on a yes/no scale to complete six basic ADLs.

Barthel Index

The Barthel Index was first published in 1965 as a quick and easy scale for measuring ADLs (Mahoney & Barthel, 1965). The measure is typically completed by the occupational therapist or other health-care worker based on observation of the person. The Barthel Index is a reliable and valid assessment (Hsieh et al., 2007; Hsueh et al., 2001).

Continuity Assessment Record and Evaluation Tool

The Continuity Assessment Record and Evaluation (CARE) Tool is a standardized assessment tool created by the Centers for Medicare & Medicaid Services (CMS) that was designed to measure the health and functioning in postacute care adults (CMS, 2021). The tool can be implemented by the care team, including rehabilitation staff across settings such as long-term care hospitals, inpatient rehabilitation, skilled nursing facilities, and home health. Measurement includes medical, cognitive, functional, and social support factors; it also predicts a person's needs pertaining to nursing, physician, and therapy services . The tool includes core items that each person is asked or completes, with supplemental items being asked to individuals with specific conditions (e.g., advanced skin ulcers).

Pediatric Evaluation of Disability Inventory-Computer Adaptive Test

The Pediatric Evaluation of Disability Inventory-Computer Adaptive Test (PEDI-CAT) is an assessment of daily activities, mobility, and social cognitive skills for children birth to 20 years of age (Haley & Coster, 2010). The assessment can be used across all patient diagnoses, conditions, and settings. A parent or clinician familiar with the person's abilities describes whether the child is able or unable to complete a variety of life activities. The PEDI-CAT leverages a computer-based algorithm to estimate a child's abilities from a minimal number of the most relevant test questions. This assessment tool requires approximately 15 minutes to administer (Dumas et al., 2012). The PEDI-CAT is a norm-referenced test with raw scores, normative standard scores, and scaled scores. It is a reliable and valid assessment (Dumas et al., 2012, 2015, 2016).

Independent Living Skills Survey

The Independent Living Skills Survey (ILSS) is a comprehensive questionnaire designed for individuals with severe and persistent mental health challenges (Wallace et al., 2000). It includes both an informant and a self-report version. The informant version rates individuals on a 5-point Likert scale

The Lived Experience

The Struggles With OCD

By Rebecca A. Grobe, Age 9

Everybody has a hard time, but some people have more than others. One thing that causes anxiety is OCD. I was diagnosed with OCD at the age of 7, but my parents started noticing things when I was a toddler. I have had troubles with organizing, being clean in order to sleep in my bed, trouble with my belongings being dirty, and so on. OCD interferes by telling me to do things that I don't want to do and thinking bad thoughts. I have put some examples in the following table to show how OCD can affect me in different ways.

Thought	Behavior	Negative Effect
There is only one hairbrush that I think is clean.	I need to brush my hair with this specific hairbrush.	When I couldn't find that brush, I couldn't brush my hair, and was late to school.
My bike was ugly.	I have an annoying tantrum demanding a new bike—NOW!	I missed a play date with a friend.
My hair needs to be wet to feel clean.	I throw a fit because I want to take another shower.	I stayed up late and was pooped in the morning.
People would think I'm ugly.	I keep searching for the right clothes to wear, but nothing is just right.	I was late to school.
Not really a thought—I just feel the urge.	I cannot stop picking at a cut on my arm and make it bleed.	My cut takes months to heal and keeps getting infected.

When I am struggling with an issue like the hairbrush, it feels like there is a bully in my mind. The bully forces me by giving me a bad feeling to do something that I don't want to do. That feeling might be strong, like a 10, but sometimes can be less intense, like a 3. The difference is that when the feeling is a lower number, I can use my strategies to fight the thoughts or feelings and I usually succeed. But when the number is high, it is hard to concentrate and be able to use my strategies. The OCD acts up and is stronger when I don't have anything to eat. One time I didn't eat all day, and when I got home my parents were worried because I had a huge fit.

Mom's Point of View

My mom has had a hard time watching me go through these difficult times and she often tries to help me, but sometimes the OCD prevents the help. My mom thinks that the OCD takes over my brain. When that happens it is hard for me to

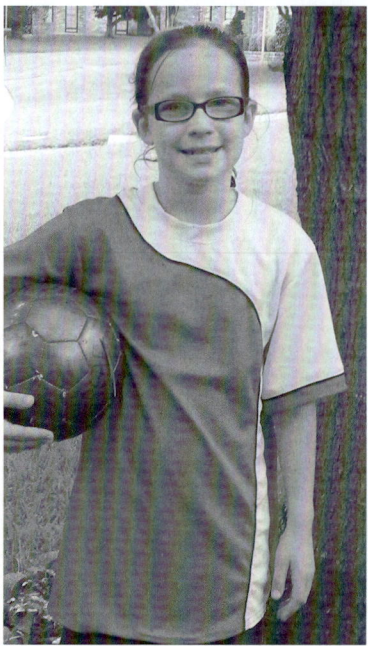

listen. When I was as young as 2, my mom learned that when she kept talking to calm me down, the talking just upset me more. So she started to repeat short phrases such as "I'm sorry you're upset," or "I love you Becca." She says my OCD attacks scared her because it could take hours to calm me down. My mom's observation was that sometimes the only way I would calm down was to exhaust myself. Once I was diagnosed, she was hopeful that we could learn about ways to defeat the OCD.

Dad's Point of View

My dad remembers times that I've missed important events because of things such as needing to organize my bag of toys. My dad has also noticed several things about my OCD. One thing is that I would get so upset that it was extremely hard to calm me down. A second thing is that when my blood sugar gets low, my OCD gets stronger. He also noticed that many of my OCD issues have to do with things being "just right." This has made it hard to tell when something is related to my OCD, because a lot of things are not just right—my clothes, my brush, my bike, my bag of toys, and so on.

Conclusion

OCD is a diagnosis that I have to live with forever, but I'm glad the doctors figured it out while I'm a kid. I have had great therapy and have continued working to beat my OCD. I have learned to use some good strategies for now and the future. But I think that living with it just makes me stronger. When I defeat the OCD, it's as if I have more power.

TABLE 46-1 | Therapeutic Reasoning Assessment Table–ADLs, IADLs, and Health Management

Which Tool?	Who Was This Tool Designed For?	Is This a Type of Tool the Person Can Do? What Is Required of the Person?	What Am I Measuring?	How Long Does It Take and Where Do I Administer This Assessment?	Is the Tool Associated With a Practice Model?
Katz Index of Independence in Activities of Daily Living Scale (Katz, 1983)	Older adults	Individuals are asked to either report their level of performance or complete a series of ADLs with skilled observation by a health professional.	Adequacy of performance in bathing, dressing, toileting, transferring, continence, and feeding	≈ 5 minutes (self-report) ≈15 minutes (direct observation)	No
Barthel Index (Mahoney & Barthel, 1965)	Adults with neurological disorders including stroke and brain injury, and older adults	Individuals are asked to either report their level of assistance needed or to complete a series of ADLs with skilled observation by a health professional.	Amount of assistance needed to complete feeding, bathing, grooming, dressing, bowel care, bladder care, toileting, transfers, ambulation, and stair climbing	≈ 5 minutes (self-report) ≈ 20 minutes (direct observation)	No
Continuity Assessment Record and Evaluation (CARE) Tool (CMS, 2021)	Adults in postacute care services (institutional and home health)	Clinician asks a series of questions regarding, or observes a person engaging in, functional, cognitive, and social/environmental tasks.	Person's medical history, prior and current functioning surrounding mobility, cognition, mood, pain, and level of assistance needed across ADLs, IADLs, and health management tasks	2-day assessment period (the day of admission and next calendar day)	No
Pediatric Evaluation of Disability Inventory–Computer Adaptive Test (PEDI-CAT; Haley & Coster, 2010)	Children birth to 20 years of age	Clinicians or parents are asked to answer a series of questions about their child's functional abilities.	Tests functional performance through time. Measures the capability and current performance in self-care, mobility, and social function.	≈15 minutes	No
Independent Living Skills Survey (ILSS; Wallace et al., 2000)	Adults with severe and persistent mental health challenges	Individuals or informants (caregivers or health-care providers) are asked to answer a questionnaire about a person's functional abilities across ADLs, IADLs, and health management tasks.	Frequency of tasks related to personal hygiene, appearance and care of clothing, care of personal possessions and living space, food preparation, health and safety, money management, transportation, leisure and recreation, work, eating behaviors, and social interaction	≈ 30 minutes	Recovery
Kohlman Evaluation of Living Skills (KELS; Thomson & Robnett, 2016)	Individuals with severe and persistent mental health challenges, brain injury, cognitive disabilities, and older adults	Individuals are asked to complete a series of ADL, IADL, and health management tasks and are evaluated on their ability to complete the tasks.	Person's accuracy in completing a series of life skills including self-care, safety and health, money management, community mobility, and telephone, employment, and leisure participation	≈ 40 minutes	No

Continued

TABLE 46-1 | **Therapeutic Reasoning Assessment Table–ADLs, IADLs, and Health Management—cont'd**

Which Tool?	Who Was This Tool Designed For?	Is This a Type of Tool the Person Can Do? What Is Required of the Person?	What Am I Measuring?	How Long Does It Take and Where Do I Administer This Assessment?	Is the Tool Associated With a Practice Model?
Milwaukee Evaluation of Daily Living Skills (MEDLS; Leonardelli, 1988)	Adult inpatients with severe and persistent mental health challenges	Individuals are asked to complete a series of ADL, IADL, and health management tasks and are evaluated on their ability to complete the tasks.	Performance in basic communication, bathing, tooth brushing, denture care, dressing, eating, eyeglass care, hair care, maintenance of clothing, makeup use, medication management, nail care, personal health care, safety in the community, safety in the home, shaving, time awareness, use of money, use of telephone, and use of transportation	≈ 2 hours Therapist can administer specific subtests only or administer assessment across sessions.	No
UCSD Performance-Based Skills Assessment (UPSA; Patterson et al., 2001)	Adults with mental health diagnoses	Individuals are asked to complete a series of ADL, IADL, and health management tasks and are evaluated on their ability to complete the tasks.	Accuracy in completing role-played household chores, communication, finance, transportation and planning, and recreational activities	≈ 30 minutes	No
Performance Assessment of Self-Care Skills (PASS; Holm & Rogers, 2008)	Adults with cardiopulmonary disease, stroke, congestive heart failure, dementia, depression, arthritis, Parkinson disease; older adults	Individuals are asked to complete a series of ADL, IADL, and health management tasks.	Independence, safety, and adequacy of task completion; 26 tasks in the following categories: functional mobility (e.g., toilet transfers), personal care (e.g., cleaning teeth), IADL with a cognitive emphasis (e.g., setting out medications according to prescription), and IADL with a physical emphasis (e.g., bed making)	≈ 2 hours Requires 1–3 hours to administer	No
Test of Grocery Shopping Skills (TOGSS; Brown et al., 2009; Hamera & Brown, 2000)	Teens and adults with serious mental health challenges	Individuals are asked to go to a grocery store and find 10 items. Individuals are scored on their time, accuracy, assistance needed, and organization with the task.	Person's ability to engage in grocery shopping	≈ 20 minutes	No
Kitchen Task Assessment (KTA; Baum & Edwards, 1993)	Adults with senile dementia, Alzheimer type	Person is instructed to make cooked pudding following written package directions; may have varied levels of verbal cues.	Initiation, organization, planning, performance, sequencing, judgment, and safety in a common food preparation task	15–20 minutes in a kitchen or clinic with access to kitchen style setup including stove, counter, refrigerator, and sink	Not developed to a specific model but may be used with several (e.g., Model of Human Occupation; Person-Environment-Occupation model)

TABLE 46-1 | Therapeutic Reasoning Assessment Table–ADLs, IADLs, and Health Management—cont'd

Which Tool?	Who Was This Tool Designed For?	Is This a Type of Tool the Person Can Do? What Is Required of the Person?	What Am I Measuring?	How Long Does It Take and Where Do I Administer This Assessment?	Is the Tool Associated With a Practice Model?
Rabideau Kitchen Evaluation–Revised (RKE-R; Neistadt, 1992)	Adults with mental health diagnoses and brain injury	Individuals are asked to make a sandwich and a hot drink.	The level of assistance needed to complete a simple cooking task	≈15 minutes	No
Eating and Meal Preparation Skills Assessment (EMPSA) Questionnaire (Lock et al., 2012)	Adolescents and adults	Individuals self-report perceived ability and motivation to perform 12 eating and meal preparation tasks on a questionnaire.	Self-perceived motivation and ability to plan menus, budget, shop, cook, pace cooking, serve portions, discard food, pace eating, eat with others, eat in public, manage distress, and eat difficult food	≈ 5 minutes	No

of frequency (always to never). The self-report version is answered yes or no. The ILSS has been found to be a reliable and valid assessment (Perivoliotis et al., 2004).

Kohlman Evaluation of Living Skills

The Kohlman Evaluation of Living Skills (KELS; Thomson & Robnett, 2016) evaluates a person's ability to complete basic living skills through a combination of interview- and performance-based items. Of note, this assessment uses tools such as a computer and cell phone to test for independence in online banking and cell phone use as appropriate. The KELS is practical to administer in a clinical setting, as it requires limited equipment. Testing with 200 individuals for the fourth version of the KELS demonstrates good reliability and validity.

Milwaukee Evaluation of Daily Living Skills

The Milwaukee Evaluation of Daily Living Skills (MEDLS) is a performance-based assessment that was designed for individuals with severe and persistent mental health challenges (Leonardelli, 1988). The assessment requires approximately 2 hours to administer, but a subset of items can be selected for use based on the concerns of an individual. The MEDLS is a reliable and valid assessment (Seyedi et al., 2016).

University of California San Diego (UCSD) Performance-Based Skills Assessment

The UCSD Performance-Based Skills Assessment (UPSA) is an assessment designed for persons with mental health diagnoses (Patterson et al., 2001). It measures the person's ability to complete different IADLs using props such as a telephone (Bowie et al., 2006). The assessment is also available as a mobile app for the iPad using virtual props. The clinician scores

the person's performance using standardized criteria. The UPSA is reliable and valid and can predict independent living status (Mausbach et al., 2008; Olsson et al., 2012).

Performance Assessment of Self-Care Skills

The Performance Assessment of Self-Care Skills (PASS; Holm & Rogers, 2008) is a performance-based assessment of ADLs and IADLs for persons with cognitive impairment, including persons with depression and dementia. The clinician observes the person performing the task and then scores their independence, safety, and outcome. The PASS describes the daily living activities in which individuals need assistance and indicates the components of the task requiring assistance (Chisholm et al., 2014). The PASS is also sensitive to persons with mild cognitive impairment (Ciro, 2014). The PASS has high reliability and validity, particularly for trained observers (Holm & Rogers, 2008).

Test of Grocery Shopping Skills

The Test of Grocery Shopping Skills (TOGSS) is a performance-based assessment that is administered in an actual grocery store (Brown et al., 2009; Hamera & Brown, 2000). The clinician evaluates the person's ability to efficiently and accurately locate 10 items on a grocery shopping list. The clinician then rates the person on their accuracy, time, and redundancy. The TOGSS is a valid and reliable assessment of executive function in a real-world setting (Hamera & Brown, 2000; Hamera et al., 2002; Zayat et al., 2011).

Kitchen Task Assessment and Children's Kitchen Task Assessment

The Kitchen Task Assessment (KTA; Baum & Edwards, 1993) is another performance-based cognitive assessment. During the KTA, the individual is instructed to make a box of pudding using the instructions on the box, and the clinician evaluates the individual's task initiation, planning and organization, safety, and appropriate task completion. The KTA was found to be a reliable and valid assessment for adults with dementia (Baum & Edwards, 1993). A modified version of the KTA was found to be reliable and valid for adults with schizophrenia (Duncombe, 2004). There is also the pediatric version of the KTA for children 8 to 12, in which the child is instructed to make playdough. The Children's KTA was found to be valid and reliable for typically developing children and individuals with sickle cell disease (Berg et al. 2012; Rocke et al., 2008).

Rabideau Kitchen Evaluation-Revised

The Rabideau Kitchen Evaluation-Revised (RKE-R; Neistadt, 1992) is a modification of the Rabideau Kitchen Evaluation (Rabideau, 1986). The RKE-R is a performance-based assessment in which a person makes a sandwich and hot drink. The clinician scores the person's ability to complete the various steps associated with the task. The RKE-R is a valid and reliable assessment and performance is related to underlying cognitive abilities (Neistadt, 1992, 1994; Yantz et al., 2010).

Eating and Meal Preparation Skills Assessment Questionnaire

The Eating and Meal Preparation Skills Assessment (EMPSA) Questionnaire is designed for persons with eating disorders (Lock et al., 2012). In the EMPSA, individuals rate their perceived ability and motivation to perform 12 eating and meal preparation tasks. The tool can be used to design interventions and to understand the effectiveness of the interventions.

Intervention

An individual's intervention plan should be developed collaboratively with the person and address the person's goals, strengths, daily routines, means, environment, and the best available evidence. Interventions, recommendations, and adaptations to individuals' ADL, IADL, and health management tasks should be feasible and acceptable to individuals for implementation into their daily routines both during admission and at discharge.

There are several different approaches to ADL, IADL, and health management intervention, with research to support their efficacy. The *OTPF* describes six types of intervention approaches (AOTA, 2020):

1. Occupations and Activities
2. Interventions to Support Occupations
3. Education and Training
4. Advocacy
5. Group Interventions
6. Virtual Interventions

Occupations and Activities

OTPs design interventions to meet the individual's goals and needs across their mind, body, and spirit (AOTA, 2020). Occupation-based interventions should be personalized.

Activity-based interventions focus on specific components of occupations, such as learning how to use the microwave as a move toward a larger cooking goal. Individuals may engage in an activity as a means to reaching a goal, such as knitting to reduce stress and promote mental well-being. Alternatively, individuals can engage in an activity with the goal of improving at that activity, such as improving financial independence by practicing budgeting and financial management skills.

Occupation as a Means to Promote General Well-Being

Engagement in cognitively demanding activities can promote general mental health and well-being. Therefore, activities with cognitive demands may be used as a means to improve general health, providing the individual with the psychological reserves to participate in ADLs, IADLs, and health management. Researchers found that college students and adults with developmental disabilities were able to decrease their stress levels when coloring complex geometric shapes such as mandalas (Curry & Kasser, 2005; Schrade et al., 2011; van der Vennet & Serice, 2012). Women with anorexia nervosa reported that knitting reduced anxiety, helped clear their mind of negative thoughts, and provided a calming effect (Clave-Brule et al., 2009).

In another study, community-dwelling older adults who learned a new cognitively demanding leisure skill (e.g., digital photography or quilting) demonstrated improved memory function after 3 months (Park et al., 2014). Geda and colleagues (2011) found that engagement in craft activities such as knitting and quilting was associated with better cognitive performance. Across studies, many of the researchers found that the creation of a craft resulted in satisfaction, pride, and a sense of accomplishment, which further contributed to psychosocial well-being. Although more research is needed, these studies suggest that OTPs can help persons with mental illness manage their symptoms by supporting engagement in cognitively demanding leisure skills. Also see Chapter 45: Self-Care and Well-Being Occupations, Chapter 50: Play, and Chapter 51: Leisure and Creative Occupations. 🤝

Activity-Based Workgroups

OTPs may also enable individuals to engage in cognitively demanding activities in a group format. In activity-based workgroups, individuals actively participate in an activity with the goal of improving interpersonal skills. For example, a group of individuals with mental health challenges or substance misuse may come together to complete a craft or cook a meal. A systematic review found three articles that investigated the effectiveness of activity-based workgroups (Bullock & Bannigan, 2011). The researchers found that persons in activity-based groups demonstrated better outcomes than individuals in verbally focused groups. The *Occupational Therapy Practice Guidelines for Adults With Serious Mental Illness* indicates that there is weak evidence to support this approach but suggest that the benefits likely outweigh the risks and drawbacks (Brown, 2012). Also see Chapter 13: Communication and Social Skills. 🤝

Interpersonal and Social Rhythm Therapy

ADLs, IADLs, and health management occupations provide a sense of order and familiarity to daily life. The disruption of routines, such as the timing of sleeping, eating,

Evidence-Based Practice

Psychoeducation Methods for Improving Engagement in Activities of Daily Living and Instrumental Activities of Daily Living

> *There is strong evidence supporting occupation-based interventions and manualized programs that use psychoeducation methods targeting ADLs and IADLs.*

RESEARCH FINDINGS

An occupational therapy systematic review evaluated interventions within the scope of occupational therapy to "improve and maintain occupational performance and participation for people with serious mental illness" (D'Amico et al., 2018, p. 7205190020p1). The results included the following:

- There is strong evidence to support the implementation of occupation-based interventions and manualized programs that use psychoeducation methods targeting ADLs and IADLs, especially when conducted within the context of person-centered goals.
- There is moderate evidence promoting the application of rest and sleep activity interventions.
- There is strong evidence available that demonstrates the utility of occupation-based social participation interventions.
- There was a dearth of research supporting animal-assisted therapy to support social participation and engagement, particularly for individuals with schizophrenia.
- There is moderate evidence surrounding the use of psychoeducation in addressing safe sexual activity.
- There is strong to moderate evidence for the use of skills training, particularly pertaining to ADL, IADL, and social skills.
- There is currently a lack of evidence surrounding the efficacy of cognitive interventions targeting ADLs and IADLs.

APPLICATIONS

➡ OTPs should ensure that ADL and IADL goals are targeted to those occupations of greatest concern to the person being served, and use psychoeducational approaches to structure engagement in those selected occupations.

➡ For ADLs and IADLs that involve social interaction with others, OTPs should help the person identify their natural social connections that support participation.

➡ When targeted skills are identified as barriers to participation, using a skills training approach, perhaps a group approach to learning, can be effective.

REFERENCES

D'Amico, M. L., Jaffe, L. E., & Gardner, J. A. (2018). Evidence for interventions to improve and maintain occupational performance and participation for people with serious mental illness: A systematic review. *The American Journal of Occupational Therapy, 72*(5), 7205190020p1–7205190020p11. https://doi.org/10.5014/ajot.2018.033332

and exercising, can lead to the onset of bipolar episodes (Swartz et al., 2012). Interpersonal and Social Rhythm Therapy (IPSRT) was developed as a psychosocial intervention for adults and adolescents with bipolar disorder (Hlastala et al., 2010). An integral part of IPSRT involves keeping a daily record of activities using the Social Rhythm Metric (Monk et al., 1990), with which individuals learn to monitor their routines and strive for regularity in the timing of their daily activities. Individuals with bipolar disorder in IPSRT identify the most unstable rhythms in their lives, set goals for change, and identify triggers that lead to disruptions. They also work to find the right balance of rest and activity.

In addition to intervention targeting daily routines, IP-SRT includes education about bipolar disorder medications and strategies to garner social support (Hlastala et al., 2010). The *Occupational Therapy Practice Guidelines for Adults With Serious Mental Illness* found fair evidence to support IPSRT and do recommend the use of this intervention approach (Brown, 2012). OTPs can use IPSRT and the theory behind this intervention approach in several ways. First, OTPs complete the IPSRT training to implement the evidence-based tool into practice. OTPs can also use themes from IPSRT in practice, such as considering the impact of routine on the performance of ADLs and symptoms of mental health diagnoses and weighing the need for rest versus activity.

A 2016 review of the literature available regarding IPSRT implementation found that the therapeutic approach demonstrates "feasible and satisfactory" outcomes to patients who have bipolar disorder (Haynes et al., 2016). Interventions for people with mood disorders (such as depression and bipolar disorder) should include strategies that promote the establishment of regularity in the timing of everyday activities (Haynes et al., 2016). Persons with bipolar disorder who received IPSRT experienced a decline in negative symptoms related to anxiety, mania, and depression (Steardo et al., 2020). Also see Chapter 14: Time Use and Habits.

Interventions to Support Occupations

Interventions to Support Occupations include methods and tasks that prepare the person for performance in occupations. They can be used as part of a treatment session in preparation for or in tandem with occupations and individual activities (AOTA, 2020). They can also be implemented with the person in the home as a method of supporting daily occupational performance (AOTA, 2020). Interventions that support occupations involve assistive technology and environmental modifications, which include self-regulation skill-building.

Assistive Technology

Using technology can be a meaningful occupation for people on the journey of mental health recovery. In addition, technology can assist individuals in better performing their daily ADL, IADL, and health management routines, particularly health management occupations. Technologies include mobile digital devices and applications (apps), video games, and global positioning devices (GPS), among others.

Mobile Digital Devices and Apps

A survey of adults with intensive mental health challenges found that 72% of people own a mobile phone, which they use for talking, texting, and accessing the internet (Ben-Zeev et al., 2013). Phone-based applications, or mobile apps, can help people reduce their mental health symptoms to enable better participation in everyday ADLs and IADLs. A systematic review found that smartphone apps can support people with mental health challenges by facilitating significant reductions in depression, stress, and substance use (Donker et al., 2013).

For example, apps can help individuals with depression self-monitor and take measures to reduce symptoms (Burns et al., 2011; Kauer et al., 2012). The "Get Happy" app delivers a form of cognitive behavioral therapy through stories and homework (Watts et al., 2013). App users decreased their symptoms of depression during a 3-month period. In persons with anxiety, app users decreased their anxiety and learned new coping skills (Grassi et al., 2010; Villani et al., 2012, 2013). For persons with substance use disorders, an app called "DBT Coach" used a dialectical behavior therapy approach to help users decrease urges to use substances (Rizvi et al., 2011).

Mobile digital devices can also help people with cognitive impairments better participate in specific ADLs and IADLs. Users can learn how to create lists, manage schedules using the calendar function, and create reminders. For example, a grocery-shopping app can help people remember their needs and avoid extraneous purchases. The alarm function can remind individuals to take their medications or engage in self-care activities. The calendar can encourage individuals to attend appointments or pay bills in a timely manner. Persons with cognitive impairment (caused by traumatic brain injury [TBI], multiple sclerosis, or autism) were able to improve their performance and satisfaction in a variety of occupations by using a digital device with training from an OTP or other health professional (Gentry et al., 2008, 2010; Patterson et al., 2001).

OTPs can help individuals improve performance of ADLs, IADLs, and health management occupations by prescribing person-centered evidence-based technologies. Although many individuals will already own smartphones, OTPs can help users who do not have a smartphone (but are interested in getting one) attain one. Lifeline is a government program that provides a discount for low-income individuals to help them better access health-care services, connect with friends and family, and call for help in an emergency (Federal Communications Commission, 2016). Once a device is acquired, OTPs can help users to identify device features (e.g., calendar or alarm) and access apps to help them achieve their goals. OTPs understand the individuals' goals, strengths, and needs, and can identify and train those they serve on how to use their mobile digital devices to improve their ADL, IADL, and health management performance.

Smartphone applications and other mobile health technologies are increasingly being used to help persons with mental health diagnoses and substance use disorders. Recent studies on health technology in mental health (e.g., Ben-Zeev et al., 2018; Donker et al., 2013) revealed that mobile apps have the potential to be effective and improve the accessibility of mental health treatment and mental health outcomes. However, most currently available apps lack scientific evidence supporting their efficacy (Moon et al., 2022). OTPs should investigate how current apps can help those individuals they are providing care to better perform their ADLs and IADLs (Donker et al., 2013). Practitioners need to understand the effectiveness of apps in the context of individuals' lives (Donker et al., 2013).

Video Games

Over 3.24 billion people play video games worldwide (Clement, 2022). Gaming can be an important IADL, and it can serve as an intervention to promote mental well-being. Video games include console games (e.g., Wii, PlayStation, Xbox), computer games, and phone-based games. Currently, in the United States, many gamers are children (24%) or adults between the ages of 18 to 34 (36%; Entertainment Software Association, 2022). Therefore, video game-based interventions are mostly targeted to the needs of children, teens, and young adults.

Video games offer three benefits over typical interventions (Wilkinson et al., 2008):

1. Video games can simulate real-life situations and learning opportunities in a manner that is efficient and engaging. For example, phobias can present a major limitation to engaging in ADLs and IADLs. Video games can provide graded exposure therapy to effectively help individuals overcome fears, particularly those difficult to create in clinical settings such as war zones and tight and crowded spaces (Cukor et al., 2015; Malbos et al., 2013).

2. Video games offer the opportunity for repeated practice. For example, TeachTown is a computer-based video game that teaches new skills related to a variety of ADL and IADL areas such as mealtime routines, dressing, and financial management using repetitive practice (Whalen et al., 2006). A preliminary study of 47 children with autism found that students who engaged with the TeachTown game improved their language and cognition better than children assigned to the control group (Whalen et al., 2010).

3. Video games can make techniques more accessible to younger users. For example, video games with biofeedback equipment were able to teach basic skills such as relaxation to people with anxiety or attention for children with attention deficit-hyperactivity disorder (ADHD; Heinrich et al., 2007; Sharry et al., 2003). Video games with biofeedback have also showed promise with use in adult populations, with a recent study finding that undergraduate students with anxiety demonstrated improvements in symptoms after engaging with a virtual reality biofeedback video game (Weerdmeester et al., 2020).

Video games can be an efficient and motivating tool in an OTP's toolbox. OTPs should consider a person's access to video games, strengths, and preferences to identify if there are video game-based interventions that can help individuals reach their goals. New video games are released daily; therefore, OTPs should routinely survey available video games anticipated to affect health and functional skills. Although many games may claim to improve health and skill acquisition, OTPs should continue to search peer-reviewed literature regarding the efficacy of a specific video game for a particular population. Little evidence informs the recommended dose and frequency of video game intervention, but OTPs should be aware that overuse of video games can have negative effects on mental health and function (Chan & Rabinowitz, 2006).

Environmental Modifications

OTPs can work with individuals using universal design principles and recommendations for changes to a person's environment or activity to support the person's ability to engage in various occupations (AOTA, 2020). OTPs can use a standardized approach, such as **Cognitive Adaptation Training (CAT)**, or implement specific modifications to meet an individual's needs.

Cognitive Adaptation Training

CAT is an intervention that uses changes to the environment, assistive technology, and other compensatory strategies to enable the adaptive behaviors needed to complete ADLs and IADLs (Velligan et al., 2008). CAT has primarily been used for people with schizophrenia and other disabling mental health challenges. CAT is based on the theory that persons with poor executive function need high levels of structure and obvious environmental cues, and persons with better executive function are able to respond to more subtle cues.

Within the CAT protocol, individuals receiving treatment undergo neuropsychological tests from a psychologist followed by a Functional Needs Assessment administered by a therapist (including OTPs; Velligan & Bow-Thomas, 2000). The Functional Needs Assessment is a 26-item performance-based measure of the individual's ability to initiate and perform basic ADLs and IADLs including grooming, shopping, home management and maintenance, and safety. During CAT, a program therapist assesses the person and their home environment to identify gaps in performance or safety risks. OTPs use the results from the cognitive testing and assessment of the home environment to create an intervention plan.

PhotoVoice

Robert

I think the calendar is a wonderful idea for the MARC Center. The calendar lets you know the different activities on different days that will be taking place at the MARC Center. What a wonderful idea for the monthly calendar to help keep me alert of certain activities that may be going on that day.

Calendars help us keep a schedule and predict upcoming activities. Are you the type of person who likes to have a routine and predictable day? How might routines support or hinder someone with a psychiatric condition?

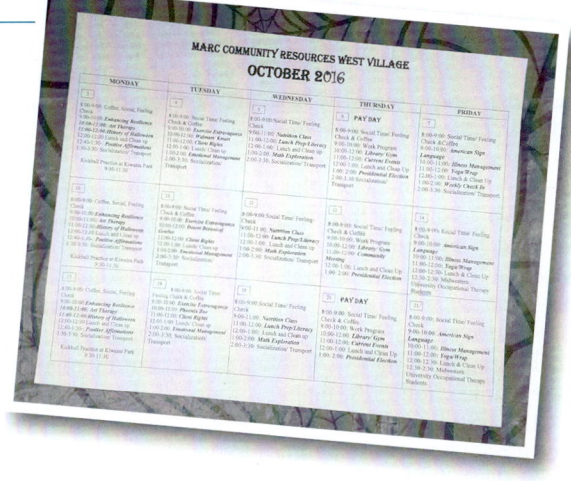

CAT interventions involve environmental supports for cueing, sequencing behavior, and removing distracting stimuli (Velligan et al., 2008). Common materials include signs, calendars, hygiene supplies, and pill containers (Velligan et al., 2006). In one case study, an individual with impairments in dressing, bathing, and grooming received CAT intervention (Velligan & Bow-Thomas, 2000). The OTP helped the person to organize his closet, placed a toothbrush and toothpaste on a basket in the bathroom mirror with a reminder sign, and posted an appearance checklist on the back of the bathroom door. Further, all signs and checklists were printed with bright bold colors to catch the individual's attention.

When implementing CAT as an intervention, individuals need environmental supports such as checklists, with environmental supports being the most impactful when implemented directly in the home (Hansen et al., 2012; Velligan et al., 2006, 2008). CAT has been shown to be an effective approach to treatment, with persons with mental health challenges demonstrating improved functional performance compared with those who received a traditional course of treatment, and with CAT demonstrating just as much effectiveness as community assertive treatment (Hansen et al., 2012; Velligan et al., 2006, 2008).

OTPs can apply the research about CAT and environmental supports in general research in several ways. First, OTPs working in an interdisciplinary setting can work with psychologists to implement the CAT intervention within their organizations. To implement formal CAT, OTPs should receive training and review the CAT manual (Velligan, 2000). OTPs can also apply the general findings of the CAT studies to their daily practice. Research suggests that individuals will benefit from person-centered adaptations to their environment (Velligan et al., 2006, 2008). OTPs can work with individuals to identify environmental supports and assistive technologies to help improve performance in ADLs and IADLs. The *Occupational Therapy Practice Guidelines for Adults With Serious Mental Illness* found strong evidence to support environmental efforts to promote adaptive functioning (Brown, 2012). The guidelines suggest that OTPs routinely provide the environmental supports to eligible individuals.

Home Environmental Skill-Building Program

The Home Environmental Skill-Building Program (ESP) is an intervention designed for people with dementia in which OTPs teach caregivers how to modify the environment (Gitlin et al., 1999). The intervention occurs during five 90-minute sessions. Three types of strategies are taught: (1) simplification of the physical environment, (2) modification of the caregiver's approach to assisting with ADL and IADL tasks, and (3) involvement of others in the caregiving process. For example, to modify the physical environment, caregivers are encouraged to eliminate clutter and use relevant assistive devices. In terms of the caregiver's approach, recommendations are made to establish daily routines and limit commands to one or two steps. Finally, caregivers are encouraged to utilize social supports, such as involving other family members in caregiving or joining a support group.

The ESP literature informs occupational therapy practice for adults with dementia and their caregivers in several ways. First, OTPs can become trained on the ESP protocol to better implement this evidence-based technique into their practice (Gitlin et al., 2001, 2003). The ESP literature also supports some general occupational therapy principles. For example, it demonstrates that OTPs can modify an individual's home environment to improve performance of ADLs and IADLs (Gitlin et al., 2001, 2003). Further, OTPs should engage in problem-solving with the individual to identify the most problematic issues and person-centered solutions (Chee et al., 2007). Lastly, the research demonstrated that role-playing with caregivers is a particularly effective strategy in working with adults with dementia (Chee et al., 2007).

Literature is available that supports the use of Home ESP as a tool for modifying the environment that can promote better performance of ADLs and IADLs for adults with dementia and their caregivers (Chee et al., 2007; Gitlin et al., 1999, 2001, 2003). In addition to caregivers creating improved physical and social environments through role-playing, benefits of the intervention approach can include decreased decline in IADL performance and decreased stress and improved well-being outcomes for caregivers (Chee et al., 2007; Gitlin et al., 1999, 2001, 2003).

Education and Training

In educational interventions, the OTP imparts knowledge and information regarding occupation, health, well-being, and overall participation that enable the person to acquire helpful behaviors, habits, and routines (AOTA, 2020). In training interventions, the OTP facilitates the acquisition of concrete skills for meeting specific goals in real-life, applied situations (AOTA, 2020). Training interventions differ from education in that the goal of such interventions is to enhance performance as opposed to education interventions, which are designed to increase understanding (AOTA, 2020). Education and training interventions can include the person, the family, and other key members of the team.

Life skills training helps individuals acquire the skills needed to live independently. Skills training can address a variety of ADLs, IADLs, and health management occupations including financial management, home management and maintenance, personal self-care (dressing, grooming, etc.), and coping skills.

Skills training interventions for individuals with serious mental health challenges are founded on learning theory. The "to be taught" skill is first broken down into its component parts. These target behaviors are taught using a variety of teaching methods designed to compensate for cognitive impairments. The skills are presented through demonstration, didactic instruction, or videotape. Individuals then practice these skills repeatedly, receiving regular feedback based on performance. Social reinforcement and other contingencies are used for motivation. Homework assignments are utilized to encourage more practice of the skills in the person's natural environment. The skills training approach can be used to teach a variety of ADLs and IADLs such as grocery shopping, health self-management, parenting, financial management, and cooking skills (Brown, 2012), as well as medication management and relaxation skills.

The UCLA Social and Independent Living Skills Program is one example of a manualized skills training program, and it is one of the most researched skills training interventions

(Eckman et al., 1992; Liberman et al., 1986, 1998; Wallace et al., 2000). In the UCLA program, modules are intended to be delivered in a small group format. It is recommended that training be provided at least twice a week in 1-hour sessions. Most of the modules take 4 months to complete, which stresses the importance of repeated practice.

The modules include content on medication management, symptoms management, leisure activities, conversation, job seeking, workplace skills, and so on. During each module, activities are graded to become more difficult. Attendees begin with an introduction to the skill and watch a video of actors modeling the target behavior. Then, participants progress to role-playing and in vivo exercises. In addition to other learning strategies, individuals are taught problem-solving approaches that can be applied to novel situations with the goal of generalizing skills from the program into real life.

Individuals with serious mental health challenges can learn new self-care, IADL, and health management skills (Brown, 2012). In addressing these areas, skills training interventions are more effective than support groups, attention control, and craft-oriented groups. Skills training has been shown to result in greater improvements in symptoms and better psychosocial functioning. These gains extend to the increase in specific skill sets, such as cooking, grocery shopping, social interactions, and health management. It is important to note that skills training is most effective when conducted in a person's natural environments, with historically effective interventions leveraging repeated practice and occurring within numerous sessions across multiple months (Brown, 2012).

In general, the *Occupational Therapy Practice Guidelines for Adults With Serious Mental Illness* recommend the use of skills training (Brown, 2012). Historically, the level of evidence has varied from fair to insufficient depending on the type of skills training, with life, cooking, and social skills training possessing fair evidence, grocery shopping and parenting having weak evidence, and financial management skills training demonstrating insufficient evidence. A more recent systematic review by D'Amico and colleagues (2018) examined the evidence for improving and maintaining occupational performance for individuals with serious mental illness. The review showed there is "moderate" to "strong" evidence supporting ADL and IADL skills training, and mixed findings on social skills training (D'Amico et al., 2018).

In building on the evidence available surrounding life skills training from a pediatric perspective, a recent literature review by Cahill and colleagues (2020) found "moderate" evidence that occupation and life skills training improve anxiety symptoms and internalizing behaviors for "children and youth" (Table 46-2). OTPs can use one of the many manualized skills training interventions (Brown et al., 2002; see Box 46-1).

Advocacy

This chapter is focused on interventions for ADLs, IADLs, and health management performance. As part of the recovery process, OTPs should help individuals improve not only their ability to perform daily activities but also their ability to engage in occupation as part of meaningful life roles and routines. For example, OTPs can build on basic activities such as bathing, grooming, dressing, and cooking to help the person better participate in meaningful roles of family life and independent living. Unfortunately, persons on the journey

TABLE 46-2 | Developing Skills Training Modules

Component	Steps
Problem identification	1. Interview individuals to identify the particular problem using open-ended questions. 2. Create a checklist based on all the problems generated by the open-ended questions. 3. Administer the checklist to a group. 4. Prioritize the most important problems.
Solution identification	1. Interview individuals to identify solutions to the problems using open-ended questions. 2. Create a checklist based on all the solutions generated by the open-ended questions. 3. Administer the checklist to a group. 4. Identify the solutions that those in the group would be most likely to use.
Module development	1. Create skills training curriculum about the problem based on the literature and individuals' input. 2. Create skills training curriculum about solutions based on the literature and individuals' input.

Holmes, E. P., Corrigan, P. W., Knight, S., & Flaxman, J. (1995). Development of a sleep management program for people with severe mental illness. Psychiatric Rehabilitation Journal, 19, 9–15. https://doi.org/10.1037/h0095445

of mental health recovery are often burdened by stigma, a lack of financial resources, and maladaptive responses to life's pressures (Smith & Kotake, 2000). Therefore, OTPs can work with individuals to transition from ADLs and IADLs to address social recovery and social inclusion (Lloyd et al., 2008).

OTPs can advocate with the person to promote occupational justice and personal empowerment in seeking and obtaining resources that support health, well-being, and occupational participation (AOTA, 2020). This could include OTP collaboration with the individual to request and establish reasonable accommodations at a person's place of employment that meet the person's mental health needs. OTPs can also empower individuals and communities to advocate for themselves and their needs through self-advocacy interventions. An example of this could include empowering an individual to independently request accommodations at work. These actions are all examples of critical health management occupations for the individuals OTPs serve.

Group Interventions

OTPs often find that setting up groups for people who are interested in learning novel ADL, IADL, and health management occupations can facilitate learning while providing a supportive and enriched occupational environment. As can be seen in the examples offered in Tables 46-3, 46-4, 46-5, and 46-6, group interventions focused on skills such as cooking, eating, financial management, and using public transportation that are facilitated by OTPs in community settings enhance participation.

Virtual Interventions

Depending on the targeted ADLs, IADLs, and health management occupations, technology offers many different approaches using virtual tools. The OTP can facilitate use

BOX 46-1 ■ Strategies for Skills Training

Motivational Strategies

- Incorporate both internal and external rewards and motivators.
- Match the motivators with the content of a program.
- Create an environment that conveys your expectations that participants will learn from the experience.
- Use certificates, graduation ceremonies, and so on, to reinforce accomplishments.

Application to Real Life

- Reflect on your personal experiences and lenses (e.g., socioeconomic status, race, education, gender and sexual identity, familial makeup, political affiliation). How might these impact your perspectives on skill training? How might you address these effects when collaborating across skills training with individuals?
- Make sure that you know what real life is for your group members.
- Practice in real-life environments whenever possible.
- Facilitate generalization by practicing in multiple real-life environments.
- Use homework so individuals can practice skills at home.
- Include other staff, families, peers, and so on, in the training.

Repeated Practice

- Teach a topic during multiple sessions.
- Incorporate several ways of teaching and practicing the same content.
- Use homework for more opportunities to practice.
- Encourage families, other staff, peers, and so on, to promote opportunities for practice.

Provide Feedback About Performance

- Make expectations clear.
- Use worksheets or quizzes and provide written or verbal feedback depending on individuals' personal factors (e.g., visual and auditory processing/abilities, learning needs, and primary language).
- Provide regular verbal feedback for performance.
- Have group members work with partners and encourage feedback among peers.

Evaluate Knowledge and Skill Acquisition

- Use quizzes or worksheets that you can review.
- Observe performance.
- Incorporate question-and-answer sessions or contests.
- Have homework that group members submit.

Match Environmental and Individual Needs

- Allow many opportunities for choice.
- Encourage group members to think of their own examples.
- Use the environments that the group members use.
- Adapt the intervention for environmental or individual differences.
- Provide multiple suggestions or techniques and help participants determine which strategy works best for them.

of these tools to meet the needs of the person, with examples offered in Tables 46-3, 46-4, 46-5, and 46-6. Also see Chapter 33: Virtual Environments.

Application of Evaluation and Intervention

This section describes five key occupations—financial management, driving and public transportation, grocery shopping, meal preparation, and medication management. For each, specific suggestions are made using a variety of evaluation and intervention approaches discussed previously.

Financial Management

Financial management and financial literacy are important IADLs in the lives of people with mental health challenges, substance use disorders, and complex health conditions. One small study of persons with dual diagnoses receiving care through the Veterans Administration found that 32% of individuals were incapable of managing their own funds (Black et al., 2008). People with mental health challenges identify better financial management and improving financial skills as one of their most important goals (Eklund, 2009). Having and managing money is instrumental for living safely in the community and ensuring adequate food, shelter, and transportation (Elbogen et al., 2011). In fact, poor financial management skills are associated with increased rates of being unhoused in persons with mental health challenges (Elbogen et al., 2013).

Persons with substance use disorders may experience challenges with financial management in particular (Rosen et al., 2009), and financial issues can be a relapse trigger. When persons with substance use disorders have money (such as the day they receive disability payments), they are prone to higher rates of drug and alcohol use; this may even result in increased rates of emergency department visits and death on payment days. Intervention on the topic of financial management can help persons with mental health conditions and substance use disorders achieve their goal related to independent living and promote better health and well-being.

Several assessment tools evaluate the ability to engage in purchasing transactions and core financial management activities. An occupational profile will help the occupational therapist understand the person's current habits, roles, and routines around financial management and to identify the person's goals and priorities. For example, the occupational profile might identify that an individual's family member currently manages all the finances, but the person's goal is to become more financially independent and to save up enough money for a deposit on an apartment.

There are a variety of performance-based measures that can be used to understand a person's current skill level. The KELS evaluates the individual's ability to identify money, make purchases with cash, pay a bill, and engage in online banking (Thomson & Robnett, 2016). The UPSA evaluates the person's ability to read, understand, and pay a bill (Patterson et al., 2001). The MEDLS evaluates the individual's ability to identify money, make change, and create a budget (Leonardelli, 1988).

TABLE 46-3 | Money Management Interventions

Intervention Approach	Description
Occupation and Activities	• Engage in purchases and banking activities in real-world settings.
Interventions to Support Occupations	• Train individuals to correctly identify coins and bills. • Use a mobile digital device to help create a budget and track spending. • Implement cognitive adaptation strategies such as a series of checklists and reminders to ensure that bills are paid correctly and on time. • Develop shopping lists to prevent overspending.
Education and Training	• Provide skills training on shopping, banking, bill pay, and money transactions. • Improve financial literacy. • Educate individuals on resources for persons with low income such as food pantries and subsidized housing. • Implement behavioral modification strategies to encourage good money management. • Engage in caregiver training to develop a social environment in which a family member assists with money management tasks.
Advocacy	• Empower individuals to increase their income such as paid employment or entitlement programs. • Empower individuals to attain appropriate money management materials such as a bank account, savings account, credit card, or debit card.
Group Interventions	• Engage group in discussions on money management strategies that have worked well for individuals in the past. • Facilitate training on creating and setting personal goals surrounding finances and money management.
Virtual Interventions	• Establish a weekly money management virtual group covering differing topics of money management each week (e.g., financial literacy, establishing tracking systems). • Explore online money management strategies in "live time" such as online banking and bill paying and money management apps.

There are a variety of evidence-based intervention approaches that OTPs can use to improve individuals' financial management skills. Table 46-3 describes intervention approaches specifically applied to the topic of financial management.

The $teps for Achieving Financial Empowerment ($AFE) intervention demonstrates the effectiveness of a person-centered combination of intervention approaches. Specifically, the $AFE program is a 2-hour person-centered intervention that includes education and skills training (Elbogen et al., 2011). The OTP educates individuals on how to save money, differentiating between wants and needs, avoiding scams, and identifying services available to low-income persons with mental health diagnoses or substance use disorders. They also engage in skills training on creating

a viable budget. In a study of 144 veterans with psychiatric disabilities and poor financial management skills, persons who implemented $AFE strategies at home were more likely to have fewer impulsive spending behaviors, to demonstrate better responsible spending behaviors, and to engage in more hours of vocational activity compared with persons who did not implement $AFE strategies (Elbogen et al., 2016).

There are additional approaches to financial management and literacy programs that are available and effective. A descriptive, mixed methods study by Gardner and colleagues (2019) found that a financial management program, Financial Management Account (FMA), improved the perceived budgeting and organizational skills of participants with substance use and mental health diagnoses, as well as aspects such as one's overall quality of life and perceptions of safety (Gardner et al., 2019). Borillo (2019) explored the use of a multiresource approach in creating a 20-lesson financial literacy program for students with learning differences (including mental health diagnoses) transitioning to work and postsecondary education opportunities. Students who participated in the study reported gaining increased financial literacy (Borillo, 2019).

These studies highlight the plethora of evidence-based resources that OTPs can draw from in addressing financial literacy and management with the people OTPs serve (Borillo, 2019; Elbogen et al., 2016; Gardner et al., 2019).

Driving and Public Transportation

For individuals to complete many aspects of ADLs, IADLs, and health management, they must have access to the community through transportation. Persons with mental health challenges and substance use disorders frequently report that a lack of transportation prevents them from doing the things they need and want to do in the community (Mojtabai et al., 2014). Persons with mental health challenges and substance misuse can drive or use public transportation to access the community. International studies suggest that about 35% of persons with mental health challenges drive (Rouleau et al., 2010).

A recent systematic review found that 31% of persons who were taking medication with schizophrenia or schizoaffective diagnoses, and 18% of individuals with unipolar and bipolar diagnoses, demonstrate increased severity of impairment in skills that are needed to effectively and safely drive (Brunnauer et al., 2021).

An individual's ability to drive may change depending on their level of wellness, medications (and their side effects), substance use status, comorbid health conditions (e.g., diabetes), and access to the financial resources needed to drive (Dun et al., 2015). Individuals may be taking medication that can impact their ability to drive (Brunnauer et al., 2021), making it important for the assessing OTP to be up to date on individuals' medications and their side effects; this helps the OTP in conducting intermittent assessment of the effect of one's medications on their ability to safely drive, and for the individual being assessed on the road to be using their medication(s) during the testing to promote the most realistic context in driving (Unsworth, 2010).

Because of the barriers to driving, many individuals with mental illness and substance use disorders use public transportation. Unfortunately, barriers also hinder public transportation use. A report by the Substance Abuse and Mental

Health Services Administration (SAMHSA, 2004) found that barriers to transportation include:

- *Affordability:* Individuals cannot afford to use public transportation regularly.
- *Accessibility:* Public transportation can be difficult to use for persons with psychiatric conditions. Specialized transportation, such as paratransit, requires individuals to schedule trips in advance and limits people's ability to get to where they need to go when they need to get there.
- *Applicability:* Many individuals with mental health challenges have a hidden disability and are not eligible for local transportation services.
- *Availability:* Individuals living in rural and suburban settings may not have access to public transportation. In urban settings, some cities have few options; this limits when and where people can travel.
- *Awareness:* Persons with mental health challenges and substance use disorders may not know how to access special transportation services or how to use public transportation.

Mental health support services such as People Incorporated (2022) note that persons with mental health challenges may not be able to afford to consistently pay for ride-share services such as Uber and Lyft when attempting to access treatment, and that people living in rural areas may have less access to transportation options. Individuals may also experience anxiety at the prospect of having to drive themselves to a health-care center to receive treatment.

Occupational therapists can evaluate individuals' community mobility. During the occupational profile, the occupational therapist can determine the person's previous driving status, main method of transportation, and any goals related to community mobility. For driving, several assessments evaluate the individual's ability to complete various components of driving. Although no one pen-and-paper test can indicate a person's ability to drive, a composite battery of assessments of different physical, cognitive, and visual domains can identify those who may be unsafe behind the wheel and would benefit from additional services (Bennett et al., 2016).

Notably, recent development of a mental health-focused screening tool, the Saskatchewan Psychiatric Occupational Driving Screen (SPOT-DS), warrants attention (Carey et al., 2018). The SPOT-DS has five categories of assessment for the OTP: cognition and perception, physical and sensation, psychosocial, medications, and an "other" category (e.g., presence of hallucinations, medication compliance, participation in electroconvulsive treatment; Carey et al., 2018).

On-road driving assessments can then be used to identify a person's appropriateness for driving (Berndt et al., 2015). There are also assessments available to identify a person's ability to take public transportation. In the MEDLS, an individual is given a local bus or train schedule and is asked to describe the number of stops between locations, to plan a trip to the grocery store, and to describe how they would get to the grocery store when there is no access to public transportation (Leonardelli, 1988). In the KELS, the occupational therapist interviews the person about their typical method of transportation and investigates their

basic knowledge of public transportation (if appropriate; Thomson & Robnett, 2016).

Once an individual's skills and priorities are determined, the OTP can develop a person-centered intervention plan to help the person reach their goals. For individuals who drive or have the capacity to drive, OTPs can provide interventions to teach driving skills. For driver training, it is important that the therapist have a dual-controlled vehicle and experience in driving instruction. Many certified driver rehabilitation specialists are occupational therapists. OTPs can also enable individuals to better use public transportation. Table 46-4 describes a variety of interventions discussed previously that are specifically applied to the topic of driving and public transportation.

Grocery Shopping, Meal Preparation, and Eating

Meal-related ADLs, IADLs, and health management are difficult for many persons with mental health diagnoses and substance use disorders. Persons with mental health challenges

TABLE 46-4 | Driving and Public Transportation Interventions

Intervention Approach	Description
Occupation and Activities	• Provide skills training on using public transportation.
Interventions to Support Occupation	• Use a mobile digital device to help navigate the community. • Use cognitive adaptation strategies to create a checklist, notes, and directions. • Practice relaxation strategies to reduce anxiety on public transportation.
Education and Training	• Provide skills training on driving. • Provide skills training on using public transportation. • Educate the person to improve knowledge of public transportation. • Implement behavioral modification strategies to encourage appropriate behaviors on public transportation. • Develop a social environment in which family members and friends can provide needed transportation.
Advocacy	• Empower individuals to partake in local programs for persons with disabilities, such as reduced fares or paratransit. • Advocate by working with public transportation providers to better understand how to serve persons with mental health challenges.
Group Interventions	• Explore local transportation options and discuss pros and cons as a group. • Examine available forms of public transportation as a group and create personalized access plan.
Virtual Interventions	• Provide skills training in "live time" using transportation apps. • Explore local transportation program support sites.

can have less nutritious diets, poor eating habits, decreased knowledge about diet and cooking, and negative attitudes toward healthy food (Bogomolova et al., 2016). Poor performance in meal-related ADLs and IADLs can result in poor weight management, nutritional deficiencies, and additional health conditions such as cardiovascular disease. Improved performance of tasks such as grocery shopping, meal preparation, and eating can help people with mental health challenges better engage in healthy and productive lives.

Several assessments evaluate the ability to complete various components of meal preparation. In the occupational profile, the occupational therapist can determine the person's habits, roles, and routines for grocery shopping, cooking, and eating. Several standardized assessments are available to help the therapist assess components of eating. For persons with eating disorders, therapists can administer the EMPSA to measure a person's perceived ability and motivation to engage in all components of grocery shopping, meal preparation, and eating (Lock et al., 2012). Therapists who wish to evaluate an individual's capacity to engage in a cooking task can administer the RKE-R (Neistadt, 1992) or the KTA (Baum & Edwards, 1993). For youth, therapists can administer the Children's KTA (Berg et al., 2012; Rocke et al., 2008). To evaluate a person's ability to grocery shop, the therapist can administer the TOGSS (Hamera et al., 2002).

A variety of evidence-based intervention approaches exist that OTPs can use to help individuals to reach their goals related to meal preparation and eating. Table 46-5 describes numerous interventions discussed previously that are specifically applied to the topics of grocery shopping, meal preparation, and eating.

Practical eating serves as an intervention approach that can be implemented in collaboration with nutrition specialists in addressing practices surrounding feeding and eating for persons with eating disorders (Biddiscombe et al., 2018). Practical eating intervention focuses on individuals being exposed to real-life situations surrounding feeding and eating, addressing cognitions surrounding meal-time engagement, and implementing strategies for cognitions and anxiety management (Sparnon & Hornyak, 1989).

Biddiscombe and colleagues (2018) implemented practical eating sessions with adults with eating disorders who were attending day programming. Sessions included "just right challenge"-based tasks including challenging cognitions and "feared" food exposure in lived environments (Biddiscombe et al., 2018). Coping strategy establishment and portion size education and "modeling" were also addressed (Biddiscombe et al., 2018). These interventions were carried out in collaboration with a dietitian (Biddiscombe et al., 2018). Participants reported that these practical eating groups were highly useful (Biddiscombe et al., 2018). This approach to care demonstrates promise in meeting the needs of individuals with eating disorders (Biddiscombe et al., 2018).

Medication Management

Psychiatric medication, when taken correctly, can reduce symptoms of mental health challenges and addiction and improve an individual's ability to live a productive life (Leucht et al., 2012), which is an important example of health management occupations. Unfortunately, many people with

TABLE 46-5	Grocery Shopping, Meal Preparation, and Eating Interventions
Intervention Approach	**Description**
Occupation and Activities	• Implement learned approaches in real-world environments, such as grocery shopping and cooking in one's own kitchen.
Interventions to Support Occupation	• Use a mobile digital device to create grocery lists, store healthy recipes, and count calories (and other nutritional information). • Use cognitive adaptation strategies to create checklists and notes for grocery shopping and cooking. • Practice cognitive-behavioral strategies to reduce distorted thoughts about weight and eating.
Education and Training	• Provide skills training on grocery shopping. • Provide skills training on cooking. • Educate the person to improve knowledge of healthy eating. • Implement behavioral modification strategies to encourage adaptive shopping and eating behaviors. • Develop a social environment in which family members support healthy eating.
Advocacy	• Work with service providers such as psychosocial clubhouses and inpatient settings to offer healthy food options and to include persons with mental illness and substance use disorders in the meal preparation process.
Group Interventions	• Facilitate education on reviewing recipes for healthy ingredients. • Engage group members in a recipe-sharing activity in which participants share their favorite healthy recipes with one another.
Virtual Interventions	• Facilitate exploration of free online resources for meal planning, preparation, and healthy recipes. • Review how to use helpful meal planning apps in "live time" (e.g., Pinterest, Paprika).

mental health challenges and substance use disorders may struggle to take their medications as prescribed. The research suggests that as many as 60% of adults with schizophrenia, 69% of adults with depression, 50% of adults with bipolar disorder, 57% of adults with anxiety disorders, and 35% of adults with alcohol use and dependence are not adherent to their medication regimens (Buckley et al., 2009).

When people with psychiatric disabilities fail to take their medications as prescribed, they experience more frequent relapses, higher intensity relapses, higher likelihood of suicidal acts, increased risk of drug dependence, increased risk of abstinence and rebound effects, and increased risk of drug toxicity (Buckley et al., 2009; Gonzalez-Pinto et al., 2006; World Health Organization [WHO], 2003).

Persons with psychiatric disabilities do not choose to be sick, but most often struggle to engage in the day-to-day management of taking their medications as prescribed. When asked about failure to take medications, persons with mental health challenges report that they do not take their medications because of stigma, lack of knowledge, adverse drug reactions, forgetfulness, insufficient environmental and social supports, and difficulty in managing complex drug regimens (Buckley et al., 2009).

Occupational therapy intervention can help persons with mental health challenges and substance use disorders achieve their goals related to health, well-being, and medication management. Several assessment tools evaluate the ability to complete various components of medication management. Many but not all individuals struggle with taking their medications as prescribed. A medication adherence screen can help OTPs to identify people at risk for poor medication adherence. The Medication Adherence Rating Scale (MARS) is a 10 yes/no question survey that investigates a person's history, beliefs, and experiences with medication. Scores lower than 10 suggest poor medication adherence and indicate that individuals may benefit from further services.

An occupational profile will help the OTP understand the person's current habits, roles, and routines concerning medication management and identify the person's goals and priorities. For example, the occupational profile may identify that the individual is responsible for remembering to take their medication every day, but the person's care team assists with monthly refills from the pharmacy.

Performance-based assessments indicate if the person has the underlying knowledge, performance skills, and abilities to complete activities associated with managing medications. The MEDLS reviews the individual's medication regimen and investigates the person's knowledge of their regimen, dosing schedule, intended effects, side effects, and problem-solving skills around running out of medication (Leonardelli, 1988). The PASS evaluates the individual's capacity for medication management by asking them to read medication information and organize fake medications in a pillbox (Holm & Rogers, 2008). Based on the evaluation, the OTP can identify who needs additional services to address medication

management, plan treatment, and evaluate the effectiveness of occupational therapy interventions.

A variety of evidence-based intervention approaches exist that OTPs can use to improve the medication management skills of those who they serve. Table 46-6 describes a variety of interventions discussed previously, specifically applied to the topic of medication management. A systematic review found that interventions providing concrete instructions and problem-solving strategies, such as reminders, self-monitoring tools, cues, and reinforcements, can be effective strategies to help people better manage their medications (Zygmunt et al., 2002).

The Integrative Medication Self-Management (IMedS) is an occupational therapy intervention that demonstrates the effectiveness of a person-centered combination of intervention approaches. The IMedS intervention is a three-step process in which the OTP (1) encourages the person to reflect on their past performance of medication management, (2) asks the individual to create a medication-related goal, and (3) helps the person generate strategies to reach their goal (Schwartz, 2015).

During the strategizing, the OTP uses Motivational Interviewing approaches to help the individual generate new strategies in six content areas as appropriate: (1) altering the activity, (2) advocacy, (3) education, (4) assistive technology, (5) environmental modifications, and (6) securing timely refills. In a small, randomized controlled trial of adults with multiple chronic physical and psychiatric conditions, the intervention helped some individuals better take their medications as prescribed (Schwartz & Smith, 2016). Persons who received the occupational therapy intervention also implemented twice as many new strategies at home to help them better manage their medication (Schwartz, 2015).

TABLE 46-6 | Medication Management Interventions

Intervention Approach	Description
Occupation and Activities	• Implement learned approaches in real-world environments, such as the pharmacy, doctors' offices, and the home.
Interventions to Support Occupation	• Use a mobile digital device to create reminders for taking medications and getting refills. • Implement cognitive adaptation strategies such as decluttering, moving medications to more visible locations, and posting visual reminders. • Use Motivational Interviewing to increase an individual's readiness to change.
Education and Training	• Provide skills training on going to the pharmacy, reading medication labels, and filling medication pill boxes. • Educate the individual to improve health literacy. • Implement behavioral modification strategies to encourage good adherence to medications. • Engage in caregiver training to develop a social environment in which a family member assists with medication management.
Advocacy	• Empower the person to better communicate with the medical team to describe medication needs and desires. • Advocate to the medical team for a medication routine that is consistent with the individual's abilities and goals. • Work with the person to create a medication list to share between health-care providers.
Group Interventions	• Facilitate group discussion on what medication management and adherence strategies have been beneficial for individuals in the past. • Explore and discuss medication management tools (e.g., pill boxes, electronic device reminders, consistent schedule).
Virtual Interventions	• Explore medication management apps in "live time." Facilitate training in online prescription renewal options.

Being a Psychosocial OT Practitioner

Managing Medications to Facilitate Community Participation

Identifying Psychosocial Strengths and Needs

Marie is a 35-year-old woman with schizophrenia who is receiving outpatient behavioral health services after a recent inpatient admission. Marie's family reached out to their local hospital because of Marie's symptom exacerbation after she stopped taking her medication and subsequently struggled to manage her home by herself. During her time in inpatient behavioral health, Marie's personal goals and occupational therapy care centered on addressing her current symptoms, creating a medication management plan, and exploring past and new leisure activities to promote stress management. Marie is highly motivated to continue engaging in her care plan at her local outpatient clinic and has goals surrounding shopping, money and long-term symptom management.

Using a Holistic Occupational Therapy Approach

Marie's outpatient OTP uses a semistructured interview format guided by the *OTPF* (AOTA, 2020) to complete Marie's initial evaluation and discuss her primary areas of concern and her personal goals pertaining to her ADL and IADL performance.

Marie wants to focus on managing her symptoms and is concerned about how they might impact her ability to engage in the shopping tasks she needs to complete each week. She continues to feel anxious about her medication management plan and has concerns that she will not be able to "stick to" her plan, leading to difficulties being able to manage shopping and home management.

In collaborating with Marie on intervention approaches that target medication management and adherence, the OTP and Marie agree to use a blended approach of CAT and psychoeducation.

First, to better understand where Marie's perceptions regarding her symptom management and medication management are and to initiate self-reflection, Marie's OTP asks her to describe factors across her environment and her personal functioning (cognitive, physical, emotional, social, cultural, etc.) that she feels might challenge her ability to consistently adhere to her medication management plan, subsequently making it difficult to engage in shopping and home management tasks. Marie discusses with her OTP that she has a very busy work schedule and often feels as though she runs out of time to take her medication in the morning (when scheduled); she does not feel comfortable taking her second dose of medication at work; and reports that if she has missed the first two doses during the day, she often questions, "What's the point?" in taking her third dose in the evening. Marie notes that she usually starts to experience negative symptoms, such as nausea, headaches, and anxiety, the day after forgoing taking a dose or multiple doses of her medication. These symptoms make it difficult to engage in her home management and shopping tasks.

Marie wants to use the skills she learned during her inpatient admission regarding medication management (creating written reminders for herself at home to take her medication and using a pill box) but is worried that these may not provide the reinforcement she needs to continue taking her medication. Marie's OTP collaborates with Marie to structure the therapy sessions shown in the following table in addressing Marie's needs.

Session 2 (after initial planning session)	Psychoeducation: Discuss benefits of consistently taking medication, even when a dose is missed. Address distorted cognitions related to taking and missing medication doses. Reframe cognitions (e.g., "Even if I miss a dose, by taking the next dose I am taking care of my health and preventing feeling ill the next day"). Homework: Track distorted cognitions that may occur throughout the week, and note when they are occurring.
Session 3	Create a daily schedule to provide structure and enhance ability to manage medications. Generate acceptable adaptive strategies for medication management during days that may deviate from Marie's normal schedule (packing extra medication using pill sorter for trips, use phone app reminders, etc.). Homework: Establish common place in the home, on Marie's phone, or other space, for visual schedule.
Session 4	Plan for environment adaptations to promote medication management, explore what has worked well as sources of reminders for Marie in the past (e.g., sticky notes, setting timers), and establish ways of removing stressors (e.g., create quiet environments at home and work). Find feasible options for Marie to take her second dose of medication at work (e.g., take a short walk at lunch during which she takes her medication, discreet packaging for medication). Create a graded plan for implementing adaptations (e.g., introducing determined strategies one by one into Marie's schedule). Homework: Implement one reminder or management strategy out of those chosen and report back on the ease of implementation during the next session.

Across each session, Marie and her OTP evaluate Marie's perception of her current medication management and symptoms. They review Marie's homework experiences and the acceptability of the environmental adaptations that Marie is gradually introducing into her daily life. Marie reports that although she continues to experience intrusive thoughts surrounding her symptoms and medication management, being able to identify them in the moment and reframing them has been beneficial. Marie also is finding that gradually introducing medication reminders into her daily schedule and using discreet containers for her medication at work have promoted her ability to consistently take her dosages at the appropriate times.

Within the intervention sessions, the OTP promotes Marie's self-efficacy and autonomy by collaborating with Marie to find adaptations and scheduling strategies that work for Marie. The OTP provides graded feedback to Marie as she creates a personal schedule and determines trial strategies for medication

management. By providing Marie with homework that she can reflect on during the next session (and adjust adaptations if necessary), the OTP is also promoting further opportunities for Marie to exercise autonomous decision-making and creating a safe space for learning through trial and error.

Reflective Questions

1. What additional psychoeducation topics or resources might be beneficial for Marie?
2. What are some ways in which the OTP could address medication management strategies regarding ordering and having prescriptions filled with Marie?
3. How would someone design an intervention that would promote Marie's autonomy and self-efficacy surrounding participating in home management or shopping tasks when experiencing negative stimuli?

Here's the Point

- Every person has a right to have consistent access to, ability in, and safety while engaging in their desired occupations, including ADLs, IADLs, and health management occupations. OTPs have a responsibility and the opportunity to serve, collaborate, and advocate alongside persons with mental health challenges to ensure and uphold these rights.
- ADLs, IADLs, and health management practices are necessary occupations that often require significant cognitive and interpersonal skills.
- Mental health challenges and substance use disorders disrupt typical cognition and emotion, limiting an individual's independence with ADLs and IADLs.
- Occupational therapists have a variety of observational and performance-based tools to help them evaluate a person's ability to complete ADLs and IADLs.

- OTPs have several evidence-based interventions to help persons with mental health challenges or substance use disorders better complete their ADLs, IADLs, and health management occupations.
- Interventions for addressing ADLs, IADLs, and health management routines may target the person, the environment, or the occupation.
- OTPs should collaboratively design the evaluation and intervention plan based on the person's strengths, preferences, and best available evidence to help individuals reach their ADL, IADL, and health management goals.

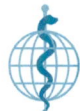

Visit the online resource center at FADavis.com to access the videos.

Apply It Now

1. Administer a Standardized Assessment

Select a performance-based standardized assessment presented in this chapter. Administer the assessment to a peer. Note that the UPSA can be accessed for free here scribd.com /document/577803862/UPSA

Reflective Questions
- How successful were you in your ability to administer the instructions and prompts in the required standardized fashion?
- Create a list of pros and cons describing the benefits and drawbacks of administering a standardized performance-based assessment versus skilled observation of a person completing a similar task. Which method of assessment will you use in the future and why?

2. Develop and Implement a Skills Training Intervention

Partner up with a peer. Identify a skill in which you have expertise, but your peer wants to learn (e.g., using chopsticks, origami, or a new social dance).

- Complete an activity analysis of the selected skill.
- Using the skills training approach described in this chapter, teach your peer to complete the new skill.

Reflective Questions

- How well was your peer able to complete the selected activity?
- What would you do differently next time to help your peer better master the skill?

3. Create an Intervention Plan

Imagine that you are working with a person with schizophrenia in their home. Ask the person to take a few pictures of

their kitchen/cooking space. Suppose the individual has a goal to be independent in cooking meals. How can you use the photos to assess the person's environment? What kinds of changes in their cooking environment might facilitate successful performance in cooking?

4. Create an Educational Handout Describing Compensatory Technology

Select a complex daily living activity such as grocery shopping, cooking, or taking medication. Create an educational handout describing different technologies (apps, assistive devices, low-tech solutions, etc.) that persons with mental health challenges can use to compensate for impairments and improve their performance of the selected IADL.

5. Video Exercise: Life Skills Groups in an Unhoused Population

Pair up with another student in your class or form a small group of students. Access and watch the "Life Skills Groups in an Unhoused Population" video at the online resource center at FADavis.com. Then, discuss and together answer the following questions.

Reflective Questions
- Kailin explains that the experience of homelessness disrupts nearly every occupation individuals engage in, from hygiene to organizing one's belongings to maintaining healthy relationships to taking public transportation. In what other settings and with what other populations might you encounter similar challenges to performing ADLs/IADLs?
- Kailin gives some examples of activities she uses in her life skills group that promote active learning. Identify another area of occupation not discussed by Kailin and provide an activity you could use that is relevant and easy to implement in this setting.

■ Kailin approaches the individuals in her life skills group openly and intentionally to "meet them where they truly are." What do you think that approach looks like, and why do you think it is successful in the life skills group?

■ Kailin found that addressing life skills in a group setting encouraged peer support opportunities. Why is peer support so crucial in this setting and with the unhoused population?

■ Why is it important for Kailin to take a collaborator role in her life skills group rather than the role as group leader? What does this allow for, and how does it better support the individuals in the group and increase their sense of autonomy?

Resources

Books

- Asher, I. E. (2014). *Occupational therapy assessment tools: An annotated index* (4th ed.). American Occupational Therapy Association.
- Frank, E. (2007). *Treating bipolar disorder: A clinician's guide to interpersonal and social rhythm therapy* (2nd ed.). Guilford Press.
- Thomson, L. K., & Robnett, R. (2016). *The Kohlman Evaluation of Living Skills* (4th ed.). American Occupational Therapy Association.
- Wallace, C. J., Liberman, R. P., Tauber, R., & Wallace, J. (2000). The Independent Living Skills Survey: A comprehensive measure of the community functioning of severely and persistently mentally ill individuals. *Schizophrenia Bulletin, 26,* 631–658. The actual instrument is appended to the article.

Websites and Articles

- Continuity Assessment Record and Evaluation Tool: https://www.cms.gov/Medicare/Quality-Initiatives-Patient-Assessment-Instruments/Post-Acute-Care-Quality-Initiatives/CARE-Item-Set-and-B-CARE
- Happify App. An evidence-based application to help people change negative cognition thinking patterns: https://www.happify.com
- Life Skills Support Group Curriculum for Los Angeles County: http://file.lacounty.gov/dmh/cms1_171974.pdf
- Pediatric Evaluation of Disability Inventory (PEDI): https://www.pearsonclinical.com/childhood/products/100000505/pediatric-evaluation-of-disability-inventory-pedi.html
- Rehabilitation Measures Database: rehabmeasures.org
- Transportation—American Occupational Therapy Association's Driving and Community Mobility Toolkit: https://www.aota.org/practice/clinical-topics/driving-community-mobility
- Transportation—Association for Driving Rehabilitation Specialists, 109 West St., Edgerton, WI 53534. 608-884-8833: www.driver-ed.org
- Transportation—Betz, M. E., Dickerson, A., Coolman, T., Davis, E. S., Jones, J., & Schwartz, R. (2014). Driving rehabilitation programs for older drivers in the United States. *Occupational Therapy in Health Care, 28*(3), 306–317. https://doi.org/10.3109/07380577.2014.908336

Videos

- Barthel Index: https://www.youtube.com/watch?v=03IsiYJSk0o
- Continuity Assessment Record and Evaluation Tool: https://www.youtube.com/watch?v=3CH0-VuBfhE
- "Cooking Group in a State Mental Hospital" video. In this video, occupational therapist Samuel Gentile describes an extremely meaningful therapeutic group he runs in a state mental hospital. Samuel's weekly cooking group allows him to assess individuals' occupational performance and physical health, as well as help them develop functional skills. He shares why the experience is so powerful for the hospital residents and what it has taught him as an OTP. Access the video at the online resource center at FADavis.com.

- Katz Index of Independence in Activities of Daily Living Scale: https://www.youtube.com/watch?v=aPLt9OjwFTk
- Kitchen Skills Sample Client Video: https://www.youtube.com/watch?v=dpJMByxf0SM&t=1s
- Kohlman Evaluation of Living Skills (4th ed.): https://www.youtube.com/watch?v=WJ7r2eNBsgo and https://www.youtube.com/watch?v=zpMPxCmvlRI
- The Test of Grocery Shopping Skills: https://www.youtube.com/watch?v=JQfIttM3p1c

References

Achterberg, W. P., Pieper, M. J., van Dalen-Kok, A. H., de Waal, M. W., Husebo, B. S., Lautenbacher, S., Kunz, M., Scherder, E. J., & Corbett, A. (2013). Pain management in patients with dementia. *Clinical Interventions in Aging, 8,* 1471–1482. https://doi.org/10.2147/CIA.S36739

American Occupational Therapy Association. (2020). Occupational therapy practice framework: Domain and process—Fourth edition. *The American Journal of Occupational Therapy, 74*(Suppl. 2), 7412410010p1–7412410010p87. https://doi.org/10.5014/ajot.2020.74S2001

Aniserowicz, A. M., Safi, F., Colquhoun, H., Stier, J., & Nowrouzi-Kia, B. (2022). Developing a profile of activities of daily living for bipolar disorder: A systematic review protocol and meta-analysis. *BMJ Open, 12*(5), e058783. https://doi.org/10.1136/bmjopen-2021-058783

Baum, C., & Edwards, D. F. (1993). Cognitive performance in senile dementia of the Alzheimer's type: The Kitchen Task Assessment. *American Journal of Occupational Therapy, 47*(5), 431–436. https://doi.org/10.5014/ajot.47.5.431

Baune, B. T., Miller, R., McAfoose, J., Johnson, M., Quirk, F., & Mitchell, D. (2010). The role of cognitive impairment in general functioning in major depression. *Psychiatry Research, 176*(2–3), 183–189. https://doi.org/10.1016/j.psychres.2008.12.001

Bennett, J. M., Chekaluk, E., & Batchelor, J. (2016). Cognitive tests and determining fitness to drive in dementia: A systematic review. *Journal of the American Geriatrics Society, 64*(9), 1904–1917. https://doi.org/10.1111/jgs.14180

Ben-Zeev, D., Brian, R. M., Jonathan, G., Razzano, L., Pashka, N., Carpenter-Song, E., Drake, R. E., & Scherer, E. A. (2018). Mobile health (mHealth) versus clinic-based group intervention for people with serious mental illness: A randomized controlled trial. *Psychiatric Services, 69*(9), 978–985. https://doi.org/10.1176/appi.ps.201800063

Ben-Zeev, D., Davis, K. E., Kaiser, S., Krzsos, I., & Drake, R. E. (2013). Mobile technologies among people with serious mental illness: Opportunities for future services. *Administration and Policy in Mental Health and Mental Health Services Research, 40*(4), 340–343. https://doi.org/10.1007/s10488-012-0424-x

Berg, C., Edwards, D. F., & King, A. (2012). Executive function performance on the Children's Kitchen Task Assessment with children with sickle cell disease and matched controls. *Child Neuropsychology, 18*(5), 432–448. https://doi.org/10.1080/09297049.2011.613813

Berndt, A. H., May, E., & Darzins, P. (2015). On-road driving assessment and route design for drivers with dementia. *The British*

Journal of Occupational Therapy, 78(2), 121–130. https://doi.org/10.1177/0308022614562397

Biddiscombe, R. J., Scanlan, J. N., Ross, J., Horsfield, S., Aradas, J., & Hart, S. (2018). Exploring the perceived usefulness of practical food groups in day treatment for individuals with eating disorders. *Australian Occupational Therapy Journal, 65*(2), 98–106. https://doi.org/10.1111/1440-1630.12442

Black, R. A., Rounsaville, B. J., Rosenheck, R. A., Conrad, K. J., Ball, S. A., & Rosen, M. I. (2008). Measuring money mismanagement among dually diagnosed clients. *The Journal of Nervous and Mental Disease, 196*(7), 576–579. https://doi.org/10.1097/NMD.0b013e31817d0535

Bogomolova, S., Zarnowiecki, D., Wilson, A., Fielder, A., Procter, N., Itsiopoulos, C., O'Dea, K., Strachan, J., Ballestrin, M., Champion, A., & Parletta, N. (2016). Dietary intervention for people with mental illness in South Australia. *Health Promotion International, 33*, 71–83. https://doi.org/10.1093/heapro/daw055

Borillo, R. (2019). *Development of a financial literacy component for a comprehensive secondary transition program for diploma-bound students with learning differences* [Doctoral project]. University of St. Augustine for Health Sciences. SOAR@USA: Student Capstone Projects Collection. https://doi.org/10.46409/sr.EOUY4396

Boulton, E. (2020). 'One dead bedroom': Exploring the impact of obsessive-compulsive disorder (OCD) on women's lived experience of sex and sexuality [Doctoral dissertation]. University of the West of England. https://uwe-repository.worktribe.com/output/1906784

Bowie, C. R., Reichenberg, A., Patterson, T. L., Heaton, R. K., & Harvey, P. D. (2006). Determinants of real-world functional performance in schizophrenia subjects: Correlations with cognition, functional capacity, and symptoms. *American Journal of Psychiatry, 163*(3), 418–425. https://doi.org/10.1176/appi.ajp.163.3.418

Bradford, R., Holliday, M., Schultz, A., & Moser, C. (2015). The role of the occupational therapist in the treatment of children with eating disorders. *Journal of Occupational Therapy, Schools, & Early Intervention, 8*(3), 196–210. https://doi.org/10.1080/19411243.2015.1077053

Brenes, G. A., Guralnik, J. M., Williamson, J. D., Fried, L. P., Simpson, C., Simonsick, E. M., & Penninx, B. W. J. H. (2005). The influence of anxiety on the progression of disability. *Journal of the American Geriatrics Society, 53*(1), 34–39. https://doi.org/10.1111/j.1532-5415.2005.53007.x

Brijnath, B., & Antoniades, J. (2016). "I'm running my depression:" Self-management of depression in neoliberal Australia. *Social Science & Medicine, 152*, 1–8. https://doi.org/10.1016/j.socscimed.2016.01.022

Brown, C. (2012). *Occupational therapy practice guidelines for adults with serious mental illness.* American Occupational Therapy Association.

Brown, C., Rempfer, M., & Hamera, E. (2002). Teaching grocery shopping skills to people with schizophrenia. *OTJR: Occupational Therapy Journal of Research, 22*(1 Suppl.), 90S–91S. https://doi.org/10.1177/15394492020220S117

Brown, C. E., Rempfer, M. V., & Hamera, E. (2009). *Test of Grocery Shopping Skills.* AOTA Press.

Brunnauer, A., Herpich, F., Zwanzger, P., & Laux, G. (2021). Driving performance under treatment of most frequently prescribed drugs for mental disorders: A systematic review of patient studies. *International Journal of Neuropsychopharmacology, 24*(9), 679–693. https://doi.org/10.1093/ijnp/pyab031

Buckley, P., Foster, A. E., Patel, N. C., & Wermert, A. (2009). *Adherence to mental health treatment.* Oxford University Press.

Bullock, A., & Bannigan, K. (2011). Effectiveness of activity-based group work in community mental health: A systematic review. *American Journal of Occupational Therapy, 65*(3), 257–266. https://doi.org/10.5014/ajot.2011.001305

Burns, M. N., Begale, M., Duffecy, J., Gergle, D., Karr, C. J., Giangrande, E., & Mohr, D. C. (2011). Harnessing context sensing to develop a mobile intervention for depression. *Journal of Medical Internet Research, 13*(3), e55. https://doi.org/10.2196/jmir.1838

Cahill, S. M., Egan, B. E., & Seber, J. (2020). Activity- and occupation-based interventions to support mental health, positive behavior, and social participation for children and youth: A systematic review. *The American Journal of Occupational Therapy, 74*(2), 7402180020p1–7402180020p28. https://doi.org/10.5014/ajot.2020.038687

Carey, A., Burton, C., Grochulski, A., Pinay, P., & Remillard, A. (2018). Development of the Saskatchewan Psychiatric Occupational Therapy Driving Screen. *British Journal of Occupational Therapy, 81*(4), 187–195. https://doi.org/10.1177/0308022617752065

Centers for Medicare & Medicaid Services. (2021). *CARE Item Set and B-CARE.* https://www.cms.gov/Medicare/Quality-Initiatives-Patient-Assessment-Instruments/Post-Acute-Care-Quality-Initiatives/CARE-Item-Set-and-B-CARE

Chan, P. A., & Rabinowitz, T. (2006). A cross-sectional analysis of video games and attention deficit hyperactivity disorder symptoms in adolescents. *Annals of General Psychiatry, 5*(1), 16. https://doi.org/10.1186/1744-859X-5-16

Chee, Y. K., Gitlin, L. N., Dennis, M. P., & Hauck, W. W. (2007). Predictors of adherence to a skill-building intervention in dementia caregivers. *Journals of Gerontology: Series A, Biological Sciences and Medical Sciences, 62*(6), 673–678. https://doi.org/10.1093/gerona/62.6.673

Chisholm, D., Toto, P., Raina, K., Holm, M., & Rogers, J. (2014). Evaluating capacity to live independently and safely in the community: Performance Assessment of Self-Care Skills. *The British Journal of Occupational Therapy, 77*(2), 59–63. https://doi.org/10.4276/030802214X13916969447038

Ciro, C. A. (2014). Maximizing ADL performance to facilitate aging in place for people with dementia. *Nursing Clinics of North America, 49*(2), 157–169. https://doi.org/10.1016/j.cnur.2014.02.004

Clave-Brule, M., Mazloum, A., Park, R. J., Harbottle, E. J., & Birmingham, C. L. (2009). Managing anxiety in eating disorders with knitting. *Eating and Weight Disorders: EWD, 14*(1), e1–e5. https://doi.org/10.1007/BF03354620

Clement, J. (2022). *Number of video gamers worldwide by region 2021.* Statista. https://www.statista.com/statistics/293304/number-video-gamers

Cloete, L. G., & Ramugondo, E. L. (2015). "I drink": Mothers' alcohol consumption as both individualised and imposed occupation. *South African Journal of Occupational Therapy, 45*(1), 34–40. https://doi.org/10.17159/2310-3833/2015/v45no1a6

Corbett, A., Husebo, B., Malcangio, M., Staniland, A., Cohen-Mansfield, J., Aarsland, D., & Ballard, C. (2012). Assessment and treatment of pain in people with dementia. *Nature Reviews Neurology, 8*(5), 264–274. https://doi.org/10.1038/nrneurol.2012.53

Cukor, J., Gerardi, M., Alley, S., Reist, C., Roy, M., Rothbaum, B. O., Difede, J., & Rizzo, A. (2015). Virtual reality exposure therapy for combat-related PTSD. In E. C. Ritchie (Ed.), *Posttraumatic stress disorder and related diseases in combat veterans* (pp. 69–83). Springer. https://doi.org/10.1007/978-3-319-22985-0_7

Curry, N. A., & Kasser, T. (2005). Can coloring mandalas reduce anxiety? *Art Therapy, 22*(2), 81–85. https://doi.org/10.1080/07421656.2005.10129441

D'Amico, M. L., Jaffe, L. E., & Gardner, J. A. (2018). Evidence for interventions to improve and maintain occupational performance and participation for people with serious mental illness: A systematic review. *The American Journal of Occupational Therapy, 72*(5), 7205190020p1–7205190020p11. https://doi.org/10.5014/ajot.2018.033332

Delva, F., Touraine, C., Joly, P., Edjolo, A., Amieva, H., Berr, C., Rouaud, O., Helmer, C., Pérès, K., & Dartigues, J. F. (2016). ADL disability and death in dementia in a French population-based cohort: New insights with an illness-death model. *Alzheimer's & Dementia, 12*, 909–916. https://doi.org/10.1016/j.jalz.2016.03.007

Donker, T., Petrie, K., Proudfoot, J., Clarke, J., Birch, M.-R., & Christensen, H. (2013). Smartphones for smarter delivery of mental health programs: A systematic review. *Journal of Medical Internet Research, 15*(11), e247. https://doi.org/10.2196/jmir.2791

Dumas, H. M., Fragala-Pinkham, M. A., Haley, S. M., Ni, P., Coster, W., Kramer, J. M., Kao, Y. C., Moed, R., & Ludlow, L. H. (2012). Computer adaptive test performance in children with and without disabilities: Prospective field study of the PEDI-CAT. *Disability and Rehabilitation, 34*(5), 393–401. https://doi.org/10.3109/09638288.2011.607217

Dumas, H. M., Fragala-Pinkham, M. A., Rosen, E. L., Lombard, K. A., & Farrell, C. (2015). Pediatric Evaluation of Disability Inventory Computer Adaptive Test (PEDI-CAT) and Alberta Infant Motor Scale (AIMS): Validity and responsiveness. *Physical Therapy, 95*(11), 1559–1568. https://doi.org/10.2522/ptj.20140339

Dumas, H. M., Fragala-Pinkham, M. A., Rosen, E. L., & O'Brien, J. E. (2016). Construct validity of the Pediatric Evaluation of Disability Inventory Computer Adaptive Test (PEDI-CAT) in children with medical complexity. *Disability and Rehabilitation, 39*, 2446–2451. https://doi.org/10.1080/09638288.2016.1226406

Dun, C., Baker, K., Swan, J., Vlachou, V., & Fossey, E. (2015). "Drive Safe" initiatives: An analysis of improvements in mental health practices (2005–2013) to support safe driving. *British Journal of Occupational Therapy, 78*(6), 364–368. https://doi.org/10.1177/0308022614562785

Duncombe, L. W. (2004). Comparing learning of cooking in home and clinic for people with schizophrenia. *American Journal of Occupational Therapy, 58*(3), 272–278. https://doi.org/10.5014/ajot.58.3.272

Eckman, T. A., Wirshing, W. C., Marder, S. R., Liberman, R. P., Johnston-Cronk, K., Zimmermann, K., & Mintz, J. (1992). Technique for training schizophrenic patients in illness self-management: A controlled trial. *American Journal of Psychiatry, 149*(11), 1549–1555. https://doi.org/10.1176/ajp.149.11.1549

Eklund, M. (2009). Work status, daily activities and quality of life among people with severe mental illness. *Quality of Life Research, 18*(2), 163–170. https://doi.org/10.1007/s11136-008-9431-5

Elbogen, E. B., Hamer, R. M., Swanson, J. W., & Swartz, M. S. (2016). A randomized clinical trial of a money management intervention for veterans with psychiatric disabilities. *Psychiatric Services, 67*(10), 1142–1145. https://doi.org/10.1176/appi.ps.201500203

Elbogen, E. B., Sullivan, C. P., Wolfe, J., Wagner, H. R., & Beckham, J. C. (2013). Homelessness and money mismanagement in Iraq and Afghanistan veterans. *American Journal of Public Health, 103*(Suppl. 2), S248–S254. https://doi.org/10.2105/AJPH.2013.301335

Elbogen, E. B., Tiegreen, J., Vaughan, C., & Bradford, D. W. (2011). Money management, mental health, and psychiatric disability: A recovery-oriented model for improving financial skills. *Psychiatric Rehabilitation Journal, 34*(3), 223–231. https://doi.org/10.2975/34.3.2011.223.231

Entertainment Software Association. (2022). *Essential facts about video game industry.* https://www.theesa.com/resource/2022-essential-facts-about-the-video-game-industry

Evans, V. C., Iverson, G. L., Yatham, L. N., & Lam, R. W. (2014). The relationship between neurocognitive and psychosocial functioning in major depressive disorder. *The Journal of Clinical Psychiatry, 75*(12), 1359–1370. https://doi.org/10.4088/JCP.13r08939

Fauth, E. B., Schwartz, S., Tschanz, J. T., Østbye, T., Corcoran, C., & Norton, M. C. (2013). Baseline disability in activities of daily living predicts dementia risk even after controlling for baseline global cognitive ability and depressive symptoms. *International Journal of Geriatric Psychiatry, 28*(6), 597–606. https://doi.org/10.1002/gps.3865

Federal Communications Commission. (2016). *Lifeline: Affordable telephone services for income-eligible subscribers.* Author. https://www.fcc.gov/lifeline-consumers

Fieo, R., Zahodne, L., Tang, M. X., Manly, J. J., Cohen, R., & Stern, Y. (2018). The historical progression from ADL scrutiny to IADL to advanced ADL: Assessing functional status in the earliest stages of dementia. *Journals of Gerontology: Series A, Biological Sciences and Medical Sciences, 73*(12), 1695–1700. https://doi.org/10.1093/gerona/glx235

Fishman, M. (2002). Treatment of HIV and addiction: Preserving therapeutic optimism. *Advanced Studies in Medicine, 2,* 189–194.

Gardner, J., Rodar, S., Ben-Baruch, M., Beronio, A., Malinak, J., Pignataro, L., Swarbrick, M., & Olker, S. (2019). Impacts of financial management programs for adults with substance-use and mental-health disorders. *The American Journal of Occupational Therapy, 73*(4 Suppl. 1), 7311520388p1. https://doi.org/10.5014/ajot.2019.73S1-PO2028

Geda, Y. E., Topazian, H. M., Roberts, L. A., Lewis, R. A., Roberts, R. O., Knopman, D. S., Pankratz, V. S., Christianson, T. J. H., Boeve, B. F., Tangaloes, E. G., Ivnik, R. J., & Petersen, R. C. (2011). Engaging in cognitive activities, aging, and mild cognitive impairment: A population-based study. *The Journal of Neuropsychiatry and Clinical Neurosciences, 23*(2), 149–154. https://doi.org/10.1176/jnp.23.2.jnp149

Gentry, T., Wallace, J., Kvarfordt, C., & Lynch, K. B. (2008). Personal digital assistants as cognitive aids for individuals with severe traumatic brain injury: A community-based trial. *Brain Injury, 22*(1), 19–24. https://doi.org/10.1080/02699050701810688

Gentry, T., Wallace, J., Kvarfordt, C., & Lynch, K. B. (2010). Personal digital assistants as cognitive aids for high school students with autism: Results of a community-based trial. *Journal of Vocational Rehabilitation, 32*(2), 101–107. https://doi.org/10.3233/JVR-2010-0499

Giebel, C. M., Sutcliffe, C., Stolt, M., Karlsson, S., Renom-Guiteras, A., Soto, M., Verbeek, H., Zabalegui, A., & Orrell, M. (2014). Deterioration of basic activities of daily living and their impact on quality of life across different cognitive stages of dementia: A European study. *International Psychogeriatrics, 26*(8), 1283–1293. https://doi.org/10.1017/S1041610214000775

Gitlin, L. N., Corcoran, M., Winter, L., Boyce, A., & Hauck, W. W. (2001). A randomized, controlled trial of a home environmental intervention: Effect on efficacy and upset in caregivers and on daily function of persons with dementia. *The Gerontologist, 41*(1), 4–14. https://doi.org/10.1093/geront/41.1.4

Gitlin, L. N., Corcoran, M., Winter, L., Boyce, A., & Marcus, S. (1999). Predicting participation and adherence to a home environmental intervention among family caregivers of persons with dementia. *Family Relations, 48*(4), 363. https://doi.org/10.2307/585243

Gitlin, L. N., Winter, L., Corcoran, M., Dennis, M. P., Schinfeld, S., & Hauck, W. W. (2003). Effects of the Home Environmental Skill-Building Program on the caregiver-care recipient dyad: 6-month outcomes from the Philadelphia REACH Initiative. *The Gerontologist, 43*(4), 532–546. https://doi.org/10.1093/geront/43.4.532

Gonzalez-Pinto, A., Mosquera, F., Alonso, M., López, P., Ramírez, F., Vieta, E., & Baldessarini, R. J. (2006). Suicidal risk in bipolar I disorder patients and adherence to long-term lithium treatment. *Bipolar Disorders, 8*(5 Pt. 2), 618–624. https://doi.org/10.1111/j.1399-5618.2006.00368.x

Grassi, A., Gaggiolo, A., & Riva, G. (2010). New technologies to manage exam anxiety. *Studies in Health Technology and Informatics, 167,* 57–62.

Haley, S. M., & Coster, W. J. (2010). *Development, standardization and administration manual. PEDI-CAT.* CRECare, LLC.

Hamera, E., & Brown, C. E. (2000). Developing a context-based performance measure for persons with schizophrenia: The Test of Grocery Shopping Skills. *American Journal of Occupational Therapy, 54,* 20–25. https://doi.org/10.5014/ajot.54.1.20

Hamera, E. K., Brown, C., Rempfer, M., & Davis, N. C. (2002). Test of Grocery Shopping Skills: Discrimination of people with and without mental illness. *Psychiatric Rehabilitation Skills, 6*(3), 296–311. https://doi.org/10.1080/10973430208408440

Hansen, J. P., Østergaard, B., Nordentoft, M., & Hounsgaard, L. (2012). Cognitive Adaptation Training combined with assertive community treatment: A randomised longitudinal trial. *Schizophrenia Research, 135*(1), 105–111. https://doi.org/10.1016/j.schres.2011.12.014

Haynes, P. L., Gengler, D., & Kelly, M. (2016). Social rhythm therapies for mood disorders: An update. *Current Psychiatry Reports, 18*(8), 75. https://doi.org/10.1007/s11920-016-0712-3

Heinrich, H., Gevensleben, H., & Strehl, U. (2007). Annotation: Neurofeedback—Train your brain to train behaviour. *Journal of Child Psychology and Psychiatry, 48,* 3–16. https://doi.org/10.1111/j.1469-7610.2006.01665.x

Hinojosa, J., Kramer, P., & Crist, P. (2014). Evaluation: Where do we begin? In J. Hinojosa & P. Kramer (Eds.), *Evaluation in occupational therapy: Obtaining and interpreting data* (4th ed., pp. 1–18). AOTA Press.

Hlastala, S. A., Kotler, J. S., McClellan, J. M., & McCauley, E. A. (2010). Interpersonal and Social Rhythm Therapy for adolescents with bipolar disorder: Treatment development and results from an open trial. *Depression and Anxiety, 27*(5), 457–464. https://doi.org/10.1002/da.20668

Holm, M. B., & Rogers, J. C. (2008). The Performance Assessment of Self-Care Skills (PASS). In B. J. Hemphill-Pearson (Ed.), *Assessments in occupational therapy mental health: An integrative approach* (2nd ed., pp. 101–112). Slack, Inc.

Holmes, E. P., Corrigan, P. W., Knight, S., & Flaxman, J. (1995). Development of a sleep management program for people with severe mental illness. *Psychiatric Rehabilitation Journal, 19*(2), 9–15. https://doi.org/10.1037/h0095445

Hsieh, Y. W., Wang, C. H., Wu, S. C., Chen, P. C., Sheu, C. F., & Hsieh, C. L. (2007). Establishing the minimal clinically important difference of the Barthel Index in stroke patients. *Neurorehabilitation and Neural Repair, 21*(3), 233–238. https://doi.org/10.1177/1545968306294729

Hsueh, I. P., Lee, M. M., & Hsieh, C. L. (2001). Psychometric characteristics of the Barthel Activities of Daily Living Index in stroke patients. *Journal of the Formosan Medical Association Taiwan Yi Zhi, 100*(8), 526–532.

Ibrahim, J. E., Anderson, L. J., MacPhail, A., Lovell, J. J., Davis, M.-C., & Winbolt, M. (2017). Chronic disease self-management support for persons with dementia, in a clinical setting. *Journal of Multidisciplinary Healthcare, 10,* 49–58. https://doi.org/10.2147/JMDH.S121626

Juniper, A. R., & Connor, L. T. (2022). Self-perceived ADL/IADL function is influenced by residual neurological impairment, aphasia, and anxiety. *Canadian Journal of Occupational Therapy, 89*(3), 307–314. https://doi.org/10.1177/00084174221098876

Katz, S. (1983). Assessing self-maintenance: Activities of daily living, mobility, and instrumental activities of daily living. *Journal of the American Geriatrics Society, 31*(12), 721–727. https://doi.org/10.1111/j.1532-5415.1983.tb03391.x

Kauer, S. D., Reid, S. C., Crooke, A. H. D., Khor, A., Hearps, S. J. C., Jorm, A. F., Sanci, L., & Patton, G. (2012). Self-monitoring using mobile phones in the early stages of adolescent depression: Randomized controlled trial. *Journal of Medical Internet Research, 14*(3), e67. https://doi.org/10.2196/jmir.1858

Keyes, C., Nolte, L., & Williams, T. I. (2018). The battle of living with obsessive compulsive disorder: A qualitative study of young people's experiences. *Child & Adolescent Mental Health, 23*(3), 177–184. https://doi.org/10.1111/camh.12216

Leonardelli, C. (1988). *The Milwaukee Evaluation of Daily Living Skills: Evaluation in long term psychiatric care.* Slack, Inc.

Leucht, S., Hierl, S., Kissling, W., Dold, M., & Davis, J. M. (2012). Putting the efficacy of psychiatric and general medicine medication into perspective: Review of meta-analyses. *British Journal of Psychiatry, 200*(2), 97–106. https://doi.org/10.1192/bjp.bp.111.096594

Liberman, R. P., Mueser, K. T., Wallace, C. J., Jacobs, H. E., Eckman, T., & Massel, H. K. (1986). Training skills in the psychiatrically disabled: Learning coping and competence. *Schizophrenia Bulletin, 12*(4), 631–647. https://doi.org/10.1093/schbul/12.4.631

Liberman, R. P., Wallace, C. J., Blackwell, G., Kopelowicz, A., Vaccaro, J. V., & Mintz, J. (1998). Skills training versus psychosocial occupational therapy for persons with persistent schizophrenia. *American Journal of Psychiatry, 155,* 1087–1091. https://doi.org/10.1176/ajp.155.8.1087

Lipskaya, L., Jarus, T., & Kotler, M. (2011). Influence of cognition and symptoms of schizophrenia on IADL performance. *Scandinavian Journal of Occupational Therapy, 18*(3), 180–187. https://doi.org/10.3109/11038128.2010.490879

Lloyd, C., Waghorn, G., & Williams, P. L. (2008). Conceptualising recovery in mental health rehabilitation. *The British Journal of Occupational Therapy, 71*(8), 321–328. https://doi.org/10.1177/030802260807100804

Lock, L., Williams, H., Bamford, B., & Lacey, J. H. (2012). The St George's eating disorders service meal preparation group for inpatients and day patients pursuing full recovery: A pilot study. *European Eating Disorders Review: The Journal of the Eating Disorders Association, 20*(3), 218–224. https://doi.org/10.1002/erv.1134

Mahoney, F. I., & Barthel, D. W. (1965). Functional evaluation: The Barthel Index. *Maryland State Medical Journal, 14,* 61–65.

Malbos, E., Rapee, R. M., & Kavakli, M. (2013). Creation of interactive virtual environments for exposure therapy through game-level editors: Comparison and tests on presence and anxiety. *International Journal of Human-Computer Interaction, 29*(12), 827–837. https://doi.org/10.1080/10447318.2013.796438

Mausbach, B. T., Bowie, C. R., Harvey, P. D., Twamley, E. W., Goldman, S. R., Jeste, D. V., & Patterson, T. L. (2008). Usefulness of the UCSD Performance-Based Skills Assessment (UPSA) for predicting residential independence in patients with chronic schizophrenia. *Journal of Psychiatric Research, 42*(4), 320–327. https://doi.org/10.1016/j.jpsychires.2006.12.008

Mojtabai, R., Cullen, B., Everett, A., Nugent, K. L., Sawa, A., Sharifi, V., Takayanagi, V., Toroney, J. S., & Eaton, W. W. (2014). Reasons for not seeking general medical care among individuals with serious mental illness. *Psychiatric Services, 65*(6), 818–821. https://doi.org/10.1176/appi.ps.201300348

Monk, T. K., Flaherty, J. F., Frank, E., Hoskinson, K., & Kupfer, D. J. (1990). The Social Rhythm Metric: An instrument to quantify the daily rhythms of life. *The Journal of Nervous and Mental Disease, 178*(2), 120–126. https://doi.org/10.1097/00005053-199002000-00007

Moon, K., Sobolev, M., & Kane, J. M. (2022). Digital and mobile health technology in collaborative behavioral health care: Scoping review. *JMIR Mental Health, 9*(2), e30810. https://doi.org/10.2196/30810

Moore, K., Merritt, B., & Doble, S. E. (2010). ADL skill profiles across three psychiatric diagnoses. *Scandinavian Journal of Occupational Therapy, 17*(1), 77–85. https://doi.org/10.3109/11038120903165115

Neistadt, M. E. (1992). The Rabideau Kitchen Evaluation—Revised: An assessment of meal preparation skill. *OTJR: Occupational Therapy Journal of Research, 12*(4), 242–255. https://doi.org/10.1177/153944929201200404

Neistadt, M. E. (1994). A meal preparation treatment protocol for adults with brain injury. *American Journal of Occupational Therapy, 48*(5), 431–438. https://doi.org/10.5014/ajot.48.5.431

Olsson, A.-K., Helldin, L., Hjärthag, F., & Norlander, T. (2012). Psychometric properties of a performance-based measurement of functional capacity, the UCSD Performance-Based Skills Assessment—Brief version. *Psychiatry Research, 197*(3), 290–294. https://doi.org/10.1016/j.psychres.2011.11.002

Park, D. C., Lodi-Smith, J., Drew, L., Haber, S., Hebrank, A., Bischof, G. N., & Aamodt, W. (2014). The impact of sustained engagement on cognitive function in older adults: The Synapse Project. *Psychological Science, 25*(1), 103–112. https://doi.org/10.1177/0956797613499592

Patterson, T. L., Goldman, S., McKibbin, C. L., Hughs, T., & Jeste, D. V. (2001). UCSD Performance-Based Skills Assessment: Development of a new measure of everyday functioning for severely mentally ill adults. *Schizophrenia Bulletin, 27*(2), 235–245. https://doi.org/10.1093/oxfordjournals.schbul.a006870

People Incorporated. (2022). *Overcoming barriers to mental health access: Transportation.* https://peopleincorporated.org/overcoming-barriers-to-mental-health-access-transportation

Perivoliotis, D., Granholm, E., & Patterson, T. L. (2004). Psychosocial functioning on the Independent Living Skills Survey in older outpatients with schizophrenia. *Schizophrenia Research, 69*(2–3), 307–316. https://doi.org/10.1016/j.schres.2003.09.012

Pisegna, J., Anderson, S., & Krok-Schoen, J. L. (2022). Occupational therapy interventions to address depressive and anxiety symptoms in the physical disability inpatient rehabilitation setting: A systematic review. *The American Journal of Occupational Therapy, 76*(1), 7601180110. https://doi.org/10.5014/ajot.2022.049068

Rabideau, G. M. (1986). *Two approaches to improving the functional performance of a cognitively impaired head injured adult* [Unpublished master's thesis]. Tufts University.

Rawat, H., Petzer, S. L., & Gurayah, T. (2021). Effects of substance use disorder on women's roles and occupational participation. *South African Journal of Occupational Therapy, 51*(1), 54–62. https://doi.org/10.17159/2310-3833/2021/vol51n1a8

Rizvi, S. L., Dimeff, L. A., Skutch, J., Carroll, D., & Linehan, M. M. (2011). A pilot study of the DBT coach: An interactive mobile phone application for individuals with borderline personality disorder and substance use disorder. *Behavior Therapy, 42*(4), 589–600. https://doi.org/10.1016/j.beth.2011.01.003

Roach, M., Lin, D., Graf, M., Pednekar, P., Chou, J. W., Benson, C., & Doshi, J. A. (2021). Schizophrenia population health management: Perspectives of and lessons learned from population health decision makers. *Journal of Managed Care & Specialty Pharmacy, 27*(10-a Suppl.), S1–S13. https://doi.org/10.18553/jmcp.2021.27.10-a.s1

Rocke, K., Hays, P., Edwards, D., & Berg, C. (2008). Development of a performance assessment of executive function: The Children's Kitchen Task Assessment. *American Journal of Occupational Therapy, 62*(5), 528–537. https://doi.org/10.5014/AJOT.62.5.528

Rosen, M. I., Carroll, K. M., Stefanovics, E., & Rosenheck, R. A. (2009). A randomized controlled trial of a money management-based substance use intervention. *Psychiatric Services (Washington, DC), 60*(4), 498–504. https://doi.org/10.1176/ps.2009.60.4.498

Rouleau, S., Mazer, B., Ménard, I., & Gautier, M. (2010). A survey on driving in clients with mental health disorders. *Occupational Therapy in Mental Health, 26*(1), 85–95. https://doi.org/10.1080/01642120903515318

Schrade, C., Tronsky, L., & Kaiser, D. H. (2011). Physiological effects of mandala making in adults with intellectual disability. *The Arts in Psychotherapy, 38*(2), 109–113. https://doi.org/10.1016/j.aip.2011.01.002

Schwartz, J. (2015). *Development and testing of an occupational therapy intervention to promote medication adherence* [Doctoral dissertation]. University of Wisconsin-Milwaukee. http://dc.uwm.edu/etd/922

Schwartz, J. K., & Smith, R. O. (2016). Intervention promoting medication adherence: A randomized, phase I, small-N study. *American Journal of Occupational Therapy, 70*, 1–11. https://doi.org/10.5014/ajot.2016.021006

Seyedi, M., Mohammadi, A., Nouri, A., & Jamshidi, F. (2016). Examining the reliability and validity of the Milwaukee Evaluation of Daily Living Skills for patients with chronic psychiatric disorders. *International Journal of Humanities and Cultural Studies (IJHCS) ISSN 2356-5926, 1*(1), 2718–2738.

Sharry, J., McDermott, M., & Condron, J. (2003). Relax to win: Treating children with anxiety problems with a biofeedback videogame. *Eisteach, 2*(25), 22–26.

Simpson, E. K., Ramirez, N. M., Branstetter, B., Reed, A., & Lines, E. (2018). Occupational therapy practitioners' perspectives of mental health practices with clients in stroke rehabilitation. *OTJR: Occupational Therapy Journal of Research, 38*(3), 181–189. https://doi.org/10.1177/1539449218759827

Smith, M. K., & Kotake, M. (2000). Recovery from a severe psychiatric disability: Findings of a qualitative study. *Psychiatric Rehabilitation Journal, 24*(2), 149–158. https://doi.org/10.1037/h0095105

Sparnon, J. L., & Hornyak, L. M. (1989). Structured eating experiences in the inpatient treatment of anorexia nervosa. In L. M. Hornyak & E. Baker (Eds.), *Experiential therapies for eating disorders* (pp. 207–233). Guilford Press.

Steardo, L., Luciano, M., Sampogna, G., Zinno, F., Saviano, P., Staltari, F., Segura Garcia, C., De Fazio, P., & Fiorillo, A. (2020). Efficacy of the Interpersonal and Social Rhythm Therapy (IPSRT) in patients with bipolar disorder: Results from a real-world, controlled trial. *Annals of General Psychiatry, 19*(1), 15. https://doi.org/10.1186/s12991-020-00266-7

Substance Abuse and Mental Health Services Administration. (2004). *Getting there: Helping people with mental illness access transportation.* DHHS Pub. No. (SMA)3948. Center for Mental Health Services, U.S. Department of Health and Human Services.

Swartz, H. A., Levenson, J. C., & Frank, E. (2012). Psychotherapy for bipolar II disorder: The role of Interpersonal and Social Rhythm Therapy. *Professional Psychology: Research and Practice, 43*(2), 145–153. https://doi.org/10.1037/a0027671

Thomson, L. K., & Robnett, R. (2016). *The Kohlman Evaluation of Living Skills* (4th ed.). American Occupational Therapy Association.

Unsworth, C. A. (2010). Issues surrounding driving and driver assessment for people with mental health problems. *Mental Health Occupational Therapy, 15*(2), 41–44. https://doi.org/10.1177/1569186119886773

van der Vennet, R., & Serice, S. (2012). Can coloring mandalas reduce anxiety? A replication study. *Art Therapy, 29*(2), 87–92. https://doi.org/10.1080/07421656.2012.680047

Velligan, D. I. (2000). *Cognitive Adaptation Training: The use of compensatory strategies in the psychosocial rehabilitation of patients with schizophrenia.* Manual for therapists. University of Texas Health Science Center at San Antonio, Department of Psychiatry.

Velligan, D. I., & Bow-Thomas, C. C. (2000). Rehab rounds: Two case studies of Cognitive Adaptation Training for outpatients with schizophrenia. *Psychiatric Services, 51*(1), 25–29. https://doi.org/10.1176/ps.51.1.25

Velligan, D. I., Diamond, P. M., Mintz, J., Maples, N., Li, X., Zeber, J., Ereshefsky, L., Lam, Y.-W. F., Castillo, D., & Miller, A. L. (2008). The use of individually tailored environmental supports to improve medication adherence and outcomes in schizophrenia. *Schizophrenia Bulletin, 34*(3), 483–493. https://doi.org/10.1093/schbul/sbm111

Velligan, D. I., Mueller, J., Wang, M., Dicocco, M., Diamond, P. M., Maples, N. J., & Davis, B. (2006). Use of environmental supports among patients with schizophrenia. *Psychiatric Services, 57*(2), 219–224. https://doi.org/10.1176/appi.ps.57.2.219

Villani, D., Grassi, A., Cognetta, C., Cipresso, P., Toniolo, D., & Riva, G. (2012). The effects of a mobile stress management protocol on nurses working with cancer patients: A preliminary controlled study. *Studies in Health Technology and Informatics, 173*, 524–528. https://doi.org/10.3233/978-1-61499-022-2-524

Villani, D., Grassi, A., Cognetta, C., Toniolo, D., Cipresso, P., & Riva, G. (2013). Self-help stress management training through mobile phones: An experience with oncology nurses. *Psychological Services, 10*(3), 315–322. https://doi.org/10.1037/a0026459

Walker, E., Kestler, L., Bollini, A., & Hochman, K. M. (2004). Schizophrenia: Etiology and course. *Annual Review of Psychology, 55*(1), 401–430. https://doi.org/10.1146/annurev.psych.55.090902.141950

Wallace, C. J., Liberman, R. P., Tauber, R., & Wallace, J. (2000). The Independent Living Skills Survey: A comprehensive measure of the community functioning of severely and persistently mentally ill individuals. *Schizophrenia Bulletin, 26*(3), 631–658. https://doi.org/10.1093/oxfordjournals.schbul.a033483

Watts, S., Mackenzie, A., Thomas, C., Griskaitis, A., Mewton, L., Williams, A., & Andrews, G. (2013). CBT for depression: A pilot RCT comparing mobile phone vs. computer. *BMC Psychiatry, 13*(1), 49. https://doi.org/10.1186/1471-244X-13-49

Weerdmeester, J., Rooij, M. M. van Engels, R. C., & Granic, I. (2020). An integrative model for the effectiveness of biofeedback interventions for anxiety regulation: Viewpoint. *Journal of Medical Internet Research, 22*(7), e14958. https://doi.org/10.2196/14958

Whalen, C., Liden, L., Ingersoll, B., Dallaire, E., & Liden, S. (2006). Behavioral improvements associated with computer-assisted instruction for children with developmental disabilities. *The Journal of Speech and Language Pathology–Applied Behavior Analysis, 1*(1), 11–26. https://doi.org/10.1037/h0100182

Whalen, C., Moss, D., Ilan, A. B., Vaupel, M., Fielding, P., Macdonald, K., Cernich, S., & Symon, J. (2010). Efficacy of TeachTown: Basic computer-assisted intervention for the Intensive Comprehensive Autism Program in Los Angeles Unified School District. *Autism: The International Journal of Research and Practice, 14*(3), 179–197. https://doi.org/10.1177/1362361310363282

Wilkinson, N., Ang, R. P., & Goh, D. H. (2008). Online video game therapy for mental health concerns: A review. *The International Journal of Social Psychiatry, 54*(4), 370–382. https://doi.org/10.1177/0020764008091659

World Health Organization. (2003). *Adherence to long-term therapies: Evidence for action.* Author.

Yantz, C. L., Johnson-Greene, D., Higginson, C., & Emmerson, L. (2010). Functional cooking skills and neuropsychological functioning in patients with stroke: An ecological validity study. *Neuropsychological Rehabilitation, 20*(5), 725–738. https://doi.org/10.1080/09602011003765690

Zayat, E., Rempfer, M., Gajewski, B., & Brown, C. E. (2011). Patterns of association between performance in a natural environment and measures of executive function in people with schizophrenia. *Psychiatry Research, 187*(1), 1–5. https://doi.org/10.1016/j.psychres.2010.11.011

Zygmunt, A., Olfson, M., Boyer, C. A., & Mechanic, D. (2002). Interventions to improve medication adherence in schizophrenia. *American Journal of Psychiatry, 159*(10), 1653–1664. https://doi.org/10.1176/appi.ajp.159.10.1653

Student

Rebecca Mannel and Janette Boney

Pursuing educational goals and engaging in all forms of available schooling can be personally and culturally relevant to an individual's mental health. This chapter describes the student role and how occupational therapy practitioners (OTPs) might assist those with lived experience of mental illnesses to pursue educational goals. It defines supported education in a higher education setting, provides an historical overview of this intervention, and describes several examples of research-based outcomes. It also profiles the role of occupational therapy in supported education, occupational therapy–supported education programs, and research on outcomes of these programs.

This chapter also describes a successful occupational therapy–supported education program conducted in a college setting and addresses the wellness model in adult education. Finally, the chapter describes the role of occupational therapy in adult learning and relates it to the *Occupational Therapy Practice Framework: Domain and Process, Fourth Edition* (*OTPF-4;* American Occupational Therapy Association [AOTA], 2020) and Person-Environment-Occupation (PEO) model. It concludes with research that has been completed on effective programs for evidence-based practice.

Overview of the Student Role

The student role transcends the traditional classroom setting and influences occupational performance across the life span. Babies learn through sensory exploration of their environments (American Academy of Pediatrics, 2021). Children, adolescents, and young adults often receive structured instruction in formal learning environments; however, education continues far beyond the classroom. Adults and older adults may choose to broaden their knowledge to prepare for, or change, employment; expand on areas of interest; learn investment strategies in preparation for retirement; or tackle new tasks that may have formerly been the responsibility of a deceased spouse. It has been shown that lifelong learning can support a fulfilling and healthy life (Kondirolli & Sunder, 2022).

Learning requires motivation and self-efficacy (Cronin-Golomb & Bauer, 2023; Schindler & Boney, 2022), areas that are often affected by the presence of mental illness (Abrams, 2022; Khalil et al., 2021). Mental health conditions are increasing on college campuses (Abrams, 2022; Jalaba, 2022). Without proper support, the student role can be affected, resulting in curtailment of desired educational levels. Educational attainment has been shown to be a social determinant of health (Kondirolli & Sunder, 2022; Zajacova &

Lawrence, 2018). OTPs recognize the importance of helping people maintain roles, including student roles, that are part of one's identity, and support future desires (AOTA, 2020). The occupational therapy profession is positioned to address the mental health crises across the life span (Jalaba, 2022).

Because Chapter 37: School Mental Health 🤝 adeptly addresses the student role in the context of the K to 12 school setting, this chapter will focus primarily on the role of the student in higher education and adult learning.

Supported Education in Higher Education

Adult education in mental health practice is most commonly referred to as **supported education**, which is defined as "the provision of individualized, practical support and instruction to assist people with psychiatric disabilities to achieve their educational goals" (Soydan, 2004, p. 227). It is an approach that provides programs and supports to help people access and complete postsecondary education (Ennals et al., 2014; Mueser & Cook, 2012; Substance Abuse and Mental Health Services Administration [SAMHSA], 2011).

Need for Supported Education With the Mental Health Population

Supported education programs are developed to meet the needs of people with the lived experience of mental illness who desire to achieve educational goals but often experience difficulty in achieving these goals (Arbesman & Logsdon, 2011; Rogers et al., 2010). These educational goals include starting, returning, or continuing in postsecondary education. In higher education, Mowbray and colleagues (2005) determined that nearly 4.29 million U.S. residents would have graduated from college if they had not experienced early-onset psychiatric illness. Compared with a 37% withdrawal rate for the general student population, 86% of students with mental illness withdraw from college before completing their degree, and they have lower graduation rates compared with general student norms (Arbesman & Logsdon, 2011; Rogers et al., 2010; Salzer, 2012; Salzer et al., 2008).

The statistics regarding the rate of mental health concerns of current students on campuses continue to grow. Up to one-third of college students reported trouble functioning because of depression. In addition, 39% of students in college experience a significant mental health issue. Every fourth student reported symptoms of depression, and every tenth student reported suicidal thoughts. In fact, suicide is the second leading cause of death among college students, claiming the lives of 1,100 students each year (Active Minds, Inc., 2023; American Psychological Association, 2013; Mackenzie et al., 2011).

In Diane Powers-Foltz Dirette's article, "Disability Services for Students in Postsecondary Education: Opportunities for Occupational Therapy" (2019), she compiled a list of potential roles for OTPs in postsecondary education:

- Develop or consult with transition or orientation programs.
- Teach self-advocacy.
- Teach study skills.
- Teach strategies for cognitive deficits, such as attention and memory.
- Address self-awareness issues and disclosure strategies.
- Teach social skills and self-regulation.
- Consult on the use of assistive technology.
- Provide life skills training.
- Teach time management skills.
- Develop or assist with mentoring or coaching programs.
- Develop support groups for psychosocial skill development (self-esteem and coping skills).
- Consult on needed accessibility—physical, visual, auditory.
- Address accommodation provisions.
- Assist with guidelines for service animals (Isaacson, 2013).
- Teach job-seeking and employment skills.
- Provide faculty training, disability education, and brain behavior relationships.
- Develop an inclusive culture and address perceptions and attitudes.
- Address stigma reduction.
- Provide training in universal design for learning (UDL).

- Serve as a consultant to disability services for students (DSS).
- Form a DSS advisory committee with members from the faculty, staff, and students (Dirette, 2019).

Another growing population of students with mental health concerns is student veterans (see Chapter 43: Serving Veterans and Service Members 🤝). Several perspectives of student veterans have to do with the tremendous differences between military and student civilian life, as noted in the PhotoVoice, the Blur, and in this chapter's The Lived Experience feature. In their most recent findings, the National Center for Education Statistics (2022) reported that approximately 26% of all undergraduates and about 17% of all graduate students were veterans or military service members. An American Council on Education (ACE) report by McBain and colleagues (2012) indicated that, although more than 500,000 veterans have enrolled in postsecondary education since 2009, graduation rates remain low (Cate, 2014).

The influx of young adult veterans with mental health challenges returning from recent wars, including Operation Enduring Freedom (OEF) and Operation Iraqi Freedom (OIF), and the low graduation rates have highlighted the need for supported education services (Ellison et al., 2012). This Lived Experience feature from Groovy's perspective provides a look at his role as it expanded from his own mental health to assisting all student veterans on his campus through the Military and Veteran Resource Center.

Students Who Benefit From Supported Education

The typical onset of psychiatric illness commonly occurs between late adolescence and early adulthood. This timing frequently disrupts entrance into and continuation of successful

PhotoVoice

Josh Collier: The Blur

The picture here is in the main lobby of the University of Wisconsin-Milwaukee. In this lobby there are posters displayed of all the different events, colleges, and groups the university has to offer. As a new veteran student it was difficult to focus. I was not in my element anymore. The structured environment of the military was a stark contrast to college life. In the military if you wanted to accomplish a task there was a definitive list of steps to take to accomplish that task and a chain of command to direct your every move. I always felt claustrophobic with the amount of control I didn't have over my life in the military, like I was crawling through a cave that had only one path to traverse. The college experience is completely different. It is like running through an open field, with hundreds of thousands of options and an abundance of free will. I was overwhelmed by the sheer amount of choices before me and things became blurry.

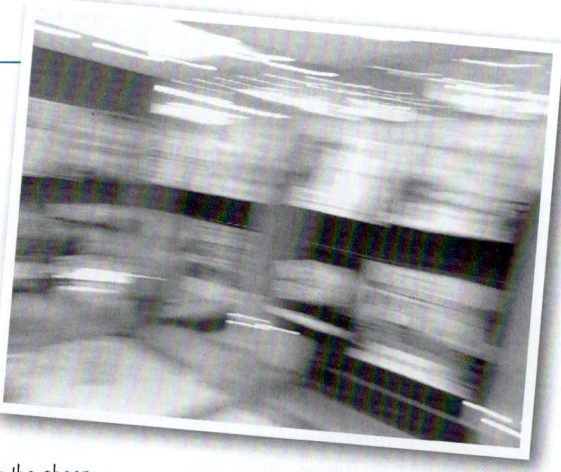

I tried to focus on what I wanted to accomplish in college to find the route I wanted to take. I came to college with a broad goal to have a career where I could help people. I wanted to grasp that feeling of knowing that I made the world a better place no matter however slight my impact. To do this I had to focus and narrow down the paths in front of me.

What aspects of the university environment can be complex for persons struggling with transition or recovery?

The Lived Experience

Student Veteran Entering Higher Education

This story demonstrates how the use of counseling (through the Veterans Administration [VA] and in the community) and student accessibility services, combined with engaging in meaningful occupations, can provide student veterans with a platform for achieving academic and career success.

My name is James M. Cocroft (better known as Groovy); as I share my story, I am 49 years old and was born and raised in Milwaukee, Wisconsin. I served in the military from 1987 until 2007 as a naval operation specialist. I evolved in that job to help link radar for surface and air, for submarines, planes, and ships. In my 20 years of experience on seven ships, several shore duties, and security patrol, I traveled from Maine to Key West, Florida; lived in Italy for 2 years, and Russia, Istanbul, Santorini, Greece, Ukraine, Romania, Bulgaria, Venice, Croatia, and Kosovo, to name a few.

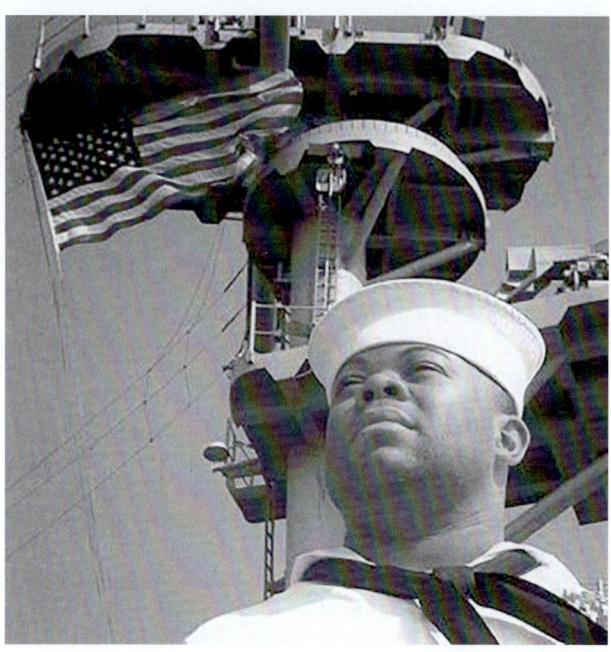

After 20 years of service, I felt I was gone long enough from my family, with a son who lived in St. Louis. I ended up retiring August 31, 2007, and came to UW-Milwaukee for a job in admissions. After 5 years of working, I decided to use my GI Bill to go to school. I had been working in the information technology (IT) field in the military, so I figured I'd get a degree in IT so I can say I have something for what I did for 20 years. I found it was kind of hard, because despite all the things I did in the military, it didn't mean anything (in the civilian world) if you didn't have a degree to go with it. I was scared to go to school; I thought, "I'm too old."

And that's when I started having some anxiety issues, had some deaths in the family, and in my transition from the military, I found I had some issues being nice. I was mean to people and I couldn't figure out why. I think one reason was fear of what was going to be happening next. In the military, you have the structure; when you get out there's no structure. . . . There's some sort of structure, but not the same as in the military. I decided to go, after some nudging from my mother and my wife, to counseling, so I went to the VA for cognitive processing therapy. That was one of the best moves I've done, because I still use those coping skills for all that I deal with in the world today. Most of the time whenever someone is around other military, guys or girls, they feel civilians do not understand what they are saying. I went in and was having the same issues with feeling my wife and my mom, and my sisters, didn't understand what I was saying or where I was coming from, only my military brothers and sisters. So my doctor said to me, "Since you figure that they don't understand you, have you ever figured out that it might be you who doesn't understand them?" That was my "aha" moment, that it isn't my way, but we have to figure out how to do this together, as a family, as human beings who coexist. I had to change my perspective, going from only my perspective.

Anger, anxiety, hypervigilance, and controlling the situation were what I was dealing with as I entered in my role as a student. I found myself shying away from really talking to people. I would always think negative about everything. Therapy taught me to think about what has happened to me in my career, think

about what I learned in the military, and to think about what I can control and what I cannot control. I learned to confront the situation after thinking through things clearly. I used to do a couple scenarios in my head and, after playing those out, picked the best solution to be able to cope. I was retaught it was OK to cry and to be vulnerable, because in the military, you never want to be vulnerable for anything. Thinking things through, controlling my breathing to relax, finding ways to do work with music on, having time to wind down, and being respectful with others, being open to their opinions instead of being combative. These were challenging because I had some school issues, anxiety and things I couldn't control; for example, I would get upset with how fast the professor would go. I would always go back to my coping skills. Having the younger generation as my classmates was a problem, but I had to change my perception, they were just at the start of their career and I was the one who was coming back to school. It was kind of irritating at first, but I had to gain a different perspective. I was aware of how people who are significantly younger than me were simply at a different time in their development. My son attended UWM with me together, so I was both a parent and a student at the same time. I found I could help students in the Black Cultural Center on campus when I gave them both perspectives, "This is what I think as a parent" and "This is what I know as a student." I found I could help others and I enjoyed that. Another source of anxiety was my struggle with thinking about my parents who are older and I was always afraid of having my parents dying. I was stressing about how can I control it, and there's nothing I can do about that. I also worked with a family therapist outside of the VA, I got put on medication, and found that I was able to focus on today and enjoying my parents today. It's a daily struggle to keep myself on my "A" game. I use my coping skills to have some sort of a normal life.

Continued

The Lived Experience—cont'd

I got my degree in 4 years. I was happy I accomplished that! With my military retirement, I was able to do school full time without working, something that single parents aren't able to do. My first semester, I got anxiety around an online class, not being able to complete so many questions in a time period, so I failed that class. Despite my thinking "there's nothing wrong with me," I decided to visit the Accessibility Resource Center on campus, and was able to get accommodations for my anxiety. The next time I took that class, I got a B and was able to navigate the system. I was scared at first to do it, but I used those tools to think it through, recognizing that if I wasn't doing well, then my family's not doing well. I graduated with a 3.2 average; at 47 years old, that is great, and I succeeded despite my struggles.

Now, 2 years after graduation, it's still a struggle; my father passed away 3 months ago, and my brother-in-law just a few weeks ago. But I have to be strong for my family, my wife, my sisters, my kids, and my mom. I'm in a grieving process myself and providing emotional support to my family. I have empathy for them, something I had before my military experience but lost for several decades while in the military and going through transition. I recommend counseling to all the military and veteran students I now work with at MAVRC (Military and Veteran Resource Center), so that you can get to love yourself more, so that you won't be scared to actually fail. Failing is a place for learning.

My mother is a master gardener, and she lives about an hour away in the country. I go out there every Sunday in the warm weather to cut the lawn, and in winter to shovel and help out. The drive out there is relaxation time, whereas shoveling the snow burns off energy; spending time with my mother and her cat, helping her with the garden, that time in nature, being right there with the river and enjoying the environment helps me de-stress. In class, I took tai chi for several semesters, which helped me with my mind and body, keeping me calm. I took a couple classes on mountain and road biking; now I ride with my wife and my daughter, so that helps me, too. I'm out and about with my little helmet on. I enjoy seeing the things you can't when you are driving, that helps me enjoy nature, and is something you don't have to pay for. I have a dog that I walk, a black lab, Koal, and that helps. Koal is one of the best things that happened to us. He keeps me calm, but I don't want him to work as a service dog, I want him to have a simple doggy life. I notice that I am now able to cope with a lot of thoughts. I let other veterans know they can get this help, too—no matter what, you have to be aware of your feelings and others' feelings, as you never know what someone else is going through.

In my job now at MAVRC, I have the opportunity to help other people in transition. I encourage others to cut down drinking to a minimum. When I see others stressing, I pull them aside, I tell them my story, and let them know how I overcame my anxiety issues. Don't jump to conclusions; take another perspective, make sure you take care of yourself. Eat right, get enough sleep if you can, go ahead and relax. Be aware that there are people out there who are struggling, maybe even more than you; make sure you are empathetic, live life to the fullest, and that you do right by people. People don't always know what's going on with you, so make sure you take the time to explain it to them so that they can be respectful. It's therapeutic in a way, to do the work I do and help other people with the help that I didn't have when I returned to school. I vowed to myself that once I get myself together, or close enough, that I would help people to navigate these pitfalls that I went through when I got out. It's good to help people know the options they have, as I didn't know. I'm here to do what wasn't done for me. Respect one another, connect because we are all human, accept our downsides, give each other support and feedback, help each other navigate, become the person you want to be. I build allies, and get things done through collaboration and teamwork. Team is how I get things done. Respect goes a long way; I try to help civilians to understand this as well.

---

postsecondary education or paid employment, affecting the individual's ability to achieve economic and social independence; the result can be cycles of poverty, isolation, homelessness, and other social and personal problems. Supported education has shown promise in assisting these individuals to achieve educational goals, thus increasing the likelihood of economic and social independence (Rogers et al., 2010; Schindler, 2019). One example is a pilot program described by Rudnick and Gover (2009) in which participants benefitted from postsecondary education leading to skilled vocation.

Supported education has expanded beyond the traditional mental health population. Supported education now addresses the needs of individuals diagnosed with autism spectrum disorder (American Psychiatric Association, 2022). Many of these students were diagnosed during their K to 12 education with autism spectrum disorder. There is a growing body of literature on supported education for these individuals (Gardner et al., 2012; Quinn et al., 2014; VanBergejik et al., 2008; Zager & Alpern, 2010).

Schindler and Boney (2022) describe a sample of students who attended a U.S. northeastern university and were enrolled in a supported education mentoring program. These students successfully graduated from the university. Primary diagnoses were depressive disorder (23%), autism spectrum disorder (20%), attention deficit-hyperactivity disorder (ADHD; 17%), learning disability (13%), anxiety disorder (13%), schizophrenia (7%), bipolar disorder (3%), and brain injury (3%). Fifty percent of the students did not have a secondary diagnosis, with anxiety as the most common secondary diagnosis (23%) followed by learning disability (7%), ADHD (7%), depressive disorder (7%), autism spectrum disorder (3%), and posttraumatic stress disorder (PTSD; 3%). It was also found that these students demonstrated internal motivation.

The Lived Experience

18-Year-Old Female First-Year College Student

If someone had come to me when I was in elementary or middle school and asked me if I thought I would ever make it to a university, I would have laughed and told them, "No!" At that age going to a college or a university was the farthest thing from my mind. I wanted to be done with school at the earliest possible time. I can remember sitting in my second-grade classroom with a trash can next to my desk because my anxiety would overcome me to the point of nausea. At that time I had no clue what was wrong and neither did anyone else. They claimed that I was just defiant and that led to a diagnosis of oppositional defiance disorder. It was not until I was entering middle school that they finally reached correct diagnoses.

I have a mixture of psychiatric disorders: obsessive-compulsive disorder, generalized anxiety disorder, and Asperger syndrome. Each of these disorders has affected me since early childhood. I felt helpless as a child because I was so confused about what was going on in my own brain, but as an adult I now understand how to accept my disabilities, and in turn accept myself.

I chose to go to college so I would be able to make a fresh start. School had always been a source of severe anxiety for me. But I was not willing to give up because I knew that I may be able to further my education and use it to help children who remind me of myself as a child. This is the reason I have chosen to major in psychology. I hope to become an art therapist so I can combine two things that I love to do.

Beginning college has brought many new and difficult challenges. For the first time in my life, I am living away from my home. My parents had always been the ones to keep me on track with school work, make sure I took care of myself, help me manage my time, and make sure I had appropriate behavior for my age. But the transition to college and living on my own caused me to become disorganized and revert back to a state of inappropriate social behavior. I knew this was likely to happen so I requested information from my psychologist about the disability services provided at my university. She recommended that I attend the Skills for Success Program before I had even set foot on campus.

The Skills for Success Program has helped me tremendously. I am paired with two graduate level occupational therapy

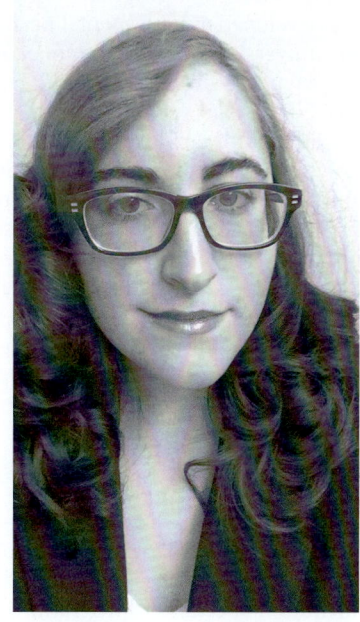

students who are my mentors and are guiding me through my transition from high school to college. They help me set goals for both my academic and social lives on campus. The overwhelming support that I have experienced through this program is amazing. Unlike some of the other programs I had tried when I was in high school, the Skills for Success Program has helped me grow. The mentors are not only here to help me meet my goals, but they also take the time to get to know me as a person and use what they know to better explain and guide me in the right direction.

The Skills for Success Program is an amazing experience, especially if you had at one point hated to ask for help or support because you felt as if it was impersonal. Because of the care and support I have received, I have been able to gain experiences that I never thought I would be able to such as going to the movies with a small group and managing my time efficiently. Even though I may still have some struggles both academically and socially, I know I can turn to my mentors and the class for the support that I need.

Barriers to Success in Higher Education

For individuals with the lived experience of mental illness, there are often many barriers to success in pursuing higher education. The most frequently cited barriers include (Belch, 2011; Hartley, 2010; Salzer et al., 2008; Schindler & Kientz, 2013):

- Symptoms of mental illness
- Side effects of medication
- Impaired cognitive functioning
- Stigma
- Inadequate assistance from college personnel

- Internal barriers, such as lost motivation, fear and anxiety, and low self-esteem

Several public laws mandate the full inclusion of people with disabilities—including psychiatric disabilities—in educational settings. These include the Americans with Disabilities Act (ADA; U.S. Department of Justice, 2016), Individuals with Disabilities Education Act (IDEA; 2004), and the Rehabilitation Act (amended 2015). However, although these laws ensure access and reasonable accommodations, they do not require the additional services needed to address barriers or provide the full level of support necessary for success.

Supported Education Models

Supported education was developed to assist individuals diagnosed with mental illness to pursue postsecondary education. Supported education programs began in the early 1990s and were developed at both mental health clinics and in colleges and universities. New programs continue to be developed at both types of sites (Arbesman & Logsdon, 2011; Mueser & Cook, 2012; Rogers et al., 2010; Thompson, 2013). Supported education programs can be found in hospitals, large public universities, community colleges, and small and large community mental health centers and provider organizations (Ringeisen et al., 2017). Models of service delivery within supported education programs were developed, and three supported education program models have been documented in the literature: (1) onsite services, (2) mobile support services, and (3) self-contained classrooms (Collins et al., 1998; Collins et al., 2000; Mowbray et al., 2005). In addition, combined models integrate features of these three service models.

Onsite Services Model

In the **onsite services model**, students attend college courses while simultaneously receiving supported education services in the form of a specialized program, counseling, or a support group (Collins et al., 1998; Gutman et al., 2009; Rudnick & Gover, 2009; Schindler & Sauerwald, 2013). In this model, academic skills such as time management, study skills, reading skills, writing skills, self-advocacy, and access to other services (e.g., tutoring and accommodations) are addressed.

Mobile Support Model

In the **mobile support model**, staff members at community-based mental health centers travel with students to provide assistance at the postsecondary educational sites where the student applies for admission or attends courses (Collins et al., 1998, 2000). The mobile support model frequently provides ongoing support, case management, and crisis intervention. Staff members meet with students in settings that students identify as the most comfortable for them (e.g., the college student center, library, coffee shop). Staff members also provide advocacy services to students and college personnel in areas such as financial aid and reasonable accommodations (Collins et al., 1998, 2000; Cook & Jonikas, 1992).

Self-Contained Classroom Model

In the **self-contained classroom model,** students attend a specialized curriculum to obtain the foundational academic, social, and psychological skills needed to enter higher education (Collins et al., 2000; Thompson, 2013; Unger et al., 1991). The self-contained classroom model is intended for students who have been out of school for a lengthy period of time and require skill building before fully entering postsecondary settings. Self-contained classrooms provide specialized instruction in study skills, basic writing and reading, basic math, and navigating the administrative aspects of an educational institution. The self-contained classroom is intended to help students reintegrate into mainstream educational classes in future semesters.

Combined Models

Many supported education programs offer programs based on combined models. These programs integrate features of each of the previously described models. Additionally, **Clubhouse Programs** have historically provided educational mentoring programs as part of the array of services offered to members. Clubhouses are community-based centers that offer members opportunities for employment, housing, education, and medical and psychiatric services. Individuals who participate in a Clubhouse are called "members" and concepts such as choice, lifetime reentry, and a sense of belonging are critical elements (Clubhouse International, 2023). Also see Chapter 35: Practice Across the Continuum of Service Needs for more detailed information about psychosocial clubhouses.

Groundbreaking Supported Education Programs and Models

In the early years of supported education, some innovative programs were developed and evaluated. These programs introduced the previously described models; they remain the important foundation for supported education and continue to be cited in the literature today. Two of these important programs are the Chicago-based Community Scholars Program (Cook & Jonikas, 1992; Cook & Solomon, 1993) and the Michigan Supported Education Program (Collins et al., 1998; Mowbray et al., 1999).

Chicago-Based Community Scholars Program

The Chicago-Based Community Scholars Program, known as the Thresholds program, combined self-contained classrooms, onsite support, and mobile-support services. This program featured a structured curriculum that addressed a variety of skills and services, such as career decision-making, study skills, library research skills, and writing skills. Participants were encouraged to enroll in regular college or technical training programs upon completion of the program (Cook & Jonikas, 1992; Cook & Solomon, 1993).

Michigan Supported Education Program

The Michigan Supported Education Program was conducted at Wayne County College in Detroit, Michigan. Both individual and group support services were provided for students enrolled in college courses (Mowbray et al., 1999). Group support meetings included a staff person and a person with lived experience who had firsthand knowledge of the experience of attending college with a psychiatric disability. Individual counseling paired a student with an assigned counselor who met with each student on a regular and as-needed basis.

Clubhouse Programs

Additional types of supported education programs have been documented in the literature. Clubhouse Programs offering educational mentoring have been documented in the literature since the early 1990s (County of San Diego Health and Human Services Agency, 2017; Dougherty et al., 1992; Macias et al., 2001). These include some mental health center–based programs that used standardized course curricula (Gutman et al., 2009; Rudnick & Gover, 2009); a program to promote the success of rural behavioral health services with an emphasis on providing assistance with registration, financial aid, and transportation (Thompson, 2013); and a program that integrated supported education with supported employment (Rudnick et al., 2013).

Skills for Success/Growth Through Occupational Therapy for Academic Learning

The Growth Through Occupational Therapy for Academic Learning (GOAL) program is an occupational therapy–based supported education program developed in a college setting in 2005 that has continued yearly. It was previously known as the Bridge Program and the Skills for Success Program. It is an example of an on-site services model. Students are referred to the program through the college's website, first-year studies program, and the office for students with disabilities.

The program is conducted during the fall and spring semesters, and students elect to attend once or twice per week for 2-hour sessions. The program consists of one-to-one mentoring that pairs master's level occupational therapy students (mentor) with undergraduate college students (mentee) under the supervision of occupational therapy faculty. The

director of the program (this chapter's author) completes an interview with each student and their parents (as applicable) before enrollment and maintains communication, as allowed by the Family Educational Rights and Privacy Act (FERPA), throughout enrollment in the program.

The goals of the program are to facilitate student success in college and, if factors overwhelmingly interfere with this goal, to identify an alternate, desirable plan. The goals of the program are addressed through the mentoring process. Mentoring is defined as the collaborative effort of the occupational therapy student and participant to develop goals and implement interventions to achieve these goals.

Mentoring begins with an assessment using the Canadian Occupational Performance Measure (COPM; Law et al., 2019), which identifies occupational performance problems in all aspects of college life, such as time management, organization of assignments, and socializing with peers. Problems are converted into long-term (semester) and short-term (monthly) goals. Common problems and goals include time management and organization, study skills, writing skills, social skills, healthy living, residential life, career planning, and leisure time. Although the activities used to address the problems and achieve goals may vary for each student, the written procedures to establish and address goals are uniform. Sample goals and interventions are shown in Table 47-1.

Goals are systematically addressed each week during the mentoring sessions using interventions implemented in a sequenced, strategic manner. (Table 47-2 shows a sample timetable for a mentoring session.) For example, the development of a goal of effective study skills begins by addressing the importance of (a) learning content presented in a class, (b) taking quizzes and tests in measuring class grades, and (c) studying as it pertains to classes in the current semester. Next, current strengths and problem areas in study skills are determined through discussion, observation, and review of previous quiz and test grades. Then, strengths are used to

TABLE 47-1 | GOAL Program Time Management and Organization Goals and Interventions

Long-Term Goals	Short-Term Goals	Initial Interventions	Weekly Interventions
D will organize and prioritize all class projects and assignments, maintain and update this system, and submit assignments on time for his Modern China and Conversational Spanish classes through the end of the semester.	D will enter all class projects and assignments in his planning system by the third week of the semester. D will independently review the calendar daily, and update and review the calendar with his mentor on a weekly basis through the end of the semester. D will break down each assignment into subcomponents and enter due dates for the subcomponents into his planning system by the fourth week of the semester. D will submit all assignments on time through the end of the semester. During each weekly mentoring session, D will provide his mentor with an update for each entry into the planning system and problem-solve any potential problems through the end of the semester.	1. Review the syllabi. 2. Input assignments into a planning system (examinations, papers, projects, homework, etc.). 3. Determine other homework that needs to be completed (reading, small group meetings, etc.) and input into a planning system. 4. Determine study and homework times and input into a planning system. 5. Break down larger assignments into subcomponents and input the subcomponents into a planning system.	1. Review the planning system. For each entry, was it completed? If so, what helped to complete this? If not, what were the obstacles? How will the obstacles be addressed? 2. Ask D if there are any updates to assignments, tests, and so on. If so, add these and their subcomponents. 3. Ask D in enough detail about reviewing his planning system as stated in the goal. If there are problems, address these. 4. Determine the plan to complete assignments due in the next week.

TABLE 47-2 | GOAL Program Timetable for Typical Mentoring Session

Timetable for Typical Mentoring Session	
2:30–2:40 p.m.	Announcements from instructor

2:40–3:00 p.m.	Time management and organization goal
	    a. Briefly review the week for any notable events.
	    b. Review and complete to-do checklist from previous session.
	    c. Review the planning system. For each entry, was it completed? If so, what helped to complete this? If not, what were the obstacles? How will the obstacles be addressed?
	    d. Are there any updates to assignments, tests, and so on? If so, add these and their subcomponents.

3:00–3:50 p.m.	Academic goal(s)
	    a. Study skills goal
	    b. Reading comprehension goal
	    c. Writing skill goal

3:50–4:10 p.m.	Self-interest goal
	    a. Social skills goal
	    b. Healthy living goal
	    c. Stress management goal

4:10–4:20 p.m.	Time management and organization goal
	    a. Determine and plan to complete assignments due in the next week.
	    b. Mentor and mentee complete weekly mentoring forms for items to be completed before the next session.
	    c. Insert items to be completed into the planning system.
	    d. Complete academic behaviors form together

address the problems. For example, if computer skills are an area of strength for the mentee, computer-based study tools are explored as a method to develop study skills.

Exploration of various study methods using trial and error continues until a sufficient quantity and quality of study methods are identified. Next, these study methods are implemented and evaluated for effectiveness. Adjustments or changes are made based on the findings. As an important standard to assess the effectiveness of study skills, the mentee explains the information under study to the mentor on a weekly basis. This sequenced, strategic method described for study skills is customized for each goal and each mentee. After each session, the mentor notes the mentee's progress or lack of progress toward the goals and makes a plan for the next session. This documentation is compiled into an in-depth progress report. At the end of each semester, the COPM is used as a reevaluation.

Occupational Therapy Student Involvement

Approximately 20 master's level occupational therapy students participate in the Skills for Success/GOAL supported education program each year. The program is embedded in two research courses and meets a Level I psychosocial fieldwork requirement. Therefore, the occupational therapy students participate in activities and complete assignments that relate to psychosocial fieldwork (mental health) or research (Schindler, 2011).

For the Level I fieldwork requirement, occupational therapy students provide mentoring to the undergraduate students (mentees) in the program. This is completed during their second year of the 2-year occupational therapy curriculum, and the occupational therapy students complete various types of instruction to develop competency as mentors before and concurrent with program implementation. During the first year of the academic program, occupational therapy students complete three mental health courses: instruction in psychiatric conditions, group dynamics and leadership, and the occupational therapy process of assessment, treatment planning, intervention, and reevaluation. They also conduct activity groups with individuals with the lived experience of mental illness at a local self-help center.

During their second year, and before their participation in the supported education program, occupational therapy students complete competency-based assignments based on written guidelines specifically related to mentoring. Assignments contain specific guidelines to ensure continuing uniformity to the approach and fidelity of the principles of the supported education model. Occupational therapy students participate in weekly small discussion groups to brainstorm activities and methods to achieve goals, discuss strengths and difficulties encountered in the mentoring process, and problem-solve in the areas experiencing difficulties. Occupational therapy students also reflect on their growth in skills and attitudes, as well as challenges encountered.

The occupational therapy students also complete research assignments related to the supported education program, which culminate in a professional poster. The students participate in the process of developing a research proposal, including introduction, literature, methodology, data collection, and data analysis. Quantitative and qualitative data are collected through the use of instruments and narratives and are analyzed and presented at the college's graduate research symposium.

Outcomes

Outcomes of the Skills for Success program have been approached from different perspectives and were described in two articles in the literature. In 2013, Schindler and

Sauerwald described results for 48 individuals with the lived experience of mental illness. The majority of these individuals were residing in the community and stated a desire to explore starting or returning to higher education. Although all participants entered the program with higher education goals, many changed their goals to employment goals after learning of the financial cost of higher education and of the level of skills required for success.

A quantitative one-group pretest-posttest survey design and posttest qualitative focus groups showed the number of participants enrolled in higher education increased from 7 to 11 (pretest = 15%; posttest = 23%), participants employed increased from 5 to 19 (pretest = 10%; posttest = 40%), and the combined category of higher education and employment increased from 12 to 30 (pretest = 25%; posttest = 63%). Statistical significance was achieved from pretest to posttest in the employment sample (p less than .000) and the combined sample of higher education and employment (p less than .000), but was not achieved in the higher education sample from pretest to posttest ($p =.125$). Quantitative and qualitative findings supported that this occupational therapy–based program, which incorporated principles of supported education and employment, could assist individuals with the lived experience of mental illness to achieve higher education and employment goals.

Another study addressed outcomes of 11 students diagnosed as children with autism (Schindler et al., 2015). These students were in their first year of college and enrolled in the supported education program. A mixed methods design with quantitative and qualitative components was used. The quantitative measures included the COPM (Law et al., 2019) and data on college retention. The qualitative measure consisted of in-depth progress note documentation throughout the program. There was a statistically significant difference between COPM pretest and posttest scores on performance ($p =.000$) and satisfaction ($p =.000$). Nine of 11 students confirmed college retention.

Three themes regarding college transition were: (1) maladaptive patterns linked to the characteristics of Asperger syndrome, (2) adaptive patterns linked to the characteristics of Asperger syndrome, and (3) parental influences. The study concluded that students with Asperger syndrome can succeed in college, especially with a combination of internal characteristics and external supports.

Both of these studies had limitations. Samples were small, and no control group was used so that all participants requesting the program could attend. Therefore, the findings cannot be generalized. Some of the outcome data was based on self-report, which has limitations (Portney, 2020).

Despite the limitations, positive components of the supported education program included that it was person-centered and occupation-based. **Person-centeredness** promotes "an approach to service which embraces a philosophy of, respect for, and partnership with, people receiving services" (Law & Mills, 2009, p. 253). A program that bases its foundation on respect for and partnership with its participants has a foundation for success from the participant's view. **Occupation-based intervention** ensured that activities used in the process were important, meaningful, and valuable to the person. Both of these components were congruent with the methods used in supported education.

Wellness Model in Adult Education

The *OTPF-4* discusses **health promotion** as an intervention approach that is appropriate for OTPs to utilize in supporting individuals, groups, and populations across the life span without the assumption of any disease process that would limit occupational performance (AOTA, 2020). By engaging in enriching experiences over various contexts, the outcome of health and wellness may be achieved (AOTA, 2020). The physical and mental health benefits of education are widely researched (Kondirolli & Sunder, 2022; Zajacova & Lawrence, 2018).

Under a wellness model, it is within occupational therapy's purview to develop programming to support the occupation of health management, assist people in developing healthy habits and routines, and educate people on the benefits of participating in community wellness programs. A variety of wellness programs are available to youth and adult learners. Some examples are described in the text that follows. See Chapter 45: Self-Care and Well-Being Occupations for more ideas on this approach.

Every Moment Counts (EMC) is one example of a mental health promotion program developed for children and youth to support mental health for success at school, home, and in the community. The multipronged and multitiered educational program was developed by OTPs to be carried out with other members of the interdisciplinary school team. The tiers in EMC have three levels utilizing the multitiered systems of support (MTSS) framework (see Chapter 37: School Mental Health for additional information on MTSS). OTPs act as change agents and promote mental health for all children, with and without known disabilities, by providing enjoyable activities and incorporating the guiding principle that small moments make big differences in how children feel and function (EMC, 2023). See Chapter 37: School Mental Health for more details about EMC.

Many college campuses are changing their approach to the mental health crisis by incorporating a wellness model and offering workshops on topics such as time management, organization, stress management, healthy living, and sleep for all college students (Abrams, 2022; Jalaba, 2022). Broadening the scope of campus-supported programs for older and nontraditional students, the Wellness Initiative for Senior Education (WISE) is an evidence-based program developed by the National Council on Aging, Inc. (NCOA). It is run by trained facilitators to improve mental health and empower older adults to advocate for their own health by providing education on the aging process, early signs of declining mental health, medication management, and making healthy lifestyle choices (NCOA, 2023).

Many college campuses also offer senior auditing programs that permit older adults to audit college courses for low or no cost, allowing adults to reap the mental health and cognitive benefits of the student role well into their senior years.

Role of Occupational Therapy in Adult Education

Although supported education is addressed in a variety of health and education professions, occupational therapy can make a distinct contribution to supported education through

Being a Psychosocial OT Practitioner

Routinizing Health Management and Daily Occupations Supporting Academic Success

Identifying Psychosocial Strengths and Needs

Occupational therapy in a higher education setting can be very rewarding but comes with unique challenges. Students may have many academic abilities but require additional support to succeed. For many students, college is the first time they are expected to develop their schedule and complete activities of daily living (ADLs) and instrumental activities of daily living (IADLs) independently. Contrary to the K to 12 setting, students at the college level must self-identify and advocate for their needs. Universities often employ support personnel such as staff in the Disability Services Office, Tutoring Center, and Wellness Center. Still, the students must take the initiative to seek out these services. Many diagnoses addressed in higher education are not new to OTPs in the K to 12 setting, but the challenges can present quite differently for young adults attending college.

Rafael is a student whose story adeptly demonstrates the challenges and successes of navigating university life with high-functioning autism spectrum disorder, which in his case includes rigid thinking, social difficulties, and emotional dysregulation, causing behavioral outbursts. Rafael was a rising college freshman at a medium-sized rural university in the northeast United States when he and his family sought the support of an occupational therapist–led weekly program designed to teach the skills needed for success in college. Rafael had never lived away from home before moving to an on-campus dormitory with an assigned new roommate. Through discussion of the occupational profile, Rafael reported that he developed adequate academic skills before college and enjoys computer gaming and drawing Pokémon characters. He has a supportive mother and one childhood friend from home with whom he communicates occasionally.

The OTP administered the COPM to measure Rafael's perceived performance and satisfaction in self-care, emotional regulation, and preparation strategies for homework and examinations. The OTP also administered the Assessment of Time Management Skills (ATMS) to determine how well Rafael implements a routine, identifies common strategies, and determines awareness of management deficits. He scored a 72 out of 120, demonstrating moderate impairment with time management skills. In supplement to this score, Rafael verbalized his desire to improve this skill, as he relies heavily on the occupational therapist–led program for structure. The OTP identifies a lack of time management skills in several areas of Rafael's life, including self-care and study habits.

Occupational Performance Problem	Importance	Initial Performance	Initial Satisfaction
Time management/organization	9	3	1
Self-care and hygiene schedule needs improvement	7	4	1
Needs emotional regulation strategies	10	3	4
Preparation strategies for examinations (study guides, etc.)	8	4	3

Based on Rafael's history and response to assessments, the OTP anticipates that support is necessary with time management, emotional regulation, and self-care.

Using a Holistic Occupational Therapy Approach

Regarding time management, Rafael's identified goals include improving time management and organization for homework and study skills. Rafael also reports he does not shower regularly; he indicates that he typically covers up with deodorant, but his appearance is impacted. His reasoning is related to further concerns regarding time management and organization difficulties, as Rafael does not make time for his showers. The OTP and Rafael explore possible strategies. Rafael chooses to develop a 24-hour color-coded schedule highlighting the time needed for classes, schoolwork/studying, sleep, meals, ADLs, and leisure with the support of the OTP. They also create a corresponding online calendar with reminder alerts and a pie chart to represent time spent visually.

When unexpected changes to Rafael's routine occur, he responds with a short temper, which elicits poor emotional regulation. Rafael's insight into his temper is a helpful tool in identifying characteristics to regulate himself better. The OTP incorporates emotional regulation strategies such as deep breathing, meditation, and journaling into treatment.

Rafael allocates most of his time to his studies and leisure participation (computer gaming and Pokémon). When discussing his typical routine during COPM administration, Rafael did not mention self-care and hygiene unless prompted. The OTP provides education on the importance of proper hygiene and how it can impact success in college and future work life. Creating a visual schedule for bathing, tooth brushing, and hair brushing, in addition to smartphone reminders, supports Rafael in improving his self-care and hygiene.

Reflective Questions

1. How might the OTP incorporate health promotion as an intervention approach for Rafael?
2. How might the OTP increase Rafael's frustration tolerance related to his college workload?
3. What other areas would be important to assess when considering Rafael's success in college?

the provision of person-centered and occupation-based approaches. Occupational therapy interventions encompass a unique combination of activities identified as relevant and important to individuals, providing meaning to everyday life and contributing to health and well-being (AOTA, 2020). These occupational therapy concepts are congruent with principles of supported education because they address the centrality of the student with real-life, relevant, and meaningful interventions to develop and accomplish higher education and lifelong learning goals.

Occupational Therapy Practice Framework

The *OTPF-4* (AOTA 2020) addresses supported education. Education and social participation are directly related to the student role. Additionally, there are several occupations that are indirectly related to the student role.

Occupations within ADLs (e.g., bathing/showering, dressing, personal hygiene and grooming, and sexual activity) impact the student role. Additionally, several occupations within the IADLs (e.g., communication management, home [dormitory or apartment] establishment and management, safety, and emergency maintenance) and health management (e.g., social and emotional health promotion and maintenance, medication management, physical activity and nutrition management) are linked to success in the student role. Another occupation, rest and sleep, is critical for success in the student role. The occupation of work may be essential for students to finance their education or their living expenses, and the occupation of leisure is important to create an appropriate balance with academics.

Several chapters are related to these occupations: Chapter 45: Self-Care and Well-Being Occupations; Chapter 46: Activities of Daily Living, Instrumental Activities of Daily Living, and Health Management Occupations; Chapter 48: Work and Volunteer Occupations; Chapter 49: Connectedness and Belonging; Chapter 51: Leisure and Creative Occupations; and Chapter 52: Sleep. 🤝

All performance skills are subcomponents of the student role including (a) motor skills, (b) process skills, and (c) social interaction skills. For a student with a psychiatric disability, process and social interaction skills may be compromised. The cognitive and social functioning needed for success in academics can be impeded by symptoms, side effects of medication, or a decrease in skills if mental illness impacts the student's functioning through time. Assessment and intervention of each of these areas within the occupations of the student role are necessary.

Performance patterns including habits, routines, roles, and rituals are integral aspects of the student role. The student role requires the development of positive habits and routines, such as efficient time management, for success. The structure of college life is significantly different from the daily structure of high school. For example, the college curriculum typically has downtime between classes with large assignments due during the course of a semester, so college students need to develop their own structure. They also need to break down large assignments and examinations, such as term papers and final examinations, into subcomponents and pace their completion of these assignments in order to achieve satisfactory grades and avoid undue stress. This requires the development of habits and routines that result in positive study skills.

All the contexts are relevant to the student role. The virtual context is especially important, because of the many varied ways that competency in electronic and digital devices is required for participation in academics and completion of assignments.

The physical and social environments, including all aspects of the college campus and interactions with professors, staff, and peers, are an intricate part of daily life as a student.

The person factors, including values, beliefs, and spirituality; body functions; and body structures represent the conscious, subconscious, and unconscious aspects that influence the role of student as a unique individual. Values, beliefs, and spirituality impact the choices some college students make, especially in areas of peer pressure including alcohol, drugs, and sexual activity. The components within the categories of body functions and body structures reverberate through the other areas of the framework. For example, challenges in the process and social interaction skills are usually also evident in the specific and global mental functions (e.g., higher-level cognitive, attention, memory, temperament, and personality).

The *OTPF-4* (AOTA, 2020) captures both the holistic and unique aspects of the individual. This is clearly evident for the student pursuing postsecondary education.

The Person-Environment-Occupation Model and Adult Learning

The PEO model is an appropriate practice model to apply to adult learning, as it considers a person's occupational performance in relation to the person, their environment, and occupation(s). Both challenges and elements that contribute to success are understood by the interplay of these three factors. This frame of reference provides OTPs with a model with which to seek an understanding of the occupational performance within adult education and the student role (Strong & Rebeiro-Gruhl, 2019). The PEO model has been applied broadly to frame evaluation and intervention in a way to help others understand the focus for, and unique contributions of, occupational therapy in educational settings (Krupa et al., 2015).

Person

As a means of beginning a conversation with a student engaging in occupational therapy, similar to all other practice settings, the occupational profile is a starting spot (AOTA, 2020). To understand the person's history of engagement in occupations across time, it is helpful to look at the student and their chosen current occupations. Related to the PEO, the "person" is considered unique, dynamic, and a participant in roles. They are viewed within contextual influences, and bring to the context a set of attributes, skills, knowledge, and experience (Brown, 2019b; Strong & Rebeiro-Gruhl, 2019). As the PEO model is applied to adult education, the "person" is viewed within their unique strengths and challenges as they relate to all aspects of the student role (academics, interpersonal, intrapersonal, etc.). The basic assumption of the PEO model is that the person is continually developing and intrinsically motivated.

The following questions can effectively assess strengths, challenges, interests, and motivation:

- What is the level of interest with the classes and courses of study?
- What is the level of comfort with class participation, discussion, small group work, and public speaking?
- What is the level of comfort in interacting with professors/teachers and peers?
- What is the level of stress management when multiple assignments and tests are due such as at midterms and finals?
- What is the reaction to receiving grades?
- What are the common emotional responses, and how do they relate to the role of student?

In addition, autonomy is also important to address:

- To what degree are assignments completed independently?
- How much assistance is required?
- What supported education model would be most beneficial?

Finally, it is important to assess performance components:

- What is the person feeling (affective), thinking (cognitive), and doing (physical)?

Environment

The "environment" is the context within which occupational performance takes place. It is considered from the unique perspective of the person (Brown, 2019a; Strong & Rebeiro-Gruhl, 2019). Within adult learning and the student role, the environment includes all aspects of the postsecondary site. For a college campus, this is not only the physical environment, but also the cultural, socioeconomic, social, and institutional environments. All aspects of the environment are assessed and addressed to promote success.

The following questions are typical questions to assess the environment:

- To what degree do the academic environments, such as classrooms, residential living spaces, and library, promote completion of assignments?
- To what degree do the social environments, such as student common areas and sports arenas (e.g., noise, level of stimulation), promote socialization?
- Do these environments promote studying and prioritizing coursework or are they distracting?
- Do these environments promote acceptance and inclusion, or do they promote peer pressure to conform to risky activities such as drug or alcohol abuse?
- For students who reside in student dormitories or apartments on the college campus, what is the level of comfort with shared or solitary living space, bedrooms, and bathroom facilities?
- For online learning, does the environment encourage or hinder learning?
- For online learning, does the student have consistent access to wi-fi and other hardware/software needed for courses?
- For online learning, does the environment encourage or hinder learning?

Occupation

The "occupations" are groups of self-directed, functional tasks and activities identified as self-care, productivity, and leisure. They are carried out within multiple contexts in fulfillment of developmentally appropriate roles. Occupations place affective, cognitive, and physical demands on the individual performing the occupation (Pizur-Barnekow & Pickens, 2019; Strong & Rebeiro-Gruhl, 2019). The occupations within adult learning are those related to the student role. These include self-care (e.g., relevant ADLs and IADLs), productivity (e.g., academics), and leisure (e.g., friendships, extracurricular activities).

When analyzing occupations, the practitioner's focus should be on the characteristics of tasks (occupation), degree of structure, duration of activity, complexity of tasks, and characteristics of task demands. For example, if the student is submitting incomplete assignments or late assignments, it is important to analyze the academic time management and organization aspects within the occupation of student.

Questions include:

- Is the student able to complete the affective, cognitive, and physical demands of this complex set of activities?
- For the affective component, how does the student plan for or respond to multiple homework assignments that may include examinations, projects, and papers? Does the student remain calm and productive or does the student experience stress that can result in behaviors that avoid or escape from the stress?
- For the cognitive component, does the student know the steps involved to set assignment priorities and organize the day or the week to complete them? To what degree can the student break down the steps of an assignment and complete them in a logical order?
- For the physical component, to what degree does the student have adequate gross motor, fine motor, posture, and vision to complete the homework assignments?

Occupational Performance

Occupational performance is the result of a dynamic relationship between the person, the environment, and their occupations. It refers to the individual's ability to choose, organize, and perform meaningful occupations that are culturally defined and age-appropriate (Strong & Rebeiro-Gruhl, 2019). Within adult education, occupational performance includes all the occupations directly or indirectly related to the student role. Occupations directly related to the student role include academic occupations, such as class attendance and participation and completion of assignments; extracurricular occupations, such as participating in college clubs and events; and occupations related to residential life, such as positive and health-promoting relationships with roommates and friends. Occupations indirectly related to the student role include those that support a healthy student role such as those related to healthy nutrition, rest and sleep, and community mobility.

When analyzing occupational performance, all three components (P, E, and O) must be considered. If occupational performance is less than productive, the OTP can collaborate with the person to identify and remove internal and external

PhotoVoice

Aaron

I am going to college in the spring semester, so I can go ahead and get my general studies degree. I want to be a sports announcer. I love talking college sports. I game plan for the game at the beginning of every week. I have to know the sports, the games, the rules, the umpires, the side judges, the players, the scouts, the colleges they came from, their diets, their stats. I have the outgoing personality for it. I am moving toward my dreams, my goals, my aspirations. As I am recovering from the problems the last 2 years, I am finding the solutions: taking it one day at a time, learning how to talk with other people, not panhandling, pretty much taking care of myself.

How does Aaron's narrative reflect his level of commitment to learning so that he can accomplish his goal of being a sports announcer? What role would you play as his OTP in helping him to follow through on this long-term goal?

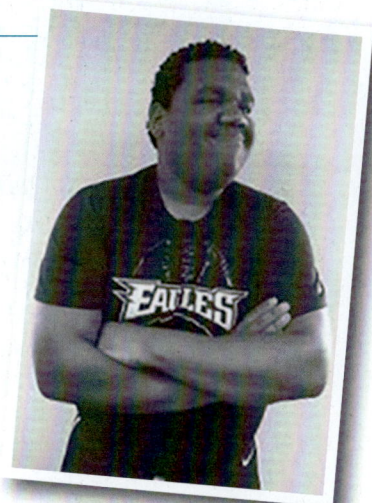

barriers or constraints and develop supports to improve the quality of the PEO fit.

Pulling Together Person, Environment, and Occupation Within Adult Learning

The PEO model is holistic and comprehensive. Supports and challenges in one area typically affect other areas. The OTP begins by addressing each area of the model as previously described and then synthesizing this information in order to develop a holistic view of the student. Based on the priorities determined from an assessment of each of the areas of the model, the OTP can focus on one area of the model or on multiple areas to facilitate change.

OTPs begin by fostering a person-centered relationship through creating a supportive social environment that demonstrates valuing the student, taking time to arrive at a common ground, and actively supporting the student's choice and decision-making. Implementation of these interventions occurs within the relevant environments. Change outcomes are measured in terms of occupational performance (Strong & Rebeiro-Gruhl, 2019).

The Evidence for Occupational Therapy–Supported Education Programs

Several occupational therapy-based supported education outcomes are described in the literature. Gutman and colleagues (2007) reported the effectiveness of an occupational therapy–based supported education program in New Jersey, and in 2009, Gutman and colleagues reported the effectiveness of an occupational therapy–based supported education program in New York. Schindler reported positive outcomes of a program for adults with mental illness that included higher education goals in 2010, provided additional outcomes with Sauerwald in 2013, and described outcomes for college students with Asperger syndrome in a supported

education program in 2015 (Schindler et al., 2015). Stoneman and Lysaght (2010) described a supported education program specific to training individuals in retail that resulted in subsequent employment in retail. Additionally, other authors describe programs specific to college students with Asperger syndrome (Gardner et al., 2012; Quinn et al., 2014).

As with the research conducted by various professional disciplines and described earlier in this chapter, the research conducted by occupational therapy researchers is minimal and shows promise, but it lacks firm evidence. Still, the holistic nature of occupational therapy makes it a good match for individuals with needs in supported education.

Fernando et al. (2017) studied the effects of a supported education program on a student's quality of life, motivation, and educational improvement, as well as if it had room for growth and success. The trio also looked to identify the strengths and weaknesses of a supported education program along with the value and impact it had on both students and staff. The study was a pilot/project case study that followed a mixed methods approach. This study took place at a psychiatric hospital with five staff members and two volunteers as student support for the program. Students were made up of both inpatients and outpatients, ages 21 and older, who were self-referred to the program with recommendations from counselors, friends, or family. Support varied from individual instruction to independent work with support when needed. The results suggest the program improved students' confidence, independence, and study skills.

It was clear that students were open and welcoming to transformative learning. The supportive environment created by staff and volunteers encouraged students to be persistent in their academics and achieve their goals. However, the program showed a low level of literary skill improvement, which suggests the need for more effective methods to teach adult learners. It is unknown if the lack of academic progress was directly related to the staff's teaching practices or if the students were setting unrealistic academic goals. Fernando et al. (2017) recommend future education programs to encourage confidence, hope, and persistence and set realistic goals and plans.

Evidence-Based Practice

Occupational Therapy Services in Supported Education

> *Supported education is an individualized process that is best delivered through a client-centered and occupation-based approach.*

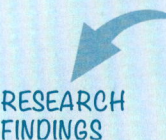

RESEARCH FINDINGS

Several research design limitations have negatively impacted the research outcomes on supported education. A systematic review of supported education literature from 1989 to 2009 (Rogers et al., 2010) found that there were very few well-controlled studies of supported education. In 2012, Mueser and Cook analyzed 20 years of supported education programs and concluded that research on different approaches has produced encouraging results regarding school-related activity, but little evidence that supported education programs are effective in helping individuals establish careers leading to personally meaningful work.

More recently, Keptner and McCarthy (2020) did a scoping review to map the literature that describes occupational therapy services provided in supported education. Keptner and McCarthy focused on the structure of occupational therapy services, the populations served, the methods of intervention, and the potential outcomes of the services. Three qualitative themes emerged from their scoping review: the focus on occupation and skills needed for success, using the campus environment, and campus collaboration. They concluded that the structure of occupational therapy services and student populations vary. They recommend future research to support the distinct value of occupational therapy in this practice area, including the scope and outcomes of occupational therapy services with different populations of students.

Correspondingly, Hofstra and colleagues (2023) systematically reviewed literature from 2009 to 2021 to find articles on the effectiveness of supported education interventions for students with psychiatric disabilities who wanted to return to or remain in education. All seven of the studies they reviewed showed positive effects of supported education on educational functioning, time spent on educational activities, sustained attention and vigilance, and interpersonal skills. Yet, only three of these studies compared the results with a control group, which has been noted in previous literature. Hofstra and colleagues (2023) suggest future research should be of higher quality (larger sample sizes, relevant outcome measures such as dropout and/or gaining a degree).

In an attempt to guide future research and programs, Hofstra and colleagues (2021) created a study protocol that combines quantitative research utilizing a randomized controlled trial with qualitative research including monitoring, interviews, and focus groups.

APPLICATIONS

➡ Using the COPM in a supported education setting allows for the identification of varied occupational performance problems in all aspects of college life. Problems such as time management, assignment organization, personal hygiene, study skills, or socializing with peers can be converted into long-term (semester) and short-term (monthly) goals.

➡ The activities used to address the problems and achieve goals will vary for each student, but keeping the written procedures to establish and address uniform goals will help with continuity.

➡ Scheduling the sessions at the same time as fellow students allows for the opportunity to work on socialization goals together.

➡ Limitations in research on occupational therapy involvement in supported education can be attributed to the fact that supported education is an individualized process. It seems to best be delivered through a client-centered and occupation-based approach.

➡ With occupational therapy's expertise in client-centered and occupation-based approaches and the use of quantitative and qualitative mixed methods research designs, OTPs have the potential to positively contribute to a growing body of literature on supported education outcomes.

Evidence-Based Practice—cont'd

REFERENCES

Hofstra, J., van der Velde, J., Farkas, M., Korevaar, L., & Büttner, S. (2023). Supported education for students with psychiatric disabilities: A systematic review of effectiveness studies from 2009 to 2021. *Psychiatric Rehabilitation Journal, 46*(3), 173–184. https://doi.org/10.1037/prj0000528

Hofstra, J., van der Velde, J., Havinga, P. J., & Korevaar, L. (2021). COMmunity PARticipation through Education (COMPARE): Effectiveness of supported education for students with mental health problems, a mixed methods study—Study protocol for a randomized controlled trial. *BMC Psychiatry, 21*(1), Article 332. https://doi.org/10.1186/s12888-021-03329-5

Keptner, K. M., & McCarthy, K. (2020). Mapping occupational therapy practice with postsecondary students: A scoping review. *The Open Journal of Occupational Therapy, 8*(1), 1–17. https://doi.org/10.15453/2168-6408.1617

Mueser, K. T., & Cook, J. A. (2012). Supported employment, supported education, and career development. *Psychiatric Rehabilitation Journal, 35*(6), 417–420. https://doi.org/10.1037/h0094573

Rogers, E. S., Kash-MacDonald, M., Bruker, D., & Maru, M. (2010). *Systematic review of supported education literature, 1989–2009.* Boston University, Sargent College, Center for Psychiatric Rehabilitation. http://www.bu.edu/drrk/research-syntheses/psychiatric-disabilities/supported-education

Here's the Point

- OTPs can assist people with lived experience of mental illnesses in pursuing educational goals.
- Supported education is an approach that provides programs and supports to help people with the lived experience of mental illness, including starting, returning, or continuing in postsecondary education such as college.
- Common barriers to success in higher education include symptoms of mental illness, medication side effects, stigma, impaired cognitive functioning, inadequate external supports, and internal barriers such as decreased motivation, anxiety, and low self-esteem.
- Supported education programs began in the early 1990s and were developed at mental health clinics, psychosocial clubhouses, and at colleges and universities. New programs continue to be developed at all types of sites. Three supported education program models are documented in the literature: (1) onsite services, (2) mobile support services, and (3) self-contained classrooms. An additional model combines two of these models.
- Supported education services have expanded beyond the traditional mental health population to include persons diagnosed with autism spectrum diagnoses and student veterans.
- The GOAL program is an example of an on-site services model that uses a mentoring approach in a suburban university. Details of the program and research outcomes were provided to facilitate understanding and application of the program.
- Research on supported education shows promise, but the majority of research reports minimal evaluation data based on weak designs with only a few well-controlled studies.
- Occupational therapy can make a distinct contribution to supported education, with the core concepts of occupational therapy interventions being person-centered and occupation-based. The *OTPF* and the PEO model demonstrate the holistic approach to supported education.

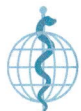 Visit the online resource center at **FADavis.com** to access the videos.

Apply It Now

1. Importance of Environment as It Relates to Completion of Homework and Studying

Go to a busy environment in your college, such as the student center or another area where a lot of students pass through during the change of classes, and begin reading a textbook chapter, studying for a test, or writing an essay. Then, go to a quiet environment, such as the library. Here, too, begin reading a textbook chapter, studying for a test, or writing an essay.

Maintain this activity for at least 5 minutes and then answer the following questions.

Reflective Questions

- In each environment, how difficult was it for you to concentrate? How much of the assignment were you able to complete?
- What were your feelings in each of the environments?
- Were you able to tune out the voices in order to attend to your reading or writing?

2. Importance of Time Management and Prioritization for Completing Assignments

This activity is intended to simulate the need to be able to plan and prioritize time in order to successfully complete classes and assignments with the least stress. Gather syllabi from at least four college courses. Use a planning system to input: (a) class schedule for attendance at all classes; (b) due dates for each assignment in each class on the correct date; (c) reading assignments on the dates to be completed; (d) two 30-minute study periods per week for each class that has examinations; and (e) two 1-hour writing periods per week for written assignments greater than 5 pages.

Reflective Questions

- Understanding that the items you scheduled still will not constitute all your obligations, how much scheduled and unscheduled waking time do you have on a weekly basis?
- Did this schedule confirm your use of time or were you surprised at the amount of time devoted to classes and schoolwork?

3. Use of Activity Analysis to Break Down Assignments Into Manageable Components and Pace Completion of Assignments for Maximum Learning

Use an example of a written paper assignment that is 5 to 10 pages and includes gathering, reading, and synthesizing journal articles. Break down the paper into five steps using the backward chaining method (i.e., start with the finished paper and work backward to determine the steps that need to be completed). Allow 1 week to complete each of the steps. Insert these subcomponent due dates into the previously described planning system.

Reflective Questions

- What are the five steps you listed?
- What are your thoughts and feelings about allowing 5 weeks to complete a paper? What are the positives? What are the negatives?
- What are your thoughts and feelings about pacing your approach to assignment completion versus working under pressure close to a deadline?
- What are your thoughts about how psychiatric symptoms would affect pacing completion of assignments versus working under pressure close to a deadline?

Resources

- Active Minds, Inc. (2023): https://www.activeminds.org
- Mental Health America. (2023). Education and recovery. https://mhanational.org/education
- Substance Abuse and Mental Health Services Administration. (2011). *Supported education: Building your program.* HHS Pub. No. SMA-11-4654. Center for Mental Health Services, U.S. Department of Health and Human Services. https://store.samhsa.gov/sites/default/files/d7/priv/sma11-4654-buildingyourprogram-sed.pdf
- Substance Abuse and Mental Health Services Administration. (2011). *Supported education: How to use the KITs.* HHS Pub. No. SMA-11-4654. Center for Mental Health Services, U.S. Department of Health and Human Services. https://store.samhsa.gov/sites/default/files/d7/priv/sma11-4654-buildingyourprogram-sed.pdf

Videos

- "Positive Mindset Creative Arts Festival" video. This video showcases the Positive Mindset Creative Arts Festival, held at the Queensland Children's Hospital in Australia. This annual children's festival promotes positive thinking about mental health and increases help-seeking behaviors with a creative arts focus. It is a notable example of how OTPs can contribute to community health efforts. The emphasis is on art as an occupation and creating space in the community to encourage and celebrate mental health. In addition, the event promotes the idea of social connection and belonging centered around self-expression of feelings across the mental health continuum and how that ultimately encourages the sense of connection and belonging with people and communities. Access the video at the online resource center at FADavis.com.
- "Occupational Therapy Collaboration in Early Head Start" video. In this video, an occupational therapist and occupational therapy assistant describe their partnership while working collaboratively at an Early Head Start program. They explain the importance of a team approach to tiered intervention services and how they work together to support children, parents, and staff. This includes strategizing on how to implement creative intervention ideas and address challenges with individual children, some of whom have experienced trauma. Access the video at the online resource center at FADavis.com.
- "Jordan's Lived Experience of Anxiety and Depression" video. In this video, occupational therapist Jordan describes her lived experience of anxiety and depression. She touches on many issues critical to recovery and occupational therapy practice, including social determinants of health, peer support, and how mental health labels can adversely affect an individual's medical treatment. Importantly, she explains how she has learned to blend her lived experience with her work as an occupational therapist, while ensuring she takes care of herself and manages her symptoms. Jordan also offers priceless words of wisdom to practitioners regarding establishing a therapeutic connection with individuals with whom they practice. Access the video at the online resource center at FADavis.com.
- "Jenny's Lived Experience of Sensory Processing Differences" video. Jenny is an occupational therapy degree (OTD) student with the lived experience of sensory differences, anxiety, and depression. In this video, she describes how she discovered her diagnosis, how it affects her in the classroom, and what interventions she uses to manage her reactions to stimuli. Importantly, she discusses the need to advocate for herself and for practitioners to help people across the life span to understand their sensory processing needs in order to improve their mental health and overall quality of life. Access the video at the online resource center at FADavis.com.
- "Aimee's Lived Experience With Substance Use and Autism" video. Aimee is an occupational therapist with the lived experience of substance use disorder. In this video, Aimee shares that she was diagnosed with childhood PTSD and that she also realized that she is autistic. She describes the behaviors that led her to that conclusion, her coping strategies, and how her lived experience affected her role as a student in graduate school. Access the video at the online resource center at FADavis.com.

Resources Specific to Student Veterans

- American Council on Education: https://www.acenet.edu/Documents/Higher-ed-spotlight-undergraduate-student-veterans.pdf
- Stockton University Military and Veteran Services: https://www.stockton.edu/veteran-affairs
- Syracuse University D'Aniello Institute for Veterans & Military Families: https://ivmf.syracuse.edu

Private Foundations

- The Aurora Foundation: http://www.snvc.com/aurora-foundation

- The Pat Tillman Foundation: https://pattillmanfoundation.org/the-foundation
- The Posse Foundation: https://www.possefoundation.org/shaping-the-future/posse-veterans-program

Government Resources
- Information for Military Families and Veterans, U.S. Department of Education: https://www.ed.gov/veterans-and-military-families/information
- U.S. Department of Veterans Affairs, Education and Training: http://www.benefits.va.gov/gibill

References

Abrams, Z. (2022). Student mental health is in crisis: Campuses are rethinking their approach. *American Psychological Association Monitor on Psychology, 53*(7), 60. https://www.apa.org/monitor/2022/10/mental-health-campus-care

Active Minds, Inc. (2023). *Statistics.* https://www.activeminds.org/about-mental-health/statistics

American Academy of Pediatrics. (2021). *How do infants learn?* https://doi.org/10.1542/peo_document355

American Occupational Therapy Association. (2020). Occupational Therapy Practice Framework: Domain and process—Fourth edition. *The American Journal of Occupational Therapy, 74*(Suppl. 2), 7412410010p1–7412410010p87. https://doi.org/10.5014/ajot.2020.74S2001

American Psychiatric Association. (2022). *Diagnostic and statistical manual of mental disorders* (5th ed., text rev.). American Psychiatric Publishing. https://doi.org/10.1176/appi.books.9780890425787

American Psychological Association. (2013). College students' mental health is a growing concern, survey finds. *Monitor on Psychology, 44*(6), 13.

Arbesman, M., & Logsdon, D. W. (2011). Occupational therapy interventions for employment and education for adults with serious mental illness: A systematic review. *American Journal of Occupational Therapy, 65*(3), 238–246. https://doi.org/10.5014/ajot.2011.001289

Belch, H. A. (2011). Understanding the experiences of students with psychiatric disabilities: A foundation for creating conditions of support and success. *New Directions for Student Services, 134*(1), 73–94. https://doi.org/10.1002/ss.396

Brown, C. (2019a). Introduction to the environment. In C. Brown, V. C. Stoffel & J. P. Muñoz (Eds.), *Occupational therapy in mental health: A vision for participation* (2nd ed., pp. 449–459). F.A. Davis.

Brown, C. (2019b). Introduction to the person. In C. Brown, V. C. Stoffel & J. P. Muñoz (Eds.), *Occupational therapy in mental health: A vision for participation* (2nd ed., pp. 85–95). F.A. Davis.

Cate, C. A. (2014). *Million records project: Research from student veterans of America.* https://studentveterans.org/wp-content/uploads/2020/08/mrp_Full_report.pdf

Clubhouse International. (2023). *How clubhouses work: The basic components of a successful clubhouse.* https://clubhouse-intl.org/resources/how-clubhouses-work

Collins, M. E., Bybee, D., & Mowbray, C. T. (1998). Effectiveness of supported education for individuals with psychiatric disabilities: Results from an experimental study. *Community Mental Health Journal, 34*, 595–613. https://doi.org/10.1023/A:1018763018186

Collins, M. E., Mowbray, C. T., & Bybee, D. (2000). Characteristics predicting successful outcomes of participants with severe mental illness in supported education. *Psychiatric Services, 51*, 774–780. https://doi.org/10.1176/appi.ps.51.6.774

Cook, J. A., & Jonikas, J. A. (1992). Models of vocational rehabilitation for youths and adults with severe mental illness. *American Rehabilitation, 18*(3), 6–12.

Cook, J. A., & Solomon, M. L. (1993). The Community Scholar Program: An outcome study of supported education for students

with severe mental illness. *Psychosocial Rehabilitation Journal, 17*, 83–87. https://doi.org/10.1037/h0095623

County of San Diego Health and Human Services Agency. (2017). *Military & veterans resource guide.* www.sandiegocounty.gov/content/dam/sdc/hhsa/programs/ais/documents/OMVA%20Resource%20Guide%20-%20March%202017-rev2.pdf

Cronin-Golomb, L. M., & Bauer, P. J. (2023). Self-motivated and directed learning across the lifespan. *Acta Psycologica, 232*, 103816. https://doi.org/10.1016/j.actpsy.2022.103816

Dirette, D. P. (2019). Disability services for students in postsecondary education: Opportunities for occupational therapy. *The Open Journal of Occupational Therapy, 7*(2), Article 1. https://doi.org/10.15453/2168-6408.1609

Dougherty, S., Hastie, C., Bernard, J., Broadhurst, S., & Marcus, L. (1992). Supported education: A clubhouse experience. *Psychosocial Rehabilitation Journal, 16*(2), 91–104. https://doi.org/10.1037/h0095698

Ellison, M. L., Mueller, L., Smelson, D., Corrigan, P. W., Stone, R. T., Bokhour, B. G., & Drebing, C. (2012). Supporting the education goals of post-9/11 veterans with self-reported PTSD symptoms: A needs assessment. *Psychiatric Rehabilitation Journal, 35*(3), 209–217. https://doi.org/10.2975/35.3.2012.209.217

Ennals, P., Fossey, E. M., Harvey, C. A., & Killackey, E. (2014). Post-secondary education: Kindling opportunities for people with mental illness. *Asia-Pacific Psychiatry, 6*(2), 115–119. https://doi.org/10.1111/appy.12091

Every Moment Counts. (2023). *Home page.* https://everymomentcounts.org

Fernando, S. I., King, A. E., & Eamer, A. (2017). Supported education practitioners: Agents of transformation. *Occupational Therapy in Mental Health, 33*(3), 279–297. https://doi.org/10.1080/0164212X.2017.1295415

Gardner, J., Mulry, C. M., & Chalik, S. (2012). Considering college? Adolescents with autism and learning disorders participate in an on-campus service-learning program. *Occupational Therapy in Health Care, 26*, 257–269. https://doi.org/10.3109/07380577.2012.720052

Gutman, S. A., Kerner, R., Zombek, I., Dulek, C., & Ramsey, C. A. (2009). Supported education for adults with psychiatric disabilities: Effectiveness of an occupational therapy program. *American Journal of Occupational Therapy, 63*(3), 245–254. https://doi.org/10.5014/ajot.63.3.245

Gutman, S. A., Schindler, V. P., Furphy, K. A., Klein, K., Lisak, J. M., & Durham, D. P. (2007). The effectiveness of a supported education program: The Bridge Program. *Occupational Therapy in Mental Health, 23*(1), 21–38. https://doi.org/10.1300/j004v23n01_02

Hartley, M. T. (2010). Increasing resilience: Strategies for reducing dropout rates for college students with psychiatric disabilities. *American Journal of Psychiatric Rehabilitation, 13*(4), 295–315. https://doi.org/10.1080/15487768.2010.523372

Hofstra, J., van der Velde, J., Farkas, M., Korevaar, L., & Büttner, S. (2023). Supported education for students with psychiatric disabilities: A systematic review of effectiveness studies from 2009 to 2021. *Psychiatric Rehabilitation Journal, 46*(3), 173–184. https://doi.org/10.1037/prj0000528

Hofstra, J., van der Velde, J., Havinga, P. J., & Korevaar, L. (2021). COMmunity PARticipation through Education (COMPARE): Effectiveness of supported education for students with mental health problems, a mixed methods study—Study protocol for a randomized controlled trial. *BMC Psychiatry, 21*(1), Article 332. https://doi.org/10.1186/s12888-021-03329-5

Individuals with Disabilities Education Act, 20 U.S.C. § 1400 (2004).

Isaacson, M. (2013). The training and use of service dogs in occupational therapy education. *Open Journal of Occupational Therapy, 1*(2), Article 6. https://doi.org/10.15453/2168-6408.1023

Jalaba, T. (2022). Occupational therapy's role in addressing the mental health crisis on college campuses. *SIS Quarterly Practice Connections, 7*(2), 18–20.

Keptner, K. M., & McCarthy, K. (2020). Mapping occupational therapy practice with postsecondary students: A scoping review. *The Open Journal of Occupational Therapy, 8*(1), 1–17. https://doi.org/10.15453/2168-6408.1617

Khalil, M., Ghayas, S., Adil, A., & Niazi, S. (2021). Self-efficacy and mental health among university students: Mediating role of assertiveness. *Rawal Medical Journal, 46*(2), 416–419.

Kondirolli, F., & Sunder, N. (2022). Mental health effects of education. *Health Economics, 31*(Suppl. 2), 22–39. https://doi.org/10.1002/hec.4565

Krupa, T., Kirsh, B., Pitts, D., & Fossey, E. (Eds.). (2015). *Bruce & Borg's psychosocial frames of reference: Theories, models and approaches for occupation-based practice* (4th ed.). Slack.

Law, M., Baptiste, S., Carswell, A., McColl, M., Polatajko, H., & Pollock, N. (2019). *The Canadian Occupational Performance Measure (COPM)* (5th ed.). CAOT Publications ACE.

Law, M., & Mills, J. (2009). Client-centered occupational therapy. In M. Law (Ed.), *Client-centered occupational therapy* (p. 253). Slack.

Macias, C., Barreira, P., Alden, M., & Boyd, J. (2001). The ICCD benchmarks for clubhouses: A practical approach to quality improvement in psychiatric rehabilitation. *Psychiatric Services (Washington, D.C.), 52*(2), 207–213. https://doi.org/10.1176/appi.ps.52.2.207

Mackenzie, S., Wiegel, J. R., Mundt, M., Brown, D., Saewyc, E., Heiligenstein, E., & Fleming, M. (2011). Depression and suicide ideation among students accessing campus health care. *American Journal of Orthopsychiatry, 81*(1), 101–107. https://doi.org/10.1111/j.1939-0025.2010.01077.x

McBain, L., Kim, Y. M., Cook, B. J., & Snead, K. M. (2012). *From soldier to student II: Assessing campus programs for veterans and service members* (Vol. 2). American Council on Education.

Mowbray, C. T., Collins, M., Bellamy, C., Megivern, D., Bybee, D., & Szilvagyi, S. (2005). Supported education for adults with psychiatric disabilities: An innovation for social work and psychosocial rehabilitation practice. *Social Work, 50*(1), 7–20. https://doi.org/10.1093/sw/50.1.7

Mowbray, C. T., Collins, M., & Bybee, D. (1999). Supported education for individuals with psychiatric disabilities: Long term outcomes from an experimental study. *Social Work Research, 23*(2), 89–100. https://doi.org/10.1093/swr/23.2.89

Mueser, K. T., & Cook, J. A. (2012). Supported employment, supported education, and career development. *Psychiatric Rehabilitation Journal, 35*(6), 417–420. https://doi.org/10.1037/h0094573

National Center for Education Statistics. (2022). *Undergraduate retention and graduation rates. Condition of education.* U.S. Department of Education, Institute of Education Sciences. https://nces.ed.gov/programs/coe/indicator/ctr

National Council on Aging, Inc. (2023). *Evidence-based program: Wellness education for senior initiative (WISE).* https://www.ncoa.org/article/evidence-based-program-wellness-initiative-for-senior-education-wise

Pizur-Barnekow, K., & Pickens, N. D. (2019). Introduction to occupation and co-occupation. In C. Brown, V. C. Stoffel & J. P. Muñoz (Eds.), *Occupational therapy in mental health: A vision for participation* (2nd ed., pp. 759–772). F.A. Davis.

Portney, L. G. (2020). *Foundations of clinical research: Applications to evidence-based practice* (4th ed.). F.A. Davis.

Quinn, S., Gleeson, C. I., & Nolan, C. (2014). An occupational therapy support service for university students with Asperger's syndrome. *Occupational Therapy in Mental Health, 30*(2), 109–125. https://doi.org/10.1080/0164212X.2014.910155

Rehabilitation Act of 1973, Pub. L. No. 93–112, 29 U.S.C. §§ 701 et seq. (amended 2015).

Ringeisen, H., Langer Ellison, M., Ryder-Burge, A., Biebel, K., Alikhan, S., & Jones, E. (2017). Supported education for individuals with psychiatric disabilities: State of the practice and policy implications. *Psychiatric Rehabilitation Journal, 40*(2), 197–206. https://doi.org/10.1037/prj0000233

Rogers, E. S., Kash-MacDonald, M., Bruker, D., & Maru, M. (2010). *Systematic review of supported education literature, 1989–2009.* Center for Psychiatric Rehabilitation.

Rudnick, A., & Gover, M. (2009). Combined supported education with supported employment. *Psychiatric Services, 60*(12), 1690. https://doi.org/10.1176/appi.ps.60.12.1690

Rudnick, A., McEwan, R. C., Pallaveshi, L., Wey, L., Lau, W., Alia, L., & Volkenburg, L. A. (2013). Integrating supported education and supported employment for people with mental illness: A pilot study. *International Journal of Psychosocial Rehabilitation, 18*(1) 5–25.

Salzer, M. S. (2012). A comparative study of campus experiences of college students with mental illness versus a general college sample. *Journal of American College Health, 60*(1), 1–7. https://doi.org/10.1080/07448481.2011.552537

Salzer, M. S., Wick, L. C., & Rogers, J. A. (2008). Familiarity with and use of accommodations and supports among postsecondary students with mental illness. *Psychiatric Services, 59*(4), 370–375. https://doi.org/10.1176/ps.59.4.370

Schindler, V. P. (2010). A client-centered, occupation-based occupational therapy programme for adults with psychiatric diagnoses. *Occupational Therapy International, 17*(3), 105–112. https://doi.org/10.1002/oti.291

Schindler, V. P. (2011). Using service-learning to teach mental health and research skills. *Occupational Therapy in Health Care, 25*(1), 54–64. https://doi.org/10.3109/07380577.2010.519430

Schindler, V. P. (2019). Student: Adult education. In C. Brown, V. C. Stoffel & J. P. Muñoz (Eds.), *Occupational therapy in mental health: A vision for participation* (2nd ed., pp. 838–852). F.A. Davis.

Schindler, V. P., & Boney, J. D. (2022). Characteristics contributing to graduation for university students with *DSM-5 d*iagnoses after completion of a mentoring program. *Mentoring & Tutoring, 30*(1), 124–141. https://doi.org/10.1080/13611267.2022.2031085

Schindler, V. P., Cajiga, A., Aaronson, R., & Salas, L. (2015). The experience of transition to college for students diagnosed with Asperger's disorder. *Open Journal of Occupational Therapy, 3*(1), Article 2. https://doi.org/10.15453/2168-6408.1129

Schindler, V. P., & Kientz, M. (2013). Supports and barriers to higher education and employment for individuals diagnosed with mental illness. *The Journal of Vocational Rehabilitation, 39*(1), 39–41. https://doi.org/10.3233/JVR-130640

Schindler, V. P., & Sauerwald, C. (2013). Outcomes of a 4-year program with higher education and employment goals for individuals diagnosed with mental illness. *Work: A Journal of Prevention, Assessment and Rehabilitation, 46*(3), 325–336. https://doi.org/10.3233/WOR-121548

Soydan, A. (2004). Supported education: A portrait of a psychiatric rehabilitation intervention. *American Journal of Psychiatric Rehabilitation, 7*, 227–248. https://doi.org/10.1080/15487760490884531

Stoneman, J., & Lysaght, R. (2010). Supported education: A means for enhancing employability for adults with mental illness. *Work (Reading, Mass.), 36*(2), 257–259. https://doi.org/10.3233/WOR-2010-1026

Strong, S., & Rebeiro-Gruhl, K. R. (2019). Person-Environment-Occupation model. In C. Brown, V. C. Stoffel & J. P. Muñoz (Eds.), *Occupational therapy in mental health: A vision for participation* (2nd ed., pp. 29–46). F.A. Davis.

Substance Abuse and Mental Health Services Administration. (2011). *Supported education: How to use the KITs.* HHS Pub. No. SMA-11-4654. Center for Mental Health Services, U.S. Department of Health and Human Services.

Thompson, C. J. (2013). Supported education as a mental health intervention. *Journal of Rural Mental Health, 37*(1), 25–36. https://doi.org/10.1037/rmh0000003

Unger, K. V., Anthony, W. A., Sciarappa, K., & Rogers, E. S. (1991). A supported education program for young adults with long-term mental illness. *Hospital and Community Psychiatry, 42*(8), 838–842. https://doi.org/10.1176/ps.42.8.838

U.S. Department of Justice. (2016, October 11). *Americans with Disabilities Act Title II Regulations.* https://www.ada.gov/law-and -regs/title-ii-2010-regulations

VanBergejik, E., Klin, A., & Volkmar, F. (2008). Supporting more able students on the autism spectrum: College and beyond. *Journal of Autism and Developmental Disorders, 38,* 1359–1370. https://doi.org/10.1007/s10803-007-0524-8

Zager, D., & Alpern, C. S. (2010). College-based inclusion programming for transition-age students with autism. *Focus on Autism and Other Developmental Disabilities, 25,* 151–157. https://doi .org/10.1177/1088357610371331

Zajacova, A., & Lawrence, E. M. (2018). The relationship between education and health: Reducing disparities through a contextual approach. *Annual Review of Public Health, 1*(39), 273–289. https://doi.org/10.1146/annurev-publhealth-031816 -044628

CHAPTER
48

Work and Volunteer Occupations

Andrew Persch and Ellie Fossey

Work is a fundamental area of human occupation. The *Occupational Therapy Practice Framework,* Fourth Edition (*OTPF-4;* American Occupational Therapy Association [AOTA], 2020) defines work as, "labor or exertion related to the development, production, delivery, or management of objects or services; benefits may be financial or nonfinancial (e.g., social connectedness, contributions to society, structure and routine to daily life)" (p. 33). Herein, "work" includes (a) employment interests and pursuits, (b) employment seeking and acquisition, (c) job performance and maintenance, (d) retirement preparation and adjustment, (e) volunteer exploration, and (f) volunteer participation.

The notion of work is so commonplace that defining it can be difficult. For example, terms such as "work," "employment," "job," "gig," "shift," and/or "labor" may be used interchangeably to reflect the construct. Yet, none of these terms adequately capture the range of unpaid occupations that may be considered work, such as domestic activities, caregiving, and volunteering.

The right to work is included in the Universal Declaration of Human Rights (United Nations [UN] General Assembly, 1948). All working-age people are entitled to employment, equitable work conditions, and safeguards against joblessness. This encompasses access to professional training and strategies to actualize the right to work (UN General Assembly, 1966). Following the declaration's publication, individuals with disabilities have gained recognition of the right to work equally with others, in voluntarily selected jobs, and in open, accessible, and inclusive work environments (UN General Assembly, 2006). All individuals have the right to access satisfactory and meaningful employment while simultaneously receiving just compensation in an environment characterized by freedom, fairness, security, and the preservation of human dignity (International Labour Organization, 2004). Unfortunately, only a small portion of the work done worldwide is paid (Gammarano, 2019).

Employment is closely tied to health and quality of life. For example, one's identity, self-worth, health, socioeconomic status, and quality of life are strongly linked to one's ability to work independently and earn a living wage (Corcoran, 2004; Pedretti & Early, 2001). For instance, the relationship between employment and health status is evident in those with disabilities (Emptage, 2005; Miller & Dishon, 2006; Petrovski & Gleeson, 1997; Waghorn et al., 2005) and those without (Benavides et al., 2000; Repetti et al., 1989; Ross & Mirowsky, 1995; Stronks et al., 1997; Virtanen et al., 2003). This research indicates that employed individuals generally enjoy better health outcomes compared with those who are unemployed, a trend that holds true for individuals with disabilities.

Given that individuals with disabilities often face lower employment rates than those without disabilities, they may be more susceptible to the negative impacts of poor health. Employment status also significantly influences the quality of life, with employed individuals typically reporting a higher quality of life than their unemployed counterparts (Clayton & Chubon, 1994; Eggleton et al., 1999; Inge, 1988; Kober & Eggleton, 2005; Miller & Dishon, 2006; Priebe et al., 1998; Sinnott-Oswald, 1991). Similar to health, the reduced quality of life stemming from unemployment or underemployment can have a more pronounced impact on individuals with disabilities compared with those without disabilities. In addition to the functional and economic implications, work provides a social-cognitive structure—the lens—through which individuals interact with and experience the world (Daston et al., 2012).

Evidence suggests that work is generally beneficial for physical and mental health, and unemployment is detrimental to health and well-being, but the nature of work and workplace characteristics can both have positive and negative influences on mental health. Many people in the workforce experience mental illness, so promoting mental health in the workplace is increasingly recognized as an important issue (Dewa et al., 2012). Current and potential workers with mental ill-health face many employment barriers that may disrupt their work participation, and those with persistent mental illness are among the most marginalized in terms of their employment patterns and economic status (Krupa, 2011b).

Underpinned by the idea that work is beneficial for one's health, the occupation of work has had a central place in the philosophy and practice of occupational therapy since its beginnings (Meyer, 1922/1977). The healing potential of work also has deep historical roots in the organization of psychiatric treatment and rehabilitation (Davidson et al., 2010; Wilcock, 2001). There are effective ways to assist people experiencing mental illness to obtain jobs and sustain employment, whether they have never worked, have not worked for a prolonged period, or are struggling to maintain work and stay well. Occupational therapy practitioners (OTPs) need to work actively to address the challenges and barriers to work participation faced by people experiencing mental illness, and to support them to pursue their vocational aspirations, access decent jobs, and develop their chosen career paths.

This chapter addresses work participation by describing how work and mental health are interconnected, the ways in which vocational development may be disrupted by mental illness, and common employment barriers faced by current and potential workers experiencing mental illness. Vocationally focused assessments, as well as individual and workplace interventions, are presented to illustrate how OTPs can promote work participation and build supports that enable people with mental ill-health to access valued work in fair and equitable conditions. The chapter also focuses on volunteer exploration and participation, activities described as a subset of "work" in the *OTPF-4* (AOTA, 2020).

Volunteering can be seen as a choice one makes when engaging in activities that serve others, the community, or organizations that matter to the person. Such activities can serve as a means for a person to connect with others, contribute or "give back" to the community, and may be a safe way to explore the world of employment. Committing to a volunteer position allows the person to explore the expectations that might accompany such a position. Exploring these choices can be an important focus of occupational therapy intervention as the person establishes goals and daily activity plans for recovery.

Overview of Work and Volunteer Occupations

In occupational therapy, work or productive occupation is acknowledged as not being restricted to paid employment; rather, it is inclusive of a broader range of occupations that make economic and social contributions, such as household work, parenting, caregiving, education, and volunteer experiences (AOTA, 2020). Work may be further distinguished from other areas of occupation, particularly activities of daily living (ADLs) and play or leisure, because of its role in facilitating identity development, as well as social and economic participation.

The belief that work is good for one's health can be traced to ancient times (Wilcock, 2001). Many studies have identified that employment is beneficial for health and well-being, depending on the nature, quality, and social context of the work (Waddell & Burton, 2006). Among its beneficial aspects, employment provides economic resources essential for material well-being and has long been recognized as imposing a time structure and predictable demand for activity in daily life, linking individuals' goals to collective purposes,

and as central to individual and social identity (Jahoda, 1981; Waddell & Burton, 2006). In comparison, strong evidence suggests unemployment is harmful to health and well-being; loss of work, prolonged unemployment, and exclusion from work may each profoundly impact the physical and mental well-being of affected persons, families, and communities, as well as their financial circumstances (Waddell & Burton, 2006). Hence, the emerging picture of positive and negative relationships between employment and mental health is complex.

Mental ill-health impacts work participation in several ways. First, many employed people in the workforce are affected by mental health issues, with approximately 10% of the working population estimated to experience a mental disorder, the most common being depression (Dewa & McDaid, 2011). These rates have risen substantially over the past decade (Torquati et al., 2019) and in the wake of the COVID-19 pandemic (Bufquin et al., 2021; Pieh et al., 2021; see this chapter's Being a Psychosocial OT Practitioner feature).

Second, mental illness often leads to use of sick days and long-term work incapacity in industrialized countries (Dewa & McDaid, 2011; Harvey et al., 2014). For the individual employee, this may have significant social and economic costs, including restricted opportunities for career development, promotion, or salary increases, whereas sickness absence because of mental illness also results in substantial loss of productivity for businesses and the economy (Dewa & McDaid, 2011).

Third, those with mental illness are less likely to be employed than other people of working age, and those adults with persistent mental illness and psychiatric disability are particularly disadvantaged in the labor market. European, U.K., and U.S. studies report 70% to 90% of persons with psychiatric disabilities are not working, more than for other disability groups (Dewa et al., 2012; Waghorn & Lloyd, 2010).

Beyond this, often the jobs that people with persistent mental ill-health get are low paying, insecure, or lack opportunities for career development, and so their employment patterns and economic status tend to be characterized by marginalization from work (Krupa, 2011b). Despite this, people experiencing mental ill-health report not only many of the same benefits from working as does the general population, but also that work is important in recovery and a source of wellness (Fossey & Harvey, 2010; van Niekerk, 2009).

The Lived Experience

Joe Crespo: Fighting a 500-Pound Bear and Gaining University Entry

Work has been an important aspect in my continued quest to recover from schizophrenia. Although my work history has been both intermittent and turbulent, just knowing that I haven't crashed signifies that there will be smoother rides in the future with fewer landings.

One of my favorite movies has a quote saying, "What one man can do another can do." Anthony Hopkins says it again,

"What one man can do another can do." He says it again, screaming at his partner to yell it with him, "WHAT ONE MAN CAN DO ANOTHER CAN DO!" The movie was The Edge. The quote is in reference to killing a bear. The characters are lost in the woods and this bear is stalking them, already having eaten their other friend. They end up killing the bear, a wild beast of 500 pounds, with a makeshift spear. This 500-pound bear is SCHIZOPHRENIA.

My mind was so disconnected to anything a person of sound body and mind could expect to experience. I saw my

Continued

The Lived Experience—cont'd

mother and father go to work every day and no matter how disconnected I was I knew that their going to work meant a roof over "our" shoulders and food to eat. No matter how bad I felt about myself I saw, knew, and hoped that one day I could go back to work and get on with my life. A few years went by after the diagnosis and onset of my illness. I was suicidal and in a state nobody in their wildest dreams could imagine. I was aware of my mental state and wanted out. This was my first thought. But how was I to get out of this state of torment? I started thinking about what had happened to me. I had had a good life, played sports, had friends, and had all the makings of a great life ahead of me. And then this blockbuster.

One day my father asked me if I wanted to type the names and addresses of business cards into his computer. I accepted the offer. No matter how messed up my head was, I was still able to type. I had taken typing in high school and still remembered how to do it. I got a job with a call center down the street and ended up staying there for 2 years. I loved going to work and I loved knowing how to type. The first day was agonizing worrying I was not going to be able to learn the job and worrying I was not going to be able to connect with other people. But smiles and laughter helped me see that I was just as capable to learn as everybody else, and oh yes, I had some money in my pocket as my dad used to emphasize. I was around others who believed in the work I did. They kept me and let others go, and I was proud of my accomplishments.

About a year into my employment, a supervisor told me that I should do data entry. They gave me more and more responsibilities doing data entry. It hit me that I was good at data entry, and I wanted to see where it would lead me. Being around supportive people made a world of difference, and my supervisor made me believe in myself with her data entry epiphany.

Along with a severe mental illness, I had a crushing dependence on alcohol. So even during this time of employment I began drinking again. It got me through each day along with my normal regime of medications that helped drown out the demons enough to let me sleep. So, I drank alone in the garage, went to bed at a reasonable time, and went to work in the morning. I did this for quite a while, and while the drinking allowed me to sleep and get up in the morning, it also gave me a horrible feeling of being dependent on something that would mask my thought disorder. Now my internal thought disorder had been externalized in my speech. As time went on, I started stuttering on the phone. It got so bad that I could barely pronounce any words at all. I was humiliated for the longest time knowing that others could hear me talk that way, but management was still on my side. They told me it was not that bad, but still I was embarrassed. I knew I did not stutter like that and it had to be the alcohol that was numbing my brain from the night before. It made me believe that I was so calm inside, when I was an utter wreck both inside and out, but I stayed on until I could no longer take it. I walked out one day and left my job. Schizophrenia had won again. Now all I had was alcohol, and a life that had gone nowhere in 2 years.

Feeling self-defeated and alone I still remembered the supervisor's words and I was revitalized. It wasn't defeat or schizophrenia that had won, it was the dark shadows that pervaded my spirit. The 500-pound bear that nobody could figure out how to kill was now mine to figure out. Freely accepting this formula to be put on my shoulders was the worst mistake I have ever made, for I was not the same as I was when I was young. I was not in high school any more playing basketball, hitting shot after shot. I was not in my prime with friends having a blast and being the life of the party. I was not Mr. Baseball Card collector, blackjack dealer, I was Joe, and I was lost. I had been through a tremendous amount of both physical and mental pain and was dealing with schizophrenia, which no single word could capture. I simply was not the same person anymore. The question now was how I was going to sustain myself while consuming alcohol, having shattered self-esteem, and trying to kill a bear as ANOTHER MAN CAN DO! The job had not paid me much. I was free to get back on track and look for a data entry position that paid more money, to start thinking about having a life of which I knew nothing about.

Around this time, I started thinking of going back to school. I had never been a really good student before, but I had always tried my hardest. I always harped to other people that it took me five times the amount of time to learn something new than a "normie." All I needed to transfer to a 4-year university was one course in mathematics. I was horrible at math. It had been 3 or 4 years of thinking about how math was keeping me from transferring. Then one day it hit me. I told myself I was going to do it. I was going to pass math. I was going to study 6 or 7 hours a day or more and I was going to pass. I was going to kill that 500-pound bear. So, I signed up to kill that bear. I knew it was going to be tough, but from the first day I studied 6 hours a day. As I was doing the problems, I was figuring out questions I had about life. I was not just doing the problems. I think this is what was different and the reason why it took me so long. Doing the problems was kind of like therapy. It was still tough, but I was learning. I showed up every day to class and when the first test came around, I ended up with a "C." I realized when I got the test back that I had not answered five questions that were on the back of the test. The teacher would write the distribution of grades on the chalkboard, and I was amazed that half of the class had failed, and I had gotten a C. I was mad at myself for not answering those questions, but I kept on studying 6 or 7 hours a day. There is no question that I was progressing. The medications must have been working because as I said before there was no way I could have even thought about math unless I was in a semistable place. Work had also helped. I do not think without the work experience at the call center I would have been able to pass math, and I did. I passed with a "B" grade. I was officially a university student. I probably cracked a real smile for the first time in my life. Something that was so deeply engraved in my brain had vanished through hard work. They say that hard work cures all. I prefer to say there is no cure, only hope of one!

Being a Psychosocial OT Practitioner

Addressing Complex Work-Related Issues After COVID-19

Identifying Psychosocial Strengths and Needs

Mental health challenges in the workplace have become increasingly prevalent, and the incidence of these challenges increased greatly during the COVID-19 pandemic. OTPs play a pivotal role in helping individuals manage and overcome these issues. Herein, OTPs use holistic assessment and intervention strategies that facilitate workplace performance.

Avery (they/them) is a single, 32-year-old project manager who works for a national information technology (IT) firm. Avery had been working in IT for over a decade when the pandemic hit. At first, the shift from the office to the virtual workplace felt natural, indeed easy. Avery had been conducting video calls with colleagues and people on a routine basis and felt comfortable using Skype and Zoom. As the months passed, Avery found themself meeting online for 8 or more hours per day, every day. After the meetings, they would order Uber Eats and code late into the night. Avery's social circle shrunk to zero; lockdowns and mask mandates precluded the valued weekly happy hour with teammates, dating, and travel to see family. Avery's physical and mental health took a turn for the worse, though they didn't recognize it at home alone. As pandemic restrictions lifted, Avery's employer decided to give up its office space and mandated that all employees work from home, indefinitely.

After a year of working from home, Avery was feeling tired. Their self-care had fallen off, they had gained 30 pounds, and they were missing deadlines. Avery's mother, who lives out of state, fell ill and was hospitalized. Suddenly, she passed. "COVID," they said. Another wave of the pandemic meant that there was no funeral, though Avery and their brother planned to hold a small ceremony when they could. Avery did not share this information with their coworkers. Avery began to dread virtual meetings that they were responsible for leading, feeling more comfortable "hiding in plain sight" on calls that were not their responsibility. At about this time, Avery's supervisor asked for a 1:1 meeting and noted the missing deadlines, and established a performance improvement plan (PIP) for them, to be reviewed in 60 days. Panic attacks followed, and Avery visited the emergency department once and urgent care once within a month. They were prescribed a limited quantity of a fast-acting antianxiety medication and directed to follow up with their primary care provider (PCP).

Avery went to see their PCP, who diagnosed them with generalized anxiety disorder (GAD). The PCP discontinued the fast-acting medication and prescribed a selective serotonin reuptake inhibitor (SSRI). Their PCP also recommended talk therapy. Knowing there would be long waits to see a social worker or counselor, the PCP encouraged Avery to use their employee assistance program (EAP) to jumpstart the process and provided a referral to occupational therapy.

Using a Holistic Occupational Therapy Approach

The OTP encounters Avery within the context of a traditional outpatient rehabilitation clinic in a private room. The OTP shares the details of the referral with Avery: occupational therapy evaluation and treatment secondary to a recent diagnosis of GAD and job-related stress. The OTP shares their goals for the initial evaluation, including developing an occupational profile and analyzing occupational performance issues with the expectation that these will inform the intervention plan for Avery. The session then proceeds within the context of a semistructured interview.

Avery shares their occupational history, current concerns, and perceived barriers. They share that they have engaged with the EAP counselor weekly for 3 weeks, have three visits remaining under this benefit, and 8 weeks yet to wait before seeing a counselor. Avery sees that their condo has become a singular

environment, a primary setting for work, self-care, and socialization. They report no recreation or leisure occupations. The OTP decided to use the COPM (Law et al., 2014) to further assess these concerns and support Avery to identify their priorities.

Avery's COPM: Initial Assessment

Occupational Performance Problems	Performance	Satisfaction
Dressing for work	5	2
Grocery shopping	3	3
Keeping and improving employment	6	3
Becoming physically active	2	5
Socializing with coworkers, family, and friends	5	2

The results of Avery's COPM, including the content of the semistructured interview, revealed much about their performance patterns, occupational engagement, and desires. Avery was clear that work performance was their primary concern but acknowledged that the other occupations identified were contributing to work difficulties, poor health, and decreased satisfaction in life. They were open to the OTP's holistic perspective about how improvements across other areas of occupation would support work performance.

Avery noted that coders are not typically regarded for their dress but shared that they had always enjoyed putting outfits together and took pride in their dress at the office. As a project manager, Avery always felt more confident when meeting with the firm's senior leadership and with outside people when they dressed professionally. Avery shared that they had the resources to buy new clothes, and the OTP suggested that Avery do so and wear them in their condo during work and waking hours.

Next, the OTP suggested that Avery truly take their lunch hour for healthy eating and some physical activity. Because Avery lives in a city, they can walk three blocks to Whole Foods, purchase a healthy lunch, eat it there, then walk back to the condo for the afternoon. This means Avery can become physically active by taking a walk every day and addresses the need to eat healthier.

Within their work-related occupations, the OTP suggested several routine changes designed to improve performance. First, Avery began to block small breaks in between meetings throughout the day, providing an opportunity to process, rest, and prepare for the next meeting. Avery blocked longer breaks before the high-stakes meetings that they were leading, which increased their preparedness and decreased anxiety. Second, the OTP assisted Avery to develop a new self-management organizational strategy to identify, review, and plan for daily, weekly, and other deadlines. Third, the OTP provided instruction in Mindfulness-Based Stress Reduction (MBSR) with the aim that these tools would allow Avery to cope with job-related stress.

Finally, the OTP encouraged Avery to reengage their social networks. Despite working from home, many of their colleagues still lived in town. Avery reinstated the weekly happy hour gathering. They also made travel plans to see their brother and plan a memorial service for their mother. Avery joined a couple of dating apps and began to attend a monthly social mixer held at Whole Foods.

Reflective Questions

1. Which other assessments might the OTP use to understand Avery's work-related performance issues?
2. Beyond MBSR, what techniques might the OTP employ to help Avery manage job-related stress?
3. What additional habit or routine-based changes would you recommend for Avery?

Workplace characteristics are also important for mental health and well-being (Kirsh & Gewurtz, 2012). For instance, poor psychosocial working conditions, such as insecure jobs, job strain (e.g., when workers have high psychological job demands but lack control over managing them), and an imbalance between the effort and reward are recognized risk factors for mental ill-health (Stansfeld & Candy, 2006). Evidence indicates a range of work-related risk and protective factors for mental health that relate not only to job design, but also at both team and organizational levels in workplaces (Harvey et al., 2014). Each workplace will have a combination of factors that interact to create working conditions that may increase the risks of employee emotional distress and mental illness or promote a mentally healthier workplace. Examples of work-related characteristics that present potential risk and protective factors for mental health in the workplace include:

- *Job design:* job content and workload, degree of discretion or choice and control within the job, work schedules and flexibility, role clarity or ambiguity, work environment, resources and feedback provided, level of work engagement, and potential exposure to trauma
- *Team factors:* social and instrumental support from colleagues and managers, quality of interpersonal relationships with coworkers and colleagues, supervision and leadership styles
- *Organizational factors:* organizational change, communication and involvement, organizational support, recognition and reward, fairness, psychosocial safety (including commitment to prevention of stress, mental health promotion, inclusive practices), a safe physical environment, support for work and life balance

OTPs need to attend to personal, health-related, social, organizational, and economic factors that influence work experiences and mental health to improve vocational and employment-related outcomes for current workers experiencing mental illness, as well as for those not presently in the workforce and those most marginalized from the world of work.

Volunteer exploration is defined as "identifying and learning about community causes, organizations, and opportunities for unpaid work consistent with personal skills, interests, location, and time available" (AOTA, 2020, p. 34). Volunteer activities may engage the person in using a variety of skills that can further strengthen other areas of occupation, especially instrumental activities of daily living (IADLs) such as care of others or pets, driving and community mobility, maintaining one's health, and safety. In addition, some volunteer positions allow the participant to explore aspects of the environment that might lead to future pursuits, such as volunteering at a welcome desk at a university and later enrolling in that university. Volunteer opportunities might reflect a leisure interest, such as being a museum docent, offering a foster home for service dogs in training, being the manager of a little league baseball team, or helping to open a community garden.

These activities offer various levels of social participation, from delivering meals on wheels and engaging in frequent one-to-one interactions to working as part of a Clubhouse culinary unit with 8 to 10 other individuals. A potential solitary occupation serving newborns might be knitting caps and blankets for homeless families.

Volunteers are people who contribute "time to helping others with no expectation of pay or other material benefit" (Wilson & Musick, 1999, p. 141). Volunteering is a common occupation, with approximately 30% of persons in the United States reported as volunteering at least once a year (Rotolo & Wilson, 2011). Volunteers participate in a variety of service opportunities from helping a friend in need, to political activism, to community representation on boards of various agencies.

Providing service to others is the hallmark of volunteer work; therefore, the title of this chapter, *Work and Volunteer Occupations,* reflects the inclusiveness of all occupations in which individuals offer their time, skills, and talents—whether in a formal volunteer role or simply as the need arises. Informal volunteerism includes helping activities such as driving a friend without transportation to the grocery store. Formal volunteerism, in contrast, involves services in which "time and effort are given for the betterment of the community in general" (Thoits & Hewitt, 2001, p. 116). Many organizations use formal volunteers to accomplish their mission. For example, individuals can volunteer with civic and political organizations, religious organizations, or organizations that address a specific issue, such as food security or environmental conservation.

Looking broadly at the landmark Rehabilitation Act of 1973, as amended in 1978, the view of disability and citizenship was captured in this congressional statement: "Disability is a natural part of the human experience and in no way diminishes the rights of individuals to . . . live independently; enjoy self-determination; make choices; contribute to society; pursue meaningful careers; and enjoy full inclusion and integration in the economic, political, social, cultural and educational mainstream of American society." For persons pursuing full participation in community life, volunteer opportunities may provide a place to belong and contribute in a manner that fulfills personal hopes and dreams.

Being engaged in volunteer activities may intersect with work and career development, a life with family and friends, and finding ways to enhance one's physical, mental, emotional, and spiritual capacity. For each person on a recovery journey, the amount of time spent in each occupation varies based on personal choice, values, and a personally defined level of optimal engagement.

Types of Work

Ross (2007) suggests the following terms to reflect the range of work and productive occupations: paid, unpaid, hidden, and substitute work.

Paid work includes all forms of employment, including self-employment, usually involving an agreement in which labor is traded for pay. It encompasses formal contracts and informal arrangements, which are often observed in developing countries (Chopra, 2009). Paid work provides structure to one's time and is of greater societal value than unpaid work. Nevertheless, the nature of paid work, working conditions, and experiences vary widely. Precarious employment, where work is time-bound or employer dependent, may offer additional income but limits employee control over hours and activities and can be detrimental to mental health (Kirsh & Gewurtz, 2012).

Unpaid work, such as domestic chores, caregiving, and volunteering, is vital to society but often goes unrecognized and unremunerated (Ross, 2007). Its economic value becomes evident when one considers replacing it with paid labor. Unpaid household and caregiving tasks are informal and typically occur within family roles, whereas volunteering often happens within community groups, fostering skill development and social connections. Some volunteer for personal growth or to gain job-related experience (Fegan & Cook, 2014). Education and training, which are also unpaid, offer personal and vocational development and, in some ways, resemble paid work by structuring one's time.

Hidden work occurs when services are exchanged for cash, goods, or other services and are not reported as income (Ross, 2007). Informal child care (i.e., baby-sitting), caring for animals, and house-sitting are common examples. Illegal activities, such as the drug trade and exploitative forced labor, often with inadequate pay and working conditions, also fall under hidden work.

Substitute work, also known as "sheltered work," historically aimed to offer structure and activity for individuals with disabilities (Ross, 2007). However, it often led to segregated, joblike settings that lacked equal rights, pay, and working conditions when compared with the mainstream workforce. Rather than serving as prevocational training as intended, it created separate employment substitutes and failed to provide the social and economic benefits of competitive integrated employment (Schneider, 2005). This type of work is considered discriminatory in terms of disabled workers' rights because of its inferior pay and conditions compared with the mainstream labor market (UN General Assembly, 2006).

The significance of investigating people's perceptions of work is evident in the diversity of the four types of work presented here (paid, unpaid, hidden, substitute). Distinguishing work solely by payment is not straightforward. The understanding of work is influenced by meanings and values attributed to various occupations by persons, communities, and cultures. Sociological, psychological, and occupational perspectives provide overlapping yet slightly distinct viewpoints (Jarman, 2010; Ross, 2007).

Evaluation and Vocationally Focused Assessment

Integrating understanding of a person's abilities and motivations into occupational therapy practice aids recovery by fostering self-efficacy and self-determination. Occupational therapy services may encompass supporting job seekers, assisting workers returning after illness or injury, suggesting workplace accommodations or modifications and strategies for managing disclosure of mental health concerns, and finding suitable volunteer and service roles.

OTPs collaborate with persons to identify occupational performance issues and then contributing factors, planning, and implementing actions to address barriers to employment. Discussing work-related concerns validates and helps to reduce the pressures to be productive and contribute to society and empowers cocreation of individualized adaptive strategies. The *OTPF-4* (AOTA, 2020) outlines the occupational therapy assessment process, which involves developing an occupational profile and analyzing occupational performance to understand persons' occupational demands and environments. Although the evaluation may involve an occupational therapy assistant, the occupational therapist holds responsibility for the overall assessment process.

The Occupational Profile

The evaluation process begins with an occupational profile, which is "a summary of a client's (person's, group's, or population's) occupational history and experiences, patterns of daily living, interests, values, needs, and relevant contexts" (AOTA, 2020, p. 21). An understanding of a person's occupational profile is most often gained through an interview between the person and practitioner, and by using an existing semistructured interview tool such as the Occupational Performance History Interview-II (OPHI-II; Kielhofner et al., 2004) or Canadian Occupational Performance Measure (COPM; Law et al., 2014). An effective beginning could involve delving into the individual's perception of work, aiming to comprehend their self-image as a worker and their professional aspirations (Fossey & Bramley, 2014).

In a vocational context, the OTP should identify the person's preferences concerning work or volunteer service opportunities through understanding their history of training, employment, volunteer service experiences, interests, values, and beliefs—all of which may help to identify motivating opportunities. For example, some may prefer to engage in service with a faith-based organization, whereas others may be more motivated by social issues such as environmental conservation.

It is also important to identify a person's habits, roles, and routines. For example, persons with mental illness may have altered sleep patterns or limited access to transportation. Therefore, a person may need experience that matches their daily schedule and available resources. Finally, the occupational profile should identify a person's goals regarding work or volunteer service. For example, some seek preemployment opportunities, whereas others are looking for social participation. The vocational profile sets the foundation for the rest of the evaluation and intervention.

The development of an occupational profile with an adolescent, young adult, or an adult later in their working life will vary in its focus. For instance, with adolescents, it is likely to focus on the young person's occupational experiences in school, leisure, and work, as well as their evolving self-knowledge about vocational interests, values, and strengths, which could support future vocational choices and decisions about job-seeking, further education, or vocational training. In comparison, in the context of looking to reenter the workforce or to transition out of the workforce, an adult's occupational profile would likely focus on prior work history; experiences of paid work, volunteering, and other forms of unpaid work; and potential sources of disruption, needs, and priorities that may influence return-to-work or retirement plans.

In each of these contexts, the OTP aims to elicit the person's views and experiences of personal and contextual barriers to work participation, as well as the resources available to support the person's pursuit of chosen work, volunteer, or other vocational options. Further conversations to identify obstacles and challenges, strengths, and support networks can facilitate shared understanding and collaborative working with the person to identify strategies for addressing issues identified.

Effective collaboration, mutual respect, a sense of hope, adaptability, and a focus on capabilities are essential for establishing a trustworthy relationship and a shared vision between the service provider (e.g., OTP) and the individual they are assisting (Johnson et al., 2009). Individuals may require substantial encouragement and assistance to develop the belief that they can consider making changes. In addition, focusing on their strengths, capabilities, and support systems can broaden their perspective about strategies and goals relating to their vocational pursuits.

Two semistructured interview tools that can guide interviews about work are the Worker Role Interview (WRI; Braveman et al., 2005) and the Work Environment Impact Scale (WEIS; Moore-Corner et al., 1998). Both are informed by Kielhofner's Model of Human Occupation (MOHO; Taylor et al., 2024), which guides OTPs to comprehend how disability, health, and life situations affect work and volunteering. MOHO emphasizes that occupations shape people's identities and abilities. Performance strengths and limitations can be analyzed by considering factors such as volition (individual interests, values, and work choices), habituation (roles, habits, and routines), and the environment (demands, relationships, and working conditions). The WRI and the WEIS are respectively used to explore work transitions and the workplace's impact on participation.

Worker Role Interview

The WRI examines the psychosocial and environmental elements that impact engagement in work and the process of returning to work. Informed by MOHO, it specifically considers the impact of volition, habituation, and perceptions of the work environment on psychosocial readiness for work (Lee & Kielhofner, 2010). The semistructured format provides occupational therapists with the flexibility to tailor questions to the individual and the context. Investigating individuals' perspectives on their self-image and their past, present, and future work experiences is valuable for pinpointing obstacles, challenges, and potential sources of support to address them.

Originally developed for use with injured workers expecting to return to a particular type of work, the current version of the WRI includes interview formats for recently injured workers and persons who have been out of the workforce for some time because of illness or disability (Braveman et al., 2005). WRI interview findings may be used to rate the extent to which 16 items related to personal causation, values, interests, roles, habits, and the environment are interfering with the person's working life. Each item in the 4-point rating scale is operationally defined (Braveman et al., 2005). Research provides evidence of the WRI's reliability and validity. The WRI measures the psychosocial ability to work of people with persistent mental illness and predicts return to work after long absences (Ekbladh et al., 2010; Sandqvist & Ekbladh, 2017). It has also been used to measure employment program outcomes (Areberg & Bejerholm, 2013).

Work Environment Impact Scale

The WEIS (Moore-Corner et al., 1998) explores the impact of workplace characteristics on work participation. It is best suited for use with workers having difficulties in current or recent jobs (Lee & Kielhofner, 2010; Williams et al., 2010). Similar in structure to the WRI, the WEIS uses a semistructured interview format to elicit the person's perception of their work environment. It can aid in constructing a comprehensive understanding of the individual's unique work circumstances and empower them to recognize and strategize for a return to work, including negotiating any necessary work adjustments. After completion of the interview, the interviewer completes a 17-item rating scale that focuses on the physical space, social contacts and supports, temporal demands, objects used, and daily job functions. Each item is rated for the degree to which that aspect of the environment supports or interferes with the person's success and satisfaction at work, using the same 4-point rating scale as the WRI.

The WEIS was developed for use with persons with physical or psychiatric disabilities. Evidence supports its construct and discriminant validity, interrater reliability, and its usefulness to identify workplace features that support workers experiencing mental ill-health to sustain employment (Sandqvist & Ekbladh, 2017; Williams et al., 2010). Its focus on workplace environments means the WEIS may be useful for assessing the occupational needs of groups of workers in particular workplaces (de las Heras de Pablo et al., 2017).

Other Assessment Tools and Concepts

In settings where learning about persons' occupational histories, interests, preferences, and abilities broadly can help to ensure their vocational issues are addressed, other MOHO-based assessment tools, such as the OPHI-II (Kielhofner et al., 2004), may be useful, even though these tools do not focus specifically on work participation.

Mental health workers, including OTPs, may not routinely discuss vocational issues with persons experiencing mental illness, or may assume that their mental health issues need to be resolved first. However, consistently posing inquiries about work from the initial assessment to every stage of service interaction and discharge planning enables OTPs to prevent reinforcing misconceptions that link employment solely with well-being and mental health issues with joblessness, lack of productivity, or incapacity for work. They can also instill hope and create opportunities for persons' vocational aspirations and capabilities to be taken seriously and enable conversations about working and supporting their self-determination (Fossey & Bramley, 2014).

Vocationally focused assessment should also focus on the critical vocational behaviors related to job choice, job acquisition, and job retention (i.e., choose, get, and keep work). The assessment of a person's job preferences and choice in the field of psychiatric rehabilitation includes consideration of work readiness based on theoretical models that propose stages of behavioral change. These models offer explanations for people's successful—and failed—attempts to eliminate problems or develop helpful habits and daily routines; they also suggest that interventions to facilitate behavioral changes must be designed to match each specific stage of change to result in positive outcomes (i.e., success in changing; Prochaska & Norcross, 2001).

The aim of a readiness assessment process is to support individuals to reflect on experiences of job-seeking and job retention and to identify lifestyle and environmental changes that they want to make in relation to work participation. Therefore, to explore work readiness and preferences, OTPs must engage the person in thoughtful discussions or values clarification activities focused on the person's satisfactions or dissatisfactions with their current situation, personal preferences, commitment to change, and sources of personal support. Using tools such as the WRI (Braveman et al., 2005) and the WEIS (Moore-Corner et al., 1998) can enable OTPs to facilitate these conversations systematically. A structured tool for identifying work accommodations and supports in the workplace (e.g., Corbière et al., 2014) may also be useful to support discussion of potential ways to manage work and mental health when issues or challenges arise.

Analysis of Occupational Performance Issues

During the analysis of occupational performance, the occupational therapist elicits more targeted information regarding the performance skills and patterns, person factors, activity demands, and contextual barriers that may need intervention to facilitate successful work participation. Assessment approaches most used to support the analysis of occupational performance in work are self-reports, observational assessments, and proxy measures of work-related functioning. Of these, observational approaches are likely to be most useful to fully understand a person's occupational performance, the impacts of sensory and cognitive disruptions on performance, and issues that may need further evaluation in vocational services.

Sensory, cognitive, and social or interpersonal domains of functioning are considered important in relation to work performance and success, but there are few well-validated tools that can be used for assessing these domains of the work performance of persons with psychiatric disabilities (Rogers & MacDonald-Wilson, 2011). Because of this, the favored approach in vocational rehabilitation has shifted toward situational assessment. This typically entails observing an individual's performance in a real or simulated setting, using rating scales to assess their skill proficiency (Rogers & MacDonald-Wilson, 2011). Therefore, practitioners need to be knowledgeable about the work tasks if they are to accurately observe and evaluate a person's performance.

Situational assessment is familiar in occupational therapy practice, including the use of established and validated measures. For example, the Assessment of Work Performance (AWP; Sandqvist et al., 2010) assesses an individual's observable skills during work performance and provides information on how efficiently and effectively the person performs a work activity. The AWP assesses 14 skills in three domains—motor skills, process skills, and communication and interaction skills. Each is rated on a 4-point ordinal rating scale. Based on studies in Sweden, evidence provides support for the content, construct, and discriminant validity of the AWP (Sandqvist & Ekbladh, 2017). Other occupational therapy–specific situational assessments for evaluating vocationally relevant skills performance include the School Version of Assessment of Motor and Process Skills (School AMPS; Fisher et al., 2007), which is used to evaluate the quality of a student's schoolwork task performance in a classroom setting.

As with most situational assessments, observation of work performance in real-life settings may be challenging and needs careful consideration. Access to work sites may not be feasible, may be too costly, or may be labor-intensive. In addition, situational assessment needs sensitive and respectful handling to ensure a worker's difficulties do not unduly draw attention in the workplace.

Occupational therapy standardized assessments evaluate many performance skills associated with work and volunteer service. Three examples are the Kohlman Evaluation of Living Skills (KELS; Kohlman Thomson & Robnett, 2016), the Executive Function Performance Test (EFPT; Baum et al., 2008), and the Cognitive Performance Test (CPT; Burns et al., 1994). See Table 48-1 for more information on these assessments.

OTPs can also use task analysis to evaluate a person's ability to complete a specific skill. For example, a person may wish to volunteer with Rebuilding Together, an organization in which volunteers work to improve the homes of people with disabilities. Volunteers complete various home improvement tasks such as painting and carpentry. The OTP may perform a task analysis by asking the person to complete a similar task, such as building a small birdhouse. By watching the person complete the task, the therapist can analyze their performance in subtasks, such as following directions, using tools, and maintaining safe behaviors. After the analysis, the practitioner can identify the person's strengths and limitations regarding a specific volunteer task.

The OTP must also assess the environment to ensure a good fit with the person's skills and preferences. For instance, an evaluation of the volunteer environment may identify barriers such as excessive noise, distractions, or safety concerns. Once a person has been placed in a volunteer service experience, the practitioner can evaluate the fit using the WEIS, which explores a variety of factors, including time demands, task demands, appeal of work tasks, work schedule, coworker interaction, supervisor interaction, rewards, sensory qualities, the physical environment, and ambience (Moore-Corner et al., 1998). Through evaluation of the environment, the OTP can help the organization make the environment more amenable to persons with lived experience or support people to address the barriers presented by the environment.

At the conclusion of the evaluation, the person and practitioner consider the identified strengths, interests, and desires for growth, and work collaboratively to determine a series of goals. The goal might be to engage in a volunteer activity or develop skills through participation as a volunteer. For example, increasing the range or amount of social participation, increasing social awareness, and spending more time in the community are goals that can be achieved through engaging in a volunteer occupation. Goals should complement intervention plans across the wellness team and reflect what matters most to the person.

Interventions That Support Work and Volunteer Performance

Facilitating entry or reentry into employment has been a focus of occupational therapy intervention since the founding of the profession (Sandqvist & Ekbladh, 2017). Many approaches have evolved since for addressing the work issues and employment barriers experienced by people with mental illness, including interventions focused on the individual level and workplace-based initiatives. OTPs may also enable

TABLE 48-1 | Therapeutic Reasoning Assessment Table: Work and Volunteer and Service Occupations

Which Tool?	Who Was This Tool Designed For?	Is This a Type of Tool This Person Can Do? What Is Required of the Person?	What Am I Measuring?	How Long Does It Take and Where Do I Administer This Assessment?	Is the Tool Associated With a Practice Model?
The Activity Card Sort (ACS; Baum & Edwards, 2008)	Adults with neurological, psychiatric, or physical dysfunction	Person describes their occupational history by sorting 89 photographs depicting people completing various daily living activities.	Participation in social, instrumental, and leisure activities	Administered in a clinical or home setting and takes approximately 20–30 minutes	The Person-Environment-Occupation (PEO) Performance model
Assessment of Work Performance (AWP; Sandqvist et al., 2010)	Persons with psychiatric disabilities interested in work	A mixed methods process of interview, observation of actual performance in real-world settings, or proxy measures. Situational assessment with rating scales is preferred.	Analysis of occupational performance regarding skills or patterns (motor, process, and communication or interaction), person factors, activity demands, and contextual barriers to successful work participation	Time varied based on self-report, observational assessment, and proxy measures of work-related functioning, with emphasis on observation of performance within sensory, cognitive, and social or interpersonal domains	Model of Human Occupation (MOHO) or PEO model
Canadian Occupational Performance Measure (COPM; Law et al., 2014)	Children older than 8 years of age to adults with mental illness; persons with neurological or orthopedic conditions	Person can communicate their difficulty in performing tasks and prioritize concerns using rating scales.	A person's perceived problems in self-care, work, and leisure; person quantitatively rates perceived occupational performance and satisfaction with performance.	Allow 20–30 minutes for initial assessment, shorter for readministration; can administer in any space where the person and practitioner can discuss privately	PEO model and the Canadian Model of Occupational Performance and Engagement
Cognitive Performance Test (CPT; Burns et al., 1994)	Adults with dementia	Occupational performance test investigates a person's ability to sort medications, shop for clothing, wash hands, prepare food, use the telephone, and travel between locations.	Person's performance in ADLs and IADLs	Administered in a clinical or home setting and takes up to 70 minutes	Cognitive Disabilities Model
Executive Function Performance Test (EFPT; Baum et al., 2008)	Adults with psychiatric disorders and people with neurological conditions	Complete four IADL tasks: paying bills, medication management, use of telephone, and a cooking task; graded cues are provided as needed.	Assesses executive function skills including safety, organization, sequencing, initiation, and judgment; used to define level of assistance for functional tasks	Typically, 60–90 minutes; requires access to a space for cooking; can be used in home, clinical, or community settings	No specific model, but consistent with several models that include an emphasis on functional performance
Kohlman Evaluation of Living Skills (KELS; Kohlman Thomson & Robnett, 2016)	Initially designed for adults within inpatient psychiatric facilities. Newest version was tested in a variety of environments and adult populations.	Requires skills of reading and writing, self-care, safety and health, money management, community mobility and telephone use, and employment and leisure.	Standardized tool to evaluate both basic ADLs and IADLs by assessing living skills grouped into categories of self-care, safety and health, money management, community mobility and telephone, and work and leisure	Typically, 30 minutes Easy to administer in table-top setting or limited space setting Requires computer to assess online banking skills	No specific model but consistent with several models that include an emphasis on functional performance

TABLE 48-1 | Therapeutic Reasoning Assessment Table: Work and Volunteer and Service Occupations—cont'd

Which Tool?	Who Was This Tool Designed For?	Is This a Type of Tool This Person Can Do? What Is Required of the Person?	What Am I Measuring?	How Long Does It Take and Where Do I Administer This Assessment?	Is the Tool Associated With a Practice Model?
Occupational Performance History Interview-II (OPHI-II; Kielhofner et al., 2004)	Adults	Semistructured interview and ratings on occupational choices, critical life events, daily routine, occupational roles, and occupational behavior setting	The person's occupational history with a focus on identity, competence, and environment	Administered in a clinical or home setting and takes 45-70 minutes	MOHO
Occupational Profile or Vocational Profile (Fossey & Bramley, 2014)	Adolescent, young adult, or adult	Tailored to developmental level, ascertains the individual's view of self as a worker, aspirations for work, perceived barriers, and resources to support person's pursuit of chosen work	Overview of goals, barriers, and supports for plans for future work	Up to ½ hour for interview and additional time for scoring Administered in a clinical or home setting	MOHO or PEO model
Vocational Fit Assessment (Persch et al., 2015)	Youth and young adults with intellectual and developmental disabilities	Provider/parent report; self-report adaptation in development	Assessment of work-related adaptive behavior and job demands. Demands and Abilities Transforming Algorithm identifies strengths and needs within the context of individual job options.	45 minutes the first time. Experienced users consistently report 20 minutes or less. Available at VocFit.com	PEO model
Work Environment Impact Scale (WEIS; Moore-Corner et al., 1998)	Adults with physical and psychosocial/psychiatric disabilities	Semistructured interview and rating of the work, physical environment, supports, temporal demands, objects used, and daily job functions	The level of fit between a person and the work environment	Up to ½ hour for interview and additional time for scoring Administered in a clinical or home setting	MOHO or PEO model
Worker Role Interview (WRI; Braveman et al., 2005; Lee & Kielhofner, 2010)	Injured workers returning to work and those out of work for a time because of illness or disability	Semistructured interview explores psychosocial and environmental factors influencing work participation and return to work; impact of volition, habituation, and perceptions of work environment on psychosocial readiness for work	Obstacles, challenges, and supports to overcome return to work	Up to ½ hour for interview and additional time for scoring Administered in clinical, home, or work setting	MOHO or PEO model

people to engage in volunteer service opportunities through interventions grounded in occupation, education, training, advocacy, and groups. In addition, volunteering can be an intervention in and of itself.

Several systematic and scoping reviews have reaffirmed the value of occupational therapy interventions that support employment of people with serious mental illness (Swarbrick & Noyes, 2018). Recent evidence reviews on this topic found strong support for the use of the Individual Placement and Support (IPS) model and for the use of cognitive interventions (McDowell et al., 2021; Noyes et al., 2018). Few of these studies were conducted by or included occupational therapists, and OTPs also find support for their use of IPS

in two literature reviews (Kirsh et al., 2019; Machingura & Lloyd, 2017). Finally, there is increasing evidence in support of the Redesigning Daily Occupations (ReDo) approach (Edgelow et al., 2020; Kirsh et al., 2019) that emphasizes occupational self-analysis, goal setting, developing and practicing strategies, and workplace implementation.

Volunteering in the community can serve several purposes. Individuals may explore their strengths and interests through activities such as tending to animals or creating art or might give back to the community by providing care and services to others. Volunteering could be an individual's primary vocational occupation, or they could choose to participate in addition to paid work (Fegan & Cook, 2014).

Individuals may seek a volunteer position before entering or reengaging with the workforce as it can help them practice job skills and implement strategies for managing their mental health before seeking employment (Farrell & Bryant, 2009; Fegan & Cook, 2014); other benefits include more social connections and developing a valued role and identity (Pérez-Corrales et al., 2019).

As with paid employment, volunteer occupations are associated with benefits to health and quality of life. Among the most relevant benefits to mental health, volunteering is associated with decreased depression. These effects have been emphasized most among older adults (Jiang et al., 2021; Musick & Wilson, 2003), though recent analyses demonstrate the benefit to adults of all ages (Yeung et al., 2018). The benefits of volunteering may be greater for those whose service is for religious causes (Musick & Wilson, 2003) or service oriented toward others (Yeung et al., 2018), although a systematic review failed to find such differential benefits (Jenkinson et al., 2013), citing the heterogeneity of the included studies.

Working Together to Support Work and Volunteerism

Working With People

Effective relationships between vocational specialists and service recipients rely on trust, collaboration, hope, flexibility, and a focus on capabilities (Johnson et al., 2009). Individuals might need support in fostering belief in their aspirations, reassurance regarding their potential for success, and assistance in considering change. It is crucial to recognize and validate each person, considering their choices, preferences, interests, and past experiences. Motivation, self-efficacy, confidence, responses to change, and individual circumstances will inevitably differ (McQueen & Turner, 2012; Royal College of Occupational Therapists [RCOT], 2017). Understanding what work means to someone is central to understanding their vocational motivations and aspirations, particularly as employment can be anxiety-inducing (Bertram & McDonald, 2015).

Partnering to Support Worker Mental Health

Collaborating with supporters and mental health workers is vital for overcoming employment barriers. Supporters can be either empowering or disempowering based on their perceptions of the person's mental health and work potential. Negative views often cite concerns about safety and well-being and may hinder progress. Collaborative planning with others can integrate coping strategies, prevention plans, and ways to identify relapse triggers. In times of change, involving others provides stability. Such teamwork enriches workers' understanding of individual strengths and impacts on work and volunteer occupations. OTPs offer insight into mental health and vocational rehabilitation. Access to their knowledge helps individuals and supports consideration of necessary risks while promoting safety.

Interagency Collaboration

Effective cooperation with various agencies is often a prerequisite for vocational success. The information necessary for pursuing vocational goals is typically scattered among different entities. For example, in the United States, this information may come from the schools, families, state departments of vocational rehabilitation, developmental disabilities, workers compensation, the Social Security Administration, and advocacy organizations, among others. Social welfare and return-to-work services are intricate and susceptible to frequent changes influenced by economic, political, and societal fluctuations. Establishing strong alliances with employment agencies allows vocational specialists to discover potential opportunities and assess their appropriateness for individuals. They may also share their insights into other services and agencies, facilitating navigation of unfamiliar systems and shared decision-making.

Establishing Relationships

Assisting individuals in securing employment or job placement may require establishing relationships with employers and line managers. This entails comprehending the work environment, employer obligations, employee rights, and the importance of approaching the matter with sensitivity and consideration for mutual rights.

OTPs may play a valuable role in providing information and support to employers to facilitate making suitable workplace accommodations for employees with mental health concerns. With the consent of both the individual and the employer, they can support the development of return-to-work plans, suggest reasonable adjustments, and facilitate discussions about how a health condition might affect workplace performance. Otherwise, the practitioner may share this information with the employee, rather than directly interacting with the employer. Regardless, a deep understanding of workplace culture and requirements is crucial to find the best fit between person, workplace, job, and employers.

Mental Health and Wellness Supports

Sustaining education or employment requires proactive use of strategies that draw on internal and external resources to manage both work and mental health (Ennals et al., 2015; Williams et al., 2016). Health management strategies assist individuals in maintaining communication with employers during crises, acute mental health episodes, substance misuse, or periods of financial and housing instability (Harris et al., 2014). Unforeseen circumstances may demand time-sensitive collaboration with other services and supporters to adapt vocational plans.

The vocational specialist reinforces effective wellness strategies, with tools such as the Wellness Recovery Action Plan (Cook et al., 2010) and mobile apps such as Working Well (Nicholson et al., 2017) for self-management and recovery support. Regular reviews of plans for employment are essential to acknowledge achievements and maintain focus. Mobile apps can help people track progress, offering a clear record of accomplishments during health fluctuations. Collaboration with service users is key to developing innovative strategies for mental health and vocational support.

Workplace Mental Health Initiatives

Initiatives to address work-related stress and promote workplace mental health may be important to decrease the prevalence of mental disorders among workers, and to reduce the

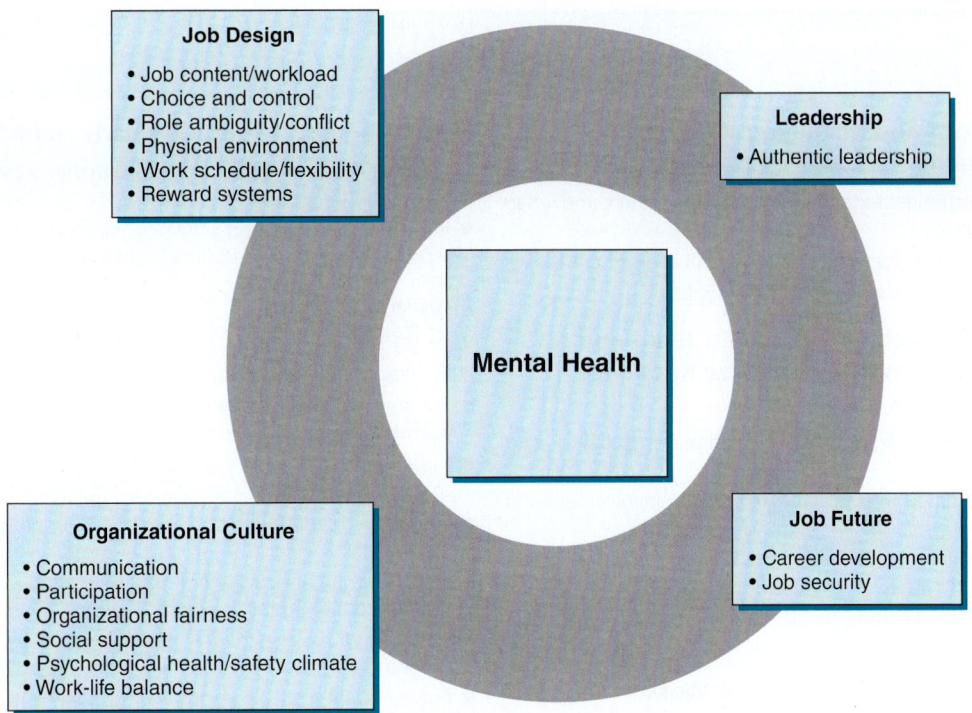

FIGURE 48-1. A framework for workplace mental health. *From Kirsh, B., & Gewurtz, R. (2012). Promoting mental health within workplaces. In R. J. Gatchel & I. Z. Schultz (Eds.),* Handbook of occupational health and wellness *(p. 244). Springer.*

work-related disability of employees who experience mental illness (Dewa et al., 2012). The framework illustrated in Figure 48-1 identifies job design, leadership, organizational culture, and job futures as key areas that could be the focus for workplace mental health promotion initiatives (Kirsh & Gewurtz, 2012). It suggests the importance of fit between the workers, work, and workplaces, as well as highlighting that workplace initiatives need to include individual, team, and organizational level strategies to promote mentally healthy workplaces.

Based on their research review, Harvey and colleagues (2014) proposed six domains of research-informed strategies for promoting workplace mental health, which are summarized in Box 48-1.

Interventions That Promote Readiness for Volunteer Occupations

Engagement in volunteer and service opportunities may include a variety of tasks from caring for animals, to completing yard work, to selling goods. When a person is unable to successfully complete an activity, OTPs work to improve their performance or select an occupation better suited to them.

Using the "just right challenge," the OTP may adjust the task to the person's current performance level and increase the complexity of the task through time until the person is independent. For example, consider a person who seeks to volunteer at the American Society for the Prevention of Cruelty to Animals but becomes anxious when caring for the needs of several animals. The person might begin by working with one animal and increase their animal care responsibilities

slowly through time. Alternatively, the OTP may adapt the environment for a person who feels anxious about engaging with new people in an unfamiliar place. They may benefit from beginning to volunteer in a local Clubhouse where staff and volunteers are familiar and welcoming to persons with mental illness, and then trying to volunteer in less familiar service environments.

Although the role of peer support specialist is a relatively new entry in the behavioral health workforce, volunteering one-on-one as a mentor to people new in their recovery process may be a meaningful way to support others. OTPs facilitate volunteer and service opportunities by engaging with the person toward meaningful positions selected by them and supporting them to find volunteer opportunities that matter to them.

Education

OTPs implement and facilitate education-based interventions to help persons in recovery engage in volunteer and service activities. In the initial stages of intervention, they educate about the benefits of volunteering, such as increased social participation, the development of new skills, and the enhancement of one's social network. Becoming familiar with local organizations allows practitioners to describe specific opportunities available in the community as a precursor to exploring what the person is aware of.

OTPs may also facilitate education sessions. For example, a practitioner may convene a panel of volunteers who also have mental illness or substance abuse to discuss volunteer and service experiences with a group of individuals interested in pursuing such work. In addition, practitioners can advise community organizations on how to better collaborate with

BOX 48-1 ■ Examples of Research-Informed Strategies for Promoting Workplace Mental Health

Designing Jobs and Managing Work to Minimize Harm

- Provide opportunities for job flexibility around where and when the work is done.
- Create opportunities for workers' involvement in decision-making.
- Ensure the physical work environment is safe.

Promoting Protective Factors at a Team and Organizational Level to Maximize Resilience

- Build a psychosocial safety climate.
- Develop policies to counteract workplace bullying and discrimination.
- Provide team-based work activities to enhance involvement and group support.
- Provide workplace mental health education for leaders, managers, and supervisors.
- Promote open communication and effective change management.

Enhancing Personal Resilience at Work

- Provide coaching and mentoring.
- Offer stress management and resilience training that uses evidence-based strategies (e.g., cognitive-behavioral strategies), especially in "high risk" occupations where workers are regularly exposed to traumatic events.
- Promote physical activity at work.

Promoting and Facilitating Early Help-Seeking

- Provide EAPs and workplace counseling that use evidence-based strategies.
- Implement peer support schemes, particularly to support those repeatedly exposed to trauma in their work.

Supporting Workers' Return to Work and Recovery From Mental Illness

- Provide supervisor support and training.
- Support partial sickness absence or "fit notes" focused on what a worker can do, so as to facilitate return to work.
- Modify jobs and make reasonable workplace accommodations to support workers' return to work or job retention.
- Encourage recruitment of workers via supported employment or IPS services.
- Increase awareness of mental well-being and mental illness as well as reduce stigma and discrimination.
- Conduct workplace mental health awareness and education programs (see the Resources section for examples).
- Provide staff with access to mental health information and resources.
- Develop work-related policies that support workers to balance the demands of their work and personal lives.

Harvey, S. B., Joyce, S., Tan, L., Johnson, A., Nguyen, H., Modini, M., & Groth, M. (2014). Developing a mentally healthy workplace: A review of the literature. National Mental Health Commission and the Mentally Healthy Workplace Alliance. https://www.headsup.org.au/docs/default-source/resources/developing-a-mentally-healthy-workplace_final-november-2014.pdf

PhotoVoice

Linda

Some ladies and I create lap blankets and jewelry to donate to people. These projects start from simple materials I have at home. I create the jewelry at the table, and I crochet the blankets in my spare time. The ladies and I volunteer our time and talent to create beautiful lap blankets and jewelry. When we all work together to give back, we can help people and bring joy to the community. No gift is too small to give back to the community.

How does social participation play a significant role in Linda's picture and narrative on the meaningfulness of her volunteer work?

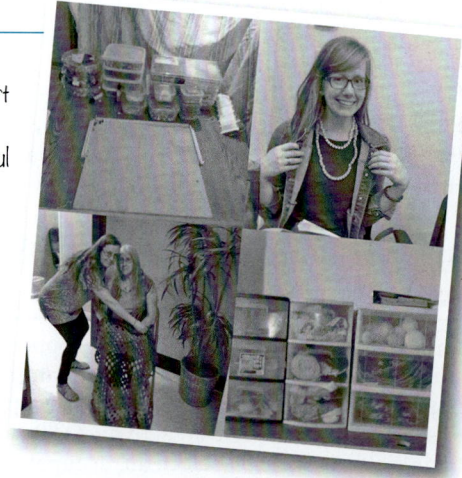

volunteers with mental and behavioral health concerns. For example, an OTP may advocate for more consumer-led positions on leadership councils or advise on policies and procedures, recommend tasks, or inform the training process to improve organizations' ability to support volunteers. OTPs educate the person and community organizations to promote volunteer service opportunities.

Skills Development

OTPs work with people to cultivate the skills and support systems necessary for successful engagement in their anticipated volunteer roles or service opportunities. In direct skills teaching, individuals with lived experience of mental illness or substance abuse are enlisted as volunteers to undertake specific activities. For example, if a person volunteers in a thrift store, they may be asked to work at the cash register, which can be a task with a high cognitive load. Using direct skills teaching, the OTP coaches the person on the variety of tasks performed by a cashier, such as scanning barcodes, entering commands into the register, and bagging items, by first talking about the skill, demonstrating the skill, and having the person practice the skill in the setting where they will be expected to carry it out (Nemec et al., 1992).

Practitioners may also educate community organization staff and volunteers about working with people with disabilities. For example, the OTP can facilitate an *In Our Own Voice* presentation from the National Alliance on Mental Illness (NAMI) or *Mental Health First Aid* from the Substance Abuse and Mental Health Services Administration (SAMHSA) to increase volunteers and service leaders' awareness and acceptance of persons living with mental illness. Improving organizational staff and peer volunteers' knowledge about recovery as it relates to mental illness and substance abuse can create a more welcoming environment for persons living with mental illness to undertake volunteering.

Advocacy

Interventions are actions intended to enhance a person's engagement in meaningful service experiences. OTPs may advocate to community organizations to increase their capacity to meet the needs and provide the best available supports for persons in recovery. For example, practitioners serving in advisory roles to programs, agencies, and community organizations can advocate to increase the number of volunteers and leaders with lived experiences. Similarly, OTPs connect community members with mental illness or substance abuse to local researchers. Connecting researchers with persons with lived experiences makes the research team stronger by encouraging participatory research, which is often endorsed by grant-funding agencies and informs what matters most to that population or community.

In self-advocacy interventions, OTPs support persons' efforts to advocate for themselves. For example, a practitioner may help a person develop strategies, such as writing and practicing a written script for requesting accommodations in volunteer service organizations. OTPs encourage persons to volunteer with organizations that advocate for the rights of persons with mental illness or substance abuse disorders. For example, across many local communities NAMI hosts an event called *NAMI Walks* to raise awareness about mental health and raise funds for the organization. OTPs can encourage persons and their families to walk in the event or serve as a volunteer, depending on their goals and preferences.

Groups

Interventions may be preparatory activities or group volunteering experiences. When occupational therapy services are delivered in inpatient settings, groups may serve as effective preparation for volunteer service participation. For example, craft and cooking groups can help persons develop interpersonal communication skills and learn how to work as a team toward a common goal or objective. In a community-based setting, groups of persons with mental illness or substance abuse can volunteer together. For example, as part of a team-building experience, a group can go to a local food pantry and work together to sort goods and make packages for food-insecure individuals. By volunteering as a group, they maintain their social support network while getting the experiences of an unfamiliar environment and current activity.

Volunteering as an Intervention

OTPs use diverse intervention approaches to facilitate involvement in volunteer positions. It is important to note that volunteering, in and of itself, can serve as a valued activity and a pathway to achieving different goals. For example, some may seek to return to work, return to their role as a parent, or become more comfortable in community environments. Volunteer service opportunities enable people to learn a variety of skills and gain exposure to a myriad of life situations. Also, volunteering allows the opportunity to give back to the community.

Persons in recovery often have good times and tough times. During tough times, a person may receive a significant level of help from family, friends, and community organizations. By transitioning to the role of volunteer, a person with mental illness can help ensure services persist to help others. For example, across the country "Warmlines," or peer-run listening phone lines, are staffed by persons in recovery to provide other persons in need with a safe place. This service supports the "pay it forward" system and provides the internal benefits of being able to help a peer.

Supported Volunteering

A supported volunteering approach incorporates resources from the community and health services to assist individuals in gaining and sustaining volunteer roles. Fegan and Cook (2014) created these guidelines for supported volunteering in the United Kingdom:

1. The volunteer actions are led by a coordinator, preferably with ample prior experience.
2. The individual's vocational goals include volunteering.
3. The experience follows standard employment processes, including applications and reviews.
4. A mentor is present and provides supervision.
5. An informal contract is in place that includes volunteer expectations, protocols for sickness and absences, codes of conduct, confidentiality, and procedures for handling grievances.
6. Orientations and role-specific trainings are provided.
7. Performance reviews are conducted to track progress and provide feedback.

Interventions That Promote Work Participation

Traditionally, rehabilitative practice required that individuals undertake prevocational preparation or training as a prerequisite to entry or reentry into employment (called a train-then-place approach). This approach has fallen out of favor, partly because of consumer and professional critiques that *prevocational* preparation imposed added barriers to work entry or reentry and failed to achieve employment outcomes for people with mental illness. Accumulated evidence through 20 years in the United States and internationally

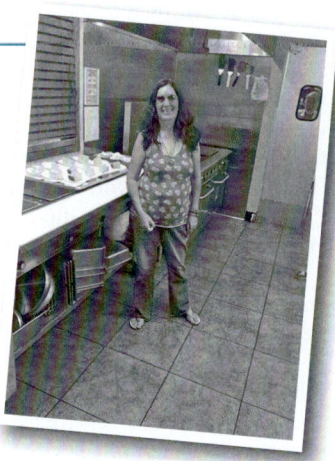

PhotoVoice

Julia

I love to volunteer in the kitchen so that it helps people be able to have someone that cares and to have someone be able to give them food to eat. It helps me to have fun serving food to other people. I like to go to "let's dish" because it helps me to be able to give people different dishes to try what we make. People like it when I volunteer because I give them the respect that I would like them to give me.

How does Julia's narrative capture the bidirectional nature of giving in her meaningful volunteer work?

has also demonstrated superior employment outcomes of an alternative place-then-train approach, in which the emphasis is reversed to focus on rapid job placement, followed by on-the-job training and support (Fioritti et al., 2014; Kinoshita et al., 2013). Originally known as IPS, this approach is further described in the text that follows.

Current best practice supports individuals to find and sustain employment of their own choosing in jobs with fair pay and working conditions, or to directly address working conditions and practices that perpetuate employment disadvantage or exclusion (Krupa, 2011a). Drawing on current accumulated evidence, Krupa (2011a) has identified eight principles of effective employment support to guide the development of employment initiatives and practices:

1. Focus on securing and sustaining employment in the community-based workforce as a desired outcome.
2. Provide a range of ongoing employment-related support.
3. Ensure that employment support practices are person-centered and collaborative.
4. Address social attitudes and structures to positively impact employment (e.g., working with employers to address workplace knowledge, practices, and policies that discriminate or exclude on grounds of mental illness).
5. Approach employment from a life-career perspective.
6. Provide early intervention to prevent employment marginalization.
7. Integrate vocational and clinical services.
8. Ensure provider competencies and practice standards are consistent with current knowledge about best practices in the field.

OTPs and researchers internationally are contributing to the body of knowledge informing the principles and practices for effective employment support. One example is The WORKS (Bramley & Mayne, 2010), a workshop-based approach using a fully resourced computer and paper-based package developed by OTPs through active collaborations with mental health service users and workers in Sheffield, England. Starting with the foundational idea that individuals possess diverse skills, experiences, and preferences, and have

encountered varied opportunities and challenges in pursuing their vocational goals, The WORKS proposes that mental health service users typically position themselves at one of three starting points concerning their vocational aspirations:

1. *Starting out.* Individuals in this category do not believe they can attain employment because of various barriers. They might have internalized negative beliefs about their skills, abilities, or societal stigmas, suggesting that individuals with mental health issues cannot or should not be employed. Low confidence and poor self-esteem may also contribute to their skepticism. Vocational specialists working with people in this situation should engage in collaborative efforts to establish a solid foundation for addressing these challenges.
2. *Moving forward.* Individuals in this category may possess some experience with or preferences regarding employment but lack confidence in their skills, abilities, or access to information to progress further. They might be interested in exploring vocational options but require support in taking the next step. In this starting point, vocational specialists collaborate with individuals to enhance their capabilities, potentially involving a graded approach to trying out new opportunities.
3. *Keeping going and growing.* Individuals in this stage are transitioning into employment but seek to identify how to address their ongoing support needs to ensure the sustainability of their employment and continued personal development. Vocational specialists should concentrate on assisting individuals in maintaining their employment during this phase.

The WORKS also offers tools and informational materials designed for use in workshops led by service users or for individual use. These resources aim to facilitate successful vocational pathways, tailored to individuals starting from different points in their journey. For example, "Starting Out" provides resources to establish the foundations of aspirational thinking, hope, and confidence. This is achieved by emphasizing existing strengths, disseminating information about choices and options, and pinpointing ongoing supports and practical needs. In Australia, occupational therapists and peer workers at a community mental health service used The WORKS to host a series of workshops targeting individuals in the "Starting Out" phase. These sessions helped participants share their experiences, identify skills, establish vocational goals, and ultimately see themselves as capable workers (Hitch et al., 2017).

Tools and activities for "Moving Forward" are designed to support capability building for job-seeking, making vocational choices, and action planning. Cassinello and Bramley (2012) utilized The WORKS framework to help examine their goals and abilities relating to work, beginning with volunteering and progressing to paid employment as a peer worker. "Keeping Going and Growing" underscores the importance of acquiring the necessary information and support to promote sustainability, which includes negotiating reasonable work adjustments and fostering employer engagement to enhance retention and support career development. Hence, OTPs may use this framework to guide working with both potential and current workers experiencing mental illness.

Supported Employment

Supported employment is an evidence-based service delivery model aimed at enhancing the employment outcomes of individuals dealing with persistent mental illness. Originating in the 1980s, it was initially developed to address the needs of individuals with developmental disabilities who had primarily been engaged in prevocational training and sheltered work settings—a situation similarly experienced by many individuals with psychiatric disabilities. As an alternative, supported employment promoted a place-then-train approach, without lengthy prior prevocational assessment or training. Originally defined as the IPS approach (Becker & Drake, 2003), it is now considered to represent general principles for evidence-based supported employment (Bond, 2004). These principles include the following:

- Competitive employment in a job consistent with the person's preferences is the goal.
- Service eligibility is based on the person's expressed desire to work; individuals are not screened out based on illness or employment history.
- Job search begins immediately upon program entry (i.e., there is no extended preparatory or assessment phase).
- Job search and job placement processes are individualized, so that job matching is consistent with the person's preferences.
- Individualized, time-unlimited follow-along support to retain employment is provided.
- Employment services are integrated and coordinated with mental health services.

When provided in a manner consistent with these principles, substantial evidence demonstrates that supported employment can assist adults with persistent mental illness and young people with psychoses to get jobs (Kinoshita et al., 2013; Krupa, 2011a; Lloyd & Waghorn, 2010). These principles can be used to provide effective services beyond the United States, although each country's policies and services may impact employment outcomes (Bond et al., 2012; Boyce et al., 2008; Waghorn et al., 2007). Recipients of supported employment services also report improved nonvocational outcomes, including better symptom control, improved self-esteem, and increased quality of life.

Supported employment based on IPS principles offers personalized employment interventions to address employment barriers (e.g., associated with symptoms, coping with illness, limited job-seeking or work experience) and support individuals to address workplace challenges (e.g., by identifying work accommodations and natural supports) at an individual level (Krupa, 2011a). Various educational, psychological, and peer support interventions may also usefully augment supported employment services (McDowell et al., 2021). Examples include the following:

- **Personalized financial counseling** regarding income support, health insurance, and other government benefits is important to assist individuals to understand, plan for, and manage the impacts of employment on income support and other benefits received as well as to make informed decisions about employment.
- **Supported education** offers individualized support for return to learning and participation in meaningful educational opportunities in a mainstream setting (Ringeisen et al., 2017). This can include attending classes with extra support for mental health and learning needs, peer support, or utilizing campuswide resources (Rudnick & Gover, 2009). An integrated approach to supported education and employment, modeled on IPS principles, may be particularly useful to minimize disruption to young people's vocational directions (Killackey et al., 2016).
- **Skills development interventions** designed to augment supported employment include cognitive enhancement strategies or social skills. One example of a combined supported employment and cognitive enhancement intervention is the Thinking Skills for Work program (McGurk et al., 2007). Developed to address cognitive difficulties that may impact work success, the Thinking Skills for Work includes participation in computer-based cognitive exercises, consultation between the cognitive specialist and employment specialist to facilitate consideration of the individual's cognitive strengths and challenges in job search planning, and support to develop strategies for coping with cognitive difficulties arising in the workplace. McGurk and colleagues found Thinking Skills for Work program participants were more likely to work, worked more hours, and earned more wages than those who only participated in the supported employment program. Training developed by Tsang and colleagues to improve social communication and problem-solving in the workplace has also been shown to enhance employment rates and job tenure (Tsang et al., 2010).

People who receive supported employment services have indicated that ongoing training and resources regarding career or financial advice, navigating disclosure processes, making informed decisions about vocational fit, having peer support, and maintaining their employment and well-being were particularly beneficial (Blank et al., 2011; Fossey & Harvey, 2010; Johnson et al., 2009; Williams et al., 2016). Acknowledging that people with lived experience are experts regarding their employment and challenges can help practitioners identify new strategies and resources to optimize their success (Boeltzig et al., 2008; Shaw & Sumsion, 2009).

Other employment initiatives, including transitional employment, self-employment, affirmative businesses and social firms, and employment in the mental health system, to varying extents, address community and systems level barriers to employment.

Transitional Employment

Transitional employment developed as part of the Clubhouse approach to psychosocial rehabilitation, along with a continuum of work opportunities that included the Clubhouse-based "work-ordered day" and community-based independent employment. Transitional employment was specifically designed for people with psychiatric disabilities to develop work readiness and to support work reentry. Transitional employment placements (TEPs) are time-limited job placements (e.g., 3 to 6 months) within mainstream workplaces at the prevailing wage. Typically, these job placements are negotiated with local businesses and "owned" by the Clubhouse, so that they may create several part-time positions for Clubhouse members with scope for others to step in if someone is temporarily unable to work.

A specific feature of transitional employment is the provision of onsite training and support from a job coach, so that transitional employment represents a means to overcome common employment barriers such as limited or no work history, lack of confidence in one's vocational skills, and the stress of job-seeking (Waghorn & Lloyd, 2010).

Because Clubhouse-based programs foster a powerful sense of mutual support among members, individuals also have a network of supports in their transition into employment. Nevertheless, the transitional employment approach has several limitations in regard to current best practices. These include the fact that TEP positions do not belong to the individual and, as with other prevocational and work preparation programs, their effectiveness to improve employment outcomes has been questioned. Although TEPs may assist some individuals with psychiatric disabilities to improve their work histories and job prospects (Henry et al., 2001; McKay et al., 2005), Clubhouses have subsequently introduced supported employment programs to achieve better employment outcomes (Macias et al., 2006).

Self-Employment

Being self-employed can offer individuals flexibility and autonomy in their work but may not traditionally be considered feasible for those with mental ill-health (Hamlet Trust et al., 2007). However, people may benefit from the freedom and healthy work–life balance that comes with being their own supervisor (Ostrow et al., 2019). Self-employment can take the form of entrepreneurship, where individuals use their strengths and creativity to create and manage a business. They can also work as an independent contractor or consultant, using their lived experience to support research, advocacy, or education initiatives (Gammon et al., 2014).

Affirmative Businesses and Social Firms

Unlike the previously noted individual level approaches to employment support, affirmative businesses and social firms address employment barriers at a community level. This is achieved by developing community businesses that create employment opportunities for people disadvantaged in the labor market. Adopting an economic development approach is widely applied to alleviate economic and labor market disadvantage because of factors that include long-term unemployment, homelessness, refugee status, disability, and mental illness.

Beginning with work cooperatives in Italy in the 1970s, affirmative businesses have been developed across Europe and internationally, although less extensively in the United States, to create employment opportunities and increase the economic self-sufficiency of persons with psychiatric disabilities (Warner & Mandiberg, 2006). Also referred to as social firms and social enterprises, they are developed to match local market gaps with the interests, talents, and resources of a particular potential workforce, and designed to create more inclusive working conditions, such as more flexible hours, job-sharing, mentorship, training, and career advancement opportunities (Krupa, 2011a).

These business ventures are developed to operate as viable community businesses; to provide community employment at market wages to individuals hired into job positions; and to create supportive, integrated workplaces (Corbière & Lecomte, 2009; Gilbert et al., 2013; Krupa, 2011a). Integration may occur at several levels: at the business level with workers engaging with the wider community through the production and sale of its goods or services, reflected in hiring a diverse workforce within the business itself, or in a business being fully owned and operated by its employees (Krupa, 2011a; Warner & Mandiberg, 2006). Some examples of affirmative businesses and social firms include a cleaning firm in Australia, food service companies in Singapore and Canada, and an organic produce initiative in the United Kingdom (Stickley & Hall, 2017).

Important assets of this approach include the creation of accessible jobs in more inclusively designed workplaces to support employees with psychiatric disabilities to sustain employment (Gilbert et al., 2013; Williams et al., 2012). It also offers possibilities for entrepreneurship to foster self-employment and small business development that may suit some people experiencing mental ill-health better than other forms of employment.

Employment Opportunities in the Mental Health Services

Hiring individuals experiencing mental ill-health within mental health services and advocacy organizations creates a distinctive work environment. In this setting, the expertise derived from the lived experience of mental health challenges and services becomes a valuable and positive qualification, serving as an asset or strength for effectively undertaking the work of recovery.

Central to the emergence and growth of specific employment positions and roles within the mental health sector is the recognition that the rights and voice of people with lived experience have been marginalized but should be central to service directions and delivery (Happell & Roper, 2006), as expressed in the phrase, "Nothing about us without us." Examples of this type of employment include the development of peer-led services and the creation of positions within mental health services focused on provision of peer support, advocacy to bring about systems change, service evaluation, and research activities (Bennetts et al., 2013; Gates & Akabas, 2007; Stoffel, 2013). Nevertheless, these employment options represent mixed opportunities; some have developed into secure jobs, yet consumer and peer workers report a range of attitudinal, organizational, and resource-related challenges in these roles.

To ensure fair and meaningful work, it is crucial to implement enhanced practices concerning employment conditions, human resources, and organizational culture. This includes establishing measures that ensure safe, sustainable, and equitable employment (Bennetts et al., 2013; Wolf et al., 2010). OTPs can play a role in facilitating access to effective workplace support within mental health services.

OTPs also work in a variety of settings where they can use strategies for promoting workplace mental health (e.g., return-to-work programs, employee assistance programs, workplace health and safety). With their frameworks for understanding the interactions between persons, their environments (such as workplaces), and occupations (such as work), OTPs are well placed to actively contribute to workplace mental health initiatives. For instance, OTPs can use this knowledge to analyze job designs from psychosocial and physical safety perspectives, to educate employers to enhance their knowledge about how to implement reasonable accommodations for workers experiencing mental illness, and to develop inclusive policies and practices at an organization level.

Here's the Point

- Mental ill-health affects many in the workforce, particularly those with persistent mental illness.
- Early development of vocational choices, skills, and identity can be profoundly affected by mental illness during adolescence and early adulthood.
- Individuals with mental illness encounter personal, social, attitudinal, and systems-level barriers to employment and these are important considerations for OTPs.
- Engaging in volunteer and service occupations can benefit the physical and mental health of those with mental illness and substance abuse disorders.
- OTPs should assess a person's experiences, interests, habits, skills, and work and volunteer environments to find suitable opportunities and targets for intervention.
- Workplace characteristics play a significant role in mental health, and strategies for promoting workplace mental health are essential.
- Best practices for improving work and volunteer outcomes are not widely available to those with mental illness or psychiatric disabilities in the United States, or elsewhere.
- OTPs can assist with interventions such as direct skills teaching, coaching, designing tailored experiences and reasonable accommodations, education, advocacy, supporting self-advocacy, and working with groups.

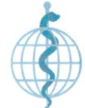 Visit the online resource center at **FADavis.com** to access the videos.

Apply It Now

1. Vocational Development

Reflect on your engagement in occupations as a child and adolescent—play, chores, school activities, hobbies, and first work experiences.

Reflective Questions
- What experiences of play and school activities prepared you for work behaviors?
- How did your family's activities and rules prepare you for work behaviors?
- What did you learn about working from your early work experiences?
- In what ways are your occupational experiences from childhood or adolescence related to your subsequent career choice?

2. Current Work and Career Choice

Reflect on your current work and decision to pursue occupational therapy as a career.

Reflective Questions
- What does work mean to you?
- How does your current work relate to your career choice?
- What influenced your decision to pursue occupational therapy as a career?

- Did you consider other careers?
- What were they, how old were you, and what influenced your thoughts about those careers?
- How does work impact other areas of your life?
- How does your work support and hinder your overall well-being and mental health?

3. Know Your Community

Research your community to identify local employment services that provide assistance and support to potential and current workers experiencing mental illness.

- Make a list of services available to job seekers experiencing mental illness.
- List any affirmative businesses or social firms in your area, and who they serve.
- Research web resources for facilitating conversations about mental health at work.
- Listen to the video-based personal stories of employees from different workplaces based on their experiences of working and mental ill-health (https://www.headsup .org.au). Write a reflection about the kinds of supports that these employees were offered by their employers— what did and did not work well, why, and what other supports might be useful.

■ Select and review one or more of the web resources listed in the text that follows to find resources that might be useful for someone considering having a conversation about mental health in the workplace. Based on your research, make a list of some potential advantages and disadvantages of talking about mental health at work.

4. Learn and Connect People to Volunteer Opportunities

Connecting people with volunteer and service opportunities requires knowledge of different volunteer opportunities and the ability to match people with optimal experiences. Complete the following steps to design a volunteer service activity for a peer.

■ Identify volunteer opportunities. Go to www.Volunteer-Match.org and identify volunteer opportunities in your community.
■ Conduct an occupational profile with a peer. Find a classmate. Conduct an occupational profile regarding volunteer and service occupations. Identify strengths, barriers, and interests related to volunteering.
■ Match your peer to a volunteer activity. Given the opportunities available in your area and the information you collected during the occupational profile, identify a volunteer opportunity that you think would be a good fit. Be sure to consider interests and skills in addition to logistical concerns such as transportation and scheduling.

Reflective Questions
■ What types of volunteer opportunities are available in your community? What kinds of opportunities are available for a diverse set of people?
■ Did you identify any volunteer experiences that would be inappropriate for people with mental illness or substance abuse? Why did you consider them to be inappropriate?
■ What type of questions might you ask during the occupational profile to explore an individual's past, current, and future volunteer service?

■ Describe the process you used to match a person with volunteer opportunities.
■ If your partner were to participate in the volunteer activity you recommended, what skills and capacities would they likely learn or gain?
■ Do you think your partner found a good volunteer or service opportunity that matched your interests and skills? Why or why not?

5. Video Exercise: Will Horowitz: Lived Experience of Autism

Pair up with another student in your class or form a small group of students. Access and watch the "Will Horowitz: Lived Experience of Autism" video at the online resource center at FADavis.com. Then, discuss and together answer the following questions:

1. As a person with lived experience, Will can see both the advantages and challenges of living with autism. From what we know about autism, what advantages and challenges might special interests present in the work setting?
2. Identify the strengths you see in Will and explain how these might be important for any productive occupations in future work and volunteer positions.
3. How has Will's insight and perspective on living with autism led to increased occupational engagement and subsequent resilience?
4. For individuals with less self-awareness than Will, how can occupational therapy practitioners support families and caregivers in shifting their perspective about their loved ones and their diagnoses and what it means for occupational engagement?
5. For nearly half of his 24 years of life, Will has found a productive way to channel his special interest in trains into volunteer and work positions in a train yard. He mentions that he may soon begin shadowing a conductor. What questions do you anticipate that administrators might have about Will's capacity to take on more responsibility in the train yard? What information might you need to gather to help support Will to answer these questions?

Resources
• Americans with Disabilities Act, Mental Health Conditions, and Workplace Accommodations: https://adata.org/factsheet/health. Straightforward information for employers, job applicants, and employees about the ADA, rights, and reasonable workplace accommodations or adjustments for mental health conditions.
• Black Dog Institute: https://www.blackdoginstitute.org.au/education-training/workplace-mental-health-and-wellbeing. Evidence-based workplace mental and well-being programs and resources, including a downloadable toolkit with information on stress, depression, and anxiety in the workplace, as well as best practice suggestions for help-seeking, supporting others, and maintaining well-being at work.
• College of Occupational Therapists/National Social Inclusion Programme. (2007). *Work matters: Vocational navigation for occupational therapy staff.* https://www.rcot.co.uk/practice-resources/rcot-publications/downloads/work-matters. Good practice information and resources for OTPs developed in the United Kingdom by the College of Occupational Therapists and National Social Inclusion Programme.
• Heads Up: https://www.headsup.org.au. Tools and resources about employer and employee rights and responsibilities; weighing up disclosure decisions and how to have conversations about mental health at work; it also addresses making reasonable adjustments and providing support when an employee or colleague is experiencing depression or anxiety.
• Incentives to Work for People on Social Security Income or Social Security Disability Insurance: http://www.ssa.gov/work. The Ticket to Work program is administered by the Social Security Administration and supports career development for working age adults who want to work and receive Social Security disability benefits. The program is free and voluntary and provides services and resources to help people with disabilities achieve their employment goals.
• Job Accommodations Network: https://askjan.org. For over 40 years, The Job Accommodation Network (JAN) has provided expert guidance and support on disability employment and job accommodations, including 1:1 consultations. These resources are meant to support employers, individuals with disabilities seeking employment or related information, and family members and providers looking to facilitate positive employment outcomes.

- Mayo Clinic Health System. (n.d.). *Helping people, changing lives: 3 health benefits of* volunteering. https://www .mayoclinichealthsystem.org/hometown-health/speaking-of -health/3-health-benefits-of-volunteering. Web story from the Mayo Clinic on the benefits of volunteering.
- MINDFUL EMPLOYER: http://www.mindfulemployer.net. Developed, led, and supported by employers in the United Kingdom, MINDFUL EMPLOYER provides businesses and organizations with information and support for staff who experience stress, anxiety, depression, or other mental health conditions. It includes downloadable tools to facilitate communication, understanding, and support between an employee and manager, and to develop well-being plans.
- Model of Human Occupation (MOHO)-Based Assessment Tools: https://moho-irm.uic.edu/default.aspx. Further information and manuals for the tools mentioned in this chapter, including WRI, WEIS, OPHI-II, MOHOST, and AWP, can be found on the MOHO website.
- National Alliance on Mental Illness (NAMI). *How volunteering improves mental health.* https://www.nami.org/Blogs/NAMI-Blog /February-2022/How-Volunteering-Improves-Mental-Health
- Repository of Employment and Vocational Recovery Resources: https://cpr.bu.edu/resources/employment. An online archive of employment materials developed by the Center for Psychiatric Rehabilitation, Boston University. It includes resources designed to guide current and potential workers with lived experiences of mental illness to think about, choose, find, and sustain work; resources for families, peer support workers, and vocational rehabilitation providers about how to support individuals in their vocational recovery; and resources for employers addressing workplace accommodations or adjustments and inclusion of employees with psychiatric disabilities.
- Supported Employment Evidence-Based Practices (EBP) Kit: https://www.samhsa.gov/resource/ebp/supported-employment -evidence-based-practices-ebp-kit. This kit provides specific information on principles, evidence, and practices for implementing supported employment services.
- Very Well Mind. *What are the mental health benefits of volunteering?* https://www.verywellmind.com/what-are-the -mental-health-benefits-of-volunteering-5248549
- Volunteer Match: http://www.volunteermatch.org
- Workplace Mental Health Promotion: https://cmhato.org. Information and how-to-guides to creating mentally healthy workplace practices and policies, developed by the Dalla Lana School of Public Health, University of Toronto and the Canadian Mental Health Association.
- "Civic Engagement Group in an Inpatient Psychiatric Unit" video. In this video, occupational therapist Jennifer speaks about her experience working as an occupational therapy assistant in an inpatient psychiatric unit for individuals with persistent mental illness. She describes a positive experience running civic engagement groups, which proved to do much more than give back to the community. In one project related to voting rights for individuals with felony histories, the group provided opportunities for the residents to practice life skills, feel empowered, and transcend the internalized stigma they faced as people living with mental illness. To access the video, visit the online resource center at FADavis.com.

References

American Occupational Therapy Association. (2020). Occupational therapy practice framework: Domain and process —Fourth edition. *American Journal of Occupational Therapy, 74*(Suppl. 2), 7412410010p1–7412410010p87. https://doi.org/10.5014/ajot .2020.74S2001

Areberg, C., & Bejerholm, U. (2013). The effect of IPS on participants' engagement, quality of life, empowerment, and motivation: A randomized controlled trial. *Scandinavian Journal of Occupational Therapy, 20,* 420–428. https://doi.org/10.3109/11038128 .2013.765911

Baum, C. M., Connor, L. T., Morrison, T., Hahn, M., Dromerick, A. W., & Edwards, D. F. (2008). Reliability, validity, and clinical utility of the Executive Function Performance Test: A measure of executive function in a sample of people with stroke. *American Journal of Occupational Therapy, 62*(4), 446–455. https://doi.org/10.5014/ajot.62.4.446

Baum, C. M., & Edwards, D. (2008). *Activity card sort* (2nd ed.). AOTA Press.

Becker, D. R., & Drake, R. E. (2003). *A working life for people with severe mental illness.* Oxford University Press.

Benavides, F. G., Benach, J., Diez-Roux, A. V., & Roman, C. (2000). How do types of employment relate to health indicators? Findings from the second European survey on working conditions. *Journal of Epidemiology and Public Health, 54*(7), 494–501. https://doi .org/10.1136/jech.54.7.494

Bennetts, W., Pinches, A., Paluch, T., & Fossey, E. (2013). Real lives, real jobs: Sustaining consumer perspective work in the mental health sector. *Advances in Mental Health, 11*(3), 308–320. https:// doi.org/10.5172/jamh.2013.11.3.313

Bertram, M., & McDonald, S. (2015). From surviving to thriving: How does that happen. *The Journal of Mental Health Training, Education and Practice, 10*(5), 337–348. https://doi.org/10.1108 /JMHTEP-06-2015-0027

Blank, A., Harries, P., & Reynolds, F. (2011). Mental health service users' perspectives of work: A review of the literature. *British Journal of Occupational Therapy, 74*(4), 191–199. https://doi.org /10.4276/030802211X13021048723336

Boeltzig, H., Timmons, J. C., & Marrone, J. (2008). Maximising potential: Innovative collaborative strategies between one-stops and mental health systems of care. *Work, 31*(2), 181–193.

Bond, G. R. (2004). Supported employment: Evidence for an evidence-based practice. *Psychiatric Rehabilitation Journal, 27*(4), 345–356. https://doi.org/10.2975/27.2004.345.359

Bond, G. R., Drake, R. E., & Becker, D. R. (2012). Generalizability of the Individual Placement and Support (IPS) model of supported employment outside the US. *World Psychiatry, 11,* 32–39. https:// doi.org/10.1016/j.wpsyc.2012.01.005

Boyce, M., Secker, J., Johnson, R., Floyd, M., Grove, B., Schneider, J., & Slade, J. (2008). Mental health service users' experiences of returning to paid employment. *Disability & Society, 23*(1), 77–88. https://doi.org/10.1080/09687590701725757

Bramley, S., & Mayne, N. (2010). *The WORKS: A resource to support you in achieving your employment ambitions.* Sheffield Health and Social Care NHS Foundation Trust.

Braveman, B., Robson, M., Velozo, C., Kielhofner, G., Fisher, G., Forsyth, K., & Kerschbaum, J. (2005). *A user's guide to Worker Role Interview.* Version 1.0. Model of Human Occupation Clearinghouse, University of Illinois at Chicago.

Bufquin, Park, J.-Y., Back, R. M., de Souza Meira, J. V., & Hight, S. K. (2021). Employee work status, mental health, substance use, and career turnover intentions: An examination of restaurant employees during COVID-19. *International Journal of Hospitality Management, 93,* 102764. https://doi.org/10.1016/j.ijhm.2020.102764

Burns, T., Mortimer, J. A., & Merchak, P. (1994). Cognitive Performance Test: A new approach to functional assessment in Alzheimer's disease. *Journal of Geriatric Psychiatry and Neurology, 7*(1), 46–54.

Cassinello, K., & Bramley, S. (2012). Keeley's journey: From service user to service provider. *Work, 43*(1), 91–97. https://doi.org /10.3233/WOR-2012-1450

Chopra, P. (2009). Mental health and the workplace: Issues for developing countries. *International Journal of Mental Health Systems, 3,* Article 4. https://doi.org/10.1186/1752-4458-3-4

Clayton, K. S., & Chubon, R. A. (1994). Factors associated with the quality of life of long-term spinal cord injured persons. *Archives of Physical Medicine and Rehabilitation, 75,* 633–638. https://doi .org/10.1016/0003-9993(94)90184-8

College of Occupational Therapists/National Social Inclusion Programme. (2007). *Work matters: Vocational navigation for occupational therapy staff.* College of Occupational Therapists, National Social Inclusion Programme and Department of Health.

Cook, J. A., Copeland, M. E., Corey, L., Buffington, E., Jonikas, J. A., Curtis, L. C., Grey, D. D., & Nichols, W. H. (2010). Developing the evidence base for peer-led services: Changes among participants following Wellness Recovery Action Planning (WRAP) education in two statewide initiatives. *Psychiatric Rehabilitation Journal, 34*(2), 113–120. https://doi.org/10.2975/34.2.2010.113.120

Corbière, M., & Lecomte, T. (2009). Vocational services offered to people with severe mental illness. *Journal of Mental Health, 18,* 38–50. https://doi.org/10.1080/09638230701677779

Corbière, M., Villotti, P., Lecomte, T., Bond, G. R., Lesage, A., & Goldner, E. M. (2014). Work accommodations and natural supports for maintaining employment. *Psychiatric Rehabilitation Journal, 37,* 90–98. https://doi.org/10.1037/prj0000033

Corcoran, M. A. (2004). Work, occupation, and occupational therapy. *American Journal of Occupational Therapy, 58,* 367–368. https://doi.org/10.5014/ajot.58.4.367

Daston, M., Riehle, J. E., & Rutkowski, S. (2012). *High school transition that works! Lessons learned from Project SEARCH.* Paul H. Brookes Publishing.

Davidson, L., Rakfeldt, J., & Strauss, J. (2010). *The roots of the recovery movement in psychiatry: Lessons learned.* John Wiley & Sons.

de las Heras de Pablo, C. G., Abelenda, J., & Parkinson, S. (2017). MOHO-based program development. In R. Taylor (Ed.), *Kielhofner's Model of Human Occupation. Theory and application* (5th ed., pp. 396–416). Wolters Kluwer.

Dewa, C. S., Corbiere, M., Durand, M., & Hensel, J. (2012). Challenges related to mental health in the workplace. In R. J. Gatchel & I. Z. Schultz (Eds.), *Handbook of occupational health and wellness* (pp. 105–129). Springer.

Dewa, C. S., & McDaid, D. (2011). Investing in the mental health of the labor force: Epidemiological and economic impact of mental health disabilities in the workplace. In I. Z. Schultz & E. S. Rogers (Eds.), *Work accommodation and retention in mental health* (pp. 33–51). Springer.

Edgelow, M., Harrison, L., Miceli, M., & Cramm, H. (2020). Occupational therapy return to work interventions for persons with trauma and stress-related mental health conditions: A scoping review. *Work, 65*(4), 821–836. https://doi.org/10.3233/WOR-203134

Eggleton, I., Robertson, S., Ryan, J., & Kober, R. (1999). The impact of employment on the quality of life of people with an intellectual disability. *Journal of Vocational Rehabilitation, 13,* 95–107.

Ekbladh, E., Thorell, L., & Haglund, L. (2010). Return to work: The predictive value of the Worker Role Interview (WRI) over two years. *Work, 35,* 163–172. https://doi.org/10.3233/WOR-2010 -0968

Emptage, N. P. (2005). Depression and comorbid pain as predictors of disability, employment, insurance status, and health care costs. *Psychiatric Services Psychiatric Services, 56,* 468–474. https://doi .org/10.1176/appi.ps.56.4.468

Ennals, P., Fossey, E., & Howie, L. (2015). Postsecondary study and mental ill-health: A meta-synthesis of qualitative research exploring students' lived experiences. *Journal of Mental Health, 24*(2), 111–119. https://doi.org/10.3109/09638237.2015.1019052

Farrell, C., & Bryant, W. (2009). Voluntary work for adults with mental health problems: A route to inclusion? A review of the literature. *British Journal of Occupational Therapy, 72*(4), 163–173. https://doi.org/10.1177/030802260907200405

Fegan, C., & Cook, S. (2014). The therapeutic power of volunteering. *Advances in Psychiatric Treatment, 20,* 217–224. https://doi.org /10.1192/apt.bp.113.011890

Fioritti, A., Burns, T., Hilarion, P., van Weeghel, J., Cappa, C., & Sunol, R. (2014). Individual placement and support in Europe.

Psychiatric Rehabilitation Journal, 37(2), 123–128. https://doi .org/10.1037/prj0000065

Fisher, A. G., Bryze, K., Hume, V., & Griswold, L. A. (2007). *School AMPS: School version of the assessment of motor and process skills* (2nd ed.). Three Star Press.

Fossey, E., & Bramley, S. (2014). Work and vocational pursuits. In K. Bannigan, W. Bryant, & J. Fieldhouse (Eds.), *Creek's occupational therapy and mental health* (5th ed., pp. 328–344). Elsevier.

Fossey, E. M., & Harvey, C. A. (2010). Finding and sustaining employment: A qualitative meta-synthesis of mental health consumer views. *Canadian Journal of Occupational Therapy, 77,* 303–314. https://doi.org/10.2182/cjot.2010.77.5.6

Gammarano, R. (2019). *Work and employment are not synonyms.* https://ilostat.ilo.org/blog/work-and-employment-are-not -synonyms

Gammon, D., Strand, M., & Eng, L. S. (2014). Service users' perspectives in the design of an online tool for assisted self-help in mental health: A case study of implications. *International Journal of Mental Health Systems, 8,* Article 2. https://doi.org/10.1186 /1752-4458-8-2

Gates, L. B., & Akabas, S. H. (2007). Developing strategies to integrate peer providers into the staff of mental health agencies. *Administration and Policy in Mental Health and Mental Health Services Research, 34,* 293–306. https://doi.org/10.1007/s10488 -006-0109-4

Gilbert, E., Marwaha, S., Milton, A., Johnson, S., Morant, N., Parsons, N., Fisher, A., Singh, S., & Cunliffe, D. (2013). Social firms as a means of vocational recovery for people with mental illness: A UK survey. *BMC Health Services Research, 13,* Article 270. https://doi.org/10.1186/1472-6963-13-270

Hamlet Trust, Project North East, and College Research & Training Unit (Royal College of Psychiatrists). (2007). *Business minds: Mainstreaming business support for mental health. Research findings from the Newcastle Demonstration Project.* http://www .hamlettrust.plus.com

Happell, B., & Roper, C. (2006). When equality is not really equal: Affirmative action and consumer participation. *Journal of Public Mental Health, 5*(3), 6–11. https://doi.org/10.1108 /17465729200600021

Harris, L. M., Matthews, L. R., Penrose-Wall, J., Alam, A., & Jaworski, A. (2014). Perspectives on barriers to employment for job seekers with mental illness and additional substance-use problems. *Health & Social Care in the Community, 22*(1), 67–77. https://doi.org/10.1111/hsc.12062

Harvey, S. B., Joyce, S., Tan, L., Johnson, A., Nguyen, H., Modini, M., & Groth, M. (2014). *Developing a mentally healthy workplace: A review of the literature.* National Mental Health Commission and the Mentally Healthy Workplace Alliance. https://www.headsup.org.au/docs/default-source /resources/developing-a-mentally-healthy-workplace_final -november-2014.pdf

Henry, A. D., Barreira, P., Banks, S., Brown, J., & McKay, C. (2001). A retrospective study of Clubhouse-based transitional employment. *Psychiatric Rehabilitation Journal, 24*(4), 344–354. https:// doi.org/10.1037/h0095070

Hitch, D., Robertson, J., Ochteco, H., McNeill, F., Williams, A., Lhuede, K., Baini, A., Hillman, A., & Fossey, E. (2017). An evaluation of a vocational group for people with mental health problems based on The WORKS framework. *British Journal of Occupational Therapy, 80*(12), 717–725. https://doi.org /10.1177/0308022617726483

Inge, K. J. (1988). Quality of life for individuals who are labeled mentally retarded: Evaluating competitive employment versus sheltered workshop employment. *Education and Training in Mental Retardation, 23,* 97–104.

International Labour Organization. (2004). *The ILO: What it is. What it does.* Author. https://www.ilo.org/publications/ilo-what -it-what-it-does

Jahoda, M. (1981). Work, employment, and unemployment values, theories, and approaches in social research. *American Psychologist, 36*(2), 184–191. https://doi.org/10.1037/0003-066X.36.2.184

Jarman, J. (2010). What is occupation? Interdisciplinary perspectives on defining and classifying human activity. In C. H. Christiansen & E. A. Townsend (Eds.), *Introduction to occupation: The art and science of living* (2nd ed., pp. 81–99). Prentice Hall.

Jenkinson, C. E., Dickens, A. P., Jones, K., Thompson-Coon, J., Taylor, R. S., Rogers, M., Bambra, C. L., Lang, I., & Richards, S. H. (2013). Is volunteering a public health intervention? A systematic review and meta-analysis of the health and survival of volunteers. *BMC Public Health, 13*(1), 1–10. https://doi.org/10.1186/1471-2458-13-773

Jiang, D., Warner, L. M., Chong, A. M. L., Li, T., Wolff, J. K., & Chou, K. L. (2021). Benefits of volunteering on psychological well-being in older adulthood: Evidence from a randomized controlled trial. *Aging & Mental Health, 25*(4), 641–649. https://doi.org/10.1080/13607863.2020.1711862

Johnson, R., Floyd, M., Pilling, D., Boyce, M., Secker, J., Grove, B., & Slade, J. (2009). Service users' perceptions of the effective ingredients in supported employment. *Journal of Mental Health, 18*(2), 121–128. https://doi.org/10.1080/09638230701879151

Kielhofner, G., Mallinson, T., Crawford, C., Nowak, M., Rigby, M., Henry, A., & Walens, D. (2004). *A user's manual for the Occupational Performance History Interview (OPHI-II)*. Version 2.1. Model of Human Occupation Clearinghouse, Department of Occupational Therapy, College of Applied Health Sciences, University of Illinois.

Killackey, E., Allott, K., Woodhead, G., Connor, S., Dragon, S., & Rong, J. (2016). Individual Placement and Support, supported education in young people with mental illness: An exploratory feasibility study. *Early Intervention in Psychiatry, 11*, 526–531. https://doi.org/10.1111/eip.12344

Kinoshita, Y., Furukawa, T. A., Kinoshita, K., Honyashiki, M., Omori, I., Marshall, M., Bond, G. R., Huxley, P., Amano, N., & Kingdon, D. (2013). Supported employment for adults with severe mental illness. *Cochrane Database of Systematic Reviews, 2013*(9), CD008297. https://doi.org/10.1002/14651858.CD008297.pub2

Kirsh, B., & Gewurtz, R. (2012). Promoting mental health within workplaces. In R. J. Gatchel & I. Z. Schultz (Eds.), *Handbook of occupational health and wellness* (pp. 243–265). Springer.

Kirsh, B., Martin, L., Hultqvist, J., & Eklund, M. (2019). Occupational therapy interventions in mental health: A literature review in search of evidence. *Occupational Therapy in Mental Health, 35*(2), 109–156. https://doi.org/10.1080/0164212X.2019.1588832

Kober, R., & Eggleton, I. R. (2005). The effect of different types of employment on quality of life. *Journal of Intellectual Disability Research, 49*, 756–760. https://doi.org/10.1111/j.1365-2788.2005.00746.x

Kohlman Thomson, L., & Robnett, R. (2016). *Kohlman Evaluation of Living Skills* (4th ed.). AOTA Press.

Krupa, T. (2011a). Approaches to improving employment outcomes for people with serious mental illness. In I. Z. Schultz & E. S. Rogers (Eds.), *Work accommodation and retention in mental health* (pp. 219–231). Springer.

Krupa, T. (2011b). Employment and serious mental health disabilities. In I. Z. Schultz & E. S. Rogers (Eds.), *Work accommodation and retention in mental health* (pp. 91–101). Springer.

Law, M., Baptiste, S., Carswell, A., McColl, M. A., Polatajko, H. J., & Pollack, N. (2014). *Canadian Occupational Performance Measure* (5th ed.). Canadian Association of Occupational Therapists.

Lee, J., & Kielhofner, G. (2010). Vocational intervention based on the Model of Human Occupation: A review of evidence. *Scandinavian Journal of Occupational Therapy, 17*, 177–190. https://doi.org/10.3109/11038120903082260

Lloyd, C., & Waghorn, G. (2010). The importance of vocation for young people with mental illness. In C. Lloyd (Ed.), *Vocational rehabilitation and mental health* (pp. 115–134). Wiley-Blackwell.

Machingura, T., & Lloyd, C. (2017). Mental health occupational therapy and supported employment. *Irish Journal of Occupational Therapy, 45*(1), 52–57. https://doi.org/10.1108/IJOT-02-2017-0004

Macias, C., Rodican, C. F., Hargreaves, W. A., Jones, D. R., Barreira, P. J., & Wang, Q. (2006). Supported employment outcomes of a randomized controlled trial of ACT and Clubhouse models. *Psychiatric Services, 57*(10), 1406–1415. https://doi.org/10.1176/ps.2006.57.10.1406

McDowell, C., Ennals, P., & Fossey, E. (2021). Vocational service models and approaches to improve job tenure of people with severe and enduring mental illness: A narrative review. *Frontiers in Psychiatry, 12*, 668716. https://doi.org/10.3389/fpsyt.2021.668716

McGurk, S. R., Mueser, K. T., Feldman, K., Wolfe, R., & Pascaris, A. (2007). Cognitive training for supported employment: 2–3 year outcomes of a randomized controlled trial. *American Journal of Psychiatry, 164*(3), 437–441. https://doi.org/10.1176/ajp.2007.164.3.437

McKay, C., Johnsen, M., & Stein, R. (2005). Employment outcomes in Massachusetts Clubhouses. *Psychiatric Rehabilitation Journal, 29*(1), 25–33. https://doi.org/10.2975/29.2005.25.33

McQueen, J. M., & Turner, J. (2012). Exploring forensic mental health service users' views on work: An interpretative phenomenological analysis. *British Journal of Forensic Practice, 14*(3), 168–179. https://doi.org/10.1108/14636641211254897

Meyer, A. (1977). Philosophy of occupation therapy. Reprinted from the Archives of Occupational Therapy, Volume 1, pp. 1-10, 1922. *American Journal of Occupational Therapy, 31*(10), 1–10.

Miller, A., & Dishon, S. (2006). Health-related quality of life in multiple sclerosis: The impact of disability, gender and employment status. *Quality of Life Research, 15*, 259–271. https://doi.org/10.1007/s11136-005-0891-6

Moore-Corner, R. A., Kielhofner, G., & Olson, L. (1998). *A user's manual for Work Environment Impact Scale*. Version 2.0. Model of Human Occupation Clearinghouse, University of Illinois at Chicago.

Musick, M. A., & Wilson, J. (2003). Volunteering and depression: The role of psychological and social resources in different age groups. *Social Science & Medicine, 56*(2), 259–269. https://doi.org/10.1016/s0277-9536(02)00025-4

Nemec, P. B., McNamara, S., & Walsh, D. (1992). Direct skill teaching. *Psychosocial Rehabilitation Journal, 16*, 13–25. https://doi.org/10.1037/h0095731

Nicholson, J., Carpenter-Song, E. A., MacPherson, L. H., Tauscher, J. S., Burns, T. C., & Lord, S. E. (2017). Developing the WorkingWell mobile app to promote job tenure for individuals with serious mental illnesses. *Psychiatric Rehabilitation Journal, 40*(3), 276–282. https://doi.org/10.1037/prj0000201

Noyes, S., Sokolow, H., & Arbesman, M. (2018). Evidence for occupational therapy intervention with employment and education for adults with serious mental illness: A systematic review. *The American Journal of Occupational Therapy, 72*(5), 7205190010p1–7205190010p10. https://doi.org/10.5014/ajot.2018.033068

Ostrow, L., Smith, C., Penney, D., & Shumway, M. (2019). "It suits my needs": Self-employed individuals with psychiatric disabilities and small businesses. *Psychiatric Rehabilitation Journal, 42*(2), 121–131. https://doi.org/10.1037/prj0000341

Pedretti, L. W., & Early, M. B. (2001). *Occupational therapy: Practice skills for physical dysfunction*. Mosby.

Pérez-Corrales, J., Pérez-de-Heredia-Torres, M., Martínez-Piedrola, R., Sánchez-Camarero, C., Parás-Bravo, P., & Palacios-Ceña, D. (2019). 'Being normal' and self-identity: The experience of volunteering in individuals with severe mental disorders—A qualitative study. *BMJ Open, 9*, e025363. https://doi.org/10.1136/bmjopen-2018-025363

Persch, A. C., Gugiu, P. C., Onate, J. A., & Cleary, D. S. (2015). Development and psychometric evaluation of the Vocational Fit Assessment (VFA). *The American Journal of Occupational Therapy, 69*(6), 6906180080p1–6906180080p8. https://doi.org/10.5014/ajot.2015.019455

Petrovski, P., & Gleeson, G. (1997). The relationship between job satisfaction and psychological health in people with an intellectual disability in competitive employment. *Journal of Intellectual & Developmental Disability, 22,* 199–211. https://doi.org/10.1080/13668259700033411

Pieh, C., Budimir, S., Delgadillo, J., Barkham, M., Fontaine, J. R. J., & Probst, T. (2021). Mental health during COVID-19 lockdown in the United Kingdom. *Psychosomatic Medicine, 83*(4), 328–337. https://doi.org/10.1097/PSY.0000000000000871

Priebe, S., Warner, R., Hubschmid, T., & Eckle, I. (1998). Employment, attitudes toward work, and quality of life among people with schizophrenia in three countries. *Schizophrenia Bulletin, 24,* 469–477. https://doi.org/10.1093/oxfordjournals.schbul.a033341

Prochaska, J. O., & Norcross, J. C. (2001). Stages of change. *Psychotherapy, 38,* 443–448. https://doi.org/10.1037/0033-3204.38.4.443

Rehabilitation Act of 1973, Pub. L. No. 93-112, 29 U.S.C. §§ 701 et seq. (1973).

Repetti, R. L., Matthews, K. A., & Waldron, I. (1989). Employment and women's health: Effects of paid employment on women's mental and physical health. *The American Psychologist, 44,* 1394–1401. https://doi.org/10.1037/0003-066X.44.11.1394

Ringeisen, H., Langer Ellison, M., Ryder-Burge, A., Biebel, K., Alikhan, S., & Jones, E. (2017). Supported education for individuals with psychiatric disabilities: State of the practice and policy implications. *Psychiatric Rehabilitation Journal, 40*(2), 197. https://doi.org/10.1037/prj0000233

Rogers, E. S., & MacDonald-Wilson, K. L. (2011). Vocational capacity among individuals with mental health disabilities. In I. Z. Schultz & E. S. Rogers (Eds.), *Work accommodation and retention in mental health* (pp. 73–89). Springer.

Ross, C. E., & Mirowsky, J. (1995). Does employment affect health? *The Journal of Health and Social Behavior, 36,* 230–243. https://doi.org/10.2307/2137340

Ross, J. (2007). *Occupational therapy and vocational rehabilitation.* Wiley & Sons.

Rotolo, T., & Wilson, J. (2011). State-level differences in volunteerism in the United States: Research based on demographic, institutional, and cultural macrolevel theories. *Nonprofit and Voluntary Sector Quarterly, 41*(3), 452–473. https://doi.org/10.1177/0899764011412383

Royal College of Occupational Therapists. (2017). *Professional standards for occupational therapy practice.* College of Occupational Therapists. https://www.rcot.co.uk/files/professional-standards-occupational-therapy-practice-2017

Rudnick, A., & Gover, M. (2009). Frontline report: Combining supported education with supported employment. *Psychiatric Services, 60*(12), 1690. https://doi.org/10.1176/ps.2009.60.12.1690

Sandqvist, J., & Ekbladh, E. (2017). Applying the Model of Human Occupation to vocational rehabilitation. In R. Taylor (Ed.), *Kielhofner's Model of Human Occupation. Theory and application* (5th ed., pp. 376–395). Wolters Kluwer.

Sandqvist, J., Lee, J., & Kielhofner, G. (2010). *Assessment of Work Performance (AWP).* Version 1.0. Model of Human Occupation Clearinghouse, University of Illinois at Chicago.

Schneider, J. (2005). Getting back to work: What do we know about what works? In B. Grove, J. Secker, & P. Seebohm (Eds.), *New thinking about mental health and employment* (pp. 37–49). Radcliffe Publishing Ltd.

Shaw, L., & Sumsion, T. (2009). There is so much more to do: Strategies and research needs to support work transitions for persons with chronic mental health conditions. *Work, 33*(4), 377–379. https://doi.org/10.3233/WOR-2009-0885

Sinnott-Oswald, M. (1991). Supported and sheltered employment: Quality of life issues among workers with disabilities. *Education and Training in Mental Retardation, 26,* 388–397.

Stansfeld, S., & Candy, B. (2006). Psychosocial work environment and mental health—A meta-analytic review. *Scandinavian Journal of Work, Environment and Health, 32*(6), 443–462. https://doi.org/10.5271/sjweh.1050

Stickley, A., & Hall, K. (2017). Social enterprise: A model of recovery and social inclusion for occupational therapy practice in the UK. *Mental Health and Social Inclusion, 21*(2), 91–101. https://doi.org/10.1108/MHSI-01-2017-0002

Stoffel, V. C. (2013). Health policy perspectives—Opportunities for occupational therapy behavioral health: A call to action. *American Journal of Occupational Therapy, 67,* 140–145. https://doi.org/10.5014/ajot.2013.672001

Stronks, K., van de Mheen, H., van den Bos, J., & Mackenbach, J. (1997). The interrelationship between income, health and employment status. *International Journal of Epidemiology, 26,* 592–600. https://doi.org/10.1093/ije/26.3.592

Swarbrick, M., & Noyes, S. (2018). Effectiveness of occupational therapy services in mental health practice. *The American Journal of Occupational Therapy, 72*(5), 7205170010p1–7205170010p4. https://doi.org/10.5014/ajot.2018.725001

Taylor, R. R., Bowyer, P., & Fisher, G. (Eds.). (2024). *Kielhofner's Model of Human Occupation: Theory and application* (6th ed.). Wolters Kluwer.

Thoits, P. A., & Hewitt, L. N. (2001). Volunteer work and well-being. *Journal of Health and Social Behavior, 42*(2), 115–131. https://doi.org/10.2307/3090173

Torquati, L., Mielke, G. I., Brown, W. J., Burton, N. W., & Kolbe-Alexander, T. L. (2019). Shift work and poor mental health: A meta-analysis of longitudinal studies. *American Journal of Public Health, 109*(11), e13–e20. https://doi.org/10.2105/AJPH.2019.305278

Tsang, H. W. H., Fung, K. M. T., Leung, A. Y., Li, S. M. Y., & Cheung, W. M. (2010). Three year follow-up study of integrated supported employment for individuals with severe mental illness. *Australian and New Zealand Journal of Psychiatry, 44,* 49–58. https://doi.org/10.3109/00048670903393613

United Nations General Assembly. (1948). *Universal Declaration of Human Rights.* https://www.un.org/en/universal-declaration-human-rights

United Nations General Assembly. (1966, December 16). *International covenant on economic, social and cultural rights.* https://www.ohchr.org/en/instruments-mechanisms/instruments/international-covenant-economic-social-and-cultural-rights

United Nations General Assembly. (2006). *Convention on the Rights of Persons with Disabilities (CRPD).* https://www.un.org/development/desa/disabilities/convention-on-the-rights-of-persons-with-disabilities.html

van Niekerk, L. (2009). Participation in work: A source of wellness for people with psychiatric disability. *Work, 32*(4), 455–465. https://doi.org/10.3233/WOR-2009-0856

Virtanen, M., Kivimäki, M., Elovainio, M., Vahtera, J., & Ferrie, J. E. (2003). From insecure to secure employment: Changes in work, health, health related behaviours, and sickness absence. *Occupational and Environmental Medicine, 60,* 948–953. https://doi.org/10.1136/oem.60.12.948

Waddell, G., & Burton, K. (2006). *Is work good for your health and wellbeing?* TSO (The Stationery Office).

Waghorn, G. R., Chant, D., White, P., & Whiteford, H. (2005). Disability, employment and work performance among people with *ICD-10* anxiety disorders. *Australian and New Zealand Journal of Psychiatry, 39,* 55–66. https://doi.org/10.1080/j.1440-1614.2005.01510.x

Waghorn, G. R., Collister, L., & Killackey, E. (2007). Challenges to implementing evidence-based supported employment in Australia. *Journal of Vocational Rehabilitation, 27,* 29–37.

Waghorn, G. R., & Lloyd, C. (2010). Employment and people with mental illness. In C. Lloyd (Ed.), *Vocational rehabilitation and mental health* (pp. 1–18). Wiley-Blackwell.

Warner, R., & Mandiberg, J. M. (2006). An update on affirmative businesses or social firms for people with mental illness.

Psychiatric Services, 57, 1488–1492. https://doi.org/10.1176/appi .ps.57.10.1488

Wilcock, A. A. (2001). *Occupation for health, Volume 1: A journey from self health to prescription.* College of Occupational Therapists.

Williams, A. E., Fossey, E., Corbiere, M., Paluch, T., & Harvey, C. (2016). Work participation for people with severe mental illnesses: An integrative review of factors impacting job tenure. *Australian Occupational Therapy Journal, 63,* 65–85. https:// doi.org/10.1111/1440-1630.12237

Williams, A. E., Fossey, E., & Harvey, C. (2010). Sustaining employment in a social firm: Use of the Work Environment Impact Scale v2.0 to explore views of employees with psychiatric disabilities. *British Journal of Occupational Therapy, 73*(11), 531–539. https:// doi.org/10.4276/030802210X12892992239279

Williams, A. E., Fossey, E., & Harvey, C. (2012). Social firms: Sustainable employment for people with mental illness. *Work, 43,* 53–62. https://doi.org/10.3233/WOR-2012-1447

Wilson, J., & Musick, M. (1999). The effects of volunteering on the volunteer. *Law and Contemporary Problems, 62,* 141–168. https:// doi.org/10.2307/1192270

Wolf, J., Lawrence, L. H., Ryan, P. M., & Hoge, M. A. (2010). Emerging practices in employment of persons in recovery in the mental health workforce. *American Journal of Psychiatric Rehabilitation, 13*(3), 189–207. https://doi.org/10.1080/15487768.2010.501294

Yeung, J. W. K., Zhang, Z., & Kim, T. Y. (2018). Volunteering and health benefits in general adults: Cumulative effects and forms. *BMC Public Health, 18,* Article 8. https://doi.org/10.1186/s12889 -017-4561-8

CHAPTER
49

Connectedness and Belonging

Carol Lambdin-Pattavina

What does it mean to belong, to feel connected; connected to self, to others, and to the world in general? There is no definitive or correct response to this question. Connectedness is a deeply personal experience and must be explored in the context of the occupational therapy process in accordance with person-centeredness. For some, connectedness is an integrated experience and might be described as easy or even second nature. For others, connectedness might be experienced as challenging, unfulfilling, or even painful. Humans are hard-wired to connect for their very survival. That reliance, however, can take on different forms, functions, and meanings.

Connection, and conversely disconnection, are part of the human experience. Those living with and without psychiatric labels may, at any given time, experience disconnection to varying degrees from situational and temporary to profound and chronic. Occupational therapy practitioners (OTPs) may bear witness to this disconnection across all practice settings and may even struggle to establish meaningful connections themselves. Supporting people to explore connectedness and the ways in which they choose to enact themselves as connected beings are foundational in the occupational therapy process.

Those working in dedicated mental health spaces may see the byproduct of disconnection even more frequently and intensely. "Social relationships, or the relative lack thereof, constitute a major risk factor for health—rivaling the effect of well-established health risk factors such as cigarette smoking, blood pressure, blood lipids, obesity and physical activity" (House et al., 1988, p. 540). In addition, disconnection is viewed by a growing number of mental health professionals as a significant contributing factor to the diagnostic labels that are collectively known as mental illness according to the *Diagnostic and Statistical Manual of Mental Disorders* (5th ed., text rev.; American Psychiatric Association, 2022).

In this chapter, the construct of connectedness and associated terms; various forms, functions, and meanings associated with connectedness; historical approaches to connection building in occupational therapy; the neuroscience of connection; and the link between connectedness and health and wellness are explored. Additionally, readers explore connectedness as it relates to the occupational therapy process from assessment to intervention. Finally, the crisis of disconnection is described against the backdrop of a global pandemic and a U.S.-based state of mental health emergency.

Definitions

An abundance of literature has aimed to gain greater clarity around, and insight into, the nature of connectedness. In time, a variety of terms have emerged, each attempting to capture the nuanced and multifaceted nature of human interaction with self, others, and the environment. Some of the frequently encountered terms include "social participation," "enacted togetherness," "belonging," and "social connectedness" (O'Rourke & Sidani, 2017). Although these definitions differ to varying degrees, this chapter extracts the commonalities that can greatly shift the focus of occupational therapy intention and intervention in this area.

Social participation is terminology that OTPs are very familiar with as it is the language used in the profession's guiding document, the *Occupational Therapy Practice Framework,* Fourth Edition (*OTPF-4*). According to the *OTPF-4,* social participation is an occupation defined as "activities that involve social interaction with others, including family, friends, peers, and community members, and that support social interdependence" (American Occupational Therapy Association [AOTA], 2020, p. 30). Under this broader category of occupation falls community, family, and peer group participation; friendships; and intimate partner relationships. Social participation and the various subcategories describe the nature of the relationship, such as "engaging in activities with others who have similar interests" (AOTA, 2020, p. 30) and "engaging in activities that result in successful interaction at the community level" (AOTA, 2020, p. 30).

What the term "social participation" does not adequately illuminate is the existential meaning and purpose of the connection for each unique person. In fact, in a recent systematic review conducted by Nastasi (2020), little evidence was found to support occupational therapy interventions targeting social participation with older adults with low vision. Although the *Occupational Therapy Practice Guidelines for Adults Living With Serious Mental Illness* indicate that there is strong evidence for occupational therapy intervention to improve social participation, the outcomes of the included studies focus primarily on symptom reduction or management related to social participation rather than the dimension of connectedness (Noyes & Lannigan, 2019). This may speak to the idea that (a) the profession has failed to adequately explore the nature of social participation, (b) the existential nature of connectedness is captured elsewhere in the *OTPF-4,* and/or (c) research in this area is focused on more concrete or objective measures of participation to the exclusion of its meaning.

Enacted togetherness is another term that has emerged in the occupational therapy literature coming out of Sweden. This term highlights the sociocultural dimensions of occupation and denotes an opportunity for meaning-making via emerging narratives that are generated in the context of *doing* together. Nyman and Isaksson (2021), who coined this term, argue that occupation is the connector, the glue that binds people together in time, place, and space to enact a togetherness that creates opportunities for life interpretation, evaluation, reevaluation, and even change. In this manner, enacted togetherness is not simply about doing but also about being and becoming, as described by Wilcock (1998), and belonging, as first described by Hammell (2004, 2014).

Belonging as a construct is familiar to many because of Maslow's work (1968) and the now famous image of the hierarchy of needs, which appears as a triangle with love and belongingness needs in the middle of a pyramid above physiological, safety, and security needs and below self-esteem and self-actualization needs. This term is reflected in the context of occupational therapy and occupational science from several authors (Hammell, 2004; Rebeiro & Cook, 1999; Wilcock, 2007). Belonging as a dimension of occupation speaks to both a literal and figurative space to go, to gather (Rebeiro et al., 2001), and represents an opportunity to give and receive mutual support, validation, and acceptance (Hammell, 2014). Belonging enhances life satisfaction and occupational engagement (Hammell, 2014; Rebeiro et al., 2001).

Critical to a sense of belonging is the opportunity to contribute to the well-being of others (Hammell, 2014). Occupational therapy practiced from a Western lens often focuses on self-reliance and independence to the exclusion of interdependence and collective ways of being. Centering the occupational therapy process around independence may be a reasonable and desired goal for some. For others, this could be perceived as irrelevant and dismissive of their lived experience. According to Hammell, relying on others, and vice versa, does, in fact, contribute to one's overall health and wellness (2014), a fact that must drive people's thinking at the individual level and one that must fuel advocacy to make systemic changes that provide space for greater emphasis on interdependence.

"Ubuntu" is an African term that originates from the Nguni cultures in South Africa and Zimbabwe (Mabele et al., 2022). This term has come to represent mutual caring, compassion, and interconnectedness and also suggests an inextricable link between all living things that must be considered and balanced for the sake of global survival and harmony. Similar to enacted togetherness, which was described earlier, Ubuntu captures the iterative process of doing, being, and becoming a person in the context of others.

Additionally, Ubuntu reflects the profound sense that the world or community of which people are a part is not static over time even as people come and go, but is a living, breathing, ever-evolving entity as individuals within that community also evolve over time (Ramugondo & Kronenberg, 2015). It is also a term that may resonate more deeply with OTPs and service users from collectivistic backgrounds than other terms to reflect and describe their personal sense of and need for interdependence (Tsatsi & Plastow, 2021). Using an Ubuntu lens invites practitioners to ask themselves, "How well are we doing together?" versus "How well is the

individual doing within the context of their community?" (Ramugondo & Kronenberg, 2015).

The last term frequently found in the literature is **social connectedness**. The key features of social connectedness include caring for others, feeling cared about, and experiencing a sense of belonging to a group or community (O'Rourke & Sidani, 2017). It is the antithesis of loneliness and reflects one's subjective assessment of the constructive nature and quality of their relationships with regard to meaning, purpose, and closeness (Ashida & Heaney, 2008). Social connectedness has been closely linked with mental wellness and many would argue that mental illness is a product of social disconnectedness (Andonian & MacRae, 2011; Bowins, 2021).

This chapter uses the term "connectedness" to encapsulate the spirit of the aforementioned terms, with an emphasis on the meaning and purpose derived from those connections and the sense of being a part of a larger collective that nurtures and can be nurtured. As discussed later in this chapter, the ways in which individuals discover connectedness may vary and include more than humans.

Birth of Connection to Self, Others, and the Environment

Mammalian survival is predicated on social connectedness. Although neurologically humans are the most developed at maturity, human offspring are the least developed when born and require the longest period of social and physical support and protection in the animal kingdom. Additionally, humans brandish no innate weaponry in the form of claws or fangs that would protect against the harsh reality of much larger predators.

From an evolutionary perspective, people have relied on those around them for their very survival. This historical reliance has created a "social brain" or one that is responsive to and impacted by those around us. Formalized in 2000, Social Cognitive Neuroscience has emerged to study just this phenomenon; how have and do people's brains change over time in the context of human interaction or social cognition to enable connectedness or disconnectedness? This field of study simultaneously researches the connections between social factors that influence behavior, cognitive processes such as information processing that allow people to interpret and ascribe meaning to these social factors, and neural processes that support these cognitive processes (Ochsner & Lieberman, 2001).

This science brings together a variety of fields including psychology, neuroscience, and sociology, and supports an integrated approach to exploring connectedness: the way in which people create, interpret, and respond to connections, how the brain becomes hard-wired to seek or avoid connection, and the meanings people ascribe to those connections. This holistic approach to connectedness can serve as a starting point for OTPs in determining how to approach and support meaningful connections of choice.

A prerequisite for connectedness is felt safety. Felt safety is a state of feeling not only physically safe but psychoemotionally safe. Felt safety is largely a product of both interoception and extero- or neuroception, which will be discussed later in greater detail. From the attachment theory literature, OTPs

---

BOX 49-1 ■ Hallmarks of Secure Versus Insecure Attachment

Secure Attachment	Insecure Attachment
■ Displays interoceptive awareness	■ Displays impaired intero- and neuroceptive awareness
■ Has ability to effectively regulate one's emotional states	■ Shows frequent emotional dysregulation
■ Shows willingness to explore the environment	■ Challenges with global and specific mental functions such as memory and executive functioning
■ Demonstrates cognitive flexibility	■ Prefers routine and familiar activities/occupations
■ Navigates relational challenges effectively	■ Engages threat response system during relational discord
■ Engages in relationships that are health-promoting	■ Engages in relationships that reenact attachments of origin
■ Develops and maintains personal boundaries	■ Experiences difficulty developing and maintaining personal boundaries
■ Feels connected to self and others	■ Feels disconnected from self and/or others
■ Will engage in novel activities/occupations	
■ Is creative and curious	

---

understand that felt safety, as well as connectedness to self and to others, is a byproduct of the attachments that people have with primary care providers, particularly those formed in utero into early childhood (Luyten et al., 2020; Pipp-Siegel et al, 1995). These attachments continue to influence connectedness to self and others for the remainder of people's lives (Kira, 2022).

These attachments are broadly categorized as secure or insecure. Secure attachments provide a foundation from which an individual can discover who they are in relationship to the world around them. Conversely, those whose attachments to primary care providers are insecure often experience the environment as frightening and adapt in ways that ensure their survival but impede personal identity development and growth (Wasmuth et al., 2019). Common hallmarks of both secure and insecure attachments can be found in Box 49-1.

For many individuals, insecure attachments with early childhood primary care providers are neurologically registered as adverse childhood experiences (ACEs) in the form of attachment trauma. Insecure attachments leave the fetus, infant, toddler, or child feeling unsafe and fearful of the environment at large. Resultingly, the threat response system automatically engages in the form of a fight-flight, freeze, fawn, or fib response. These responses are adaptive; they support perceived self-preservation and create a sense of safety. Trauma responses or adaptations are many and varied and can have a profound impact on occupational performance and participation over the course of the life span. Given that attachment trauma occurs in the context of a relationship, the core challenges often center around connectedness to self and others. Not all individuals who have experienced an insecure attachment will manifest with the challenges noted in Box 49-1, but it is an area of exploration for OTPs when considering both the barriers and supports to connectedness.

Secure attachments serve as the foundation for the differentiation of self from the mother and the development of selfhood by serving as a safe container from which to explore. Just as in Ubuntu, a person's identity is developed and shaped by those around them (Adams & Casteleijn, 2014). In the context of an insecure attachment that may be rooted in fear, distrust, disorganization, or disinterest, selfhood is secondary to adapting in ways that secure survival.

Historical Approaches to Connectedness in Occupational Therapy

As previously discussed, occupational therapy has traditionally utilized the term "social participation" when describing how people interact with others and with groups in various contexts. As people have seen, however, the term "social participation" does not fully embody the form, function, and meaning of connectedness. As enacted in occupational therapy, social participation reflects a colonized understanding of the ways in which individuals are expected to engage with others in context. In the *OTPF-4,* communication and interaction skills undergird social participation. From making eye contact to shaking someone's hand to turning toward someone as they speak to sustaining a conversation, many OTPs have spent countless hours engaged in social interaction skill development to ready them for social participation.

Skill development of any kind has merit as long as the individual has the desire to gain or enhance the skills in question to support their engagement in occupations. People must ask themselves, however, does this individual feel connected to self, others, and the world around them in ways that augment their overall health and wellness? This is the question that shifts the conversation from expectations of what skills might be "appropriate" from a Western, white-centric perspective regarding acceptable social participation to one that better reflects an existential need for connectedness.

Social participation and the more encompassing term "connectedness" can be particularly challenging for those bearing psychiatric labels. Connectedness is predicated on felt safety, which is a byproduct of having secure attachments. Many people living with mental illness experienced insecure attachments in early childhood (Herstell et al., 2021; Mullen, 2019; Pearse et al., 2020). Therefore, bonding with self and others can be challenging because of inherent fear, mistrust, and challenges related to self-identity. Skill development devoid of understanding the true nature of the relational difficulties can intensify the disconnection.

OTPs frequently work within traditional systems of mental health care. It is important to note that these systems were not historically designed to promote connectedness;

TABLE 49-1 | **Advocating for Connectedness**

Individual	Community	Population
• Utilize a connection menu in all settings so that persons have a choice about the ways in which they want to connect and the frequency and duration of that connection. • Increase your professional knowledge of the connection between attachment trauma and mental illness. • Prioritize the development of a secure attachment with each person in the occupational therapy process. • Assess the practice environment for supports and barriers to creating secure attachments with staff.	• Develop intergenerational community programs that target secure attachment, safety, and connectedness. • Provide educational programs that target care providers regarding the centrality of secure attachments to neurodevelopment. • Educate school-based providers regarding attachment trauma and its manifestations that can result in behavioral labels. • Engage in continuing education regarding generational trauma and its intersectionality with racism that fuels disconnection.	• Advocate for and support legislation that creates more time and space in school systems for social-emotional development. • Advocate for the expansion of community mental health services that allow for more and varied connection-building opportunities. • Explore alternative systems of care that allow for greater connection and are not predicated on traditional reimbursement models. • Utilize OTP skills in the context of other employment titles such as legislator where changes can be effected more directly.

in fact, they are often oppressive and retraumatize the individuals they purport to help. Brief stays, hyperfocus on medical reductionism in the form of psychotropic medications, and limits on the type, frequency, and duration of intervention can all interfere with developing connectedness, which many with lived experience report as the most important aspect of their recovery journey (Aga et al., 2021; Saeri et al., 2018).

Influencing change in the systems of mental health care is a key responsibility of every OTP. If disconnection is responsible in part for the development of a mental illness (Dawson-Rose et al., 2020; Longden et al., 2012; MacIntosh et al., 2015), then it is the OTPs' moral and ethical duty to advocate for systemic changes across the continuum of care from acute to community-based that place connectedness at the center of care. Suggestions for advocacy at the individual, community, and population levels can be found in Table 49-1.

Connectedness and Health and Wellness

What is it about connectedness that is so beneficial aside from procuring people's survival? Connectedness, particularly social connection, has been shown to improve both physical and mental health and wellness across diverse populations (Beatson & Taryan, 2003; Begun et al., 2018; John-Henderson et al., 2020). Factors such as body mass index, blood glucose levels, blood pressure, heart rate, and psychological state have all been shown to improve in the context of social connectedness (Blum et al., 2022; Martino et al., 2017).

Conversely, those who do not experience a sense of connectedness often have more mental health challenges including depression, anxiety, psychosis, and loneliness, and have higher incidences of diabetes, obesity, cardiovascular disease, and cancer (Martino et al., 2017). The evidence is clear that connectedness is central to health and wellness. Exclusionary practices even in health care can highlight the issue that inclusion is a basic necessity and therefore a human right (Hocking, 2019). Excluding individuals or groups of people can result in disconnections that have far-reaching consequences.

Crisis of Disconnectedness

The United States is currently amid what might be described as a crisis of disconnection. This disconnectedness is reflected in major and long-lasting societal events and trends.

Some of these notable societal trends and events include the rise in diagnosed mental health conditions (Mental Health America, 2021), skyrocketing suicide rates (American Foundation for Suicide Prevention, 2022), incidences of substance use and associated overdose deaths that are higher than ever in many age and ethnic groups (National Institute on Drug Abuse [NIDA], 2023; Substance Abuse and Mental Health Services Administration [SAMHSA], 2021), daily mass shootings (Gun Violence Archive, 2023), negative fallout of excessive exposure to social media (Huang, 2022), an epidemic of loneliness (McGinty et al., 2020), the long-term psychological and social implications of a recent global pandemic (World Health Organization [WHO], 2022), climate change that is gradually rendering the planet uninhabitable (National Aeronautics and Space Administration, 2023), and a health-care workforce that is dwindling because of burnout and compassion fatigue (Cavanagh et al., 2020).

In people's rush to solve these problems, they often granularize and pathologize societal challenges versus taking a bigger and more humanistic approach to sustainable solutions. If people were to step back to collectively assess these societal trends and events, they might recognize that even though they manifest differently, all roads generally lead back to a fundamental and profound disconnection with self, others, and/or the environment.

The current trend in gun violence, for example, and in particular mass shootings, is that they are perpetrated by late adolescents and emerging adults. People understandably ponder the *why* after such events and often land quickly on the rationale that the perpetrator is mentally ill. If someone examines the occupational history of these individuals, they will consistently find that the shooters experienced many ACEs and circumstances including attachment trauma, foster care placement, and bullying, and typically lacked adequate care to address these gaps in basic survival and developmental needs.

Without a secure and reliable connection to primary care providers or a sense of belonging to a community

(Weiss, 1973), it is difficult at best to develop a connection to self and subsequently others. The following quote comes from a note left by a recent school shooter: "I don't have any friends. I don't have any family. I've never had a girlfriend. I've never had a social life. I've been an isolated loner my entire life. This was the perfect storm for a mass shooter" (Rieck et al., 2022). These words reflect a depth of disconnectedness that was long-standing and potentially preventable. Developing a deeper understanding of the roots of these behaviors does not condone these actions but rather gives people food for thought with regard to how they can contribute to a framework of connection that catches people before they fall into the river.

A less talked about but strong contributor to the mental health challenges and ultimate disconnectedness in the United States is the use and impact of technology, particularly social media. Although there are benefits to using technology to support connection, evidence consistently shows that excessive social media use in particular negatively impacts self-esteem and life satisfaction and positively correlates with depression and loneliness (Huang, 2022). Social media poses a threat to those whose connection to self and others is already at risk. Filters, controlling narratives that may or may not closely resemble reality, and cyberbullying are just a few of the pitfalls associated with excessive social media use (Cover, 2022; Weinstein et al., 2021).

Another issue of grave concern that relates directly to connectedness is loneliness. It may well be the newest human epidemic. In fact, Surgeon General Dr. Vivek Murthy (2020) penned a book titled, *Together: The Healing Power of Human Connection in a Sometimes Lonely World.* In it, he highlights the global implications of loneliness from heart disease, stroke, and high blood pressure to dementia, anxiety, depression (Murthy, 2020), and suicidal behaviors (Stickley & Koyanagi, 2018).

A survey conducted by Cigna indicates that more than half of U.S. adults are considered lonely (2018). Young adults are twice as likely as seniors to be lonely, and 42% of adults ages 18 to 34 report always feeling left out (Cigna, 2018). A more recent report from the National Academies of Sciences, Engineering, and Medicine indicates that one-third of adults ages 45 and older feel lonely (2020). Resultingly, there is a 30% increase in the likelihood of dying if one is lonely, socially isolated, and living alone for extended periods (Holt-Lunstad et al., 2015).

Perhaps the most recent event to highlight the centrality of connectedness to health and wellness is the COVID-19 pandemic. The pandemic and its aftermath have wreaked havoc on the state of mental health and mental health care in the United States because of collective isolation, occupational deprivation, and fear of pandemic-related unknowns, as well as heightened societal concerns including political discord and racism (Mukhtar, 2020; Pai & Vella, 2021). WHO indicates that rates of anxiety and depression increased by 25% in the first year of the COVID-19 pandemic. So significant was this rise that the U.S. Preventive Services Task Force is currently developing a recommendation that all adults, whether or not they exhibit signs or symptoms, undergo anxiety screening in the context of primary care visits. Substance use has also increased since the beginning of the pandemic (NIDA, 2022).

To self-regulate in the face of anxiety, depression, loneliness, and other psychiatric labels, many people turn to drugs and alcohol. The SAMHSA reports that substance use is up among substance users by a "little" or "much more" (2020) and more U.S. citizens are becoming acutely aware of the growing opioid crisis in the country. In fact, deaths resulting from opioid-related overdoses are up nearly 520% since 1999 (National Center for Drug Abuse Statistics, 2023).

Core disconnection impacts all aspects of people's individual and collective experiences. It impacts them socially, economically, politically, culturally, and environmentally. Although this crisis of disconnection may seem insurmountable because of the sheer magnitude of how disconnection manifests, as has been previously explored, it must be addressed in people's everyday practice.

Evaluation: Assessing Connectedness

How then do OTPs intervene when the person is experiencing a level of disconnection that is impacting mental and/or physical health and wellness and results in occupational disruption? As discussed earlier, social participation may not reflect a level of engagement that holds meaning and purpose for the person. It is critical that, from the initial occupational profile to assessment, intervention, and discharge, OTPs are exploring in tandem with the person how a meaningful connection looks and how the OTP can support them in sustaining that connection.

The occupational profile has become a required first step in the occupational therapy process based on Medicare standards. The occupational profile provides a very broad picture of the person from occupational history to performance patterns and person factors that might be supporting and hindering a person's current occupational circumstance.

The mention of connectedness in the profile can be seen in the form of "support and relationships" and "social background," both of which fall under the area of contexts. How connectedness is approached by the clinician is up to the clinician to determine based upon their knowledge of the centrality of connection and skill in mining useful information. Although questions such as "Do you have friends?" or "Do you engage in activities with others?" might speak to the quantity of social interaction, they do not necessarily capture the more existential notion of belongingness that encapsulates the many meanings that people ascribe to how, when, and why they connect with themselves, others, and their environment. Questions that better target connectedness might include, "When do you feel most connected to yourself, to others, and to the world around you?" or "What stands in the way of you feeling connected to yourself, others, or the environment?" This line of questioning moves the conversation away from a hyperfocus on doing and into the realm of being, becoming, and ultimately belonging.

Once an occupational profile has been gathered, additional exploration of connectedness may be warranted in the form of additional structured or unstructured, standardized, or nonstandardized assessments. Several instruments that directly or indirectly support the exploration of connectedness are described in the text that follows, and more can be found in Table 49-2.

The Personal Recovery Outcome Measure (PROM) was developed by a Canadian occupational therapist, Skye

The Lived Experience

D.M.

I've dealt with mental health issues since I was a kid. I was very disruptive and was held back in first grade because of developmental issues. I made it to sixth grade with help from a lot of teachers. My mental health got worse when my little cousin passed away and at that same time, I was diagnosed with a life-altering disease.

Diabetes really changed my life; that's when my first suicide attempts happened. Shortly after that, I was admitted to a children's psychiatric unit for a week. In the following months, I was learning how to live with needles, lancets, and test strips, which made me feel really different from other people who didn't have the disease. My dad, who already lived separately from us, left for good one day, leaving us with a house debt. Shortly after my dad left, the bank took my childhood home from us and I felt more disconnected than ever. We were homeless for the summer. Also, during this summer, I was on my way to a psychiatric facility for youth, because of my behavior during middle school. I was tutored for the rest of my eighth-grade year, which separated me even more from my peer group.

In ninth grade, I started attending a school for kids with behavioral issues. My mental health only got worse there; I was out of control and felt so alone. During one incident, the police were called and I was maced and then asked to leave the school. After I was expelled, I went to another program; this is when things started to change for me. It was here that I met a lot of great people who helped me to feel like I was part of a community. I became very close with one person. Unfortunately, this person left the facility and a week later took their life by suicide. This loss caused my mental health to get worse for a few months because I started to feel really alone again. I was coming to the end of my time in the program because I was about to age out.

I went back to my hometown my senior year and graduated with my friends, which was great. After my senior year, I already had a job lined up—I was going to be a day-care teacher. My mental health was doing rather well. I was a day-care teacher for 2 years but got burnt out. I also worked part-time at a roller rink, sometimes working 50 to 60 hours. When the place was sold, my mental health took a turn for the worse because I was jobless and I had lost my work community. I turned to things to numb my feelings and anything I thought would work didn't. I did a lot of bad things over the years.

During that time, I dated a girl for a bit. Things were good until she discovered I was an addict. When she was pregnant, I chose drugs over her and the baby. I still regret that. For a couple more years, I hung around people who didn't care about me. When I watched a friend of mine smoking an empty meth pipe because he was so high, I realized this time in my life needed to end. I stopped using hard drugs and have been sober for 15 years. I am very proud of that! After using drugs for years, I met a lady who was in a bad relationship. I helped her out of it and we started dating. Things were great. She had three kids that I got along with and we got married after 8 or so years of being together. My mental health was doing really well, and she knew most of my past. But also being with her, I was secluded from people for years. My anxiety got worse, I got worse, and she didn't know how to handle it.

We argued a lot; a lot of saying "sorry" but not fixing things. So, in December of 2018, she kicked me out. There were multiple reasons she gave me. Around this time my dad got very sick. My dad passed away and that sent me into a spiral of emotions. This is where I get pushed to my limits. She was all I knew for 11 years and it was all gone: the dogs, cats, the kids—all of it. I felt very alone and disconnected. I instantly thought, "What can kill the pain?" My second thought was suicide, so I tried and ended up in the hospital. Then I ended up in a crisis stabilization unit (CSU); this happened four or five times. I then connected with a case worker who has helped me out a lot. This is when I found the Clubhouse–a place to go, do things, get out of my head, meet new people, and feel like I am a part of something. Even so, I kept going in and out of hospitals following suicide attempts and suicidal thinking and had multiple stays at different CSUs. For a while, I was trying to end my life literally every week.

I remember one phone call that changed my life. It was with a former staff member at the Clubhouse. It was a 2-hour phone call. During that call, this staff member talked to me on her own time (outside of Clubhouse hours). I was able to be honest with her about my feelings of being better off dead. She listened to me and made sure I was safe before hanging up. This was a reminder that even when I don't feel it, people do care about me.

Since then, I have done two different jobs. I worked as a dishwasher at a major hotel chain and as a prep worker at a restaurant. I really enjoyed both of these positions. It's taken a lot of hard work to have made it out of my most recent mental health issues.

In all, I tried to end my life 30 times and thought about it a hundred times. I have been through dozens of intensive outpatient programs. I've had a ton of therapists. What really helped me is really changing my thought process. Like "Is it a bad day or a bad 5 minutes?" I started journaling about 3 years ago, and it's amazing to read everything I wrote down. So right now, in life, I'm doing well. It's been 2 years since I've been in a CSU. I go to the Clubhouse 5 days a week to stay busy and connect with a community that makes me feel seen and valued. I stay late on Fridays to hang out with other members of our extended day program. I've had my ups and downs with a lot in life. I now know it's ok to have my feelings and emotions and thoughts; it's what we do with them that counts and sharing them with others can form connections that can save lives.

TABLE 49-2 | Therapeutic Reasoning Assessment Table: Connectedness and Belonging

Which Tool?	Who Was This Tool Designed For?	What Is Required of the Person? Can They Use the Tool?	What Am I Measuring?	How Long Does It Take and Where Do I Administer This Assessment?	Is the Tool Associated With a Practice Model?
Canadian Personal Recovery Outcome Measure (Barbic & Rennie, 2016; Barbic et al., 2018)	Adults (18+ years)	30-item self-report that indicates how frequently a person experienced the item; can be read to the person	A measure of recovery in adults with mental health disorders	10–12 minutes	Recovery Model (Jacob, 2015; SAMHSA, 2012)
Occupational Self-Assessment (OSA; Baron et al., 2006)	Adults (18+ years)	Can be completed as a self-report or in a format of a semistructured interview with support from an OTP	Self-reported competency and value across various occupations	30–60 minutes	Model of Human Occupation (MOHO)
Social and Community Opportunities Profile–Short (SCOPE; Huxley et al., 2012)	Adults (18+ years)	48-item instrument	Social, leisure, and community participation	30–45 minutes	Doing, being, belonging, and becoming (Hammell, 2004; Wilcock, 1998, 2006)
Social Inclusion Questionnaire User Experience (SInQUE; Mezey et al., 2013, 2020)	Adults (18+ years)	Structured interview around productivity, consumption, access to services, social integration, and political engagement	Objective and subjective aspects of social inclusion for persons with mental health concerns	30–45 minutes	No specific model but consistent with models emphasizing social participation and belonging
Social Connectedness Scale (SCS; Lee & Robbins, 1995)	12+ years	20 items that can be completed as a self-report or via interview	Extent to which a person feels connected to others in their social environment	10–12 minutes	No specific model but consistent with models emphasizing social participation and belonging
Activity Card Sort–Advancing Inclusive Participation (Baum & Edwards, 2008; Tyminski et al., 2020)	Community dwelling adults	76 cards representing social, home management, nonsanctioned (i.e., smoking, drinking alcohol), work, education, daily living, physical activity, leisure, health management, and community independence activities	Overview of previous, current, or desired engagement in the occupations	15 minutes	Person-Environment-Occupation Model

Barbic (Barbic & Rennie, 2016). The PROM is a 30-question self-report measure that asks persons to indicate how often they have experienced each item in the past week (i.e., ranging from none of the time to all of the time). The items progress from those related to self, to those related to meaning and purpose in one's life, to connectedness with the environment. The adjusted score is used to locate the item related to one of the three areas where dialogue can further the exploration of self, meaning, or connectedness with the person for the purposes of planning intervention.

Self-reports are extremely pertinent to the construct of connectedness because they support a person's perspective of the form, function, and meaning of existing and/or desired

connections. In a recent study regarding the Canadian Personal Recovery Outcome Measure (C-PROM), researchers found that the area of social connectedness was one of deprivation, and a third of study participants reported that they felt isolated rather than a part of society (Barbic et al., 2018).

Another assessment that comes from the profession is the Occupational Self-Assessment (OSA; Baron et al., 2006). This assessment is a self-report measure and targets a better understanding of the individual's perceived competence with items related to aspects of themselves and their environment as well as the value of and satisfaction with these items. Although not directly assessing connectedness, there are several items on both subscales titled "myself" and "my environment" that relate to connectedness, including "expressing myself to others," "getting along with others," "people who support and encourage me," and "people who do things with me."

The Model of Human Occupation (MOHO) serves as the theoretical foundation upon which the OSA was built (Kielhofner & Burke, 1980). The MOHO is predicated on person-centeredness and, as such, the OTP is invited to explore the OSA responses in collaboration with the person. This exploration, specifically around the aforementioned items, can serve to better understand the ways in which, and in what contexts and environments, the person feels connected in order to codesign an intervention plan that is tailored to the individual.

The Social and Community Opportunities Profile–Short (SCOPE), the Social Inclusion Questionnaire User Experience (SInQUE), the Social Connectedness Scale (SCS), and the Activity Card Sort–Advancing Inclusive Participation (ACS-AIP; Tyminski et al., 2020) are instruments that specifically target one or more constructs related to connectedness. Each of these scales is a self-report measure. The short version of the SCOPE is a 42-item instrument that targets inclusion and measures perceived opportunities for inclusion and satisfaction with those opportunities as well as more objective items related to participation opportunities such as opportunities for work, housing, education, and leisure (Huxley et al., 2012). The SCOPE is particularly useful in demonstrating how choice and opportunity in tandem with subjective experiences of inclusion result in participation and engagement (Baumgartner & Burns, 2014).

The SInQUE, developed by Mezey and colleagues (2013), is specific to the mental health population and is a 75-item instrument. The two-part instrument gathers information regarding inclusion for (a) the year before the current hospitalization and (b) the person's current situation. The SInQUE captures both objective and subjective information and perceptions related to productivity, consumption, access to services, political engagement, and social integration (Baumgartner & Burns, 2014). Unique to this instrument is that it captures reasons for nonparticipation yet does not penalize the individual who chooses not to participate in various activities.

Finally, the SCS was developed by Lee and Robbins and measures aspects of belongingness including connectedness, affiliation, and companionship (1995). Since its initial development, the SCS has been revised and currently contains 20 statements that are rated based on the degree to which respondents agree or disagree with each item.

The ACS-AIP is based on the original Activity Card Sort, Second Edition (ACS) developed by Baum and Edwards (2008). The ACS-AIP (Tyminski et al., 2020) was developed to specifically target individuals who are unhoused but can be used with a variety of individuals who are marginalized because of its flexibility and adaptability. It consists of 76 cards of individuals engaged in a variety of activities and instrumental activities of daily living (IADLs) common to those who are unhoused. The images on the cards are black-and-white ink drawings of actual pictures. This was done to expand inclusivity as the gender, ethnicity, and environment of the people represented in the drawings are nondescript and could represent any number of the aforementioned identities and contexts.

The ACS-AIP is based upon Q-sort methodology and thus persons are asked to sort the cards based upon the five categories: "do now," "do less," "want to do," "never did," and "given up." Aside from the ink drawings, the ACS-AIP differs from the original ACS in two other important ways. The first way is that the ACS-AIP includes "nonsanctioned" occupations or those that, in some ways, do not contribute to one's overall health and wellness such as alcohol and drug use and theft. The stigma associated with many of these nonsanctioned occupations tends to fuel disconnection between those who engage in these occupations and the larger society. Another critical way in which this version differs from the original is that the ACS-AIP includes a series of follow-up questions for each card.

The authors of this assessment highlight the importance of the therapist–person relationship and that without a secure attachment to the person responses to the ACS may be compromised and the connectedness needed for engagement in the occupational therapy process will not develop. Table 49-2 summarizes instruments that can be used by OTPs to capture various aspects of connectedness. Other tools that might be considered as a part of the assessment process are listed in Table 49-3.

Once the OTP has gained a comprehensive understanding of the person's challenges related to connection with self, others, and/or the environment, the cocreation of an intervention plan commences. The depth and breadth of intervention may vary based upon variables such as identified areas to be addressed in the occupational therapy process, the nature of the setting (e.g., acute vs. community), and subsequent time afforded to work with the person; focus, however, should remain on ways in which OTPs can support persons to strengthen connections as identified and desired. The following interventions are evidence-informed and speak to strengthening connections with self, others, and the environment based on the desired form, function, and meaning of those connections.

Interventions

A variety of interventions might be selected to promote social connectedness and belonging. This section provides an overview of interventions targeting the person and their environments.

Interventions Targeting the Person

As discussed earlier in this chapter, connection via early primary care providers often sets the stage for connection, or conversely disconnection, from self. If the connection to early primary care providers is insecure, attachment trauma can result (Streeck-Fischer & van der Kolk, 2000; Teicher et al., 2002). Attachment trauma can lead to the development of insecure attachment styles that often reflect a generalized fear and distrust both of others and self. Disconnection from self can result in and bear the label of a psychiatric illness such as borderline personality disorder, substance use disorder, and schizophrenia, among many others. Healing the connection with self can seem daunting not only to the individual but to the practitioner as well, and even though there are any number of approaches, the basic principles of this work are relatively simple.

The first goal of therapy should be the development of a trusting relationship with the person, for without it, nothing

TABLE 49-3 | Additional Assessments Measuring Aspects of Social Connectedness

Assessment	Type/ Administration	Constructs Measured/ Additional Information
Watts Connectedness Scale (Watts, et al., 2022)	Pen-and-paper/self-report	Assesses the degree to which an individual perceives connectedness to themselves, others, and the world. The assessment contains 19 items. Persons read and rate each statement on a scale that ranges from "not at all" to entirely based on how they have felt over the past 2 weeks.
The Occupational Performance History Interview II (OPHI-II; Kielhofner et al., 2004)	Semistructured interview with an option for pencil-and-paper self-report of narrative slope	Assesses occupational competence and the influence of the environment on occupational functioning as well as occupational identity. These constructs are assessed through the lens of capturing information related to daily routines, roles, settings, activity, and occupational choices as well as critical life events. The interviewer has latitude to explore ways in which the individual feels/does not feel connected to themselves, others, and their environment that support or detract from occupational functioning.
The General Belongingness Scale (Malone et al., 2012)	Pen-and-paper/self-report	Persons rate 12 statements based on a Likert 7-point scale ranging from strongly agree to strongly disagree. Half of the items relate to acceptance and inclusion, whereas the other six relate to rejection and exclusion.
Self-Connection Scale (SCS; Klussman et al., 2022)	Pen and paper/self-report	This 12-item instrument assesses an individual's connection to self; a construct comprising self-awareness, self-acceptance, and self-alignment. Respondents answer each question based on the degree to which they agree or disagree with each statement.
Pet Owner Connectedness Scale (POCS; Oliva & Johnston, 2022)	Pen-and-paper/self-report	This instrument consists of two subscales including the owner–pet connection subscale and the connectedness through pet subscale. Respondents indicate the degree to which they agree or disagree with statements such as "My pet provides comfort and reassurance."

else can be accomplished. Acceptance of a person's authentic self can fuel their connection with self and ability to make decisions that are in closer alignment with their values and goals. If a person is experiencing an active threat response it is imperative that people work neurologically from the bottom up versus the top down. Showing up and being consistent lessens environmental threat and allows space for reconnection. Disconnection happened over time; conversely, connection will not happen overnight. Respect for neurodiversity is paramount, and people must assess their own biases with regard to how people might connect with self. It is enough to be in a relationship with a person without the need to create a product or develop a skill.

Most frequently, disconnection from self happens early in life and continues to manifest throughout the life span in the absence of intervention. Several useful approaches have been developed in the pediatric world as that is where and when people begin to see the fallout from insecure attachments. Bruce Perry's Neurosequential Model of Therapeutics (NMT; 2006) and the Attachment, Regulation, and Competency (ARC) framework (Kinniburgh et al., 2005) are frameworks that can be useful even with an adult population. Both are predicated on a bottom-up approach; supporting the nervous system to disengage the threat response must occur first before engagement of higher-order cognitive processes such as executive functioning becomes available.

The NMT is an approach to intervention rather than a specific clinical intervention. The model brings together principles from both neurodevelopment and traumatology to shape assessment, intervention, interprofessional care, and family involvement (Perry & Hambrick, 2008). The manifestation of trauma is a direct reflection of when the trauma began and what regions of the brain and neural networks were forming

or developing at the time; the manifestations of trauma that occurred preverbally, even in utero, are often widespread because brain development was in full swing and, consequently, globally impacted. Healing the brain must occur in a neurosequential order from the primitive or reptilian brain to the limbic or mammalian brain and finally to the neocortex. Assessment will determine where to begin (primitive to neocortex) based upon the neural markers reflected in behavior.

Similar to the NMT, the ARC Model provides an approach to intervention that is based upon the development of secure attachments, the ability to self-regulate, and the development of cognitive, emotional, intrapersonal, and interpersonal competencies that are often derailed in the context of developmental trauma (Kinniburgh et al., 2005). Unique to NMT is the intentional focus on systems of care and how these systems can support the development of the three ARC components. Although both ARC and NMT were developed with children and adolescents in mind, they can be a useful lens through which to view adult disconnection where there is a trauma history and difficulties with emotional regulation, executive functioning, and intrapersonal and interpersonal functioning, for example, are evident.

Another target area for intervention that is commonly impacted in the context of developmental trauma is interoception. As previously discussed, interoception is the newest identified sensory system and it is the system responsible for registering and responding to cues related to internal states such as hunger, temperature, and even feeling states (Ceunen et al., 2016). In the midst of developmental trauma, any number of neurodevelopmental processes can be disrupted or even derailed, and the development of the ability to process sensory information from both external and internal sources is no exception. Interoception was first described by Sherrington (1906). Understanding interoception and the ramifications of interoceptive challenges within occupational therapy has been much more recent, however (Mahler, 2015).

Much of people's knowledge has come from other fields with regard to the intersections between interoception, disconnection with self (often in the form of alexithymia), and even psychiatric labels (Desdentado et al., 2023; Edwards & Lowe, 2021). Kelly Mahler, OTR/L, has been instrumental in translating this knowledge for the profession in terms of the occupational implications of interoceptive challenges and, specifically, how to address these challenges in the context of the occupational therapy process. With the understanding that every person is unique, the general approach to interoceptive challenges includes supporting people to first notice and explore internal states via sensory-based activities such as spelling words with different body parts or noticing how different body parts feel in cold versus hot water.

People are habituated to using the Westernized feelings lexicon that includes descriptions such as happy, sad, angry, and anxious. In Mahler's approach, it is critical that the person describes the internal state using language and phrasing that makes sense to them. In doing so, they are able to make sense of and connection to self that is self-generated and therefore more meaningful in the context of their personal narrative. For example, people might engage a person in a preferred physical activity and subsequently process their internal states using the previously described approach. Once the individual has established their unique language, it is imperative that their support team, including their OTP, use that language to sustain the connections made.

In concert with interoceptive work, grounding and mindfulness techniques are also evidence-informed approaches that can enhance connection with self. Grounding falls under the umbrella of somatic therapy, which seeks to bring mind and body into closer alignment by supporting the individual to discharge the physiological remnants of trauma from the body (Bisson et al., 2020; Mavranezouli et al., 2020). Grounding specifically supports the individual in bringing their awareness back to their physical body in the physical environment in which they find themselves. This technique is frequently used with individuals who are experiencing a panic attack, active threat response, and a dissociative episode, and often includes asking the individual to connect with their sensory world by stating things they see, hear, feel, and smell, for example.

Mindfulness originated in Eastern Buddhist practices and refers to "the awareness that emerges through paying attention on purpose: in the present moment and non-judgmentally" (Kabat Zinn, 2003, p. 145). Remaining present or *mindful,* which encourages awareness and merging of somatic, psychological, and emotional experiences, can help to mitigate depersonalization. This is a hallmark of many mental health diagnoses, including borderline personality disorder, dissociative identity disorder, and trauma-related disorders such as posttraumatic stress disorder (PTSD; Gilmartin et al., 2017; Polusny et al., 2015).

Although the gold standard of mindfulness is **mindfulness-based stress reduction (MBSR)**, which typically includes 2- to 3-hour sessions 1 ×/week for 8 weeks (Heeter et al., 2017), success is also being seen with smaller dosing, frequency, and duration (Heeter et al., 2017; Horner et al., 2014; Sevilla-Llewellyn-Jones et al., 2018). Mindfulness

simultaneously requires and enhances attention regulation, body awareness, emotional regulation, interoception or experience of self, and cognitive flexibility (Fani et al., 2023; Hölzel et al., 2011).

Mindfulness at its core is a spiritual practice, a fact that should not go unnoticed or unappreciated. Being in tune with the self and connecting in a meaningful and deeply spiritual way to the universe to discover one's truth and existential purpose is a personal experience and journey that cannot be relegated to objective markers of competency. Some would argue that mindfulness is not a practice at all but rather a natural state that becomes clouded by thoughts (Kelley et al., 2015).

The aforementioned interventions support the individual in calming their threat response and returning to a state of homeostasis; this includes reconnection to self in both body and mind. At this point, the cerebral cortex and its associated functions once again become available for use by the individual. Cognitive behavioral approaches historically have relied on the person being able to engage the neocortex to gain insight and think metacognitively about their situation and the relationship between thoughts, feelings, and behaviors. **Cognitive Behavioral Therapy (CBT)** has been in use for over 100 years, and for the past 60 has been the gold standard for use with those labeled with any number of psychiatric illnesses.

Newer iterations of a CBT approach include Dialectical Behavioral Therapy (DBT) and Acceptance and Commitment Therapy (ACT). Both of these therapies are frequently adapted for use by OTPs and focus on supporting the individual to develop a deeper understanding of and connection to themselves by focusing on enhancement of self-acceptance, engagement in metacognitive activities, and development of skills necessary to live authentically.

Dr. Marsha Linehan developed DBT in response to the difficulty she experienced when treating those diagnosed with borderline personality disorder who presented with parasuicidality (Shearin & Linehan, 1994). She identified that her persons' dichotomous thinking prevented them from being able to connect with themselves and subsequently others as well. DBT is a manualized program based on four core skills: mindfulness, distress tolerance, emotional regulation, and interpersonal effectiveness.

Mindfulness, as previously described, is a newer addition to CBT approaches and enables persons to notice their thoughts without becoming consumed by their thoughts. Distress tolerance training helps people cope with situations that may not be in their control and move on from them. Emotional regulation enables people to manage big feeling states before they become all-consuming. Interpersonal skills are those building blocks needed to relate to others that many bearing psychiatric labels never had the opportunity to develop secondary to developmental trauma.

As is common with many CBT approaches, DBT therapists utilize readings and worksheets in addition to talk therapy to effect change in their people. OTPs can also use these readings and worksheets as interventions to support occupation and are then invited to practice the DBT skills learned in the context of occupation. It is recommended that OTPs obtain additional training in both ACT and DBT before incorporating them into daily practice. Examples of DBT in action are provided in Box 49-2.

BOX 49-2 ■ Dialectical Behavioral Therapy in Action

Dialectical Behavioral Therapy

Core mindfulness: Engage in practices that invite the person to attune to their internal and external world in the present moment.

Interpersonal effectiveness: Role-play scenarios that include the need for conflict resolution. Debrief to ensure that boundaries of self and others were respected during the role-play.

Emotional regulation: Engage in interoceptive activities to enhance awareness of internal states including emotional states.

Distress tolerance: Introduce an activity of interest such as origami in which the probability of making a mistake is high. Ask the person to describe the feelings as they move through the activity to reinforce that these feelings can be uncoupled from self-harming or defeating behaviors.

ACT, developed by Dr. Steven Hayes, is another present-oriented approach to enhancing psychological flexibility and supporting a more authentic existence (Hayes, 2004). The approach is based upon six core principles: cognitive defusion, acceptance, connection with the present moment, values, self as context, and committed action.

Cognitive defusion invites the person to detach from their thoughts and view them objectively and without judgment. Acceptance reflects a stance of openness to the present and future. Connection with the present moment parallels mindfulness and the connection that brings to the self and the current context and environment. Values reflect what is meaningful and important to an individual. Self as context reflects the holding space for both self as content and self as process. The content of the self is made up of thoughts and feelings, as well as actions that ebb and flow, start, and stop, which reflects the process of the self. Self as context is the ability to witness self in real-time as though an observer in one's own life. Finally, committed action involves the steps one is willing to take to move toward greater psychological flexibility and authenticity.

ACT and DBT differ significantly from earlier CBT interventions in that these newer approaches embrace the understanding that cognitive, affective, and behavioral change is difficult and does not generally happen quickly. The acceptance piece that each brings to the process is essential in reconnecting with self in ways that are nonjudgmental, more realistic, and nurturing, which, in turn, enables the individual to feel safer and more secure in exploring their environment and engaging occupationally.

Metacognitive Reflection and Insight Therapy (MERIT) is another manualized approach to supporting those with psychiatric labels by targeting the development of metacognition. Developed by Dr. Paul Lysaker and colleagues, MERIT is a form of psychotherapy (De Jong et al., 2013). According to MERIT, metacognition is the ability to form an integrated schema of oneself and others and use this ability to effectively respond to circumstances that arise in the context of everyday living.

There are eight core elements of this model: detecting and clarifying the agenda, inserting the therapist's mind, eliciting the narrative episode, defining the psychological problem, reflecting on the therapeutic relationship, reflecting on progress, stimulating self-reflection and awareness of the other, and stimulating mastery. The MERIT-Therapist Adherence Scale (MERIT-TAS) accompanies the model and supports the clinician in self-reflection on their own practice by capturing information related to the degree they adhered to each of the eight elements. MERIT has been more widely used by OTPs in Canada and is currently migrating to the United States (Wasmuth et al., 2022). MERIT elements will feel familiar to OTPs as the crux of the approach rests on connection and meaning-making for the person. When using MERIT as a psychotherapy approach, OTPs will need to reimagine their use in an occupation-centered practice.

Interventions Targeting the Environment

The following broad interventions target the environment. According to the *OTPF-4*, environment factors fall under the broader category of context. These factors include natural and humanmade environments that feature flora and fauna; products such as those related to technology; and people and animals that serve to enhance physical, emotional, and relational well-being. Although it is common to conjure up images of people when considering connection and belongingness, it is imperative that individuals broaden their thinking to include additional ways in which people find a connection; these might include pets, service animals, nature, and even a metaverse.

Although readers will not find the term "connection menu" in the literature, it is a helpful concept to consider. A connection menu can be likened to a sensory diet, which is described as a menu and routine of sensory activities developed specifically for an individual based upon their sensory needs and the types and dosing of sensory activities that will help them maintain an optimum level of arousal and engagement with their environment (Wilbarger 1984). Similarly, OTPs can support persons in developing their own connection menu replete with types and dosing of connection opportunities that support a global sense of connectedness (see Fig. 49-1).

The connection menu also provides the OTP with a lens through which to view their work and the system in which this work is conducted. For example, does the facility support voice and choice by providing persons with a menu of professional and paraprofessional services, as well as volunteers from which they can pick? Is 1:1 and/or group attendance mandatory? Are persons able to engage in ways that support their felt connection, such as sitting on the periphery of a group? These and other questions are those OTPs must be asking themselves if they are to consistently and intentionally lead with connection.

Environmental Interventions Related to Support and Relationships

As described earlier, connection goes beyond engagement in activities and occupations with others. To experience authentic connection and a sense of belongingness, the individual typically perceives that they are cared for, that they are

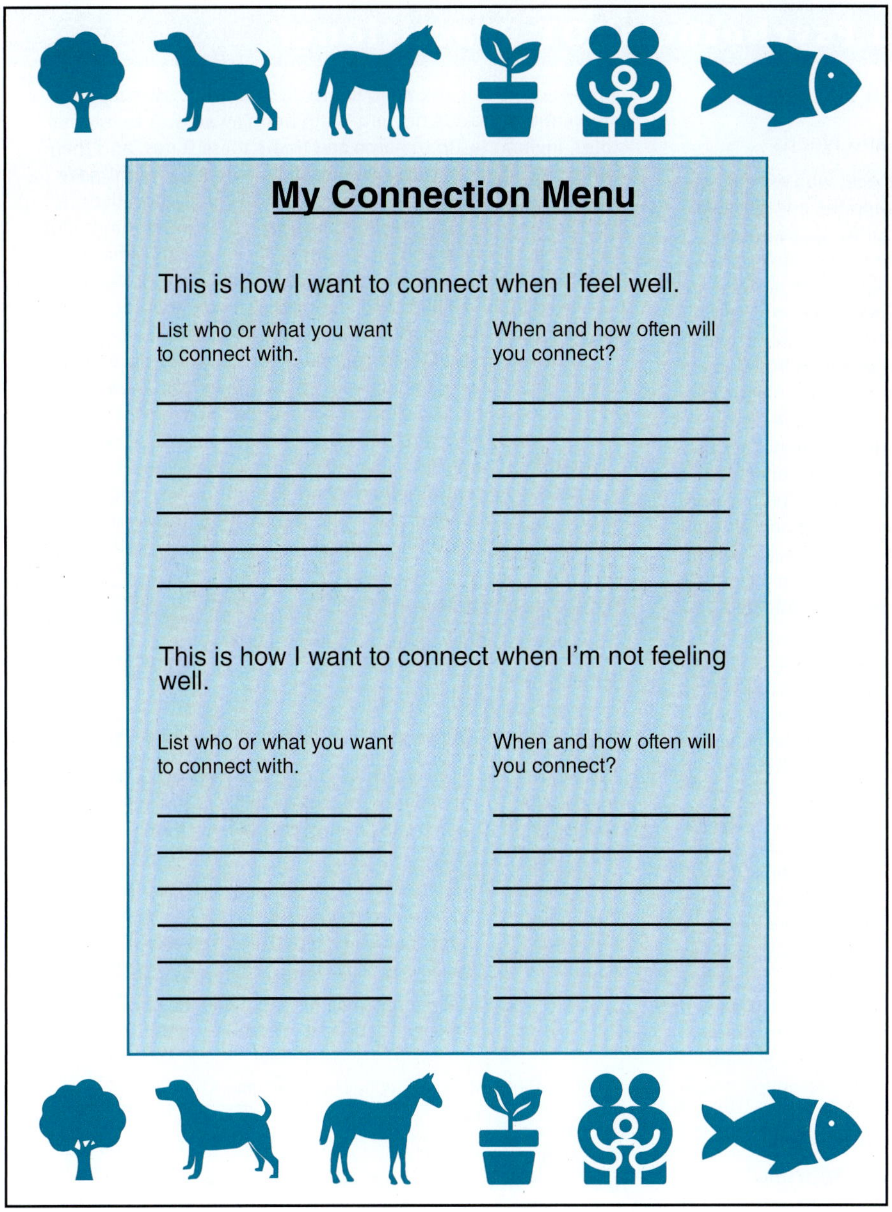

My Connection Menu

This is how I want to connect when I feel well.

List who or what you want
to connect with.

When and how often will
you connect?

_____

_____

_____

_____

_____

_____

_____

_____

_____

_____

This is how I want to connect when I'm not feeling
well.

List who or what you want
to connect with.

When and how often will
you connect?

_____

_____

_____

_____

_____

_____

_____

_____

_____

_____

FIGURE 49-1. Sample connection menu worksheet.

able to enact caring for others, believe that they are part of a larger community, and find meaning in shared experiences. Hence, interventions and programming that target connection must be grounded in the constructs of caring, inclusion, and meaning-making.

OTPs often deliver interventions in a group format, particularly in dedicated mental health spaces. Groupwork dates back to the beginning of the profession. How and why groups are facilitated in occupational therapy practice has morphed over time as they reflected shifts in health-care paradigms and theory. OTPs develop and facilitate different types of groups including task, education, topical, sensory groups, and more. Aside from the content delivered, what is it about the nature of groupwork that has the potential to heal disconnection?

In a recent meta-ethnography, researchers identified nine occupational therapy group-related articles for study inclusion spanning 1999 to 2019 (Zedel & Chen, 2021). Three overarching themes were identified: (1) Occupational

therapy groups facilitate transformative change via meaningful occupation, (2) the transformative process elicits positive experiences such as enhanced self-esteem and development of life skills, and (3) not all participant needs were met in the context of a group because of being at different stages in their recovery.

Multiple subthemes were also identified, and those most relevant to connection included the idea that occupational therapy groups foster interpersonal connections and a sense of belonging (moving from feeling alone to feeling connected and feeling accepted and supported). Groups afford an opportunity for members to engage in meaningful activities with those who have shared experiences and who, because of these shared experiences, can offer nonjudgmental support and acceptance (Lund et al., 2019; Rouse & Hitch, 2014). It is also important to note that there were participants across studies in this meta-ethnography who did not benefit from occupational therapy groups, as evidenced by theme 3. This

Being a Psychosocial OT Practitioner

Connection as a Lifeline: Justin's Story

Identifying Psychosocial Strengths and Needs

OTPs encounter people in all therapeutic spaces who experience feelings of disconnection from self, others, and the environment; it is not a human experience unique to those with a diagnosed mental health condition. Disconnection can be the result of, or lead to, any number of physical and mental health challenges and significantly impact occupational performance and participation.

Consider the story of Justin. Justin was born to parents who were using substances at the time. He was removed from his biological parents' care at the age of 22 months and placed in state custody. Throughout Justin's childhood, he moved more than 13 times to various foster homes. Justin's academic performance was average, and he typically kept to himself and spent most of his free time playing online video games. Justin became increasingly withdrawn and angry as he moved through his teenage years. The public school recommended a full psychological assessment, the results of which indicated that he had a learning disability and a mood dysregulation disorder. Justin initiated several school fights and was eventually removed and placed in a school for youth with behavioral challenges. Justin quit school before graduating, left his foster home, and was unhoused for several years. Justin began to use substances, including alcohol and opiates, that were shared with him by some of the older men in the encampment, where he set up a makeshift home.

Justin is now 28 years old and has been dropping by the day shelter for showers, food, and "just to sit somewhere I don't have to worry about being safe." The OTP employed at the shelter has begun to engage Justin in conversation regularly to establish a trusting and secure therapeutic relationship. Justin demonstrates a desire to improve his circumstances but often makes self-deprecating statements such as, "Clearly, I'm not worthy of anything good as no one, not even my birth parents, wanted me" and "I just feel so all alone, even disconnected to myself." The OTP determines that Justin's significant trauma history, rooted in insecure attachments and ACEs, has led to Justin's disconnection from self and others. They believe that occupational therapy intervention is warranted to establish connection and safety, which will support Justin in exploring his environment through occupational participation.

Using a Holistic Occupational Therapy Approach

The OTP initially gathered an occupational profile. As this process unfolded, Justin described the depth of his disconnection and how that disconnection had impacted every facet of his occupational life, from making friends and performing in school to developing health-promoting habits and routines. Justin indicated that he felt safe in the online space but lost connection to other gamers when he became unhoused. Based on this information, the OTP asked Justin to complete the PROM, a measure of personal recovery. The results were analyzed through the CHIME framework for recovery (Connectedness, Hope, Identity, Meaning, and Empowerment). The results indicated that intervention might begin with establishing connectedness, hope, and identity. Justin corroborated the results, indicating that he felt disconnected from everyone and everything, including himself. He described not being in touch with internal states, making it very difficult to relate to the feelings of self and others.

Given these initial concerns, the OTP asks Justin if he would collaborate with them on developing his interoceptive awareness and completing a connection menu. Justin agreed and stated he was already "feeling more positive" about his future.

Together, the OTP and Justin explore a variety of interventions to support occupation and activities related to building interoceptive awareness. Each session begins with a grounding activity to support Justin in being present in his own body to develop an awareness of internal states that can enhance his connection to self and build his sense of identity. Interoceptive interventions include helping Justin bring awareness to internal states, inviting Justin to name and frame these states, and then connecting them to other circumstances when he might have experienced similar internal states. The OTP uses cognitive behavioral interventions to help Justin become more mindful of the connection between his thoughts, feelings, and behaviors. Justin has been developing strategies he can use to better support his identified values and vision for recovery that focus on the person, the occupation, and the environment.

Additionally, the OTP collaborates with Justin to develop a connection menu to enhance his ability to identify where he is on the continuum and support connection choices that will be effective based on that continuum. Throughout the sessions, the OTP assumes a trauma-informed stance, titrates choices to support empowerment based on where Justin is on the languishing versus flourishing continuum, and leads with a deep sense of what could be to Justin to support posttraumatic growth.

My Connection Menu

This is how I want to connect when I feel *well*.

List who or what you want to connect with.	When and how often will you connect?
"People here at the shelter, especially staff who I trust."	"I think I should come over here every day and spend most of the day when I can. I feel better when I am around people I trust who care about me."
"People in the gaming community."	"Every day if I can get a hold of a computer. I know we can only stay on for half an hour at a time, but it'll be nice to get back into it."
"Dogs."	"I really like dogs—they like me no matter what. I saw a staff member had a dog the other day, and I hope they bring it in every day. Makes me smile."

This is how I want to connect when I feel *unwell*.

List who or what you want to connect with.	When and how often will you connect?
"People in the gaming community."	"When I start to withdraw before it gets really bad, and I don't want to play at all. Like at least once a week at the shelter if I can get on a computer."
"Dogs."	"I think having a dog around would help me from getting so down in the dumps. I hope that staff member can bring the dog back at least once a week."
"People at the shelter."	"The social worker said they were going to help me get a phone, so if you haven't seen me in a while, it might be nice for someone to call me every couple of days so I don't feel so lonely, or maybe I'll even come back around."

Reflective Questions

1. Describe the connection between Justin's trauma history and secure versus insecure attachment.
2. How might you respond to Justin if he begins to describe aspects of his trauma history?
3. How would you design a treatment session to strengthen Justin's awareness of the link between decreased interoceptive awareness and difficulties with occupational performance and participation that align with his desire to be more connected to self, others, and the environment?

speaks to the concept of the connection menu mentioned previously and that OTPs must be asking persons whether or not they currently want to include groups as part of this diet.

Additional research has also highlighted the centrality of inclusion and how that can be incorporated in the context of occupational therapy services. According to the United Nations (UN), inclusion is a human right, and the profession of occupational therapy is in concert with this perspective (Chibaya et al., 2021; Hocking, 2019; Hocking et al., 2022). According to the World Federation of Occupational Therapists' position statement titled "Occupational Therapy and Human Rights," inclusion is a matter of occupational injustice; therefore, exclusion is a human rights violation (Hocking et al., 2022).

Enactment of inclusivity must be present in all facets of the profession, from academia to research to clinical practice to advocacy and beyond. In academia, that inclusivity might manifest as students with lived experience leading school-based mental health initiatives. In research, this means including researchers with lived experience as primary researchers or consultants. In clinical practice, this might translate to the inclusion of those with lived experience on advisory boards. And in advocacy, this means that those with lived experience must inform those processes either directly or by proxy.

Principles of self-advocacy would dictate that the ways and extent to which people choose to be included must be a personal choice as an expression of their connection menu (SAMHSA, 2012). Being included in spaces in which people do not experience a sense of connection with others may be as isolating as not being included at all. This is the premise for the creation of psychosocial Clubhouses that began in the mid-1940s in the United States. A group of ex-patients or self-identified psychiatric survivors coalesced around feeling "othered," having no voice and choice, and being stigmatized to the point of societal exclusion. Initially known as We Are Not Alone (WANA), the original 10 members began the first psychosocial Clubhouse in New York City, which they named Fountain House (Doyle et al., 2013).

There are more than 300 Clubhouses worldwide, and 40 states currently have Clubhouses. The Clubhouse model is based upon a work-ordered day in which Clubhouse colleagues and staff work side by side to manage the daily operations. Membership is voluntary and colleagues can come and go as they choose. A variety of vocational models are used including Clubhouse-specific work opportunities, transitional employment (TE), and Individual Placement and Support (IPS). According to Clubhouse International (2022), Clubhouses focus on strengths, provide educational and vocational opportunities, and invite the development of supportive friendships through a caring and committed community. The fundamental tenets upon which both occupational therapy and Clubhouses were founded, including person-centered and directed care, naturally intersect.

OTPs are becoming more involved in Clubhouse work either directly or via academic clinical rotations. These are opportunities to align the profession with those who have lived experience to enhance occupational participation and justice. Psychosocial Clubhouses may not be a good fit for everyone's connection menu; those with lived experience may appreciate that these spaces are occupied by people who shared similar psychiatric experiences, whereas others may

reject a Clubhouse setting for the same reason. What is important is that those with lived experience have the choice to easily move in and out of spaces according to their connection needs and desires.

The COVID-19 pandemic highlighted another avenue for connectedness: virtual platforms. Imposed restrictions on community movement and physical interactions called for human creativity and ingenuity in terms of how people might connect even with those closest to them. Before the pandemic, virtual platforms such as Zoom, Google Meet, and Go To Meeting were not widely utilized as a standard form of connecting with others in business, health care, or a personal context; the pandemic rapidly changed all of that. Most work-related meetings, health-care visits, and social gatherings of nearly every kind were now, in the midst of a pandemic, relegated to a screen.

The use of technology to communicate about health-related conditions dates back to the discovery of the telephone (Baumann & Scales, 2016), although its historical use was sporadic and poorly integrated. That all changed when COVID-19 swept across the globe. Restrictions on movement to minimize the spread of the virus, along with a real fear of contracting the illness, accelerated the use of technology to communicate by and with all health professionals exponentially.

According to the WHO International Telecommunication Union (WHO-ITU, 2022), telehealth incorporates the use of information and communication technologies to deliver health-care services that include diagnosis, evaluation, treatment, research, and education when patients and providers are separated by distance. Because of the COVID-19 pandemic, telehealth became an accepted and more standardized method of service delivery for both physical and mental health care. Telehealth enables those who may not have resources such as time, finances, or transportation to access needed care.

Telecommunications allows a provider to connect with anyone anywhere as long as that individual has access to the needed technology and that provider is licensed in the state in which the individual resides. This was not typically the case at the start of the pandemic, but the profession of occupational therapy quickly pivoted; nearly 31 states (at the time of this printing) have signed a compact with one another allowing OTPs to practice in states that have licensure reciprocity.

For many, decreased social connectivity and an inability to share a physical space while connecting had immediate and devastating consequences in terms of mental health and wellness and connectedness. The prevalence of anxiety, depression, sleep disturbances, distress, and suicidality increased as a direct result of COVID-19 (COVID-19 Mental Disorders Collaborators, 2021; Mahmud et al., 2023). This was not true for everyone, however. Many people actually preferred the decreased pressure for connectivity and found greater connection via virtual platforms as they perceived the virtual space to be less of a threat and one in which they felt they had greater control over the process of connection.

Pets come in all shapes and sizes, from dogs and cats to mice, pigs, snakes, ferrets, and more. Humans have been domesticating animals for consumption and use as early as 30,000 BCE (Zeder, 2008). Because many of these animals are no longer widely consumed or used in the context of labor, such as dogs, they can often be found in relationships with their owners. Nearly 70% of U.S. households include a pet (Spots.com, 2022). Anecdotal evidence suggests people prefer animal over human companionship, because of perceptions of unconditional love, acceptance, and positive regard, as well as the fact that animals cannot talk back. There is some scientific evidence, however, that supports many people's love for their furry and not-so-furry friends.

Allen (2003) first described what is now known as the "pet effect" or the positive implications of pet ownership. Positive implications include improved cardiovascular functioning (Hughes et al., 2020), motivation and purpose (Zablan et al., 2023), decreased perceived loneliness (Cleary et al., 2021; Martos Martinez-Caja et al., 2022), and decreased stress (Allen, 2003; Beetz et al., 2012). OTPs may work in settings where pet ownership is possible, such as home health, or they may work in settings where interaction with pets via animal-assisted therapy (AAT) or animal-assisted activities (AAA), such as a justice-based or residential setting, is the only viable option. In either case, interaction with animals appears to be beneficial if the person chooses animals as part of their connection menu (National Institutes of Health, 2018).

Studies have shown that interventions that utilize animals have therapeutic benefits in the occupational therapy process. OTPs have employed animals to effect positive changes in settings such as in higher education to reduce stress and anxiety (Kivlen, Quevillon et al., 2022); elementary education to support attention, initiation, and emotional regulation (Mendonca et al., 2017); and in the context of a burn center to reduce pain and anxiety (Pruskowski et al., 2020), to name a few. Animals have also been used specifically to enhance constructs related to connectedness such as forming attachments, helping others, and relating (Williams & Metz, 2014).

Why is it easier for some people to connect to an animal, particularly those that become their pets, rather than another person? Qualitative evidence indicates that pets can (a) mitigate against feelings of isolation and loneliness, (b) support physical health by engaging in activities associated with the occupation of caring for pets and animals, (c) serve as conduits for additional human connection, and (d) bring meaning and a sense of self-worth to the care provider (Brooks et al., 2018;

Obradović et al., 2020). People report that they perceive a sense of unconditional positive regard by their pets and animals (Obradović et al., 2020) and a sense of ease about the relationship, both of which create a sense of safety and trust (Ein et al., 2018) that can be missing from human connection for those with lived experience of a psychiatric illness.

Although a lesser-known practice in the United States, "care farming" has gained popularity in places such as the United Kingdom and Scandinavia. Care farming is an intervention situated in agricultural contexts in which farm-related activities are utilized as a means to promote health and wellness for vulnerable populations. Examples of activities might include feeding cows, grooming horses, collecting chicken eggs, and milking goats. Care farming in these and other countries reflects a burgeoning sense of community responsibility for the care of these populations that are incrementally being withdrawn from large government entities (Gorman, 2019).

Care farming goes beyond the aforementioned activities; it encompasses the relationships and practices that emerge in the context of agricultural space. Research utilizing this intervention approach has been conducted with a wide array of conditions and circumstances, such as people with mental illness, those experiencing trauma, those who are unhoused, and veterans.

These studies have yielded positive results including decreased perceived loneliness (Greenleaf & Roessger, 2017), perceived acceptance and empathy, creation of a secure attachment with the farm community, and enhanced ability to connect with others as a byproduct of connection with the animals (Cacciatore et al., 2020; Elsey et al., 2016).

The evidence for the use of pet interventions to enhance a sense of connectedness is mixed (Scoresby et al., 2021; see Table 49-4 for a summary of current evidence). Pet interaction, similar to human interaction, is multidimensional and the effects are far-reaching and varied for each individual. Use of interventions, whether pet ownership, AAT, animal-related engagement, or caring farming, must be person-driven and dosed according to their preferred connection menu (see Table 49-5 for terms related to therapeutic animal interactions).

PhotoVoice

Izzy

"I used to curse being awake. I dreaded being conscious. My days entailed waking up, taking medication, and falling back asleep only to wake up again. Although I longed to be unconscious, I sought to be loved and love something. Ra'ahmi opened the door to recovery. He brought me to the park which led to social contact. Social contact led to renewing my relationship with my case manager. Renewing my relationship with my case manager led me to Recovery Innovations. This led ME to looking beyond my diagnosis."

—Izzy

Reflect on the healing power of social connectedness with animals, such as that expressed in Izzy's PhotoVoice. How can you use this as an exemplar for encouraging and activating those you work with as an OTP?

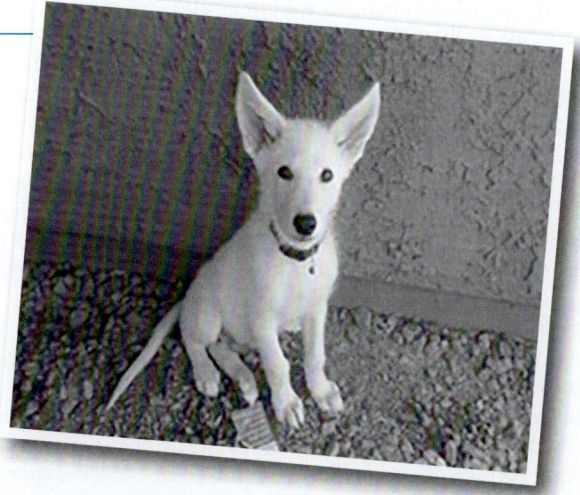

TABLE 49-4 | **Current Occupational Therapy Evidence Supporting Use of Pets/Animals to Facilitate Connection**

Authors (see Reference List for Full Citation)	Summary
Meredith et al. (2023)	The study surveyed 97 dog owners regarding the level of care provided and adult attachment styles. Findings indicate that the more care provided, the stronger the bond with the pet and that separation from the pet caused distress to varying degrees based on the adult attachment style. OTPs have a role in understanding the nature of this attachment and how to facilitate these relationships.
Højgaard-Bøytler & Argentzell (2022)	Eleven participants living with psychiatric labels were interviewed regarding their experiences with equine-assisted therapy (EAT). The overarching theme gleaned from data analysis was that the participants' relationship with the horse led to a sense of togetherness that supported personal development and facilitated occupational engagement. Pertinent subthemes included not feeling alone, feeling comforted and building a friendship with the animal, and creating relationships and togetherness with people because of the EAT. EAT can be used to support the generalization of the experience to everyday life and human relationships.
Kivlen, Winston et al. (2022)	Participants ($n = 104$) were randomly assigned to either a control or treatment group. The treatment group received canine-assisted intervention for 35 minutes each week for 6 consecutive weeks. Quality of life (QoL) indicators improved for the treatment group including mood, well-being, energy level, and happiness. Satisfaction with social relationships also improved as a measure of QoL.
McLaughlin & Hamilton (2019)	Semistructured focus groups were conducted with seven ex-serving military personnel diagnosed with PTSD who also utilized a service dog. Five themes emerged from the data related to having the service animal: feeling less isolated, feeling more connected and less alone, feeling safer, improvement in mood and ability to self-manage, and service dog as a lifeline or reason to live.
Williams & Metz (2014)	The study was conducted at a community-based program and included six male participants deemed "at risk." Participants used cameras (PhotoVoice) to capture their experience of training rescue animals. Six themes emerged: forming an attachment to the animal, helping others, relating to the animal, gaining patience, wanting to better themselves, and teaching. The use of rescue animals may be effective in developing responsibility, trust, and a secure attachment for those who historically have challenges connecting to others in their environment.

Humans are inextricably linked to the natural environment but modernization has begun to impact this connection. Industrialization and the shift in occupations from those primarily centered around farming to those centered around industry and now technology, population growth, and the current climate crisis have fundamentally altered how people interact with and connect to the natural environment. Nearly 70% of the world's population is projected to live in urban areas by the year 2050 (UN, 2019).

Although one might argue whether occupations have shifted over the past 125 years for better or worse, the reality is that people's current performance patterns and occupational forms and functions have widened the chasm between humans and nature. People are no longer as reliant on direct contact with the natural world to meet their daily occupational needs, such as foraging the land for food to prepare a daily meal or collecting pebbles to design a game to play with friends. Research indicates that those who are more connected to the natural environment report higher well-being (Pritchard et al., 2020), vitality, life satisfaction, happiness, the inclusion of nature in self (Capaldi et al., 2014), improved cognition, social skills, and mental and physical health (Barragan-Jason et al., 2023), yet opportunities to interact directly with nature continue to diminish.

Engagement with the natural environment can serve as a protective factor against mental unwellness (Piccininni et al., 2018). Both Pinel and Tuke, whose work can be traced to the origins of occupational therapy, understood this as their approaches included routine interaction with nature (Cutcliffe & Travale, 2016). Yet many dedicated places and spaces for those labeled with a psychiatric illness continue to be sparse and often devoid of access to the natural environment (Shepley et al., 2016), which is known to be a source of potential connection. For those who choose to find or augment their connection menu, as measured via links with the natural environment, OTPs can facilitate this connection in everyday practice.

Because of the combination of a shrinking natural environment and an innate desire to know one's place relative to the world around them (Cutcliffe & Travale, 2016), many with and without lived experience are yearning to connect with the natural environment. This connection has emerged in various forms including forest bathing (shinrin-yoku in Japanese), green care, gardening, and earthing or grounding.

Forest bathing is an ancient and meditative practice of leisurely walking through a forest and periodically taking breaks to contemplate one's surroundings, engage in breathing exercises, and rest (Antonelli et al., 2019). The recommended time spent bathing is 2 to 4 hours and should be supervised by a trained guide or prefaced with educational materials such that participants can maximize their experience. During the bathing, participants typically select one of the traditional five senses on which to focus during their session, such as vision, and the colors and shapes of the leaves or sounds, such as the swaying of trees or the wind through branches. Forest bathing has been found to improve mental well-being through stress and anxiety reduction, emotional balance, and improvement in mood (Antonelli et al., 2022) and heart rate variability (Lucius, 2023).

Although there is limited evidence relative to forest bathing and connectedness, the practice is rooted in a Japanese worldview that is collectivistic and intertwined with nature.

TABLE 49-5 | Therapeutic Use of Animals to Promote Connectedness: Terminology

Term	Definition	Additional Information
Animal-assisted therapy (AAT)	An umbrella term for structured and goal-oriented services that are delivered by professionals who have expertise in their scope of practice and incorporate animals to achieve therapeutic outcomes for their persons. AAT includes AAI, AAA, and AAE.	Administered by a professional who has received training related to the therapy animals in addition to their profession-specific training
Animal-assisted intervention (AAI)	A structured intervention that utilizes an animal(s) to assist or support the person in addressing person-specific goals	The use of AAI for persons should be developed and implemented as an interprofessional team.
Animal-assisted activities (AAA)	Less formal than intervention, these activities are intended to target motivation and enhance quality of life	Activities are delivered by volunteers, paraprofessionals, or professionals who have received training regarding the delivery of these activities and an animal deemed suitable.
Animal-assisted education (AAE)	Structured and intentional use of animals facilitated by general or special education staff to support the achievement of academic-related goals	OTPs may suggest the inclusion of an animal for certain persons in the general or special education classroom to enhance felt safety and subsequent ability to learn.
Animal-assisted crisis response (AACR)	Use of animals to provide comfort and safety during natural, human-caused, or technological disasters	Animals can help professionals build connections with those who have experienced trauma because of these disasters.
Animal-assisted workplace well-being (AAWW)	Use of animals in a work environment to support well-being, decrease stress, and enhance morale and productivity	Workplace wellness programs developed by OTPs might include the periodic or consistent presence of an animal.
Animal-related engagement (ARE)	Remembrance of thoughts and feelings associated with animal interaction by methods other than face-to-face contact	OTPs might utilize ARE in the context of a reminiscence group or show images of animals to elicit thoughts and emotions that may enhance connection-building among group members.
Therapy animal	Animals such as dogs, cats, horses, rabbits, and so on, that have been assessed for their ability to provide physical, emotional, and psychological benefits to those engaged in activities related to AAI and AAA, for example	These animals must abide by "no pet" policies and are not granted special access.
Assistance animal (also commonly called service animal)	Dogs or miniature horses that are individually trained to perform certain tasks for their humans to assist with the performance of daily occupations and to help maintain safety	These animals are considered working animals as opposed to pets although the bond between the human and animal can be quite strong. These animals are granted full access to places and spaces where the general public is allowed to go.
Emotional support animal/comfort animal	An animal that provides support to an individual who has a mental health condition	Animals must be prescribed by a mental health professional. They are not granted access commensurate with service animals although they may live with their owners in residences covered by the Fair Housing Amendments Act despite a "no pet" policy.
Facility animal	Animals such as dogs, cats, fish, and birds that are regularly present in a health-care setting	These animals should be properly trained/vetted if they will also be used for extended periods of time in the context of AAT.

Adapted from International Association of Human-Animal Interaction Organizations. (2018). The IAHAIO definitions for animal assisted intervention and guidelines for wellness of animals involved in AAI. IAHAIO White Paper. https://iahaio.org/wp/wp-content/uploads/2021/01/iahaio-white-paper-2018-english.pdf; Pet Partners. (n.d.). Glossary. https://petpartners.org/learn/terminology

Forest bathing has also been linked to spirituality, which is a construct that reflects the degree to which people feel connected to themselves, their values, and their meaning and purpose while in human form (Hansen & Jones, 2020).

Green care is an approach to mental health care that intentionally includes interaction with the natural environment, often in the form of farming or gardening. Farming and gardening for those living with a mental illness have been practiced for centuries. Occupational therapy was a part of this movement at the inception of the profession when persons would be taken out to the grounds of the facility to farm and garden to reap the crops to feed those in the institution.

Although there was a secondary benefit of communing with nature, the primary intent was the engagement in work activities that benefited the institution (Sempik, 2010). One of the primary purposes of green care, as people know it today, is to promote connectedness to nature (Cutcliffe & Travale, 2016).

Pretty (2004) identified various levels of contact with nature, including (a) viewing nature through a window, (b) being in nature such as forest bathing, and (c) active interaction with the environment such as gardening or farming. Although dosing in terms of frequency and intensity of green care has not been established, the benefits of improved well-being and connectedness are clear.

Gardening is a familiar occupation to many OTPs and has long been used therapeutically across most practice areas (Patil et al., 2019; Sinnott & Rowlis, 2021; Vibholm et al., 2020). Traditional gardening evokes images of being immersed in nature and tending plots of land from which fruits, vegetables, and flora are to be cultivated. Urbanization and a faster-paced health-care environment have driven OTPs in some cases to contemplate gardening in smaller spaces and places.

Despite the smaller scale, results have been similar, with persons reporting improved mental well-being (Mourão et al., 2022), improvements in needed and desired skill acquisition (Patil et al., 2019), and goal attainment (Sinott & Rowlis, 2021). Gardening also promotes perceived connectedness to the natural environment. As both a means and an end, gardening has been used successfully as an occupational therapy approach to promoting social inclusion, belongingness, motivation, and a sense of accomplishment (Cipriani et al., 2018; Suto et al., 2021), Watching plants grow because of being nurtured provides a tangible experience for persons.

Both the process of routine care as well as the product of watching a plant grow because of that care can be grounding and beneficial to those who have difficulty with connectedness, self-worth, agency, and purpose. If nurtured properly and provided the resources to flourish, plants will grow. This process can serve as a powerful metaphor for persons in the context of their own lives; if they take care of themselves as well as the others in their lives, they too may grow and flourish.

Here's the Point

- A sense of connectedness often holds deeper meaning than the term social participation.
- Connectedness is central to overall health and wellness.
- Disconnection often occurs as the result of early childhood trauma and insecure attachment as well as systemic occupational and social injustices.
- Connectedness is an ongoing human process, and OTPs must challenge themselves to fully explore and support connectedness throughout the occupational therapy process from the occupational profile to discharge planning. Creating a sense of connection may look different for everyone. Discovering ways that enhance a sense of connection is central to healing and recovery.
- Individuals must have voice and choice related to how they want to connect with self, others, and the world around them.

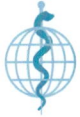 Visit the online resource center at **FADavis.com** to access the videos.

Apply It Now

1. Attachments

Consider your own early childhood attachments. Would you broadly classify them as secure or insecure? Whether these attachments were generally secure or insecure, how have they impacted your ability to connect with yourself, others, and the world around you?

2. Your Sense of Connectedness

Take a moment to consider your own sense of connectedness. Under what circumstances do you feel most connected to yourself, to others, and to the world around you? Conversely, under what circumstances do you feel least connected to yourself, to others, and to the world around you? If you are comfortable, share these self-observations with a peer. How are your experiences of connectedness similar and how do they differ?

3. My Connection Menu

Complete the "My Connection Menu" for yourself. Compare and contrast ways of connecting that might be similar and different from your peers. How and when can we use the "My Connection Menu" in the occupational therapy process?

Resources

Websites

- Amy Wagenfeld Design: https://amywagenfelddesign.com
- Care Farming Network: https://carefarmingnetwork.org
- Clubhouse International: https://clubhouse-intl.org
- COVID-19 and the Isolation Pandemic: https://covid19.ssri.psu.edu/articles/covid-19-and-isolation-pandemic
- Green Care Coalition: https://greencarecoalition.org.uk/about
- How Attachment Styles Affect Adult Relationships: https://www.helpguide.org/articles/relationships-communication/attachment-and-adult-relationships.htm
- Indigenous Women and Their Connection to the Earth and Her Waters: https://www.theindigenousfoundation.org/articles/indigenous-women-and-their-connections-to-earth-and-water
- Keynote: ACEs to Assets 2019–Dr. Gabor Maté–Trauma As Disconnection From the Self: https://www.bing.com/videos/riverview/relatedvideo?&q=trauma+and+disconnection
- Occupational Narratives Database: https://occupational-narratives.wfot.org
- Pet Partners: https://petpartners.org
- Social Connectedness: https://www.cdc.gov/social-connectedness/about/; https://www.cdc.gov/emotional-wellbeing/social-connectedness/index.htm
- Surgeon General Discusses Health Risks of Loneliness and Steps to Help Connect With Others: https://youtu.be/vSbxMkRYb6o
- The Foundation for Art & Healing Project Unlonely: https://www.artandhealing.org/unlonely-project

Assessments

- General Belongingness Scale: https://www.sciencedirect.com/science/article/pii/S019188691100482X
- Occupational Performance History Interview II (OPHI-II): https://moho-irm.uic.edu
- Occupational Self-Assessment (OSA): https://moho-irm.uic.edu
- Personal Recovery Outcome Measure (PROM): https://mentalhealthcommission.ca/resource/a-new-way-of-measuring-recovery-personal-recovery-outcome-measure
- Pet Owner Connectedness Scale (POCS): https://www.tandfonline.com/doi/epdf/10.1080/08927936.2022.2027095
- Self-Connection Scale (SCS): https://connectionlab.com/wp-content/uploads/2021/11/Self-Connection-Scale.pdf
- Watts Connectedness Scale: https://link.springer.com/article/10.1007/s00213-022-06187-5

Videos

- "Positive Mindset Creative Arts Festival" video. This video showcases the Positive Mindset Creative Arts Festival, held at the Queensland Children's Hospital in Australia. This annual children's festival promotes positive thinking about mental health and increases help-seeking behaviors with a creative arts focus. It is a notable example of how OTPs can contribute to community health efforts. The emphasis is on art as an occupation and creating space in the community to encourage and celebrate mental health. In addition, the event promotes the idea of social connection and belonging centered around self-expression of feelings across the mental health continuum and how that ultimately encourages the sense of connection and belonging with people and communities. To access the video, visit the online resource center at FADavis.com.
- "Prioritizing Family During a Mother's Cancer Treatment" video. Marylein Serrano is a mother of two children and a speech language therapist who has had several cancer diagnoses. In this video, she discusses how she worked to prioritize her family during cancer treatment, with the help of friends and extended family. She also shares her fears and how she made the most of her time with her husband and children. To access the video, visit the online resource center at FADavis.com.
- "Two Practitioners Discuss Their Work in Suicide Prevention" video. In this video, two occupational therapists, Nadine and Kim, discuss their work in suicide prevention. They share reflections and pearls of wisdom gained in years of practice in this area–both observations about people in crisis and how they have responded as practitioners. They express the role that the occupational lives of these individuals have in their recovery and crisis plans, as well as serving as a springboard for interventions. Nadine and Kim also describe what is rewarding about this work and the crucial need to meet their self-care and well-being needs in order to stay connected to this work. To access the video, visit the online resource center at FADavis.com.
- "Jordan's Lived Experience of Recovery as an Occupational Therapy Practitioner" video. In this video, occupational therapist Jordan describes her lived experience of anxiety and depression. She touches on many issues critical to recovery and occupational therapy practice, including social determinants of health, peer support, and how mental health labels can adversely affect an individual's medical treatment. Importantly, she explains how she has learned to blend her lived experience with her work as an occupational therapist, while ensuring she takes care of herself and manages her symptoms. Jordan also offers priceless words of wisdom to practitioners regarding establishing a therapeutic connection with individuals with whom they practice. To access the video, visit the online resource center at FADavis.com.
- "Nicholas's Lived Experience of Schizophrenia" video. Nicholas is an occupational therapist living with the lived experience of schizophrenia. In this video, he describes his first episode of psychosis and the crucial role that occupational therapy played in his recovery. Nicholas emphasizes the importance of engaging with other people during rehabilitation and how, through occupational engagement, he discovered reconnection, felt loved, and found a sense of meaning and purpose. To access the video, visit the online resource center at FADavis.com.
- "Aster's Lived Experience of Suicidality" video. Aster is an occupational therapist, educator, and disability researcher who shares their experience with major depression and suicidality. In this video, Aster openly and courageously describes an episode of suicidality that resulted in taking a leave of absence from work. They discuss the actions and resources that helped them get through the crisis, including creating a psychiatric advance directive, planning for their safety, and stopping an asthma medication that was worsening their symptoms. Aster's video also addresses the topics of social connectedness, stigma, and trauma recovery following a mental health crisis. To access the video, visit the online resource center at FADavis.com.

References

Adams, F., & Casteleijn, D. (2014). New insights in collective participation: A South African perspective. *South African Journal of Occupational Therapy, 44*(1), 81–87.

Aga, N., Rowaert, S., Vander Laenen, F., Vandevelde, S., Vander Beken, T., Audenaert, K., & Vanderplasschen, W. (2021). Connectedness in recovery narratives of persons labeled not criminally responsible: A qualitative study. *International Journal of Forensic Mental Health, 20*(3), 303–316. https://doi.org/10.1080/14999013.2021.1880503

Allen, K. (2003). Are pets a healthy pleasure? The influence of pets on blood pressure. *Current Directions in Psychological Science, 12*(6), 236–239. https://doi.org/10.1046/j.0963-7214.2003.01269.x

American Foundation for Suicide Prevention. (2022). *Suicide statistics.* https://afsp.org/suicide-statistics

American Occupational Therapy Association. (2020). Occupational therapy practice framework: Domain and process—Fourth edition. *American Journal of Occupational Therapy, 74*(Suppl. 2), 7412410010p1–7412410010p87. https://doi.org/10.5014/ajot.2020.74S2001

American Psychiatric Association. (2022). *Diagnostic and statistical manual of mental disorders* (5th ed., text rev.). American Psychiatric Publishing. https://doi.org/10.1176/appi.books.9780890425787

Andonian, L., & MacRae, A. (2011). Well older adults within an urban context: Strategies to create and maintain social participation. *British Journal of Occupational Therapy, 74*(1), 2–11. https://doi.org/10.4276/030802211X12947686093486

Antonelli, M., Barbieri, G., & Donelli, D. (2019). Effects of forest bathing (shinrin-yoku) on levels of cortisol as a stress biomarker: A systematic review and meta-analysis. *International Journal of Biometeorology, 63*(8), 1117–1134. https://doi.org/10.1007/s00484-019-01717-x

Antonelli, M., Donelli, D., Carlone, L., Maggini, V., Firenzuoli, F., & Bedeschi, E. (2022). Effects of forest bathing (shinrin-yoku) on individual well-being: An umbrella review. *International Journal of Environmental Health Research, 32*(8), 1842–1867. https://doi.org/10.1080/09603123.2021.1919293

Ashida, S., & Heaney, C. A. (2008). Differential associations of social support and social connectedness with structural features of social networks and the health status of older adults. *Journal of Aging and Health, 20*(7), 872–893. https://doi.org/10.1177/0898264308324626

Barbic, S. P., Kidd, S. A., Durisko, Z. T., Yachouh, R., Rathitharan, G., & McKenzie, K. (2018). What are the personal recovery needs of community-dwelling individuals with mental illness? Preliminary findings from the Canadian Personal Recovery Outcome

Measurement (C-PROM) study. *Canadian Journal of Community Mental Health, 37*(1), 29–47. https://doi.org/10.7870/cjcmh-2018-005

Barbic, S. P., & Rennie, M. (2016). *A new way of measuring recovery: Personal Recovery Outcome Measure.* https://mentalhealthcommission.ca/resource/a-new-way-of-measuring-recovery-personal-recovery-outcome-measure

Baron, K., Kielhofner, G., Iyenger, A., Goldhammer, V., & Wolenski, J. (2006). *A user's manual for the Occupational Self Assessment (OS).* Model of Human Occupation Clearinghouse, University of Illinois Chicago.

Barragan-Jason, G., Loreau, M., de Mazancourt, C., Singer, M. C., & Parmesan, C. (2023). Psychological and physical connections with nature improve both human well-being and nature conservation: A systematic review of meta-analyses. *Biological Conservation, 277,* Article 109842. https://doi.org/10.1016/j.biocon.2022.109842

Baum, C., & Edwards, D. (2008). *Activity Card Sort* (2nd ed.). AOTA Press.

Baumann, P. K., & Scales, T. (2016). History of information communication technology and telehealth. *Academy of Business Research Journal, 3,* 48–52. https://une.idm.oclc.org/login?url=https://www.proquest.com/scholarly-journals/history-information-communication-technology/docview/1863562170/se-2

Baumgartner, J. N., & Burns, J. K. (2014). Measuring social inclusion—A key outcome in global mental health. *International Journal of Epidemiology, 43*(2), 354–364. https://doi.org/10.1093/ije/dyt224

Beatson, J., & Taryan, S. (2003). Predisposition to depression: The role of attachment. *Australian & New Zealand Journal of Psychiatry, 37*(2), 219–225. https://doi.org.une.idm.oclc.org/10.1046/j.1440-1614.2003.01126.x

Beetz, A., Uvnäs-Moberg, K., Julius, H., & Kotrschal, K. (2012). Psychosocial and psychophysiological effects of human-animal interactions: The possible role of oxytocin. *Frontiers in Psychology, 3,* 234. https://doi.org/10.3389/fpsyg.2012.00234

Begun, S., Bender, K. A., Brown, S. M., Barman-Adhikari, A., & Ferguson, K. (2018). Social connectedness, self-efficacy, and mental health outcomes among homeless youth. *Youth & Society, 50*(7), 989–1014. https://doi.org/10.1177/0044118X16650459

Bisson, J. I., van Gelderen, M., Roberts, N. P., & Lewis, C. (2020). Non-pharmacological and non-psychological approaches to the treatment of PTSD: Results of a systematic review and meta-analyses. *European Journal of Psychotraumatology, 11*(1), 1795361. https://doi.org/10.1080/20008198.2020.1795361

Blum, R. W., Lai, J., Martinez, M., & Jessee, C. (2022). Adolescent connectedness: Cornerstone for health and wellbeing. *British Medical Journal, 379,* e069213. https://doi.org/10.1136/bmj-2021-069213

Bowins, B. (2021). *States and processes for mental health: Advancing psychotherapy effectiveness* (pp. 41–47). Elsevier. https://doi.org/10.1016/C2020-0-00574-8

Brooks, H., Rushton, K., Lovell, K., Bee, P., Walker, L., Grant, L., & Rogers, A. (2018). The power of support from companion animals for people living with mental health problems: A systematic review and narrative synthesis of the evidence. *BMC Psychiatry, 18*(1), 1–12. https://doi.org/10.1186/s12888-018-1613-2

Cacciatore, J., Gorman, R., & Thieleman, K. (2020). Evaluating care farming as a means to care for those in trauma and grief. *Health & Place, 62,* 102281. https://doi.org/10.1016/j.healthplace.2019.102281

Capaldi, C. A., Dopko, R. L., & Zelenski, J. M. (2014). The relationship between nature connectedness and happiness: A meta-analysis. *Frontiers in Psychology, 5,* Article 976. https://doi.org/10.3389/fpsyg.2014.00976

Cavanagh, N., Cockett, G., Heinrich, C., Doig, L., Fiest, K., Guichon, J. R., Page, S., Mitchell, I., & Doig, C. J. (2020). Compassion fatigue in healthcare providers: A systematic review and meta-analysis. *Nursing Ethics, 27*(3), 639–665. https://doi.org/10.1177/0969733019889400

Ceunen, E., Vlaeyen, J. W. S., & Van Diest, I. (2016). On the origin of interoception. *Frontiers in Psychology, 7,* 743. https://doi.org/10.3389/fpsyg.2016.00743

Chibaya, G., Govender, P., & Naidoo, D. (2021). United Nations Convention on the Rights of Person with Disabilities (UNCRPD) implementation: Perspectives of persons with disabilities in Namibia. *Occupational Therapy International, 2021,* 1–17. https://doi.org/10.1155/2021/6693141

Cigna. (2018). *Cigna U.S. loneliness index.* https://www.cigna.com/static/www-cigna-com/docs/about-us/newsroom/studies-and-reports/combatting-loneliness/loneliness-survey-2018-full-report.pdf

Cipriani, J., Georgia, J., McChesney, M., Swanson, J., Zigon, J., & Stabler, M. (2018). Uncovering the value and meaning of a horticulture therapy program for persons at a long-term adult inpatient psychiatric facility. *Occupational Therapy in Mental Health, 34*(3), 242–257. https://doi.org/10.1080/0164212X.2017.1416323

Cleary, M., West, S., Visentin, D., Phipps, M., Westman, M., Vesk, K., & Kornhaber, R. (2021). The Unbreakable Bond: The mental health benefits and challenges of pet ownership for people experiencing homelessness. *Issues in Mental Health Nursing, 42*(8), 741–746. https://doi.org/10.1080/01612840.2020.1843096

Clubhouse International. (2022). *What we do–Clubhouse International.* https://clubhouse-intl.org/what-we-do/overview

Cover, R. (2022). Digital hostility: Contemporary crisis, disrupted belonging and self-care practices. *Media International Australia, 184*(1), 79–91. https://doi.org/10.1177/1329878X221088048

COVID-19 Mental Disorders Collaborators. (2021). Global prevalence and burden of depressive and anxiety disorders in 204 countries and territories in 2020 due to the COVID-19 pandemic. *Lancet (London, England), 398*(10312), 1700–1712. https://doi.org/10.1016/S0140-6736(21)02143-7

Cutcliffe, J. R., & Travale, R. (2016). Unearthing the theoretical underpinnings of "Green Care" in mental health and substance misuse care: Theoretical underpinnings and contemporary clinical examples. *Issues in Mental Health Nursing, 37*(3), 137–147. https://doi.org/10.3109/01612840.2015.1119220

Dawson-Rose, C., Shehadeh, D., Hao, J., Barnard, J., Khoddam-Khorasani, L. L., Leonard, A., Clark, K., Kersey, E., Mousseau, H., Frank, J., Miller, A., Carrico, A., Schustack, A., & Cuca, Y. P. (2020). Trauma, substance use, and mental health symptoms in transitional age youth experiencing homelessness. *Public Health Nursing (Boston, Mass.), 37*(3), 363–370. https://doi.org/10.1111/phn.12727

De Jong, S., Van Donkersgoed, R., Arends, J., Buck, K. D., Lysaker, P. H., Wunderink, L., Van Der Gaag, M., Aleman, A., & Pijnenborg, M. (2013). MERIT: A multi-center randomized controlled trial to study the effects of a new metacognitive therapy. *Schizophrenia Bulletin, 39,* S327. https://doi.org/10.1093/schbul/sbt011

Desdentado, L., Miragall, M., Llorens, R., & Baños, R. M. (2023). Disentangling the role of interoceptive sensibility in alexithymia, emotion dysregulation, and depression in healthy individuals. *Current Psychology, 42,* 20570–20582. https://doi.org/10.1007/s12144-022-03153-4

Doyle, A., Lanoil, J., & Dudek, K. J. (2013). *Fountain House: Creating community in mental health practice.* Columbia University Press.

Edwards, D. J., & Lowe, R. (2021). Associations between mental health, interoception, psychological flexibility, and self-as-context, as predictors for alexithymia: A deep artificial neural network approach. *Frontiers in Psychology, 12,* 637802. https://doi.org/10.3389/fpsyg.2021.637802

Ein, N., Li, L., & Vickers, K. (2018). The effect of pet therapy on the physiological and subjective stress response: A meta-analysis. *Stress & Health, 34*(4), 477–489. https://doi.org/10.1002/smi.2812

Elsey, H., Murray, J., & Bragg, R. (2016). Green fingers and clear minds: Prescribing "care farming" for mental illness. *The British Journal of General Practice, 66*(643), 99–100. https://doi.org/10.3399/bjgp16X683749

Fani, N., Guelfo, A., La Barrie, D. L., Teer, A. P., Clendinen, C., Karimzadeh, L., Jain, J., Ely, T. D., Powers, A., Kaslow, N. J., Bradley, B., & Siegle, G. J. (2023). Neurophysiological changes associated with vibroacoustically-augmented breath-focused mindfulness for dissociation: Targeting interoception and attention. *Psychological Medicine, 53*(16), 7550–7560. https://doi.org/10.1017/S0033291723001277

Gilmartin, H., Goyal, A., Hamati, M. C., Mann, J., Saint, S., & Chopra, V. (2017). Brief mindfulness practices for healthcare providers—A systematic literature review. *American Journal of Medicine, 130*(10), 1219.e1–1219.e17. https://doi.org/10.1016/j.amjmed.2017.05.041

Gorman, R. (2019). Thinking critically about health and human-animal relations: Therapeutic affect within spaces of care farming. *Social Science & Medicine, 231*, 6–12. https://doi.org/10.1016/j.socscimed.2017.11.047

Greenleaf, A. T., & Roessger, K. M. (2017). Effectiveness of care farming on veterans' life satisfaction, optimism, and perceived loneliness. *Journal of Humanistic Counseling, 56*(2), 86–110. https://doi.org/10.1002/johc.12046

Gun Violence Archive. (2023). *Mass shootings in 2023.* https://www.gunviolencearchive.org/reports/mass-shooting

Hammell, K. W. (2004). Dimensions of meaning in the occupations of daily life. *Canadian Journal of Occupational Therapy, 71*, 296–305. https://doi.org/10.1177/000841740407100509

Hammell, K. W. (2014). Belonging, occupation, and human well-being: An exploration. *Canadian Journal of Occupational Therapy, 81*(1), 39–50. https://doi.org/10.1177/0008417413520489

Hansen, M. M., & Jones, R. (2020). The interrelationship of Shinrin-Yoku and spirituality: A scoping review. *Journal of Alternative & Complementary Medicine, 26*(12), 1093–1104. https://doi.org/10.1089/acm.2020.0193

Hayes, S. C. (2004). Acceptance and Commitment Therapy and the new behavior therapies: Mindfulness, acceptance and relationship. In S. C. Hayes, V. M. Follette, & M. Linehan (Eds.), *Mindfulness and acceptance: Expanding the cognitive behavioral tradition* (pp. 1–29). Guilford.

Heeter, C., Lehto, R., Allbritton, M., Day, T., & Wiseman, M. (2017). Effects of a technology-assisted meditation program on healthcare providers' interoceptive awareness, compassion fatigue, and burnout. *Journal of Hospice & Palliative Nursing, 19*(4), 314–322. https://doi.org/10.1097/NJH.0000000000000349

Herstell, S., Betz, L. T., Penzel, N., Chechelnizki, R., Filihagh, L., Antonucci, L., & Kambeitz, J. (2021). Insecure attachment as a transdiagnostic risk factor for major psychiatric conditions: A meta-analysis in bipolar disorder, depression and schizophrenia spectrum disorder. *Journal of Psychiatric Research, 144*(1), 190–201. https://doi.org/10.1016/j.jpsychires.2021.10.002

Hocking, C. (2019). A reflection on inclusion and human rights for occupational therapists. *New Zealand Journal of Occupational Therapy, 66*(2), 24–28.

Hocking, C., Townsend, E. (Liz), & Mace, J. (2022). World Federation of Occupational Therapists position statement: Occupational therapy and human rights (revised 2019)—The backstory and future challenges. *World Federation of Occupational Therapists Bulletin, 78*(2), 83–89. https://doi.org/10.1080/14473828.2021.1915608

Højgaard-Bøytler, J., & Argentzell, E. (2022). Experiences of equine assisted therapy and its influence on occupational engagement among people with mental health problems. *Occupational Therapy in Mental Health, 39*(4), 394–418. https://doi.org/10.1080/0164212x.2022.2156428

Holt-Lunstad, J., Smith, T. B., Baker, M., Harris, T., & Stephenson, D. (2015). Loneliness and social isolation as risk factors for mortality: A meta-analytic review. *Perspectives on Psychological Science, 10*(2), 227–237. https://doi.org/10.1177/1745691614568352

Hölzel, B. K., Carmody, J., Vangel, M., Congleton, C., Yerramsetti, S. M., Gard, T., & Lazar, S. W. (2011). Mindfulness practice leads to increases in regional brain gray matter density. *Psychiatry Research, 191*(1), 36–43. https://doi.org/10.1016/j.pscychresns.2010.08.006

Horner, J. K., Piercy, B. S., Eure, L., & Woodard, E. K. (2014). A pilot study to evaluate mindfulness as a strategy to improve inpatient nurse and patient experiences. *Applied Nursing Research, 27*(3), 198–201. https://doi.org/10.1016/j.apnr.2014.01.003

House, J. S., Landis, K. R., & Umberson, D. (1988). Social relationships and health. *Science, 241*, 540–545. https://doi.org/10.1126/science.3399889

Huang, C. (2022). A meta-analysis of the problematic social media use and mental health. *International Journal of Social Psychiatry, 68*(1), 12–33. https://doi.org/10.1177/0020764020978434

Hughes, M. J., Verreynne, M.-L., Harpur, P., & Pachana, N. A. (2020). Companion animals and health in older populations: A systematic review. *Clinical Gerontologist, 43*(4), 365–377. https://doi.org/10.1080/07317115.2019.1650863

Huxley, P., Evans, S., Madge, S., Webber, M., Burchardt, T., McDaid, D., & Knapp, M. (2012). Development of a social inclusion index to capture subjective and objective life domains (phase II): Psychometric development study. *Health Technology Assessment, 16*(1), 1–248. https://doi.org/10.3310/hta16010

Jacob, K. S. (2015). Recovery model of mental illness: A complementary approach to psychiatric care. *Indian Journal of Psychological Medicine, 37*, 117–119. https://doi.org/10.4103/0253-7176.155605

John-Henderson, N. A., Henderson-Matthews, B., Ollinger, S. R., Racine, J., Gordon, M. R., Higgins, A. A., Horn, W. C., Reevis, S. A., Running Wolf, J. A., Grant, D., & Rynda-Apple, A. (2020). Adverse childhood experiences and immune system inflammation in adults residing on the Blackfeet reservation: The moderating role of sense of belonging to the community. *Annals of Behavioral Medicine, 54*(2), 87–93. https://doi.org/10.1093/abm/kaz029

Kabat-Zinn, J. (2003). Mindfulness-based interventions in context: Past, present, and future. *Clinical Psychology: Science and Practice, 10*(2), 144–156. https://doi.org/10.1093/clipsy.bpg016

Kelley, T. M., Pransky, J., & Lambert, E. G. (2015). Realizing improved mental health through understanding three spiritual principles. *Spirituality in Clinical Practice, 2*(4), 267–281. https://doi.org/10.1037/scp0000077

Kielhofner, G., & Burke, J. P. (1980). A Model of Human Occupation, Part 1. Conceptual framework and content. *American Journal of Occupational Therapy, 34*(9), 572–581. https://doi.org/10.5014/ajot.34.9.572

Kielhofner, G., Mallinson, T., Crawford, C., Nowak, M., Rigby, M., Henry, A., & Walens, D. (2004). *The Occupational Performance History Interview II.* Model of Human Occupation Clearinghouse.

Kinniburgh, K. J., Blaustein, M., Spinazzola, J., & van der Kolk, B. A. (2005). Attachment, self-regulation, and competency. *Psychiatric Annals, 35*(5), 424–430. https://doi.org/10.3928/00485713-20050501-08

Kira, I. A. (2022). Taxonomy of stressors and traumas: An update of the development-based trauma framework (DBTF): A life-course perspective on stress and trauma. *Traumatology, 28*(1), 84–97. https://doi.org/10.1037/trm0000305

Kivlen, C. A., Quevillon, A., & Pasquarelli, D. (2022). Should dogs have a seat in the classroom? The effects of canine assisted education on college student mental health. *Open Journal of Occupational Therapy (OJOT), 10*(1), 1–14. https://doi.org/10.15453/2168-6408.1816

Kivlen, C., Winston, K., Mills, D., DiZazzo-Miller, R., Davenport, R., & Binfet, J.-T. (2022). Canine-assisted intervention effects on the well-being of health science graduate students: A randomized controlled trial. *American Journal of Occupational Therapy, 76*(6), 7606205120. https://doi.org/10.5014/ajot.2022.049508

Klussman, K., Nichols, A. L., Curtin, N., Langer, J., & Orehek, E. (2022). Self-connection and well-being: Development and validation of a self-connection scale. *European Journal of Social Psychology, 52*(1), 18–45. https://doi.org/10.1002/ejsp.2812

Lee, R. M., & Robbins, S. B. (1995). Measuring belongingness: The Social Connectedness and the Social Assurance scales. *Journal of Counseling Psychology, 42*(2), 232–241. https://doi.org/10.1037/0022-0167.42.2.232

Longden, E., Madill, A., & Waterman, M. G. (2012). Dissociation, trauma, and the role of lived experience: Toward a new conceptualization of voice hearing. *Psychological Bulletin, 138*(1), 28–76. https://doi.org/10.1037/a0025995

Lucius, K. (2023). Heart rate variability and integrative therapies. *Integrative & Complementary Therapies, 29*(1), 40–48. https://doi.org/10.1089/ict.2023.29060.klu

Lund, K., Argentzell, E., Leufstadius, C., Tjörnstrand, C., & Eklund, M. (2019). Joining, belonging, and re-valuing: A process of meaning-making through group participation in a mental health lifestyle intervention. *Scandinavian Journal of Occupational Therapy, 26*(1), 55–68. https://doi.org/10.1080/11038128.2017.1409266

Luyten, P., Campbell, C., & Fonagy, P. (2020). Borderline personality disorder, complex trauma, and problems with self and identity: A social-communicative approach. *Journal of Personality, 88*(1), 88–105. https://doi.org/10.1111/jopy.12483

Mabele, M., Krauss, J., & Kiwango, W. (2022). Going back to the roots: Ubuntu and just conservation in Southern Africa. *Conservation & Society, 20*(2), 92–102. https://doi.org/10.4103/cs.cs_33_21

MacIntosh, H. B., Godbout, N., & Dubash, N. (2015). Borderline personality disorder: Disorder of trauma or personality, a review of the empirical literature. *Canadian Psychology/Psychologie Canadienne, 56*(2), 227–241. https://doi.org/10.1037/cap0000028

Mahler, K. (2015). *Interoception: The eighth sensory system: Practical solutions for improving self-regulation, self-awareness and social understanding.* AAPC Publishing.

Mahmud, S., Mohsin, M., Dewan, M. N., & Muyeed, A. (2023). The global prevalence of depression, anxiety, stress, and insomnia among general population during COVID-19 pandemic: A systematic review and meta-analysis. *Trends in Psychology, 31*(1), 143–170. https://doi.org/10.1007/s43076-021-00116-9

Malone, G. P., Pillow, D. R., & Osman, A. (2012). The General Belongingness Scale (GBS): Assessing achieved belongingness. *Personality and Individual Differences, 52*(3), 311–316. https://doi.org/10.1016/j.paid.2011.10.027

Martino, J., Pegg, J., & Frates, E. P. (2017). The connection prescription: Using the power of social interactions and the deep desire for connectedness to empower health and wellness. *American Journal of Lifestyle Medicine, 11*(6), 466–475. https://doi.org/10.1177/1559827615608788

Martos Martinez-Caja, A., De Herdt, V., Enders-Slegers, M.-J., & Moons, C. P. H. (2022). Pet ownership, feelings of loneliness, and mood in people affected by the first COVID-19 lockdown. *Journal of Veterinary Behavior, 57*, 52–63. https://doi.org/10.1016/j.jveb.2022.09.008

Maslow, A. (1968). *Toward a psychology of being* (2nd ed.). Van Nostrand Reinhold.

Mavranezouli, I., Megnin-Viggars, O., Daly, C., Dias, S., Welton, N. J., Stockton, S., Bhutani, G., Grey, N., Leach, J., Greenberg, N., Katona, C., El-Leithy, S., & Pilling, S. (2020). Psychological treatments for post-traumatic stress disorder in adults: A network meta-analysis. *Psychological Medicine, 50*(4), 542–555. https://doi.org/10.1017/S0033291720000070

McGinty, E., Presskreischer, R., Han, H., & Barry, C. (2020). Psychological distress and loneliness reported by US adults in 2018 and April 2020. *Journal of the American Medical Association, 324*(1), 93–94. https://doi.org/10.1001/jama.2020.9740

McLaughlin, K., & Hamilton, A. L. (2019). Exploring the influence of service dogs on participation in daily occupations by veterans with PTSD: A pilot study. *Australian Occupational Therapy Journal, 66*(5), 648–655. https://doi.org/10.1111/1440-1630.12606

Mendonca, R., Yhost, S., Santalucia, S., & Ideishi, S. (2017). Evaluation of the impact of animal assistive intervention on attention, social initiation, and regulation skills of children with disabilities. *American Journal of Occupational Therapy, 71*(4 Suppl. 1), 7111515217p1. https://doi.org/10.5014/ajot.2017.71S1-PO1157

Mental Health America. (2021). *Mental health needs in the U.S. grew dramatically in 2020.* https://mhanational.org/mental-health-needs-us-grew-dramatically-2020

Meredith, P., Strong, J., Condon, L., Lindstrom, D., & Hill, J. (2023). Understanding the occupational role of dog ownership through the lens of attachment theory: A survey study. *British Journal of Occupational Therapy, 86*(3), 205–214. https://doi.org/10.1177/03080226221133036

Mezey, G., White, S., Harrison, I., Bousfield, J., Lloyd-Evans, B., Payne, S., & Killaspy, H. (2020). Validity, reliability, acceptability, and utility of the Social Inclusion Questionnaire User Experience (SInQUE): A clinical tool to facilitate social inclusion amongst people with severe mental health problems. *Social Psychiatry Psychiatric Epidemiology, 55*, 953–964. https://doi.org/10.1007/s00127-019-01826-3

Mezey, G., White, S., Thachil, A., Berg, R., Kallumparam, S., Nasiruddin, O., Wright, C., & Killaspy, H. (2013). Development and preliminary validation of a measure of social inclusion for use in people with mental health problems: The SInQUE. *International Journal of Social Psychiatry, 59*(5), 501–507. https://doi.org/10.1177/0020764012443752

Mourão, I., Mouro, C. V., Brito, L. M., Costa, S. R., & Almeida, T. C. (2022). Impacts of therapeutic horticulture on happiness and loneliness in institutionalized persons with mental health conditions. *British Journal of Occupational Therapy, 85*(2), 111–119. https://doi.org/10.1177/03080226211008719

Mukhtar, S. (2020). Psychological health during the coronavirus disease 2019 pandemic outbreak. *International Journal of Social Psychiatry, 66*(5), 512–516. https://doi.org/10.1177/0020764020925835

Mullen, G. (2019). Mapping evidence from systematic reviews regarding adult attachment and mental health difficulties: A scoping review. *Irish Journal of Psychological Medicine, 36*(3), 207–229. https://doi.org/10.1017/ipm.2017.27

Murthy, V. (2020). *Together: The healing power of human connection in a sometimes lonely world.* Harper Wave.

Nastasi, J. A. (2020). Occupational therapy interventions supporting leisure and social participation for older adults with low vision: A systematic review. *American Journal of Occupational Therapy, 74*(1), 1–9. https://doi.org/10.5014/ajot.2020.038521

National Academies of Sciences, Engineering, and Medicine. (2020). *Social isolation and loneliness in older adults: Opportunities for the health care system.* National Academies Press. https://doi.org/10.17226/25663

National Aeronautics and Space Administration. (2023). *Understanding our planet to benefit humankind.* https://climate.nasa.gov

National Center for Drug Abuse Statistics. (2023). *Opioid epidemic: Addiction statistics.* https://drugabusestatistics.org/opioid-epidemic

National Institute on Drug Abuse. (2022). *COVID-19 & substance use.* https://nida.nih.gov/research-topics/comorbidity/covid-19-substance-use

National Institute on Drug Abuse. (2023). *Drug overdose death rates.* https://nida.nih.gov/research-topics/trends-statistics/overdose-death-rates

National Institutes of Health. (2018). The power of pets: Health benefits of human-animal interactions. *NIH News in Health.* https://newsinhealth.nih.gov/2018/02/power-pets

Noyes, S., & Lannigan, E. G. (2019). *Occupational therapy practice guidelines for adults living with serious mental illness.* AOTA Press.

Nyman, A., & Isaksson, G. (2021). Enacted togetherness—A concept to understand occupation as socio-culturally situated. *Scandinavian Journal of Occupational Therapy, 28*(1), 41–45. https://doi.org/10.1080/11038128.2020.1720283

Obradović, N., Lagueux, É., Michaud, F., & Provencher, V. (2020). Pros and cons of pet ownership in sustaining independence in community-dwelling older adults: A scoping review. *Ageing & Society, 40*(9), 2061–2076. https://doi.org/10.1017/S0144686X19000382

Ochsner, K. N., & Lieberman, M. D. (2001). The emergence of Social Cognitive Neuroscience. *American Psychologist, 56*(9), 717–734. https://doi.org/10.1037/0003-066X.56.9.717

Oliva, J. L., & Johnston, K. L. (2022). Development of the Pet Owner Connectedness Scale (POCS). *Anthrozoos, 35*(4), 545–557. https://doi.org/10.1080/08927936.2022.2027095

O'Rourke, H. M., & Sidani, S. (2017). Definition, determinants, and outcomes of social connectedness for older adults: A scoping review. *Journal of Gerontological Nursing, 43*(7), 43–52. https://doi.org/10.3928/00989134-20170223-03

Pai, N., & Vella, S.-L. (2021). COVID-19 and loneliness: A rapid systematic review. *Australian and New Zealand Journal of Psychiatry, 55*(12), 1144–1156. https://doi.org/10.1177/00048674211031489

Patil, G., Asbjørnslett, M., Aurlien, K., & Levin, N. (2019). Gardening as a meaningful occupation in initial stroke rehabilitation: An occupational therapist perspective. *Open Journal of Occupational Therapy (OJOT), 7*(3), 1–15. https://doi.org/10.15453/2168-6408.1561

Pearse, E., Bucci, S., Raphael, J., & Berry, K. (2020). The relationship between attachment and functioning for people with serious mental illness: A systematic review. *Nordic Journal of Psychiatry, 74*(8), 545–557. https://doi.org/10.1080/08039488.2020.1767687

Perry, B. D. (2006). Applying principles of neurodevelopment to clinical work with maltreated and traumatized children: The Neurosequential Model of Therapeutics. In N. B. Webb (Ed.), *Working with traumatized youth in child welfare* (pp. 27–52). Guilford Press.

Perry, B. D., & Hambrick, E. P. (2008). The Neurosequential Model of Therapeutics. *Reclaiming Children and Youth, 17*(3), 38–43.

Piccininni, C., Michaelson, V., Janssen, I., & Pickett, W. (2018). Outdoor play and nature connectedness as potential correlates of internalized mental health symptoms among Canadian adolescents. *Preventive Medicine, 112*, 168–175. https://doi.org/10.1016/j.ypmed.2018.04.020

Pipp-Siegel, S., Brown, S. R., Easterbrooks, M. A., & Harmon, R. J. (1995). The relation between infants' self/mother knowledge and three attachment categories. *Infant Mental Health Journal, 16*(3), 221–232. https://doi.org/10.1002/1097-0355(199523)16:33.0.CO;2-B

Polusny, M. A., Erbes, C. R., Thuras, P., Moran, A., Lamberty, G. J., Collins, R. C., Rodman, J. L., & Lim, K. O. (2015). Mindfulness-Based Stress Reduction for posttraumatic stress disorder among veterans: A randomized clinical trial. *Journal of the American Medical Association, 314*(5), 456–465. https://doi.org/10.1001/jama.2015.8361

Pretty, J. (2004). How nature contributes to mental and physical health. *Spirituality and Health International, 5*, 68–78. https://doi.org/10.1002/shi.220

Pritchard, A., Richardson, M., Sheffield, D., & McEwan, K. (2020). The relationship between nature connectedness and eudaimonic well-being: A meta-analysis. *Journal of Happiness Studies, 21*(3), 1145–1167. https://doi.org/10.1007/s10902-019-00118-6

Pruskowski, K. A., Gurney, J. M., & Cancio, L. C. (2020). Impact of the implementation of a therapy dog program on burn center patients and staff. *Burns: Journal of the International Society for Burn Injuries, 46*(2), 293–297. https://doi.org/10.1016/j.burns.2019.11.024

Ramugondo, E. L., & Kronenberg, F. (2015). Explaining collective occupations from a human relations perspective: Bridging the individual-collective dichotomy. *Journal of Occupational Science, 22*(1), 3–16. https://doi.org/10.1080/14427591.2013.781920

Rebeiro, K. L., & Cook, J. V. (1999). Opportunity, not prescription: An exploratory study of the experience of occupational engagement. *Canadian Journal of Occupational Therapy, 66*(4), 176–187. https://doi.org/10.1177/000841749906600405

Rebeiro, K. L., Day, D. G., Semeniuk, B., O'Brien, M. C., & Wilson, B. (2001). Northern Initiative for Social Action: An occupation-based mental health program. *The American Journal of Occupational Therapy, 55*(5), 493–500. https://doi.org/10.5014/ajot.55.5.493

Rieck, D., Bell, K., & Neman, D. (2022, October 26). St. Louis school gunman left note describing lonely life, 'perfect storm' for mass shooting. *St. Louis Post-Dispatch.* https://stltoday.com/news/local/crime-and-courts/st-louis-school-gunman-left-note-describing-lonely-life-perfect-storm-for-mass-shooting/article_607b33cc-2402-55a7-94c9-f0c2214bec5c.html

Rouse, J., & Hitch, D. (2014). Occupational therapy led activity based group interventions for young people with mental illness: A literature review. *New Zealand Journal of Occupational Therapy, 61*(2), 58–63.

Saeri, A. K., Cruwys, T., Barlow, F. K., Stronge, S., & Sibley, C. G. (2018). Social connectedness improves public mental health: Investigating bidirectional relationships in the New Zealand attitudes and values survey. *Australian and New Zealand Journal of Psychiatry, 52*(4), 365–374. https://doi.org/10.1177/0004867417723990

Scoresby, K. J., Strand, E. B., Ng, Z., Brown, K. C., Stilz, C. R., Strobel, K., Barroso, C. S., & Souza, M. (2021). Pet ownership and quality of life: A systematic review of the literature. *Veterinary Sciences, 8*(12), 332. https://doi.org/10.3390/vetsci8120332

Sempik, J. (2010). Green care and mental health: Gardening and farming as health and social care. *Mental Health & Social Inclusion, 14*(3), 15–22. https://doi.org/10.5042/mhsi.2010.0440

Sevilla-Llewellyn-Jones, J., Santesteban-Echarri, O., Pryor, I., McGorry, P., & Alvarez-Jimenez, M. (2018). Web-based mindfulness interventions for mental health treatment: Systematic review and meta-analysis. *JMIR Mental Health, 5*(3), e10278. https://doi.org/10.2196/10278

Shearin, E. N., & Linehan, M. M. (1994). Dialectical behavior therapy for borderline personality disorder: Theoretical and empirical foundations. *Acta Psychiatrica Scandinavica. Supplementum, 379*, 61–68. https://doi.org/10.1111/j.1600-0447.1994.tb05820.x

Shepley, M. M., Watson, A., Pitts, F., Garrity, A., Spelman, E., Kelkar, J., & Fronsman, A. (2016). Mental and behavioral health environments: Critical considerations for facility design. *General Hospital Psychiatry, 42*, 15–21. https://doi.org/10.1016/j.genhosppsych.2016.06.003

Sherrington, C. S. (1906). *The integrative action of the nervous system.* Yale University Press.

Sinnott, R., & Rowlís, M. (2021). A gardening and woodwork group in mental health: A step towards recovery. *Irish Journal of Occupational Therapy, 49*(2), 96–103. https://doi.org/10.1108/IJOT-08-2021-0018

Spots.com. (2022). *Pet ownership statistics.* https://spots.com/pet-ownership-statistics

Stickley, A., & Koyanagi, A. (2018). Physical multimorbidity and loneliness: A population-based study. *PloS One, 13*(1), e0191651. https://doi.org/10.1371/journal.pone.0191651

Streeck-Fischer, A., & van der Kolk, B. (2000). Down will come baby cradle and all; Diagnostic and therapeutic implications of chronic trauma on child development. *Australian and New Zealand Journal of Psychiatry, 34*, 903–918. https://doi.org/10.1080/000486700265

Substance Abuse and Mental Health Services Administration. (2012). *SAMHSA's working definition of recovery.* Publication ID PEP12-RECDEF. https://store.samhsa.gov/sites/default/files/d7/priv/pep12-recdef.pdf

Substance Abuse and Mental Health Services Administration. (2020). *National survey on drug use and health (NSDUH).* https://www.samhsa.gov/data/data-we-collect/nsduh-national-survey-drug-use-and-health

Substance Abuse and Mental Health Services Administration. (2021). *National survey on drug use and health* (NSDUH). https://www.samhsa.gov/data/data-we-collect/nsduh-national-survey-drug-use-and-health

Suto, M. J., Smith, S., Damiano, N., & Channe, S. (2021). Participation in community gardening: Sowing the seeds of well-being. *Canadian Journal of Occupational Therapy, 88*(2), 142–152. https://doi.org/10.1177/0008417421994385

Teicher, M. H., Andersen, S. L., Polcari, A., Anderson, C. M., & Navalta, C. P. (2002). Developmental neurobiology of childhood stress and trauma. *Psychiatric Clinics of North America, 25*(2), 397–426. https://doi.org/10.1016/S0193-953X(01)00003-X

Tsatsi, I. A., & Plastow, N. A. (2021). Optimizing a halfway house to meet mental health care users' occupational needs. *Canadian Journal of Occupational Therapy, 88*(4), 352–364. https://doi.org/10.1177/00084174211044896

Tyminski, Q. P., Drummond, R. R., Heisey, C. F., Evans, S. K., Hendrix, A., Jaegers, L. A., & Baum, C. M. (2020). Initial development of the Activity Card Sort–Advancing Inclusive Participation from a homeless population perspective. *Occupational Therapy International, 2020,* Article 9083082. https://doi.org/10.1155/2020/9083082

United Nations, Department of Economic and Social Affairs, Population Division. (2019). *World urbanization prospects: The 2018 revision.* United Nations. https://www.un-ilibrary.org/content/books/9789210043144

Vibholm, A. P., Christensen, J. R., & Pallesen, H. (2020). Nature-based rehabilitation for adults with acquired brain injury: A scoping review. *International Journal of Environmental Health Research, 30*(6), 661–676. https://doi.org/10.1080/09603123.2019.1620183

Wasmuth, S., Horsford, C., Mahaffey, L., & Lysaker, P. H. (2022). "Metacognitive Reflection and Insight Therapy" (MERIT) for the occupational therapy practitioner. *Canadian Journal of Occupational Therapy, 90*(4), 333–343. https://doi.org/10.1177/00084174221142172

Wasmuth, S., Luther, L., Hamm, J., & Lysaker, P. (2019). Relationships between occupational participation and ontological security in persons with schizophrenia. *American Journal of Psychiatric Rehabilitation, 22*(3), 179–200. https://www.muse.jhu.edu/article/797608

Watts, R., Kettner, H., Geerts, D., Gandy, S., Kartner, L., Mertens, L., Timmermann, C., Nour, M. M., Kaelen, M., Nutt, D., Carhart-Harris, R., & Roseman, L. (2022). The Watts Connectedness Scale: A new scale for measuring a sense of connectedness to self, others, and world. *Psychopharmacology, 239*(11), 3461–3483. https://doi.org/10.1007/s00213-022-06187-5

Weinstein, E., Kleiman, E. M., Franz, P. J., Joyce, V. W., Nash, C. C., Buonopane, R. J., & Nock, M. K. (2021). Positive and negative uses of social media among adolescents hospitalized for suicidal behavior. *Journal of Adolescence, 87*(1), 63–73. https://doi.org/10.1016/j.adolescence.2020.12.003

Weiss, R. S. (1973). *Loneliness: The experience of emotional and social isolation.* The MIT Press.

Wilbarger, P. (1984). Planning an adequate sensory diet: Application of sensory processing theory during the first year of life. *Zero to Three, 5*(1), 7–12.

Wilcock, A. (1998). Reflections on doing, being and becoming. *Canadian Journal of Occupational Therapy, 65*(5), 248–256. https://doi.org/10.1177/000841749806500501

Wilcock, A. A. (2006). *An occupational perspective of health* (2nd ed.). Slack, Inc.

Wilcock, A. A. (2007). Occupation and health: Are they one and the same? *Journal of Occupational Science, 14,* 3–8. https://doi.org/10.1080/14427591.2007.9686577

Williams, R. L., & Metz, A. E. (2014). Examining the meaning of training animals: A PhotoVoice study with at-risk youth. *Occupational Therapy in Mental Health, 30*(4), 337–357. https://doi.org/10.1080/0164212X.2014.938563

World Health Organization. (2022). *COVID-19 pandemic triggers 25% increase in prevalence of anxiety and depression worldwide.* https://www.who.int/news/item/02-03-2022-covid-19-pandemic-triggers-25-increase-in-prevalence-of-anxiety-and-depression-worldwide

World Health Organization-International Telecommunication Union. (2022). *WHO-ITU global standard for accessibility of telehealth services.* https://www.who.int/publications/i/item/9789240050464

Zablan, K., Melvin, G., & Hayley, A. (2023). Older adult companion animal-owner wellbeing during the COVID-19 pandemic: A qualitative exploration. *Anthrozoös, 36*(2), 237–256. https://doi.org/10.1080/08927936.2022.2125198

Zedel, J., & Chen, S.-P. (2021). Person's experiences of occupational therapy group interventions in mental health settings: A meta-ethnography. *Occupational Therapy in Mental Health, 37*(3), 278–302. https://doi.org/10.1080/0164212X.2021.1900763

Zeder, M. A. (2008). Domestication and early agriculture in the Mediterranean Basin: Origins, diffusion, and impact. *Proceedings of the National Academy of Sciences of the United States of America, 105*(33), 11597–11604. https://doi.org/10.1073/pnas.0801317105

Anita C. Bundy, Rosa Román-Oyola, and Shelly J. Lane

This chapter addresses the key aspects of play and its association with mental health. It defines play and playfulness and describes their characteristics. A sense of belonging is an important benefit of play; in fact, belonging links play and playfulness to mental health. The chapter also explains the neural pathways, networks, and neurotransmitters that enable play and playfulness. The role of play in occupational participation is important to occupational therapy practitioners (OTPs), and their use of the relevant assessments and interventions is explored.

Overview of Play and Playfulness

Play comprises some of the most meaningful activities in which both children and adults engage. But play is a paradox. On the one hand, it is the primary occupation of children and an important lifelong occupation. On the other hand, even though occupational performance is fundamental to occupational therapy, improved play is rarely a goal of intervention—even for children.

It is important to distinguish between the related concepts of play and playfulness. Play is what a person *does* (i.e., an activity), whereas *playfulness* is the way one approaches a situation. Play activities take the form of transactions between the player and the physical and social environments. Playfulness is an aspect of personality that is present even in infancy, but the environment affects its manifestation. Very restrictive environments dampen an individual's playfulness, and very supportive environments promote it. Thus, playfulness is both a state and a trait.

Similar to many constructs in occupational therapy, there are multiple definitions of play, but no consensus on any (Hurd & Anderson, 2010). Probably the most common way of defining play is by listing characteristics that, when present, separate play from nonplay or other occupations. Whether considering an activity/transaction or approach to everyday life, play and playfulness share common characteristics. Both are relatively internally controlled, intrinsically motivated, and free of unnecessary constraints of reality (Skard & Bundy, 2008). Skard and Bundy added **framing** (i.e., the cues that separate play from "reality") as a fourth defining characteristic of play and playfulness.

Neither play/playfulness nor nonplay/nonplayfulness are either-or phenomena. That is, an activity is not *either* play *or* nonplay, and a person is not *either* playful *or* not playful. Play and nonplay, playfulness and nonplayfulness represent continua. The same is true of each of the characteristics, or elements, that contribute to play and playfulness. That is, one's perception of control ranges from internal to external; the source of motivation from intrinsic to extrinsic; and the extent to which one can suspend reality from free to not free. Figure 50-1 is a schematic representation of the play/nonplay continuum and the continua associated with each of the contributing elements. Similar to play and playfulness, the four defining characteristics of play are abstract and beg to be defined. How does someone know them when they see them? To enable therapists to evaluate play and playfulness and target them in intervention, Skard and Bundy (2008) operationalized these elements in the Test of Playfulness (ToP).

Internal Control

Internal control refers to an individual's feeling of being "in charge" of their actions and at least some aspects of an activity's outcome. One can see internal control in players' actions: they are free to choose whether to engage and when to leave; they are free to modify the rules; and they have the needed skills to engage. When engaged with others, players must share control; otherwise, not everyone can be playing. People see shared control in behaviors such as negotiation and supporting one another (Skard & Bundy, 2008). Neumann (1971) indicated that internal control was the most important play characteristic because, when individuals feel control, they can change aspects of the situation (e.g., who to include, what to do) to make it more enjoyable.

Intrinsic Motivation

When players engage in an activity purely because they want to and not primarily for extrinsic gain, **intrinsic motivation** is exhibited. Of course, extrinsic motivators (e.g., winning a game) often are a part of play, but they are not the driving force. Intrinsic motivation exists when an individual is totally engaged, persists with the activity in the face of obstacles, and feels enjoyment (Skard & Bundy, 2008). Intrinsic motivation is the most cited characteristic of play (e.g., American Occupational Therapy Association [AOTA], 2020; Parham & Fazio, 2008).

However, to say that motivation is intrinsic does not identify the *source* of the motivation (i.e., what the player gets from the activity). Common play motivations include socialization and mastery, but there are many others—and motivation is always determined by the player. The text that follows features a description of play motivations inherent to the categories of play Caillois (2001) described.

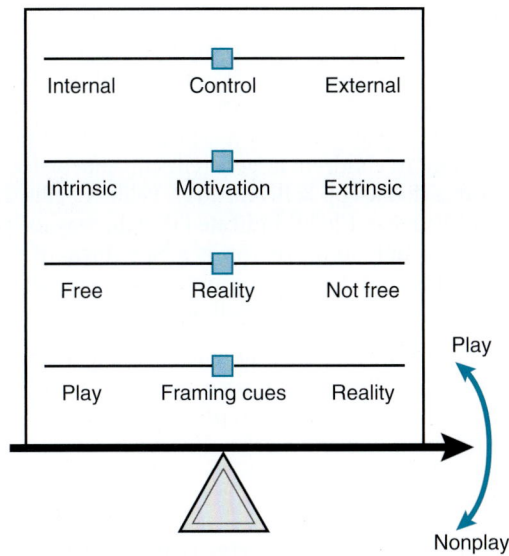

FIGURE 50-1. Characteristics of play and playfulness.

Freedom From Unnecessary Constraints of Reality

To be **free from unnecessary constraints of reality** means that individuals leave behind some of the everyday tasks and worries that preclude their engagement; they are free to choose how close to objective reality a transaction will be. Often this latter description suggests pretending—to be someone they are not, to do something they are not doing, that an object or person is something/someone other than what they actually are. For example, a child on a swing can choose to assume a superhero persona or simply to swing, enjoying the sensation of the air and the movement or challenging oneself to go as high as possible. Although pretending commonly comes to mind when one thinks of suspending reality, this play element also takes other forms, including joking, teasing, clowning, and playful mischief (Skard & Bundy, 2008).

Framing

Framing refers to the ability to give and read social cues about how to interact with one another and maintain a play theme over time. Because play is, by definition, buffered from real life consequences (Bruner et al., 1976), it is important that players give others clear cues about how they wish to be treated (Skard & Bundy, 2008).

There is a lack of consensus on the definition of play, but the four mentioned play characteristics serve as cohesive elements when reflecting on play and its distinctiveness from other occupations. Another point of consensus regarding play is its relevance as the primary occupation of children and an important lifelong occupation. Play evolves with maturity, but people of all ages play. Certainly, the fastest rate of brain development occurs within the first 3 years of life (Hudspeth & Matthews, 2015). However, the brain continues to develop within the context of life opportunities. Of course, play, and particularly social play, is one of the wonderful opportunities that life presents for advancing brain development.

How the Brain Promotes Play

What is the neuroscience of play? It might seem that having these two words in the same sentence is itself contradictory. Does thinking of play in the context of neuroscience take the playfulness away? Or does it offer people an opportunity to develop a richer understanding of the complexity of play?

This section assumes the latter; it considers the evidence in the literature and links it to the knowledge base on play and playfulness. This linkage provides a foundation for clinical reasoning when working with individuals who have mental health challenges. First, this section considers the neural functions related to motor play, social interactions, emotional regulation, and cognition and links these functions to mental health and belonging. *For readers who are interested in understanding neural structures, systems, and neurochemistry, please access additional content at the online resource center at FADavis.com for a deeper look at these constructs.*

Who Plays? Play and the Brain

Play and playful behavior have been documented in many mammals and birds. Burghardt (2005, 2010) and Bateson (2014) indicated that fish, reptiles and, potentially, invertebrates evidence instances of play. Playful interactions vary from species to species. Not surprisingly, primates in particular show high levels of playfulness (Kerney et al., 2017), with humans showing the greatest variety of these behaviors. The characteristics of playfulness relative to human interactions are delineated earlier in this chapter, but the literature on animal playfulness is less specific. However, recall that playfulness is an approach to a situation, one that reflects a positive mood and intrinsic motivation (Bateson, 2014). These features of interaction are readily observable in animal interactions.

Do play and playfulness have evolutionary or developmental benefits for the brain? Some evidence suggests that the most playful animals show slower brain maturation and generally have larger brains, although the relationship between brain size and playful behavior has been questioned (Iwaniuk et al., 2001; Montgomery, 2014; Pellis et al., 2019). In fact, Pellis and Pellis (2009) indicated that, rather than overall brain size, researchers should look at enlargement of specific areas of the brain related to playfulness.

The basis for this stance rests, in part, on the fact that there is insufficient data on the complexity and variability of play across species. Consistent with this, early primate researchers linked engagement in social play to the larger neocortex of primates. They speculated that engagement with larger social groups contributed to increased cortex size, potentially because of the need to maintain multiple social relationships (Dunbar, 1992, 1995; Lewis, 2000). Further, Lewis and Barton (2004, 2006) indicated that a larger cerebellum and cortex are associated with more play, and a bigger amygdala and hypothalamus are associated with more social play. The cerebellum is important to many aspects of play.

Is Animal Play a Basis for Understanding Human Play and Playfulness?

Play and playfulness are not as clearly defined in animals as in humans, but there is ample evidence that many animals are playful. For instance, dogs "invite" play through playful bowing, which frames the interaction as play. Dogs demonstrate a wealth of other playful behaviors, such as play biting, which is a means of framing such that biting is not interpreted as actual fighting. A relaxed, open mouth is another demonstration of framing. Dogs also use "rapid mimicry" during play, a fast but involuntary imitation of the emotional expression of another, which is a way of giving and reading cues (framing; Bradshaw et al., 2015; Palagi et al., 2015.)

Several nonhuman primates also show this response during playful interactions, as do some nonprimate mammals. Many primates are noted to be highly playful. For instance, squirrel monkeys and rhesus macaques are highly social; their play begins at a young age, very similar to how it does in humans, and follows a similar course, reaching a peak in "childhood" and diminishing as they reach adulthood (Burghardt, 2005; Lafreniere, 2011). Gender differences in play behaviors have been widely identified across species (Burghardt, 2005). However, this chapter does not explore these differences.

Much of what people know about play comes from the study of rats, a species of mammal that plays extensively throughout childhood and adolescence. Rat play is limited in scope and somewhat stereotypical, making it easier to study than primate play. Rats engage in what is termed rough and tumble play or play fighting, a physical/motor and social play that is highly predictable and easily studied. Most mammals engage in physically playful social interactions, making this type of play meaningful for understanding the neural underpinnings of play and playfulness (Siviy, 2016). Chasing is another form of rough and tumble play seen across humans and animals, although not necessarily in rats.

Although it is necessary to rely on literature reflecting animal play, this chapter presents information on humans when possible. Panksepp and Biven (2012) explained that researchers begin to understand the neuroscience of human play by looking at play research because neural structures supporting play are largely subcortical, and subcortical structures across species are more similar than cortical structures.

Neural Connections Supporting Play

The earlier discussion concerning literature on play and playful behaviors in animals provides insight into the neural bases for playful actions and attitudes. Literature also links these attitudes and behaviors more specifically to human neural functions. This helps to deconstruct play into some component themes that consider multiple aspects of behavior, including sensory, motor, motivational, cognitive, social, and emotional. Aligning these themes with brain structures and regions is a task that is fraught with error, because brain structures do not function independently of one another. This is especially true for complex behaviors and attitudes such as play and playfulness. Nonetheless, some brain structures are core to play, playing, and playfulness and can be linked to neural networks that better reflect how the brain functions.

Cerebellar-Cortical Connections Supporting Movement and Play

Movement is at the center of many aspects of play. It has been called the "gas" behind social interactions, a foundation for learning, and a key factor in brain growth (Brown &

Vaughan, 2009). Although not always playful, physical activity has been suggested as one of the important factors supporting mental health (Hosker et al., 2019; Rodriguez-Ayllon et al., 2019; Vankim & Nelson, 2013).

Play fighting or physical play, typical of animal play but also important to children, largely relies on subcortical neural structures (Panksepp & Biven, 2012; Pellis & Pellis, 2009). Brown and Vaughan (2009) indicated that the way to "jump-start" play is simply to move; this is a basic form of play. In considering the foundations of movement as core to play, it is important to look to the cerebellum.

For readers who are interested in understanding neural structures, systems, and neurochemistry, please access additional content at the online resource center at FADavis.com for a deeper understanding of how the cerebellum supports movement and play.

Cerebellar-Cortical Connections Supporting Emotion, Social Interaction, Cognition, and Play

Play clearly taps into the emotional functions of limbic structures. According to Neale (2018), engagement in play and playful behaviors lead to neuroplastic changes in many brain regions; notable here are limbic structures that mediate the expression of social behaviors. Earlier, cognition, emotion, and social interaction were identified as central to internal control, intrinsic motivation, and the ability to give and read social cues. Functions associated with the cerebellum were also described. In fact, prolonged periods of play associated with childhood have been linked to rate of growth of the cerebellum, not just for its role in movement but also for its role in cognition (Brown & Vaughan, 2009). Thus, although basic and stereotypical playful interactions do not rely on cortical influences, other aspects of play do.

Thinking back to the remaining feature of playfulness, freedom from unnecessary constraints of reality also requires examining the link between the cerebellum and cognition. The cerebellum influences higher level functions through widespread links to the frontal and prefrontal cortices.

For readers who are interested in understanding neural structures, systems, and neurochemistry, please access additional content at the online resource center at FADavis.com for a deeper understanding of how the cerebellum supports emotions, social interaction, cognition, and play.

Other Functions of the Brain That Support Play

Although the cerebellum and its interconnectivity with multiple neural structures and regions is central to play and playfulness, some additional details on neural function are important. As noted, intrinsic motivation, reflected in part in enjoyment, is a core feature of play. As Vandervert (2017) noted, fun is an inherent reward for play. In fact, the capacity to find joy in life is essential to well-being. In considering the neural underpinnings of fun and enjoyment, it helps to understand emotional regulation and reward. These functions have been associated with limbic structures, the neurotransmitter dopamine, and endogenous opioid peptides that modulate neurotransmitter actions, along with other neurotransmitters. This section briefly considers the role of dopamine and opioids in mediating pleasure, thus implicating these substances in play and playfulness.

Reward and pleasure come from many sources. In addition to play, eating tasty food, engaging in sex, and social interactions all are reward-driven activities. Berridge and Kringelbach (2015) indicated that all these forms of pleasure activate regions of the brain similarly, allowing people to generalize about the overall experience of pleasure. Implicated in people's ability to experience pleasure are regions of the prefrontal cortex associated with limbic functions (i.e., orbitofrontal, insula, anterior cingulate cortices) and other limbic structures (i.e., nucleus accumbens, amygdala, and the ventral pallidum; Berridge & Kringelbach, 2015), all structures previously associated with play and playfulness.

Related to social interaction, the social reward system involves the ventral tegmentum, pituitary, hypothalamus, and regions of the orbitofrontal cortex. And what has been termed the "social brain" includes regions of the prefrontal cortex, limbic structures, and parietal structures (Pellis et al., 2023; Schneider et al., 2022). Thus, an individual's ability to experience pleasure relies on both cortical and subcortical brain regions.

For readers who are interested in understanding neural structures, systems, and neurochemistry, please access additional content at the online resource center at FADavis.com for a deeper understanding of other functions of the brain that support play.

Developmental Benefits of Play

Play is essential to "typical" motor, social, emotional, and cognitive development (Baarendse et al., 2013; Siviy, 2016; Spinka et al., 2001; Van Den Berg et al., 1999; Vanderschuren & Trezza, 2014; Von Frijtag et al., 2002). Relative to the impact on social and emotional development, play is associated with social competence (Siviy & Panksepp, 2011; Van Den Berg et al., 1999); is a foundation for the development of socioemotional intelligence (Panksepp & Biven, 2012; Van Den Berg et al., 1999); and has high reward value (Trezza et al., 2010). In support of emotional well-being, Howard and McInnes (2013) showed that engaging children in "play," rather than "not play," activities led to greater involvement on the part of the player and, importantly, to behaviors reflecting emotional well-being.

Play is also crucial for maintaining social relationships (Bekoff, 1976). Beyond a direct impact on social skills, the social interactions associated with play can reduce stress and support maintenance of social groups (Pellis & Pellis, 2009). These play features seem to apply to humans and animals (Lafreniere, 2011).

Playing has also been shown to support young animals (including humans) to acquire the skills they need to become efficient adults (Andersen et al., 2022) by promoting the development of behavioral flexibility to meet the demands of an ever-changing environment (Vanderschuren & Trezza, 2014). Bateson (2014) suggested that play supports the ability to create new and unique solutions to social and physical challenges. Consistent with this view, humans experience long developmental periods during which play is one primary occupation that supports adaptability and flexibility

as they encounter and construct play situations (Brown & Vaughan, 2009).

Investigators have shown that preventing play in young rats during a time when social play is highly evident leads to lasting impairments in social interactions (Van Den Berg et al., 1999; Von Frijtag et al., 2002), emotional regulation (Von Frijtag et al., 2002), and cognitive development (Baarendse et al., 2013; Van Den Berg et al., 1999; Vanderschuren & Trezza, 2014). Even short-term play deprivation in rats leads to intense bouts of animal play considered "rebound play" (Lafreniere, 2011; Panksepp & Beatty, 1980; Siviy & Panksepp, 2011). The long-range effects of play and social interaction deprivation include diminished social interactions in adult rats, such as reduced tolerance to social approaches from other rats, which is expressed as aggressive or excessively timid behavior (Lafreniere, 2011).

More profound effects of play deprivation have been shown in primates; social isolation has been linked to deficits in regulation of emotional arousal (Lafreniere, 2011) and nonverbal communication of emotions (Miller et al., 1967). Brown and Vaughan (2009) suggested that preschool children with limited play opportunities can develop difficulties in reading the play cues of playmates. According to Lafreniere (2011), play deprivation in children also results in a rebound effect. Pelligrini and colleagues further suggested that increasing the wait time before recess can lead to rebound activity as children take back control of activity levels and seek a variety of sensory inputs (Pellegrini et al., 1995; Smith & Hagan, 1980). Intrinsic motivation might also be a part of this rebound play. These investigators also suggested that contextual factors influence rebound, such as the environmental temperature and location (inside or outside) of recess.

The current emphasis on indoor, more sedentary, play activities can lead to longer, vigorous bouts of play once children are given the opportunity to play. There is some suggestion that the current parenting practices of structuring and scheduling play experiences for children could actually impair playfulness, either because it interferes with opportunities to create play and discover (Brown & Vaughan, 2009) or because the imposed structure limits the more spontaneous occurrence of physical play (Siviy & Panksepp, 2011). In a recent systematic review of unstructured play interventions, Lee and colleagues (2020) found that positive outcomes were noted in children's physical activity levels, social engagement, and emotional well-being.

Although in many mammals play is a lifelong occupation, as noted earlier, compared with the young members of a variety of species, adults play less. However, continued play and exploration into adulthood in humans is important and can be linked to a reduced likelihood of common disorders associated with aging, such as dementia, neurological disorders, and cardiovascular disease (Brown & Vaughan, 2009). For adults, very similar to how they are for children, long periods of no play have been linked to changes in mental health such as darkened mood, anhedonia, and loss of optimism (Brown & Vaughan, 2009).

Both genetics and the environment affect play. Relative to genetics, rats bred for features that reflect greater playful behavior (e.g., responsiveness to tickle) are themselves more playful (Siviy & Panksepp, 2011). Early environments, specifically the interactions and early social bonds between mother and child or mother and rat pup, are crucial for

The Lived Experience

Play to Deal With the Unexpected: Let's Go to "Vacaciones Mágicas"!

In the middle of the COVID-19 lockdown, Rocío, the daughter of one of the chapter authors, was very disappointed that the family could not go on vacation. What follows is a compelling story of how, through play, Rocío managed the occupational disruption stemming from lockdown—and brought her family along with her.

One day, Rocío came to us very excited with an idea: "Let's go to "Vacaciones Mágicas"! My husband and I were surprised and asked her to explain. She did. Our response: "No way!" We felt like all we could think about were the many things we must handle: our own work responsibilities, duplicated by remote work; our new roles as teacher's assistants at home; caring for the needs of some of the elder family members. . . . However, she insisted on it several times every day until she convinced us.

What was "Vacaciones Mágicas"? It was an imaginary hotel located in our own home! A few days before our "departure" for the hotel, we got involved in the preparation of the hotel's sign using markers and a big and colorful piece of trace paper. The day before we left, we took a suitcase out of the closet and packed some clothes. The next day (a Friday), after work, we placed the suitcase in the car and, literally, left for a brief trip around the nearest two or three blocks. A few minutes later, when we returned, we were not at home anymore! We were at "Vacaciones Mágicas!" Immediately, after we arrived at the

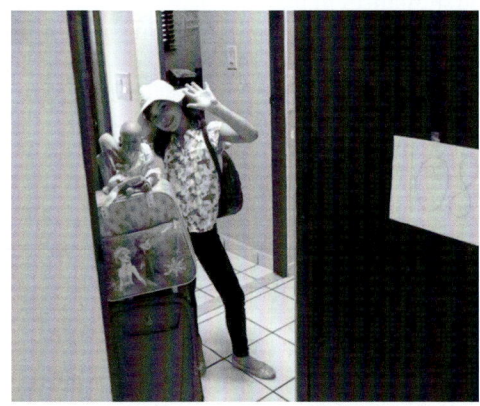

"hotel," Rocío put on a sun hat and became the host. She received us, completed the registry, and gave us the "room key" she had prepared a few days before. Then, she took off the sun hat and, magically, turned into our daughter again. We entered the hotel room and officially began our one day and a half joyful vacation. Various tours were included with our stay (e.g., a climbing tour to the roof, a walking tour to the park, a picnic in the backyard). There was a lot to do and much fun to have! After returning home on Sunday, we realized that, more than just making Rocío happy, "Vacaciones Mágicas" was a precious time in which we reconnected with each other through play, while creating an invaluable memory for all of us.

overall well-being and survival (Baumeister & Leary, 1995) and form a foundation for play and interaction. In addition, mother–infant bonding or attunement is a basis for play and, as development unfolds, lays a foundation for emotional regulation, future brain development (Brown & Vaughan, 2009), and a sense of belonging and survival (Baumeister & Leary, 1995). In fact, human mothers' responsiveness to their infant during play at 10 months of age positively predicts higher cognitive capacities and skills (e.g., problem-solving, knowledge, and memory) at 18 months. This effect is independent of maternal education, home adversity, and infant advanced object play (Neale et al., 2018).

Relative to context, the expression of play behaviors is subject to environment, as well as emotional and physical state. Researchers have shown that play behaviors are not seen when people are stressed, anxious, hungry, or unwell. Playing requires a positive mood, supporting engagement in activities that are both spontaneous and flexible (Bateson, 2014). As such, play itself is an indicator of psychological and physical well-being (Held & Špinka, 2011).

Play and Well-Being in Times of Occupational Disruption

Occupational disruption occurs in the face of significant life events that provoke an interruption of the normal patterns of occupational engagement (Whiteford, 2000). Such

interruptions can affect physical and mental health. Because of its global impact, COVID-19 is a familiar example of the consequences of occupational disruption to health. Researchers (Luck et al., 2021; Sangster Jokić & Jokić-Begić, 2022) linked the occupational disruption that accompanied the pandemic to an increase in loneliness, anxiety, depression, distress, and stress. Indeed, various systematic reviews (de Sousa et al., 2021; Racine et al., 2021; Stracke et al., 2023; Xiong et al., 2020) evidenced the effects of COVID-19 on the mental health of populations around the world.

However, many other circumstances contribute to occupational disruption and the challenges it causes (e.g., natural and humanmade disasters, migration, the diagnosis of a disease, an injury, and life transitions [e.g., retirement; being a first-time parent]). Engaging in play is one means by which people manage occupational disruption.

Play and Mental Health, Belonging and Relatedness

The story of Rocío and her family demonstrates that the occupational disruption meted out by COVID-19 can be managed. But why and how does occupational disruption impact mental health? And how and why does play mitigate occupational disruption and positively influence mental health? The concept of belonging provides a potential explanation for the relationship between occupational disruption and mental health. See Chapter 49: Connectedness and Belonging for more emphasis on these constructs. 🤝

Play is a fundamentally social occupation (e.g., Caillois, 2001; Pellis et al., 2010; Powrie, 2019; Sutton-Smith, 1997). Although one *can* identify independent play activities, Caillois (2001) argued persuasively that "play lacks something when it is reduced to a mere solitary exercise" (p. 37). The relationship between players is more than simply social; it is one of "belonging." Of course, play is only one context in which belonging is prominent; close friendships and intimate relationships are others. Nonetheless, belonging is *always* present in genuine play, and a sense of belonging ties play intimately to mental health.

A second factor linking play and mental health is that, because it is freely chosen and done for its own sake rather than for extrinsic reward (e.g., Brown & Vaughan, 2009; Caillois, 2001; Sutton-Smith 1997), play makes important statements about identity. In fact, Plato is credited with saying that someone can learn more about a person in an hour of play than in a year of conversation. It follows, then, that in play, players reveal their most honest selves to one another. Further, for play to be genuine, playmates must accept one another unconditionally. Ryan and Deci (2017) indicated that when individuals (read here as playmates) accept one another unconditionally, each is more able to be authentic. They further indicated that *all* people sense when another's support is genuine. This statement is true of playmates of all ages—from infants to older adults.

Conversely, Deci and Ryan (2017) suggested that authentic participation as playmates contributes to psychological well-being in both players. When social connectedness is missing, when individuals lack a sense of belonging, Eisenberger (2012) suggested that they experience "social pain," presenting evidence that the sense of social pain or social disconnection is processed through the same neural pathways as is physical pain. In this review, Eisenberger suggested that this helps explain why physical pain seems to be reduced when people experience social connectedness. Thus, engaging in authentic play with an engaged playmate can enhance a sense of belonging.

Play is an excellent medium for interventions to promote mental health. In addition, the neural overlap between physical and social pain pathways helps practitioners understand how social connection and support, both inherent in play and playful interactions, can reduce physical pain (Eisenberger, 2012). Being playful and engaging in play helps preserve identity in the face of adverse circumstances (Berk et al., 2006; Casey et al., 2017; Clark, 2006; Moore et al., 2020), including threats to mental health (e.g., Dodd & Lester, 2021; Gray, 2011). Further, by promoting empathy, negotiation, problem-solving, creativity, and cooperation (Vazquez, 2020; Yogman et al., 2018), play contributes to the development of prosocial behavior, another reflection of mental health (World Health Organization, 2022).

Gisela's The Lived Experience story is a clear example about how engaging in play in the middle of an adverse situation (i.e., breast cancer) can contribute to reinforce belongingness through relatedness and benefit mental health.

Allen, Kern, and colleagues (2021) offered a tentative framework that could serve as a basis for developing interventions to support belonging and, ultimately, well-being. Although they did not address play as a medium for

intervention, the framework in Figure 50-2 suggests play as an ideal context for building interrelationships and ultimately belonging, and illustrates the interrelationships among components of belonging facilitated through play. Allen, Kern, and colleagues suggested that belonging reflects four interrelated components set within social, cultural, environmental, and temporal contexts: (1) competencies (i.e., skills and abilities); (2) opportunities (i.e., enablers, reduction of barriers); (3) motivation (i.e., inner drive to belong); and (4) positive and negative perceptions derived from experience.

The case of Jerad and Jon in Box 50-1 illustrates how the four interrelated components of Allen, Kern, and colleagues' (2021) model can work together to build a sense of belonging in play. The case of Marco in Box 50-2 delineates a time when altering the components increased Marco's playfulness and ability to play, which, in turn, increased his sense of belonging.

The Lived Experiences of Rocío and Gisela and the play narratives of Jerad and Jon and Marco provide rich examples of the power of play as a medium for universal growth in social, emotional, and cognitive processing, leading to goal-oriented behaviors that satisfy basic needs, including belonging. The Apply It Now activity suggestions at the end of the chapter will help readers analyze these cases more deeply.

Assessment

Linking Play and Playfulness to Belonging in Assessment

The ToP (Skard & Bundy, 2008) is an observational assessment that operationally defines the four elements of playfulness proposed at the opening of this chapter (i.e., internal control, intrinsic motivation, freedom from unnecessary constraints of reality, and framing). Table 50-1 provides details about the ToP and the evidence for reliability and validity of results gathered with it.

In the ToP, internal control, which Neumann (1971) named as the most important element of play, comprises many of the same concepts Ryan and Deci (2017) included in their description of autonomy. In fact, Ryan and Deci indicated explicitly that autonomy involves an *internal perceived locus of causality*. In reference to relatedness (i.e., belonging), Ryan and Deci cited previous reporting (Deci & Ryan, 2014; Ryan, 1993) focusing on autonomy support involving empathy and respect that, in turn, facilitates a [play] partner's desire for more relatedness—and subsequent actions to achieve relatedness. When partners encourage one another, implicitly or explicitly, they convey a message that their partner is competent, thus establishing a greater sense of belonging.

On the ToP, internal control has two components: actions that pertain primarily to the self and, more germane to this discussion, actions that reflect shared control. Shared control occurs in the context of social play. It involves negotiating, sharing, initiating play with others, entering an existing group, and, importantly, supporting playmates. Framing also is relevant to this discussion. Players who achieve high scores on supporting the play of others and reading social cues exhibit autonomy support and increase the sense of belonging. Players who fail to support or respond to a playmate's cues

The Lived Experience

Mothering, Playing, and Breast Cancer: Gisela's Story

When diagnosed with breast cancer, Gisela was 32 years old and lived in Puerto Rico with her 2- and 1-year-old daughters and her partner. Three days after the diagnosis, she moved to the U.S. mainland for medical treatment. After 3 weeks, her partner and daughters joined her. At the time of Gisela's interview, the family had lived in Massachusetts for a year, and Gisela was near the end of her adjuvant chemotherapy. The following are some of the memories Gisela remembered so vividly.

About Her Daughters and the Moving Process, Gisela Shared

Moving was so hard [for her daughters] because they left behind their lives—their day care, the house, and Coffee (their dog) to come to a whole different place: a smaller space—an apartment. . . . Even the weather was different. We couldn't just go to the park whenever we wanted. And Coffee. . . . My older daughter still asks about him and says that she will soon go to her Puerto Rico home to get him. It was so hard. They both regressed regarding things that they had overcome. They both asked to use baby bottles again, the oldest one wanted to wear diapers, and the youngest one began to pull her hair out, literally. Indeed, when I shaved my head, we decided to shave hers too, so she stopped doing it. All that made my heart broken, but we didn't know what else to do. Our nearest support to deal with these things were ourselves, a cousin that lived here in MA (who was recovering from her own cancer process), and our family in Puerto Rico.

About Playing Before and During the Disease Process

Before the disease, I was stricter. Indeed, I can say that, before the diagnosis, my oldest daughter was Daddy's girl because he was more playful than me. I was more like: "Keep things cleaned!" or "No more running or jumping!" I didn't want them to get hurt. But, when we moved, I knew that they were dealing with a lot of changes, so I was always looking for alternatives to keep them busy. We used brown paper to draw and paint, we played bubbles, play doh. . . .

However, when the chemo treatment began, I turned off a little because I didn't have the same strength. My mood was too down, and after the first chemo I experienced some panic attacks. Especially, the next 3 days after every chemo were awful. Fortunately, by the time I shaved my head (which was much earlier than the beginning of the treatment), we bought a toy doctor kit for the girls. They came with me to some of my medical appointments and saw the nurses work. So, when I came back from every chemo, they got their kit and checked me up: put me on some bandages, took my blood pressure, and gave me healing kisses. Also, there were times when my cousin took care of them while I was in chemo. When I came back home, there was always a welcoming poster that they had prepared for me, and they had different themes. I remember I once had a Wonder Woman poster. And truth is that I was feeling terrible, but all those things made me feel full. I was feeling terrible, but full at the same time. I indeed enjoyed having them with me in bed, even when I knew that after a while, they would begin jumping on bed.

Still, I feel like I missed much of those months with them because there were times when I just felt I was absent because of the treatment. My strength, my creativity were low. It wasn't until after the surgery that I began to feel that I could be like I was before. However, I believe that without my daughters, the process would have been much harder. Many times, they woke me up either because they wanted to take care of me by using their doctor kit, or because they wanted to go to the park. Playing with them has been therapeutic to all of us. I laugh at their occurrences, and we all get connected by having a good time. We go to the park, and I become a monster that chases them; play with the dolls and we all become dolls' mommies. I accept to play, not only because of them, but also because of me. It gives me strength, energy, a moment to forget about all that's happening, a time to enjoy my daughters, and a reason to look ahead and continue this battle.

---

thwart their playmate's desires for relatedness. As Ryan and Deci (2017) suggested, if a play partner requires their playmate to relinquish autonomy, ostensibly for the sake of relatedness, both will experience a reduced sense of belonging and, consequently, lower levels of wellness.

Using the ToP, Cordier and colleagues (2010a, 2010b) observed 112 children with attention deficit-hyperactivity disorder (ADHD) playing with a typically developing usual playmate (often a sibling) and compared the play of the children with ADHD with that of 126 typically developing dyads (252 children total). Cordier and colleagues established characteristic patterns of playfulness in the participants with ADHD *and* their typically developing playmates. Although expressing good ideas for play and skillfully negotiating to get their own needs met, the children with ADHD had significantly less ability to respond to playmates' play cues, support playmates in their play, engage intensely and skillfully in social play, or take another's perspective (i.e., share, transition between activities, pretend skillfully). Drawing from Feshbach's (1997) seminal work, Cordier and colleagues (2010a) attributed this pattern to decreased empathy.

Although significantly better at items that measured modifying and persisting with play activities and responding to play cues, many of the typically developing playmates' other ToP scores were similar to those of the children with ADHD. When playing with a child with ADHD, the playmates had difficulty with the intensity and skill of social play, sharing, supporting their playmate, transitioning, and pretending

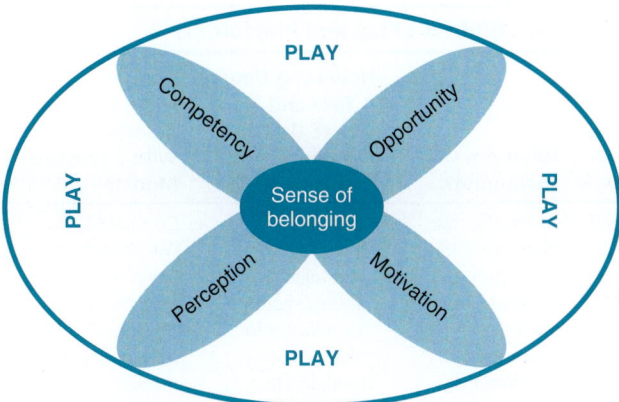

FIGURE 50-2. Interrelationships among components and context of belonging. *Adapted from Allen, K-A., Kern, M. L., Rozek, C. S., McInerney, D. M., & Slavich, G. M. (2021). Belonging: A review of conceptual issues, an integrative framework, and directions for future research.* Australian Journal of Psychology, 73, *87–102. https://doi.org /10.1080/00049530.2021.1883409*

BOX 50-1 ■ Jerad and Jon

Jerad and Jon are 9-year-old third graders and best friends. Similar to many boys their age, both say that recess is the best part of school. Playing tag is one of their favorite playground activities. The school playground is genuinely inclusive of children, such as Jerad and Jon, who use power wheelchairs. On the day they were observed, Jon and Jerad played tag on and around a very large, fully ramped wooden structure. The two moved as fast as they could, navigating the narrow paths and tight turns on the structure, both laughing and screeching. Jerad began in the lead with Jon close behind. At one point, Jon turned around and left the structure, hiding in a shadow and yelling, "Come and get me!" Jerad, in pursuit, yelled at the top of his lungs, "I'm gonna' get you! You little chicken!" Jerad caught Jon and then turned around, yelling for Jon to catch *him.* "Come and get me. Nah nah boo boo." A lot of negotiation followed. Both boys took up the chants. They left the structure and began chasing each other on the paved pathways threading through the playground. They continued to wheel on and off and around the structure, screeching at the tops of their lungs. At one point, Jerad engaged the playground aid, asking her to save him. She responded in a playful voice that she would not. Jon then played a trick on Jerad. He stopped and fell silent. "I'm not your friend," he said. Jerad, hearing the change in Jon's tone, turned around and approached his friend. And Jon tagged him—which led to a renewal of chase and tag.

Jon and Jerad clearly were playing. And just as clearly, they felt a sense of belonging. According to their teachers, this play session was typical of the boys' interactions. The games changed but the evidence of their sense of belonging did not. The social interactions between the boys were an integral component of their play. Jon's and Jerad's play provided a context for their feelings of belonging and, more importantly, their desire for belonging fulfilled a basic psychological need. Play is a common context yielding a sense of belonging. All the criteria Baumeister and Leary (1995) cited as necessary to fundamental human motivations are readily seen in the sense of belonging engendered in play.

BOX 50-2 ■ Marco

Marco is 7 years old and a first grader in a Catholic school not far from his home. Marco is of above average intelligence; his favorite subjects at school are math and music. When asked, Marco reported that he does not have any friends at school. His teacher indicated that he often spends recess in the bathroom; that way he avoids having to play with classmates. At home, Marco says he plays with his 5-year-old brother, Jeremy, but his mother reports that he mostly plays alone. He particularly enjoys playing with his model train set although, again, his mother indicated that his play is quite repetitive. When he was 4, Marco was diagnosed as autistic.

Marco's school enrolled in research implemented by an interdisciplinary team in Sydney, Australia. The project was known as the Sydney Playground Project. Collaborating with school personnel, the research team placed recycled materials on school playgrounds. To be included, materials could not have any obvious play value. They included such things as car tires, milk crates, bread crates, buckets, crash mats, conduit piping, and pool noodles. Children used the materials in many ways, but one of the most popular was to build new structures. Marco was intrigued by the materials and their possibilities. Not long after they appeared on the playground, Marco spent a whole recess period creating a very lifelike motorcycle from crates and tires. Other children saw the motorcycle and began inviting Marco to build it with them. He became part of a small group of boys who routinely played together, gathering up as many loose parts as they could each recess period and constructing something new. During one recess, the boys built a truck and Marco became the driver. He had a steering wheel and a seat belt and could be heard speaking over the truck radio—giving instructions to the other boys in the group.

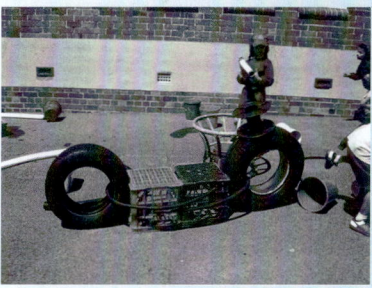

Marco never again spent a recess period in the bathroom. For the first time, Marco went home with stories about what he did with his friends at school; his parents were thrilled. His teacher noted she had never realized Marco had such skills for pretending.

skillfully, although their scores on these items were somewhat less extreme than those of the participants with ADHD. Cordier and colleagues suggested that, similar to the participants with ADHD, the pattern of the playmates' scores reflected lack of empathy. Cordier and colleagues proposed that the playmates might have mirrored some of the negative behaviors of the children with ADHD but, to keep the play flowing, the playmates became more adaptive and flexible (Cordier et al., 2010b).

In a proposition of their Relationships Motivation Theory, Ryan and Deci (2017) offered a plausible explanation for the playmates' apparent lack of empathy when playing with

TABLE 50-1 | Therapeutic Reasoning Assessment Table: Measures of Children's Play and Playfulness

Which Tool?	Who Was This Tool Designed For?	Is This a Type of Tool This Person Can Use? What Is Required of the Person?	What Am I Measuring?	How Long Does It Take and Where Do I Administer This Assessment?	Is the Tool Associated With a Practice Model?
Test of Playfulness (ToP; Bundy et al., 2001; Skard & Bundy, 2008)	Ages 6 months to 18 years old Typically developing children (Serrada-Tejeda et al., 2021; Waldman-Levi et al., 2022) Children on the autism spectrum (Kent et al., 2020; Muys et al., 2006) Children with physical disabilities (Bulgarelli et al., 2018; Harkness & Bundy, 2001) Children with ADHD (Wilkes-Gillan et al., 2022) Mothers and children victims of domestic violence (Waldman-Levi & Weintraub, 2015)	Child/adolescent is observed during free play for about 15 minutes. Observation-based assessment using a 4-point scale. Items are scored in terms of extent, intensity, and skillfulness.	Assess the four characteristics of playfulness: internal control, intrinsic motivation, freedom from unnecessary constraints of reality, and framing.	Administered in any setting and takes approximately 15 minutes for observation Translated to Spanish, Danish, German	Compatible with Person-Environment-Occupation (PEO) and developmental models
My Child's Play Questionnaire (MCP; Schneider & Rosenblum, 2014)	Parents of children ages 3–9 years old Parents of children with neurodevelopmental disorders (Romero-Ayuso et al., 2021) Parents of school-age children (Vigil-Dopico et al., 2022)	Parent questionnaire with 50 items with a 5-point Likert scale to indicate the frequency in which the child shows the behavior in the item.	Assess parents' perception about child's play performance. Includes four factors: executive functions, interpersonal relationships, play choices and preferences, and opportunities in the environment.	Administered in any setting and is reported to be a short, simple, and easy questionnaire for parents Translated in Spanish	Compatible with PEO and developmental models
Child Behavior Inventory of Playfulness (CBI; Rogers et al., 1998)	Mothers of Chinese preschool children (Tun et al., 2020) Teachers of Japanese preschool children (Taylor & Rogers, 2001)	Questionnaire that can be completed by parents or teachers. The playfulness factor consists of 21 items about overall playfulness, orientation to a task, intrinsic motivation, nonlinearity, freedom from externally imposed rules, and active involvement during the task. The externality factor consists of seven items related to behaviors that could reduce a child's ability to play. Items are scored with a 5-point Likert scale to indicate to what extent the item characterizes the child.	Assess playfulness as a trait characteristic. Includes two factors: general playfulness and externality.	Administered in school or home setting and takes approximately 15 minutes Translated in Greek and Japanese	

Evidence-Based Practice

Play Intervention for Children With Attention Deficit-Hyperactivity Disorder and Their Playmates

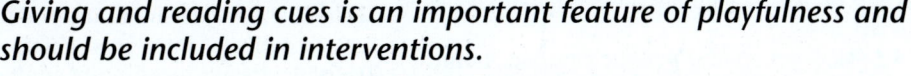

Giving and reading cues is an important feature of playfulness and should be included in interventions.

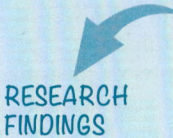

RESEARCH FINDINGS

Building on Cordier's work identifying common patterns of playfulness with children with ADHD, Wilkes-Gillan and colleagues (Barnes et al., 2017; Wilkes-Gillan et al., 2014a, 2014b, 2016, 2017) developed an intervention in which they convinced both the children with ADHD and their playmates that they would have more fun if their playmates also were having fun. They taught the children to read the cues of their playmates and to figure out how to better support their playmates' play. They employed video and live modeling and a home program featuring Oober, a fictional alien who required assistance from an earthling to learn how to fit in and belong. The result was that participants attained significantly higher ToP scores at the end of the intervention that were generalized to their homes and maintained for at least 18 months.

APPLICATIONS

➡ Giving and reading cues is an important feature of playfulness; take time in intervention to guide children to develop these skills.
➡ Playing and playfulness require social interactions with others; peer modeling, in this case around giving and reading cues, is a tool worth considering.

REFERENCES

Barnes, G., Wilkes-Gillan, S., Cordier, R., & Bundy, A. (2017). The social play, social skills and parent-child relationships of children with ADHD 12 months following a RCT of a play-based intervention. *Australian Occupational Therapy Journal, 64,* 1–9. https://doi.org/10.1111/1440-1630.12417

Wilkes-Gillan, S., Bundy, A., Cordier, R., Lincoln, M., & Hancock, N. (2014a). Child outcomes of a pilot parent-delivered intervention for improving the social play skills of children with ADHD and their playmates. *Developmental Neurorehabilitation, 19,* 238–245. https://doi.org/10.3109/17518423.2014.948639

Wilkes-Gillan, S., Bundy, A., Cordier, R., & Lincoln, M. (2014b). Eighteen month follow-up of a play-based intervention to improve the social play skills of children with ADHD. *Australian Occupational Therapy Journal, 61,* 299–307. https://doi.org/10.1111/1440-1630.12124

Wilkes-Gillan, S., Bundy, A., Cordier, R., Lincoln, M., & Chen, Y.-W. (2016). A randomised controlled trial of a play-based intervention to improve the social play skills of children with attention deficit hyperactivity disorder (ADHD). *PLoS One, 11*(8), 1–22. https://doi.org/10.1371/journal.pone.0160558

Wilkes-Gillan, S., Cantrill, A., Cordier, R., Barnes, G., Hancock, N., & Bundy, A. (2017). The use of video-modelling as a method for improving the social play skills of children with attention deficit hyperactivity disorder (ADHD) and their playmates. *British Journal of Occupational Therapy, 80,* 196–207. https://doi.org/10.1177/0308022617692819

children with ADHD. "To the degree that an individual in a relationship relates to the partner more as an object, stereotype, or thing, rather than as a person intrinsically worthy of respect, the partner will accordingly experience thwarting of the basic psychological needs, resulting in a lower quality relationship and poorer well-being" (p. 314). The Evidence-Based Practice box describes an evidence-based intervention that focused on building the components of playfulness in children with ADHD and later with autism.

Considering play in the delivery of mental health services is pertinent. The question is: When? The identification of a diminished sense of belongingness is a main indicator that

play can be considered as a part of the assessment and/or intervention process. Recall the previously highlighted link between belonging and mental health. As a fundamental human motivation (Allen, Kern, et al., 2021; Baumeister & Leary, 1995), a sense of belonging entails the need to relate to others; failure to satisfy this need threatens health and well-being (Ryan & Deci, 2017). In addition, there are links between the elements of belonging and the elements of play and playfulness, which were previously discussed. Interviewing and listening carefully to the stories shared by persons related to their sense of belonging can be an important part of the assessment process. Some examples of the questions that might elicit stories about belonging and planning include:

- Who are the most significant people in your life? Why?
- Who are the people toward whom you feel closest or trust?
- What are the kinds of groups in your community with whom you regularly participate (e.g., a sports team, church group, book club, gaming club)? What motivates you to do so?
- Among the places you routinely participate (e.g., home, school, work), where do you feel most involved? Why?
- As you consider the people around you, who are the ones who form your main support network? What made you think about them?

See Chapter 49: Connectedness and Belonging for more measures of belonging, both formal and informal. 🤝

Assessment of Play and Playfulness in Mental Health

Recognizing motivation as a primary component of playfulness, this section emphasizes the importance of interviews and tools that provide the opportunity to gain knowledge about a person's interests and motivations. Interviewing is essential to any evaluation. Getting information about the person's interests, use of time, participation in diverse occupations, and enjoyment of activities can determine if play or playfulness is appropriate as part of the treatment plan. OTPs can assess both play and playfulness using structured and unstructured strategies. Verbal interviewing and completion of graphics or tables depicting the person's use of time are examples of unstructured or informal strategies that can provide valuable information about the person's interests.

Caillois's (2001) categorization of play can be useful for helping to understand *why* a player chooses particular play activities. That is, what are players seeking in their play? What are their motivations? What about particular play activities give them enjoyment? Identifying the sources of motivation can be particularly useful for helping individuals select the play activities that will best meet their needs.

Caillois (2001) named four types of play that reflect the motive for the play and apply across the life span: agon (i.e., competition), alea (i.e., chance), mimicry (i.e., pretend, simulation), and ilinx (i.e., the pursuit of pure sensation or "vertigo"). Caillois went on to say that any one play activity can represent more than one play type. He placed play activities on continua according to how purely each reflects its primary category and how much it also reflects another category. Caillois further defined two additional terms: paidia (the spontaneous manifestation of play characterized by disturbance and tumult) and ludus (a taste for difficulty). These terms, at opposite ends of another continuum, describe the degree to which rules and order are present in each of the four categories of play. For example, children swinging or twirling fall more toward the paidia end of the ilinx continuum, and skiing and mountain climbing fall toward the ludic end.

Specific information about a person's participation in playful occupations can also be collected through instruments such as the Occupational Experience Profile (e.g., Atler, 2016; Atler et al., 2016, 2017) or Experience Sampling Methodology (Hektner et al., 2007). Other structured or more formal strategies include interest profiles such as the Kid Play Profile, Preteen Play Profile, and the Adolescent Leisure Interest Profile (Henry, 2008). Other examples include the Children's Assessment of Participation and Enjoyment (CAPE), which can be used along with the Preferences for Activities of Children (PAC; King et al., 2004). Although these latter tools are not direct assessments of play, they include related content. Table 50-2 provides more information about tools to measure activities of interest in children and adolescents, and Table 50-3 details measures of adult playfulness.

Tables 50-1 and 50-3 include examples of measures of play and playfulness for children and measures of playfulness for adults that focus on playfulness or its components. A systematic review (Romli & Wan Yunus, 2020) on the evidence of psychometric properties and clinical utility of play instruments in occupational therapy identified the use of the ToP in combination with the Test of Environmental Supportiveness as observation-based instruments to obtain useful information about intrinsic aspects of play. The My Child's Play (MCP) questionnaire also was identified as a useful questionnaire-based play instrument (Romli & Wan Yunus, 2020).

Identifying evaluation tools related to play and playfulness for children can be easier than identifying instruments targeted to adolescents and, especially, to adults. Indeed, research about adult play and playfulness is still scarce. Most of the tools available assess adults' playfulness as a personality trait (see selected examples in Table 50-3). However, it is possible to find in them, at minimum, some of the elements of playfulness. As an example, the Adult Playfulness Trait Scale (APTS; Shen et al., 2014a, 2014b) includes the dimensions of fun-seeking motivation, uninhibitedness, and spontaneity. Fun-seeking motivation includes the areas of fun belief, initiative, and reactivity. Aspects of intrinsic motivation are embedded in these dimensions of the APTS, in items such as "I think fun is a very important part in life." Also, aspects related to control and freedom from unnecessary constraints of reality are depicted in items of the uninhibitedness dimension (e.g., I understand social rules but most of the time I am not restricted by them).

It is important to note that the APTS, as well as the Other-directed, Lighthearted, Intellectual, and Whimsical measure (OLIW playfulness questionnaire) and most measures of adult playfulness, conceptualize playfulness as a personality trait. This can be an advantage when considering play as part of occupational therapy mental health services for adults. Tools such as these might help the person to gain awareness about their overall attitude/state/trait when approaching life situations. However, using this type of measure should not replace strategies to get information about the person's interests, preferences, and occupational participation. This knowledge is critical and can be gained using either informal or formal strategies (e.g., interviews, interest profiles).

An additional consideration when evaluating play in mental health is the environment. Play environments can make important differences in the participation and performance of those involved. Indeed, concepts such as playful work design and playful learning environments or gamification of learning have become more common in research (Bakker & van Woerkom, 2017; Koeners & Francis, 2020). However,

TABLE 50-2 | Therapeutic Reasoning Assessment Table: Tools to Measure Activities of Interest in Children and Adolescents

Which Tool?	Who Was This Tool Designed For?	Is This a Type of Tool This Person Can Use? What Is Required of the Person?	What Am I Measuring?	How Long Does It Take and Where Do I Administer This Assessment?	Is the Tool Associated With a Practice Model?
Pediatric Interest Profiles: Kid Play Profile, Preteen Play Profile, and the Adolescent Leisure Interest Profile (Henry, 2008)	Children, preteens, and adolescents with and without disabilities (Henry, 2008) Children with no disabilities (Lugton et al., 2020)	Children/adolescents are asked multiple questions addressing feelings of enjoyment and competence in the activities, and whether the activities are done alone or with others. Categories of activities for the Kid and Preteen Profiles are Sports, Outdoor, Summer, Winter, Indoor, Creative, Socializing Activities, and Lessons and Classes. The Adolescent Leisure Profile substitutes the Summer, Winter, and Indoor categories for Relaxation, Intellectual, and Club/Community Activities. Drawings are used to depict play and leisure activities (Henry, 2008).	Play and leisure interests and participation of children, preteens, and adolescents	Administered in any setting and takes approximately 10–20 minutes	Not specifically but compatible with PEO, Model of Human Occupation (MOHO), and developmental models
Children's Assessment of Participation and Enjoyment and Preferences for Activities of Children (CAPE/PAC; King et al., 2004, 2007)	Ages 6–21 years of age Children with intellectual disabilities (King et al., 2013) Children with cerebral palsy (Imms et al., 2017) Children with autism (Potvin et al., 2013)	Children self-report (self-administered or interviewer-assisted) about participation and preferences for 55 activities (without parental assistance). Activities are classified into two categories (Formal and Informal) and five types: Recreational, Active Physical, Social, Skill-Based, and Self-Improvement/Educational.	The CAPE assesses children's participation in recreation and leisure activities outside of mandated school activities. The PAC assesses child's preferences for those activities. Together they assess six dimensions of participation: Diversity, Intensity, Where, With whom, Enjoyment, and Preferences	Administered in home, school, or community setting CAPE: 30–45 minutes PAC: 15–20 minutes Translations in Portuguese, Arabic, German, Norwegian, Swedish, Dutch, and Spanish	PEO model

available tools about playful environments relate mainly to the extent to which aspects of the environment (e.g., other people, space, and/or available materials) support or hinder children's play. This is the case of the Test of Environmental Supportiveness (Skard & Bundy, 2008) and the Parent/Caregiver's Support of Young Children's Playfulness Scale (Waldman-Levy & Bundy, 2016).

As of this writing, a generic measure of playful environments has not been developed. Nonetheless, practitioners can collect valuable information about the environment by interviewing and through careful observation. Very likely the observation of natural environments is more feasible when working with younger individuals, as adults might be uncomfortably aware when being observed. This can impact their behavior negatively, even though the focus of the evaluation is environmental support rather than the adult's behavior or performance.

Clinical Reasoning to Guide Assessment of Play and Playfulness

As is the case in any service delivery, the specifics related to the assessment of play in mental health must match the needs of individuals and their situations. This section describes a clinical reasoning pathway using the cases of Marco (see Box 50-2) and Sonia, a youth transitioning from high school to college who is experiencing significant anxiety. This method of reasoning can guide decision-making when considering play as part of an assessment process.

Suppose an OTP receives a referral to evaluate Marco, a 7-year-old first grader who avoids playing with classmates (or just being with them) during school recess. The OTP begins to analyze this situation, looking at the information communicated by Marco's parents and teacher and thinking in terms

TABLE 50-3 | Therapeutic Reasoning Assessment Table: Measures of Adult Playfulness

Which Tool?	Who Was This Tool Designed For?	Is This a Type of Tool This Person Can Use? What Is Required of the Person?	What Am I Measuring?	How Long Does It Take and Where Do I Administer This Assessment?	Is the Tool Associated With a Practice Model?
Adult Playfulness Trait Scale (APTS; Shen et al., 2014a, 2014b)	College students to older adults (Saliba & Barden, 2021; Shen et al., 2014a, 2014b)	Person responds to 19 items on a 7-point Likert scale to indicate level of agreement with statements formulated around fun-seeking motivation, uninhibitedness, and spontaneity.	Measures the level to which the person aligns with playfulness; main scale looks at fun-seeking motivation (with subscales of fun belief, initiative, and reactivity), uninhibitedness, and spontaneity	Administered in any setting and takes approximately 30 minutes	No
Other-directed, Lighthearted, Intellectual, and Whimsical (OLIW) Playfulness Scale (Proyer, 2017)	Adolescents (Proyer & Tandler, 2020) College students (Proyer, 2017) Various studies have used it with adults in general (e.g., Brauer et al., 2021; Brauer & Proyer, 2017; Farley et al., 2021)	Person responds to a questionnaire consisting of 28 items; seven per each of the four facets, using a 7-level response scale based on level of agreement. Examples are: Other-directed: "I have close friends with whom I can just fool around and be silly." Lighthearted: "Many people take their lives too seriously; when things do not work you just have to improvise." Intellectual: "If I want to develop a new idea further and think about it, I like to do this in a playful manner." Whimsical: "I have the reputation of being somewhat unusual or flamboyant." A short version (OLIW-S) of 12 items was developed with initial validity evidence (Proyer et al., 2020).	Assesses four facets of playfulness: Other-directed, Lighthearted, Intellectual, and Whimsical	Administered in any setting and takes 10–12 minutes	No

of belonging, and identifies Marco's lack of connectedness to his classmates and difficulty contributing to them in a way that they would value.

Intuitively, the OTP might think that obtaining an interest profile would be a good starting point to assess Marco. However, having obtained information from his parents and teacher and acknowledging that the main reason for Marco's referral is inherently attached to a specific context (i.e., school recess), the OTP must look for an opportunity to evaluate the school recess environment and, if possible, Marco's participation in it. Ideally, this would occur through direct observation, either unstructured (by observing general aspects serving as facilitators or barriers to play) or structured. For example, using the ToP together with the Test of Environmental Supportiveness (TOES) can provide useful information about the environment and Marco's playfulness. After obtaining the best information possible about the environment and Marco's participation, the OTP can decide whether to administer an interest profile, always keeping in mind that the core of Marco's assessment should be to get the necessary information to determine an intervention pathway to promote his participation in school recess.

Now, imagine a referral to evaluate Sonia, a youth transitioning from high school to college, who is experiencing significant anxiety and reporting that she feels as if she does not fit in this new environment. She reports feeling lonely, having sleeping problems, being unusually irritable, being unable to concentrate when studying, and feeling hopeless about her future. As a first step, the OTP considers whether any of her concerns suggest a lack of the sense of belonging.

The OTP knows that life transitions can affect a sense of belonging, and this seems to be an important factor in Sonia's situation (e.g., she reports feeling as if she does not fit in). Of course, the OTP would want to obtain more information about Sonia's health history (e.g., Is this the first time she has experienced this level of anxiety?). Depending on the context of service delivery, the OTP might be able to get that information in advance (e.g., from a discussion with other members of the interdisciplinary team) or by asking her during the initial occupational therapy interview.

The initial interview could be an opportunity to obtain more information about Sonia's sense of belonging, either through informal questions (such as the ones presented previously, which can be adapted to her situation) or by using a belongingness questionnaire. Also, the OTP needs to gather information about Sonia's interests, time use, and occupational participation. Together, this information will help the OTP determine if play and playfulness could be an important piece in Sonia's treatment plan. If so, the OTP could consider the pertinence of administering an adult playfulness scale to further guide the decision process.

Recall the important overall considerations during assessment:

1. Analyze the sense of belonging to determine the pertinence of play and playfulness as part of the assessment and intervention processes.
2. Identify the adequacy of components that contribute to a sense of belonging—competencies, opportunities, motivations, and perceptions—through interview or standard assessment.
3. Consider how play fits into the individual's life. Practitioners can include various areas when considering play as part of the assessment process in mental health, including the person's interests, use of time, and occupational participation; the person's playfulness; and the playfulness of the environment. The decision about which areas to emphasize as part of the assessment process must intrinsically respond to the individual's situation and reported main needs.
4. Consider whether play is a potential medium for, or desired outcome of, intervention.

Intervention: Enhancing Mental Health Through Play

Finding evidence-based occupational therapy interventions employing play as a means or an outcome for children is much easier than identifying research about play and playfulness in adulthood. Van Vleet and Feeney (2015) proposed a model about the immediate and long-term outcomes of play behavior (Fig. 50-3), which comprises three core components of play behaviors in adulthood: (1) goal of amusement/fun, (2) enthusiastic and in-the-moment attitude, and (3) highly interactive. These three are in line with the components of the Model of Playfulness (Skard & Bundy, 2008). For example, the goal of amusement/fun can be paralleled with a component of intrinsic motivation in Skard and Bundy's model.

According to Van Vleet and Feeney (2015), playfulness can lead to personal and relational outcomes. Positive affect and reduced daily stress are among the immediate personal outcomes. Feeling accepted, valued, and compatible (i.e., as though one belongs) during play as well as in intimate relationships, reduced conflict, and effective communication are relational outcomes. In the long term, reduced chronic stress, flexible thinking patterns, and psychological and physical health are important personal outcomes (Van Vleet & Feeney, 2015).

Considering playfulness as an aspect of intervention with the potential to contribute to concrete personal and relational outcomes is an important affirmation of its value to occupational therapy interventions with people of all ages. Integrating play in therapy from a mental health perspective entails one or both of the following key aspects: (a) the potential of *personal playful moments* to contribute to the individual's well-being, and/or (b) the potential of playful environments to contribute to the individual's well-being. These must be considered in light of the person's history and evaluation results.

Personal Playful Moments

Personal playful moments refer to periods of time, however brief, in which a person is actively engaged in a playful situation. These situations vary widely, such as playing hide and seek, joyfully dancing with a partner, and engaging in playful teasing with friends. Identifying opportunities for individuals to get involved in playful moments can enhance health and well-being. This section describes examples of the use of personal playful moments with children and adults.

As mentioned, research about play-focused interventions with adults is still very young. One example is based on a work under development and relates to the use of play to intervene with mothers in cancer treatment having young children. A second example involves the potential use of play to help adults who experience clinical levels of anxiety.

Based on a phenomenological study (Román-Oyola et al., 2023) about play between mothers who were breast cancer survivors and who also had young children during their treatment, Román-Oyola and colleagues (2022) proposed the development of a play-based coaching intervention to improve well-being of dyads of mothers with cancer and their children. Narratives of cancer survivors indicated that they indeed wished to engage in playful interaction with their children; however, while in treatment, various external factors hindered the ability to have those playful moments with their children. The main external factors identified were side effects associated either with the condition or the treatment, especially physical and mental fatigue; differences between the child's and adult's interests and abilities; and lack of time (because of the many health-care requirements added to their ordinary routines and responsibilities).

The common barriers to mothers experiencing personal playful moments led to a play-based coaching intervention consisting of three blocks: (1) "potential modifications to activities and/or environment," (2) "matching the adult's and the child's way of playing," and (3) "making play part of the routine." Each block includes an in-person session followed by a virtual session. Coaching should reflect the theme of the block.

During in-person sessions, the practitioner assumes the role of a coaching partner, discussing the mother's play moments with the child and additional areas of interest. The intent is to help mothers gain awareness of the elements of playfulness (i.e., intrinsic motivation, shared control, suspension of reality, and framing) and find ways to help them create moments of playful interactions with their young children. As suggested by previous exploratory researchers (Román-Oyola et al., 2022) and by Van Vleet and Feeney (2015), such playful interactions entail important personal and relational benefits that can impact health outcomes of cancer patients and, indeed, of patients with other chronic conditions.

The second example relates to anxiety among college students. Prevalence of anxiety in this population is documented, with 66% reporting feeling overwhelmingly anxious (American College Health Association, 2019). Interventions for common mental health problems among college students

Being a Psychosocial OT Practitioner

Overcoming Anxiety Through Occupations That Enhance Belonging

Identifying Psychosocial Strengths and Needs

OTPs frequently encounter people whose psychosocial challenges, such as anxiety, impair participation. Consider the story of Sonia, who has just transitioned from high school to college. Sonia was very sociable in high school and had several good friends. However, she is now experiencing significant anxiety and fears she will never belong at college and might even flunk out. She reports feeling lonely, having sleeping problems, being unusually irritable, being unable to concentrate when studying, and feeling hopeless about her future. Sonia is described further in the chapter.

Sonia's anxiety and lack of a sense of belonging have led her to avoid going out and socializing. The OTP believes that, with intervention, Sonia will recapture the self she was in high school. However, without intervention, Sonia's fears and social isolation may spiral into more significant anxiety and lead to self-fulfilling prophecies about not belonging and flunking out of college.

Using a Holistic Occupational Therapy Approach

Through a semistructured interview about her feelings of loneliness and fear of not fitting in and failing coursework, Sonia's OTP helped her identify how her beliefs affect her participation. To encourage self-reflection, the OTP asked Sonia about her history with school, friends, and anxiety and how things were different or the same now that she is in college.

Sonia shared a history of anxiety that began when she was a young teen. She felt the same fear of not fitting in when she started high school, although those fears resolved as she became more involved in school and with friends. She also had similar difficulties with sleeping and studying and felt angry and irritable at times during high school.

Together, Sonia and the OTP explored barriers contributing to Sonia's anxiety and interfering with her ability to develop a sense of belonging in college. Most of the barriers were negative self-perceptions. The OTP hypothesized that helping Sonia reframe her self-perceptions would increase her willingness to socialize and engage in activities to improve her sense of belonging. Feeling a greater sense of belonging would also contribute to reducing Sonia's anxiety. With the OTP's encouragement, Sonia identified cognitive strategies to help her change her negative self-perceptions and feel a greater sense of belonging in her new environment. Sonia kept a log of the barriers and strategies identified during the session.

Barriers: Negative (self) perceptions interfering with Sonia's ability to develop a sense of belonging	**Strategies** to help Sonia develop a better sense of belonging
"I can't stop thinking that my social skills will never be enough or that I will never have the right clothes or hairstyle for others to like me."	"In high school, my best friends were in the choir, and we had so much fun together. I really enjoy singing and am good at it." (Competency; Perception) "The college choir is holding tryouts next month. If I make the choir, I might also make new friends." (Motivation; Opportunity)
"I'm sure I will never make friends or fit in here."	"There is a girl on my floor who often sits alone in the cafeteria. I wonder if she is lonely, too. I'll ask if I can sit with her the next time I see her there." (Perception; Opportunity) "Maybe she would also go shopping with me for some new clothes. And I really like her hairstyle; I wonder where she gets it done." (Motivation; Opportunity)
"I will probably flunk out of college, so none of this matters anyway."	"I've always been good at school. My close friends in high school were also straight-A students. If I schedule enough time to study, the same things will happen at college." (Competency, Opportunity) "I know that feeling like a good student helps me feel better about myself overall. When I feel better about myself, I'm a much better friend." (Perception, Competency)

Sonia and the OTP create weekly goals and a daily schedule with time for studying and socializing. The OTP asks Sonia to continue writing down any thoughts and perceptions that may interfere with her goal of developing a sense of belonging at college and identify additional reframing strategies to review at future sessions. Sonia and the OTP also role-play scenarios where Sonia introduces herself to others to help her consider and prepare for multiple social situations that have caused her anxiety in the past. Sonia plans to meet with the OTP monthly to monitor her progress.

Reflective Questions

1. What other assessments might the OTP consider for Sonia? Provide a rationale for the chosen assessments.
2. Sonia indicated that she has trouble sleeping. How might her sleep difficulties impact her mental health and social participation? How might the OTP help Sonia with rest and sleep?
3. Design role-play activities to help Sonia develop skills and self-confidence in making new friends.

(i.e., anxiety and depression) are based mainly on cognitive behavioral and mindfulness therapy (Huang et al., 2018; Worsley et al., 2022). Although these have demonstrated effectiveness, according to a meta-analysis by Huang and colleagues (2018), other interventions such as art, exercise, and peer support showed the highest effect sizes regarding the reduction of anxiety in university and college students with generalized anxiety disorder.

Recall the case of Sonia, a youth transitioning from high school to college who reported feeling as if she did not fit the college environment. During an initial interview, the OTP got additional information about her. She is enrolled in her first semester in pursuit of a bachelor's degree in biology. Sonia has always been an outstanding student. Indeed, she is the first one in her family able to go to college after getting a scholarship that covered all her tuition.

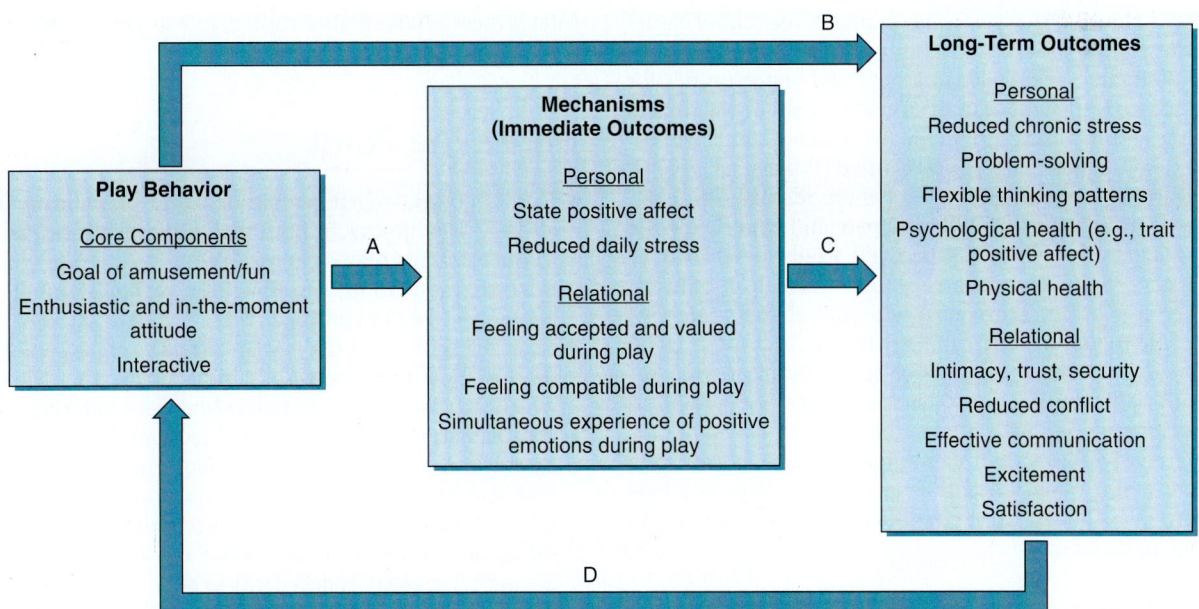

FIGURE 50-3. Model of the effects of play in adulthood. *Reprinted with permission from Van Vleet, M., & Feeney, B. C. (2015). Young at heart: A perspective for advancing research on play in adulthood.* Perspectives on Psychological Science, 10(5), 639–645. https://doi.org/10.1177/1745691615596789

As soon as she moved to her lodging, she found work as a cashier in a community pharmacy during the weekends, which she thought would be perfect to combine with the earnings from the university's work-study program. However, she says she just can't understand what is happening to her. During high school, she used to be much busier than now, but that never affected her academic performance. Sonia used to participate in the school choir, offered math tutoring as a volunteer to elementary school students Mondays to Thursdays, assisted with house chores, did some outdoor activities with friends during weekends, and worked as a cashier in a local store twice a week. Now, everything is so different. She is feeling lonely, very irritable, hopeless, and unable to concentrate when studying. Indeed, the last time she was supposed to attend an examination, she did not show up because she felt so tense that she thought she would be unable to be successful. That's what made her decide to seek help.

If play has not been the subject of research about helping college students experiencing anxiety, the question is: How could playfulness help Sonia with the management of her anxiety? Acknowledge that Sonia is going through a life transition, which inherently can affect a person's sense of belonging. Furthermore, she used to enjoy outdoor activities with friends, participated in a choir, and was a math tutor volunteer for children. Based on this, steps to help Sonia could include:

1. Join Sonia in an analysis of the use of her time and occupational balance.
2. Orient Sonia to the components of playfulness and its benefits.
3. Help Sonia identify ordinary ways in which she could use and take advantage of a playful attitude.
4. Help Sonia identify a few activities, preferably at the university, in which she could participate while experiencing, at least to some extent, the components of playfulness.

Of course, additional approaches could help Sonia, such as applying strategies to improve her study skills and modifying her physical and sensory environments to improve focus during studying. However, your focus here is on approaches that involve the value of playfulness. Although presented as steps, the previous examples would not necessarily need to be applied in sequence. For example, steps two and three can potentially be intertwined. The OTP might work with Sonia to identify ordinary ways to use playfulness while orienting her about the components of playfulness.

Individuals will be involved in a playful activity to the extent that they feel intrinsically motivated toward the activity, perceive that they have some degree of control over it, feel free from the constraints of reality, and find themselves in a context characterized by cues that contribute to keeping them immersed in what is occurring (Skard & Bundy, 2008). Ordinary ways in which a person might feel this way are while participating with others in a competitive game and while involved in something they enjoy so much that they feel intrinsically motivated and skillful enough to perceive themselves as being in control. Further, they can get immersed in it to the point of feeling some freedom from reality constraints.

For example, people might enjoy going snorkeling with friends for reasons that go beyond its benefits as a recreational activity. Snorkeling may also satisfy their curiosity and provide them with joyful unexpected moments, such as finding a fish cave for the first time. Every time something similar to this happens, an "Aquaman" feeling (suspension of reality) invades them, driving them to continue enjoying snorkeling. The same "feeling" might occur while dancing, during humorous teasing with friends, or when enacting a scene while telling a personal story to a close friend or family member (Van Vleet & Feeney, 2015).

In Sonia's case, it would be pertinent to join her in thinking of her interests and reflecting on her feelings while engaged in those activities. What made her enjoy being a math tutor for children? How did she feel while singing in the school choir? Was she able to sing "as if nobody listens"? The goal is to guide Sonia into acknowledging potential opportunities for playfulness. Despite the scarcity of evidence about playfulness in adults, a study using a randomized placebo-controlled intervention suggests that it can be learned (Proyer et al., 2021).

Regarding step 4, helping the person identify some activities in which they could participate and experience the components of playfulness, the OTP would need to offer guidance to Sonia about how to find information of available services or extracurricular activities at the university. Being able to identify such an activity (e.g., a choir, a group dedicated to some sort of outdoor activity) can provide Sonia with opportunities of ordinary moments of playfulness, whereas interacting with others, sharing positive emotions, feeling compatibility, and gaining acceptance as part of a group can affirm her sense of belonging to college as a new place to her. This, in turn, could help Sonia to reduce and manage her anxiety.

Playful Environments

Physical and social aspects of the environment can facilitate or hinder playfulness. This is true when referring to children and adults. As explained in Marco's case, an evaluation of the environment and opportunities for playfulness within it could lead to important modifications that would facilitate playful moments not only for a single person, but for an entire group or community.

The benefits of playful environments have been studied in a variety of contexts, including some typically frequented by adults, such as higher education and workspaces. Bakker and van Woerkom (2017) introduced the concept of playful work design to refer to the process through which employees proactively create conditions within work activities to foster enjoyment and challenge without altering the design of the work itself. Playful work design helps employees be more engaged and creative, and counteracts a lack of enthusiasm and energy associated with emotionally draining or repetitive and tedious tasks (Bakker et al., 2020).

Koeners and Francis (2020) referred to "Playful Universities" and stated that playful environments within higher education counteract a fear of failing and avoidance of risk and promote a true cocreation of knowledge. Playful educational approaches provide opportunities to create and experience the joy associated with discovery of knowledge in safe and failure-free environments (Heljakka, 2023). Therefore, playful resilience, "a quality of individuals who deliberately and determinedly employ their playfulness in order to relate, react, and pro-act in overcoming mental stress" (Heljakka, 2023, p. 2), is enhanced. Participants in a phenomenological study about play as a foundation to learning identified the following benefits of playful learning in higher education: relational safety and warm classroom environments, removal of barriers to learning, awakening of positive affect and motivation, and ignition of an open and engaged learning stance (Forbes, 2021).

Although research about ways to infuse playfulness into environments is relatively scarce, OTPs can analyze social and physical aspects of diverse contexts (e.g., home, community areas, schoolyards) to increase playfulness.

Interprofessional collaboration also can be a great advantage for this purpose.

Here's the Point

- Play is action—what people do—and playfulness is an attitude—an approach. Both play and playfulness, as well as the elements that compose them (i.e., internal control, intrinsic motivation, freedom from reality, framing), are best considered as continua.

- Research shows that the neural correlates of play and playfulness show that almost all animals play. The degree to which they play seems to reflect brain or brain region size and the nature of their social interactions. In humans, the cerebellum as well as multiple neural networks support play and playfulness. Further, reward and pleasure, sensations linked to play, are associated with the neurotransmitter dopamine; the brain's use of dopamine is increased during play. Deep engagement in play, sometimes called flow, is linked to a norepinephrine pathway that underlies task engagement and motivation, implicating norepinephrine in play and playfulness.

- Engaging in play yields many benefits including supporting overall development, learning to establish and maintain social relationships, developing emotional regulation, and acquiring skills for coping with engagement in an ever-changing environment. In contrast, play deprivation can have long-term negative effects on health and development. Play also serves as practice for the unexpected; through play, people develop flexibility to deal with the unexpected. Thus, play is core to a person's ability to adapt.

- The relationship between play and mental health is complex. Mental health-related conditions can impair social relationships and inadequate social connectedness is linked to mental health concerns. Through play, people establish social bonds and develop a sense of belonging that is core to mental well-being. In playing, one can genuinely connect with a "playmate," supporting a sense of belonging and developing empathy, problem-solving, creativity, cooperation, and others. Although engaging in play is challenged in stressful situations, such as those that disrupt daily life, playing may be exactly what is needed to manage occupational disruption and support mental health.

- In considering play to promote mental health, when an individual does not experience a sense of belonging, practitioners should examine their playfulness and involvement in meaningful play. Thus, it may be helpful to begin the intervention process by assessing a person's sense of belonging through interview or careful observation. Depending on the findings, practitioners may move on to assessing elements of play and playfulness.

- Assessing playfulness involves examining intrinsic motivation for play (what is the individual seeking). This can be accomplished through interview and structured assessment of interests, time use, and participation. Assessing playfulness also necessitates considering skills reflecting internal control and giving and reading cues in support of engaging in and maintaining play transactions in the human and nonhuman environment. Interventions designed around cue reading have been shown to be effective in supporting playfulness in children with ADHD.

- Context is core to playfulness. A foundation for intervention was suggested, using a framework developed by Allen, Kern, and colleagues (2021) comprising four interrelated components: competencies, opportunities, motivations, and perceptions. Integrating play in therapy with the intent to increase well-being and mental health entails addressing (a) personal playful moments and (b) playful environments in light of the person's history and evaluation results.

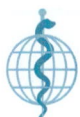 Visit the online resource center at FADavis.com to access the videos.

Apply It Now

1. You Learn More in an Hour of Play Than a Year of Conversation

Conjure up an image of one of your best friends: someone with whom you feel a genuine sense of belonging. How does play contribute to your relationship and your sense of belonging? Relive and describe some play transactions that stick out in your mind. Do you believe that Plato was correct in saying that you learn more in an hour of play than a year of conversation? Why or why not? Discuss with a friend.

2. Video Exercise: Playing for Mother Undergoing Cancer Treatment

Pair up with another student in your class or form a small group of students. Access and watch the "Playing for Mother Undergoing Cancer Treatment" video at the online resource center at FADavis.com. Then, discuss and together answer the following questions.

Reflective Questions
- We often think of play as an occupation for children and youth; however, this video reminds us of play as a co-occupation. How can OTPs support adults in this important co-occupation? What barriers might be present, and how could you address them?
- OTPs understand that the various roles individuals play are an important part of their identity as occupational beings. How can we support individuals living with chronic conditions and/or physical disabilities to reconnect with their previous roles and identities, despite their limitations and/or the barriers that might be present?
- Through her experience, Marylein learned to cope with her fears and anxieties and came to terms with her limitations, ultimately learning to ask for help when she needed it. When working with people in similar situations, how can we facilitate and foster this sense of resilience and help individuals recognize that asking for help is not admitting to failure or weakness, but rather that depending on others is an avenue in which we can thrive, heal, and live?

3. Brain Hat

Ellen McHenry's Basement Workshop offers free educational interventions and downloads (https://ellenjmchenry.com), one of which is the "Brain Hat." As you construct your brain hat, study the cortical regions and functions that are noted. Based on the material presented in this chapter, think more specifically about the functions associated with play and playful behavior. Identify the regions associated with the social brain, emotion regulation, creativity, and imagination; all are core characteristics supporting play and maintaining play and playful interactions. Note that Ellen has included cerebellar hemispheres; given how much time has been devoted to cerebellar complexity, this area of the brain is one on which you would clearly want to delineate the expanded functions. Keep your paper brain as a handy reminder of regional brain structures and functions that can help you understand the neuroscience underlying play and playful behavior.

4. Combining Motivation, Social Interaction, and Neural Processing

Many games involve thinking and doing, along with engaging with others. You may recall the game of spoons. Some aspects of this interactive game, pertinent to the content in this chapter, include social interaction, motivation, control, and the giving and reading of cues that keep the game fun. There are other considerations, but this is a start. Find some friends and have a game of spoons. As you do, think about the features of playfulness (intrinsic motivation, internal control, freedom to suspend reality, framing) and associate these with brain structures and networks.

How to Play Spoons: To play, you need at least four players, a deck of cards, and spoons for each player, minus one. Spoons are arranged in a circle in the center of the table and each player is dealt four cards to start. The goal is to collect four-of-a-kind (e.g., four hearts, four 8s). The dealer begins the game by taking a card from the top of the remaining cards in the deck and decides whether to keep it or pass it to the left, seeking to get four of a kind. The player to the left picks up the card and makes the same decision. Players examine cards and decide whether to keep or pass along. Once someone gets four of a kind, they take a spoon. As soon as this happens, everyone tries to grab a spoon. The person left "spoonless" is out and the game begins again. The winner is the last person still in the game. There are other nuances of this game, but this will get you started!

5. Find Playful Opportunities in Your Educational Environment

Think about your interests and those activities in which you experience to a greater or lesser extent the components of playfulness (i.e., intrinsic motivation, perception of control, freedom from reality constraints, and social cues characteristic of play). Join a partner to identify up to three opportunities (e.g., specific activities/services or established groups) available at your institution in which both of you might potentially experience playfulness. What makes you think that participating in such activities will be a playful experience for you?

Which benefits (if any) can you anticipate from participating? Attend one of those activities with your partner during the upcoming days. Discuss together how you felt after participating. Was it as playful as you expected? Why?

Resources

- Ellen McHenry's Basement Workshop: https://ellenjmchenry.com. Ellen has a wealth of information and several free downloads included in her "World of Educational Inventions." Note that her materials are available in multiple languages as well. The one included in this chapter is the "Brain Hat."
- The Genius of Play: https://thegeniusofplay.org. This website, developed by The Toy Association, is aimed to provide families with information and inspiration to promote play as an important part of their day. It comprises a variety of resources including useful brief reports and articles, and the "Once Upon a Playtime Podcast." Although the website is focused mostly on children's play in the family context, there is a section about Parent's Play Perspective (see the six benefits of play tab). Various resources are available in English and Spanish. They can be excellent tools to integrate when educating or coaching families to engage in play and playful situations with their children.
- Neuroscience Online, an Open-Access Neuroscience Electronic Textbook: https://nba.uth.tmc.edu/neuroscience. This site provides an online, interactive "text" for the study of neuroscience. It is provided in open-access format through the Department of Neurobiology and Anatomy at The University of Texas Health Science Center at Houston, McGovern Medical School.
- "Occupational Therapy and Music Therapy in Early Head Start" video. In this video, an occupational therapist and music therapist discuss their unique and effective collaboration in a Head Start program. Running an 8-week group for infants and toddlers, the therapists assessed the children and established preventive goals linked to developmental milestones in areas such as self-regulation, awareness of self and others, attention, language, and motor movements. Access the video at the online resource center at FADavis.com.
- "Tricks and Techniques From the Mother of an Autistic Son" video. In this video, Laura describes her and her family's creative and adaptive ways of helping their autistic son, Will, succeed. Giving several specific examples of solutions to common problem behaviors and challenges, Laura shares practical wisdom, "tricks and techniques" from 20 years of experience as the mother of an autistic son, with a focus on recognizing and focusing on Will's strengths. Access the video at the online resource center at FADavis.com.

References

Allen, K-A., Kern, M. L., Rozek, C. S., McInerney, D. M., & Slavich, G. M. (2021). Belonging: A review of conceptual issues, an integrative framework, and directions for future research. *Australian Journal of Psychology, 73,* 87–102. https://doi.org/10.1080/00049530.2021.1883409

American College Health Association. (2019). *American College Health Association-National College Health Assessment II: Reference group executive summary spring 2019.* Author. https://www.acha.org/documents/ncha/NCHA-II_SPRING_2019_US_REFERENCE_GROUP_EXECUTIVE_SUMMARY.pdf

American Occupational Therapy Association. (2020). Occupational therapy practice framework: Domain and process—Fourth edition. *American Journal of Occupational Therapy, 74*(Suppl. 2), 7412410010p1–7412410010p87. https://doi.org/10.5014/ajot.2020.74S2001

Andersen, M. M., Kiverstein, J., Miller, M., & Roepstorff, A. (2022). Play in predictive minds: A cognitive theory of play. *Psychological Review, 130*(2), 462–479. https://doi.org/10.1037/rev0000369

Atler, K. (2016). The experiences of everyday activities post-stroke. *Disability and Rehabilitation, 38,* 781–788. https://doi.org/10.3109/09638288.2015.1061603

Atler, K. E., Barney, L., Moravec, A., Sample, P. L., & Fruhauf, C. A. (2017). The daily experiences of pleasure, productivity, and restoration profile: A case study. *Canadian Journal of Occupational Therapy, 84*(4-5), 262–272. https://doi.org/10.1177/0008417417723119

Atler, K., Moravec, A., Silver-Seidle, J., Manns, A., & Stephans, L. (2016). Caregivers' experiences derived from everyday occupations. *Physical and Occupational Therapy in Geriatrics, 34,* 71–87. https://doi.org/10.3109/02703181.2015.1120843

Baarendse, P. J. J., Counotte, D. S., O'Donnell, P., & Vanderschuren, L. J. M. J. (2013). Early social experience is critical for the development of cognitive control and dopamine modulation of prefrontal cortex function. *Neuropsychopharmacology, 38,* 1485–1494. https://doi.org/10.1038/npp.2013.47

Bakker, A. B., Scharp, Y., Breevaart, K., & de Vries, J. (2020). Playful work design: Introduction of a new concept. *The Spanish Journal of Psychology, 23,* E19. https://doi.org/10.1017/SJP.2020.20

Bakker, A. B., & van Woerkom, M. (2017). Flow at work: A self-determination perspective. *Occupational Health Science, 1*(1–2), 47–65. https://doi.org/10.1007/s41542-017-0003-3

Barnes, G., Wilkes-Gillan, S., Cordier, R., & Bundy, A. (2017). The social play, social skills and parent-child relationships of children with ADHD 12 months following a RCT of a play-based intervention. *Australian Occupational Therapy Journal, 64,* 1–9. https://doi.org/10.1111/1440-1630.12417

Bateson, P. (2014). Play, playfulness, creativity and innovation. *Animal Behavior and Cognition, 2*(2), 99–112. https://doi.org/10.12966/abc.05.02.2014

Baumeister, R. F. & Leary, M. R. (1995). The need to belong: Desire for interpersonal attachments as a fundamental human motivation. *Psychological Bulletin, 117,* 497–529. https//doi.org/10.1037/0033-2909.117.3.497

Bekoff, M. (1976). Animal play: Problems and perspectives. In P. P. G. Bateson & P. H. Klopfer (Eds.), *Perspectives in ethology* (pp. 165–188). Springer. https://doi.org/10.1007/978-1-4615-7572-6_4

Berk, L. E., Mann, T. D., & Ogan, A. T. (2006). Make-believe play: Wellspring for development of self-regulation. In D. G. Singer, R. M. Golinkoff, & K. Hirsh-Pasek (Eds.), *Play=Learning: How play motivates and enhances children's cognitive and social-emotional growth* (pp. 74–100). Oxford University Press.

Berridge, K. C., & Kringelbach, M. L. (2015). Pleasure systems in the brain. *Neuron, 86*(3), 646–664. https://doi.org/10.1016/j.neuron.2015.02.018

Bradshaw, J. W. S., Pullen, A. J., & Rooney, N. J. (2015). Why do adult dogs "play"? *Behavioural Processes, 110,* 82–87. https://doi.org/10.1016/j.beproc.2014.09.023

Brauer, K., & Proyer, R. T. (2017). Are impostors playful? Testing the association of adult playfulness with the Impostor Phenomenon. *Personality & Individual Differences, 116,* 57–62. https://doi.org/10.1016/j.paid.2017.04.029

Brauer, K., Proyer, R. T., & Chick, G. (2021), Adult playfulness: An update on an understudied individual differences variable and its role in romantic life. *Social and Personality Psychology Compass, 15,* e12589. https://doi.org/10.1111/spc3.12589

Brown, S., & Vaughan, C. (2009). *Play: How it shapes the brain, opens the imagination, and invigorates the soul.* Avery.

Bruner, J. S., Jolly, A., & Sylva, K. (Eds.). (1976). *Play: Its role in development and evolution*. Basic Books.

Bulgarelli, D., Bianquin, N., Besio, S., & Molina, P. (2018). Children with cerebral palsy playing with mainstream robotic toys: Playfulness and environmental supportiveness. *Frontiers in Psychology, 9*, 1814. https://doi.org/10.3389/fpsyg.2018.01814

Bundy, A., Nelson, L., Metzger, M., & Bingaman, K. (2001). Validity and reliability of a Test of Playfulness. *The Occupational Therapy Journal of Research, 21*(4), 276–292. https://doi.org/10.1177/153944920102100405

Burghardt, G. M. (2005). *The genesis of animal play: Testing the limits*. MIT Press.

Burghardt, G. M. (2010). The comparative reach of play and brain: Perspective, evidence, and implications. *American Journal of Play, 2*, 339–356.

Caillois, R. (2001). *Man, play and games*. University of Illinois Press.

Casey, T., Chatterjee, S., Assi, M., Maharjan, S., Wirunrapan, K., & Gupta, S. (2017, September). *Unleashing the power of play in situations of crisis*. Paper presented at the 20th International Play Association Triennial World Conference, Calgary, Alberta, Canada.

Clark, C. D. (2006). Therapeutic advantages of play. In A. Göncü & S. Gaskins (Eds.), *Play and development: Evolutionary, sociocultural and functional perspectives* (pp. 275–293). Lawrence Erlbaum.

Cordier, R., Bundy, A. C., Hocking, C., & Einfeld, S. (2010a). Empathy in the play of children with ADHD. *Occupational Therapy Journal of Research, 30*, 122–132. https://doi.org/10.3928/15394492-20090518-02

Cordier, R., Bundy, A. C., Hocking, C., & Einfeld, S. (2010b). Playing with a child with ADHD: A focus on the playmates. *Scandinavian Journal of Occupational Therapy, 17*, 191–199. https://doi.org/10.3109/11038120903156619

de Sousa, G. M., Tavares, V. D. O., de Meiroz Grilo, M. L. P., Coelho, M. L. G., de Lima-Araújo, G. L., Schuch, F. B., & Galvão-Coelho, N. L. (2021). Mental health in COVID-19 pandemic: A meta-review of prevalence meta-analyses. *Frontiers in Psychology, 12*, 703838. https://doi.org/10.3389/fpsyg.2021.703838

Deci, E. L., & Ryan, R. M. (2014). Autonomy and need satisfaction in close relationships: Relationship motivation theory. In N. Weinstein (Ed.), *Human motivation and interpersonal relationships: Theory, research and applications* (pp. 53–73). Springer.

Dodd, H. F., & Lester, K. J. (2021). Adventurous play as a mechanism for reducing risk for childhood anxiety: A conceptual model. *Clinical Child and Family Psychology Review, 24*, 164–181. https://doi.org/10.1007/s10567-020-00338-w

Dunbar, R. I. M. (1992). Neocortex size group size primates. *Journal of Human Evolution, 20*, 469–493. https://doi.org/10.1016/0047-2484(92)90081-J

Dunbar, R. I. M. (1995). Neocortex size group size hypothesis. *Journal of Human Evolution, 28*, 287–296. https://doi.org/10.1006/jhev.1995.1021

Eisenberger, N. I. (2012). The neural bases of social pain: Evidence for shared representations with physical pain. *Psychosomatic Medicine, 74*, 126–135. https://doi.org/10.1097/PSY.0b013e3182464dd1

Farley, A., Kennedy-Behr, A., & Brown, T. (2021). An investigation into the relationship between playfulness and well-being in Australian adults: An exploratory study. *OTJR: Occupational Therapy Journal of Research, 41*, 56–64. https://doi.org/10.1177/1539449220945311

Feshbach, N. D. (1997). Empathy: The formative years: Implications for clinical practice. In A. C. Bohart & L. S. Greenberg (Eds.), *Empathy reconsidered: New directions in psychotherapy* (pp. 33–59). American Psychological Association.

Forbes, L. (2021). The process of playful learning in higher education: A phenomenological study. *Journal of Teaching and Learning, 15*, 57–73. https://doi.org/10.22329/jtl.v15i1.6515

Gray, P. (2011). The decline of play and the rise of psychopathology. *American Journal of Play, 3*, 443–463.

Harkness, L., & Bundy, A. (2001). The Test of Playfulness and children with physical disabilities. *Occupational Therapy Journal of Research, 21*(2), 73–89. https://doi.org/10.1177/153944920102100203

Hektner, J. M., Schmidt, J. A., & Csikszentmihalyi, M. (2007). *Experience sampling method. Measuring the quality of everyday life*. Sage.

Held, S. D. E., & Špinka, M. (2011). Animal play and animal welfare. *Animal Behaviour, 8*, 891–899. https://doi.org/10.1016/j.anbehav.2011.01.007

Heljakka, K. (2023). Building playful resilience in higher education: Learning by doing and doing by playing. *Frontiers in Education, 8*, 1071552. https://doi.org/10.3389/feduc.2023.1071552

Henry, A. (2008). Assessment of play and leisure in children and adolescents. In L. D. Parham & L. S. Fazio (Eds.), *Play in occupational therapy for children* (2nd ed., pp. 95–193). Mosby.

Hosker, D. K., Elkins, R. M., & Potter, M. P. (2019). Promoting mental health and wellness in youth through physical activity, nutrition, and sleep. *Child and Adolescent Psychiatric Clinics of North America, 28*(2), 171–193. https://doi.org/10.1016/j.chc.2018.11.010

Howard, J., & McInnes, K. (2013). The impact of children's perception of an activity as play rather than not play on emotional well-being. *Child: Care, Health & Development, 39*, 737–742. https://doi.org/10.1111/j.1365-2214.2012.01405.x

Huang, J., Nigatu, Y. T., Smail-Crevier, R., Zhang, X., & Wang, J. (2018). Interventions for common mental health problems among university and college students: A systematic review and meta-analysis of randomized controlled trials. *Journal of Psychiatric Research, 107*, 1–10. https://doi.org/10.1016/j.jpsychires.2018.09.018

Hudspeth, E., & Matthews, K. (2015). Neuroscience and play therapy: The neurobiologically-informed play therapist. In K. J. O'Connor, C. E. Schaefer, & L. D. Braverman (Eds.), *Handbook of play therapy* (2nd ed., pp. 583–597). John Wiley & Sons.

Hurd, A. R., & Anderson, D. M. (2010). *The park and recreation professional's handbook*. Human Kinetics.

Imms, C., King, G., Majnemer, A., Avery, L., Chiarello, L., Palisano, R., Orlin, M., & Law, M. (2017). Leisure participation–preference congruence of children with cerebral palsy: A Children's Assessment of Participation and Enjoyment International Network descriptive study. *Developmental Medicine and Child Neurology, 59*, 380–387. https://doi.org/10.1111/dmcn.13302

Iwaniuk, A. N., Nelson, J. E., & Pellis, S. M. (2001). Do big-brained animals play more? Comparative analyses of play and relative brain size in mammals. *Journal of Comparative Psychology, 115*, 29–41. https://doi.org/10.1037/0735-7036.115.1.29

Kent, C., Cordier, R., Joosten, A., Wilkes-Gillan, S., & Bundy, A. (2020). Can we play together? A closer look at the peers of a peer-mediated intervention to improve play in children with autism spectrum disorder. *Journal of Autism and Developmental Disorders, 50*, 2860–2873. https://doi.org/10.1007/s10803-020-04387-6

Kerney, M., Smaers, J. B., Schoenemann, P. T., & Dunn, J. C. (2017). The coevolution of play and the cortico-cerebellar system in primates. *Primates, 58*(4), 485–491. https://doi.org/10.1007/s10329-017-0615-x

King, G. A., Law, M., King, S., Hurley, P., Hanna, S., Kertoy, M., & Rosenbaum, P. (2007). Measuring children's participation in recreation and leisure activities: Construct validation of the CAPE and PAC. *Child: Care, Health and Development, 33*, 28–39. https://doi.org/10.1111/J.1365-2214.2006.00613.X

King, G. A., Law, M., King, S., Hurley, P., Hanna, S., Kertoy, M., Rosenbaum, P., & Young, N. (2004). *Children's Assessment of Participation and Enjoyment (CAPE) and Preferences for Activities of Children (PAC)*. Harcourt Assessment.

King, M., Shields, N., Imms, C., Black, M., & Ardern, C. (2013). Participation of children with intellectual disability compared with typically developing children. *Research in Developmental Disabilities, 34*, 1854–1862. doi.org/10.1016/j.ridd.2013.02.029

Koeners, M. P., & Francis, J. (2020). The physiology of play: Potential relevance for higher education. *International Journal of Play, 9,* 143–159. https://doi.org/10.1080/21594937.2020.1720128

Lafreniere, P. (2011). Evolutionary functions of social play life histories, sex differences, and emotion regulation. *American Journal of Play, 3,* 464–488.

Lee, R. L. T., Lane, S., Brown, G., Leung, C., Kwok, S. W. H., & Chan, S. W. C. (2020). Systematic review of the impact of unstructured play interventions to improve young children's physical, social, and emotional wellbeing. *Nursing & Health Sciences, 22,* 184–196. https://doi.org/10.1111/nhs.12732

Lewis, K. P. (2000). A comparative study of primate play behaviour: Implications for the study of cognition. *Folia Primatologica, 71,* 417–421. https://doi.org/10.1159/000052740

Lewis, K. P., & Barton, R. A. (2004). Playing for keeps. Evolutionary relationships between social play and the cerebellum in nonhuman primates. *Human Nature, 15*(1), 5–21. https://doi.org/10.1007/s12110-004-1001-0

Lewis, K. P., & Barton, R. A. (2006). Amygdala size and hypothalamus size predict social play frequency in nonhuman primates: A comparative analysis using independent contrasts. *Journal of Comparative Psychology, 120*(1), 31–37. https://doi.org/10.1037/0735-7036.120.1.31

Luck, K., Luke, A., & Doucet, S. (2021). Occupational disruption during pandemic: Exploring the experiences of individuals living with chronic disease. *Journal of Occupational Science, 22,* 352–367. https://doi.org/10.1080/14427591.2020.1871401

Lugton, E., Brown, T., & Stagnitti, K. (2020). Convergent validity between three self-report measures of children's play and activity interests, *Journal of Occupational Therapy, Schools, & Early Intervention, 13,* 374–394. https://doi.org/10.1080/19411243.2020.1769001

Miller, R. E., Caul, W. F., & Mirsky, I. A. (1967). Communication of affects between feral and socially isolated monkeys 1. *Journal of Personality and Social Psychology, 7,* 231–239. https://doi.org/10.1037/h0025065

Montgomery, S. H. (2014). The relationship between play, brain growth and behavioural flexibility in primates. *Animal Behaviour, 90,* 281–286. https://doi.org/10.1016/j.anbehav.2014.02.004

Moore, S. A., Faulkner, G., Rhodes, R. E., Brussoni, M., Chulak-Bozzer, T., Ferguson, L. J., Mitra, R., O'Reilly, N., Spence, J. C., Vanderloo, L. M., & Tremblay, M. S. (2020). Impact of COVID-19 virus outbreak on movement and play behaviors of Canadian children and youth: A national survey. *International Journal of Behavioral Nutrition and Physical Activity, 17,* 85. https://doi.org/10.1186/s12966-020-00987-8

Muys, V., Rodger, S., & Bundy, A. (2006). Assessment of playfulness in children with autistic disorder: A comparison of the Children's Playfulness Scale and the Test of Playfulness. *OTJR: Occupational Therapy Journal of Research, 26,* 159–170. https://doi.org/10.1177/153944920602600406

Neale, D., Clackson, K., Georgieva, S., Dedetas, H., Scarpate, M., Wass, S., & Leong, V. (2018). Toward a neuroscientific understanding of play: A dimensional coding framework for analyzing infant-adult play patterns. *Frontiers in Psychology, 9,* Article 273. https://doi.org/10.3389/fpsyg.2018.00273

Neumann, E. A. (1971). *The elements of play.* MSS Information.

Palagi, E., Nicotra, V., & Cordoni, G. (2015). Rapid mimicry and emotional contagion in domestic dogs. *Royal Society Open Science, 2,* 150505. https://doi.org/10.1098/rsos.150505

Panksepp, J., & Beatty, W. W. (1980). Social deprivation and play in rats. *Behavioral and Neural Biology, 30,* 197–206. https://doi.org/10.1016/S0163-1047(80)91077-8

Panksepp, J., & Biven, L. (2012). *The archeology of mind: Neuroevolutionary origins of human emotions.* Norton.

Parham, L. D., & Fazio, L. S. (Eds.). (2008). *Play in occupational therapy for children* (2nd ed.). Mosby.

Pellegrini, A. D., Huberty, P. D., & Jones, I. (1995). The effects of recess timing on children's playground and classroom behaviors. *American Educational Research Journal, 32,* 845–864. https://doi.org/10.2307/1163338

Pellis, S. M., & Pellis, V. C. (2009). *The playful brain. Venturing to the limits of neuroscience.* Oneworld Press.

Pellis, S. M., Pellis, V. C., & Bell, H. C. (2010). The function of play in the development of the social brain. *American Journal of Play, 2,* 278–296.

Pellis, S. M., Pellis, V. C., Ham, J. R., & Stark, R. A. (2023). Play fighting and the development of the social brain: The rat's tale. In *Neuroscience & Biobehavioral Reviews, 145,* 105037. https://doi.org/10.1016/j.neubiorev.2023.105037

Pellis, S. M., Pellis, V. C., Pelletier, A., & Leca, J. B. (2019). Is play a behavior system, and, if so, what kind? *Behavioural Processes, 160,* 1–9. https://doi.org/10.1016/j.beproc.2018.12.011

Potvin, M. C., Snider, L., Prelock, P., Kehayia, E., & Wood-Dauphinee, S. (2013). Children's Assessment of Participation and Enjoyment/Preference for Activities of Children: Psychometric properties in a population with high-functioning autism. *American Journal of Occupational Therapy, 67,* 209–217. https://doi.org/10.5014/ajot.2013.006288

Powrie, B. (2019). *The meaning of leisure participation: Perspectives of children and young people with significant physical disabilities* [Unpublished doctoral dissertation]. The University of Queensland. https://doi.org/10.14264/uql.2019.275

Proyer, R. T. (2017). A new structural model for the study of adult playfulness: Assessment and exploration of an understudied individual differences variable. *Personality and Individual Differences, 108,* 113–122. https://doi.org/10.1016/J.PAID.2016.12.011

Proyer, R. T., Brauer, K., & Wolf, A. (2020). Assessing Other-directed, Lighthearted, Intellectual, and Whimsical playfulness in adults. *European Journal of Psychological Assessment, 36,* 624–634. https://doi.org/10.1027/1015-5759/a000531

Proyer, R. T., Gander, F., Brauer, K., & Chick, G. (2021). Can playfulness be stimulated? A randomised placebo-controlled online playfulness intervention study on effects on trait playfulness, well-being, and depression. *Applied Psychology: Health and Well-Being, 13,* 129–151. https://doi.org/10.1111/aphw.12220

Proyer, R. T., & Tandler, N. (2020). An update on the study of playfulness in adolescents: Its relationship with academic performance, well-being, anxiety, and roles in bullying-type-situations. *Social Psychology of Education, 23,* 73–99. https://doi.org/10.1007/s11218-019-09526-1

Racine, N., McArthur, B. A., Cooke, J. E., Eirich, R., Zhu, J., & Madigan, S. (2021). Global prevalence of depressive and anxiety symptoms in children and adolescents during COVID-19: A meta-analysis. *JAMA Pediatrics, 175*(11), 1142–1150. https://doi:10.1001/jamapediatrics.2021.2482

Rodriguez-Ayllon, M., Cadenas-Sánchez, C., Estévez-López, F., Muñoz, N. E., Mora-Gonzalez, J., Migueles, J. H., Molina-García, P., Henriksson, H., Mena-Molina, A., Martínez-Vizcaíno, V., Catena, A., Löf, M., Erickson, K. I., Lubans, D. R., Ortega, F. B., & Esteban-Cornejo, I. (2019). Role of physical activity and sedentary behavior in the mental health of preschoolers, children and adolescents: A systematic review and meta-analysis. *Sports Medicine, 49,* 1383–1410. https://doi.org/10.1007/s40279-019-01099-5

Rogers, C. S., Impara, J. C., Frary, R. B., Harris, T., Meeks, A., Semanic-Lauth, S., & Reynolds, M. (1998). Measuring playfulness: Development of the Child Behavior Inventory of Playfulness. In M. Duncan, G. Chick, & A. Aycock (Eds.), *Play and Culture Studies, 4,* 121–135. Ablex Publishing.

Román-Oyola, R., Bundy, A., Castro, E., Castrillo, O., Morel, K. Y., Molina-Martínez, R., Montes-Burgos, A., Rodríguez-Santiago, A., & Rosado-Torres, D. (2023). Play and mothers' relationships with children in the context of breast cancer. *OTJR: Occupational Therapy Journal of Research, 43*(1), 43–51. https://doi.org/10.1177/15394492221093996

Román-Oyola, R., Bundy, A., Castro, E., Castrillo, O., & Sala, A. C. (2022, February 23–25). *Development and acceptability of a play-based intervention to improve QoL and wellbeing of mothers with cancer and their young children* [Poster presentation]. Advancing the Science of Cancer in Latinos, San Antonio, Texas.

Romero-Ayuso, D., Ruiz-Salcedo, M., Barrios-Fernández, S., Triviño-Juárez, J. M., Maciver, D., Richmond, J., & Muñoz, M. A. (2021). Play in children with neurodevelopmental disorders: Psychometric properties of a parent report measure 'My Child's Play.' *Children, 8*(1), 25. https://doi.org/10.3390/children8010025

Romli, M. H., & Wan Yunus, F. (2020). A systematic review on clinimetric properties of play instruments for occupational therapy practice. *Occupational Therapy International, 2020,* 2490519. https://doi.org/10.1155/2020/2490519

Ryan, R. M. (1993). Agency and organization: Intrinsic motivation, autonomy and the self in psychological development. In J. Jacobs (Ed.), *Nebraska Symposium on Motivation: Vol 40. Developmental perspectives on motivation* (pp. 1–56). University of Nebraska Press.

Ryan, R. M., & Deci, E. L. (2017). *Self-determination theory: Basic psychological needs in motivation, development, and wellness.* Guilford. https://doi.org/10.1521/978.14625/28806

Saliba, Y. C., & Barden, S. M. (2021). Playfulness and older adults: Implications for quality of life. *Journal of Mental Health Counseling, 43,* 157–171. https://doi.org/10.17744/mehc.43.2.05

Sangster Jokić, C. A., & Jokić-Begić, N. (2022). Occupational disruption during the COVID-19 pandemic: Exploring changes to daily routines and their potential impact on mental health. *Journal of Occupational Science, 29,* 336–351. https://doi.org/10.1080/14427591.2021.2018024

Schneider, E., & Rosenblum, S. (2014). Development, reliability, and validity of the My Child's Play (MCP) Questionnaire. *American Journal of Occupational Therapy, 68,* 277–285. https://doi.org/10.5014/ajot.2014.009159

Schneider, N., Greenstreet, E., & Deoni, S. C. L. (2022). Connecting inside out: Development of the social brain in infants and toddlers with a focus on myelination as a marker of brain maturation. *Child Development, 93*(2), 359–371. https://doi.org/10.1111/cdev.13649

Serrada-Tejeda, S., Santos-del-Riego, S., Bundy, A., & Pérez-de-Heredia-Torres, M. (2021). Spanish cultural adaptation and inter-rater reliability of the Test of Playfulness. *Physical and Occupational Therapy in Pediatrics, 41,* 555–565. https://doi.org/10.1080/01942638.2021.1881199

Shen, X. S., Chick, G., & Zinn, H. (2014a). Playfulness in adulthood as a personality trait: A reconceptualization and a new measurement. *Journal of Leisure Research, 46,* 58–83. doi.org/10.1080/00222216.2014.11950313

Shen, X. S., Chick, G., & Zinn, H. (2014b). Validating the Adult Playfulness Trait Scale (APTS): An examination of personality, behavior, attitude, and perception in the nomological network of playfulness. *American Journal of Play, 6,* 345–369.

Siviy, S. M. (2016). A brain motivated to play: Insights into the neurobiology of playfulness. *Behaviour, 153*(6–7), 819–844. https://doi.org/10.1163/1568539X-00003349

Siviy, S. M., & Panksepp, J. (2011). In search of the neurobiological substrates for social playfulness in mammalian brains. *Neuroscience & Biobehavioral Reviews, 35*(9), 1821–1830. https://doi.org/10.1016/j.neubiorev.2011.03.006

Skard, G., & Bundy, A. C. (2008). Test of Playfulness. In L. D. Parham & L. S. Fazio (Eds.), *Play in occupational therapy for children* (2nd ed., pp. 71–94). Mosby.

Smith, P. K., & Hagan, T. (1980). Effects of deprivation on exercise play in nursery school children. *American Educational Research Journal, 28,* 922–928. https://doi.org/10.3102/00028312032004

Spinka, M., Newberry, R. C., & Bekoff, M. (2001). Mammalian play: Training for the unexpected. *The Quarterly Review of Biology, 76,* 141–168. https://doi.org/10.1086/393866

Stracke, M., Heinzl, M., Müller, A. D., Gilbert, K., Thorup, A. A. E., Paul, J. L., & Christiansen, H. (2023). Mental health is a family affair—Systematic review and meta-analysis on the associations between mental health problems in parents and children during the COVID-19 pandemic. *International Journal of Environmental Research and Public Health, 20*(5), 4485. https://doi.org/10.3390/ijerph20054485

Sutton-Smith, B. (1997). *The ambiguity of play.* Harvard University Press.

Taylor, S. I., & Rogers, C. S. (2001). The relationship between playfulness and creativity of Japanese preschool children. *International Journal of Early Childhood, 33,* 43–49. https://doi.org/10.1007/BF03174447

Trezza, V., Baarendse, P. J. J., & Vanderschuren, L. J. M. J. (2010). The pleasures of play: Pharmacological insights into social reward mechanisms. *Trends in Pharmacological Sciences, 31,* 463–469. https://doi.org/10.1016/j.tips.2010.06.008

Tun, J. E., Arshat, Z., & Ismail, N. (2020). Playfulness and emotional intelligence of Chinese preschool children: Is it parental monitoring so important? *Test Engineering & Management, 83,* 3025–3037.

Van Den Berg, C. L., Hol, T., Van Ree, J. M., Spruijt, B. M., Everts, H., & Koolhaas, J. M. (1999). Play is indispensable for an adequate development of coping with social challenges in the rat. *Developmental Psychobiology, 34,* 129–138. https://doi.org/10.1002/(SICI)1098-2302(199903)34:2<129::AID-DEV6>3.0.CO;2-L

Van Vleet, M., & Feeney, B. C. (2015). Young at heart: A perspective for advancing research on play in adulthood. *Perspectives on Psychological Science, 10,* 639–645. https://doi.org/10.1177/1745691615596789

Vanderschuren, L. J. M. J., & Trezza, V. (2014). What the laboratory rat has taught us about social play behavior: Role in behavioral development and neural mechanisms. *Current Topics in Behavioral Neurosciences, 16,* 189–212. https://doi.org/10.1007/7854_2013_268

Vandervert, L. (2017). Vygotsky meets neuroscience: The cerebellum and the rise of culture through play. *American Journal of Play, 9*(2), 202–227.

Vankim, N. A., & Nelson, T. F. (2013). Vigorous physical activity, mental health, perceived stress, and socializing among college students. *American Journal of Health Promotion, 28,* 7–15. https://doi.org/10.4278/ajhp.111101-QUAN-395

Vazquez, C. (2020). *Play's role in the development of antisocial behavior.* Williams Honors College, Honors Research Projects. https://ideaexchange.uakron.edu/honors_research_projects/1075

Vigil-Dopico, R., Delgado-Lobete, L., Montes-Montes, R., & Prieto-Saborit, J. A. (2022). A comprehensive analysis of the relationship between play performance and psychosocial problems in school-aged children. *Children, 9,* 1110. https://doi.org/10.3390/children9081110

Von Frijtag, J. C., Schot, M., Van Den Bos, R., & Spruijt, B. M. (2002). Individual housing during the play period results in changed responses to and consequences of a psychosocial stress situation in rats. *Developmental Psychobiology, 41,* 58–69. https://doi.org/10.1002/dev.10057

Waldman-Levi, A., & Bundy, A. (2016). A glimpse into co-occupations: Parent/Caregiver's Support of Young Children's Playfulness Scale. *Occupational Therapy in Mental Health, 32,* 217–227. https://doi.org/10.1080/0164212X.2015.1116420

Waldman-Levi, A., Bundy, A., & Shai, D. (2022). Cognition mediates playfulness development in early childhood: A longitudinal study of typically developing children. *The American Journal of Occupational Therapy, 76*(5), 7605205020. https://doi.org/10.5014/ajot.2022.049120

Waldman-Levi, A., & Weintraub, N. (2015). Efficacy of a crisis intervention in improving mother–child interaction and children's play functioning. *The American Journal of Occupational Therapy, 69*(1), 6901220020p1–6901220020p11. https://doi.org/10.5014/ajot.2015.013375

Whiteford, G. (2000). Occupational deprivation: Global challenge in the new millennium. *British Journal of Occupational Therapy, 63,* 200–204. https://doi.org/10.1177/030802260006300503

Wilkes-Gillan, S., Bundy, A., Cordier, R., & Lincoln, M. (2014a). Child outcomes of a pilot parent-delivered intervention for improving the social play skills of children with ADHD and their playmates. *Developmental Neurorehabilitation, 19,* 238–245. https://doi.org/10.3109/17518423.2014.948639

Wilkes-Gillan, S., Bundy, A., Cordier, R., & Lincoln, M. (2014b). Eighteen month follow-up of a play-based intervention to improve the social play skills of children with ADHD. *Australian Occupational Therapy Journal, 61,* 299–307. https://doi:10.1111/1440-1630.12124

Wilkes-Gillan, S., Bundy, A., Cordier, R., Lincoln, M., & Chen, Y.-W. (2016). A randomised controlled trial of a play-based intervention to improve the social play skills of children with attention deficit hyperactivity disorder (ADHD). *PLoS One, 11*(8), 1–22. https://doi.org/10.1371/journal.pone.0160558

Wilkes-Gillan, S., Cantrill, A., Cordier, R., Barnes, G., Hancock, N., & Bundy, A. (2017). The use of video-modelling as a method for improving the social play skills of children with attention deficit hyperactivity disorder (ADHD) and their playmates. *British Journal of Occupational Therapy, 80,* 196–207. https://10.1177/0308022617692819

Wilkes-Gillan, S., Cordier, R., Bundy, A., Lincoln, M., Chen, Y.-W., Parsons, L., & Cantrill, A. (2022). A pairwise randomised controlled trial of a peer-mediated play-based intervention to improve the social play skills of children with ADHD: Outcomes of the typically-developing playmates. *PLoS One, 17*(10), e0276444. https://doi.org/10.1371/journal.pone.0276444

World Health Organization. (2022). *World mental health report: Transforming mental health for all.* Author. https://www.who.int/publications/i/item/9789240049338

Worsley, J. D., Pennington, A., & Corcoran, R. (2022). Supporting mental health and wellbeing of university and college students: A systematic review of review-level evidence of interventions. *PLoS One, 17*(7), e0266725. https://doi.org/10.1371/journal.pone.0266725

Xiong, J., Lipsitz, O., Nasri, F., Lui, L. M., Gill, H., Phan, L., Chen-Li, D., Iacobucci, M., Ho, R., Majeed, A., & McIntyre, R. S. (2020). Impact of COVID-19 pandemic on mental health in the general population: A systematic review. *Journal of Affective Disorders, 277,* 55–64. https://doi.org/10.1016/j.jad.2020.08.001

Yogman, M., Garner, A., Hutchinson, J., Hirsh-Pasek, K., Michnick Golinkoff, R., & Committees on Psychosocial Aspects of Child and Family Health, Council on Communications and Media. (2018). The power of play: A pediatric role in enhancing development in young children. *Pediatrics, 142*(3), e20182058. https://doi.org/10.1542/peds.2018-2058

Leisure and Creative Occupations

Virginia C. Stoffel

During one's lifetime, their engagement across the occupations of everyday life goes through shifts, with expected changes in roles and role expectations, priorities, and motivations. This chapter focuses on engagement in leisure and creative occupations, terms that are likely best defined by the person or group engaging in particular activities.

For example, take cooking as an occupation. As children, people often play in child-sized kitchens, pretending to make and serve tea and cookies to their friends and dolls. Cooking as a play activity might morph into cooking and baking as a leisure interest in school-age children, perhaps becoming something they do with parents, grandparents, or siblings. Depending on their life contexts and expectations from others, cooking and baking might remain a leisure interest for their lifetime. However, if cooking is a primary contribution to their family or a paid or volunteer job, their view of cooking and baking can evolve over time from a leisure activity to employment, for example. Cooking might also be considered a creative activity, especially when experimenting with various recipes, spices, and ingredients, as well as methods of cooking (stove, oven, microwave, outdoor grill or smoker, open fire).

Asking about the meaning of selected occupations is an important part of the occupational therapy practitioners' (OTPs') process. This helps OTPs recognize that meanings can be shaped by culture, norms, and diversity of life experiences. Checking out barriers and facilitators to carrying out occupations based on skills, emerging skills, interests, and aspects of the available environment to safely engage in varied occupations is part of the Person-Environment-Occupation (PEO) approach emphasized throughout this text (see Chapter 3: Person-Environment-Occupation Model for additional examples 🤝). OTPs might also reflect on their own leisure interests and creative pursuits, and their meaningfulness to everyday life.

As occupational beings who serve others through occupational therapy, the lessons OTPs learn about themselves through the lens of engagement in meaningful leisure and creative occupations and these lessons can bring insights that will strengthen their impact as practitioners in the lives of those they serve.

Given that OTPs carry out their professional roles in a wide variety of settings and environments, where people live (homes, neighborhoods, communities), learn (day care, school, training, enrichment programs offered in virtual and face-to-face formats), work (paid and unpaid, volunteer), play (environments for play, recreation, and leisure pursuits), and pray (religious and spiritual environments) influence those

roles. The practitioner must attend to the match between the person, their environments, and the occupations they intend to pursue, so as to achieve the desired outcomes.

The importance of engagement in play for brain development, as well as the attitudinal aspects of being playful for engaging socially with others and enhancing one's mental well-being through the sense of belonging through play, is emphasized in Chapter 50: Play. 🤝 It is likely that practitioners can extend their understanding of the brain healing benefits of leisure and creative occupations, in addition to the benefits of a playful and creative spirit, from infants and toddlers to youth and throughout adulthood. Play might be considered a prime occupation for children, whereas leisure and creative occupations might be considered prime for older adults, especially as they relinquish work and family obligations when moving into retirement.

The importance of life balance is often cited as a wellness strategy for school-age populations (see Chapter 37: School Mental Health 🤝 and Chapter 47: Student 🤝), as well as adults carrying employment and family/caregiving as prime roles. Chapter 45: Self-Care and Well-Being Occupations frames a multidimensional approach to self-care and wellness, which includes the importance of balancing life across self-care, productive, and leisure occupations. 🤝

This chapter starts by exploring the link between engagement in leisure and creative occupations and their impact on health and well-being. Then the chapter describes and characterizes basic concepts associated with leisure and creative occupations, providing an overview of the wide variety of activities that make up these domains. Examples of real-world perspectives are highlighted using the chapter's The Lived Experience, PhotoVoice, and Being a Psychosocial OT Practitioner features. Evidence is provided throughout the chapter, including significant literature around measuring and facilitating engagement in leisure and creative occupations believed to impact health and well-being.

Leisure and Creative Occupations for Promoting Health and Well-Being

In their editorial on leisure and well-being, Mansfield, Daykin, and Kay (2020) reflect on the two perspectives commonly used in studying well-being—the eudaimonic perspective (such as positive psychological functioning, meaning, and flourishing) and the hedonic perspective (such as happiness,

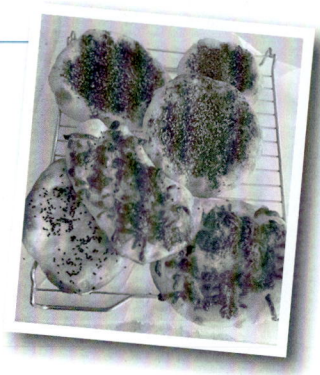

PhotoVoice

Making Manaqeesh (Middle Eastern Pastries)

In my culture, making food for others is a form of love, connectedness, and trust. People who eat together will never betray one another. Making Manaqeesh (Middle Eastern pastries) is one activity I do for well-being and self-care, as it reminds me of collective love. Making Zaatar Manaqeesh (thyme pastries) in particular reminds me of my father, who used to have it for breakfast for over 20 years. He believed thyme makes you smarter (he was wicked smart!). Making it for my kids and telling them that it was his favorite pastry brings peace and comfort to my heart, as it reminds me of him and the happy memories we had together.

How could you learn more about this person's culturally connected occupations and ensure that they find time and space to practice them as they build healthy routines?

positive emotions, and life satisfaction)—and consider how they might be associated with engagement in varied activities. They note that the World Happiness Report (Helliwell et al., 2024) highlights the importance of leisure engagement to people's well-being, suggesting strategies for enhancing the availability of urban woodlands and forests for engaging in meaningful activities, participatory activities such as music-making, and leisure activities that enhance spiritual well-being (see Chapter 53: Spiritual Occupations 🤝). They encourage critical thinking about impoverished populations, in which access to environments and occupations considered ideal for experiencing well-being are inequitable.

In 2020, the Robert Wood Johnson Foundation in the United States assembled insights from practitioners, researchers, and innovators from around the globe to define how progress might look if well-being for all people, communities, and environments was adopted (Plough, 2020). The multidimensional goals of improving health, expanding economic means, and meeting basic needs, along with social connectedness, belonging and purpose, moments of joy and happiness, deep satisfaction with life based on equity and human rights, and connecting people with the planet are included in a thoughtful collection of essays, which is part of the Culture of Health Series (Plough, 2020).

In occupational therapy, various researchers have emphasized different aspects. For example, Reilly (1974) focused on how creative activities impact human development across the life span by enhancing exploration and skill acquisition in a playful manner. Hasselkus (2011) framed creativity as the mundane moments in life that get sparked by passion, spirit, and electricity, highlighting the attitudinal element contributing to creativity. Gillam (2018) framed creativity as a "healing, life-affirming activity" (p. 21) emphasizing the "doing" impact. Perruzza and Kinsella (2010) described the link between engagement in creative arts to multiple aspects of health and well-being, such as perceived control, sense of self, expression, transforming an illness experience, purpose in life, and social support.

Hansen and colleagues (2020) explored both creativity and creative occupations to clarify these concepts when considering how creative activity is implemented as an occupational therapy intervention in studies disseminated across the world. In this chapter's The Lived Experience feature, readers will hear from Jan Kobe about her experiences of leisure and creative activities as a part of her mental health recovery, meaningful work, and how, in retirement, she is reclaiming her identity as an artist.

Defining Leisure Occupations

The *Occupational Therapy Practice Framework,* Fourth Edition (*OTPF-4;* American Occupational Therapy Association [AOTA], 2020) includes leisure as a category among eight other occupations common to everyday life. The *OTPF-4* offers this definition of **leisure:** "Nonobligatory activity that is intrinsically motivated and engaged in during discretionary time, that is, time not committed to obligatory occupations such as work, self-care, or sleep" (Parham & Fazio, 1997, p. 250, as cited in AOTA, 2020).

Each of these words suggests important features required for an activity to be considered leisure—an activity that is done because the person wants to engage in it (nonobligatory and intrinsically motivated) during their free time. What the definition fails to point out, at least explicitly, is the level of meaningfulness that might be imbued in the activity, how leisure might be a factor in helping people achieve life balance with their obligatory occupations, and whether the concept of time not committed to obligatory occupations is actually possible across all populations. Do all people have equal access to "free time"?

Judith Friedland, a Canadian occupational therapy historical scholar, noted in her Muriel Driver Memorial Lecture in 2003 that the use of arts and crafts in occupational therapy between 1890 and 1930 was shaped by three movements (Arts and Crafts Movement, Settlement House Movement, and the Mental Hygiene Movement) present in North America and the United Kingdom. William Morris, one of several leaders in the Arts and Crafts Movement, advocated that engaging people in arts and crafts was a means of restoring a sense of community, bringing great joy and beauty to all (including those challenged by mental illness, and those dealing with immigration and displacement).

Friedland highlights how Clifford Beers, a leader in the Mental Hygiene Movement, promoted the awareness of the therapeutic qualities inherent in engagement in arts and crafts by promoting identity and self-image, offering people skills for work, invoking the "art spirit" for promoting health

The Lived Experience

Jan Kobe, an Artist With a Passion for Creative Expression

Editor's Note: In May 2023, I interviewed Jan Kobe, an artist who contributed to the first edition of this text by cofacilitating Photo-Voice workshops. We spent time together in Kansas City in August of 2005 (the same days that Hurricane Katrina hit) to go through PhotoVoice training, and Jan agreed to be interviewed to share her stories about engagement in art as a piece of her mental health recovery and as meaningful to her everyday life, in her career and now in her retirement.

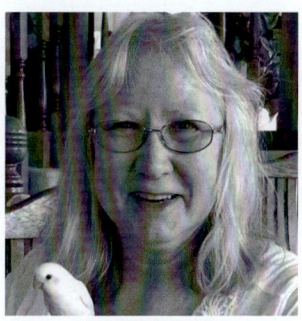

Jan shared with me that she was gifted with feedback about being wise, blessed, and a gifted person. She reflected first on her job at the Wyandotte Mental Health Center in August of 2022, a position that was created for her as a peer and an artist, given her degree in art. Here are her words:

I created an art program 23 years ago, and I remember the first day on the job, I walked into the space where the program would take place and there were several large black cabinets, and I was asked to organize, neatly label, and put things back in. I took it on like a duck to water; it was a very natural fit. I am a nurturer and given that I have no children of my own, I took people under my wing as a caring nurturer. I provided people with art supplies and it was healing to sit at the table with them and see them get involved in doing art—it was introduced more as a play activity and I saw how therapeutic it was for them. Totally based on art and the creative process.

Our studio was called "Art Makers Place" and I created a curriculum for three different art groups a week. One was called "New Horizons" for young people, another was called "Fabric Expression" for sewing groups, and the third group was called "Open Studio" for mural painting. We just opened it up to any patient of Wyandotte who wanted to participate. Art is healing. Doing art is a safe method to be in a group setting and to express without touching on trauma or deep-rooted psychosis. This is what I did for my career. Other people totally valued this; they would come in and just sit at a table. They knew it was a play activity and they could decide if they wanted to interrupt others to be involved in creating the mural. Somebody would pass the paint bottle, or somebody else would look over their shoulder, and say "Wow, I like that piece." I always called the art process a safe haven, a place where nobody would experience harm. The arts program was fully backed by our CEO of the mental health center, and he believes in the arts program.

When I left my position at the mental health center, my lifetime goal was to explore my own work, fulltime, before I got too old. So now I'm exploring my work. I have two pieces in an art gallery right now, and two others that will be going to the gallery at the end of this month. I have some of my art online, and I've written and designed a children's book. It is about a little bird that was born differently, he was navy blue, unlike other birds around him. At the end of the book, he learns how to fly and be open to the world that is around him. So while it's not directly about mental illness, it provides a way to understand being different. That you can still explore the world and enjoy the beauty of it. I am hopeful to find a publisher who will print it in my lifetime.

When I was in high school, planning for college, I thought I'd like to be an occupational therapist. I told my career counselor at the high school that I thought with my art skills and my interest in healing professions that would be a good match. I was told by a college counselor that my science grades were not high enough. So, I went into illustrations. I was a good student, but not necessarily in science. I always wanted to give back through my art. I worked for 3 years at Hallmark in Kansas City and then took on a job at their Hallmark Studio in San Francisco. After another 2 years, I found myself burned out. This was before my first onset. I knew I wanted to work with people who were mentally ill. I had run into a woman who was homeless and on the streets, and I hoped to work with people like her. There were some mental disturbances in my family, so I was aware of the needs. When I had the insight that I wanted to use art to work with people with mental illness, shortly thereafter, I had my own experience with psychosis. You tell me there is a God in heaven watching out for you—I was hospitalized for psychosis of unknown origin while in San Francisco and came back home to Kansas to get treatment. And I've been here ever since, just like Dorothy in the Wizard of Oz! My hometown and family are here—it is a comfort to me.

Now, I am moving slowly in my art and always have something on the drawing board. I am slowly reaching out to the community and trying to be part of an exhibit with other members of the community. These are not art exhibits as an explicit part of the mental health community, just as part of the community overall. I am working with three galleries and am excited about fulfilling my dream to get my work out before I'm too old to be productive.

This is a new chapter in my career, this is a major shift, from my 23 years doing art as a healing practice with people affected by mental illness, and now being out on my own as an artist. It is scary leaving the protective umbrella. I'm helping at a food pantry at church as a volunteer, and lots of my time is now freed up for me to do my artwork at this stage of life.

You know when it is time to turn over the torch in your life. At the mental health center, a creative wellness group was run by two younger peer support workers, and I shared with them that I have every confidence in you that you will flourish in your work. I was able to share that with them before I retired. I turned it over to good hands.

Continued

The Lived Experience—cont'd

At the time I retired, I transferred my meds from one pharmacy to another and relapsed given the medication changes and insurance limitations. I needed hospitalization for about a month to overcome my stress and anxiety and they needed to change my medications. It was a dark chapter of my retirement. But I am back on solid ground again. It was a scary time to be back in the hospital after 40 years of recovery. And I am thankful for the medication doctors who were able to figure out, after trial and error, what would work for me, and what was acceptable to those who insure me. The chemistry of the brain—I thank God for what they have done for me, given my chemical imbalance. So much more research needs to be done in the field.

There are so many people in the outside world who only see the stigma and don't know what help is needed and how they can be involved. I love the beautiful vision of your mental health text. I just wish that more people could learn from it and share the vision to put this into practice. It gives me hope to hear your vision for recovery—keep sharing it with the world!

and well-being, and, on a practical level, lessening the need for physical restraints (Friedland, 2003).

The *OTPF-4* (AOTA, 2020) also provides examples of leisure done at the individual level, as well as the group level (e.g., reading a book/being part of a book club; independently cooking/engaging in a cooking class or culinary arts group). Leisure occupations flexibly offer people the opportunity to engage in solitary and social activities; these choices can hold different meanings as well as motivations for people. Note the kinds of leisure occupations people engage in when alone versus with others. What kind of meaning does each offer to them? What is the just right amount of social connectivity in a person's daily social needs? These questions offer the OTP a way of helping those they serve plan for their health and well-being.

Another concept in the leisure studies literature is that of **serious leisure** (Stebbins, 1996), when engagement in a particular leisure activity might take on greater importance and a higher level of obligation regarding the pursuit of perseverance, acquisition of specialist skills, and entry into new social worlds. That is, what started as a leisure pursuit might start resembling work, insofar as making a deeper commitment to building capacity, using time, and connecting with others who share the same passion for the activity.

Consider the recent growth of pickleball across the United States and the world in the past 5 years. At the amateur level, this activity encourages healthy engagement in a physical activity that is accessible to not only older adults but increasingly people of all ages. It is enjoyable to engage in matches with others who enjoy the sport. However, within a relatively short time period, those amateurs may find themselves seeking out daily matches in varied venues, indoor and out, depending on the climate and access to pickleball courts. The strong desire to play can lead to some interesting accommodations. For example, in northern cities, it is not unheard of to change an indoor ballroom into a place where people can learn to play pickleball and host tournaments until the outdoor weather permits play. In these cases, what once was simply an enjoyable pastime evolves in a driving need to play.

PhotoVoice

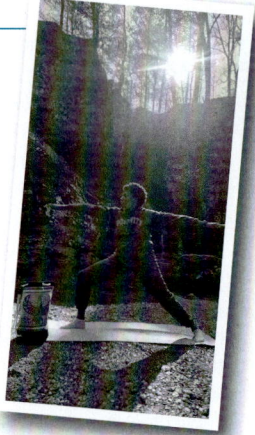

Well-Being Warrior

Yoga is a leisure occupation that allows me to be creative and practice self-care. This is a photo of me in my element as a well-being warrior in Warrior II pose. I first practiced yoga while in occupational therapy school at a community center with my mother, experiencing the best night's sleep afterwards. However, it didn't feel native to me or my body until I learned about Kemetic yoga, which predates Indic yoga practices and originates from Kemet/Ancient Egypt. As a Kemetic and Vinyasa yoga instructor, I can craft my own practice and enjoy being outdoors in nature, especially near water.

How does this narrative clue you to the fact that yoga has become a "serious leisure" occupation for this person? What can you learn about yoga that will help you as an OTP and others who want to learn?

considerations as how relaxing the activity is, the developmental match for the person/group participating, the social aspects of the activity, the environment within which the activity takes place and how appealing that is for participants, the aesthetic features of the activity, how fun and entertaining the activity is, whether productive life skills might be built by engaging in the activity, and how exciting people find the activity (Şimşek & Çevik, 2020).

Dimensions of Leisure

In the process of developing measurement tools around leisure and leisure time use, researchers have defined various dimensions of leisure that provide a deeper look at the ways leisure activities can be analyzed. These include such

Categories of Leisure Activities

The researchers who developed the Leisure Participation Assessment Tool for the Elderly (Jeong et al., 2020) assigned leisure activities into eight major categories: (1) sports/exercise, (2) games (involving two or more people using a game board, cards, or video), (3) social (visiting; gathering; volunteering; communicating via text, phone, or email), (4) cultural (arts and creative activities, gardening, watching performances, reading), (5) learning (formal and informal), (6) refresh (relaxation, meditation, prayer, meeting someone for tea), (7) outings (travel, camping, shopping, driving), and (8) information communication (TV, radio, internet). These categories offer OTPs the opportunity to engage in exploring varied types of leisure occupations that might bring enjoyment and fulfillment to a person's life.

Motivation for Engagement in Leisure

Several researchers consider motivation for leisure to be critical for understanding the link between sustained engagement in leisure and life satisfaction. Several studies (Morris & Rogers, 2004; Morris & Roychowdhury, 2020; Roychowdhury, 2018) have identified factors impacting choices around engaging in any physical activity by studying adults as well as children ages 9 and older. Intrinsic factors include the motivation to master and enjoy the activity. Social factors include the opportunities for affiliation, competition, and meeting others' expectations. Body/mind factors include the motivation to improve one's physical health, psychological health, and appearance.

Collectively, understanding the dimensions of leisure, the varied categories of leisure, and the varied motivations for engaging in leisure activities lay a foundation for the OTP, who may find that the person/group they are serving is interested in exploring leisure pursuits as well as participating in leisure activities that will enhance their life satisfaction and well-being. Identifying potential barriers or interferences in leisure engagement will be important as well. These barriers can involve physical (inaccessibility, location), economic (too costly, not available nearby), time (finding and creating time), information (not well marketed to all), environmental (challenges in natural environment, clean water and air, safety), or attitudinal constraints (unwelcoming to diverse or stigmatized populations). OTPs must address these factors to assure that occupational justice, engagement, and belonging can be a reality. Also see Chapter 11: Motivation. 🤝

Creativity and Creative Occupations

Although creative occupations are not explicitly included in the *OTPF-4* (AOTA, 2020; some may view creative activities as a subcategory of leisure), the interest in and preponderance of evidence around the health-promoting aspects of creative activities is growing at the individual, group, community, and population levels. As noted earlier, Hasselkus (2011) identified creativity as being part of everyday life when mundane moments are filled with spirit, electricity, and passion. In addition, Gillam (2018) noted creativity was both healing and life-affirming.

Several more definitive descriptions of creativity are offered as well. Schmid (2005) defined **creativity** as the "innate capacity to think and act in original ways, to be inventive,

to be imaginative and to find new and original solutions to needs, problems and forms of expression" (p. 6). Villanova and Cunha (2021) offered an expanded view of **everyday creativity** as "a phenomenon in which a person habitually responds to daily tasks in an original and meaningful way . . . everyday creativity can either be a creative product which is communicated to and assessed by the creator's immediate society, or a creative experience that is often personal and assessed by only the individual" (p. 691). Hence, one can be seen as creative based on formal and informal means, as viewed by others or as viewed by self.

OTPs in South Africa (Van der Reyden et al., 2019) framed the term **creative** as including a person's ability to create themselves through responding to the challenges of everyday life and creating tangible objects as well as potential solutions. Given the emphasis in occupational therapy to focus on everyday life, these definitions give broad space for what is considered "creative" as OTPs explore creativity and creative occupations with those they serve.

Creative activities have been explored related to the occupational value they bring to the participant (Hansen et al., 2022; Persson & Erlandsson, 2010) using the Value and Meaning in Occupation (ValMO) Model (Erlandsson & Persson, 2020). Persson and colleagues' earlier work (2001) described the experience of engaging in occupations with a core concept around three parallel dimensions of occupational value (also called the Occupational Value Triad): (1) concrete (tangible and visible), (2) sociosymbolic (social, cultural, universally valued when doing), and (3) self-rewarding (immediate rewards inherent in doing certain occupations). These potentially present with varied intensity levels.

In a study regarding the experience of occupational value when doing creative activities in a mental health context (Hansen et al., 2022), researchers found interventions that included creative activities were of high value to the lived experiences of participants across all three dimensions (Table 51-1). The value dimensions were studied to identify the kinds of value experienced by the participants (return to everyday life, new meaningful activity, having work and a possibility to develop as an artist, strengthened identity and recognition, belonging, self-expression, positive emotions and well-being, distraction, and creating a "free space"). The subcategories reflect the perspectives of the participants as they engage in the creative activity interventions. The Occupational Value Triad in Table 51-1 was extracted from participants' perspectives after engaging in a creative activity of their choice involving leather, jewelry, recycling shop, drawing/painting, pottery, metal, and carpentry.

Creative arts include five categories (Davies et al., 2012):

1. Visual arts, such as design and crafts (e.g., drawing; painting; crafting; coloring; making jewelry; designing fashion; creating ceramics; molding sculpture; developing origami; painting murals; visiting a gallery; attending an exhibition, pottery class, or knitting group)
2. Online, digital and electronic arts (e.g., art websites, digital photography, digital film making, animation, viewing e-concerts, viewing e-galleries, e-arts)
3. Community and cultural festivals (e.g., festivals related to national holidays, community events, religious dates, or events of cultural significance)

TABLE 51-1 | **Experiences of Occupational Value When Doing Creative Activities Interventions (Cal) in a Mental Health Context**

Value Dimensions	Subcategories: Participant Perspectives on Their Experiences	Categories
Concrete occupational value	• Cal creates daily rhythm and structure. • Cal provides energy and motivation for activities of everyday life.	Return to everyday life
	• Working professionally with arts and crafts creates meaningful content and activity in everyday life. • Cal gives something to do and look forward to. • Experiences with Cal have meant new activity in everyday life outside of the hospital.	New meaningful activity
	• Doing Cal involves serious work making marketable products in appropriate facilities. • Cal developed possibilities for creative expression and technical artistic processes.	Having work and a possibility to develop as an artist
Sociosymbolic occupational value	• Doing Cal creates an experience of having a "normal" identity. • Recognition of the creative product leads to recognition of the person behind. • Doing Cal leads to a feeling of social recognition and of "being someone."	Strengthened identity and recognition
	• Contact with peers means reflection, expressing oneself, and seeing your own situation in another and new perspective. "You are not alone." • The stories of others create hope. • People can be part of a creative and social community. • People can be part of the tradition and culture in the family.	Belonging
	• The creative product is a reflection of the personality. • Expression of emotions, identity, and mental status is shown through the therapeutic expression. • It creates a visible physical form which helps deal with negative energy.	Self-expression
Self-rewarding occupational value	Doing Cal: • Creates positive emotions and development, self-confidence, well-being and joy • Is relaxing, calming, and stress reducing	Positive emotions and well-being
	Doing Cal: • The brain gets a "break," forgetting time and place • Creates peace, diversion, and refuge • Creates a break from everyday trivial activities	Distraction and creating a "free space"

Hansen, B. W., Leufstadius, C., Pedersen, H. A., Berring, L. L., & Erlandsson, L. (2022). Experiences of occupational value when doing creative activities in a mental health context. Occupational Therapy in Mental Health, 38(4), 383–402. https://doi.org/10.1080/0164212X.2022.2067285

4. Performing arts (e.g., singing, playing a musical instrument, dancing, drama, composing, jamming, busking, sound art, listening to music, listening to a concert, attending the theater, dance classes, music lessons)
5. Literature (e.g., creative writing, storytelling, reading novels, writing poetry, journaling, attending a book launch, attending an author's talk, participating in a writing workshop, book clubs)

Davies and colleagues (2023) conducted research on the art of aging well and found those who voluntarily engaged in any recreational arts occupations for enjoyment, as entertainment, or as a hobby experienced better physical and mental health when compared with those who did not engage in such activities. These findings are important for OTPs when offering creative occupations as an essential part of health promotion.

Occupational Therapy to Enable Leisure and Creative Occupations

The International Creative Abilities Network (ICAN) provides information about the Vona du Toit Model of Creative Ability (VdTMoCA; Van der Reyden et al., 2019).

This occupational therapy practice model originated from the theory of creative ability developed by South African occupational therapist Vona du Toit, a WFOT leader and theorist who died in 1974 (du Toit, 1974). This model is being used across the world, from South Africa (for the past 50 years) to more recently Japan and the United Kingdom. International Conferences have been held in South Africa, Japan, Australia, the United Arab Emirates, Namibia, Mauritius, and Singapore.

The following description from the ICAN website provides a glimpse of the Model of Creative Ability (https://www.ican-uk.com/all-about-the-vdtmoca/overview-of-the-vdtmoca-and-ican):

The model's unique contribution to the occupational therapy profession is understanding people in terms of sequential levels of creative ability. The term creative refers to one's ability to change in response to life's demands (the creation of oneself), as well as creation of tangible things and solutions to problems. From a developmental perspective, each level of creative ability is comprised of interrelated volition, motivation and action (behaviours, skills, performance). Identifying and understanding a person's level of creative ability enables therapists to understand and provide therapeutic intervention for people of all degrees of volition, motivation and ability (Van der Reyden et al. 2019). Such knowledge can also guide intervention by other disciplines, family, carers and health and social care support staff (Van der Reyden & Sherwood, 2019).

The VdTMoCA is client-centered, ability and recovery focused. Occupational therapy is offered to match what the person has volition, motivation and ability for, but which also poses a challenge, mastery of which has the potential to result in growth in volition, motivation and ability. The individual's experience of having their motivation (needs) met, and experiencing ability to do activities of daily living, both motivates and enables them to engage. Through engagement, behavior and skills are developed toward the next level. Equally, the model informs intervention to maintain and/or prevent decline in ability, e.g., when improvement and growth into higher levels is not possible, or a person has a progressive condition such as dementia.

The model provides a detailed guide to the selection, structuring and presentation of intervention (Casteleijn & Holsten, 2019). This includes the use of activity, activity groups, and differing situations as the core of occupational therapy treatment, but informs all interactions with the individual, including how to approach the person, structure self-care intervention, and develop a meaningful routine that attends to all aspects of daily living including use of free time (leisure).

The Resources section at the end of this chapter provides more information regarding ICAN, as well as materials and interactive community data available from VdTMoCA.

The upcoming sections of this chapter review concrete ways for OTPs to address and enable leisure and creative occupations.

Assessment

Assessment begins with an occupational profile (AOTA, 2020) to gain a perspective on the person's life occupations; the environments in which they engage; and their goals, values, and interests, as well as the challenges they face as they pursue a path to health, recovery, and well-being. Identifying what matters most to the person will shape the initial intervention plan and targeted outcomes. Working collaboratively, OTPs are guided by the person, their goals, and the occupations they want and need to do as they embark on their journey of health and well-being, including those leisure and creative occupations that will provide a strong foundation for their journey.

Table 51-2 provides an overview of a variety of tools that can be used to get a perspective on how the person views the meaningful occupations they want and need to engage in, and their interest in exploring and participating in occupations that will strengthen their engagement in healthy and meaningful occupations, including those associated with leisure and creativity.

The Canadian Occupational Performance Measure (Law et al., 2019) provides an overview of satisfaction with and performance across all three areas of self-care, leisure, and productivity. This will provide the person and their OTP with a sense of where targeted barriers might be addressed by using the person's strengths to build motivation, skill, and self-efficacy to explore and carry out the occupations they consider most important to them.

PhotoVoice

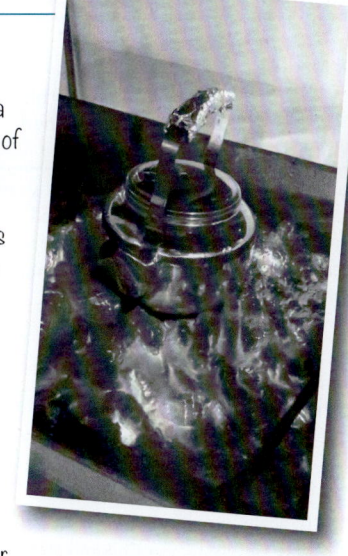

Sage-Infused Tea on Burning Coal

Making sage-infused tea over burning coal is one of the most joyful, relaxing activities that I do to ease my heart. The tea is delicious and the sage is very calming. Sage has significant cultural and religious roots in Arab culture. It is a sacred herb that is believed to expel evil and heal the body and heart. The Arabic name (Marymia) is named after Mary the mother of Issa (Jesus) who was told by God to drink some sage to ease labor pains. Marymia is usually consumed in the cold days of winter to bring warmth to the body and solace to broken hearts.

Identify all of the dimensions of leisure in this PhotoVoice.

The Activity Card Sort (Baum & Edwards, 2008) and the Modified Interest Checklist (Klyczek et al., 1997) can help OTPs identify the full range of occupations that might stimulate a person's interest and motivation to address the challenges they face when engaging in healthy and productive occupations consistent with their recovery goals. Using the cards/checklist, the OTP and person can also evaluate the balance of social connections, environmental contexts, and novel activities that would be optimal for matching their strengths, interests, and vulnerabilities as they work to establish healthy routines of everyday life.

Insights can be gained around the features and motivations associated with physical activities, leisure activities, community participation, and meaningfulness of activities using the other tools listed in Table 51-2. In particular, the Leisure Participation Assessment Tool for the Elderly might help persons over the age of 65 best match the activities they want to frequently engage in while eliminating or lessening interferences to participation.

Intervention

The person and their OTP will develop a plan identifying targeted activities based on the person's level of independence in implementing the steps to achieve their goals. The literature highlights approaches to working with individuals and groups to activate their engagement by using strategies that encourage planning and experimenting with varied activities, environments, and people so that the person can build their repertoire of choices around what, when, where, and how

TABLE 51-2 | Therapeutic Reasoning Assessment Table: Leisure and Creative Occupations Measures

Which Tool?	Who Was This Tool Designed For?	Is This a Type of Tool This Person Can Use? What Is Required of the Person?	What Am I Measuring?	How Long Does It Take and Where Do I Administer This Assessment?	Is the Tool Associated With a Practice Model?
Canadian Occupational Performance Measure (COPM; Law et al., 2019)	• Adults (18+ years) • Children and youth 8+ years • Parents of young children (0–8 years)	The assessment is completed as a semistructured interview with support from an OTP.	A measure of occupational satisfaction and performance in self-care, leisure, and productivity	Administered in any setting and takes 30–60 minutes	Canadian Model of Occupational Performance (CMOP-E; Townsend & Polatajko, 2007)
The Activity Card Sort (ACS; Baum & Edwards, 2008)	Adults with neurological, psychiatric, or physical dysfunction	Person describes their occupational history by sorting 89 photographs depicting people completing various daily living and leisure activities.	Participation in social, instrumental, and leisure activities	Administered in a clinical or home setting and takes approximately 20–30 minutes	The PEO Performance model
The Physical Activity & Leisure Motivation Scales (PALMS; Morris & Roychowdhury, 2020; Roychowdhury, 2018)	• Adults (18+) • Children and youth 9+ years	Person identifies their motivation for engaging in varied physical and leisure activities.	Motivations include intrinsic (mastery, enjoyment) and extrinsic (social such as affiliation, competition, and meeting others' expectations; and body/mind motives such as physical and psychological health and appearance)	Administered in any setting, typically less than 30 minutes	Compatible with PEO and Model of Human Occupation (MOHO)
Leisure Activity Participation Scale (LAPS; Şimşek & Çevik, 2020)	Adults (18+)	Person responds to statements about leisure activities (relaxing, training, socialization, impressive environment, productive activity, aesthetic, fun, exciting) reflecting their lived experiences.	Dimensions of leisure activities that can be measured by those who participate in them, revealing motivations	Administered in any setting; time to complete not reported	Compatible with PEO and MOHO
Community Participation Indicators (CPI; Heinemann et al., 2011)	Adults 18–65 and 66+ with a wide variety of self-identified disabilities	Person identifies how often, how important, and if the person feels they are doing the activity enough in their home and community across 48 items, which include activities of daily living (ADLs), instrumental activities of daily living (IADLs), leisure and social events, and reflections on the control they have over their participation.	Examines two domains of community participation: engagement in activities the person holds to be important, and control over their participation	Can be administered in any setting using pencil and paper or via a computer; takes 10–15 minutes	Activity choice and desire for change gained from the measure consistent with PEO and MOHO
Leisure Participation Assessment Tool for the Elderly (Jeong et al., 2020)	Older adults (65+) who are community dwelling	Person responds to 81 items across eight categories of leisure activities, indicating the frequency of participation (quantitatively) and their satisfaction and interest (qualitatively) in the activities.	A measure of leisure participation and exploration in community dwelling elderly, including their perspective on what interferes with participation	Can be administered in any setting; time to complete not reported	Consistent with PEO and MOHO

TABLE 51-2 | Therapeutic Reasoning Assessment Table: Leisure and Creative Occupations Measures—cont'd

Which Tool?	Who Was This Tool Designed For?	Is This a Type of Tool This Person Can Use? What Is Required of the Person?	What Am I Measuring?	How Long Does It Take and Where Do I Administer This Assessment?	Is the Tool Associated With a Practice Model?
Meaningful Activity Participation Assessment (MAPA; Eakman, 2007; Eakman et al., 2010)	Older adults (65+) who are community dwelling	Person responds to a checklist-type survey consisting of 28 diverse activity items, recording the frequency of participation and the degree of personal meaningfulness experienced with each activity.	Frequency and ascribed meaning are intended to reflect a person's overall level of meaningful activity participation, with higher scores indicative of greater perceived meaningful activity participation (0–672 possible range of scores).	Can be administered in groups of 3–15 people, allowing as much time as needed to complete the questionnaire (average was 45 minutes)	Consistent with PEO and MOHO models
Modified Interest Checklist (Klyczek et al., 1997)	Adolescents and adults	Person indicates strength of interest for 68 activities.	Assesses the person's strength of interest in 68 activities related to past, present, and future to inform activity choices.	Can be done in any environment (home, school, community, clinical settings); time to complete not specified	Consistent with PEO model and MOHO MOHO-IRM website provides versions for diverse learners and people from Ireland and the United Kingdom

they will engage. OTPs find that using creative activities as an intervention for persons with mental illness is commonly used, at least weekly because of the diverse objectives that it can address and its usefulness for both 1:1 and group interactions (Griffiths & Corr, 2007).

The manual *Action Over Inertia: Addressing the Activity-Health Needs of Individuals With Serious Mental Illness* (Krupa et al., 2010) features worksheets designed by a team of occupational therapists across Canada to give structure to the process of exploring a person's activity patterns, creating daily time logs, exploring an analysis of occupational balance, monitoring daily routines and structure, finding meaning and satisfaction, engaging in social interactions, and accessing community environments. This helps OTPs and people when planning for future ways to experiment with new occupations or creative interests, finding quick activity changes (such as finishing a project, listening to music, playing an instrument, writing a poem, singing in the shower, visiting a new website on the computer), and beginning to make an intentional path for the future around leisure and creative activities as part of an overall plan for activity engagement linked to health and well-being. Enabling sustained commitment to building a rich and engaged menu of options is ultimately part of the structured approach to Action Over Inertia.

Psychologists call **activity scheduling**, which is considered a cognitive behavioral tool, **behavioral activation**. Multiple websites offer worksheets and guidelines for building 7-day-a-week plans emphasizing positive and mood-lifting activities to overcome depression in children and adults. Ultimately,

the goal is to help the person formulate a plan they believe will work for them and will commit to following through on (Starkman, 2021). See the Resources list at the end of this chapter to access an example of a manualized intervention using Behavioral Activation for Depression.

Farhadian and colleagues (2024) developed a leisure activity group intervention for persons recovering from substance use disorders. Consisting of 12 sessions offered twice a week, the intervention showed positive effects on occupational performance and balance, leisure participation, quality of life, and a decrease in drug craving. Sessions 1, 2, and 12 were focused on leisure education, exploration, planning, and creating individualized leisure plans, whereas sessions 3 to 11 involved actual engagement in the chosen leisure occupations as a group. Selected activities included going to a theater, experiencing escape rooms, taking walks, attending a museum, bowling, playing paintball, shooting, and karting.

Table 51-3 includes interventions reflected in the occupational therapy literature offering examples of the varied ways engagement in leisure and creative occupations impact individuals and groups. In addition, this chapter's Being a Psychosocial OT Practitioner feature shows best practices for using leisure and creative activities to meet a person's psychosocial needs. Chapter 50: Play 🤝 offers insights on facilitating play and playfulness to enhance mental health and a sense of belonging, and Chapter 37: School Mental Health provides direction to afterschool programming that enhances participation in leisure and recreational activities as a part of the student role. 🤝

TABLE 51-3 | A Sampling of Leisure and Creative Occupation Interventions Featured in AOTA's *OT Practice Magazine*, 2017–2023

Type of Leisure/Creative Occupation; How Structured; Collaborators	Targeted Population	Outcomes Achieved and Participant Perspectives	Author(s), Date of Publication
Songwriting as an occupation structured as a group, met 2x per week for 4 weeks. Occupational therapists collaborated with performing musicians and music therapists.	Homeless men with mental illness living in an emergency transitional homeless shelter	All participants completed one song and rated positive changes in both performance and satisfaction scores on the COPM. Themes included love, spirituality, longing, and grief. "It opened my mind to others' perspectives and helped me overcome some mental and emotional struggles" (p. 23).	Raphael-Greenfield et al. (2017)
Grow Bag zoom gardening together during the pandemic, virtually. Lead occupational therapist was also a master gardener. Each received a 7-gallon Grow Bag kit with rich porous soil, starter plants, tools, and laminated care instructions.	Eight participants who were developmentally and/or intellectually disabled engaged in this program that promotes health through gardening.	Participants were engaged in Zoom sessions, and home visits were conducted by the adult services director. A reflection by a participant and support team: "Tending to his garden and tracking its progress is something that has contributed to Trevor's summer quarantine routine. And as many of us know, a routine is very important right now" (p. 17).	Colucci & Kowalski (2020)
Building blocks for social participation: Fostering friendship and collaboration through play-based clubs. Lego Clubs were implemented in three settings: an afterschool program at a public school, a private school for children with special needs, and a pro bono outpatient clinic staffed by graduate students and supervised by occupational therapy faculty.	Children ages 5–12 with two siblings as peer models of varying abilities. Program included a snack, warmup activity, and a Lego building session. Sessions were cofacilitated by occupational therapy students and an occupational therapy faculty supervisor, who had access to speech language pathologist. Ten children participated in the group that occurred over 10 weeks.	Recommendations for future facilitation of sessions included practical tips to handle sensory issues, social anxiety, visual perceptual issues, and management of challenging behaviors. The parent of a participant said, "My oldest had a hard time socially at school. He was much more aware of the other children around him. He wasn't just doing his own thing—it was a great improvement!" (p. 20).	Matthews et al. (2021)
Art with a heart: A creative fundraiser for a clinic run by occupational therapy students and faculty, where artwork was created by children receiving occupational therapy services using paint, crayons, feathers, beads, fabric, pipe cleaners, and so on.	An online art show and auction was held with 75 pieces of work from children and artists, and an ability to share about the services offered at the clinic. They raised more than $10,000 for the occupational therapy services offered at the clinic.	The clinic has served more than 400 children, trained 200 students and 225 teachers, and works with around 200 parents. An occupational therapy student reflected, "It's really cool to see how excited they are, and their families are really excited and can't wait to see the artwork on the website. It's just really inspiring" (p. 37).	Zachry et al. (2022)
Practitioner Health and Wellness: What are you doing on the weekends?	Factors that support the psychological well-being of health providers during SARs-CoV-2 were explored.	High occupational balance, positive psychological working conditions, low workload, and high sense of community control and justice were associated with little to no symptoms of stress. Weekend activities that affected overall well-being such as voluntary engagement in reading a book, low effort activities such as watching TV, social activities, and physical activities showed higher levels of psychological well-being and lower levels of work-related stress.	Cahill (2022)
Riding the Wave: Occupational Therapy's Role in Surf Therapy: an occupational therapy degree capstone project involving a trained facilitator of surfing with an occupational therapy background	Descriptions of individual interventions for two children that were tailored to their particular needs were shared.	"Surf therapy is more than just building the skills needed to surf a wave on your own; it's also about building confidence and self-esteem, trusting someone new to help you succeed, learning to pay attention and sustain that attention, developing skills for regulating your emotions of fear and excitement, and discovering how to fail and fail—and get right back on the surfboard."	Tubbs & Folan (2023)

TABLE 51-3 | **A Sampling of Leisure and Creative Occupation Interventions Featured in AOTA's** *OT Practice Magazine,* **2017–2023—cont'd**

Type of Leisure/Creative Occupation; How Structured; Collaborators	Targeted Population	Outcomes Achieved and Participant Perspectives	Author(s), Date of Publication
Overcoming the Barriers to Aquatic Recreation: A Training Program for Adults With Physical Disabilities: an adaptive aquatics doctoral capstone project, where in three sessions in a large therapy pool the focus was on learning safe transfers into and out of the pool, using and modifying flotation devices to meet individual needs, and learning techniques for completing dressing and showering in the locker room.	Five participants were highlighted, including persons with spinal cord injuries, multiple sclerosis, or Kniest syndrome, and a person with an unknown neurological condition.	Individual goals were set in addition to the previously described goals. All achieved varied goals related to swimming, water play, practicing breathing exercises, and training caregivers in ways to support community participation for future swimming. Participants gained a better understanding of their ability to engage in an aquatic environment and to better address barriers in accessing community pools.	Adams & Wingrat (2023)

Evidence on Creative Activity Intervention With Individuals and Groups

Hansen, Erlandsson, and Leufstadius (2020) sought a common way to identify the essential components of using creative activities as intervention (CaI) in occupational therapy. The five common elements identified were that the intervention:

1. Often consisted of arts and crafts activities using mind and body (examples included paint, fabric, clay, paper- and wood-based projects, drama and music)
2. Was experienced by the person as meaningful and carried out in a safe, facilitating environment
3. Enhanced creative processes, inherent experiences, and opportunities for self-expression and reflection
4. Facilitated development of skills that transfer over to enhancing occupational performance and managing everyday life
5. Can be flexibly implemented with individuals and groups using different approaches to allow for varied goals and settings

The varied approaches included experiencing joy in the process and production of creation; using psychosocial strategies to enhance social connections and belonging; increasing personal knowledge and skills that build psychological, social, and emotional capacities to manage everyday life more effectively; and using creative media to enhance self-expression and development, thereby finding novel ways to look at oneself and one's life circumstances as a means of overcoming challenge and despair.

This concept analysis clarified that the actual activity selected is less important because it is the participant who selects and builds meaning based on their experience with the creative process and product. The therapeutic context is understood as a creative space within which exploration and an unfolding of one's natural creative processes occurs in a playful manner. Understanding these essential components of creative activities as intervention, accompanied by the approach that matches the person's goals and needs, provides OTPs with the tools for using their therapeutic use of self to facilitate the creative processes.

Nonintervention Creative Activity for Individuals and Groups

In a scoping review, Ludowyke et al. (2023) investigated the meaning and purpose of creativity experienced in daily life occupations for persons with mental health conditions. Because these creative acts were distinct from creativity experienced in creative activity interventions, they were called nonintervention creative experiences and activities. Their focus was on those activities chosen by the person in their home, community, and neighborhoods, not those structured as occupational therapy mental health interventions. The person selected and engaged in everyday activities and processes based on their subjective motivation.

Based on content analysis and qualitative thematic analysis, Ludowyke and colleagues (2023) found that these kinds of creative activities occurred in participatory arts-based programs such as choir singing, theater, art media, and creative writing, which occurred in places such as museums and other specifically designated areas for the arts. They also noted informal drop-in activity spaces and programs where people engaged in crafts, gardening/horticulture, table-top games, and puzzles. A third location of creative activities occurred in an individual's homes where they self-initiated creative activities of their interest.

Themes around people's engagement in nonintervention activities were clustered into the impacts made on the person (mental and physical health benefit; increased confidence and feelings of achievement); the environment (social environments where they felt connected and belonging; safe and accommodating places to be); the occupations (meaning; purpose that fit into routines; experiences of flow, safety, and

Being a Psychosocial OT Practitioner

Overcoming Depression After Spinal Cord Injury

Contributed by John Rider, PhD, OTR/L, MSCS, CEAS

Identifying Psychosocial Strengths and Needs

OTPs can address leisure occupational engagement to improve health and well-being across practice settings and diagnoses. Consider the story of Liam, a young adult attending an outpatient neurorehabilitation clinic after a motor vehicle accident resulting in a C7 spinal cord injury. Upon returning home after inpatient rehabilitation, Liam was reluctant to start outpatient therapy. His parents report that he has been severely depressed since the accident and has refused to attend any social events despite persistent invitations from his friends. Liam is 24 years old, graduated with a degree in accounting a year ago, and lives with his parents in a single-story home. Fortunately, his home only needed a ramp to make it wheelchair accessible. Liam worked virtually when the accident occurred and wants to continue working from home.

Liam is considered a quadriplegic because his upper extremities are affected by the spinal cord injury, with impaired elbow extension, finger extension, fine motor coordination, and grasp/pinch strength. He has been in a custom manual wheelchair for a month and is completing most ADLs with increased time and adapted equipment. He requires minimum assistance with transfers and is still hesitant to propel his wheelchair over uneven surfaces and up/down curbs. He is independent with dressing and self-care but reports that he has not resumed cooking or housekeeping because he lives with his parents, who have been doing that for him since the accident. However, upon further discussion, Liam reported that he did enjoy grilling on his patio with his dad, and his family frequently hosted barbecues with extended family and friends.

During the occupational profile, Liam gave short answers, displayed limited engagement, and reported that he was only there because his parents wanted him to be. When asked about goals, Liam shared that he wants to be independent in all transfers and to be able to work from home again. He indicated he wasn't interested in learning to drive an adapted vehicle because he "had nowhere to go." When asked about interests and what he does for fun, Liam stated, "I used to do a lot of things for fun, but I can't do them anymore." The OTP spent time exploring Liam's past interests, occupations he wanted to pursue in the future, and his perspectives on barriers to participation. Liam identified going to the gym and playing sports as a preferred leisure occupation but felt those were no longer options because of the wheelchair and his upper extremity impairments. Liam also mentioned cooking for himself again, but it was lower on his priorities.

Using a Holistic Occupational Therapy Approach

The OTP and Liam created goals to address transfers, ensure wheelchair skills, and explore leisure occupations. Between working on transfers and wheelchair skills, the OTP and Liam looked online at wheelchair-accessible venues, events, activities, and transportation options. The OTP shared some newer apps designed for wheelchair users where other wheelchair users review locations and businesses on their accessibility and share tips and tricks for traveling. Liam was excited to show the apps to his dad when he came to pick him up.

Given that Liam used to play sports and enjoyed going to the gym, at their next session, the OTP provided Liam with information on adaptive sports and clubs in the area. Liam's "homework" was to review them and identify one he wanted to learn more about and possibly try.

At the next session, Liam had a grin on his face. He said he wanted to look into wheelchair rugby (also known as quad rugby). He was especially excited because he had always wanted to try rugby, but his high school didn't have a team. The OTP had volunteered with the local wheelchair rugby team as a student, and a few times as a clinician, so he had a few friends on the team. They watched some videos online about the game and started learning the rules. The OTP incorporated throwing and catching with wheelchair skills training to simulate wheelchair rugby, which made Liam even more excited.

With Liam's permission, the OTP invited the local wheelchair rugby team captain to their next session to discuss the game, team, and practices. The OTP and Liam also invited his parents to come and learn more about the game. The team captain shared that an OTP comes to their practices and assists with their training to ensure each player's exercises and drills are safe. They practice one night a week, and anyone who is available attends an adapted gym every Saturday to work out together. The gym has equipment designed for wheelchair users. Liam exchanges contact information with the team captain and gets the team schedule for the next month.

For the first time, Liam is all smiles. However, he shares that he is nervous because this is the first social endeavor since his accident outside of therapy. The OTP and Liam discuss his initial concerns and fears and make a detailed plan on what he needs to do to take the next steps toward participating in wheelchair rugby. The plan includes scheduling an appointment with his doctor to get clearance to play; learning the rules; creating a home program for conditioning; learning about precautions, such as autonomic dysreflexia; figuring out transportation; planning for bowel and bladder management outside of the home, and so on. Together, they start addressing each item until they can schedule an occupational therapy session at the adapted gym and a session at a wheelchair rugby practice. At the end of the first practice, while debriefing, Liam mentions that he wants to learn more about adapted driving now that he has "somewhere to go." Liam continues to play with the team after being discharged from occupational therapy and competes in his first wheelchair rugby tournament later that year with his OTP in attendance.

Reflective Questions

1. What standardized assessments might have been useful with Liam when he had difficulty identifying preferred leisure occupations?
2. What other benefits might Liam gain by participating in a leisure activity with other individuals with spinal cord injuries?
3. How would you design a treatment session to explore or engage in creative activities with Liam in an outpatient setting?

Evidence-Based Practice

Creative Art Occupations in People With Chronic Disabling Conditions

Making art helps individuals socially connect and reclaim a positive identity.

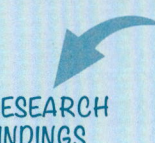

RESEARCH FINDINGS

Reynolds (2003); Reynolds and Prior (2006); and Reynolds, Vivat, and Prior (2008) conducted a series of qualitative studies involving persons with chronic disabling conditions and their motivation for and engagement in creative art occupations. The impact on identity, coping, personal growth, achievement, and status was uncovered, as well as the adoption of a more positive view of self as an artist, a person who lived with hope and who resisted being dominated by labels associated with their illness. The process of moving toward a new identity takes time, even years, and involves acceptance of their chronic condition, as well as finding ways to live with their limitations and reprioritizing their occupations. Art-making was manageable within their abilities and a way to socially connect with others and reclaim a positive identity.

APPLICATIONS

➡ Offering opportunities to find meaningful activities is an important part of the adaptation and identity-making process.
➡ Finding creative activities that also allow the person to express grief and loss are healing ways to cope with chronic disabling conditions.
➡ Even when a person has not engaged in creative activities earlier in life, the process of learning and engaging in novel creative occupations facilitates building supportive social networks and a wider cultural milieu.
➡ Persons involved in these studies recommended that the opportunities for creative engagement be offered early in the recovery process, as many took years to find meaningful occupations as a means to health and daily life satisfaction.

REFERENCES

Reynolds, F. (2003). Reclaiming a positive identity in chronic illness through artistic occupation. *OTJR: Occupational Therapy Journal of Research, 23*(3), 118–127. https://doi.org/10.1177/153944920302300305
Reynolds, F., & Prior, S. (2006). The role of art-making in identity maintenance: Case studies of people living with cancer. *European Journal of Cancer Care, 15,* 333–341. https://doi.org/10.1111/j.1365-2354.2006.00663.x
Reynolds, F., Vivat, B., & Prior, S. (2008). Women's experiences of increasing subjective well-being in CFS/ME through leisure-based arts and crafts activities: A qualitative study. *Disability and Rehabilitation, 30*(17), 1279–1288. https://doi.org/10.1080/09638280701654518

stability); spirituality and creating an identity (being oneself and moving toward the future, transformation, self-discovery toward recovery); barriers and challenges experienced (stigma and attitudes, systemic challenges in biomedical and institutional stances, economic barriers); and perceived personal limitations associated with the person's mental abilities connected with their mental illness and other health factors such as pain and fatigue (Fig. 51-1).

Ludowyke and colleagues (2023) encourage OTPs to consider how the community can support accessible, inclusive arts programming as healthy and safe places for people in recovery to carry out their meaningful occupations. For example, nonclinical public spaces such as churches, schools, libraries, community centers, parks, and galleries are ideal for creating meaningful places where community-dwelling citizens with mental health challenges can engage and fully participate in meaningful occupations of their choice.

Arts and Health Programs for Communities and Populations

A final area in which future growth in meaningful leisure and creative activity participation might take place is as part of a public health and large-scale focus on arts and health.

Participatory arts programs offered in communities and across populations since the 1990s are adding to the evidence

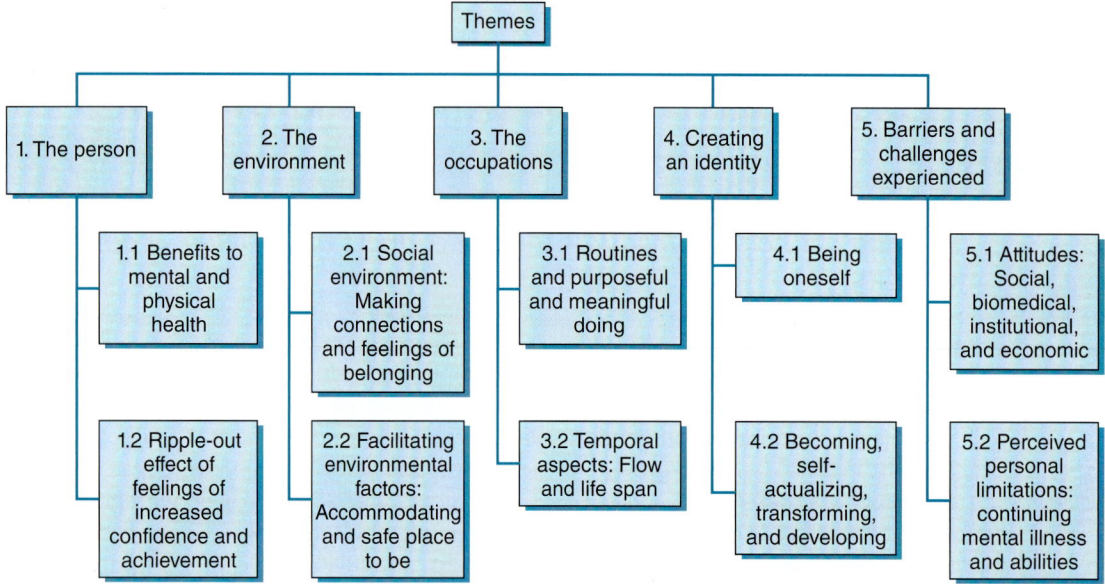

FIGURE 51-1. Themes and subthemes from a scoping review of meaning and purpose of creativity in daily life occupations. *From Ludowyke, L., Lentin, P., & Brown, T. (2023). The meaning and purpose of creativity in the daily life occupations, activities, acts and behaviors amongst adults living with mental health conditions: A scoping review.* Occupational Therapy in Mental Health, 40*(1), 45–85. https://doi.org/10.1080/0164212X.2023.2218121*

around individuals' health impacts, especially on mental health and well-being (White, 2009). Davies and Clift (2022) suggest that "arts and health" has become a new discipline informing policy, practice, and programs, and they developed a glossary so that the language of these health initiatives for both the general population and specific populations (e.g., young people, older adults, people with disabilities) can be communicated clearly across the world.

As an example of one country's efforts to implement an arts and health program, Laitinen and colleagues (2022) describe how grassroots activities moved to influence national policies in Finland. In 2019, the Finnish government acknowledged the intersection of arts, culture, health, and well-being, given nearly a decade of programs implemented beginning in 2010. They passed an act (Municipal Cultural Activities Act, 166/2019) where one aim was to promote art and culture as part of health and well-being. The act emphasized inclusion and communality for all residents, noting that the varied systems needed to cooperate across health care, national social welfare, economic and regional policies, and art and cultural policies.

For example, professional dancers have served as dance ambassadors in eldercare settings, nursery schools, and disability units in the community. Citizens volunteer as art and culture companions to those who have not been exposed to these venues in over 20 cities in Finland. In addition, financially pressed family can access funds to experience art and cultural events (Laitinen et al., 2022).

These provide OTPs with an emerging set of opportunities to help all people participate in and advocate for expanded opportunities in support of community health and well-being. With the primary domain of the profession being "achieving health, well-being, and participation in life through engagement in occupation" (AOTA, 2020, p. 5), advocacy and leadership at the societal level are critical to strengthen the impact worldwide.

Here's the Point

- Leisure and creative occupations may be highly meaningful ways to help people regain a sense of self after an injury or trauma.
- Successful engagement in leisure and creative occupations may stimulate motivation to work on other important occupations, offering hope and a reason to engage despite challenges.
- Across one's life span, leisure and creative occupations may constrict or expand depending on a person's life circumstances and expected performance of other occupational roles. During times where school, work, and family responsibilities dominate, leisure and creative occupations may offer life balance.
- As one moves toward retirement, the time available for leisure and creative occupations may expand and engagement may become even more meaningful to one's identity, health, and mental health.
- Assessments help the person to explore with their OTP the varied opportunities, facilitators, and barriers to engagement.
- Activity sampling, activity scheduling, and reflecting on dimensions of leisure and creative occupations all serve as potential interventions for engagement.
- Use of creative activity engagement as an intervention and pursuit of creative occupations independent of intervention both impact health and well-being.
- Exploration of the impact of cultural, recreational, and creative programming to impact public health has shown promising results in several countries (Finland, Italy, Australia, United Kingdom, Africa) and deserves more attention.

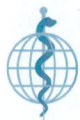 Visit the online resource center at FADavis.com to access the videos.

Apply It Now

1. Leisure and Creative Occupation Exploration and Participation

Select a novel leisure or creative occupation to learn. Spend 8 weeks engaged in the occupation, devoting time each week to performing this occupation. Record your experience in a journal including the dates you participated, the amount of time spent, what you did, and the meaning of the experience to you. Respond to the following focused questions at the end of each week. At the conclusion of the learning activity, reflect on how you could employ your new knowledge when you approach leisure and creative occupations with the people you will serve as an OTP.

Reflective Questions

■ Week 1: How did you decide which occupation you would do? In what ways does your culture influence your choices? What facilitates your options? What limits your options? How did you begin engaging in your selected occupation? How does it feel to do something new and unfamiliar?
■ Week 2: Have you experienced problems with occupational participation? Occupational deprivation? Occupational alienation? If so, how have these challenges impacted your experience? If not, how might some of these issues serve as potential problems for someone who desires to be engaged in the same occupation? How does what you do shape society, and how does society shape what you do?
■ Week 3: Consider other people who also engage in this occupation. In what ways are you connected to them? If the occupation you engage in occurs as a part of a group, how has the group affected your participation and experience? If your occupation is done as a solitary activity, how has that affected your participation and experience?
■ Week 4: Where does your occupation fit in your own development? What experiences in your past affect your present experience? How does your experience compare with cultural expectations for a person of your age and situation? What do you feel or think about this? How does your occupational choice reflect your family history? What potential does this occupation have to affect your future?
■ Week 5: Consider your entire routine of occupations. In what ways does your selected occupation affect you (your health, well-being, feelings of competency, self-esteem, etc.)? How do you presently use time in your life? How has adding this occupation affected your occupational balance?
■ Week 6: Have you had any moments when you experienced flow in this occupation? If so, think about the factors that led to this experience. If not, try to determine what prevents flow.
■ Week 7: Describe the "therapeutic" aspects of the occupation for you. Are there "limitations"? How might you modify or grade the experience? For whom would this occupation be optimal?
■ Week 8: What have you learned about yourself while doing this occupation across time? How can you apply your knowledge to your future role as an OTP?

(The previous assignment was adapted from one designed by Virginia A. Dickie.)

2. Identifying Community Resources for Leisure and Creative Occupations

Review weekly newspaper offerings and internet resources for free and low-cost leisure and creative activities in your area. Try to find two to three activities you could recommend for people with the following interests and conditions and explain your choices.

■ Middle school child with autism and an interest in trains
■ Young woman with posttraumatic stress disorder who has difficulty with crowds but enjoys hip-hop music
■ Older man with mild dementia who enjoys birdwatching

3. Video Exercise: Leisure Occupations for Unhoused Individuals

Pair up with another student in your class or form a small group of students. Access and watch the "Leisure Occupations for Unhoused Individuals" video at the online resource center at FADavis.com. Then, discuss and together answer the following questions.

Reflective Questions

■ What kinds of barriers do you think the unhoused population with whom Kailin works face when it comes to accessing and participating in leisure occupations in their daily lives? How did she work to overcome the barriers?
■ What approach did Kailin take to identifying what leisure activities might be enjoyable for specific individuals?
■ Which of the specific activities Kailin described resonates most with you in light of the population you work with or envision working with? What steps would you need to take to facilitate those activities?
■ How would you "sell" an individual with mental illness on the "power of fun," as described by Kailin?

Resources

• *Behavioral Activation for Depression* is a manualized guide from the University of Michigan: https://medicine.umich.edu/sites/default/files/content/downloads/Behavioral-Activation-for-Depression.pdf
• International Creative Ability Network: Vona du Toit Model of Creative Ability: https://www.ican-uk.com. This website contains information, training materials, and resources highlighting the work of the VdTMoCA and the ICAN.
• Model of Human Occupation-Intentional Relationship Model. https://moho-irm.uic.edu

- Special Olympics: SpecialOlympics.org. Visit this site to gain an awareness of the organization's sports, games, and competition; inclusive health activities; and how youth and schools can build leadership and inclusion across people of all abilities. The site also highlights volunteer opportunities and options for supporting Special Olympics at the local, state, national, and international levels.

Creative Arts Programs

- Friendship Circle: friendshipcircle.org
- National Endowment for the Arts: arts.gov/impact/accessibility/careers-in-the-arts-for-people-with-disabilities
- New Horizons Un-Limited: new-horizons.org/adparp.html
- ReelAbilities (film festivals advancing accessibility through film): https://reelabilities.org

Videos

- "Caregiver of Spouse With Alzheimer Disease on Challenges" video. Nancy is the wife and caregiver of a man with early-onset Alzheimer disease. Her husband, Bill, had an exciting civilian career as well as one with the U.S. Navy. In this video, she describes the challenges they face now that he is unable to work, particularly because he has few hobbies or friends. Nancy shares her struggle maintaining a schedule and filling his time, and describes how she encourages occupations that are meaningful to him. Access the video at the online resource center at FADavis.com.
- "Occupational Therapy Approaches in a Shelter for Unaccompanied Refugee Youth" video. In this video, occupational therapist Claudette Fette shares the impactful work she, volunteer students, and staff performed in a massive unaccompanied minor shelter in Texas in 2021. Many of the minors, mostly from Central America, had histories of trauma, and the conditions in the shelter were dismal—lack of meaningful occupations, bullying, untrained staff, and so on. Claudette describes her approach to assessing the environment, training staff, recruiting volunteers, responding to the minors' trauma responses, and creating and supporting occupations and leisure activities. Access the video at the online resource center at FADavis.com.
- "Positive Mindset Creative Arts Festival" video. This video showcases the Positive Mindset Creative Arts Festival, held at the Queensland Children's Hospital in Australia. This annual children's festival promotes positive thinking about mental health and increases help-seeking behaviors with a creative arts focus. It is a notable example of how OTPs can contribute to community health efforts. The emphasis is on art as an occupation and creating space in the community to encourage and celebrate mental health. In addition, the event promotes the idea of social connection and belonging centered around self-expression of feelings across the mental health continuum and how that ultimately encourages the sense of connection and belonging with people and communities. Access the video at the online resource center at FADavis.com.
- "Will Horowitz: Lived Experience of Autism" video. In this video, a young autistic adult describes his childhood interest in trains and how it has translated into an adult volunteer opportunity. He explains that, although an autistic individual can seem to have a "one-track mind" about a subject, it can also become an advantage in that they can become very specialized, as has been true for him with the Steam Into History project at a local railroad. Access the video at the online resource center at FADavis.com.

References

Adams, A., & Wingrat, J. (2023, June). Overcoming the barriers to aquatic recreation. *OT Practice, 28,* 14–17. https://www.aota.org/publications/ot-practice/ot-practice-issues/2023/overcoming-the-barriers-to-aquatic-recreation

American Occupational Therapy Association. (2020). Occupational therapy practice framework: Domain and process —Fourth edition. *American Journal of Occupational Therapy, 74*(Suppl. 2), 7412410010p1–7412410010p87. https://doi.org/10.5014/ajot.2020.74S2001

Baum, C., & Edwards D. F. (2008). *Activity Card Sort* (2nd ed.). AOTA Press.

Cahill, S. (2022, October 1). Research update: Practitioner health and wellness. *OT Practice.* https://www.aota.org/publications/ot-practice/ot-practice-issues/2022/research-update-practitioner-health-wellness

Casteleijn, D., & Holsten, E. (2019). Creative ability—Its emergence and manifestation. In D. Van der Reyden, D. Casteleijn, W. Sherwood, & P. deWitt (Eds.), *The Vona du Toit Model of Creative Ability: Origins, constructs, principles and application in occupational therapy* (pp. 119–124). The Vona and Marie du Toit Foundation.

Colucci, C. N., & Kowalski, K. Z. (2020, December 23). Grow bag zoom gardening: Together during the pandemic, virtually. *OT Practice.* https://www.aota.org/publications/ot-practice/ot-practice-issues/2020/pandemic-virtual-gardening

Davies, C. R., Budgeon, C. A., Murray, K., Hunter, M., & Knuiman, M. (2023). The art of aging well: A study of the relationship between recreational arts engagement, general health and mental wellbeing in cohort of Australian older adults. *Frontiers in Public Health, 11,* 1288760. https://doi.org/10.3389/fpubh.2023.1288760

Davies, C. R., & Clift, S. (2022). Arts and health glossary— A summary of definitions for use in research, policy and practice. *Frontiers in Psychology, 13,* 949685. https://doi.org/10.3389/fpsyg.2022.949685

Davies, C. R., Rosenberg, M., Knuiman, M., Ferguson, R., Pikora, T., & Slatter, N. (2012). Defining arts engagement for population-based health research: Art forms, activities and level of engagement. *Arts Health, 4,* 203–216. https://doi.org/10.1080/17533015.2012.656201

du Toit, V. (1974). An investigation into the correlation between volition and its expression in action. *South African Journal of Occupational Therapy, 6–9.*

Eakman, A. M. (2007). *A reliability and validity study of the Meaningful Activity Participation Assessment.* University Microfilms International.

Eakman, A. M., Carlson, M. E., & Clark, F. A. (2010). The Meaningful Activity Participation Assessment: A measure of engagement in personally valued activities. *International Journal of Aging and Human Development, 70*(4), 299–317. https://doi.org/10.2190/AG.70.4.b

Erlandsson, L.-K., & Persson, D. (2020). *The ValMO model: Occupational therapy for a healthy life by doing.* Studentlitteratur AB.

Farhadian, M., Akbarfahimi, M., Abharian, P. H., Khalafbeigi, M., & Yazdani, F. (2024). The effect of leisure intervention on occupational performance and occupational balance in individuals with substance use disorder: A pilot study. *Occupational Therapy International, 2024,* Article 6299073. https://doi.org/10.1155/2024/6299073

Friedland, J. (2003). Why crafts? Influences on the development of occupational therapy in Canada from 1890 to 1930. *Canadian Journal of Occupational Therapy, 70*(4), 204–212. https://doi.org/10.1177/000841740307000403

Gillam, T. (2018). *Creativity, wellbeing and mental health practice.* Palgrave Pivot.

Griffiths, S., & Corr, S. (2007). The use of creative activities with people with mental health problems: A survey of occupational therapists. *British Journal of Occupational Therapy, 70*(3), 107–114. https://doi.org/10.1177/030802260707000303

Hansen, B. W., Erlandsson, L., & Leufstadius, C. (2020). A concept analysis of creative activities as intervention in occupational therapy. *Scandinavian Journal of Occupational Therapy, 28*(1), 63–77. https://doi.org/10.1080/11038128.2020.1775884

Hansen, B. W., Leufstadius, C., Pedersen, H. A., Berring, L. L., & Erlandsson, L. (2022). Experiences of occupational value when doing creative activities in a mental health context. *Occupational Therapy in Mental Health, 38*(4), 383–402. https://doi.org/10.1080/0164212X.2022.2067285

Hasselkus, B. R. (2011). *The meaning of everyday occupation* (2nd ed.). Slack, Inc.

Heinemann, A. W., Lai, J., Magasi, S., Hammel, J., Corrigan, J. D., Bogner, J. A., & Whiteneck, G. G. (2011). Measuring participation enfranchisement. *Archives of Physical Medicine and Rehabilitation, 92*, 564–571. https://doi.org/10.1016/j.apmr.2010.07.220

Helliwell, J. F., Layard, R., Sachs, J. D., De Neve, J.-E., Aknin, L. B., & Wang, S. (Eds.). (2024). *World Happiness Report 2024.* University of Oxford: Wellbeing Research Centre. https://worldhappiness.report

Jeong, E., Yoo, E., Kim, J.-B., Kim, J.-R., Han, D., & Park, J. (2020). The development of Leisure Participation Assessment Tool for the Elderly. *Occupational Therapy International, 2020,* Article 9395629. https://doi.org/10.1155/2020/9395629

Klyczek, J. P., Bauer-Yox, N., & Fiedler, R. C. (1997). The Interest Checklist: A factor analysis. *American Journal of Occupational Therapy, 51*(10), 815–823. https://doi.org/10.5014/ajot.51.10.815

Krupa, T., Edgelow, M., Chen, S., Mieras, C., Almas, A., Perry, A., Radloff-Gabriel, D., Jackson, J., & Bransfield, M. (2010). *Action Over Inertia: Addressing the activity-health needs of individuals with serious mental illness.* CAOT Publications ACE.

Laitinen, L., Jakonen, O., Lahtinen, E., & Lilja-Viherlampi, L-M. (2022). From grass-roots activities to national policies—The state of arts and health in Finland. *Arts & Health, 14*(1), 14–31. https://doi.org/10.1080/17533015.2020.1827275

Law, M., Baptiste, S., Carswell, A., McColl, M. A., Polatajko, H., & Pollock, N. (2019). *Canadian Occupational Performance Measure* (5th ed. rev.). COPM Inc.

Ludowyke, L., Lentin, P., & Brown, T. (2023). The meaning and purpose of creativity in the daily life occupations, activities, acts and behaviors amongst adults living with mental health conditions: A scoping review. *Occupational Therapy in Mental Health, 40*(1), 45–85. https://doi.org/10.1080/0164212X.2023.2218121

Mansfield, L., Daykin, N., & Kay, T. (2020). Leisure and wellbeing. *Leisure Studies, 39*(1), 1–10. https://doi.org/10.1080/02614367.2020.1713195

Matthews, A., Buteau, E., & Fairman, A. (2021, July 21). Building blocks for social participation: Fostering friendship and collaboration through play-based clubs. *OT Practice.* https://www.aota.org/publications/ot-practice/ot-practice-issues/2021/building-blocks

Morris, T., & Rogers, H. (2004). *Measuring motives for physical activity.* Sport and chance of life: Proceedings of 2004 International Sport Science Congress (pp. 242–250), Seoul. Kansas Association for Health, Physical Education, Recreation, and Dance.

Morris, T., & Roychowdhury, D. (2020). Physical activity for health and wellbeing: The role of motives for participation. *Health Psychology Report, 8*(4), 391–407. https://doi.org/10.5114/hpr.2020.100111

Parham, L. D., & Fazio, L. S. (Eds.). (1997). *Play in occupational therapy for children.* Mosby

Perruzza, N., & Kinsella, E. A. (2010). Creative arts occupations in therapeutic practice: A review of the literature. *British Journal of Occupational Therapy, 73*(6), 261–268. https://doi.org/10.4276/030802210X12759925468943

Persson, D., & Erlandsson, L.-K. (2010). Evaluating OVal-9, an instrument for detecting experiences of value in daily occupations. *Occupational Therapy in Mental Health, 26*(1), 32–50. https://doi.org/10.1080/01642120903515284

Persson, D., Erlandsson, L.-K., Eklund, M., & Iwarsson, S. (2001). Value dimensions, meaning, and complexity in human occupation: A tentative structure for analysis. *Scandinavian Journal of Occupational Therapy, 8*, 7–18. https://doi.org/10.1080/11038120119727

Plough, A. L. (Ed.). (2020). *Well-being: Expanding the definition of progress: Insights from practitioners, researchers, and innovators from around the globe.* The Robert Wood Johnson Foundation Culture of Health Series. Oxford University Press. https://doi.org/10.1093/oso/9780190080495.001.0001

Raphael-Greenfield, E., Westover, L. A., & Winterbottom, L. (2017, October 30). Songwriting as an occupation: A medium for occupational goal attainment for homeless men with mental illness. *OT Practice, 22*(19), 21–23.

Reilly, M. (1974). *Play as exploratory learning: Studies of curiosity behavior.* Sage.

Reynolds, F. (2003). Reclaiming a positive identity in chronic illness through artistic occupation. *OTJR: Occupational Therapy Journal of Research, 23*(3), 118–127. https://doi.org/10.1177/153944920302300305

Reynolds, F., & Prior, S. (2006). The role of art-making in identity maintenance: Case studies of people living with cancer. *European Journal of Cancer Care, 15*, 333–341. https://doi.org/10.1111/j.1365-2354.2006.00663.x

Reynolds, F., Vivat, B., & Prior, S. (2008). Women's experiences of increasing subjective well-being in CFS/ME through leisure-based arts and crafts activities: A qualitative study. *Disability and Rehabilitation, 30*(17), 1279–1288. https://doi.org/10.1080/09638280701654518

Roychowdhury, D. (2018). A comprehensive measure of participation motivation: Examining and validating the Physical Activity and Leisure Motivation Scale (PALMS). *Journal of Human Sport and Exercise, 13*(1), 231–247. https://doi.org/10.14198/jhse.2018.131.20

Schmid, T. (2005). *Promoting health through creativity: For professionals in health, arts and education.* John Wiley & Sons.

Şimşek, K. Y., & Çevik, H. (2020). Development of the Leisure Activity Participation Scale (LAPS). *Loisir et Société / Society and Leisure, 43*(1), 98–115. https://doi.org/10.1080/07053436.2020.1727661

Starkman, E. (2021). *Behavioral activation and how to use it.* WebMD. Accessed February 7, 2004, at https://www.webmd.com/mental-health/behavioral-activation-how-to-use-it

Stebbins, R. A. (1992). *Amateurs, professionals and serious leisure.* McGill University Press.

Stebbins, R. A. (1996). *The barbershop singer: Inside the social world of a musical hobby.* University of Toronto Press.

Townsend, E., & Polatajko, H. (2007). *Enabling occupation II: Advancing an occupational therapy vision for health, well-being, and justice through occupation.* CAOT Publications ACE.

Tubbs, B., & Folan, R. (2023). Riding the wave: Occupational therapy's role in surf therapy. *OT Practice, 28*, 12–17. https://www.aota.org/publications/ot-practice/ot-practice-issues/2023/riding-the-wave-ots-role-in-surf-therapy

Van der Reyden, D., Casteleijn, D., Sherwood, W., & de Witt, P. (Eds.). (2019). *The Vona du Toit Model of Creative Ability: Origins, constructs, principles and application in occupational therapy.* Vona and Marie du Toit Foundation.

Van der Reyden, D., & Sherwood, W. (2019). The Vona du Toit Model of Creative Ability core constructs and concepts. In D. Van der Reyden, D. Casteleijn, W. Sherwood, & P. de Witt (Eds.), *The Vona du Toit Model of Creative Ability: Origins, constructs, principles and application in occupational therapy* (pp. 58–104). Vona and Marie du Toit Foundation.

Villanova, A. L. I., & Cunha, M. P. E. (2021). Everyday creativity: A systematic literature review. *Journal of Creative Behavior, 55*(3), 673–695. https://doi.org/10.1002/jocb.481

White, M. (2009). *Arts development in community health: A social tonic.* Radcliffe Publishing.

Zachry, A. H., Saucer, C., & Wilson, M. (2022). Art with a heart: The Rachel Kay Stevens Art Show & Auction. *OT Practice, 27*(1), 36–37.

Sleep is the occupation that takes up approximately one-third of people's lives and serves as a foundation of all their waking occupations. The quantity and quality of a person's sleep impact everything they do each day (Leive & Morrison, 2020). Disruptions to sleep, including insufficient sleep duration, negatively affects people's health and development, cognition, mood, and life quality. Understanding the nature of sleep and sleep problems offers occupational therapy practitioners (OTPs) the opportunity to help people with problems in this foundational occupation. Fortunately, the occupational therapy profession is rapidly expanding its capacity to identify and improve sleep health through an array of effective approaches (Eakman et al., 2022; Faulkner et al., 2022; Ho & Siu, 2018).

This chapter offers an overview of sleep including its role in human health and development, the neurophysiological underpinnings of effective sleep and its regulation, and impacts of sleep problems upon people's mental and behavioral health, as well as approaches OTPs might employ to improve sleep health in the persons that they serve. **Insomnia**, one of many sleep disorders, is highlighted for two key reasons. First, insomnia is the most common sleep disorder that frequently co-occurs in persons with mental and behavioral health challenges (Aernout et al., 2021; Pappa et al., 2020). Second, there are effective behavioral interventions such as multicomponent Cognitive Behavioral Therapy for Insomnia (CBT-I) which are within the OTP's scope of practice.

Role of Sleep in Health and Growth

Sleep Debt

People's bodies have a biological need for sleep that must be satisfied. Most adults have a sleep "need" of between 7 and 9 hours in a 24-hour period (Hirshkowitz et al., 2015), though individual needs vary regarding how much sleep allows them to participate optimally during the day. Sleep need varies based on one's age, with a newborn needing as much as 17 hours of sleep per 24-hour period, whereas an older adult typically requires 7 hours. When a person's sleep falls below these levels for an extended period of time, they go into **sleep debt**. Sleep debt and insomnia are common problems in modern society that can lead to health-related problems such as depression.

Adults ages 18 to 60 years need a minimum of 7 hours of sleep in a 24-hour period to promote optimal health (Watson et al., 2015). These authors had determined that sleeping less than 7 hours per night on a regular basis was associated with a host of adverse health outcomes including obesity, diabetes, hypertension, heart disease and stroke, depression, and increased risk of death. Insufficient sleep quantity creates cognitive performance limitations in executive functioning, attention, concentration, and working memory (Durmer & Dinges, 2005). Tissue healing and immune functioning can be impaired, and inadequate sleep can also lead to increased pain sensitivity. In addition, persons living with Alzheimer and Parkinson diseases typically have sleep disturbances, and sleep problems appear to be a risk factor in the development and worsening of these neurodegenerative diseases (Hale et al., 2020).

Sleep debt is an increasing problem in children. With more mothers in the workforce, children often stretch the length of their waking day into the evening in order to have needed time with their parents. Family and work demands have been associated with parental stress and sleep problems which can result in sleep difficulties in children. So, although a child in the classroom who is disruptive and overly active may be challenged by attention deficits, those deficits may be compounded by insufficient sleep because of the routines within their home environment (Martin et al., 2019).

Development, Functioning, and Well-Being

Recently, the idea of **sleep health** emerged, honoring the role of promoting effective sleep regulation to maintain or improve health. Buysse (2014) stated, "Good sleep is essential to good health" (p. 9). This approach builds on past research that has identified factors that contribute to poor sleep and ill-health. Alternatively, a sleep health perspective encourages people to consider factors that might support effective sleep regulation and duration. Briefly, promotion of sleep health includes attention to five core factors: satisfaction with one's sleep, feeling alert and well-rested, timing of sleep (e.g., regular sleep/wake times), high sleep efficiency (e.g., sleeping greater than 90% of the time one is in bed), and finally sufficient sleep duration (e.g., most adults do well with 7 to 9 hours daily).

Poor sleep has been consistently associated with poor health and disease risk such as cardiovascular disease, obesity, depression, and other mental health challenges. Yet as people seek to understand factors capable of improving sleep health, it is important to note that sleep health is not solely a personal behavioral responsibility.

Factors at multiple social levels can lead to poor sleep. A careful review (Hale et al., 2020) indicates multiple interacting factors. For example, black Americans may have poorer sleep on average, perhaps because of greater levels of stress compared with white Americans. In addition, poor social relationships can create feelings of being unsafe within the sleeping environment, thereby limiting effective sleep quality and quantity. Community-level factors such as school start times or work demands can influence effective sleep regulation and duration. OTPs can consider interventions aimed at the individual and their daily round of activities; however, they should also consider the person's social environment including the social policies that can perpetuate sleep–health disparities.

Sleep, Cognition, and Mood

It is common knowledge that a good night's sleep is an important preparation for any significant cognitive challenge, such as taking a test. Studies have shown that decreased sleep results in slower reaction times, lowered academic performance, irritability, and poorer problem-solving (Walker, 2009). Evidence also points to the importance of maintaining consistency in sleep patterns, such as keeping a consistent waking time. For example, college students who wake up early a few days a week, then sleep in on the other days, are at greater risk for insomnia and poor academic performance (Hershner, 2020).

Sufficient sleep appears to be essential for the consolidation of memories, enabling effective engagement with one's world and promoting emotional processing. In the face of poor sleep, it can be difficult to solve the daily problems people inevitably face, which in turn can lead to chronic stress. There appears to be a feedback loop in which chronic stress and associated activation of the hypothalamic-pituitary-adrenal (HPA) system can lead to poor sleep (Nollet et al., 2020).

Sleep disturbances, especially with co-occurring stress and anxiety, are intimately linked to mood. Chronic sleep deprivation has been related to the development of mood disorders via neurochemical pathways including decreased production of dopamine and serotonin (Palagini et al., 2019). Further, poor sleep has been shown to increase the risk for developing a mood disorder such as depression and suicidality (Riemann et al., 2020). It is important for the OTP to develop systematic approaches for evaluating and targeting sleep disturbances, especially sleep debt and insomnia, as part of their clinical practice when working with persons with mood disorders. Without sufficient sleep, especially in the face of chronic stress and HPA activation, a person may be unable to competently navigate day-to-day responsibilities, thereby limiting experiences of meaning and purpose in life (Eakman, 2015). Breaking this cycle through sleep health promotion is essential to optimize occupational performance and well-being.

The Physiology of Sleep: Two-Process Model of Sleep Regulation

Sleep generally occurs in a predictable way from day to day, offering routines that help people to predict and manage their daily lives. An understanding of sleep and its effective regulation is essential to promote sleep quality and quantity. The Two-Process Model of Sleep Regulation proposed by Borbély (1982) is a conceptual framework informing research and clinical practice in sleep and insomnia. This model indicates that sleep–wake regularity is controlled by two interacting processes, Process S, the **sleep-driver system**, and Process C, the **circadian system**. Effective behavioral interventions for improving sleep require understanding of the interactions of these processes.

First, the sleep-driver system (Process S) is a homeostatic system that depends on the amount of time an individual remains awake versus asleep from day to day. During a typical day, the "pressure" to feel sleepy and fall asleep steadily increases as people are active and engaged in their day-to-day activities. As their typical bedtime approaches, they feel sleepiness as sleep pressure continues to build. During a "good night's sleep," sleep pressure is gradually lowered, and is at its lowest upon waking (Dijk & Lazar, 2012).

Second, the circadian system (Process C) is the body's "internal clock" or pacemaker, which operates on a 24-hour schedule. Exposure to daylight is the system's most powerful cue. This process controls biochemical, physiological, and behavioral systems, which oscillate regularly. For example, a person's body temperature rises then falls as part of Process C; rising body temperature promotes a person's alertness, whereas falling body temperature reduces alerting cues to the brain, thereby promoting sleepiness.

Waking daily at a consistent time and exposing yourself to light and activity helps to entrain Process C. Staying active and engaged during the day steadily builds sleep pressure as part of Process S. Toward evening when light levels fall, Process C triggers a release of melatonin which promotes lowering of the body temperature. When the S and C processes are well coordinated, people fall asleep more quickly, sleep more deeply, and therefore feel well rested following their sleep (Dijk & Lazar, 2012). In Figure 52-1 (Angelhoff, 2017), the "sleep gate" indicates when sleep pressure is at its highest and cuing from the circadian system has substantially decreased. When people's sleep is well regulated, falling asleep is most likely to occur during the "sleep gate" in a recurring pattern from night to night. The following will offer an overview of Process S, Process C, and their roles in the effective regulation of sleep.

Homeostatic Sleep-Driver System

The sleep-driver system (Process S) is a homeostatic process that plays an essential role in the effective regulation of sleep (Borbély et al., 2016). This regulatory system is sleep–wake dependent such that the longer a person is awake during the day or across multiple days, the more there is a "pressure" or "drive" to fall asleep. Said in another way, the longer a person remains awake the more they feel the need to sleep. Sufficient sleep duration and quality (i.e., slow wave sleep) serves to

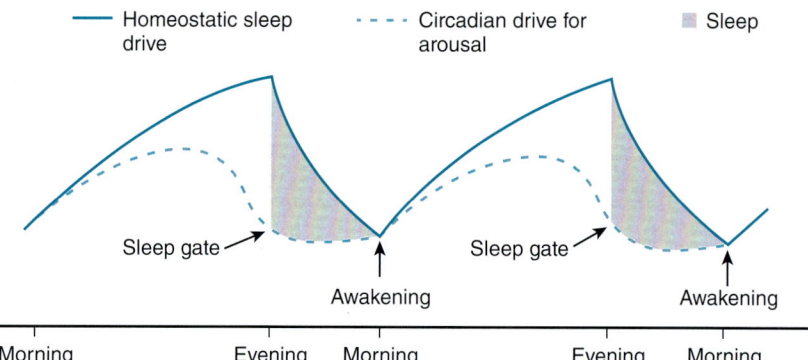

FIGURE 52-1. The sleep gate. *Courtesy of Angelhoff, C. (2017). What about the parents? Sleep quality, mood, saliva cortisol response and sense of coherence in parents with a child admitted to pediatric care. Linköping University Electronic Press.*

reset the S system. Individuals typically need between 7 and 9 hours of sleep each 24-hour period. Sleep pressure is at its lowest level after a "good night's sleep."

Human activity during the day has been associated with an increasing concentration of adenosine, a byproduct of the adenosine triphosphate (ATP) system, the workhorse of the body's cells. Adenosine binds to receptors in the forebrain area, which inhibits wakefulness and promotes falling asleep (Dijk & Lazar, 2012); therefore, adenosine may be an essential regulatory chemical within Process S.

Evidence supporting some common sleep hygiene recommendations seem to have their basis in Process S. Napping, for example, is effective in minimizing sleep debt and lowering sleep drive. Napping can be useful in making up for lost sleep. However, napping can also limit the sufficient accumulation of sleep pressure, contributing to insomnia by making falling asleep and staying asleep more difficult, which can lead to less restorative slow wave sleep (Werth et al., 1996).

Caffeine is found in many drinks (e.g., coffee and energy drinks) which are known to promote wakefulness. The caffeine molecule has a similar shape to the adenosine molecule, and caffeine can bind to the brain's adenosine receptors; this process activates the brain and promotes wakefulness (Riemann & Nissen, 2012). Occasional caffeine use may be fine when someone wants to promote alertness and stay focused during an afternoon of studying. But caffeine consumed later in the day will block adenosine binding, making falling asleep and staying asleep more difficult.

Napping can be used as an important way to promote sleep health, especially if a person's lifestyle demands lead to sleep debt by reducing their opportunity to meet their ongoing need for sleep. A useful balance of sleeping and napping can support an individual's need for sleep from day to day. Napping can also deplete the building of sleep drive, thereby making falling asleep at a regular time more difficult, as well as making it less likely the person has a sufficient amount of restorative slow wave sleep. Napping can also perpetuate and worsen sleep disorders such as insomnia, leading to poorer sleep quality (Mazza et al., 2020). Insomnia and how napping may interfere with effective sleep regulation are addressed later in this chapter.

Circadian System

Sleep is a daily occupation that occurs in a predictable way, nested within an individual's circadian rhythm. This regularity can promote well-being because it offers a familiar pattern to daily life. The circadian rhythm is the physiological 24-hour time pattern of human life (Turek & Zee, 2017). It includes usual periods of being alert and awake when people engage in their daily activities followed by a period of unconsciousness during sleep. Light, especially exposure to sunlight, is the most powerful external cue to the circadian system. The suprachiasmatic nucleus (SCN), known as the body's "master clock," sits within the brain's hypothalamus, just above the optic chiasma. Light-sensitive ganglia in the retina of a person's eyes project to the SCN via the retinohypothalamic track. Light and dark cycles based on a 24-hour cycle help to entrain, or regulate, the timing of the human circadian system to promote effective sleep.

The circadian rhythm is the physiological and temporal structure around which everyday routines are built. The role of the circadian system includes, in part, body temperature changes through a 24-hour period. Lower light levels near the end of the day are sensed by the SCN and cue the pineal gland to release melatonin. Melatonin, commonly known as the sleep hormone, promotes a decrease in core body temperature and slows body activities and brain functions, thereby promoting sleep (Rosenwasser & Turek, 2017). However, the circadian system also influences an abundance of processes such as glucose metabolism, autonomic nervous system activity, immune functioning, inflammation, and tissue healing.

In addition, human organs and their accompanying cells have their own "peripheral clock," which the SCN helps to orchestrate. These peripheral clocks influence a person's feeding and fasting, heart rate and muscle strength, liver functioning, and insulin production (Grossbellet & Etienne, 2017). Disruptions in circadian rhythms because of shift work can lead to sleep loss and metabolic risks to physical health such as cancer. Sleep loss can also lead to performance limitations, which can contribute to the onset of anxiety and depression (Abbott et al., 2017). OTPs who promote sleep health can use evidence-based therapeutic tools to help a person regulate their sleep–wake cycles and promote sleep quantity and quality, thereby fostering well-being.

People's circadian rhythms can be influenced by external factors, such as light, and by their daily activities. Exposure to sunlight and routine activity can serve as Zeitgebers, or "time givers," and can cue people's bodies to promote effective sleep regulation. Building routines into people's days, including waking at a consistent time followed by breakfast, then school, work, or social activities, can entrain their circadian system, as well as build sleep drive.

Bipolar disorder, a chronic mood disorder, features significant disruptions to circadian rhythm regularity. Sleep disturbances, sleep deprivation, and circadian rhythm disruptions are a key feature of the condition, and these factors are known to precede the onset of symptoms (Murray & Harvey, 2010). Zeitgebers are now used as essential aspects of treatment, both in the acute phase of the disorder and in recovery. Based on a social Zeitgeber hypothesis, the regularity of routines, including sleep and waking, and stability of interpersonal relationships have a protective effect in persons with mood disorders. Treatment focuses on regularizing routines to promote circadian regularity, normalizing sleep–wake cycles, fostering self-acceptance, and building interpersonal relationships (Frank et al., 2000; Gold & Kinrys, 2019).

People may even have a preferred chronotype, often referred to as "morningness" (or a "Lark") or "eveningness" (or an "Owl"). Most people are somewhere in the middle, though about one-fifth are Larks, which is a mild advance of the sleep phase. Larks prefer to go to bed early and wake early. About one-fifth are "Owls" who have a mild sleep phase delay and prefer to stay up later and sleep in. These chronotypes or forms of circadian rhythm preferences have a genetic basis; nearly 50% of chronotype preference may be inherited, though chronotype can also be influenced by environmental (light exposure), activity (mealtimes), and social cues (Pack et al., 2017).

Sleep Neurochemistry

There is an intricate balance of arousal or alerting mechanisms, which facilitate people being awake, that work together with sleep-promoting mechanisms, which help people fall and stay asleep (McGinty & Szymusiak, 2017). The stress hormone *cortisol* acts to promote wakefulness and serves a key role in regulating circadian processes (Mohd Azmi et al., 2021).

Neurochemicals that promote wakefulness also include serotonin, norepinephrine, histamine, orexin, acetylcholine, dopamine, and glutamate. *Serotonin,* which is released in the midbrain during exercise, for example, has an immediate alerting effect promoting wakefulness. However, some medications for treating depression and anxiety, such as selective serotonin reuptake inhibitors (SSRIs), can block reabsorption of serotonin, which can make falling and staying asleep more difficult. *Orexin*-containing neurons in the hypothalamus also have an arousing effect with significant implications for the sleep–wake system (Pizza et al., 2022). Narcolepsy, which results in excessive sleepiness, happens because of a disruption within orexin neurons. Newer sleep-promoting medicines (e.g., suvorexant) work by blocking the binding of orexin, which limits cognitive arousal and promotes sleep onset.

Alternatively, there are processes at work that serve to downregulate or calm both body and brain, thereby promoting falling and staying asleep. As previously mentioned, *melatonin* is released from the light-sensitive pineal gland near the optic chiasma. When melatonin is released, body temperature and alerting signals to the body decrease, which promotes sleep onset. Also, *adenosine* builds in the brain as a person is awake and engaged in daily activities, and adenosine binding with receptors in the basal forebrain promotes falling asleep and staying asleep.

Gamma-aminobutyric acid (GABA) is a neurotransmitter that is well-known for its calming effect against anxiety as well as slowing down a person's brain to promote sleep onset (Hepsomali et al., 2020). Sleep medications such as zolpidem or Ambien increase the activity of the GABA receptors, thereby promoting sleep onset. Substances such as alcohol and benzodiazepines (for example, Xanax) also increase GABA receptor activity and promote sleep, though with greater negative side effects compared with nonbenzodiazepine medications.

Other sleep-promoting substances linked to falling and staying asleep include *cytokines, prostaglandins,* and *growth hormone releasing hormones,* which regulate healing and growth in the body (McGinty & Szymusiak, 2017). Concentrations of proinflammatory *cytokines,* such as interleukin-1 (IL-1), build during the day and play a role in sleep regulation. During active infection processes, greater amounts of IL-1 are released, which help to promote healing, sleep onset, and sleep maintenance. Persistently elevated levels of cytokines, however, are associated with chronic disease processes such as type 2 diabetes.

Sleep Architecture, Types, and Phases

Sleep occurs in a pattern that is phased and rhythmic, repeating itself multiple times during the night. This pattern is often referred to as *sleep architecture,* because a hypnogram produced by a sleep laboratory resembles a city skyline (Carskadon & Dement, 2017). During sleep, brain activity can be tracked by an electroencephalograph (EEG). Typically, a hypnogram shows the brain waves during a full night's sleep. The brain activity changes from one type to another as the sleep type changes.

The Stages of NREM Sleep

Non–rapid eye movement (NREM) sleep constitutes the greatest proportion of adult human sleep. During NREM sleep, the body is active. People can turn and adjust their body and coverings for comfort without fully waking. NREM includes three stages of sleep that descend from very light sleep to the deepest dreamless sleep—slow wave sleep. Healthy sleep begins with stage 1, when a person begins to doze off, yet they would notice if something happened in the room. Stage 2 is a transitional stage, during which brain waves slow and the body moves toward deep sleep. Slow wave sleep (also referred to as stages 3 and 4) is the deepest sleep phase, in which the body gets its most restorative rest. During slow wave sleep, adenosine is slowly cleared from around the brain, the immune system produces its protective metabolic components, and glucose is stored to provide optimal brain functioning upon waking.

REM Sleep

Rapid eye movement (REM) sleep involves high brain activity levels (Carskadon & Dement, 2017). REM sleep typically occurs five or six times during the night and accounts for 25% of sleep in a healthy adult. Dreams occur during REM sleep. There are many theories regarding why humans dream, but the consensus is that dreams help the brain to consolidate, integrate, and analyze recent memories during sleep (Stickgold & Wamsley, 2017). Dreaming is associated with memory consolidation, especially emotional memories and motor learning.

Typical Sleep Patterns

For healthy adults, a typical sleep pattern includes several cycles that begin with stage 1 NREM sleep, progress to NREM slow wave sleep, and then move into REM sleep, then repeat. Typically, individuals gain the deeper, more restorative slow wave sleep during the early portion of their sleep period. These NREM–REM cycles last about 90 minutes. People often awaken for brief periods between cycles and then doze off again. Generally, toward the end of the sleep period, the proportion of REM sleep increases.

Sleep Across the Life Span

Just as the body changes with age, so does sleep. The amount of sleep time and the amount of time spent in different sleep stages also changes throughout the life span. As shown in Table 52-1, people require the greatest amount of sleep at birth, after which the amount of sleep decreases until they reach adulthood (Carskadon & Dement, 2017). The guidelines in Table 52-1 are a recommendation only. Some individuals need more sleep than is suggested to function at their best, whereas others may function well with less than the recommended time. As noted in a joint statement from the American Academy of Sleep Medicine and the Sleep Research Society, adults should sleep at least 7 hours per night to prevent adverse health outcomes.

Infancy and Childhood Sleep and Napping

Newborns tend to sleep 16 to 18 hours a day. Fifty percent of their sleep is REM sleep, which is the highest percentage of REM sleep humans experience throughout their lifetime.

TABLE 52-1 | Sleep Requirements Throughout the Life Span

Age	Hours of Sleep Recommended
0–3 months	14–17 hours
4–11 months	12–15 hours
1–2 years	11–14 hours
3–5 years	10–13 hours
6–13 years	9–11 hours
14–17 years	8–10 hours
18–25 years	7–9 hours
26–64 years	7–9 hours
65+ years	7–8 hours

Hirshkowitz, M., Whiton, K., Albert, S. M., Alessi, C., Bruni, O., DonCarlos, L., Hazen, N., Herman, J., Katz, E. S., Kheirandish-Gozal, L., Neubauer, D. N., O'Donnell, A. E., Ohayon, M., Peever, J., Rawding, R., Sachdeva, R. C., Setters, B., Vitiello, M. V., Ware, J. C., & Adams Hillard, P. J. (2015). National Sleep Foundation's sleep time duration recommendation: Methodology and results summary. Sleep Health, 1(1), 40–43. https://doi.org/10.1016/j.sleh.2014.12.010

Newborns have the shortest sleep cycles, lasting about 55 minutes, and wake frequently, even at night. Infants slowly begin to stabilize their melatonin levels during their first 3 months, after which a more stable sleep pattern may emerge (Carskadon & Dement, 2017).

As children grow, the amount of sleep they require decreases. At 3 to 5 years old, 11 to 13 hours of sleep are needed in each 24-hour cycle. Naps have shortened in length and frequency, the amount of REM sleep decreases, and the length of the sleep cycle increases. Sleep also plays a role in the child's health, as a child's immune system works to fight off disease while they sleep (Opp & Krueger, 2017). Lack of sleep can be attributed to the overscheduling of today's child and their caregivers. Instead of appearing drowsy, the child may instead appear "hyperactive," moving and fidgeting to stay awake, which can make attending to tasks in school difficult. Also, sensory sensitivities in neurodiverse children may contribute to resistance to going to bed as well as longer times to fall asleep once in bed (Hartman et al., 2022).

Napping behaviors differ between children and adults because their need for sleep changes as they age and develop. According to Jones and Spencer (2020), young infants' sleep is considered polyphasic, with napping occurring four or more times during the day. Toddlers' sleep tends to become biphasic, and napping occurs less frequently as they age. Napping does influence child development and has been shown to promote learning, memory, and language (Hupbach et al., 2009). For example, napping in toddlers was associated with improved ability to learn novel language skills compared with toddlers who had not napped. Napping during the daytime can influence children's circadian rhythms, leading to later bedtimes compared with toddlers who are not typical nappers (Akacem et al., 2015).

Teen Sleep and Napping

Teenagers have busy schedules, including academics, extracurricular activities, recreation, and jobs, and they are often chronically sleep deprived (Seton & Fitzgerald, 2021). In addition, teenagers typically prefer to stay up late and sleep later in the morning, leading to a form of "social jet lag" attributed to circadian rhythm delays (Crowley et al., 2007). Chronic poor sleep can lead to difficulty with mood regulation, including anxiety and depression, school absenteeism, and reduced academic success. Fortunately, later school start times appear to be having some beneficial effects on sleep health and academic performance (Groen & Pabilonia, 2019). Monitoring teen sleep patterns when difficulties with mood and occupational performance arise may help determine if poor sleep is a contributing factor.

Napping behaviors tend to change in adolescents and young adults (Jones & Spencer, 2020). Sleep and napping are influenced heavily by activity schedules in industrialized societies, which may limit sufficient opportunities for sleep. Adolescents and young adults tend to report napping for recovery because they had not been receiving enough sleep. Individuals nap to allow time for recovery during bouts of illness, though people report napping just because it feels good. Recovery naps can promote alertness, improve cognitive performance, and ensure memory consolidation, so napping can have a clear benefit by meeting an individual's sleep need and improving performance in day-to-day activities (Jones & Spencer, 2020).

Adult and Older Adult Sleep and Napping

Adults should be getting between 7 and 9 hours of sleep a night, although many do not reach this threshold because of busy schedules. When adults reach their senior years, sleep patterns continue to change, with more light stage 1 NREM sleep and less deep NREM sleep (Scullin et al., 2017). Therefore, older adults often rouse from sleep throughout the night. This effect can be worsened by health-related conditions that compound their sleep issues, such as nocturia, cardiovascular disease, chronic pain, and disordered breathing. In addition, Alzheimer disease and Parkinson disease occur more frequently in the older population and are both linked to sleep disturbances. Thus, difficulty maintaining healthy sleep through the night, a form of insomnia, is highly prevalent in the older adult population (Barczi & Teodorescu, 2017).

The prevalence of daytime napping in older adulthood is often as high as 60%, accompanied by age-related chronic conditions, changes in sleep patterns, and lifestyle changes. A recent study found that habitual short naps (e.g., 30 minutes) were associated with better health outcomes compared with longer naps (e.g., greater than 90 minutes). People who napped for longer periods of time were more likely to have cardiovascular and metabolic diseases, declining cognitive function, and increased rates of mortality (Zhang et al., 2020). The pattern between nighttime sleeping, napping, and health is complex, and likely varies because of differences in cultural beliefs, though persons who habitually nap and report poor nighttime sleep may be more likely to experience elevated levels of stress and depression (Devine & Wolf, 2016).

Insomnia Disorder

Insomnia is recognized as difficulty with falling asleep or staying asleep, co-occurring with impairments in or distress regarding daytime performance. Insomnia occurs despite having sufficient opportunity for sleeping. This often differs from insufficient sleep syndrome, for example, which occurs because of lack of opportunity for sleep (e.g., a single parent working two jobs while raising children). Acute insomnia lasting for a few days is a common reaction to stressful events, and typically resolves without intervention. However, when insomnia persists for months and longer there can be negative consequences for an individual's well-being and health. An OTP can simply ask, "Do you have difficulty sleeping?" or "Do you have difficulty falling or staying asleep?" which can help identify if the individual is concerned about the quality or quantity of their sleep (Roth, 2007, p. S7).

According to the *Diagnostic and Statistical Manual of Mental Disorders* (5th ed.; *DSM-5;* American Psychiatric Association, 2013), insomnia is often accompanied by anxiety and depression. Importantly, ongoing difficulties with falling or staying asleep lead to cognitive and emotional difficulties, which limit skills needed for living one's coveted life. Nearly 30% of adults report insomnia symptoms (Morin et al., 2006); and these numbers have increased worldwide to nearly 53% during the COVID-19 pandemic (AlRasheed et al., 2022).

Diagnosis

Diagnostic criteria for insomnia include a person's report of (a) difficulty falling asleep or staying asleep, taking more than 30 minutes to fall asleep; and/or (b) associated fatigue/sleepiness or concerns about sleep or impairments in attention/concentration/memory or impairments in social, family, occupational, or academic performance (American Academy of Sleep Medicine, 2014). Chronic insomnia disorder (National Center for Health Statistics, 2024: ICD 10) requires that the difficulties with sleep are not because of an inadequate opportunity for sleep, and that symptoms occur at least 3 days per week and have continued for at least 3 months. Importantly, insomnia symptoms should not be better explained by another sleep disorder (e.g., obstructive sleep apnea [OSA]).

Given the prevalence of insomnia in the general population, it is not surprising that insomnia is a common co-occurring condition for individuals experiencing mental and behavioral health challenges. For example, estimates indicate about 40% to 70% of persons with depression report complaints about sleeping and circadian disruptions (Staner, 2010). Present understanding is that the relationship between depression and insomnia is likely bidirectional. Depression can lead to chronic insomnia, though chronic insomnia can increase the chance that a person will develop depression or worsen their depression symptoms (Baglioni et al., 2011).

Additional evidence about the relationship between insomnia and mood disorders comes from nonpharmacological treatments of insomnia such as CBT-I. Improvements in insomnia symptoms following completion of CBT-I, for example, have resulted in clinically meaningful improvements in depression symptoms (Cunningham & Shapiro, 2018). Furthermore, a study of CBT-I delivered by OTPs found that anxiety, depression, and stress symptoms improved, along with insomnia symptoms, in post-9/11 military veterans (Eakman et al., 2022). Kendrick's experience with receiving CBT-I, and the process of CBT-I delivered by an OTP, are highlighted in this chapter (Lovell, 2023).

Models of Insomnia

Important questions regarding insomnia include, "Why does insomnia occur?" and "Which factors contribute to developing or worsening insomnia symptoms?" This is because by understanding how insomnia occurs, it may be possible to reduce or eliminate symptoms and promote well-being. The following brief review offers a few of the more prominent models of insomnia and their relationships with nonpharmacological sleep improvement strategies such as multicomponent CBT-I.

The *Stimulus Control Model* (Bootzin, 1972) is a behavioral model indicating that pairing of just a few cues for sleep (e.g., bedtime and bedroom) can promote the association of these cues with the onset of sleep. The concern in insomnia may be that individuals add additional cues at bedtime or in bed such as smartphone or computer use, television watching, working, worrying in bed, eating in bed, and so on. These additional cues weaken the association of the bed with sleep.

A classical conditioning perspective was added to this model, indicating that the additional activities occurring in bed (e.g., working, smartphone use, worrying) actually condition arousal or wakefulness when in bed (Perlis et al., 2017); this increases time spent in bed awake and the time it takes to fall asleep, resulting in less time sleeping. This model has led to common sleep improvement instructions within CBT-I including the following: (a) use the bed only for sleep, sex, and sickness; (b) get out of bed if not sleeping; and (c) return to bed only when sleepy. Such instructions, if followed by a person, will likely result in increased daytime sleepiness, which can increase risks for accidents; therefore, careful education and monitoring by the therapist is required. More details on this can be found later in this chapter within the intervention section.

The *Three-Factor Model* (Spielman et al., 1987), also known as the *Spielman* or *3P Model,* is another behavioral model of insomnia informed from a biopsychosocial perspective. This model uses a vulnerability-stressor perspective to understand how insomnia can occur and become chronic.

The individual may have *predisposing* factors that can increase the risk for developing insomnia; these may be biological (e.g., hyperarousal), psychological (e.g., excessive worrying), and social (e.g., child rearing). *Precipitating* factors are seen as "triggers" for insomnia; these may be traumatic events or the onset of a physical or psychological illness. In working with veterans with insomnia, it was found that these triggers were often basic training, service in a combat zone, and service-connected injuries. *Perpetuating* factors are "self-reinforcing" behaviors adopted by the individual to cope with their poor sleep. For example, individuals will engage in behaviors to make up for lost sleep, such as going to bed early, staying in bed longer, and opting out of activities during daytime for napping. However, these behaviors tend to lead to extended time in bed, which limits building of sleep drive and often disrupts effective regulation of the circadian system.

The 3P Model has led to sleep restriction therapy as an active component of CBT-I, which involves limiting the amount of time a person is in bed (sleep opportunity) and the amount of time they can reliably generate sleep in a 24-hour period (sleep ability; Perlis et al., 2017).

The *Microanalytic Model* (Morin, 1993) or *Cognitive-Behavioral Model* builds upon the maladaptive behaviors identified within both the *Stimulus Control* and *3P* Models, such as extended time in bed, irregular sleep–wake timing, and napping as contributing factors to chronic insomnia. According to Morin (1993), these maladaptive behaviors are self-reinforcing and lead to poor sleep. Intervention is required to address them directly and target a person's level of pre-sleep arousal, comprising emotional, cognitive, and physiological forms of arousal. A sense of worry or anxiety can make sleep onset difficult, or impossible, even if sufficient sleep drive has accumulated during the day and alerting cues from the circadian system have decreased.

Rumination, especially about daily stressors and the impacts of poor sleep upon the next day's occupational performance, greatly disrupts effective sleep regulation and contributes to insomnia and sleep debt (Åkerstedt et al., 2017). These worries may also reflect inaccurate beliefs (e.g., "When I am having difficulty falling asleep, I must try harder to sleep."). Arousal is seen as a key concern in chronic insomnia, and strategies such as mindfulness practice and effective strategies for worrying have been integrated as part of multicomponent CBT-I, along with the previously mentioned stimulus control and sleep restriction therapies mentioned earlier (Carney & Manber, 2009; Maurer & Kyle, 2022; Ong, 2017).

Populations at Risk for Insomnia

Most populations seen by OTPs will be at risk for insomnia, in large part because of the stress and anxiety they face because of challenges with occupational performance and uncertainty regarding their futures. Insomnia is common in persons with cancer, heart failure, chronic pain, Alzheimer disease, multiple sclerosis, alcoholism, and chronic obstructive pulmonary disease. Treatments such as CBT-I are effective in treating insomnia (Muench et al., 2022). Screening for and addressing sleep problems such as insomnia are becoming standard practice for OTPs.

Anxiety and Posttraumatic Stress

If individuals managing their anxiety disorders do not get enough restorative sleep, the lack of sleep can increase their arousal level and anxiety and make falling asleep and staying asleep more difficult; this can lead to a self-perpetuating cycle of insomnia and anxiety (Krystal et al., 2017). Challenges in childhood and adolescence such as separation anxiety disorder, generalized anxiety disorder, social phobia, obsessive-compulsive disorder, and posttraumatic stress disorder (PTSD) can persist into adulthood, so understanding a person's history is essential to effective sleep-related intervention (Victor & Bernstein, 2009).

Anxiety and posttraumatic stress commonly occur with depression and sleep disturbances such as insomnia. The prevalence of insomnia in persons with PTSD has been estimated at 63% (Ahmadi et al., 2022), and up to 90% among military veterans exposed to combat. PTSD symptoms such as reexperiencing trauma, hypervigilance, and nightmares contribute to insomnia and sleep debt in this population. See Chapter 18: Anxiety Disorders. 🤝

Mood Disorders

Insomnia and hypersomnia (extended time sleeping) are features of major depressive disorder (American Psychiatric Association, 2013). Sleep disturbances such as insomnia can contribute to depression severity, lower the effectiveness of mental health treatment, and lead to relapse in depression symptoms (Manber & Chambers, 2009). Effective treatments for insomnia such as CBT-I can improve insomnia and depression symptoms and complement antidepressant medication therapies (Cunningham & Shapiro, 2018). OTPs should consider screening for depression co-occurring with insomnia symptoms.

Individuals experiencing bipolar disorder often report a reduced need for sleep during manic episodes, and insomnia or hypersomnia may present during depressive episodes (Kaplan, 2020). Sleep-related difficulties include longer time to fall asleep (e.g., more than 30 minutes), problems with falling and staying asleep, and poorer sleep efficiency. These often co-occur with more frequent and longer daytime napping (Meyer et al., 2020; Ritter et al., 2012). Individuals who display high day-to-day variability in total sleep time often report mood instability and impaired information processing speed, thereby making daily life more difficult (Bradley et al., 2020). See Chapter 20: Mood Disorders. 🤝

Schizophrenia Spectrum Disorders

Individuals experiencing schizophrenia spectrum disorders have frequent complaints of insomnia and hypersomnia. There is evidence of biological changes in an individual's circadian rhythms and melatonin production, extended total sleep time and time in bed, and difficulties with falling and staying asleep (Meyer et al., 2020). Sleep disturbances associated with schizophrenia also have negative impacts upon day-to-day functioning. Difficulties with sleep regulation and sleep quality contribute to a loss of control over one's life by limiting opportunities to participate in valued activities. Sleep can be used by the individual as an escape from life's difficulties. Individualized approaches are important; for example, interventions addressing activity routines and the environment should be considered to improve effective sleep regulation as well as a means of gaining a sense of control over day-to-day life. See Chapter 23: Schizophrenia Spectrum and Psychotic Disorders. 🤝

Shift Workers

Shift workers often have disturbed sleep patterns because of the unusual timing of their daily occupations and sleep, resulting in a misalignment between their circadian and homeostatic sleep-driver systems. They negotiate between their shift work schedule and the more typical schedules of their families, friends, and community services, leading to excessive sleepiness, which can cause driving and workplace accidents. Shift workers are at increased risk for cardiovascular disease and cancer, as well as depression (especially women; Torquati et al., 2019). Nonpharmacological interventions are being trialed for shift workers (Crowther et al., 2021), including changes in shift scheduling, light exposure therapies, and behavioral adjustments to sleep and social activity timing.

Because sleep issues can signal a mental health disorder, OTPs need to screen for sleep problems in their practice. Kendrick's case in this chapter's The Lived Experience feature illustrates how his experience with shift work may have contributed to his insomnia when he entered college.

Evidence-Based Practice

Approaches to Improving Sleep in People With Schizophrenia Spectrum Disorders

Occupational therapists should recommend intervention approaches that are aligned with each individual's unique circumstances.

RESEARCH FINDINGS

A group of clinical experts, practitioners, caregivers, and service users recommended intervention approaches for improving sleep in persons with schizophrenia spectrum disorders (Faulkner et al., 2022). The following recommendations reflect general agreement regarding the intervention approach. Intervention approaches should be applied considering each individual's unique circumstances.

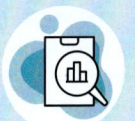

APPLICATIONS

The following recommendations should be considered by the OTP when working with a person's sleep issues:
➡ Maintain a consistent sleep schedule (time to bed and rise time).
➡ Limit nonsleep activities in bed (only sleep and sex in bed).
➡ Create consistent morning routines (sunlight-exposed activities, use alarm to wake).
➡ Create consistent evening routine (calming activities to relax and wind down).
➡ Engage in daytime activities (goal-directed, productive activities of interest to person).
➡ Increase sun (light) exposure in morning and daytime (limit light exposure at night).
➡ Modify sleeping environment (reduce light exposure, sounds, nonsleep activity).

REFERENCES

Faulkner, S. M., Drake, R. J., Ogden, M., Gardani, M., & Bee, P. E. (2022). A mixed methods expert opinion study on the optimal content and format for an occupational therapy intervention to improve sleep in schizophrenia spectrum disorders. *PLoS One, 17*(6), e0269453. https://doi.org/10.1371/journal.pone.0269453

The Lived Experience

Kendrick

My problems with sleeping have been present most of my life. I recall often being awake until the early morning when I was in high school. I had a feeling of "being revved up" that would start in the evening and last for hours. This feeling gave me a sense of focus, and I would play video games while others in the house slept. I felt like the time was my own, and I liked this opportunity to be alone.

After graduating from high school I knew I had to do something with my life and military service seemed like my best option. My second bout with sleep problems began during my 8 years of service in the U.S. Air Force. I was trained as an F-16 fighter aircraft mechanic and traveled the world, including deployments in Europe, and South and East Asia. I noticed I wasn't getting enough sleep because of a constantly rotating work schedule, including day shift (5 a.m. to 3 p.m.), swing shift (2 p.m. to midnight), and mid-shift (11 p.m. to 6 a.m.).

After an honorable discharge, I used my veterans benefit to attend college. The transition to civilian life was stressful for me. The COVID-19 pandemic was in full swing, I was a first-generation student, and I quickly realized I was unlike the other college freshmen who had just graduated from high school. My sleep difficulties quickly reemerged. I was napping 2 to 3 hours about every other day but was always sleepy during the day, and I felt like I was losing track of time. I was going through a lot, and it was a stressful time, so I guess I needed the naps. I believed that I had no control over my life, and I was increasingly worried about my emotional instability. I sought help from the Veterans Health Administration, and a mood stabilizer was prescribed for bipolar disorder. Later, I contacted the sleep services program within the university's occupational therapy program because I was waking up exhausted and having difficulties in my classes.

I recall the OTP in the sleep services program asked me to complete some forms and record my sleep routines for a couple of weeks using a sleep diary. The therapist soon let me know that she could help me, but she told me that the treatment would not be easy, and that my sleep would likely get worse before it got better. I was getting less than 6 hours of sleep each night on average, and I was willing to put up with more poor sleep in the short term if it could help me sleep better by the end of therapy. I soon began to experience how CBT-I could improve my sleep and my life.

The OTP and I discussed my daily activity routines, and it was recommended that I try sleep scheduling as part of CBT-I. I actually just wanted to sleep for 8 hours. That's about it. And so we started off at like 2:00 a.m. for my bedtime and waking up at 10:00 a.m. I didn't start classes until 11. To wake at the same time every day, I used my cell phone as an alarm. I put my phone across the room, and then I just got up and started my day. A routine of activities helped me have a purpose for getting up each morning. I would take a shower. That's the first thing I always do—take a shower and do some self-care stuff, wash my face, brush my teeth, you know, stuff like that. I'd make lunch if I wanted a lunch, fill my water bottle up, and get ready for class.

The experience with the OTP helped me understand my circadian preference to go to bed late and wake up later in the day and the importance of my circadian rhythm in regulating

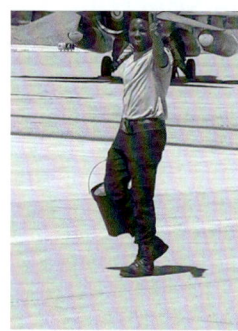

my sleep. That's how I learned about my personal circadian rhythm. I'm a night owl one hundred percent. I like to wake up later in the morning than earlier in the morning. That's a big help, so I try not to plan any events before 10.

The first couple of weeks of CBT-I were the most difficult for me. The hard part is committing; getting up in the morning was super hard, even though I was super consistent about it. It was so difficult. I understood that sleep scheduling also involved getting to bed at 2 a.m. each night, and it was recommended that I build in a "buffer zone" before my agreed-upon bedtime to help me fall asleep faster. I would do something super mundane like wash dishes or chill out on the balcony and just relax or go for a walk or read a book.

I also practiced stimulus control, which involved me getting out of bed when I was not able to sleep. I recalled the advice from my OTP to pair my bed with sleeping and to get out of bed when I could not sleep. I would just lay down and try and fall back asleep, but if not, I'd just get up and just pace or something for like 15 to 20 minutes, which helped calm me down. Then I just go back to sleep. But practicing stimulus control had its hard days too. There were some days where I couldn't sleep at all. I would just stay up. So, like, yeah, I'll just stay up all night sometimes.

As my CBT-I treatment progressed, I also used activities during the day to help build my sleep drive and entrain my circadian system. By trying to be more active during the day when I could, without forcing it, just expending more energy and stuff, so a lot more thinking, a lot more writing and creative exercises or working out a little bit more or spending more time outside in the sun. Within a few weeks, I noticed these strategies were having an effect on my sleep. I was falling asleep pretty quickly, like within 15 minutes instead of 30 or an hour. I also noticed that my consistency in maintaining my sleep schedule helped me feel sleepy before bedtime. My body would start to get tired, and by around 11 or 12, the gears started slowing down. I knew I'd be able to fall asleep soon.

Months later, after successfully completing CBT-I, I was getting 8 hours of sleep on average compared with less than 6 hours before I started working with the occupational therapist. CBT-I was absolutely fantastic because it helped me regulate my day, which is like the most important part about CBT-I. I wanted to regulate my day because I was pretty much sleeping through most of my day, and I didn't have a very clear schedule. CBT-I helped me move forward and helped me get closer to regulating my time. I continue to notice improved daytime functioning. I am still feeling really well-rested. I have a lot more focus when I wake up now too. It's because I've been waking up at a consistent time each morning.

Threats to Women's Sleep

Females experience more disturbed sleep and report insomnia more often than men (Zeng et al., 2020). Women's risk for insomnia also increases during menstruation, pregnancy, and menopause (Baker et al., 2018). Cultural factors can also impair women's sleep. Women are typically the primary caregivers for children as well as for older adult parents who may require assistance during the night.

Other Sleep Disorders

Sleep disorders are highly variable and they can co-occur with insomnia. The following are sleep disorder categories identified within the most recent version of the International Classification of Sleep Disorders (American Academy of Sleep Medicine, 2014). OTPs should consider referring a person to a sleep specialist if they suspect the presence of these disorders.

Sleep-Related Breathing Disorders

Sleep-related breathing disorders involve impaired respiration while sleeping, with OSA being the most common (Sateia & Thorpy, 2017). OSA in adults is characterized by frequent periods when breathing stops (apneas), often because muscle tone in the tongue and soft palate lessens and these structures interrupt airflow. Individuals with OSA have frequent brief awakenings during the night and along with reductions in both NREM and REM sleep. These conditions can impair the bed partner's ability to maintain peaceful sleep. Central sleep apnea falls in this category, a condition in which central nervous system dysfunction impairs breathing (Baillieul et al., 2019).

Hypersomnolence Disorders

In hypersomnolence disorders, an individual demonstrates excessive daytime sleepiness and difficulty staying awake during the day despite not having another sleep disorder (Sateia & Thorpy, 2017). Narcolepsy is a well-known hypersomnolence disorder (Bassetti et al., 2019) because of a selective loss or dysfunction in orexin-producing neurons in the brain. Narcolepsy can present with cataplexy (a sudden, brief loss of voluntary muscle control triggered by strong emotions) along with sleep paralysis and disturbed sleep.

Circadian Rhythm Sleep–Wake Disorders

Circadian rhythm disorders present as individual sleep patterns that are out of sync with society's expectations for sleep timing (Sateia & Thorpy, 2017). Delayed sleep phase happens when sleep occurs later than the desired societal norms and is frequently seen in adolescents and young adults. In contrast, advanced sleep phase is more commonly seen in older adults. In these cases the individual's body (i.e., circadian system) is not entrained to the rising and setting of the sun. Night-shift workers are especially prone to circadian rhythm sleep disorders. "Social jet lag" can even occur when individuals choose later waking times on the weekends, compared with weekdays (Roach & Sargent, 2019).

Parasomnias

Parasomnias can include bruxism (teeth grinding), sleep terrors, and sleep walking. Because the individual is unaware of their actions, the results can be worrisome and even dangerous. For example, people with parasomnias may eat during their sleep and not remember it the next day or may leave their home in the middle of the night (Hirshkowitz & Smith, 2004). Sleep terrors, a form of parasomnia that usually occurs in children, is especially frightening because children have difficulty separating their dreams from real life. This can be confusing for them and their caregivers. Another parasomnia that frequently occurs in children is sleep-related enuresis, otherwise known as bedwetting during sleep (Gu et al., 2016).

Sleep-Related Movement Disorders

Sleep-related movement disorders occur when the body moves involuntarily during sleep (Sateia & Thorpy, 2017). Restless legs syndrome (RLS) is a common example of this condition. RLS symptoms can include sensations of something crawling inside the person's legs or arms, making falling asleep more difficult. RLS occurs more often in women compared with men (Trotti, 2017). Periodic leg movement disorder (PLMD) is another type of sleep-related movement disorder. This involuntary movement of the legs and sometimes arms usually occurs in a regular pattern of movements. Unlike RLS movements, which can occur while awake, the movements related to PLMD occur only during sleep. Sleep-related movement disorders also include sleep-related leg cramps and benign sleep myoclonus in infants.

Role of Occupational Therapy

Screening and Assessment

OTPs offer a needed perspective on sleep health within the care teams in which they serve. Screening for sleep disturbances should be a standard aspect of occupational therapy practice. Screening can identify sleep disturbances that often go undetected by other professions. When found, the OTP can pursue referrals to sleep-medicine specialists in support of the person's sleep health. Screening can be as simple as asking a couple of questions: "Do you have any difficulties with falling or staying asleep?" as well as "Are you dissatisfied with the amount or quality of your sleep?" Responses to these questions can be followed up with questions to clarify the nature of the person's sleep-related concerns.

The OTP should determine the person's daily demands and life roles (e.g., caregiver, worker, student), and confirm the nature of the sleep difficulties (e.g., difficulties falling or staying asleep). During assessment, the OTP should develop an occupational profile, as recommended by the American Occupational Therapy Association (AOTA, 2020), to ensure the "occupational" nature of the people's concerns are well understood. Through interview and chart review, the practitioner should seek to understand when and how long the sleep difficulties have been occurring as well as the person's most pressing sleep-related concerns. A brief medical history can uncover co-occurring concerns, past treatments for sleep disturbances, and use of prescription or over-the-counter medications that may interfere with sleep.

The Insomnia Severity Index (ISI: Bastien et al., 2001) is a widely used tool to assess insomnia symptom severity, including difficulties with falling and staying asleep, dissatisfaction with sleep, the extent to which sleep problems interfere with daily performance, and worries about poor sleep. The ISI includes just seven questions, and scores between 8 and 14 indicate subthreshold insomnia for which sleep health promotion strategies would be a warranted approach to support sleep health. If chronic insomnia can be confirmed, CBT-I may be warranted.

The Sleep Hygiene Index (SHI; Mastin et al., 2006) assesses behaviors and environmental factors that contribute to poor sleep. In this way, the SHI is predictive of sleep disturbance. The items in the SHI represent three general areas of poor sleep hygiene that should offer insight into tailoring treatment approaches. Questions related to sleep timing such as going to bed and waking at different times have implications for regulating the circadian system. Questions related to the sleep environment such as having too much light in the room or worrying in bed can uncover targets for interventions to promote sleep health.

The Pittsburgh Sleep Quality Index (Buysse et al., 1989) offers a detailed look at sleep disturbing factors. Scores of 6 or greater indicate poor sleep, often reflecting insufficient sleep duration and quality, as well as lifestyle factors contributing to poor sleep. The Epworth Sleepiness Scale (Johns, 1991) can be used to determine if the person has difficulties with daytime functioning because it asks the likelihood of falling asleep during daily activities. The Karolinska Sleepiness Scale (Shahid et al., 2012) can also be used to assess daytime

sleepiness and is available from its authors (Torbjorn. Akerstedt@ki.se). Scales such as this establish the daytime effects of sleep disturbances and are used weekly in monitoring sleepiness in response to sleep-related treatments such as CBT-I.

After the therapist has determined that difficulties with poor or insufficient sleep exist, more thorough assessments can help to identify the presence of chronic insomnia as well as other sleep-related diagnoses. An essential assessment tool for OTPs addressing sleep is the Consensus Sleep Diary (Carney et al., 2012). The person or their caregiver completes a daily record of sleep-related behaviors across one or more weeks. This offers insight into the time a person goes to bed, how long it takes them to fall asleep, whether or not they wake during the night, and the time of their final waking in the morning. The OTP can determine specific patterns in sleep timing (e.g., time to bed and waking), and can monitor the person's total sleep time and their total time in bed.

The OTP working with Kendrick in this chapter's The Lived Experience feature used the recommended minimum of 2 weeks of sleep diary data to determine his sleep patterns and average total sleep time. This data was used to establish his treatment plan, and weekly sleep diary use served to monitor his progress throughout treatment.

These tools are summarized in Table 52-2. In addition to conducting an occupational profile as noted in the text that follows, several other tools might be helpful in identifying the barriers and facilitators to addressing sleep behaviors as a part of the person's health and well-being plan.

A recently developed assessment used in CBT-I is the Sleep Disorders Symptoms Checklist (SDS-CL-25; Klingman et al., 2017). Please note that the OTP should receive advanced education and training in CBT-I (see Resources at

---

TABLE 52-2 | Therapeutic Reasoning Assessment Table: Sleep

Which Tool?	Whom Was This Tool Designed For?	What Is Required of the Person? Can They Use the Tool?	What Am I Measuring?	How Long Does It Take, and Where Do I Administer This Assessment?	Is the Tool Associated With a Practice Model?
Insomnia Severity Index (ISI; Bastien et al., 2001)	Ages 17+	Person must be capable of accurate self-report using a simple scale.	Rating the nature and symptoms related to insomnia symptoms and the impact of sleep disturbances on daily function	Quick seven-item screening can be completed in a few minutes in any quiet space	No specific occupational therapy model but consistent with Person-Environment-Occupation (PEO) perspectives
Sleep Hygiene Index (SHI; Mastin et al., 2006)	Ages 18+	Person must be capable of accurate self-report using a simple scale.	Rating the frequency of behaviors and environmental factors associated with sleep habits	13 items related to sleep habits completed in 5 minutes in any quiet space	No specific occupational therapy model but consistent with PEO perspectives
Pittsburgh Sleep Quality Index (Buysse et al., 1989)	Ages 24+	Person must be capable of accurate self-report using a simple scale.	Rating of sleep quality and sleep disturbance over a 1-month period	19 items can be completed within 5–10 minutes in any quiet space	No specific occupational therapy model but consistent with PEO perspectives
Consensus Sleep Diary (Carney et al., 2012)	Ages 18+	Person or their caregiver must be capable of accurate self-report using a simple scale/ item response.	Information about daily sleep patterns— completed daily across a time period such as 2 weeks	Each day, the person must complete their report regarding 14 items within 1 hour of awakening.	No specific occupational therapy model but consistent with PEO perspectives

the end of this chapter) before its use. The SDS-CL-25 offers information to confirm the presence of insomnia, concerns with insufficient sleep and circadian preference, as well as screening for additional sleep-related diagnoses such as OSA, circadian rhythm disorder, RLS, narcolepsy, and parasomnias that may warrant referral to a sleep-medicine specialist.

Other assessment tools may be implemented to deepen the OTP's understanding of a person's sleep disturbance and its impacts upon daily life. The Morningness-Eveningness questionnaire (Horne & Ostberg, 1976) assesses an individual's circadian preference; this information can be useful for understanding why, for example, falling asleep at 10:00 p.m. and waking by 6:00 a.m. may be difficult for a person who habitually prefers to go to bed later and wake later in the day. The Functional Outcomes of Sleep Questionnaire (FOSQ; Chasens et al., 2009) reflects the impact of excessive daytime sleepiness on daily activities and offers a useful "occupational" perspective on poor sleep. Areas of occupation are related to engagement in home, leisure, and social activities.

The Motivation for Change Index (Perlis et al., 2008) offers information regarding how sleep disturbances impact a person's life and their willingness to endure a nonpharmacological/behavioral treatment. CBT-I may initially worsen insomnia symptoms before they improve, and the person should be made aware of this. Sleep environment assessments can help in determining how the home environment may hinder sleep, including nonsleep-related activities in bed, the presence of cosleepers (human and animal), excess light and sound, and perceptions of safety and security when sleeping. Such assessments are critically important given that low socioeconomic status and living in urban environments can independently predict poor sleep health (Johnson et al., 2021).

Finally, assessments of depression, such as the Patient Health Questionnaire-9 (Kroenke et al., 2001), and anxiety, such as the Generalized Anxiety Disorders Screener (Lowe et al., 2008), offer insight into the presence of co-occurring mental health challenges that can contribute to poor sleep.

Intervention

Intervention planning should proceed following completion of an occupational profile (AOTA, 2020), as well as after developing a thorough understanding of the nature of the sleep-related concerns, their likely causes, and their impacts upon occupational performance. It is recommended that the OTP use a person-centered approach to collaboratively develop treatment goals. Goal setting will often include changes in the person's typical routines so as to improve their sleep-health. Careful use of assessments will aid in establishing realistic goals and monitor a person's response to intervention.

There is a range of intervention approaches and outcomes within the occupational therapy profession's scope of practice (Smallfield & Molitor, 2018). The more effective interventions are multicomponent (i.e., integrating a few complementary approaches) consistent with aspects of CBT-I, many of which are presented in the text that follows.

Sleep Hygiene Education Interventions

Sleep hygiene education is commonly reported as an area of nonpharmacological intervention delivered by OTPs. Providing sleep hygiene education can improve related knowledge, though with inconsistent improvements in insomnia

symptoms and sleep health (e.g., sleep efficiency; Chung et al., 2018; Dietrich et al., 2016; Gutman et al., 2017). This may be caused by large variations is what is considered "sleep hygiene" (Posner & Gehrman, 2011). Sleep hygiene education targeted to an individual's unique circumstances (e.g., limiting caffeine in the evening for those who engage in this behavior), combined with weekly monitoring of sleep-promoting routines, may be more likely to generate a therapeutic effect.

The SHI and an environment-based assessment can be used to identify if sleep hygiene concerns are present. A metaphor of a ladder linking sleep hygiene to good sleep can be a useful clinical tool. Each rung on the ladder can represent useful sleep hygiene behaviors/environments that contribute to optimal sleep health. When the ladder has all its "rungs," then optimal sleep is more likely. As more of the "rungs" of the ladder are missing because of poor sleep hygiene, then optimal sleep quality is at greater risk. A therapeutic approach could entail identifying ineffective sleep hygiene concerns and developing behavior/environment change goals to improve sleep health. Individualized approaches are important for addressing difficulties with sleep. For individuals with schizophrenia, for example, addressing evening routines, daytime activity, and environmental interventions may improve effective sleep regulation as well as provide a means of gaining a sense of control over day-to-day life (Faulkner et al., 2022).

The OTP should clearly explain how "sleep works," and that sleep hygiene behaviors can degrade or contribute to effective sleep regulation (e.g., synchrony between the circadian and homeostatic sleep-driver systems). Sleep diary data can be used to make the person more aware of existing routines that may impair sleep health such as frequent napping or irregular waking times. Given stress and worry can make falling and staying asleep difficult, OTPs should also consider how hyperarousal, including anxiety and stress related to fulfilling expected life roles, could inhibit sleep health. If the person's sleep hygiene is not improving, then the practitioner should reevaluate the most pressing concerns contributing to ineffective sleep regulation. A referral to a CBT-I practitioner or sleep specialist may be necessary to improve sleep health, especially if chronic insomnia is present (Chung et al., 2018).

Sleep Hygiene and the Sleep Environment

OTPs are well aware of the transactions between the person, their occupations, and their environment. The following text addresses some approaches to environmental modifications that may support a person's sleep health; these approaches should target those sleep hygiene risks noted by the person.

Ideally, a dark, cool, and quiet room is likely to promote sleep. The visual system cues the body to recognize day and night by responding to environmental light. For sleep, a room should be completely dark, with no television or technology on (i.e., computers, e-readers, telephones) because light triggers the brain to believe it is "daytime." Light-blocking curtains or eye masks may be needed to block light from registering on the retina. Before bedtime, consider blue blocking glasses for those exposed to light-emitting diodes (LED). These glasses can block LED blue light (i.e., 400–525 nanometers), which may promote subjective sleep quality (Bigalke et al., 2021). Exposure to daylight upon awakening and maintaining higher light levels during the day (350–500 lux) can promote effective circadian rhythmicity. The OTP should become familiar with recently developed guidelines (Brown et al., 2022).

A comfortable bed or sleeping area supports effective sleep, in part through limiting cognitive or somatic arousal because of pain and discomfort. Consider a mattress that is firm and supportive as well as a pillow that supports the head with good spinal alignment. This may be especially important for individuals who experience chronic pain (Ancuelle et al., 2015). Of course, in non-Western countries, other sleeping places might be used, such as an individual or family hammock.

Linens and bed coverings should be comfortable, and the weight of blankets is an important factor to consider. Some people prefer a heavy blanket, providing calming proprioceptive input, whereas others prefer only a light cover. Recent evidence has shown weighted blankets may improve symptoms of anxiety and hyperarousal, though connections to improved sleep are less clear (Eron et al., 2020). A cool, though not cold, room can promote sleep because it supports decreases in core body temperature associated with the circadian system regulation. A room that is too cold or hot, however, can promote unwanted arousal, thereby limiting sleep quality (Lan et al., 2017).

In order to sleep, the sleep environment should be as quiet as possible. Quiet environments can promote effective sleep because they limit auditory stimulation, which can promote arousal, especially during NREM stage 1 and 2. Consider earplugs and turning off noise from cell phones, televisions, computers, or radios. A white noise machine or fan could be used to drown out unavoidable noises in the sleep environment, though their effectiveness is not well established (Riedy et al., 2021). Limit waking the person during the evening to promote better sleep. Keep voice volume low and minimize noisy machines, which can lessen sleep disturbances and reduce the need for prescribing sedatives (Bartick et al., 2010).

Sleep Hygiene: Sleep Timing and Participation

Waking the same time every day and engaging in personal routines can promote circadian rhythmicity, build sleep drive, and add purpose and meaning to one's daily life. Western industrialized nations have a monophasic sleep pattern, which typically includes being awake for 16 hours during the day, then sleeping for 8 hours during the night (Steger, 2012).

Some daily variation in routine bedtimes and rise-times are common and likely not a problem. However, larger (e.g., 2 hours) daily variations can create a form of "social jet lag," limit sleep duration and quality, degrade daytime functioning, and increase risks for mood disorders in adults

(Bei et al., 2016) and adolescents (Castiglione-Fontanellaz et al., 2023). Middle and high school students who sleep in on weekends and then return to an early rise-time during the week are most susceptible to this form of social jet lag. Building in morning weekend activities and limiting exposure to electronics before bedtime may promote sleep health and reduce risk for mood disorders (Cain & Gradisar, 2010; Gradisar et al., 2022).

To limit the development of insomnia, sleep hygiene education commonly recommends leaving the bed if not sleeping, engaging in a relaxing activity, then returning to bed when feeling sleepy. This recommendation is related to the Stimulus Control Model presented earlier and seeks to help the individual associate the bed with sleeping. This aspect of sleep hygiene includes instructions not to engage in activities that are not related to sleep (e.g., cell phone/computer use) in bed. These activities can lead to presleep arousal and create an unconscious association between the bed and not sleeping. Recommendations to leave the bedroom will limit total sleep time and can increase sleepiness, which can increase risk of injury. Careful monitoring of sleep timing and sleepiness, along with risk mitigation because of sleepiness, is recommended to evaluate response to this form of sleep hygiene education.

Napping, which was reviewed earlier, is a common activity, often socially appropriate, and it can be supportive of growth and development. A brief nap can be used to limit feeling sleepy during the day, which may promote daily performance. Napping, however, can deplete the building of sleep drive during the day, and habitual napping may ultimately contribute to the development of insomnia. The OTP should be aware of age-related, cultural, and personal variability in napping beliefs and behaviors.

The timing of meals can degrade or promote sleep quality. Having a high calorie meal closer to one's typical bedtime (within 60 minutes) can make falling and staying asleep more difficult (Crispim et al., 2011). In addition, moving habitual mealtimes later in the evening can create a circadian shift in sleep timing and lead to sleep debt, difficulty waking, and increased risk for obesity (Spaeth et al., 2019). Alternatively, individuals should be encouraged to have routine mealtimes that can be used to promote effective sleep regulation (Boege et al., 2021).

Limiting caffeine in the evening is important so that adenosine binding can occur in promotion of falling and staying asleep. Restricting alcohol, nicotine, and other substances can also support sleep health. For example, though alcohol's sedative effects may promote falling asleep, they can also lead to fragmented sleep and poor sleep quality (Stepanski & Wyatt, 2003).

Being a Psychosocial OT Practitioner

Overcoming Sleep Issues From College to the Military and Back

Identifying Psychosocial Strengths and Needs

Transitioning from military service into civilian life can present significant life challenges, including mood instability and difficulties with sleep participation because of significant changes in the demands and temporal structure of day-to-day life. Kendrick had recently ended a commitment with the U.S. Air Force and started

undergraduate classes using his veteran's benefits. He noticed his poor sleep routines from his shiftwork in the Air Force were negatively affecting his sleep. Specifically, Kendrick had difficulties falling and staying asleep, and he was not getting enough sleep most nights, which limited his effective participation in college. This, combined with a recently diagnosed mood disorder (i.e., bipolar II), convinced Kendrick to seek assistance from occupational therapists who specialize in behavioral treatments for insomnia.

Upon screening, the OTP determined that Kendrick likely had chronic insomnia. The OTP therefore asked Kendrick to complete more thorough sleep-related assessments about his daytime sleepiness, his sleep hygiene practices and sleep environment, his beliefs about his sleep difficulties, and his mood (i.e., anxiety and depression), as well as keep a daily sleep diary which he completed for a couple of weeks. The daily sleep diary was essential to the process because it helped the OTP identify the patterns in Kendrick's sleep, such as when he would go to bed and wake for the day. Following a clinical interview and review of the assessment data, the OTP confirmed Kendrick was experiencing chronic insomnia, insufficient sleep (i.e., less than 6 hours per night on average), and a mood disorder that was stable when Kendrick was taking his prescribed medication. The OTP also identified that Kendrick was highly motivated to adopt new sleep preparation and sleep participation behaviors in hopes of improving the quality and quantity of his sleep.

The OTP, who had advanced education and training in CBT-I, completed a conceptualization of Kendrick's case, in which the OTP identified factors that were likely perpetuating his insomnia. Sleep drive concerns included extended lingering in bed for 46 minutes on average and occasional napping. Circadian concerns included inconsistent time to bed ranging from 10:20 p.m. to 7:45 a.m. and time out of bed ranging from 7:45 a.m. to 12:15 p.m. He set his alarm clock only 3 days a week to wake up in time for classes. General arousal concerns included worrying and ruminating about his future as well as experiences of feeling "revved up" when trying to fall asleep. Maladaptive sleep behaviors included playing video games, using his cell phone until bedtime, and consuming caffeine in the evening. Sleep environment concerns included exposure to excess light and a messy/cluttered studio apartment. Of benefit to sleep, Kendrick reported walking most places and doing light calisthenics in the morning upon waking, which promoted circadian entrainment and building his sleep drive.

Using a Holistic Occupational Therapy Approach

The OTP consulted with the Veterans Health Administration nurse practitioner who oversaw the medical management of Kendrick's mood disorder. The consensus was to proceed with multicomponent CBT-I and replace sleep restriction therapy with sleep scheduling, which was less likely to worsen mood symptoms.

CBT-I included Kendrick's ongoing daily use of a sleep diary, sleep scheduling, stimulus control, psychoeducation, and cognitive therapy, as well as relaxation training. The OTP educated Kendrick on how his inconsistent sleep schedule was weakening his sleep drive and circadian system alignment and that naps further made falling and staying asleep more difficult. Sleep scheduling involved agreeing to and setting a consistent daily rise time that allowed Kendrick to meet his activity demands (e.g., attending classes and studying). This involved setting an alarm for the same time each morning, and it was paired with going to bed at a consistent bedtime. Kendrick was educated about stimulus control therapy, and he agreed to leave the bed if he could not sleep, and to return to the bed when sleepy. At each following session, the OTP reviewed Kendrick's sleep diary with him to evaluate his average sleep efficiency, including the time it took to fall asleep and his total sleep time. The OTP also monitored his mood, daytime sleepiness, and sleep hygiene behaviors. The OTP combined these daily sessions with behavior change approaches such as supporting his decision-making, self-monitoring, providing feedback on behavioral goals, and problem-solving, which helped to establish effective sleep-related behaviors. For example, one aspect of problem-solving involved establishing consistent mealtimes so that meals served as additional cues to entrain Kendrick's circadian rhythm.

Sessions occurred about every week to every other week. Kendrick continued to be highly motivated to "adhere" to the agreed time to bed and time out of bed, as well as leaving the bed when he couldn't sleep. About 1 month into his treatment, Kendrick noted that it was becoming easier to fall asleep and stay asleep. Kendrick and the OTP noted that he was developing a more consistent routine of activities, for example, getting up at the same time and either going to class or exercising. Immediately before his time to bed, he would practice a brief meditation, which helped to calm him down. This consistency was associated with Kendrick feeling sleepy at the scheduled time to bed, and he was rarely experiencing that "revved up" feeling he had before treatment had begun. These experiences motivated Kendrick to continue with his sleep schedule, his napping had stopped, and he would consistently leave the bed when he couldn't sleep. By the time therapy was nearing its end, Kendrick was realizing 8 hours of sleep each night on average, compared with less than 6 hours when therapy had begun. He reported a greater ability to focus on his studies, and his mood was improving consistently across the few months of treatment.

Multicomponent Cognitive Behavioral Therapy for Insomnia (CBT-I)

Activities: Sleep Preparation and Sleep Participation

Sleep restriction therapy	Limiting a person's time in bed to their average sleep ability (i.e., total sleep time) combined with consistent time to go to bed and time to get out of bed; limit napping. Caution: This can result in increased daytime sleepiness, thereby increasing risk of accidents.
Sleep scheduling	Person to use a consistent time to bed and time out of bed based on the person's typical (average) time in bed; limit napping.
Stimulus control therapy	Person to leave the bed (bedroom) when not sleeping for 15 minutes and return to bed only when sleepy. Caution: This can result in increased daytime sleepiness, thereby increasing risk of accidents.
Psychoeducation	Person is educated on factors supporting effective sleep regulation (e.g., homeostatic sleep-driver system, circadian system, cognitive/emotional arousal).
Cognitive therapy	Person is engaged in discussions or behavioral experiments to adapt an inaccurate sleep-related belief (e.g., if I have difficulty sleeping, I should try harder) to one that is more accurate (e.g., sleep will "come to me").
Relaxation therapy	Person engages in activities that help to decrease cognitive and emotional arousal (e.g., mindfulness meditation, yoga, body scan).
Behavior change techniques	Strategies adopted by an OTP to develop consistency in a person's behavior change (e.g., self-monitoring, feedback on behaviors, and behavioral experiments).

Reflective Questions

1. Which specific assessments would you use to determine if Kendrick was experiencing chronic insomnia? How would you justify from the assessments that Kendrick had insomnia?
2. How might the OTP specifically address Kendrick's daily routines beyond mealtimes and attending class in order to build sleep drive?
3. How would you design a treatment session that supports Kendrick's understanding of how his sleep is regulated (i.e., building on the Two-Process Model of Sleep Regulation)?

Multicomponent CBT-I for Insomnia

CBT-I is the recommended first-line treatment for insomnia by the American Academy of Sleep Medicine and the American College of Physicians (Qaseem et al., 2016; Schutte-Rodin et al., 2008). First-line treatment means that the treatment is the preferred and best available for addressing a medical concern, such as insomnia disorder in this case.

There is overwhelming evidence that CBT-I is more effective in the treatment of chronic insomnia than sleep medications such as sedative-hypnotics, and CBT-I has much lower side effects (Muench et al., 2022). The challenge, however, is that there is a lack of providers who have received sufficient education and training in the delivery of CBT-I. CBT-I is increasingly being delivered in community-based and primary care settings by a range of professionals such as nurses, nurse practitioners, social workers, psychologists, and occupational therapists (Davidson et al., 2019; Muench et al., 2022). Well-trained occupational therapists are now beginning to safely and effectively deliver CBT-I, though it is the practitioner's responsibility to access proper education, supervision, and/or consultation (Eakman et al., 2022; Green & Hicks, 2015).

Briefly, CBT-I is delivered when an individual presents with a diagnosis of chronic insomnia. Other medical and sleep-related conditions should be stable. The person should understand that CBT-I is a behavioral, nonpharmacological intervention and that it may not be easy to endure in the first couple weeks of therapy (as shown in Kendrick's experience). CBT-I requires 2 weeks of pretreatment daily sleep diary data and is typically delivered weekly across 8 weeks, though it can be briefly delivered in 4 weeks or extended over a longer period as needed (Bramoweth et al., 2020).

CBT-I typically includes a combination of sleep restriction and stimulus control therapies (Baglioni et al., 2022; Manber & Carney, 2015; Perlis et al., 2008). Sleep restriction therapy serves to limit the time a person is in bed (sleep opportunity) to the average time they are capable of generating consolidated sleep (sleep ability). For example, a person sleeps on average 6 hours each night, though they spend nearly 8 hours in bed trying to get the sleep they feel they desperately need. In this example, the person's sleep efficiency (SE) is calculated using weekly averages of their total sleep time (TST) divided by their total time in bed (TIB) multiplied by 100 (SE = TST/TIB × 100). For example, 6 hours of total sleep time divided by 8 hours of time in bed, multiplied by 100 = 75% sleep efficiency, indicating poor sleep quality. The therapist and person agree to a time the person will get out of bed for the day (e.g., 7:00 a.m.) to entrain the circadian system, and to an initial time to go to bed (1:00 a.m. in this case) to match the person's sleep ability (e.g., 6 hours).

In subsequent meetings, if the person's sleep efficiency improves to 90% or greater, then they are given an earlier time to bed (e.g., 12:45). The goal is to gradually build the individual's total sleep time progressively across the weeks of therapy while maintaining high sleep efficiency. Daily sleep diary data are essential to this treatment; treatment should not occur without it. The challenges to sleep restriction therapy include difficulty staying awake until a person's prescribed time to bed and staying in bed after their prescribed time out of bed. Sleep restriction therapy leads to increasing sleepiness during the day, which can promote falling and staying asleep. Increasing daytime sleepiness indicates increasing sleep

pressure, which may present risks for accidents. The OTP is responsible for this increased safety risk and must establish ways to reduce injury risk.

Stimulus control therapy builds can improve sleep by pairing the cue of one's bed and bedroom with sleep (Bootzin & Perlis, 2011). If the person is having difficulty falling asleep, they should leave their bedroom and return only when sleepy. If a person is typically on their cell phone or laptop watching videos in bed while trying to fall asleep, those activities should be moved to a different location before bedtime. If a person wakes during the night and has difficulty falling back asleep, they should engage in a relaxing activity and return to bed only when sleepy. Sleep restriction therapy and stimulus control therapies include a set time to wake to entrain the circadian system. Napping during the day, especially longer naps later in the day, are discouraged because they can deplete sleep drive, making falling asleep in the evening more difficult.

Another common component of CBT-I includes techniques for managing stress and cognitive arousal as bedtime approaches or during the night when a person is having difficulties sleeping. Jason Ong (2017) has developed a specialized approach to CBT-I by incorporating mindfulness-based approaches with sleep restriction and stimulus control therapies; meditations, yoga, and tai chi are commonly used. This approach works by minimizing cognitive and emotional arousal, thereby promoting falling and staying asleep. Another approach, used by Kendrick in this chapter's The Lived Experience feature, included creating a "buffer zone"; in Kendrick's case, he engaged in calming activities to quiet his mind and help create a routine to help him fall asleep faster. Journaling and creating "to-do" lists can be helpful to process the day, make plans for the next day, and then let those concerns go in preparation for sleep (Manber & Carney, 2015).

Psychoeducation and cognitive therapies are also used within CBT-I. A main component of psychoeducation is education about sleep regulation and insomnia. People should understand factors that can promote and hinder effective sleep based upon the Two-Process Model of Sleep Regulation. Education on models of insomnia can help the person know which factors (e.g., napping, using electronic devices in bed) may be perpetuating their insomnia. Cognitive therapies can challenge ineffective sleep beliefs that contribute to excessive worrying, and behavioral experiments can be used to establish new activity routines that can promote sleep health (Baglioni et al., 2022)

Sleep hygiene education and goal setting should address individualized concerns (Posner & Gehrman, 2011). For example, avoiding caffeine close to bedtime can allow more adenosine binding, thereby promoting falling and staying asleep. Exercising regularly would help build sleep drive, whereas managing stress and reducing bedroom noise could reduce arousal concerns. Further, decreasing light exposure at night and keeping the room temperature cool (59.9°F–67.1°F [15.5°C–19.5°C]) yet comfortable can help entrain the person's circadian system and promote effective sleep regulation.

Sleep Medicine Professionals

OTPs interested in supporting persons' sleep health will certainly interact with sleep medicine practitioners. This field is vast, including specialists in sleep physiology, genetics, chronobiology, occupational sleep medicine, and pharmacology, to name just a few (Kryger et al., 2017). OTPs addressing insomnia concerns are encouraged to collaborate with a person's primary care physician to ensure medical issues are stable and consider referral to a sleep specialist who can identify and address co-occurring sleep disorders. OSA and its treatment using continuous positive airway pressure (CPAP) during sleep is common in adults and children (Levert et al., 2022). OTPs could develop health management routines to support the use and care of the CPAP machine.

Behavioral sleep medicine is an expanding practice area most concerned with the evaluation and treatment of sleep disorders using behavioral and cognitive approaches. This specialty would be a perfect match for an OTP or researcher wishing to specialize in sleep. Behavioral sleep medicine leverages cognitive behavioral therapies to address thoughts and behaviors that may interfere with effective sleep. OTPs and researchers are encouraged to look further into this specialty and consider obtaining advanced training.

OTPs should also collaborate with allied medical practitioners to address medications and their routine use. Medicines used to treat mood disorders can have negative effects on sleep architecture. SSRIs used to treat mood disorders, for example, can lead to a loss in total REM sleep early in treatment (Hutka et al., 2021). Timing of medications could also influence falling and staying asleep; therefore, it is important to monitor a person's sleep including their sleep preparation and medication routines through use of a sleep diary. In addition, OTPs should become familiar with sleep disorders that may co-occur in common disease processes such as RLS and REM sleep behavior disorders in Parkinson disease (Lajoie et al., 2021) or insomnia, sleep phase delay, and hypersomnia in persons experiencing schizophrenia spectrum and bipolar disorders (Laskemoen et al., 2019).

Technology, Culture, and Sleep

The advent of the lightbulb and the proliferation of its use changed the way humans experienced the night. Access to artificial light and industrialization have led to increases in sleep deprivation across the globe. In Western nations, there has been a change from "biphasic" sleep in which sleep occurred in two 3- to 4-hour segments in the night to "monophasic" sleep, which is now pervasive across industrialized nations (Ekirch, 2018). Cultural and personal differences are also associated with where and how people might sleep. Bed sharing, for example, is common in parents and children, couples, siblings, and with pets. Subjective reports of sleep quality have been found to be higher on average when persons cosleep, perhaps indicating a relative sense of safety and security (Andre et al., 2021). Objective measures, however, often indicate poorer sleep quality during cosleeping. The OTP must take care in understanding cosleeping behaviors and their impact on sleep for their people.

Sleep health has often been seen as an individual behavioral concern in which a person does not adopt behaviors that promote their sleep quality and quantity. Yet sleep difficulties are often tied to physical and social conditions such as poverty and racial disparities. Sleep for those in poverty and in urban settings is associated with low sleep quality and quantity and low quality of life (Simonelli et al., 2013).

Within the United States, racial discrimination continues to be a pervasive concern, often co-occurring with poverty and unsafe living environments, which negatively impact sleep health and human development (El-Sheikh et al., 2022; Hart et al., 2021). The term "sleep desert" has even been proposed to indicate how structural racism and socioeconomic inequality have contributed to poor sleep, which together with poor nutrition and inadequate exercise can exacerbate racial health disparities (Attarian et al., 2022).

Technological changes have continued to influence people's daily lives as well as the quantity and quality of their sleep. Electronic devices (e.g., laptops, smartphones, and tablets) used throughout the day are also used excessively well into the night, leading to an epidemic of sleep problems and sleep debt (Mei et al., 2018). Children, adolescents, and adults are going to bed and sleeping with their electronic devices. These behaviors appear to degrade overall sleep quality and have been found to contribute to the development of depression and anxiety (Dinis & Bragança, 2018).

Consumer technologies, however, can also assist in monitoring people's activity levels and sleep health. Applications can monitor how long people sleep and how much they move (Fig. 52-2). Although collecting data on sleep time does not improve people's sleep directly, collecting this information can provide a sleep baseline for goal setting and to monitor progress in therapy. Technology can be used to provide white noise, music, or guided meditations to help with falling asleep. Apps also exist for keeping a sleep log or reminding people to start their sleep preparation routine. Because technology continues to evolve, OTPs may want to explore and try the technology themselves to see what may work for their people.

The practice of sleep medicine is changing because of both commercially available monitoring technologies and electronically mediated interventions for insomnia. Cognitive behavioral therapies (including CBT-I) have developed electronically mediated or digitized approaches, referred to as "dCBT," reflecting a move to digital medicine (Luik et al., 2017). There are variations including fully automated interventions without clinical support, automated interventions with the guidance of a trained practitioner, and elements of automation (e.g., use of application-based sleep diary), yet intervention is fully guided by the practitioner. Digital CBT-I outcomes are typically not inferior to face-to-face CBT-I, indicating these forms of intervention will continue to be developed and employed to those who can access and use digital media (Soh et al., 2020).

Here's the Point

- Sleep is the occupation that occupies the largest percentage of human life. Sleep is engaged in by all human beings, is foundational to the quality of all other occupations, and is essential to human health and well-being.
- Effective sleep regulation occurs through achieving synchrony between the circadian system, which operates on a 24-hour cycle for which light exposure is a key driver, and the homeostatic sleep-driver system, in which sleep pressure builds during the waking hours to promote falling and staying asleep.

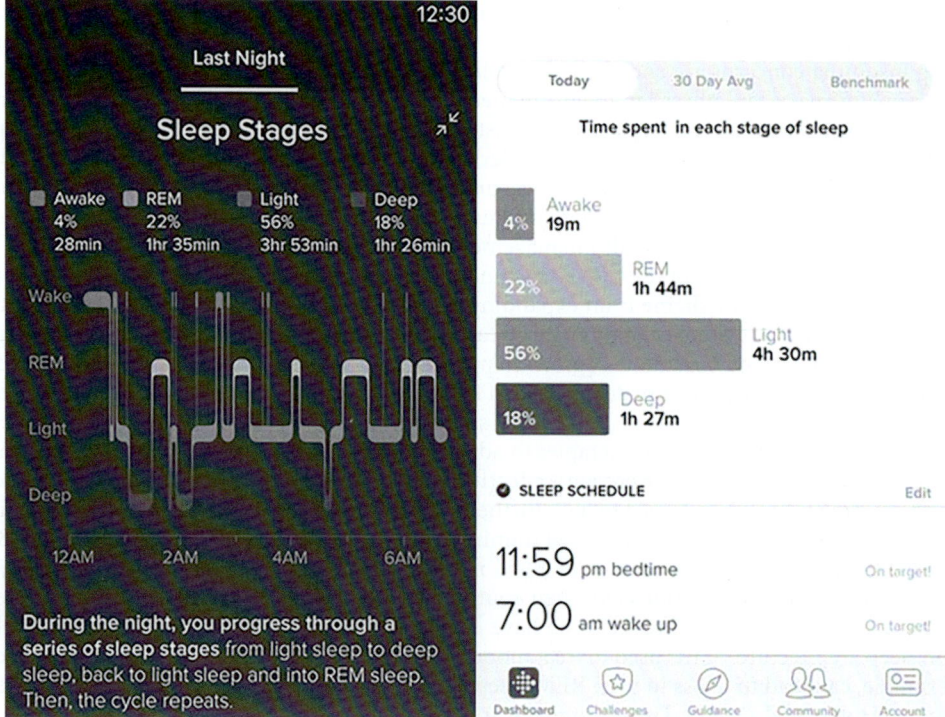

FIGURE 52-2. Data on how much time was spent in each of the four stages of sleep using Fitbit.

- The alternating stages of sleep are referred to as sleep architecture, with slow wave NREM sleep being the most restorative.
- Individuals have a daily sleep need that varies with age; insufficient quality and quantity of sleep (sleep debt) can impair optimal human performance, development, health, and well-being.
- Insomnia, the most common sleep disorder, is highly prevalent in populations regularly served by OTPs, and insomnia can worsen mental and behavioral health conditions.
- Multicomponent CBT-I is the first-line treatment for insomnia and can be safely and effectively delivered by OTPs with advanced education and training.

- OTPs can support people's effective sleep regulation through the occupational therapy process, including screening, evaluation, treatment involving collaborative goal setting, and monitoring a person's response to intervention.
- Collaboration with a person's primary care physician, and a sleep medicine practitioner should co-occurring sleep disorders be present, is recommended.

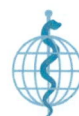 Visit the online resource center at FADavis.com to access the video.

Apply It Now

1. Sleep Diary

Keep a sleep diary for 2 weeks (14 days). Use the consensus sleep diary (Carney et al., 2012) or download CBT-i Coach from the U.S. Department of Veterans Affairs (https://mobile.va.gov/app/cbt-i-coach).

Reflective Questions
- Which days did you have your highest versus your lowest sleep efficiency [(TIB/TST) × 100 = SE]?
- Which days did you have the most versus the least sleep? What was going on in your life?

- Can you describe the daily activities that most influence the C and S systems according to the Two-Process Model of Sleep Regulation?
- What changes to your daily occupations might improve your sleep health?

2. Two in a Bed

If you regularly share a bed, read *Two in a Bed* by Paul Rosenblatt (2012), which is a study of the social context of sleep. Describe or discuss how the points made in this study are congruent or incongruent with your own experiences of bed-sharing.

3. Community Resources

Do some research on sleep medicine in your community. Seek recommendations from colleagues regarding reputable sleep laboratories and specialists. If you are treating a population at risk for sleep issues, it may be useful to prepare an information page on sleep problems that you can provide to people.

4. An Educational Intervention

Work with someone you know, a friend or relative, who experiences some sleep challenges and wants to enjoy higher quality sleep. Use this chapter, internet sites, or other resources to gather information about the sleep issue that is of most concern to the person. Organize it in a way that you think will fit their learning style and then discuss it together.

Resources

Books on Multicomponent CBT-I and Nonpharmacological Insomnia Interventions

- Baglioni, C., Espie, C. A., & Riemann, D. (2022). *Cognitive-behavioural therapy for insomnia (CBT-I) across the life span.* John Wiley & Sons (updated review of CBT-I approaches and outcomes from children through older adults).
- Carney, C. E., & Manber, R. (2009). *Quiet your mind and get to sleep: Solutions to insomnia for those with depression, anxiety, or chronic pain.* New Harbinger Publications (self-help style book for improving insomnia in persons with co-occurring conditions).
- Green, A., & Brown, C. (2015). *An occupational therapist's guide to sleep and sleep problems.* Jessica Kingsley Publishers (an occupational therapy perspective on sleep and sleep Problems).
- Manber, R., & Carney, C. E. (2015). *Treatment plans and interventions for insomnia: A case formulation approach.* Guilford Press (comprehensive guide for evaluation and treatment using CBT-I).
- Nowakowski, S., Garland, S., Grandner, M. A., & Cuddihy, L. (2021). *Adapting cognitive behavioral therapy for insomnia.* Elsevier (CBT-I treatment guidelines for advanced CBT-I practitioners).
- Ong, J. C. (2017). *Mindfulness-based therapy for insomnia.* American Psychological Association (approaches for integrating mindfulness within CBT-I).
- Perlis, M., Aloia, M., & Kuhn, B. (2011). *Behavioral treatments for sleep disorders.* Elsevier (overview of behavioral treatments often used within CBT-I).
- Perlis, M. L., Jungquist, C., Smith, M. T., & Posner, D. (2008). *Cognitive Behavioral Treatment of Insomnia: A session-by-session guide.* Springer (classic guide for insomnia assessment and intervention using CBT-I).

Continuing Education and Training in Multicomponent CBT-I

- It is essential that the occupational therapy profession develops resources for education, training, and practice to promote sleep health in those OTPs serve. Presently, there are advanced education opportunities the OTP could consider in developing deeper understandings of insomnia. Given sleep preparation and sleep participation is within the OTP's scope of practice, it is strongly recommended they complete a "basic" CBT-I course, along with peer-mentorship, supervision, and/or consultation, before attempting delivery of a multicomponent CBT-I. Please consider "basic" training courses from the list that follows:
  - 3-day Basic CBT-I Course/3-day Advanced CBT-I face-to-face courses delivered through the University of Pennsylvania Perelman School of Medicine: http://www.med.upenn.edu/bsm/cbt.html
  - Assessment and Treatment of Sleep Disturbances in Military Populations: Cognitive-Behavioral Therapy for Insomnia (CBT-I) online course with Uniformed Services University: http://deploymentpsych.org/training

- Cognitive Behavioral Therapy for Insomnia (CBT-I) Evidence-based insomnia interventions for trauma, anxiety, depression, chronic pain, and more online course with PESI: https://catalog.pesi.com/sales/bh_c_001249_cbti_041718_organic-85242
- Cognitive-Behavioral Therapy for Insomnia for Occupational Therapists (CBT-I for OT) online course with Colorado State University: https://www.chhs.colostate.edu/ot/research/restoring-effective-sleep-tranquility/cognitive-behavioral-therapy-for-insomnia-for-occupational-therapy

Video

- "Fieldwork Experience in Juvenile Correction Setting" video. In this video, occupational therapist Maggie reflects on how she felt prepared and unprepared for her fieldwork experience. She touches on topics such as trauma, emotional regulation, and sensory processing, and emphasizes the need to be aware of her own self-care by setting boundaries. Access the video at the online resource center at FADavis.com.

Organizations and Web-Based Resources

- Centers for Disease Control and Prevention: https://www.cdc.gov/sleep/resources.html. This site from the Centers for Disease Control and Prevention offers information about sleep, patient organizations, and other resources, including information about drowsy driving.
- Massachusetts Institute of Technology: https://medical.mit.edu/community/sleep/resources. The Massachusetts Institute of Technology has this resource site with print and downloadable audio guides for insomnia and sleep problems.
- National Alliance on Mental Illness: https://www.nami.org/Learn-More/Mental-Health-Conditions/Related-Conditions/sleep-disorders. The National Alliance on Mental Illness offers information about the connection between sleep and mental health.
- National Sleep Foundation: https://sleepfoundation.org. The National Sleep Foundation has a plethora of resources to help you learn about sleep and your state of health.
- Sleep Health Foundation: https://www.sleephealthfoundation.org.au. This site has, among its many resources, fact sheets about sleep and many mental health conditions across the life span.
- Society of Behavioral Sleep Medicine: https://www.behavioralsleep.org. This interdisciplinary organization is committed to advancing the scientific approach to studying the behavioral, psychological, and physiological dimensions of sleep and sleep disorders.

References

Abbott, S. M., Malkani, R. G., & Zee, P. C. (2017). Circadian dysregulation in mental and physical health. In M. Kryger, T. Roth, & W. Dement (Eds.), *Principles and practice of sleep medicine* (6th ed., pp. 405–413). Elsevier.

Aernout, E., Benradia, I., Hazo, J.-B., Sy, A., Askevis-Leherpeux, F., Sebbane, D., & Roelandt, J.-L. (2021). International study of the prevalence and factors associated with insomnia in the general population. *Sleep Medicine, 82,* 186–192. https://doi.org/10.1016/j.sleep.2021.03.028

Ahmadi, R., Rahimi, S., Olfati, M., Javaheripour, N., Emamian, F., Ghadami, M. R., Khazaie, H., Knight, D. C., Tahmasian, M., & Sepehry, A. A. (2022). Insomnia and post-traumatic stress disorder: A meta-analysis on interrelated association (n= 57,618) and prevalence (n= 573,665). *Neuroscience & Biobehavioral Reviews, 141,* 104850. https://doi.org/10.1016/j.neubiorev.2022.104850

Akacem, L. D., Simpkin, C. T., Carskadon, M. A., Wright, K. P., Jr., Jenni, O. G., Achermann, P., & LeBourgeois, M. K. (2015). The timing of the circadian clock and sleep differ between napping and non-napping toddlers. *PLoS One, 10*(4), e0125181. https://doi.org/10.1371/journal.pone.0125181

Åkerstedt, T., Perski, A., & Kecklund, G. (2017). Sleep, occupational stress, and burnout. In M. Kryger, T. Roth, & W. Dement (Eds.), *Principles and practice of sleep medicine* (6th ed., pp. 736–741). Elsevier.

AlRasheed, M. M., Fekih-Romdhane, F., Jahrami, H., Pires, G. N., Saif, Z., Alenezi, A. F., Humood, A., Chen, W., Dai, H., Bragazzi, N., Pandi-Perumal, S. R., BaHammam, A. S., & Vitiello, M. V. (2022). The prevalence and severity of insomnia symptoms during COVID-19: A global systematic review and individual participant data meta-analysis. *Sleep Medicine, 100,* 7–23. https://doi.org/10.1016/j.sleep.2022.06.020

American Academy of Sleep Medicine. (2014). *International classification of sleep disorders* (3rd ed.). Author.

American Occupational Therapy Association. (2020). Occupational therapy practice framework: Domain and process—Fourth edition. *American Journal of Occupational Therapy, 74,* 7412410010p1–7412410010p87. https://doi.org/10.5014/ajot.2020.74S2001

American Psychiatric Association. (2013). *Diagnostic and statistical manual of mental disorders* (5th ed.). American Psychiatric Publishing. https://doi.org/10.1176/appi.books.9780890425596

Ancuelle, V., Zamudio, R., Mendiola, A., Guillen, D., Ortiz, P. J., Tello, T., & Vizcarra, D. (2015). Effects of an adapted mattress in musculoskeletal pain and sleep quality in institutionalized elders. *Sleep Science, 8*(3), 115–120. https://doi.org/10.1016/j.slsci.2015.08.004

Andre, C. J., Lovallo, V., & Spencer, R. M. C. (2021). The effects of bed sharing on sleep: From partners to pets. *Sleep Health, 7*(3), 314–323. https://doi.org/10.1016/j.sleh.2020.11.011

Angelhoff, C. (2017). *What about the parents? Sleep quality, mood, saliva cortisol response and sense of coherence in parents with a child admitted to pediatric care.* Linköping University Electronic Press.

Attarian, H., Mallampalli, M., & Johnson, D. (2022). Sleep deserts: A key determinant of sleep inequities. *Journal of Clinical Sleep Medicine, 18*(8), 2079–2080. https://doi.org/10.5664/jcsm.10072

Baglioni, C., Battagliese, G., Feige, B., Spiegelhalder, K., Nissen, C., Voderholzer, U., Lombardo, C., & Riemann, D. (2011). Insomnia as a predictor of depression: A meta-analytic evaluation of longitudinal epidemiological studies. *Journal of Affective Disorders, 135*(1), 10–19. https://doi.org/10.1016/j.jad.2011.01.011

Baglioni, C., Espie, C. A., & Riemann, D. (2022). *Cognitive-Behavioural Therapy for Insomnia (CBT-I) across the life span: Guidelines and clinical protocols for health professionals.* John Wiley & Sons.

Baillieul, S., Revol, B., Jullian-Desayes, I., Joyeux-Faure, M., Tamisier, R., & Pépin, J.-L. (2019). Diagnosis and management of central sleep apnea syndrome. *Expert Review of Respiratory Medicine, 13*(6), 545–557. https://doi.org/10.1080/17476348.2019.1604226

Baker, F. C., de Zambotti, M., Colrain, I. M., & Bei, B. (2018). Sleep problems during the menopausal transition: Prevalence, impact, and management challenges. *Nature and Science of Sleep, 10,* 73–95. https://doi.org/10.2147/nss.S125807

Barczi, S. R., & Teodorescu, M. C. (2017). Psychiatric and medical comorbidities and effects of medications in older adults. In M. Kryger, T. Roth, & W. Dement (Eds.), *Principles and practice of sleep medicine* (6th ed., pp. 1484–1495). Elsevier.

Bartick, M. C., Thai, X., Schmidt, T., Altaye, A., & Solet, J. M. (2010). Decrease in as-needed sedative use by limiting nighttime sleep disruptions from hospital staff. *Journal of Hospital Medicine, 5*(3), E20–E24. https://doi.org/10.1002/jhm.549

Bassetti, C. L., Adamantidis, A., Burdakov, D., Han, F., Gay, S., Kallweit, U., Khatami, R., Koning, F., Kornum, B. R., & Lammers, G. J. (2019). Narcolepsy—Clinical spectrum, aetiopathophysiology, diagnosis and treatment. *Nature Reviews Neurology, 15*(9), 519–539. https://doi.org/10.1038/s41582-019-0226-9

Bastien, C. H., Vallieres, A., & Morin, C. M. (2001). Validation of the Insomnia Severity Index as an outcome measure for insomnia research. *Sleep Medicine, 2,* 297–307. https://doi.org/10.1016/s1389-9457(00)00065-4

Bei, B., Wiley, J. F., Trinder, J., & Manber, R. (2016). Beyond the mean: A systematic review on the correlates of daily intraindividual variability of sleep/wake patterns. *Sleep Medicine Reviews, 28,* 108–124. https://doi.org/10.1016/j.smrv.2015.06.003

Bigalke, J. A., Greenlund, I. M., Nicevski, J. R., & Carter, J. R. (2021). Effect of evening blue light blocking glasses on subjective and objective sleep in healthy adults: A randomized control trial. *Sleep Health, 7*(4), 485–490. https://doi.org/10.1016/j.sleh.2021.02.004

Boege, H. L., Bhatti, M. Z., & St-Onge, M.-P. (2021). Circadian rhythms and meal timing: Impact on energy balance and body weight. *Current Opinion in Biotechnology, 70,* 1–6. https://doi.org/10.1016/j.copbio.2020.08.009

Bootzin, R. R. (1972). *Stimulus control treatment for insomnia.* Proceedings of the 80th Annual Convention of American Psychological Association.

Bootzin, R. R., & Perlis, M. L. (2011). Stimulus control therapy. In M. L. Perlis, M. Aloia, & B. Kuhn (Eds.), *Behavioral treatments for sleep disorders* (pp. 21–30). Elsevier.

Borbély, A. A. (1982). A two process model of sleep regulation. *Human Neurobiology, 1,* 195–204.

Borbély, A. A., Daan, S., Wirz-Justice, A., & Deboer, T. (2016). The Two-Process Model of Sleep Regulation: A reappraisal. *Journal of Sleep Research, 25,* 131–143. https://doi.org/10.1111/jsr.12371

Bradley, A. J., Anderson, K. N., Gallagher, P., & McAllister-Williams, R. H. (2020). The association between sleep and cognitive abnormalities in bipolar disorder. *Psychological Medicine, 50*(1), 125–132. https://doi.org/10.1017/S0033291718004038

Bramoweth, A. D., Lederer, L. G., Youk, A. O., Germain, A., & Chinman, M. J. (2020). Brief behavioral treatment for insomnia vs. cognitive behavioral therapy for insomnia: Results of a randomized noninferiority clinical trial among veterans. *Behavior Therapy, 51*(4), 535–547. https://doi.org/10.1016/j.beth.2020.02.002

Brown, T. M., Brainard, G. C., Cajochen, C., Czeisler, C. A., Hanifin, J. P., Lockley, S. W., Lucas, R. J., Münch, M., O'Hagan, J. B., & Peirson, S. N. (2022). Recommendations for daytime, evening, and nighttime indoor light exposure to best support physiology, sleep, and wakefulness in healthy adults. *PLoS Biology, 20*(3), e3001571. https://doi.org/10.1371/journal.pbio.3001571

Buysse, D. J. (2014). Sleep health: Can we define it? Does it matter? *Sleep, 37*(1), 9–17. https://doi.org/10.5665/sleep.3298

Buysse, D. J., Reynolds, C. F., Monk, T. H., Berman, S. R., & Kupfer, D. J. (1989). The Pittsburgh Sleep Quality Index: A new instrument for psychiatric practice and research. *Psychiatry Research, 28,* 193–213. https://doi.org/10.1016/0165-1781(89)90047-4

Cain, N., & Gradisar, M. (2010). Electronic media use and sleep in school-aged children and adolescents: A review. *Sleep Medicine, 11*(8), 735–742. https://doi.org/10.1016/j.sleep.2010.02.006

Carney, C. E., Buysse, D. J., Ancoli-Israel, S., Edinger, J. D., Krystal, A. D., Lichstein, K. L., & Morin, C. M. (2012). The

Consensus Sleep Diary: Standardizing prospective sleep self-monitoring. *Sleep, 35,* 287–302. https://doi.org/10.5665/sleep.1642

Carney, C. E., & Manber, R. (2009). *Quiet your mind and get to sleep: Solutions to insomnia for those with depression, anxiety, or chronic pain.* New Harbinger Publications, Inc.

Carskadon, M., & Dement, W. (2017). Normal human sleep: An overview, section 1 normal sleep and its variants. In M. Kryger, T. Roth, & W. Dement (Eds.), *Principles and Practice of Sleep Medicine* (6th ed., pp. 15–24). Elsevier.

Castiglione-Fontanellaz, C. E., Schaufler, S., Wild, S., Hamann, C., Kaess, M., & Tarokh, L. (2023). Sleep regularity in healthy adolescents: Associations with sleep duration, sleep quality, and mental health. *Journal of Sleep Research, 32*(4), e13865. https://doi.org/10.1111/jsr.13865

Chasens, E. R., Ratcliffe, S. J., & Weaver, T. E. (2009). Development of the FOSQ-10: A short version of the Functional Outcomes of Sleep Questionnaire. *Sleep, 32*(7), 915–919. https://doi.org/10.1093/sleep/32.7.915

Chung, K.-F., Lee, C.-T., Yeung, W.-F., Chan, M.-S., Chung, E. W.-Y., & Lin, W.-L. (2018). Sleep hygiene education as a treatment of insomnia: A systematic review and meta-analysis. *Family Practice, 35*(4), 365–375. https://doi.org/10.1093/fampra/cmx122

Crispim, C. A., Zimberg, I. Z., dos Reis, B. G., Diniz, R. M., Tufik, S., & de Mello, M. T. (2011). Relationship between food intake and sleep pattern in healthy individuals. *Journal of Clinical Sleep Medicine, 7*(6), 659–664. https://doi.org/10.5664/jcsm.1476

Crowley, S. J., Acebo, C., & Carskadon, M. A. (2007). Sleep, circadian rhythms, and delayed phase in adolescence. *Sleep Medicine, 8*(6), 602–612. https://doi.org/10.1016/j.sleep.2006.12.002

Crowther, M. E., Ferguson, S. A., Vincent, G. E., & Reynolds, A. C. (2021). Non-pharmacological interventions to improve chronic disease risk factors and sleep in shift workers: A systematic review and meta-analysis. *Clocks & Sleep, 3*(1), 132–178. https://doi.org/10.3390/clockssleep3010009

Cunningham, J. E. A., & Shapiro, C. M. (2018). Cognitive Behavioural Therapy for Insomnia (CBT-I) to treat depression: A systematic review. *Journal of Psychosomatic Research, 106,* 1–12. https://doi.org/10.1016/j.jpsychores.2017.12.012

Davidson, J. R., Dickson, C., & Han, H. (2019). Cognitive Behavioural Treatment for Insomnia in primary care: A systematic review of sleep outcomes. *British Journal of General Practice, 69*(686), e657–e664. https://doi.org/10.3399/bjgp19X705065

Devine, J. K., & Wolf, J. M. (2016). Integrating nap and night-time sleep into sleep patterns reveals differential links to health-relevant outcomes. *Journal of Sleep Research, 25*(2), 225–233. https://doi.org/10.1111/jsr.12369

Dietrich, S. K., Francis-Jimenez, C. M., Knibbs, M. D., Umali, I. L., & Truglio-Londrigan, M. (2016). Effectiveness of sleep education programs to improve sleep hygiene and/or sleep quality in college students: A systematic review. *JBI Evidence Synthesis, 14*(9), 108–134. https://doi.org/10.11124/JBISRIR-2016-003088

Dijk, D.-J., & Lazar, A. S. (2012). The regulation of human sleep and wakefulness: Sleep homeostasis and circadian rhythmicity. In C. M. Morin & C. A. Espie (Eds.), *The Oxford handbook of sleep and sleep disorders* (pp. 39–60). Oxford University Press. https://doi.org/10.1093/oxfordhb/9780195376203.013.0003

Dinis, J., & Bragança, M. (2018). Quality of sleep and depression in college students: A systematic review. *Sleep Science, 11*(4), 290. https://doi.org/10.5935/1984-0063.20180045

Durmer, J. S., & Dinges, D. F. (2005). Neurocognitive consequences of sleep deprivation. *Seminars in Neurology, 25*(1), 117–129. https://doi.org/10.1055/s-2005-867080

Eakman, A. M. (2015). Meaning, sense-making and spirituality. In C. H. Christiansen, C. M. Baum, & J. Bass (Eds.), *Occupational therapy: Performance, participation, and well-being* (4th ed., pp. 313–331). Slack.

Eakman, A. M., Schmid, A. A., Rolle, N. R., Kinney, A. R., & Henry, K. L. (2022). Follow-up analyses from a waitlist control trial of occupational therapist-delivered Cognitive-Behavioral Therapy for Insomnia among military veterans with chronic insomnia. *American Journal of Occupational Therapy, 76*(2), 7602205110. https://doi.org/10.5014/ajot.2022.045682

Ekirch, A. R. (2018). What sleep research can learn from history. *Sleep Health, 4*(6), 515–518. https://doi.org/10.1016/j.sleh.2018.10.004

El-Sheikh, M., Gillis, B. T., Saini, E. K., Erath, S. A., & Buckhalt, J. A. (2022). Sleep and disparities in child and adolescent development. *Child Development Perspectives, 16*(4), 200–207. https://doi.org/10.1111/cdep.12465

Eron, K., Kohnert, L., Watters, A., Logan, C., Weisner-Rose, M., & Mehler, P. S. (2020). Weighted blanket use: A systematic review. *The American Journal of Occupational Therapy, 74*(2), 7402205010p1–7402205010p14. https://doi.org/10.5014/ajot.2020.037358

Faulkner, S. M., Drake, R. J., Ogden, M., Gardani, M., & Bee, P. E. (2022). A mixed methods expert opinion study on the optimal content and format for an occupational therapy intervention to improve sleep in schizophrenia spectrum disorders. *PLoS One, 17*(6), e0269453. https://doi.org/10.1371/journal.pone.0269453

Frank, E., Swartz, H. A., & Kupfer, D. J. (2000). Interpersonal and social rhythm therapy: Managing the chaos of bipolar disorder. *Biological Psychiatry, 48*(6), 593–604. https://doi.org/10.1016/S0006-3223(00)00969-0

Gold, A. K., & Kinrys, G. (2019). Treating circadian rhythm disruption in bipolar disorder. *Current Psychiatry Reports, 21,* 1–8. https://doi.org/10.1007/s11920-019-1001-8

Gradisar, M., Kahn, M., Micic, G., Short, M., Reynolds, C., Orchard, F., Bauducco, S., Bartel, K., & Richardson, C. (2022). Sleep's role in the development and resolution of adolescent depression. *Nature Reviews Psychology, 1*(9), 512–523. https://doi.org/10.1038/s44159-022-00074-8

Green, A., & Hicks, J. (2015). Assessment and non-pharmocological management of insufficient and excessive sleep. In A. Green & C. Brown (Eds.), *An occupational therapist's guide to sleep and sleep problems* (pp. 131–159). Jessica Kingsley Publishers.

Groen, J. A., & Pabilonia, S. W. (2019). Snooze or lose: High school start times and academic achievement. *Economics of Education Review, 72,* 204–218. https://doi.org/10.1016/j.econedurev.2019.05.011

Grossbellet, E., & Etienne, C. (2017). Central and peripheral circadian clocks. In M. Kryger, T. Roth, & W. Dement (Eds.), *Principles and practice of sleep medicine* (6th ed., pp. 396–404). Elsevier. https://doi.org/10.1016/B978-0-323-24288-2.00038-6

Gu, Y.-M., Kwon, J. E., Lee, G., Lee, S. J., Suh, H. R., Min, S., Roh, D. E., Jo, T. K., Baek, H. S., Hong, S. J., Seo, H., & Cho, M. H. (2016, October 30). Sleep problems and daytime sleepiness in children with nocturnal enuresis. *Childhood Kidney Diseases, 20*(2), 50–56. https://doi.org/10.3339/jkspn.2016.20.2.50

Gutman, S. A., Gregory, K. A., Sadlier-Brown, M. M., Schlissel, M. A., Schubert, A. M., Westover, L. A., & Miller, R. C. (2017). Comparative effectiveness of three occupational therapy sleep interventions: A randomized controlled study. *OTJR: Occupational Therapy Journal of Research, 37*(1), 5–13. https://doi.org/10.1177/1539449216673045

Hale, L., Troxel, W., & Buysse, D. J. (2020). Sleep health: An opportunity for public health to address health equity. *Annual Review of Public Health, 41,* 81–99. https://doi.org/10.1146/annurev-publhealth-040119-094412

Hart, A. R., Lavner, J. A., Carter, S. E., & Beach, S. R. (2021). Racial discrimination, depressive symptoms, and sleep problems among Blacks in the rural South. *Cultural Diversity and Ethnic Minority Psychology, 27*(1), 123. https://doi.org/10.1037/cdp0000365

Hartman, A. G., McKendry, S., Soehner, A., Bodison, S., Akcakaya, M., DeAlmeida, D., & Bendixen, R. (2022). Characterizing sleep differences in children with and without sensory sensitivities. *Frontiers in Psychology, 13,* 875766. https://doi.org/10.3389/fpsyg.2022.875766

Hepsomali, P., Groeger, J. A., Nishihira, J., & Scholey, A. (2020). Effects of oral gamma-aminobutyric acid (GABA) administration on stress and sleep in humans: A systematic review. *Frontiers in Neuroscience, 14,* 923. https://doi.org/10.3389/fnins.2020.00923

Hershner, S. (2020). Sleep and academic performance: Measuring the impact of sleep. *Current Opinion in Behavioral Sciences, 33,* 51–56. https://doi.org/10.1016/j.cobeha.2019.11.009

Hirshkowitz, M., & Smith, P. B. (2004). *Sleep disorders for dummies.* John Wiley & Sons.

Hirshkowitz, M., Whiton, K., Albert, S. M., Alessi, C., Bruni, O., DonCarlos, L., Hazen, N., Herman, J., Adams Hillard, P. J., Katz, E. S., Kheirandish-Gozal, L., Neubauer, D. N., O'Donnell, A. E., Ohayon, M., Peever, J., Rawding, R., Sachdeva, R. C., Setters, B., Vitiello, M. V., & Ware, J. C. (2015). National Sleep Foundation's updated sleep duration recommendations: Final report. *Sleep Health, 1*(4), 233–243. https://doi.org/10.1016/j.sleh.2015.10.004

Ho, E. C. M., & Siu, A. M. H. (2018). Occupational therapy practice in sleep management: A review of conceptual models and research evidence. *Occupational Therapy International, 2018,* 8637498. https://doi.org/10.1155/2018/8637498

Horne, J. A., & Ostberg, O. (1976). A self-assessment questionnaire to determine morningness-eveningness in human circadian rhythms. *International Journal of Chronobiology, 4*(2), 97–110.

Hupbach, A., Gomez, R. L., Bootzin, R. R., & Nadel, L. (2009). Nap-dependent learning in infants. *Developmental Science, 12*(6), 1007–1012. https://doi.org/10.1111/j.1467-7687.2009.00837.x

Hutka, P., Krivosova, M., Muchova, Z., Tonhajzerova, I., Hamrakova, A., Mlyncekova, Z., Mokry, J., & Ondrejka, I. (2021). Association of sleep architecture and physiology with depressive disorder and antidepressants treatment. *International Journal of Molecular Sciences, 22*(3), 1333. https://doi.org/10.3390/ijms22031333

Johns, M. W. (1991). A new method for measuring daytime sleepiness: The Epworth Sleepiness Scale. *Sleep, 14*(6), 540–545. https://doi.org/10.1093/sleep/14.6.540

Johnson, D. A., Jackson, C. L., Guo, N., Sofer, T., Laden, F., & Redline, S. (2021). Perceived home sleep environment: Associations of household-level factors and in-bed behaviors with actigraphy-based sleep duration and continuity in the Jackson Heart Sleep Study. *Sleep, 44*(11), zsab163. https://doi.org/10.1093/sleep/zsab163

Jones, B. J., & Spencer, R. M. C. (2020, Deember). Role of napping for learning across the lifespan. *Current Sleep Medicine Reports, 6*(4), 290–297. https://doi.org/10.1007/s40675-020-00193-9

Kaplan, K. A. (2020). Sleep and sleep treatments in bipolar disorder. *Current Opinion in Psychology, 34,* 117–122. https://doi.org/10.1016/j.copsyc.2020.02.001

Klingman, K. J., Jungquist, C. R., & Perlis, M. L. (2017). Introducing the Sleep Disorders Symptom Checklist-25: A primary care friendly and comprehensive screener for sleep disorders. *Sleep Medicine Research, 8*(1), 17–25. https://doi.org/10.17241/smr.2017.00010

Kroenke, K., Spitzer, R. L., & Williams, J. B. W. (2001). The PHQ-9 validity of a brief depression severity measure. *Journal of General Internal Medicine, 16*(9), 606–613. https://doi.org/10.1046/j.1525-1497.2001.016009606.x

Kryger, M., Roth, T., & Dement, W. (2017). *Principles and practice of sleep medicine* (6th ed.). Elsevier.

Krystal, A. D., Stein, M. B., & Szabo, S. T. (2017). Anxiety disorders and posttraumatic stress disorder. In M. Kryger, T. Roth, & W. C. Dement (Eds.), *Principles and practice of sleep medicine* (pp. 1341–1351). Elsevier.

Lajoie, A. C., Lafontaine, A.-L., & Kaminska, M. (2021). The spectrum of sleep disorders in Parkinson disease: A review. *Chest, 159*(2), 818–827. https://doi.org/10.1016/j.chest.2020.09.099

Lan, L., Tsuzuki, K., Liu, Y. F., & Lian, Z. W. (2017). Thermal environment and sleep quality: A review. *Energy and Buildings, 149,* 101–113. https://doi.org/10.1016/j.enbuild.2017.05.043

Laskemoen, J. F., Simonsen, C., Büchmann, C., Barrett, E. A., Bjella, T., Lagerberg, T. V., Vedal, T. J., Andreassen, O. A., Melle, I., & Aas, M. (2019). Sleep disturbances in schizophrenia spectrum and bipolar disorders—A transdiagnostic perspective. *Comprehensive Psychiatry, 91,* 6–12. https://doi.org/10.1016/j.comppsych.2019.02.006

Leive, L., & Morrison, R. (2020). Essential characteristics of sleep from the occupational science perspective. *Brazilian Journal of Occupational Therapy, 28*(3), 1072–1092. https://doi.org/10.4322/2526-8910.ctoarf1954

Levert, D., Maniaci, J., Tapia, I. E., & Xanthopoulos, M. S. (2022). An overview and application of evidence-based interventions to improve adherence to positive airway pressure for the treatment of pediatric obstructive sleep apnea. *Clinical Practice in Pediatric Psychology, 10*(4), 384. https://doi.org/10.1037/cpp0000465

Lovell, E. (2023). *Promoting adherence to Cognitive-Behavioral Therapy for Insomnia in the medically complex case.* Colorado State University.

Lowe, B., Decker, O., Muller, S., Brahler, E., Schellberg, D., Herzog, W., & Herzberg, P. (2008). Validation and standardization of the Generalized Anxiety Disorder Screener (GAD-7) in the general population. *Medical Care, 46,* 266–274. https://doi.org/10.1097/MLR.0b013e318160d093

Luik, A. I., Kyle, S. D., & Espie, C. A. (2017). Digital cognitive behavioral therapy (dCBT) for insomnia: A state-of-the-science review. *Current Sleep Medicine Reports, 3,* 48–56. https://doi.org/10.1007/s40675-017-0065-4

Manber, R., & Carney, C. E. (2015). *Treatment plans and interventions for insomnia: A case formulation approach.* Guilford Press.

Manber, R., & Chambers, A. S. (2009). Insomnia and depression: A multifaceted interplay. *Current Psychiatry Reports, 11*(6), 437–442. https://doi.org/10.1007/s11920-009-0066-1

Martin, C. A., Papadopoulos, N., Chellew, T., Rinehart, N. J., & Sciberras, E. (2019). Associations between parenting stress, parent mental health and child sleep problems for children with ADHD and ASD: Systematic review. *Research in Developmental Disabilities, 93,* 103463. https://doi.org/10.1016/j.ridd.2019.103463

Mastin, D. F., Bryson, J., & Corwyn, R. (2006). Assessment of sleep hygiene using the Sleep Hygiene Index. *Journal of Behavioral Medicine, 29,* 223–227. https://doi.org/10.1007/s10865-006-9047-6

Maurer, L. F., & Kyle, S. D. (2022). Efficacy of multicomponent CBT-I and its single components. In C. Baglioni, C. A. Espie, & D. Riemann (Eds.), *Cognitive-Behavioural Therapy for Insomnia (CBT-I) across the life span* (pp. 42–50). John Wiley & Sons. https://doi.org/10.1002/9781119891192.ch3

Mazza, M., Lapenta, L., Losurdo, A., Marano, G., Testani, E., Janiri, L., Mazza, S., & Della Marca, G. (2020). Polysomnographic and psychometric correlates of napping in primary insomnia patients. *Nordic Journal of Psychiatry, 74*(4), 244–250. https://doi.org/10.1080/08039488.2019.1695285

McGinty, D., & Szymusiak, R. (2017). Neural control of sleep in mammals. In M. Kryger, T. Roth, & W. Dement (Eds.), *Principles and practice of sleep medicine* (6th ed., pp. 62–77). Elsevier.

Mei, X., Zhou, Q., Li, X., Jing, P., Wang, X., & Hu, Z. (2018). Sleep problems in excessive technology use among adolescent: A systemic review and meta-analysis. *Sleep Science and Practice, 2*(1), 1–10. https://doi.org/10.1186/s41606-018-0028-9

Meyer, N., Faulkner, S. M., McCutcheon, R. A., Pillinger, T., Dijk, D.-J., & MacCabe, J. H. (2020). Sleep and circadian rhythm disturbance in remitted schizophrenia and bipolar disorder: A systematic review and meta-analysis. *Schizophrenia Bulletin, 46*(5), 1126–1143. https://doi.org/10.1093/schbul/sbaa024

Mohd Azmi, N. A. S., Juliana, N., Azmani, S., Mohd Effendy, N., Abu, I. F., Mohd Fahmi Teng, N. I., & Das, S. (2021, January 14). Cortisol on circadian rhythm and its effect on cardiovascular system. *International Journal of Environmental Research and Public Health, 18*(2), 676. https://doi.org/10.3390/ijerph18020676

Morin, C. M. (1993). *Insomnia: Psychological assessment and management*. Guilford Press.

Morin, C. M., LeBlanc, M., Daley, M., Gregoire, J., & Merette, C. (2006). Epidemiology of insomnia: Prevalence, self-help treatments, consultations, and determinants of help-seeking behaviors. *Sleep Medicine, 7*(2), 123–130. https://doi.org/10.1016/j.sleep.2005.08.008

Muench, A., Vargas, I., Grandner, M. A., Ellis, J., Posner, D., Bastien, C. H., Drummond, S. P. A., & Perlis, M. L. (2022). We know CBT-I works, now what? *Faculty Reviews, 11*(4), 1–22. https://doi.org/10.12703/r/11-4

Murray, G., & Harvey, A. (2010). Circadian rhythms and sleep in bipolar disorder. *Bipolar Disorders, 12*(5), 459–472. https://doi.org/10.1111/j.1399-5618.2010.00843.x

National Center for Health Statistics. (2024). *ICD-10-CM: International classification of diseases, 10th revision, clinical modification.* Centers for Disease Control and Prevention.

Nollet, M., Wisden, W., & Franks, N. P. (2020). Sleep deprivation and stress: A reciprocal relationship. *Interface Focus, 10*(3), 20190092. https://doi.org/10.1098/rsfs.2019.0092

Ong, J. C. (2017). *Mindfulness-based therapy for insomnia*. American Psychological Association.

Opp, M. R., & Krueger, J. M. (2017). Sleep and host defense. In M. Kryger, T. Roth, & W. C. Dement (Eds.), *Principles and practice of sleep medicine* (6th ed., pp. 193–201). Elsevier.

Pack, A. I., Keenan, B. T., Byrne, E. M., & Gehrman, P. R. (2017). Genetics and genomic basis of sleep disorders in humans. In M. H. Kryger, T. Roth, & W. Dement (Eds.), *Principles and practice of sleep medicine* (6th ed., pp. 322–339). Elsevier.

Palagini, L., Bastien, C. H., Marazziti, D., Ellis, J. G., & Riemann, D. (2019). The key role of insomnia and sleep loss in the dysregulation of multiple systems involved in mood disorders: A proposed model. *Journal of Sleep Research, 28*(6), e12841. https://doi.org/10.1111/jsr.12841

Pappa, S., Ntella, V., Giannakas, T., Giannakoulis, V. G., Papoutsi, E., & Katsaounou, P. (2020). Prevalence of depression, anxiety, and insomnia among healthcare workers during the COVID-19 pandemic: A systematic review and meta-analysis. *Brain, Behavior, and Immunity, 88*, 901–907. https://doi.org/10.1016/j.bbi.2020.05.026

Perlis, M. L., Ellis, J. G., Kloss, J. D., & Rieman, D. W. (2017). Etiology and pathophysiology of insomnia. In M. Kryger, T. Roth, & W. C. Dement (Eds.), *Principles and practice of sleep medicine* (6th ed., pp. 769–784). Elsevier.

Perlis, M. L., Jungquist, C., Smith, M. T., & Posner, D. (2008). *Cognitive Behavioral Treatment of Insomnia: A session-by-session guide.* Springer.

Pizza, F., Barateau, L., Dauvilliers, Y., & Plazzi, G. (2022). The orexin story, sleep and sleep disturbances. *Journal of Sleep Research, 31*(4), e13665. https://doi.org/10.1111/jsr.13665

Posner, D., & Gehrman, P. R. (2011). Sleep hygiene. In M. Perlis, M. Aloia, & B. Kuhn (Eds.), *Behavioral treatments for sleep disorders* (pp. 31–43). Academic Press.

Qaseem, A., Kansagara, D., Forciea, M. A., Cooke, M., & Denberg, T. D. (2016). Management of chronic insomnia disorder in adults: A clinical practice guideline from the American College of Physicians. *Annals of Internal Medicine, 165*(2), 125–133. https://doi.org/10.7326/M15-2175

Riedy, S. M., Smith, M. G., Rocha, S., & Basner, M. (2021). Noise as a sleep aid: A systematic review. *Sleep Medicine Reviews, 55*, 101385. https://doi.org/10.1016/j.smrv.2020.101385

Riemann, D., Krone, L. B., Wulff, K., & Nissen, C. (2020). Sleep, insomnia, and depression. *Neuropsychopharmacology, 45*(1), 74–89. https://doi.org/10.1038/s41386-019-0411-y

Riemann, D., & Nissen, C. (2012). Sleep and psychotropic drugs. In C. M. Morin & C. A. Espie (Eds.), *The Oxford handbook of sleep and sleep disorders* (pp. 190–222). Oxford University Press.

Ritter, P. S., Marx, C., Lewtschenko, N., Pfeiffer, S., Leopold, K., Bauer, M., & Pfennig, A. (2012). The characteristics of sleep in patients with manifest bipolar disorder, subjects at high risk of developing the disease and healthy controls. *Journal of Neural Transmission, 119*(10), 1173–1184. https://doi.org/10.1007/s00702-012-0883-y

Roach, G. D., & Sargent, C. (2019). Interventions to minimize jet lag after westward and eastward flight. *Frontiers in Physiology, 10*, 927. https://doi.org/10.3389/fphys.2019.00927

Rosenblatt, P. C. (2012). *Two in a bed: The social system of couple bed sharing.* State University of New York Press.

Rosenwasser, A. M., & Turek, F. W. (2017). Physiology of the mammalian circadian system. In M. Kryger, T. Roth, & W. C. Dement (Eds.), *Principles and practice of sleep medicine* (6th ed., pp. 351–361). Elsevier.

Roth, T. (2007). Insomnia: Definition, prevalence, etiology, and consequences. *Journal of Clinical Sleep Medicine, 3*(5 Suppl.), S7–S10. https://doi.org/10.5664/jcsm.26929

Sateia, M. J., & Thorpy, M. J. (2017). Classification of sleep disorders. In M. Kryger, T. Roth, & W. Dement (Eds.), *Principles and practice of sleep medicine* (6th ed., pp. 618–626). Elsevier.

Schutte-Rodin, S., Broch, L., Buysse, D. J., Dorsey, C., & Sateia, M. (2008). Clinical guideline for the evaluation and management of chronic insomnia in adults. *Journal of Clinical Sleep Medicine, 4*(5), 487–504.

Scullin, M. K., Fairley, J., Decker, M. J., & Bliwise, D. L. (2017, May 1). The effects of an afternoon nap on episodic memory in young and older adults, *Sleep, 40*(5), zsx035. https://doi.org/10.1093/sleep/zsx035

Seton, C., & Fitzgerald, D. A. (2021). Chronic sleep deprivation in teenagers: Practical ways to help. *Paediatric Respiratory Reviews, 40*, 73–79. https://doi.org/10.1016/j.prrv.2021.05.001

Shahid, A., Wilkinson, K., Marcu, S., & Shapiro, C. M. (2012). Karolinska Sleepiness Scale (KSS). In A. Shahid, K. Wilkinson, S. Marcu, & C. M. Shapiro (Eds.), *STOP, THAT and one hundred other sleep scales* (pp. 209–210). Springer. https://doi.org/10.1007/978-1-4419-9893-4

Simonelli, G., Leanza, Y., Boilard, A., Hyland, M., Augustinavicius, J. L., Cardinali, D. P., Vallières, A., Pérez-Chada, D., & Vigo, D. E. (2013). Sleep and quality of life in urban poverty: The effect of a slum housing upgrading program. *Sleep, 36*(11), 1669–1676. https://doi.org/10.5665/sleep.3124

Smallfield, S., & Molitor, W. L. (2018). Occupational therapy interventions addressing sleep for community-dwelling older adults: A systematic review. *The American Journal of Occupational Therapy, 72*(4), 7204190030p1–7204190030p9. https://doi.org/10.5014/ajot.2018.031211

Soh, H. L., Ho, R. C., Ho, C. S., & Tam, W. W. (2020). Efficacy of digital cognitive behavioural therapy for insomnia: A meta-analysis of randomised controlled trials. *Sleep Medicine, 75*, 315–325. https://doi.org/10.1016/j.sleep.2020.08.020

Spaeth, A. M., Hawley, N. L., Raynor, H. A., Jelalian, E., Greer, A., Crouter, S. E., Coffman, D. L., Carskadon, M. A., Owens, J. A., Wing, R. R., & Hart, C. N. (2019). Sleep, energy balance, and meal timing in school-aged children. *Sleep Medicine, 60*, 139–144. https://doi.org/10.1016/j.sleep.2019.02.003

Spielman, A. J., Caruso, L. S., & Glovinsky, P. B. (1987). A behavioral perspective on insomnia treatment. *Psychiatric Clinics of North America, 10*(4), 541–553. https://doi.org/10.1016/S0193-953X(18)30532-X

Staner, L. (2010). Comorbidity of insomnia and depression. *Sleep Medicine Reviews, 14*(1), 35–46. https://doi.org/10.1016/j.smrv.2009.09.003

Steger, B. (2012). Cultures of sleep. In A. Green & A. Westcombe (Eds.), *Sleep: Multi-professional perspectives* (pp. 68–85). Jessica Kingsley Publishers.

Stepanski, E. J., & Wyatt, J. K. (2003). Use of sleep hygiene in the treatment of insomnia. *Sleep Medicine Reviews, 7*(3), 215–225. https://doi.org/10.1053/smrv.2001.0246

Stickgold, R., & Wamsley, E. J. (2017). Why we dream. In M. Kryger, T. Roth, & W. Dement (Eds.), *Principles and practice of sleep medicine* (6th ed., pp. 509–514). Elsevier.

Torquati, L., Mielke, G. I., Brown, W. J., Burton, N. W., & Kolbe-Alexander, T. L. (2019). Shift work and poor mental health: A meta-analysis of longitudinal studies. *American Journal of Public Health, 109*(11), e13–e20. https://doi.org/10.2105/AJPH.2019.305278

Trotti, L. M. (2017). Restless legs syndrome and sleep-related movement disorders. *Continuum, 23*(4, Sleep Neurology), 1005–1016. https://doi.org/10.1212/CON.0000000000000488

Turek, F. W., & Zee, P. C. (2017). Introduction: Master circadian clock and master circadian rhythm. In M. Kryger, T. Roth, & W. Dement (Eds.), *Principles and practice of sleep medicine* (6th ed., pp. 340–350). Elsevier.

Victor, A. M., & Bernstein, G. A. (2009). Anxiety disorders and posttraumatic stress disorder update. *Psychiatric Clinics of North America, 32*(1), 57–69. https://doi.org/10.1016/j.psc.2008.11.004

Walker, M. P. (2009). The role of sleep in cognition and emotion. *Annals of the New York Academy of Sciences, 1156*(1), 168–197. https://doi.org/10.1111/j.1749-6632.2009.04416.x

Watson, N. F., Badr, M. S., Belenky, G., Bliwise, D. L., Buxton, O. M., Buysse, D., Dinges, D. F., Gangwisch, J., Grandner, M. A., Kushida, C., Malhotra, R. K., Martin, J. L., Patel, S. R., Quan, S. F., Tasali, E., Twery, M., Croft, J. B., Maher, E., Barrett, J. A., . . . Heald, J. L. (2015). Recommended amount of sleep for a healthy adult: A Joint Consensus Statement of the American Academy of Sleep Medicine and Sleep Research Society. *Journal of Clinical Sleep Medicine, 11*(6), 591–592. https://doi.org/10.5664/jcsm.4758

Werth, E., Achermann, P., & Borbély, A. A. (1996). Brain topography of the human sleep EEG: Antero-posterior shifts of spectral power. *Neuroreport, 8*(1), 123–127. https://doi.org/10.1097/00001756-199612200-00025

Zeng, L.-N., Zong, Q.-Q., Yang, Y., Zhang, L., Xiang, Y.-F., Ng, C. H., Chen, L.-G., & Xiang, Y.-T. (2020). Gender difference in the prevalence of insomnia: A meta-analysis of observational studies. *Frontiers in Psychiatry, 11*, 577429. https://doi.org/10.3389/fpsyt.2020.577429

Zhang, Z., Xiao, X., Ma, W., & Li, J. (2020, September). Napping in older adults: A review of current literature. *Current Sleep Medicine Reports, 6*(3), 129–135. https://doi.org/10.1007/s40675-020-00183-x

Spiritual Occupations

Sharon Gartland

Occupational therapy has long valued everyday human activity as a source of meaning that impacts the lives of people and supports them to thrive. Spiritual occupations fall squarely in the category of meaningful occupations. Although overtly spiritual and religious activities such as attendance at religious services, prayer, and meditation are clearly identified as spiritual occupations, there are a variety of additional meaningful tasks that support individuals in living full and healthy lives. Most individuals can identify preferred occupations that serve to "ground" or "center" them in their identity (i.e., who they are, what their values are, and who they want to align themselves with in the process of life). Zimmer and colleagues (2016) state that "some form of spiritual-like thinking as it is ordinarily defined is quite common among people in countries around the world characterized by different dominant religious traditions and different degrees of secularism" (p. 375).

This chapter describes how occupational therapy practitioners (OTPs) can support people in identifying these significant occupations in their lives and enable satisfactory participation in them. Although there is considerable support for recognizing the importance of spirituality within occupational therapy (American Occupational Therapy Association [AOTA], 2020; Polatajko et al., 2007), there is a long history of confusion and debate concerning definitions and the placement of spirituality within frameworks and conceptual models (Humbert, 2016). Within four editions of the *Occupational Therapy Practice Framework (OTPF),* an official document of the AOTA (2014, 2020), the concept of spirituality has been moved and redefined in an attempt to bring clarity to this complex concept.

The current definition for **spirituality** adopted within the fourth edition of the *OTPF (OTPF-4;* AOTA, 2020), taken from Billock (2005), is "a deep experience of meaning brought about by engaging in occupations that involve the enacting of personal values and beliefs, reflections, and intention within a supportive contextual environment" (p. 83). This definition shifts the focus for occupational therapy practice to engagement in spiritual occupations rather than a more generic definition of spirituality.

The Canadian Model of Occupational Performance and Engagement (CMOP-E), which is published and endorsed by the Canadian Association of Occupational Therapists (CAOT), places spirituality as the core of the person and was one of the first conceptual models to highlight this important area of focus for occupational therapy (Polatajko et al., 2007). Along with the explicit naming of the concept of spirituality from formal occupational therapy professional organizations

such as AOTA and CAOT, a limited but growing amount of evidence in the occupational therapy literature shows that individuals look to their spiritual practices to support them through difficult life challenges such as health crises (Humbert, 2016).

Religion and Spirituality in Mental Health Practice

The importance of acknowledging the spiritual and religious practices of individuals who receive mental health services is increasingly recognized. There is growing evidence of the appreciation for the role of religion and spirituality as a positive source of support and coping for individuals with a variety of mental health diagnoses (Lucchetti et al., 2021; Milner et al., 2020). Lucchetti and colleagues (2021) summarize that the evidence for a positive connection with higher levels of spirituality and religious involvement is strongest with depression, suicidality, and substance use disorder, particularly in the U.S. population. Most scientific studies on spirituality have centered around spirituality impacted by depression, suicidality, and substance use disorder.

There are mixed findings associating spirituality with anxiety, obsessive-compulsive disorder, bipolar disorder, and eating disorders. Psychotic disorders with religious delusions are associated with poorer outcomes, but in the absence of those delusions, spiritual and religious involvement can contribute to better outcomes. Despite robust evidence for a positive impact in the United States for many diagnoses, research on spirituality and religion in other cultures demonstrates variable data in relation to mental health outcomes. This is a strong reminder to all clinicians to recognize the cultural impact of work in this area.

A systematic review of the literature on religion and spirituality in relationship to mental disorders found that higher religious/spiritual involvement was linked to fewer mental disorders in 72% of the studies, whereas only 4.7% of the studies found a negative impact on mental disorder for those involved in religious/spiritual activities (Bonelli & Koenig, 2013). There is mild supporting evidence for a link between religious/spiritual involvement and positive health outcomes with stress-related disorders and other organic mental disorders (Bonelli & Koenig, 2013).

Wilding (2007) found themes of spirituality providing meaning to life and increased coping ability with mental illness during interviews with six individuals with a variety of mental health conditions. As an occupational scientist, she also notes the value of supporting meaningful everyday occupations and occupations shared with others as part of incorporating spirituality into work with people. Overall, the theme of spirituality as life-sustaining was found during the interviews, which supports the importance of OTPs attending to this concept during practice.

Persons receiving occupational therapy may use an individual definition of spirituality or may link it to more formal communal religious practices. In a review of research on the impact of Western and Middle Eastern religious practices on mental health, beneficial outcomes included greater overall well-being, hope and optimism, and a greater sense of meaning and purpose for both the Western and Middle Eastern traditions (Koenig et al., 2012).

Better outcomes in individuals with depression, suicide, anxiety, and substance abuse were also linked with religious and spiritual involvement in culturally embedded faith traditions of Christianity and Islam (Koenig et al., 2012). Shilo et al. (2016) studied Jewish males who self-identified as gay or bisexual as well as religious. They found that positive religious coping strategies resulted in better mental health outcomes for this cohort. Religious practices they characterized as creating identity conflict with their sexual identity functioned as negative religious coping, resulting in poorer mental health outcomes.

Several studies have found a positive impact of religious attendance on individuals with a variety of mental health conditions. One study of 47 persons with psychiatric disabilities found that religious attendance was an important factor in contributing to spiritual well-being, despite the severity of symptoms (Fukui et al., 2012). In a 14-year follow-up study conducted with a large Canadian population, attending religious services every few weeks was found to decrease the incidence of major depression (Balbuena et al., 2013).

Involvement in religious institutions provided an important social community for support and interaction in older adults, preventing loneliness and social isolation that contribute to poor mental health outcomes (Rote et al., 2012). Twenty young people with autism and other developmental disabilities were interviewed about their expressions of faith, revealing that congregational activities performed with others was an important avenue of spiritual expression for this population, and the social connections made within faith communities provided a source of enjoyment for most of the participants (Liu et al., 2014).

The global pandemic in March 2020, which moved most of the world into social isolation, impacted what opportunities were available for spiritual and religious engagement. Many communal activities were limited, which impeded or changed many individuals' spiritual occupations. It also provided an opportunity to look at the role religious/spiritual coping plays in coping with traumatic events. Zhang and colleagues (2021) looked at a construct called spiritual fortitude (SF). In a systematic review, they found that SF provided many positive health benefits related to coping and posttraumatic growth.

The preponderance of evidence supports a focus for OTPs on enabling involvement in individual spiritually meaningful occupations as well as participation in religious/spiritual communities and the practices connected to those communities as a means of facilitating health and well-being for persons seeking mental health recovery. Whether embedded in more formal organized practices or individually defined and practiced, spirituality is shown to be an important factor within mental health practice for OTPs and other mental health providers. As person-centered practitioners, OTPs can and should identify and enable the spiritual occupations that support mental health and well-being for all persons they serve.

Spiritual Occupations

Occupations connected to a person's spirituality fall into two categories: (1) secular but infused with meaning, and (2) traditionally religious. These occupations can be as varied as each person involved and may include creative, nature-based, social, mindful and reflective, and formal religious practices. OTPs should encourage people to identify their own definitions of spirituality and religion and choose the meaningful occupations that support their spirituality.

Spiritual occupations are a significant category of human occupations and OTPs need training and clarity about this area of focus. The highly personal nature and amorphous concept of spiritual occupations can feel daunting to new or unfamiliar practitioners and may result in a lack of attention to this health-enhancing area of human occupation (Humbert, 2016). Additionally, clinicians may feel concerned about inadvertently imposing their own beliefs and spirituality on a vulnerable population when broaching this topic while conducting initial interviews and goal setting (Humbert, 2016). Appropriate caution is important but should not prevent the addressing of this significantly beneficial part of many lives.

This section provides a framework from which OTPs can identify occupations that have been shown to support spiritual growth and flourishing in some individuals. However, it is important to remain open to new and unexpected ways of participating in spiritual activities as defined by those served.

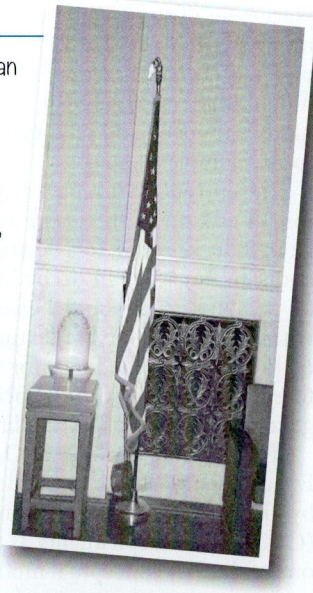

PhotoVoice

This is a picture of an American flag in church with a holy water font next to it. Having the freedom as an American citizen to fully participate in my community and my church, and get the help I need for my mental illness, helps me realize what America has done and is doing for people like me.

OTPs encourage those being served to be empowered to use all programs and services that support their vision of their own recovery through building habits and routines. How might an OTP help a person reflect on their own spiritual habits and routines?

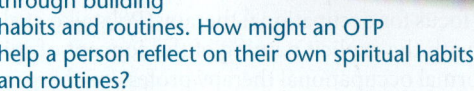

Creative Occupations

Creativity, beauty, and artistic expression have been historically significant in spiritual expression and are often linked to spirituality for some people (Nesbit, 2006). However, this linkage has not been widely studied. Occupations such as drawing, painting, singing, playing musical instruments, journaling, writing poetry and/or fiction, and dancing can all play a role in helping a person discover meaning or connect with the sacred or transcendent aspects of themselves and others. Although typically categorized as leisure occupations in occupational therapy practice, these creative pursuits often fulfill a much more significant function in the lives of people. Creating art in many forms can be a hobby for some, and a deeply significant spiritual activity for others.

In addition to art creation, enjoying and consuming art, literature, and music, both sacred and otherwise, can serve a significant and meaningful purpose for an individual beyond pleasant diversions. Exploring the role and meaning of the arts in a person's life is a key aspect of addressing spiritual occupations.

Many persons with mental illness see a connection between making art and their own spirituality (Van Lith, 2013, 2015). Participating in the creation of art supported their health and healing and allowed them to find mental space to process deep life questions about their illness and more broad spiritual questions. Malviya and coworkers (2022) found that religious/spiritual singing and movement has a positive impact on mental health. Some art-making activities such as quilting, writing, and painting are especially conducive to storytelling and can be cathartic for the person in their journey through trauma or illness. Sharing their art then becomes part of wellness, healing, and empowerment as they express their own narrative with others.

Being an appreciative consumer of the arts is also a source of spiritual succor for many persons. Songs, poems, and artwork that resonate with others have long been seen as a pathway to the soul, and gifted artists can bring clarity to others' internal chaos through their gifts shared with the world. Encouraging nonartists to identify what art says to them or note how it opens them up to new ways of viewing their life is one way to explore creative occupations.

Traditional faith communities often incorporate art and beauty as a pathway to worship and spirituality. The worship spaces can vary from architectural masterpieces to more humble, simplistic contexts, which nonetheless provide support for spiritual growth and encounters. How sacred space draws the attention of a visitor to look in certain directions (often upward) and respond in certain emotional ways is part of the significance of these buildings to promoting spiritual growth. Sacred music, both performative and participatory, is a key feature of many faith traditions. Poetry, spoken word, rhetoric, and readings from ancient texts (which are often a form of art themselves) endure as traditions in many mainstream religions. Finally, art in the form of paintings, stained glass, sculptures, weavings, banners, and more continues to highlight the use of beauty in sacred spaces to move humans to more lofty thoughts. The topic of creativity is explored in more detail in Chapter 51: Leisure and Creative Occupations.

Nature-Based Occupations

Occupations that promote sensory and physical contact with nature are also traditionally cited as important to the spirituality of persons (Capaldi et al., 2015). A sense of connectedness to nature during outdoor activities was found to impact psychological well-being (Kamitsis & Francis, 2013). Hiking, rock climbing, camping, running, biking, sailing, swimming, and gardening are examples of common ways in which people connect with nature and are affected spiritually by their participation in these activities. Many organized faith communities encourage retreats and camping experiences in nature to provide time for reflection and connection with the natural world and its divine creator (Heintzman, 2009).

Gardening has been identified as a spiritual experience that supports stress management in persons with a variety of health challenges (Unruh & Hutchinson, 2011). In this study, researchers discovered that gardening was particularly important to the spiritual life of individuals who did not identify as having a formal religious orientation. Beavers and colleagues (2022) looked at a racial and ethnic minority

PhotoVoice

Billy

Here you can see music and notes. This represents my passion for singing music. It brings me joy because God gave me this special talent. Recognizing a higher power in my life reminds me to be joyful each day. I know when I sing He hears me just like David.

Reflect on how meaningful occupations such as singing and listening to music influence active engagement in spiritual occupations.

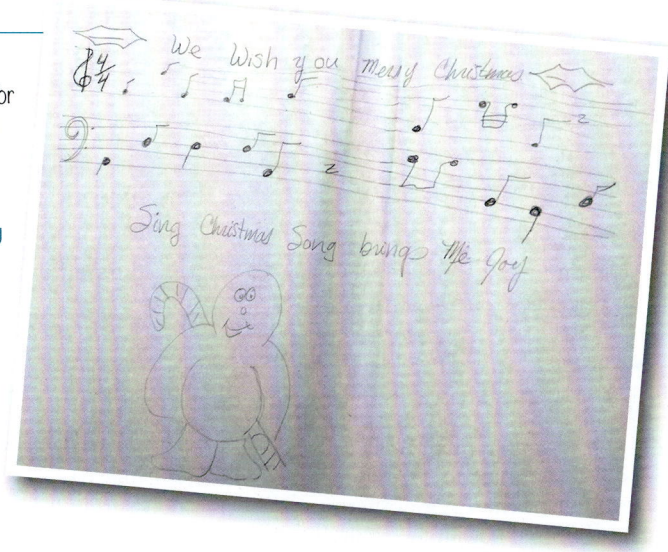

PhotoVoice

Sacred Trees

Enjoying the sunset over the fields of sacred olive trees is an activity that gives me comfort and boosts my mental peace. Olive trees are holy in my culture and being around them feels like being closer to God. In my culture, some believe that sunset is the time when angels go to sleep and demons come out for the night. So being closer to a sacred tree when the sun goes down calms the nerves and protects from evil. Although I am not religious, the cross-generational beliefs about olive trees find their way to my heart and mind.

How might you use this reflection to further explore other healing practices that hold cultural significance for this person?

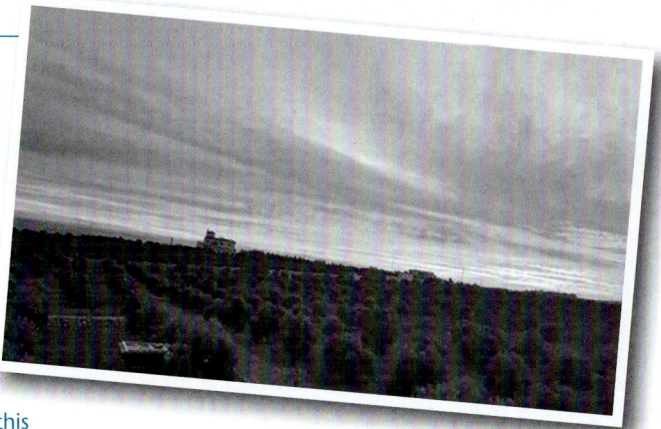

PhotoVoice

Doesha

I am singing to God. When I am getting too hard on myself I get to worshipping my higher power because it brings peace and enjoyment over me. It also reminds me that I am still loved by Him despite my shortcomings.

For some, spirituality offers a path to life balance. As an OTP, how will you help those you serve to find ways to enhance their spiritual well-being?

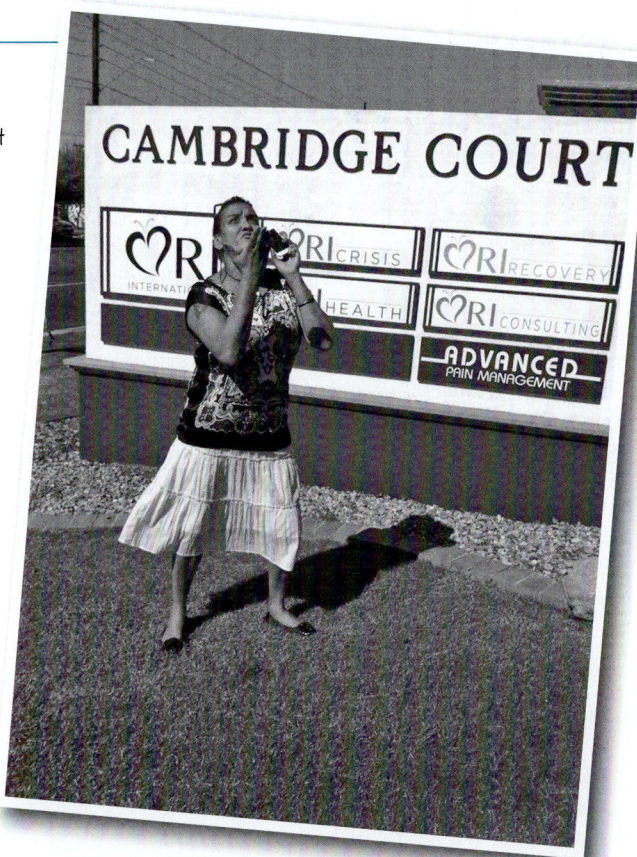

population of 28 gardeners who reported improved mood, stress relief, and personal growth. Some runners experience both the benefits of mastery over their body and the meditative experience of being outdoors, which supports a transcendent experience (Simpson et al., 2014).

Probing thoughtfully into an enjoyable activity to explore a deeper meaning for a particular person is one way to identify spiritual occupations. Swimming for one person may be a healthy habit, whereas for others it may be how they sort out their existential questions regularly. Identifying which occupations provide solace, space to think, and opportunities to

right-size various concerns, as well as to remind individuals to get out of their own heads, is an important process to offer persons on their path to health and well-being.

Social Participation: In-Person and Virtual

Spirituality can be deeply linked to relationships with other individuals. Supporting persons receiving occupational therapy to identify friends, mentors, and spiritual guides and then initiate relationships with them may be one way to enable healthy spiritual growth (Humbert, 2016). Formal and informal support groups centered around shared challenges and experiences can assist people in finding answers to deeper questions, such as, "Why did this happen? How do I cope? Where can I turn for help and guidance?" The 12-step program within Alcoholics Anonymous is one example of a formal structured support group that has a long history of supporting individuals who struggle with substance abuse and other addictions by using a spiritual framework (Kelly & Greene, 2014). Support groups also offer opportunities to share wisdom and guide others, which may be meaningful to persons as part of their spiritual philosophy of life.

Altruism, generosity, and care for others are shared values within many faith traditions. If persons are able to identify spiritual practices that can be done in the community, these activities offer an added social component that can deepen the value of the experience and help them to grow spiritually while participating with others. Examples include yoga and tai chi classes, meditation and prayer groups, and mindfulness practices in the community.

Traditional and formalized faith communities offer a wide array of social participation opportunities that are designed to deepen the religious and spiritual life of participants. Attending worship services, volunteering in the children's program, singing in the choir, and visiting the sick are all ways that one might participate in a local congregation. If a person is comfortable with the belief structures of these communities, they offer a rich resource for meaningful religious and spiritual occupations that may serve to promote their well-being. The topic of social participation is explored in more detail in Chapter 49: Connectedness and Belonging.

The expansion of online opportunities in recent years has created another place for spiritual support and connection for many individuals. Support groups for individuals with specific mental health diagnoses exist on several social media platforms and can provide a safe and potentially anonymous place to give and receive emotional and spiritual support, particularly around mental health challenges. Support groups that are more overtly connected to faith traditions are also available on social media platforms or may be made available more privately through the monitored websites of individual faith communities.

Guiding persons receiving occupational therapy toward well-moderated sites that reduce risk for harm and distress to the participants is key in enabling social participation in an online format. In a 2020 study exploring social media and spirituality conducted by Barnes and Hollingsworth, participants noted the strong need for safe spaces, genuine relationships, and spiritual connection. Social media offers some protected space for those wrestling with stigma felt during in-person gatherings yet still longing for spiritual community (Barnes & Hollingsworth, 2020).

For regular attenders at religious services, the COVID-19 pandemic in 2020 produced a surge of online faith-based opportunities at many faith communities because in-person gatherings were limited for a time. This has expanded opportunities for virtual participation in spiritual occupations. Papadopoulos and colleagues (2021), in a survey of online sources, noted that during COVID-19, digital technologies were inadequate in meeting the spiritual needs of many persons receiving health care. Since those early days, increasing expectation and demand for virtual spiritual support and connection has expanded the opportunities for those seeking them as well as the skills of participants in accessing them.

Mindfulness and Reflective Practices

Mindfulness practices are spiritual occupations that can help busy minds and people experiencing stress to slow down and focus on what they are doing in the present. These practices, which have emerged from Buddhist meditative traditions, are gaining much attention within occupational therapy literature and education (Hardison & Roll, 2016; Reid et al., 2013). Examples of mindfulness practices include setting aside regular time within daily routines to focus on the present, tuning in to body sensations, and learning to objectively observe emotions and responses in the moment (Reid et al., 2013).

Many people today are turning to mindfulness practices to support them in managing stress and anxiety and practice being fully present throughout their day. There are many books, videos, and mobile apps available to guide individuals through mindfulness practices at their convenience. One recent randomized controlled trial study showed that group mindfulness meditation practices were effective in reducing anxiety, depression, and stress in adults with mental health diagnoses (Sundquist et al., 2015). Combining mindfulness practices with daily routines is one way to support deeper meaning and significance within everyday occupations.

Chapter 12: Emotion Regulation includes additional information on mindfulness and a descriptive box regarding mindfulness practices.

Mindfulness-Based Stress Reduction (MBSR) is a secular evidence-based approach rooted in Buddhist spirituality that is used to support health and well-being for several conditions and by several disciplines, including occupational therapy. Grossman et al. (2004) conducted a meta-analysis on MBSR that indicated that it was an effective strategy for enhancing coping abilities for individuals with a variety of chronic conditions and challenges. A systematic review and meta-analysis conducted by Burton and colleagues (2016) found mindfulness-based interventions were useful in reducing stress in health-care professionals. Luken and Sammons (2016) found strong evidence for reducing job burnout, characterized by stress and depression, through mindfulness techniques.

Klatt et al. (2015) designed and studied a mindfulness-based intervention called Mindfulness in Motion (MIM) designed to be delivered onsite for workers in high stress jobs. This intervention, conducted in a group for 8 weeks, was found to increase resiliency and work engagement and was reported to be well received with a 97% retention rate. Increasing interest in mindfulness has emerged in the occupational therapy literature. It is considered a natural adjunct to occupation-based practice.

Reflective journaling is a quiet occupation that some individuals link with enhanced spirituality and mental health (Davidson & Robison, 2008; Ullrich & Lutgendorf, 2002). The person's act of writing out their story or purposely reflecting on reasons for gratitude is experienced by some as a spiritually centering activity. Including cognitive processing along with emotional expression yields better outcomes from journaling among individuals with posttraumatic stress disorder (PTSD). Cognitive processing involves describing thought processes in addition to identifying feelings about a situation or narrative (Ullrich & Lutgendorf, 2002).

Yoga is another calming and centering practice that has been increasing in popularity within occupational therapy. Practicing yoga was shown to be helpful in reducing anxiety

PhotoVoice

Nancy

My morning routine—candle, coffee, Buddhist reading, to-do list, puppy by my side—is CRUCIAL to my well-being. At best, I am able to calm my mind, stop the racing thoughts, and even meditate. This starts my day in a healthy way, and I feel the difference all day—maybe a little more patience, maybe more contentment.

When my LOWD (loved one with dementia) gets up early and disrupts this routine, it feels like an intrusion. In fact, it's irritating and frustrating, although I'm careful not to show it. He interrupts me constantly, so I often give up on reading, and meditation is impossible.

In the scheme of things, missing my morning routine is a small thing. But when many small things compound throughout the day, I feel exhausted.

How could you explore backup routines with this caregiver so they could be implemented when typical routines get disrupted?

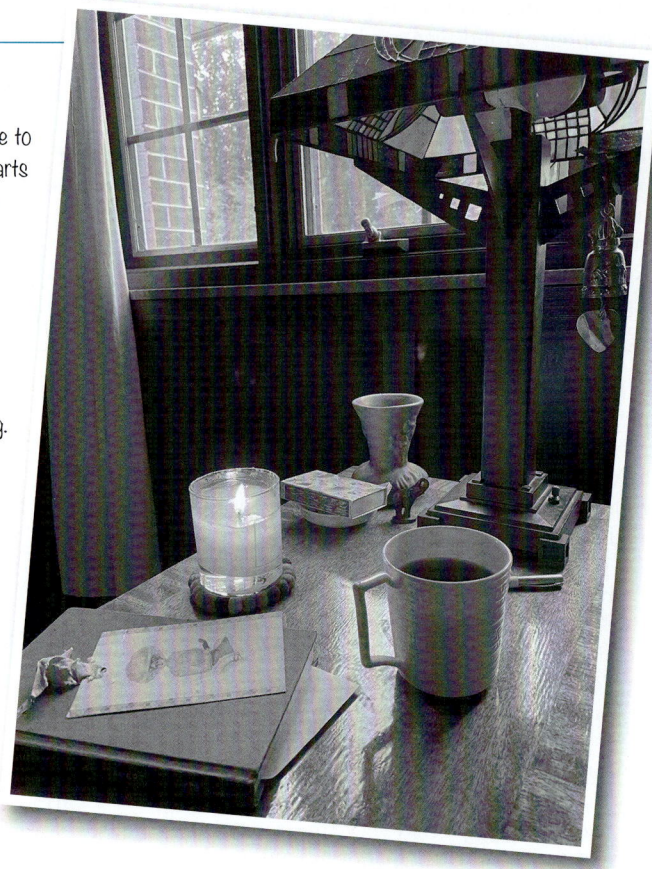

in children and youths with anxiety disorders (Weaver & Darragh, 2015). For many, yoga is considered a spiritual occupation that supports mental health and well-being. The systematic review done by Weaver and Darragh (2015) indicates support for encouraging this occupation as a means for improving overall health and well-being for young people with anxiety disorders. It is another example of an occupation that many may participate in as part of a wellness goal; however, with some probing questions, it may be identified as spiritually significant to a person.

Formal Religious Practices

Many of the spiritual occupations described thus far are also present or compatible within faith community structures. These and other context-specific spiritual occupations are typically aligned with a specific belief system and come with deep meaning and significance attached to them. Although OTPs do not need to become experts in all the various religions and faith practices that they might encounter, it is important to recognize the high significance and specific meaning that might be attached to these experiences and practices.

Common aspects of formal religion include communal worship and social gatherings, prayer/meditation, meaningful rituals, rites of passage and holy days, study of sacred texts, and service to others, among others. However, even the rituals and activities that seem similar across contexts can vary in how they are performed and conducted in a specific faith tradition.

Dimensions such as temporality and physical environment as well as habits and routines are all important to explore with a person in relation to their formal religious practices. What part of these have flexibility? What is a requirement of their faith community? What options are available for adaptation and modification? An example of this is the important Roman Catholic sacrament of the Eucharist. There are certain places and times where this occurs, certain requirements for participating in this sacrament, and a high degree of spiritual significance attached to this sacred activity. This practice varies significantly from some Protestant Christian traditions of communion or Lord's Supper but may look similar from an outsider's viewpoint. Taking the time both to identify spiritual occupations for which a person may want assistance as well as conducting a thorough analysis to understand the task and its spiritual meaning and significance is important in this category of spiritual occupation.

A ritual that is important within many religious traditions is a day or time set apart for rest, meditation, or restoration. Smith-Gabai and Ludwig (2011) explore the concept of the Jewish Sabbath as a meaningful ritual that may support spiritual health in the midst of a modern culture that moves at a fast pace. Helping people identify a need for a regular rhythm of rest in their routines might be framed as part of their spiritual traditions. Seeking out whether there are supports within their community of faith to help establish this health-giving routine, such as identifying specific gathering times, retreat guides, or spiritual leaders/facilitators, may be part of the role an OTP could play in facilitating participation in this form of spiritual occupation. The language and resources used to discuss participation should be supplied or recommended by the person themself through respectful clinical inquiry.

Even within the Jewish faith, the practice of Sabbath can vary significantly depending on the form of Judaism being practiced and the preferences of the person involved. Working with this type of spiritual occupation goal would be an excellent opportunity to learn more about varied religious traditions and practices so that all can be well supported.

Grief Rituals and Hospice Care

Spirituality is often a core human feature that emerges during times of grief, death, and dying. Even for individuals who do not typically identify as spiritual, being confronted with mortality in themselves or others often stirs up deeper life questions. Supporting persons receiving occupational therapy to process their grief in meaningful ways is an underexplored area of practice.

Grief rituals, whether formally connected to organized faith practices or not, are historically relied upon during times of loss. One hospice center practices a ritual of the staff quietly and respectfully lining the hallway as the body of a recently deceased patient is wheeled out of the building. The family is encouraged to walk along with the loved one's body and they can choose music that is meaningful to them during this brief procession. The concept of a "sacred pause," which includes family and staff, is a simple one that can provide closure and lessen distress for family members as well as healthcare staff (Kapoor et al., 2018).

Funeral services are traditionally used to process grief and honor the dead in a variety of cultures, religions, or value

The Lived Experience

Michelle

Editor's Note: Michelle is a 46-year-old mother of two teenagers. She spends much of her time caring for her family and extended family as well as running a small pottery business. Michelle was diagnosed with rheumatoid arthritis as a young adult. Her caregiving roles are complicated by a teen with significant mental illness struggles for the past 4 years; a family history of attention deficit-hyperactivity disorder (ADHD), which affects her husband and both children; and a father with senile dementia.

Seven years ago I started a journey to find out who I am and what I want from this life, so I have been using lots of my time to honor that and figure that out, to figure out who I am. Because of my rheumatoid arthritis, I have to be very careful about respecting my body and managing my stress, which is hard to do. I mostly wanted to address that I was just generally unhappy in my life. I sought out yoga instruction to help me start this process.

When I first started yoga practice, my instructor asked, "Why do you want to start doing yoga?" and the first thing out of my mouth without even thinking about it was "I need enlightenment," and I thought, where did that come from? When I am on the mat, there is a spotlight on myself, on my true soul and there is no avoiding it. I am learning to carry that spotlight off the mat as well in my practice. I've noticed when I have waned away from my practice, I lose myself again.

If I am not feeding or building my spirituality, I am not a centered person. I am lost as to who I am and why I am here. I find on the flip side when I am feeding it, it is very clear to me why I am here, who I am and what I should be doing. My mental health is directly connected—I have had long bouts of time where I am completely disconnected from myself, not taking care of myself, where I feel horrible, I feel worthless and like I have nothing to offer anyone.

I am having some scary clarity right now. These last few months I was stuck, with my head in the sand, depressed, sleeping in a lot, lethargic, not productive, and then I went to a pottery workshop which gave me a week away from my life, and I began to get clarity. So, I have been doing a ton of yoga

since I got back, and writing, and making art. I feel suddenly called to make really good work. I'm believing in myself as an artist, unlike ever before.

Every summer I get the brochures for this ceramics camp, and I always put it aside saying "I just can't do that. I don't deserve this. I'm needed around here. It's too much money," all those stupid excuses you tell yourself. But this time I decided I had to do it. I was stalled and needed to do something to break out of the sadness. I was really sad. I finally realized that I was worth it, that it was a bargain if it helped me to break the stuckness, to clear it out.

Other ways that I nurture myself spiritually include my volunteer work with my dog which helps me bring calmness to people at the suicide prevention center on campus, connecting with my friends, honoring my body by eating well, and of course making my art work. Selling my art can be a connection to feeling valued, as a person and as an artist.

My church community and my pastor have been important in the past but are not so much right now. I have been hiding out a bit the last few years of crisis, avoiding the church ladies who I can't face right now with their questions and comments. I just don't want to talk about things right now, maybe because I don't have the answers, maybe I am ashamed, I don't know. Sometimes you feel a little attacked when you go back to your church family after being away so long.

I have spent so much time caring for family members, to get them to help themselves. Some of them have been so stuck for so long, I've realized, I can't carry them. It's killing me. I've decided I'm done. Peace out. I have had daily neck pain which I directly connect to everybody else's problems on my shoulder. Everybody off! My time at Clay Camp was when I realized that I didn't have to carry that anymore.

Spirituality is the only way, it's the entrance to the path to happiness. It's the start to uncovering the things that feed your soul and is key to living your life as your authentic self and being who you were meant to be on this earth and being the best you can be. I need to do the things that refill my well so I can care well for others.

systems (Mitima-Verloop et al., 2021). These formal rituals are highly personal and specific to each family and their traditions. There is a role for OTPs to support the participation in these rituals and to explore what they prefer as they approach end of life for themselves or a loved one. Although uncomfortable for some to discuss, pondering what supports a good death in a hospice setting or nursing home is a fact of life for those facing their mortality. Selecting what daily occupations are prioritized as someone approaches death as well as encouraging a time of discussion and planning for post-death rituals is an emergent role for OTPs in these settings (Chow et al., 2023).

For people who have experienced loss, particularly unexpected loss, many of the spiritual occupations mentioned earlier may provide a time for processing grief and working through the trauma of loss. Exploring participation in specific activities such as creating a roadside shrine after a car accident, joining a group paddle-out for surfers, taking flowers or other mementos to a grave site, or planting a tree in honor of a loved one may facilitate spiritual healing. Occupational therapy's emphasis on doing as well as talking provides a unique perspective to the processing of grief. Exploring meaningful activities or rituals that help to mourn and bring closure for those experiencing loss is an important contribution to supporting mental health and well-being.

Role of Occupational Therapy in Enabling Spiritual Occupations

OTPs have a primary responsibility to support meaningful engagement in daily occupations when working with persons who have mental health conditions. That includes identifying and facilitating participation in spiritual and religious occupations such as those discussed previously. It does not mean that OTPs are expected to function as clergy or any other form of spiritual expert. As with other practice foci, knowing when to partner with or refer a person to another appropriate profession or discipline is important for achieving goals that are outside the OTP's expertise and training in occupational therapy. Hospital chaplains are an especially helpful resource when addressing issues of spirituality. Certified chaplains have specific training in pastoral care and are skilled in working with health issues in individuals from a variety of faith traditions (Humbert, 2016).

There can be a complex relationship between faith communities and individuals with mental health conditions, as well as a potential conflict between personal spiritual beliefs and the non-faith–based interventions being used to support health and well-being (Sabry & Vohra, 2013; Sullivan et al., 2014). This conflict is often a result of poor training and competing theories, explanations, and treatment approaches for mental health symptoms. The lack of comfort and training for mental health providers (including OTPs) in incorporating religion/spirituality in treatment is matched by the lack of comfort and training for clergy and faith communities on issues of mental health and mental illness (Sabry & Vohra, 2013). Best practice for OTPs is to take the initiative to educate themselves as providers and to potentially play a role in education about mental health conditions and inclusion within spiritual/religious contexts.

Initial Assessment

Questions concerning spirituality and/or spiritual occupations are not always consistently included in initial occupational history-taking and development of occupational profiles. However, the addition of some simple questions when first interviewing persons in a mental health setting can ensure that they are given the opportunity to receive the support and problem-solving needed to engage in healthy and meaningful spiritual occupations. The following sample questions can be used to briefly screen for the importance of religious or spiritual practices and/or occupations in the life of a person (Culliford, 2007):

- "What spiritual or religious activities, if any, are important to you?"
- "What helps you most when things are difficult, when times are hard?"

Open-ended follow-up questions such as, "Would you like to say more about that?" can build on initial information and can help uncover more details about spiritual identities, religious affiliations, and common spiritual practices. Some specific prompting related to common religious and secular spiritual practices may be an important follow-up to the initial brief screening and will assist the person in setting goals for themselves.

Another tool for taking a spiritual history is the mnemonic FICA (Culliford, 2007, p. 215; Puchalski & Romer, 2000):

- F—Faith and belief (What gives the person's life meaning?)
- I—Importance (How important is this to their life situation?)
- C—Community (Do they have a place in any social or religious group?)
- A—Address in care (How would they like their beliefs to be addressed in health care?)

Taking care to explain the role of occupational therapy and the broad scope of human occupation that falls within its domain may help the conversation to feel more comfortable and less intrusive. Use of the Canadian Occupational Performance Measure (COPM) is recommended for helping formulate goals that are occupation-based and meaningful to the person, including ones that fall in the category of spiritual occupations (Law et al., 2014).

The Occupational Therapy Quality of Experience and Spirituality Assessment Tool (OT-Quest) is an assessment tool designed specifically to gather information about the spirituality of the person completing it. OTPs may find this tool useful to further explore and identify spiritual occupations and help set goals for therapy. The tool is based on a three-dimensional model of spirituality (Schulz, 2008). See Figure 53-1.

Intervention

The practitioner and person work collaboratively to identify appropriate and specific goals, which may or may not include spiritual occupations, for occupational therapy to address. Caution must be exercised when supporting engagement in spiritual and religious activities so that respect and humility are conveyed. Being aware of the OTP's own background,

Three-Dimensional Spirituality Model

The Mystery That Is Spirituality

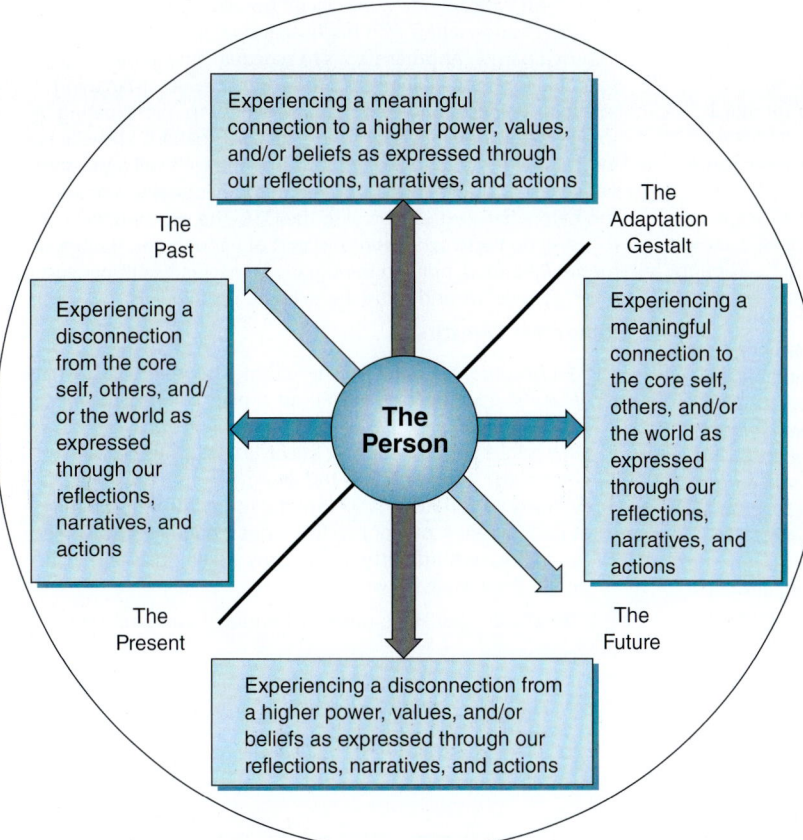

FIGURE 53-1. Three-Dimensional Spirituality Model. Connectedness to spirituality can be conceptualized as having a vertical element (a greater power—such as the Divine, values, or beliefs) and a horizontal element (self, others, and the world). *From Schulz, E. (2008). Three dimensional spirituality model. In B. J. Hemphill-Pearson (Ed.),* Assessments in occupational therapy mental health: An integrated approach *(2nd ed., Fig. 17-1, p. 265). Slack.*

Being a Psychosocial OT Practitioner

When Depression Accompanies Rheumatoid Arthritis: Reactivating Engagement in Spiritual Occupations

Identifying Psychosocial Strengths and Needs

OTPs in outpatient clinics addressing physical disabilities encounter people whose psychosocial needs, such as depression and anxiety, can also impair their participation and lead to further functional challenges. Consider the story of Michelle, a wife and stay-at-home mom with rheumatoid arthritis (RA) and a formal depression diagnosis. The stress of caregiving for two teenage children with mental health and learning challenges, an aging parent, and the workload around household chores causes her to have regular painful flare-ups, limiting her ability to carry out many of her instrumental activities of daily living.

Michelle is seeing an OTP for her RA diagnosis. The OTP provided custom splints and educated Michelle on nonpharmacological pain management techniques and energy conservation strategies. She has been working with her physician on the pharmacological management side but is concerned about the RA medications she has had to take for the last 20 years and the effect they may have on her as she ages. She is aware of the link between stress and RA symptoms but doesn't feel she has many options to reduce the many stressors in her life.

The OTP determines that Michelle would benefit from stress management techniques and wellness strategies. She believes Michelle is at high risk for further disability, loss of function, and worsening depression symptoms.

Using a Holistic Occupational Therapy Approach

The OTP conducts an occupational profile interview with Michelle to identify what occupations help relieve her stress and promote wellness. She shares a long history of involvement in her neighborhood church, which has recently stopped for various reasons. She also notes the significance of yoga practices and ceramics, which spiritually center her when she can participate in them. It is clear that Michelle considers herself a very spiritual person, which is vital to her overall well-being, but she has not been able to nurture that aspect of herself. The OTP uses the FICA questions to gain insight into Michelle's spiritual history.

To encourage self-reflection, the OTP asks Michelle for more details about how each activity contributes to her well-being and the barriers to returning to those occupations. She shares that a barrier to all of them has been increased depression and lack of motivation to participate because of her role as a primary caregiver. She also feels guilty about spending money on her activities as she does not currently contribute to the household

Continued

Being a Psychosocial OT Practitioner—cont'd

income. She has been unable to produce or sell pottery for a while. She also has not prioritized her health and well-being, and it is taking a toll.

Specific details from the FICA include the following:

Yoga: This is a practice Michelle has engaged in for at least the past 6 years. Michelle knows she is at her best when she takes a regular yoga class, but she stopped a while ago because of the expense, time, and pain limitations.

Ceramics: As a gifted artist, Michelle often finds solace in creating beautiful things out of clay. The sensory experience and act of manipulating the clay never fail to "settle her soul." Although she has a studio in her home and a small pottery business, she has not worked there for a few years.

Faith community involvement: This community has significantly supported Michelle over the years. She does not attend services, partly because her family does not want to go and because of her own shifting spiritual needs. She also has been sleeping poorly, so getting up on Sundays when she could sleep in is not appealing.

Michelle and her OTP prioritize which of her identified spiritual occupations she wants to start again, and which would have the most impact on her well-being and stress reduction. She chooses ceramics first and then yoga. She isn't sure about returning to her church. Using a solution-focused coaching approach, the OTP supports Michelle in identifying the steps to return to these two valued occupations. The first step is to address her

discomfort with spending money on herself. Michelle initiates a budget conversation with her husband to address this self-imposed barrier. Another step is to schedule time in her weekly schedule for these vital health-producing activities. Managing safe joint practices and pain management while participating in these tasks is imperative for successful participation. Michelle has long wanted to attend a clay camp that she feels will jump-start her ceramics again, and she picked this as her goal to sign up for this before her next session with the OTP. The accountability of focusing on these occupations as part of her ongoing treatment for her RA and identifying the significant overall health benefits is a way to redefine and value these leisure pursuits.

Reflective Questions

1. As it becomes clear that Michelle values her spirituality, what are some additional areas you can explore to find other occupations that support her well-being in this way?
2. How might the OTP support Michelle's return to her faith community if she indicates this as a goal?
3. How would you justify addressing these spiritual occupations as part of your scope of practice if questioned by a coworker, supervisor, or third-party payer? How would goals that incorporate these areas be written?

See The Lived Experience: Michelle for more information on this case.

Evidence-Based Practice

Enabling Religious Attendance

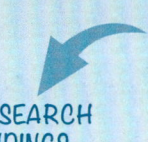

RESEARCH FINDINGS

> *OTPs should support and enable regular participation in religious activities for individuals who identify this as a meaningful occupation.*

Available evidence supports that attendance in regular church services and faith community gatherings enhances mental health. In a large population-based, 14-year longitudinal study, attending monthly services was found to have a protective effect on preventing major depression (Balbuena et al., 2013). Compared with individuals who did not have church attendance, monthly attendees were at 22% lower risk to develop depression. These findings were supported in another large longitudinal study by Li and colleagues (2016), who found that regular religious attendance lowered the risk for depression in women. This study also identified a decrease in religious attendance for individuals with depression. Barton and colleagues (2013) found that religious attendance served as a protective factor for individuals who were at-risk for depression.

Based on available evidence, OTPs should support and enable regular participation in religious activities such as weekly religious services for those who identify this as a meaningful occupation. Analyzing the barriers to attendance and the supports available to participate is a standard skill in occupational therapy. Unfortunately, there is little specific research available to guide intervention in enabling religious participation. Eyres and colleagues (2019) suggest that use of familiar occupational therapy strategies such as those mentioned previously to support engagement in occupation should be applied in support of "religious doing." One evidence-based intervention approach used to support individuals with participation goals is Occupational Performance Coaching (OPC).

Evidence-Based Practice—cont'd

Enabling Religious Attendance

Graham et al. (2020) provide a manual for the use of this coaching method that has been successfully applied to a variety of populations. One of its strongest features is that it is a solution-focused coaching intervention centered on the person's self-identified participation goals. It encourages a collaborative approach with the eventual goal of self-efficacy on the part of the person. This results in skill development and confidence that can carry over to addressing future goals. Key points are noted in the following list.

APPLICATIONS

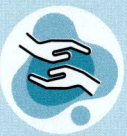

➡ OTPs should identify the spiritual occupations the person reports as important to them.
➡ Interventions used to support occupational participation such as OPC will help individuals meet goals for religious attendance.
➡ OTPs involved in wellness and prevention practice should also consider supporting religious participation goals for their patient as a prevention strategy.

REFERENCES

Balbuena, L., Baetz, M., & Bowen, R. (2013). Religious attendance, spirituality, and major depression in Canada: A 14-year follow-up study. *Canadian Journal of Psychiatry, 58*(4), 225–232. https://doi.org/10.1177/070674371305800408

Barton, Y. A., Miller, L., Wickramaratne, P., Gameroff, M. J., & Weissman, M. M. (2013). Religious attendance and social adjustment as protective against depression: A 10-year prospective study. *Journal of Affective Disorders, 146*(1), 53–57. https://doi.org/10.1016/j.jad.2012.08.037

Eyres, P., Bannigan, K., & Letherby, G. (2019). An understanding of religious doing: A PhotoVoice study. *Religions, 10*(4), Article 269. https://doi.org/10.3390/rel10040269

Graham, F., Kennedy-Behr, A., & Ziviani, J. (2020). *Occupational Performance Coaching: A manual for practitioners and researchers.* Routledge. https://doi.org/10.4324/9780429055805

Li, S., Okereke, O. I., Chang, S. C., Kawachi, I., & VanderWeele, T. J. (2016). Religious service attendance and lower depression among women—A prospective cohort study. *Annals of Behavioral Medicine, 50*(6), 876-884. https://doi.org/10.1007/s12160-016-9813-9

experience, and beliefs will support more sensitive and successful intervention around spiritual occupations.

As with all occupational performance goals, further occupational analysis is necessary to identify the barriers and supports to occupational performance in a spiritually significant activity. For example, a person may have expressed the desire to participate in meditative practices to help them to cope better with stress and anxiety. A skilled clinician will assist the person in identifying specifically what they are looking for. For example, do they want this in a specific faith tradition? Have they done it before? Is it important that it be done alone or with others? The practitioner also pursues inquiries concerning how to move forward with a goal: What kind of support and training is needed? What are the reasons they are not doing this already? What barriers do they anticipate? Intervention might involve collaborative problem-solving, skills training, environmental adaptation, emotional support, or accountability.

Interventions can involve addressing the person, environment, or occupation—or a combination of these categories. For example, person-level interventions for spiritual occupations could include providing social skills training to enhance success in social participation within a faith community. Training in social communication, personal hygiene, social space, and proper adherence to relevant rituals and routines

could be provided or sought out from others (such as clergy) if needed. Alternatively, training and advocacy could be offered at the environment level by an OTP to a faith community to increase acceptance of disability and introduce supports for a person within that specific context. Finally, the occupation itself can be adapted as needed if there are constraints on participation for any number of reasons. For example, a person with severe social anxiety or PTSD may access worship services online as an alternative to in-person participation when symptoms are flaring.

Here's the Point

■ Spirituality and spiritual occupations are incorporated into the *OTPF-4* (AOTA, 2020) and recognized as an integral part of human flourishing.

■ As mental health-care providers, OTPs need to be intentional in seeking training and education on how to best support persons who identify specific religious and spiritual involvement (i.e., spiritual occupations), within and outside of faith traditions, as an important part of their life.

■ Persons may identify traditional religious occupations, such as involvement in a faith community, or meaningful secular occupations that promote their own spiritual growth, such as spending time in nature, exercising, or creating art.

■ As with all occupational performance goals, further occupational analysis is necessary to identify the barriers and supports to occupational performance in a spiritually significant activity.

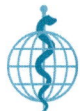 Visit the online resource center at **FADavis.com** to access the video.

Apply It Now

1. Exploring Your Own Spiritual Lens

■ Consider your own experiences of spirituality. How do you define it in your own life, if at all? What occupations would you point to as supporting your religious/spiritual well-being? What role would you want someone else to play in encouraging or facilitating you in your spiritual occupations?

■ Now consider future service recipients or others you have interacted with in the past. Have you experienced discomfort with the ways others define their spirituality? Have you ever experienced others trying to impose their definition and practices of religion or spirituality on you? How did that feel?

■ How might your spiritual belief system affect your thinking about mental illness or disability?

■ Discuss your responses with others and find out how similar/different your reactions are. Talk about how you would apply your awareness to potential occupational therapy practice situations.

2. Through the Lens of the Person Receiving Occupational Therapy

Read over The Lived Experience of Michelle. Consider the following questions:

■ What do you learn about her view of spirituality?

■ What occupations are most important to supporting her spiritual health and how do they contribute to her overall well-being?

■ What factors have contributed to successful participation in those spiritual occupations and what has served as barriers?

Reflective Questions

■ Given the evidence about religious attendance serving as a protective factor for mental health, if you were working as Michelle's OTP, would you address her current lack of church attendance? Why or why not? If yes, what might you do to facilitate reengaging with her formal faith community?

3. Expanding Your Lens

What faith traditions or spiritual practices are popular in your geographic region of practice? Consider ways to familiarize and better understand this identified spiritual topic. Examples might be to interview someone, explore official websites, attend an event such as a faith community gathering, or read a relevant book.

Resources

Books

• Carter, E. W. (2007). *Including people with disabilities in faith communities: A guide for service providers, families, & congregations.* Paul H. Brookes Publishing.
• Humbert, T. (2016). *Spirituality and occupational therapy.* AOTA Press.

Video

• "Caregiver of Spouse With Alzheimer Disease on Challenges" video. Nancy is the wife and caregiver of a man with early-onset Alzheimer disease. Her husband, Bill, had an exciting civilian career and U.S. Navy career. In this video, she describes the challenges they face now that he is unable to work, particularly because he has few hobbies or friends. Nancy shares her struggle maintaining a schedule and filling his time, and describes how she encourages occupations that are meaningful to him. Access the video at the online resource center at FADavis.com.

Online Resources

• Blue Dove Foundation: https://thebluedovefoundation.org /jewish-mental-health-values. This foundation is working to remove stigma and increase understanding around mental illness in Jewish communities.

• Disability and Faith: http://www.disabilityandfaith.org. Disability and Faith is an organization that trains faith-based organizations on how to be more welcoming and accessible.

• Faith for All: http://www.faithforall.org. This is a nondenominational organization interested in accelerating congregational accessibility.

• *Health Care Provider's Handbook on Hindu Patients*: https://aahiinfo.org/wp-content/uploads/2023/04/Healthcare -Handbook_Hindu.pdf. This handbook was originally created by Queensland Health (Government of Australia) and covers a range of topics and aims to inform health-care providers about the religious beliefs and practices of Hindu patients that can affect health care.

• Institute for Muslim Mental Health: https://muslimmentalhealth .com. This site provides an overview of mental health and Islam.

• Kay Warren: Mental Health & the Church: https://kaywarren .com/mentalhealthandthechurch. This site provides resources to implement a Church-initiated mental health strategy.

• Mental Health: A Guide for Faith Leaders: https://www .psychiatry.org/File%20Library/Psychiatrists/Cultural -Competency/Mental_Health_Guide_Tool_Kit_2018.pdf

• Mindful Living Programs: http://www.mindfullivingprograms .com/index.php. This is an example of mindful living training (Mindfulness), which is available online.

- National Alliance of Mental Illness: Faith & Spirituality: http://www.nami.org/Find-Support/Living-with-a-Mental-Health-Condition/Faith-Spirituality. This is a summary of spiritual practices that help support those living with a mental health condition.
- National Alliance of Mental Illness FaithNet: http://www.nami.org/faithnet. This is part of the National Association of Mental Illness and provides support for inclusion in faith organizations.
- National Catholic Partnership on Disability: https://ncpd.org/resources_and_toolkits/association-catholic-mental-health-ministers
- Pew Research Center: The Global Religious Landscape: http://www.pewforum.org/2012/12/18/global-religious-landscape-exec. This site provides information on the global religious landscape
- Pew Research Center: Religious Landscape Study: http://www.pewforum.org/religious-landscape-study. This details a large-scale study of the religious landscape in the United States.
- Tip Sheets and Resources: https://tipsheets.vkcsites.org/inclusion-in-a-faith-community-tip-sheet-for-religious-and-spiritual-leaders. This site offers a tip sheet for religious leaders to support inclusion.
- Vanderbilt Kennedy Center: https://vkc.vumc.org/vkc. This company's mission is to facilitate discoveries and best practices to improve the lives of persons with developmental disabilities and their families.

References

American Occupational Therapy Association. (2014). Occupational therapy practice framework: Domain and process (3rd ed.). *American Journal of Occupational Therapy, 68*(Suppl. 1), S1–S48. https://doi.org/10.5014/ajot.2014.682006

American Occupational Therapy Association. (2020). Occupational therapy practice framework: Domain and process —Fourth edition. *American Journal of Occupational Therapy, 74*(Suppl._2), 7412410010p1–7412410010p87. https://doi.org/10.5014/ajot.2020.74S2001

Balbuena, L., Baetz, M., & Bowen, R. (2013). Religious attendance, spirituality, and major depression in Canada: A 14-year follow-up study. *Canadian Journal of Psychiatry, 58,* 225–232. https://doi.org/10.1177/070674371305800408

Barnes, S. L., & Hollingsworth, C. (2020). Spirituality and social media: The search for support among Black men who have sex with men in Tennessee. *Journal of Homosexuality, 67*(1), 79–103. https://doi.org/10.1080/00918369.2018.1525945

Barton, Y. A., Miller, L., Wickramaratne, P., Gameroff, M. J., & Weissman, M. M. (2013). Religious attendance and social adjustment as protective against depression: A 10-year prospective study. *Journal of Affective Disorders, 146*(1), 53–57. https://doi.org/10.1016/j.jad.2012.08.037

Beavers, A. W., Atkinson, A., Varvatos, L. M., Connolly, M., & Alaimo, K. (2022). How gardening in Detroit influences physical and mental health. *International Journal of Environmental Research and Public Health, 19*(13), 7899. https://doi.org/10.3390/ijerph19137899

Billock, C. (2005). *Delving into the center: Women's lived experience of spirituality through occupation* (Publication No. AAT 3219812) [Doctoral dissertation, University of Southern California]. ProQuest Dissertations and Theses Global.

Bonelli, R. M., & Koenig, H. G. (2013). Mental disorders, religion and spirituality 1990 to 2010: A systematic evidence-based review. *Journal of Religion and Health, 52,* 657–673. https://doi.org/10.1007/s10943-013-9691-4

Burton, A., Burgess, C., Dean, S., Koutsopoulou, G. Z., & Hugh-Jones, S. (2016). How effective are mindfulness-based interventions for reducing stress among healthcare professionals? A systematic review and meta-analysis. *Stress and Health, 33*(1), 1–11. https://doi.org/10.1002/smi.2673

Capaldi, C. A., Passmore, H. A., Nisbet, E. K., Zelenski, J. M., & Dopko, R. L. (2015). Flourishing in nature: A review of the benefits of connecting with nature and its application as a wellbeing intervention. *International Journal of Wellbeing, 5*(4), 1–16. https://doi.org/10.5502/ijw.v5i4.449

Chow, J. K., Pickens, N. D., Fletcher, T., Bowyer, P., & Thompson, M. (2023). Missed opportunities to ease suffering: An explanatory model of occupational therapy utilization in end-of-life care. *American Journal of Hospice and Palliative Medicine, 40*(9), 1004–1012. https://doi.org/10.1177/10499091221143917

Culliford, L. (2007). Taking a spiritual history. *Advances in Psychiatric Treatment, 13,* 212–219. https://doi.org/10.1192/apt.bp.106.002774

Davidson, J. U., & Robison, B. (2008). Scrapbooking and journaling interventions for chronic illness: A triangulated investigation of approaches in the treatment of PTSD. *The Kansas Nurse, 83*(3), 6–11.

Eyres, P., Bannigan, K., & Letherby, G. (2019). An understanding of religious doing: A PhotoVoice study. *Religions, 10*(4), Article 269. https://doi.org/10.3390/rel10040269

Fukui, S., Starnino, V. R., & Nelson-Becker, H. B. (2012). Spiritual well-being of people with psychiatric disabilities: The role of religious attendance, social network size and sense of control. *Community Mental Health Journal, 48,* 202–211. https://doi.org/10.1007/s10597-011-9375-z

Graham, F., Kennedy-Behr, A., & Ziviani, J. (2020). *Occupational Performance Coaching: A manual for practitioners and researchers.* Routledge. https://doi.org/10.4324/9780429055805

Grossman, P., Niemann, L., Schmidt, S., & Walach, H. (2004). Mindfulness-Based Stress Reduction and health benefits: A meta-analysis. *Journal of Psychosomatic Research, 57*(1), 35–43. https://doi.org/10.1016/S0022-3999(03)00573-7

Hardison, M. E., & Roll, S. C. (2016). Mindfulness interventions in physical rehabilitation: A scoping review. *The American Journal of Occupational Therapy, 70*(3), 7003290030p1–7003290030p9. https://doi.org/10.5014/ajot.2016.018069

Heintzman, P. (2009). Nature-based recreation and spirituality: A complex relationship. *Leisure Sciences, 32*(1), 72–89. https://doi.org/10.1080/01490400903430897

Humbert, T. K. (2016). *Spirituality and occupational therapy: A model for practice and research.* AOTA Press.

Kamitsis, I., & Francis, A. J. (2013). Spirituality mediates the relationship between engagement with nature and psychological wellbeing. *Journal of Environmental Psychology, 36,* 136–143. https://doi.org/10.1016/j.jenvp.2013.07.013

Kapoor, S., Morgan, C. K., Siddique, M. A., & Guntupalli, K. K. (2018). "Sacred pause" in the ICU: Evaluation of a ritual and intervention to lower distress and burnout. *American Journal of Hospice and Palliative Medicine®, 35*(10), 1337–1341. https://doi.org/10.1177/1049909118768247

Kelly, J. F., & Greene, M. C. (2014). Toward an enhanced understanding of the psychological mechanisms by which spirituality aids recovery in Alcoholics Anonymous. *Alcoholism Treatment Quarterly, 32*(2-3), 299–318. https://doi.org/10.1080/07347324.2014.907015

Klatt, M., Steinberg, B., & Duchemin, A. M. (2015). Mindfulness in Motion (MIM): An onsite mindfulness based intervention (MBI) for chronically high stress work environments to increase resiliency and work engagement. *Journal of Visualized Experiments: JoVE, 2015*(101), e52359. https://doi.org/10.3791/52359

Koenig, H. G., Al Zaben, F., & Khalifa, D. A. (2012). Religion, spirituality and mental health in the West and the Middle East. *Asian Journal of Psychiatry, 5*(2), 180–182. https://doi.org/10.1016/j.ajp.2012.04.004

Law, M., Baptiste, S., Carswell, A., McColl, M., Polatajko, H., & Pollock, N. (2014). *Canadian Occupational Performance Measure* (5th ed.). CAOT Publication ACE.

Li, S., Okereke, O. I., Chang, S. C., Kawachi, I., & VanderWeele, T. J. (2016). Religious service attendance and lower depression among women—A prospective cohort study. *Annals of Behavioral Medicine, 50*(6), 876–884. https://doi.org/10.1007/s12160-016-9813-9

Liu, E. X., Carter, E. W., Boehm, T. L., Annandale, N. H., & Taylor, C. E. (2014). In their own words: The place of faith in the lives of young people with autism and intellectual disability. *Intellectual and Developmental Disabilities, 52*(5), 388–404. https://doi.org/10.1352/1934-9556-52.5.388

Lucchetti, G., Koenig, H. G., & Lucchetti, A. L. G. (2021). Spirituality, religiousness, and mental health: A review of the current scientific evidence. *World Journal of Clinical Cases, 9*(26), 7620–7631. https://doi.org/10.12998/wjcc.v9.i26.7620

Luken, M., & Sammons, A. (2016). Systematic review of mindfulness practice for reducing job burnout. *American Journal of Occupational Therapy, 70*(2), 7002250020p1–7002250020p10. https://doi.org/10.5014/ajot.2016.016956

Malviya, S., Zupan, B., & Meredith, P. (2022). Evidence of religious/spiritual singing and movement in mental health: A systematic review. *Complementary Therapies in Clinical Practice, 47*, 101567. https://doi.org/10.1016/j.ctcp.2022.101567

Milner, K., Crawford, P., Edgley, A., Hare-Duke, L., & Slade, M. (2020). The experiences of spirituality among adults with mental health difficulties: A qualitative systematic review. *Epidemiology and Psychiatric Sciences, 29*, e34. https://doi.org/10.1017/S2045796019000234

Mitima-Verloop, H. B., Mooren, T. T. M., & Boelen, P. A. (2021). Facilitating grief: An exploration of the function of funerals and rituals in relation to grief reactions. *Death Studies, 45*(9), 735–745. https://doi.org/10.1080/07481187.2019.1686090

Nesbit, S. G. (2006). Using creativity to experience flow on my journey with breast cancer. *Occupational Therapy in Mental Health, 22*, 61–79. https://doi.org/10.1300/J004v22n02_03

Papadopoulos, I., Lazzarino, R., Wright, S., Ellis Logan, P., & Koulouglioti, C. (2021). Spiritual support during COVID-19 in England: A scoping study of online sources. *Journal of Religion and Health, 60*, 2209–2230. https://doi.org/10.1007/s10943-021-01254-1

Polatajko, H. J., Townsend, E. A., & Craik, J. (2007). Canadian Model of Occupational Performance and Engagement (CMOP-E). In E. A. Townsend & H. J. Polatajko (Eds.), *Enabling Occupation II: Advancing an occupational therapy vision for health, well-being, & justice through occupation* (pp. 22–36). CAOT Publications ACE.

Puchalski, C., & Romer, A. L. (2000). Taking a spiritual history allows clinicians to understand patients more fully. *Journal of Palliative Medicine, 3*, 129–137. https://doi.org/10.1089/jpm.2000.3.129

Reid, D., Farragher, J., & Ok, C. (2013). Exploring mindfulness with occupational therapists practicing in mental health contexts. *Occupational Therapy in Mental Health, 29*, 279–292. https://doi.org/10.1080/0164212X.2013.819727

Rote, S., Hill, T. D., & Ellison, C. G. (2012). Religious attendance and loneliness in later life. *The Gerontologist, 53*, 39–50. https://doi.org/10.1093/geront/gns063

Sabry, W. M., & Vohra, A. (2013). Role of Islam in the management of psychiatric disorders. *Indian Journal of Psychiatry, 55*(Suppl. 2), S205–S214. https://doi.org/10.4103/0019-5545.105534

Schulz, E. (2008). OT-Quest assessment. In B. J. Hemphill-Pearson (Ed.), *Assessments in occupational therapy mental health: An integrated approach* (2nd ed., pp. 263–289). Slack.

Shilo, G., Yossef, I., & Savaya, R. (2016). Religious coping strategies and mental health among religious Jewish gay and bisexual men. *Archives of Sexual Behavior, 45*, 1551–1561. https://doi.org/10.1007/s10508-015-0567-4

Simpson, D., Post, P. G., Young, G., & Jensen, P. R. (2014). "It's not about taking the easy road": The experiences of ultramarathon runners. *Sport Psychologist, 28*, 176–185. https://doi.org/10.1123/tsp.2013-0064

Smith-Gabai, H., & Ludwig, F. (2011). Observing the Jewish Sabbath: A meaningful restorative ritual for modern times. *Journal of Occupational Science, 18*(4), 347–355. https://doi.org/10.1080/14427591.2011.595891

Sullivan, S., Pyne, J. M., Cheney, A. M., Hunt, J., Haynes, T. F., & Sullivan, G. (2014). The pew versus the couch: Relationship between mental health and faith communities and lessons learned from a VA/clergy partnership project. *Journal of Religion and Health, 53*(2), 1267–1282. https://doi.org/10.1007/s10943-013-9731-0

Sundquist, J., Lilja, Å., Palmér, K., Memon, A. A., Wang, X., Johansson, L. M., & Sundquist, K. (2015). Mindfulness group therapy in primary care patients with depression, anxiety and stress and adjustment disorders: Randomised controlled trial. *The British Journal of Psychiatry, 206*, 128–135. https://doi.org/10.1192/bjp.bp.114.150243

Ullrich, P. M., & Lutgendorf, S. K. (2002). Journaling about stressful events: Effects of cognitive processing and emotional expression. *Annals of Behavioral Medicine, 24*, 244–250. https://doi.org/10.1207/S15324796ABM2403_10

Unruh, A., & Hutchinson, S. (2011). Embedded spirituality: Gardening in daily life and stressful life experiences. *Scandinavian Journal of Caring Sciences, 25*, 567–574. https://doi.org/10.1111/j.1471-6712.2010.00865.x

Van Lith, T. (2013). "Painting to find my spirit." Art making as the vehicle to find meaning and connection in the mental health recovery process. *Journal of Spirituality in Mental Health, 16*, 19–36. https://doi.org/10.1080/19349637.2013.864542

Van Lith, T. (2015). Art making as a mental health recovery tool for change and coping. *Art Therapy, 32*(1), 5–12. https://doi.org/10.1080/07421656.2015.992826

Weaver, L. L., & Darragh, A. R. (2015). Systematic review of yoga interventions for anxiety reduction among children and adolescents. *American Journal of Occupational Therapy, 69*, 6906180070p1–6906180070p9. https://doi.org/10.5014/ajot.2015.020115

Wilding, C. (2007). Spirituality as sustenance for mental health and meaningful doing: A case illustration. *Medical Journal of Australia, 186*, S67–S69. https://doi.org/10.5694/j.1326-5377.2007.tb01046.x

Zhang, H., Hook, J. N., Van Tongeren, D. R., Davis, E. B., Aten, J. D., McElroy-Heltzel, S., Davis, D. E., Shannonhouse, L., Hodge, A. S., & Captari, L. E. (2021). Spiritual fortitude: A systematic review of the literature and implications for COVID-19 coping. *Spirituality in Clinical Practice, 8*(4), 229–244. https://doi.org/10.1037/scp0000267

Zimmer, Z., Jagger, C., Chiu, C. T., Ofstedal, M. B., Rojo, F., & Saito, Y. (2016). Spirituality, religiosity, aging and health in global perspective: A review. *SSM Population Health, 2*, 373–381. https://doi.org/10.1016/j.ssmph.2016.04.009

Template for Person-Environment-Occupation (PEO) Analysis

Occupational Participation Issue(s) Identified by the Person

Assessment of Main Components Impacting Occupational Participation

Occupation

Consider:

- Access to valued occupations
- Cultural and societal meanings and developmental expectations of this occupation
- Reviewing the steps involved and identifying the physical, cognitive, affective, and social demands
- Requirements for space, time, materials, and resources

Person

Consider:

- Personal values, preferences, and interests
- Illnesses and effect on body functions and structures, especially regarding affective, cognitive, and physical functions
- Person's relationship with health condition, sense of self, and personal resources
- Life experiences, developmental stage
- Spirituality, connection with the world
- Personality, habits, routines

Environment

Consider:

- Cultural (beliefs, customs, traditions)
- Social (friends, family, social network)
- Institutional structures and policies (legislative bodies, education and employment organizations, health and social services)
- Physical (natural, human-built)
- Social determinants (non medical factors impacting health outcomes, such as environmental conditions in which people grow, work, live, and age; stigma and social norms; and policies and political systems)

Assessment of Person-Environment-Occupation (PEO) Transactions

Person-Occupation (P x O)

Consider:

- Person's perception of the occupation; meaning ascribed; motivation
- Person's abilities and limitations to perform the occupation's tasks or activities
- Implications for learning

Occupation-Environment (O x E)

Consider:

- Equitable opportunities for participation in occupations in the environment
- Support for occupation in this environment
- Occupational demands when performed in this environment
- How tasks are organized, reinforced, and formal and informal rules applied

Person-Environment (P x E)

Consider:

- Support for this individual in this environment
- Person's perception of the environment; meaning ascribed
- Disabling factors

Formulation of Occupational Participation Issue (P x E x O)

What is supporting and constraining occupational participation for this person to engage in the identified occupation within the given environment?

Theoretical Approaches to Guide Intervention

Based on the underlying issues and the target(s) for intervention, select theoretical approach(es) to guide your intervention(s).

Recommendations or Plan to Improve Occupational Participation (the PEO Fit)

Template for Person-Environment-Occupation (PEO) Analysis

Appendix B

Index of Assessments

Because this textbook is organized according to the Person-Environment-Occupation (PEO) model rather than assessments, different assessment measures are interspersed throughout the chapters. This index was developed as a reference tool to enable readers to quickly identify the chapters in which a particular assessment is addressed. Entries refer to the chapter(s), and not the page number, where the content on the relevant assessment is found. In some cases, an assessment is discussed in detail, whereas in other cases, it is simply identified as a relevant measure.

Index of Interventions

This index outlines occupational therapy intervention approaches for individuals with psychosocial concerns. In occupational therapy, the ultimate outcome is always occupational participation, but this table designates the target of intervention that leads to more effective and satisfying occupational participation. It also provides a brief synopsis of the intervention and identifies the accompanying chapter(s) in this text that provide more detailed information about those approaches.

Approach	Target(s) of Intervention	Brief Synopsis	Chapters With Additional Information
Acceptance and Commitment Therapy	Psychological flexibility	Acceptance of difficult feelings and mindfulness combined with identification of personal values and concrete steps toward action	• Chapter 8: Cognitive Beliefs • Chapter 10: Coping and Resilience • Chapter 15: Pain • Chapter 49: Connectedness and Belonging
Action Over Inertia	Meaningful and productive activity	Manualized intervention with workbook to increase engagement in meaningful and productive activity	• Chapter 14: Time Use and Habits • Chapter 31: The Home Environment: Permanent Supportive Housing • Chapter 51: Leisure and Creative Occupations
Activity Scheduling	Engagement/Participation	Scheduling activities that provide pleasure and a sense of achievement	• Chapter 8: Cognitive Beliefs
Adapting the Environment	Features of the environment	Aspects of the environment that act as barriers are changed to promote occupational participation	• Chapter 7: Cognition • Chapter 12: Emotion Regulation • Chapter 46: Activities of Daily Living, Instrumental Activities of Daily Living, and Health Management Occupations
ADL, IADL, and Life Skills Training	ADLs and IADLs	Application of learning and behavioral strategies to promote acquisition of new skills	• Chapter 31: The Home Environment: Permanent Supportive Housing • Chapter 41: State Hospitals • Chapter 42: Homelessness and Housing Insecurity • Chapter 43: Serving Veterans and Service Members • Chapter 46: Activities of Daily Living, Instrumental Activities of Daily Living, and Health Management Occupations
Advocacy and Self-Advocacy	Reducing stigma and misunderstanding	Developing knowledge of rights and skills to advocate for full inclusion and education/awareness of mental health issues. Also includes advocacy organizations such as Fireweed Collective, Institute for Development of Human Arts, Project LETS, and Hearing Voices Network	• Chapter 27: Mental Health Stigma and Sanism • Chapter 29: Families • Chapter 32: The Neighborhood and Community • Chapter 38: Early Psychosis Programs for Adolescents and Young Adults • Chapter 44: Addressing Suicide Across the Continuum • Chapter 46: Activities of Daily Living, Instrumental Activities of Daily Living, and Health Management Occupations • Chapter 48: Work and Volunteer Occupations
Affect Regulation Training (ART)	Affect regulation	The use of cognitive and somatic approaches to regulate affect when confronted with challenging situations and triggers	• Chapter 12: Emotion Regulation

Continued

Approach	Target(s) of Intervention	Brief Synopsis	Chapters With Additional Information
Affirmative Businesses and Social Firms	Work	Community businesses created to offer employment opportunities to disadvantaged persons such as individuals with psychiatric disabilities	• Chapter 48: Work and Volunteer Occupations
ALERT Program	Attention/Arousal	Use of sensory strategies to maintain optimal levels of arousal	• Chapter 37: School Mental Health
Arts and Crafts Activities and Community Arts	Leisure, social, and spiritual connection	Using arts and crafts as media to promote leisure participation, social inclusion, and wellness	• Chapter 10: Coping and Resilience • Chapter 12: Emotion Regulation • Chapter 45: Self-Care and Well-Being Occupations • Chapter 51: Leisure and Creative Occupations • Chapter 53: Spiritual Occupations
Arts and Health Programs	Well-being and health	Public health programs that utilize exposure and participation to arts for well-being and health	• Chapter 51: Leisure and Creative Occupations
Assertive Community Treatment	Community living	Team approach to providing rehabilitation and support to promote community living	• Chapter 35: Practice Across the Continuum of Service Needs
Assistive Technology	Participation	Devices and products that allow a person with a disability to participate in daily life	• Chapter 14: Time Use and Habits • Chapter 33: Virtual Environments • Chapter 46: Activities of Daily Living, Instrumental Activities of Daily Living, and Health Management Occupations
Attachment, Regulation, and Competency (ARC)	Person's trauma and attachment history, self-regulation skills, and safety	Strengthening the caregiver system and teaching skills for self-regulation	• Chapter 12: Emotion Regulation • Chapter 36: Early Intervention: A Practice Setting for Early Childhood Mental Health • Chapter 49: Connectedness and Belonging
Balancing Everyday Life (BEL)	Activity balance and engagement	Group-based manualized intervention focused on making lifestyle changes and achieving balanced engagement in meaningful activities	• Chapter 14: Time Use and Habits
Behavioral Activation	Engaging in positive activities	Identifying activities that provide positive feedback and developing strategies for participation	• Chapter 51: Leisure and Creative Occupations
Behavioral Approaches	Positive behaviors	Using rewards and reinforcements to develop positive behaviors	• Chapter 12: Emotion Regulation • Chapter 15: Pain
Bridging the Transition From Homelessness to Housed	Stable housing	Providing opportunities and skill building based on the level of transition the person is in	• Chapter 42: Homelessness and Housing Insecurity
Building Healthy Routines and Habits	Time use and habit development	Learning to reduce engagement in unhealthy routines and increase engagement in healthy routines	• Chapter 14: Time Use and Habits
Calm Moment Cards	Reduce stress	Informational sheets with strategies and activities to reduce stress in school setting	• Chapter 37: School Mental Health
Capabilities, Opportunities, Resources, and Environments (CORE)	Occupational participation	Identifying or creating opportunities, resources, and environments to provide the individual with agency and choice for occupational participation	• Chapter 28: Social Determinants and Mental Health
Caring for Yourself	Support for family and friends	Workbook for family and friends to support someone with mental health challenges	• Chapter 29: Families
Children of Parents With Mental Illness	Support and well-being for the child	Web-based support with resources for children who have a parent with a mental health challenge	• Chapter 29: Families

Approach	Target(s) of Intervention	Brief Synopsis	Chapters With Additional Information
Cognitive Adaptation Training	Environmental features that pose cognitive barriers	A manualized intervention using compensatory strategies is implemented that reduces cognitive demands that interfere with ADL and IADL performance	• Chapter 7: Cognition • Chapter 46: Activities of Daily Living, Instrumental Activities of Daily Living, and Health Management Occupations
Cognitive Behavioral Therapy	Distorted beliefs	Distorted beliefs are identified and then challenged by providing evidence to the contrary	• Chapter 8: Cognitive Beliefs • Chapter 10: Coping and Resilience • Chapter 15: Pain • Chapter 43: Serving Veterans and Service Members • Chapter 49: Connectedness and Belonging
Cognitive Behavioral Therapy–Insomnia	Sleep	Combines cognitive therapy with sleep restriction and sleep hygiene strategies	• Chapter 43: Serving Veterans and Service Members • Chapter 52: Sleep
Cognitive Disabilities Model and Cognitive Disabilities Model Reconsidered	Activity and environmental modification	Based on cognitive level, the activity and environment are modified to promote successful occupational participation	• Chapter 7: Cognition
Cognitive Functional (Cog-Fun) Therapy for Children With Attention Deficit Hyperactivity Disorder (ADHD)	Executive strategies	Manualized program that involves teaching executive strategies, enabling the therapeutic environment, and creating supports	• Chapter 7: Cognition
Cognitive Orientation to Daily Occupational Performance (CO-OP)	Problem-solving in the context of occupational performance	A four-step strategy of goal, plan, do, check is taught to help the individual problem-solve a particular occupational goal	• Chapter 7: Cognition
Cognitive Remediation	Cognitive skills	Restoring specific cognitive skills through repetition and feedback in the context of occupational performance	• Chapter 7: Cognition
Comfortable Cafeteria	Positive cafeteria environment	Staff and cafeteria employees provided with strategies and resources to create a positive environment in the cafeteria for students	• Chapter 37: School Mental Health
Community Case Management	Community integration	Building on strengths of the individual and community supports to promote community integration	• Chapter 35: Practice Across the Continuum of Service Needs
Community Clutter and Hoarding Toolkit	Hoarding	Reducing clutter to maintain housing using Motivational Interviewing and goal setting; targets older adults	• Chapter 31: The Home Environment: Permanent Supportive Housing
Compulsive Hoarding–Frontline Worker's Toolkit	Hoarding	Reducing clutter to maintain housing	• Chapter 31: The Home Environment: Permanent Supportive Housing
Connection Menu	Connection	Identify and provide supports to create connections to people, pets, and nature	• Chapter 49: Connectedness and Belonging
Coping Internalized Stigma Program (PAREI)	Self-stigma	Cognitive behavioral therapy and mutual support	• Chapter 27: Mental Health Stigma and Sanism
Developmental Individual Differences Relationship-Based (DIR) Floortime™	Social emotional development	Using the child's interest to motivate the child to learn what they need to learn	• Chapter 13: Communication and Social Skills
Dialectical Behavior Therapy Skills Training	Emotion regulation	Skills targeting mindfulness meditation, interpersonal effectiveness, emotion regulation, and distress tolerance	• Chapter 12: Emotion Regulation • Chapter 49: Connectedness and Belonging

Continued

Approach	Target(s) of Intervention	Brief Synopsis	Chapters With Additional Information
Drive Thru Menus for Attention and Strength	Attention	Activities to keep the body quiet during classroom activities	• Chapter 37: School Mental Health
Drive Thru Menus for Relaxation and Stress Busters	Stress reduction	Visualization, meditation, and movement activities used in the school system	• Chapter 37: School Mental Health
Dunn Model of Sensory Processing	Adapting or matching the environment to meet sensory processing needs	Creating or matching environments or materials that meet sensory processing needs based on a four-quadrant model of sensory sensitivity, sensation avoiding, low registration, and sensation seeking	• Chapter 9: Sensory Processing and the Lived Sensory Experience • Chapter 12: Emotion Regulation
Dynamic Interactional Approach	Processing strategies	Strategies that compensate for executive function impairments are taught; these strategies can be used across different occupations	• Chapter 7: Cognition
Education for Stigma Reduction	Public stigma	Sharing of evidence and lived experience to counteract stigmatizing attitudes	• Chapter 27: Mental Health Stigma and Sanism
Ending Self-Stigma	Self-stigma	Psychoeducation and cognitive behavioral therapy	• Chapter 27: Mental Health Stigma and Sanism
Errorless Learning	Learning	Training that occurs in such a way that mistakes are minimized or not allowed	• Chapter 7: Cognition • Chapter 41: State Hospitals
Expressive Writing	Stress reduction and coping	Writing about difficult situations to process the experience	• Chapter 10: Coping and Resilience
Faith Communities	Spiritual and social connections	Structured opportunities to express spiritual connections and practice rituals with others	• Chapter 53: Spiritual Occupations
Families Overcoming Under Stress (FOCUS)	Resilience	Intervention for military families; family creates its own story to build on strengths	• Chapter 10: Coping and Resilience
Family Psychoeducation/ Family to Family	Relationships between family members and individuals with psychiatric disability	A family group approach where individuals can develop supportive relationships and receive education and develop problem-solving skills to address specific family concerns	• Chapter 10: Coping and Resilience • Chapter 39: Peer-Led Services
Federally Qualified Health Centers	Access to care for underserved populations	Comprehensive health-care services offered at a sliding scale	• Chapter 34: Integrated Behavioral Health and Primary Care
Gardening (Healing/ Therapeutic)	Improved physical and mental well-being	Exposure to nature and opportunities to take care/grow plants	• Chapter 30: Natural Environments
Gatekeeper Training	Reducing suicide risk	Screening for suicide risk and education on risk and protective factors and referral strategies/resource	• Chapter 44: Addressing Suicide Across the Continuum
Get Ready to Learn	Stress reduction and attention	Yoga-based curriculum to use in the classroom	• Chapter 37: School Mental Health
Graded Exposure	Reduction of fear and anxiety	Gradual exposure to feared situations typically combined with relaxation/ mindfulness	• Chapter 15: Pain
Grief Rituals	Grief and loss	Formal or informal practices to express grief and acknowledge person that was lost	• Chapter 53: Spiritual Occupations
Growth Through Occupational Therapy for Academic Learning	Higher education	1:1 mentoring provided by occupational therapy students to support undergraduate colleges students with mental health conditions	• Chapter 47: Student
Healthy Navigators	Health services	A person who is knowledgeable about existing services becomes a liaison to link persons to existing services; peer navigators may serve this role	• Chapter 34: Integrated Behavioral Health and Primary Care

Approach	Target(s) of Intervention	Brief Synopsis	Chapters With Additional Information
Home Environmental Skill Building	ADLs and IADLs	Teaching caregivers how to modify the environment to facilitate ADL and IADL performance in people with dementia	• Chapter 46: Activities of Daily Living, Instrumental Activities of Daily Living, and Health Management Occupations
Identity Development Evolution and Sharing (IDEAS)	Public stigma	Plays are created based on interviews of people with lived experience and shared for viewing and discussion	• Chapter 27: Mental Health Stigma and Sanism
Integrative Medication Self-Management	Medication management	Person sets goal for medication management and therapist creates strategies to meet goal	• Chapter 46: Activities of Daily Living, Instrumental Activities of Daily Living, and Health Management Occupations
Interoception Activity Cards	Interoceptive awareness	100 activities to practice interoceptive awareness	• Chapter 37: School Mental Health
Interoceptive Awareness Training/ Interoceptive Curriculum	Interoceptive awareness	Activities to help individual recognize and respond to body signals and develop healthy habits	• Chapter 12: Emotion Regulation • Chapter 37: School Mental Health • Chapter 49: Connectedness and Belonging
Interpersonal and Social Rhythm Therapy (IPSRT)	Routines	Teaching individuals how to monitor routines and create stability in daily schedules	• Chapter 14: Time Use and Habits • Chapter 46: Activities of Daily Living, Instrumental Activities of Daily Living, and Health Management Occupations
Interpersonal Effectiveness Training	Interpersonal relationships	Education and practice of effective skills for relating to others	• Chapter 12: Emotion Regulation
Joint Attention Training	Reciprocal communication	Setting up play situations and then modeling and prompting joint attention	• Chapter 13: Communication and Social Skills
Leisure Activity Groups	Leisure	Leisure education and exploration followed by engagement in leisure activities	• Chapter 51: Leisure and Creative Occupations
Leisure Exploration	Leisure	Identifying and pursuing leisure activities	• Chapter 43: Serving Veterans and Service Members • Chapter 45: Self-Care and Well-Being Occupations
Lifestyle Redesign	Health and wellness	Creation of habits and routines that are personally meaningful and promote health	• Chapter 45: Self-Care and Well-Being Occupations
LIVE LIFE	Suicide prevention	A public health program that includes awareness raising and capacity building	• Chapter 44: Addressing Suicide Across the Continuum
Making Leisure Matters	Hobbies and interests	Leisure coaching to explore and promote participation in leisure activities for children and youth	• Chapter 37: School Mental Health
Managing Overweight Veterans Everywhere Program	Weight management	Individual counseling and groups to develop healthy habits related to nutrition and physical activity	• Chapter 43: Serving Veterans and Service Members
Meaningful Activities and Recovery (MA&R)	Activity engagement	Uses the Profile of Occupational Engagement in People With Severe Mental Illness (POES-S) to help individuals with mental illness to incorporate meaningful activities into daily life	• Chapter 14: Time Use and Habits
Mental Health/Drug Courts	Alternatives to incarceration	Mental health/substance abuse services, employment, and social services as alternatives to incarceration	• Chapter 40: Criminal Justice Systems
Metacognitive Reflection and Insight Therapy (MERIT)	Metacognition/Insight	Uses relationship between therapist and person to create narratives that help person to increase awareness and metacognition	• Chapter 7: Cognition • Chapter 49: Connectedness and Belonging
Michigan Supported Education	Higher education	Support group led by person with lived experience and individual school counseling	• Chapter 47: Student

Continued

Approach	Target(s) of Intervention	Brief Synopsis	Chapters With Additional Information
Mindfulness Meditation/ Mindfulness-Based Stress Reduction/ Grounding	Enhancing emotional well-being	A form of meditation practice that focuses awareness nonjudgmentally on the present	• Chapter 8: Cognitive Beliefs • Chapter 10: Coping and Resilience • Chapter 12: Emotion Regulation • Chapter 43: Serving Veterans and Service Members • Chapter 45: Self-Care and Well-Being Occupations • Chapter 49: Connectedness and Belonging • Chapter 53: Spiritual Occupations
Mobile Support Model	Higher education	Mental health professionals provide supportive services to students with psychiatric disabilities in a college setting	• Chapter 47: Student
Motivational Interviewing	Engagement in health-promoting behaviors	A person-centered manner of interacting that helps the person self-identify reasons for changing behaviors	• Chapter 11: Motivation
Multifamily Group Therapy	Better family functioning	Family members learn problem-solving strategies to manage everyday challenges	• Chapter 38: Early Psychosis Programs for Adolescents and Young Adults
Narrative Enhancement and Cognitive Therapy	Self-stigma	Cognitive restricting and development of narratives with a positive identity	• Chapter 27: Mental Health Stigma and Sanism
Nature-Based Interventions	Spiritual connection	Spending time in outdoor activities for spiritual connection	• Chapter 53: Spiritual Occupations
Non-Intervention Creative Activity	Participation in creative activity	Community or home-based participation in creative activities such as choir, creative writing, and crafts	• Chapter 51: Leisure and Creative Occupations
Nonsequential Model of Therapeutics™	Creating safety for those who have experienced trauma	Hierarchical approach that addresses neurological networks beginning with regulation, progressing to relationships with others, and finally advancing to reasoning	• Chapter 5: Trauma-Informed Practice
Occupation-Based Community Development (OBCD) Framework	Occupational participation	Involving the community in action-oriented problem-solving to address structural inequities	• Chapter 28: Social Determinants and Mental Health
On-Site Services Model	Higher education	Existing services on college campus are used to support people with mental health conditions	• Chapter 47: Student
Outdoor Play	Child development, health, and well-being	Play that takes place outdoors and is often unstructured	• Chapter 30: Natural Environments
Pain Neuroscience Education	Pain management	Teaching about biological and physiological processes of pain	• Chapter 15: Pain
Parents and Teachers as Allies	Awareness of mental health issues in the school	National Alliance on Mental Health (NAMI) program led by parent, a youth with mental health issues, and a teacher to increase awareness of mental health issues in the school	• Chapter 29: Families
Partial Hospitalization/ Intensive Outpatient Programs	Transition from intensive to less intensive mental health services	Group-based services for community reintegration	• Chapter 35: Practice Across the Continuum of Service Needs
Patient-Centered Medical Home	Quality and satisfaction with health-care services	Patient-driven interdisciplinary, coordinated health care	• Chapter 34: Integrated Behavioral Health and Primary Care
Peer-Bridgers	Transition from hospital to community	Use of trained peers to help person navigate system and successfully transition to the community	• Chapter 39: Peer-Led Services
Peer-Coaching/ Mentoring	Socialization and quality of life	Peer with good emotion regulation and socialization skills provides modeling and support	• Chapter 12: Emotion Regulation

Approach	Target(s) of Intervention	Brief Synopsis	Chapters With Additional Information
Peer-Mediated Intervention	Social skills	Typically developing peers are trained to facilitate interactions with another child with social needs	• Chapter 13: Communication and Social Skills
Peer Support Programs	Social connectedness and support	Education, socialization, and advocacy services provided by a person with a lived experience of mental illness	• Chapter 32: The Neighborhood and Community • Chapter 39: Peer-Led Services
Personal Playful Moments	Play	Teach person about benefits of play, then identify opportunities and facilitate engagement in playful activities	• Chapter 50: Play
Picture Exchange Communication Systems (PECS)	Communication	Using a set of pictures to develop skills in communication	• Chapter 13: Communication and Social Skills
Play-Based Coaching	Play	Using a coaching approach to match child's and parent's ways of playing and help parent to modify activity and environment to facilitate play and employ strategies to make play part of daily routine	• Chapter 50: Play
Playful Environments	Play	Modifying the social and physical aspects of environments to promote play	• Chapter 50: Play
Problem-Solving Courts	Alternatives to incarceration	Nonadversarial judge problem-solves approach to the offense that does not involve incarceration	• Chapter 40: Criminal Justice Systems
Program for the Education and Enrichment of Relational Skills	Making and keeping friends	Social skills training along with caregivers acting as coaches	• Chapter 13: Communication and Social Skills
Psychosocial Clubhouses	Social inclusion	Membership in an organization structured around a work-ordered day to address functions of the clubhouse	• Chapter 35: Practice Across the Continuum of Service Needs
Quiet Contemplation in Nature	Stress reduction, cognition	Spending time in nature may be combined with meditation or other forms of reflection	• Chapter 30: Natural Environments
Recovery College	Public and self-stigma	People with and without mental illness learn about mental illness together	• Chapter 27: Mental Health Stigma and Sanism • Chapter 32: The Neighborhood and Community
Recovery Through Activity	Engagement in meaningful activity	Identifying interests and motivators to increase participation	• Chapter 31: The Home Environment: Permanent Supportive Housing
Redesigning Daily Occupations (ReDO)	Balance of restful and reviving occupations	Manualized program analyzing activity patterns and then setting goals and developing strategies to change patterns of time use	• Chapter 14: Time Use and Habits
Refreshing Recess	Positive recess experience	Strategies for fostering friendships, resolving conflicts, and engaging children in play	• Chapter 37: School Mental Health
Reintegration for Persons in Criminal Justice Systems	Transition to community	Skill development often focused on vocational skills	• Chapter 40: Criminal Justice Systems
Relapse Prevention (for pain)	Pain management	Identify goals and strategies for when one encounters difficulties that might result in pain	• Chapter 15: Pain
Relaxation and Refocusing Strategies	Stress management	Abdominal breathing, progressive muscle relaxation, autogenic techniques, mindfulness meditation, guided imagery, and virtual reality to promote state of calm	• Chapter 15: Pain

Continued

Approach	Target(s) of Intervention	Brief Synopsis	Chapters With Additional Information
Remotivation Process	Motivation	Uses Model of Human Occupation to foster development to next stage of motivation	• Chapter 11: Motivation
Safety Plan	Reducing suicide risk	Creating a plan with the person at risk of suicide to reduce lethal means and increase use of coping strategies	• Chapter 44: Addressing Suicide Across the Continuum
Self-Contained Classroom	Higher education	People with psychiatric disabilities meet in own class on a college campus to develop skills for success in college	• Chapter 47: Student
Self-Monitoring	Thoughts, emotions, and behaviors	Persons observe and record specific targets related to thoughts, feelings, and behaviors	• Chapter 8: Cognitive Beliefs
Self-Talk and Affirmations	Positive thinking	Using self-directed statement to develop more positive thinking	• Chapter 8: Cognitive Beliefs
Sensory Integration	Specific sensory systems	Person-directed approach that uses play and activity to target specific senses to elicit an adaptive response	• Chapter 9: Sensory Processing and the Lived Sensory Experience
Sensory Processing	Participation in daily life	Creating sensory supportive environments to promote participation	• Chapter 9: Sensory Processing and the Lived Sensory Experience • Chapter 31: The Home Environment: Permanent Supportive Housing • Chapter 36: Early Intervention: A Practice Setting for Early Childhood Mental Health • Chapter 38: Early Psychosis Programs for Adolescents and Young Adults • Chapter 41: State Hospitals
Sensory Rooms/ Sensory Diet	Self-regulation	Using sensory stimuli to meet unique sensory needs. In treatment settings, a room or objects are available that contain calming sensory input; individuals can use the room whenever they feel agitated, angry, frustrated, and so on	• Chapter 9: Sensory Processing and the Lived Sensory Experience • Chapter 41: State Hospitals
Shared Decision-Making	Professional reasoning	Process for partnering with the person receiving services to make decisions about care	• Chapter 6: Evidence-Based Practice
Skills for Safer Living	Reducing suicide risk	Cognitive behavioral and dialectical behavioral strategies to describe feelings as an alternative to suicidal thinking	• Chapter 44: Addressing Suicide Across the Continuum
Sleep Hygiene Education	Sleep	Develop and monitor routines and create an environment that promotes sleep	• Chapter 52: Sleep
Social Network Sites	Connection and communication with others	Websites or apps that allow users to communicate	• Chapter 33: Virtual Environments
Social Skills Training and Cognitive Behavioral Social Skills Training	Social skills	Behavioral and learning theories used with feedback and practice to teach social skills	• Chapter 13: Communication and Social Skills
Social Stories	Social skills	Stories are used to introduce and teach appropriate behaviors for specific situations	• Chapter 13: Communication and Social Skills
$teps for Achieving Financial Empowerment (SAFE)	Money management	Education and skills training related to financial independence	• Chapter 46: Activities of Daily Living, Instrumental Activities of Daily Living, and Health Management Occupations
Stress Management and Resiliency Training	Resilience and coping strategies	A manualized intervention using mindfulness and cognitive retraining	• Chapter 10: Coping and Resilience
Supported Education	Adult education	Support and skills training to enable engagement in postsecondary education	• Chapter 38: Early Psychosis Programs for Adolescents and Young Adults • Chapter 47: Student

Approach	Target(s) of Intervention	Brief Synopsis	Chapters With Additional Information
Supported Employment	Work	Rapid placement in competitive employment consistent with person's preferences with on-the-job training and follow along supports as long as necessary	• Chapter 14: Time Use and Habits • Chapter 38: Early Psychosis Programs for Adolescents and Young Adults • Chapter 48: Work and Volunteer Occupations
Supported Housing/Permanent Supportive Housing	Independent living	Adaptations, supports, and skills training to facilitate successful home management and independent living	• Chapter 31: The Home Environment: Permanent Supportive Housing
Supported Self-Management	Pain and chronic disease management	Teaching skills for daily management of symptoms	• Chapter 15: Pain
Supported Volunteering	Volunteer work	Mentorship with clear guidelines and skills training for specific volunteer positions	• Chapter 48: Work and Volunteer Occupations
Support Groups	Social and spiritual connections	People with shared experience offering support and counseling	• Chapter 53: Spiritual Occupations
Telehealth	Access to services	Method of delivering services virtually	• Chapter 33: Virtual Environments • Chapter 36: Early Intervention: A Practice Setting for Early Childhood Mental Health
Therapeutic Writing and Other Creative Media	Coping methods and personal understanding and coming to terms with trauma	Use of writing (e.g., journaling) and other creative media (e.g., painting, dance, and music) to explore losses and sources of resilience	• Chapter 10: Coping and Resilience • Chapter 12: Emotion Regulation
The WORKS	Work	Workshop approach to address process of pursuing and attaining vocational aspirations	• Chapter 48: Work and Volunteer Occupations
This Is My Brave	Public stigma	Storytelling performance by people with lived experience	• Chapter 27: Mental Health Stigma and Sanism
Thought Record	Negative beliefs	Identify situations that prompted negative thoughts and create evidence to counteract thoughts	• Chapter 8: Cognitive Beliefs
Thresholds	Higher education	Mixed model of supported education that provides preparation for college/technical programs	• Chapter 47: Student
Transitional Employment	Work	Time-limited job placements in mainstream workplaces with on-site training and job coach	• Chapter 48: Work and Volunteer Occupations
Trauma-Informed Care/Practice	Honoring a person's trauma history and promoting safety	Acknowledges the prevalence of trauma, creating safe environments, and promoting the individual's resources and resiliency	• Chapter 5: Trauma-Informed Practice • Chapter 12: Emotion Regulation • Chapter 42: Homelessness and Housing Insecurity
Treatment Mall	Life skills and participation in productive activity	A decentralized state hospital program whereby participants create their own schedule from a choice of large selection of treatment groups	• Chapter 41: State Hospitals
Tree Theme Method	Coping with everyday occupations	Uses creative media to tell a story about the self	• Chapter 10: Coping and Resilience
Unstuck and On Target	Executive function	A manualized cognitive intervention with activities designed to improve flexibility and develop scripts and routines.	• Chapter 7: Cognition
Vet to Vet	Support and well-being	Peer providers with lived experience as veterans provide counseling	• Chapter 39: Peer-Led Services
Video and Gaming Systems	Skill development and occupational participation	Use of video and gaming technology as a means of delivering services	• Chapter 33: Virtual Environments • Chapter 46: Activities of Daily Living, Instrumental Activities of Daily Living, and Health Management Occupations
Virtual Reality	Skill development and occupational participation	Use of computer-produced images and sounds representing a place or situation as a means of delivering services	• Chapter 33: Virtual Environments

Continued

Approach	Target(s) of Intervention	Brief Synopsis	Chapters With Additional Information
Warm line	Precrisis support	Phone line managed by peers with a lived experience to offer support	• Chapter 39: Peer-Led Services
Wellness Coach	Wellness/health	A peer provides education and resources to link person to primary care provider and achieve wellness goals	• Chapter 39: Peer-Led Services
Wellness Recovery Action Plan	Wellness/Well-being	A manualized self-management program for identifying goals and strategies to improve health and manage crises	• Chapter 39: Peer-Led Services • Chapter 48: Work and Volunteer Occupations
Whole School Services for Mental Health Promotion	Academic and social participation	Strategies that target the entire student body by creating social, emotional, and physical activities that are enjoyable for all students (e.g., Comfortable Cafeteria, Relaxing Recess)	• Chapter 37: School Mental Health
Wilderness Programs	Enhanced coping, self-confidence, autonomy	Goal-directed challenges in a group setting outdoors	• Chapter 30: Natural Environments
Workplace Mental Health Initiatives	Wellness in the workplace	Promotion of workplace mental health through education, reasonable accommodations, and wellness activities	• Chapter 48: Work and Volunteer Occupations
Zones of Regulation and Alert Program	Develop self-regulation strategies for managing states of alertness	Programs provide systems to help the individual identify state of alertness so that they can apply strategies to achieve the desired level of alertness	• Chapter 9: Sensory Processing and the Lived Sensory Experience • Chapter 12: Emotion Regulation • Chapter 37: School Mental Health

Index of Practice Models and Theories

Although this textbook is organized around the Person-Environment-Occupation (PEO) model, many other practice models and theoretical approaches are also described and referenced throughout the chapters. While compiling this list, it became clear that there was a continuum from broader theories to more specific models of practice, and that distinguishing between the two is sometimes difficult. This list includes theories that provide a framework for understanding phenomena, as well as practice models that describe particular intervention approaches with a theoretical underpinning. The chapter cross references allow the user to find related content about the practice models and theoretical approaches.

Model	Chapters
ABC Model	8
Acceptance and Commitment Therapy (ACT)	8, 12
Action Over Inertia	14, 31, 51
Acute Stress Response (Fight, Flight, Freeze, Fawn)	10
Adult Learning	47
Arts and Crafts Movement	1
Assertive Community Treatment/Program for Assertive Community Treatment	14, 35
Attachment Regulation and Competency Framework	49
Attachment Theory/Psychobiological Attachment Theory	13, 22, 36, 49
Attention Restoration Theory	30
Behavioral Activation	8, 12, 51
Bioecological Systems Theory	36
Biophilia	30
Canadian Model of Occupational Performance and Engagement (CMOP-E)	11, 53
Capabilities, Opportunities, Resources, and Environments (CORE) Approach	28
Care Coordination/Collaborative Care Model	35
Clinical Staging Model	38
Cognitive Adaptation (includes Cognitive Adaptation Training)	7
Cognitive Behavioral Theory	8, 12, 37
Cognitive Disabilities Model	7
Cognitive Disabilities Reconsidered Model	7
Cognitive Functional Therapy	7
Cognitive Orientation to Daily Occupational Performance	7
Cognitive Remediation	7
Community Case Management	35
Cultural Humility	28
Dialectical Behavior Therapy	12
Diathesis Stress Model	10, 23
Do-Live-Well Framework	28
Dunn's Model of Sensory Processing/Sensory Processing	9, 20, 38
Dynamic Interactional Approach	7
Ecological Model of Human Performance (EHP)	11, 36

Continued

Model	Chapters
Positive Behavioral Interventions and Supports	37
Positive Youth Development	37
Posttraumatic Growth	5
Process Model of Emotional Regulation	12
Pryor and Reeder Model of Stigma	27
Psychoeducation	8
Rational Emotive Behavior Therapy	8
Recognize Privilege, Acknowledge Injustice, and Reframe Perspective to Reach Equity (PAIRE) Model	28
Recovery Model	1, 2, 29, 41
Redesigning Daily Occupations	14
Relationships Motivation Theory	50
Relevance Theory	13
Salutogenesis and Sense of Coherence	10
Sanism, Mad Movement, Mad Studies	27
Schema Theory	22
Self-Contained Classroom Model	47
Self-Determination Theory	11
Self-Efficacy Theory	11
Sensory-Based Interventions	9
Sensory Integration	9
Sensory Processing Model	9, 12, 36, 37
SHARE Framework (Lived Sensory Experience)	9
Situated Learning Theory	42
Skills Training	12, 46
Social and Emotional Learning	12, 37
Social Cognition Theory	13
Social Determinants of Health	29, 32, 34, 36
Social Learning Theory	13
Social Skills Training	13
Social Stories	13
Speech Act Theory	13
Stimulus Control Model	52
Strengths-Based Approach	5
Stress Reduction Theory	30
Structured Leisure Participation	37
Supported Education	47
Supported Housing/Permanent Supportive Housing	31
Supported Life Approaches	31
Supported Work/Supported Volunteering	48
Systems of Care	2, 29
Three-Dimensional Spirituality Model	53
Three-Factor Model	52
Transactional Model of Occupation	14
Transactional Model of Stress and Coping	10
Transtheoretical Model (of change)	11
Trauma-Informed Care/Practice	5, 25, 41, 42
Trauma-Informed Oregon	5
Treatment Mall Approach	41
Two-Process Model of Sleep Regulation	52
Value and Meaning in Occupation Model	51
Von du Toit Model of Creative Ability	51
Wraparound Model	2, 29

ABC model—from Albert Ellis's Rational Emotive Behavior Therapy, the idea that activating events lead to beliefs that result in consequences (feelings and behaviors).

Acceptance—accepting people as they are; this includes absolute worth, or the sincere belief and respect for a person's natural desire to change in a positive direction. It also includes empathy, or the practitioner's capacity to take the person's perspective and collaborate truthfully with them.

Access to housing—a core element of permanent supportive housing that is intended to make housing available by addressing both the discriminatory protections that have been established and the readiness perspective maintained by older housing models.

Accommodations—changes that allow greater access to successful participation.

Acculturation—a multidimensional process that occurs when people from different cultural groups have continuous contact, which results in changes to cultural norms, values, language, attitudes, behaviors, cognition, and identities in either or both groups.

Acquired physical disability—a wide range of disabilities that can result from trauma or disease, including but not limited to spinal cord injuries, traumatic brain injuries, stroke, and significant musculoskeletal injuries such as limb amputation, multiple trauma, and burn injuries.

Active leisure—activities, sports, or hobbies where the individual exerts physical or mental energy.

Activities of daily living (ADLs)—the simple and not-so-simple things that individuals do every day to care for themselves.

Activity scheduling—the process of arranging activities so that one has a balance of work, restoration, and leisure.

Activity space—the physical area that people traverse as they engage in daily activities.

Acute pain—a type of pain that comes quickly, can be severe, but lasts a relatively short time. Often caused by tissue irritation or damage in relation to injury, disease, disability, or medical procedures.

Acute stress—the type of stress that comes and goes quickly.

Adaptation—the achievement of a good fit between a person and their environment.

Adaptation energy—as defined in the Occupational Adaptation Model, this is the amount of resources one expends to engage in occupations.

Adaptive paranoia—refers to a healthy suspicion in Black individuals that develops because of police profiling and experiences of racism in everyday environments.

Adaptive response behaviors—the third and final piece of the adaptive response generation subprocess.

Adaptive response mechanism—as defined in the Occupational Adaptation Model, this is the response to challenge that is classified as either primitive (hyperstable), transitional (hypermobile), or blended (mature).

Adaptive response modes—in the Occupational Adaptation framework, behavior is identified as an existing, modified, or new adaptive response mode.

Adjudication—the formal delivery of judgment about whether a law was broken and, if so, the sentence for the person convicted of the crime.

Adverse childhood experiences (ACEs)—potentially traumatic events experienced before the age of 18 that may include physical, sexual, or emotional abuse; parental divorce; domestic violence; or the incarceration of a parent.

Aesthetic—repeated sensory experiences that are coupled with memories and can create preferences and orientations to the world.

Affirmations—written or oral statements that confirm or reinforce something as true and are a form of positive self-talk that helps to counteract negative self-scripts or beliefs.

Agoraphobia—symptoms of marked fear or anxiety in at least two of the following five situations—using public transportation, being in open spaces (e.g., parking lots and marketplaces), being in enclosed spaces (e.g., shops and theaters), standing in line or being in a crowd, and being outside the home alone.

Alert Program—a program that helps children manage their levels of alertness or arousal; uses the metaphor of "How does your engine run?"

Alexithymia—difficulty with awareness of emotions.

Allodynia—pain caused by a stimulus that does not normally provoke pain.

Alterations in arousal and reactivity—being irritable and having angry outbursts, behaving recklessly and self-destructively, being hypervigilant, being easily startled, or having difficulty concentrating or sleeping.

Americans with Disabilities Act of 1990—a landmark civil rights law passed to address the basic human rights of people living with disabilities. The law is meant to protect people from discrimination based on disability in employment, state and federal government services, commercial facilities, telecommunications, and transportation.

Amplitude—refers to a sound's loudness and is measured by the height of a sound wave.

Amygdala—part of the brain associated with emotional responses and the consolidation of memories.

Analysis of occupational performance—the evaluative process of determining the barriers and facilitators of occupational performance.

Analysis of occupational performance issues—during the analysis of occupational performance, the occupational therapist elicits more targeted information regarding the performance skills and patterns, person factors, activity demands, and contextual barriers that may need intervention to facilitate successful work participation.

Anchoring and adjustment heuristic—a decision-making strategy that involves starting with a primary piece of information and then making adjustments with additional information.

Anhedonia—absence of pleasure from those activities that would ordinarily be enjoyable.

Animal hoarding—a type of hoarding disorder in which the individual accumulates animals while failing to provide minimal standards of care.

Anorexia nervosa (AN)—a condition characterized by extremely low weight, a fear of gaining weight, and a distorted body image.

Anorexia nervosa, binge-eating/purging type—a subtype of AN in which the individual counteracts excessive eating by self-induced vomiting or other means of purging the food.

Anorexia nervosa, restricting type—a subtype of AN in which the individual severely limits their food intake.

Anticipatory beliefs—an expectation of reward.

Antiracism—actively working to dismantle and eliminate racism nationally, locally, and in interactions with individuals people treat and those they encounter and work with.

Antisocial personality disorder—a condition characterized by a pervasive pattern of disregard for, and a violation of, the rights of others.

Anxiety—an emotion that can range from relatively mild feelings of uneasiness to immobilizing terror.

Anxious distress—a subtype of major depressive disorder with high levels of anxiety symptoms.

Apps—abbreviated term for applications, which are software programs designed to perform a specific function for a user. They are typically used in smartphones, tablets, and computers to run software.

Arts and crafts movement—an aesthetic development in the late 19th and early 20th centuries in reaction to the Industrial Revolution that strove for a greater emphasis and appreciation for decorative arts.

Assessment research—a type of evidence that examines the reliability, validity, and other psychometric properties of assessments.

Assistive technology—any item, piece of equipment, or product system, whether acquired commercially off the shelf, modified, or customized, that is used to increase, maintain, or improve functional capabilities of individuals with disabilities.

Assistive technology resource center (ATRC)—a center designed to demonstrate assistive technology resources to consumers that offers the opportunity to loan devices to determine whether they will fit the consumer's needs.

Assistive technology service—any service that provides an individual with a disability who uses an assistive technology device with assistance in the selection, acquisition, or use of an assistive technology device.

At risk—refers to children who are more likely to develop a delay if early intervention services were not provided.

Attachment theory—posits that the initial emotional and physical connection between an infant and a primary caregiver has a long-lasting impact on the individual's personal growth into adulthood.

Attention—efficiently using cognitive resources to take in the information needed to accomplish a task.

Attention restoration theory—explains the ability of the brain to relax in nature and thereby reduce stress and anxiety.

Attentional deployment—describes how individuals pay attention to aspects of the situation that trigger a specific emotional response.

Attenuated psychotic symptoms (APSs)—psychotic symptoms that are below the threshold required for diagnosis.

Atypical features—a subtype of depression characterized by an improvement in mood with positive events, excessive sleep, an increase in appetite, leaden paralysis, worsening of symptoms at night, and rejection sensitivity.

Audio Visual Assisted Therapy Aid for Refractory (AVATAR) therapy—therapist-assisted computerized treatment program designed to target distressing auditory verbal hallucinations (voices) in participants whose symptoms have typically been resistant to medication.

Audit trails—the process of creating documentation of the data collection process in qualitative research.

Auditory system—important for locating objects in the environment and plays a critical role in detecting and deciphering the auditory stimuli that constitute speech including variations in tone that also communicate meaning.

Automatic thoughts—mental activity that comprises the outermost or surface level of a person's thoughts that occur in response to an event or action.

Autonomy—capacity of the person for self-direction and the making of their own choices as opposed to authority, in which the therapist tells the person what to do.

Availability heuristic—a decision-making strategy whereby people estimate frequency or make decisions based on how easy it is to think of an example.

Avoidance—a coping method that involves withdrawal, distraction, use of substances, or other methods of staying away from a stressor.

Avoidant personality disorder—a condition characterized by a pervasive pattern of social inhibition, feelings of inadequacies and hypersensitivity, criticism, and rejection.

Avoidant/restrictive food intake disorder (ARFID)—a disorder of restricting food intake because of the perception of food as unappetizing, uninteresting, or because of the fear of an aversive consequence of eating.

Avolition—a decrease in motivation to initiate and perform self-directed purposeful activities.

Becoming—relates to a person's sense of future or potential, transformation, and self-actualization. Practitioners can explore the process of occupational adaptation and the influence of the person's context on their capacity to engage in valued well-being occupations.

Behavioral activation (BA)—a strategy that aims to increase engagement in positive activity, counteract avoidance behavior, and increase the individual's access to positive reinforcers.

Behavioral approach system (BAS)—activated in response to a desirable stimulus; the BAS is activated when the person experiences a rewarding event, and deactivated when rewards are lost or when failures occur.

Behavioral experiments (BEs)—a collaborative strategy in which the therapist and person create opportunities for the person to actively test thoughts, attitudes, beliefs, and related behaviors as part of discovering their relative utility or validity.

Being—a person's state that allows for reflection, contemplation, and discovery. Practitioners can consider the person's performance of well-being occupations, including values, motivations, and roles associated with the occupation.

Being at home—being in an environment that is stable and a safe place to live.

Belonging—being a member of a group or organization. Practitioners can explore the person's connectedness to others in their family, friends, and people in the wider community associated with the well-being occupations.

Binge-eating disorders—a condition characterized by eating large amounts of food along with the feeling of being unable to control the eating.

Binocular vision—ability in which the visual field of each eye overlaps and enables humans to see depth and three-dimensional images.

Biophilia—an instinctive bond that humans develop with other living organisms; a propensity to affiliate with the natural world.

Biosocial theory of borderline personality disorder—asserts that this personality disorder is primarily characterized by emotional dysregulation, which emerges from transactions between individuals with biological vulnerabilities (poor impulse control and emotional sensitivity) and specific environmental influences of repeated invalidation experiences associated with the expression of emotions.

Bipolar disorder—a mood disorder characterized by the elevated, elated, and energized mood of mania; frequently, but not always, includes episodes of depression.

Bipolar I disorder—characterized by one or more manic episodes or mixed episodes (i.e., frequent fluctuations between low and expansive mood).

Bipolar II disorder—characterized by one or more major depressive episodes and at least one hypomanic episode.

Board and care home—a living arrangement often within someone's home that provides shelter, food, and 24-hour supervision or protective oversight and personal care services to residents.

Body dysmorphic disorder—a condition characterized by a preoccupation with perceived flaws or defects in physical appearance that are not apparent to others.

Body posture—nonverbal means of conveying emotion or adding emphasis to the verbal language tools people use to communicate; the position of one's body in space.

Bolstering—effect that occurs when people act to maintain mental health despite a crisis.

Borderline personality disorder (BPD)—personality disorder most associated with emotional dysregulation; individuals with BPD have difficulties with emotional sensitivity, greater intensity of negative emotions, greater lability of negative emotions, a lack of appropriate regulation strategies, and an excess of maladaptive regulation strategies.

Borderline personality organization—characterized by identity diffusion, severe distortions in interpersonal relations, lack of direction in life goals and work, manifestations of primitive defensive mechanisms, lack of anxiety tolerance, difficulties in impulse control, and

varying degrees of superego deterioration (antisocial behavior).

Bouncing back—recovering from adversities or adapting and "bouncing back" to previous levels of health.

Buffering—effect that occurs when positive emotions, processes, conditions, and/or relationships act to lessen the chance of psychological illness during a crisis.

Building—effect that occurs after facing adversity in which the individual responds in a positive transformative way that builds new processes and outlooks.

Bulimia nervosa—a condition characterized by a distorted body image and periods of overeating followed by purging.

Capacity—the sum total of resources and abilities that a patient can draw on; it includes physical, mental, social, financial, personal, and environmental domains.

Care coordination—deliberately organizing care activities and sharing information among all the participants concerned with a person's care to achieve safer and more effective care.

Case control design—a type of research design that examines risk factors by comparing people with and without a condition.

Case management—a person-centric, collaborative process of assessment, planning, facilitation, and advocacy to meet the individual's health needs and promote population health management goals.

Catastrophizing—making unrealistic and excessive negative self-statements in response to pain. It is related to poorer outcomes including greater pain intensity, greater psychological distress, decreased functional independence, depression, and psychosocial dysfunction.

Catatonia—specifier that is applied when the individual experiences marked psychomotor disturbances and exhibits symptomology such as, but not limited to, stupor, mutism, negativism, or agitation.

Categorization—the cognitive process of organizing items into groups.

Ceiling effect—an assessment in which the scoring is flawed such that many individuals receive the highest score possible.

Central coherence—the ability to take in data and assess the gestalt or big picture meaning.

Central executive network—use of cortical regions for sustained attention, problem-solving, and working memory, also known as executive functions.

Choice of housing—a core element of permanent supportive housing. It distinguishes permanent supportive housing from other approaches by its fundamental commitment to providing consumers with a personal choice of living arrangements such as the neighborhood in which they wish to reside and the particular dwelling.

Chronic diseases—medical conditions that are ongoing, lasting for a year or longer, and limit engagement in activities of daily living.

Chronic health conditions—disease processes that generally persist over the course of a lifetime and include conditions such as diabetes, heart disease, chronic lung disease, cancer, and arthritis.

Chronic homelessness—when a person has been unhoused for 1 year or multiple episodes within a 3-year period.

Chronic pain—pain that persists beyond its typical course of recovery; chronic pain does not appear to serve a biological purpose and is often experienced in the presence of minimal or no apparent tissue damage.

Cilia—microscopic hairlike structures in the inner ear that send sound waves to the brain for interpretation.

Circadian system—process C of the sleep–wake cycle; the body's "internal clock" or pacemaker, which operates on a 24-hour schedule.

Civil commitment—when an individual is court-ordered to be treated for mental illness against their wishes after being deemed a danger to themself or others.

Clinical high risk—someone at high risk for psychosis and who experiences a brief intermittent psychotic episode, or has a significant decline in functioning, or a close relative with a psychotic disorder.

Clinical recovery—method focused on reducing the symptoms associated with the disorder.

Clinical staging model—breaks down early psychosis into stages (0–4), from high risk with no symptoms and seeking help, to severe and persistent mental illness, and is meant to inform appropriate interventions based on each stage.

Clubhouse programs—community-based centers that offer members opportunities for employment, housing, education, and medical and psychiatric services.

Cochlea—fluid-filled, spiral-like structure in the inner ear that responds to vibration from sounds by producing nerve impulses.

Cognition—mental processes that are associated with perceiving, making sense of, and using information.

Cognitive adaptation—strategies that adapt the environment or task to compensate for cognitive impairments.

Cognitive Adaptation Training (CAT)—an intervention that uses changes to the environment, assistive technology, and other compensatory strategies to enable the adaptive behaviors needed to complete activities of daily living and instrumental activities of daily living; uses a different set of strategies for apathetic versus disinhibited behaviors.

Cognitive-Behavioral Social Skills Training (CBSST)—a manualized intervention designed to improve cognition and facilitate the acquisition of social skills for individuals with schizophrenia.

Cognitive Behavioral Therapy (CBT)—an active, problem-oriented intervention that seeks to identify and change maladaptive beliefs, attitudes, and behaviors that contribute to emotional distress.

Cognitive beliefs—mental system that an individual holds to be true to evaluate themself, others, and the environment.

Cognitive Disabilities Model—a hierarchical model used to create interventions in which individuals with cognitive impairments can be successful. Modifications to the activity and environment form the basis for intervention.

Cognitive Disabilities Model for Dementia—focuses on the individual's capacities and strengths to promote the highest level of functioning for people with dementia. It is based on Allen's Cognitive Levels.

Cognitive-Functional (Cog-Fun) Therapy—designed to help young people with attention deficit hyperactivity disorder acquire executive strategies and self-efficacy so that they can engage more successfully in occupational performance. It is a manualized intervention that uses four main change mechanisms: (1) metacognitive learning, (2) environmental supports, (3) occupation-centered assessment and intervention, and (4) positive engagement.

Cognitive functions—mental processes used for reasoning such as planning, mental flexibility, judgment and impulse control, perspective taking, attention, and memory; they contribute to an individual's ability to communicate socially.

Cognitive load—the amount of information working memory can handle at any given time.

Cognitive neuroscience—supports the argument that the quality and type of environment affect human health and well-being, can reduce stress and anxiety, and impact human behavior and performance.

Cognitive Orientation to Daily Occupational Performance (CO-OP)—an occupational therapy model that uses an individualized approach to help the person problem-solve the steps needed to perform a desired occupation.

Cognitive reappraisal—refers to deliberately challenging and reinterpreting people's automatic emotional response to a situation.

Cognitive remediation—an intervention aimed at improving or restoring specific cognitive skills, such as attention, memory, and problem-solving, so that the individual can more successfully engage in everyday occupations.

Cognitive restructuring methods—any psychological method used to remove negative thoughts or irrational roadblocks that harm a person's emotional health and replace those thoughts with neutral or more positive perspectives.

Collaborative care—situation in which patients are getting services from a specialist who collaborates with their primary care physician to provide care to the patient.

Combat and Operational Stress Control (COSC) Unit—battlefield military mental health-care setting that provides restoration, reconditioning, reconstitution, and stabilization focusing on returning service members to duty.

Combat Operational Stress Reaction (COSR)—temporary behavioral, cognitive, emotional, and physical changes resulting from the experiences or consequences of repeated exposure to a single stressor, or multiple stressors, in combat or noncombat operational settings.

Community—a term oriented to people and relationships. The people and relationships that comprise a community may be in one's neighborhood, but may also be located in other neighborhoods, regions, or beyond.

Community development—a process that promotes social justice and economic opportunity by involving community members to participate in the process.

Community integration—when individuals with psychiatric conditions or other disabilities are part of the day-to-day life of their community.

Compassion—an essential component of the spirit of Motivational Interviewing; a compassionate attitude is the therapist's genuine dedication to promote and prioritize the person's welfare and well-being.

Compassion fatigue—also known as caregiver burnout, it is characterized by a state of physical, emotional, and mental exhaustion in response to the unending demands of caring for a dependent family member. Compassion fatigue can also be experienced by individuals in the helping professions.

Compensatory approach—intervention approach whereby the therapist adapts the environment, task, or teaching method to compensate for an impairment.

Competence—a belief in an individual's own capability, which motivates them to act, similar to self-efficacy.

Comprehensibility—the degree to which a situation is understandable and predictable for the person.

Compulsions—repetitive behaviors or mental acts that are done in response to an obsessive thought.

Concept formation—learning to conceive and respond in terms of abstract ideas based on an action or object.

Conduct disorder—a condition seen in children who engage in deceit, theft, and other serious violations of conduct.

Cones—sensors on the retina that allow for the perception of color and produce sharp images in bright light.

Confirmability—the process of verifying qualitative data.

Connection or relatedness—the need to experience a sense of belonging and connectedness to other people.

Construct validity—when an assessment measures the construct it is intended to measure.

Consultant—a person who provides expert advice to an individual or organization.

Context—refers to the environmental conditions surrounding a person.

Co-occupation—refers to two people performing a task, each influencing the other, involving aspects of shared physicality, shared emotionality, shared communication, and shared intentionality.

Co-occurring disorder (COD)—the condition of having one or more substance-use disorders or one or more mental disorders.

Coping—used more specifically to describe the explicit actions taken by individuals as they encounter difficult conditions in their daily lives; occurs in response to situations that are perceived as relevant or vital to an individual's well-being.

Core beliefs—deep level beliefs that describe how the individual sees the self, the world, and others.

Core cognitive distortions—errors in thinking that reflect dysfunctional cognitive beliefs.

Correctional officer (CO)—a person who maintains custody and security of justice-involved individuals, usually within the confines of a correctional institution.

Correlational study designs—a type of research design that describes the relationship between two or more variables that are associated with each other.

Co-teaching—involves two or more school providers providing instruction.

Creative—an ability to think and respond in new ways.

Creativity—the innate capacity to think and act in original ways, to be inventive, to be imaginative, and to find new and original solutions to needs, problems, and forms of expression.

Credibility—refers to the integrity of qualitative data; the data accurately reflects the reality of the participants.

Criminal justice system—typically includes law enforcement agencies, courts, lawyers, and institutions to supervise and detain individuals who are convicted of crimes and to provide rehabilitation that may prevent future crimes.

Cross-sectional—data that is collected at one point in time.

Cultural hegemony—refers to the idea that in a culturally diverse society the ruling class dominates and shapes culture and ideology through social structures, systems, and institutions to ensure that their worldview (e.g., beliefs, perceptions, values, mores) are the accepted cultural norm.

Cultural humility—refers to both attitudes and processes that are grounded in a respectful approach toward others. It requires practitioners to employ critical reflexivity, challenge their biases, recognize and address power differentials between themselves and those they work with, and engage in life long learning and reflective practice.

Culturally responsive practice—a practice that creates a supportive, inviting environment where persons, particularly those who have been marginalized, feel a sense of belonging.

Cyclothymic disorder—a chronic (at least 2-year period) mood disturbance that is characterized by fluctuating hypomanic symptoms and depressive symptoms that are not of sufficient number or severity to reach the criteria for either manic episodes or major depressive episodes.

Dayroom—a common space or community room in the hospital that encourages socialization and relaxation; the dayroom has a daily schedule of activities to provide structure and therapeutic engagement, including group treatment, social interactions, and leisure activities for the individual.

Decent, safe, and affordable housing—a core element of permanent supportive housing that addresses the critical importance of the quality of the living environment to recovery, as well as how the common experience of poverty can make this element of supportive housing so challenging to achieve.

Decision-making—process of making choices when several options are available.

Deep brain stimulation—a treatment for which a device is implanted in the brain that generates electrical impulses to specific brain regions.

Deep pressure—tactile sensory input such as firm holding, hugging, and squeezing that provides a calming sensation by activating the parasympathetic nervous system.

Deep processing—finding meaning in facts, which results in better remembering.

Default mode network—brain areas that are activated during wakeful rest when people are not actively engaged in a specific task.

Deflection—typically occurs before a person is arrested or has contact with the justice system. Intended to provide a path for treatment that averts the need for action by law enforcement agencies.

DEI—abbreviation that stands for diversity, equity, and inclusion.

Deinstitutionalization—the process by which long-term hospitals for persons living with mental illness and other disabling conditions were closed beginning in the 1980s to the present day. Before this event, persons living with mental illness and other disabling conditions were largely cared for in long-term (i.e., potentially decades) institutional settings. This approach was abandoned in favor of community-based models of care.

Delusions—distortions in thought or false beliefs.

Department of Housing and Urban Development (HUD)—federal agency that serves as the primary source of public funds for financing new housing construction and rehabilitation of existing properties and provides rental assistance in the United States.

Dependability—the stability of qualitative data over time and conditions.

Dependent personality disorder—condition characterized by a pervasive and excessive need to be taken care of that leads to submissive and clinging behaviors and the fear of separation.

Depression—a temporary mood state or chronic mental disorder characterized by feelings of sadness, loneliness, despair, low self-esteem, and self-reproach; accompanying signs may include psychomotor retardation or less frequently agitation, withdrawal from social contact, and vegetative states such as loss of appetite and insomnia.

Depressive episode—the period characterized by a depressed mood and loss of interest or pleasure in life activities for at least 2 weeks.

Diabetes distress—the emotional response to the stress of managing and living with diabetes, including treatment, symptoms, and the social impact of chronic illness.

Diagnostic overshadowing—overfixation on the mental condition resulting in overlooking symptoms or concerns related to other medical conditions.

Dialectic—the core of Dialectical Behavior Therapy; it involves considering and integrating contradictory facts and ideas.

Diathesis stress model—a psychological theory that attempts to explain psychiatric conditions as the result of an interaction between a susceptible biological vulnerability and environmental stress.

Diathesis stress theory—originally used to explain schizophrenia but since applied to other psychiatric conditions; proposes that exposure to stress and a biological predisposition are necessary for the expression of a condition.

Direct service provider—an occupational therapy practitioner whose primary role is to provide services directly to the person. The interventions can include the full scope of interventions, including individual and group sessions, that address the occupational needs identified by the people on their caseload.

Discriminant validity—when an assessment is capable of distinguishing groups of individuals in the expected direction.

Discriminative touch—light touch that indicates to the individual where they are being touched and what they are touching.

Disruptive mood dysregulation disorder—symptoms of the disorder present as persistent irritability and frequent episodes of extreme behavior dysregulation.

Diversion—typically occurs after a person is arrested and can take place before charges are filed, before a person appears in court, and before adjudication. Individuals complete work, rehabilitation, or educational diversion programs instead of being incarcerated.

Divided attention—the ability to focus on more than one task at a time.

Doing—acting on the environment and interacting with other people.

Double depression—a combination of major depressive disorder and persistent depressive disorder.

Drug court—a specialized court for individuals with substance use disorders who commit crimes. The court partners with providers offering drug treatment and rehabilitation services and the person may be diverted from incarceration and/or serve reduced jail time.

Duration of untreated psychosis (DUP)—the period of time between a person beginning to experience psychotic symptoms and the initiation of treatment.

Dysesthesia—unpleasant abnormal sensations that can become intense and/or painful.

Eardrum—body part that separates the outer ear from the middle ear; it vibrates in response to sound waves and transfers vibrations to the bones of the middle ear.

Early intervention—a multidisciplinary, coordinated, natural environment-based system for young children birth to 3 years old who have developmental delays or specific health conditions. Services address developmental delays and at-risk situations of the child or family. These services are provided under Part C of the Individuals with Disabilities Education Act.

Early psychosis programs—programs designed to provide early intervention during either the prodrome period or the first episode psychosis period and promote improved functional status and improve lifelong functioning.

Early relational health—a framework that explores the role of early relationships and experiences in healthy development across a child's lifetime.

Eating disorders—conditions in which eating habits or behaviors are influenced by thoughts and feelings about weight and body shape.

Ecological systems theory—theory that looks at health behaviors and conditions within the context of a system of relationships in a person's environment. A person's environment is proposed to include complex "layers"—intrapersonal, interpersonal, communities and organizations, policies and laws, and socioenvironmental context—each of which has an impact on health outcomes.

Ecosocial occupational therapy—the intersection between occupation, occupational justice, and ecology.

Efficacy research—studies that examine the usefulness of an intervention.

Eight dimensions of wellness—emotional/mental, environmental, financial, intellectual, occupational, physical, social, and spiritual.

Electroconvulsive therapy—a treatment in which electricity is used to induce a seizure.

Embodied and emplaced—as a person repeatedly performs occupations in similar contexts, recurring sensory experiences become embodied as sensory expectations.

Emotion—reflects subjective thoughts that are associated with expressive behaviors, including the facial expressions people make and the words that they say, as well as physiological and neurological changes. It is dependent on the person's mood, relationships, and circumstance.

Emotion dysregulation—emotional responses that are not adaptive to the particular situation.

Emotion-focused coping—managing the feelings provoked by a crisis.

Emotion perception—the recognition and interpretation of emotional signals that make up social communication.

Emotion regulation—actions or behaviors an individual uses to identify, manage, and express feelings while engaging in activities or interacting with others.

Emotion-regulation failures—occur when an individual fails to engage in a strategy that would be helpful in the situation, resulting in behaviors such as acting out or behavioral problems.

Emotional dysregulation—responses that are not adapted to fit the situation.

Emotional function—necessary for communication and socialization and includes emotion perception, empathy, and emotional regulation.

Emotional misregulation—occurs when an individual uses an emotional regulation strategy that is poorly matched to the current situation.

Emotional performance—identified as a person factor relevant to occupational therapy practice and includes the regulation and range of emotions, appropriateness of emotions, and lability of emotions.

Emotional regulation—ability to maintain control over one's emotional state and emotional expression.

Empathic inquiry—a type of interviewing style that seeks to understand a person's experiences, concerns, and perspectives. A way of communicating compassionately and prioritizing making human connections during interactions between a health-care professional and an individual seeking services.

Empathy—a complex construct of emotion perception that encompasses the ability of a person to perceive emotion in both themselves and other people, the ability to understand what another person is thinking or feeling, self-awareness, and the ability to regulate one's own emotional state.

Enacted togetherness—highlights the sociocultural dimensions of occupation and denotes an opportunity for meaning-making via emerging narratives that are generated in the context of *doing* together.

Engagement in occupation—performance of occupations as the result of choice, motivation, and meaning within a supportive context (including environmental and personal factors).

Environment—refers to the surroundings where an individual operates.

Environmental contexts—external conditions or surroundings in which an individual lives or works.

Environmental press—the demands that the environment places upon the individual.

Epidemiology—branch of medicine that studies the factors that contribute to the presence or absence of medical and psychiatric conditions or events.

Episodic memory—the ability to recall events that have happened to the individual. Episodic memory is organized temporally, or by when it occurred.

Errorless learning—an approach to learning new information that avoids making mistakes, compensates for self-monitoring problems, and prevents intrusive errors.

Evaluate the evidence—the process of assessing the quality of a study or studies to determine the strength of the research evidence.

Evaluation—the process of data gathering.

Every Student Succeeds Act (ESSA)—passed in 2015, the ESSA is the primary education law in the United States. The intent of the law is to support innovation in education and to provide evidence for high-quality, evidence-based education programs.

Everyday creativity—a phenomenon in which a person habitually responds to daily tasks in an original and meaningful way; everyday creativity can either be a creative product or a creative experience.

Evidence-based medicine—the use of the current best evidence to make the best medical decisions for a patient.

Evidence-based practice—the use of the current best evidence to make the best practice decisions for an individual.

Evocation—during Motivational Interviewing, eliciting from the person their own goals and values toward change.

Excoriation disorder—condition in which skin picking is used as a coping mechanism to reduce anxiety and create a sense of relief.

Executive function—a cognitive system that controls and manages other cognitive processes and includes higher order processes such as planning, cognitive flexibility, problem-solving, and abstract thinking.

Exosystem—component of the Ecological Systems Model that the individual does not directly interact with but still has an impact on the individual such as a neighborhood, friends' parents, and mass media.

Experimental designs—a type of research design that includes random assignment to an experimental and control group for the purpose of determining whether the intervention caused the outcome.

Expresses emotions—identified as a necessary social interaction performance skill that is defined as displays affect and emotions in a socially appropriate manner.

Facial expression—nonverbal means of conveying emotion or adding emphasis to the verbal language tools people use to communicate; movements of muscles on the face to convey an individual's emotional state.

Facilitative beliefs—attitudes that are permissive and view substance use as acceptable in spite of the potential consequences.

Fair Housing Act (Title VIII of the Civil Rights Act of 1968)—an act of Congress that prohibits discrimination in the sale, rental, and financing of dwellings based on race, color, religion, sex, or national origin.

Family-centered care—a way of providing services that assures the health and well-being of children and their families through respectful family/professional partnerships.

Family-driven—when families are drivers of their own plans and pivotal in shaping agencies and systems.

Family-focused care—taking the perspective of the whole family rather than a collection of individuals.

Family-focused practice—broadens perspectives from a narrow focus on the mental health consumer to one that includes their family and caregivers.

Fawn—a response to threat in which the threatened person tries to please the person who is triggering the fear.

Feelings—conscious mental understanding of an emotional state that occurs when an individual recognizes that their physiology, behavior, and subjective thought processes involve a specific emotion.

Fight—response to fear that involves confronting the threat with a physical reaction.

Filter theory—a model of attention that suggests there is a limit to the amount of information a person can attend to at any one point in time.

First episode psychosis (FEP)—refers to the first time that an individual reaches diagnostic criteria for psychosis and includes the first 2 to 5 years after the diagnosis.

First-generation antipsychotics—the first class of drugs used to treat psychotic symptoms. Also called typical antipsychotics, these medications work as dopamine antagonists.

Flexible, voluntary, and recovery-focused services—a core element of permanent supportive housing that refers to the importance of individualized services that meet the particular needs of the person seeking housing.

Flight—response to fear; avoiding danger when unable to fight.

Floor effect—an assessment that is limited by not allowing for the full range of scores, as too many individuals scored at the bottom range of the scale.

Flourishing—a high level of psychological and social functioning.

Flow—a state of consciousness involving full immersion, focus, and enjoyment that occurs when someone is involved in an activity with high but manageable challenges that requires the full use of their skills.

Focusing events—incidents or a series of incidents that impact a significant group of people and may lead to a response from local, state, or federal governments in the form of policy change.

Forensic commitment—when an individual is court-ordered to be treated for mental illness after being charged with or convicted of criminal behavior related to their mental state.

Framing—the platform by which play is enacted; it sets the ground rules for play; cues that separate play from reality.

Free from unnecessary constraints of reality—individuals leave behind some of the everyday tasks and worries that preclude their engagement; they are free to choose how close to objective reality a transaction will be.

Freeze—response to fear; remaining quiet until the threat has passed.

Frequency—refers to a sound's pitch and is measured by the total number of waves produced in 1 second.

Functional cognition—application of cognition within the context of everyday activities.

Functional recovery—recovery is aimed at improvement in occupational, social, and adaptive functioning.

Functional separation of housing and services—a core element of permanent supportive housing that ensures that the tenant with mental illness is the primary lessee or mortgage holder, not a mental health or social service agency.

Gatekeeper training—an approach to suicide prevention, which teaches gatekeepers (individuals who have primary contact with those at risk for suicide) how to identify people at risk for suicide.

Generalizability—also referred to as external validity, it is the degree to which a study or studies can be applied to different populations.

Generalized anxiety disorder (GAD)—a condition characterized by excessive fear or anxiety about several everyday life circumstances.

Generativity—the different ways people attempt to "leave their mark" on the world, perhaps by creating or nurturing things that will outlast them, caring for others, or contributing to society in a positive way.

Gestures—used to convey emotional state to another individual; movement from part of the body to indicate a desire.

Golgi tendon—organs that provide information at the site where the tendon meets the muscle; they act with muscle spindles to provide proprioceptive information.

Grave disability—when a person is unable to provide for their basic needs because of a mental illness.

Gravely disabled—a legal status used for involuntary mental health hospitalization (definition varies by state), in which a person, because of a mental or physical condition, is unable to provide for their basic personal needs for food, clothing, or shelter.

Grounded theory—a qualitative research design that explores phenomena with the goal of theory development.

Group comparison design—a research design in which at least two groups are compared for differences on some outcome variable(s).

Guided discovery—the process of asking questions that leads to self-awareness.

Habit training—attributed to Eleanor Clarke Slagle as an effort to overcome disorganized habits as a major problem of mental disorders, this process involves exposing persons to a well-balanced day with work, games, and recreation, creating routines that allow the person to return to community life.

Habits—behaviors or patterns of activity that are relatively familiar and may be practically automatic.

Habituation—the internalized patterns or ways people do things and organize their participation.

Halfway house—an institution available for individuals to reintegrate from an institution to the community by learning the necessary skills. This type of housing is temporary.

Hallucinations—distortions in perception.

Harm reduction—practices and policies that reduce the consequences of behaviors such as drug use.

Have housing—housing is available, but conditions are frequently substandard and often temporary.

Health—overcoming or managing one's disease(s) or symptoms.

Health equity—an ideal that strives to ensure that every person, regardless of race, ethnicity, socioeconomic status, disability, gender identity, sexual orientation, geographic location, preferred language, or any other characteristic, has fair and equal access to health care.

Health management—includes activities related to developing, managing, and maintaining health and wellness routines, including self-management, with the goal of improving or maintaining health to support participation in other occupations.

Health navigator—a person trained to help others manage and coordinate their physical health care, mental health care, and wellness needs.

Health promotion—intervention approaches to improve health knowledge, attitudes, skills, and behavior.

Heuristics—simple "rules of thumb" that help people make decisions quickly.

Hidden work—when services are exchanged for cash, goods, or other services but are not reported as income.

Hippocampus—part of the brain associated with emotional responses and the consolidation of memories.

Histrionic personality disorder—a condition characterized by superficial relationships and a desire to be the center of attention.

Hoarding disorder—a condition in which the individual has difficulty discarding their possessions, resulting in the accumulation of excessive clutter.

Holistic—a view that looks at the whole person and considers the mind, body, and spirit.

Home—a stable and safe place to live.

Homeless shelters—a facility that provides temporary and safe housing to individuals experiencing homelessness.

Homelessness—a condition of lacking safe, stable, and affordable housing.

Homework—assignments outside of therapy sessions that encourage individuals to experiment with, apply, practice, and supplement what is addressed in therapy.

Hope—one of the recovery principles; it is a catalyst to recovery and can be fostered by peers, practitioners, and family.

Housed identity—supporting the development of new daily routines that offer structure and are tied to the role of tenant.

Housing First—an approach to permanent supportive housing that provides unconditional, permanent housing as quickly as possible.

Housing First Model—a social services model prioritizing permanent housing over other services.

Housing integration—a core element of permanent supportive housing that ensures that people with a psychiatric diagnosis live alongside individuals without diagnosis, rather than clustered together in predominantly psychiatric communities.

Hyperalgesia—pain caused by a stimulus that does not normally provoke pain.

Hyperresponsive—intense or overexaggerated response to stimuli.

Hypomanic episodes—although similar to manic episodes, with periods of elevated, expansive, or irritable mood, the symptoms are at a lower intensity and without marked impairment in social or occupational functioning.

Hyporesponsive—diminished response to stimuli.

Hypothalamic-pituitary-adrenal (HPA) axis—a regulatory network that includes the hypothalamus, pituitary, and adrenal glands; it operates in response to stress and consists of chemical messengers that prepare the body for the "fight-or-flight response," as well as a return to homeostasis, or relaxation, when the threat has been removed.

Hypotheses testing—the research process of designing a study, collecting data, and analyzing the results to determine whether or not a hypothesis is supported.

Hypothesis—a proposed explanation of facts that has not yet been proved.

Identifying a problem—the first step in evidence-based practice that involves specifying the question to be answered by the available research.

Identifying the relevant evidence—a step in evidence-based practice that involves searching the research evidence for studies that can answer the research question.

Illness burden—impact of medical symptoms such as pain or fatigue.

Implement this information into practice—the step of evidence-based practice that involves applying the evidence to clinical situations.

Incidence—the number of new cases of a condition within a period of time.

Individualized—having a plan based on the specific needs of the individual; resources are generated based on their strengths and needs rather than from a set list of strategies or options to choose from.

Individualized Family Service Plan (IFSP)—a plan of care that identifies the family's resources, desired outcomes for their child, activities to achieve the noted outcomes, developmental strengths and needs of their child, and plans for transition if the child is approaching their third birthday.

Individuals with Disabilities Act—the primary federal education legislation, which governs education for children with disabilities.

Inertia—resistance to changing the way one has been doing things.

Insomnia—a major category of sleep disorders that occurs when an individual has difficulty initiating sleep, maintaining sleep, getting enough sleep, or has impaired sleep quality.

Instrumental activities of daily living (IADLs)—tasks that are not necessary for fundamental functioning and are used to help an individual live independently in a community and move within a community; they include care of others, care of pets and animals, child rearing, communication management, driving and community mobility, financial management, home establishment and management, meal preparation and cleanup, religious and spiritual expression, safety and emergency maintenance, and shopping.

Integrated behavioral health care—the consideration of mental health and substance abuse conditions, along with any other health conditions within the same episode of care, as well as across the person's life span.

Integrated care—patients receive related services such as behavioral health services and physical health services as a routine part of their health care.

Integrated services—involves providing occupational therapy in the student's natural environment, emphasizing nonintrusive methods and common goals.

Intensive individualized interventions—concentrated services that are directed at the specific needs of the individual.

Interactive reevaluation—informal but systematic observation of a person during therapy as part of the ongoing process of assessment.

Interests—things that give an individual pleasure and satisfaction.

Internal control—an individual's feeling of being "in charge" of their actions and at least some aspects of an activity's outcome.

Internal locus of control—the extent to which an individual believes they can influence or make a difference in the circumstances in life.

Internalized stigma—when a person with mental or physical illness comes to believe the assumptions and stereotypes surrounding their disorder.

Interoception—sensory perception of internal bodily states and organ function.

Interprofessional teams—health-care teams that include members from different disciplines who work together toward common goals to meet the needs of a population.

Interrater reliability—the degree to which two or more testers will score an assessment in the same way.

Intersecting identities—concept that an individual's identity is multifactorial and can be impacted by things such as an individual's race, gender, language, sexuality, culture, poverty, employment and housing status, ableism and paternalism; these impact a person's disability experience and human rights, including access to meaningful occupational opportunities and ongoing participation.

Intersectional lens—recognition for how a person's environment and occupational engagement bring into focus all forms of oppression including ableism, ageism, racism, and colonialism.

Intersectionality—addresses how an individual's social, political, and occupational differences may overlap to create systemic oppression and inequities in occupational opportunities.

Intervention—a form of treatment or action that is deliberately taken to prevent or treat a disease.

Intrinsic motivation—behavior that is driven by internal rewards that are naturally satisfying.

Intrusion—intrusive thoughts such as distressing dreams, involuntary memories, or flashbacks of the event.

JEDI—justice, equity, diversity, and inclusion.

Jurisdiction—refers to the court that has the power and authority to make legal decisions and/or the territory where the court exercises these powers.

Just right challenge—a situation in which the task requirements and the individual's performance skills are at the same level.

Languishing—refers to a state in which low levels of subjective well-being are combined with low levels of psychological and social well-being.

Laws—actions that provide legal and institutional frameworks with which to implement policy. Ultimately, laws outline the process of enforcement for public policy.

Leisure—a nonobligatory activity that is intrinsically motivated and engaged in during discretionary time, that is, time not committed to obligatory occupations such as work, self-care, or sleep.

Level I evidence—the highest level of evidence for efficacy research based in systematic reviews with at least two randomized controlled trials.

Level II evidence—the second highest level of evidence for efficacy research derived from randomized controlled trials.

Level III evidence—the third highest level of evidence for efficacy research derived from nonrandomized controlled trials.

Level IV evidence—the fourth highest level of evidence for efficacy research derived from pre- and posttest designs without a control group.

Level V evidence—the fifth highest level of evidence for efficacy research derived from case studies or expert opinion.

Lifestyle balance—a satisfying congruence between actual participation and desired participation of daily occupation that is healthful, meaningful, and sustainable to an individual within the context of their current life circumstances.

Light touch—an alerting stimulus; it can be perceived as painful and bothersome, and might elicit negative emotions.

Linear continuum paradigm—an early model of housing for persons with psychiatric disabilities that provided sequential and graded reintroduction into community life, primarily from institutions. The goal is to match the needs of the consumer with the level of housing.

Lived experience—firsthand accounts based on personal experience.

Lived Sensory Experience—the unique experience of the individual that involves more than one sensation and reflects a dynamic intersection of numerous stimuli that are mutually affecting the person's experience of the stimulus.

Long-term memory—phase of the memory process considered as the permanent storehouse of information that has been registered, encoded, rehearsed, and stored for future retrieval.

Low barrier shelters—a shelter that provides immediate and easy access.

Low registration—a pattern of sensory processing characterized by high threshold and passive response; individuals tend to miss input that others take in, yet they are highly flexible because they are not bothered by sensory stimuli and can typically manage distracting environments well.

Macrosystem—component of the Ecological Systems Model that focuses on the institutions within society such as government, the education system, and the legal system.

Major depressive disorder—characterized by one or more instances of a major depressive episode, but no occurrence of a manic episode.

Major depressive episode—occurs when a depressed mood or absence of interest or engagement in all or mostly all activities occurs almost daily, for at least 2 weeks.

Maladaptive behavior—behaviors that interfere with an individual's ability to engage in their activities of daily living that result from "the just right challenge" not being met.

Maladaptive coping—ineffective coping strategies characterized by an external locus of control, worry, magical thinking (i.e., wishing the problem would just go away), denial, blaming oneself or others, use of escape and avoidance strategies (such as overeating, overdrinking, smoking, or medication), and keeping to oneself.

Manage—handle something with a degree of skill.

Manageability—degree to which a person believes they can handle a situation and have the necessary resources to do so.

Manic episodes—the period characterized by an abnormally elevated, expansive, or irritable mood for at least 1 week, in conjunction with other criteria, such as inflated self-esteem or grandiosity, decreased need for sleep, rapid speech, psychomotor agitation, and involvement in high-risk activities.

Many pathways—recovery pathways are highly personalized. Recovery is nonlinear, characterized by continual growth and improved functioning that may involve setbacks.

Massive open online courses—free web-based distance learning programs that are designed for large numbers of geographically dispersed students.

Massively multiplayer online (MMO) gaming—online video game with a large number of players on the same server.

Mastery—an aspect of self-efficacy that reflects possession of the consummate skill.

Mastery experiences—having a successful experience when engaged in an activity. Mastery experiences lead to a sense of self-efficacy.

Meaningfulness—belief that a situation is worth engaging in and that the person cares about what will happen.

Medicaid—a government-funded health-care program for people with low income that is funded through a combination of state and federal funding. Eligibility for Medicaid varies by state.

Medicaid buy-in program—a program that allows people who would otherwise lose eligibility for Medicaid because of financial gains from employment to maintain coverage by payment of a premium or copayment for services.

Medical respite care programs—acute and postacute medical care for people experiencing homelessness who are too ill or frail to recover from a physical illness or injury on the streets, but who are not ill enough to be in a hospital.

Medicare—a government-funded health insurance program that provides health insurance for all people eligible for Social Security benefits over the age of 65 and to people under the age of 65 with qualifying disabilities.

Medication-assisted treatment (MAT)—a developing approach to substance use disorder (SUD) treatment that supports the safety, health, and well-being of individuals experiencing SUDs; this harm-reduction approach to recovery combines medications with counseling and behavior therapies.

Melancholic—a subtype of depression characterized by anhedonia, early morning awakening, guilt, severe loss of appetite, and depression that is worse in the morning.

Mental functions—cognitive, affective, and perceptual skills that influence performance in occupations.

Mental health—a state of positive emotional, psychological, and social well-being.

Mental health continuum—model that describes the different states of mental health that a person can experience over time.

Mental health court—a specialized court that partners with mental health providers to divert people with severe mental illness from incarceration to judicially supervised programs usually provided in community-based settings.

Mental health prevention—strategies aimed at reducing the incidence and seriousness of problem behaviors and mental health conditions.

Mental health promotion—efforts to support positive mental health, such as developing social, emotional, and coping skills; creating supportive school, home, and community environments; reducing stigma and discrimination, and providing education.

Mental health recovery—a highly individual process of change toward reaching one's full potential and living a self-directed life.

Mental Hygiene Movement—a 20th-century perspective about the responsibility that states and communities have for providing needed services to their citizens with mental health issues.

Mental ill-health—a state of poor mental functioning and performance.

Mental wellness—an asset or resource that enables positive states of well-being and provides the capability for people to achieve their full potential.

Mentalization—the act of understanding the experiences and actions of oneself and others, such as assumptions, attitudes, wishes, hopes, intentions, or plans, consciously or unconsciously.

Mentalizing—a subprocess of social cognition related to understanding the mental states of others; also described as theory of mind.

Mesosystem—component of the Ecological Systems Model that focuses on the interactions of two or more microsystems such as the relationship between a child's home and school environment.

Metacognition—a self-awareness of what one knows and doesn't know. It includes anticipating one's abilities to cognitively manage situations and recognizing errors as they occur.

Metacognitive reasoning abilities—the ability to reflect on and evaluate one's own thinking.

Metacognitive Reflection and Insight Therapy (MERIT)—designed as a metacognitive approach for schizophrenia to improve one's ability to form complex ideas about the self and others; it is focused on the therapeutic relationship as a means for addressing everyday problems.

Microsystem—the center of the Ecological Systems Model that focuses on the individual's immediate setting and persons with which the individual has direct contact such as family, friends, and school.

Military culture—a unique set of values, beliefs, symbols, language, dress, behaviors, relationships, and work that is inherent to service members and veterans, though these elements can vary between military branches.

Military Sexual Trauma (MST)—sexual assault or sexual harassment that occurs during one's military service. Those with MST may experience nightmares and difficulty feeling safe or expressing strong emotions such as anger, self-blame, and reduced self-esteem.

Mindfulness-based cognitive therapy (MBCT)—a modified form of cognitive therapy that integrates mindfulness practices such as breathing exercises and meditation.

Mindfulness-based occupational therapy (MBOT)—an emerging approach that seeks to integrate mindful approaches into occupational therapy practice.

Mindfulness-based stress reduction (MBSR)—a program that supports people with stress, anxiety, depression, and chronic pain and uses a process of focusing on the present in a nonjudgmental way.

Mindfulness meditation—a technique that focuses on the present in a nonjudgmental way, attending to what "is."

Minority stress theory—stigma associated with being in a minority group; results in an increased exposure to stressful life situations.

Mismatch negativity—occurs when a repetitive sound stimulus is interrupted by another sound of different frequency or duration.

Mobile support model—a supported education model in which staff members at community-based mental health centers travel with students to provide assistance at the postsecondary educational sites where the student applies for admission or attends courses.

Modal Model of Emotions—a representation of emotions as a recursive process between the person and situation, with four basic phases of a transactional sequence—situation, attention, appraisal, and response.

Modeling—acquiring and learning a new skill by observing and imitating behavior being performed by another.

Money Follows the Person demonstration project—a program that provides funding specifically for costs associated with transitioning to the community from an institutional setting such as a nursing home.

Mood disorder—an umbrella term that encompasses conditions in which individuals experience an extreme in the continuum of typical moods.

Mood state—a more comprehensive emotional state that persists for a long period of time, such as cheerfulness and depression.

Moral treatment—a philosophy and approach to psychiatric care that emphasizes respect for individuals and improved treatment in psychiatric hospitals.

Multicontext approach—a cognitive intervention focused on strategy training and the ability to use these strategies in real-world occupation participation; it considers the interplay of the person, activity, and environment.

Multitiered approach to mental health—a tiered public health approach for children and youth that prepares *all* school personnel (e.g., teachers, administrators, psychologists, social workers, and related service providers) to proactively address the mental health needs of all students.

Multi-User Virtual Environment (MUVE)—a computer, server, or internet-based virtual environment that can be accessed by multiple users simultaneously.

Muscle dysmorphia—a type of body dysmorphic disorder in which the preoccupation focuses on being insufficiently muscular.

Muscle spindles—body parts that act as sensory receptors and provide information about muscle length and velocity of stretch; they act with Golgi tendons to provide proprioceptive information.

Narcissistic personality disorder—a condition characterized by a pervasive pattern of grandiosity (in fantasy and behavior), need for admiration, and lack of empathy.

Narrative enhancement and cognitive therapy (NECT)—a group-based intervention that uses cognitive behavioral techniques and empowering approaches to reduce the self-stigma associated with mental illness.

Narrative research—a group of approaches that use a person's story or account of experiences or events as the primary data in the research. This type of research often focuses on the experiences of individuals as portrayed in their own words and stories, including visual representations of those experiences.

Nature—the physical world as opposed to human-made creations.

Nature prescribing—a form of drug-free health care that involves recommendations to spend time in nature to improve health.

Negative alterations in cognitions and mood—negative thoughts and feelings such as distorted thoughts, ongoing fear, anger, horror, shame or guilt, decreased interest in activities previously enjoyed, feeling detached from others, or being unable to experience positive emotions.

Negative symptoms—symptoms of schizophrenia characterized by the absence of typical function, such as flat affect, social withdrawal, and difficulty initiating activity.

Neighborhood—conceptualized as the loosely bound physical space that surrounds the area in close proximity to an individual's place of residence.

Neighborhood Profile—an assessment of the physical and social structure of a neighborhood, which can be used to inform neighborhood regeneration efforts.

Nested social systems—the basis of the Ecological Systems Model, which states that there are many influences on an individual such as their microsystem, mesosystem, exosystem, and macrosystem.

Neurodiversity-affirming practice—a strengths-based approach that recognizes the value and uniqueness of neurodivergent individuals.

Neuropathic pain—sensation that arises from an identifiable lesion or disease of the somatosensory system. It can involve peripheral nerve impingement or lesion, spinal cord lesion, and lesions or damage in the somatosensory parts of the cortex.

Neurotic personality organization—less severely impaired personality structure as compared to borderline and psychotic and tends to be characterized by rigidity, self-doubt, and irritability.

Nocebo effect—the adverse effect that follows an inert treatment, diagnosis, education, or care plan because of negative expectations.

Nociception—neural process of encoding noxious stimuli.

Nociceptive pain—arises from actual or threatened damage to nonneural tissue from the activation of nociceptors. Nociceptive pain warns of potential damage.

Nociplastic pain—sensation that arises from altered nociception, despite no clear evidence of actual or threatened tissue damage, causing activation of peripheral nociceptors. It is thought to result from alterations in central nervous system processing.

Nonexperimental—in research, a nonexperimental study is one in which an independent variable such as a participant characteristic, condition, or type of intervention cannot be manipulated and thus cannot provide evidence of change in a dependent variable.

Nonrandomized controlled trial—a type of experimental study in which subjects in the study are assigned to different intervention conditions in a manner that is not random.

Non–rapid eye movement (NREM)—stages 1 to 3 of sleep that do not include rapid eye movement sleep and constitute the greatest proportion of adult human sleep; during NREM sleep, dreaming does not occur, and the body is active.

Not guilty by reason of insanity or guilty except for insanity—a legal finding, depending on the state, indicating an individual is either not responsible for their actions, or lacked the capacity to understand their actions because of a mental illness at the time of the crime.

Nurturing care—a stable environment that promotes health and optimal nutrition, protects children from threats, and provides opportunities for early learning through affectionate interactions and relationships.

Obsessions—recurrent and persistent thoughts, urges, and/or images that are experienced as intrusive and unwanted.

Obsessive-compulsive personality disorder (OCPD)—a condition characterized by a preoccupation with orderliness, perfectionism, and mental and interpersonal control at the expense of flexibility, openness, and efficiency.

Occupational adaptation—the process of internal adaptation that occurs when a person engages in meaningful activity.

Occupational balance—a satisfactory variety of activities and occupations that meet an individual's various needs.

Occupational choice—a recognition that choice can be contextually situated, such that opportunities for occupation are inequitably distributed and influenced by the lifestyles, expectations, resources, and dominant values of social groups in social contexts.

Occupational competence—the degree to which one sustains a pattern of occupational participation that reflects one's occupational identity. Competence appears to begin with organizing one's life to meet basic responsibilities and personal standards and extends to meeting role obligations and then achieving a satisfying and interesting life.

Occupational consciousness—an ongoing awareness of cultural hegemony and recognition that dominant practices are sustained through what people do every day.

Occupational deprivation—a state of prolonged exclusion from engagement in occupations of necessity or meaning because of factors that stand outside the control of the individual.

Occupational enrichment—the deliberate manipulation of environments to aid and support engagement in a range of occupations congruent with those that the individual might normally perform.

Occupational identity—sense of oneself in regard to an occupation (i.e., one's sense of self as a worker).

Occupational load—the number of roles, tasks, and occupations that an individual undertakes in the course of a specific time span.

Occupational possibilities—refers to the idea that occupation is situated. Specifically, that ways and types of doing that are available to a person must be viewed within a sociohistorical and socioenvironmental lens.

Occupational profile—a summary of a person's occupational history, obtained by formal and informal interview techniques, which helps the practitioner develop an understanding of a person's history, life experiences, values, interests, and needs that may be addressed in occupational therapy interventions.

Occupational transition—the process of negotiating life changes.

Occupation-based intervention—approaches that use engagement in occupation as the process or therapeutic agent of change.

Olfactory system—chemical sensory system perceiving smell that is highly connected with the gustatory system.

Olmstead Decision—a ruling of the Supreme Court of the United States which decided that people with disabilities have a right to live and receive services in a community of their choosing.

Olmstead Integration Mandate—based on a Supreme Court ruling, the requirement that individuals with disabilities should be offered community-based housing as opposed to unnecessary institutionalization regardless of cost.

Online self-help support groups—virtual gatherings of people who share common ground in some way and can offer emotional support to one another. Participants may share a similar experience, or they may share a common identity.

Onsite services model—a supported education model in which students attend college courses while simultaneously receiving supported education services in the form of a specialized program, counseling, or a support group. In this model, academic skills such as time management, study skills, reading skills, writing skills, self-advocacy, and access to other services are addressed.

Operant conditioning—an approach developed by B. F. Skinner in which a spontaneously emitted behavior (operant behavior) is either rewarded (reinforced) or punished and then either increases or decreases in frequency, respectively.

Orbitofrontal cortex (OFC)—a key component of the emotional circuit responsible for inhibiting impulsive behaviors, it is associated with insula functioning and the ability to integrate internal feelings with the external context to guide behavior.

Ossicles—three small bones in the middle ear.

Outcome—the result of an intervention. It can be the measurement of whether a program or a specific intervention strategy produced the intended changes.

Overresponsivity—a sensory modulation challenge characterized by having responses to sensory stimuli that can be faster, last longer, or be more intense than the expected sensory responsivity.

Overwhelm—general term often used in health-care settings when persons have difficulty managing the combined challenges of their illness.

Paid work—all forms of employment, including self-employment, usually involving an agreement whereby labor is traded for pay.

Pain—an unpleasant sensory and emotional experience associated with actual or potential tissue damage or described in terms of such damage.

Pain behaviors—what a person says or does—or does not do—which communicates to others the presence of pain.

Pain self-efficacy—beliefs about one's ability to perform a range of tasks despite pain or to cope with pain.

Panic attack—an abrupt surge of intense fear that peaks within minutes and includes physical symptoms such as palpitations, sweating, trembling, chest pain, and nausea.

Panic disorder—a condition diagnosed when an individual experiences recurrent, unexpected panic attacks.

Paranoid personality disorder—a condition characterized by a pervasive lack of trust and suspiciousness of others.

Paresthesia—pain characterized by numbness, tingling, "pins and needles," or electric shocklike pain.

Parole—a period of control and monitoring that occurs after a person's release from incarceration.

Participation—the act of doing the occupation, planning for the occupation, maintaining a balance with other areas of occupation, and obtaining and appropriately using related tools and supplies.

Participatory action research—an approach to research that emphasizes participation and action by individuals and/or members of communities who are affected by that research. The approach gives agency to those being researched by providing meaningful opportunities to be engaged in all parts of the research process from design to analysis and dissemination.

Participatory design workshopping—engaging end users in creative strategies to elicit feedback about their desires and vision for a designed space.

Participatory research—fact-gathering system in which efforts are made to equalize the positions of research and participants; participants take on more of an active role in research and typically use qualitative methods.

Partnership—in the therapeutic relationship, the collaboration between the therapist and person.

Passive leisure—activities in which an individual does not exert physical or mental energy; sometimes referred to as "quiet leisure."

Patient-centered medical home (PCMH)—a primary care model based on patient-centered, coordinated, team-driven care and supported by strong health information technology.

Patient-centered practice/Patient centeredness—a therapeutic relationship in which the person is empowered to act as the primary decision-maker in their treatment.

Patient factors—capacities that reside within the individual that influence their performance in occupations.

Patterns of interest—a preference for certain ways of carrying out activities; for example, a tendency to prefer solitary or social activities or tendency to prefer physical or intellectual activities.

Peer-led services—mental health services in which people in recovery assume a lead role in the development, control, and provision of services. These services are offered by people with a lived experience who are hopeful and open minded, and who seek to facilitate change through person-driven, strengths-focused services.

Peer-mediated interventions (PMIs)—an approach developed to improve the social and communication skills of children with disabilities by training peers to act as models.

Peer respite center—a voluntary, short-term overnight program that provides safe spaces for individuals experiencing a mental health crisis; designed as an alternative to inpatient psychiatric hospitalization.

Peer support—occurs when people provide knowledge, experience, and/or emotional, social, or practical help to each other based upon a shared experience.

Peer support worker (PSW)—individual with lived experience of recovery from a mental health condition, substance use disorder, or both, who is trained to support other individuals and their families in recovery. Also known as a peer support specialist.

Peer-to-peer support—a way of giving and receiving help in which peers provide services to other peers.

Peers for Progress—program designed to accelerate the availability of best practices in peer support, which is done by conducting and disseminating research, creating networks to share knowledge and experience, and advocating for more peer support services.

Perception of social cues—involves the nuanced and complicated process of perceiving and making sense of the information provided through facial expressions, voice inflection, gestures, and physical proximity.

Performance capacity—considers the extent to which underlying abilities facilitate or inhibit occupational performance and participation including the subjective mind-body experience.

Peripartum onset—depression that occurs during pregnancy or within 4 weeks after childbirth.

Permanent supportive housing—an evidence-based model of housing that allows individuals with psychiatric conditions or individuals who are homeless to receive housing for as long as they desire with the necessary support to maintain independent living.

Persistent depressive disorder—formerly known as dysthymic disorder, a condition that shares similar features with major depressive disorder, but symptoms are less severe and must be present chronically (a period of at least 2 years) rather than episodically.

Person-centeredness—promotes "an approach to service which embraces a philosophy of, respect for, and partnership with, people receiving services" (Law & Mills, 2009, p. 253).

Person-driven—approach in which self-determination and self-direction are the foundations for recovery as individuals define their own life goals and design their unique path(s) toward those goals.

Person-Environment-Occupation (PEO) model—a conceptual framework developed by a group of Canadian occupational therapy clinicians and researchers to provide a systematic way to analyze complex occupational performance issues within the context of occupational therapy practice.

Personal causation—one of the components of the volitional system in the Model of Human Occupation, which involves the personal assessment of abilities leading to the belief that the individual can change their situation.

Personal recovery—recovery that is aimed at development of personally valued goals and identity.

Personality—individual differences in thinking, feeling, and behaving that are present across situations and time. Personality is derived from both biological (temperament) and environmental factors (character).

Personalized financial counseling—offered to augment supported employment services regarding income support, health insurance, and other governmental benefits to assist individuals to understand, plan for, and manage the impacts of employment on such benefits.

Phenomenology—a qualitative research method that studies how people experience phenomena, as described from their subjective, first-person point of view.

Phobia—a marked fear or anxiety about a specific object or situation, such as flying, heights, animals, or receiving an injection.

Photoreceptors—parts of the eye that convert light into electrical signals and are connected to the optic nerve; two types: cones and rods.

PhotoVoice—participatory approach that uses photographs and brief narratives to give voice directly to the research participants whose voices are often unheard.

Picture Exchange Communication System (PECS)—a protocol-driven method that allows individuals with autism or other communication disorders to use pictures to express their wants or needs.

Place-train perspective—an approach that allows individuals to quickly be placed in the settings they desire (work, housing, education) and then receive the necessary training to remain in that setting as opposed to the approach of receiving preparatory or transitional services.

Placebo effect—situation in which persons experience a positive effect after a course of action because of positive expectations about what the intervention will do and not the intervention per se.

Politics—activities by individuals or groups that influence the policies of government, including the resolution of debate or conflict between competing interests.

Polysensorial—understanding that the meaning and experience of any particular stimulus is affected by the intersection of that stimulus with other stimuli the person experiences in that situation; sensory stimuli are never experienced in isolation.

Positive childhood experiences (PCEs)—events that occur during a child's early development that help shape the child's sense of belonging.

Positive symptoms—symptoms in schizophrenia that represent aberrations in behavior or behaviors that are not typically present in other individuals, such as hallucinations, delusions, disorganized thinking, and disorganized behavior.

Posttraumatic growth (PTG)—positive psychological changes experienced because of the struggle with trauma or highly challenging situations.

Posttraumatic stress symptoms—symptoms similar to those experienced with posttraumatic stress disorder (PTSD) but do not meet the full criteria for PTSD diagnosis. People may still experience symptoms such as nervousness, fear, intrusive dreams, and anxious thoughts.

Pragmatics—used to refer to the social interaction skills that combine to facilitate participation in social interactions. They encompass behaviors related to the communicative, social, and emotional aspects of social communication.

Predictive research—research design in which the purpose is to determine what factors predict some other variable or outcome.

Predictive validity—the extent to which performance on a test is related to later performance that the test was designed to predict. For example, if an activities of daily living/instrumental activities of daily living assessment can be used to accurately predict a person's future ability to live independently, that test would be said to have good predictive validity.

Predisposing factors—variables that can increase the individual's vulnerability to develop a particular condition.

Prereflective and habitual—a stage of development wherein the individual acquires habits for sensing their environment.

Pretest–posttest design without a control—a quasi-experimental research design in which participants are not assigned randomly, and measurements are taken both before and after a treatment; often used to determine whether treatment had an impact.

Prevalence—an epidemiological term that refers to the proportion of the population who have a specific condition.

Probation—a judicial sentence of community-based supervision or a requirement that a person fulfill certain conditions of behavior in lieu of incarceration; can include a fine, a jail sentence, or both.

Problem-focused coping—an adaptive coping strategy in which individuals deal directly with a challenging situation either by obtaining more information, acquiring new skills to manage the situation, or by altering the situation or environment.

Problem-solving—cognitive processes used to reach a certain goal when the best pathway to that goal is not immediately discernable.

Problem-solving courts—courts designed to address a defendant's underlying problems and assign remediation, restitution, or rehabilitation as alternatives to incarceration (see drug court, mental health court, and veterans court).

Procedural memory—recollections about how to do something, such as how to ride a bike or bake a cake. Procedural memory takes longer to create and is less susceptible to errors.

Process Model of Emotional Regulation—a model that identifies five processes or strategies used to regulate emotions.

Processing speed—the amount of time required to perceive information, process that information, and carry out a response.

Prodrome period—the time between the emergence of early signs of the illness and the point at which the diagnostic criteria for the disorder are met.

Program for the Education and Enrichment of Relational Skills (PEERS)—a social skills training program focused on the making and keeping of friends for adolescents and young adults with autism.

Proprioception—the awareness of the physical body's position in space.

Prospective cohort study—a study planned in advance and carried out over a period of time. These studies follow groups of individuals who share some characteristics and differ on others to investigate causal factors for illnesses and to establish links between risk factors and health outcomes.

Protective factors—characteristics that can reduce the risk of poor mental health and increase a person's resilience; these can be biological (temperament), psychological (self-control), familial (good parental monitoring), or community (peer-group).

Psychoeducation—the process of teaching relevant psychological principles, knowledge, and skills to persons with a mental health condition.

Psychosis—a mental health condition that is characterized by a misunderstanding of the nature of reality, changes in the brain's ability to process/organize information, and experiences such as hallucinations, delusions, disorganized behavior/thoughts, and negative symptoms.

Psychotic personality organization—characterized by lack of integration of the concept of self and significant others, that is, identity diffusion, a predominance of primitive defensive mechanisms centering on splitting, and loss of reality testing.

Public health—practices that work to promote the health and well-being of populations and the communities they are in.

Public policy—actions that local, state, or federal governments choose to do—or not to do. Such policies are often informed by the values and objectives of citizens as well as the values and priorities of those in power.

Public stigma—endorsement of negative stereotypes by others such as family members and the general population; includes prejudice and can lead to discriminatory behaviors.

Purpose—the reason an activity assumes meaning.

Qualitative research—a scientific method of naturalistic inquiry that gathers nonnumerical data in an effort to gain in-depth understanding of social phenomenon within a natural setting; in occupational therapy, the focus is often on the lived experiences of humans and the meaning of their experiences when participating in daily occupations.

Quality of life—the general well-being of individuals that includes a person's subjective sense of health, comfort, and enjoyment of life.

Quantitative research—a scientific method that emphasizes objective measurement of numerical data and analysis using statistical analysis of the data.

Randomized controlled trial—a type of experimental study that randomly assigns subjects into experimental and control groups, and which is conducted so that as many sources of bias are removed from the process as possible such that the only expected difference between the control and experimental groups is the outcome variable being studied.

Rapid cycling—specifier for bipolar disorders that is given when four or more episodes occur in 12 months.

Rapid eye movement (REM) sleep—stage of sleep that involves high brain activity levels and accounts for 25% of sleep in healthy adults. Dreaming occurs when REM sleep is reached.

Rational emotive behavior therapy (REBT)—a cognitive model of emotional response where irrational beliefs about how things "must" and "should" be for persons to be happy interfere with well-being. The intervention works to change irrational beliefs and develop unconditional acceptance of self, others, and life.

Realize—be aware of something and understand what that means.

Reason—to understand and justify actions and events.

Reassessment—the use of a specific assessment tool at another point in time to measure change.

Recognize—to identify that something has occurred.

Recovery—a process of achieving life's ambitions and dreams whether or not mental health symptoms exist.

Recovery principles—tenets that practitioners can use to transform mental health systems from a medical to recovery paradigm.

Regression analysis—a statistical method used to examine the relationship between two or more variables of interest; this helps a researcher understand which of various independent variables are related to the dependent variable.

Regulate—the control and management of an individual's reactions to stimuli.

Regulations—detailed rules for enforcing laws, including the responsibilities and constraints that constitute what it means to follow laws, and the process for monitoring enforcement.

Relate—making a connection between or relating to something or someone.

Related services—services such as occupational therapy that are mandated in U.S. school districts when students with disabilities require such services to benefit from special education.

Relational—method in which sensory habits are often developed through participation in the social world.

Relational support—assistance that comes from others, often peers, to help individuals achieve their goals and have their needs met.

Relevance theory—theory that attempts to explain how people interpret and understand language in communication. Communication is most effective when the information conveyed is relevant to the listener's goals and expectations.

Reliability—the degree to which a measure is stable and consistent across time, and between testers and forms.

Relief-oriented beliefs—assumption that using a substance will alleviate discomfort.

Remediation approach—an intervention in which the impairment is targeted, and intervention is directed at improving the targeted skill.

Repetitive transcranial electromagnetic stimulation—a treatment in which magnets are used to excite or inhibit specific brain areas.

Representativeness heuristic—a decision-making approach in which choices are based on models or prototypes the individual has come to expect.

Resident mobility—the degree to which residents move in and out of a neighborhood over time.

Residential reentry centers (RRCs)—settings that provide safe, structured, and supervised transitional housing offering various programs and services for individuals serving probation or who may require pretrial detention.

Resilience—an individual's ability to endure stressful situations without suffering the physiological or psychological consequences that can be associated with such adversity.

Resist—refrain from doing something.

Respect—community, systems, and societal acceptance and appreciation for people affected by mental health and substance use problems—including protecting their rights and eliminating discrimination.

Respond—saying or doing something as a reply.

Response modulation—occurs after the emotion has unfolded and typically involves efforts to suppress the emotion.

Response rate—the percentage of individuals that respond to a survey.

Responsiveness—the degree to which a measure is able to detect a change.

Retrospective cohort study—a study in which data that was collected previously are examined to compare two groups: one that experiences a condition and one that does not.

Risk factors—variables that increase the likelihood that someone will experience a condition.

Rods—component of the eye best at detecting motion; they are more prominent on the periphery of the retina.

Role-playing game—while engaging in a game, the individual participating takes on the role of a fictional character for the duration of the game and plays as if they were that character.

Routines—patterns of activity that comprise habits and the typical sequence in which they are undertaken. Routines are observable, regular, and repetitive and provide structure for daily life.

Safe—protection from harm or danger.

Safe, stable, and nurturing relationships (SSNRs)—relationships free of physical or psychological harm. These relationships are essential to prevent child maltreatment and to assure that children reach their full potential.

Safety plan—specific strategies that focus on reducing the risk of suicide.

Salience network—comprises linked brain regions important in filtering the vast amount of sensation received and determining what deserves attention.

Salutogenic Model—focuses on understanding health instead of disease to explain how some people adapt and survive in the face of adversity.

Sample size—the total number of participants in a study.

Sanism—systematic discrimination and oppression against individuals with a mental health condition.

Scattered-site housing—the practice of having individuals with psychiatric disabilities reside in apartment buildings in which the majority of tenants are not other people with psychiatric disabilities.

Schema—mental representation that creates structure out of related concepts.

Schema theory—a cognitive theory that explains how individuals develop cognitive frameworks based on experience to explain their world.

Schizoaffective disorder—a condition characterized by a combination of psychotic and mood symptoms.

Schizoid personality disorder—a condition characterized by a pervasive pattern of social detachment and a restricted range of emotional expression in interpersonal settings.

Schizophrenia—a condition characterized by psychotic symptoms, flat affect, social withdrawal, and impairments in functioning.

Schizotypal personality disorder—a condition characterized by a pervasive pattern of social and interpersonal deficits along with cognitive and perceptual distortions.

School mental health (SMH)—mental health programs or services for children in the school setting.

Screening, Brief Intervention, and Referral to Treatment (SBIRT)—an evidence-based practice used to identify, reduce, and prevent problematic use, abuse, and dependence on alcohol and illicit drugs.

Script—a type of schema that describes the sequence of events that one expects to occur in a familiar activity.

Seasonal affective disorder (SAD)—condition in which one's mood and how one thinks or functions is altered with the changing of the seasons.

Seasonal pattern—a specifier used when the major depressive disorder is recurrent and the onset occurs at a particular time of year.

Second-generation antipsychotics—also known as atypical antipsychotics, these work as a dopamine antagonist but tend to have fewer motor-related side effects than first-generation antipsychotics.

Section 504 of the Rehabilitation Act—a civil rights law that offers protection for people with disabilities.

Section 8 housing voucher system—a program designed to play a role in assisting low-income individuals and families in obtaining housing. With Section 8 vouchers, renters typically pay no more than 30% of their income toward rent.

Selective and focused—belief that people are not passive recipients to sensory stimuli; rather, people are active sensory beings who are already engaged with a sensory environment that is overflowing with stimuli. The body orients itself to different features of that sensory environment.

Selective attention—the process of sorting out and focusing on the relevant sensory stimuli in the environment.

Selective mutism—the consistent failure to speak in social situations in which it is warranted, despite the ability to speak in other situations.

Self-accountability—a person taking responsibility for the way they respond to something and the way they act.

Self-appraisal—ability to determine one's strengths and weaknesses while performing different tasks.

Self-contained classroom model—a special education classroom that is separated from general education classrooms in which students attend a specialized curriculum to obtain the foundational academic, social, and psychological skills needed to enter higher education.

Self-determination—a basic human right of individuals to have autonomous decision-making over their own bodies and life; the right to independently decide in matters such as medical treatment, family life, public life, and so on.

Self-determination theory (SDT)—theory of human motivation, personality development, and well-being that focuses on self-determined behavior and the social and cultural conditions that promote it.

Self-efficacy—the belief in one's ability to succeed in specific situations or to accomplish a task.

Self-efficacy beliefs—beliefs people have regarding their capabilities to succeed in a specific situation or in accomplishing a desired task.

Self-harm—deliberate self-injurious actions without an intent to die.

Self-help/mutual-aid/mutual-help support groups—an approach that recognizes people facing the same problem learn from and support one another when they share their experiences and strengths with an understanding and accepting community of peers.

Self-management—the tasks that an individual must undertake to live well with one or more chronic conditions. These tasks include gaining confidence to deal with medical management, role management, and emotional management.

Self-management support—when a health professional or peer collaborates to teach self-management skills.

Self-monitoring—a cognitive behavioral self-regulatory or self-management process that involves paying deliberate attention to specific aspects of one's thoughts, emotions, and behavior.

Self-report tool—any method involving asking a participant about their feelings, experiences, perceptions, attitudes, or beliefs. It can take multiple forms such as a survey, questionnaire, or poll in which respondents read the question and select a response by themselves without researcher interference.

Self-stigma—occurs when stigmatized individuals agree with and internalize negative stereotypes (e.g., the person believes that they are deviant or shamefully different).

Self-talk—the process in which human beings talk to themselves out loud or as part of an inner dialogue stream that is used to monitor behavior and accomplish a task.

Semantic memory—memory for facts.

Semicircular canals—three fluid-filled tubes in the inner ear that contain vestibular receptors.

Sensation avoiding—a pattern of sensory processing characterized by a low threshold and active response; an individual may create or choose environments that reduce sensory input and may do well in low stimulus situations but be distressed in situations in which they cannot control the environment.

Sensation seeking—a pattern of sensory processing characterized by a high threshold and active response; individuals engage with their environment to meet their sensory needs and change the environment to obtain higher levels of sensory input. Individuals are easily bored or frustrated in environments that do not meet their elevated needs for sensation.

Sense of capacity—the personal acknowledgment of one's abilities.

Sense of coherence—construct in the Salutogenic Model where people can better manage stress when they can make sense of and have confidence that they can deal with the stressful situation.

Sensory-based interventions (SBIs)—interventions that are provided in the individual's natural environment and use sensory input as a way to organize the individual's level of arousal to meet the needs of the situation.

Sensory gating deficiencies—an impairment characterized by difficulty screening out irrelevant information.

Sensory integration—the neurobiological process involved in organizing multiple sensations from the environment and the person's own body. Sensory integration is followed by an adaptive response, which involves a purposeful, goal-directed response to a sensory experience.

Sensory modalities—independent sensory systems, including visual, auditory, tactile, gustatory, olfactory, proprioceptive, and vestibular systems, that perceive stimuli of the outside world.

Sensory processing—the interpretation of sensory information into meaningful and usable constructs for action.

Sensory processing measure—a behavioral rating scale assessing sensory processing in different environments.

Sensory profiles (SPs)—an assessment of an individual's response to sensory events in their daily life that categorizes these responses into four sensory preferences—low registration, sensory seeking, sensation sensitivity, and sensation avoiding.

Sensory rooms—areas utilized in treatment settings to provide desired sensory stimuli to individuals with atypical sensory needs; they are often used to manage anxiety and reduce disruptive behaviors.

Sensory sensitivity—a pattern of sensory processing characterized by a low threshold and passive response. This pattern can lead to a heightened awareness of the environment and more information with which to make decisions; in contrast, individuals may be highly distractible and more likely to experience discomfort in high-intensity environments.

Separation anxiety disorder—a condition characterized by excessive fear or anxiety about separation from home or primary attachment figures.

Serious leisure—engagement in a particular leisure activity that might take on importance and a higher level of obligation to the pursuit of, perseverance with, and acquisition of specialist skills and entry into new social worlds.

Severe emotional disturbance (SED)—generally refers to children and youth with significant mental health needs.

Shared decision-making—a model for making health-care decisions where the practitioner and person contribute jointly to the decision-making process.

Short-term memory—memories held for only a matter of seconds or minutes.

Single-subject design—a research design that does not combine data across individuals but instead examines how one individual responds to different conditions with the purpose of examining the efficacy of an intervention.

Situation modification—process in which environmental and social factors can be modified as the situation unfolds to impact the resulting emotional experience.

Situation selection—process that occurs before an emotional event that is used to increase the likelihood of a specific emotion occurring.

Skills development interventions—approaches whereby individuals acquire specific skills, often focusing on cognitive, social, and emotional regulation skills.

Sleep debt—the physical condition of tiredness because of inadequate sleep.

Sleep-driver system—process S of the sleep–wake cycle; it is a homeostatic system that depends on the amount of time an individual remains awake versus asleep from day to day.

Sleep health—honoring the role of promoting effective sleep regulation to maintain or improve health.

Small group interventions—treatment or actions that target a small number of individuals.

Social anxiety disorder—a condition characterized by intense fear or anxiety of social situations in which the person may be judged or scrutinized by others.

Social capital—the power that individuals hold in society that are afforded to them through the social locations that they occupy (i.e., race, gender, sexual orientation, class), and the relationships that they develop in their communities and society.

Social cognition—refers to the psychological and cognitive processes that are involved in interpreting and responding to social information.

Social cognitive theory—also referred to as social learning theory, this theory emphasizes the critical roles of social and cognitive factors, as well as behavior and environment, in the process of human learning and behavior change.

Social connectedness—belonging to a group or community; feeling cared about and caring for others.

Social context—environments that involve relationships with individuals, groups, and organizations.

Social determinants of health—the conditions in which people are born, grow, work, live, and age, and the wider set of forces and systems shaping the conditions of daily life and resulting health status.

Social distance—the degree to which a person wants to exclude others; can apply to the exclusion of persons with mental illness in various social situations.

Social learning theory—the process of learning that occurs by observing others in a social context.

Social media—interactive technologies that facilitate the creation and sharing of information, ideas, interests, and other forms of expression through virtual communities and networks.

Social modeling—learning that occurs by watching the behavior of others.

Social network sites (SNS)—any websites with a personal profile of the individual, whether that be public or semi-public, that allows for engagement with others.

Social participation—the interweaving of occupations to support desired engagement in community and family activities as well as those involving peers.

Social persuasion—direct verbal encouragement from another person.

Social rhythms—patterns that refer to an individual's daily routines.

Social Security Disability Insurance (SSDI)—a public assistance program designed to provide a financial safety net for workers who become disabled and are unable to continue working.

Social skills training (SST)—based on principles from social learning theory, an intervention in which social skills are learned from observation, modeling, reinforcement, and generalization.

Social stories—a learning tool that uses stories to introduce and teach interpersonal behaviors to children with autism.

Social support—assistance that comes from other people or groups of people.

Socratic questioning—strategically using open-ended questions to gather information.

Socratic questioning with guided discovery—the process of asking a series of questions that promotes reflection and self-awareness.

Somatic/emotional states—the physical and emotional responses to an activity.

Sound waves—vibrations that move through elastic mediums in response to auditory stimuli.

Specific mental functions—the designation in the *Occupational Therapy Practice Framework* that encompasses cognitive skills and executive functions.

Speech act theory—belief that language is used to achieve goals or tasks, and speech acts are units of communication with specific intentions.

Spirituality—the aspect of humanity that refers to the way individuals seek and express meaning and purpose and the way they experience their connectedness to the moment, to self, to others, to nature, and to the significant or sacred.

Stable—something that is unlikely to change.

Stagnation—one's failure to find a way to contribute, which may cause a person to feel unproductive, disconnected, or uninvolved with others, the community, or society in general.

Stigma—negative attitudes and a behavioral chain that begins by applying a stigmatizing mark to a person, progresses through the attitude structures, and results in discrimination.

Stigma by association—when family members and friends of the person with the stigmatized condition may also feel the devaluation of being stigmatized.

Strengths-based—an approach that focuses and builds upon the person's strengths, looking at what the person can do as opposed to what they cannot do.

Stress reduction theory—posits physiological stress is relieved through contact with nature.

Stressors—conditions that create demands on a person and may contribute to a stress response, a state of physiological alertness that may help achieve a goal or assist with survival.

Structural stigma—when society and societal institutions operate in ways that weave inequities and injustices into laws, policies, or practices.

Subacute pain—pain that typically remains present from 6 weeks to 3 months.

Substance use disorder (SUD)—condition that involves the use of psychoactive substances for the purpose of their effect on the central nervous system or to prevent or reduce withdrawal symptoms. In SUDs, the individual continues to take the substance despite negative consequences.

Substantial Gainful Activity—a monthly earned income amount determined by the federal government to be sufficient for self-support; used to determine eligibility for Social Security Disability Insurance.

Substitute work—also known as "sheltered work," activities historically aimed to offer structure and activity for individuals with disabilities.

Suicidal ideation—thoughts about suicide; it can include determining the method, having a plan, and/or possessing an intent to act, or it can be passive thoughts about death without intent or plan.

Suicide—death caused by self-directed injurious behavior with any intent to die because of the behavior.

Suicide intervention—the focus of this stage is to address the risk of suicide, focusing on how best to respond early when someone has thoughts of suicide or suicide-related actions. All thoughts of suicide require a response.

Suicide postvention—in this phase, support is provided to those affected after a suicide attempt or loss, with follow-up education/prevention to reduce the risk of future crises. It includes support for family and friends after a death by suicide, as well as the staff involved.

Suicide prevention—also known as the life promotion phase, the focus of this stage of the continuum is early detection and acting on collective high-risk factors.

Suicide prevention continuum—refers to the interconnectedness of prevention-intervention-postvention work, thereby providing an overarching framework for how to approach suicide at all levels.

Supplemental Security Income (SSI)—a public assistance program designed to provide monetary income to citizens and qualified noncitizens of the United States who are over the age of 65, blind, or disabled. Unlike Social Security Disability Insurance, funds are provided to people who have not been adequately employed and consequently have not paid sufficient Social Security taxes to qualify for other Social Security benefits.

Supported education—support and instruction specifically meant for adults with psychiatric disabilities and intended to meet the unique postsecondary educational goals of each individual.

Supported employment (SE)—refers to an evidence-based employment service delivery model for improving competitive employment outcomes of people with disabilities.

Survey research—a research design that uses surveys as the means of collecting data.

Survivor's guilt—an experience that occurs when an individual assumes responsibility for the death or injury of another person, even when the survivor had no control over the outcome of the situation.

Systematic reviews—a summary of the results of available well-designed controlled trials that assesses the level of evidence on the effectiveness of an intervention, and which can inform a practitioner's therapeutic reasoning.

Systemic trauma—experience of being systemically minoritized, and not a minority status itself, that results in negative health outcomes.

Systems of care (SoC)—services offered to families who are involved with child service agencies. It consists of three core values: being family-driven and youth guided, community based with local child/youth/family services and support working together, and culturally and linguistically competent.

Tactile system—consists of a variety of sensory receptors in the skin that respond to different forms of touch.

Telehealth—the use of information and communication technologies to deliver health-related services when the provider and person are in different physical locations.

Telescoping effect—describes how women experience stronger responses to substances and accelerated disease progression, initially using substances in smaller amounts, but more quickly progressing to addiction.

Teletherapy in early intervention—the use of communication technologies to deliver early intervention services.

Temperament—how an infant is predisposed to react to their environment and ability to self-regulate responses to the stimulus.

Test–retest reliability—a measure of consistency of a test; obtained by administering the same test twice over a period of time to a group of individuals.

Thalamus—part of the brain that acts to relay sensory information from the body; also plays a role in sleep and consciousness as well as learning and memory.

The outcomes of the implementation should be evaluated—a component of evidence-based practice that involves determining the success of implementing practices based on the evidence.

Therapeutic milieu—the therapeutic milieu extends beyond the physical features of the environment to include group treatment, and allows the individual to practice shaping behaviors and social interactions in a community setting.

Therapeutic reasoning—the process by which practitioners obtain a comprehensive understanding of the person and use practice models to inform their decision-making.

Threats to validity—factors that impact the rigor of quantitative research. These include threats to internal validity that can compromise the confidence with which one can draw conclusions of causality and threats to external validity, which impact confidence in stating the generalizability of the results to other groups.

Thrive—realizing one's strengths, feeling good, finding purpose, and striving for well-being.

Thriving and rising—moving beyond just coping with adversities by finding meaning in adversities in order to enhance health and well-being.

Ticket-to-Work program—a program that allows people with disabilities to enter work rehabilitation programs and earn an income for a trial period before losing their Medicaid benefits.

TIC-TOC technique—a strategy used in cognitive behavioral therapy that focuses on identifying and reframing task-interfering cognitions (TICs) and replacing them with task-oriented cognitions (TOCs).

Time diaries—a tool used to assess how an individual spends their time each day by keeping a detailed record.

Transactional Model of Stress and Coping—describes the process by which people deal with stressful situations.

Transactive model—the belief that relationships are multidirectional and mutually influential across multiple intersections. A change in the occupation can influence change in the person and environment, and iteratively each element can influence each other.

Transferability—refers to the degree to which the results of a qualitative research study can be applied or transferred to similar settings, situations, or populations.

Transitional housing—programs that are designed to promote housing stability and provide temporary housing for up to 2 years. In addition to offering housing, they typically offer varied services, and some programs address the specific needs of persons with mental illness, individuals in substance abuse recovery, and women and children who are survivors of domestic violence.

Trauma—a single event, multiple events, or a set of circumstances that is experienced by an individual as physically and emotionally harmful or threatening and that has lasting adverse effects on the individual's physical, social, emotional, or spiritual well-being.

Trauma-informed approaches—strengths-based service delivery approaches emphasizing physical, psychological, and emotional safety for survivors of trauma and their providers. It considers the impact of trauma and creates opportunities for survivors to rebuild a sense of control and empowerment.

Trauma-informed care (TIC)—an organizational structure that involves understanding, recognizing, and responding to the effects of all types of trauma in all types of settings. TIC considers the impact of trauma and creates opportunities for survivors to rebuild a sense of control and empowerment.

Trauma Informed Oregon (TIO)—a model that outlines steps to progress a workplace, health-care setting, community center, school, or any system to a trauma-informed culture.

Trauma sensitive—taking into account individuals' past traumas and creating a safe and respectful environment that enables them to regulate their emotions and behaviors to succeed in all areas of functioning.

Treatment burden—time, energy, and cognitive load required to adhere to treatment regimens.

Triple Aim—related to the passage of the Affordable Care Act, the Triple Aim prioritizes improvement of the personal experience of health-care services, improvement of the health of the population, and a reduction of the per capita health-care expenses.

Trustworthiness—refers to the degree to which the qualitative researcher applies methods that help establish that the results of a study are credible and believable; have transferability to similar settings, situations, or populations; and that the processes of data collection and analysis are dependable and confirmable.

Underresponsivity—a sensory modulation difference characterized by having responses to sensory stimuli that can be slower, shorter, or less intense than the expected sensory responsivity.

Unipolar depression—a mood disorder characterized by recurrent episodes of depression, which is the low, sad, unpleasant mood of an extreme in the continuum of typical moods.

Unipolar disorder—term used synonymously with major depressive disorder. It is characterized by one or more instances of a major depressive episode, but no occurrence of a manic episode.

Unpaid work—activities such as domestic chores, caregiving, and volunteering that go unremunerated. Unpaid work is vital to society but often goes unrecognized.

Unstuck and on Target—a manualized intervention designed to improve flexibility, planning, and organization in autistic children.

Utility—as an aspect of evaluation, utility refers to the usefulness of a measure in everyday practice. This can include an assessment of whether the assessment is appropriate, accessible, practical, and acceptable to the person.

Validity—refers to how well a test measures what it sets out to measure; a test of cognition should measure cognition and not something else such as fine motor control. There are various types of validity in research.

Values—one of the components of the volitional system as part of the Model of Human Occupation; something that is important, useful, or of worth.

Verbal fluency—associated with memory; the ability to recall and retrieve verbal information from your memory.

Vestibular system—sensory system responsible for sense of balance and spatial orientation for coordinating movement through detection of the position and movement of the head in space.

Veterans court—a specialized court that assists veterans who are struggling with addiction, mental illness, or co-occurring disorders who are charged with a crime. Veterans often receive a peer mentor who is a veteran and attend judicially supervised programs usually provided by the Veterans Administration.

Veterans Health Administration (VHA)—U.S. health-care system serving military personnel who have separated from the service. The VHA offers comprehensive mental health services to veterans through inpatient, outpatient, and community-based settings.

Vet-to-Vet program—a partnership program that utilizes veterans in recovery in a peer-counseling capacity to help other veterans.

Vicarious experience—an indirect experience or an experience that is not firsthand. One may have a vicarious experience by watching, reading about, or listening to another's story.

Video gaming—the act of engaging in a video game whether on a console, computer, web browser, or virtual reality.

Vigilance—the ability to sustain attention through time.

Virtual environment—refers to the internet, text messaging, social media, video messaging, and other forms of virtual communication that provide opportunities for social connection, information gathering, and leisure pursuits.

Virtual health—the use of technology including phones, videos, apps, text messaging, and other platforms for the delivery of health care to a patient outside of a health system.

Virtual learning—an environment where students study a curriculum that is digital based and taught by instructors who lecture online. It can take place through either synchronous or asynchronous methods.

Virtual Mental Health Communities (VMHC)—communities that meet through a virtual platform or social media and are virtual spaces where individuals with similar interests can connect and offer support.

Virtual reality (VR)—a simulated experience that employs pose tracking and 3D near eye displays to give the user an immersive feel of a virtual world.

Visual field—the area an individual can see from their position in an environment.

Visual supports—use of pictures or text to promote communication with individuals who have limited verbal language.

Visual system—the sensory system that provides information about the physical properties of the environment and the objects in it, such as their shape, size, color, and proximity to the person and other objects.

Vocal prosody—refers to linguistic functions such as intonation, tone, stress, and rhythm.

Volition—a pattern of thoughts and feelings that provides motivation for occupation; it influences an individual's choice of occupation and persistence when engaging in that occupation.

Volitional process—the continuous cycle of experiencing, interpreting, anticipating, and choosing.

Volunteer exploration—determining volunteer opportunities available that meet an individual's personal skills, interests, location, and time restrictions.

Volunteering—a choice one makes to engage in activities that serve others, the community, or organizations.

Warmline—a variation on the idea of a crisis hotline, the warmline is a telephone line that can provide support to a person who may need assistance but whose needs are not urgent.

Well-being—positive psychological functioning, including the dimensions of acceptance of self, positive relations with others, autonomy, environmental mastery, purpose in life, and personal growth.

Wellness—a conscious, deliberate process that requires a person to become aware of and make choices for a more satisfying lifestyle.

Wellness coach—a specialized type of peer–professional partnership in which peer support workers help an individual to link to a primary health-care professional and provide support and encouragement to help that individual set and achieve a desired short-term wellness or health-related goal.

Wellness Recovery Action Plan (WRAP)—an individualized plan developed by a person in recovery to identify strategies for maintaining wellness and addressing concerns as they arise.

Work—labor or exertion related to the development, production, delivery, or management of objects or services; benefits may be financial or nonfinancial.

Workers—individuals who participate in some form of work.

Working memory—involves short-term memory storage and active manipulation of new information; that is, the person is temporarily "working with" the information.

Workload—encompasses the many tasks related to a specific job responsibility or life role.

World Health Organization (WHO)—United Nations agency that promotes worldwide health and well-being to make health accessible for everyone worldwide.

Wraparound—a planning process that brings people together from different parts of the whole family's life. With help from one or more facilitators, people from the family's life work together, coordinate their activities, and blend their perspectives on the family situation.

Zones of Regulation—an intervention designed to help individuals with sensory modulation difficulties develop skills in consciously regulating their actions.

Index

References followed by the letter "f" are for figures, "t" are tables, and "b" are boxes.

O

Practice Models and Theoretical Approaches Index

Although this textbook is organized according to the person-environment-occupation model rather than theoretical models, different theoretical models are interspersed throughout the chapters. This index was developed as a reference tool to enable readers to quickly identify the chapters in which a particular theoretical model is addressed. Entries refer to the chapter(s), and not the page number, where the content on the relevant theoretical model is found. In some cases, the theoretical model is discussed in detail, whereas in other cases, it is simply identified as a relevant method.